HEART
FAILURE

A COMPANION TO **BRAUNWALD'S HEART DISEASE**

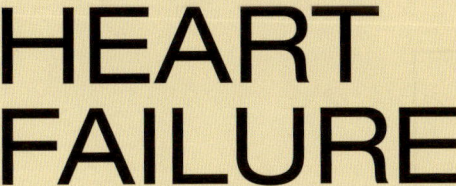

HEART
FAILURE

A COMPANION TO **BRAUNWALD'S HEART DISEASE**

FOURTH EDITION

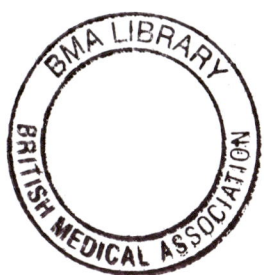

G. MICHAEL **FELKER,** MD, MHS

Professor of Medicine
Division of Cardiology
Chief, Heart Failure Section
Duke University School of Medicine
Durham, North Carolina

DOUGLAS L. **MANN,** MD

Lewin Chair and Professor of Medicine, Cell Biology, and Physiology
Chief, Division of Cardiology
Washington University School of Medicine in St. Louis
Cardiologist-in-Chief
Barnes-Jewish Hospital
St. Louis, Missouri

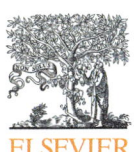

ELSEVIER

HEART FAILURE: A COMPANION TO BRAUNWALD'S HEART DISEASE, FOURTH EDITION   ISBN: 978-0-323-60987-6

Copyright © 2020 by Elsevier, Inc. All rights reserved.

Notices

Knowledge and best practice in this field are constantly changing. As new research and experience broaden our understanding, changes in research methods, professional practices, or medical treatment may become necessary.

Practitioners and researchers must always rely on their own experience and knowledge in evaluating and using any information, methods, compounds, or experiments described herein. In using such information or methods they should be mindful of their own safety and the safety of others, including parties for whom they have a professional responsibility.

With respect to any drug or pharmaceutical products identified, readers are advised to check the most current information provided (i) on procedures featured or (ii) by the manufacturer of each product to be administered, to verify the recommended dose or formula, the method and duration of administration, and contraindications. It is the responsibility of practitioners, relying on their own experience and knowledge of their patients, to make diagnoses, to determine dosages and the best treatment for each individual patient, and to take all appropriate safety precautions.

To the fullest extent of the law, neither the Publisher nor the authors, contributors, or editors, assume any liability for any injury and/or damage to persons or property as a matter of products liability, negligence or otherwise, or from any use or operation of any methods, products, instructions, or ideas contained in the material herein.

Previous editions copyrighted 2016, 2011, and 2004.

International Standard Book Number: 978-0-323-60987-6

Publishing Director: Dolores Meloni
Senior Content Development Specialist: Anne Snyder
Publishing Services Manager: Catherine Albright Jackson
Senior Project Manager: Claire Kramer
Design Direction: Renee Duenow

Printed in China.

Last digit is the print number: 9   8   7   6   5   4   3   2   1

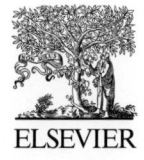

ELSEVIER

1600 John F. Kennedy Blvd.
Ste 1600
Philadelphia, PA 19103-2899

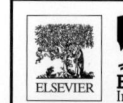

To

Claire, William, Caroline, and my parents

Laura, Erica, Jonathan and Stephanie, and
Dr. Nicholas Davidson (for being there)

CONTRIBUTORS

E. Dale Abel, MD, PhD
Francois M. Abboud Chair in Internal Medicine
John B. Stokes III Chair in Diabetes Research
Chair and Department Executive Officer
Department of Internal Medicine
Director, Fraternal Order of Eagles Diabetes Research Center
Director, Division of Endocrinology and Metabolism
Professor of Medicine, Biochemistry, and Biomedical
    Engineering
University of Iowa
Carver College of Medicine
Iowa City, Iowa
Chapter 17: Alterations in Cardiac Metabolism in Heart Failure

Luigi Adamo, MD, PhD
Advanced Heart Failure and Cardiac Transplant Specialist
Instructor of Medicine
Barnes-Jewish Hospital
Washington University School of Medicine
St. Louis, Missouri
*Chapter 12: Alterations in Ventricular Structure: Role of
    Left Ventricular Remodeling and Reverse Remodeling
    in Heart Failure*

Shah R. Ali, MD
Cardiology Fellow
Department of Internal Medicine
Division of Cardiology
University of Texas Southwestern Medical Center
Dallas, Texas
Chapter 3: Cellular Basis for Myocardial Regeneration and Repair

Larry A. Allen, MD, MHS
Professor of Medicine
Division of Cardiology
Department of Medicine
Medical Director, Advanced Heart Failure
University of Colorado
School of Medicine
Aurora, Colorado
*Chapter 50: Decision Making and Palliative Care in Advanced
    Heart Failure*

George L. Bakris, MD
Professor of Medicine
Director, American Society of Hypertension Comprehensive
    Hypertension Center
The University of Chicago Medicine
Chicago, Illinois
*Chapter 15: Alterations in Kidney Function Associated with
    Heart Failure*

Gerald S. Bloomfield, MD, MPH
Associate Professor of Medicine and Global Health
Duke Clinical Research Institute
Duke Global Health Institute and Department of Medicine
Duke University
Durham, North Carolina
Chapter 30: Heart Failure and Human Immunodeficiency Virus

Robert O. Bonow, MD, MS
Max and Lilly Goldberg Distinguished Professor of Cardiology
Vice Chair for Development and Innovation
Department of Medicine
Northwestern University Feinberg School of Medicine
Chicago, Illinois
*Chapter 19: Heart Failure as a Consequence of Ischemic Heart
    Disease*

Biykem Bozkurt, MD, PhD, FACC, FAHA, FHFSA, FACP
The Mary and Gordon Cain Chair and W. A. "Tex" and
    Deborah Moncrief, Jr., Chair
Professor of Medicine and Vice Chair of Medicine
Medicine Chief, DeBakey VA Medical Center
Associate Director, Cardiovascular Research Institute
Director, Winters Center for Heart Failure
Baylor College of Medicine
Houston, Texas
*Chapter 20: Heart Failure as a Consequence of Dilated
    Cardiomyopathy*

Michael R. Bristow, MD, PhD
Professor of Medicine
Division of Cardiology
University of Colorado Health Sciences Center
Aurora, Colorado
Chapter 6: Adrenergic Receptor Signaling in Heart Failure

Angela L. Brown, MD
Associate Professor
Department of Medicine
Division of Cardiology
Washington University School of Medicine
St. Louis, Missouri
*Chapter 40: Management of Heart Failure in Special
    Populations: Older Patients, Women, and Racial/Ethnic
    Minority Groups*

Heiko Bugger, PD Dr med, FESC
Attending Cardiologist
Department of Cardiology
Medical University of Graz
Graz, Austria
Chapter 17: Alterations in Cardiac Metabolism in Heart Failure

John C. Burnett, MD
Marriott Family Professor of Cardiovascular Research
Professor of Medicine and Physiology
Cardiorenal Research Laboratory
Department of Cardiovascular Medicine
Department of Physiology and Bioengineering
College of Medicine
Mayo Clinic
Rochester, Minnesota
*Chapter 9: Natriuretic Peptides in Heart Failure:
    Pathophysiologic and Therapeutic Implications*

Javed Butler, MD, MPH, MBA
Patrick Lehan Professor and Chairman
Department of Medicine
University of Mississippi School of Medicine
Jackson, Mississippi
Chapter 18: Epidemiology of Heart Failure

John D. Carroll, MD
Professor of Medicine
Director of Interventional Cardiology
Division of Cardiology
University of Colorado School of Medicine
Aurora, Colorado
*Chapter 26: Heart Failure as a Consequence of Valvular
    Heart Disease*

Adam Castaño, MD, MS
Division of Cardiology
Center for Cardiac Amyloidosis
Columbia University College of Physicians and Surgeons
New York, New York
Chapter 22: Cardiac Amyloidosis

Anna Marie Chang, MD
Assistant Professor, Emergency Medicine
Sidney Kimmel Medical College at Thomas Jefferson
    University
Philadelphia, Pennsylvania
*Chapter 47: Disease Management and Telemedicine in
    Heart Failure*

Jay N. Cohn, MD
Professor of Medicine
Rasmussen Center for Cardiovascular Disease Prevention
University of Minnesota Medical School
Minneapolis, Minnesota
Chapter 35: Disease Prevention in Heart Failure

Wilson S. Colucci, MD
Professor of Medicine and Physiology
Boston University School of Medicine
Chief, Section of Cardiovascular Medicine
Co-Director, Cardiovascular Center
Boston Medical Center
Boston, Massachusetts
Chapter 8: Oxidative Stress in Heart Failure

Louis J. Dell'Italia, MD
Birmingham VA Medical Center
University of Alabama at Birmingham School of Medicine
Birmingham, Alabama
*Chapter 5: Molecular Signaling Mechanisms of the
    Renin-Angiotensin System in Heart Failure*

Anita Deswal, MD, MPH
Professor of Medicine
Baylor College of Medicine
Chief, Section of Cardiology
Michael E. Debakey VA Medical Center
Houston, Texas
*Chapter 39: Treatment of Heart Failure with Preserved
    Ejection Fraction*

Adam D. DeVore, MD, MHS
Assistant Professor of Medicine
Duke University School of Medicine
The Duke Clinical Research Institute
Durham, North Carolina
Chapter 49: Quality and Outcomes in Heart Failure

Abhinav Diwan, MD
Associate Professor of Medicine
Cell Biology and Physiolgoy
Center for Cardiovascular Research
Division of Cardiology and Department of Internal Medicine
Washington University School of Medicine
Staff Physician, John Cochran Veterans Affairs Medical Center
St. Louis, Missouri
Chapter 1: Molecular Basis for Heart Failure

Hilary M. DuBrock, MD, MMSc
Assistant Professor
Division of Pulmonary and Critical Care
Mayo Clinic
Rochester Minnesota
Chapter 43: Pulmonary Hypertension

Shannon M. Dunlay, MD, MSc
Associate Professor of Medicine
Department of Cardiovascular Diseases
Mayo Clinic
Rochester Minnesota
Chapter 43: Pulmonary Hypertension

Nina Dzhoyashvili, MD, PhD
Research Fellow
Cardiorenal Research Laboratory
Department of Cardiovascular Medicine
Department of Physiology and Bioengineering
College of Medicine
Mayo Clinic
Rochester, Minnesota
*Chapter 9: Natriuretic Peptides in Heart Failure:
    Pathophysiologic and Therapeutic Implications*

Gregory A. Ewald, MD
Professor of Medicine
Associate Chief of Cardiology
Medical Director, Cardiac Transplant and Mechanical
    Circulatory Support Program
Washington University School of Medicine
St. Louis, Missouri
Chapter 45: Circulatory Assist Devices in Heart Failure

Justin A. Ezekowitz, MBBCh, MSc
Professor, Department of Medicine
University of Alberta
Co-Director, Canadian VIGOUR Centre
Cardiologist, Mazankowski Alberta Heart Institute
Edmonton, Alberta, Canada
Chapter 48: Management of Comorbidities in Heart Failure

James C. Fang, MD, FACC
Professor of Medicine
Chief, Division of Cardiovascular Medicine
University of Utah Health
Salt Lake City, Utah
Chapter 34: Hemodynamics in Heart Failure

Savitri Fedson, MD, MA
Associate Professor
Center for Medical Ethics and Health Policy
Baylor College of Medicine
Associate Professor
Section of Cardiology
Michael E. DeBakey VA Medical Center
Houston, Texas
*Chapter 39: Treatment of Heart Failure with Preserved
    Ejection Fraction*

Matthew J. Feinstein, MD, MS
Assistant Professor of Medicine
Division of Cardiology
Department of Medicine
Northwestern University Feinberg School of Medicine
Chicago, Illinois
Chapter 30: Heart Failure and Human Immunodeficiency Virus

G. Michael Felker, MD, MHS
Professor of Medicine
Division of Cardiology
Chief, Heart Failure Section
Duke University School of Medicine
Durham, North Carolina
*Chapter 19: Heart Failure as a Consequence of Ischemic
    Heart Disease*
*Chapter 37: Contemporary Medical Therapy for Heart
    Failure Patients with Reduced Ejection Fraction*

John D. Ferguson, MD
Professor of Medicine
Director of Electrophysiology
University of Virginia Medical Center
Charlottesville, Virginia
*Chapter 38: Management of Arrhythmias and Device
    Therapy in Heart Failure*

Victor A. Ferrari, MD
Professor of Medicine and Radiology
Chair, Penn Cardiovascular Imaging Council
Department of Medicine
Cardiovascular Medicine Division
Penn Cardiovascular Institute
Perelman School of Medicine at the University of Pennsylvania
    Hospital
Philadelphia, Pennsylvania
Chapter 32: Cardiac Imaging in Heart Failure

Carlos M. Ferrario, MD
Dewitt-Cordell Professor of Surgical Sciences
Department of Surgery
Wake Forest University School of Medicine
Winston Salem, North Carolina
*Chapter 5: Molecular Signaling Mechanisms of the
    Renin-Angiotensin System in Heart Failure*

James D. Flaherty, MD, MS
Associate Professor of Medicine
Division of Cardiology
Northwestern University Feinberg School of Medicine
Chicago, Illinois
*Chapter 19: Heart Failure as a Consequence of Ischemic
    Heart Disease*

John S. Floras, MD, DPhil, FRCPC
Canada Research Chair in Integrative Cardiovacular Biology
University Health Network and Sinai Health System
Division of Cardiology
Peter Munk Cardiac Centre
Professor, Faculty of Medicine
University of Toronto
Toronto, Ontario, Canada
*Chapter 13: Alterations in the Sympathetic and Parasympathetic
    Nervous Systems in Heart Failure*

Viorel G. Florea, MD, PhD, DSc
Associate Professor of Medicine
University of Minnesota Medical School
Minneapolis Veterans Affairs Health Care System
Minneapolis, Minnesota
Chapter 35: Disease Prevention in Heart Failure

Hanna K. Gaggin, MD, MPH
Assistant Physician, Cardiology Division
Massachusetts General Hospital
Assistant Professor of Medicine
Harvard Medical School
Boston, Massachusetts
Chapter 33: Biomarkers and Precision Medicine in Heart Failure

Barry Greenberg, MD
Distinguished Professor of Medicine
Director, Advanced Heart Failure Treatment Program
Division of Cardiovascular Medicine
University of California, San Diego
La Jolla, California
Chapter 31: Clinical Evaluation of Heart Failure

Joshua M. Hare, MD
Louis Lemberg Professor of Medicine
Cardiovascular Division
Director, Interdisciplinary Stem Cell Institute
Leonard M. Miller School of Medicine
Miami, Florida
*Chapter 21: Restrictive and Infiltrative
    Cardiomyopathies and Arrhythmogenic Right
    Ventricular Dysplasia/Cardiomyopathy*

Adrian F. Hernandez, MD, MHS
Professor of Medicine
Duke University School of Medicine
The Duke Clinical Research Institute
Durham, North Carolina
Chapter 49: Quality and Outcomes in Heart Failure

Joseph A. Hill, MD, PhD
Professor of Medicine and Molecular Biology
James T. Willerson MD Distinguished Chair in Cardiovascular
    Diseases
Frank M. Ryburn, Jr., Chair in Heart Research
Director, Harry S. Moss Heart Center
Chief of Cardiology
University of Texas Southwestern Medical Center
Dallas, Texas
Chapter 1: Molecular Basis for Heart Failure

Nasrien E. Ibrahim, MD
Assistant in Medicine
Cardiology Division
Section of Advanced Heart Failure and Transplant
Massachusetts General Hospital
Instructor of Medicine
Harvard Medical School
Boston, Massachusetts
Chapter 33: Biomarkers and Precision Medicine in Heart Failure

James L. Januzzi, Jr., MD
Physician, Cardiology Division
Massachusetts General Hospital
Hutter Family Professor of Medicine
Harvard Medical School
Boston, Massachusetts
Chapter 33: Biomarkers and Precision Medicine in Heart Failure

Susan M. Joseph, MD
Center for Advanced Heart and Lung Disease
Baylor University Medical Center
Dallas, Texas
*Chapter 40: Management of Heart Failure in Special
    Populations: Older Patients, Women, and Racial/Ethnic
    Minority Groups*

Daniel P. Judge, MD
Professor of Medicine
Division of Cardiology
Medical University of South Carolina
Director, Cardiovascular Genetics
Charleston, South Carolina
*Chapter 24: Heart Failure as a Consequence of Genetic
    Cardiomyopathy*

Andrew M. Kahn, MD, PhD
Professor of Medicine
Division of Cardiovascular Medicine
University of California, San Diego
La Jolla, California
Chapter 31: Clinical Evaluation of Heart Failure

Andreas P. Kalogeropoulos, MD, MPH, PhD
Associate Professor of Medicine
Division of Cardiology
Stony Brook University School of Medicine
Stony Brook, New York
Chapter 18: Epidemiology of Heart Failure

David A. Kass, MD
Abraham and Virginia Weiss Professor of Cardiology
Professor of Medicine
Professor of Biomedical Engineering
Professor of Pharmacology and Molecular Sciences
Director, Institute for CardioScience
The Johns Hopkins Medical Institutions
Baltimore, Maryland
Chapter 10: Systolic Dysfunction in Heart Failure

John Keaney, MB BCh BAO
Electrophysiologist
Mater Misericordiae University Hospital
Dublin, Ireland
Chapter 42: Neuromodulation in Heart Failure

Ahsan A. Khan, MBChB, MRCP
Clinical Research Fellow in Cardiology
Institute of Cardiovascular Sciences
University of Birmingham
City Hospital
Birmingham, United Kingdom
*Chapter 14: Alterations in the Peripheral Circulation in
    Heart Failure*

Paul J. Kim, MD
Assistant Professor of Medicine
Division of Cardiovascular Medicine
University of California, San Diego
La Jolla, California
Chapter 31: Clinical Evaluation of Heart Failure

Jon A. Kobashigawa, MD
Professor of Medicine
Associate Director, Cedars-Sinai Heart Institute
Director, Advanced Heart Disease Section
Director, Heart Transplant Program
Cedars-Sinai Medical Center
Clinical Professor of Medicine
The David Geffen School of Medicine at UCLA
Los Angeles, California
Chapter 44: Heart Transplantation

Evan P. Kransdorf, MD, PhD
Assistant Professor of Medicine
Smidt Heart Institute
Cedars-Sinai Medical Center
Los Angeles California
Chapter 44: Heart Transplantation

Eric V. Krieger, MD
Adult Congenital Heart Service
University of Washington Medical Center and Seattle
    Children's Hospital
Department of Medicine
Division of Cardiology
University of Washington School of Medicine
Seattle, Washington
*Chapter 27: Heart Failure as a Consequence of Congenital
    Heart Disease*

Nicholas T. Lam, PhD
Postdoctoral Researcher
Department of Internal Medicine
Division of Cardiology
University of Texas Southwestern Medical Center
Dallas, Texas
Chapter 3: Cellular Basis for Myocardial Regeneration and Repair

Daniel J. Lenihan, MD
Professor of Medicine
Director, Cardio-Oncology Center of Excellence
Cardiovascular Division
Washington University School of Medicine
St. Louis, Missouri
Chapter 46: Cardio-Oncology and Heart Failure

Gregory Y.H. Lip, MD, FRCP, FACC, FESC
Professor of Cardiovascular Medicine
Liverpool Centre for Cardiovascular Science
University of Liverpool and Liverpool Heart and Chest Hospital
Liverpool, United Kingdom
Aalborg Thrombosis Research Unit
Department of Clinical Medicine
Aalborg University
Aalborg, Denmark
Chapter 14: Alterations in the Peripheral Circulation in Heart Failure

Chris T. Longenecker, MD
Assistant Professor
Division of Cardiovascular Medicine
Department of Medicine
Case Western Reserve University School of Medicine
University Hospitals Harrington Heart and Vascular Institute
Cleveland, Ohio
Chapter 30: Heart Failure and Human Immunodeficiency Virus

W. Robb MacLellan, MD
Professor of Medicine
Robert A. Bruce Endowed Chair in Cardiovascular Research
Head, Division of Cardiology
University of Washington
Seattle, Washington
Chapter 41: Stem Cell-Based and Gene Therapies in Heart Failure

Douglas L. Mann, MD
Lewin Chair and Professor of Medicine, Cell Biology, and Physiology
Chief, Division of Cardiology
Washington University School of Medicine in St. Louis
Cardiologist-in-Chief
Barnes-Jewish Hospital
St. Louis, Missouri
Chapter 7: Role of Innate Immunity in Heart Failure
Chapter 12: Alterations in Ventricular Structure: Role of Left Ventricular Remodeling and Reverse Remodeling in Heart Failure
Chapter 19: Heart Failure as a Consequence of Ischemic Heart Disease

Ali J. Marian, MD
Professor of Molecular Medicine (Genetics) and Internal Medicine (Cardiology)
Director, Center for Cardiovascular Genetics
James T. Willerson, MD, Distinguished Chair in Cardiovascular Research
Institute of Molecular Medicine
University of Texas Health Sciences Center
Houston, Texas
Chapter 23: Heart Failure as a Consequence of Hypertrophic Cardiomyopathy

Daniel D. Matlock, MD, MPH
Associate Professor
Division of Geriatrics
Department of Medicine
University of Colorado
Anschutz Medical Center
Aurora, Colorado
Chapter 50: Decision Making and Palliative Care in Advanced Heart Failure

Mathew S. Maurer, MD
Arnold and Arlene Goldstein Professor of Cardiology
Professor of Medicine
Division of Cardiology
Columbia University Medical Center
New York, New York
Chapter 22: Cardiac Amyloidosis

Dennis M. McNamara, MD, MS
Director, Center for Heart Failure Research
Professor of Medicine
University of Pittsburgh Medical Center
Pittsburgh, Pennsylvania
Chapter 28: Heart Failure as a Consequence of Viral and Nonviral Myocarditis

Robert J. Mentz, MD, FAHA, FACC, FHFSA
Associate Professor of Medicine
Division of Cardiology
Duke University School of Medicine
Durham, North Carolina
Chapter 37: Contemporary Medical Therapy for Heart Failure Patients with Reduced Ejection Fraction

Marco Metra, MD
Professor, Division of Cardiology
Department of Medical and Surgical Specialties, Radiological Sciences, and Public Health
University of Brescia
Brescia, Italy
Chapter 36: Acute Heart Failure

Carmelo A. Milano, MD
Professor of Surgery
Chief, Section of Adult Cardiac Surgery
Surgical Director for LVAD Program
Division of Cardiothoracic Surgery
Duke University Medical Center
Durham, North Carolina
Chapter 45: Circulatory Assist Devices in Heart Failure

Arunima Misra, MD
Associate Professor of Medicine
Baylor College of Medicine
Houston, Texas
Chapter 39: Treatment of Heart Failure with Preserved Ejection Fraction

Joshua D. Mitchell, MD
Assistant Professor of Medicine
Director, Cardio-Oncology Fellowship
Washington University School of Medicine
St. Louis, Missouri
Chapter 46: Cardio-Oncology and Heart Failure

Alan R. Morrison, MD, PhD
Assistant Professor of Medicine
Section of Cardiovascular Medicine
Providence VA Medical Center
Alpert Medical School at Brown University
Providence, Rhode Island
Chapter 32: Cardiac Imaging in Heart Failure

Adam Nabeebaccus, PhD, MBChB, BSc
School of Cardiovascular Medicine and Sciences
King's College London
London, United Kingdom
Chapter 2: Cellular Basis for Heart Failure

Kenta Nakamura, MD
Acting Instructor
Department of Medicine
Division of Cardiology
University of Washington
Seattle, Washington
Chapter 41: Stem Cell-Based and Gene Therapies in Heart Failure

Jose Nativi-Nicolau, MD
Assistant Professor of Medicine
University of Utah Health
Salt Lake City, Utah
Chapter 34: Hemodynamics in Heart Failure

Doan T. M. Ngo, BPham, PhD
Associate Professor
School of Biomedical Sciences and Pharmacy
University of Newcastle
Newcastle, New South Wales, Australia
Chapter 8: Oxidative Stress in Heart Failure

Kelsie E. Oatmen, BS
Research Technician
University of South Carolina School of Medicine
Columbia, South Carolina
MD Candidate
University of Michigan Medical School
Ann Arbor, Michigan
Chapter 4: Myocardial Basis for Heart Failure: Role of Cardiac Interstitium

Peter S. Pang, MD
Associate Professor of Emergency Medicine and Medicine
Indiana University School of Medicine
Indianapolis, Indiana
Chapter 36: Acute Heart Failure

Lampros Papadimitriou, MD, PhD
Assistant Professor of Medicine
Division of Cardiology
Stony Brook University School of Medicine
Stony Brook, New York
Chapter 18: Epidemiology of Heart Failure

Walter J. Paulus, MD, PhD
Cardiologist and Professor of Cardiovascular Physiology
Department of Physiology
Institute for Cardiovascular Research VU
VU University Medical Center
Amsterdam, The Netherlands
Chapter 11: Alterations in Ventricular Function: Diastolic Heart Failure

Tamar S. Polonsky, MD, MSCI
Assistant Professor of Medicine
Director, Cardiovascular Prevention
The University of Chicago Medicine
Chicago, Illinois
Chapter 15: Alterations in Kidney Function Associated with Heart Failure

J. David Port, PhD
Professor of Medicine and Pharmacology
Division of Cardiology
University of Colorado Health Sciences Center
Aurora, Colorado
Chapter 6: Adrenergic Receptor Signaling in Heart Failure

Florian Rader, MD, MSc
Co-Director, Clinic for Hypertrophic Cardiomyopathy and Aortopathies
Assistant Director, Non-invasive Laboratory
Hypertension Center of Excellence
Critical Cardiac Care
Smidt Heart Institute
Cedars-Sinai Medical Center
Los Angeles, California
Chapter 25: Heart Failure as a Consequence of Hypertension

Loheetha Ragupathi, MD
Cardiology Fellow
Thomas Jefferson University Hospitals
Philadelphia, Pennsylvania
Chapter 47: Disease Management and Telemedicine in Heart Failure

Margaret M. Redfield, MD
Professor of Medicine
Department of Cardiovascular Diseases
Mayo Clinic
Rochester Minnesota
Chapter 43: Pulmonary Hypertension

Michael W. Rich, MD
Professor of Medicine
Department of Medicine
Division of Cardiology
Washington University School of Medicine
St. Louis, Missouri
Chapter 40: Management of Heart Failure in Special Populations: Older Patients, Women, and Racial/Ethnic Minority Groups

Joseph G. Rogers, MD
Professor of Medicine
Division of Cardiology
Duke University School of Medicine
Durham, North Carolina
Chapter 45: Circulatory Assist Devices in Heart Failure

John J. Ryan, MD
Assistant Professor of Medicine
University of Utah Health
Salt Lake City, Utah
Chapter 34: Hemodynamics in Heart Failure

Hesham A. Sadek, MD, PhD
Associate Professor
Department of Internal Medicine
Division of Cardiology
Associate Director
Center for Regenerative Science and Medicine
University of Texas Southwestern Medical Center
Dallas, Texas
Chapter 3: Cellular Basis for Myocardial Regeneration and Repair

Can Martin Sag, MD
Clinic and Polyclonic for Internal Medicine II
University Hospital Regensburg
Regensburg, Germany
Chapter 2: Cellular Basis for Heart Failure

Ashley A. Sapp, BA
Administrative Coordinator
Research and Graduate Education
University of South Carolina School of Medicine
Columbia, South Carolina
Chapter 4: Myocardial Basis for Heart Failure: Role of Cardiac Interstitium

Douglas B. Sawyer, MD, PhD
Chief, Cardiovascular Services
Maine Medical Center
Scarborough, Maine
Chapter 46: Cardio-Oncology and Heart Failure

P. Christian Schulze, MD, PhD
Professor of Medicine
Department of Medicine
Division of Cardiology
University Hospital Jena
Friedrich-Schiller-University Jena
Jena, Germany
Chapter 16: Alterations in Skeletal Muscle in Heart Failure

Ajay M. Shah, MD, FMedSci
British Heart Foundation Professor of Cardiology
School of Cardiovascular Medicine and Sciences
King's College London
London, United Kingdom
Chapter 2: Cellular Basis for Heart Failure

Eduard Shantsila, PhD
Clinical Research Fellow in Cardiology
University of Birmingham Institute of Cardiovascular Sciences
City Hospital
Birmingham, United Kingdom
Chapter 14: Alterations in the Peripheral Circulation in Heart Failure

Jagmeet P. Singh, MD, DPhil
Professor of Medicine
Roman W. DeSanctis Endowed Chair in Cardiology
Harvard Medical School
Associate Chief
Cardiology Division
Massachusetts General Hospital
Boston, Massachusetts
Chapter 42: Neuromodulation in Heart Failure

Albert J. Sinusas, MD
Professor of Medicine and Radiology and Biomedical Imaging
Section of Cardiovascular Medicine
Department of Medicine
Yale University School of Medicine
New Haven, Connecticut
Chapter 32: Cardiac Imaging in Heart Failure

Karen Sliwa, MD, PhD
Professor, Hatter Institute for Cardiovascular Research in Africa
Department of Cardiology and Medicine
Faculty of Health Sciences
University of Cape Town
Cape Town, South Africa
Chapter 29: Heart Failure in the Developing World

Francis G. Spinale, MD, PhD
Associate Dean, Research and Graduate Education
Director, Cardiovascular Translational Research Center
Professor, Departments of Surgery and Cell Biology and Anatomy
University of South Carolina School of Medicine
WJB Dorn Veteran Affairs Medical Center
Columbia, South Carolina
Chapter 4: Myocardial Basis for Heart Failure: Role of Cardiac Interstitium

Simon Stewart, PhD, FESC, FAHA
Professor, Hatter Institute for Cardiovascular Research in Africa
Department of Cardiology and Medicine
Faculty of Health Sciences
University of Cape Town
Cape Town, South Africa
Chapter 29: Heart Failure in the Developing World

Carmen Sucharov, PhD
Associate Professor of Medicine
Division of Cardiology
University of Colorado Health Sciences Center
Aurora, Colorado
Chapter 6: Adrenergic Receptor Signaling in Heart Failure

Martin St. John Sutton, MBBS
John Bryfogle Professor of Medicine
Division of Cardiovascular Medicine
Perelman School of Medicine
University of Pennsylvania Medical Center
Philadelphia, Pennsylvania
Chapter 32: Cardiac Imaging in Heart Failure

Aaron L. Sverdlov, MBBS, PhD, FRACP
Associate Professor
Director of Heart Failure
School of Medicine and Public Health
University of Newcastle
Newcastle, New South Wales, Australia
Chapter 8: Oxidative Stress in Heart Failure

Michael J. Toth, PhD
Professor, Departments of Medicine and Molecular Physiology
   and Biophysics
University of Vermont College of Medicine
Burlington, Vermont
Chapter 16: Alterations in Skeletal Muscle in Heart Failure

Anne Marie Valente, MD
Boston Adult Congenital Heart and Pulmonary Hypertension
   Program
Brigham & Women's Hospital
Boston Children's Hospital
Departments of Medicine and Pediatrics
Harvard Medical School
Boston, Massachusetts
*Chapter 27: Heart Failure as a Consequence of Congenital
   Heart Disease*

Loek van Heerebeek, MD, PhD
Cardiologist
Department of Physiology
Institute for Cardiovascular Research VU
VU University Medical Center
Department of Cardiology
Onze Lieve Vrouwe Gasthuis
Amsterdam, The Netherlands
*Chapter 11: Alterations in Ventricular Function: Diastolic
   Heart Failure*

Jasmina Varagic, MD, PhD
Associate Professor
Cardiovascular Science Center
Hypertension and Vascular Research
Wake Forest University School of Medicine
Winston Salem, North Carolina
*Chapter 5: Molecular Signaling Mechanisms of the
   Renin-Angiotensin System in Heart Failure*

†**Ronald G. Victor, MD**
Research Director, Burns and Allen Chair in Cardiology
Associate Director, Hypertension Center of Excellence
Cedars-Sinai Smidt Heart Institute
Cedars-Sinai Medical Center
Los Angeles, California
Chapter 25: Heart Failure as a Consequence of Hypertension

Ian Webb, MRCP, PhD
Consultant Cardiologist
King's College Hospital
King's College London British Heart Foundation Centre of
   Excellence
London, United Kingdom
Chapter 2: Cellular Basis for Heart Failure

Adam R. Wende, PhD
Associate Professor
Department of Pathology
Division of Molecular and Cellular Pathology
University of Alabama at Birmingham
Birmingham, Alabama
Chapter 17: Alterations in Cardiac Metabolism in Heart Failure

David Whellan, MD, MHS
James C. Wilson Professor of Medicine
Senior Associate Provost for Clinical Research
Associate Dean for Clinical Research
Sidney Kimmel Medical College
Executive Director, Jefferson Clinical Research Institute
Philadelphia University and Thomas Jefferson University
Philadelphia, Pennsylvania
*Chapter 47: Disease Management and Telemedicine in Heart
   Failure*

Dominik M. Wiktor, MD
Assistant Professor of Medicine
Division of Cardiology
University of Colorado School of Medicine
Aurora, Colorado
*Chapter 26: Heart Failure as a Consequence of Valvular
   Heart Disease*

† Deceased.

FOREWORD

Heart failure is an important global health problem, with an estimated 38 million patients worldwide. Despite striking advances in the diagnosis and treatment of a variety of cardiovascular disorders during the past three decades, the prevalence of heart failure is increasing. Indeed, heart failure may be considered to be the price of successful management of congenital, valvular and coronary disease, hypertension, and arrhythmias. While both the morbidity and mortality in patients with these disorders have improved markedly, they are often associated with myocardial damage, which, if prolonged, often leads to heart failure.

With the progressive aging of the population, the incidence and prevalence of this condition are continuing to rise. In high-income countries, heart failure is now the most common diagnosis in patients over the age of 65 admitted to hospitals. In medium- and low-income countries, the case fatality rates of heart failure are two to three times greater than in high-income countries. The costs of caring for these patients are immense, in large part because of their hospitalizations, which, paradoxically, are increasing as their lives are prolonged.

On a more positive note, there has been enormous progress in this field, with important new information obtained about the disordered pathobiology, diagnosis, and treatment of heart failure; this has now become a well-recognized subspecialty of cardiovascular medicine and surgery.

This fourth edition of *Heart Failure* is a magnificent text that covers every important aspect of the field. It represents the efforts of 111 authors, who are experienced and recognized experts. G. Michael Felker and Douglas Mann, the coeditors, bring enormous clinical expertise, basic and clinical investigative experience, and energy to this effort.

Heart Failure will be of enormous interest and value to clinicians, investigators, and trainees who are concerned with enriching their understanding of and caring for the ever-growing number of patients with this condition. We are proud of this important companion to *Heart Disease: A Textbook of Cardiovascular Medicine.*

Eugene Braunwald, MD
Douglas P. Zipes, MD
Peter Libby, MD
Robert O. Bonow, MD
Gordon F. Tomaselli, MD

The editors are pleased to present the fourth edition of *Heart Failure: A Companion to Braunwald's Heart Disease*. The field of heart failure continues to rapidly evolve, with new breakthroughs in our understanding of both underlying biology and novel diagnostic and therapeutic approaches. Our goal in this fourth edition is to provide a comprehensive source for practitioners, nurses, physicians-in-training, and students at all levels for a state-of-the-art view of the field of heart failure, from its scientific underpinnings to the latest clinical advances. The print version of the fourth edition, which has been revised extensively, is complemented by a online version that is updated frequently with the results of late-breaking clinical trials, reviews of important new research publications, and updates on clinical practice authored by leaders in the field. These online supplements are selected and edited superbly by Dr. Eugene Braunwald.

As with the earlier editions, the goal in organizing this textbook was to summarize the current understanding of the field of heart failure in a comprehensive bench-to-bedside textbook that would be broadly useful to practitioners, researchers, and students. The field of heart failure has increasingly become a well-defined subspecialty within cardiovascular medicine, with its own advanced training pathway and board certification. In this context, we have substantially revised the book from the prior edition to reflect emerging areas of both scientific and clinical impact.

Sixteen of the 50 chapters in this edition are new, including 4 chapters covering topics that were not addressed in prior editions. We have 42 **new authors**, who are highly accomplished and recognized in their respective disciplines. All chapters carried over from the prior edition have been thoroughly updated and extensively revised. Finally, given the increasing importance of clinical practice guidelines in contemporary cardiovascular practice, we have continued to include updated summaries of practice guidelines for acute heart failure, heart failure with reduced ejection fraction, heart failure with preserved ejection fraction, and the use of cardiac devices at the end of the appropriate chapters.

A detailed rendering of all of the changes in the new edition is not feasible within the limitations of a preface. However, the editors would like to highlight several of the exciting changes in the fourth edition. The sections on the basic mechanism of disease in heart failure (Section I) and on mechanisms of disease progression in heart failure (Section II) contain entirely new chapters on the cellular basis for myocardial regeneration, the renin-angiotensin system, oxidative stress, natriuretic peptide biology (completely new for this edition), and cardiac metabolism. Section III, which is on the etiologic basis for heart failure, features new chapters on ischemic heart failure and heart failure and valvular heart disease, as well as completely new chapters on heart failure and HIV infection and cardiac amyloidosis not covered in the prior editions of the book. The sections on the clinical assessment of heart failure (Section IV) and therapy for heart failure (Section V) include new chapters on acute heart failure, cardiac transplantation, arrhythmias, and device therapy, and there is a completely new chapter on neuromodulation in heart failure.

The extent to which this fourth edition of *Heart Failure: A Companion to Braunwald's Heart Disease* proves useful to those who seek to broaden their knowledge base in an effort to improve clinical outcomes for patients with heart failure reflects the expertise and scholarship of the many talented and dedicated individuals who contributed to the preparation of this edition. It has been a great pleasure to work with them, and it has been our great fortune to learn from them throughout this process. In closing, the editors recognize that a single text cannot adequately cover every aspect of a subject as dynamic or as expansive as heart failure. Accordingly, we apologize in advance for any omissions and shortcomings in the fourth edition.

G. Michael Felker, MD, MHS
Douglas L. Mann, MD

ACKNOWLEDGMENTS

No textbook of the size and complexity of *Heart Failure: A Companion to Braunwald's Heart Disease* can come about without support from a great many individuals. We would like to begin, first and foremost, by thanking Dr. Eugene Braunwald for providing us with the inspiration, as well as the opportunity, to edit the fourth edition of the *Heart Failure Companion*. We would also like to extend our thanks to Drs. Bonow, Libby, and Tomaselli, whose continued guidance is sincerely appreciated. The editors also acknowledge the unswerving support of Elsevier, who approved of the concept of publishing a comprehensive heart failure textbook in 2001 and who has continued to provide support to allow the editors to refine the original vision with each subsequent edition of the *Heart Failure Companion*. We would like to formally acknowledge and thank the following members of the Elsevier staff without whom the fourth edition would not have happened: Dolores Meloni, Publishing Director, for always believing in and championing the *Heart Failure Companion;* Anne Snyder, Senior Content Development Specialist, for quietly holding everything (mainly the editors) together and keeping everything on time; and Claire Kramer, senior project manager. Dr. Mann would also like to thank his administrative assistant, the indefatigable Ms. Mary Wingate, for making all aspects of his professional life possible.

CONTENTS

BRAUNWALD'S HEART DISEASE
FAMILY OF BOOKS

BRAUNWALD'S HEART DISEASE COMPANIONS

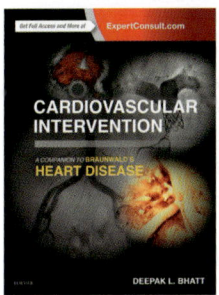

BHATT
Cardiovascular Intervention

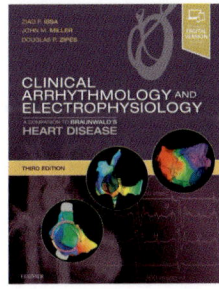

ISSA, MILLER, AND ZIPES
Clinical Arrhythmology and Electrophysiology

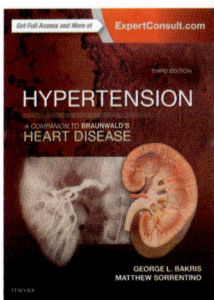

BAKRIS AND SORRENTINO
Hypertension

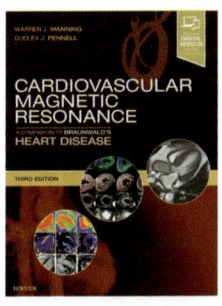

MANNING AND PENNELL
Cardiovascular Magnetic Resonance

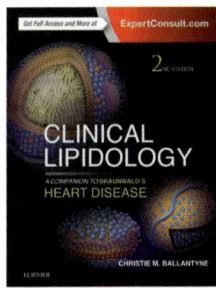

BALLANTYNE
Clinical Lipidology

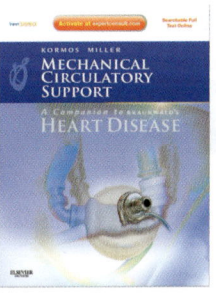

KORMOS AND MILLER
Mechanical Circulatory Support

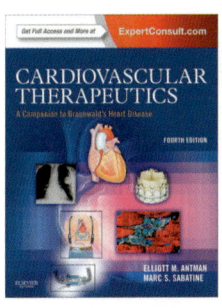

ANTMAN AND SABATINE
Cardiovascular Therapeutics

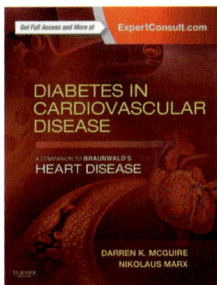

MCGUIRE AND MARX
Diabetes in Cardiovascular Disease

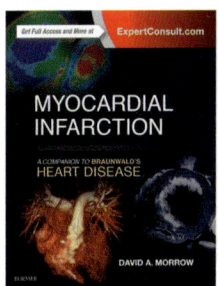

MORROW
Myocardial Infarction

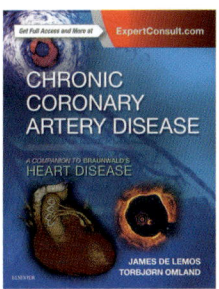

DE LEMOS AND OMLAND
Chronic Coronary Artery Disease

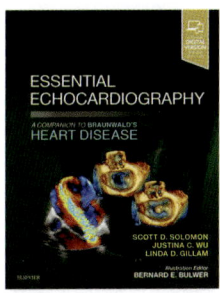

SOLOMON, WU, AND GILLAM
Essential Echocardiography

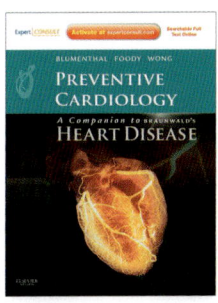

BLUMENTHAL, FOODY, AND WONG
Preventive Cardiology

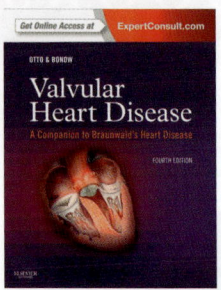

OTTO AND BONOW
Valvular Heart Disease

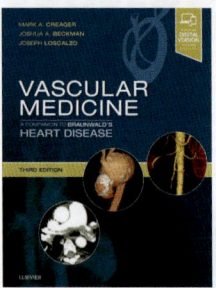

CREAGER, BECKMAN, AND LOSCALZO
Vascular Medicine

BRAUNWALD'S HEART DISEASE REVIEW AND ASSESSMENT

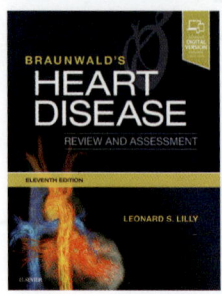

LILLY
Braunwald's Heart Disease Review and Assessment

BRAUNWALD'S HEART DISEASE IMAGING COMPANIONS

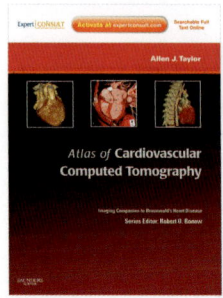

TAYLOR
Atlas of Cardiovascular Computer Tomography

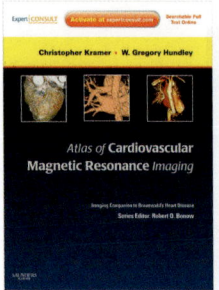

KRAMER AND HUNDLEY
Atlas of Cardiovascular Magnetic Resonance Imaging

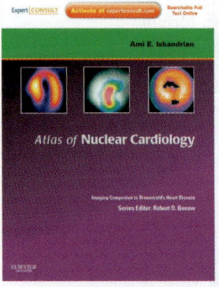

ISKANDRIAN AND GARCIA
Atlas of Nuclear Cardiology

Molecular Basis of Heart Failure

Abhinav Diwan, Joseph A. Hill

OUTLINE

TYPES OF HEART FAILURE

Heart failure (HF) is a multisystemic disorder characterized by profound disturbances in circulatory physiology and a plethora of myocardial structural and functional changes that adversely affect the systolic pumping capacity and diastolic filling of the heart. A discrete inciting event, such as myocardial infarction (MI) or administration of a chemotherapeutic agent, may be identifiable as a proximate trigger in some cases. However, in the vast majority of instances, contributory risk factors (e.g., hypertension, obesity, ischemic heart disease, valvular disease, or diabetes) or genetic and environmental cues are uncovered during the diagnostic workup. These processes adversely affect myocardial biology and trigger cardiomyocyte hypertrophy, dysfunction, and cell death. They also provoke alterations in the extracellular matrix and vasculature, promoting neurohormonal signaling as an adaptive response that paradoxically worsens the pathophysiology. At the cellular level, loss of cardiomyocytes occurs focally with an acute MI or diffusely with some chemotherapeutic agents and with viral myocarditis. This leads to sustained hemodynamic stress, which results in increased hemodynamic load on the surviving myocardium. Simultaneously,

molecular changes are triggered in various cardiac cell types, either in response to the inciting stress or as a secondary consequence of increased hemodynamic load, culminating in contractile dysfunction, altered relaxation and stiffness, fibrosis, and vascular rarefaction.

Evolution of the disease process entails inexorable progression of these cellular and molecular changes in the face of unremitting stress, often despite state-of-the-art antiremodeling therapies. When the process reaches its end stage, mechanical circulatory support or heart transplantation is required. Elucidation of the molecular and cellular bases of these changes during the course of HF pathogenesis is therefore paramount in developing the next generation of therapeutic approaches to address the growing epidemic of HF. For the convenience of the reader, a glossary of abbreviations used in this discussion is presented at the end of this chapter.

HFrEF Versus HFpEF: Ramifications for Understanding the Underlying Biology (see also Chapters 9, 10, and 18)

Left ventricular (LV) ejection fraction (EF), assessed as the fraction of the end-diastolic volume that is ejected upon contraction, has been the cornerstone metric for characterization of LV systolic function in patients with HF. Despite meaningful limitations, including being affected by loading conditions and masking critical information on changes in LV dimensions, EF demonstrates a strong inverse relationship with clinical outcomes in HF in patients with reduced EF.[1] Accordingly, guidelines from national societies for the management of patients with HF recommend their classification into HF with reduced ejection fraction (≤40%; HFrEF) and HF with preserved ejection fraction (≥50%, HFpEF); patients with an EF in the range of 41% to 49% are denoted as being in the "midrange" (HFmEF).[2] Epidemiologic studies have shown that HFpEF patients constitute approximately half of all patients with HF (**see also Chapter 10**).[3] Subsequent outcomes analyses of these subsets have revealed that patients with HFpEF (and HFmEF) also have markedly increased mortality and morbidity mirroring that of patients with HFrEF.[4] As a result, an understanding of the molecular basis for the development and progression of HFpEF is critical, as all current clinical therapeutics for HF are based exclusively on data from clinical trials that enrolled HFrEF patients; subsequent clinical trials in HFpEF patients have failed to replicate the mortality benefits observed with therapies targeting the neurohormonal axes in HFrEF patients. Specifically, clinical trials testing angiotensin antagonism (angiotensin-converting–enzyme [ACE] inhibitors or angiotensin-receptor antagonists [ARB]), mineralocorticoid antagonism, or beta blockers have demonstrated mortality and morbidity benefits in patients in HFrEF. In contrast, targeting these signaling pathways in patients with HFpEF has demonstrated limited benefits with a decrease in heart failure hospitalizations with mineralocorticoid antagonism, underscoring the limited therapeutic options in the clinical armamentarium for this condition (discussed in Shah et al.[5]).

The pathobiology of HFpEF has largely been informed by studies in humans owing to a paucity of animal models that mimic the multifaceted cardiac and systemic abnormalities observed in the human syndrome. Hypertension, advanced age, obesity, type 2 diabetes mellitus, sleep apnea, and renal dysfunction are major risk factors—a reality that points to the need for novel approaches for modeling this condition in animals above and beyond the approaches employed to date. The myocardial pathophysiology in HFpEF is characterized by ventricular diastolic dysfunction with impairment of relaxation and/or ventricular compliance, both of which alter ventricular filling and manifest as elevated left atrial pressures and pulmonary congestion either at rest or under stress, as with exercise, tachycardia, or hypertension. Studies have shown that alterations in ventricular filling are coupled with impaired augmentation of ventricular systolic performance under stress, often in the setting of multisystem abnormalities in the vasculature (endothelial dysfunction [**see Chapter 11**], inflammation [**see Chapter 7**], and increased arterial stiffness) and in skeletal muscle (impaired oxygen uptake and utilization [**see Chapter 16**])—with accompanying renal dysfunction. In cardiomyocytes, evidence has been uncovered for alterations in the phosphorylation of titin (**see also Chapter 11**), a giant sarcomeric spring protein that determines cardiomyocyte passive stiffness, as well as in total collagen volume fraction in the extracellular space in the setting of increased passive cardiomyocyte stiffness.[6]

Age-related increases in myocardial mass (cardiac hypertrophy) have also been ascribed a prominent role in the pathogenesis of HFpEF. Indeed, parabiosis studies indicate that establishing a shared circulation between young and old mice leads to a reduction in cardiomyocyte size and changes in gene expression (downregulation of atrial natriuretic peptide [ANP] and upregulation of sarcoplasmic reticulum Ca^{2+} ATPase [SERCA], see discussion further on).[7] In this study, mechanistic experiments implicated aging-dependent downregulation of GDF-11, a circulating signaling protein member of the transforming growth factor beta (TGF-β) family, in fostering cardiomyocyte changes

that could predispose to HFpEF. Evidence has also been uncovered for increased circulating inflammatory markers, myocardial macrophage infiltration, and coronary microvascular endothelial dysfunction, pointing to a role for inappropriate and sustained activation of inflammatory signaling in the pathogenesis of HFpEF.[8] The increasing prevalence of HFpEF has also been attributed in part to the obesity epidemic occurring in both the developed and developing world, with studies beginning to elucidate metabolic abnormalities that predispose to myocardial diastolic dysfunction. Indeed, calorie restriction and exercise have been documented to be effective in reducing morbidity in this population.[9] Taken together, the multitude of predisposing conditions and the multisystemic abnormalities uncovered thus far in patients with HFpEF have led to the notion that HF in the setting of preserved ejection fraction is triggered by diverse pathophysiologic drivers that may have common manifestations but require individualized therapeutic strategies.[5] The exploration of the biology of HFpEF will require the development and validation of animal models that incorporate these diverse pathophysiologic inputs in order to unveil unique molecular mechanisms involved and develop rational therapies to deal with them.

INVESTIGATIVE TECHNIQUES AND MOLECULAR MODELING

Contemporary investigation into the molecular pathogenesis of heart disease has been driven by parallel advances in preclinical modeling, genetic manipulation, and imaging technologies coupled with rapid refinements in high-throughput sequencing technology. Together, these developments have permitted the integration of unbiased approaches with candidate gene–based reductionist strategies to interrogate cellular pathways in animal models of HF and in specimens from patients with HF. Simultaneously, the framework for understanding normal cardiac growth and development as well as physiologic myocardial function has been refined. With these advances, insights gained from genome-wide analyses of human disease and small animal preclinical studies can be tested in large animal models. As a consequence, a pipeline-based approach for the development and evaluation of therapeutic strategies has emerged.

The existing paradigm for deciphering the molecular basis of HF is based on a reductionist strategy to define events in myocyte and nonmyocyte cell types triggered by disease-related injury (e.g., ischemia and reperfusion, viral infection, chemotherapeutic agents) or biomechanically transduced due to changes in hemodynamic load (either pressure or volume overload). These stimuli elicit specific changes in gene expression, resulting in perturbations in proteins and signaling pathways that affect the structure and function of the heart. Preclinical model systems ranging from in vitro experimentation in isolated cardiomyocytes to in vivo studies in large animal models have been employed to dissect the molecular and cellular pathways involved. A clear advantage of large animal models is the close resemblance of the cardiac structure and function and coronary vasculature in these animals to those of the human heart. On the other hand, small mammals, such as mice, zebrafish, and invertebrates (e.g., *Drosophila*), allow for genetic manipulation with progressive ease as one moves down the evolutionary tree.[10] Investigative approaches have evolved from an early focus on the pharmacologic manipulation of specific pathways in large animals to experimentation involving gain of function and loss of function of candidate genes and/or proteins in small animals in order to recapitulate human pathology.

In vitro techniques in isolated cardiomyocytes have evolved from the development of isolated neonatal rat cardiomyocytes to studies in isolated adult cardiomyocytes and in reprogrammed induced pluripotent stem (iPS) cells differentiated into beating cardiomyocytes and cardiac microtissues.[10–12] Neonatal rat and mouse cardiomyocytes continue to be widely used, as these cells are easily isolated and cultured. Also, they respond to hypertrophic stimuli with an increase in cell size associated with increased protein synthesis and changes in gene expression, mimicking the cardiomyocyte hypertrophic response in vivo. This model system allows the study of cellular changes occurring in hemodynamic overload–induced hypertrophy. A major shortcoming of neonatal cardiomyocytes, however, is the incompletely developed sarcomeric architecture and sarcoplasmic reticulum network. To overcome these limitations, techniques to isolate calcium-tolerant adult cardiomyocytes have been developed to allow for the measurement of contraction, relaxation, and calcium transients. These cells are also amenable to gene transfer with viral vectors. Given that the mouse is the predominant mammalian model for genetic manipulations, isolated field-paced cultured adult myocytes are an attractive model system for assessing the effects of genetic manipulations on cardiomyocyte function.

A major breakthrough in defining patient- and disease-specific alterations in cardiomyocytes was achieved with the observation that isolated somatic cells, such as fibroblasts obtained from a skin biopsy, can be reprogrammed with a cocktail of transcription factors to acquire the characteristics of stem cells.[13] These induced pluripotent stem cells (iPS cells) can subsequently be transdifferentiated into beating cardiomyocytes in vitro, with the structural and functional characteristics of adult cardiomyocytes. When they are transdifferentiated from iPSCs derived from a human, these cardiomyocytes are uniquely suited to deciphering the biology of human cardiomyocytes and to dissecting the unique effects of human disease-causing mutations therein. Indeed, as this technology has become technically more accessible, there has been an explosion of studies that have utilized the iPSC platform to begin to elucidate the basis of human cardiac disease.[11,14–19]

The ability to conduct genome editing with the CRISPR-Cas9 system (see further on), zinc-finger nucleases, and transcription activator–like effector nucleases (TALENs)[20,21] offers tremendous promise for manipulating molecular pathways in patient-specific iPS cells (reviewed in Hockemeyer and Jaenisch[22])s. Also, given their extensive potential for self-renewal and differentiation as well as for reduced immunogenicity in an autologous setting, these cells have been investigated to determine their potential for developing cellular therapy for cardiac disease.[23] Another exciting development has been the direct reprogramming of resident cardiac fibroblasts into cardiomyocytes with delivery of a cocktail of transcription factors in vivo and the discovery of RNA processing and splicing factors that regulate this process (**see also Chapter 2**).[24] This has set the stage for novel strategies for the in vivo manipulation of cardiac regeneration with contemporary genetic targeting techniques (**see also Chapter 3**).

Although in vitro systems are well suited to the study of myocyte cell biology, in vivo modeling is required to determine the effect of disease processes on organ structure and function. The prerequisites for an ideal model system are as follows: (1) a high degree of similarity to human cardiac structure and function, (2) ease of surgical manipulation with development of structural and functional changes that mimic human pathology, (3) superior fidelity to the implementation of targeted genetic interventions to perturb molecular pathways and mimic human genetic alterations, and (4) suitability for application of analytic assays in the live organism to permit serial evaluation in a high-throughput fashion. None of the currently available model systems offers all these advantages, thus necessitating the use of combinations to interrogate the wide range of pathophysiologic, molecular, and cellular changes observed in cardiovascular disease.

Large animal models are well suited to studies involving disease-related stresses, such as valvular stenosis or insufficiency, ischemia/reperfusion, pressure overload, and cardiomyopathy (e.g.,

pacing-induced HF or coronary microembolization).[10] These allow for evaluation of hemodynamic and neurohormonal events in disease progression; however, such animal models do not allow for genetic manipulation. Small mammals, particularly mice, have served as an almost ideal system for experimental in vivo studies. Techniques for genetic perturbations, surgical intervention, and the assessment of cardiac structure and function with noninvasive and invasive approaches have been developed over the last three decades. Despite persistent concerns regarding the translation of findings from the mouse to the human, many observations regarding disease pathophysiology mimic those noted in human disease. Indeed, data obtained in murine models are the backbone of our contemporary understanding of the molecular basis of HF. At the other extreme, model systems such as zebrafish and *Drosophila* are ideally suited for rapid and high-throughput modeling to unveil the effects of genetic perturbations; these models, however, can be less informative with respect to alterations in myocardial structure and function or circulatory pathophysiology.

A transgenic gain-of-function approach is typically employed to evaluate whether a gene or its product, by virtue of its structure or its functional involvement in a particular signaling pathway, is *sufficient* to stimulate myocardial pathophysiology. Forced expression in cardiomyocytes of proteins is conventionally achieved by driving their expression with cardiomyocyte-specific promoters, such as Mlc2v and αMHC.[25] This strategy achieves a high level of gene expression in the early embryonic heart or starting at birth, respectively. For proteins that may have lethal effects following forced expression or when temporal evaluation of the effects of forced expression are to be studied, conditional bitransgenic systems are employed, whereby the expression of the protein of interest can be switched on or off with drug administration, typically tetracycline derivatives or mifepristone.

A loss-of-function approach is designed to determine whether a certain gene (or its product) is *necessary* for a specific phenotype. One approach is to forcibly overexpress a modified protein that has dominant-negative effects by virtue of its structure or function. The potential limitations of this methodology stem from the unpredictable effects of a modified protein, which may be difficult to discern experimentally, and the possibility of noncanonical effects of high-level protein expression, whereby even otherwise inert proteins may induce pathology.[25] A more scientifically robust strategy is gene ablation, which has been achieved using homologous recombination in embryonic stem cells. This strategy has permitted the evaluation of nonredundant functional roles of mammalian proteins in normal development and homeostasis and in pathophysiologic processes relevant to human disease states. To overcome limitations pertaining to the systemic effects of germline gene ablation, tissue-specific ablation has been achieved in the heart using cre-lox (or flp-FRT: flippase, flippase recognition target) technology.[25] Cardiomyocyte-specific gene deletion may be achieved in the embryo with Cre expression driven by the Nkx2.5 promoter (knocked into the Nkx locus) or conditionally at any age with Cre expression induced by tamoxifen treatment in Cre-ER (mutant estrogen receptor)–expressing (αMHC promoter driven) Mer-Cre-Mer transgenic mice. Simultaneously, a "tool box" has been developed to target diverse cell types at various developmental stages, driving an explosion of knowledge in cardiac development and regeneration.[26]

In parallel, there have been exciting developments in tools to target resident cardiac fibroblasts, which form 10% of all cells in the heart[27] and can be activated to transform into myofibroblasts to drive the fibrotic response. Specifically, tamoxifen-inducible systems have been generated driven by promoters for genes expressed in fibroblasts of epicardial origin with persistent expression in mature fibroblasts, namely encoding transcription factor 21 (Tcf21) and platelet-derived growth factor receptor-α (Pdgfr-α), as well as with periostin (Postn gene), which is expressed in activated cardiac fibroblasts (reviewed by

Tallquist and Molkentin[28]). Coordinated international efforts have created repositories of targeted genes with an ever-expanding list of available targets. This is likely to facilitate further expansion of experimentation with these technologies in the future.

The discovery of the CRISPR-Cas9 system, a bacterial system for adaptive immunity, has spurred major breakthroughs in gene editing technologies, enabling precise targeting of the mammalian genome.[29,30] Specificity is achieved in this system by small RNAs termed *guide RNAs* (gRNAs) that direct Cas-9 to a specific site in genomic DNA for inducing cleavage, which is subsequently repaired by nonhomologous end-joining and homology-directed repair mechanisms to result in deletions or specific targeted mutations directed by a homology repair template that is coadministered, respectively. This technique has been rapidly applied to facilitate gene targeting in iPSCs to discern the mechanistic basis of human cardiac disease[31] and to correct mutations in engineered human tissue as a proof of principle of its therapeutic potential in a future human application.[32] This technology has essentially become the preferred approach to rapidly and efficiently target genes for generating knockouts, knockins, and transgenic mice.

With the development of this technology, genetic manipulation offered a powerful experimental strategy to clarify the role of specific genes and proteins in cardiovascular homeostasis. Interactions among genetic changes and various stressors could be examined with the advent of microsurgical techniques to mimic human cardiovascular disease.[10] Examples of such approaches include the induction of ventricular pressure overload or MI. Pressure overload can be induced by thoracic aortic constriction or pulmonary artery banding. Induction of MI can be performed either by reversible ligation or permanent occlusion of murine coronary arteries to simulate ischemia-reperfusion injury or permanent infarction, respectively. This can also be performed in a closed-chest model to minimize inflammatory changes related to open surgery, thereby more closely mimicking human disease. Miniaturization of invasive hemodynamic monitoring has been achieved with the development of micromanometer-tipped catheters for pressure measurement and conductance catheters for pressure-volume loop assessment of load-independent indices. Noninvasive assessment by echocardiography and magnetic resonance imaging has also advanced significantly for myocardial function and tissue characterization, and high-resolution positron emission tomography with computed tomography imaging has been miniaturized to evaluate various facets of cardiac metabolism in the mouse heart. Finally, telemetry-based cardiac rhythm monitoring has permitted rapid throughput evaluation of arrhythmic phenotypes in mutant mouse models.

The isolated perfused working heart preparation and the ejecting heart model are experimental approaches well suited to investigating cardiac function and metabolism in the setting of disease (e.g., ischemia-reperfusion injury) coupled with pharmacologic perturbations in genetically manipulated mice.[10] Together, these approaches comprise a comprehensive "tool kit" that allows for the detailed evaluation of molecular pathways in the context of pathologic stress.

MOLECULAR DETERMINANTS OF PHYSIOLOGIC CARDIAC GROWTH, HYPERTROPHY, AND ATROPHY

Based on early studies in rodents, cardiomyocytes have traditionally been regarded as terminally differentiated cells that rapidly exit the cell cycle early in the postnatal period. Cardiomyocytes manifest increases in cell size and nuclear division, leading to bi- and even multinucleated mature cells, but true cell division appears to occur at a low frequency.[33] As a consequence, cardiomyocyte hypertrophy has been understood as the dominant response of adult cardiomyocytes to injury, as opposed to the hyperplasia observed in tissues with robust

regenerative capabilities. Indeed, cardiomyocyte loss due to cell death has been considered largely irreplaceable. Recent work has challenged these notions, and accumulating evidence indicates that adult cardiomyocytes retain a modest capability of reentering the cell cycle for replication, occurring at a rate much lower than that observed prior to the early postnatal period (**see also Chapter 3**).[34,35]

Cardiac hypertrophy has been conceptualized as "physiologic" to indicate normal postnatal growth and the cardiac enlargement observed with the increased workload demands of pregnancy or exercise conditioning; conversely, "pathologic" hypertrophy is observed in response to disease-related stress, such as hemodynamic overload or myocardial injury.[36,37] Hypertrophy serves to normalize wall stress occurring with increased hemodynamic load, thereby diminishing oxygen consumption, and is traditionally viewed as an "adaptive" response. In pathologic states, however, hypertrophy may be considered maladaptive, as it often progresses to a decompensated state, with the development of cardiomyopathy and HF.

Although these descriptive terms reflect the nature of the inciting stimulus and the probable outcome, it is the specific intracellular signaling events that are closely correlated with outcome. Indeed, the hypertrophic response may match the stimulus but not track its pathologic characteristics. In a study where intermittent pressure overload was induced with reversible transverse aortic constriction, quantitatively less severe hypertrophy was observed as compared with persistent pressure overload.[38] However, the key pathologic characteristics of maladaptive pressure overload hypertrophy were comparable and resulted in functional decompensation with both intermittent and persistent pressure overload, suggesting that it is the nature of the inciting stress, not its frequency or intermittency, that is most relevant.

Normal embryonic and postnatal cardiac growth, termed *cardiac eutrophy*, and physiologic hypertrophy of the adult heart share important traits that distinguish physiologic from pathologic hypertrophy.[36] Physiologic hypertrophy is associated with normal contractile function and normal relaxation. Myocardial collagen deposition is not observed, and capillary density is increased in proportion to the increase in myocardial mass. Additionally, favorable bioenergetic alterations are observed with enhanced fatty acid metabolism and mitochondrial biogenesis. Also, the characteristic expression of a "fetal gene program" seen in pathologic hypertrophy is not observed with physiologic hypertrophy. Physiologic hypertrophy is typically mild (~10%–20% increase in mass over baseline) and regresses without permanent sequelae upon termination of increased hemodynamic demand. Indeed, induction of physiologic hypertrophy by exercise and molecular manipulation of cardiac growth signaling pathways induced primarily in physiologic hypertrophy (see further on) have been reported to prevent or ameliorate the effects of pathologic hypertrophy and HF.[39]

Eutrophy occurs via activation of signaling pathways similar to those observed in exercise-induced hypertrophy (Fig. 1.1). At birth, a dramatic increase in circulating thyroid hormone levels transcriptionally upregulates the synthesis of contractile and calcium handling proteins in the heart and induces a myosin heavy chain isoform shift.[36] Concomitantly, the peptide growth factor IGF-1 is secreted primarily from the liver in response to growth hormone released from the pituitary gland, stimulating physiologic growth. An essential role for IGF-1 in normal growth is evidenced by growth retardation and perinatal lethality in IGF-1 and IGF receptor (IGFR)-1 null mice.[36]

Development of physiologic cardiac hypertrophy in response to exercise is also triggered by IGF-1, levels of which are increased in trained athletes and in cardiomyocytes in response to hemodynamic stress.[36] Indeed, IGF-1 signaling is required for exercise-induced hypertrophy; the hypertrophic response to swimming was completely suppressed in mice with cardiomyocyte-targeted ablation of the IGF-1

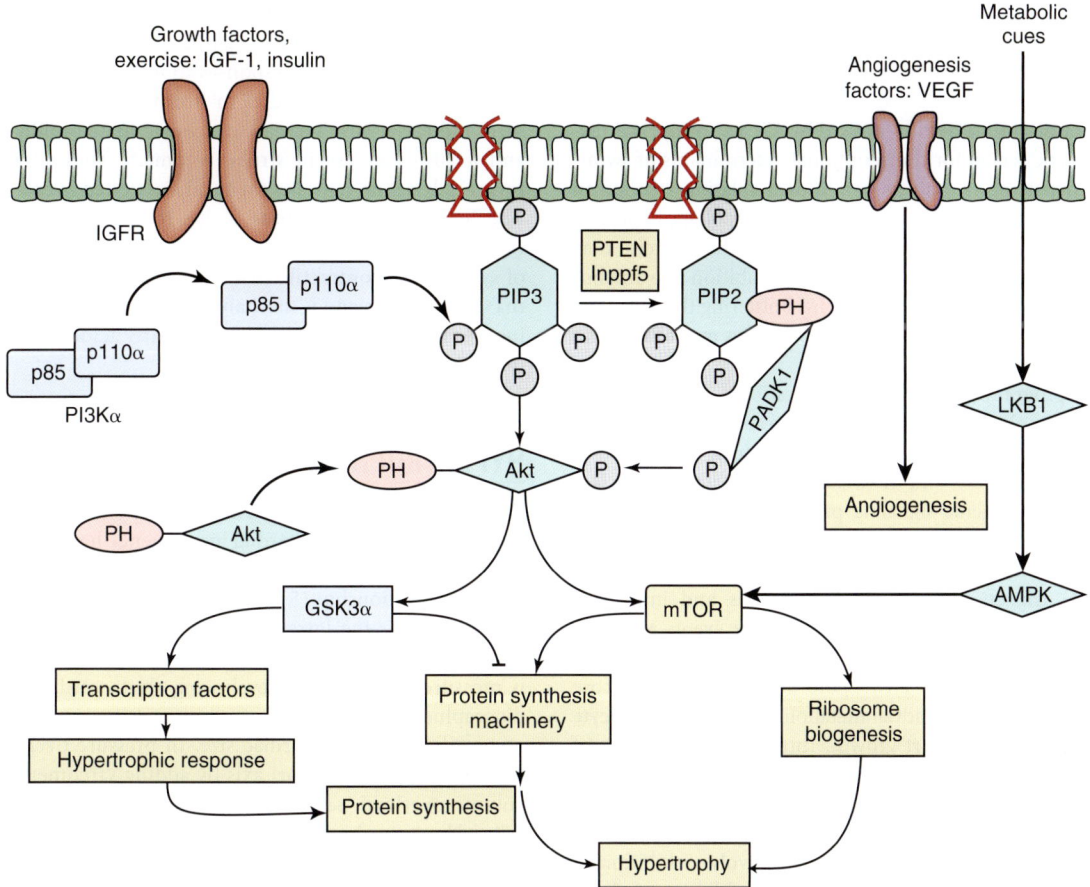

Fig. 1.1 Molecular Signaling in Physiologic Hypertrophy. Normal growth and exercise induce cardiac hypertrophic signaling via IGF-1 release. IGF-1 binds the membrane-bound IGF receptor *(IGFR)*, leading to autophosphorylation and the recruitment of PI3K isoform p110α to the cell membrane. PI3Kα phosphorylates phosphatidylinositols in the membrane at the 3' position in the inositol ring, generating PIP3. Protein kinase B (Akt) and its activator PDK1 associate with PIP3, resulting in Akt activation, which also requires phosphorylation by PDK2 (mTORC2) for full activity (not shown). Activated Akt phosphorylates and activates mTOR, resulting in ribosome biogenesis and stimulation of protein synthesis. Akt also phosphorylates GSK3 (both α and β isoforms), resulting in repression of its antihypertrophic signaling (see later in the chapter). The phosphatases, PTEN and Inpp5f, dephosphorylate PIP3 to generate phosphatidyl PIP2 and shut off the signaling pathway. Physiologic hypertrophy may be triggered by metabolic cues (circulating fatty acids) and requires coordinated induction of angiogenesis.

receptor. Interestingly, induction of IGF-1 production and secretion by cardiac fibroblasts is observed in pressure overload–induced hypertrophy mediated via the activation of the Kruppel-like transcription factor KLF5.[40] This has been implicated in provoking cardiomyocyte hypertrophy by paracrine signaling to preserve cardiac function in the short term, possibly by maintaining an adequate "adaptive" hypertrophic response.[40] Insulin signaling also transduces physiologic cardiac growth, in addition to governing metabolism, as mice with ablation of the insulin receptor manifest reduced cardiomyocyte size with depressed myocardial contractile function. Insulin receptor ablation as well as ablation of insulin receptor substrates IRS1 and IRS2, individually in cardiomyocytes,[41] attenuate development of exercise-induced hypertrophy.[36] Additionally, ablation of the insulin receptor exacerbates pathologic hypertrophy, suggesting an increased propensity for decompensation in the absence of protective physiologic hypertrophic signaling.[36]

IGF-1 and insulin signaling converge on heterodimeric lipid kinases, termed *PI3Ks* (**see** Fig. 1.1), and class I PI3Ks catalyze the formation of phosphatidylinositol-3,4,5-trisphosphate. PI3P recruits downstream effectors such as Akt via a PH-3 domain. Phosphoinositide

phosphatases, namely phosphatase and tensin homolog (PTEN) and Inpp5f, extinguish PI3P signaling. Class IA PI3 kinases (PI3Kα, β, and δ) mediate signaling downstream of receptor tyrosine kinases, namely IGFR, the insulin receptor, and integrins (see further on). Class IA PI3Ks are heterodimers composed of a regulatory subunit (p85α or p85β, or their truncated splice variants p50α or p55α) and a catalytic subunit (p110α, p110β or p110δ). PI3Kγ, a class IB PI3 kinase, is composed of the p110γ catalytic subunit bound to either p84/87 or p101 regulatory adaptor and primarily signals downstream of G protein–coupled receptors (such as the β-adrenergic receptor) in cardiomyocytes. Although genomic ablation of PI3K (p110α) is embryonic lethal in a murine model at day 9.5 of gestation, expression of a dominant-negative mutant of p110α in the postnatal heart reduces adult heart size and blunts development of swimming-induced cardiac hypertrophy.[36] Additionally, a gain-of-function approach with forced cardiomyocyte expression of p110α results in cardiac growth with characteristics of physiologic hypertrophy; ablation of PTEN kinase promotes cardiac growth,[36] confirming a role for this pathway in physiologic cardiac hypertrophy. PI3K (p110α) is also essential for maintaining ventricular function via membrane recruitment of protein kinase B/Akt (**see** Fig. 1.1). Ablation of Akt1 and/or Akt2 downstream of PI3K activation, as well as its activator PDK1, reduces cardiac mass, further emphasizing the essential role of this signaling pathway in normal cardiac growth.[36]

C/EBPβ, a transcription factor repressed by Akt activation, was discovered in a genetic screen for transcriptional determinants of swimming-induced hypertrophy, and its conditional ablation resulted in increased cardiomyocyte proliferation and mild physiologic hypertrophy.[36] This study suggested the exciting possibility that exercise may promote cardiomyocyte proliferation. C/EBPβ inhibition also ameliorated pressure overload induced hypertrophy, bolstering the paradigm that stimulation of physiologic hypertrophy pathways may offer benefits by hitherto undiscovered mechanisms.

Metabolic reprogramming and angiogenesis are other essential components of the physiologic hypertrophic response. Indeed, targeted ablation of LKB1 (an activator of AMPK, which is activated in response to energy deficit)[42] and of vascular endothelial growth factor (VEGF), a proangiogenic signaling protein (in *vegfb*-null mice), provokes reduced postnatal cardiac size and vascular rarefaction.[36] Remarkably, cardiomyocyte-specific ablation of the glucose transporter (GLUT4) triggers cardiomyocyte apoptosis and interstitial fibrosis in the setting of swimming exercise. These events are associated with Akt dephosphorylation by increased levels of phosphatase protein phosphatase 2A (PP2A),[43] pointing to a role for glucose uptake in maintaining mitochondrial metabolism and cardiomyocyte survival during physiologic heart growth. Intriguingly, activation of AMPK (which senses the ratio of AMP/ATP and ADP/ATP, i.e., the energetic state of the cell) is observed with physiologic hypertrophy and has been demonstrated to inhibit pathologic hypertrophy.[36,42] The mechanism for this observation appears to involve inhibition of O-GlcNAcylation of proteins by AMPK-mediated inhibition of glutamine:fructose-6-phosphate aminotransferase (GFAT), which reduces the supply of N-acetylglucosamine.[44]

Despite these observations, it is critical to proceed cautiously with strategies to stimulate physiologic hypertrophy in hopes of ameliorating pathologic hypertrophy. This is underscored by the observations that forced cardiac expression of IGF-1 initially produces functionally compensated ventricular hypertrophy that evolves, over time, into pathologic hypertrophy with fibrosis and systolic dysfunction.[36] Also, forced cardiomyocyte expression of Akt, its pivotal downstream signaling effector, results in compensated hypertrophy, which transitions to cardiac failure due to inadequate angiogenesis.[42] Mechanistically, it is plausible that exuberant cardiomyocyte hypertrophy, whether initially physiologic or pathologic, may outstrip concordant angiogenesis and exceed the individual's capacity for oxygen and nutrient delivery sufficient to meet the demands of the hypertrophied myocyte. This may explain the rare clinical observations of irreversible ventricular hypertrophy and dilation observed in athletes after long-term participation in endurance sports with a strength component, such as rowing and cycling.[45]

Cardiomyocyte size is remarkably plastic[46]; the heart undergoes atrophy with a reduction in hemodynamic load or metabolic demand, as may occur in conditions of weightlessness and extended bed rest, as with spinal cord injury. This may involve the inhibition of growth pathways, as seen with suppression of insulin signaling in cancer-induced cardiac cachexia in mice, which was reversible with exogenous insulin treatment.[47] A parallel induction of proteolytic and catabolic pathways, such as activation of the ubiquitin-proteasome system, facilitates the atrophic response. Indeed, activation of muscle ring finger1 (Murf 1) ligase has been demonstrated to be essential for the regression of pressure-overload hypertrophy, and loss of function of Murf1 and Murf2 in the heart lead to spontaneous cardiac hypertrophy and HF via the downregulation of E2F transcription factor signaling.[48] Cardiac growth and atrophy are also observed as physiologic responses to metabolic demand, as demonstrated in fascinating studies in Burmese pythons, wherein a large meal induces a 40% increase in cardiac mass rapidly over 48 hours and a 50% increase in stroke volume.[49] These dramatic changes revert to baseline values as the meal is digested over a period of days. The increased cardiac mass is due to cardiomyocyte hypertrophy (and not hyperplasia); it is associated with transcriptional induction of synthesis of contractile elements with activation of PI3K-Akt and mTOR pathways and is mechanistically driven by increased circulating free fatty acids and stimulation of fatty acid uptake and oxidation in the myocardium.

MOLECULAR DETERMINANTS OF PATHOLOGIC HYPERTROPHY

Cardiac hypertrophy occurring in response to injury, hemodynamic overload, or myocardial insufficiency has been conceptualized as a compensatory response to normalize wall stress as defined by LaPlace's relationship ($S = PR/2H$, where S is wall stress [force per unit area], P is the intraventricular pressure, R is the radius of the ventricular chamber, and H is the wall thickness).[50] Hypertrophy is measured at the organ level using electrocardiographic, echocardiographic, and/or magnetic resonance imaging (MRI) indices of myocardial mass and cardiac size. In pressure overload, cardiomyocytes enlarge in the short axis by adding sarcomeres in parallel. In volume overload, sarcomeres are added in series, lengthening the cell.[51] Hypertrophic remodeling is then characterized as concentric (increased wall thickness without dilation) or eccentric (chamber dilation with a mild increase in wall thickness), respectively, with pressure and volume overload stress.

Is Load-Induced Hypertrophy Ever Compensatory?

A purely physical perspective on the mechanics of hypertrophy conceptualizes the primary change in ventricular geometry (i.e., wall thickening) as helpful in normalizing wall stress and postponing the inevitable functional decompensation and adverse remodeling (wall thinning and chamber dilation) per initial concepts proposed in the 1960s by Meerson and assessed by Grossman et al. (reviewed in Schiattarella et al.[52]). Interestingly, studies in animal models have suggested that reactive hypertrophy after hemodynamic overloading may be entirely dispensable to functional compensation and even undesirable.[53,54] Indeed, epidemiologic evidence from humans with hypertension and LV hypertrophy (LVH) unequivocally demonstrates marked increases in HF, coronary heart disease, and sudden cardiac death[52,55]; moreover, reversal of LVH with neurohormonal blockade has firmly established a strong correlation between regression of LVH and prevention of clinical outcomes.[52] These observations have led to the characterization of load-induced hypertrophy as pathologic based on the development of HF and cardiomyopathic decompensation. Indeed, these observations indicate that the "quality of the myocardium" rather than its "quantity" may be a more important determinant of development of HF; this underscores the need for large animal studies to determine whether load-induced hypertrophy is compensatory or detrimental.[52] Indeed, in pathologic hypertrophy, the characteristic gene expression changes, cardiomyocyte dysfunction, and altered neurohormonal responsiveness (reviewed in Nakamura et al.[42]) are in striking contrast to those observed during normal cardiac growth and physiologic hypertrophy, and they portend adverse outcomes. Therefore the interruption of pathologic hypertrophic signaling may be a desirable therapeutic endpoint in HF.

Transcriptional Regulation of Pathologic Cardiac Hypertrophy

A hallmark of pathologic hypertrophy in the adult heart is reexpression of embryonic cardiac genes, a process often referred to as the "fetal gene program," as this aspect of the cardiac response to stress or injury recapitulates aspects of cardiac development.[42] The earliest detectable change (within hours of increasing afterload or stimulating cultured cardiomyocytes to hypertrophy with norepinephrine) is induction of regulatory transcription factors c-fos, c-jun, jun-B, c-myc, and Egr-1/nur77, and heat shock protein (hsp) 70, thereby mimicking changes observed with cell cycle entry. Induction of these "early response genes" drives expression of other genes in the fetal program. The prototypical gene, atrial natriuretic factor (ANF), is expressed early during heart development through the coordinated interactions of Nkx2.5, GATA-4, and PTX transcription factors, but only in the atria of normal adult hearts. A robust induction of ventricular ANF expression (and related brain natriuretic peptide [BNP]) is observed in pathologic hypertrophy and HF. In fact, increased BNP secretion from the stressed heart is used widely as a biomarker of HF. Other elements of the fetal gene program induced in pathologic hypertrophy and HF encode sarcomeric genes, such as βMHC, MLC2v, α-skeletal actin, and β-tropomyosin, proteins that are prominent in embryonic, but not adult, ventricle.

Cardiac gene expression in pathologic hypertrophy is driven by the reactivation of many developmentally regulated transcription factors (Fig. 1.2). GATA4 and GATA6 are two such zinc finger DNA-binding transcription factors that are individually essential for heart tube development and myocyte proliferation during embryogenesis.[42] Both of these transcription factors are also essential for homeostatic expression of various cardiomyocyte genes in the adult heart, including ANF,

BNP, ET-1, α-skeletal actin, αMHC, βMHC, cardiac troponin c, and AT1Ra; their individual or combinatorial ablation results in progressive cardiomyopathy. In pressure-overload hypertrophy, cardiomyocyte-specific deletion of either GATA4 or GATA6 markedly attenuates development of pressure-overload hypertrophy, resulting in accelerated decompensation. Importantly, GATA4 signaling may be essential for sustaining angiogenic responses in pressure-overload hypertrophy via VEGF activation,[36] underscoring its critical role in this setting.

Prohypertrophic signaling pathways, such as activation of MAP kinase cascades downstream of Gαq-coupled α-adrenergic (α1A) receptors, trigger activation of GATA4. GATA4 also complexes with other transcription factors such as Nkx2.5, Mef2, a coactivator, p300, SRF, and nuclear factor of activated T-cells (NFAT) to effect cardiac gene expression (see Fig. 1.2).[39] Serum response factor (SRF) is another cardiac-enriched transcription factor that coordinately induces sarcomerogenesis with other transcription factors, including SMAD1/3, Nkx2–5, and GATA4. Cardiomyocyte-specific ablation of SRF in the adult heart results in progressive development of cardiomyopathy with disorganization of the sarcomeres and HF. SRF also interacts with myocardin and HOP transcription factors. HOP antagonizes SRF signaling, and conditional ablation of HOP results in aberrant cardiac growth with evidence of both lack of myocyte formation and excess cardiomyocyte proliferation. Myocardin acts as a cardiac and smooth muscle–specific coactivator of SRF and is essential for embryonic cardiomyocyte proliferation[39] and the maintenance of normal sarcomeric organization in the adult heart.

There has been much speculation about the functional impact of reexpression of the fetal gene program in pathologic hypertrophy.[56] It has been postulated that an increased ratio of β-MHC/α-MHC isoforms impairs myocardial contractility due to relative inefficiency of

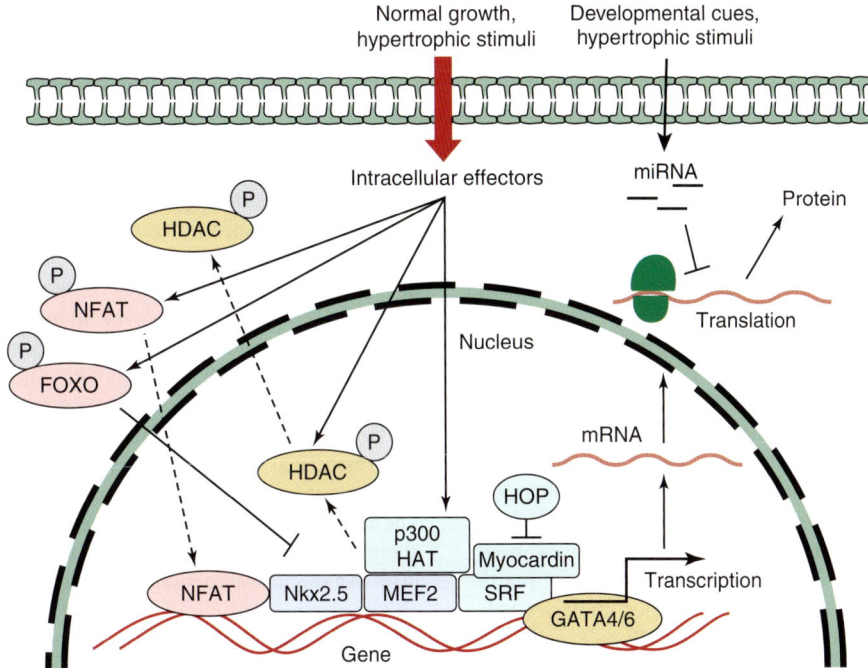

Fig. 1.2 Regulation of Gene Expression in Normal Growth and Pathologic Hypertrophy. A common set of transcription factors determines normal cardiac growth and pathologic hypertrophy, such as GATA4, Nkx2.5, SRF, MEF2 and NFATs. Hypertrophic signaling pathways result in phosphorylation of HDACs with export out of the nucleus, permitting histone acetylation by HATs, with activation of gene transcription to generate messenger RNA (mRNA). mRNA is spliced to yield a mature form, which recruits the protein synthesis machinery leading to protein translation. miRNAs inhibit mRNA translation and/or enhance mRNA degradation to negatively regulate translation. FoxO3 family and Wnt transcription factors (not shown) negatively regulate hypertrophic growth.

the β-isoform, culminating in reduced sarcomeric shortening, prolonged relaxation, and adverse remodeling. Although this may have a major impact in the adult mouse ventricle, which predominantly expresses the faster α-isoform, its relevance in the adult human heart, in which 90% of the myosin heavy chain is the β-isoform, is less clear. In contrast, downregulation of the gene encoding the SERCA affects the activity of this important Ca^{2+} pump, which is responsible for the rapid diastolic reuptake of calcium into the sarcoplasmic reticulum.[39] This has been established as an important mechanism for the contractile dysfunction observed in human HF.

Multiple studies focusing on transcriptome profiling of cardiac pathology have identified a panoply of gene expression changes in both human HF and animal models of pathologic hypertrophy (http://www.cardiogenomics.org).[57] These myocardial mRNA signatures and the different patterns of gene expression in normal, early-failing, late-failing, and recovering hearts might be useful as prognostic biomarkers and could help guide therapeutics. Also, in the past decade, there have been dramatic advances in sequencing technologies. A rapidly accumulating list of individual variations in genetic sequence (termed *single-nucleotide polymorphisms*) and their combinations, through genome-wide association studies (GWAS), holds promise to uncover novel targets for further mechanistic exploration in HF.[58]

Another layer of complexity in gene regulation has been revealed by studies of microRNAs (miRNAs). These are short, noncoding, naturally occurring single-stranded RNAs that regulate gene expression negatively by promoting the degradation of mRNAs and/or inhibiting mRNA translation, thereby suppressing protein synthesis (see Fig. 1.2). miRNAs are abundantly expressed in the myocardium and differentially regulated in animal models and human HF.[44] miRNAs are essential for homeostatic gene regulation, as targeted cardiomyocyte-specific ablation of Dicer, an enzyme essential for miRNA processing, causes HF with profound transcriptional dysregulation of cardiac contractile proteins.[59] Upstream signaling pathways alter miRNA expression in response to developmental cues and hypertrophic stimuli, such as the regulation of miR-1 and miR-133 from a common precursor by SRF and MEF2. These transcription factors control cardiomyocyte proliferation during development and downregulate miR-1 and miR-133, facilitating prohypertrophic pathways in swimming-induced and pressure overload hypertrophy. Another group of miRNAs is localized to the myosin heavy chain genes, miR-208a, miR-208b, and miR-499 (termed MyomiRs). These have been shown to regulate transcriptional repressors and thyroid hormone signaling to transduce the changes in myosin heavy chain gene expression observed in pathologic hypertrophy. Importantly, targeted deletion of miR-208a prevented reexpression of the fetal gene program and attenuated pathologic remodeling with pressure overload. Upregulation of the miR-15 family at birth plays an important role in suppressing cardiomyocyte proliferation in the immediate postnatal period.[60] Indeed, miR-15 inhibition with locked nucleic acids stimulates continued cardiomyocyte proliferation after birth and induces the regeneration of myocardium when administered post-MI in adult mice. This restores the regenerative capacity otherwise observed only in 1-day-old pups. Therefore targeting the regulation of gene expression with miRNA-targeted strategies holds promise in developing novel therapeutics to treat HF.

Cellular Mechanisms of Impaired Cardiomyocyte Viability

Hypertrophy of the ventricular myocardium is an independent risk factor for cardiac death[55] and is observed with near-universal prevalence in patients with HF. LV hypertrophy may, in part, underlie the diastolic dysfunction observed in HFpEF.[3] In addition, in patients with HFrEF, pathologic LV hypertrophy progresses inexorably from a compensated or nonfailing state to dilated cardiomyopathy and overt failure.[42] It is important to recognize that although the essential feature of cardiac hypertrophy is increased cardiomyocyte size/volume, other myocardial alterations—such as fibroblast hyperplasia, deposition of extracellular matrix proteins, and a relative decrease in vascular smooth muscle and capillary density[42]—also contribute to the progression from functionally compensated pathologic hypertrophy to overt HF.

Activation of Cell Death Pathways (see also Chapter 2)

Evidence for cardiomyocyte "dropout" due to death or degeneration is observed in failing hearts and in pathologic hypertrophy before the development of cardiomyopathy. The extant literature indicates that hypertrophied cardiomyocytes are likely to die from a number of different processes, and cardiomyocyte death can be a causal factor in cardiomyopathic decompensation, although the relative contribution of specific pathways appears to vary with pathologic context.[61] Cardiomyocyte death may be programmed (i.e., cell suicide) by apoptosis, necrosis, or autophagy or it may be accidental (as in conventional necrosis due to interruption of vascular supply). Histologic evidence for all forms of death is seen in end-stage human cardiomyopathy.[62]

The term *apoptosis* is derived from the Greek expression for "the deciduous autumnal falling of leaves" (*apo* means "away from" and *ptosis* means "falling"); it is an orderly and highly regulated energy-requiring process that mediates targeted removal of individual cells during development without provoking an immune response. The rates of apoptosis, measured as apoptotic indices (e.g., the number of TUNEL-positive nuclei/total nuclei), parallel the rates of cell division and are highest in the outflow tract (~50%); intermediate in the endocardial cushions, which are sites of valve formation, and in the LV myocardium (10%–20%); and lowest in the right ventricular myocardium (~0.1% at birth).[61] Both cardiomyocyte apoptosis and mitosis in the LV myocardium virtually cease soon after birth and within the first 2 weeks of life in the right ventricle. Abnormal persistence of apoptosis in right ventricular myocardium contributes to the pathogenesis of arrhythmogenic right ventricular dysplasia, a disorder caused by mutations provoking abnormal localization of desmosomal proteins leading to the suppression of Wnt signaling. This stimulates de novo adipogenesis from resident cardiac stem cells to cause right ventricle–specific cardiomyocyte apoptosis and fibrofatty replacement associated with arrhythmias and sudden death.[63] Apoptotic cardiomyocytes are extremely rare in normal adult myocardium (1 apoptotic cell per 10,000–100,000 cardiomyocytes). Together with reactivation of the "fetal gene program" in hypertrophied and failing hearts, the prevalence of cardiomyocyte apoptosis is markedly increased in chronic cardiomyopathies.[64] Apoptotic cardiomyocyte death may also play a role in the transition of pressure overload hypertrophy to dilated cardiomyopathy. Emerging evidence suggests that necrosis, a form of cell death associated with rupture of the plasma membrane and inflammatory infiltration, may be programmed and controlled by the cell.[61] The death machinery that orchestrates these processes exhibits cross talk at multiple levels, whereby features of either or both forms may be dominant in a specific pathophysiologic setting.

Cell death may be initiated by ligand-dependent signaling from the cell exterior through the extrinsic or receptor-mediated pathways; conversely, it may occur by induction of the death machinery within the cell through mitochondrial pathways (Fig. 1.3).[61] Sustained experimental pressure overload is sufficient to induce expression of the prototypical death-promoting cytokine, TNF. This molecule signals via the type 1 TNF receptor (TNFR1) to stimulate cardiomyocyte hypertrophy and apoptosis and provoke contractile dysfunction.[65] A potentially causal role for elevated levels of this cytokine is suggested by elevated TNFα plasma levels that are correlated with the degree of

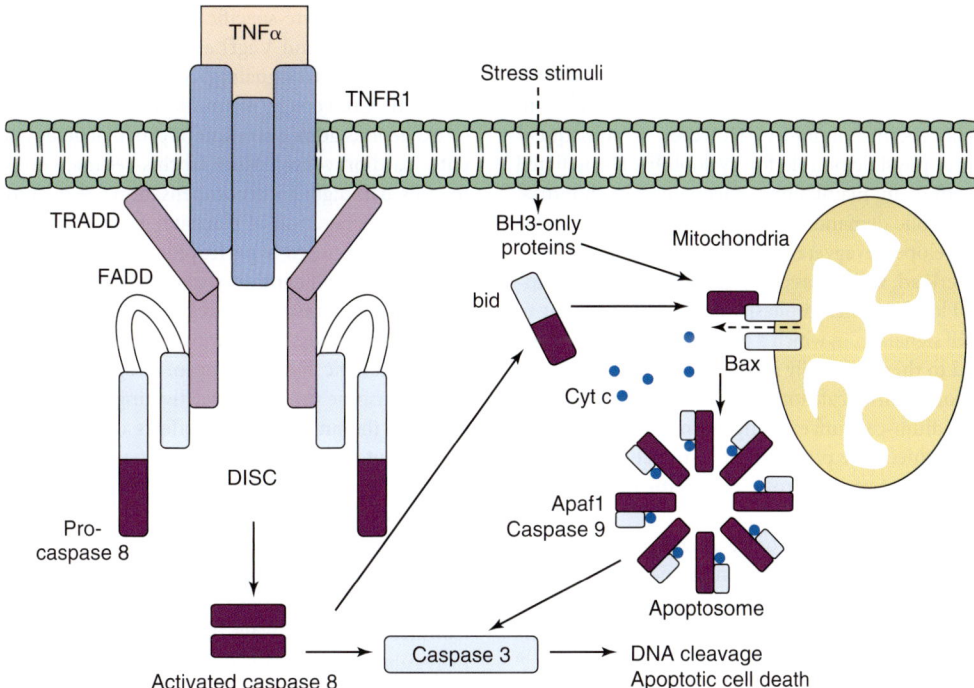

Fig. 1.3 Cell Death Signaling in Heart Failure. Cell death machinery is activated via an "extrinsic pathway," when death-inducing ligands such as TNF/Fas engage cognate receptors, or an "intrinsic pathway" triggered by stress-mediated transcriptional induction or activation of prodeath BH3 domain-only proteins. TNFα binds the TNF receptor 1 (TNFR1) homotrimer, resulting in the recruitment of proteins via the death domains TRADD and FADD and procaspase 8 and assembly of DISC (death-inducing signaling complex). This causes cleavage activation of caspase 8, which cleaves and activates the effector caspase, caspase 3. Activated caspase 3 proteolyses cellular substrates and causes cell death. BH3 domain-only Bcl2 family proteins get activated in response to stress stimuli (as with transcriptional induction of BNIP3L/Nix with pathologic hypertrophic signaling; see text for details) to permeabilize mitochondria. The extrinsic pathway is also amplified by the caspase 8-induced cleavage of bid, the truncated form of which, t-bid, interacts with multidomain proapoptotic Bcl2 proteins Bax and Bak (not shown) to engage the intrinsic pathway. This results in mitochondrial outer membrane permeabilization and release of cytochrome c (cyt c), which associates with the adapter protein Apaf-1, ATP, and procaspase 9, forming the apoptosome, with activation of caspase 9. Activated caspase 9, in turn, activates caspase 3. This process is opposed by Bcl2 and Bcl-xl (not shown), and by inhibitor protein XIAP. Smac/DIABLO and Omi/HtrA2 are released during mitochondrial permeabilization (not shown) and bind to XIAP, relieving its inhibitory effect. Also released are DNAses: AIF (apoptosis-inducing factor) and EndoG, which cause internucleosomal DNA cleavage.

cardiac cachexia in end-stage HF.[66] Death receptor signaling downstream of TNFR1 is triggered by TNF binding to a receptor homodimer, resulting in formation of the death-inducing signaling complex (DISC) with recruitment of adaptor protein FADD and caspase 8 (an upstream member of a family of executioner cysteine proteases). Activated caspase 8 then cleaves caspase 3 and Bid, a proapoptotic Bcl2 family member. Activated caspase 3, the effector caspase, activates a nuclear DNAase (CAD-caspase activated DNAse), resulting in internucleosomal cleavage of DNA and chromatin condensation. The generation of truncated tBid links the extrinsic pathway to activation of the intrinsic pathway. This leads to their simultaneous activation in TNF-induced cardiomyocyte apoptosis in the setting of TNF-induced depletion of antiapoptotic signaling proteins in the mitochondria.[65] Although elevated TNF levels signal to provoke myocardial hypertrophy with increased cardiomyocyte apoptosis, adverse ventricular remodeling, and systolic dysfunction in rodent models, endogenous TNF signaling is cytoprotective in ischemia-reperfusion injury. This indicates that precise context-dependent modulation of TNF signaling may be required to attenuate cell death in pathologic hypertrophy.

The intrinsic mitochondrial pathway of programmed cell death is triggered by stress-induced upregulation or activation of BH3 domain-only prodeath proteins (see Fig. 1.3),[61] such as with Gαq/PKC/SP-1–mediated transcriptional induction of BNIP3L/Nix in pathologic hypertrophy. Nix targets and permeabilizes mitochondria to induce the release of prodeath mediators such as cytochrome c. Nix-induced mitochondrial permeabilization may be direct via outer membrane permeabilization (MOMP) or may occur via Nix targeting to the ER, triggering ER-mitochondrial cross talk to provoke calcium overload and opening of the mitochondrial permeability transition pore (MPTP). In the cytosol, cytochrome c binds to the adaptor protein Apaf-1 (apoptotic protease activating factor-1), resulting in sequential recruitment and cleavage-mediated activation of caspase 9 and caspase 3. Together with the release of AIF (apoptosis inducing factor) and endoG from the mitochondrial intermembranous space, this results in activation of PARP and DNA cleavage in the nucleus (see Fig. 1.3) and cell death. Stress-induced cardiomyocyte death is an important determinant of pathologic hypertrophy and decompensation, as cardiomyocyte-specific ablation of Nix attenuates pressure overload–induced ventricular remodeling and programmed cell death.[61]

Calcium overload–induced opening of MPTP is also implicated in programmed necrosis. Inhibition of MPTP formation with mitochondrial ablation of *ppif* (the gene encoding cyclophilin D), a critical mitochondrial matrix component of the MPTP, reduces cell death provoked by ischemia-reperfusion injury. However, a subsequent study reported a critical physiologic role for cyclophilin D-mediated mitochondrial Ca²⁺ efflux in maintaining adequate mitochondrial function to match metabolic demand. In this study, mice with cyclophilin D deficiency developed exaggerated hypertrophy and HF with exercise or pressure overload, which was corrected by transgenic restoration of cyclophilin D levels.[67] This emphasizes a paradigm similar to that observed with TNF signaling, in which a precise modulation of the MPTP will be required to therapeutically address programmed necrosis in HF. Indeed, mitochondrial calcium overload can be countered by the mitochondrial sodium-calcium exchanger (encoded by Slcb81); stimulating its activity reduced the propensity for mitochondrial permeability transition and prevented necrotic cell death in models of HF.[68]

In pathologic hypertrophy, cardiomyocyte necrosis may also be triggered by ischemia due to mismatch between the degree of hypertrophy and vascular supply. An adequate blood supply for growing myocardium is critical to normal cardiac function, and capillary density is closely coupled to myocardial growth during development.[36] As discussed earlier, pathologic hypertrophy is associated with relative vascular rarefaction (as compared with normal capillary density observed with physiologic hypertrophy), with decreased capillary density, decreased coronary flow reserve, and increased diffusion distance to myocytes. There is a temporal correlation between decreased capillary density and cardiomyocyte "dropout" during decompensation in both human disease and experimental animal models. Indeed, in pressure overload–induced hypertrophy, impairment of angiogenesis

with cardiomyocyte-specific GATA4 ablation (and resultant deficiency of angiopoietin and Vegf) and sustained increases in p53 (with suppression of HIF1α signaling) accelerate the progression to decompensated HF. Conversely, restoration of angiogenesis with p53 inhibition or exogenous administration of proangiogenic agents markedly attenuates cardiomyocyte death in this setting, confirming a central role for this paradigm in decompensation. Also, studies have shown that enhanced generation of placental growth factor (PGF) by various cell types in response to hypertrophic stress in the myocardium stimulates angiogenesis and cardiomyocyte hypertrophy via IL6 generation, and this angiogenic response can be stimulated further to prevent decompensation of pressure-overload hypertrophy.[69] Additionally, during the physiologic hypertrophy of pregnancy, proangiogenic signaling via peroxisome proliferator activating factor γ coactivator α (PGC1α) counters the antiangiogenic effects of a VEGF inhibitor secreted by the placenta, termed sFLT-1.[70] Deficiency of the angiogenic response provokes peripartum cardiomyopathy, pointing to a critical need for coordinated increases in angiogenesis and myocyte size to maintain physiologic hypertrophy.

Cell Survival Pathways

Countervailing pathways that promote cell survival play critical roles in regulating cell death during pathologic cardiac remodeling. One such pathway is elicited by the IL-6 family of cytokines, comprising IL-6, cardiotrophin, and LIF and signaling via a shared membrane receptor, namely the gp130 glycoprotein, which has intrinsic tyrosine kinase activity (Fig. 1.4). Binding of ligand induces gp130 homodimerization or oligomerization with β-subunits of other cytokine receptors, stimulating autophosphorylation on receptor cytoplasmic tails and activating intrinsic tyrosine kinase activity. This permits the binding of adaptor proteins Grb2 and Shc to SH2 binding domains

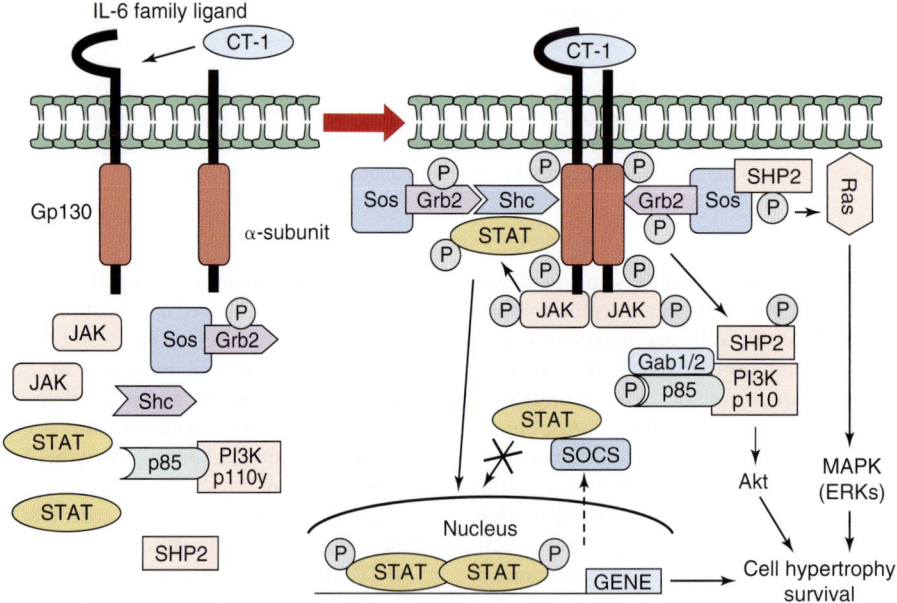

Fig. 1.4 Gp130-Mediated Survival Signaling in Heart Failure. Ligand-induced homodimerization of Gp130, a transmembrane receptor protein, or heterodimerization with α-receptor subunits for IL-6 cytokine family members such as CT-1, LIF, or oncostatin M, causes tyrosine autophosphorylation and recruitment and activation of JAK1/2. Subsequently, two major intracellular signaling cascades are triggered: (1) Signal transducer and activator of transcription (STAT)-1/3 pathway with STAT dimerization and translocation to the nucleus with activation of gene transcription. This pathway is opposed by induction of SOCS proteins, which bind to and prevent STAT translocation. (2) SH2-domain–containing cytoplasmic protein phosphatase (SHP2)/ MEK/extracellular signal-regulated kinase (ERK) pathway. Additionally, Grb2 binding with Gab1/2 causes PI3K mediated Akt activation. These pathways signal to promote cardiomyocyte hypertrophy and survival.

to activate Janus kinases (JAKs), which phosphorylate STAT transcription factors. Activated STAT dimers then migrate to the nucleus to (1) regulate gene expression; (2) activate SH2 domain-containing cytoplasmic protein tyrosine phosphatase (SHP2), which subsequently activates the MEK/ERK pathway; and (3) activate the Ras/mitogen-activated protein kinase, leading to MAPK activation and extracellular signal-regulated kinase (ERK) signaling (see Fig. 1.4). A simultaneous transcriptional upregulation of SOCS family proteins via STAT signaling provides for feedback inhibition of these pathways (see Fig. 1.4). Gp130 activation is transiently observed early after the onset of pressure overload, and this survival pathway is deactivated during the transition to failure, possibly related to interruption of gp130-JAK-STAT signaling by stress-induced SOCS3 and the resulting suppression of STAT3 signaling. Importantly, ablation of gp130 provokes exaggerated cardiomyocyte apoptosis with fulminant HF and pressure overload hypertrophy.[61]

Autophagy (in Greek, meaning to eat oneself) is a lysosomal degradative pathway essential for breaking down intracellular constituents to recycle defective proteins and mitochondria and to replenish nutrients during periods of deprivation. Autophagy of intracellular constituents is critical for cardiomyocyte survival during the early perinatal period of starvation, as mice deficient of key autophagy proteins, such as ATG5 and ATG7 (both essential for the initial step of autophagosome formation), develop fatal myocardial deterioration.[71] Autophagy is also essential for cardiomyocyte homeostasis in adult mice, as adult-onset cardiomyocyte-specific ablation of ATG5 results in fulminant HF, and postnatal onset of ATG7 deficiency leads to the insidious development of cardiomyopathy with aging.[71] Stimulation of autophagy enhances cardiomyocyte survival during myocardial ischemia, as mice expressing a dominant-negative mutant of AMPK are unable to mount an effective autophagic response to ischemia and manifest larger infarct sizes as compared with controls. Interestingly, perinatal onset of ATG5 deficiency is well tolerated yet induces rapid decompensation in the setting of pressure overload. Foci of degenerated cardiomyocytes with autophagic vacuoles are observed in human dilated cardiomyopathy and aortic stenosis,[62] suggesting that this pathway plays an important role in human pathophysiology.

Interestingly, other studies have suggested that the induction of autophagy may be potentially deleterious in certain forms of cardiac injury. In particular, mice with haplo-insufficiency of Beclin-1 demonstrate decreased infarct size with ischemia-reperfusion injury and attenuation of pressure overload–induced adverse ventricular remodeling.[71] Whether these effects are due to a role for Beclin-1 in autophagy or involve Beclin-1–induced signaling via other mechanisms remains to be fully delineated. Therefore, whereas evidence suggests a predominantly pro-survival role for autophagy, the therapeutic targeting of autophagy in HF will require careful experimental validation in large animal models.

Mitochondria and Metabolic Remodeling in Pathologic Hypertrophy

The heart is a mitochondria-rich organ that depends on oxidative phosphorylation via the Krebs cycle to satiate its massive demands for the energy it needs for its continuous mechanical contraction (see also Chapter 17). At birth, a metabolic shift in substrate preference occurs, moving from reliance on glucose to fatty acids and accompanied by a surge in mitochondrial biogenesis. This surge in postnatal mitochondrial biogenesis is required to permit normal cardiac growth and function, as mice deficient in both PGC1α and β isoforms (which play redundant roles in induction of the mitochondrial biogenesis program) manifest a rapid development of cardiomyopathy in the early neonatal period, accompanied by marked mitochondrial structural

derangements.[72] Activation of PGC1α and stimulation of mitochondrial biogenesis occur with exercise-induced physiologic hypertrophy via PI3K (but not Akt) activation. PGC1α and β are transcriptional coactivators that drive activation of the transcription factors NRF1, NRF2, and ERRα. These proteins, in turn, stimulate the biogenesis of nuclear DNA-encoded mitochondrial proteins and TFAM, which drives transcription in the mitochondrial genome. They also function in concert with PPAR transcription factors to regulate metabolic gene expression in the heart. Cardiomyocyte-specific ablation of TFAM mimics the phenotype observed with combinatorial PGC1α and β ablation, with increased ROS generation leading to lethal cardiomyopathy.[73] The transcription factor KLF4 binds to the estrogen-related receptor/PPARγ coactivator 1 (ERR/PGC-1) complex. Its cardiomyocyte-specific ablation provokes a lethal cardiomyopathy, revealing that KLF4 is another critical modulator of mitochondrial biogenesis in the heart. These findings lend further support to the premise that the maintenance of a "normal" mass of properly functioning mitochondria is critical for cardiac homeostasis.

Pathologic cardiac hypertrophy is associated with a shift in cardiac metabolism back to glucose, with transcriptional downregulation of the fatty acid metabolic machinery associated with the repression of both PGCα and β (see also Chapter 17). Importantly, in these studies, genetic ablation of the PGC1α/PPAR/ERR signaling axis accelerated decompensation in pressure-overload hypertrophy.[74] Multiple mitochondrial abnormalities were observed with transition from a compensated to decompensated state, and magnetic resonance spectroscopy demonstrated reduced "high-energy" phosphate stores (phosphocreatine or PCr) in pressure overload–induced ventricular hypertrophy; these stores progressively decline during the transition to HF.[74]

Damaged and dysfunctional mitochondria are separated from the mitochondrial network by fission, and mitochondrial proteins are ubiquitinated to sequester these mitochondria in autophagosomes for removal via lysosomal degradation. This process, termed *mitophagy*, plays a critical role in mitochondrial quality control in the heart; ablation of key mediators such as PINK1 and PARKIN resulted in cardiomyopathy at baseline or under stress, respectively.[75] Inadequate mitophagy as well as impaired mitochondrial biogenesis result in impaired mitochondrial quality control and an inability to maintain a normal complement of mitochondria, provoking decompensation and HF. Accordingly, simultaneous stimulation of mitophagy and mitochondrial biogenesis is currently being evaluated as a strategy to treat HF.

Neurohormonal Signaling and Cardiomyocyte Dysfunction

Activation of the sympathetic nervous system in HF commences early as an adaptive response to maintain cardiac function and adequate cardiac output (see also Chapters 6 and 13). Persistent sympathetic activation, however, becomes progressively maladaptive over time, as catecholamines are toxic to cardiomyocytes (see also Chapter 6).[76] In vivo, persistent activation of catecholamine signaling pathways, such as by chronic infusion of isoproterenol, causes cardiomyopathy associated with cardiomyocyte loss.[42] These effects are largely blocked by pharmacologic inhibition of the β1-receptor and the L-type calcium channel.

There are nine subtypes of adrenergic receptors (three each of α1, α2, and β), and β1 receptors are the most abundant subtype in the myocardium, present in a 10:1 ratio as compared with α receptors. Catecholamine signaling via cardiomyocyte β-adrenoceptors regulates increases in myocardial contractility by modulating inotropy and chronotropy. The β1-adrenoreceptor signals via the stimulatory G protein (Gαs) to activate adenyl cyclase, resulting in cyclic AMP production, which acts as a second messenger to activate protein kinase A (Fig. 1.5). In comparison, signaling downstream of the β2-adrenoreceptor couples to both Gαs and the

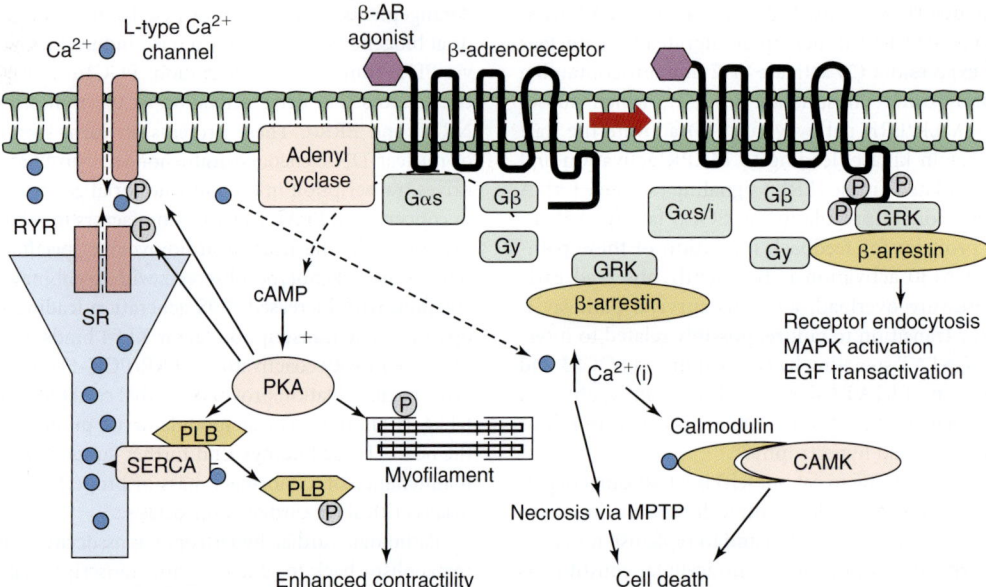

Fig. 1.5 β-Adrenoreceptor Signaling in Heart Failure. Catecholamine binding to the seven transmembrane myocardial β1-adrenoreceptors activates Gsα signaling, with displacement of bound GDP by GTP, and association with Gβ and Gγ forming the heterotrimer at the receptor. This causes cyclic AMP generation via stimulation of adenyl cyclase, which activates PKA. PKA phosphorylates the L-type calcium channel, enhancing Ca²⁺ entry, and RYR enhancing calcium release from the SR, increasing intracellular calcium (Ca²⁺[i]) available for excitation contraction coupling. PKA phosphorylates phospholamban, derepressing SERCA activity with enhanced SR Ca²⁺ reuptake, and phosphorylates troponin on the myofilaments, with the net effect of enhancing contractility. Termination of G protein signaling occurs with GTPase activity of Gsα, causing GDP formation and cAMP being degraded by phosphodiesterases (not shown). Additionally, activated β-adrenoreceptors are phosphorylated at their cytoplasmic tails by G protein–receptor kinases, causing receptor endocytosis. Increased Ca²⁺(i) with chronic adrenoreceptor signaling causes necrotic cell death via calmodulin-mediated CaM kinase activation and mitochondrial permeability transition pore (MPTP) formation (see text). β2-Adrenoreceptor activation stimulates Giα with inhibition of adenyl cyclase (not shown). A delayed phase of signaling downstream of β1-adrenoreceptor may also be activated by GRK-mediated recruitment of β-arrestin with transactivation of EGF and enhanced survival signaling (see text).

inhibitory G protein (Gαi), but results primarily in inhibition of adenyl cyclase and the downregulation of cAMP levels. In normal myocardium, β1 receptors constitute approximately 80% of all β-adrenoreceptors.[77] However, HF is associated with desensitization of β1 adrenoreceptor signaling, preferential internalization and degradation of β1 receptors, and a proportionate increase in β2-adrenoceptor-mediated inhibitory G(i) signaling. The latter occurs via redistribution of β2-adrenergic receptors from T tubules to the cell surface, an event that shifts the localized compartmentalization of G(i)-mediated cAMP responses to diffuse intracellular effects. Gα subunit signaling is suppressed via GTPase activation, which is enhanced by regulators of G-protein signaling (RGS) proteins. Recent studies implicate an important role for a G-protein interacting protein, nucleoside diphosphate kinase C (NDPK-C), which is upregulated in human HF; this occurs in switching Gαs to Gαi signaling to lower cAMP levels in response to β-adrenoceptor stimulation.[78] In another exciting discovery, the beneficial effects of cardiac resynchronization therapy in the failing myocardium were found to be transduced by an increase in RGS2/RGS3 protein levels and a shift from G(i) to G(s) signaling. Interestingly, a burst of β2-receptor–mediated inhibitory G(i) signaling may also transduce the reversible myocardial dysfunction of the middle and apical segments of the LV myocardium (which harbor a proportionately greater abundance of β2 receptors as compared with basal segments) observed in catecholamine-mediated stress cardiomyopathy (also referred to as Takotsubo cardiomyopathy).[79] Together these studies underscore the potential for therapeutically targeting G(i) signaling in various forms of HF.

In cardiomyocytes, membrane depolarization induces rapid calcium entry into the cytoplasm through L-type Ca²⁺ channels, triggering Ca²⁺-induced Ca²⁺ release from the sarcoplasmic reticulum through the ryanodine receptor and culminating in mechanical contraction. During diastole, membrane repolarization is associated with the rapid reuptake of Ca²⁺ through SR uptake mediated by the SERCA. The β1-adrenoceptor/Gsα/PKA signaling axis increases contractility via PKA-mediated phosphorylation of phospholamban to relieve inhibition on SERCA and promote diastolic calcium uptake into the SR. This results in increased SR Ca²⁺ loading and larger systolic Ca²⁺ transients that augment contractility. PKA also phosphorylates both L-type Ca²⁺ channels to enhance Ca²⁺ entry and ryanodine receptors, acting at multiple levels to increase Ca²⁺ availability for excitation-contraction coupling. PKA-mediated phosphorylation also enhances relaxation by activating type-1 protein phosphatase (PP1) inhibitor-1 protein to prevent dephosphorylation of phospholamban at Ser16, and via phosphorylation of contractile proteins such as troponin I and myosin-binding protein C. In addition, PKA phosphorylates phosphodiesterases (PDEs), which are located in the same membrane subcompartment as the β-receptor signaling complex and mediate the hydrolysis of cAMP. This, in turn, potentiates cAMP-mediated signaling events by preventing its feedback inhibition (see Fig. 1.5).

Genetic manipulation of adrenergic receptors and their effectors have uncovered mechanisms underlying catecholamine toxicity.[77] Although forced expression of low levels of β2 receptors enhances cardiac function, expression at much higher levels provokes dilated and fibrotic cardiomyopathy. In contrast, forced expression of the β1 receptor provokes hypertrophy progressing to failure. Signaling via β receptors does not appear to transduce pressure overload hypertrophy, as it progresses similarly in combined β1- and β2-receptor knockout mice relative to wild-type controls. Importantly, targeted ablation of β1 receptors results in the absence of a contractile response to adrenergic agonists, underscoring an essential role for β1 receptors in transducing the effects of catecholamines to govern contractility. In contrast, disruption of β2 receptors has minimal consequences, such as impaired isoproterenol-mediated vasodilation and differences in energy metabolism.

β1 and β2 receptors have distinct effects on cardiomyocyte apoptotic cell death related to the specifics of each G-protein coupling pathway. Signaling via the Gαs-coupled β1 receptors (but not β2 receptors) stimulates cell death via reactive oxygen species and activation of the JNK family of MAP kinases, leading to mitochondrial cytochrome c release and MPTP opening. Sustained β1 signaling also increases intracellular free Ca^{2+} via the L-type Ca^{2+} channel, resulting in activation of CaMKIIδ and cardiomyocyte apoptosis.[80] Indeed, CaMK inhibition with forced expression of a dominant-negative CaMKIIδ mutant attenuates cardiomyocyte apoptosis, prevents hypertrophy and LV remodeling, and protects against isoproterenol-induced cardiomyopathy. At physiologic levels, activation of β2 adrenoceptor signaling switches from the stimulatory Gsα pathway to the inhibitory Giα signaling by means of receptor phosphorylation by PKA activated downstream of the Gsα subunit. This, in turn, triggers dissociation of the Gβγ subunit from Giα, resulting in activation of the PI3K-Akt survival pathway (see Fig. 1.5).

Cyclic AMP generation also activates transcription. Indeed, a counterbalance among cAMP response element binding ATF/CREB family transcription factors, namely CREB2 and CREM, appears to regulate transcription downstream of β1-adrenergic receptors. CREB2 antagonism with forced cardiac expression of a dominant-negative isoform results in dilated cardiomyopathy with progressive LV remodeling, cardiac dysfunction, and HF, whereas CREM inactivation rescues cardiomyocyte hypertrophy, fibrosis, and LV dysfunction in β1-adrenoceptor-overexpressing mice.[42] Also, enhanced β1-adrenergic signaling results in activation of NGF1a-binding protein (Nab1), a transcriptional repressor of early growth response (Egr) transcription factors, which attenuates pressure-overload hypertrophy and prevents its decompensation. These studies point to a fine balance in transcriptional activation that determines cell fate with β1-adrenergic receptor signaling.

Activation of the β1 receptor leads to recruitment of G-protein kinases (GRKs), which phosphorylate the cytoplasmic tail of the receptor and inhibit receptor signaling (see Fig. 1.5).[81] GRK-mediated recruitment of β-arrestins 1 and 2 also mediates internalization of the receptors in clathrin-coated pits resulting in downregulation of signaling. The internalized receptors can either be recycled back to the plasma membrane upon cessation of stimulus or targeted for lysosomal and ubiquitin-proteasome–mediated degradation by ubiquitination of β-arrestin. However, the GRK-β-arrestin complex also acts as a scaffold for recruitment of tyrosine kinases of the Src family, resulting in activation of the MEK1-ERK signaling cascade to mediate prohypertrophic effects. The complex nature of the temporal and spatial consequences of activation of this pathway is highlighted by divergent pathways that are activated downstream (discussed further on).

GRKs 2, 5, and 6 are predominantly expressed in the myocardium.[81] Activation of GRK2 and GRK5 modulates cardiac function, as forced cardiac expression of either is sufficient to attenuate isoproterenol-mediated increases in contractility. Conversely, their cardiac ablation or dominant-negative inhibition results in enhancement of the contractile response. GRK2 plays a critical role in cardiac development, and its activation has differential effects depending upon the chronicity of the inciting stimulus. Indeed, loss of GRK2 prevents adverse ventricular remodeling in the setting of chronic isoproterenol infusion by downregulating β1 receptor signaling, but its inhibition prevents HF after MI, likely by preventing receptor downregulation in the acute setting. In pressure-overload hypertrophy, GRK2 expression increases with stimulation of β2-receptor phosphorylation to enhance inhibitory G(i) signaling. In this setting, inhibition of G(i) with pertussis toxin rescues contractile dysfunction and prevents cardiac decompensation. The protective effects of nitric oxide stimulation in this setting may also be transduced by preventing GRK2-mediated downregulation of β1-adrenergic receptors. Interestingly, enhanced GRK2 signaling in the adrenal gland has been implicated as the culprit in provoking sympathetic hyperactivation in HF by downregulating adrenal α2-adrenoreceptors and preventing the feedback inhibition of catecholamine release. These studies suggest that GRK2 inhibition may be a therapeutic strategy, targeting multiple elements of HF pathophysiology. Activation and nuclear localization of GRK5 is observed downstream of Gαq signaling in pressure-overload hypertrophy, where it functions as a histone deacetylase to activate the transcription factor MEF2 and provoke pathologic hypertrophic signaling.[39]

Biased Agonism as a Novel Concept in Cardiac Therapeutics

A novel survival pathway is triggered by GRK-mediated recruitment of β-arrestin to adrenergic receptors, which leads to cleavage of heparin-binding EGF ligand by a membrane-bound matrix metalloprotease.[81] EGF receptor transactivation protects against catecholamine-induced cardiomyopathy by enhancing survival signaling. Indeed, β-adrenergic blockers may vary in their clinical efficacy in patients with HF owing to their ability to provoke signaling through this novel pathway. This observation among others has spurred interest in understanding signaling via GPCRs leading to biased agonism,[82] where GPCRs are regarded to be in "multistate" conformations such that a ligand may transduce signaling via a particular signal transduction pathway without activating others downstream of the same receptor, permitting modulation of the signaling effects that can be targeted for therapeutic benefit in HF.

For example, distinct populations of phosphorylation sites have bene identified on the β2-adrenergic receptor such that carvedilol binding resulted in interaction of the receptor primarily with GRK2, whereas isoproterenol (a stronger agonist than carvedilol) resulted in binding and activation of both GRK2 and GRK6 signaling downstream.[83] TRV120027, a β-arrestin-biased ligand at the AT1A receptor, demonstrates biased agonism via a β-arrestin–dependent mechanism promoting myofilament responsiveness to calcium via altered protein phosphorylation to increase contractility without inducing hypertrophy.[84]

Another example of GPCR signaling where biased agonism is being exploited for its therapeutic potential is signaling via the apelin receptor, which was demonstrated to be critical for maintaining cardiac contractility and preventing decompensation under pressure overload.[85] Novel agonists are being developed to activate the apelin receptor with reduced β-arrestin recruitment and receptor internalization to attenuate detrimental β-arrestin signaling. Structural insights are being revealed at an explosive pace to clarify the interaction between ligands and GPCRs and their downstream signaling adaptors, which has generated much excitement in the field of cardiovascular therapeutic development.[82] Emerging evidence points to increased S-nitrosylation of β-arrestins 1 and 2 at a single cysteine in patients with HF and in a murine model of pressure overload–induced hypertrophy and

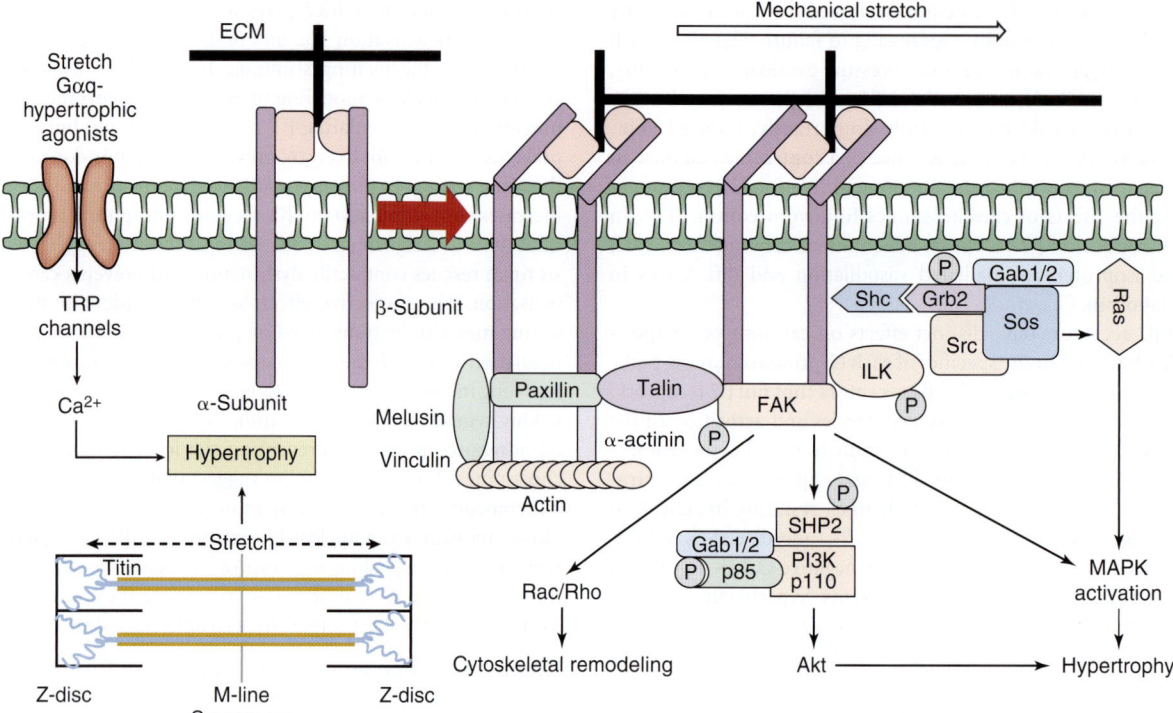

Fig. 1.6 Cellular Transduction of Biomechanical Stress. Integrins are heterodimeric proteins formed by the association of various combinations of single-transmembrane α- and β-subunits, which are attached to the extracellular matrix proteins such as laminin and fibronectin. Biomechanical stress induces changes in conformation and integrin clustering, resulting in assembly of the focal adhesion complex comprising the kinases FAK, Src, and ILK, along with adaptor proteins vinculin, paxillin, talin, α-actinin, and melusin, which connect the integrins to the cytoskeletal elements (actin). Stretch-mediated phosphorylation and activation of FAK and ILK causes MAPK (ERK) and Akt activation via the SHP2/PI3K pathway, resulting in hypertrophic signaling. Additionally, FAK activates the small G proteins Rac and Rho (see further on), which transduce cytoskeletal reorganization in hypertrophy. Integrin signaling also activates Ras via Shc/Grb2/Gab1/2-mediated Src kinase activation, which transduces hypertrophic signaling via MAPK (ERK) activation. Stretch and hypertrophic agonists also cause the activation of transient receptor potential (TRP) channels, resulting in Ca^{2+} entry, which stimulates progrowth signaling. Titin (blue) is a giant sarcomeric protein that acts as a molecular spring to connect the Z-disc to the M-line and senses stretch to activate signaling via interaction with multiple proteins and its C-terminal kinase domain. Additionally, mechanosensing also occurs at the intercalated disc via protein complexes—termed *desmosome, fascia adherens,* and *area composite*—which link proteins at the intercalated disc to the sarcomere (not shown; see text).

decompensation.[86] This inhibits β2-adrenoceptor signaling but results in increased interaction with Mdm2, a proto-oncogene that inhibits HIF1α signaling in a biased fashion. Accordingly, mice with a point mutation in the cysteine demonstrated increased β2-adrenoceptor signaling in response to TAC as well as rapid β-arrestin–mediated desensitization, demonstrating that targeting the nitrosylation of β-arrestins may be a strategy to achieve biased agonism in the setting of HF.

CASCADES THAT TRANSDUCE HYPERTROPHIC SIGNALING

As discussed previously, pathologic cardiomyocyte hypertrophy is a central event in the pathogenesis of cardiac failure such that persistent and progressive activation of hypertrophic signaling cascades in hypertrophied myocytes can lead to failure. Reactive hypertrophy with cardiac injury results in decreased intrinsic contractility of hypertrophied myocytes due to changes in contractile protein isoforms, the calcium cycling apparatus, and metabolic efficiency. This further impairs global cardiac function, stimulating more hypertrophy and ultimately cardiomyocyte death, accelerating decompensation and the transition to dilated cardiomyopathy. This section examines the current state of

knowledge regarding biochemical and molecular events that promote, transduce, and ultimately produce HF.

Biomechanical Sensors of Hypertrophic Stimuli

It is widely accepted that the major stimulus for hypertrophy is increased wall stress resulting from elevated hemodynamic load, which occurs globally or regionally in response to injury as sensed by individual myocytes and perhaps by other resident cell types in the heart. In vivo, cardiomyocytes are intricately connected to the extracellular matrix (ECM), such that stretch is transduced via the intercellular and ECM connections via stretch-sensing proteins at the sarcolemma within the sarcomere and at the intercalated disc (Fig. 1.6).

Mechanotransduction at the sarcolemma is transduced via transient receptor potential (TRP) channels through stretch-activated Ca^{2+} current in cardiomyocytes (**see** Fig. 1.6).[87] A subset of these channels is also activated by diacyl glycerol (DAG), a key signaling molecule downstream of prohypertrophic Gαq signaling. Studies have confirmed an important role for two family members, TRPC1 and TRP6, in transducing pressure-overload hypertrophy in mouse models, and a role for the TRP vanilloid 4 (TRPV4) channel in transducing pulmonary edema in HF.[87] In this study, TRPV4 expression was found to be increased in lungs from patients with HF-induced pulmonary edema, and blockade of these channels by an orally administered chemical inhibitor prevented increases in vascular permeability and pulmonary edema. Integrins, a diverse family of cell-surface receptors, are also implicated as key mechanotransducers at the sarcolemma.[87] Integrins comprise α and β subunits in various combinations, each with an extracellular domain that interacts with extracellular matrix proteins and a short cytoplasmic tail that interacts with the cytoskeleton at the focal adhesion complex (**see** Fig. 1.6). Accordingly, studies have established that stretch and neurohormonal signaling activate hypertrophic pathways downstream of integrin signaling through multiple pathways, including (1) the recruitment and activation of focal adhesion kinase (FAK), a tyrosine kinase; (2) activation of Src family members, which are membrane-bound SH2 domain–containing tyrosine kinases; (3) tyrosine phosphorylation of Grb2-associated binder (Gab) family proteins, with docking and activation of PI3K/Akt and ERK1/2 signaling; (4) activation of the serine/threonine kinase integrin-linked-kinase (ILK); and (5) recruitment of adaptor proteins, such as melusin and vinculin.

Shp2, (Src homology region 2, phosphatase 2) a phosphatase that tonically inhibits prohypertrophic FAK signaling, is inactivated by stretch to stimulate hypertrophy. The following lines of evidence[87] suggest that the integrin-costamere signaling axis plays an essential role in cardiac homeostasis and transduction of hypertrophic stress, as follows: (1) Cardiomyocyte-specific ablation of FAK prevents pressure overload-induced hypertrophy and induction of ANF, and in vivo siRNA–mediated FAK antagonism prevented and even reversed established pressure-overload hypertrophy with transverse aortic constriction. (2) Cardiomyocyte-specific gene targeting of ILK or the β1 subunit resulted in spontaneous cardiomyopathy. (3) Ablation of melusin, a striated muscle-specific protein that interacts with the cytoplasmic tail of β1-integrin, prevented the myocardial hypertrophic response to pressure overload. (4) Talin, a protein located in costameres, is observed to be upregulated with pressure overload, and cardiomyocyte-specific Talin-2 ablation attenuated pressure-overload hypertrophy and contractile dysfunction.

Mechanotransduction at the intercalated disc is postulated to occur via protein complexes termed the *fascia adherens* (comprising an N-cadherin complex that links to the actin proteins in sarcomeres by α-catenins, vinculin and F-actin), the desmosome (comprising desmocollin and desmoglein, both cadherin family members and desmoplakin complexes that link to the Z-discs via desmin) and the area composite, wherein both desmosome and N-cadherin complexes come together to link with various elements of the sarcomere.[87] Both α-E-catenin and N-cadherin knockout mice demonstrate cardiomyopathy, indicating a critical role for these proteins at the intercalated disc. Mutations in all desmosomal proteins have been implicated in the pathogenesis of arrhythmogenic right ventricular cardiomyopathy in humans, with mechanistic involvement of excessive Wnt signaling implicated in mouse models targeting these proteins in cardiomyocytes.[87]

Titin, a large sarcomeric protein component of the thin filament, anchors the Z-disk at one end and extends to the M line at the other; it is postulated to function as a molecular spring providing passive stiffness to the cell and acting as a biomechanical sensor with stretch-induced activation of its C-terminal kinase domain at the M-line[87] (**see** Fig. 1.6). Mutations in the gene coding for titin have been implicated as the most common cause of familial dilated cardiomyopathy (observed in 25% of all cases).[88] Titin is also a major determinant of resting cardiomyocyte elasticity, and hypophosphorylation of its more compliant isoform N2B (which is transcriptionally induced as an adaptive response in pathologic hypertrophy) has been implicated as a cause of diastolic stiffness in patients with HFpEF (**see**

also Chapter 11).[6] Titin also binds to MARP family of proteins and FHL-1 through its N2A and N2B regions, respectively, and targeting these proteins individually has resulted in cardiomyopathy implicating a central role for these complexes.[87] Of note, telethonin, a titin-associated protein localized to the Z-disc in normal cardiomyocytes, can be mislocalized within the nucleus in human HF, and its ablation in cardiomyocytes prevents hypertrophy and induces massive apoptosis in response to pressure overload.[87] Another sensing apparatus for mechanical stretch is postulated to exist within structural proteins in the Z-disc, where the small LIM-domain protein muscle LIM protein (MLP) is anchored and transduces stress stimuli.[87] Calsarcin-1 is another Z-disc protein, mutations in which have been linked to human hypertrophic cardiomyopathy and its ablation in mice results in increased calcineurin activity under pressure overload hypertrophic stress leading to decompensation.[87]

Neurohormonal and Growth Factor Signaling (see also Chapters 5 and 6)

Pathologic hypertrophy is also transduced via autocrine and paracrine release of neurohormones and growth factors that signal through highly specialized cognate receptors.[56] Mechanical stretch induces autocrine secretion of angiotensin II, endothelin 1, and peptide growth factors such as FGF. Also, conditioned medium from stretched myocytes provokes hypertrophy in unstretched cardiomyocytes, attesting to the presence of a paracrine and/or autocrine signaling pathway for hypertrophy. Interestingly, pressure-overload hypertrophy may be transduced by stretch-triggered signaling via activation of the angiotensin I (AT1) receptor without the need for angiotensin, suggesting redundancy at the cell membrane level in transduction of mechanical load to the cardiomyocyte.[42] In addition, mechanical stretch provokes production of neurohormones, growth factors, and cytokines by nonmyocytes in the heart, leading to the proliferation cardiac fibroblasts and acting as an amplification loop to increase neurohormonal effects on cardiomyocytes.

Neurohormones, such as epinephrine, angiotensin II, and endothelin, signal via heptahelical transmembrane receptors coupled to heterotrimeric G proteins. G proteins comprise three polypeptide chains: α, β, and γ (Fig. 1.7). The α subunits are organized into four primary groups, Gαs, Gαi, Gαq, and Gα12/13, and are largely responsible for determining activation of downstream signaling effectors. Signaling through Gαq-coupled receptors by Ang II and other neurohormones activates phospholipase C, which catalyzes hydrolysis of phosphatidyl inositol 4,5 bis-phosphate (PIP2) to inositol 1,4,5-trisphosphate (IP3) and diacylglycerol (DAG). DAG and IP3 activate protein kinase C (PKC), a family of powerful growth-stimulating serine/threonine kinases. IP3 also interacts with IP3 receptors (IP3Rs) to trigger intracellular Ca^{2+} release, which can activate signaling through Ca^{2+}-dependent PKCs, Ca^{2+}-calmodulin dependent kinases (CaMKs), and calcineurin. Cytosolic Ca^{2+} also interacts with DAG to activate PKC (**see** Fig. 1.7). PTEN is a phosphatase that dephosphorylates the 3' position on IP3 and shuts down this signaling pathway. Another arm of signaling is triggered by the dissociated (free) Gβγ subunits, leading to recruitment and activation of PI3Kγ to the sarcolemma to facilitate interaction with phosphoinositides (**see** Fig. 1.7).

α-Adrenergic Receptors (see also Chapter 6)

As discussed earlier, HF is associated with sympathetic activation and increased circulating proliferation levels of catecholamines, which activate α1-adrenergic receptors, leading to Gαq activation. There are three subtypes: α1A/C, α1B, and α1D, of which the first two are present in the human and mouse myocardium but are not observed to be differentially regulated in HF.[89] In vitro, norepinephrine and

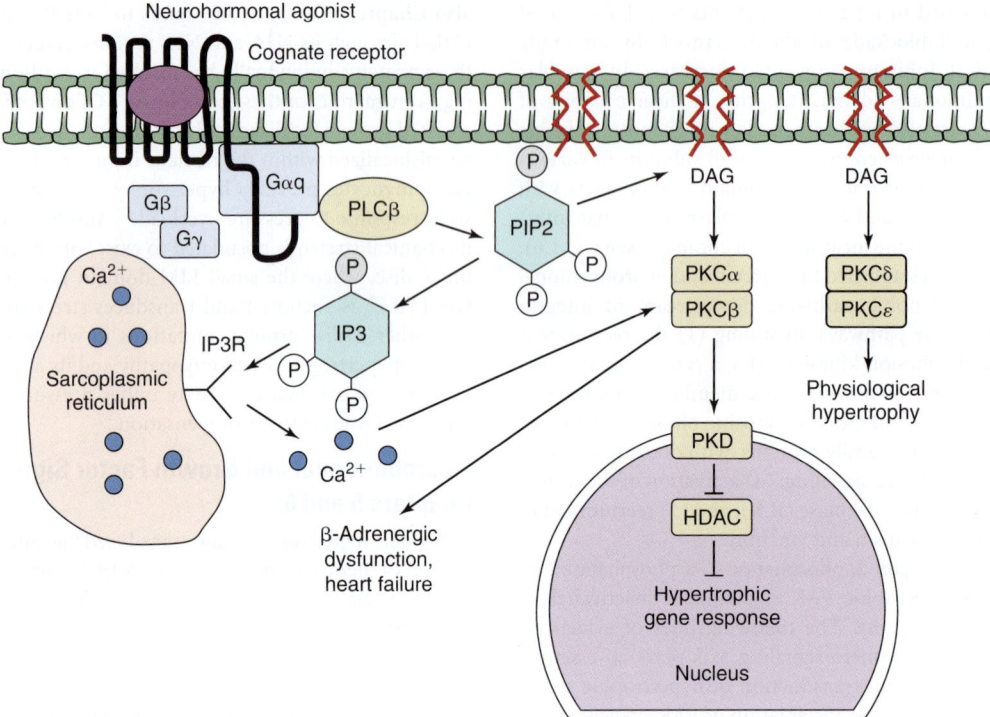

Fig. 1.7 Neurohormonal Signaling via Gαq in Pathologic Cardiac Hypertrophy. Binding of neurohormones to the cognate neurohormonal receptor causes GTP exchange and activation of the Gα subunit, with dissociation from the Gβγ subunit and recruitment of PLCβ to the cell membrane. PLCβ causes hydrolysis of PIP2 with generation of IP3 and DAG. IP3 binds to IP3 receptors (IP3Rs) on the sarcoplasmic reticulum triggering Ca^{2+} release, which elicits PKC activation along with DAG for classic PKCs (α and β). Novel PKCs (δ and ε) are activated by DAG alone. See text for details of PKC signaling in heart failure. Classic PKCs activate PKD, which phosphorylates class II HDACs (5 and 9), resulting in export from the nucleus and derepression of hypertrophic gene transcription.

phenylephrine stimulate cardiomyocyte hypertrophy, which is marked by increases in protein synthesis, induction of early-response genes, reactivation of the fetal gene program, and increases in cell size. Studies investigating the in vivo role of these receptors in hypertrophy point to redundancy in signaling via the two cardiac-expressed α1 adrenergic receptor subtypes, as individual genetic ablation of the α1A/C or α1B receptors alone reveals a role in blood pressure modulation without an effect on cardiac hypertrophy. In contrast, combinatorial ablation of both subtypes together points to an essential role for α1 receptor signaling in normal postnatal cardiac growth and hypertrophy.[36] Indeed, the double knockout hearts were 40% smaller than wild type, with reduced cardiomyocyte cross-sectional area and mRNA content, decreased ERK (but not Akt) activation, and a lack of reduction in blood pressure (i.e., at similar afterload). Interestingly, mice with combinatorial α1A and α1B ablation manifest an equivalent hypertrophic response with pressure overload compared with controls, along with markedly decreased survival, decreased upregulation of "fetal genes," and increased cell death and fibrosis. These findings may stem from lack of prosurvival signaling via the ERK pathway. Together, these studies indicate that α-adrenergic receptors play a crucial role in normal cardiac growth but are redundant for pathologic hypertrophic signaling, primarily regulating cell survival in this setting.

Angiotensin Signaling (see also Chapter 6)

Angiotensin II (Ang II), a powerful vasoconstrictor, derives from sequential cleavage of circulating angiotensinogen by renin and angiotensin converting enzyme (ACE). Reducing Ang II levels via pharmacologic inhibition of ACE is a cornerstone of therapy for cardiomyopathy

and HF in humans (**see also Chapter 37**). The ACE2 enzyme converts angiotensin II to angiotensin 1-7 (Ang 1-7) peptide and accumulating evidence indicates that Ang 1-7 peptide signals via AT2 receptor and Mas (a $G^{q/11}$ coupled receptor) in the central nervous system to lower blood pressure. Also, Ang 1-7 peptide signaling antagonizes Ang II actions at the tissue level to attenuate myocardial remodeling under stress. Neprilysin, a neutral endopeptidase, breaks down Ang 1-7 as well as bradykinin and natriuretic peptides in the circulation; combined neprilysin and AT1R inhibition has emerged as a promising clinical strategy to lower mortality in patients with HF.[90]

Endothelin

Endothelin-1 (ET-1) is a 21–amino acid polypeptide cleaved from a larger precursor by endothelin-converting enzyme primarily by endothelial cells and to a smaller extent in cardiomyocytes and fibroblasts. ET-1signals via the ET1A and ET1B receptors, which are both coupled to Gαq, such that ET1 is sufficient to induce cardiomyocyte hypertrophy in vitro. Although ET1 appears to be a part of the autoregulatory loop with Ang II, as ET1 receptor blockade antagonizes AngII-mediated hypertrophy, it does not play a nonredundant role in transducing pathologic hypertrophy.[89]

The Gαq/Phospholipase C/Protein Kinase C Signaling Axis

Redundancy in signal transduction at the receptor level in pathologic hypertrophy has prompted evaluation of Gαq and G11, heterotrimeric G proteins, as potential nodal points for targeting pathologic signaling. Indeed, Gαq and G11 are critical mediators of pathologic hypertrophic signaling, as combined cardiomyocyte-specific ablation of Gαq and G11 prevents development of pressure-overload hypertrophy and attenuates fetal gene expression and fibrosis with preservation of myocardial function. The importance of this pathway to human HF is further demonstrated by the observation that polymorphisms in the gnaq (Gαq) gene, with a single base-pair change from GC to TT at positions -694/-695 in the promoter, results in increased Gαq promoter activity. This is associated with the increased prevalence of LV hypertrophy in normal subjects and increased mortality in African American patients with HF.

Gαq signaling is terminated by GTPase activity, which is markedly enhanced by RGS proteins, thereby acting as negative regulators of G proteins. Several RGS proteins are expressed in the heart. RGS2 downregulates Gαq/G11 signaling, and transgenic expression of the RGS domain of GRK2 prevents the development of pressure-overload hypertrophy and fibrosis via inhibition of Gαq signaling.[91] Conversely, RGS2 ablation worsens pressure-overload hypertrophy without affecting the physiologic hypertrophic response to swimming exercise. Importantly, activation of protein kinase G1 via inhibition of phosphodiesterase 5 (PDE5) as well as inhibition of its oxidation caused sustained localization of RGS2 to the Gαq receptors and prevented development of pressure-overload hypertrophy.[92] Recent studies have also found upregulation of the PDE9A isoform in patients with HFpEF, and ablation of PDE9A was sufficient to rescue established pressure overload–induced pathologic hypertrophy and myocardial dysfunction by enhancing natriuretic peptide–induced cGMP signaling.[93]

Phospholipase Cβ (PLCβ) is a prototypical downstream effector of Gαq and Gβγ signaling (see Fig. 1.7). Activation of PLCβ via Gαq receptors has been observed in pathologic hypertrophy in vivo. Of the four isoforms, PLCβ1 and β3 are expressed in the heart. While in vitro studies suggest an essential role for PLC1β isoforms in transducing Gαq-mediated hypertrophic signals, in vivo confirmation of this will require tissue-specific targeting. This is due to the observation that germline PLCβ1 knockout mice develop seizure activity, and PLCβ3 knockout mice harbor abnormalities in neutrophil chemotaxis and skin ulcers, but no apparent abnormalities in normal cardiac development. Levels of PLCε, another cardiac-expressed phospholipase (which is downstream of nonreceptor tyrosine kinase signaling such as with Ras), are observed to be elevated in human dilated cardiomyopathy and in response to isoproterenol treatment and pressure overload.[39] Germline ablation of PLCε results in contractile dysfunction with reduced β-adrenergic responsiveness and exaggerated catecholamine-induced cardiomyopathy and decompensation, indicating an essential role in modulating β-adrenoceptor signaling in HF.

Activation of PKCs downstream of Gαq/PLCβ has emerged as a key mediator of altered myocardial contractility and cardiomyocyte survival in pathologic hypertrophic signaling (see Fig. 1.7). In the heart, the functionally important PKC isoforms are PKCα and β ("conventional" PKCs that are activated by DAG with a requirement for Ca²⁺); PKC δ and ε ("novel" PKCs that are activated by DAG without a requirement for Ca²⁺); and PKC ζ and ι/λ ("atypical" PKCs that bind PIP3 and ceramide but not DAG or PMA. Upon activation, PKCs translocate to specific subcellular locations, such as PKCα to the membrane, PKCβ1to the nucleus, PKCε to the myofibrils, and PKCδ redistributing in a perinuclear localization. In the rodent heart, Gαq signaling in pressure-overload hypertrophy and HF upregulates PKCα and translocates PKCε to the membrane. PKCα activation negatively regulates myocardial contractility but not the hypertrophic response.[89] Indeed, inhibition of PKCα prevents contractile dysfunction without affecting the degree of hypertrophy in pathologic hypertrophic states. PKCβ signaling is also not required for transducing hypertrophy with pressure overload or phenylephrine. Mice with combined genetic ablation of the novel PKCs, PKCδ and PKCε, in embryonic

cardiomyocytes demonstrate cardiomyocyte hyperplasia, whereas their combined postnatal ablation did not affect LV mass but induced gene expression changes characteristic of pathologic hypertrophy.[94] Additionally, PKCε-mediated activation of aldehyde dehydrogenase in ischemia facilitates removal of ROS-induced toxic aldehydes and offers cardioprotection in this setting. Ca²⁺ dependent, nonconventional PKCs also activate protein kinase D (PKD) (Fig. 1.8). Protein kinase D directly phosphorylates class II HDACs (histone deacetylases), resulting in their export from the nucleus and derepression of transcription. PKD1 activation is involved in transducing hypertrophy, as siRNA-mediated knockdown of PKD1 prevents hypertrophic cardiomyocyte growth by agonists that signal via Gαq and Rho GTPase. Also, cardiomyocyte-specific deletion of PKD, prevents pressure-overload hypertrophy with preserved cardiac function and prevention of remodeling.[39] In myocardial ischemia, calpain-mediated cleavage of PKCα releases a constitutively active fragment PKMα, which activates PKD with nuclear to cytoplasmic transport of the transcriptional repressor HDAC5 and activation of pathologic gene transcription.[39] These studies involving modulation of PKC pathways highlight the qualitative nature of hypertrophic signaling, wherein differential activation of divergent pathways downstream of common nodal points determines its adaptive or pathologic nature.

Mitogen-Activated/Stress-Activated Protein Kinase Signaling Cascades

Activation of G protein–coupled receptors generates dissociated Gβγ subunits, which cross talk with small GTPase proteins (see further on) or directly activate mitogen-activated protein kinases (MAPKs).[39] Multiple other signaling pathways—such as receptor tyrosine kinases, serine/threonine kinases (e.g., downstream of TGFβ) signaling), Janus-activated kinases (JAK-STAT activation via the gp130 receptor), and stress stimuli such as stretch—activate MAPK pathways. MAPKs are three-tiered cascades consisting of a MAPKKK (MAP3K or MEKK), a MAPKK (MEK), and a MAPK, the transducer of the signal downstream from the cascade. There are three major groups of MAPKs: extracellular signal regulated kinases (ERK), c-Jun N-terminal kinases JNKs (also known as stress-activated protein kinase and/or SAPKs and p38s. Specific MAPKKs activate specific MAPKs: MAPKK1/2 for ERK1/2, MAPKK3/6 for p38s and MAPKK4/7 for JNKs. At the next tier, each MAPKKK can activate different MAPKK-MAPK pathways, suggesting a mechanism for integration of upstream signaling. MAPKs phosphorylate multiple substrates, including enzymes and transcription factors with overlapping specificity that regulate cardiac gene expression ("immediate early response" factors), cell survival, mRNA translation (eIF4E), and mRNA stability. Specificity for downstream substrates is primarily determined via docking interactions to integrate downstream signaling. For example, although p90RSKs are phosphorylated primarily by ERK1/2, MAPKAPK2 is phosphorylated by p38-MAPK; and Msk1/2 may be phosphorylated by either ERK1/2 or p38-MAPK.

At the top tier of kinases are the MAPKKKs (see Fig. 1.8), such as mammalian sterile 20-like kinase 1 (Mst1), which is a mammalian homolog of Hippo, a master regulator of cell death, proliferation, and organ size in *Drosophila* (Fig. 1.9). Mst kinases complex with the scaffold protein, Salvador (Sav) to phosphorylate the large tumor suppressor homolog (Lats) kinases; which phosphorylate Yap and Taz, two related transcriptional coactivators that are excluded from the nucleus and thereby inactivated. In a dephosphorylated state, Yap and Taz partner with the transcription factor Tead to regulate gene expression. Activated Yap1 activates the IGF and Wnt signaling pathways to increase cardiomyocyte proliferation and embryonic heart size. Mst1 is activated by cardiac stress, and forced expression of Mst1 inhibits autophagy and mitophagy survival pathways to provoke an

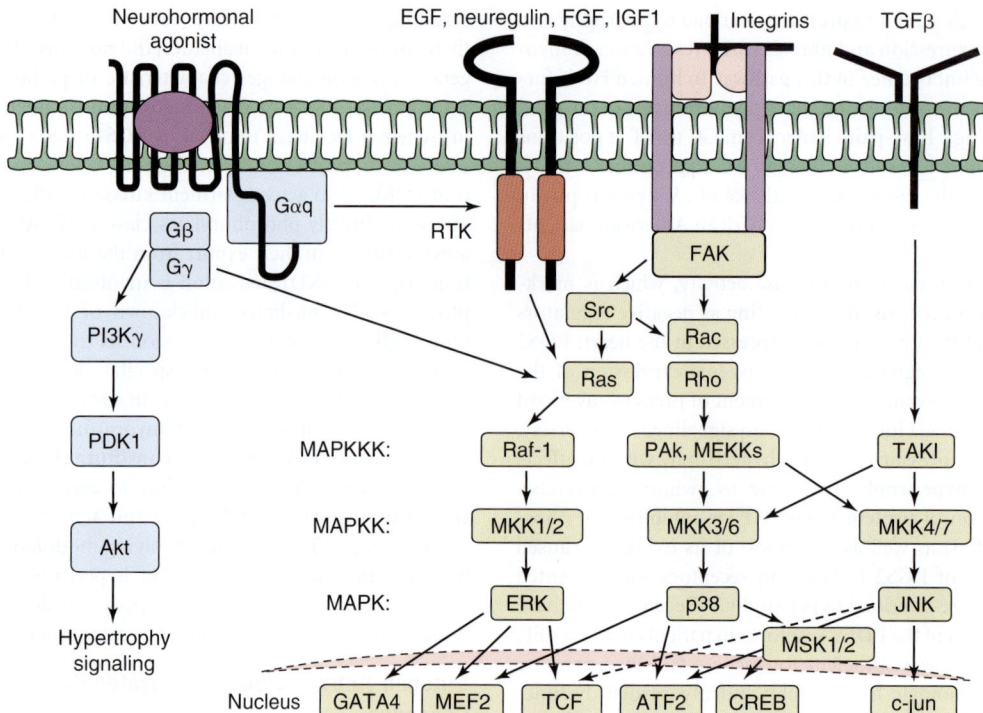

Fig. 1.8 Neurohormonal Activation of MAPK Signaling in Pathologic Hypertrophy. Activated Gαq protein causes activation of small G proteins such as Ras either directly via the released Gβγ subunits or via cross-talk with RTKs, which are activated by growth factors such as EGF, neuregulin, FGF, and IGF-1 (see later in text). This leads to stimulation of the MAPK signaling cascades. MAPKs are also activated by integrin signaling and TGF receptor–mediated activation of TAK1. MAPK cascades are organized into three tiers: MAPKKKs, which activate MAPKKs, which subsequently activate MAPKinases. MAPKs signal redundantly via multiple transcription factors (see details in text). Gβγ subunits of the Gαq signaling complex also activate PI3Kγ, resulting in Akt activation and hypertrophy signaling.

apoptotic cardiomyopathy.[42] Ras-association domain family 1 isoform A (Rassf1A), a Ras-GTP binding protein, acts as an activator of Mst1 and appears to play divergent roles in cardiomyocytes and fibroblasts.[95] Whereas cardiomyocyte-specific ablation of Rassf1A protects against pressure overload–induced hypertrophy and decompensation, germline ablation of Raasf1A results in markedly enhanced myocardial fibrosis with cardiac pressure overload. These discrepant findings were resolved by the observation that loss of Rassf1A in cardiac fibroblasts results in enhanced TNF generation with increased cell death and fibrosis in the heart. Another upstream serine threonine kinase, Lats2, activates Mst1, and its transgenic expression results in reduced heart size. Conversely, expression of a dominant-negative Lats2 mutant results in hypertrophy, indicating that the Lats2-Mst1 pathway is also a negative regulator of cardiomyocyte size. In aggregate, these studies illustrate how the same pathway may promote cardiomyocyte apoptosis but suppress fibroblast activation, highlighting the need for targeting specific cell types for desirable effects. The Hippo signaling pathway is also a negative regulator of cardiomyocyte proliferation[96] as cardiomyocyte-specific ablation of Salvador (Sav; see Fig. 1.9), the scaffolding protein, activated canonical Wnt signaling to increase cardiomyocyte proliferation and resulted in a 2.5-fold increase in cardiac mass accompanied by cardiomyopathy and early lethality. Inducible ablation of Salvador scaffolding protein 3 weeks after MI stimulated cardiac myocyte proliferation from preexisting cardiac myocytes in a regulated manner coordinately with reduced fibrosis and vascularization, to reverse established cardiomyopathy.[97] In this study, Hippo-deficient cardiac myocytes demonstrated upregulation of proliferative genes as well as stress-response genes such as Park2 (encoding for Parkin), pointing to a role for enhanced mitochondrial quality control in the regenerative myocardium.

Subsequent stepwise activation of kinases culminates in the activation of the effector kinases (see Fig. 1.8). ERK1/2 is activated via Gαq signaling in response to hypertrophic agonists (e.g., Ang II, PE, ET1, and stretch) in vitro and by pressure overload in vivo.[39] Accumulated evidence suggests a predominant role for the ERK signaling axis in promoting hypertrophy, and the p38 and JNK axes in regulating cell death and fibrosis. A role for the ERK pathway in hypertrophic signaling was interrogated with combinatorial gene ablation studies, wherein ERK2 was silenced in a cardiomyocyte-specific manner, or inferred from studies with transgenic expression of MEK1. Interestingly, although MEK1 activation provoked concentric hypertrophy, ablation of both ERK1/2 did not affect normal cardiac growth or development of pressure overload hypertrophy.[39] Rather, it resulted in dilated, eccentrically hypertrophied chamber morphology with lengthening of myocytes and contractile dysfunction mimicking observations with volume overload–induced hypertrophy. ERK1/2-mediated phosphorylation of GATA4 at serine 105 is critical for its ability to transduce pathologic cardiac growth, as knockin mice homozygous for a nonphosphorylatable mutant at this locus did not manifest hypertrophy in response to pressure overload or angiotensin II infusion. Rather, these stimuli led to rapid development of cardiac failure, indicating that ERK1/2-GATA4-mediated cardiac growth is predominantly consistent with "physiologically hypertrophied myocardium."[36]

p38 and JNK kinases were originally discovered as "stress-responsive kinases" on account of their rapid activation in response to stressful stimuli.[39] Of the four genes encoding p38s, p38α is the most abundant in the heart, with minimal p38β detected. p38 and JNK signal via transcription factors c-jun, ATF2, ATF6, Elk-1, p53, and NFAT4. Loss-of-function modeling with transgenic expression of dominant-negative mutants of

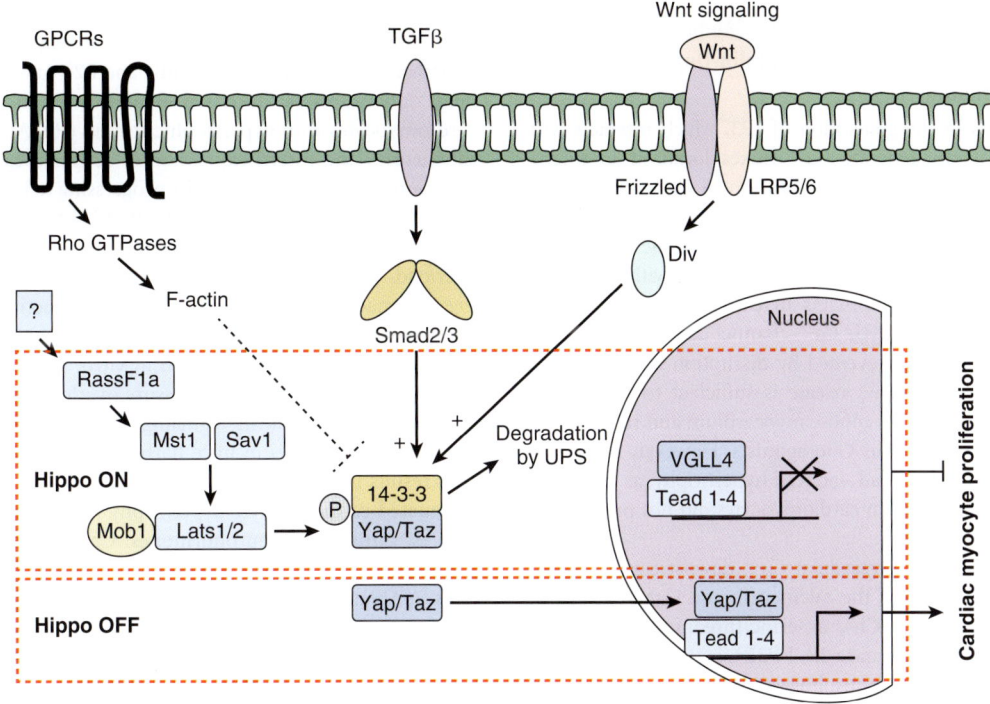

Fig. 1.9 Signaling via the Hippo Pathway. The Yap and Taz proteins are two related transcriptional coactivators that serve as the downstream mammalian effectors in a pathway that is homologous with the *Drosophila* Hippo signaling pathway. The upstream regulators of this pathway are yet to be identified in cardiomyocytes but could involve signaling through G protein–coupled receptors via F-actin, which is postulated to inhibit Hippo signaling; inputs through the TGFβ and Wnt signaling pathway bind to phosphorylated Yap/Taz and increase its sequestration in the cytosol. When the Hippo signaling pathway is turned on, Rassf1a, a Ras GTPase–binding protein activates a MAPKKK called Mst1. Mst kinases complex with the scaffold protein Salvador (Sav) to phosphorylate the large tumor suppressor homolog (Lats) kinases, which phosphorylate Yap and Taz. Phosphorylated Yap/Taz bind to 14-3-3 proteins and are retained in the cytosol—that is, excluded from the nucleus and targeted for degradation. In this state, the repressor protein VGLL4 binds to the Tead family of transcription factors in the nucleus to suppress transcription. When Hippo signaling is turned off, Yap/Taz are dephosphorylated and translocate to the nucleus, where they bind to the Tead proteins to activate transcription. The Yap/Taz proteins also act as coactivators of Notch signaling (via NICD downstream of the Notch receptor processing), Smad 1 and 4 (downstream of TGFβ signaling) and β-catenin/TCF/LEF complex downstream of activated Wnt signaling. The Hippo pathway negatively regulates cardiomyocyte proliferation.

p38α or p38β, as well as p38α gene ablation, revealed an antihypertrophic effect in exercise-induced and pathologic hypertrophy. Similarly, stress-induced JNK signaling (c-Jun N-terminal kinases) appears to be antihypertrophic, as mice with either dominant-negative repression or combined ablation of JNK1 and 2, exhibit increased basal and pressure overload–induced cardiac mass with depressed calcineurin-NFAT signaling. Combinatorial ablation JNK1, 2, and 3 increases cardiomyocyte apoptosis in response to pressure overload with rapid cardiomyopathic decompensation, indicating a prominent role for these stress-induced kinases in cell survival signaling.

The terminal MAPKs, ERK, JNK, and p38 are inactivated by dephosphorylation at serine/threonine residues by a family of dual-specificity phosphatases. This feedback inhibition is critical for maintaining basal cardiac function, as combinatorial ablation of DUSP1 and DUSP4 provokes cardiomyopathy with unrestrained activation of p38.[39] This progressive cardiomyopathy and cardiac dysfunction was prevented with pharmacologic p38 inhibition, indicating a redundant role for these two phosphatases (as individual knockout was of no consequence) in cardiac homeostasis.[98]

Ask-1 is a MAPKKK that is upregulated in the myocardium by angiotensin stimulation via AT1R-induced oxidative stress and NFkB activation. Activation of Ste20/oxidant stress response kinase 1 (SOK-1), an Mst family member known to be activated by oxidant stress, mediates Ask-1 activation in this setting. Ask-1 ablation significantly attenuates cardiomyocyte apoptosis and cardiomyopathic decompensation induced by angiotensin infusion, in response to pressure overload or coronary artery ligation, yet without an effect on hypertrophic signaling. Conversely, overexpression of Ask1 induces cardiomyocyte apoptosis and accelerates development of HF via activation of the calcineurin axis. Indeed, Ask1 physically interacts with subunit B of calcineurin (PP2B), resulting in enhancement of Ask1 activity by calcineurin-induced dephosphorylation. Ask1-p38α signaling is a negative regulator of adaptive hypertrophy, as mice with Ask1 ablation display increased cardiomyocyte hypertrophy when subjected to swimming exercise, as is also observed in p38α-deficient mice subjected to the same stimulus.[36,42] One of the central kinases upstream of ERKs is Raf-1 (and the related B-Raf).[39] Deletion of Raf-1 led to increased cardiomyocyte death with LV dysfunction and dilation in mice. However, this did not appear to be due to ERK inhibition. Rather, the apoptosis signal regulating kinase (ASK1) was activated (as were JNKs and p38), and deleting ASK1 rescued the LV dilatation and dysfunction. Thus Raf-1 is a critical regulator of cell death in the heart, acting through ASK1.

Inositol 1,4,5-Trisphosphate-Induced Ca²⁺-Mediated Signaling, Calcineurin/NFAT Axis, and Ca²⁺/Calmodulin-Dependent Protein Kinase Signaling

Gαq signaling results in the generation of IP3, which interacts with intracellular receptors to generate Ca^{2+} fluxes localized to microdomains, leading to the compartmentalization of Ca^{2+}-induced signaling (Fig. 1.10).[39] This segregates the signaling effects of local Ca^{2+} alterations from the global Ca^{2+} transients that determine contraction. For example, β2-adrenergic receptors are associated with caveolin-3 protein within caveolar microdomains in cardiomyocytes, and this allows for the regulation of L-type Ca^{2+}-channel activity with β2-dependent activation, which is prevented by disruption of the caveolar architecture. IP3R-mediated Ca^{2+} release is sufficient to transduce a mild hypertrophic phenotype in mouse myocardium and regulates the hypertrophic response to various Gαq agonists. However, this axis is not required for pressure overload–induced hypertrophy, as transgenic expression of an IP3 "sponge" in cardiomyocytes did not prevent this response in a murine model.[42]

IP3- mediated release of intracellular Ca^{2+} downstream of hypertrophic Gαq signaling activates the calcineurin and CaMK pathways (**see** Fig. 1.10). Calcineurin (Cn), a serine/threonine phosphatase (also known as protein phosphatase 2B, PP2B), is stimulated by Ca^{2+} binding to calmodulin and dephosphorylates the transcription factor NFAT at an N-terminal serine residue.[39] This allows for NFAT

translocation to the nucleus. The functional protein is a dimer comprising two subunits, A and B. Cn is encoded by three genes (CnA α, β, and γ) and CnB by two genes (CnB1 and B2), of which the mammalian heart only expresses CnAα, CnAβ, and CnB1. In vitro stimulation of cardiomyocytes with hypertrophic stimuli (PE, AngII, ET-1) activates calcineurin, and forced expression of activated calcineurin results in pronounced cardiac hypertrophy progressing to HF. Calcineurin activity is increased in human compensated LV hypertrophy, in the myocardium of patients with HF, and in animal models of both pressure overload– and exercise-induced cardiac hypertrophy. Studies employing pharmacologic inhibition of calcineurin activity with FK506 and cyclosporine have demonstrated that calcineurin transduces pathologic hypertrophic signaling both in vitro, in response to PE, Ang II and ET1, and in response to pressure overload in vivo. Confirmatory evidence for calcineurin signaling in pathologic hypertrophy has emerged from studies in mice harboring ablation of the CnAβ gene. This results in an 80% reduction in calcineurin activity and results in attenuated cardiomyocyte hypertrophy in response to pressure overload or infusion of neurohormones. Calcineurin is localized at the Z-disc in a complex with calsarcins, providing access to NFAT proteins.[87] Ablation of calsarcin-1 increases pressure overload–induced calcineurin signaling, resulting in a rapid progression to HF. Signaling via FGF23 with activation of the calcineurin-NFAT pathway has also been implicated in development of LV hypertrophy in patients with chronic kidney disease, who often develop HF with preserved ejection

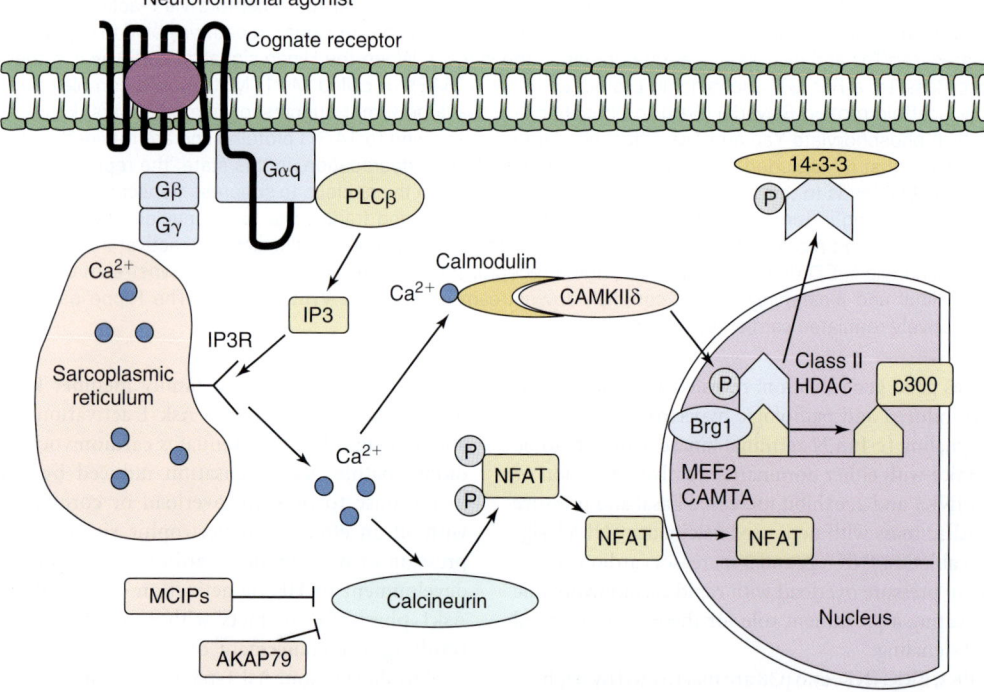

Fig. 1.10 **Neurohormonal Activation of Calcineurin and CAMK Signaling.** Gαq/Gα11-mediated production of IP3 via PLCβ causes the release of intracellular Ca²⁺ from the SR via the IP3Rs, leading to activation of protein phosphatase and calcineurin. Calcineurin dephosphorylates the NFAT transcription factor, resulting in its nuclear translocation and activation of hypertrophy gene transcription. AKAP79 and MCIPs are endogenous inhibitors of calcineurin activity. The increased cytoplasmic calcium concentration (Ca²⁺ [i]) also causes activation of CAMKs via interaction with calmodulin. CAMKs phosphorylate class II HDACs, resulting in HDAC's translocation out of the nucleus and binding to 14-3-3 protein in the cytoplasm. This allows histone acetylation by HAT p300, derepressing hypertrophic gene transcription mediated by transcription factors such as MEF2 and CAMTA. Brg1 is a transcriptional modulator that associates with HDACs on the MHC gene promoters to enhance βMHC (MYH7) and suppress αMHC (MYH6) transcription. Brg1 gets turned off at birth during normal growth and is reactivated in pathologic hypertrophic signaling to effect the shift in myosin heavy chain gene expression.

fraction (HFpEF).[99] This could be a significant step forward in our understanding of mechanisms in this population.

Activation of calcineurin (and the NFAT axis) is triggered by elevated cytosolic Ca^{2+}, and the source of the elevated Ca^{2+} levels has been the subject of extensive investigation.[100] Potential candidates include the L-type Ca^{2+} channel (LTCC), the T-type Ca^{2+} channel, and transient receptor potential channels (TRPCs). The LTCC mediates Ca^{2+}-induced Ca^{2+} release during each depolarization, which drives excitation-contraction coupling. Mice with heterozygous germline deletion or cardiomyocyte-specific ablation of the α1c subunit of the LTCC manifest mild reductions in LTCC current in adulthood, with mild impairment in cardiac function and development of cardiac hypertrophy with aging. When these mice were subjected to swimming (physiologic exercise) or pathologic stress (pressure overload or isoproterenol infusion) in young adulthood, exaggerated hypertrophy and rapid development of HF was observed. This was driven by activation of the calcineurin-NFAT axis due to elevated cytosolic Ca^{2+}. A subsequent study, which selectively targeted LTCCs located only in caveolin-3 microdomains, ablated Ca^{2+} influx–mediated NFAT activation with minimal reduction in basal Ca^{2+} current, indicating that focal LTCC-mediated Ca^{2+} release in microdomains may trigger pathologic signaling via calcineurin-NFAT pathway.

In the heart, all four NFAT isoforms are present, and NFAT transcription factors are essential for normal cardiac development.[100] Ablation of NFATc2 and NFATc3, but not NFATc4, protects against pressure overload–and angiotensin-induced hypertrophy with attenuated expression of "fetal genes" without affecting development of exercise-induced adaptive hypertrophy.[39] The upstream regulators of NFAT signaling reflect the extensive cross talk between various signaling pathways and include GSK3β (which is discussed further on), p38, and JNK MAP kinases. These factors phosphorylate and inactivate NFAT by facilitating nuclear export, accounting for some of the observed antihypertrophic actions.

Calcineurin signaling is restrained by modulatory calcineurin inhibitory proteins, or MCIPs, which bind to calcineurin to inhibit its activity.[100] MCIP1 gene transcription is activated in the heart by calcineurin-mediated NFAT signaling, providing a negative feedback loop for repression of calcineurin signaling, whereas MCIP2 expression is induced by thyroid hormone signaling. Forced expression of MCIP1 is antihypertrophic and results in a reduction in unstressed adult heart weight (by 5%–10%), and attenuates both physiologic hypertrophy induced by swimming and pathologic hypertrophy induced by calcineurin activation or pressure overload. MCIP1 overexpression also attenuates the development of pathologic hypertrophy after MI with preservation of systolic function. This suggests a beneficial effect of preventing pathologic hypertrophy signaling in the surviving myocardium. Although these studies indicate that enhanced MCIP1 signaling is primarily antihypertrophic, loss of function by MCIP1 gene ablation did not lead to overt phenotypic abnormalities, indicating that basal MCIP1 levels do not regulate eutrophic cardiac growth. Rather, MCIP1 ablation paradoxically attenuated the hypertrophic response to pressure overload, and combinatorial ablation of both MCIP1 and MCIP2 attenuated both swimming-induced and pressure overload–induced hypertrophy. This indicates that regulation of hypertrophy via MCIP1 may be bimodal, wherein endogenous levels are required for hypertrophic signaling, and elevated levels can inhibit other prohypertrophic pathways. A small EF hand domain–containing protein and integrin-binding protein-1 (CIB1) was recently discovered in a screen for mediators of calcineurin-induced pathology and identified as another critical mediator of calcineurin-mediated pathology in pressure-overload hypertrophy and dysfunction.[101]

Signaling via Ca^{2+}/Calmodulin-Dependent Protein Kinase

Increased cytosolic Ca^{2+} also activates CaMKs, a family of enzymes that phosphorylate multiple Ca^{2+} handling proteins to regulate myocardial contractility (see Fig. 1.10). All four CaMKs, I-IV, can activate MEF2-mediated transcription of fetal genes in vivo.[100] CaMKIIδ, the predominant cardiac isoform, phosphorylates HDAC4, a class II histone deacetylase, resulting in its export from the nucleus, leading to de-repression of fetal cardiac gene expression. Ablation of CaMKIIδ attenuates pressure overload–induced hypertrophy via inhibition of HDAC4. Aldosterone-mediated ROS generation causes oxidation and activation of CaMKII, which may explain its deleterious cellular effects in cardiomyocytes, as myocardial CaMKII inhibition prevented aldosterone-induced activation of MMPs and cardiac rupture after MI. Additionally, mitochondria-localized CaMKII modulates mitochondrial calcium uniporter activity and regulates susceptibility to mitochondrial permeability transition under stress. Accordingly, inhibition of mitochondrial CaMKII prevents MPTP-driven mitochondrial Ca^{2+} overload and cell death in ischemia-reperfusion injury.[80]

Epigenetic Regulation of Transcription in Cardiac Hypertrophy

Reversible acetylation of histone proteins governs steric access of transcription factors to DNA. Histones are nuclear proteins within the nucleosome, a compact structure consisting of chromatin genomic DNA tightly coiled around histone octamers. This structure prevents access of transcription factors to DNA and represses gene expression. Histone acetyltransferases (HATs) acetylate conserved lysine residues in histone tails, neutralizing their positive charge, resulting in destabilization of histone-histone and histone-DNA interactions (see Fig. 1.10). Thus HATs generally stimulate gene expression. In contrast, histone deacetylases (HDACs) counter this effect, promoting chromatin condensation and repressing transcription (see Fig. 1.10). Recent studies indicate that chromatin conformation is altered in failing human hearts and pressure-overloaded mouse hearts, to reveal increased enhancer–gene interactions that promote gene transcription. This can be mimicked by inducible ablation of CTCF, a structural protein that maintains chromatin conformation, levels of which are observed to be reduced in failing hearts and restored toward normal after mechanical LVAD support.[102]

HATs belong to five families, and p300 and CREB binding protein (CBP) are the most abundant HAT family members in cardiac muscle.[103] P300 binds to and acts as a transcriptional coactivator for GATA4, MEF2, and SRF, and dominant-negative p300 prevents the acetylation and coactivation of GATA-4 downstream of G signaling, resulting in a cardiomyopathy. Evidence supporting therapeutic targeting of p300 in prevention and treatment of pathologic hypertrophy has emerged from studies of p300 HAT inhibition by curcumin (a polyphenol abundant in the spice turmeric).[103] Pretreatment with curcumin prevented development of hypertrophy and cardiac decompensation in response to pressure overload or phenylephrine infusion in vivo in mice. Treatment of mice with curcumin resulted in compensated myocardial hypertrophy after induction of pressure overload or phenylephrine infusion and was sufficient to cause regression of cardiomyocyte and cardiac hypertrophy.

HDACs are classified into three categories based on homology with yeast HDACs.[103] Class I HDACs comprise primarily a catalytic domain, whereas class II HDACs have phosphorylation sites that serve as targets for signaling pathways and interact with transcription factors. Class III HDACs require NAD for activity. Class II HDACs (HDAC4, HDAC5, HDAC7, and HDAC9) control cardiac growth by translocation across the nuclear membrane to the cytoplasm. HDACs are commonly associated with MEF2 proteins in the nucleoplasm.

MEF2 activity is held in check in the adult myocardium by binding to class II HDACs (HDAC4, 5, and 7). This repression is relieved by phosphorylation of HDACs by Ca^{2+}/calmodulin kinases (CaMK), which causes HDAC export out of the nucleus, and enhances association of p300 with MEF2, promoting gene transcription. By this mechanism, multiple hypertrophic signaling pathways—including MAPKs, calcineurin, CaMKII, and protein kinase D—converge on MEF2 activation by class II HDAC export, relieving transcriptional repression. Indeed, MEF2D-mediated transcriptional activation plays an essential role in stress-induced "fetal gene regulation" with cardiomyocyte-specific MEF2D deletion preventing development of hypertrophic ventricular remodeling in response to pressure-overload stress.

Forced expression of class II HDACs, HDAC5 and HDAC9, prevents hypertrophy in response to agonists such as phenylephrine or serum in vitro. In contrast, HDAC5- and HDAC9-null hearts develop spontaneous cardiac hypertrophy with derepression of MEF2 activity as well as profoundly exaggerated hypertrophy in response to pressure overload. Their response to swimming-induced hypertrophy is not altered, suggesting these HDACs predominantly regulate pathologic hypertrophy. Spatial regulation of this signaling occurs through local inositol 1,4,5-trisphosphate receptors (InsP3Rs) situated in the nuclear envelope, where IP3 produced in response to $G\alpha q$-coupled endothelin (ET1) receptor activation causes local Ca^{2+} release, CaMKII activation, and HDAC5 export. This provides a mechanism to separate Ca^{2+}-mediated transcriptional changes from the beat-to-beat cycling that determines contractility. Recent studies ascribe a key role to the N-terminus of HDAC4, levels of which are increased with exercise and downregulated in failing hearts.[104] An N-terminal peptide of HDAC4 controls metabolism by driving expression of transcription factor Nr4a1-mediated O-GlcNAcylation of STIM1, a store-operated calcium channel protein.

In contrast to class II HDACs, class I HDACs (HDACs 1, 2, 3, and 8) stimulate cardiac growth. HDAC2-null mice are resistant to myocardial hypertrophic stimuli, and HDAC2 transgenic mice manifest an exaggerated hypertrophic response involving HDAC2-mediated suppression of the gene encoding inositol polyphosphate-5-phosphatase f (Inpp5f), resulting in activation of Akt-PDK1 signaling with constitutive activation of GSK-3β.[103] Additionally, chemical inhibition of GSK3β (see below) results in re-sensitization to the hypertrophic response *in vivo* in HDAC2-deficient hearts, implicating increased GSK3β-mediated antihypertrophic signaling in the absence of HDAC2 as the mechanism for suppression of hypertrophy. Recent studies have implicated a critical role for class I HDACs 1 and 2 in transducing pressure overload hypertrophy via mTOR activation.[105] Cardiomyocyte-specific ablation of HDAC1 and 2, combinatorially, activated TSC2 signaling which inhibited mTOR activity. Pharmacologic inhibition of histone deacetylases by trichostatin A and scriptaid, two broad-spectrum HDAC inhibitors, or SK7041, an HDAC class 1- specific inhibitor, suppresses hypertrophy by a dominant effect on class I HDACs, in part via inhibition of autophagy signaling.[103]

Deacetylation mediated by class III HDACs (Sir2 family of kinases) requires NAD^+ and produces 2'-O-acetyl-ADP-ribose (O-AADPR) and nicotinamide. Both Sirt1 and Sirt2 are induced by ischemia/reperfusion injury in the heart, but although ablation of Sirt1 protects against cardiomyocyte death,[39] Sirt2 signaling is cardioprotective by deacetylation of LKB1 and AMPK activation and protects against Ang II-induced pathologic hypertrophy as well as hypertrophy in the aging heart.[106] Mice with Sir2 ablation are relatively protected against programmed necrosis in ischemia-reperfusion injury.[107] Sirt3 activation in the myocardium confers antihypertrophic signaling via FoxO3-mediated induction of ROS scavenging enzymes, and mice with Sirt3 ablation developed spontaneous hypertrophy with dysfunction and fibrosis at 10 weeks of age.[103]

Epigenetic regulation by Brg1, a chromatin-remodeling protein, has been assigned an important role in maintaining fetal gene expression in the myocardium prior to birth.[103] Brg1 associates with HDAC2 and HDAC9 on the αMHC promoter and with PARP on the βMHC promoter to suppress or activate transcription, respectively, in the fetal state. Expression of Brg-1 is extinguished soon after birth to depress transcription in the postnatal period but is rapidly reactivated with pressure overload and other hypertrophic stresses to provoke reexpression of the fetal gene program. Intriguingly, Brg1 cooperatively signals with Forkhead box M1 (FoxM1) transcription factor in endothelial cells to mediate the switch from the ACE isoform, Ace to Ace2, in pressure-overload hypertrophy[108] and contributes to pathologic hypertrophy signaling and fibrosis. Furthermore, pharmacologically targeting the activity of BET (bromodomain and extraterminal) family of proteins that bind to acetylated DNA and facilitate transcriptional activation by recruitment of coregulatory complexes such as mediator and the transcription elongation factor b (P-TEFb), blocked transcriptional elongation of genes implicated in pathologic hypertrophy and markedly attenuated pressure overload–induced cardiac remodeling and decompensation.[109]

Cross Talk Between Gαq and PI3K/Akt/mTOR/GSK3 Hypertrophic Signaling Pathways

$G\alpha q$/phospholipase C pathways also cross talk with the PI3K/Akt signaling axis in transducing pathologic hypertrophy signals (Fig. 1.11). $G\alpha q$-coupled receptors activate PI3Kγ, an isoform that is different from the α-isoform, which is activated in physiologic hypertrophy mediated by the IGF-1 pathway. The mechanism of activation also differs. PI3Kα is activated by receptor tyrosine kinase–mediated phosphorylation. PI3Kγ binds to G$\beta\gamma$ dissociated from $G\alpha q$ after ligand interaction, providing access to membrane phosphoinositides (**see** Figs. 1.8 and 1.11). PI3Kγ (p110γ) signals through Akt and is required for pressure overload–induced hypertrophy.[39] Also, in contrast to brief activation of p110α by exercise in stimulating physiologic hypertrophy, activation of p110γ is sustained downstream of $G\alpha q$ signaling and recruits additional signaling pathways, namely the phospholipase Cβ and calcineurin/NFAT axis, to determine the pathologic nature of hypertrophy.[36,42] PI3Kγ-null mice develop rapid cardiac dilation despite maintaining preserved ventricular contractility in response to pressure-overload stress. This is due to increased β-adrenorecetor-CREB-mediated transcriptional activation of MMPs and extracellular matrix breakdown.

Signaling downstream of Akt is divergent (**see** Fig. 1.11), which may also determine whether the hypertrophy is adaptive or maladaptive. One axis involves activation of mTOR (mechanistic target of rapamycin), a serine-threonine kinase that controls protein synthesis. mTOR exists in two complexes, mTORC1 or mTORC2.[110] mTORC1 primarily comprises mTOR along with Raptor (regulatory-associated protein of mTOR), is rapamycin-sensitive, and is the primary driver of cellular growth. mTORC1 also comprises mLST8 (mammalian lethal with SEC13 protein 8), which is necessary for kinase activity; proline-rich Akt substrate of 40 kDa (PRAS40) and DEPTOR (DEP domain-containing mTOR-interacting protein), which are the inhibitory subunits; and Tel2 (Tel 2 interacting protein 1). mTORC2 contains the same proteins except that Rictor is substituted for Raptor; it controls the actin cytoskeleton and determines cell shape. Signaling downstream of mTOR plays a central role in mediating hypertrophic signaling, as conditional ablation of mTOR in the adult myocardium provokes the rapid onset of cardiomyopathy with widespread apoptosis, altered mitochondrial ultrastructure, and accumulation of eukaryotic translation initiation factor 4E-binding protein 1.[110] Also, cardiomyocyte-specific ablation of Raptor results in the inhibition

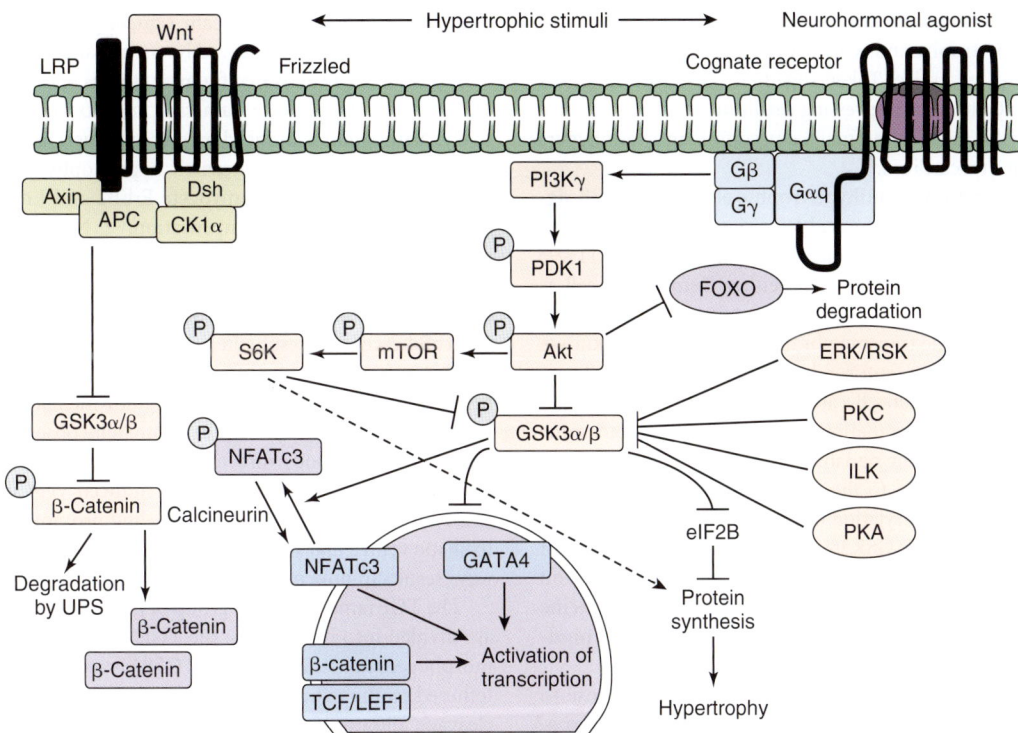

Fig. 1.11 Regulation of Hypertrophy via Wnt/β-Catenin and Akt/mTOR/GSK3β Signaling. Wnt signaling is activated by hypertrophic stimuli to assemble the LRP-Frizzled-Dishevelled receptor signaling complex together with other proteins—Axin, APC, and CK1α—which induces dephosphorylation of GSK3α/β to relieve the tonic inhibition and prevent degradation of β-catenin by the ubiquitin-proteasome system. This causes the accumulation of β-catenin, which translocates to the nucleus to associate with transcription factor TCF/LEF1 and initiate hypertrophic gene transcription. In response to neurohormonal receptor activation, Gαq and Gβγ subunits dissociate. Subsequently Gβγ-mediated PI3Kγ activation leads to Akt activation and the stimulation of protein synthesis via mTOR and suppresses antihypertrophic signaling via GSK3β. Akt also phosphorylates and causes the export of FoxO transcription factors from nucleus-suppressing protein degradation via the ubiquitin-proteasome pathway. GSK3α/β exerts tonic inhibition on multiple prohypertrophic transcription factors and its phosphorylation relieves this inhibition, resulting in hypertrophic signaling. Inhibition of GSK3α/β is a nodal point for convergence of hypertrophic signaling pathways and also occurs via phosphorylation by PKA (downstream of Gsα), PKCs (downstream of Gαq), ERK/ribosomal S6 kinases (downstream of small G protein signaling), and ILK (downstream of integrin signaling).

of mTORC1 and spontaneous development of cardiomyopathy with lack of hypertrophy in response to pressure overload.[111] mTORC1 signaling also appears to be required for the development of pathologic hypertrophy in response to pressure overload, as mice with inducible cardiomyocyte–specific mTOR and the raptor gene deletion develop cardiac dysfunction and HF without hypertrophy in response to transverse aortic constriction.[110] Whether this lack of hypertrophy reflects a lack of compensation in response to the pressure overload or whether mTORC1 ablation affects the quality of the hypertrophy remains to be characterized. These findings suggest a primary role for mTOR in facilitating cardiomyocyte hypertrophy and the survival in response to stress.

A second Akt pathway leads to phosphorylation and suppression of glycogen synthase kinase (GSK3β) with disinhibition of hypertrophic signaling (**see** Fig. 1.11).[112] GSK3β is tonically active in the myocardium and its phosphorylation by Akt relieves downstream antihypertrophic signaling. GSK3β is also phosphorylated and activated by protein kinase A (PKA) and in response to activation of the Gαq/PKC/ERK/p90 ribosomal S6kinase axis, thereby derepressing downstream hypertrophic signaling.[113] In vivo, pressure overload causes rapid phosphorylation of GSK3β within 10 minutes after transverse aortic constriction is applied, pointing to early recruitment of the kinase

in the hypertrophic response. Germline ablation of GSK3β results in embryonic lethality with lack of cardiac differentiation of embryoid bodies, congenital defects, and a markedly hypertrophied ventricular chamber resulting from increased cardiomyocyte proliferation. This indicates a prominent developmental role for GSK3β. In myocardial ischemia, GSK3β activation, via a constitutively active knockin, reduced infarct size, whereas dominant-negative GSK-3β expression or heterozygous ablation worsened ischemia-induced cell death with parallel modulation of ischemia-induced autophagy. In contrast, virtually opposite observations were made with reperfusion injury, the reasons for which are not clear. GSK3β may play a prominent role in suppressing cardiomyocyte proliferation in response to stress, as adult-onset inducible GSK-3β-null mice with ischemia/reperfusion injury demonstrate less ventricular dilation and postinfarct remodeling associated with increased cardiomyocyte proliferation.

Just as occurs with GSK-3β, GSK3α signaling is antihypertrophic.[112] In contrast to GSK3β, germline ablation of GSK3α did not elicit developmental abnormalities but resulted in progressive cardiomyocyte hypertrophy and dysfunction. Pressure overload was associated with a markedly enhanced hypertrophic response that rapidly transitioned to dilation, along with markedly impaired β-adrenergic responsiveness. GSK3α mice subjected to ischemia/reperfusion injury prior to spontaneous development of hypertrophy also manifest exaggerated hypertrophy and worse postinfarction remodeling as compared with wild-type mice. Taken together, these data suggest a prominent role for GSK3β in suppressing cardiomyocyte proliferative capacity, whereas GSK3α signaling may be predominantly antihypertrophic in the adult myocardium.

A novel mechanism for the antihypertrophic effects of GSK3β signaling may occur through the canonical Wnt signaling axis, which is under tonic repression by GSK3β-mediated signaling (see Fig. 1.11).[112] Wnts are extracellular proteins that signal either from cell to cell as membrane-bound proteins or as secreted proteins via heptahelical Frizzled receptors and single transmembrane-pass coreceptors known as low-density lipoprotein receptor–related proteins (LRPs). Tonic activity of GSK3β phosphorylates β-catenin, a transcription factor, at three sites, targeting it for degradation by the ubiquitin-proteasome system. With activation of Wnt signaling via Frizzled-LRP receptors, the entire complex is recruited to the receptor with scaffolding proteins, resulting in the phosphorylation of LRP and Dishevelled, which inhibits GSK3β and prevents GSK3β-mediated phosphorylation of β-catenin. In this form, β-catenin accumulates in the nucleus and forms a complex with a transcription factor TCF/LEF1 (T-cell–specific transcription factor/lymphoid enhancer factor 1) by displacing a binding protein, Groucho, thereby activating gene transcription.

Wnt signaling plays an important role in the cardiac response to hypertrophic stimuli, as mice with adult-onset cardiomyocyte-specific β-catenin ablation displayed marked attenuation of hypertrophy in response to pressure overload with reduced expression of c-fos and c-jun and without adverse consequences on myocardial function. Furthermore, mice with cardiomyocyte-specific overexpression of a dominant inhibitory mutant of Lef-1 manifest profound cardiomyocyte growth impairment with reduced heart weight, contractile dysfunction, and early death.[112] In contrast, β-catenin stabilization leads to decreased cardiomyocyte size, with upregulation of the atrophy-related protein IGFBP5. The signaling pathways connecting hypertrophic stimuli to β-catenin signaling appear complex. This is because, in contrast to the insights gained from β-catenin ablation in pressure overload, it was the gain of function of β-catenin with stabilization and increased expression, and not cardiomyocyte-specific ablation, that attenuated angiotensin II–mediated hypertrophy.[112]

In addition to stimulating protein synthesis, Akt suppresses protein degradation via phosphorylation of FoxO (O family of forkhead/winged-helix) transcription factors.[112] Akt-mediated phosphorylation of FoxOs suppresses their transcriptional activity by facilitating interaction with 14-3-3 proteins, leading to export from the nucleus and targeting for ubiquitin-proteasomal degradation (see Fig. 1.11). This prevents the expression of proapoptotic genes and the upregulation of the E3-ligase atrogin-1/MAFbx. Atrogin-1 is a cardiac- and skeletal muscle–specific F-box protein that binds to Skp1, Cul1, and Roc1 (the common components of SCF ubiquitin ligase complexes) and regulates muscle atrophy. Atrogin-1 also ubiquitinates and activates FOXO to suppress Akt-mediated hypertrophy signaling. Therefore suppression of atrogin-1 may provide another explanation for Akt-mediated pathologic hypertrophic signaling when Akt is activated via Gαq signaling (see later).

Non–Insulin-Like Growth Factor Signaling in Hypertrophy

Cardiomyocytes elaborate peptide growth factors in response to stress, including the prototypical growth factors neuregulin, EGF, and TGFβ (Fig. 1.12). Neuregulin, a member of the epidermal growth factor (EGF) signaling pathway, activates tyrosine kinase receptors (ErbB2, ErbB3, and ErbB4), leading to dimerization, tyrosine autophosphorylation, and recruitment of downstream signaling effectors.[114] All three isoforms of neuregulin are cleaved by membrane-bound metalloproteinases, producing an activated fragment that is released or associates with EGF receptor to provoke paracrine and juxtacrine signaling, respectively. Neuregulin is induced by pressure overload in the endothelium during development of concentric hypertrophy, and its levels decline along with those of cardiomyocyte ErbB2 and ErbB4 with transition to cardiomyopathic decompensation.[114] Neuregulin signaling primarily regulates cardiomyocyte survival, as endothelial cell–derived neuregulin protects cardiomyocytes against ischemic injury but not hypertrophy. Importantly, cardiomyocyte-specific ablation of ErbB2 or ErbB4 receptors results in spontaneous development of cardiomyopathy, accompanied by increased cardiomyocyte apoptosis.[114] These findings implicate the loss of neuregulin-mediated survival signaling as a major mechanism for the cardiotoxicity observed with use of trastuzumab, an antibody directed against the ErbB2 receptor, as a chemotherapeutic agent. Neuregulin-1 induced Vegf signaling promotes ECM synthesis, whereas Notch signaling promotes ECM degradation to shape ventricular trabeculae, and abnormal signaling in these pathways results in noncompaction cardiomyopathy.

The TGF family is a large group of polypeptide growth factors. They are divided into two groups: the TGF/activin subfamily and the bone morphogenic proteins (BMPs). TGFβ1 is secreted in a latent form and tethered to the extracellular matrix. Its stimulus-induced proteolytic cleavage allows interactions with TGFβRI and TGFβRII, its cognate cell-surface receptors, serine-threonine kinases that phosphorylate and activate downstream signaling proteins called Smads. Upon activation, Smad transcription factors translocate to the nucleus and activate gene transcription. TGFβ signaling also activates MAPKs (see later), such as the TAK1 (TGF-activated kinase)-MEK4-JNK1 and TAK1-MEK3/6-p38 axes, and tyrosine kinase pathways such as Ras/ and RhoA/p160 Rho-associated kinase (ROCK). TGFβ1 signaling mediates angiotensin-induced hypertrophy, as TGFβ1-null mice manifest a markedly attenuated hypertrophic response with minimal fibrosis and ANF gene induction with preservation of myocardial function. TAK1 is a MAPKKKinase activated downstream of TGFβ and transduces p38 activation.[39] Smad4 is the canonical transcription factor downstream of TGFβ signaling; given the prohypertrophic effects of TGFβ1 and its downstream MAPK kinase TAK1, it was unexpected that cardiomyocyte-specific gene ablation of Smad4 would result in spontaneous cardiac hypertrophy with reexpression of fetal genes and activation of the MEK1-ERK1/2 pathway. This suggests that Smad4 signaling acts in an antihypertrophic manner in opposition to TGFβ-induced MAPK activation. Genetic ablation of BMP9 resulted in marked increase in pressure overload–induced fibrosis and worsened adverse ventricular remodeling; administration of recombinant BMP9 or disruption of endoglin signaling limits cardiac fibrosis and attenuates LV remodeling, pointing to BMP9 as an endogenous inhibitor of cardiac fibrosis.

Role of Small G Proteins

Peptide growth factors and G protein–coupled receptors also transduce neurohormonal and stretch-induced hypertrophy via nonreceptor tyrosine kinases such as Src, serine-threonine kinases such as Raf, and small G proteins such as Ras.[39,115] Ras is the prototypical signaling molecule downstream of receptor tyrosine kinases (RTKs), causing MAPK activation by recruitment of the adaptor proteins Shc and Grb2, which bind the guanine nucleotide exchange factor (GEF) named Sos (Son of Sevenless), and activate Ras. The phosphotyrosine residues on the RTKs also interact with other proteins that have intrinsic catalytic activity, such as Src family tyrosine kinases, PI3Kγ, and PLCγ, thereby mediating cross talk between these signaling pathways (see Fig. 1.8). Ras, along with Rac, Rho, and Rab, is a member

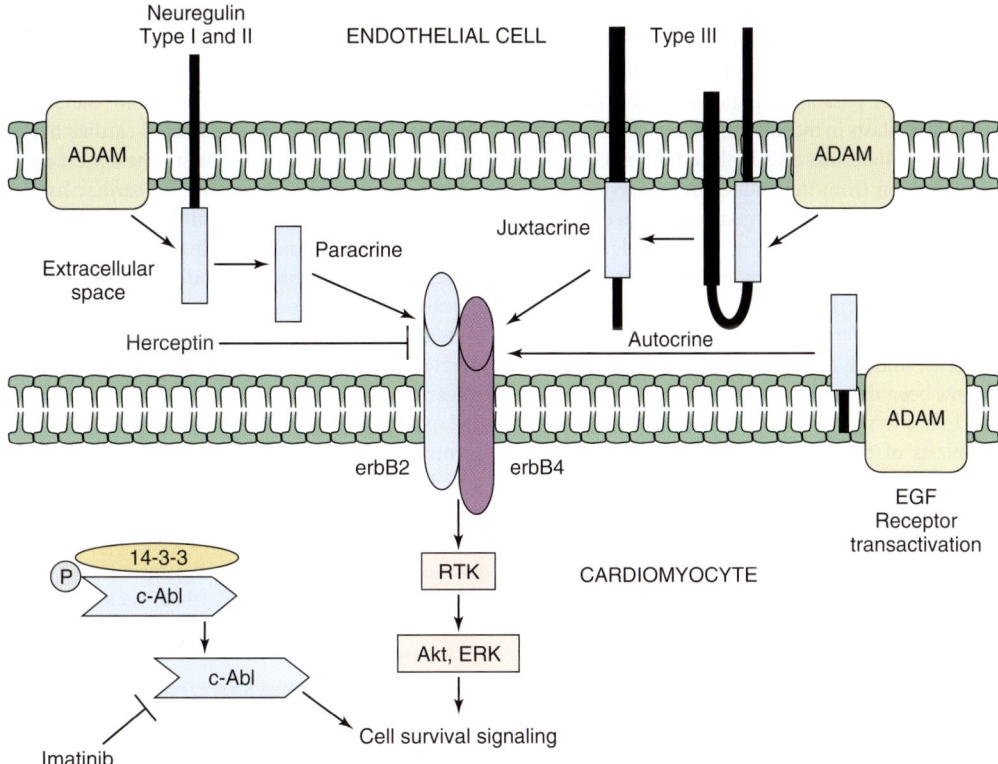

Fig. 1.12 Neuregulin/EGF/c-Abl Signaling in Hypertrophy. Neuregulins are transmembrane proteins of the EGF family, present mainly on endothelial cells as three different types (I, II, and III). Proteolytic cleavage by A disintegrin and the metalloproteinase (ADAM) family enzyme provokes exposure of an EGF-like signaling domain, which interacts with erbB2 and erbB4 receptors, resulting in receptor tyrosine kinase activation. EGF signaling is also activated by GRK-β-arrestin-mediated EGF cleavage by ligand-occupied seven transmembrane neurohormonal receptors. Neuregulins and EGF activate Akt and ERK signaling pathways to promote cell survival in the heart. Chromosomal translocation with formation of Bcr-cAbl fusion protein is implicated in the pathogenesis of chronic myeloid leukemia. Inhibition of endogenous c-Abl protein by imatinib (an antibody directed against the c-Abl protein [Imatinib]) and antagonism of the ErbB2/4 receptor by trastuzumab (an antibody-based chemotherapeutic agent used to treat breast cancer) antagonizes c-Abl and neuregulin-mediated survival signaling, respectively, resulting in cardiomyocyte death and heart failure.

of the small G protein family that exists bound to GDP in the inactive state. Upon stimulation, GDP is exchanged for GTP and followed by a conformational change resulting in stimulation of mitogen-activated protein kinase (MAPK) cascades. Intrinsic GTPase activity then extinguishes the signal, returning the G protein to its basal state. GEFs are proteins that facilitate GTP exchange, and GAPs promote inactivation by activating the GTPase activity. Ras and Rac1 are activated by Gαq agonists (PE, Ang II, endothelin-1, and mechanical stretch) and are sufficient to induce hypertrophy. In contrast, mice with forced cardiomyocyte expression of Rho A do not develop hypertrophy and instead develop fatal cardiomyopathy. RhoA activates Rho kinases, namely ROCK1 and ROCK2. Interestingly, ROCK1 deletion markedly reduces fibrosis in mice subjected to pressure overload, suggesting activation of maladaptive signaling pathways downstream of Rho in pressure overload hypertrophy. Rac1 also transduces hypertrophic signaling via increased generation of reactive oxygen species by NADPH oxidase signaling. Indeed, cardiomyocyte-specific gene ablation of Rac1 attenuates myocardial oxidative stress and hypertrophy in response to Ang II infusion.

The rapid development of therapeutics targeting various malignancies has uncovered numerous reports of cardiotoxicity with these drugs, spurring development of the cardio-oncology field.[116]A plethora of potential mechanisms exists for the cardiotoxicity observed with targeting tyrosine kinases downstream of growth factors to inhibit cell growth and division and angiogenesis to interrupt the tumor blood supply or microtubule network for destabilization. Early studies are beginning to delineate underlying mechanisms to develop targeted preventive and therapeutic approaches. A specific mechanism was identified with an essential role for c-Abl, a nonreceptor tyrosine kinase, in cardiomyocyte homeostasis (see Fig. 1.12). This was based on the observations that some patients with chronic myelogenous leukemia who were treated with imatinib (Gleevec), a small molecular inhibitor of the fusion protein Bcr-Abl, developed LV dysfunction. Modeling of this process in mice revealed imatinib-induced cardiomyocyte death due to both apoptotic and necrotic pathways leading to myocardial dysfunction. Activation of ER stress and JNK activation were implicated in this process.

CARDIAC FIBROSIS

Deposition of excess and disorganized fibrous tissue in the myocardium in the interstitial and perivascular space is a sine qua non myocardial histologic change observed in HF, often preceding its clinical manifestation in animal models. Cardiac fibrosis is variously characterized as a form of repair or replacement when it occurs in response to cardiomyocyte death (as in MI) or reactive, which is speculated to be primarily driven by activation of signaling pathways that stimulate fibroblast proliferation and deposition of extracellular matrix. The past decade has witnessed rapid advances in our understanding of molecular pathways that regulate cardiac fibroblast function and their role in myocardial fibrosis. Extensive experimentation from multiple groups using lineage tracing as well as parabiosis paradigms have demonstrated that adult cardiac fibroblasts in the unstressed and injured heart are primarily derived from mesodermal cells in the embryonic epicardium with a small contribution from the endocardium (reviewed in Tallquist and Molkentin[28]). Recent studies targeting ablation of Hippo signaling pathway kinases Lats1/2 implicate a central role for this pathway in the transition of epicardial mesenchymal cells to cardiac fibroblasts and for extracellular matrix remodeling to sustain coronary vascular development.[117] Transdifferentiation of other cell types such as circulating immune cells, smooth cells, pericytes, and endothelial to fibroblast lineage has now been demonstrated to be a rare event in the settings of myocardial infarction or pressure overload stress. Indeed, Tcf21-expressing fibroblasts of embryonic origin were shown to be the primary cell type that were marked by periostin-promoter driven Cre expression in "activated myofibroblasts" post-MI, exclusively in the area of injury.[118] Ablation of these activated myofibroblasts with diphtheria toxin–induced cytotoxicity prevented post-MI scar formation leading to ventricular rupture and markedly increased lethality. Interestingly, these periostin-expressing myofibroblasts demonstrated plasticity, with regression to a less activated state after removal of the AngII/PE stimulus.[118]

Elegant lineage tracing studies have examined the dynamics of fibroblast proliferation and phenotypic change post-MI.[119] In the immediate post-MI period, Tcf21-labeled resident cardiac fibroblasts start proliferating and activate periostin as well as α-smooth muscle actin (αSMA) expression transiently; rates of cell death are also upregulated in the activated fibroblasts as a likely attempt to shape the stable scar. With deposition of collagen and maturation of the extracellular matrix, these myofibroblasts lose the αSMA expression and become incorporated in the stable scar as matrifibrocytes. Fibroblast-specific ablation of the protein kinase p38α (Mapk14 gene) attenuated the differentiation of resident fibroblasts into myofibroblasts, whereas transgenic gain of function of p38α accelerated the development of interstitial and perivascular fibrosis in multiple tissues, indicating that p38α signaling is a key regulator of fibroblast responses postinjury.[120] A genome-wide screen for other factors that regulate myofibroblast differentiation uncovered an important role for a RNA-binding protein muscleblind-like1 (MBNL1) in regulating a network of transcripts including SRF and calcineurin in regulating myofibroblast differentiation.[121] Secretion of Follistatin-like 1 (Fstl1), a secreted glycoprotein, is upregulated in the immediate postinjury period and fibroblast-specific ablation of Fstl1 attenuated transition to myofibroblasts with increased cardiac rupture post-MI, pointing to a critical role for this signaling pathway in ensuring a stable scar.[122] Levels of Fstl1 were found to decline in the epicardium post-MI, and epicardial application of human Fstl1 stimulated cardiac myocyte regeneration in mouse and swine models of MI to improve survival and attenuate post-MI remodeling.[123]

Studies demonstrate that fibroblasts proliferate and coalesce in three-dimensional arrangements in the area of injury, and aggregation in this network is responsible for global changes in gene expression as well as release of a specific secretome of proteins that drives cardiomyocyte hypertrophy.[124] Remarkably, these changes are reversible, raising hopes for therapies targeting fibroblast aggregation in preventing cardiac hypertrophy and failure. Indeed, pharmacologic inhibition of fibroblast-derived fibronectin polymerization in the extracellular space attenuates post-IR remodeling in mice.[125] Expression of thioredoxin domain containing 5 (TXNDC5), a cardiac fibroblast (CF)-enriched endoplasmic reticulum protein, was observed to be upregulated in failing human hearts and genetic ablation of TXNDC5 attenuated isoproterenol-induced cardiac hypertrophy, reduced fibrosis, and improved left ventricle function.[126] Recent studies implicate osteopontin among other proteins in the secretome from visceral adipose tissue in driving age-related cardiac hypertrophy and fibrosis in mice, by inhibiting fibroblast senescence; and removal of visceral adipose tissue caused regression of cardiac hypertrophy and fibrosis. Similarly, ablation of β-catenin specifically in fibroblasts prevented pressure overload–induced fibrosis as well as reduced cardiomyocyte hypertrophy.[127] A long noncoding RNA, Meg3, was found to be specifically expressed in cardiac fibroblasts and inhibition of Meg3 prevented matrix metalloproteinase-2 (MMP2) induction with pressure overload hypertrophy and attenuated cardiac fibrosis.[128] A series of elegant experiments demonstrated upregulation of Lysyl oxidase-like 2 (Loxl2), an enzyme that cross-links collagen in the myocardium and serum of patients with both HFrEF and HFpEF; and treatment with anti-Loxl2 antibodies or fibroblast-specific targeted ablation of the Loxl2 gene prevented excessive myofibroblast formation and fibrosis and rescued both systolic and diastolic dysfunction under pressure overload stress.[129] These studies raise hopes for developing targeted therapies to counter HFpEF, which is characterized by cardiomyocyte hypertrophy and increase myocardial fibrosis.[130]

CARDIAC INFLAMMATION

The rapidly expanding state of knowledge in deciphering the role of the immune system in HF is reviewed extensively in **Chapter 7**. Herein, we will focus on the molecular pathways that have been implicated in driving cardiac inflammation during injury and disease states. Myocardial injury incites inflammation with activation of both innate and adaptive immune pathways to orchestrate myocardial repair. This involves release of conserved endogenous mediators with stimulation of cytokine and chemokine production that recruits infiltrating cells. Dysregulated or excessive inflammation is implicated mechanistically in driving adverse remodeling (reviewed in Epelman et al.[131]).

Upon cardiac injury, resident cardiac immune cells are activated by release of damage-associated molecular patterns (DAMPs) via signaling through a fixed number of germline-encoded pattern recognition receptors (PRRs). PPRs include toll-like receptors (TLRs) and C-type lectin receptors on plasma membrane and endosomes and retinoic acid-inducible gene I (RIG-I)-like receptors (RLRs), NOD-like receptors (NLRs) and absent-in-melanoma 2 (AIM2) receptors located in intracellular membranes. PRRs trigger signaling cascades to activate nuclear factor-κB (NF-κB), activator protein 1 (AP-1), and interferon regulatory factor (IRF) transcription factors, which drive cytokine and chemokine production. PRRs also trigger assembly of the inflammasome, a cytosolic protein complex that converts pro-caspase 1 into the catalytically active caspase 1 protease and drives production of interleukin-1β (IL-1β) and IL-18; and activation of inflammasome has been implicated in driving adverse cardiac remodeling after MI.[132] TLR4 signaling has been implicated in activation of mesenchymal stromal cells[133] and ablation of TLR4 results in reduced ischemia injury,[131] but its role in specific immune cell types remains to be characterized. Epicardial Hippo signaling also regulates cardiac inflammation in response to injury as epicardium-specific ablation (with Wt1 promoter-driven Cre) of Yap and Taz, two core Hippo signaling mediators resulted in attenuated recruitment of T-regulatory cells (T-regs) with increased pericardial inflammation and fibrosis extending into the myocardium resulting in cardiomyopathy and death.[134]

Mast cells degranulate to recruit neutrophils acutely after MI. This is followed by a wave of monocyte-derived macrophage recruitment, and macrophages phagocytose dead cells by efferocytosis to facilitate repair.

Macrophage-specific ablation of Mertk, a tyrosine kinase that plays an important role in phagocytosis results in persistence of neutrophils and systolic dysfunction[135] indicating a critical role for macrophages in resolution of inflammation. Elegant studies have defined differential roles for resident cardiac macrophages (which are of embryonic origin and identified by the lack of CCR2 expression) in promoting tissue healing and for recruited monocyte-derived macrophages (which are bone marrow–derived and identified by high expression of CCR2) in driving sustained inflammation and adverse cardiac remodeling.[136] These paradigms continue to be refined through elucidation of cell type–specific transcriptional profiles that will permit targeting specific subsets to elucidate their roles.

Another fascinating development has been the discovery of the role of clonal hematopoiesis in cardiovascular pathology. Accumulation of somatic mutations in hematopoietic cells in aging individuals attributed to mutations in the gene encoding the epigenetic modifier enzyme Ten-Eleven Translocation-2 (TET2) has been implicated in promoting clonal expansion of mutant cells; and TET2-deficient myeloid cells accelerated atherosclerosis progression in mouse models[137] and worsened maladaptive cardiac remodeling after pressure overload driven by excess activation of the inflammasome and IL1β generation.[138] Macrophages have also been assigned a role in promoting ventricular diastolic dysfunction, as studies in aged mice and in humans with HFpEF demonstrate increased myelopoiesis in the bone marrow and spleen resulting in myocardial macrophage expansion in mice.[139] These cardiac macrophages were shown to produce IL-10 which induces fibroblast proliferation, and IL-10 ablation improved diastolic function, suggesting a therapeutic target to disrupt a link between myocardial inflammation and fibrosis leading to diastolic dysfunction with hypertension and aging. Another inflammatory mediator, IL-11, has been identified as a fibroblast-restricted (and a dominant) transcriptional target of TGFβ signaling, and ablation of IL-11 receptor (IL11RA) attenuated cardiac fibrosis in response to angiotensin II infusion and pressure overload–induced hypertrophy.

Accumulation of T and B lymphocytes has been observed in failing human hearts and in mouse myocardium subjected to pressure-overload stress, with enlarged mediastinal lymph nodes as a source of these lymphocytes migrating into the heart.[140] Ablation of recombination-activating gene 2 expression (RAG2KO) in mice results in a lack of B and T lymphocytes as well as ablation of CD4+ T cells (but not CD8+ T cells) and attenuated LV dilation and LV dysfunction with pressure overload.[140] Recent studies demonstrate increased recruitment of Th1 effector T cells in myocardium of patients with nonischemic cardiomyopathy as well as with pressure overload, and these cells are implicated in driving conversion of fibroblasts to myofibroblasts resulting in cardiac fibrosis.[141] The interplay between cardiac inflammation and fibrosis continues to be an area of active investigation, with potential for uncovering novel therapeutic targets to treat HF.

SUMMARY AND FUTURE DIRECTIONS

We have witnessed a breathtaking emergence of discoveries in the elucidation of the molecular basis of HF. Although the information presented here is inadequate to fully chronicle all the developments, we have tried to present a framework for understanding the complex and intricate signaling processes that govern cardiac growth, development, and pathology. Investigators and clinicians alike are acutely aware of the current limitations of HF therapeutics, with persistent high morbidity and mortality, and the nature of investigation has been increasingly refocused toward evaluating and developing therapeutic targets. Simultaneously, ground breaking basic discoveries continue to emerge, which often challenge the existing dogma and stimulate innovation to tackle fundamental questions. One such discovery in recent years has been the appreciation that cardiomyocytes may continue to be replenished in the adult myocardium, which harbors a complement of resident cardiac cells that can be expanded and recruited to assist with cardiac repair. Another exciting possibility is the potential to predict disease risk and response to therapy based on an individual's genetic makeup. Given recent advances in sequencing technology and systems biology approaches, "big data," with its unbiased approaches to understanding disease, is rapidly taking center stage.

We are poised to enter an era of increased risk for cardiovascular diseases, driven by the current epidemic of obesity and westernization of cultures all over the world. The next generation of cardiac investigators will likely redirect their research efforts to tackle these challenges while continuing to invest in understanding the molecular underpinnings of cardiac development and homeostasis. With rapid advances in our understanding of the molecular basis for HF continuing, the future holds exciting prospects that some of the therapeutic strategies highlighted in this chapter will be translated into clinical use in a safe and cost-effective manner.

KEY REFERENCES

5. Shah SJ, Kitzman DW, Borlaug BA, et al. Phenotype-specific treatment of heart failure with preserved ejection fraction: a multiorgan roadmap. *Circulation*. 2016;134:73–90.
7. Loffredo FS, Steinhauser ML, Jay SM, et al. Growth differentiation factor 11 is a circulating factor that reverses age-related cardiac hypertrophy. *Cell*. 2013;153:828–839.
11. Hinson JT, Chopra A, Nafissi N, HEART DISEASE, et al. Titin mutations in iPS cells define sarcomere insufficiency as a cause of dilated cardiomyopathy. *Science*. 2015;349:982–986.
24. Liu Z, Wang L, Welch JD, et al. Single-cell transcriptomics reconstructs fate conversion from fibroblast to cardiomyocyte. *Nature*. 2017;551:100–104.
27. Pinto AR, Ilinykh A, Ivey MJ, et al. Revisiting cardiac cellular composition. *Circ Res*. 2016;118:400–409.
28. Tallquist MD, Molkentin JD. Redefining the identity of cardiac fibroblasts. *Nat Rev Cardiol*. 2017;14:484–491.
52. Schiattarella GG, Hill TM, Hill JA. Is load-induced ventricular hypertrophy ever compensatory? *Circulation*. 2017;136:1273–1275.
82. Wisler JW, Xiao K, Thomsen AR, Lefkowitz RJ. Recent developments in biased agonism. *Curr Opin Cell Biol*. 2014;27:18–24.
131. Epelman S, Liu PP, Mann DL. Role of innate and adaptive immune mechanisms in cardiac injury and repair. *Nat Rev Immunol*. 2015;15:117–129.
137. Fuster JJ, MacLauchlan S, Zuriaga MA, et al. Clonal hematopoiesis associated with TET2 deficiency accelerates atherosclerosis development in mice. *Science*. 2017;355:842–847.

The full reference list is available online at ExpertConsult.

Abbreviations Used in this Chapter

Abbreviation	Name	Note
AngII	Angiotensin II	Hypertrophic agonist
AMPK	Adenosine monophosphate kinase	
ANF	Atrial natriuretic factor	"Early" response gene
AP-1	Activator protein 1	Transcription factor
AT1Ra, AT1Rb	Angiotensin II receptor type Ia or Ib	
Ask-1	Apoptosis signal regulating kinase 1	MAP kinase kinase
ATF1	Activating transcription factor 1	
βARK (GRK2)	β-Adrenergic receptor kinase (G-protein receptor kinase 2)	Gβγ-dependent, phosphorylates β-adrenergic receptors
BNP	Brain natriuretic peptide	TGFβ superfamily ligands
BMP	Bone morphogenic proteins	
CAD	Caspase associated DNAase	
CaMK	Ca^{2+} calmodulin dependent kinase	
cAMP	Cyclic adenosine monophosphate	
cAMP Kinase	Cyclic 3′,5′-adenosine monophosphate kinase	
CREB	cAMP response element–binding protein	cAMP-responsive transcription factor
CREM	Cyclic AMP response element modulator	cAMP-responsive transcription factor
CRISPR-Cas9	Clustered regularly interspaced short palindromic repeats (CRISPR)–associated (protein) 9	Bacteria-derived enzymatic system for genetic editing
CT-1	Cardiotrophin-1	IL-6 family cytokine
DAG	Diacyl glycerol	Endogenous PKC agonist
DISC	Death-induced signaling complex	Signaling complex downstream of death receptor.
4E-BP	4E-binding protein	
EGF	Epidermal growth factor	
egr-1	Early growth response gene 1	Transcription factor
eIF4F	Eukaryotic initiation factor 4F	Stimulates initiation of translation at a subset of transcripts
ErbB2-4	EGF family tyrosine kinase receptors	Receptors for neuregulins
ET-1	Endothelin 1	
ET_A, ET_B	Endothelin receptors A and B	
ECM	Extracellular matrix	
EGF	Epidermal growth factor	
Elk-1	TCF family transcription factor	
Ets1	TCF family transcription factor	
ERK	Extracellular receptor kinase	MAP kinase
FAK	Focal adhesion kinase	Nonreceptor tyrosine kinase
FGF	Fibroblast growth factor	Growth factor
c-fos	c-fos oncogene	Component of transcription factor AP-1
FoxO	O family of forkhead/winged-helix transcription factors	
Gα, Gβγ	Subunits of heterotrimeric G proteins	
GAP	GTPase activating proteins	
GATA4	GATA binding protein 4	
GDP	Guanosine diphosphate	
GDF-11	Growth differentiation factor 11	TGF-β superfamily protein.
GEF	Guanine exchange factor	Activators of small G proteins
gp130	Glycoprotein 130	Receptor for IL6-family cytokines
GPCR	Heterotrimeric G protein–coupled receptor	
Grb2	Growth factor receptor–bound protein 2	Adaptor protein linking RTKs and Ras
GRK	G protein receptor kinase	Inhibits G protein signaling and recruits adaptor proteins to stimulate alternate pathways.
GSK3β	Glycogen synthase kinase 3β	Kinase downregulated by hypertrophic stimuli
GTP	Guanosine triphosphate	
HB-EGF	Heparin-binding EGF-like growth factor	
HAT	Histone acetyltransferase	Induces histone acetylation with activation of transcription
HDAC	Histone deacetylase	Represses transcription by inducing histone de-acetylation
IGF-1	Insulin-like growth factor	Growth factor
IL-6	Interleukin 6	cytokine
IP3	Inositol 1,4,5 trisphosphate	
ILK	Integrin-linked kinase	Serine threonine kinase associated with β-integrin
JAK	Janus activating kinase	Tyrosine kinase activated by gp130
JNK	Jun N terminal kinase	MAP Kinase

Abbreviations Used in this Chapter—cont'd

Abbreviation	Name	Note
c-jun	jun oncogene	Component of AP-1 transcription factor
KLF-5	Kruppel-like transcription factor	
LIF	Leukemia inhibitory factor	IL6 cytokine
MADS domain	DNA binding motif	Present in SRF and MEF2 transcription factors
MAPK	Mitogen activated protein kinase	
MAPKK	MAPK kinase	Also known as MEK or MK
MAPKKK	MAPK kinase kinase	Also known as MEKK or MKK
MEF2	Myocyte enhancer factor 2	Transcription factor
MEK-1	MAP kinase kinase 1	Activator of ERK MAPKs
MCIP	Modularity calcineurin-inhibitory proteins	Endogenous inhibitor of calcineurin
MHC	Myosin heavy chain	
miRNAs	MicroRNAs	Endogenous RNAs that inhibit mRNA translation/enhance degradation
MLC	Myosin light chain	
MLP	Muscle LIM protein	
mRNA	messenger RNA	
mTOR	Mechanistic target of rapamycin	Kinase involved in regulation of protein synthesis
c-myc	myc oncogene	Transcription factor
NE	Norepinephrine	catecholamine
Nab1	NGF1a-binding protein	Transcriptional repressor
NFAT	Nuclear factor of activated T cells	Transcription factor
PDK1	Phosphoinositide-dependent kinase 1	Downstream effector of PI3K
PDGFRα	Platelet-derived growth factor receptor-α	Fibroblast-expressed growth factor receptor
PE	Phenylephrine	α-adrenergic agonist
PI3K	Phosphoinositide 3-kinase	
PIP2	Phosphatidyl inositol 4,5-bisphosphate	
PIP3	Phosphatidyl inositol 3,4,5-trisphosphate	
PITX2	Paired-like homeodomain transcription factor 2	Transcription factor
PKA	Protein kinase A	
PKB	Protein kinase B	Also known as Akt
PKC	Protein kinase C	
PKD	Protein kinase D	
PLC	Phospholipase C	
PMA	Phorbol 12-myristate 13-acetate	PKC agonist
PTEN	Phosphatase and tensin homolog	
p53	Tumor suppressor gene	Transcription factor
p70S6K	Ribosomal p70 S6 kinase	Protein kinase involved in protein synthesis
Ras	ras oncogene	Small G protein
RTK	Receptor tyrosine kinase	
ROCK	Rho kinases	
RYR	Ryanodine receptor	
SERCA	Sarcoplasmic reticulum Ca^{2+} ATPase	Pumps Ca^{2+} from cytoplasm to sarcoplasmic reticulum
SH2	Src homology domain 2	Binds phosphotyrosine residues
SHP2	SH2 domain-containing cytoplasmic protein tyrosine phosphatase	
siRNAs	Short interfering RNAs	Inhibit mRNA translation
SOCS	Suppressors of cytokine signaling	Endogenous repressor of STATs.
c-src	src oncogene	Nonreceptor tyrosine kinase
SRF	Serum response factor	Transcription factor
STAT	Signal transducer and activator of transcription	Transcription factor regulated by JAKs
TALEN	Transcription activator–like effector nuclease	Genetic editing tool
TRPCs	Transient receptor potential channels	Ion channels
Tcf21	Transcription factor 21	Transcription factor that drives embryonic fibroblast commitment
TCF/LEF1	T-cell–specific transcription factor/lymphoid enhancer factor 1	Transcription factor
TAK1	TGFβ-activated kinase 1	MAPKK activated by TGFβ
TGFβ	Transforming growth factor β	cytokine
TNF	Tumor necrosis factor	cytokine
TRP	Transient receptor potential channel	Store operated calcium channels
TUNEL	Terminal deoxynucleotidyl transferase dUTP nick end labeling	
VEGF	Vascular endothelial growth factor	Angiogenic cytokine

2

Cellular Basis for Heart Failure

Adam Nabeebaccus, Can Martin Sag, Ian Webb, Ajay M. Shah

The development of heart failure in the context of chronic disease stresses such as hypertension or myocardial infarction (MI) is characterized initially by complex changes in the structure and function of the heart at the molecular (**see also Chapter 1**), cellular, and organ levels. This dynamic process, termed *cardiac remodeling* (**see also Chapter 12**), leads to contractile dysfunction, chamber dilatation, ventricular dyssynchrony, and arrhythmias. At the cellular level, the remodeling heart manifests significant alterations both in the cardiac myocytes and in nonmyocyte cells, such as fibroblasts, endothelial cells, and immune cells. In addition, there are significant changes in the myocardial vasculature and the composition of the extracellular matrix.

Progressive changes in the cardiac myocyte phenotype are a central abnormality in the chronically stressed and failing heart. The phenotype comprises multiple components including cell hypertrophy (**see Chapter 1**) and alterations in calcium handling, sarcomeric function, electrical properties, redox homeostasis, metabolism, energetics, and cell viability that collectively make a major contribution to the global cardiac phenotype. Cardiomyocyte hypertrophy is also observed in physiologic settings (e.g., pregnancy or in athletes) but in this case is not accompanied by detrimental changes such as contractile impairment. This divergence in phenotypes indicates that different components of the cardiomyocyte phenotype are capable of being regulated independently, at least to some extent. Even in a disease setting (e.g., early during pressure overload), the heart may hypertrophy but maintain contractile function (*adaptive* remodeling), whereas with more chronic disease stress it begins to fail. Thus the overall phenotype may be determined by the balance between potentially adaptive and maladaptive processes that occur within the cardiac myocyte.

In this chapter, we review the main cardiomyocyte cellular alterations that contribute to the pathogenesis of heart failure. We start by discussing the cellular basis for contractile dysfunction (**see also Chapter 10**), the key cardiac manifestation of heart failure. The contribution of changes in excitation-contraction coupling (particularly calcium handling and sarcomeric function) to contractile dysfunction and arrhythmogenesis is considered. We next discuss several global alterations within cardiomyocytes that also impact on contractile function and cell viability, such as changes in redox homeostasis and signaling, cellular stress responses, and macromolecular and protein turnover. As will become evident, these global processes interact with each other and have complex effects on the remodeling process (e.g., redox homeostasis and signaling modulate excitation-contraction coupling, as well as stress responses). The cardiomyocyte phenotype in the failing heart may also be affected by other cardiac cell types and, in turn, influence those cell types. The role of cardiomyocyte interactions with other cell types—in particular fibroblasts, endothelial cells, and immune/inflammatory cells—is therefore discussed. Finally, we review the role of regulation by noncoding mRNAs such as microRNAs (miRNAs), which often have global effects on cellular signaling pathways in the failing heart. The signaling pathways that underlie the development of myocyte hypertrophy per se are discussed elsewhere in this edition. Likewise, the important role of alterations in myocardial energetics and metabolism, which, for example, may have a major impact on contractile function during heart failure, is covered in other chapters.

CONTRACTILE DYSFUNCTION

Cardiac myocytes in the failing heart exhibit several abnormalities of contractile function, including a reduction in contractile amplitude and force of contraction, a slowing of contraction and relaxation, an increase in diastolic force, and altered responses to changes in heart rate and β-adrenergic stimulation. Perturbations in both excitation-contraction coupling and sarcomere properties contribute to these abnormalities. We provide a brief overview of normal excitation-contraction coupling and sarcomeric function and then address the distinct abnormalities that occur in heart failure.

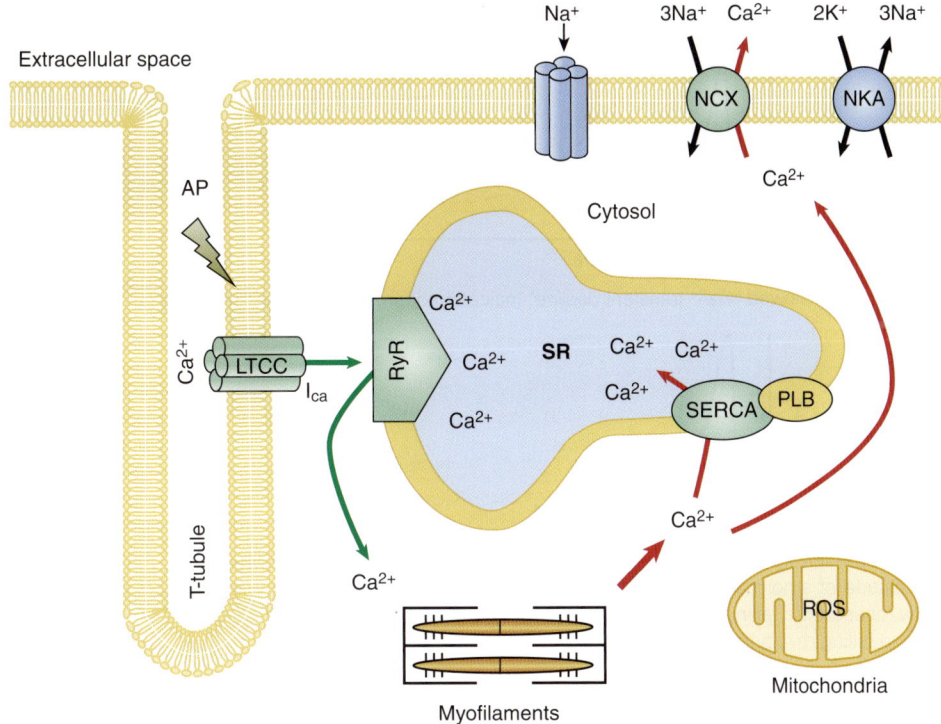

Fig. 2.1 Normal Excitation-Contraction Coupling. On systolic depolarization of the membrane potential, L-type Ca^{2+} channels (LTCC)-mediated Ca^{2+} (I_{Ca}) induces Ca^{2+} release from the SR via the ryanodine receptor (RyR). Ca^{2+} binds to the myofilaments and initiates contraction *(green arrow)*. During diastole *(red arrows)*, Ca^{2+} is actively taken up into the SR via SERCA2a and also partly extruded to the extracellular space via NCX. *AP,* Action potential; *NKA,* Na^+/K^+ ATPase; *PLB,* phospholamban; *ROS,* reactive oxygen species, *SR,* sarcoplasmic reticulum.

Normal Excitation-Contraction Coupling

Physiologic cardiac function requires the coordinated temporal and spatial activation of the heart. At a cellular level, this finely tuned process is regulated mainly by accurately synchronized Ca^{2+} fluxes in every cardiomyocyte (**Fig. 2.1**).[1] When an action potential depolarizes the cell, voltage-dependent L-type Ca^{2+} channels (LTCCs) located mainly in the transverse tubules (T-tubules) open to generate an inward Ca^{2+} current (I_{Ca}), which induces a localized increase of Ca^{2+} in the "dyadic cleft" in close neighborhood to the Ca^{2+} release or ryanodine receptor channels (RyR2) of the sarcoplasmic reticulum (SR). This transsarcolemmal Ca^{2+} influx activates the RyR2 and results in so-called Ca^{2+}-induced Ca^{2+} release from the SR, which provides the major component of the increase in cytosolic Ca^{2+} during systole (i.e., the "Ca^{2+} transient"). Intracellular Ca^{2+} concentration increases from approximately 100 nmol/L during diastole to approximately 1 μmol/L during systole and causes myofilament activation and contraction. Repolarization of the membrane potential is induced by inactivation of I_{Ca} and the activation of delayed rectifying K^+ currents. During diastole, Ca^{2+} is removed from the cytosol via two major pathways: (1) the SR Ca^{2+} ATPase (SERCA2a) located in the membrane of the SR, which pumps Ca^{2+} back into the SR lumen; (2) the sarcolemmal Na^+/Ca^{2+} exchanger (NCX1), which transfers Ca^{2+} into the extracellular space. Through these two Ca^{2+} transport mechanisms, $[Ca^{2+}]_i$ decreases to physiologic resting concentrations of approximately 100 nmol/L, allowing the cell to relax and to regain its physiologic diastolic resting cell length.

Impaired Ca^{2+} Handling in Failing Cardiac Myocytes

Prolongation of the action potential duration, depressed force generating capacity, and slowed contraction and relaxation rates are the hallmark functional changes of the failing human heart. Impaired Ca^{2+} handling is a key feature of the failing cardiac myocyte, with great pathophysiologic relevance for the progressive deterioration in contractile function of the failing heart. Distinct alterations in the expression levels, as well as posttranslational modifications of important cardiac Ca^{2+}-handling proteins, causatively contribute to systolic and diastolic contractile dysfunction and to an increased propensity for cardiac arrhythmias.[2] The posttranslational modifications that alter the function of key Ca^{2+}-handling proteins include alterations in phosphorylation,[3] nitrosylation,[4] oxidation status,[5] and sumoylation.[6] Altered protein phosphorylation occurs secondary to changes in the activity of various kinases (e.g., cAMP-dependent protein kinase [PKA], calcium-calmodulin-dependent kinase II [CaMKII]), as well as perturbations in phosphatase (e.g., protein phosphatase 1 [PP1]) activity.[7]

The failing cardiac myocyte has a significantly diminished amplitude of the systolic Ca^{2+} transient as compared with nonfailing control myocytes (**Fig. 2.2**), which is a major factor responsible for the reduced contractile amplitude of the failing cell (*systolic* dysfunction, **see Chapter 10**). Failing myocytes typically also exhibit a slowed decay of the Ca^{2+} transient during diastole, which is a major contributor to abnormal (delayed) relaxation. In addition, the normal increase in amplitude of Ca^{2+} transient (and therefore force of contraction) that occurs with faster heart rate is blunted or even reversed in the failing heart (i.e., the normal positive force-frequency relationship [FFR] is converted to a flat or a negative FFR). It is generally accepted that a reduction in the Ca^{2+} content of the SR is a major reason for the diminished amplitude of the systolic Ca^{2+} transient and the abnormal FFR. A decreased SR Ca^{2+} content has been consistently observed in myocytes isolated from failing human and animal hearts, whereas alterations in

Decreased "systolic Ca²⁺ transient" in failing cardiac myocytes

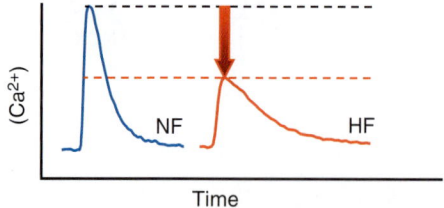

Slowed "Ca²⁺ transient decline" indicating depressed SR Ca²⁺ reuptake

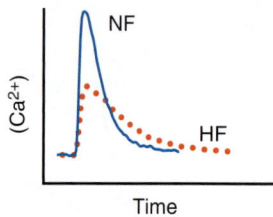

Fig. 2.2 Representative Ca²⁺ Transients of Failing and Nonfailing Cardiac Myocytes. In the upper panel, the amplitude of a normal nonfailing *(NF)* Ca²⁺ transient *(blue)* is compared with the Ca²⁺ transient that is typically measured in failing myocytes *(HF, red)*. The bottom panel illustrates the slowed Ca²⁺ transient decay kinetics in failing myocytes *(red)*.

LTTC-mediated Ca²⁺ influx appear to be less relevant.[1,2] From a mechanistic point of view, a reduction in SR Ca²⁺ content can result either from insufficient diastolic Ca²⁺ refilling (or loading) of the SR or from an increased loss of Ca²⁺ via the RyR2 Ca²⁺ release channels during diastole and may also be influenced by changes in NCX activity. In fact, all three mechanisms may contribute to the reduction in SR Ca²⁺ content and contractile phenotype of the failing myocyte (**Fig. 2.3**).

Reduced SR Ca²⁺ Reuptake in Heart Failure (see also Chapter 1)

During diastole, SERCA2a pumps Ca²⁺ into the SR lumen and provides a sufficient Ca²⁺ content to be released during the subsequent systolic heartbeat. SERCA2a-dependent diastolic Ca²⁺ uptake into the SR normally dominates over transsarcolemmal Ca²⁺ extrusion via the NCX. SERCA2a is subject to regulation by the phosphoprotein phospholamban (PLB), which on phosphorylation by CaMKII (at Thr-17) and/or PKA (at Ser-16) releases its inhibitory effect on SERCA2a because of a dissociation of the PLB/SERCA2a complex.[8] SERCA2a protein levels are reduced in failing myocardium, which is paralleled by a reduction in SERCA2a sumoylation,[6] and results in an impairment of diastolic Ca²⁺ reuptake into the SR. Moreover, the levels of PLB are unaltered and its phosphorylation state may be reduced, so that there is greater relative inhibition of SERCA2a by nonphosphorylated PLB, thereby aggravating the impairment of Ca²⁺ reuptake (**see Fig. 2.3**).[9] The decrease in SR Ca²⁺ content results in less Ca²⁺ available for the subsequent systolic Ca²⁺ transient and impairs systolic function.

Decreased SERCA2a expression may also affect diastolic function of the failing heart. If no other mechanism (such as an increased NCX activity [see later discussion]) compensates for the reduction in SERCA2a function with respect to removal of Ca²⁺ from the cytosol during diastole, then there is diastolic cytosolic Ca²⁺ overload. Myocytes that have increased diastolic Ca²⁺ levels will have persistent low-level myofilament activation at a time when the myofilaments should be fully relaxed, resulting in increased diastolic force and diastolic dysfunction. This failure to relax fully during diastole impairs the filling of the heart and thereby may also worsen systolic dysfunction.[10] Moreover, the abnormally elevated diastolic Ca²⁺ levels may have multiple other effects, such as changes in gene transcription,

cell viability, and mitochondrial function through altered activation of Ca²⁺-dependent kinases (e.g., CaMKII), phosphatases (e.g., calcineurin), mitochondrial enzymes, caspases, and other mechanisms.

In view of these effects on contractile function, as well as other aspects of the failing heart phenotype, restoring SERCA2a function in heart failure might represent a promising therapeutic approach.[11] Experimental studies showed that adenoviral overexpression of SERCA2a in human cardiomyocytes can improve cardiac contractility because it restores SR Ca²⁺ content and the systolic Ca²⁺ transient, whereas reduced cytosolic Ca²⁺ levels preserve diastolic function. In addition, SERCA2a overexpression was shown to improve myocardial energetics and endothelial function and to have antiarrhythmic effects.[9] The potential clinical relevance of SERCA2a stimulation has been addressed in the CUPID trials (Calcium Up-Regulation by Percutaneous Administration of Gene Therapy in Cardiac Disease) in which patients with heart failure were treated with a single infusion of an adeno-associated viral (AAV) vector delivering SERCA2a versus placebo. Although this initial study suggested potential efficacy, the larger study CUPID2 trial failed to show efficacy in advanced heart failure.[12]

Increased NCX Activity in the Failing Heart

The NCX is localized at the cardiomyocyte sarcolemma where, in its "forward mode," it transfers one Ca²⁺ ion into the extracellular space in exchange for three Na⁺ ions using the transmembrane gradient for Na⁺ (**see Fig. 2.1**). This mechanism is electrogenic because it results in the net movement of one positive charge into the cytosol and can therefore depolarize the membrane potential and even have arrhythmogenic effects under conditions of spontaneous and localized rises in [Ca²⁺]ᵢ (see later discussion). NCX expression and activity are found to be increased in human and experimental heart failure, which may have complex functional effects depending on the mode of NCX activity and stage of heart failure. In the face of downregulated SERCA2a function, enhanced NCX activity competes with SERCA2a for Ca²⁺ elimination during diastole. This may further aggravate the decrease in SR Ca²⁺ content because less cytosolic Ca²⁺ is available for SERCA2a-mediated SR Ca²⁺ loading. However, the increase in NCX function can also partly protect cardiac myocytes against severe diastolic Ca²⁺ overload and diastolic dysfunction. Indeed, an increase in NCX levels in explanted human myocardial samples was found to correlate with a preservation of diastolic function, whereas patients with diastolic dysfunction had decreased NCX levels.[2] On the other hand, NCX activity can contribute to Ca^{2+} overload in settings where there is intracellular Na^+ overload. The reason is that at high $[Na^+]_i$, NCX switches to a "reverse mode" and pumps out Na^+ in exchange for Ca^{2+}. The increased contribution of NCX-dependent Ca^{2+} influx, as opposed to SR Ca^{2+} release during systole in failing myocytes, has adverse effects on mitochondrial Ca^{2+} uptake (which relies on high Ca^{2+} gradients), and promotes increased mitochondrial reactive oxygen species (ROS) levels because of reduced activity of Ca^{2+}-dependent Krebs cycle dehydrogenases that normally maintain antioxidant reserves.[13] This detrimental mechanism can become further aggravated in a ROS-dependent manner and lead to a vicious cycle of impaired cytosolic and mitochondrial Ca^{2+} fluxes and increased oxidative stress because ROS induce further cytosolic Na^+ overload.[14]

"Leaky" RyR2 Cause Diastolic SR Ca^{2+} Loss in Heart Failure

Diastolic "leak" of Ca^{2+} from the SR due to a pathologic increase in RyR2 open probability is an important mechanism that contributes to the lowering of SR Ca^{2+} content in heart failure. Ca^{2+} leaks from the SR through spontaneous and uncoordinated Ca^{2+} release events or "Ca^{2+} sparks." The expression of RyR2 itself appears to be unchanged in heart failure, but its functional regulation is dramatically altered by complex posttranslational modifications. These alterations involve an increase in RyR2 phosphorylation as a result of hyperactive protein

kinases, such as CaMKII[15] and PKA,[16] and possibly reduced RyR2 dephosphorylation.[17] An increase in RyR2 oxidation or nitrosylation as a consequence of increased oxidative and nitrosative stress in heart failure may also be important.[5] Although transient phosphorylation- and redox-dependent regulation of RyR2 gating may fulfill physiologic functions in healthy myocytes, in the failing myocyte the hyperphosphorylation and/or oxidation of RyR2 leads to severe diastolic SR Ca^{2+} leakage. Furthermore, the coupling of LTCC to RyR is also impaired in heart failure because of T-tubule remodeling, such that some RyR are "orphaned" and contribute to dyssynchronous Ca^{2+} release.[18]

The precise mechanisms of RyR2 hyperphosphorylation and the kinases responsible for this abnormality are important to establish because they may represent therapeutic targets but are still a matter of debate. Although one laboratory reported strong evidence for a PKA-mediated dysregulation of the RyR2 in heart failure,[3,16] others failed to show an increase in PKA-dependent hyperphosphorylation.[19] There is also evidence for an involvement of CaMKII-dependent RyR2 phosphorylation in inducing SR Ca^{2+} leak.[20] Redox-related dysregulation of RyR2 opening in the failing heart[5] may involve increased ROS produced by mitochondria or other sources such as nicotinamide adenine dinucleotide phosphate (NADPH) oxidases (**see also Chapter 8**), and is related to the oxidation of specific cysteine residues within the RyR2.[5] Interestingly, both the protein kinases implicated in RyR2 hyperphosphorylation (i.e., CaMKII and PKA) are subject to redox activation,[21] so that alterations in the redox milieu of failing myocytes may also exert indirect effects on RyR2. In this regard, it is interesting to note that increased ROS in heart failure also impact adversely on

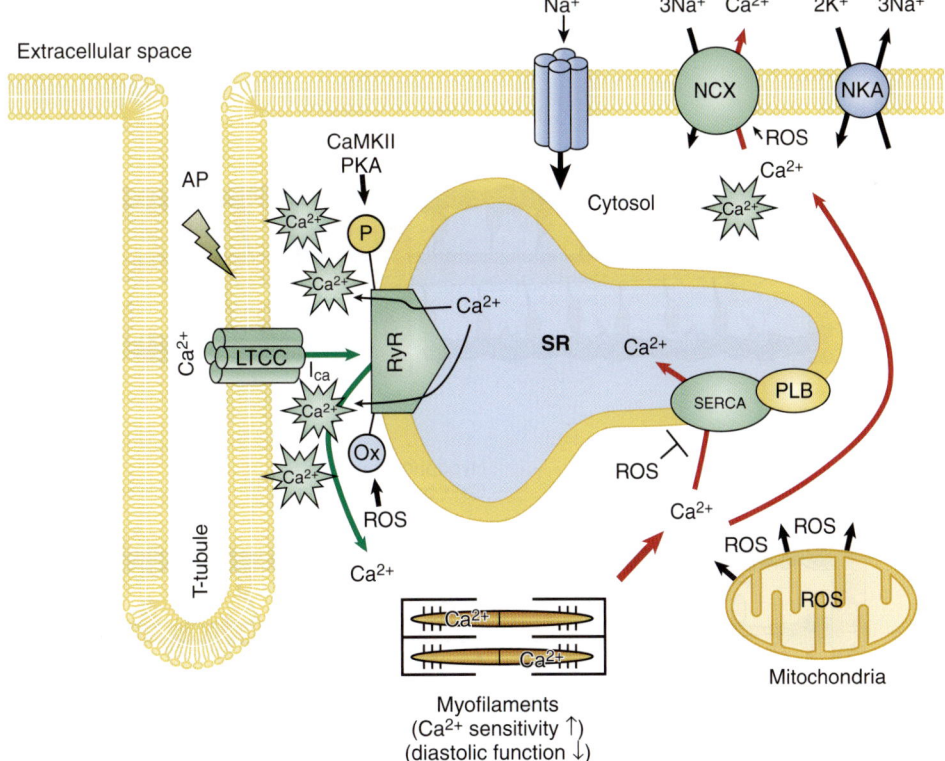

Fig. 2.3 Abnormalities of Cardiac Ca^{2+} Handling in Heart Failure. Sarcoplasmic reticulum *(SR)* Ca^{2+} content is typically diminished in failing myocytes because of (1) increased diastolic SR Ca^{2+} leak induced by RyR hyperphosphorylation *(orange arrow)* or oxidation *(light blue arrow)*; (2) decreased SR Ca^{2+} reuptake because of reduced SERCA expression; (3) increased NCX expression and activity that removes Ca^{2+} to the extracellular space. Note that increased oxidative stress in heart failure (e.g., because of increased mitochondrial reactive oxygen species *[ROS]* or other sources) can further aggravate these abnormalities. Myofilament dysfunction also contributes to the contractile abnormalities. *AP,* Action potential; *NKA,* Na^+/K^+ ATPase; *PLB,* phospholamban.

SERCA2a function and other aspects of Ca^{2+} handling in the failing cell (**see Fig. 2.2**). More recently it has been shown that an increase in calcium leak from RyR2 results in mitochondrial calcium overload, which in turn has been linked to heart failure progression.[22]

Contribution of Impaired Ca^{2+} Handling to Arrhythmia

Impaired cardiomyocyte Ca^{2+} handling not only leads to systolic and diastolic dysfunction but also contributes to the development of arrhythmias in heart failure. The dysregulation of RyR2 Ca^{2+} release is of particular relevance in this regard.[23-25] The enhanced diastolic SR Ca^{2+} leak in failing cells and the accompanying spatially and temporally uncoordinated increases in intracellular Ca^{2+} may drive the NCX to exchange Ca^{2+} for Na$^+$, thereby inducing an influx of positive charge (I_{ti}) that partly depolarizes the cell during phase 4 of the action potential (**see Fig. 2.3**). These spontaneous depolarizations of the membrane potential are termed *delayed afterdepolarizations (DADs)* and are arrhythmogenic. Because NCX expression and activity are increased in heart failure, the depolarizing influx of positive charge (I_{ti}) will be greater for any given spontaneous Ca^{2+} release from the SR. Thus the combination of leaky RyR2 and increased NCX activity synergizes to enhance ventricular arrhythmogenesis. Similar mechanisms may also contribute to the development of atrial fibrillation,[26] the occurrence of which is higher in heart failure. There is a significant potential for feedback among the different ionic mechanisms that contribute to arrhythmogenesis in the failing cardiomyocyte and therefore the possibility of a self-sustaining vicious cycle of hampered Ca^{2+} and Na$^+$ handling that contributes to contractile dysfunction and arrhythmia. For example, if the NCX starts to function in reverse mode because of elevated intracellular [Na$^+$], the resulting increase in Ca^{2+} influx may activate proarrhythmogenic kinases such as CaMKII and lead to further arrhythmogenic SR Ca^{2+} leakage through phosphorylation of RyR2.

Sarcomeric Dysfunction in Heart Failure

Cardiac mechanical activity occurs as a result of the interaction between changes in cytosolic Ca^{2+} concentration and the contractile myofilaments (**Fig. 2.4**). Contractile function is influenced not only by

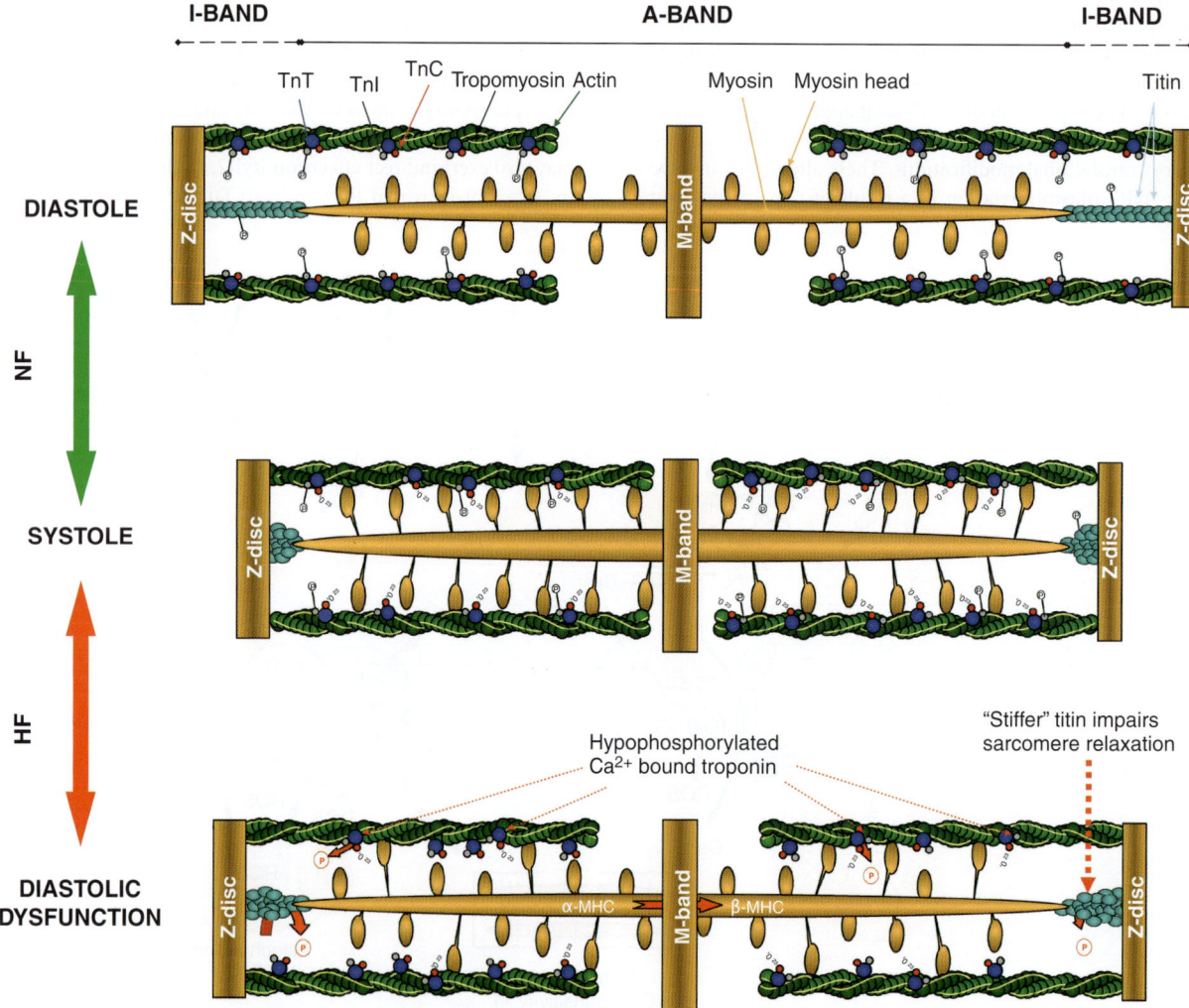

Fig. 2.4 **Main Aspects of Sarcomeric Dysfunction in Heart Failure.** During diastole *(upper panel)*, mechanical interaction of myosin *(light brown)* and actin *(green)* is inhibited by tropomyosin *(yellow)* and troponin I *(gray)*. Titin *(light blue)* is elongated and exerts restraint on diastolic relaxation of the sarcomeres. During systole *(middle panel)*, Ca^{2+} binds to troponin C *(red)*, which causes a conformational change of the tropomyosin-troponin complex *(blue)* and allows the myosin heads to interact with actin. The subsequent sliding movement of myosin and actin relative to each other causes sarcomere shortening and contraction. In heart failure *(HF, bottom panel)*, hypophosphorylation of troponin I and titin results in impaired sarcomere relaxation because of a persistently Ca^{2+}-activated tropomyosin-troponin complex and increased titin-dependent stiffness, respectively. *NF*, nonfailing.

changes in Ca^{2+} concentration but also by the intrinsic myofilament responsiveness to Ca^{2+}, which is dependent on the properties of the actomyosin complex and regulatory proteins such as the troponin complex and myosin-binding protein C. During diastole, the mechanical interaction between actin and myosin is inhibited by the tropomyosin-troponin complex. When cytosolic Ca^{2+} concentration increases during systole, the binding of Ca^{2+} to troponin C (cTnC) relieves this inhibitory effect and allows actomyosin interaction and contraction to occur. A subsequent decrease in cytosolic Ca^{2+} leads to its release from cTnC and muscle relaxation. Other components of the sarcomere also affect the mechanical properties of heart muscle. In particular, the giant filamentous protein titin—which connects the Z disc to the M band and confers significant "elasticity" to the sarcomere—has an important influence on passive muscle stiffness,[27] which in turn is an important determinant of diastolic function.

Significant evidence suggests that alterations in myofilament properties contribute to systolic and diastolic contractile dysfunction in heart failure.[10,28] Perhaps the best-known contribution of myofilament properties to contractile changes in the stressed and failing heart is the shift of myosin heavy chain (MHC) from the fast α-MHC to a slower β-MHC isoform. The significantly lower ATPase activity of β-MHC is beneficial in that it is more energetically efficient but at the same time may result in slower relaxation and lower contractility. This isoform shift is a prominent feature in rodent models, where α-MHC is the dominant isoform in healthy myocardium, but may be less important in human heart failure because β-MHC dominates over α-MHC in healthy human ventricular myocardium. Nevertheless, a small impact of such an MHC isoform shift is suggested in failing human ventricular tissue.[10]

A major regulator of myofilament Ca^{2+} sensitivity in the normal heart is the PKA-mediated phosphorylation of troponin I (cTnI), which results in a lower affinity for Ca^{2+} and contributes to faster kinetics of myofilament cross-bridge cycling (i.e., faster contraction and relaxation of myocytes). In the failing heart, PKA-dependent phosphorylation of cTnI is generally decreased (related to reduced β-adrenergic responsiveness) and results in increased myofilament Ca^{2+} sensitivity.[10] The major effect of such an increase in myofilament Ca^{2+} sensitivity is thought to be to impair relaxation and aggravate the slowed kinetics of Ca^{2+} transient decay in the failing myocyte (see Fig. 2.4). Similar functional effects on myofilament Ca^{2+} sensitivity have been reported when there is C-terminal truncation of cTnI after myocardial ischemia/reperfusion injury, and these could play a particular role in ischemic heart failure. The phosphorylation of myosin-binding protein C is thought to play a role in the physiologic enhancement of rate of contraction and relaxation observed after β-adrenergic stimulation. Therefore hypophosphorylation of myosin-binding protein C may also contribute to contractile dysfunction.[28,29]

Another shift in protein isoform that is reported in failing hearts is a shift from the stiffer (i.e., less elastic) *N2B* titin isoform to a more compliant *N2BA* isoform.[30] It is suggested that this shift may counterbalance the decreased phosphorylation status of titin in the failing human heart,[31] which functionally results in an increased passive stiffness. The underlying defect in titin phosphorylation is thought to be PKA dependent (as with reduced cTnI and myosin-binding protein C phosphorylation), but dysfunctional CaMKII-dependent phosphorylation of titin is also reported.[28] Cyclic GMP-dependent protein kinase (PKG), activated by nitric oxide (NO), may also phosphorylate cTnI and titin and have similar effects to PKA. In heart failure, there is usually a reduction in NO/PKG activity, which promotes increased titin-dependent passive stiffness.[32] Finally, changes in the redox milieu within the failing myocytes may also contribute to contractile dysfunction (e.g., through specific oxidative modifications in titin that lead to increased passive stiffness).[33]

GLOBAL MECHANISMS AFFECTING CARDIOMYOCYTE FUNCTION IN HEART FAILURE

Redox Homeostasis in the Heart (see also Chapter 8)

ROS are generated in cardiac myocytes (as in other cell types) either as a by-product of cellular respiration and metabolism or through specialized enzymes. An important physiologic function of ROS is in redox signaling (i.e., the highly specific, usually reversible oxidation/reduction modification of signaling molecules involved in various homeostatic processes).[34] Redox signaling is tightly regulated in a spatially and temporally confined manner and depends on appropriate inactivation or scavenging of ROS by cellular antioxidants to terminate the ROS signal. Another critical function of ROS is their involvement in oxidative protein folding in the endoplasmic reticulum (ER). In pathologic settings such as heart failure, physiologic redox signaling pathways may be perturbed or different redox-sensitive signaling pathways may be activated. Altered redox homeostasis in the ER may have a major impact on protein synthesis and stress responses (see later). In addition, an imbalance between ROS production and antioxidant reserves (i.e., oxidative stress) can result in nonspecific detrimental effects because of the irreversible oxidation of macromolecules, membranes, and DNA. Therefore alterations in redox homeostasis in the failing cardiomyocyte have a profound impact on many aspects of the myocyte phenotype.

Major sources of ROS in failing cardiac myocytes include the mitochondrial electron transport chain (ETC), NADPH oxidase proteins (NOXs), monoamine oxidases, uncoupled NO synthases (NOSs), and xanthine oxidases.[21] Pathophysiologically important ROS species include superoxide, hydrogen peroxide (produced by dismutation of superoxide), hydroxyl ions, and peroxynitrite generated by the reaction of superoxide with NO. Electron leak from the mitochondrial ETC generates superoxide, and this becomes quantitatively more important in heart failure as a result of ETC dysfunction, uncoupling, and an impairment of mitochondrial antioxidants. Mitochondrial ROS generation can lead to opening of the mitochondrial permeability transition pore (MPTP) and loss of cell viability. Furthermore, such ROS production may also induce further mitochondrial ROS production, termed *ROS-induced ROS release*.[35] Monoamine oxidases, which catabolize the neurotransmitters noradrenaline and serotonin, have recently been recognized as additional important mitochondrial sources of ROS in the failing heart.[36] Nonmitochondrial ROS sources, such as NOXs and xanthine oxidase, may also stimulate mitochondrial ROS production. Xanthine oxidase–derived ROS may be particularly important in the setting of ischemia-reperfusion.[37] The inhibition of mitochondrial ROS using various mitochondrially targeted agents is considered to be a promising therapeutic approach in heart failure.[38]

NOX proteins are especially important for redox signaling, being the only source that has a primary ROS-generating function. They catalyze electron transfer from NADPH to molecular O_2, thereby generating superoxide and/or hydrogen peroxide. Among seven distinct NOX family members, NOX2 and NOX4 are expressed in cardiomyocytes and other cardiac cells (e.g., endothelial cells, fibroblasts, inflammatory cells).[21,39] Although both isoforms generate ROS, there are significant differences in their structure, activation, and subcellular localization that contribute to important differences in function. NOX2 has been shown to have a physiologic function in stretch-induced excitation-contraction coupling,[40] whereas NOX4 may regulate cardiomyocyte differentiation.[41] The activities of both NOX2 and NOX4 are increased in heart failure, the former mainly as a result of increased activation by stimuli, such as angiotensin II and cytokines, and the latter largely because of increased expression levels. An additional Ca^{2+}-sensitive isoform, NOX5, may be important in the human heart.

NOS enzymes normally catalyze the production of NO from L-arginine. Cardiomyocytes constitutively express neuronal (nNOS) and endothelial (eNOS) isoforms, which have distinct physiologic actions, notably in regulating excitation-contraction coupling and inotropic responsiveness.[42] An inducible iNOS isoform is upregulated in response to cytokine stimulation. During heart failure, NOSs can become "uncoupled" and switch from NO to superoxide generation, resulting in loss of the normal NO-mediated effects, as well as detrimental effects related to ROS production. Partial uncoupling results in the simultaneous generation of NO and superoxide, leading to peroxynitrite production. Uncoupling of NOSs is usually related to a reduction in the availability of the cofactor tetrahydrobiopterin.[42] In the case of eNOS, there additionally is S-glutathionylation of specific cysteine residues in the reductase domain.[43] Importantly, both these mechanisms are enhanced by oxidative stress so that NOS uncoupling can often act to amplify ROS generation by other sources.

Alterations in antioxidant balance are an important contributor to altered redox homeostasis in the failing heart. These include changes in antioxidant enzymes, such as superoxide dismutases, catalase, glutathione peroxidase, thioredoxin, peroxiredoxin, glutathione S-transferases, and others. A crucial factor for redox homeostasis is the level of NADPH in different cellular compartments, with this nucleotide being required for the regeneration of reduced pools of major cellular antioxidants, such as glutathione, glutaredoxin, and thioredoxin. Therefore metabolic reactions that generate NADPH have a potentially broad impact on the myocyte phenotype. In the mitochondria, the activity of Ca^{2+}-dependent dehydrogenases is important in this regard, and this is inhibited by cytosolic Na^+ overload in heart failure as mentioned earlier.[14] In the cytosol, glucose-6-phosphate dehydrogenase (G6PD) is a key rate-limiting enzyme involved in NADPH production and has been shown to affect cardiomyocyte calcium homeostasis and contractile dysfunction in ischemia-reperfusion.[44] Interestingly, excessively high levels of NADPH and glutathione can be detrimental by inducing so-called reductive stress. In a mouse model of mutant αB-crystallin (CryAB) cardiomyopathy, such reductive stress is associated with abnormal protein folding and the accumulation of protein aggregates in cardiomyocytes.[45]

Altered redox homeostasis affects an extensive range of molecular targets in the failing cardiomyocyte, including kinases, phosphatases, ion transporters and channels, myofilaments, and transcription factors, as reviewed in detail elsewhere.[21] Here we discuss a few examples where the mechanisms of such redox modifications and their impact on the myocyte phenotype have been addressed in sufficient depth to offer the promise of therapeutically tractable targets. Redox dysregulation affects several proteins involved in abnormal excitation-contraction coupling, as discussed earlier. NOX2 appears to be an important ROS source in this regard and may act both through direct oxidation of proteins critical in excitation-contraction coupling such as RyR2 and via the modulation of redox-sensitive kinases or phosphatases that regulate such proteins.[21,46] NOX2 is also implicated in the genesis of atrial fibrillation.[47] Several signaling pathways involved in cardiomyocyte hypertrophy are in part redox-regulated (e.g., the activation of ASK-1, ERK1/2, NF-κB, and Akt). NOX2 is again an important ROS source responsible for such regulation, especially in the setting of increased renin-angiotensin system activation.[21,48] Class II histone deacetylases (HDACs) are key regulators of hypertrophic gene expression, allowing this to occur when they are exported from the cardiomyocyte nucleus. A thioredoxin 1–sensitive pathway for the specific oxidation and subsequent nuclear export of HDAC4 is reported to be important in adrenergic-mediated cardiomyocyte hypertrophy.[49,50] Cardiomyocyte viability may be adversely affected by an altered redox balance (e.g., leading to increased mitochondrial ROS production). In addition, the specific oxidative activation of kinases such as CaMKII has been found to be important.[21] PKG is also oxidatively activated and was shown to be physiologically important in stretch-induced tuning of the Frank-Starling response via the phosphorylation of phospholamban,[51] but persistent oxidation during chronic pressure overload was found to be detrimental.[52] Not all ROS effects are detrimental in the stressed cardiomyocyte. For example, an increase in NOX4 has been shown to be cardioprotective during chronic pressure overload or ischemic stress by enhancing beneficial signaling mechanisms including myocyte hypoxia-inducible factor 1-alpha (HIF1α) signaling leading to paracrine effects on myocardial capillary density,[53] enhancement of the activating transcription factor 4 (ATF4)-mediated integrated stress response[54] and alterations in myocardial substrate use.[55] This underscores the concept that the effects of altered redox homeostasis may vary depending on the ROS source and its subcellular location.

Protein Synthesis, Turnover, Quality Control, and Stress Responses

The dynamic cellular remodeling that occurs in the stressed and failing heart involves substantial changes in protein synthesis and turnover and requires robust quality control mechanisms to ensure the degradation or clearance of abnormal proteins (e.g., misfolded proteins and protein aggregates). Several organelles and systems are important for these functions, including the ER, the ubiquitin-proteasome system (UPS), and autophagy. The cell can mount specific stress responses designed to facilitate the maintenance of some of these functions (e.g., the unfolded protein response [UPR] or an enhancement of autophagy). These systems make a major contribution to the cellular phenotype in the failing heart and may represent targets for therapeutic modulation. We next discuss in more detail the role of some of these systems in the failing heart.

Endoplasmic Reticulum and the Unfolded Protein Response

The cardiac myocyte SR is a specialized ER that is especially important for intracellular Ca^{2+} regulation, and this is known to become dysfunctional in heart failure, as discussed earlier in this chapter. In addition to Ca^{2+} homeostasis, the ER coordinates other important functions such as the correct folding, posttranslational modification, and quality control of membrane and secreted proteins, gluconeogenesis, lipid, and steroid synthesis.[56] It also interacts with and influences mitochondrial function (e.g., through transfer of Ca^{2+} from the ER). These functions are important in cardiac myocytes as in other cell types, although the distinction and/or overlap between the SR and ER remain poorly defined. The requirement for protein folding, quality control, and related functions in the ER changes significantly in the remodeling heart where there are significant alterations in protein turnover (e.g., due to hypertrophy), metabolism, and energetics. The maintenance of appropriate ER function therefore becomes an important factor in cellular homeostasis.

The ER stress response or UPR is a conserved mechanism that senses the status of ER protein folding by detecting the accumulation of misfolded proteins and inducing a program of changes that affects both the ER and other cellular organelles and processes.[57] The UPR encompasses homeostatic mechanisms that include the increased synthesis of chaperones, which assist the refolding of misfolded proteins, inhibition of further protein translation that may aggravate misfolding and ER overload, and the activation of degradation pathways to break down misfolded proteins. Many different stressors can induce the UPR, including glucose or amino acid deprivation, oxidative stress, hypoxia, and ionic imbalance. Induction of the UPR is mediated through three transmembrane ER stress sensors, namely protein kinase RNA-like

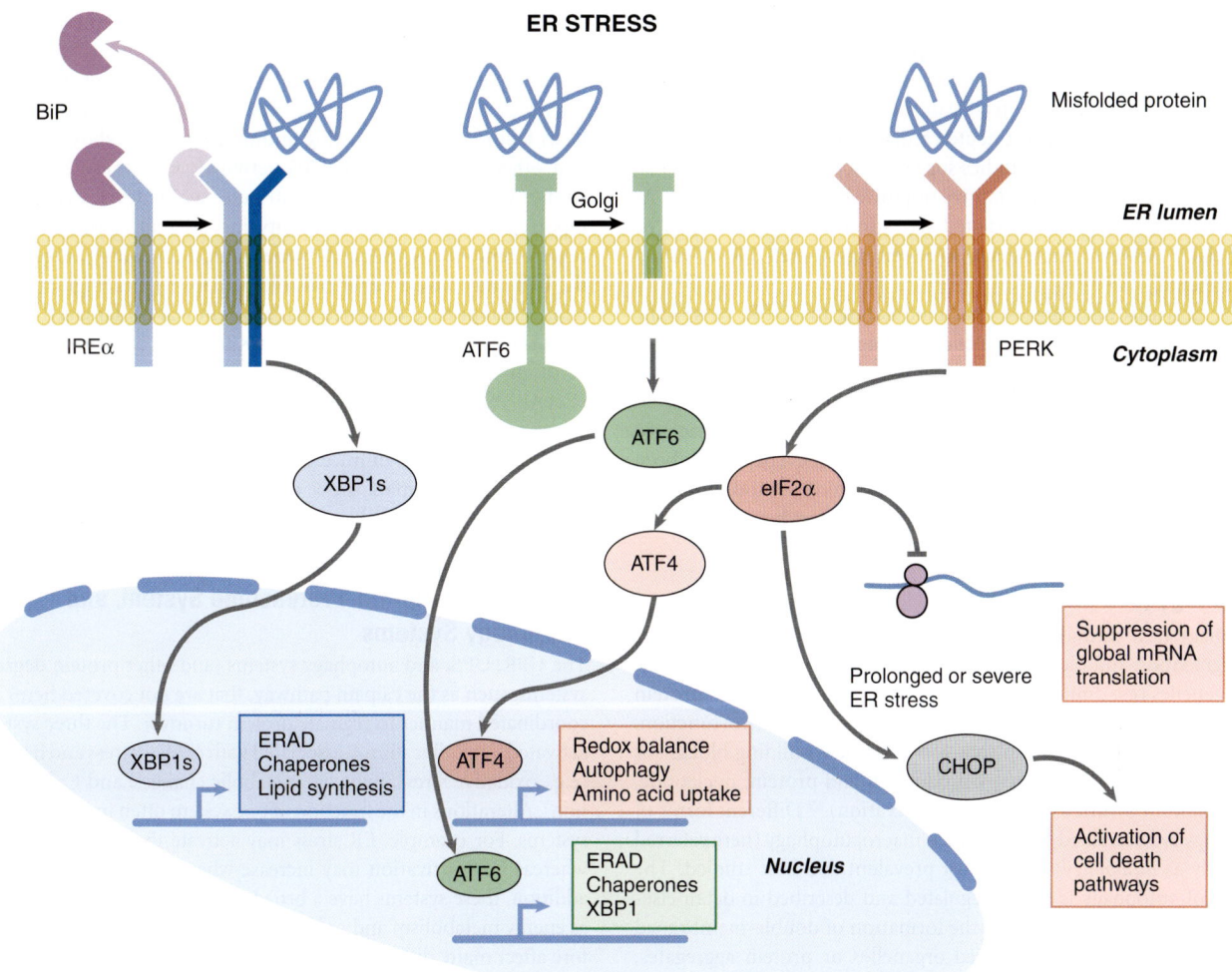

Fig. 2.5 Endoplasmic Reticulum (ER) Stress Leading to Activation of the Unfolded Protein Response. ER stress triggers a set of homeostatic cellular changes termed the *unfolded protein response (UPR)*. This involves the activation of three ER-resident transmembrane proteins: protein kinase RNA-like ER kinase *(PERK)*, inositol-requiring kinase 1 (IRE1), and activating transcription factor 6 *(ATF6)*. ER stress activation of the UPR is an adaptive response to cardiac stress; however, prolonged or more severe stress can lead to the activation of apoptotic pathways and a maladaptive ER stress response. PERK and IRE1 are activated either by dissociation of BiP/GRP78, allowing dimerization and activation by autophosphorylation, or misfolded proteins can directly bind to PERK and IRE1 and cause dimerization and activation. ATF6 is activated through a protease mechanism. Downstream of ATF6 and the transcription factor XBP1s (which is activated by IRE), multiple chaperones and ER-associated degradation *(ERAD)* proteins are induced, which help to fold proteins and to target misfolded proteins for degradation. In addition, global protein translation is inhibited by PERK-induced phosphorylation of eIF2α, thus reducing protein load to the ER. However, ATF4 translation is upregulated and induces genes involved in adaptive responses (e.g., redox balance, angiogenesis, amino acid uptake, autophagy). Prolonged ER stress can cause ATF4 to activate proapoptotic pathways via C/EBP-homologous protein *(CHOP)*-mediated signaling.

ER kinase (PERK), inositol-requiring kinase 1 (IRE1), and activating transcription factor 6 (ATF6), that "sense" luminal ER stress and respond by activating specific transcriptional pathways while inhibiting global protein translation (**Fig. 2.5**). Such activation of the UPR has the potential to be an adaptive response that restores homeostasis or a detrimental response that triggers cell death pathways, depending on its strength, duration, and context.

Recent research indicates that the UPR is activated in the ischemic, hypertrophic, and failing heart and contributes to the cellular phenotype through effects on cell protein turnover, metabolism, function, and viability.[56] Myocardial tissue from patients with dilated or ischemic cardiomyopathy shows increased expression of many proteins involved in the UPR, such as the three stress sensors and ER chaperones.[58,59] A similar activation of the UPR is found in animal models of heart failure (e.g., mice subjected to chronic pressure overload or in models of salt-sensitive hypertension and failure).[56,60] The transgenic expression of a mutant KDEL receptor, whose normal function is to retrieve ER chaperones and misfolded proteins with KDEL (Lys-Asp-Glu-Leu) sequences from intracellular compartments, such as the Golgi to the ER, as part of a quality control mechanism, results in dilated cardiomyopathy in a mouse model—indicating the importance of the ER chaperone function.[61] More direct evidence of the role of the UPR in heart failure comes from mouse studies in which heart-specific expression of a dominant negative mutant of ATF6 resulted in adverse cardiac remodeling and heart failure, whereas mice expressing a constitutively active ATF6 had reduced post-MI cardiac remodeling.[62] The activation of an ATF6-dependent gene program by thrombospondin 4 was found to be protective during myocardial injury.[63] ATF6 also seems to protect against acute cardiac stress, such as ischemia-reperfusion injury.[64] These studies suggest that activation of the ATF6 limb of the UPR may be an adaptive response during heart failure. As mentioned earlier, NOX4-mediated activation of ATF4 may also be beneficial.[54] However, there may also be settings where UPR activation is detrimental.

The previous data suggest that modulating the UPR, or specific limbs of the UPR, could be a beneficial therapeutic approach to tackle cellular dysfunction in heart failure. For example, approaches could be designed to augment ATF6 activation. An alternative approach could be to use artificial chemical chaperones such as 4-phenylbutyric acid (4-PBA) and tauroursodeoxycholic acid (TUDCA). These have been shown to reduce ER stress and have beneficial effects in models of insulin resistance,[65] and preliminary studies also suggest beneficial effects in mouse models of chronic pressure overload.[66,67]

Autophagy (see also Chapter 1)

Autophagy (self-eating) is an important homeostatic mechanism for the degradation and recycling of various cellular components, including organelles (e.g., mitochondria, ER), macromolecules (e.g., protein aggregates), and lipids.[68] It serves an important quality control function, as well as being a mechanism that generates new building blocks for cellular processes such as energy production and protein, nucleotide, and membrane synthesis (e.g., during starvation).[69] Different forms of autophagy are described, among which macroautophagy (here referred to simply as *autophagy*) is the most prevalent and best studied. The process of autophagy is highly regulated and described in detail elsewhere.[68-70] It is characterized by the formation of double-membraned autophagosomes around damaged organelles or protein aggregates, which then fuse with lysosomes to form autophagolysosomes within which the contents are degraded by lysosomal hydrolases.[70] A family of proteins encoded by *autophagy*-related (Atg) genes is involved in the different steps of the autophagic process.[70] The mammalian target of rapamycin complex 1 (mTORC1) is a key activator of autophagy in response to "nutrient stress" (e.g., hypoxia or nutrient deprivation).

Increased levels of autophagy are found in human failing hearts,[71,72] and studies in gene-modified mouse models have provided mechanistic insights regarding the physiologic and pathologic roles of autophagy in the heart. Mice lacking lysosome-associated membrane protein 2 (LAMP2), which is required for autophagic degradation, develop cardiomyopathy.[73] Similarly, mice with cardiac-specific deficiency of Atg5 develop cardiac dysfunction accompanied by increased levels of ubiquitinated proteins, ER stress, and apoptosis[74] and die prematurely after approximately 6 months of age.[75] Furthermore, these animals have an impaired response to imposition of pressure overload, suggesting that autophagy is an adaptive protective mechanism. However, there may some settings in which autophagy could be detrimental.[76]

Ubiquitin-Proteasome System

The UPS is the major cellular system for the degradation of proteins, both as a physiologic pathway (e.g., in various cell signaling responses) and in settings where there is an increase in misfolded or damaged proteins (e.g., ER stress or oxidative stress). As with autophagy, UPS-dependent protein degradation is a highly regulated process. Proteins are targeted for ATP-dependent degradation in the 26S proteasome after they have been polyubiquitinated on lysine residues via specific ubiquitin-activating, ubiquitin-conjugating, and ubiquitin ligase enzymes.

Ubiquitinated proteins are found to accumulate in human failing myocardium,[71,77] and proteasomal catalytic activities were markedly reduced compared with nonfailing hearts.[78] However, the functional impact is not clear from these studies. Studies in animal models of heart failure report conflicting findings, with some showing a decrease and others an increase in UPS activity.[77] Of clinical interest, small studies in patients with left ventricular assist devices (LVADs) have reported that proteasomal activity increases in association with the reverse remodeling induced by mechanical unloading, suggesting that the UPS may have a beneficial role perhaps by clearing damaged proteins.[79] Supportive evidence that the removal of damaged proteins is important in the failing heart comes from models of desmin-related cardiomyopathy and of mutations in the chaperone αB-crystallin (CryAB),[80] where the accumulation of protein aggregates appears to be proteotoxic to the heart. Human desmin-related cardiomyopathy can be recapitulated in mice expressing a cardiac-specific CryAB[R120G] mutant; these animals show evidence of protein aggregation, UPS impairment, and dilated cardiomyopathy.[81]

Coordinated Functions of the Unfolded Protein Response, Ubiquitin-Proteasome System, and Autophagy Systems

The UPR, UPS, and autophagy systems (and other protein degradation systems, such as the calpain pathway, that are not covered here) act in a coordinated manner to regulate protein turnover. The three systems are activated by similar stimuli associated with cardiac stress and heart failure (e.g., oxidative stress, hypoxia, metabolic changes, and Ca^{2+} dysregulation). Alterations in the function of one system often impact on the other systems. For example, ER stress may activate the UPS and autophagy, whereas UPS activation may increase when autophagy is impaired. In addition, these systems have a broader impact on other processes, such as energy metabolism and redox, and ionic homeostasis, and may therefore affect many different aspects of the cellular phenotype in the failing heart. As discussed earlier, appropriate function of these pathways seems to be required for adaptation to chronic cardiac stress and the maintenance of normal cardiac function. On the other hand, an insufficient activation or an excessive activation of these pathways may contribute to maladaptive remodeling and the development of heart failure (**Fig. 2.6**).

CARDIOMYOCYTE INTERACTIONS WITH OTHER CELL TYPES

The number of nonmyocytes (e.g., fibroblasts, endothelial cells) in the heart outnumbers the contractile cell population, and interactions between cardiomyocytes and nonmyocytes are important not only physiologically but also in the setting of heart failure. We focus here on intercellular paracrine signaling involving cardiomyocytes during the development of cardiac remodeling and failure.

Paracrine Effects of Endothelial Cells

Coronary microvascular and endocardial endothelial cells are known to exert paracrine effects on cardiomyocytes through the secretion of factors such as NO, endothelin, and neuregulin, affecting both contractile function and growth.[82,83] For example, NO modulates myocardial relaxation, the Frank-Starling response, β-adrenergic inotropic responsiveness, and myocardial energetics.[45] Endothelial NO-dependent effects on myocardial function may become impaired during chronic pressure overload and failure (e.g., due to increased endothelial ROS production) and thereby affect contractile function, substrate metabolism, and hypertrophy.[84,85] Endothelial production of endothelin-1 (ET-1) acts as a stimulus for cardiomyocyte hypertrophy during pressure overload.

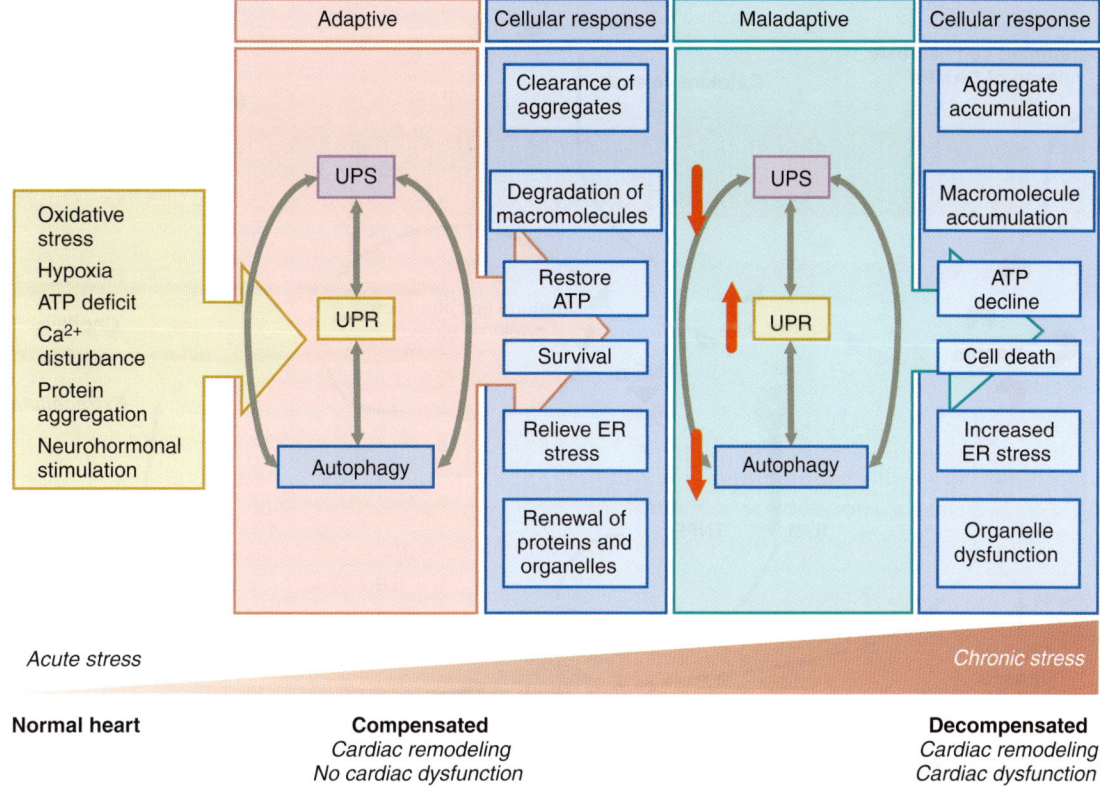

Fig. 2.6 Coordinated activation of the unfolded protein response *(UPR)*, ubiquitin-proteasome system *(UPS)*, and autophagy systems in response to cardiac stress. Diverse stimuli that result in cardiac stress activate the UPR, autophagy, and UPS systems. Initially these systems serve to reestablish cellular homeostasis and maintain adaptive remodeling and function. Prolonged or more severe stress may override the coordinated and balanced action of these systems and culminate in a maladaptive remodeling process and cardiac dysfunction.

Paracrine Effects of Fibroblasts

Cardiac fibroblasts are key players not only in fibrosis but also in the regulation of cardiomyocyte hypertrophy. Their phenotype changes in response to stress, and they transform into myofibroblasts that secrete cardioactive paracrine factors.[86] Experimental evidence suggests that a significant component of angiotensin II–mediated cardiac hypertrophic effects may be mediated by fibroblast factors, such as ET-1 and transforming grown factor-β (TGF-β).[87] Other important growth factors in the paracrine and autocrine interplay between cardiomyocytes and myofibroblasts include fibroblast growth factor-2 (FGF-2), platelet-derived growth factor (PDGF)–A/B, insulin-like growth factor 1 (IGF-1), and interleukin 6 (IL-6) family of interleukins, which include leukemia inhibitory factor (LIF) and cardiotrophin-1 (CT-1). Some of these are cardioprotective, but many act to stimulate fibrosis in the primary "healing" response to injury.

Cardiomyocyte Angiogenic Signaling

There is an important relationship between cardiomyocyte hypertrophy and myocardial capillary density and angiogenesis, especially during chronic pressure overload. Recent experimental work indicates that a matching between capillary density and hypertrophy helps to preserve cardiac contractile function and reduce adverse remodeling. Hypertrophic stimuli induce cardiomyocyte expression of the angiogenic growth factors such as VEGF, angiopoietin-2, and platelet-derived growth factor (PDGF), which promote angiogenesis and act to maintain myocardial blood flow.[88] Cardiomyocyte VEGF production is regulated both by hypoxic and nonhypoxic signaling pathways

through the transcription factors HIF1 and GATA4, respectively.[89,90] It has been found that an inhibition of cardiomyocyte HIF1 activation during chronic pressure overload promotes decompensation and the development of heart failure, whereas exogenous VEGF is protective.[90] Recently, a NOX4-dependent enhancement of cardiomyocyte HIF1 activation and subsequent VEGF release was identified as an important endogenous cardioprotective mechanism during chronic pressure overload.[53]

Activation of Inflammatory Pathways (see also Chapter 7)

The activation of the innate immune system is an important player in the progression toward heart failure. It has been recognized for many years that proinflammatory and antiinflammatory cytokines produced within the heart itself under conditions of hemodynamic stress are involved in the inflammatory cell influx into the myocardium and that this contributes to cardiomyocyte contractile dysfunction and damage, as well as extracellular matrix remodeling. The proinflammatory cytokine tumor necrosis factor (TNF) has been extensively studied in heart failure progression. Mouse models of cardiac-specific TNF overexpression develop accelerated ventricular hypertrophy, fibrosis, dilation, and failure during chronic pressure overload.[91] Both TNF and IL-1 activate detrimental NF-κB-dependent remodeling in the heart.[92] Despite the delineation of these pathways, therapies targeted at cytokines such as TNF-α have not led to effective therapies so far.

Recent studies indicate that an important mechanism for the development of "sterile" (i.e., noninfective) inflammation during

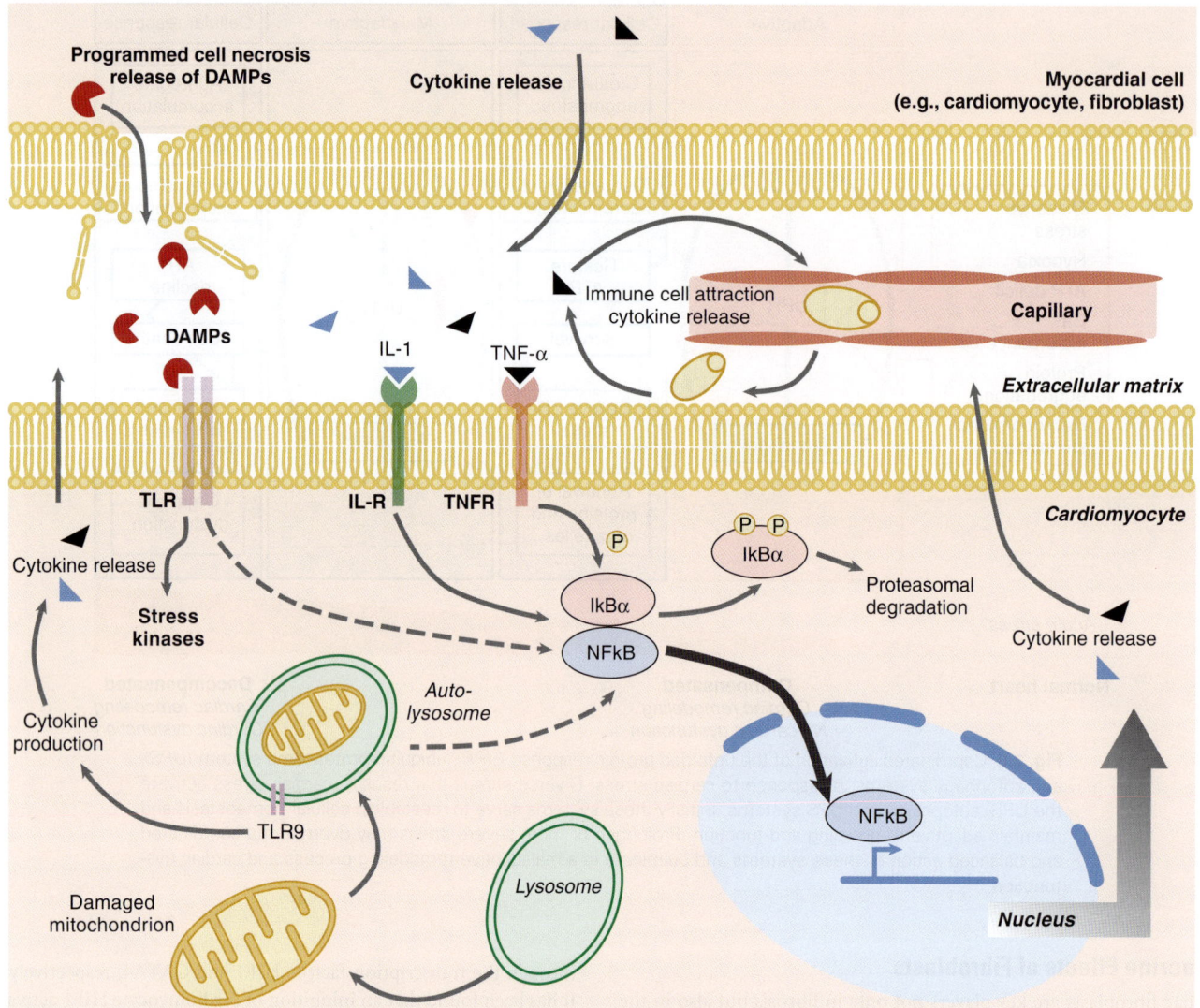

Fig. 2.7 Overview of the Innate Immune Response in the Myocardium During Chronic Cardiac Stress and Heart Failure. In response to chronic stress, proinflammatory cytokines including interleukin-1β (IL-1β) and tumor necrosis factor α (TNF-α) can be released from myocytes, fibroblasts, or immune cells. They can signal to myocytes, resulting in activation of signaling pathways leading to cardiac remodeling. Activation of the nuclear factor κB (NF-κB) pathway promotes further cytokine production, cell death pathway activation, and prohypertrophic and fibrotic pathways. Cytokines can trigger cells to undergo programmed necrosis, resulting in the release of damage-associated molecular patterns *(DAMPs)* that signal via toll-like receptors *(TLRs)* on the surface of cardiomyocytes to potentiate cytokine production and other stress kinase signaling. Impaired autophagy of damaged mitochondria during cardiac stress can also activate endolysosomal TLR9 through binding to released mitochondrial DNA, thereby triggering proinflammatory cytokine production, macrophage, and immune cell recruitment and further inflammation.

heart failure may be damage-associated molecular patterns (DAMPs) released from damaged myocardial cells (**Fig. 2.7**). DAMPs consist of released intracellular proteins, such as heat shock proteins, oxidized LDLs, and free fatty acids, or extracellular matrix components such as fibronectin.[93] They are recognized by immune cells through cell surface receptors that include Toll-like receptors (TLRs) and nucleotide-oligomerization domain (NOD)-like receptors, resulting in the triggering of inflammatory responses. TLRs may also be activated on cardiomyocytes themselves to induce production of cytokines, which then amplify the inflammatory response. Indeed, TLR4 is reported to be upregulated in the failing human heart. Recently, a novel mechanism was reported that links mitochondrial dysfunction, autophagy,

and sterile inflammation in the chronic pressure-overloaded heart.[94] Oka and associates discovered that during mitophagy (autophagy of dysfunctional mitochondria) in pressure-overloaded hearts, fragments of mitochondrial DNA are released that stimulate the activation of cardiomyocyte TLR9 receptors and evoke inflammation. The genetic inactivation of cardiomyocyte DNAse-II, which degrades mitochondrial DNA, resulted in a marked accumulation of mitochondrial DNA in autolysosomes and a profound myocarditis and dilated cardiomyopathy. Importantly, treatment with a TLR9 antagonist could reduce myocardial inflammation both in DNAse-II knockout mice and wild-type mice, suggesting this may be a suitable therapeutic target in heart failure.

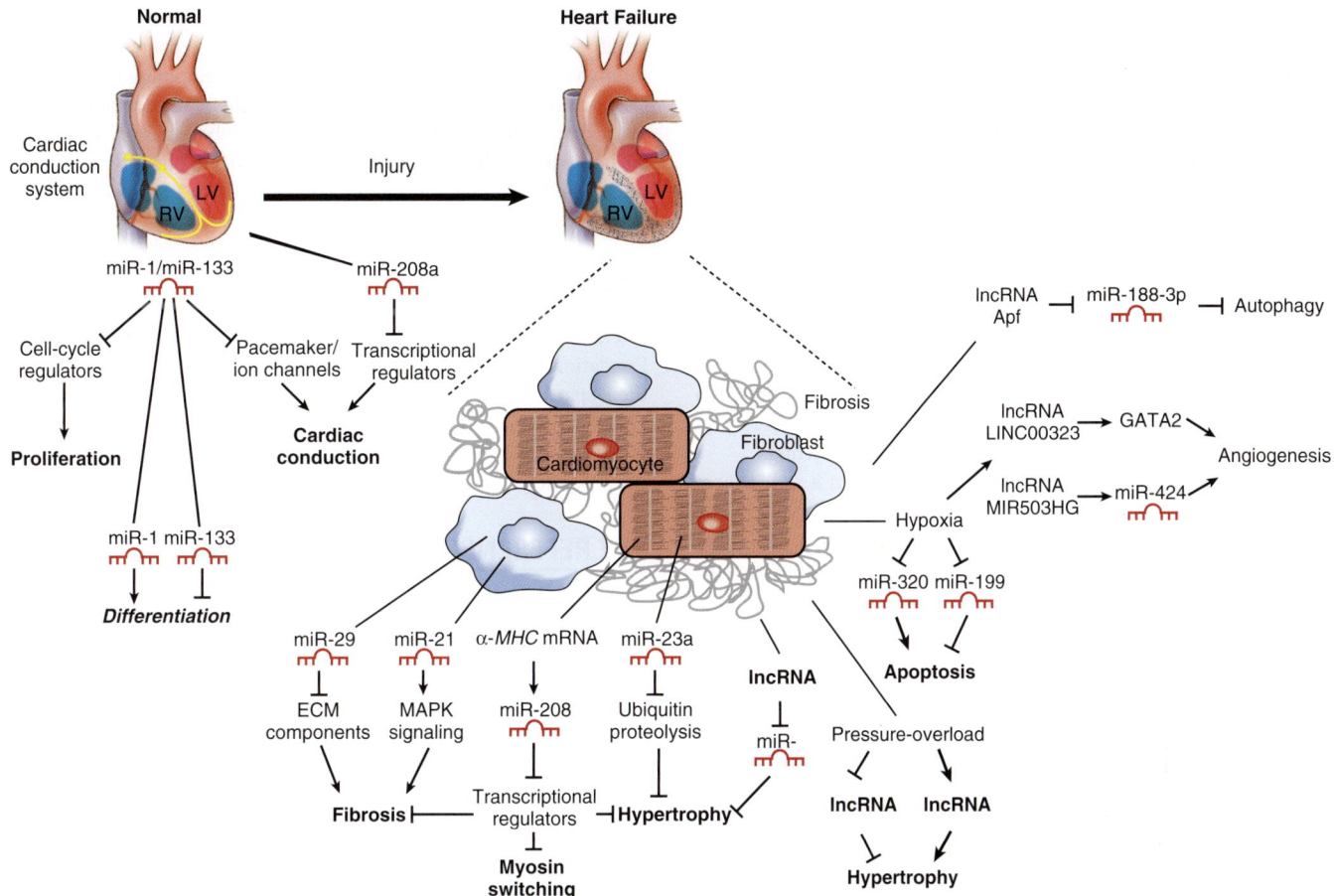

Fig. 2.8 Functional Role of microRNAs (miRNAs) and Long Noncoding RNAs (lncRNAs) in the Normal and Failing Heart. A normal and a hypertrophic/failing heart are shown in schematic form, depicting miR-NAs and lncRNAs that contribute to normal function or pathologic remodeling. All arrows denote the normal action of each component or process. miR-1 and miR-133 are involved in the development of a normal heart *(left)* by regulating proliferation, differentiation, and cardiac conduction. After cardiac injury *(right)*, various miRNAs and lncRNAs contribute to pathologic remodeling and the progression to heart failure. miR-29 blocks fibrosis by inhibiting the expression of ECM components, whereas miR-21 promotes it. miR-208 controls myosin isoform switching, cardiac hypertrophy, and fibrosis. miR-23a promotes cardiac hypertrophy by inhibiting ubiquitin proteolysis, which itself inhibits hypertrophy. Hypoxia results in the repression of miR-320 and miR-199, which promote and block apoptosis, respectively. lncRNA Chrf (cardiac hypertrophy related factor) inhibits miR-489 which itself is antihypertrophic. During pressure-overload stress, lncRNA Mhrt is reduced and disinhibits the hypertrophic response, whereas the lncRNA Chast is upregulated and promotes hypertrophy. Hypoxia stimulates endothelial cells to produce two lncRNAs, LINC00323 and MIR503HG, which both regulate angiogenesis. In pathologic stress, lncRNA Apf drives autophagy by inhibiting mir-188-3p. *ECM,* extracellular matrix; *LV,* left ventricle; *MAPK,* mitogen-activated protein kinase; *MHC,* myosin heavy chain. Modified from Small EM, Olson EN. Pervasive roles of microRNAs in cardiovascular biology. *Nature.* 2011;469:336–342; lncRNA functional roles adapted from Bär C, Chatterjee S, Thum T. Long noncoding RNAs in cardiovascular pathology, diagnosis, and therapy. *Circulation.* 2016;134:1484–1499.

MICRORNA AND LONG NONCODING RNA-DEPENDENT PATHWAYS

miRNAs are highly conserved endogenous nucleotide segments of noncoding RNA (typically around 22 nucleotides long) that regulate the stability and translation of mRNA transcripts. miRNAs function by base pairing with 3′ untranslated regions within a transcript, resulting in gene silencing via translational repression and/or target mRNA degradation. Individual miRNAs can act as "master regulators" of cellular signaling processes through their ability to regulate multiple genes within signaling pathways. As such, they may have a major impact on cellular phenotypes. Recent work in animal models, supported by studies in human tissue, indicates that alterations in miRNA expression

have a significant influence on the cardiomyocyte phenotype in the failing heart (**Fig. 2.8**).[95] Moreover, these effects extend to an impact on nonmyocyte cells and on cell-cell interactions within the heart.

Numerous miRNAs can influence the cardiomyocyte hypertrophic response to stress, including antihypertrophic (e.g., miR-1, miR-9, miR-26, miR-29, miR-98, miR-133) and pro-hypertrophic (e.g., miR-21, miR-23a, miR-143, miR-199a, miR-199b, miR-208, miR-499) effects. Some of these act primarily within nonmyocytes in the remodeling and failing heart (e.g., miR-21 and miR-29 within fibroblasts). Changes in miRNA profiles play an important part in the reexpression of fetal gene profiles in the stressed and failing heart. Interestingly, miRNA transcription may be regulated by certain stress-activated transcription factors (e.g., NFAT, STAT3, SRF), suggesting that global regulatory circuits coordinate the molecular remodeling that underpins the development of the cellular phenotype in the failing heart.[95] The specific molecular targets of miRNAs that are altered in heart failure include proteins involved in cardiomyocyte growth, sarcomere function, excitation-contraction coupling, cell-cycle regulation, protein turnover, redox homeostasis, paracrine regulation, fibrosis, inflammation, angiogenesis, and other processes, illustrating the potentially profound effects of these master regulators.

Increases in miRNA expression can in principle be therapeutically targeted (e.g., with antagomirs), and studies in animal models suggest that such approaches offer significant potential.[95] The concept of targeting multiple pathologic components with a single antagomir is intuitively attractive, but there are significant challenges to overcome, in particular the need to specifically target the heart. In principle, miRNAs could also be delivered as a therapeutic, but again there are challenges with respect to pharmacokinetics, pharmacodynamics, and specific targeting.

miRNAs are also found circulating in the blood in a stable form both in the healthy setting and in diseases. Plasma miRNA profiles change specifically and significantly in different diseases, including heart failure.[96] The pathophysiologic relevance of this finding remains to be fully established (e.g., do circulating miRNAs facilitate signaling between different cells or tissues or do they simply represent a "spillover"?). Regardless of the answer, there is great interest in the potential for changes in plasma miRNA profiles to serve as biomarkers for disease diagnosis, prognosis, and/or monitoring.

In a similar vein, another class of highly abundant noncoding RNAs called long noncoding RNAs (lncRNAs) are emerging as potential regulators of remodeling in the failing heart.[97] These are typically greater than 200 nucleotides in length and can subserve diverse regulatory roles in gene expression and translation (e.g., epigenetic modulation, acting as molecular sponges, and modulating alternative splicing of genes signal). lncRNAs have been shown to have important functions in cardiac development, but investigation of their roles in the cardiac responses to stress and in heart failure is still in its infancy. Nevertheless, early studies suggest that individual lncRNAs may have important roles in epigenetic regulation during cardiac hypertrophy,[98] and human genome–wide association studies also support a key role.[99]

CONCLUSIONS AND FUTURE DIRECTIONS

Profound alterations in gene and protein expression, molecular regulation, and signaling occur in the cardiomyocytes in a heart under chronic stress and largely underpin the complex changes in cellular phenotype that gradually develop. These changes in cardiomyocyte phenotype, along with associated changes in other cardiac cell types and in the extracellular matrix, play a major role in overall cardiac remodeling and the subsequent development of the multiorgan heart failure syndrome. In this chapter, we have discussed alterations in cardiomyocyte function that contribute to the development of pathologic cardiac remodeling and failure. These include specific abnormalities in cardiac contractile function, as well as global alterations in cellular homeostasis that also impact on the myocyte phenotype. A better understanding of these complex changes offers the potential to identify new therapeutic targets for use in heart failure.

ACKNOWLEDGMENTS

The authors' work is supported by the British Heart Foundation; a Fondation Leducq Transatlantic Network of Excellence award; and the Department of Health via a National Institute for Health Research (NIHR) Biomedical Research Centre award to Guy's & St Thomas' NHS Foundation Trust in partnership with King's College London and King's College Hospital NHS Foundation Trust.

KEY REFERENCES

2. Lehnart SE, Maier LS, Hasenfuss G. Abnormalities of calcium metabolism and myocardial contractility depression in the failing heart. *Heart Fail Rev.* 2009;14:213–224.
12. Greenberg B, Butler J, Felker GM, et al. Calcium upregulation by percutaneous administration of gene therapy in patients with cardiac disease (CUPID 2): a randomised, multinational, double-blind, placebo-controlled, phase 2b trial. *Lancet.* 2016;387:1178–1186.
21. Burgoyne JR, Mongue-Din H, Eaton P, et al. Redox signaling in cardiac physiology and pathology. *Circ Res.* 2012;111:1091–1106.
42. Carnicer R, Crabtree MJ, Sivakumaran V, et al. Nitric oxide synthases in heart failure. *Antioxid Redox Signal.* 2013;18:1078–1099.
56. Doroudgar S, Glembotski CC. New concepts of endoplasmic reticulum function in the heart: programmed to conserve. *J Mol Cell Cardiol.* 2013;55:85–91.
74. Nakai A, Yamaguchi O, Takeda T, et al. The role of autophagy in cardiomyocytes in the basal state and in response to hemodynamic stress. *Nat Med.* 2007;13:619–624.
78. Predmore JM, Wang P, Davis F, et al. Ubiquitin proteasome dysfunction in human hypertrophic and dilated cardiomyopathies. *Circulation.* 2010;121:997–1004.
91. Mann DL. Stress-activated cytokines and the heart: from adaptation to maladaptation. *Annu Rev Physiol.* 2003;65:81–101.
95. Quiat D, Olson EN. MicroRNAs in cardiovascular disease: from pathogenesis to prevention and treatment. *J Clin Invest.* 2013;123:11–18.
97. Bär C, Chatterjee S, Thum T. Long noncoding RNAs in cardiovascular pathology, diagnosis, and therapy. *Circulation.* 2016;134:1484–1499.

The full reference list is available on ExpertConsult.

Cellular Basis for Myocardial Regeneration and Repair

Shah R. Ali, Nicholas T. Lam, Hesham A. Sadek

Cardiac regeneration refers to the process of heart repair after an injury through repopulation of specific cell types to replace the damaged tissue, to regain functional capacity. Although credible evidence existed for this phenomenon in lower vertebrates, the belief in the potential for cardiac regeneration in mammals is a recent development. It was previously believed that the heart is a "postmitotic" organ whose workhorse cell, the cardiomyocyte, is incapable of cell division. In the past two decades, the heart's reputation dramatically changed from a postmitotic organ to a highly proliferative one and, more recently, to an organ with only modest turnover capacity. These opposing views of cellular turnover in the mammalian heart generated a number of exciting and precise studies that provide significant and novel insights into heart regeneration. Indeed, we now have stringent evidence that the adult mammal heart is capable of a low rate of turnover throughout life, with a notable window for complete regenerative potential restricted to the early neonatal period. In this chapter, we will describe the physiologic and pathologic cardiomyogenesis that occurs in mammals, and we will discuss different classes of investigative therapies with the potential to stimulate cardiac regeneration in the adult heart.

THE POSTNATAL HEART IS NOT A POSTMITOTIC ORGAN

The foundations for the notion that the heart is a static organ incapable of regeneration were established in the mid-1920s. A significant publication in 1925 claimed that mitotic figures are not detectable in human cardiomyocytes,[1] which thereby were considered cells irreversibly withdrawn from the cell cycle: this study effectively introduced the concept that the heart is a terminally differentiated, postmitotic organ.

The notion that the pool of myocytes present at birth is irreplaceable during the life span of the organism gained further support from a series of autoradiographic studies conducted in the 1960s that delivered tritiated thymidine to the myocardium during postnatal development and pathologic overload to quantify DNA replication. The degree of DNA synthesis in myocyte nuclei was negligible, and therefore the increase in heart size that occurs with age was correlated to cardiomyocyte cell size growth from increased cell volume (i.e., hypertrophy rather than hyperplasia was thought to be the predominant mechanism for the postnatal gain in heart weight).[1a]

In the late 1990s and early 2000s, a highly publicized series of publications from the Piero Anversa group directly challenged the dogma of the heart as a postmitotic organ.[2-7] They evaluated hearts from patients who died a few days after a myocardial infarction (MI) (as well as control hearts), and they observed expression of Ki-67, a cell cycle–associated nuclear antigen, in the border zone of the infarct and the remote zones.[3] They found putative evidence of mitotic spindles, formation of contractile rings, karyokinesis, and cytokinesis in tissue sections by immunofluorescence in injured hearts. From these observations, they concluded that there is significant cardiomyogenic potential in the human heart and that "regeneration of myocytes may be a critical component of the increase in muscle mass of the myocardium." This report spurred intense investigation into further characterization of postnatal cardiac growth and raised important questions about the parent cell of origin of new cardiomyocytes. However, another study raised doubts regarding the use of Ki-67 to prove cell division, because it showed that Ki-67 expression after human MI may be due to polyploidization rather than bona fide mitosis.[8]

In subsequent reports the Anversa group provocatively claimed that on average 22% new myocytes were generated every year in humans, suggestive of a life span of 4.5 years for this cell type.[9,10] Independent efforts to replicate these results using different techniques could not corroborate this degree of cardiomyocyte turnover. In the past few years, clonal analysis[11,12] and radioisotope labeling methods[13-15] have provided the most reliable data for cardiac growth and its dynamics after birth in mammals. It is now believed that the mammalian heart experiences a very low—albeit not zero—rate of turnover mediated by preexisting cardiomyocytes, with a possible small increase in cardiomyogenesis after MI which has tangential clinical impact.

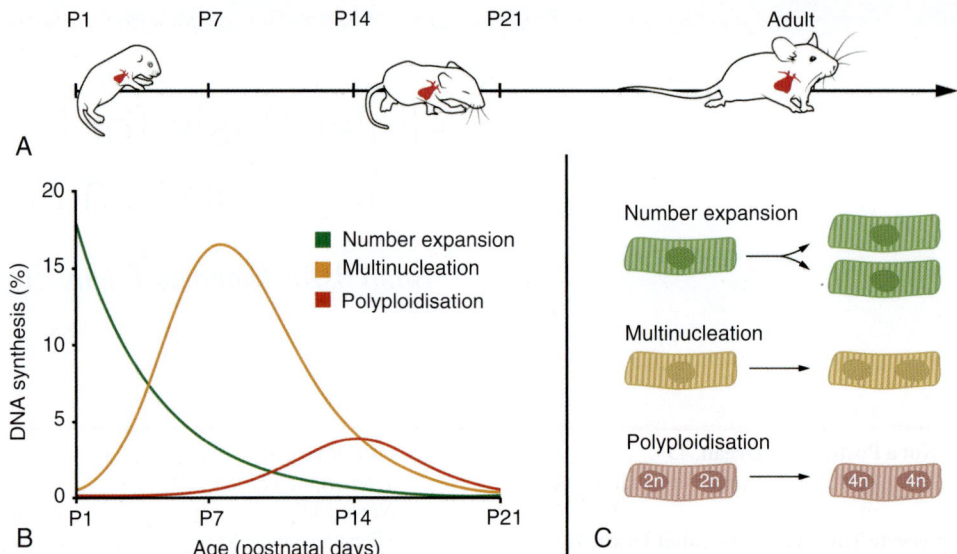

Fig. 3.1 Cardiomyocyte DNA Synthesis in Growing Mouse Hearts. (A–C) The time course and quantification of postnatal cardiomyocyte DNA synthesis. (B and C) Cardiomyocyte proliferation, multinucleation, and polyploidization were observed in the postnatal murine heart. The magnitude and time course of the cardiomyocyte number expansion, multinucleation, and polyploidization were related. The graphs depict the DNA content changes per unit time based on stereological estimates and flow cytometric measurements of the cardiomyocyte number expansion, multinucleation, and polyploidization. The changes in DNA synthesis were related to the time around birth (P2). *2n,* Diploid nuclei; *4n,* tetraploid nuclei. From Alkass K, Panula J, Westman M, Wu TD, Guerquin-Kern JL, Bergmann O. No evidence for cardiomyocyte number expansion in preadolescent mice. *Cell.* 2015;163:1026–1036.

Sources of Controversy in Postnatal Mammalian Cardiomyocyte Proliferation

To understand the basis for conflicting results and the wide range of myocyte proliferation rates in the field, it is important to understand the cardiomyocyte cell cycle. The fundamental basis for controversy in the field is the uncoupling of DNA synthesis, nuclear division (karyokinesis), and abscission (cytokinesis)—leading to multinucleated and polyploid cells—that occurs in mammalian cardiomyocytes, which confounds interpretation of traditional cell turnover assays based on DNA replication.

Nearly 20 years ago, the administration of thymidine analogues to mice revealed two temporally distinct phases of DNA synthesis that characterize the prenatal and early postnatal growth of the myocyte compartment.[16] The first peak in DNA synthesis was observed in the fetal heart and attributed to cardiomyocyte proliferation. Conversely, the second phase of DNA synthesis, which was detected 4 days after birth, primarily occurs due to binucleation without cytokinesis. These fundamental findings have been reproduced numerous times using other methodologies to identify replicating nuclei in cardiomyocytes in rodents (Fig. 3.1). These findings also illuminate the challenge of measuring cardiomyocyte turnover: not all DNA synthesis results in cytokinesis. In fact, there is a progressive decline in the rate of cardiomyocyte cell proliferation concomitantly with a rise in DNA synthesis. In mice, around postnatal day 7 (P7) there is a peak in cardiomyocyte binucleation and around P14 there is a peak in polyploidy (DNA replication without nuclear division), leading to 4n, 8n, 16n, etc. chromosome copy numbers. These consistent results cast a penumbra of uncertainty over any method that relies exclusively on DNA or nuclear division as a proxy for cell division in cardiomyocytes. In addition, markers of S phase of the cell cycle may be incorporated during DNA repair, leading to a false-positive interpretation. Ultimately, there is no marker of mitosis that *prima facie* confirms that cytokinesis has occurred/will occur: even cytokinesis-associated proteins may moonlight in other phases of the cell cycle, thus limiting their utility to specifically denote abscission.[8,17,18]

Another factor that complicates interpretation of proliferation assays in cardiomyocytes is the difficulty to distinguish cardiomyocyte/cardiomyocyte nuclei from nonmyocyte cell types in tissue sections histologically. Sophisticated methodologies like lineage tracing and fate-mapping mouse models have provided significant insights into postnatal cardiomyocyte turnover, but they carry their own shortcomings such as questions about promoter fidelity, inefficient reporter gene expression, and cellular fusion or transfer of reporter proteins.[19]

Collectively, these considerable caveats impede use of routine assays to confirm or quantify cardiomyocyte mitosis. As such, it became imperative for the field of cardiovascular biology to turn to more rigorous techniques to prove occurrence of new cardiomyocyte generation, such as the use of multiple mitotic markers and analysis of cell size and cell number quantification within the same study. In addition, the field has increasingly relied on clonal analysis because it enables precise determination of parent-progeny relationships and relies on completion of cytokinesis. However, this highly rigorous approach also carries many of the fate-mapping caveats outlined earlier. Finally, radioisotope labeling–based methods combined with sophisticated mathematical modeling in mice and in humans buttress the clonal analysis findings and have provided us the most meticulous calculations of the rate of cardiac growth in mammals.

Evidence of Cardiomyocyte Turnover in the Adult Heart

Frisen and coworkers used a carbon-14 (^{14}C)-based methodology to calculate the precise rate of cardiomyocyte turnover in the human heart in 2009.[13] In brief, they obtained autopsied human heart samples and isolated cardiomyocyte nuclei using specific antibodies. Then they retrospectively determined the birth date of cardiomyocytes by measuring and correlating ^{14}C levels in cardiomyocyte genomic DNA with atmospheric ^{14}C levels. The characteristic exponential decay of atmospheric ^{14}C after the 1963 Limited Nuclear Test Ban Treaty allowed them to ascribe a date mark to each cardiomyocyte. They operated on key assumptions that the ^{14}C level in a cell's DNA remains stable after its last cell division and reflects the concentration of ^{14}C in the atmosphere at the time of last cell division. Thus the rise and decay of ^{14}C in the Earth's atmosphere due to historical nuclear weapons testing facilitated precise calculations of cardiomyocyte turnover kinetics in humans.

These ^{14}C radioisotope label measurements convincingly demonstrated that the heart indeed is not a postmitotic organ. Frisen and colleagues showed that the annual birth rate of cardiomyocytes in humans is highest in the first decade and after that decreases to less than 1% throughout life. In fact, the pattern is very similar to that observed in mice (see Fig. 3.1**B**). Due to differing interpretations of the ^{14}C data, Frisen and coworkers performed additional stereological analysis to further validate their results.[14] They obtained tissue from 29 human postmortem samples with no history or evidence of heart disease and measured the proliferation kinetics of cardiomyocytes, endothelial cells, and mesenchymal cells in the heart. Due to the use of stereology, they were also able to measure total cell numbers and cell volumes in a given tissue sample. They confirmed that the cardiomyocyte cell volume increases with age (Fig. 3.2E) but the total number of cardiomyocytes remains relatively constant (see Fig. 3.2B). After modeling for binucleation and ploidy that occurs in the first three decades of life (Fig. 3.3A; also see Fig. 3.2C), they confirmed their initial findings that the cardiomyocyte proliferation rate in humans is less than 1% after age 10, and this rate continues to decline with aging (see Fig. 3.3**C**). They further investigated proliferation rates in specific regions of the heart and found no differences in cardiomyocyte renewal kinetics among the myocardial layers (e.g., endocardium, myocardium, epicardium), zones (e.g., apex, base), or chambers, arguing against the existence of a region-specific progenitor population.[20]

Senyo and colleagues extended the aforementioned findings to mice by combining genetic fate-mapping with multi-isotope imaging mass spectrometry (MIMS), which requires administration of [^{15}N]thymidine and is analogous to the ^{14}C radiolabel technique (Fig. 3.4).[15] They calculated an annual rate of turnover of murine cardiomyocytes from preexisting cardiomyocytes at 0.76%. They also found that 8 weeks after an MI in adult mice, 3.2% of the cardiomyocytes in the infarct border zone had undergone division. However, as with the work of Frisen and coworkers, certain assumptions have to be made about the fraction of DNA synthesis that occurs due to multinucleation and polyploidy as opposed to completion of the cell cycle through abscission. For example, only mononuclear diploid cardiomyocytes were counted as true newborn daughter cells, whereas polyploid or multinucleate cardiomyocytes with nuclear ^{15}N were presumed to be the result of DNA synthesis without cytokinesis.

Although these radioisotope labeling–based analytical methods provided meticulous insights into cardiomyocyte renewal dynamics that corroborated across mammalian species, these techniques could not prove the ontogeny of postnatal cardiomyogenesis at the single cell level. Because the source of new cardiomyocytes was a key question in the field, clonal and nonclonal fate-mapping techniques were used to definitively provide an answer.

The "Mosaic Analysis of Double Markers" (MADM) model is ideally suited to the study of the heart because Cre recombination in replicating cells can result in asymmetric inheritance of fluorescent labels in the two daughter cells: one nucleus obtains the tdTomato gene and the other nucleus receives the green fluorescent protein (GFP) gene.[20a] If there is no nuclear division or no cytokinesis, then the parent cell will remain double-positive for the two fluorescent proteins. However, if the dividing parent cell undergoes mitosis with cytokinesis, the two

daughter cells will become asymmetrically fluorescent (Fig. 3.5A). Thus cytokinesis is necessary and sufficient to generate single-labeled cells, and the sibling relationship of daughter cells can be ascertained due to the asymmetric label. Moreover, because the labeling is indelible, MADM permits clonal analysis of daughter cells (i.e., assessment of the proliferative capacity of individual cells over time).

Using MADM, Ali and coworkers directly showed that existing cardiomyocytes that express the sarcomeric protein α-myosin heavy chain are the parent cells of postnatal newborn cardiomyocytes (see Fig. 3.5).[11] Cardiomyocytes that underwent division appeared to divide only once over the time course analyzed, arguing against a small pool of highly proliferative cardiomyocytes. Moreover, all sibling daughter cells were both cardiomyocytes; there were no instances of nonmyocyte and myocyte sibling cells, arguing against the existence of a bipotent or multipotent cardiac progenitor. However, a shortcoming of MADM is that, owing to inefficient Cre recombination, it underestimates the rate of cardiomyocyte proliferation and cannot directly *disprove* the existence of a progenitor parent cell. Nonetheless, other lineage tracing models estimate the contribution to cardiomyogenesis from resident stem/progenitor cells at less than 0.01% per year.[21]

These prior studies left open the question as to whether all cardiomyocytes are able to participate in postnatal cardiomyogenesis or whether a unique subset of cardiomyocytes boasts this potential. Based on their findings that exposure to normoxia after fetal life is associated with postnatal cardiomyocyte cell cycle arrest, Kimura and colleagues developed a novel hypoxia fate-mapping model to ascertain the mitotic potential of hypoxic cardiomyocytes (Fig. 3.6).[12] They showed that hypoxic cardiomyocytes, as marked by Hif-1α expression, comprise the predominant subtype of adult cardiomyocytes that undergoes postnatal division during physiologic aging; these cells also proliferate after an MI injury. The majority of newborn cardiomyocytes—as identified by nuclear BrdU incorporation—appear to arise from this cohort of hypoxic cardiomyocytes, which are smaller, predominantly mononuclear, and accumulate less oxidative DNA damage than the remaining cardiomyocytes. These findings strengthen the claim that the majority of mammalian adult cardiomyocytes are postmitotic and denote hypoxia signaling as an important player in postnatal cardiomyogenesis.

The combination of lineage tracing, radioisotope labeling, and clonal analysis has provided the most meticulous assessments of both cardiomyocytes renewal rates and ontogeny in the mammalian heart. These studies clearly demonstrate that, although the majority of mammalian adult cardiomyocytes do not participate in cell division during aging or with injury, a small subset retains mitotic potential that may be targeted for therapeutic purposes.

Molecular Basis of the Terminally Differentiated State of Cardiomyocytes

Evidence from animal models showed that only a very small fraction of cardiomyocytes undergoes turnover in the mammalian heart, whereas the remainder appears to be cell cycle arrested. The search for the molecular control underlying withdrawal of most postnatal cardiomyocytes from the cell cycle resulted in the compilation of a list of genes that are known to promote growth arrest in multiple systems. Cessation of myocyte proliferation at birth has been linked to the downregulation of cyclins, cyclin-dependent kinases (CDKs), and E2F transcription factors[22-25] and to the upregulation of the negative modulators of cell cycle progression: Cdkn1a, Cdkn1b, Cdkn1c, and Cdkn2c.[26] The presence of functional growth factor receptors on the plasma membrane of mature myocytes endows them with the capacity for physiologic and/or pathologic hypertrophy needed in response to pathologic loads in combination with reexpression of the fetal gene program.[27]

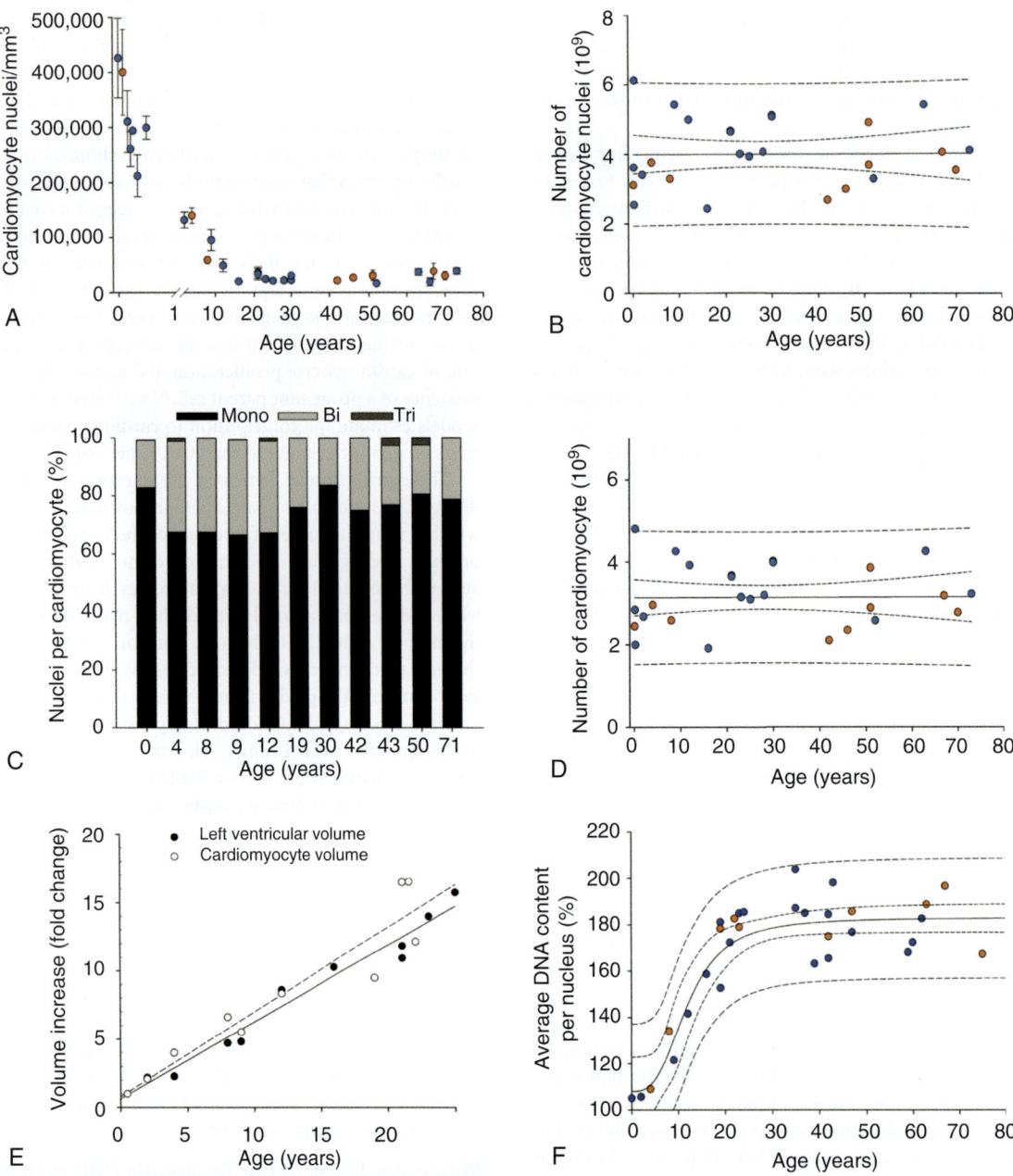

Fig. 3.2 Cardiomyocyte Number, Volume, and DNA Content in Growing and Adult Hearts. (A) The density of cardiomyocyte nuclei declines in growing hearts and remains constant during aging. (B) The number of cardiomyocyte nuclei in the left ventricle, calculated using the reference volume (see the Experimental Procedures), is stable postnatally. (C) The ratio of mononucleated to multinucleated cardiomyocytes is already established at birth. (D) Based on the number of cardiomyocyte nuclei and the level of multinucleation, the number of cardiomyocytes does not change significantly in growing hearts or with age (R = .01; P = .96). (E) Comparison between left ventricular volume increase *(black dots and black regression line)* and average increase in cardiomyocyte volume *(white dots and dashed regression line)*. Regression curves do not show any significant difference between the groups (P = .67; ANCOVA). (F) Human cardiomyocyte nuclei are mostly diploid at birth and start to ploidize mainly in the second decade of life (100% corresponds to diploid nuclei; 200% corresponds to tetraploid nuclei). *Red data points* indicate females, and *blue data points* indicate male subjects. *Dashed lines* indicate the prediction interval *(long dashes)* and the confidence interval *(short dashes)*. From Bergmann O, Zdunek S, Felker A, et al. Dynamics of cell generation and turnover in the human heart. *Cell.* 2015;161:1566–1575.

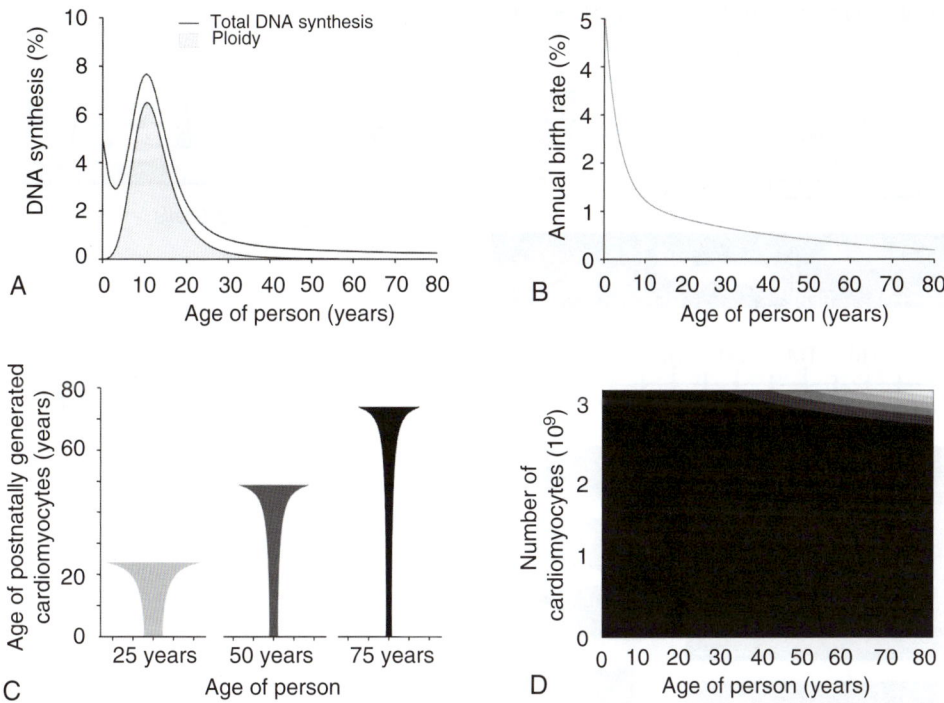

Fig. 3.3 (A) Total DNA synthesis inferred from genomic carbon-14 concentration in cardiomyocytes at different ages *(black)* with that associated with polyploidization indicated *(pattern fill)*. (B) Annual birth rates of cardiomyocytes in the left ventricle decline in an exponential fashion in the growing heart and adult heart. Cardiomyocytes renew at a rate of 0.8% at the age of 20, whereas in old subjects this rate declines to values less than 0.3%. (C) Age distribution of adult-born cardiomyocytes at 25, 50, and 75 years of age. (D) The total number of cardiomyocytes is already established at birth and remains constant with age. For a given age of the person, postnatally generated cells are shown with different shades of gray, indicating the decade in which they were generated. During a lifetime, approximately 35% of all cardiomyocytes are exchanges postnatally, with most cardiomyocytes already generated at birth and in the first years of life. Cardiomyocyte renewal is based on the cumulative survival model. From Bergmann O, Zdunek S, Felker A, et al. Dynamics of cell generation and turnover in the human heart. *Cell.* 2015;161:1566–1575.

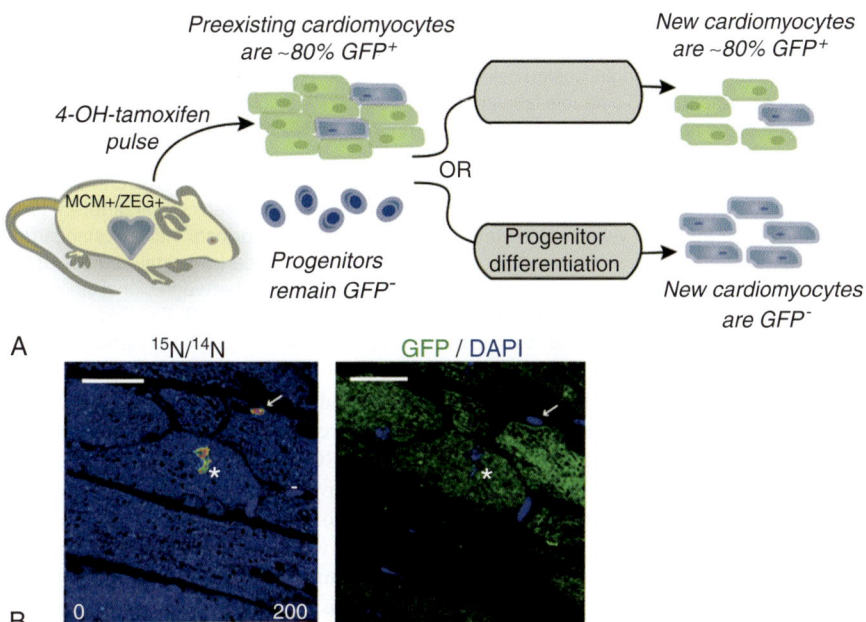

Fig. 3.4 New Cardiomyocytes are Derived From Preexisting Cardiomyocytes During Aging. (A) Experimental strategy. MerCreMer+/ZEG+ (MCM+ZEG+) mice (n = 4) were treated for 2 weeks with 4-OH-tamoxifen to induce cardiomyocyte-specific green fluorescent protein *(GFP)* expression. [15N]Thymidine was administered continuously during a 10-week chase, then cycling cells were identified by 15N labeling. New cardiomyocytes (15N+) derived from preexisting cardiomyocytes should express GFP at a rate similar to that of the surrounding quiescent (15N−) cardiomyocytes. New cardiomyocytes (15N+) derived from progenitors should be GFP−. (B) Left, 15N:14N hue–saturation–intensity image showing a [15N]thymidine-labeled cardiomyocyte nucleus *(white asterisk)* and a 15N+ noncardiomyocyte *(white arrow)*. Right, immunofluorescent image showing that the 15N+ cardiomyocyte is GFP+. Scale bars, 15 μm. From Senyo SE, Steinhauser ML, Pizzimenti CL, et al. Mammalian heart renewal by pre-existing cardiomyocytes. *Nature* 2013;493:433–436.

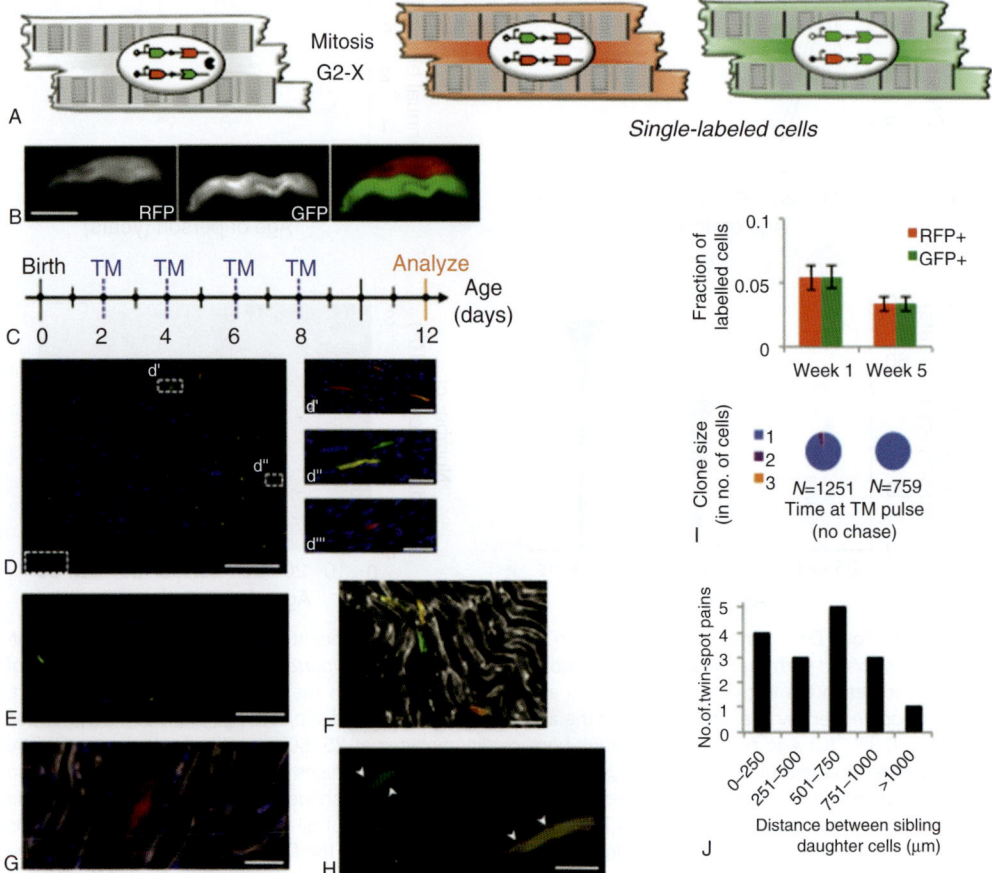

Fig. 3.5 Cardiomyocytes Divide Postnatally in Mice. (A) Mosaic analysis of double markers *(MADM)* recombination in a parent cardiomyocyte in Myh6-expressing cells leads to red fluorescent protein (RFP+) and green fluorescent protein (GFP+) single-labeled daughter cardiomyocytes *(arrowheads)*. (B) Example of an alternate-label sibling pair (scale bar, 15 μm). (C) Tamoxifen (TM) delivery strategy for D–H. (D) Section through P12 heart reveals double-labeled and sparse single-labeled cells (scale bar, 100 μm). (d′) RFP+ single-labeled cell along with its partner GFP+ single-labeled cell and double-labeled cells. (d″) GFP+ single-labeled cell (with evident sarcomeric elements) and a double-labeled cell. (d‴) An RFP+ single-labeled cell (scale bars, 10 μm). (E) MADM labeling in the atria (scale bar, 50 μm). (F) Example of GFP+ cell and double-labeled cell that stain positive for troponin *(white)* (scale bar, 10 μm). (G) α-Actinin staining *(white)* reveals sarcomeric structures of an RFP+ cardiomyocyte (scale bar, 5 μm). (H) GFP+ cardiomyocyte forms gap junctions (Connexin43, *white*) with underlying syncytium (scale bar, 5 μm). (I, Upper) Frequency of single-labeled cells at different timepoints after TM administration (n = 3; *P* values calculated with Student t test; error bars indicate standard error of the mean *[SEM]*). (Lower) Analysis of same-color clones for the above mice (n = total number of single-labeled cells observed per group). (J) Histogram of the distribution of distance between clonal sibling cells (n = 5 mice). From Ali SR, Hippenmeyer S, Saadat LV, Luo L, Weissman IL, Ardehali R. Existing cardiomyocytes generate cardiomyocytes at a low rate after birth in mice. *Proc Nat Acad Sci.* 2014;111:8850–8855.

Based on observations in skeletal myoblasts,[28] it was hypothesized that the retinoblastoma (Rb) protein permanently inhibits the transition of cardiomyocytes from the G_1 to the S phase of the cell cycle. For example, the neonatal heart harbors inactive (hyperphosphorylated) Rb, coincident with myocyte renewal, whereas adult and hypertrophied hearts are characterized by high levels of hypophosphorylated, active Rb, which opposes myocyte division.[29] Similarly, the cell cycle regulators cyclins A, D1, D2, and D3 are highly expressed in the developing heart and rapidly downregulate after birth.[22-25]

Recent evidence supports the hypothesis that activation of the DNA damage response (DDR) pathway in the postnatal period leads to cell cycle arrest in mammalian cardiomyocytes. The relative hypoxemia of fetal circulation is replaced with normoxia after birth upon exposure to environmental oxygen.[30] Concomitant with this rise in circulating oxygen tension is a transition in the neonatal mouse heart from glycolysis to aerobic metabolism, which is a metabolic switch that leads to reliance on

mitochondria for energy generation and therefore leads to high levels of reactive oxygen species (ROS). Puente and colleagues showed that high levels of ROS in the postnatal heart generates oxidative DNA damage, which activates the DDR pathway.[30] They showed that exposure to postnatal hypoxemia, inhibition of DDR, and ROS attenuation extend the postnatal window of cardiomyocyte proliferation. On the other hand, hyperoxemia and ROS generators shorten the window. In further support of this hypothesis, Nakada and colleagues were able to partially ameliorate the postmitotic phenotype of adult cardiomyocytes by exposing mice to environmental hypoxia.[31] They showed that there is increased proliferation of cardiomyocytes at 7% atmospheric oxygen level due to a decrease in ROS and oxidative DNA, compared with normoxic control mice that experience 21% environmental oxygen (Fig. 3.7).[31]

The polyploidization of mammalian cardiomyocytes has also been associated with the loss of proliferative potential, although polyploid liver cells are capable of division and contribute to hepatocyte

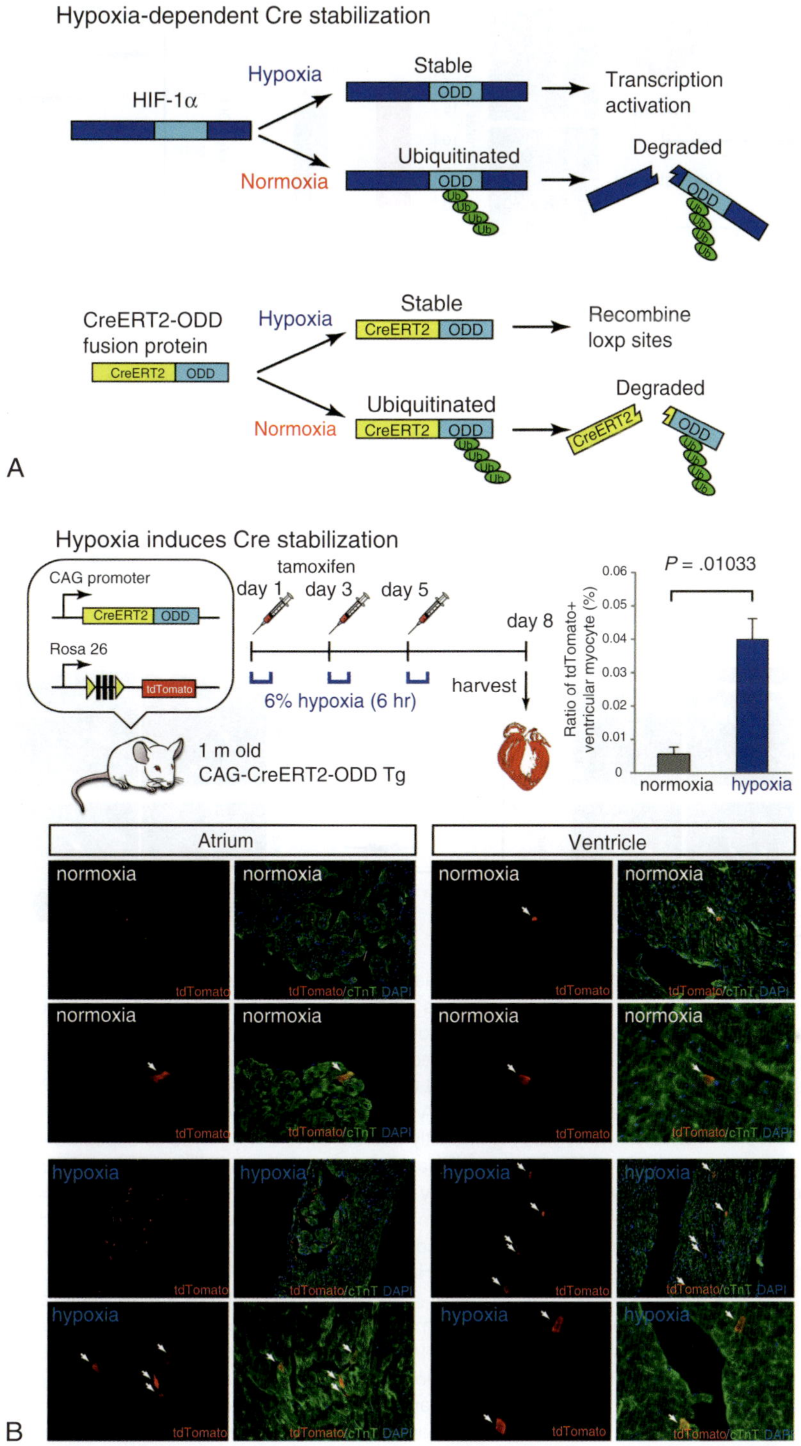

Fig. 3.6 Generation of Hif-1α–Dependent Fate-Mapping Model. (A) Schematic diagram of a strategy to activate Cre protein in a Hif-1α stability–dependent manner. Under normoxic conditions, the oxygen-dependent degradation (ODD) domain of Hif-1α is hydroxylated and ubiquitylated leading to E3 ubiquitin proteasome–dependent protein degradation, whereas under hypoxic conditions, the ODD domain is not hydroxylated and avoids protein degradation. To activate Cre in hypoxic conditions, we generated transgenic mice in which the CAG-promoter-driven CreERT2–ODD fusion protein is expressed so that the CreERT2 protein is only stabilized in Hif-1α–expressing hypoxic cells. (B) Validation of the hypoxia-dependent model was performed by exposing mice to intermittent hypoxia (6% O$_2$ for 6 h every other day) at the same time as tamoxifen pulse, before hearts were harvested 3 days later. Images and graph show a significant increase in the number of both atrial and ventricular cardiomyocytes with tdTomato fluorescence after hypoxia exposure in CAG-creERT2-ODD;R26R/tdTomato transgenic hearts. A two-tailed unpaired t-test was used for statistical analysis. From Kimura W, Xiao F, Canseco DC, et al. Hypoxia fate mapping identifies cycling cardiomyocytes in the adult heart. *Nature.* 2015;523:226–230.

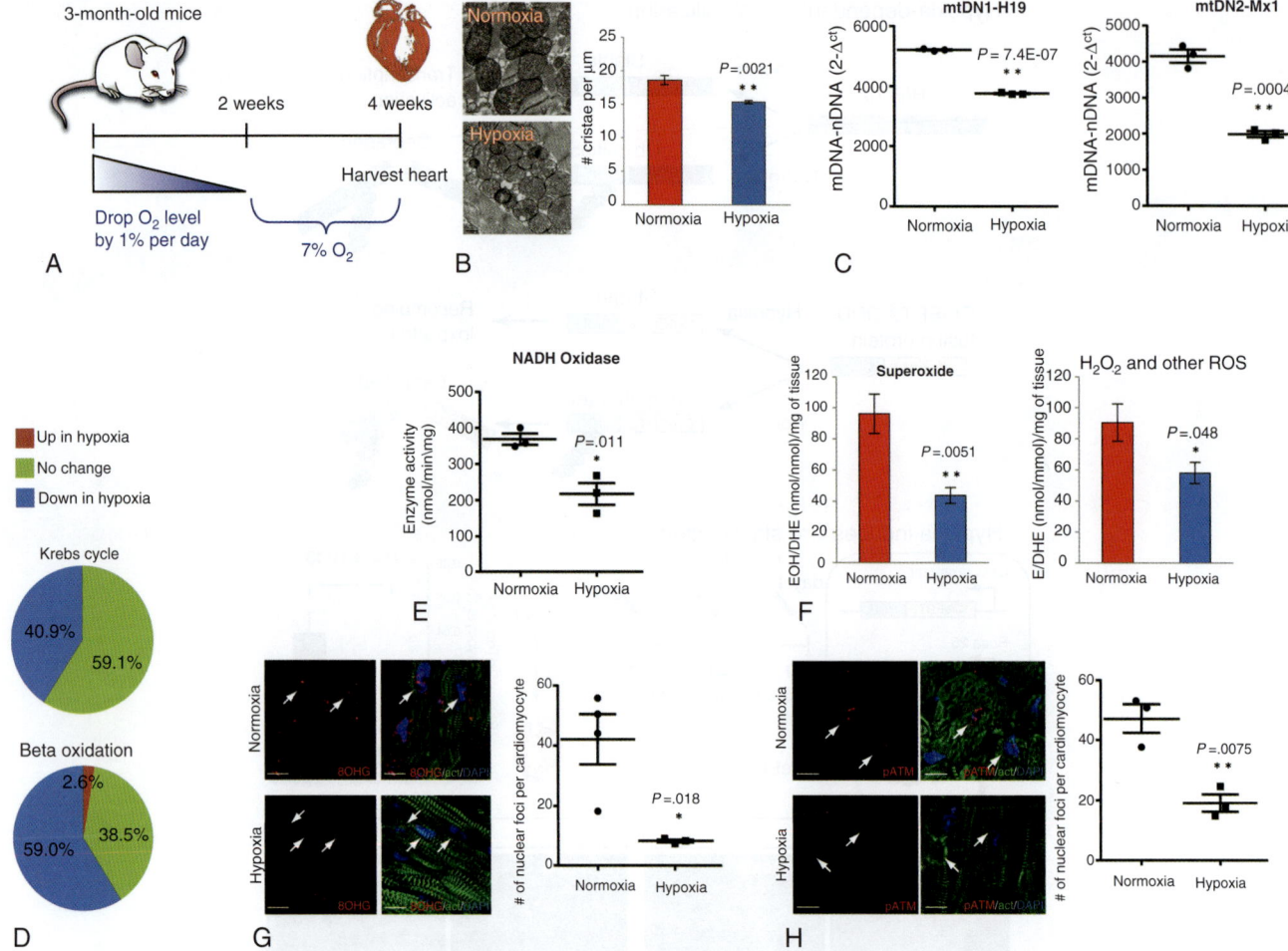

Fig. 3.7 Chronic hypoxia exposure leads to decreased mitochondrial reactive oxygen species *(ROS)* and decreased oxidative DNA damage in cardiomyocytes. (A) Schematic of gradual induction of severe hypoxemia. (B) Transmission electron microscopy images of mitochondria in ventricular cardiomyocytes and quantification of average number of cristae per micrometer showed a significantly less dense cristae structure in cardiomyocytes in the hypoxia-exposed heart (n = 5 each). (C) Quantitative polymerase chain reaction (PCR) analysis of mitochondrial DNA showed that mitochondrial DNA copy number normalized to nuclear DNA copy number (mtDN1 vs. H19 or mtDN2 vs. Mx1) was significantly decreased following hypoxia exposure (n = 3 each). (D) Quantitative mass spectrometry analysis showed that a large proportion of enzymes involved in mitochondrial Krebs cycle and fatty acid β oxidation was significantly decreased following hypoxia exposure (n = 3 each; values rounded to the nearest decimal place). (E) The enzymatic activity of nicotinamide adenine dinucleotide (NADH) oxidase (normalized to mitochondrial protein) showed a significant decrease in electron transport chain activity following chronic hypoxia exposure (n = 3 each). (F) High-performance liquid chromatography–based measurement of superoxide *(left side)*, and H_2O_2 and other ROS *(right side)* both indicated a significant decrease in ROS level in the heart after an exposure to hypoxia (n = 5 each). (G) Immunofluorescence using anti-8OHG antibody showed a significant decrease in oxidative DNA damage in cardiomyocytes from hypoxia-treated mice (n = 4 for normoxia, and 3 for hypoxia). (H) Immunofluorescence using an anti-phosphorylated-ATM (ataxia telangiectasia mutated) antibody showed a significant decrease in the activation of DNA damage response pathway in cardiomyocytes from hypoxia-treated hearts (n = 3 each). Scale bars, 10 μm. Data are presented as mean ± SEM. *DHE*, Dihydroethidium; *EOH*, 2-hydroxyethidium. *$P < .05$, **$P < .01$. From Nakada Y, Canseco DC, Thet S, et al. Hypoxia induces heart regeneration in adult mice. *Nature* 2017;541:222–227.

regeneration.[32] A recent comprehensive survey of the cardiomyocyte nucleation status in 120 inbred mouse strains found a wide variation in the frequency of mononuclear diploid cardiomyocytes, ranging from 2.3% to 17.0% of all cardiomyocytes.[33] Intriguingly, it was observed that strains with more mononuclear diploid cardiomyocytes had increased cardiomyocyte proliferation and regeneration after adult MI injury. This hypothesis was directly tested in zebrafish, in which 99% of adult cardiomyocytes are mononuclear diploid and retain the capacity to regenerate after injury. Transient gene perturbation resulted in polyploidy in half of the zebrafish cardiomyocytes (upon activation of

a dominant-negative version of a key cytokinesis protein, ECT2).[34] In this model, mononuclear diploid cardiomyocytes proliferated at higher rates than polyploid cardiomyocytes after amputation of the ventricular apex in adult zebrafish.[34] Intriguingly, when the fraction of polyploid cells rises to approximately 50% of the entire cardiomyocyte cohort, the regenerative ability of adult zebrafish was significantly impaired. It remains to be seen whether such a mechanism applies also to the mammalian heart. Moreover, whether binuclear and polyploid mammalian cardiomyocytes may undergo abscission during aging or after a pathologic insult remains an open question.

Another challenge to the ability of postnatal cardiomyocytes to divide may lie outside the cell: a recent report documented a change in extracellular matrix composition in the first week of life in neonatal mice that correlates with the loss of significant proliferative capacity.[35] Specifically, the extracellular matrix proteoglycan agrin is present in neonatal mouse hearts and is necessary for neonatal cardiac regeneration. Agrin expression is lost in the first week of life, but a single myocardial injection of agrin after MI in adult mice increased cardiomyocyte proliferation, reduced fibrosis, and improved systolic function.

The mechanism by which the extracellular matrix plays in a role in cardiomyocyte proliferation could be through transduction of mechanical load, which has been shown to influence the cardiomyocyte nuclear and mitochondrial state in the human heart. A natural model for unloading the left ventricle is the left ventricular assist device (LVAD), which is implanted in advanced heart failure patients as a bridge to orthotopic heart transplant or as a destination therapy.[36] LVADs are mechanical pumps that increase cardiac output and systemic perfusion and thereby improve end-organ function. Notably, a small subset of LVAD patients has experienced sufficient myocardial recovery to be able to undergo LVAD explantation. The functional recovery in these patients suggests a salutary effect of pressure unloading of the left ventricle as accomplished by an LVAD. Cardiac biopsies from LVAD patients showed a decrease in global cardiomyocyte polyploidy (which is increased in failing hearts) and an increase in the number of diploid cardiomyocytes, which suggests that mitosis of cardiomyocytes and/or abscission of polyploid cardiomyocytes may be occurring in unloaded hearts.[37] Moreover, post-LVAD hearts have reduced mitochondrial DNA copy number, smaller cardiomyocytes, and reduced activity in the DDR pathway.[38] Consistent with prior findings that activation of the DDR pathway dampens cardiomyocyte division, post-LVAD hearts have increased expression of mitosis- and cytokinesis-associated proteins (Fig. 3.8). These findings imply that mechanical unloading may lead to cardiomyocyte cell division and thus may represent another means to achieve cardiac regeneration.

Viewed together, these studies demonstrate that a number of cell autonomous as well as non–cell autonomous mechanisms underlie the terminally differentiated state that characterizes the majority of cardiomyocytes in the mammalian heart. It remains unclear at this time if all the previously described mechanisms apply to all cardiomyocytes or whether subpopulations of cardiomyocytes are differentially affected. Further evaluation and manipulation of these pathways will be necessary to optimize therapies that undergird cardiac regeneration.

MECHANISMS OF CARDIAC REGENERATION

Endogenous Heart Regeneration in Lower Vertebrates and Mammals

There are few known species with the capacity to substantially regenerate the heart. In 2002 Poss and colleagues first demonstrated that surgical resection of 20% of the zebrafish single ventricle was followed by full regeneration without fibrotic scarring within 60 days (Fig. 3.9).[39,40] Fate mapping confirmed that cardiac regeneration is primarily mediated by proliferation of preexisting cardiomyocytes in adult zebrafish.[41,42]

The demonstration that vertebrates like teleost fish could regenerate the heart raised the exciting possibility that mammals may also possess this capability. In 2011 Sadek and colleagues adapted the zebrafish ventricular apical resection model to neonatal mice to assess for cardiac regeneration.[43] This landmark study revealed that 1 day postpartum (P1) mice retain a capacity to regenerate their hearts following cardiac resection (Fig. 3.10). P1 mice underwent surgical resection of 15% of the left ventricle, and within 21 days the myocardium was completely replaced, with normalization of the left ventricular ejection fraction at 2 months after resection.

Genetic fate mapping suggested that the primary source of regeneration is expansion of existing cardiomyocytes. Notably, apical resection did not result in cardiomyocyte hypertrophy or significant fibrosis.

In contrast, the ability to regenerate the heart is lost by P7 in mice. Despite a proportionally smaller surgical amputation in P7 mice (owing to higher surgical mortality), their myocardium failed to regenerate and instead showed fibrotic changes. This loss of cardiac regenerative potential within the first week of postnatal life coincides with cardiomyocyte binucleation and withdrawal from the cell cycle (i.e., a switch from hyperplasia to hypertrophy) in rodents.[44] A more physiologically relevant model of myocardial infarction, by ligation of the left anterior descending coronary artery, validated the narrow intrinsic regenerative window to the first week of life in mice.[45] Numerous studies have since used the apical resection model[35,46-59] and myocardial infarction neonatal mouse heart models[46,50,60-66] to better understand factors that promote or inhibit cardiac regeneration.[66a] These surgical models continue to provide mechanistic insights into mammalian cardiac regeneration that can occur upon repopulation of lost or damaged tissue, even in the face of residual extracellular matrix deposition or a minor amount of fibrin deposition.

The exposition of cardiac regeneration in newborn mice leads to the inference that higher mammals may also boast such a potential. It is interesting to speculate the possibility that after cardiac injury, human neonatal hearts may also be able to regenerate. Apart from anecdotal reports of improvement in ejection fraction following MI of a newborn infant,[67] it is difficult to comment on the ability of the newborn human heart to regenerate: in the absence of viability studies documenting reversal of nonviable myocardium, an improvement of systolic function could be attributed to reversal of transient contractile dysfunction such as in cases of myocardial stunning or hibernation.

Induction of Cardiomyocyte Proliferation

Adult mammalian hearts exhibit a low rate of cardiomyocyte proliferation under physiologic conditions to maintain cardiomyocyte renewal.[11,13,15,68] Furthermore, the prevailing predominant mechanism of cardiac regeneration in zebrafish and neonatal mice is proliferation of preexisting cardiomyocytes.[41,43,45] Therefore it is of great interest to identify mechanisms that promote proliferation of adult cardiomyocytes as a potential strategy to restore cardiac tissue after injury.[69]

Cyclins and Cyclin-Dependent Kinases

Cell cycle progression is positively modulated by cyclin/cyclin-dependent kinase (CDK) complexes, and cyclins are downregulated in cardiomyocytes postnatally. Combined overexpression of CDK1, CDK4, cyclin B1, and cyclin D1 caused replication of adult cardiomyocytes.[70] Induction of these four factors after surgically induced MI led to an improvement in ejection fraction and a smaller scar size.

microRNAs

microRNA (miR)-195 is the most upregulated miR in the murine heart from P1 to P10 and, through inhibition of key mitotic genes such as checkpoint kinase 1, it contributes to cardiomyocyte cell cycle withdrawal that occurs over this time frame.[45] Transgenic cardiac overexpression of miR-195 impairs cardiomyocyte proliferation and yields smaller hearts, and knockdown of miR-195 increases the number of mitotic cardiomyocytes. On the other hand, multiple miRs may positively upregulate neonatal cardiomyocyte proliferation in culture.[71] Of note, miR-590 and miR-199a increase cardiomyocyte division in animal models and, when delivered into the adult mouse heart at time of MI, can lead to an improvement in systolic function and reduction in infarct size. These and other reports demonstrate that perturbation of critical miRs may enable cardiac regeneration.[72,73]

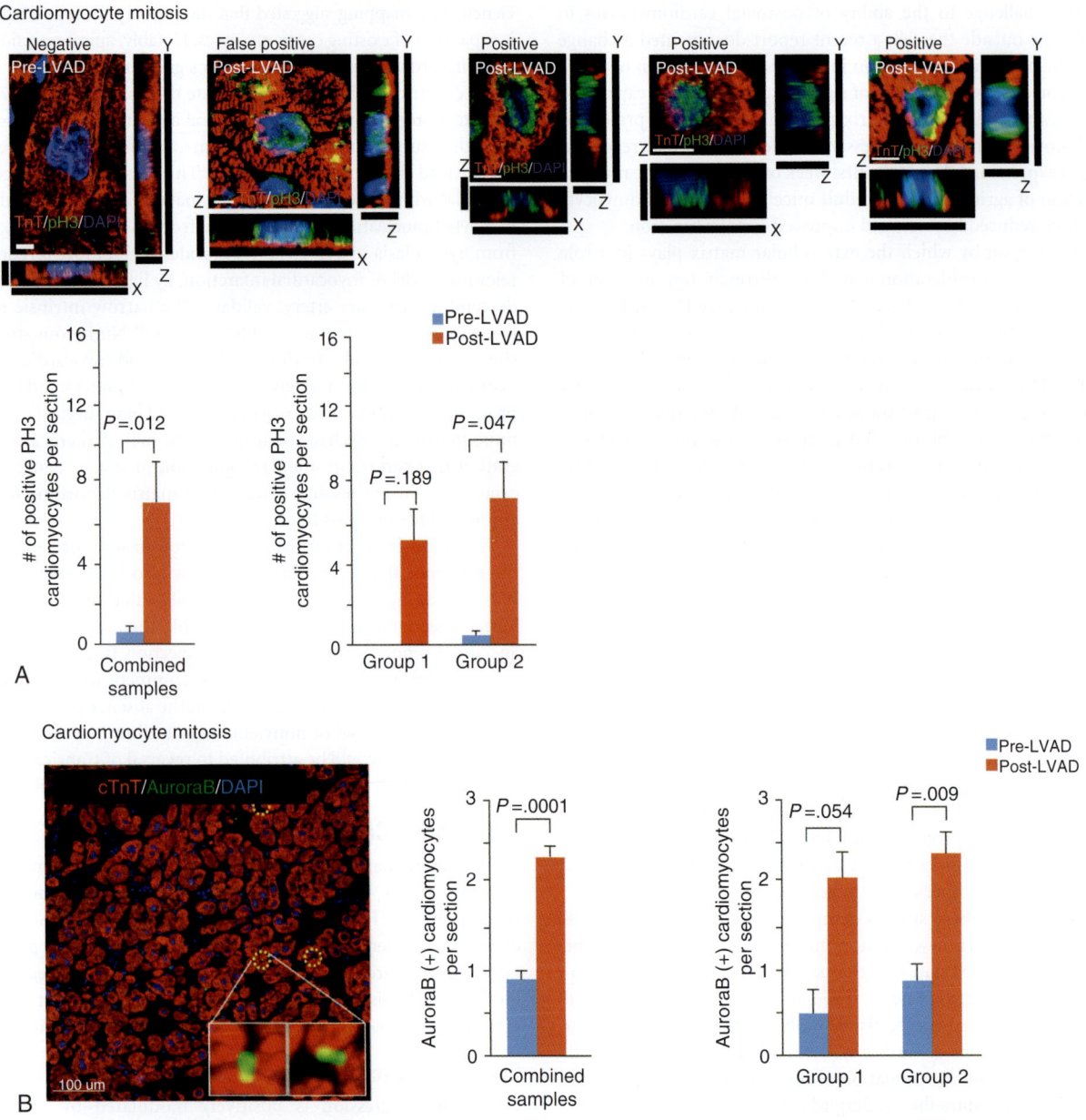

Fig. 3.8 Left Ventricular Assist Device *(LVAD)*-Mediated Pressure Unloading Induces Cardiomyocyte Proliferation in Adult Human Heart. (A) Confocal z-stack imaging after PH_3 antibody staining showed a significant increase in cardiomyocyte mitosis in the longer-duration group 2 LVAD hearts (scale bar, 5 μm). Note that stringent criteria were used for localization of PH_3 staining to cardiomyocytes. True- and false-positive examples are provided. (B) Confocal z-stack imaging of Aurora B kinase showed a marked increase in cardiomyocyte cytokinesis in the longer-duration group 2 LVAD hearts (scale bar, 100 μm). Note the localization of Aurora B kinase to the cleavage following between 2 cardiomyocytes *(right inset)*. *cTnT,* Cardiac troponin T; *PH_3,* phosphorylated histone H3. From Canseco DC, Kimura W, Garg S, et al. Human ventricular unloading induces cardiomyocyte proliferation. *J Am Coll Cardiol.* 2015;65:892–900.

Transcription Factors

The perturbation of FOXO and MEF2 transcription factor activity in cultured cardiomyocytes demonstrated their role in modulating cardiomyocyte cell cycle in vitro.[74,75] Further insights into the effects of various transcription factors on the cardiac postmitotic state in animal models may have therapeutic implications. MEIS1 is a homeodomain transcription factor that regulates cardiac differentiation during development. During the first week of life in mouse, MEIS1 protein is expressed, but it does not localize to the nucleus. At P7, MEIS1 nuclear translocation correlates with cardiomyocyte withdrawal from the cell cycle, in part mediated through its activation of CDK inhibitors p15, p16, and p21. Transgenic mice with enforced cardiomyocyte-specific MEIS1 expression lose the ability to regenerate after P1 MI. In contrast, the normal proliferation window is extended beyond P7 when Meis1 is deleted in cardiomyocytes (Fig. 3.11).[61]

In contrast to MEIS1, transcription factor GATA4 loses its expression after the first week of life in mice.[76] Adenoviral-mediated increase in GATA4 levels after P7 cryoinjury increases cardiomyocyte proliferation and improves cardiac function.[76] In contrast, abrogation of neonatal GATA4 activity impaired regeneration after P0 cryoinjury.

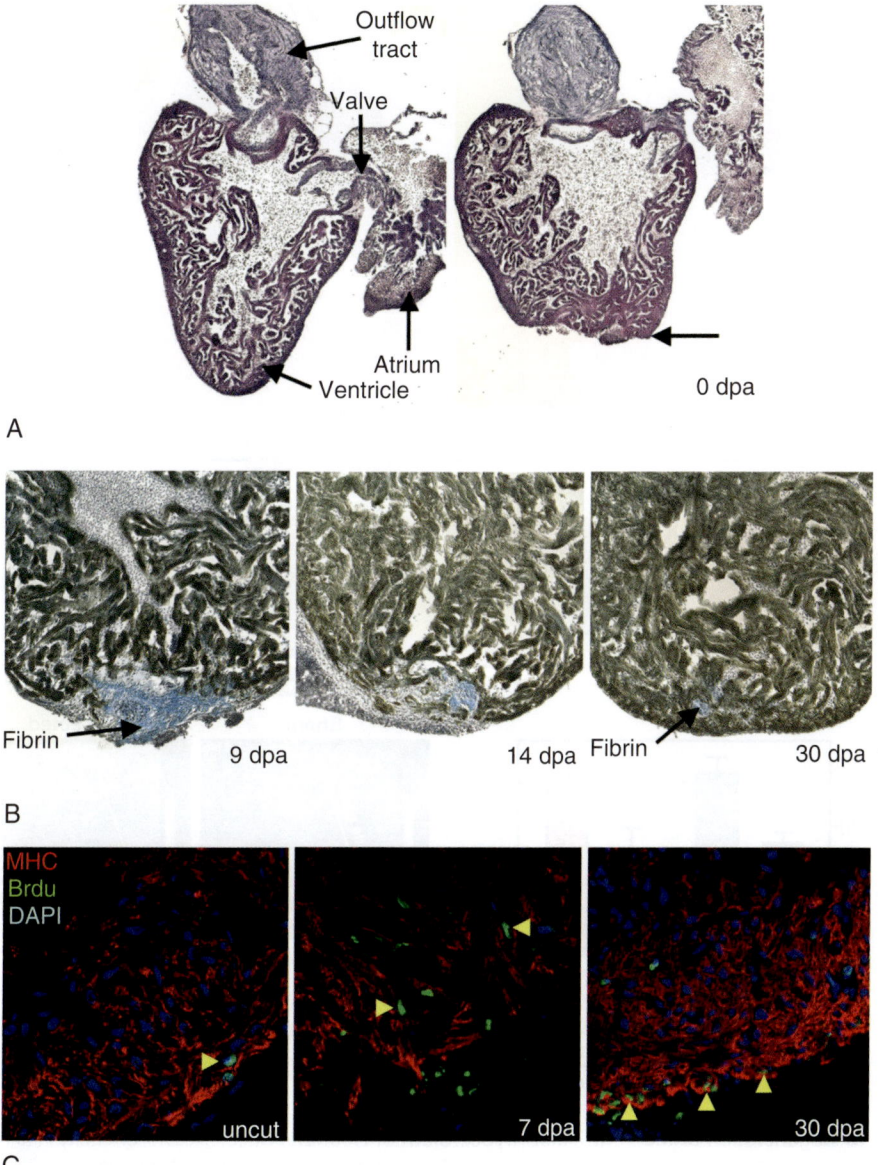

Fig. 3.9 Cardiac Regeneration in Zebrafish. (A) Hematoxylin and eosin stain of the adult zebrafish heart before and after 20% ventricular resection. (B) Ventricular sections stained for myosin heavy chain to identify cardiac muscle *(brown)* and aniline blue to identify fibrin *(blue)*. Mature fibrin seals the wound by 7 dpa and is gradually replaced by cardiac muscle. The wall is typically restored by 30 days post amputation (dpa). (C) BrdU incorporation, a marker of DNA synthesis and cellular proliferation, is activated in cardiomyocytes by 7 dpa *(yellow)*. The ventricular wall is restored by proliferation at the leading edge of cardiomyocytes. From Poss, KD. Getting to the heart of regeneration in zebrafish. *Semin Cell Dev Biol.* 2007;18(1):36–45, 2007.

Nerves

An important cardiac-neural axis may underlie neonatal heart regeneration: P1 mouse hearts treated with atropine at time of apical resection had decreased cardiomyocyte proliferation compared with controls, likely due to inhibition of cholinergic transmission. [50] Apical resection at P1 in combination with left-sided vagotomy also decreased cardiomyocyte proliferation. These findings suggest a role for cholinergic signaling in regulating mammalian heart regeneration. In a separate study, chemical sympathectomy of P2 mice that underwent apical resection led to fibrosis and impaired regeneration of the myocardium.[77] These observations may be mediated by nerve growth factor, which was shown to indirectly increase cardiomyocyte proliferation in larval zebrafish. [78]

Hippo Signaling

Discovered in Drosophila, the Hippo signaling pathway has an evolutionarily conserved role in regulating organ size by controlling cell proliferation and apoptosis.[79] Perturbation of Hippo signaling in the mouse heart can increase cardiomyocyte proliferation and lead to cardiomegaly, indicating that Hippo is involved in cardiac development and injury (Fig. 3.12).[80–83] Yap, the most downstream Hippo signaling component in mice, is a transcriptional coactivator that is sequestered in the cytoplasm upon phosphorylation. Once dephosphorylated, the active form of Yap accumulates in the nucleus and interacts with TEA domain transcription factors to promote cardiomyocyte division.[81] Mice with cardiac-specific

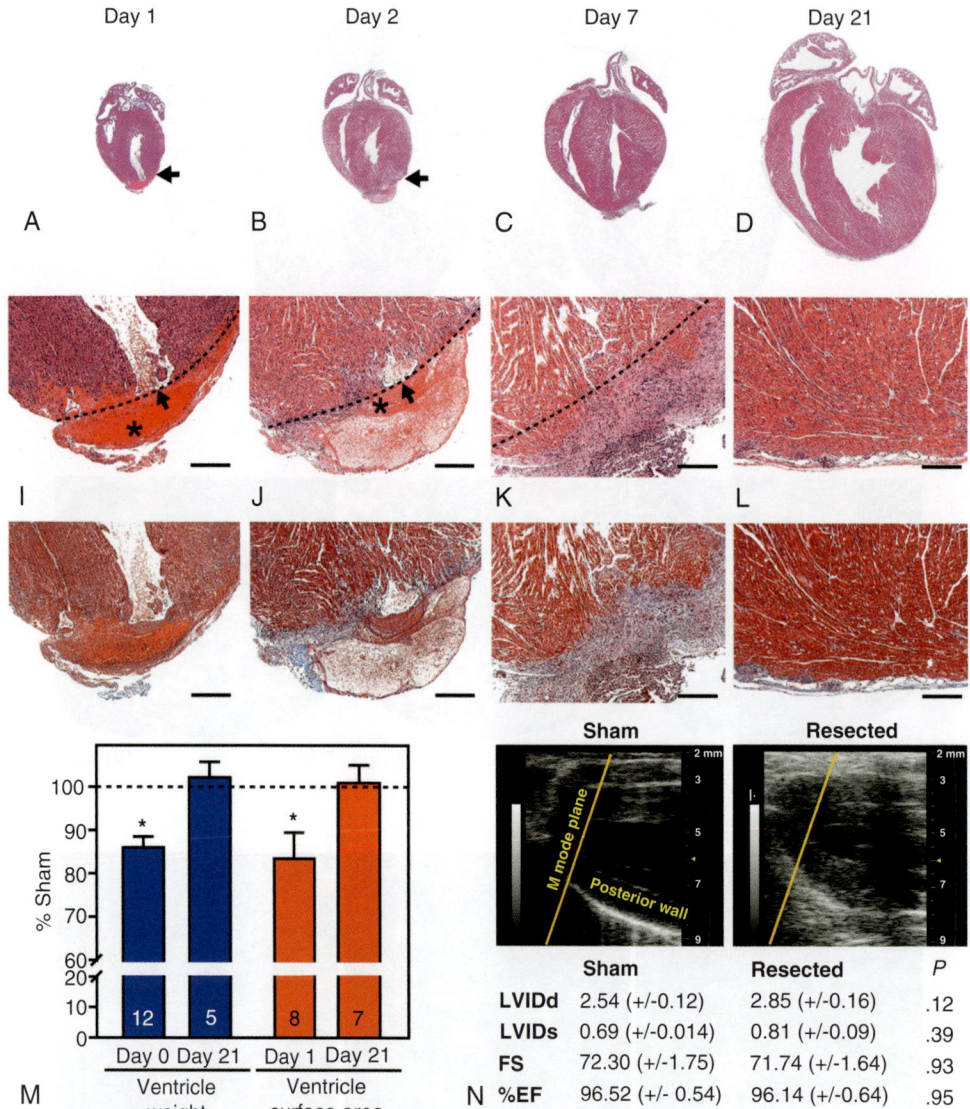

Fig. 3.10 Regeneration of the Ventricular Myocardium of Neonatal Mice. (A–D) Hematoxylin and eosin (H&E) staining of the mouse heart at 1, 2, 7, and 21 days post resection *(dpr)*. *Arrow* denotes injury site. (E–H) H&E-stained sections at higher magnification. The *asterisk* marks a large blood clot adjacent to the left ventricular chamber *(arrow)* at 1 and 2 dpr. *Dashed line* indicates the resection plane. Scale bars, 200 μm. (I–L) Trichrome-stained serial sections showing early deposition of epicardial extracellular matrix *(blue staining)* at 7 dpr, with minimal evidence of cardiac fibrosis by day 21 (scale bars, 200 μm). (M) Quantification of surgical reproducibility and regeneration. Ventricle weights and sagittal section surface area are presented as percentages of sham-operated controls. Numbers of samples analyzed are indicated within the bars. Values are presented as means ± SEM; *$P < .05$. (N) Images of two-dimensional echocardiogram in the parasternal long axis view. *Yellow line* indicates motion *(M)* mode plane. Lower panel shows left ventricular *(LV)* dimensions and function of sham-operated and resected hearts at 60 dpr. Left ventricular internal diameter at end systole *(LVIDs)* and end diastole *(LVIDd)* were used for calculating fractional shortening *(FS)* and ejection fraction (EF). Values are presented as means ± SEM; n = 3 per group. From Porrello ER, Mahmoud AI, Simpson E, Hill JA, Richardson JA, Olson EN, Sadek HA. Transient regenerative potential of the neonatal mouse heart. *Science.* 2011;331:1078–1080.

mutant, constitutively active YAP exhibit enhanced cardiomyocyte proliferation and increased heart size, as well as prolongation of the neonatal cardiac regenerative window via activation of Wnt and IGF signaling pathways.[81,83] In contrast, Yap deletion in cardiomyocytes leads to thinner myocardium and compromised heart function from 6 to 12 weeks of life and results in premature death between 11 and 20 weeks.[83]

Ventricular Unloading

Ventricular unloading increases cell cycle progression in cardiomyocytes and improves heart function.[38,84] A case study of an infant with severe heart failure who received a heterotopic heart transplant provides a natural example of ventricular unloading, as the native heart remained in place without the exclusive role to provide circulatory support.[84] Remarkably, the patient's birth heart recovered function

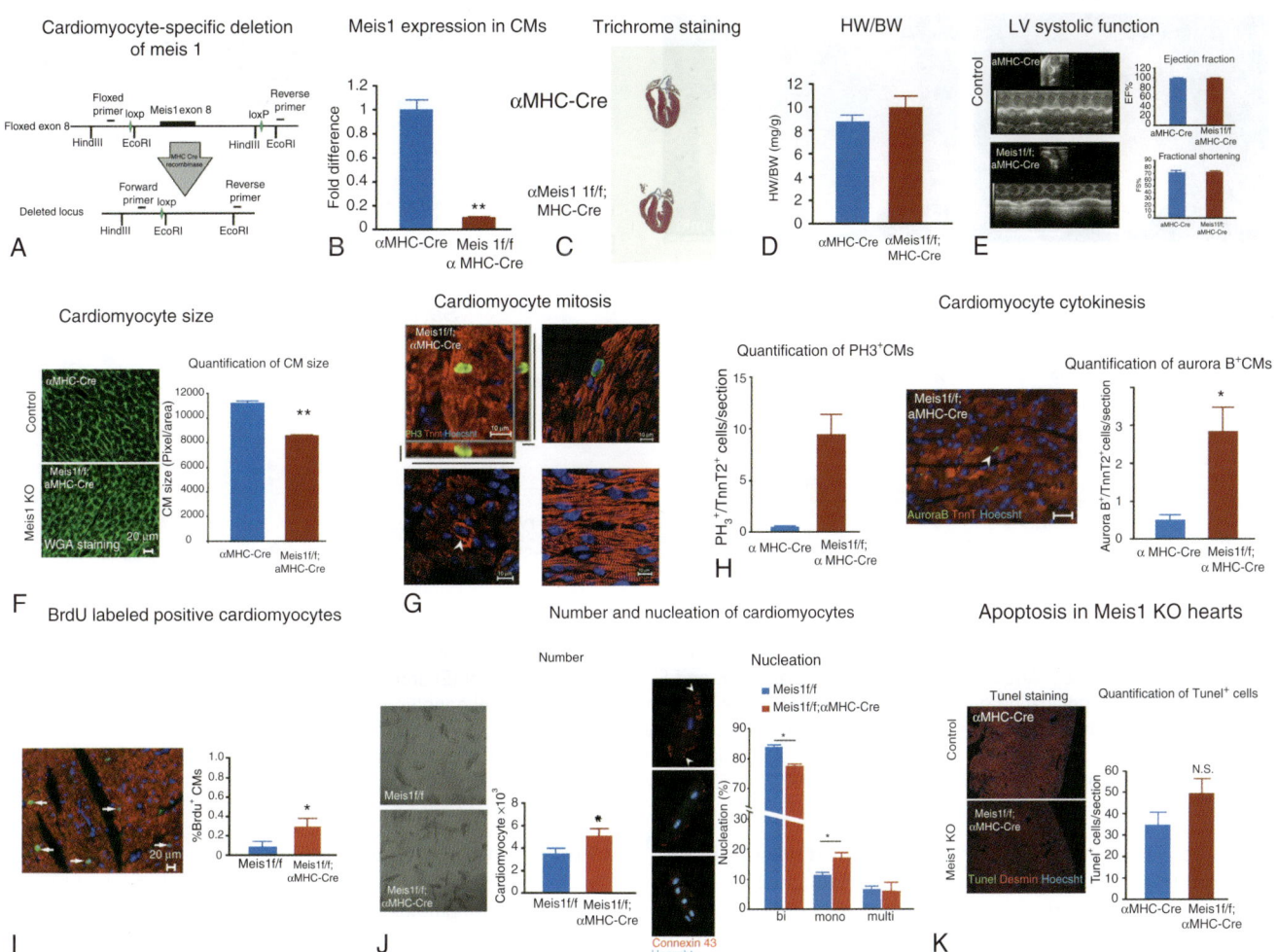

Fig. 3.11 Cardiomyocyte Proliferation at P14 Following Meis1 Deletion. (A) Schematic of Meis1 floxed allele. Control mice were α-myosin heavy chain (αMHC)–Cre, Meis1 knockout (KO) mice were Meis1f/f αMHC-Cre. (B) Quantitative real-time PCR (qRT-PCR) demonstrates deletion of Meis1 in isolated cardiomyocytes at P14 (n = 3). (C) Trichrome staining of wild-type and Meis1 KO hearts at P14. (D) Heart weight *(HW)* to body weight *(BW)* ratio in wild-type and Meis1 KO hearts (n = 4–7 per group). (E) Left ventricular systolic function quantified by ejection fraction and fractional shortening (n = 4–7 per group). (F) Wheat germ agglutinin *(WGA)* staining and cell size quantification. Quantitative analyses represent counting of multiple fields from three independent samples per group (~50 cells per field assessed, total ~250 cells per group). (G) Confocal image with z-stacking showing colocalization of PH_3, TnnT2, and Hoechst in a Meis1 KO heart at P14 *(top left)*. Confocal image of a PH_3+ cardiomyocyte in a Meis1 KO heart *(top right)*. Immunostaining showing sarcomere disassembly in Meis1 KO hearts *(arrowhead, bottom left)*. Normal sarcomeric structure of Meis1 KO myocardium *(bottom right)*. Graph shows quantification of the number of PH_3+ TnnT2+ nuclei. (H) Immunostaining showing expression of Aurora B in Meis1 KO cardiomyocytes at P14 and quantification of the number of Aurora B+ TnnT2+ cardiomyocytes. Quantitative analysis of PH_3 and Aurora B+ cardiomyocytes represents counting of multiple sections from three independent samples per heart (~3 sections per heart) (G and H). (I) Immunostaining showing colocalization of BrdU, α-actinin, and Hoechst in Meis1 KO heart at P14 and quantification of the number of BrdU+ cardiomyocytes *(arrows)*. Quantification represents counting of several sections from (3–6) independent samples per group. Total number of cardiomyocytes counted for proliferation indices was $2 \times 10^3 - 2.5 \times 10^3$ myocytes per section. (J) Representative images of control and Meis1 KO isolated cardiomyocytes, and quantification of the number of myocytes from control and Meis1 KO hearts. Approximately $1 \times 10^3 - 1.5 \times 10^3$ cardiomyocytes were counted using a hemocytometer per group, using three independent samples *(left)*. Immunostaining of isolated cardiomyocytes with Connexin 43, and quantification of the number of nuclei in control and Meis1 KO hearts. For nucleation, approximately 1×10^3 cardiomyocytes were counted per sample, using three independent samples per group *(right)*. (K) Apoptosis analysis. Image showing colocalization of TUNEL, Desmin, and Hoechst in a control and Meis1 KO heart. Quantification of TUNEL-positive cells (n = 3). Values presented as mean ± SEM, *P < .05, **P < .01. From Mahmoud AI, Kocabas F, Muralidhar SA, et al. Meis1 regulates postnatal cardiomyocyte cell cycle arrest. *Nature.* 2013;497:249–253.

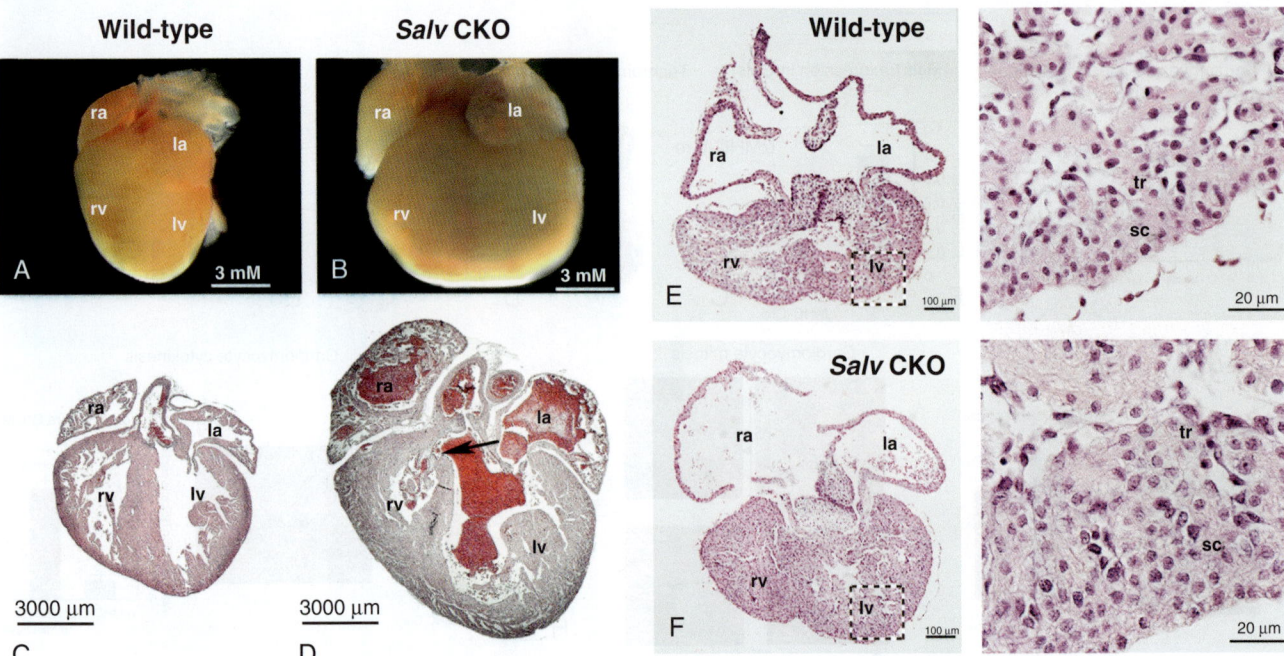

Fig. 3.12 Salvador Mutant Cardiomegaly. (A–D) Control (A and C) and Salv CKO (B and D) P2 neonate hearts. Hearts in (A) and (B) were sectioned and stained with hematoxylin and eosin (H&E), as shown in (C) and (D). Arrow, ventricular septum defect. (E and F) H&E-stained control (E) and Salv CKO (F) hearts. High magnification of (E) and (F) are shown in the right-hand images. Control genotype is Nkx2.5cre; Salvf/+. *la*, Left atrium; *lv*, left ventricle; *ra*, Right atrium; *rv*, right ventricle; *sc*, subcompact; *tr*, trabecular myocardium. From Heallen T, Zhang M, Wang J, et al. Hippo pathway inhibits Wnt signaling to restrain cardiomyocyte proliferation and heart size. *Science*. 2011;332:458–461.

over this period. Owing in part to transplant-related side effects, the donor heart was removed: the patient's own heart resumed full circulatory function. The underlying mechanism in this report is unknown, but it is hypothesized that reducing the heart's workload may help with recovery of heart function. Analogously, mechanical support by LVADs may promote the ability of the heart to regenerate, possibly due to pressure unloading of the native heart by the pump device.[38]

EXOGENOUS CARDIOMYOCYTES FOR CELL THERAPY (SEE ALSO CHAPTER 41)

Since the generation of human embryonic stem cell (hESC) lines and discovery of induced pluripotent stem cells (iPSCs) in 2006 by Yamanaka and colleagues,[85] the ability of these collective pluripotent stem cells (PSCs) to generate cells and tissues to potentially treat human diseases has been highly esteemed. The promise of pluripotent cells in the treatment of heart disease is in part through their ability to generate substrates for cell transplantation therapy, the founding premise for which is the hypothesis that an increase in cardiomyocyte number after myocardial injury benefits cardiac function.[41,43]

Over the past decade, significant progress has been made in identification of differentiation conditions that give rise to purified cardiomyocyte populations at a high yield. Use of certain cytokines markedly enhances the cardiac differentiation efficiency of PSCs.[86-88] Although it is now readily possible to derive cardiomyocyte-like cells from PSCs, a challenge for the field—especially as it relates to potential cell transplantation—relates to precise characterization of these cells. Transcriptional analysis of PSC-derived cardiomyocytes (CMs) has shown that they express genes associated with contractile apparatus components, calcium handling machinery, and electrical connectivity and therefore phenotypically appear to be CMs. However,

the resemblance is closer to immature, embryonic CMs than to adult CMs.[89] To this end, recent work used a functional screen of hESC-derived cardiac organoids to identify a metabolic-based method to "mature" PSC-derived CMs.[90] Furthermore, although current protocols to differentiate PSCs to CMs are not contaminated by derivation of other cell types, the population nevertheless is heterogeneous as ventricular, nodal, and atrial subtypes of CMs are obtained, which have distinct electrophysiologic properties.[91,92] More work is therefore needed to specifically purify different subtypes of cardiomyocytes.

Several groups have transplanted PSC-derived cells into animal models, with promising results that also raise some concerns. One of the earliest examples of hESC-derived CM implantation in a rodent model was reported in 2005: a mixed population of cardiac-enriched hESC-derived cells was injected into rat hearts with demonstration of long-term engraftment of the hESC-CMs.[93,94] Subsequently, this group transplanted purified hESC-derived CMs into a guinea pig heart model and showed that addition of donor cells improved mechanical function after cryoinjury and reduced spontaneous arrhythmias.[95] Ardehali and colleagues extended these observations by showing that hESC-derived cardiovascular progenitors can engraft in fetal *human* tissue (that was surgically transplanted into the mouse pinna) and generate cardiomyocytes, vascular smooth muscle cells, and endothelial cells.[96] One of the first primate studies used macaque hosts and showed that hESC-derived CMs electromechanically engraft and couple into the primate heart after myocardial ischemia with reperfusion injury (Fig. 3.13).[97] However, the hESC-CMs remained immature 3 months after transplantation and, opposed to data from small animal studies, nonfatal ventricular arrhythmias were observed.

Animal studies have also revealed that transplanted cells are often unviable after direct intramyocardial injection, which may be due to high injection pressures and/or a nonsalutary local tissue microenvironment.

GFP (Human) α-Actinin (Human+Monkey) Nuclei

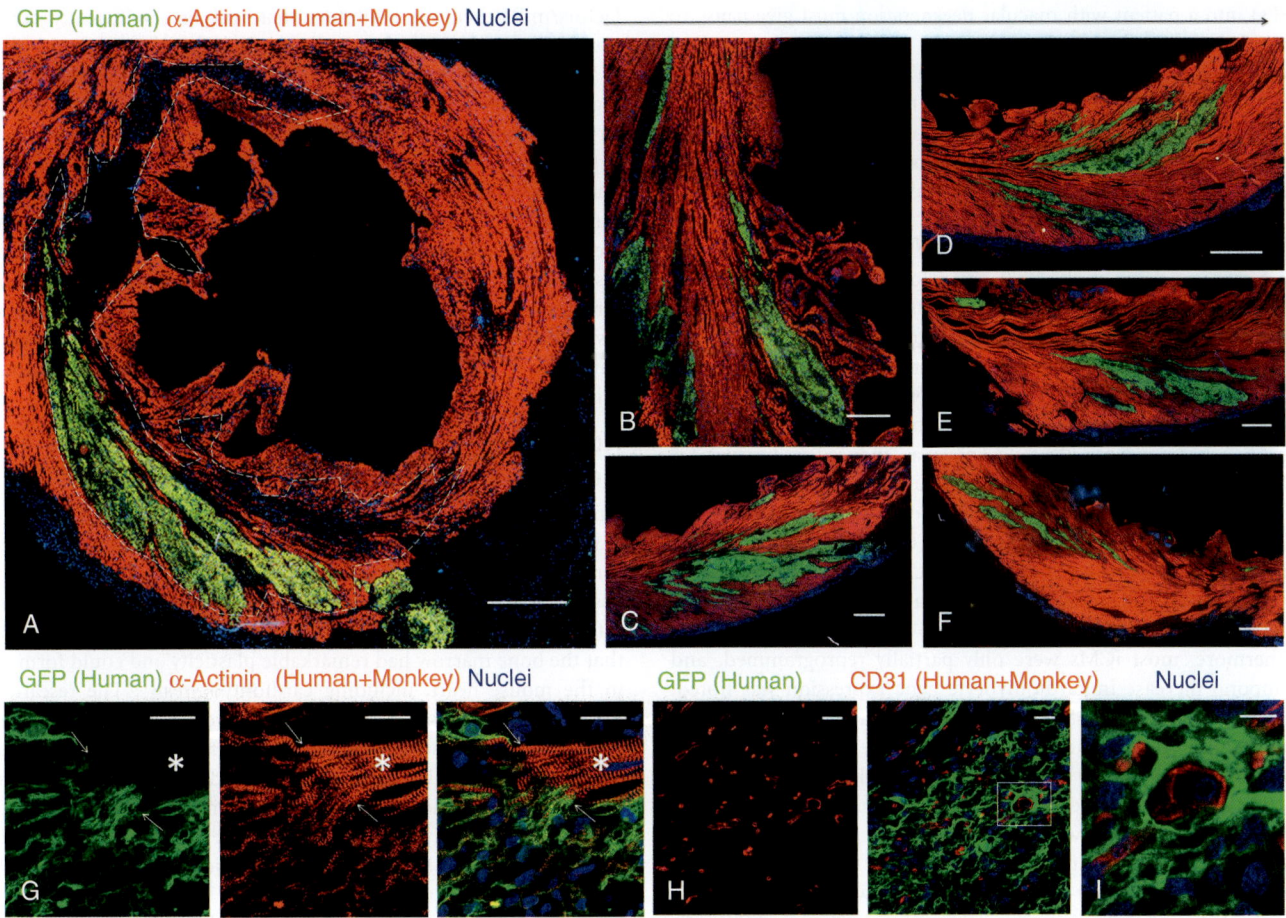

GFP (Human) α-Actinin (Human+Monkey) Nuclei   GFP (Human)   CD31 (Human+Monkey)   Nuclei

Fig. 3.13 Confocal Immunofluorescence of Macaque Hearts Subjected to Myocardial Infarction and Transplantation of Human Embryonic Stem Cell Cardiomyocytes (hESC-CM). Grafts studied at 14 days (A–G) and 84 days post engraftment (H and I). (A) Remuscularization of a substantial portion of the infarct region (dashed line) with hESC-CM coexpressing green fluorescent protein (GFP). The contractile protein α-Actinin (red) is expressed by both monkey and human cardiomyocytes (scale bar, 1000 μm). (B–F) Images from the periinfarct region of the same heart shown in (A), demonstrating significant hESC-CM engraftment (scale bar, 1000 μm). (G) Graft-host interface at 14 days with interconnected α-Actinin (red) expressing cardiomyocytes (arrows). Note host sarcomeric cross-striations (asterisk) show greater alignment than hESC-CM graft (scale bar 25 μm). (H and I) Day-84 hESC-CM grafts contain host-derived blood vessels lined by CD31+ endothelial cells (scale bar, 20 μm; inset scale bar, 10 μm). From Chong JJ, Yang X, Don CW, et al. Human embryonic-stem-cell-derived cardiomyocytes regenerate non-human primate hearts. Nature. 2014;510:273–277.

Therefore bioengineering approaches are being explored to improve cell viability. Use of hydrogel-based tissue that contains extracellular matrix (ECM) proteins as a scaffold material for PSC-derived cells has had inconsistent results when transplanted collectively into various animal models.[98] Detachable, three-dimensional (3D) cell sheets of iPSC-CMs have been developed as a substrate for cell transplantation, with a more durable effect on transplant cell viability.[99] Another innovative scaffold that most closely resembles native human myocardium is decellularized cadaveric heart tissue, obtained from primary tissue or via a 3D printing approach.[100,101] It is becoming increasingly clear that the delivery mechanism for transplanted PSC-derived cells is an important aspect of the challenge of cell transplantation therapy.

The first case report of PSC-CMs transplantation into humans was published in 2015; cardiac-committed cells differentiated from an hESC line were sorted on the basis of their surface markers and embedded into a fibrin scaffold patch.[102] The patch was surgically delivered into a middle-aged man with advanced heart failure at the time of coronary artery bypass grafting onto the epicardial surface of a nonrevascularized, infarcted, akinetic region of the heart. The patient was initiated on immunosuppressive drugs after cell transplantation. Three months after the surgery, there was echocardiographic evidence of contractility in the patch-treated area, the patient improved in his New York Heart Association (NYHA) functional class, and there were no arrhythmias and no evidence of tumor formation. In 2018, the same group reported the transplantation of cardiovascular progenitors derived from hESCs into six patients with advanced ischemic cardiomyopathy at time of coronary artery bypass graft surgery.[103] Although patients did not have arrhythmias or cardiac tumors at 18-month follow-up, half of the patients developed clinically silent alloimmunization. The clinical benefits in these patients were not large in magnitude, but there was in increase in systolic motion of the transplanted myocardial segments, and all patients had symptomatic improvement. This trial demonstrates the short- and intermediate-term safety of cell transplantation using PSC-derived cardiac cells.

In spite of the encouraging findings from these human trials, experiences from transplantation of iPSC-derived retinal epithelial cells

(RPEs) into a patient with macular degeneration must give pause to the PSC-derived cell transplantation field. Takahashi and coworkers observed two genetic changes in both the patient's iPSCs and RPEs differentiated from those iPSCs.[104] Neither mutation is associated with tumor formation, yet it is clear from this incident that the field of cell transplantation therapy for the treatment of heart diseases remains in its infancy, with a number of vital issues waiting to be addressed.

Direct Reprogramming to Cardiomyocyte Fate

Although it was shown in the 1980s that ectopic, enforced expression of the transcription factor MyoD in fibroblasts could "transdifferentiate" them into skeletal muscle cells,[105] the search for a single transcription factor that could convert one somatic cell type into another had been unfruitful for other cell types. In 2010, the "cellular reprogramming" advance was extended to the heart[106]: a small fraction of fibroblasts in culture was converted to a cardiomyocyte-like state, known as "induced cardiomyocyte" (iCM), upon addition of a combination of transcription factors.[107,108]

The initial reports used the key cardiac developmental transcription factors GATA4, Mef2c, and Tbx5 (GMT), which were delivered by retroviral vectors to cardiac fibroblasts in culture.[107] As with induced pluripotency using the Yamanka factors,[109] the efficiency of iCM generation was low, at 6.5% of cultured fibroblasts. Furthermore, most iCMs were only partially reprogrammed, and a temporal increase in cardiomyocyte gene expression was noted. Transcriptional analysis of iCM cells showed an upregulation in functionally important cardiac genes and a decrease in fibroblast genes, consistent with a change in phenotype and cell identity. However, functional analysis of these cells revealed that only approximately a third of the iCMs showed spontaneous Ca^{2+} oscillations, whose pattern was most similar to that observed in neonatal myocytes. Interestingly, genetic fate-mapping studies showed that reprogramming leads to a direct conversion from one committed, differentiated cell type to another of a different embryonic origin. Two weeks after induction of the three transcription factors, the converted cells retained a cardiomyocyte phenotype with no further need for GMT expression, indicating that lineage conversion is a stable process.

Next, landmark studies demonstrated that fibroblasts (and other nonmyocyte populations) in the mouse heart could be directly converted to cardiomyocytes in situ using retroviral delivery of GMT: lineage conversion after an MI improved cardiac function in mice (Fig. 3.14).[110,111] The efficiency of reprogramming in vivo was also low: 2.4% to 6.5% of the cardiomyocytes were derived from fibroblasts. Transcriptional assessment showed that iCMs most closely resemble neonatal and adult ventricular cardiomyocytes. Analyses of gap junction protein expression, dye transfer, and patch clamping in iCMs suggest that they electrically couple with endogenous cardiomyocytes. These proof-of-principle studies lend further support to the hypothesis that increasing cardiomyocyte quantity after an MI has a beneficial effect on overall cardiac systolic function.

The mechanism by which cellular reprogramming causes lineage conversion to the myocyte fate is change in the epigenetic status of the cell upon enforced expression of the GMT cardiac developmental transcription factors. The various cocktails of transcription factors, miRs, small molecule inhibitors, etc. turn on a cardiomyocyte-specific family of genes and, concomitantly, turn off fibroblast-specific genes. Analysis of histone modifications in iCMs showed that they acquire a chromatin pattern similar to endogenous cardiomyocytes at some cardiac specific genes. Modulation of transforming growth factor β (TGF-β) and Wnt pathways by chemical inhibition improved reprogramming efficiency, highlighting the important role of signaling pathways during lineage conversion.[112]

Currently, studies within the field of direct reprogramming aim to determine the optimal stoichiometric ratio of transcription factors/miRs/chemical inhibitors that will most efficiently convert noncardiomyocytes into cardiomyocytes.[113,114] Although direct in vivo reprogramming for the in situ conversion of cells is an exciting therapeutic possibility, many questions remain prior to testing in larger animals and, ultimately, in humans. For example, as with iPS-derived cardiomyocytes, it remains imperative to fully characterize the phenotypic similarities and differences between native endogenous cardiomyocytes and iCMs. The basic GMT combination can generate multiple different cardiomyocyte subtypes, including conduction system cells.[90] It may be important therefore to identify a specific combination of reprogramming factors and relative dosages that leads to a singular subset of cardiomyocytes. Overall, the promising results to date of direct reprogramming of iCMs in mice generate much hope for this technique as a potential therapy for humans.

Noncardiomyocyte Cell Therapy: Where We Stand (see also Chapter 41)

One of the most controversial questions in the field of cardiac regeneration has been whether there is a resident cardiac stem or progenitor cell. An organ-specific stem cell divides asymmetrically, generates tissue-restricted daughter cells, is multipotent, and generally has significant regenerative potential. The Anversa group claimed in 2001 that the bone marrow had remarkable plasticity and could form cells in the mouse heart, including cardiomyocytes.[115] The researchers isolated c-kit-expressing, lineage-negative cells from the bone marrow of GFP mice and transplanted them into wild-type adult mouse hearts at time of MI, and they identified de novo myocardium and blood vessel formation directly arising from the donor bone marrow cells.[115] Subsequently, clinical trials were performed in which various cell types from the bone marrow were injected into patients either intravenously or directly into the heart. There was no significant improvement in hard outcomes, and any beneficial effects are now thought to be due to a paracrine effect.[116-119] Independent investigations of this remarkable transdifferentiation hypothesis indicate cell fusion and suboptimal analytic technique occurred, rather than lineage conversion.[120,121]

A well-studied cell population that has been used extensively for heart regeneration studies is cardiac-resident c-kit–expressing cells.[122,123] In mouse models c-kit–positive cardiac stem cells were shown to replenish the heart after MI.[124,125] However, rigorous lineage-tracing of c-kit–derived cells in mouse models showed that these cells do not significantly contribute to the cardiomyocyte lineage during development, aging, or following cardiac injury (Fig. 3.15).[21,126,127] Importantly, a randomized-control clinical trial, SCIPIO, was performed in which c-kit–expressing cells were isolated from the atria of patients with ischemic cardiomyopathy, expanded in culture, and autologously delivered to patients by intracoronary injection.[128] Results from this small, phase I trial showed an improvement in ejection fraction for the c-kit–recipient group, but this report was given an "Expression of Concern" notification by *The Lancet* in 2014 due to ongoing investigations at the host institution into the integrity of the published data.[129]

Another well-described putative progenitor population isolated from the heart is the set of cardiosphere-derived cells (CDCs).[130] These cells are obtained by forming 3D cardiospheres from human heart tissue. In a small-scale phase I trial, CADUCEUS, autologous CDCs were delivered into patients with ischemic cardiomyopathy via intracoronary injection resulting in an improvement in systolic function.[131] However, Marban and coworkers have determined that paracrine effects rather than direct cardiomyogenesis underlie the benefit of CDCs.

A recent National Heart, Lung, and Blood Institute (NHLBI)-funded early phase trial (POSEIDON-HF) of bone marrow–derived

MYOCARDIAL EXTRACELLULAR MATRIX STRUCTURE AND COMPOSITION

The myocardial ECM contains a fibrillar collagen network, a basement membrane, proteoglycans and glycosaminoglycans, and bioactive signaling molecules. The myocardial fibrillar collagens, such as collagen types I and III, ensure the structural integrity of adjoining myocytes, provide the means by which myocyte shortening is translated into overall LV pump function, and are essential for maintaining the alignment of myofibrils within the myocyte through a collagen-integrin-cytoskeletal-myofibril relation.[38-42,55,56] While the fibrillar collagen matrix was initially considered to form a relatively static complex, it is now recognized that these structural proteins can undergo rapid degradation and fairly rapid turnover. Collagen fibril formation entails posttranslational modification. The carboxyterminal of the procollagen fibril is cleaved by a proteolytic reaction that results in a conformational change necessary for collagen fibril cross-linking and triple helix formation.[43] A critical step in the proper formation and structural orientation of the fibrillar collagen matrix is collagen cross-linking. Interruption of collagen cross-linking has been clearly demonstrated to alter myocardial ECM structure and in turn LV geometry and function.[44-46] Furthermore, alterations in fibrillar collagen cross-linking have been identified in myocardial samples taken from patients with end-stage HF.[29] While the newly formed, uncross-linked collagen fibrils are vulnerable to degradation, the triple helical collagen fiber is resistant to nonspecific proteolysis, and further degradation requires specific enzymatic cleavage. During collagen cross-link formation, the carboxyterminal peptide is released into the vascular space.[52,57] Collagen type I fiber formation results in the release of a 100-kDa procollagen type I carboxyterminal propeptide (PIP).[58,59] Similarly, the formation of mature collagen III fibers results in the release of a 42 kDa procollagen peptide (PIIIP).[53,58] As will be discussed, a number of associated proteins are necessary for the proper transport, assembly, and stability of the collagen fibril, and monitoring these collagen peptides and associated proteins has been demonstrated to provide diagnostic utility in terms of ECM remodeling and HF progression.

The integrins are a family of transmembrane proteins that serve multiple functions with respect to myocardial structure and function.[38,40,41] The integrins form the binding interface with proteins comprising the basement membrane and therefore directly influencing myocyte growth and geometry. Moreover, the integrins coalesce at important structural sites within the myocyte, called costameres, which are composed of cytoskeletal proteins, such as alpha-actinin and vinculin, which form a key intracellular support network for contractile protein assembly and maintaining sarcomeric alignment.[38,40,41,60,61] The myocyte costamere is also where the integrins appear to cluster and interdigitate with an intracellular signaling cascade system, such as focal adhesion kinase. Thus, disruptions of normal integrin–ECM interactions will likely result in significant changes in myocyte structure and function.

There are a number of extracellular proteins that comprise the basement membrane, such as collagen IV, fibronectin, and laminin. Thus, while fibrillar collagen has been the focus of most past studies, both basic and clinical, collagen is actually a modest component of the ECM. Thus, studies that evaluate both collagen content as well as other constituents of the ECM are beginning to emerge. For example, patients with DCM and mechanical assist devices demonstrate marked shifts in both fibrillar collagen and the basement membrane component, laminin.[62] Representative images from this study are shown in Fig. 4.1. It is the basement membrane that forms the anchoring points for the fibrillar matrix and contact points for other proteoglycans, such as chondroitin sulfate within the ECM. For example, the abundant binding of negatively charged unbranched glycosaminoglycans within chondroitin sulfate results in a molecule with a high osmotic activity.[63] Accordingly, changes in the content and distribution of these proteoglycan will affect hydration within the extracellular space, and in turn directly influence myocardial compliance characteristics. Moreover, these highly charged molecules within the ECM result in the formation of a hydrated gel that serves as a reservoir for signaling molecules and bioactive peptides. Therefore, the ECM is an important determinant of extracellular receptor–ligand interactions. Another important function of the myocardial ECM is that it serves as a reservoir for critical biological signaling molecules that regulate myocardial structure and function. For example, tumor necrosis factor (TNF) is initially a membrane-bound molecule that requires proteolytic processing and release into the interstitial space in order to form ligand complexes with cognate receptors.[54,64,65] Another example is transforming growth factor (TGF)-β, which exists in a latent form bound to the ECM, and requires proteolytic processing within the myocardial interstitium to become a competent signaling molecule.[66-68] TGF signaling produces multiple cellular responses—most importantly, the stimulation of ECM protein synthesis.[69-71] Thus, while this chapter will primarily focus upon the collagen fibrillar network, it is becoming recognized that the myocardial interstitium is a complex environment, which contains structural and signaling molecules that directly affect overall myocardial form and function.

THE MYOCARDIAL FIBROBLAST

The most abundant cell type within the LV myocardium is the fibroblast. This is the predominant cell type that is responsible for maintaining ECM homeostasis in terms of collagen synthesis and degradation. This does not imply that the fibroblast is operative in isolation, as significant biomechanical and bioactive signals between the cardiocyte-fibroblast and endothelial cell–fibroblast interactions likely dictate the rate and type of ECM synthesis and degradation. What appears to occur in disease states, whereby enhanced fibrosis and/or ECM remodeling occurs, is a significant change in the fibroblast phenotype. This process, whereby a significant population of phenotypically differentiated fibroblasts arises with ECM remodeling, can been termed as a transdifferentiation process, and the resultant cell type has been defined as the myofibroblast.[72-75] However, this does not imply that the normal fibroblast phenotype is extinguished, but rather there is likely increased proliferation of fibroblasts that do not express the myofibroblast phenotype. Thus, in ECM remodeling there is likely expansion and proliferation of both fibroblasts and myofibroblasts, which in turn will significantly affect the balance between collagen synthesis and degradation. In terms of myocardial ECM remodeling in HFrEF, changes in the synthesis-degradation axis occur, resulting in ECM instability (Fig. 4.2). In contrast, with HFpEF, robust expansion of myofibroblasts occurs, resulting in increased ECM synthesis and accumulation (see Fig. 4.2). The specific cell type of origin with respect to the myofibroblast remains unclear and may arise from a stem-cell type, pericyte, or a clonal expansion of endogenous fibroblasts. Whatever the case, the myofibroblast is not found in normal LV myocardium but is readily identifiable in the context of LV remodeling. The myofibroblast is typically identified through cellular constituents and by function.[72-75] Specifically, the mature myofibroblast expresses alpha smooth muscle actin (SMA), whereas normal fibroblasts do not. In addition, cultured myofibroblasts demonstrate much higher proliferation, margination, invasion, and ECM contractile behavior.

One of the more active areas of research in the cancer field is that of mesenchymal cell transdifferentiation (MET), whereby mesenchymal cells under control of the local environment will transdifferentiate

| Nonfailing | HFrEF | HFrEF-LVAD |

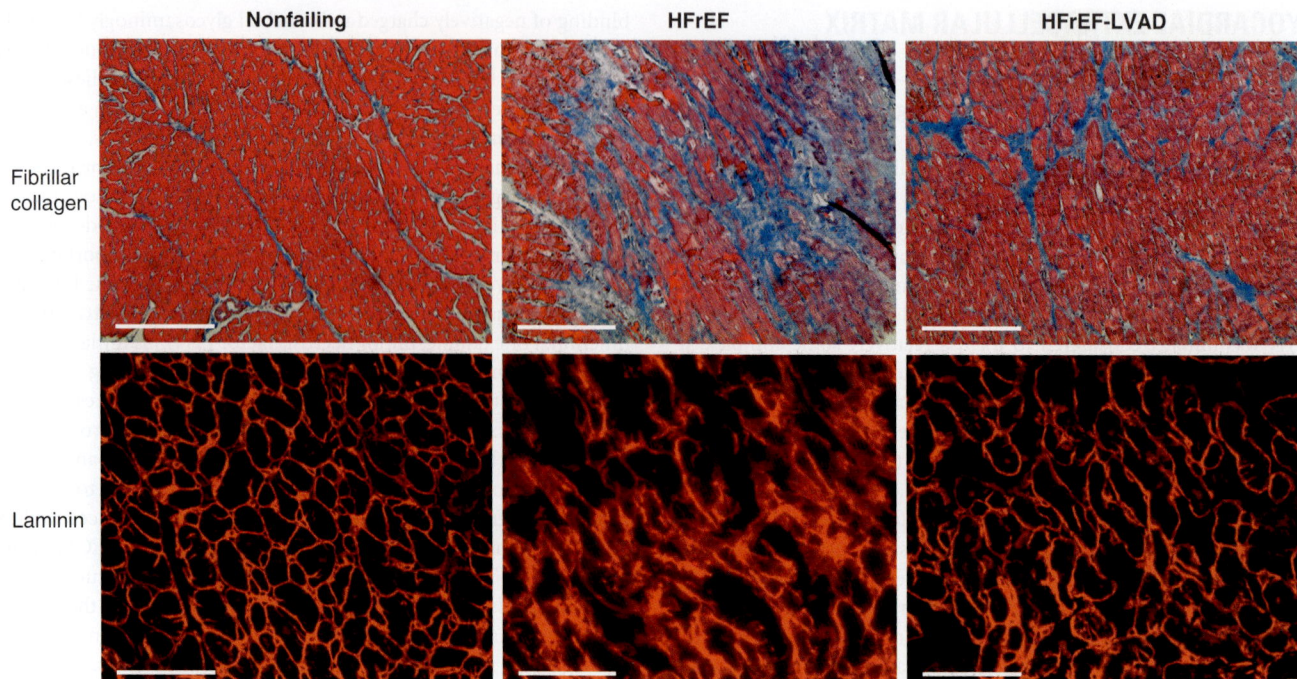

Fig. 4.1 Representative left ventricular *(LV)* sections taken from biopsies of nonfailing referent patients, patients with heart failure with reduced ejection fraction *(HFrEF)* dilated cardiomyopathy *(DCM)*, and HFrEF patients receiving LV assist devices *(LVAD)* with respect to histological changes in fibrillar collagen content *(top panels)* and laminin *(bottom panels)*. Histological staining for increased collagen accumulation ("fibrosis") is evident by the blue staining pattern and is increased with HFrEF and reduced with LVAD support. In terms of the basement membrane laminin, which plays a critical role in myocyte binding and transduction to the extracellular matrix (ECM), shifts in the relative distribution occurred with HFrEF and again with LVAD support. Thus, dynamic changes in both fibrillar collagen and other key constituents of the ECM occur with HFrEF, which are modifiable by mechanical support. Bars indicate 100 μm. From Sakamuri SS, Takawale A, Basu R, et al. Differential impact of mechanical unloading on structural and nonstructural components of the extracellular matrix in advanced human heart failure. *Transl Res.* 2016;172:30–44.

into a proliferative cancer type.[73,75] There are significant similarities in the signaling pathways that are evoked during this mesenchymal transdifferentiation process to that of fibroblast–myofibroblast transdifferentiation.[72-75] Since the myocardial fibroblast is a cell type of mesenchymal origin, it follows that the expression of specific transcription factors and cell markers would be operative similar to that of MET. There is compelling evidence to suggest that this fibroblast transdifferentiation is accompanied by an intermediate step or cell type, the proto-myofibroblast. This proto-myofibroblast will express unique cell markers, such as a splice variant of fibronectin—the extra-domain A (fibronectin ED-A).[72-75] What is clear is that the canonical thought that the fibroblast is a single phenotypic entity must be revisited, and changes in the type, proliferation, and function of sub populations of fibroblasts likely contribute to specific forms of ECM remodeling, and in turn will influence myocardial form and function with HF.

MYOCARDIAL EXTRACELLULAR MATRIX PROTEOLYTIC DEGRADATION: THE MATRIX METALLOPROTEINASES

The matrix metalloproteinase (MMP) are a diverse family of zinc-dependent proteases that play a role in normal ECM turnover as well as in pathological tissue remodeling processes.[25,26,47-51,76-84] Currently, over 25 distinct human MMPs have been identified and characterized. While initially thought to only cause ECM proteolysis, a highly diverse set of biological functions have been identified, which include cytokine processing and activation of pro-fibrotic signaling molecules.[25,26,50,51]

Moreover, MMP activity is highly dynamic within the human myocardial ECM. Specifically, using microdialysis techniques coupled with MMP fluorescent substrates, it has been identified that continuous MMP activity exists within the human myocardium under ambient conditions, which can increase significantly in a matter of seconds.[26] The MMPs were historically classified into sub groups based upon substrate specificity and/or structure, and an informal nomenclature for some of the individual MMPs arose from these initial substrate studies. However, there is significant overlap in MMP proteolytic substrates, and a more rigid numerical classification is now utilized. Important MMPs in the context of myocardial ECM remodeling include the collagenases, such as MMP-1 and MMP-13; the stromelysins/matrilysins, which include MMP-3/MMP-7; the gelatinases, which include MMP-9 and MMP-2; and the membrane-type MMPs (MT-MMPs). Taken together, once the MMPs are activated, these enzymes can degrade all ECM components; therefore it is important that the activity of these enzymes is kept under tight control and interaction.[48,85] The regulation of MMPs can take place at the level of transcription, posttranscription, posttranslation, and endogenous inhibition. These levels of control are briefly outlined in the next few paragraphs with examples of how this regulation is operative in the context of myocardial ECM remodeling.

Transcriptional Regulation of Extracellular Matrix Degradation; Matrix Metalloproteinase Polymorphisms

Transcriptional regulation of MMPs is primarily determined by upstream gene promoter activity whereby a number of intracellular signaling factors bind to specific sequences within the MMP promoter

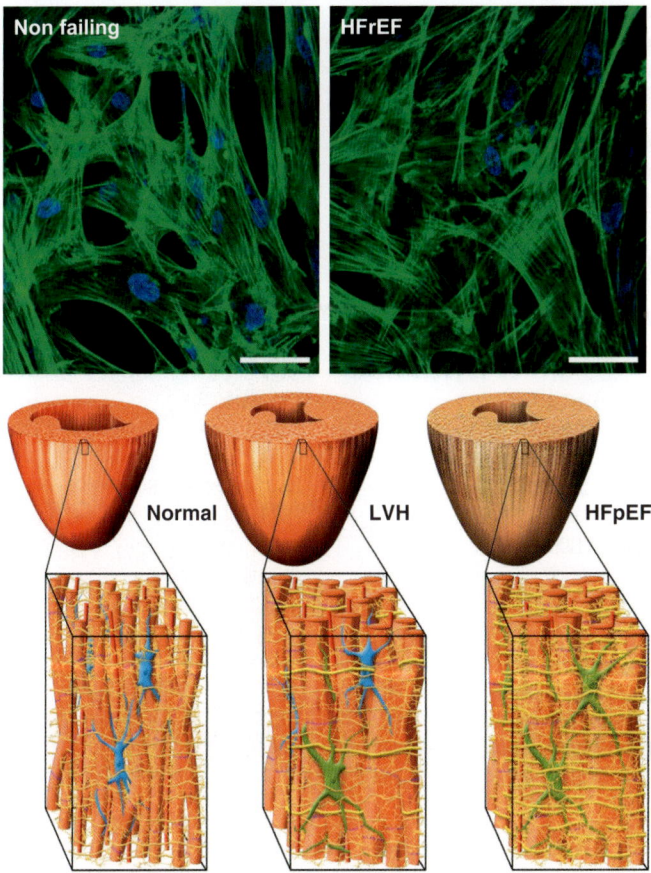

Fig. 4.2 *TOP*: In patients with heart failure with reduced ejection fraction *(HFrEF)*, in this case end-stage dilated cardiomyopathy requiring transplantation, left ventricular (LV) myocardial fibroblast growth patterns and phenotype were altered when compared to referent nonfailing LV biopsy specimens. [187] Bars indicate 25 µm. *BOTTOM*: In patients with LV hypertrophy *(LVH)*, fibroblast proliferation occurs but is also associated with shifts in myocardial fibroblast phenotype, as defined by patterns of cell surface and contractile protein markers. In heart failure with preserved ejection fraction *(HFpEF)* secondary to LVH, the emergence of this proliferative and differentiated fibroblast occurs and is associated with shifts in extracellular matrix synthetic and degradative pathways. Courtesy of Dr. Adam Hartstone-Rose, Cell Biology and Anatomy, University of South Carolina School of Medicine.

sequence. As such, there has been considerable interest in nucleic acid substitutions (i.e., polymorphisms) that occur within the MMP promoter regions and in relation to overall MMP levels, and most importantly in relation to cardiovascular outcomes. There have been a number of MMP polymorphisms identified in key MMP types, which include the collagenases (MMP-1, MMP-8), the gelatinases (MMP-2, MMP-9), and stromelysins (MMP-3). A brief synopsis of MMP polymorphisms with respect to cardiovascular remodeling processes and selected citations are provided in Table 4.1.[1-12,19-24,86-108] This summary table is by no means exhaustive but underscores the fact that several polymorphisms, primarily within the MMP promoter regions, have been identified and associated with subsets of patients at risk for cardiovascular events.

Several of the MMP types identified in Table 4.1 are associated with acute/chronic inflammation in that these proteases are expressed by inflammatory cells as well as being induced by mediators of inflammation, such as through cytokine signaling. For example, MMP-8 and MMP-9 are highly expressed by neutrophils and macrophages, and rapid

induction of these MMP types through inflammatory signaling pathways has been well established. Coronary artery disease, and more specifically vulnerable coronary plaques, has been associated with inflammation and local activation of MMP-9 and MMP-8. With respect to MMP-9, a variant has been identified, which is a single base substitution between cytosine (C) and thymidine (T).[2,3,90] The T allele results in a higher relative level of promoter activity when compared to the C allele. The presence of the MMP-9 T allele resulted in increased plasma levels of MMP-9.[90] A naturally occurring variant in the MMP-3 promoter region are the 5A and 6A alleles; the 5A allele has been associated with increased MMP-3 promoter activity, and in turn, increased relative MMP-3 protein levels.[4-8] In a study performed in over 2800 Japanese patients, the 5A polymorphism was associated with increased risk of MI, particularly in women.[6] Mizon-Gerad and colleagues reported that homozygosity for the 5A allele in patients with nonischemic cardiomyopathy was associated with poor survival.[3] In a preliminary clinical study, the addition of a guanine within the MMP-1 promoter region (-1607 1G/2G) was associated within an acceleration of adverse LV myocardial remodeling in patients post-MI.[9,10] With respect to MMP-8, increased local MMP-8 levels and polymorphisms within the MMP-8 promoter region have been identified with coronary plaque progression and acute events.[107,109] For example, Salminen and colleagues performed a genome-wide association study (GWAS) to that of plasma MMP-8 levels as well as overall cardiovascular events in a large cohort of patients.[109] These investigators identified that in certain subsets of patients, polymorphisms within the MMP-8 promoter region were associated with different plasma MMP-8 levels. Past studies have identified that polymorphisms within the MMP-9 promoter region would also result in higher plasma MMP-9 levels and in turn impart increased risk for cardiovascular events.[2,90] More importantly, however, Salminen and colleagues identified several important polymorphisms distal to that of MMP-8 itself using a GWAS approach: that of complement factor-H and in a specific member of the S100A family, both of which directly or indirectly may have influenced MMP-8 levels.[109] While this is an oversimplification, these findings add to the body of evidence regarding an inter relationship between inflammatory signaling pathways, MMP induction, and cardiovascular risk.

Past studies of MMP polymorphisms and cardiovascular risk have identified both gender and ethnicity as important independent confounding variables in predictive cardiovascular risk models.[19,87,107,110,111] Indeed, a past study reported that polymorphisms contained within the MMP-8 promoter region conferred increased risk for the progression of carotid artery disease, specifically in women.[107] In another study, the severity of carotid artery disease was most strongly associated with a common MMP-9 polymorphism (-1562T) in women.[19] With respect to ethnicity, specific MMP polymorphisms have been identified to confer increased risk of cardiovascular disease progression and cardiovascular events in Asians and in blacks of African descent.[87,111,112] For example, a polymorphism within the MMP-9 promoter is more frequent in African-Americans and is associated with higher MMP-9 plasma levels.[111,112] Since MMP-9 has been implicated to promote adverse cardiovascular remodeling, then this would imply a higher relative risk for disease progression with this MMP-9 polymorphism.

Specific MMP polymorphisms confer additive risk for cardiovascular events in subjects with other risk factors, such as diabetes and obesity.[111,113] For example, MMP-9 polymorphisms identified in patients with metabolic syndrome appear to be synergistic with respect to cardiovascular events.[70] Of potentially greater significance, MMP-2 and MMP-9 polymorphisms, which have been associated with cardiovascular disease progression (**see** Table 4.1), have been more commonly identified in childhood obesity.[114,115] While remaining speculative, these MMP polymorphisms may confer an increased risk for adverse

TABLE 4.1   Polymorphisms in Matrix Metalloproteinase Promoters

Polymorphism	Biologic Effect	Clinical Association	References
MMP-9			
-1562 C/T	Promoter activity	Post-MI remodeling	1, 2, 19–22, 87, 90
		Remodeling in DCM	3
-279 R/Q	Catalytic activity	Remodeling in DCM	1, 3
		Risk of post-MI remodeling	86, 91
		Differing pharmacologic response in CVD	88
	Promoter Activity	CAD	86, 101
		TAA/AAA	100, 103
MMP-2			
-790 T/G	Transcription factor binding	CAD, HF, CVD, HTN, TAA	23, 24, 92–94
MMP-3			
1171-5A/6A	Promoter activity	Post-MI remodeling	4-7, 11, 22, 87, 96
1612-5A/6A		MVP	97
		Remodeling in DCM	4, 89
	Promoter	CAD	100, 104
		HTN	104
		AAA	105, 106
MMP-1			
-1607 1G/2G	Transcription factor binding	Risk of post-MI remodeling, HF, CVA	9, 10, 89, 108
-519-340 A/G-C/T	Promoter activity	Risk of post-MI remodeling, BAV	12, 98, 99
MMP-8			
	Promoter	CVD	107
		TAA	107
MMP-12			
	Promoter	CVD	88

AAA, Abdominal aortic aneurysm; *CAD*, coronary artery disease; *CVA*, cerebrovascular accident; *CVD*, cardiovascular disease; *DCM*, dilated cardiomyopathy; *HTN*, hypertension; *MI*, myocardial infarction; *MVP*, mitral valve prolapse; *TAA*, thoracic aortic aneurysm.

cardiovascular remodeling at a much younger age. In a robust sample size of hypertensive patients (>42,000), Tanner and colleagues identified interactions between antihypertensive agents to that of MMP-9 and MMP-12 polymorphisms and subsequent cardiovascular events.[88] This suggests that identifying specific MMP polymorphisms, particularly in more vulnerable patient populations, may provide additional guidance for specific pharmacotherapy. For example, MMP-1 polymorphisms have been shown to provide additive prognostic value in patients with acute coronary syndromes, and thus may identify a subset of patients for more intensive pharmacotherapy.[98] Of course, simple sequence substitutions within the MMP gene or the promoter region provide only a partial picture into the complex regulation of MMPs within the cardiovascular system. Nevertheless, there is growing evidence that polymorphisms that affect MMP transcriptional control may play a critical role in how these proteases contribute to cardiovascular remodeling and, ultimately, cardiovascular outcomes.

Matrix Metalloproteinase Posttranscriptional Regulation

Posttranscriptional events are directly influenced by small noncoding RNA molecules (**see also Chapter 2**) termed microRNAs (miRs). miRs can bind to mRNA and interfere with the initiation of translation and/or accelerate mRNA degradation. As depicted in Fig. 4.3, it is becoming apparent that specific miRs will cause posttranscriptional alterations in functional clusters of proteins that would be relevant to LV remodeling and to the ECM in particular. Largely utilizing mouse models of MI and aortic constriction, preclinical studies have investigated the effects of specific miRs, as well as the associated mechanisms on ECM remodeling and myocardial fibrosis. For example, miR-328 was found to upregulate TGF-beta and increase fibrillary collagen deposition.[116] Other miRs, such as miR-19b, advance myocardial fibrosis by promoting fibroblast proliferation and migration.[117] Furthermore, miR-21 and miR-155 are among a subset of miRs that contribute to fibrosis by both increasing profibrotic growth factors and promoting fibroblast survival.[118-122] Conversely, a robust group of miRs, such as miR-29,[123,124] miR-214,[125,126] or miR-133,[127-130] have been associated with antifibrotic outcomes. However, there are not always clear categorical distinctions between pro- and antifibrotic miRs. For instance, miR-15 has been observed to influence all of the aforementioned pathways.[131,132] As the complex relationships between miRs and LV remodeling have become better understood, the clinical potential of miRs in cardiovascular disease has become apparent as well.

Clinical studies are demonstrating the prognostic potential of these miRs to identify those patients at increased risk for HF and to diagnose HF and monitor disease progression. miRs can be actively transported into the interstitial space,[133] and thus, a pool of miRs exist within the ECM. These miRs can egress to the systemic circulation allowing for detection in patient plasma. For example, miR-34a

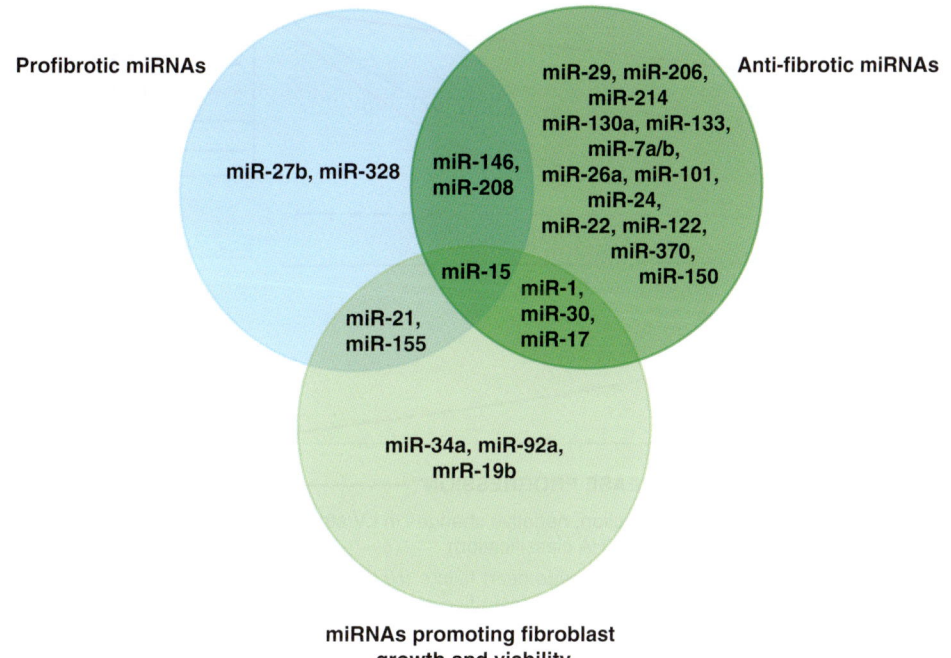

Fig. 4.3 A Venn diagram depiction of microRNAs *(miRs)* and functional domains relevant to extracellular matrix remodeling. A number of these miRs cross over to more than one generalized functional domain and is reflective of the fact that miRs have more than one target sequence. The miRs designated herein have been identified from the published literature (PubMed Search, March 2017) and a number of these references have been cited in the text.

promotes fibroblast survival, and plasma levels can predict patient development of ischemic HF after an MI.[134] In patients with chronic HFrEF and HFpEF, the temporal trends of miR-22 correlated with the composite primary outcome of HF hospitalization, cardiovascular mortality, cardiac transplant, or LV assist device placement.[135] Additionally, miR concentrations in the plasma of patients with various etiologies of HF have been screened against those in healthy controls to detect miR patterns unique to HF. From these studies, miR-21 was identified as being consistently upregulated in the plasma of HFrEF patients and can make a diagnosis of HFrEF with high sensitivity and specificity.[136-140] miR-21,[140] along with miR-208[141] and miR-1,[137] also correlate with measurements of disease severity and may aid in identification of disease progression. These trends are further depicted graphically in Fig. 4.4.

Similar screening studies have compared plasma miRs in patients with HFrEF to those in patients with HFpEF. Beber et al. reported that co-testing of five miRs present in the plasma could distinguish between HFrEF and HFpEF.[94] Included in this group of miRs are three that are known to regulate ECM remodeling: miR-30, miR-146, and miR-328.[142] Patterns in HFrEF and HFpEF of these and additional miRs involved in ECM remodeling are presented in Table 4.2. The discovery that miRs can influence ECM remodeling in patients with HFrEF and HFpEF has led to efforts to harness the potential of miR expression as a therapeutic. This concept has been investigated in mouse models of aortic constriction[123] and hypertension.[124] Overexpression of the antifibrotic miR-29 decreased LV fibrosis,[123] and reduced expression of profibrotic mediators such as TGF beta.[124] miR-214 has also been implicated as a potential therapeutic as infusion in angiotensin II treated mice attenuated cardiac fibrosis[125] and decreased the expression of TGF beta and fibrillary collagen in mouse models of acute MI.[126] Additionally, transgenic overexpression of miR-133 in mice undergoing transverse aortic

constriction improved myocardial fibrosis as well as diastolic dysfunction.[128] Translating these concepts from animal models to clinical research has the potential to introduce a novel strategy for treating both HFrEF and HFpEF.

Matrix Metalloproteinase Posttranslational Regulation

While the level of MMP synthesis is an important determinant of matrix degradation, the true degradative capacity of the MMPs is dependent upon the activation of the MMP pro-enzyme. After being synthesized in a latent, pro-enzyme, or zymogen form, the MMPs are secreted into the extracellular space. In order for MMP zymogen activation to occur, a sequence of proteolytic events must take place. Thus, an important control point or MMP activity is proteolytic cleavage by other enzymes (e.g., serine proteases and other MMP species), or by exposure to certain physical and chemical effectors.[48,49,85] It has been demonstrated that serine proteases, such as plasmin, can generate active MMPs. In addition, MMP activation can also occur at the cell surface involving the MT-MMPs.[143,151] At the cell membrane, MT-MMP is already in an active state, so it can then activate other MMP species at the cell surface. It has been clearly established that MT1-MMP activates MMP-2, and in fact may be the predominant pathway for MMP-2 activation.[144-150] Moreover, it appears that a very wide proteolytic portfolio for MT1-MMP exists, which would imply that this MMP type may participate in a number of enzymatic and signaling cascades within the myocardial ECM. [25,50,51] This is likely to hold particular relevance since robust levels of MT1-MMP have been identified within both experimental and clinical forms of HF.[28,34,151-154]

Endogenous Matrix Metalloproteinase Inhibition

Another important control point of MMP activity is in the inhibition of the activated enzyme by the action of a group of specific

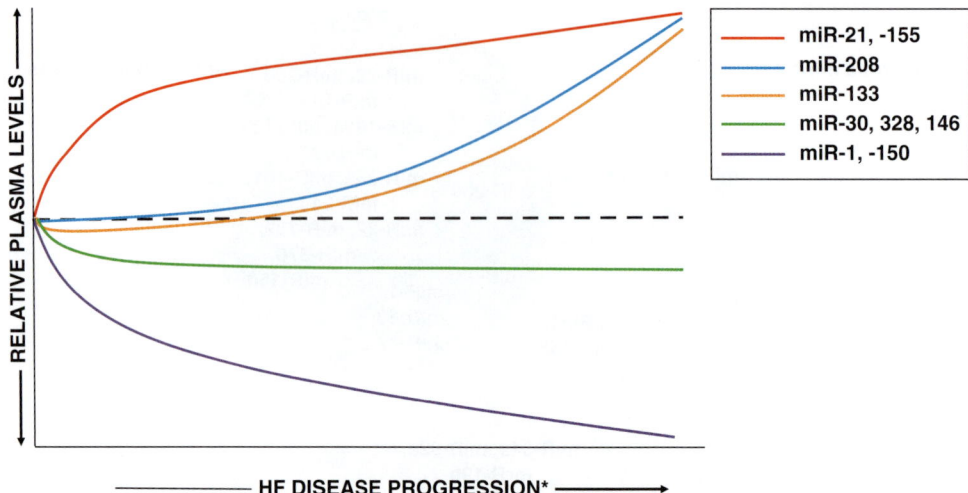

(*as defined by decline in ejection fraction, negative changes in LV structure, and worsening NYHA classification)

Fig. 4.4 Schematic of the relationship between heart failure *(HF)* progression and changes in plasma levels for specific microRNAs *(miRs)* that have been identified to regulate key pathways in extracellular matrix *(ECM)* remodeling. It is notable that certain miRs that can modulate pro-fibrotic pathways actually fall with HF progression, indicating that increased transcription of ECM proteins and signaling molecules likely occur. Thus, unlike classical biomarker profiles, which most often rise as a function of disease progression, a relative fall in plasma levels for certain miRs may hold relevant prognostic as well as mechanistic insight into adverse ECM remodeling with HF. In addition, the pattern and time course of these changes in plasma miRs may be specific to HF phenotype, and examples of this are shown in Table 4.2. *LV*, Left ventricular. Schematic produced from data reported from references 1–10, 86–90, 116–142, 245, 256.

MMP inhibitors, termed tissue inhibitors of matrix metalloproteinases (TIMPs).[47-49,76,77,84] There are four known TIMP species of which TIMP-1 and TIMP-2 are the best characterized. The TIMPs are low-molecular-weight proteins that can complex noncovalently with high efficiency to MMPs in a 1:1 molar ratio. Therefore, these inhibitory proteins are an important endogenous system for regulating MMP activity in vivo. While the TIMPs are expressed in a variety of cells, TIMP-4 shows a high level of expression in cardiovascular tissue.[155,156] While a predominant characteristic of the TIMPs is in the inhibition of active enzymes, this is likely to be an overly simplistic view of the function of these proteins. For example, studies have demonstrated TIMPs to be involved in the process of MMP activation, to exhibit growth factor–like properties, and to participate in apoptosis.[157-160] For example, the over-expression of TIMP-1, -2, -3, -4 was induced in murine myocardial fibroblasts by adenoviral mediated transduction.[158] In this study, a number of differential biological effects were observed by TIMP induction, which included the effects on collagen synthesis and apoptosis. These effects were not due to MMP inhibition since pharmacological MMP inhibition did not recapitulate these effects; therefore this indicated a direct action of TIMPs on fibroblast function. Moreover, TIMP-specific effects were observed in which TIMP-2 caused a robust increase in collagen synthesis, whereas TIMP-3 accelerated fibroblast apoptosis. Using transgenic constructs, differential effects of TIMP-3 have been observed in terms of LV remodeling and progression to HF, whether due to MI or pressure overload.[62,161] More recent studies have identified that delivering a recombinant TIMP-3 post-MI can reduce adverse ECM remodeling and the progression of LV failure.[162,163] These results underscore the highly diverse and complex nature of these TIMPs that exists within the myocardial interstitium and not only holds potential diagnostic/prognostic potential but also therapeutic relevance.

HEART FAILURE WITH REDUCED EJECTION FRACTION AND EXTRACELLULAR MATRIX REMODELING—MYOCARDIAL INFARCTION (SEE ALSO CHAPTERS 34 AND 19)

A prolonged ischemic event, with or without reperfusion, causes a cascade of biological events that can be considered a wound-healing process and thus the canonical phases of wound healing are often utilized, which consist of three overlapping phases: inflammation, proliferation, and maturation. The first phase is the acute period in which reactive oxygen species, bioactive signaling molecules, and peptides released from the local environment cause inflammatory cell recruitment and invasion. The initiation of the inflammatory phase is likely due to the release of molecules as a result of myocyte death, and in turn induce the expression of cytokines, such as TNF alpha and the interleukins. A more comprehensive examination of cell viability and inflammation are found elsewhere in this text. Some key aspects of the early post-MI inflammatory process include: (a) activation of the intracellular transduction pathway, nuclear factor kappa B; (b) induction of a diverse family of chemokines; and (c) neutrophil recruitment and margination. While initially considered a rather monochromatic cell type in terms of form and function, the macrophages within the MI region appear to be quite heterogeneous and may ultimately influence the magnitude and direction of the localized inflammatory process.[164-168] While this inflammatory process is critical to initiate a reparative response following myocardial injury, it appears that unlike other sites of tissue injury, the inflammatory response is prolonged within the MI region. The second phase is heralded by proliferation and transdifferentiation of myocardial fibroblasts into myofibroblasts.[169,170] Further, released matrix structural proteins, such as fibrillar collagens, and matrix–integrin–cytoskeletal interactions facilitate contraction of the wound. The

TABLE 4.2 Plasma miR Patterns in Heart Failure With Reduced Ejection Fraction and Heart Failure With Preserved Ejection Fraction in Extracellular Matrix Remodeling

miR	Effect	Pattern in HFrEF	Pattern in HFpEF	Citations
miR-21	Fibroblast survival and growth, ECM deposition	Increased, correlated with disease severity	Increased	46, 52, 53, 55, 57–60, 152, 153, 177
miR-155	Fibroblast proliferation and inflammation, collagen deposition	Increased	?	61, 72
miR-208	Regulate collagen deposition	Increased in end stage HFrEF	?	29, 30, 56, 75
miR-133	Reduce collagen expression and cardiomyocytes apoptosis	Decreased after cardiac injury, increased in end stage HFrEF	?	56
miR-30	Decrease collagen deposition and regulate apoptosis	Decreased	Decreased	31, 63, 76
miR-328	Regulate profibrotic pathways	Decreased	Decreased	76
miR-146	Regulate collagen deposition	Decreased	Decreased	27, 28, 76
miR-1	Reduce ECM deposition	Decreased, correlated with disease severity	?	70, 71, 153
miR-150	Inhibit activation of cardiac fibroblasts	Decreased in end stage HFrEF	?	73

ECM, Extracellular matrix; *HFpEF,* heart failure with preserved ejection fraction; *HFrEF,* heart failure with reduced ejection fraction; *miR,* microRNA.

third phase of the wound-healing process normally results in complete contraction of the wound, apoptosis of the myofibroblasts, and the formation of a relatively acellular scar. However, in the context of post-MI remodeling, this canonical set of events does not necessarily occur. Rather, there is a continued proliferation and transdifferentiation of fibroblasts within the MI and border regions accompanied by a shift in matrix proliferative/degradative pathways within these transformed cells.

Significant changes within the ECM occur during all time points post-MI and likely contribute to the overall adverse LV remodeling process.[41,171-174] First, the inflammatory response causes the release of MMPs as well as other proteases to degrade the ECM and allow for margination of inflammatory cells.[174-176] However, with a persistent inflammatory state, MMP induction will also destabilize the newly formed ECM and the nascent scar. Second, the continued proliferation and altered expression of myofibroblasts within the MI region in terms of the balance between MMP and TIMP levels cause ECM instability and infarct expansion. Specifically, the transformed fibroblast population within the MI region likely results in a shift in the relative balance of MMPs and TIMPs,[177,178] favoring accelerated ECM turnover and the failure of mature scar formation.[177-179] Third, a robust expression of "profibrotic" signaling molecules occurs within the myofibroblasts and the residual myocyte populations, such as TGF, but this does not result in a well-formed ECM.[150,166,180] Specifically, TGF signaling is enhanced within the MI region and causes significantly higher fibrillar collagen transcription;[150,167,181] however, a number of critical posttranslational events involving collagen assembly are likely to be defective.[180] For example, a loss of the matricellular protein, secreted protein acidic and rich in cysteine (SPARC), which is involved in procollagen processing to a mature collagen fibril, resulted in impaired collagen maturation and MI scar formation.[182] Further, the interactions of the glycoproteins fibronectin and tenascin C may directly alter cell–ECM interactions, whereby other bioactive molecules, such as osteopontin, can directly influence ECM biosynthesis through a number of signaling pathways. Transmembrane receptors and co-receptors, such as endoglin and syndecan, which can modify profibrotic signaling through TGF and other growth factors, also likely play an important role not only in ECM synthesis and degradation but also in terms of myofibroblast transformation. Thus, abnormalities in fibroblast phenotype coupled with defects in both ECM synthesis and degradation pathways possibly converge to cause a feed-forward

process in terms of MI wall thinning and dyskinesis, increased radial wall stress, and local strain patterns, and ultimately contribute to overall infarct expansion, LV remodeling, and HFrEF. These pathways and processes, as they may relate to the prognosis and diagnosis of HFrEF, are presented in a subsequent section.

HEART FAILURE WITH REDUCED EJECTION FRACTION AND EXTRACELLULAR MATRIX REMODELING-DILATED CARDIOMYOPATHY (SEE ALSO CHAPTER 20)

DCM constitutes a broad classification of primary myocardial disease states, which contribute to a significant proportion of patients with HFrEF, and several chapters within this text examine in detail the several animal models of DCM that have identified increased MMPs within the myocardium.[32-34,183,184] In the rapid pacing DCM model, increased abundance of several MMP types occurred, with a loss of ECM structural integrity that coincided with the onset of LV remodeling and dilatation.[33,34] Moreover, these changes in MMP myocardial levels and LV geometry preceded significant alterations in cardiomyocyte contractile function, which underscored the functional importance of MMP-mediated ECM disruption as an early event in this model of DCM. More definitive cause–effect relationships between LV myocardial remodeling and MMP induction have been established through the use of pharmacological MMP inhibitors.[32,34] For example, MMP inhibition in the pacing DCM model attenuated the degree of LV dilation and dysfunction.[32] In the canine model of ischemic DCM, pharmacological MMP inhibition attenuated the progression of LV dilation and systolic dysfunction.[133] Thus, a contributory mechanism for the LV remodeling that occurs during the experimental form of DCM is MMP induction and heightened MMP activity within the LV myocardium.

A number of studies have examined relative MMP and TIMP expression in end-stage human DCM.[27-31] Uniformly, these past studies have demonstrated an increase in certain MMP species in end-stage human HF. One of the first studies was by Gunja-Smith and colleagues in which increased myocardial MMP gelatinolytic activity was reported in DCM.[29] Using immunoblotting procedures, subsequent studies identified that several MMP species were increased in LV myocardial extracts taken from patients with end-stage DCM.[27,28]

For example, increased MMP-3 and MMP-9 levels were observed in the DCM myocardial extracts. While MMP-13 was barely detected in the normal myocardium, a robust immunoreactive signal for MMP-13 was observed in DCM myocardium.[28] Interestingly, MMP-13 has been associated with pathological remodeling states, such as breast carcinomas.[185,186] The most robust change in MMP types within the DCM myocardium was that of MT1-MMP.[28] A persistent induction and expression of MT1-MMP occurred in DCM fibroblasts when compared to myocardial fibroblasts harvested from nonfailing patients.[187] Li et al. provided evidence to suggest that changes in the MMP/TIMP stoichiometric ratio occurred with end-stage DCM disease.[30] In DCM, an absolute reduction in MMP-1/TIMP-1 complex formation has been observed.[28] In a transgenic model of TIMP-3 deletion, a DCM phenotype was reported as a function of age.[161] In DCM patients, chronic unloading of the LV through the use of ventricular assist devices was associated with a reduction in LV chamber dilation and myocardial MMP levels.[35] Taken together, these results suggest that reduced MMP/TIMP complex formation may occur in cardiomyopathic disease states, which in turn would contribute to increased myocardial MMP activity and ECM remodeling.

Heart Failure With Reduced Ejection Fraction and Extracellular Matrix Remodeling—Hypertensive Heart Disease (see also Chapter 25)

The fundamental milestone in the development and progression of HFpEF is that of concentric LV hypertrophy, which is due to accelerated growth of both the myocyte and ECM compartments. The stimulus for LV hypertrophy is that of a prolonged pressure overload, which can arise as a function of hypertension, aortic stenosis, and arterial stiffening as a utility of age.[28-30,55,56] While LV hypertrophy is initially an appropriate adaptive response, continued myocyte growth and expansion of the ECM will eventually lead to fundamental defects in LV diastolic performance. The physiology and pathophysiology of diastolic performance and clinical considerations of HFpEF are the subjects of a subsequent chapter. While a number of active and passive properties of the myocardium are altered in HFpEF, a predominant determinant is changes in ECM structure and content. Specifically, increased fibrillar collagen content as well as the accumulation of other nonstructural ECM proteins are invariable structural events in progressive LV hypertrophy and diastolic dysfunction. The continuous and potentially accelerated accumulation collagen within the ECM will reduce LV myocardial compliance and thereby impair the passive LV filling phase of diastole, and present as a resistance to flow with atrial contraction.[188-191] The summation of these changes in both myocyte and ECM structure and function with progressive LV hypertrophy is a rise in LV filling pressures and, by extension, increased pulmonary capillary wedge pressure (PCWP). The increased PCWP will in turn contribute to higher pulmonary venous pressures and ultimately yield two of the more consistent and severe symptoms associated with HFpEF: exercise intolerance and pulmonary congestion.[171,192-194] Finally, with persistently increased LV stiffness (both active and passive) and a higher PCWP, left atrial (LA) enlargement occurs, and thus measures of atrial size can also be indicative of worsening LV diastolic function and progression of HFpEF. Clinical studies have demonstrated that both direct and indirect measurements of ECM remodeling, particularly myocardial collagen accumulation, are directly related to increased PCWP as well as LA volumes.[171,188-194]

As shown in Fig. 4.2, key changes in ECM structure and function include fibroblast proliferation/transdifferentiation as well as fibrillar collagen accumulation. In pressure overload secondary to aortic stenosis, the significant myocardial collagen accumulation was associated with a concomitant increase in relative myocardial TIMP levels.[195,196]

Experimental studies support the concept that diminished myocardial MMP activity can facilitate collagen accumulation in developing hypertrophy.[197,198] In the spontaneously hypertensive rat, the development of compensated hypertrophy is associated with increased myocardial TIMP levels, which would imply reduced MMP activity.[197,198] The changes in myocardial MMP activation is likely to be time dependent and may not be constant throughout the development of pressure overload hypertrophy.[199] Furthermore, the utilization of a microdialysis method to directly measure MMP interstitial activity demonstrated that MMP activity was reduced as a function of LV afterload.[37] In a large animal model of progressive aortic stenosis that recapitulated features of HFpEF, changes were induced in MMP and TIMP profiles, which would favor ECM accumulation.[200] In a murine model of LV pressure overload, genetic deletion of MMP-2 reduced the degree of myocardial fibrillar collagen accumulation and improved the indices of LV diastolic function.[201] Since the primary mechanism for conversion of pro-MMP-2 to active MMP-2 is through complex formation with MT1-MMP, the induction of this MMP type may be pivotal in the changes in ECM structure and content that occur in HFpEF.[85,202-204] MT1-MMP expression is sensitive to changes in mechanical load, whereby increased wall tension proliferated MT1-MMP promoter activity in vitro.[175] Increased myocardial MT1-MMP expression has been identified in patients with LV pressure overload.[205] In animal models of LV pressure overload, an early and sustained induction of MT1-MMP has been identified.[176,200,206] For example, increased MT1-MMP promoter activity, and subsequently MT1-MMP proteolytic activity, has been reported following the induction of LV pressure overload in mice.[176] The pathways by which MT1-MMP contributes to adverse ECM remodeling likely include facilitating proteolysis of interstitial molecules directly (such as integrins), amplification of active MMP-2 causing ECM instability, and abnormal architecture, as well as through enhancing profibrotic signaling pathways. Specifically, an important proteolytic relationship possibly exists between MT1-MMP and the subsequent activation of the profibrotic signaling molecule TGF,[85,172,175,176,200,201,206,207] which would hold particular relevance in the context of LV pressure overload. Competent signaling of TGF requires release from a latency-bound state, binding to the TGF receptor complex, and induction of the transduction elements-Smads. TGF activation through Smads not only will induce fibrillar collagen expression, but also will facilitate fibroblast transformation/transdifferentiation. Thus, a likely important proteolytic interaction exists between certain MMP types, such as MT1-MMP, and the TGF signaling axis in terms of ECM accumulation and the progression to HFpEF.

While certain MMP types, such as MMP-2 and MT1-MMP, appear to be uniformly increased with LV pressure overload, other MMP types, such as the interstitial collagenase MMP-13, have been reported to be decreased.[79,196] Other MMP types, such as MMP-1 and MMP-3, appear to be either unchanged or reduced with LV pressure overload.[79,85,173,174,189,196,205,208] Interestingly, transgenic expression of human MMP-1 in mice (this MMP type is absent in rodents) and induction of LV pressure overload resulted in a relative reduction in myocardial fibrillar collagen content and improved indices of LV function.[209] These findings suggest that the loss of normal constitutive levels of certain MMP types, or failure of an induction of certain MMP types with LV pressure overload, may facilitate abnormal ECM accumulation and adverse myocardial remodeling. This process does not occur in isolation, and key matricellular proteins and signaling molecules, such as thrombospondin and osteopontin, are also likely to play a key role in abnormal ECM composition with LV pressure overload and progression to HFpEF. These determinants of ECM regulation with HFpEF are examined further in the context of diagnostic/prognostic potential.

MYOCARDIAL EXTRACELLULAR MATRIX REMODELING IN HEART FAILURE—DIAGNOSTIC POTENTIAL

Chapter 33 has been dedicated to biomarker profiling and HF, and thus the focus herein will be to examine specific biomarkers that hold relevance to ECM remodeling, with particular attention to those that hold diagnostic/prognostic potential. In terms of plasma biomarker profiling with HFrEF and a post-MI etiology, plasma troponin levels and other biomarkers are obviously relevant; thus it is likely that a specific portfolio of ECM biomarkers will provide specific prognostic information in the post-MI period. For example, past studies have demonstrated that increased plasma levels of collagen peptide fragments occur following MI and in progressive HFrEF.[188,210-212] In keeping with ECM degradation, the induction of ECM proteases, such as the MMPs, occur in patients following MI and likely hold predictive value in terms of identifying those patients at greatest risk for the early development of HFrEF.[188,212-217] For example, the magnitude of plasma MMP-9 levels that occur within the early post-MI period is associated with a greater degree of LV dilation at 6 months post-MI.[214] In a study by Wagner and colleagues, the early increase in MMP-9 levels was associated with an increased risk of the later development of HF (odds ratio of 6.5).[213] In a recent report that compiled the results from approximately 60 studies in patients post-MI,[218] those that were most consistently present in prediction models included indices of neurohormonal activation, such as brain natriuretic peptide and indices of ECM degradation, such as MMP-9.[212] Cytokine/chemokine release that would cause the induction of pathways relevant to ECM degradation and fibroblast transformation, as well as the release of matrikines, all occur in patients in the post-MI period.[219-223] Other matrix-related molecules, such as galectin-3, have been associated with determinants of ECM remodeling but are not necessarily independently predictive of HFrEF.[224-226] In addition to plasma biomarkers for ECM degradation, increased markers for ECM synthesis have also been identified, which include the TGF co-receptor endoglin and the matrikines tenascin-C, osteopontin, and syndecan-4.[227-232] In large survey studies that included subjects with MI and DCM, plasma levels of MMPs and TIMPs have provided clear prognostic information with respect to cardiovascular events and mortality.[233-236] Finally, plasma profiling of these determinants of ECM remodeling may hold value as both a diagnostic and a therapeutic predictor, that is, theragnostic. For example, retrospective plasma samples taken from HFrEF patients with a 12-month follow-up after cardiac resynchronization therapy (CRT) identified that TIMP-1 levels may hold predictive value in terms of CRT response.[237]

Since the ECM likely plays a critical role in the pathophysiology of HFpEF, strategies that can evaluate and quantify changes in this entity hold prognostic relevance. A summary of representative plasma biomarkers that have been evaluated in the context of HFpEF that may hold relevance to ECM remodeling is presented in Table 4.3. For example, plasma profiles of peptide fragments of fibrillar collagens (types I and III) have been used in patients with developing and established HFpEF.[189,192-194,219,238] The collagen fibril may undergo posttranslational modification by enzyme mediated cross-link reactions as well as nonenzyme mediated cross-link formation. Of note, nonenzymatic cross-link formation can be mediated by advanced glycation end products (AGEs).[239,240] AGEs bind to specific cell membrane receptors that include the receptor for AGE (RAGE). Since increased fibrillar collagen stability can occur through increased RAGE interactions, profiling plasma levels of soluble RAGE (sRAGE) as well as indices of AGE formation may hold prognostic/functional relevance in HFpEF.[239,240] A biologically relevant consequence of increased collagen AGEs is reduced susceptibility to MMP-mediated degradation and turnover. Significant and directional changes in the plasma profiles of MMPs and TIMPs occur in patients with developing HFpEF and have been shown to hold potential prognostic utility.[79,208,241,242] For example, a specific cassette of MMPs and TIMPs, coupled with N-terminal pro b-type natriuretic peptide (NT-BNP), provided significant prediction in terms of patients at risk for the development of HFpEF.[208] Other ECM chemokines/matrikines, such as cardiotrophin, have been associated with the development and progression of HFpEF.[243-245] It is notable that the recent American Heart Association scientific position statement regarding the use of biomarkers for HFpEF identified a number of ECM-related proteins and pathways, which are those prominently identified in Table 4.3.[246]

Imaging

While plasma profiling changes in determinants of ECM structure and function likely hold diagnostic and prognostic relevance in terms of HF progression, advanced imaging approaches that target the ECM also will likely play an important role in providing mechanistic insight into this process. Cardiac imaging in HF is a focus of other chapters within this text, but important advances in imaging relevant to ECM remodeling and HF progression will be briefly discussed here. First is specific three-dimensional imaging of the ECM using advanced microscopy methods. Second is continued advancements and refinements of LV imaging, such as cardiac magnetic resonance imaging (cMRI) and that of hybrid computed tomography (CT) and single-photon emission computed tomography (SPECT/CT). Some examples of each of these approaches, which continue to provide new insight into the complex nature of the myocardial ECM, is presented in the following paragraphs.

In the majority of past studies examining the ECM in cardiac disease states, the focus has been on the quantitation of fibrillar collagen content. This is most commonly performed by histochemical or biochemical methods, and while informative, it does not provide a comprehensive evaluation of the ECM in terms of nonfibrillar collagen composition as well as a more detailed analysis of ECM structure. In terms of the latter, an approach that has been advanced and continues to be refined is that of second harmonic generation (SHG) microscopy.[247,248] SHG imaging provides a method to examine more closely the three-dimensional architecture of the fibrillary collagen matrix through optical sectioning. The SHG signal is generated by photons interacting with the tight alignment of the repeating structures found within the triple helices of fibrillary collagen.[247] The second harmonic wave produced in this manner can then be analyzed with respect to collagen fibril alignment, fiber angles, and other parameters that cannot be examined using conventional histochemistry and histological sectioning. As an example, Fig. 4.5 presents porcine referent normal and post-MI optical sections using three-dimensional stacking and subsequent analysis using SHG. This porcine MI model has been described previously, which produces a uniform LV anterior MI,[162] and the LV sections shown are at 4 weeks post-MI. While significant accumulation of fibrillar collagen within the MI region was evident, using SHG moved beyond simple collagen content assessment and demonstrated a shift in the alignment and distribution of the collagen network within the MI region. While fibrillar collagen can impart significant resistance to deformation, the biophysical properties of the collagen network are dependent upon the highly organized helical structure of the mature collagen fibril. Thus, while collagen accumulation or "fibrosis" has occurred at this late post-MI time point, the uniform architecture found in normal myocardium is lost and as such will alter mechanical properties accordingly. The assessment of the ECM using these optical imaging and processing algorithms will likely not only yield new insight into the structure of this myocardial entity, but also provide for potentially novel therapeutic targets.

TABLE 4.3 Plasma Profiles of Determinants of Extracellular Matrix Remodeling in Patients With Heart Failure With Persevered Ejection Fraction

Subjects (n)	Biomarker (s)	Primary Observation	References
156	MMP-1, TIMP-1, PINP	TIMP-1 levels were highest in patients with elevated PCWP, whereas relative MMP-1 levels were lower and PINP levels higher	192
171	PICP, PINP, CITP, PIIINP, MMP-1, MMP-2, MMP-9; CTX, serum carboxy-terminal, amino-terminal	A combinatorial predictive model of collagen peptides and MMP-2 levels in patients with indices of worsening diastolic function	214, 215
880	PICP, ICTP, PIIINP	PICP and ICTP elevated in elderly patients with HF	193
153	PICP	Collagen I peptide associated with worsening diastolic function	223
334	PINP, PIIINP, OPN	Stepped increases in pro-collagen and osteopontin caused incremental increases in the hazard ratio for cardiovascular events	238
580	AGEs, sRAGE	Indices of AGEs, such as pentosidine and soluble receptor for AGE, increased in plasma in HFpEF and in univariate models associated with clinical outcomes	239
880	PIP, CITP, PIIINP	CITP specifically associated with worsening HF and hospitalization in patients with HFpEF, but not HFrEF	193
26	AGEs	Indices of increased AGEs associated with diastolic dysfunction	240
103	MMP-2, -9, -13, TIMP-1, -2	Patients with LV hypertrophy and HF demonstrated specific reductions in MMPs and increased TIMP-1.	246, 281
28	MMP-1	MMP-1 levels reduced in HFpEF	241, 281
120	TIMP-1	Elevated TIMP-1 associated with reduced early LV filling velocity	242

AGEs, Advanced glycation end products; *CITP,* carboxy-terminal telopeptide of collagen type I ; *CTX,* C-terminal telopeptides; *HF,* heart failure; *ICTP,* I collagen telopeptide; *LV,* left ventricle; *MMP,* matrix metalloproteinase; *OPN,* osteopontin; *PCWP,* pulmonary capillary wedge pressure; *PICP,* pro-I collagen peptide; *PIP,* procollagen type I carboxyterminal propeptide; *PIIINP,* N-terminal procollagen III propeptide; *sRAGE,* soluble RAGE; *TIMP,* tissue inhibitors of matrix metalloproteinase.

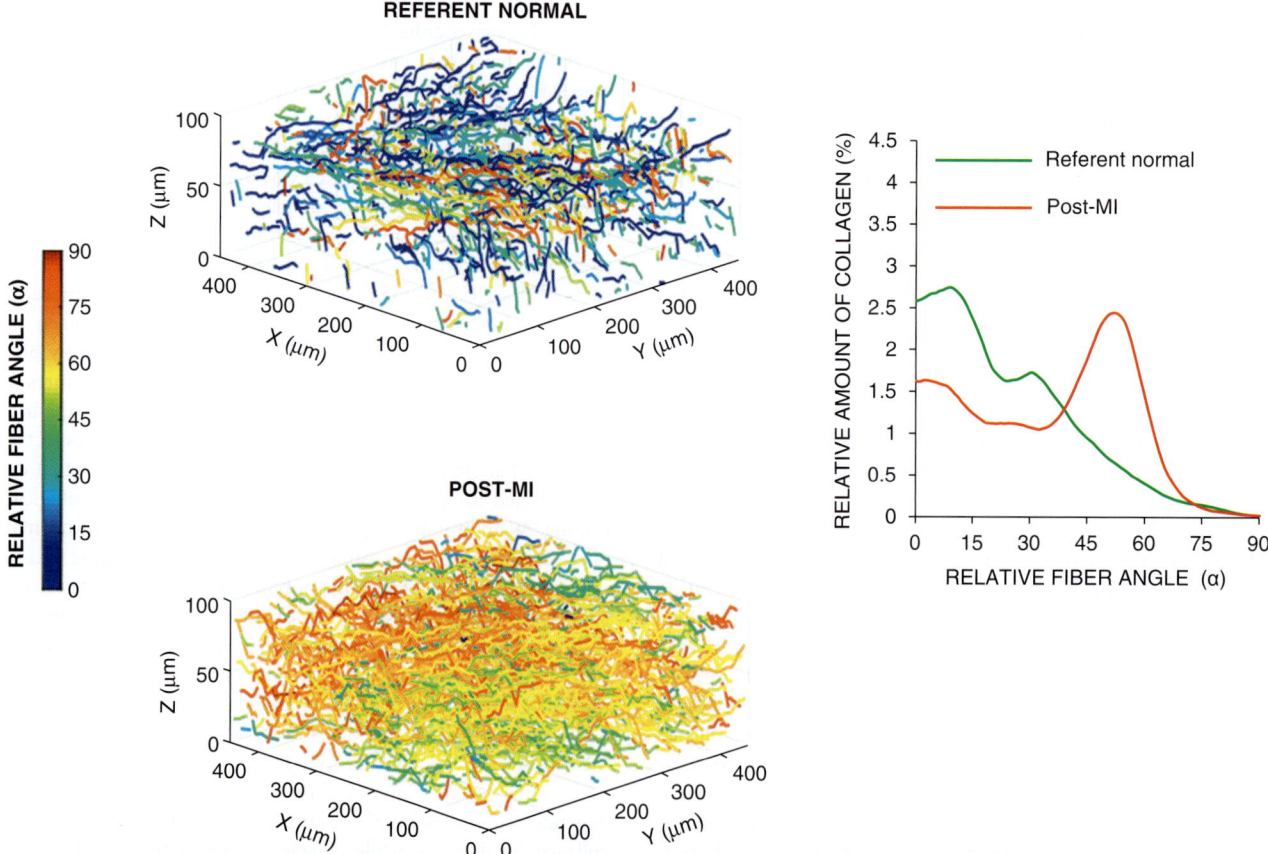

Fig. 4.5 Representative left ventricular *(LV)* sections taken from referent normal and post-myocardial infarction *(MI)* porcine myocardium, whereby optical sectioning has been performed and subjected to second harmonic generation *(SHG)* analysis. LV full thickness, unfixed sections were imaged at 10 μm intervals up to a 200 μm image depth (40× magnification, Leica TCS SP8, Leica Microsystems, Germany) and then reconstructed. The relative content of the fibrillar collagen matrix increased, as expected within the MI region, but in addition, analysis of the return SHG signal allowed for quantifiable assessment of fibrillar collagen geometry. In this instance, the distribution of fibrillar collagen fiber angles shifted to the right post-MI and would in turn alter the biophysical characteristics of the extracellular matrix.

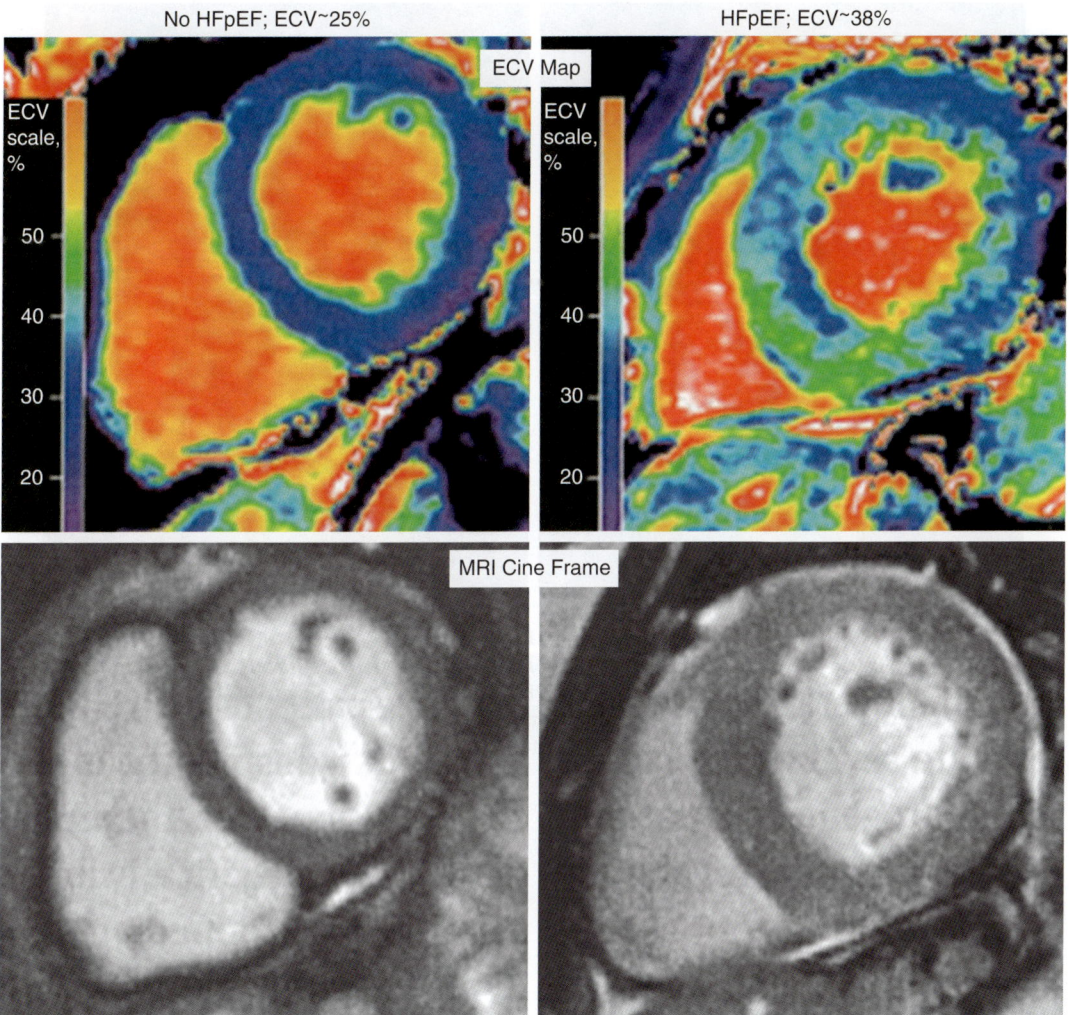

Fig. 4.6 *TOP*: Representative cardiac magnetic resonance imaging *(cMRI)* images and late gadolinium enhancement at end-diastole in a patient with no heart failure with preserved ejection fraction *(HFpEF)* and in a patient with HFpEF. The extracellular volume *(ECV)* index was increased in the HFpEF patient, and in a cohort of HFpEF patients, the ECV index was associated with more rapid progression of heart failure and greater cardiovascular events. *BOTTOM*: The representative left ventricular cine cMRI images in which the ECV computations were obtained is shown. Modified from Schelbert EB, Fridman Y, Wong TC, et al. Temporal relation between myocardial fibrosis and heart failure with preserved ejection fraction: association with baseline disease severity and subsequent outcome. *JAMA Cardiol.* 2017;2(9):995–1006.

At the organ level, continued advancements in quantifying the ECM, or more precisely quantifying the extracellular volume (ECV) using cMRI and late gadolinium enhancement, has occurred.[248-253] While ECV is a composite index of the ECM in terms of structural and fluid components, clear changes in this ECV index have been identified where increased ECM deposition is a key pathophysiological event. For example, in a large cohort of HFpEF patients, the cMRI computed ECV index was associated with progression of the HF process and increased cardiovascular events.[249,250] Representative cMRI images for this study are shown in Fig. 4.6 whereby the increased ECV coincident with LV hypertrophy and HFpEF is evident. In patients with HFrEF secondary to DCM, increased ECV computations, reflecting a diffuse fibrotic process, were directly correlated with biopsy-derived measurements of fibrillary collagen content.[249,251] In patients with LV hypertrophy due to severe aortic stenosis, ECV computations following aortic valve replacement were reported to be increased.[252] This apparent paradoxical finding is due to the fact that LV cellular volumes regressed much more rapidly following relief of the pressure overload, and thus the relative proportion of

the LV myocardial ECV will appear increased.[252] This observation is not dissimilar to previous LV biopsy studies performed before and after aortic valve replacement identified a relative increase in fibrillar collagen content.[254-256] While the clinical utilization and interpretation of cMRI-derived ECV measurements remains to be fully established, the fact that these noninvasive measurements can identify dynamic changes within the ECM and appear to correlate with biopsy-derived measurements holds promise. In terms of visualizing the determinants of ECM structure and composition, the use of SPECT/CT and radiolabeled ligands also continues to mature. For example, a radiotracer that binds to active MMPs has been successfully used in the porcine post-MI model and identified region- and time-dependent changes in MMP activity.[249] Using multiple slice CT and SPECT image registration, a distinct region of heightened MMP activity post-MI can be visualized and is shown in Fig. 4.7. The use of multimodal imaging and advanced algorithms, such as those briefly outlined here, will likely yield important mechanistic insights into ECM remodeling and the progression of both HFrEF and HFpEF as the instrumentation and imaging agents continue to improve.

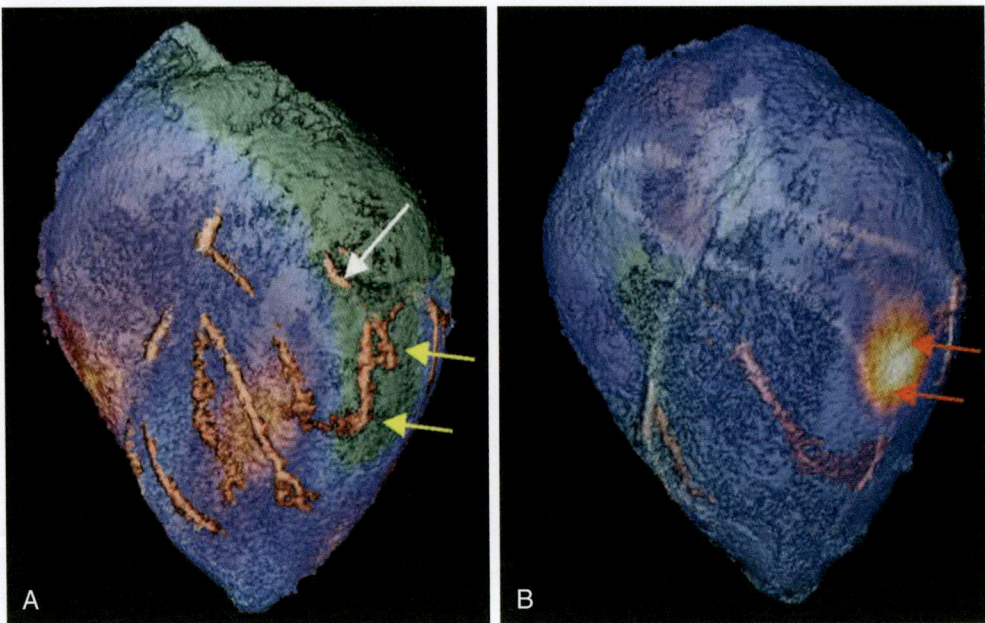

Fig. 4.7 Representative hybrid SPECT/CT image of a porcine heart following a 90-minute balloon occlusion of a marginal branch of the left circumflex artery *(white arrow)*, demonstrating a 99mTc-Tetrofosmin perfusion defect *(yellow arrows)* (A). Follow-up SPECT/CT image 3 days post-MI after injection of an MMP-targeted radiotracer (99mTc-RP805), demonstrating MMP activation *(red arrows)* in risk area previously defined with 99mTc-Tetrofosmin (B). (Courtesy Drs. Stephanie Thorn and Albert Sinusas, Yale University).

SUMMARY AND FUTURE DIRECTIONS

The Extracellular Matrix and Diagnostics

There is no question that biomarkers will play an even greater role in identifying the relative risk, presence, and progression of ECM remodeling in both HFrEF and HFpEF.[246] It is also clear that no single biomarker will be sufficient to provide critical insight into the complex ECM remodeling process. What remains to be established and defined is the optimal "cassette" of clinical variables and ECM biomarker measurements, which will provide useful and actionable predictive value in patients with a high risk for the development of HFrEF or HFpEF. It is most likely that a multimodality approach will be utilized, which is both HF and temporally specific. Indeed, as outlined in previous sections of this chapter, there are important parallelisms between cancer and the underlying myocardial remodeling process in terms of fibroblast transformation/transdifferentiation and the use of biomarker signatures to define the aggressiveness and potential acceleration of the disease process. For example, the use of markers from several functional domains, such as neurohormonal pathways, indices of cell viability and phenotype, as well as determinants of ECM remodeling, will likely yield a specific cassette of biomarkers that will differentiate HFrEF and HFpEF and also allow "staging" of the underlying myocardial remodeling process. It is further likely that profiling ECM remodeling will entail measurements at the transcriptional, posttranscriptional, and posttranslational levels. For example, there is possibly a cluster of miRs that regulate key ECM translational pathways, and profiling these across time would hold prognostic utility in terms of identifying those patients at increased risk for HF as well as potentially monitoring the progression of this disease process. Finally, integrating biomarker profiles of ECM remodeling and imaging modalities also holds future promise whereby biomarker screening would be followed by more specific cardiac imaging studies and would allow for more accurate identification of the HF phenotype as well as staging disease progression.

The Extracellular Matrix and Therapeutics

Targeting downstream mediators of ECM remodeling, such as the MMPs, has encountered difficulty in terms of targeting the specific MMP types that are causative in adverse LV remodeling. For example, broad-spectrum MMP inhibition demonstrated favorable effects with short-term dosing in large animal models of MI and HFrEF,[178] but concerns regarding systemic toxicity of broad-spectrum MMP inhibition and difficulties in dosing strategies yielded equivocal clinical results. Nevertheless, since the role of MMP induction and activation in adverse post-MI remodeling is likely significant, the identification of the specific MMP types and selective MMP inhibitors will remain an important area for research and development. Renewed interest in alternative strategies to interrupt MMP activity has occurred due to the initial favorable clinical results using doxycycline in post-MI patients.[257-259] Specifically, the TIPTOP trial identified that doxycycline treatment in the early post-MI period was associated with a relative reduction in LV dilation and shifts in the plasma MMP/TIMP ratios.[257,258] In terms of the activated fibroblasts within the MI region, this appears to be a TGF-dependent process[150,169-171]; therefore strategies that disrupt TGF signaling are likely to alter this fibroblast transdifferentiation process.[150,180,260-262] For example, membrane-bound MMPs likely contribute to the activation of TGF within the ECM, and this proteolytic-activation cascade may yield a number of potential targets.[263] In other studies, direct interference with TGF by genetic, neutralizing antibodies, or oral pharmacological inhibitors have demonstrated early favorable results in animal models of HFrEF.[260-262,264] In terms of proteases, the ECM and the fibroblast—a serine protease termed fibroblast activation protein (FAP)—have been identified to contribute to the activation and transdifferentiation of cancer-associated fibroblasts, and recent studies have identified FAP in animal models of

HF.[263,264] The finding that the induction of FAP is associated with ECM remodeling and the emergence of a more malignant fibroblast phenotype is all the more relevant as pharmacological FAP inhibitors have been developed.[265-267]

The use of biomaterials derived from the ECM or the mimic of a specific composite of the ECM have been the subject of a number of past translational studies, with a particular focus upon post-MI remodeling and the progression to HFrEF.[256,268-273] The predominant approach has been to directly inject these ECM biomaterials into the MI region, whereby interruption of MI wall thinning and changes in local stress-strain patterns have been realized.[256,268,269,271,272] For example, a purified bovine collagen containing predominantly type I collagen increased LV wall thickness and relative function in a post-MI rat model.[268] Using a polyacrylamide-based hydrogel containing fibroblast growth factor, targeted injections within the MI region in rats improved LV pump function.[270] In more recent studies, hyaluronic acid-based hydrogels (a common constituent of the ECM) with sequestered therapeutic peptides or miRs have been injected into animal models post-MI.[162,274] Initial clinical feasibility studies utilized the injection of an ECM biomaterial seeded with bone marrow cells (the MAGNUM trial) and demonstrated that relative MI thickness was augmented up to 1 year postinjection.[275] Using an alginate-based hydrogel, direct myocardial injections in HFrEF patients with DCM have identified positive effects.[276,277] Using a decellularized ECM, implantation in post-LV device patients has identified increased myocardial stability.[278] In a bioabsorbable form of ECM, intracoronary injections in patients with post-MI remodeling has been reported with no early adverse events.[279] Thus ECM biomaterials alone or as an adjunctive approach to local pharmacological or cell-based therapies in the context of post-MI remodeling hold potential therapeutic relevance in the context of developing HFrEF.

From the first report of the importance of collagenase by Gross and colleagues[280] regarding the resorption of a tadpole tail, it is now clearly recognized that ECM remodeling plays a critical role in tissue structure and function. The myocardial ECM is not a passive entity, but rather a complex and dynamic microenvironment, which represents an important structural and signaling system within the myocardium. Significant advancements have been made in the use of ECM profiling for the purposes of prognosis in both HFrEF and HFpEF. Future translational and clinical research focused on the molecular and cellular mechanisms that regulate ECM structure and function will likely contribute to an improved understanding of the LV remodeling process in both of these forms of HF, and yield important diagnostic and therapeutic targets.

Acknowledgments

Dr. Francis Spinale is supported by the Research Service of the Department of Veterans Affairs. The author wishes to recognize the significant contributions of past MUSC and USC medical and graduate students that participated in our cardiovascular research program over the past two decades.

KEY REFERENCES

94. Beber AR, Polina ER, Biolo A, et al. Matrix Metalloproteinase-2 polymorphisms in chronic heart failure: relationship with susceptibility and long-term survival. *PLoS One*. 2016;11(8):e0161666.

109. Salminen A, Vlachopoulou E, Havulinna AS, et al. Genetic variants contributing to circulating matrix metalloproteinase 8 levels and their association with cardiovascular diseases: a genome-wide analysis. *Circ Cardiovasc Genet*. 2017;10(6).

189. Martos R, Baugh J, Ledwidge M, et al. Diastolic heart failure: evidence of increased myocardial collagen turnover linked to diastolic dysfunction. *Circulation*. 2007;115(7):888–895.

208. Zile MR, Desantis SM, Baicu CF, et al. Plasma biomarkers that reflect determinants of matrix composition identify the presence of left ventricular hypertrophy and diastolic heart failure. *Circ Heart Fail*. 2011;4(3):246–256.

231. Rosenberg M, Zugck C, Nelles M, et al. Osteopontin, a new prognostic biomarker in patients with chronic heart failure. *Circ Heart Fail*. 2008;1(1):43–49.

246. Chow SL, Maisel AS, Anand I, et al. Role of biomarkers for the prevention, assessment, and management of heart failure: a scientific statement from the American Heart Association. *Circulation*. 2017;135(22):e1054–e1091.

249. Schelbert EB, Fridman Y, Wong TC, et al. Temporal relation between myocardial fibrosis and heart failure with preserved ejection fraction: association with baseline disease severity and subsequent outcome. *JAMA Cardiol*. 2017;2(9):995–1006.

251. Nakamori S, Dohi K, Ishida M, et al. Native T1 Mapping and extracellular volume mapping for the assessment of diffuse myocardial fibrosis in dilated cardiomyopathy. *JACC Cardiovasc Imaging*. 2018;11(1):48–59.

257. Cerisano G, Buonamici P, Valenti R, et al. Early short-term doxycycline therapy in patients with acute myocardial infarction and left ventricular dysfunction to prevent the ominous progression to adverse remodelling: the TIPTOP trial. *Eur Heart J*. 2014;35(3):184–191.

276. Mann DL, Lee RJ, Coats AJ, et al. One-year follow-up results from AUGMENT-HF: a multicentre randomized controlled clinical trial of the efficacy of left ventricular augmentation with Algisyl in the treatment of heart failure. *Eur J Heart Fail*. 2016;18(3):314–325.

The full reference list for this chapter is available on ExpertConsult.

5

Molecular Signaling Mechanisms of the Renin-Angiotensin System in Heart Failure

Carlos M. Ferrario, Louis J. Dell'Italia, Jasmina Varagic

A PERSPECTIVE ON THE RENIN ANGIOTENSIN ALDOSTERONE SYSTEM

Although Bright (1827) first associated kidney hardness with a strong arterial pulse, current knowledge regarding the role of the renin angiotensin aldosterone system to homeostasis has been gained over the last 50 years. It is not to be denied that the discoveries associated with characterization of this critically important circulating and tissue-borne hormonal system transcended the field of cardiovascular medicine, having a major impact on the research and treatment of renal, neurological, hepatic, and skeletal diseases. The broad role of the hormone angiotensin II (Ang II) and its biologically related main peptides—angiotensin-(1-7) (Ang-[1-7]), angiotensin III (Ang III), and angiotensin-(1-9) (Ang-[1-9])—in modulating immune and inflammation responses is a reason why drugs acting to inhibit, or block renin-angiotensin system effectors are showing benefits above and beyond their original indication. Antitumoral actions are documented for drugs preventing Ang II actions[1] or increasing Ang-(1-7) activity.[2,3] The ubiquitous mechanisms accounting for such a diverse spectrum of actions involve multifactorial signaling pathways.[4]

This chapter reviews the molecular mechanisms of the renin-angiotensin system, and underscores a major opportunity to develop a new generation of drugs with an increased capacity to reach the intracellular sites at which locally borne angiotensins modulate organ function. The clinical applications of antagonizing the renin-angiotensin system are reviewed in Chapter 37. For the convenience of the reviewer, a summary of the abbreviations used is presented at the end of this chapter.

THE BIOCHEMICAL PHYSIOLOGY OF THE RENIN ANGIOTENSIN SYSTEM

Initial studies of Ang II formation and action were influenced by the prevailing assumption that this peptide acted as a circulating hormone

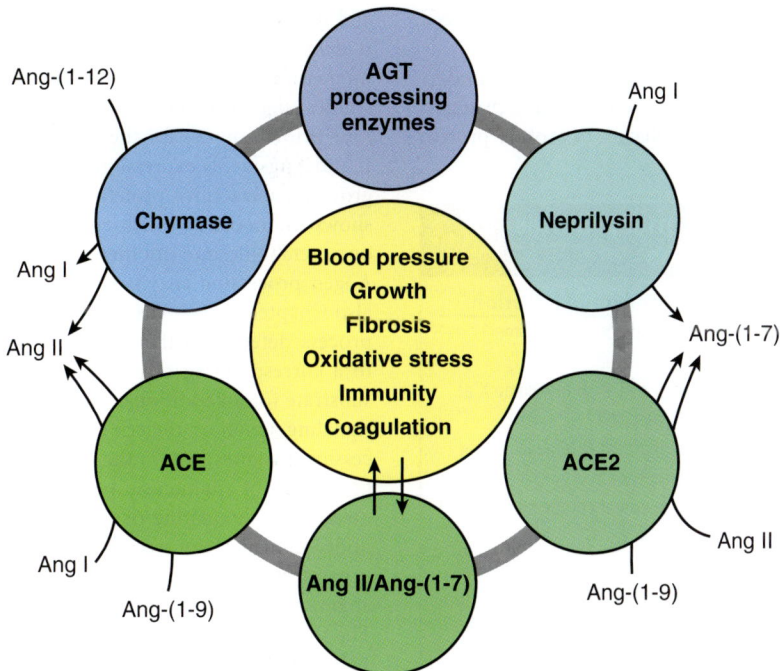

Fig. 5.1 Counterbalancing arms of the renin-angiotensin system.

originating from the action of renal renin on the angiotensinogen (AGT) released from the liver. During the decades preceding the current millennium, enzymological studies were driven to answer how renal renin acted on the rate limiting step protein substrate that accounted for the generation of angiotensin peptides. Over a span of probably two decades, the accepted view of the system was that renal renin generated angiotensin I (Ang I) by splitting the bond between leucine ^{10} (Leu^{10}) and leucine ^{11} (Leu^{11}) from the liver derived AGT substrate. The early conclusions were partly misleading, as they failed to realize that valine ^{11} (Val^{11}) is substituted for Leu^{11} in the human AGT molecule. Circulating Ang I was then further processed into Ang II by the action of angiotensin-converting enzyme (ACE), which hydrolyzed the bond between phenylalanine ^{8} (Phe^8) and histidine ^{9} (His^9) in the C-terminus of the Ang I molecule. The resulting molecule was Ang II, the main bioactive peptide of the renin angiotensin system. This conceptual understanding of the biochemical pathways for Ang II production implies the existence of a linear system in which the hydrolytic activity of renin and ACE sequentially cleaved Ang I from AGT and Ang II from Ang I. The 1980s began to force a reconsideration of these concepts as identification of Ang-(1-7) in Ferrario's research program,[5] and the heptapeptide fragment angiotensin IV (Ang IV)[6] challenged the prevailing simplistic understanding of Ang II singularity in the regulation of blood pressure and fluid balances (Fig. 5.1). A diagram of the family of angiotensin peptides derived from the N-terminal end of AGT is documented in Table 5.1. Table 5.2 illustrates the location of the extended number of humans' genes now recognized to account for the expression and function of the renin angiotensin system.

As illustrated in Table 5.1, humans and rodents differ in the molecular sequence of the amino terminal end of the AGT molecule as valine replaces leucine in position 11. Additional significant differences exist in the amino acid sequence of human AGT beyond valine^{11} (Val^{11}). Table 5.1 shows that the human amino acid chain beyond Val^{11} is composed of Ile^{12}-His^{13}-Asn^{14}-Glu^1, while in the rat the amino acid sequence contains Tyr^{12}-Tyr^{13}-Ser^{14}-Lys^{15}. These amino acid differences influence the identity and affinity of the enzymes cleaving the biologically active angiotensins from AGT.[7] Indeed, it has been well documented that rat renin has no hydrolytic activity on human AGT.

TABLE 5.1 The Family of Recognized Biologically Active Angiotensins Sequences in Humans

Peptide	Amino Acid Sequence
Angiotensinogen (AGT)	H$_2$N-Asp^1-Arg^2-Val^3-Tyr^4-Ile^5-His^6-Pro^7-Phe^8-His^9-Leu^{10}-Val^{11}-Ile^{12}-His^{13}-Asn^{14}-Glu^{15}-COOH
Angiotensin-(1-12)	H$_2$N-Asp^1-Arg^2-Val^3-Tyr^4-Ile^5-His^6-Pro^7-Phe^8-His^9-Leu^{10}-Val^{11}-Ile^{12}-COOH
Angiotensin-(1-10) (Ang I)	H$_2$N-Asp^1-Arg^2-Val^3-Tyr^4-Ile^5-His^6-Pro^7-Phe^8-His^9-Leu^{10}-COOH
Angiotensin-(1-9)	H$_2$N-Asp^1-Arg^2-Val^3-Tyr^4-Ile^5-His^6-Pro^7-Phe^8-His^9-COOH
Angiotensin-(1-8) (Ang II)	H$_2$N-Asp^1-Arg^2-Val^3-Tyr^4-Ile^5-His^6-Pro^7-Phe^8-COOH
Angiotensin A	H$_2$N-Ala^1-Arg^2-Val^3-Tyr^4-Ile^5-His^6-Pro^7-Phe-COOH^8
Angiotensin-(1-7) [Ang-(1-7)]	H$_2$N-Asp^1-Arg^2-Val^3-Tyr^4-Ile^5-His^6-Pro^7-COOH
Almandine	H$_2$N-Ala^1-Arg^2-Val^3-Tyr^4-Ile^5-His^6-Pro^7-COOH
Angiotensin-(1-5)	H$_2$N-Asp^1-Arg^2-Val^3-Tyr^4-Ile^5-COOH
Angiotensin-(2-8) (Ang III)	H$_2$N- Arg^2-Val^3-Tyr^4-Ile^5-His^6-Pro^7-Phe^8-COOH
Angiotensin-(3-8) (Ang IV)	H$_2$N- Val^3-Tyr^4-Ile^5-His^6-Pro^7-Phe^8-COOH

Valine in position 11 (Val^{11}) is present in the human angiotensinogen sequence while Leucine is the amino acid contained in rodents.

Contemporary research affirms the view that the renin angiotensin system is a complex system in which biological diversity is revealed not only by the different effects of the products generated from either Ang I or Ang II but also through its receptors and peptide-forming and degrading enzymes. That the renin angiotensin system was far more complex than generally accepted, and that this complexity guarantees a well-tuned adaptation of the blood supply of the body compartments to all physiological conditions, was advanced as early as 1991.[8]

The principles of network biology allow a more precise understanding of the complex interactions between enzymes and products within the renin angiotensin system. The behavior of protein-protein

and molecular interactions of the renin angiotensin system network is determined by the orchestrated activity of several components interacting with each other through pair-wise interactions. Our studies suggest the existence within the renin angiotensin system of four primary nodes for the deterministic control of hormone (Ang II and Ang-[1-7]) expression signaling cellular functions in terms of growth, contractility, protein synthesis, and gene expression. Fig. 5.2 shows the nodes at which enzymes catalyze reactions transforming one metabolite into another. The four nodes are represented as (a) Aogen processing enzymes; (b) neutral endopeptidases (NEPs; see also Chapter 9); (c) ACE; and (d) ACE2. At each node, a regulated process determines the secondary processing of a protein/peptide to a corresponding shorter fragment destined to serve as either a substrate for an additional processing at a secondary node or a final signaling action on the cell's receptor. At the first node (Aogen processing enzymes), AGT, the sole known identified substrate for the generation of angiotensin peptides, is catalyzed into forming Ang I directly via circulating or tissue expressed renin. Within this same node, however, our recent studies show that AGT is a substrate generating another Ang I-forming precursor, the dodecapeptide angiotensin-(1-12) (Ang-[1-12]), by an enzyme that is not renin. The intermediate products upstream from Ang I (Ang I or Ang-[1-12]) now become substrates to be acted upon by either the neprilysin (NEPs node; see also Chapter 9) or the ACE node where these enzymes cleave Ang I to generate Ang II (ACE node) or transform Ang I into Ang-(1-7) (NEPs node). Importantly, the ACE node also functions to regulate the concentration of Ang-(1-7), since ACE degrades this heptapeptide into Ang-(1-5) (not shown). The fourth node (ACE2) cleaves Ang II into Ang-(1-7).

Establishing the characteristics of the factors regulating the activity of each node is not a trivial matter, as each component of the system can exert a regulatory influence on either the enzymes' expression or activity and the product generated at each node. For example, Ang II plasma or tissue concentrations shows a feed forward interaction with the Ang I-forming enzyme node as the peptide stimulates the expression of AGT transcripts in the liver, heart, and kidneys.[9,10] Interestingly,

TABLE 5.2 Location of Primary Genes Accounting for RAS Functions

Gene	Chromosomal Location
Angiotensin-converting enzyme (ACE)	long (q) arm of chromosome 17 at position 23.3
Angiotensin-converting enzyme 2 (ACE2)	long (q) arm of chromosome X at position 22.2
Angiotensin II type 1 receptor (AGTR1)	long (q) arm of chromosome 3 at position 24
Angiotensin II type 2 receptor (AGTR2)	long (q) arm of chromosome X at position 23
Angiotensinogen (AGT)	long (q) arm of chromosome 1 at position 42.2
Carboxypeptidase A1	long (q) arm of chromosome 7 at position 32.2
Chymase (CMA1)	long (q) arm of chromosome 14 at position 12
Elastase-2 (ELA2)	short arm (p) of chromosome 19 at position 13.3
Mas receptor (MAS1)	long (q) arm of chromosome 6 at position 25.3
MrgD Receptor	long (q) arm of chromosome 11 at position 13.3
Renin (REN)	long (q) arm of chromosome 1 at position 32.1

Data reported for genes expressed in *Homo sapiens* (human) as compiled by the National Center for Biotechnology Information (https://www.ncbi.nlm.nih.gov/).

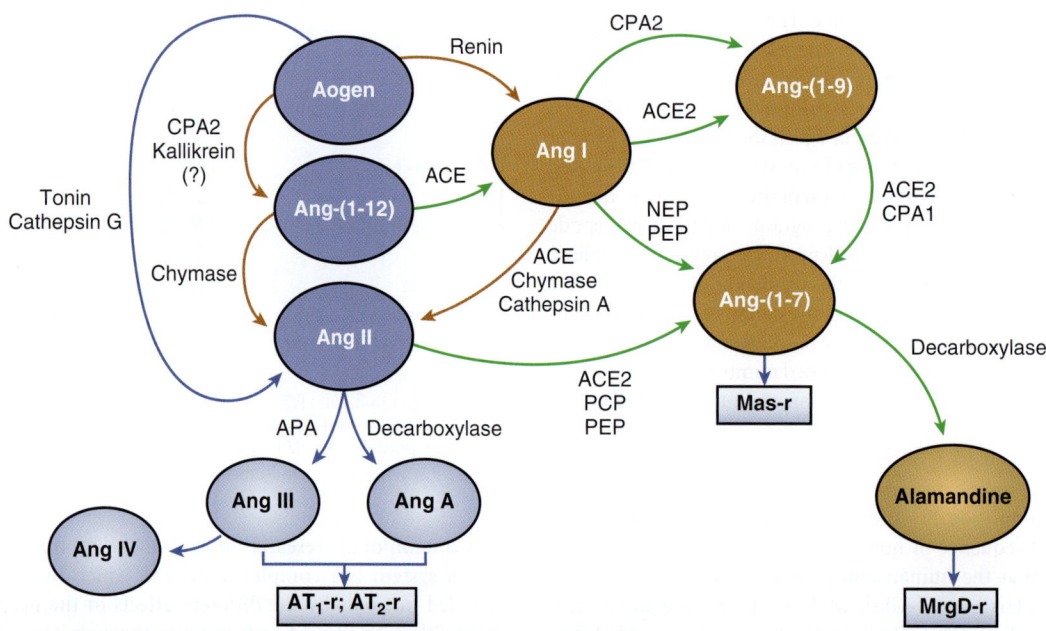

Fig. 5.2 A detailed summary of the biotransformation pathways generating biologically active angiotensins comprises enzymes from distinct endopeptidase and carboxypeptidase families. *ACE,* Angiotensin-converting enzyme; *ACE2,* angiotensin-converting enzyme 2; *APA,* aminopeptidase A; *CPA1 and CPA2,* carboxypeptidase A1 and A2; *PCP,* prolyl-carboxypeptidase; *PEP,* prolyl endopeptidase.

Ang-(1-7) modulates the activity of the ACE node by acting as a weak endogenous inhibitor of the C-terminal domain of the enzyme.[11] In addition, Ang II exerts a negative regulatory interaction on ACE2 gene expression, a feedback interaction that is neutralized by Ang-(1-7).

Renin and Pro-Renin

The enzyme renin can be ubiquitously expressed by a variety of cells, as new evidence suggests its critical evolutionary involvement in tissue homeostasis only in part through its role in regulating body fluid volumes.[12] Although renin is found in many different tissues, its highest expression in the juxtaglomerular cells of renal afferent arterioles constitutes the pivotal sensory mechanism that determines its release into the circulation. Importantly, other renal locations for renin synthesis and release are found in a subset of mesangial cells, arteriolar smooth muscle cells, interstitial pericytes,[12] and distal nephrons and renal collecting duct.[13,14] Studies reporting the existence of renin and pro-renin in distal nephrons and collecting ducts substantiate the potential for renal tubular Ang II formation as an alternative mechanism that, independent of the blood pressure and sodium sensory mechanisms of the juxtaglomerular apparatus and the macula densa, could contribute to the pathogenesis of essential hypertension.[15,16.] The active renin enzyme synthesized as preprorenin is converted into the active releasable form through loss of the signal peptide and removal of the 43-amino-acid pro-segment contained in prorenin. The discovery of a prorenin receptor (PPR) revealed a nonproteolytic mechanism for the activation of renin through the exposure of its catalytic site.[17] Deletion of 10 bp in exon 5 of the Ren gene in the rat caused inactivation of the renin gene, loss of renin granules in juxtaglomerular cells, and significant alterations in renal morphology[18] comparable to those obtained with renin cells ablation in mice.[19]

It has not been possible to find sufficient discriminative renin activity by assay procedures in the circulation as a superior biomarker of an overactive renin angiotensin system. This failure contributed to the search for renin expression and action within the tissue environment, particularly within the vascular wall and the heart. It was assumed that renin present in the extracellular milieu of the heart and blood vessels could generate Ang I from the plasma substrate, leading to Ang II formation by the action of ACE contained by vascular endothelial cells or perivascular tissue. No definitive conclusion has been reached as to whether renin is synthesized by cells in tissues other than the kidneys or its presence in nonrenal tissues reflects a cellular uptake mechanism.[20]

Renin release from juxtaglomerular cells is modulated by the renal baroreceptor through changes in renal perfusion pressure, the sensory of sodium (Na^+) by the macula densa, and renal sympathetic nerve activity. Additional regulation of active renin secretion is exerted by Ang II through renal AT_1 receptors, the primary intracellular second messenger cAMP, and arachidonic acid (AA) derivatives.

Other Nonrenin Enzymes

Over the years, several renin-like enzymes were postulated to release Ang I from either AGT or the model synthetic substrate tetradecapeptide angiotensin-(1-14) (Ang-[1-14]). Cathepsin D and cathepsin G,[21] acid and neutral proteases, tonin,[22] the serine protease Esterase B,[23] kallikrein-like serine proteases,[24] and mouse gamma-nerve growth factor (γ-NGF) are among the enzymes implicated as Ang l-forming enzymes. Tonin forms Ang II directly from a plasma protein, from the tetradecapeptide substrate Ang-(1-14), and from Ang I. Tonin is present in most tissues, but in highest concentration it is found in submaxillary glands. A neutral protease with Ang l-forming activity that could readily be separated from acid proteases and both plasma and renal renin was identified in the dog brain.[25] Findings of extended forms of Ang I, Ang-(1-25),[26] and the dodecapeptide angiotensin-(1-12)[7,27]

in human and rodents raise additional issues as to whether nonrenin mechanisms may be more critical than anticipated previously.

Angiotensinogen

This 452-amino acid protein is the only known forming precursor of angiotensin peptides. The liver is the primary site for its synthesis, although in more recent years extrahepatic sources of generation exist in visceral fat, renal tubules, brain, heart, and reproductive organs. The AGT protein is produced through the cleavage of a single gene pre-pro-AGT (see Table 5.1).[10,28] Synthesis, processing, and glycosylation changes vary in relation to species and site of tissue generation. The levels of the AGT protein are influenced by glucocorticoids, estrogen, thyroid hormone, insulin, and Ang II.[29] A positive feedback in which Ang II augments AGT production has been demonstrated in the kidney and the liver. This mechanism may act to prevent depletion of substrate during excess Ang II production. On the other hand, Ang II reduces AGT mRNA in adrenal glands. Genetic studies underscore the critical role for the substrate in contributing to hypertension pathogenesis. Studies in transgenic mice show that arterial pressure increases in proportion to the number of AGT gene copies. Likewise, deletion of the AGT gene[30] is associated with lower resting blood pressure, while the Lu et al.[31] recent study shows that hypo-expression of the gene in a low-density lipoprotein receptor$^{-/-}$ background is associated with reduced blood pressure, less atherosclerosis, decreased body weight gain, and liver steatosis. Emerging evidence regarding an interplay among radical oxygen species (ROS), inflammation, and Ang II is strengthened by the observation that oxidative stress exposes the cleavage site of the AGT molecule to renin.[32] Single nucleotide polymorphisms (SNPs) in the AGT gene have been explored for hypertension linkage. Data suggest that T174 and M235T associates with hypertension.[33,34] We showed that genetic variation of the M235T, but not the ACE (I/D), genotype contributes to the presence of coronary heart disease independently of blood pressure.[35]

Angiotensin I and II Forming Enzymes

The past decade has forced a revision of accepted tenets regarding the enzymatic pathways forming Ang II and other biologically active renin angiotensin system peptides. The classic view that ACE (EC 3.4.15.1) is the critical enzymatic fulcrum for the generation of Ang II has been challenged by the finding that chymase (CMA1; EC 3.4.21.39) forms Ang II directly from Ang-(1-12).[36,37] Neprilysin and thimet oligopeptidase (EC 3.4.24.15) cleave Ang I to produce Ang-(1-7) in the circulation,[38] while renal neprilysin generates Ang-(1-7) from either locally contained Ang-(1-12) or Ang I.[39] Less appreciated are potential roles of (a) carboxypeptidase A (EC 3.4.17) forming angiotensin-(1-9) from Ang-(1-12) or Ang-(1-7) from Ang II; and (b) the Ang II generating ability of elastase-2 (EC 3.4.21.37).[40] The variety of alternate pathways for angiotensin peptide formation may explain the failure to sustain Ang II suppression in patients chronically dosed with effective amounts of ACE inhibitors.[41,42] The importance of these alternate pathways, primarily at the tissue level, may explain why the actual quantitative reduction in cardiovascular endpoints obtained with this drug class is less than predicted on the basis of their mode of action and physiological actions.[7,43,44]

Angiotensin-Converting Enzyme

Renin catalytic action on human AGT generates angiotensin I (Ang I) through the cleavage of the amino acid bond between leucine and valine at positions 10 and 11. ACE, a di-carboxy peptidyl peptidase with a molecular weight of 150 to 180 kDa, cleaves Ang I to generate Ang II by removing the last two amino acids of the decapeptide (see Table 5.1). Although the role of ACE in forming Ang II was first identified by

Skeggs, Marsh, Khan, and Shumway in 1954, recognition of its critical role in the renin angiotensin system cascade awaited the development of the solid-phase method of peptide synthesis by Merrifield in 1964. Ng and Vance's identification of the lung as a critical physiological locus for the processing of circulating Ang I into Ang II set the stage for the development of ACE inhibitors, the first landmark clinically successful approach to blockade of the renin angiotensin system.

ACE can act on other substrates, including bradykinin, substance P, and the tetrapeptide N-acetyl-Ser-Asp-Lys-Pro (Ac-SDKP). ACE-mediated inhibition of bradykinin and Ac-SDKP metabolism are implicated in contributing to the mode of action of ACE inhibitors through potentiation of bradykinin vasodilator responses or antifibrotic mechanisms. The occurrence of angioedema, a side effect of ACE inhibitors more frequent in women and black patients, has also been linked to prevention of bradykinin and substance P metabolism.[45,46]

ACE is ubiquitously found in cardiovascular tissues, primarily expressed in epithelial and endothelial cells. ACE activity found in blood, lymph, and cerebrospinal fluid represents a form of the enzyme that has lost its anchoring to the cell's membranes by the cleavage of its C-terminus hydrophobic region. The process accounting for the shedding of ACE from the vascular endothelium remains to be characterized. Recently, lysozyme and bilirubin have been identified as contributing to ACE-shedding.[47] Another feature of ACE that bears importance for its role within the renin angiotensin system arises from the fact that its extracellular loop contains two catalytic sites termed the C- and N-domains. While the catalytic activity of the C-domain has been linked to the processing of Ang I into Ang II, the N-domain cleaves Ang-(1-7) into Ang-(1-5).[48]

The variety of substrates on which ACE can express its hydrolytic activity implicate its role in the regulation of multiple organ and cellular functions. Since human kidneys contain large proportions of ACE compared with other organs other than the lung, it has been argued that renal ACE-mediated Ang II formation acts as a master switch in the control of nephron sodium transport and the development of hypertension.

Chymase

Chymases are a group of chymotrypsin-like serine proteinases that have multiple functions in tissue injury and remodeling. Phylogenetic studies have divided chymases into two isoenzyme groups, α and β. An α-chymase gene has been identified in all mammals, including humans, while β-chymases exist only in several rodent species. β-Chymases are not expressed in humans. This is an important distinction because α-chymase forms Ang II, while β-chymases can both form and degrade Ang II.[49] Chymase is elaborated by mast cells, vascular endothelial cells, and other interstitial cells within the human heart.[50] The identification of other cellular sources, including cardiac fibroblasts and vascular endothelial cells, demonstrates a more widely dispersed production and distribution system that accounts for its relatively high protein abundance (about 1.3 μg/g in human heart tissue). Evidence for its intracellular presence in cardiomyocytes in the human heart opens an entirely new compartment of chymase-mediated actions that were previously thought to be limited to the extracellular space.[51]

Chymase is 20 times more catalytically efficient than ACE in Ang I conversion to Ang II in the human heart. With ACE largely located on endothelial cells with its catalytic site exposed to the vascular lumen and chymase activity largely located in tissue, there is a compartmentalization of ACE- and chymase-mediated Ang II formation in the tissue and vascular space.[52] The presence of chymase in tissue has been invoked in the mechanism of "ACE escape" and in a more indirect means through ACE inhibitor increase in bradykinin, causing mast cell degranulation and chymase release. Most recently, AGT has been shown to be a substrate for Ang-(1-12) generation in the human heart that is independent of renin and ACE.[36,37,53]

In addition to its very potent Ang II-forming capacity, chymase protease actions also mediate cleavage of matricellular proteins and peptides, including laminin and fibronectin, important in cell survival; chymase activates peptide and enzyme precursors including matrix metalloproteinases (MMPs), transforming growth factor-β (TGF-β), stem cell factor (SCF) (causing further mast cell degranulation and chemotaxis), interleukin-6 (IL-6) and IL-1β, and conversion of pre-pro-endothelin I (pre-proET1).[51] All these mechanisms of action are crucial factors in cardiovascular injury and remodeling (see also Chapters 1, 2, 4, and 12). Taken together, chymase mediates a critical balance of (1) profibrotic ET-1 and Ang II formation, myofibroblast formation, and TGF-β activation; (2) antifibrotic protease activation of MMPs, direct digestion of matricellular proteins, and formation of bradykinin (BK); and (3) inflammatory cytokines and SCF activation and chemotaxis of inflammatory cells.[51] These multiple protease actions in addition to its Ang II-forming capacity are complemented by chymase upregulation in the human myocardial infarction heart and vulnerable atherosclerotic plaque, aortic aneurysm, atherosclerosis, and diabetic kidney.[51]

Angiotensin-Converting Enzyme 2

ACE2 is a type 1 integral membrane glycoprotein that functions as a mono carboxypeptidase–converting Ang I into Ang-(1-9) and Ang II into Ang-(1-7). The affinity of the enzyme for Ang-(1-7) formation from Ang II is higher than its affinity for Ang I. Although ACE2 is a close ACE homologue, ACE2 catalytic activity is not blocked by drugs that inhibit ACE. Like many other enzymes, ACE2 displays hydrolytic activity for other proteins such as vasoactive bradykinin (1–8), des-Arg-kallidin, Apelin-13, and Apelin-36. Additional features of the enzyme include 48% sequence identity with collectrin at the noncatalytic C-terminal domain of the enzyme and the demonstration that ACE2 is the receptor for SARS virus. While ACE2 is most abundant in heart, kidney, the retina, and the utero-placenta complex, a secreted form of ACE2 generated from the hydrolytic activity of a disintegrin and metalloprotease domain 17 (ADAM17) is present in blood.

The Crackower et al.[54] landmark study demonstrated ACE2's role in the regulation of cardiac function. That Ang II influenced ACE2 gene expression in the heart[55] provided evidence for the existence of a regulatory control of Ang II expression by the opposing actions of ACE as an Ang II-forming enzyme versus the ACE2 Ang II-degrading mechanism.[56] Additional studies directed to understand the signaling mechanisms by which Ang-(1-7) acts as a negative regulator of Ang II actions identified a primary role of ACE2 in the formation of the heptapeptide from Ang II in the heart. These studies showed that cardiac overexpression of ACE2 reversed cardiac hypertrophy in SHR, identified the mas receptor as the site at which Ang-(1-7) acts to inhibit myocyte hypertrophy,[57] demonstrated a role of ACE2 in modulating the central neurogenic actions of Ang-(1-7), and revealed a critical role of the ACE2/Ang-(1-7)/mas-receptor axis in the regulation of fetal development and pregnancy. These data now constitute the foundation for a more precise mechanistic analysis of the biological and signaling processes by which the ACE2/Ang-(1-7)/mas receptor axis counteracts the actions of Ang II on blood pressure, cardiac and vascular remodeling, and metabolic and renal function.[58,59]

Other Angiotensin-Forming Enzymes

Because proteolytic enzymes participate in multiple regulated cellular processes, alternate biotransformation pathways within the renin angiotensin system need not be restricted to classic canonical and non-canonical pathways. The molecular basis for the effector hormonal and tissue actions of angiotensins in maintaining the normalcy of the internal environment transcends their function in the control of fluid volumes and tissue perfusion. The tissular actions of Ang II as a growth factor, a stimulant of fibrosis, and its prothrombotic mechanisms need not be identical in the heart, brain, kidneys, and bone marrow. The demonstration of the existence of renin angiotensin system genes in the intracellular environment[60] need not reflect a functional processing of biologically active angiotensins through enzymatic pathways previously characterized in the circulation or even the extracellular compartments. Ang II participation in innate and adaptive immune mechanisms,[61] modulation of hematopoiesis, and progenitor cell expression and function may result from biochemical biotransformation of precursor peptides where neither renin nor ACE play a role. In the context of this discussion, emerging studies demonstrating novel roles for carboxypeptidase A and B (see Table 5.2), elastase, cathepsin G, proteinase 3, caspase-1, and chymase in angiotensin peptide metabolism or processing of inflammatory cytokines such as IL-1β[62] deserve future attention.

Main Angiotensin Products

The demonstration that the renin angiotensin system contains both a pressor and depressor arm is now well accepted, and the source of potential therapeutic approaches based on augmenting the activity of the depressor arm. Since these concepts were advanced by Ferrario's laboratory,[63] others have taken to exploring the dynamics of these mechanisms mostly in laboratory animals. The pressor arm of the system is defined as being composed of the enzyme ACE, the Ang II product, and the Ang II type 1 (AT_1) receptor (ACE/Ang II/AT_1-R axis). The opposing arm of the system is defined as including the enzyme ACE2, the Ang-(1-7) product, and the mas receptor [ACE2/Ang-(1-7)/mas axis]. Since the original description of the two opposing arms by Ferrario,[54,60] Ang-(1-9) cardio renal protective actions should be included as a component of the opposing arm of the system, while a resurgence of the importance of chymase as the major Ang II-forming enzyme in humans[51] needs similar inclusion.

Angiotensin-(1-12)

There has been a paucity of research regarding the potential existence of intermediate peptides derived from AGT with molecular sequences larger than Ang I (see Fig. 5.2). Earlier studies identified low and high molecular forms of circulating AGT in plasma. A high-molecular-weight AGT is present in human plasma at concentrations amounting to no more than 5% of the total circulating substrate. The high-molecular-weight form of the substrate is increased in normal pregnancy and pregnancy-induced hypertension. In 2006, Nagata et al. reported the presence of proangiotensin 2 (currently renamed as Ang-[1-12]) in the plasma and tissues of a Japanese strain of Wistar rats.[27] The peptide was shown to generate Ang II, as the pressor response induced by its injection into the systemic circulation could be abrogated by pretreatment with captopril or candesartan.[27] The discovery of this extended Ang I form was confirmed to function as an endogenous source for Ang II production in rodent hearts and kidneys, human left ventricular tissue, and left atrial tissue obtained from humans undergoing heart surgery.[64] Overall, the accumulating evidence demonstrates that Ang-(1-12) may be an intracellular substrate accounting for Ang II actions through the hydrolytic activity of chymase.[7,36,43,53] A second peptide composed of 25 amino acids has been identified in human urine. Like Ang-(1-12), big angiotensin-25 (Ang-[1-25]) generates Ang II through the catalytic action of chymase. The existence of intermediate forms of AGT that generate Ang II independent of renin uncovers non-canonical mechanisms for interstitial or intracellular Ang II production.

Angiotensin-(1-9)

The nonapeptide Ang-(1-9) is a relatively new addition to the active renin angiotensin system effector molecules, possessing actions like those associated with Ang-(1-7) in terms of systemic vasodilation, cardiac hypertrophy, and hyperplasia.[65,66] Ang-(1-9) actions are mediated through binding of the peptide to AT_2 receptors. Although there is a tendency to consider Ang-(1-9) as a product of Ang I by ACE2, Ocaranza et al.[66] report a greater affinity of carboxypeptidase A and cathepsin A in processing Ang I into Ang-(1-9). Ang-(1-9) metabolism into Ang-(1-7) occurs via the action of ACE, although prolyl endopeptidase, neprilysin, and thimet oligopeptidase have been reported to have comparable hydrolytic actions. It is of interest to note that the antihypertensive cardio-renal protective actions of ACE inhibition may be amplified through inhibition of Ang-(1-7) and Ang-(1-9) metabolism. Since neurolysin (E.C. 3.4.24.16), a cytosolic enzyme, has moderate binding affinity for Ang-(1-9), it has been suggested that this mechanism may downregulate binding of Ang II to AT_1-R. Ang-(1-9) has been detected in human blood and heart tissue, and the nonapeptide shows significant ability to stimulate atrial natriuretic peptide. Further work should be pursued to determine the potential ability of Ang-(1-9) to counteract the neurohormonal mechanisms accompanying chronic heart failure. Comparative studies of the action of Ang-(1-7) versus Ang-(1-9) are needed.

Angiotensin I and Angiotensin II

There is no evidence of biological actions of Ang I other than to serve as the substrate for the generation of Ang II via ACE in rodents and chymase in humans or Ang-(1-9) production from ACE2. Ang II biological actions, primarily mediated through binding of the agonist to AT_1 receptors, represent the major effector pathway of the renin angiotensin system with pleotropic physiological and pathological actions that contribute to chronic diseases, inflammation, metabolic abnormalities, and cancer. Ang II catabolism is mediated by aminopeptidases (angiotensinase A) or through processing of the peptide into Ang-(1-7) by ACE2. The hydrolytic activity of aminopeptidase A through the cleavage of Asp^1 in the amino-terminal end of the molecule accounts for the generation of Ang III, which is the preferred agonist of renal AT_2 receptors. Aminopeptidase N converts Ang III into Ang IV. Thus aminopeptidase activities can have significant effects on the catabolism of the amino terminal end of Ang II.

Angiotensin III and Angiotensin IV

Since the pioneer studies of Goodfriend and Peach,[67] the heptapeptide [des-Asp^1] Ang II (angiotensin III; see Table 5.2) has been reported to reproduce all of Ang II effects, although with lower potency. Studies exploring Ang III mechanisms of action in the brain suggested that Ang II needed to be converted into Ang III for selective binding to AT_1 receptors (Ang III hypothesis). No conclusive evidence in support of this hypothesis has become available.[68] On the other hand, recent studies demonstrate that Ang III inhibits renal proximal tubule sodium (Na^+) reabsorption by AT_2 receptors.[69] These studies affirm a natriuretic role for renal AT_2 receptors. Whether similar differential actions of Ang III versus Ang II in other organs exist remains undetermined, although Ang III was shown to induce phosphorylation of extracellular signal-regulated kinases (ERK1/2) and stress-activated protein kinase (SAPK)/c-jun N-terminal kinase (JNK) pathways with a potency comparable to Ang II.[70]

Ang IV is another peptide fragment, with a truncated amino terminal end that was originally thought to bind to another G-couple subtype angiotensin receptor (AT_4). In-depth studies of its actions in neural tissues revealed the specific, high-affinity binding site to be the insulin-regulated aminopeptidase (IRAP), a protein highly expressed in vesicles containing the insulin-sensitive glucose transporter GLUT4.[71] A soluble form of IRAP is reported to degrade oxytocin and vasopressin. Main biological actions of Ang IV appear to target the brain, where the hexapeptide enhances learning and memory.[71] While Ang IV may act as a weak vasodilator agonist in the circulation, it is able to augment renal blood flow and inhibit tubular sodium transport.

Angiotensin-(1-7)

The 1988 demonstration that a heptapeptide fragment of Ang I, lacking the sequence of Phe^8-His^9-Leu^{10} (see Table 5.1), was biologically active[72] accounts for the radical change of thinking regarding the biochemical physiology and function of the renin angiotensin system.[73] Characterization of the biochemical pathways responsible for the formation of Ang-(1-7) from Ang I revealed the role of several tissue-specific endopeptidases prolyl oligopeptidase 24.26 (brain, vascular endothelium, and kidney), neutral endopeptidase 24.11 ([neprilysin] circulation and kidney), and metalol-endopeptidase 24.15 (brain, vascular smooth muscle).[74] The activity of these enzymes in Ang-(1-7) formation is dependent in part on the relative concentration of the enzyme in tissues, since in the kidney neprilysin plays a predominant role in the hydrolysis of Ang-(1-7) into Ang-(1-4). In contrast, ACE cleaves Ang-(1-7) into Ang-(1-5) in the circulation, the vascular endothelium, and the lung. There is now agreement that Ang-(1-7) binds to the mas receptor in conveying the signal to account for most of Ang-(1-7)'s biological actions.

While Ang-(1-7) was initially shown to be a vasodilator peptide functioning to oppose Ang II vasoconstrictor actions (see Fig. 5.1), Ferrario and colleagues[73,75] first advanced the hypothesis that hypertension and aging, as well as impaired cardiac, renal, vascular, and metabolic function, was the result of a deficiency in the expression of the ACE2/Ang-(1-7)/mas-receptor axis rather than simply an increased expression of Ang II pressor and proliferative actions. This hypothesis was buttressed by original studies showing low urinary excretion rates of Ang-(1-7) in untreated essential hypertensive subjects[76] restored by chronic treatment with an ACE inhibitor[77] or a dual vasopeptidase inhibitor.[78] A turning point in the validation of Ang-(1-7) critical counterregulatory function was achieved by the physiological and molecular characterization of the role of ACE2 in regulating Ang-(1-7) endogenous production from Ang II.[54] Ang-(1-7)'s mechanism of action in terms of inhibiting myocyte hypertrophy, exhibiting antiproliferative actions, counteracting inflammatory signals and expression of ROS, facilitating nitric oxide (NO) release, and inhibiting platelet aggregation and low-density lipoprotein cholesterol deposition in the subendothelial region of large arterial vessels are summarized in multiple publications.[56,73] Signal transduction pathways in which Ang-(1-7) acts as a ligand are complex, engaging not only the mas receptor but also through the binding of the heptapeptide to AT_2-R and possibly bradykinin B2 receptors. Since the original studies by Loot et al.,[79] Ang-(1-7) has been reported to act as a cardioprotective agent in myocardial infarction and heart failure.[80] Newer studies document that Ang-(1-7) restores myocyte L-type calcium current (ICa^{++},L) responses in experimentally induced heart failure through a mas receptor signaling mechanism involving activation of NO/bradykinin pathways.[81] Ang-(1-7) increases in (Ca^{++})I transients induces positive inotropic and lusitropic effects in left ventricular function and myocyte contractility in heart failure.[82]

Ala[1]-Angiotensin II and Almandine

An intriguing 2007 investigation reported the detection of an Ang II-like peptide in human plasma, in which the amino acid Aspartic acid (Asp) had been replaced by Alanine (Ala) in position 1 of the N-terminus of the molecule.[83] The peptide, named angiotensin A

($Des[Asp^1]$-$[Ala^1]$-Ang II; Ang A), possessed biological activity comparable to Ang II but with a higher affinity for AT_2 receptors.[83] On the other hand, the active metabolite of losartan (EXP-3174) abolished the vasoconstrictor response induced by Ang A, while PD123319 (AT_2 receptor antagonist) had no effect.[83] The discrepancy between high Ang A AT_2 receptor affinity, and persistence of a biological effect following blockade of this receptor remains unexplained. Ang A formation was interpreted by Jankowski et al.[83] to be the result of the enzymatic activity of mononuclear leukocyte-derived aspartate decarboxylase.

In the steps of the German investigators, a group of researchers working under the tutelage of the Brazilian investigator Robson Santos reported in 2017 a comparable decarboxylase process that results in the formation of a ($Des[Asp^1]$-$[Ala^1]$-Ang-[1-7]).[84] The heptapeptide Ala^1-Ang-(1-7) is named almandine.[84] Fig. 5.2 outlines the various proposed pathways associated with the generation of almandine. Another potentially distinctive feature of almandine is that the transformed heptapeptide appears to show higher affinity for a subclass of mas-related proteins, the MrgD receptors.[85] The mas-related G-protein coupled receptor member D (see Table 5.2) is a protooncogene previously associated with functioning as a specific receptor for beta-alanine.[86-88] The significance of Ang A and almandine as secondary tissue-alternates regulating the cardiovascular actions of the renin angiotensin remains to be understood.[89]

ANGIOTENSIN II MEDIATED SIGNALING PATHWAYS

Angiotensin II Receptors

Ang II exerts its biological function through two major Ang II receptors: AT_1-R and AT_2-R. AT_3-R and AT_4-R are also described in cardiovascular organs. Since their biological functions are not well characterized, this chapter will focus primarily on the signaling pathways transduced by AT_1-R and AT_2-R. While AT_1-R is widely expressed in many organs including kidney, brain, heart, and vasculature, expression of AT_2-R in healthy subjects declines in these tissues after birth but could be upregulated under pathological conditions.[90] Both receptors are seven transmembrane receptors and belong to the superfamily of G protein-coupled receptors (GPCR), sharing only 34% sequence identity. In general, AT_1-R mediates Ang II regulation of blood pressure, cell growth and proliferation, cardiac contractility, and salt/water balance. However, an excessive Ang II stimulation of AT_1-R results in a variety of deleterious cardiovascular effects reflected by AT_1-R-mediated vasoconstriction, hypertrophy, apoptosis, fibrosis, oxidative stress, inflammation, enhancement of sympathetic outflow, and aldosterone release. On the other hand, a growing body of evidence testifies that activation of AT_2-R counterbalances the effects of Ang II on AT_1-R inducing vasodilation, decreasing cell proliferation, and fibrosis.[91] It is also suggested that Ang II action on unopposed AT_2-R may contribute to the beneficial cardiovascular effects of AT_1-R pharmacological blockade.[92] Additionally, inhibition of AT_1-R signaling may be also caused by dimerization of the two receptors.[93,94] However, the significance of AT_2-R-mediated effects in cardiovascular pathology still remains unclear, since conflicting studies point to their deleterious cardiovascular effects as well.[95]

Besides AT_1-R/AT_2-R interactions, these receptors may undergo dimerization with other receptors as well. It has been suggested that heterodimerization with the bradykinin B_2[96] or adrenergic receptors[97] potentiates AT_1-R signaling. Importantly, valsartan, an AT_1-R antagonist, blocks signaling pathways of both AT_1-R and adrenergic receptors in mice, whereas β-adrenergic receptor blockers restrict Ang II signaling cascade in heart failure.[97] AT_1-R can also heterodimer with apelin, mas, and several dopamine receptors to alter receptor signaling.[98,99]

On the other hand, AT_2-R may dimer with the mas receptor,[100] and AT_2 receptor blockers may cancel beneficial effects of mas activation in the brain of hypertensive animals.[101] Moreover, to enhance their biological activities, both Ang II receptors can form homodimers before being translocated to the cell membrane.[102]

Like many GPCRs, Ang II mediated AT_1-R activation is subject to desensitization and internalization due to decreased receptor responsiveness. In this process, several serine/threonine residues on the cytoplasmic part of the receptors undergo phosphorylation by G-protein receptor kinases (GRK).[103] Ang II can also phosphorylate AT_1-R,[104] providing a mechanism of how chronic Ang II activation of AT_1-R downregulates its own receptor. Following phosphorylation, recruitment of β-arrestin[105] dissociates AT_1-R from G proteins and starts receptor internalization into clathrin-coated pits or noncoated specialized microdomains called caveolae. Most recently, it has been demonstrated that β-arrestin has a role not only in heterologous AT_1-R desensitization, but also in mediating G protein-independent signaling of AT_1-R (see also Chapter 13). These findings reveal an additional layer of GPCRs interaction without forming receptor heteromers.[106] Most of the internalized receptors are degraded in lysosomes, while roughly one-fourth of them recycle to the plasma membrane. A recent study showed that AT_2-R do not undergo desensitization due to the lack of ability to recruit β-arrestin.[94] Thus it is possible that, upon activation, AT_2-R may mediate a prolonged signaling response.

Ang II interaction with AT_1-R involves G protein-dependent and G protein-independent signaling cascades that trigger a series of pathophysiological effects of Ang II. AT_1-R mostly couples with G proteins (Gαq/11, Gαi/o, Gα12/13) to induce classic G-protein mediated pathways.[107] The AT_1-R-coupled G-protein mediated signaling also involves transactivation of growth factor receptors, as well as activation of several tyrosine kinases, mitogen-activated protein kinases (MAPKs), small GTP-binding proteins, and nicotinamide adenine dinucleotide phosphate (NADPH) oxidases (NOXs). In addition, AT_1-R signaling involves G protein-independent pathways as well, through activation of tyrosine kinases and β-arrestin recruitment. It is important to note that the later mechanism may represent a cardioprotective signaling response. On the other hand, the beneficial cardiovascular effects of AT_2-R predominately reflect its coupling to Giα, leading to activation of protein phosphatases and the NO-cyclic guanosine monophosphate (cGMP) system.

Ang II/AT_1-R-Mediated G Protein-Coupled Pathways

Ang II activation of AT_1-R involves dissociation of heterotrimeric G proteins (Gα, Gβγ) by replacing guanosine diphosphate (GDP) in the Gα subunit with guanosine triphosphate (GTP). There are several subfamilies of Gα and Ang II/AT_1-R signals through Gαq/11, Gαi/0, and Gα12/13. The Gβγ complex also transduces Ang II/AT_1-R cellular effects. In addition to GTPase, which restores the original association of the inactivate states of Gα and Gβγ complex, several GRKs and regulators of G protein signaling (RGS) contribute to the restriction of GPCR activation[108,109] and may be potential targets for novel therapeutic approaches.

Ang II/AT_1-R-Mediated Classic G Protein-Coupled Signaling Pathways

Ang II/AT_1-R interaction involving Gαq/11 protein activates several signaling cascades important for regulation of blood pressure, cardiac growth, and contractility (Fig. 5.3). One of the Gαq/11-mediated downstream signaling pathways involves activation of phospholipase C (PLC-β), leading to hydrolysis of phosphatidylinositol-4,5-bisphosphate (PIP_2) into two key second messengers:

inositol trisphosphate (IP3) and diacylglycerol (DAG).[110] IP3, binding to its receptor on the sarcoplasmic reticulum, releases Ca^{2+} into the cytoplasm. Additional Ca^{2+} influx resulting from Ang II coupling to Gα12/13[107] and activation of plasma membrane L-type Ca^{2+} channels further promotes Ca^{2+} binding to calcium binding proteins, calmodulin/troponin, and activation of myosin light chain kinase (MLCK). Phosphorylation of the myosin light chain by MLCK enhances the interaction between actin and myosin, promoting vascular and cardiac contraction.[111] Negative regulation of contractility is imposed by myosin light chain phosphatase (MLCP), which deactivates MLCK. In contrast, MLCP inhibition by Rho kinase results in enhanced contraction.[112]

In addition to IP_3, DAG also serves as a second messenger in Ang II induced vasoconstriction and hypertrophy by activating downstream protein kinase C (PKC) and Ras, Raf, and MEK/ERK1/2 pathways. Diacylglycerol kinases (DGK) deplete intracellular DAG by converting it to phosphatidic acid (PA) and in that way may negatively regulate Ang II hypertrophic effects through this signaling pathway. However, different DGK isoforms may exert different functional roles on cardiac structure and function. Thus cardiac specific overexpression of DGKξ in mice prevents Ang II-induced cardiac hypertrophy, suggesting a potential for DGKξ to inhibit the Gαq/11-PLC-DAG pathway.[113] Conversely, DGKα overexpression in mouse cardiomyocytes exacerbated systolic dysfunction following ischemia/reperfusion damage.[114] It seems that these detrimental effects reflect the DGKα-mediated inhibition of cardioprotective effects of PKCε, ERK1/2, and p70s6 kinase activation. Thus further studies are warranted for establishing specific DGK isoforms as potential therapeutic targets in the treatment of cardiac hypertrophy and dysfunction.

AT_1-R coupling to Gβγ induces phospholipase D (PLD) activation generating PA, which rapidly converts to DAG, cross-bridging to PKC-dependent downstream signaling activation (see Fig. 5.3). Several studies show that PLC/PLD signaling pathways are augmented in hypertensive rats, supporting a concept of their critical role in the development of hypertensive disease.[115] Moreover, Gαq/11-dependent AT_1-R-mediated activation of phospholipase A_2 (PLA$_2$) results in the production of AA, whose metabolites are important regulators of vasculature and cardiac growth and contraction. An additional layer in Ang II/AT_1-R positive regulation of vascular and cardiac contraction reflects AT_1-R coupling to Gα12/13. This interaction not only mediates Ca^{2+} influx through activation of L-type Ca^{2+} channels but also negatively regulates MLCP through GTPase Rho (see Fig. 5.3).[112] It has been shown that vascular injury and hypertension were associated with increased vascular Rho/Rho kinase activation.[116] In contrast, AT_1-R coupling to pertussis toxin-sensitive Gαi protein negatively regulates cardiac contraction by inhibiting adenylyl cyclase, thereby attenuating cAMP production. In agreement with these findings, upregulation of Gαi protein in human heart tissue from patients with heart failure has been demonstrated.[117] Since decreased cAMP production in vascular smooth muscle cells (VSMCs) results in vasoconstriction, these two mechanisms acting in concert may contribute to the development and progression of heart failure.

Ang II/AT_1-R-Mediated Transactivation of Receptor Tyrosine Kinases

It is currently well accepted that Ang II transactivates several receptor tyrosine kinases, including epidermal growth factor receptor (EGFR), platelet-derived growth factor receptor (PDGFR), and insulin-like growth factor 1 receptor (IGF-1R). Most of the Ang II/AT_1-R-mediated growth effects in the cardiovascular system depend on

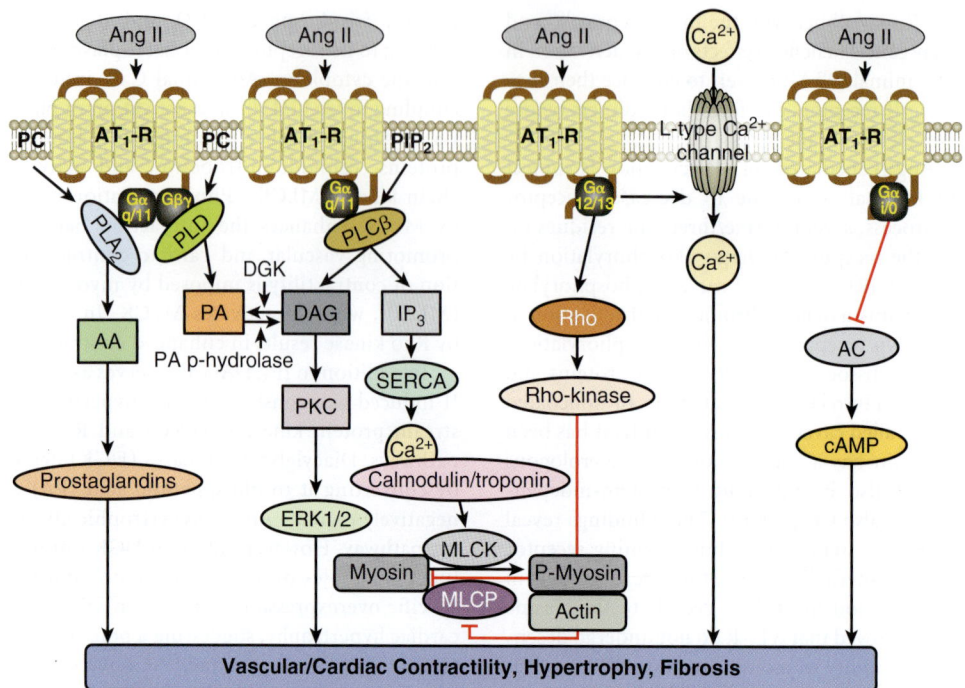

Fig. 5.3 Ang II/AT1-R-Mediated Classic G Protein-Coupled Signaling Pathways. Ang II signaling through AT1-R mostly involves Gαq/11 protein. This activates PLC leading to DAG and IP3 formation and consequent activation of PKC and releases of Ca2+ from SERCA, respectively. PKC activates ERK1/2 and contributes to hypertrophy, while Ca2+ binding to calmodulin/troponin activates MLCK to phosphorylate myosin light chain and induces contraction. AT1-R also couples with Gαq/11 to produce AA and its metabolites prostaglandins implicated in regulation of contraction and vascular and cardiac growth. Activation of PLD in Gβγ-dependent ways leads to production of PA, which rapidly converts to DAG, cross-bridging to PKC-dependent downstream signaling activation. AT1-R coupling with Gα12/13 activates plasma membrane L-type Ca2+ channels and increases Ca2+ influx while negatively regulating MLCP through GTPase Rho. AT1-R coupling to pertussis toxin-sensitive Gαi protein negatively regulates cardiac contraction by inhibiting AC, thereby attenuating cAMP production. *AA,* Arachidonic acid; *AC,* adenylyl cyclase; *ERK,* extracellular signal-regulated kinases; *PC,* protein C; *PKC,* protein kinase C.

the transactivation of EGFR. Indeed, both pharmacological inhibition and genetic silencing of EGFR significantly reduced Ang II-induced Akt/ERK1/2 signaling pathway activation, hypertrophic marker overexpression, and cell hypertrophy of cardio-myoblast cell line H9c2. Likewise, in a complimentary in vivo study, EGFR inhibition attenuated cardiac remodeling in Ang II infused mice.[118] The activation cascade starts with stimulation of ADAM in a PKC-, Ca2+-, and ROS-dependent manner through sequential activation of the nonreceptor protein tyrosine kinases Src and Pyk2 to shed heparin-binding EGF (HB-EGF) (Fig. 5.4), which induces EGFR dimerization and autophosphorylation.[119-121] Recent evidence suggests that ADAM17 has a critical role in EGFR transactivation mediating Ang II-induced myocyte hypertrophy[121] and that caveolin-1, the major structural protein of caveolae, negatively regulates Ang II-induced ADAM17-dependent EGFR transactivation in VSMCs.[122] Indeed, infection of an adenovirus encoding caveolin-1 significantly reduced Ang II-induced EGFR transactivation and subsequent ERK1/2 activation, and consequent VSMC hypertrophy and migration. After activation, EGFR recruits adapter proteins Grb2/Shc/Sos to induce the Ras/Raf/ERK1/2 pathway leading to cell growth and hypertrophy, as well as phosphoinositide 3-OH kinase (PI3K)/Akt, signaling implicated in cell survival and growth. Thus EGFR may exert cardioprotective effects against acute cardiac load and myocardial ischemia.[123] However, accumulating evidence from experimental studies suggest that EGFR activation may be detrimental as well. The occurrence of ischemia/reperfusion-induced arrhythmia depends on EGFR activation[124] and, if chronically

activated after myocardial infarction, the EGFR-mediated decrease in myofibroblast proliferation and collagen synthesis may lead to cardiac rupture.[125] Thus further studies are needed in careful consideration of the therapeutic potential of AT1-R-mediated EGFR signaling pathways. In addition to EGFR, Ang II/AT1-R transactivates PDGFR through its adapter molecule Shc, and sequential activation of MAPK is implicated in cardiovascular growth and hypertrophy.[126,127] On the other hand, IGF-1R transactivation leads to activation of PI3K and ERK/1/2, signaling cascades in regulation of cell growth, proliferation, and survival.[128,129]

Ang II/AT1-R-Mediated Nonreceptor Tyrosine Kinases Activation

Pluripotent effects of Ang II in the cardiovascular system also reflect its ability to activate numerous nonreceptor tyrosine kinases involved in several pathways that are implicated in regulation of cell growth, survival, and adhesion (see Fig. 5.4). Thus Ang II/AT1-R signaling involves Src family kinase, Janus kinases (JAKs), focal adhesion kinase (FAK), Ca2+-dependent tyrosine kinase Pyk2, p130Cas, and PI3K.

A growing body of evidence points to c-Src as a critical contributor to various Ang II cellular effects. This tyrosine kinase is activated by Gβγ complex in an ROS-dependent manner and activates several downstream signaling molecules such as Ras, FAK, JAK/STAT (Fig. 5.5). Recent studies demonstrated that enhanced activation of vascular c-Src, ERK1/2, and JNK in Ang II-infused mice was normalized in mice with partial deletion of c-Src or in

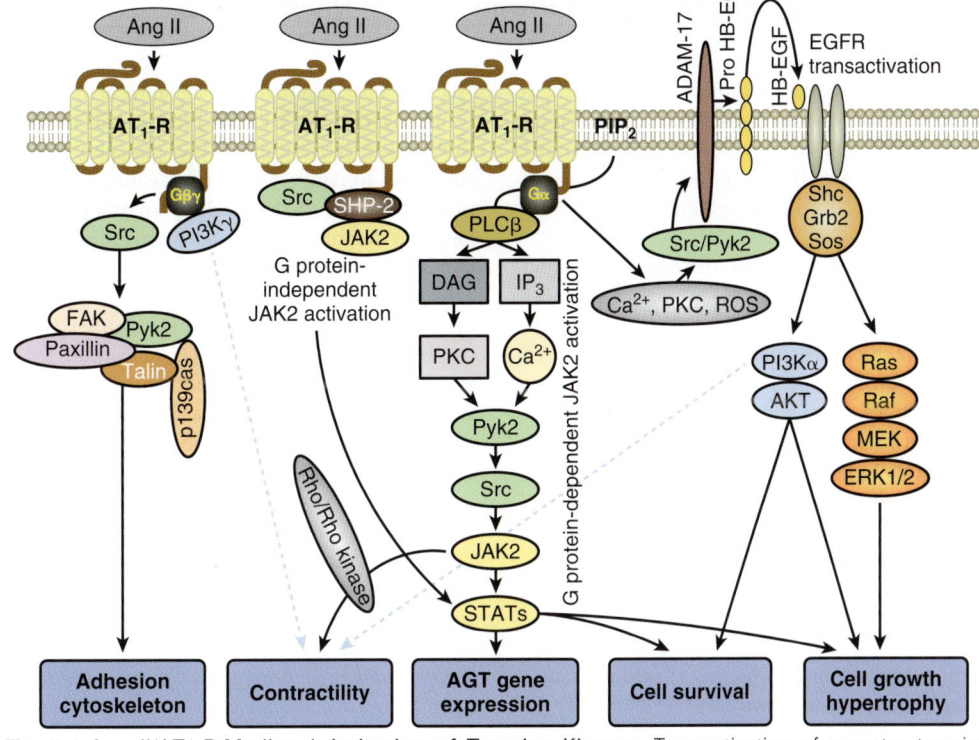

Fig. 5.4 Ang II/AT1-R-Mediated Activation of Tyrosine Kinases. Transactivation of receptor tyrosine kinase EGFR starts with stimulation of ADAM in a PKC-, Ca²⁺-, and ROS-dependent manner through sequential activation of the nonreceptor protein tyrosine kinases Src and Pyk2 to shed HB-EGF, which induces EGFR dimerization and autophosphorylation. Activated EGFR then recruits adapter proteins Grb2/Shc/Sos to induce the Ras/Raf/ERK1/2 pathway, leading to cell growth and hypertrophy as well as PI3K/Akt signaling implicated in cell survival and growth. Ang II/AT1-R signaling also includes numerous nonreceptor tyrosine kinases (Src family kinase, JAKs, FAK, Pyk2, p130Cas, and PI3K) involved in several pathways that are implicated in regulation of cell growth, survival, adhesion, and contractility. Ang II/AT1-R activates JAK2 via both G protein-dependent and independent signaling connected to various cardiovascular pathologies. *ADAM,* A disintegrin and metalloprotease; *ERK,* extracellular signal-regulated kinases; *JAK,* Janus kinases; *PKC,* protein kinase C; *STAT,* signal transducer and activator of transcription

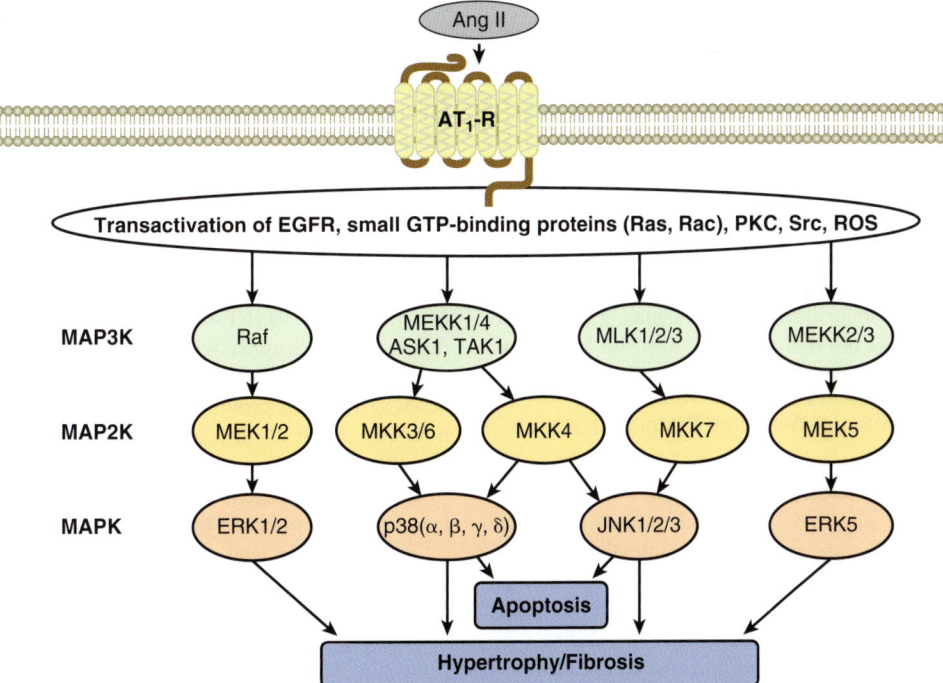

Figure 5.5 Ang II/AT1-R-Mediated Mitogen-Activated Protein Kinases *(MAPK)* Activation. Ang II/AT1-R signaling activates the MAPK cascade by transactivation of EGFR, by PKC and GTP-binding proteins, and by ROS. The MAPK pathway is a three-step cascade consisting of MAP kinase kinase kinase *(MAP3K)*, MAP kinase kinase *(MAP2K)*, and MAPK. At least four differently regulated MAPKs are present in mammalian tissues, including ERK1/2, JNK1/2/3, p38 proteins, and ERK5. *ERK,* Extracellular signal-regulated kinases; *PKC,* protein kinase C.

mice treated concomitantly with c-Src inhibitor. These changes resulted in a decrease in blood pressure, normalized cardiac function, and attenuation of endothelial dysfunction caused by Ang II infusion.[130] By activating c-Src, Ang II also induces association of FAK, Pyk2, paxillin, talin, and p130Cas that regulates cell shape and movement (see Fig. 5.4).

Ang II regulates cardiovascular growth through JAK/signal transducer and activator of transcription (STAT) signaling pathway as well. The JAK family includes several cytoplasmic tyrosine kinases (JAK1, JAK2, JAK3, Tyk2), which, when stimulated, initiate STAT protein dimerization and translocation to the nucleus to regulate the transcription of target genes. It has been shown that losartan, an AT1-R antagonist, reduced interstitial fibrosis and improved cardiac function in diabetic rats by inhibiting the JAK/STAT singling pathway.[131]. In VSMC, AT1-R-mediated JAK2 activation involves Gαq protein and secondary messengers IP3 and DAG that increase intracellular Ca^{2+} and activate PKC-δ, respectively (see Fig. 5.4). Both Ca^{2+} and PKC-δ are necessary for c-Src activation, which ultimately activates JAK.[132] While nuclear translocation of phosphorylated STAT1, STAT2, and STAT3 by JAK2 and TYK2 has been shown as a critical event in transducing Ang II cardiovascular growth and remodeling effects,[133] activation of STAT3 and STAT5 is a crucial step in inducing AGT gene expression.[134] The latter mechanism underlines a detrimental amplifying effect of a positive feedback loop between Ang II and its substrate. In addition, a recent study demonstrated that in normal human cardiomyocytes Ang II preferentially activates JAK2/STAT3/B-cell lymphoma-extra large (Bcl-xL) pathway implicated in cardiac survival and growth while in failing cardiomyocytes JAK2/STAT5 activation without Bcl-xL change was observed.[135] The authors concluded that the altered JAK2-induced STATs response in human failing cardiomyocytes may be relevant for the progression of cardiac dysfunction in heart failure. Importantly, activated JAK2 also promotes vasoconstriction and hypertension through the Rho/Rho-kinase pathway by reducing MLCP activity.

A family of PI3Ks is another tyrosine kinase activation pathway involved in wide array of Ang II/AT1-R-mediated cellular functions (see Fig. 5.4). PI3Kγ requires activation by Gβγ complex, whereas PI3Kα is activated by receptor tyrosine kinase. Regarding the effects on contractility, the role of specific PI3Ks is still controversial. While early work showed that PI3Kγ negatively regulates cardiac contractility by depleting cAMP levels,[136] PI3Kα enhanced cardiac contraction strength and L-type Ca^{2+} currents.[137] However, a more recent report suggests that PI3Kα, not PI3Kγ, was required for the negative inotropic effects of Ang II[138] suggesting its potential role in development of heart failure. PI3K transduction also includes Akt/PKB signaling implicated in not only protein syntheses through activation of p70s6-kinase but also in cell survival by promoting Bcl-2 and inhibiting caspase.

Ang II/AT₁-R-Mediated Mitogen-Activated Protein Kinases Activation

Activation of MAPKs is an established mechanism in numerous biological effects mediated by Ang II/AT1-R stimulation. At least four differently regulated MAPKs are present in mammalian tissues, including ERK1/2, JNK1/2/3, p38 proteins, and ERK5. The MAPK activation cascade involves upstream kinases, MAP kinase kinase (MAP2K), and MAP kinase kinase kinase (MAP3K), MEKK1-4, TGF β-activated kinase (TAK1), thousand-and-one amino acid 1-3 (TAO1-3), mixed-lineage kinase 2/3 (MLK2/3), apoptosis signal regulating kinase 1/2 (ASK1/2), and Raf at the MAP3K level, and MEK1/2, and 5, as well as MKK 3, 4, 6 and 7 at the MAP2K level

(see Fig. 5.5). Ang II/AT1-R signaling activates the MAPK cascade by transactivation of EGFR, by PKC and GTP-binding proteins, and by ROS. Upon activation, MAPKs phosphorylate various downstream substrates to regulate gene expression, cellular metabolism, growth, programmed death, extracellular matrix proteins, and contraction. It has been described that ERK1/2 activation could mediate both adaptive and maladaptive responses in the heart[139]. Thus while ERK1/2 activation mediated by Gαq was associated with phosphorylation of cytosolic targets inducing protein synthesis in physiological hypertrophy, Gβγ-mediated ERK1/2 activation led to nuclear position and transcription of the genes associated with pathological hypertrophy.[140] A recent study described that enhanced ERK1/2 signaling also promoted Ang II-induced fibroblast proliferation and extracellular matrix deposition.[141] Furthermore, Ang II activation of JNK appears to have a role in the development of cardiac hypertrophy and apoptosis, two major features of early-stage heart failure.[142,143] Finally, like the role of ERK, activation of p38 may lead to development of cardiac remodeling and dysfunction, while it may be beneficial following ischemic preconditioning.[144] Therefore, further studies are warranted in a quest to comprehensively understand the role of MAPKs and their potential as therapeutic targets for treatment of heart failure.

Ang II/AT₁-R-Mediated Reactive Oxygen Species Signaling

Many well-established Ang II contributions to the development of heart failure, including cardiac hypertrophy and remodeling as well as abnormalities in contraction and electrical function, have been shown to be dependent on ROS production and activation of redox signaling. It has been demonstrated that cardiac ROS generated by mitochondria, xanthine oxidase, NADPH oxidase proteins (NOX; NOX-2 and NOX-4 are the most predominant isoforms in heart tissue), and uncoupled NOS is regulated by Ang II/AT1-R signaling (Fig. 5.6). NADPH oxidase is critically involved in promoting diverse detrimental effects of Ang II in cardiomyocytes and its activation of involves a small GTP-binding protein Rac1. A growing body of evidence suggests that experimental and clinical heart failure are associated with an increase in both NADPH oxidase and xanthine oxidase.[145] Importantly, AT1-R blockade reversed structural and functional cardiac derangement by reducing the activities of these ROS-generating enzymes.[146] Similarly, Ang II-mediated mitochondrial ROS production leads to the development of experimental heart failure.[147] Numerous downstream molecules and pathways are modulated by ROS, such as protein tyrosine kinases, MAPK, transcription factors, and ion channels. Thus redox-sensitive regulation of downstream ERK, ASK-1, and nuclear factor kappa-light-chain-enhancer of activated B cells (NF-κB) is involved in Ang II-promoted cardiomyocyte hypertrophy, whereas enhanced cardiomyocyte apoptosis via ROS-dependent activation of calcium calmodulin kinase II (CaMKII) follows prolonged Ang II stimulation and may cause pronounced cell death in heart failure.[148] Redox-sensitive modulation of p38MAPK, JNK, and PI3K pathways has also been implicated in cardiomyocyte programmed death, leading to progressive ventricular remodeling in heart failure.

In addition, several proteins involved in excitation contraction coupling, such as L-type Ca^{2+} channels, sarcoplasmic reticulum Ca^{2+}-ATPase, and phospholamban, are either direct or indirect targets of ROS in pathological conditions contributing to contractile dysfunction.[149] It was also demonstrated that ROS modulates sodium, potassium, and calcium handling linking oxidative stress and development of arrhythmia.[150] On the other hand, a growing body of evidence suggests that redox-dependent Ang II-mediated signaling induces cardiac fibrosis by

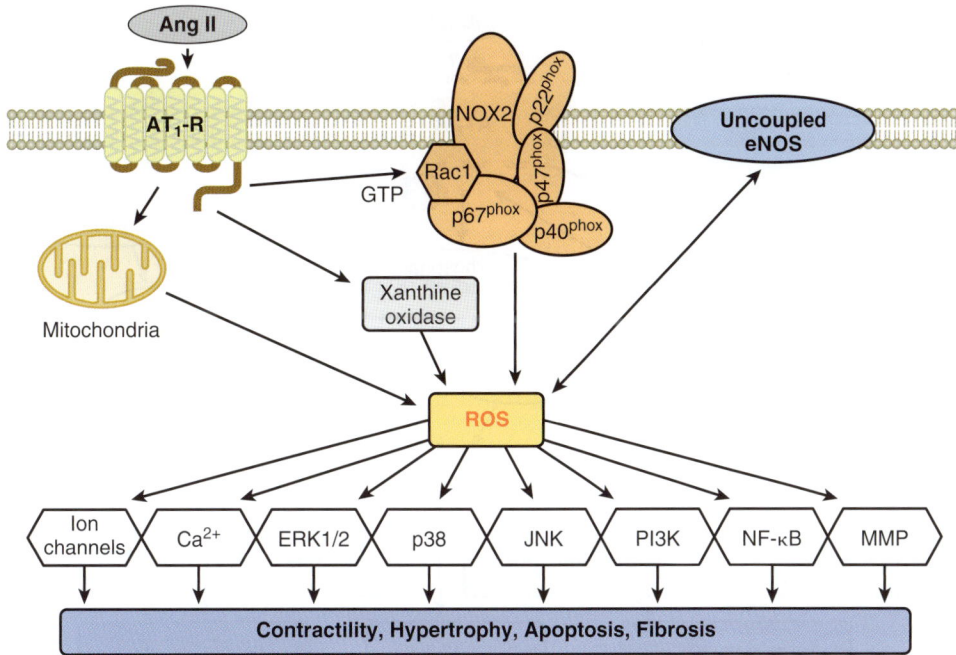

Fig. 5.6 Ang II/AT1-R-Mediated Reactive Oxygen Species Signaling. ROS generated by mitochondria, xanthine oxidase, NADPH oxidase proteins (NOX), and uncoupled NOS are regulated by Ang II/AT1-R signaling. The redox-sensitive modulation of downstream molecules and pathways including protein tyrosine kinases, MAPKs, Ca^{2+} handling proteins, transcription factors, and ion channels are implicated in development of cardiac hypertrophy, fibrosis, apoptosis, and contractile dysfunction. *ERK*, extracellular signal-regulated kinases.

promoting NOX2-dependent fibroblast proliferation. Indeed, NOX2-null mice exhibit reduced fibrosis following Ang II infusion.[151] Especially important for the pathogenesis of ventricular dilation in heart failure are studies showing that NADPH oxidase mediates Ang II/aldosterone-induced MMP activation.[151,152] Thus Ang II-mediated redox signaling pathways are well-accepted contributors to the development and progression of heart failure and are increasingly recognized as targets for development of novel therapeutic approaches.

G-Protein-Independent AT₁-R Signaling Pathways

It is recognized that, in addition to AT₁-R-mediated G protein-dependent stimulation of the JAK/STAT signaling cascade described previously, Ang II may exert its pathological effects in fibroblasts and VSMC through G protein-independent JAK/STAT activation by c-Src homology phosphatase-2 (see Fig. 5.4).[153,154]

Besides nonreceptor tyrosine kinases, Ang II/AT₁-R signaling independent of G protein involves direct association with an adapter protein β-arrestin. As mentioned before, β-arrestins have a distinctive role in AT₁-R desensitization and internalization. However, numerous studies suggested that after G protein uncoupling, receptor-bound β-arrestin may initiate several downstream pathways, including MAPK, c-Src family kinases, JNK, and PI3K.[155-157] Some of these signaling cascades promote cardiac survival by inhibiting apoptosis and inflammation. Therefore it seems that β-arrestin could be considered as a novel therapeutic target because of its dual role in inhibiting pathological G protein-dependent signaling while simultaneously stimulating beneficial β-arrestin-mediated cardioprotective pathways. However, since there are two β-arrestin isoforms, and several studies suggest they may have opposing cardiac effects,[158] it will be important to unravel their precise mechanism of action before β-arrestins are considered as additional targets for therapeutic intervention.

Ang II/AT₂-R-Mediated Signaling Pathways

In contrast to AT₁-R, AT₂-R generally couples to Gαi protein, leading to distinctly different intracellular signaling mechanisms (Fig. 5.7). Accumulated evidence documents that Ang II stimulation of AT₂-R induces vasodilation in isolated resistance vessels.[159,160] In concert with this in vitro data, in vivo studies, in which expression or activity of AT₂-R was manipulated genetically or pharmacologically, support the concept that AT₂-R is vasodilatory and counteracts the pressor effects of AT₁-R stimulation by Ang II. Most of this effect is mediated through the NO/cGMP pathway by release of bradykinin and NOS activation.[90] Importantly, a recent study showed that NO donors upregulated AT₂-R expression in endothelial cells through activation of cGMP, protein kinase G (PKG), and p38MAPK.[161] This positive feedback mechanism might be important in maintaining blood pressure in response to long-term agonist stimulation. An additional signaling cascade in AT₂-R-mediated vascular effects may reflect the ability of AT₂-R to inhibit JNK activity affecting Pyk2 in a SHP-1 dependent manner in VSMC.[162] Others reported that AT₂-R attenuated AT₁-R-induced PLD.[163]

Over the past decade, a growing body of evidence suggests that Ang II/AT₂-R-mediated activation of several phosphatases (MAPK phosphatase 1 [MKP-1], Src homology 2 domain-containing phosphatase 1 [SHP-1], and protein phosphatase 2 [PP2A]) could halt the Ang II/AT₁-R-mediated activation of downstream protein kinases involved in AT₁-R effects on cell proliferation and growth as well as inflammation, apoptosis, and oxidative stress.[164-166] It has also been known that AT₂-R-mediated antiproliferative effects of Ang II could involve AT₂-R interacting protein (ATIP) (also called AT₂ binding protein of 50 kDa [ATBP50]) which facilitates AT₂-R trafficking to plasma membrane.[167] Moreover, trans-inactivation of receptor tyrosine kinases by

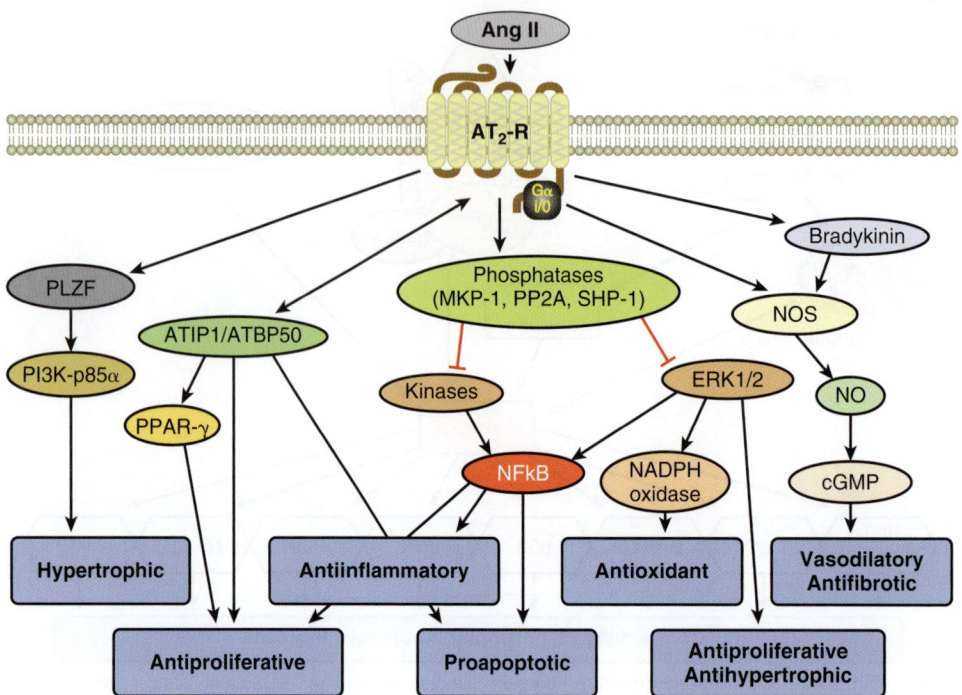

Fig. 5.7 Schematic Diagram of the Major AT$_2$-R-Mediated Signaling Pathways. Majority of vasodilatory effects of AT$_2$-R activation are mediated through NO/cGMP pathway by release of bradykinin and NOS activation. Antioxidant, anti-inflammatory, proapoptotic, and growth and proliferation inhibition of AT$_2$-R involve activation of several phosphatases (MKP-1, PP2A, SHP-1) to dephosphorylate ERK1/2 and other kinases. Interaction with ATIP1 is implicated in the AT$_2$-R-mediating antiproliferative and proapoptotic effects of Ang II. On the other hand, recruitment of PLZF to AT$_2$-R induces hypertrophic response. *ATIP*, AT$_2$-R interacting protein; *ERK*, extracellular signal-regulated kinases.

AT$_2$-R has also been associated with AT$_2$-R alliance with its interacting protein.[168] More recent studies further implicated the interaction of ATIP1 with peroxisome proliferator-activated receptor γ (PPARγ) in AT$_2$-R-mediating attenuation of vascular intimal proliferation.[169]

Conflicting results involving AT$_2$-R signaling in cardiovascular pathology have been described also. Thus a vasoconstrictor effect mediated by increased expression of AT$_2$-R in resistant arteries was observed in old but not young rats.[170] Furthermore, adenovirus-mediated overexpression of human AT$_2$-R in porcine cardiac fibroblasts inhibited protein tyrosine phosphatases, although it did not affect fibroblast proliferation.[171] It has also been reported that promyelocytic leukemia zinc finger protein (PLZF) interacts with AT$_2$-R in promoting cardiac hypertrophy and fibrosis by increasing transcription of regulatory subunit p85α of PI3K.[172] However, additional studies revealed that AT$_2$-R itself does not promote hypertrophic effects, and that certain cell conditions facilitate the PLZF recruitment to AT$_2$-R to induce hypertrophic response.[95] Because of these and other controversial data, further studies to elucidate the pathophysiological role of AT$_2$-R activation are warranted.

SUMMARY AND CONCLUSIONS

The discoveries reviewed herein support the view that the renin angiotensin system is a complex system in which biological diversity is not only demonstrated by the different effects of the products generated from either Ang I or Ang II but also through its receptors and peptide-forming and degrading enzymes. That the renin angiotensin system was far more complex than generally accepted, and that this complexity guarantees a well-tuned adaptation of the blood supply of the body compartments to all physiological conditions, were advanced

as early as 1991.[8] Today, these tissue-specific mechanisms exerted by a host of small peptides, all derived from one single gene producing the protein AGT, are the basis for attempting new therapies for halting or regressing the consequences of chronic heart failure (see Chapter 37), essential hypertension, type 2 diabetes, chronic renal disease, and cerebrovascular events.[43]

ACKNOWLEDGMENTS

We thank Ms. Jessica VonCannon, B.Sc., for her careful proofreading of this chapter. Work described here from the authors' laboratories was funded by a Program Project Grant 2P01HL051952 from the National Heart, Lung, and Blood Institute of the National Institutes of Health.

KEY REFERENCES

4. Kumar R, Baker KM, Pan J. Molecular signaling mechanisms of the renin-angiotensin system in heart failure. In: Mann DL, Felker GM, eds. *Heart Failure: a Companion to Braunwald's Heart Disease*. Philadelphia, PA: Elsevier-Saunders; 2015:79–93.

7. Ferrario CM, Ahmad S, Varagic J, et al. Intracrine angiotensin II functions originate from noncanonical pathways in the human heart. *Am J Physiol Heart Circ Physiol*. 2016;311(2):H404–414.

43. Ferrario CM, Mullick AE. Renin angiotensin aldosterone inhibition in the treatment of cardiovascular disease. *Pharmacol Res*. 2017;125(Pt A):57–71.

51. Dell'Italia LJ, Collawn JF, Ferrario CM. Multifunctional role of chymase in acute and chronic tissue injury and remodeling. *Circ Res*. 2018;122(2):319–336.

84. Lautner RQ, Villela DC, Fraga-Silva RA, et al. Discovery and characterization of alamandine: a novel component of the renin-angiotensin system. *Circ Res*. 2013;112(8):1104–1411.

FURTHER READING

da Silva Novaes A, Ribeiro RS, Pereira LG, et al. Intracrine action of angiotensin II in mesangial cells: subcellular distribution of angiotensin II receptor subtypes AT1 and AT2. *Mol Cell Biochem*. 2018.

Messerli FH, Bangalore S, Bavishi C, Rimoldi SF. angiotensin-converting enzyme inhibitors in hypertension: to use or not to use? *J Am Coll Cardiol*. 2018;71:1474–1482.

Miyoshi T, Nakamura K, Miura D, et al. Effect of LCZ696, a dual angiotensin receptor neprilysin inhibitor, on isoproterenol-induced cardiac hypertrophy, fibrosis, and hemodynamic change in rats. *Cardiol J*. 2018.

Patel S, Hussain T. Dimerization of AT2 and Mas receptors in control of blood pressure. *Curr Hypertens Rep*. 2018;20:41.

Whelton PK, Carey RM. The 2017 American College of Cardiology/American Heart Association clinical practice guideline for high blood pressure in adults. *JAMA Cardiol*. 2018;3:352–353.

The full reference list is available on ExpertConsult.

Abbreviations Used in This Chapter

Abbreviation	Full Name
ACE	Angiotensin-converting enzyme
ACE2	Angiotensin-converting enzyme 2
Ac-SDKP	N-acetyl-Ser-Asp-Lys-Pro tetrapeptide
Almandine	[Des[Asp1]-[Ala1]-angiotensin-(1-7)
Ang	Angiotensin
Ang (1-5)	Angiotensin-(1-5)
Ang A	Angiotensin A or [Des[Asp^1]-[Ala^1]-angiotensin II
Ang I	Angiotensin I
Ang II	Angiotensin II
Ang III	Angiotensin III
Ang IV	Angiotensin IV
Ang-(1-12)	Angiotensin-(1-12)
Ang-(1-14)	Angiotensin-(1-14)
Ang-(1-25)	Angiotensin-(1-25)
Ang-(1-7)	Angiotensin-(1-7)
Ang-(1-9)	Angiotensin-(1-9)
AT$_1$-R	Angiotensin II type 1 receptor
AT$_2$-R	Angiotensin II type 2 receptor
AGT	Angiotensinogen
CaMKII	Calcium calmodulin kinase II
cAMP	Cyclic adenosine monophosphate
DAG	diacylglycerol
DGK	Diacylglycerol kinases
EGF	Epidermal growth factor
EGFR	Epidermal growth factor receptor
FAK	Focal adhesion kinase
Gamma NGF	Gamma-nerve growth factor
GDP	Guanosine diphosphate
GLUT4	Insulin-sensitive glucose transporter
GPCR	G protein-coupled receptors
GRK	G-protein receptor kinases
GRS	Regulators of G protein signaling
GTP	Guanosine triphosphate
IGF-1R	Insulin-like growth factor 1 receptor
IL-6	Interleukin-6
IL-1β	Interleukin-1β

Abbreviation	Full Name
IP3	inositol trisphosphate
IRAP	Insulin-regulated aminopeptidase
GLUT4	Insulin-sensitive glucose transporter
JNK	Janus kinases
MAP	Mitogen-activated protein kinase
MAP2K	MAP kinase kinase
MAP3K	MAP kinase kinase kinase
MAPKs	Mitogen-activated protein kinases
MLCK	myosin light chain kinase
MLCP	Myosin light-chain phosphatase
MLK2/3	Mixed-lineage kinase 2/3
MMPs	Metalloproteinases
NADPH	Nicotinamide adenine dinucleotide phosphate
NEP	Neprilysin
NO	Nitric oxide
PDGFR	Platelet derived growth factor receptor
PA	Phosphatidic acid
PI3K	Phosphoinositide 3-OH kinase
PIP2	Phosphatidylinositol-4,5-bisphosphate
PLA2	Phospholipase A2
PLC-β	Phospholipase C
PLD	Phospholipase D
PP2A	Protein phosphatase 2
PPARγ	Peroxisome proliferator-activated receptor γ
PPR	Prorenin receptor
pre-proET1	Pre-pro-endothelin I
ROS	Radical oxygen species
SAPK	Stress-activated protein kinase
SHP-1	Src homology 2 domain-containing phosphatase
SHR	Spontaneously hypertensive rats
SCF	Stem cell factor
TAK1	TGF β-activated kinase
TAO1-3	Thousand-and-one amino acid 1-3
TGF-β	Transforming growth factor-β
VSMC	Vascular smooth muscle cells

Adrenergic Receptor Signaling in Heart Failure

J. David Port, Carmen Sucharov, Michael R. Bristow

Normal and pathophysiological stresses result in increased myocardial demand that is met by a commensurate increase in cardiac adrenergic drive. To facilitate this increase, the neurotransmitter norepinephrine (NE) is released from adrenergic (sympathetic) nerve endings within the heart. Upon binding to β-adrenergic receptors (β-ARs), multiple signaling pathways are activated, resulting in increases in heart rate, force of contraction, and rate of relaxation. Increased adrenergic drive also results in metabolic adjustments (glucose vs. lipid) as well as in a multitude of changes in posttranslational modifications of proteins, gene expression patterns, and epigenetic modifications—notably to the acetylome and methylome. The immediate result of increased adrenergic drive is an increase in blood pressure and cardiac output. In the setting of acute heart failure, adrenergic activation occurs in response to hemodynamic overload and/or to an intrinsic reduction in pump function. However, in the setting of chronic decompensated heart failure, a response that is normally physiologic and transient is instead sustained in an attempt to maintain myocardial performance at a homeostatic level. Under these conditions, the initially beneficial adrenergic support mechanisms become manifestly maladaptive and contribute directly to the progressive natural history of heart failure.

In this chapter, the long-term consequences of sustained adrenergic activation in chronic heart failure (CHF) from reduced left ventricular ejection fraction (heart failure with reduced ejection fraction [HFrEF]), or CHF with pathologic eccentric remodeling and systolic dysfunction, will be reviewed. Particular emphasis will be placed on alterations in β-adrenergic signal transduction and gene expression patterns that occur in the context of the failing human heart, and the impact of these changes on myocardial disease progression. Adrenergic receptor pharmacology relevant to heart failure, as well as recent data from transgenic animals and model systems that demonstrate the myopathic potential of individual components of the adrenergic signaling cascade, will also be reviewed. These changes are likely to be applicable to CHF with preserved left ventricular ejection fraction ("HFpEF"); however, in human heart failure or animal models, HFpEF has not been investigated sufficiently to arrive at a firm conclusion. Therefore, in this discussion, CHF implies chronic HFrEF.

ROLE OF INCREASED ADRENERGIC DRIVE IN THE NATURAL HISTORY OF HEART FAILURE

In patients with CHF, the adrenergic nervous system is critical to the support of myocardial function. However, chronic activation contributes to progressive myocardial *dys*function and left ventricular pathological remodeling. Regardless of etiology, a decrease in myocardial function results in activation of afferent signaling from baroreceptors and chemoreceptors to the central nervous system, such that efferent cardiac adrenergic nerves release more NE,[1,2] activating β-ARs, increasing heart rate and, depending on the degree of functional reserve, increasing myocardial contractility. The increases in heart rate and contractility favorably affect both systolic and diastolic function, thereby increasing cardiac output. As heart failure worsens, adrenergic drive continues to increase in an attempt to compensate for the progressive loss of cardiac function (**Fig. 6.1**).[1,2] However, long-term exposure to high concentrations of NE has marked adverse effects on myocardial and cardiac myocyte biology (**Fig. 6.2**).[3,4] Conversely, inhibitors of adrenergic signaling that have demonstrated favorable effects on heart failure natural history include β-blocking agents and inhibitors of the renin–angiotensin–aldosterone system, which indirectly lower adrenergic drive. There is extensive clinical trials literature supporting the use of these classes of agents as well as definitive guidelines (American Heart Association/American College of Cardiology [AHA/ACC]) for their optimal administration (**see Chapter 37**).[5-10]

Although the "cardiotoxic" effects of catecholamines, in particular NE, have been recognized for more than a century,[11] we have only recently begun to understand the detailed molecular mechanisms by which sustained increases in cardiac adrenergic drive adversely affect myocardial biology and structure/function phenotype. Treatment of isolated cardiac myocytes with concentrations of NE equivalent to those in the failing human heart cause dramatic changes in cell morphology and, within a matter of days, up to a 60% loss of myocyte viability.[3] This effect is mimicked by exposing myocytes to the nonselective β-agonist isoproterenol, an effect that is inhibited pharmacologically by the β-blocker, propranolol, suggesting that the acute toxic effects of NE are mediated almost exclusively through β-ARs rather than through α-ARs.[12] As described below, signaling via the β₁-AR is generally considered to be more biologically harmful than via the β₂-AR.[12,13] This finding is supported by clinical trial data, where differences in β₁-AR blocking doses and enrollment criteria are considered[5,14]; further, β₁-AR selective blockade[7,15,16] appears equally efficacious as treatment with nonselective β-blockers,[8,16] meaning that β₁-AR signaling is the key general mechanism mediating reversible pathobiologic effects in the failing heart.

As stated above, elevated plasma concentrations of NE reflecting overflow from adrenergically activated organs including the heart[2,17,18] are a well-recognized biomarker of CHF.[19] However, as adrenergic activation persists, cardiac NE stores become depleted.[20] Ultimately, other tissue sources of catecholamines (i.e., the adrenal medulla) are stimulated, leading to generalized adrenergic activation and spillover of cardiac derived NE into the systemic circulation.[2,4] As systemic[19,21] or cardiac[22] NE levels increase, so does mortality in patients with heart

failure. These observations have been validated further by evidence from numerous clinical trials of β-blocker therapy, demonstrating reverse remodeling (improved systolic function and decreased left ventricular volumes, typically measured as the ejection fraction)[23-25] and improved survival[7,15,26] in patients with heart failure who receive β-blocker therapy, long term.

Interestingly, in marked contrast to adults with HFrEF, β-blocker therapy does not appear to be particularly efficacious in pediatric heart failure patients.[27] Although the findings are somewhat anecdotal, pediatric patients with systolic heart failure appear to respond more favorably than adults to type 3 phosphodiesterase (PDE) inhibitors.[28] Underlying this difference are markedly different gene expression patterns and adrenergic receptor biology in adult versus pediatric populations.[29]

A recent realization is that *insufficient* adrenergic drive in individuals with CHF can also increase mortality.[5,30] In contrast to β-blocking agents, sympatholytic agents (agents that lower adrenergic activity) can actually increase mortality, presumably via excessive withdrawal of adrenergic support to the failing heart. In contrast, β-blocking agents are pharmacologically reversible mass-action agents, and in their presence adrenergic support to the failing heart can be accessed if needed simply by increasing cardiac adrenergic drive. One β-blocker in clinical development, bucindolol, is both a nonselective β-blocker and a mild sympatholytic agent.[8,21] When NE lowering from bucindolol is mild, the result is an enhancement of efficacy. However, in some patients, the degree of sympatholysis produced by bucindolol can be excessive, obviating any benefit realized from the β-blockade.[21] It is now understood that the sympatholytic effects of bucindolol are under control of prejunctional α₂C adrenergic receptors, the implication being that exaggerated/adverse NE lowering can be avoided by not treating patients who have a loss of function α₂C polymorphism in combination with a decreased function β₁-AR genetic variant (see below).

Historical studies suggested that one underlying mechanism of NE toxicity involves cyclic adenosine monophosphate (cAMP)-mediated increases in intracellular calcium.[3] Increased formation of the second messenger cAMP leads to activation of protein kinase A (PKA), which in turn phosphorylates a variety of target proteins involved in regulating intracellular calcium, including key targets such as phospholamban (PLB), L-type calcium channels (LTCCs, CaV₁.₂), and ryanodine

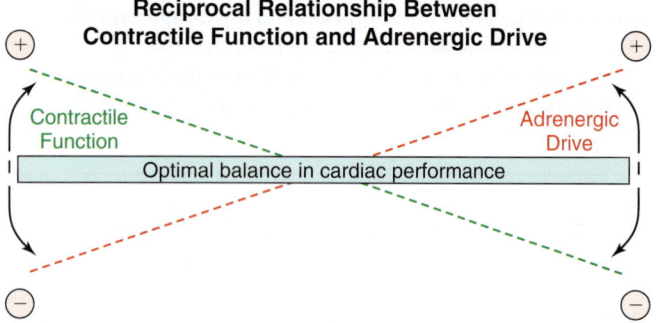

Reciprocal Relationship Between Contractile Function and Adrenergic Drive

Contractile Function

Adrenergic Drive

Optimal balance in cardiac performance

Fig. 6.1 Homeostatic regulation of contractile function. Adrenergic drive acts as a servo-control regulator of normal cardiac contractile function. When cardiac contractile function is adequate to sustain normal homeostasis, adrenergic drive is low or reduced. In contrast, when contractile function is inadequate to support homeostasis, cardiac adrenergic drives increases to a commensurate degree. (Adapted from Port JD, Bristow MR. Altered β-adrenergic receptor gene regulation and signaling in chronic heart failure. *J Mol Cell Cardiol.* 2001;33:887–905, Academic Press.)

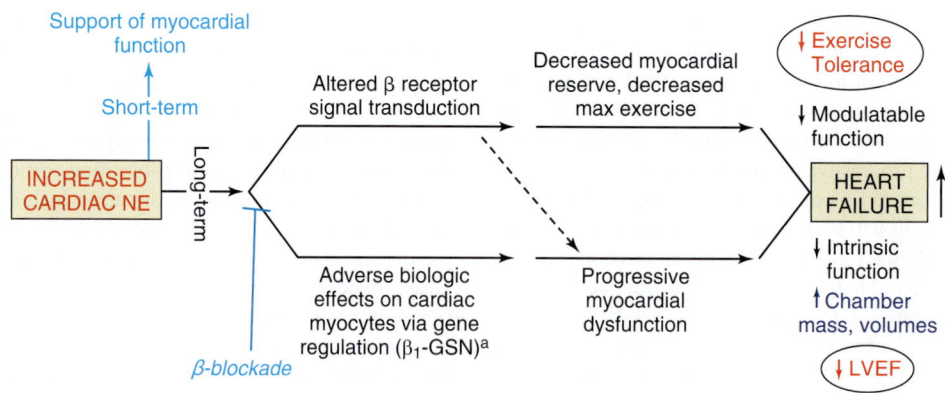

ᵃβ₁ adrenergic receptor Gene Signaling Network

Fig. 6.2 Role of increased adrenergic drive in the natural history of heart failure. A primary maladaptive response to chronic heart failure is a net increase in cardiac interstitial norepinephrine *(NE)* concentration, resulting from increased release and/or decreased reuptake. Increased NE results in a second maladaptive response to heart failure that of altered β-adrenergic receptors signaling. These changes, in combination with the direct adverse biological effects of catecholamines, result in decreased myocardial reserve and progressive myocardial dysfunction, the ultimate result being decreases in both "modulatable" and intrinsic myocardial function.

receptors (RyR2). Enhanced phosphorylation of calcium channels leads to an increased flux of extracellular calcium into the cell, activating downstream effectors including proteases, kinases, and phosphatases. Activation of the β_1-AR subtype also appears to promote increased calcium influx via cAMP-independent mechanisms.[31] Importantly, β_1-ARs can be cAMP-independent activators of CaMKII,[32] a signaling pathway known to have particularly adverse effects on cardiac myocytes.[33] Regardless of the exact mechanism(s) invoked, excessive β-AR stimulation results in oxidative stress and calcium overload, conditions promoting cell death through a number of mechanisms, including necrosis and apoptosis. Long-term adrenergic activation has also been shown to cause changes in the gene expression profile of cardiac myocytes, the general response being activation of the so-called fetal gene program[34] that is under β_1-adrenergic control via membership in a larger gene signaling network.[35,36] As discussed in Chapter 1, the fetal gene program, which is a molecular surrogate for hypertrophy/heart failure, includes downregulation in the gene expression of the fast-contracting α-isoform of myosin heavy chain (MHC) (MYH6) and SR Ca^{2+} ATPase (ATP2A2), upregulation of the slow contracting β-MHC isoform (MYH7), and upregulation of ANP (NPPA) and BNP (NPPB).

In the failing heart, β-ARs and certain downstream PKA-dependent effectors in the β-adrenergic signaling cascade undergo agonist-mediated, time-dependent downregulation and desensitization, presumably in an attempt to withdraw the heart from an excess of deleterious signaling. These changes result in a marked attenuation of the failing heart's ability to respond to either endogenous or exogenous catecholamines. Consequently, the amount of cAMP generated in response to a given amount of adrenergic stimulation can be significantly decreased. Evidence has been provided through experiments using isolated, denervated preparations of human heart tissue revealing that failing hearts have a reduced cAMP content compared to nonfailing controls.[37,38] Extending this observation to the clinical standpoint, reduced responsiveness to catecholamines translates into a decrease in myocardial reserve, which is most commonly manifested as an impaired ability to exercise and means less ability to respond to any form of circulatory stress. In contrast, PKA-independent signaling pathways, such as CaMKII, may undergo upregulation.[5]

In summary, the role of increased adrenergic drive in the natural history of heart failure is a seemingly a paradoxical one. On the one hand, adrenergic activation is essential to meeting the demands of increased physiological and pathological stress in the failing heart; on the other hand, chronic adrenergic stimulation is a major contributor to progressive myocardial dysfunction and remodeling that characterizes heart failure. However, from an evolutionary biology standpoint, this situation is entirely plausible; adrenergic mechanisms have evolved to allow reproductive-age individuals to cope with and escape from highly stressful short-term situations; they are not particularly well suited to chronic support of the failing heart that typically occurs beyond the reproductive years.

ADRENERGIC RECEPTOR PHARMACOLOGY

In the 1940s, Ahlquist[39] recognized that adrenergic receptors could be subdivided into two major classes, α- and β-ARs (**Fig. 6.3**), both of which serve as binding sites for the endogenous catecholamines, epinephrine and NE. Almost 20 years later, Lands and colleagues,[40] using rank orders of agonists, proposed that β-ARs could be divided into β_1- and β_2-AR subtypes. A few years later, use of selective β_1- and other β-AR antagonists formalized this classification and expanded it to include an additional β-AR subtype,[41] later named the β_3-AR.[42] Building on this basic pharmacology was work in the 1970s and 1980s centered on direct identification of receptors by radioligand binding

and the biochemistry of signaling pathways.[43,44] Based on the groundbreaking peptide biochemistry work of Khorana and colleagues on rhodopsin,[45] subsequent work by Lefkowitz and colleagues described the molecular cloning of a number of G-protein coupled receptors (GPCRs) including α_1-, α_2-ARs, and the β_1- and β_2-ARs.[46-50] Perhaps more than any other previous advance in the field, this knowledge permitted the analysis of adrenergic receptor biology in exquisite detail and allowed for an appreciation of the true complexity of adrenergic receptor signaling, including the definition of a multitude of gene regulatory motifs and the recognition of highly organized multi-protein signaling complexes. Ultimately, the combined work of Lefkowitz and Kobilka on GPCR pharmacology, biochemistry, and molecular biology, as well as Kobilka's subsequent work on GPCR structural biology, resulted in their being awarded the Nobel Prize in Chemistry in 2012.

Relevant to the human heart, there are two major subclasses of α-ARs, α_1- and α_2-ARs, of which there are several subtypes (**see Fig. 6.3**).[51] These α_1-AR subtypes are coupled to the Gq/G11-family of G-proteins, linked to stimulation of phospholipase C (PLC), which in turn promotes phosphoinositide (PIP$_2$) turnover. The two primary products of this reaction are inositol triphosphate (IP$_3$), which stimulates the release of intracellular calcium, and diacylglycerol (DAG), which stimulates protein kinase-C (PKC) activity.[52] Increases in intracellular calcium and PKC-mediated phosphorylation of target proteins both activate signaling pathways and gene expression patterns which, depending on the PKC subtype, result in a hypertrophic myocardial phenotype as well as vasoconstriction.[53] Examples of other Gq-coupled receptors whose stimulation also results in a hypertrophic phenotype are the angiotensin II AT1 and endothelin-1 receptors. Each of these receptor pathways represents pharmacological targets central to the management of heart failure and/or its precursors, such as systemic or pulmonary hypertension.

In contrast to α_1-, α_2-ARs are generally described as inhibitory presynaptic or prejunctional neuronal receptors functioning to suppress the release of NE from the synapse. The potential importance of this function in the setting of heart failure has been emphasized in a study by Small and colleagues,[54] wherein a naturally occurring "loss of function" polymorphism of the $\alpha2C$-AR, when present in combination with a "gain of function" polymorphism of the β_1-AR, produced a significantly increased risk of heart failure in certain populations. These and other β-AR polymorphisms, and their relevance to CHF, are discussed in greater detail below.

β-ARs are also subdivided, with three distinct receptor subtypes encoded by separate genes β_1-(ADRB1), β_2- (ADRB2), and β_3-(ADRB3). β_1- and β_2-ARs were first described by agonist[40] or antagonist[41] pharmacologic responses, and then by molecular cloning.[46,47] In contrast, β_3-ARs were first definitively identified by molecular cloning[42] after being classified as beyond the β_1, β_2 paradigm[41]

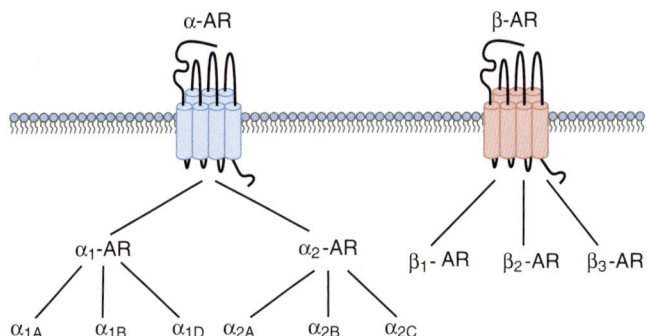

Fig. 6.3 Adrenergic signaling pathways. Adrenergic receptor (AR) subtypes.

or "atypical"[55] in various organs, as determined by pharmacologic response. β3-ARs are generally associated with regulation of metabolic rate, modulation of nitric oxide (NO) formation, gut and urinary tract smooth muscle relaxation and, to a lesser degree, with changes in cardiac contractility.[56] β3 receptors are expressed at low abundance but are coupled via a nitric oxide synthase (NOS)/NO/soluble guanylate cyclase/cGMP mechanism to a negative inotropic response in human ventricular myocardium,[57] where they may play a cardioprotective role.[56] In contrast, β1- and β2-ARs have the clear functional role of increasing myocardial performance,[5] and both are expressed at a substantial abundance in human ventricular myocardium with β1-AR density greater than β2.[58]

β1- and β2-ARs, respond equally well to the full agonist isoproterenol, and are distinguished primarily by their affinity for NE. β1-ARs have 10- to 30-fold greater affinity for NE than β2-ARs.[14,40] An even greater degree of distinction is achieved through the relative affinities of selective antagonists.[58,59] In the context of heart failure, the most clinically relevant compounds differentiating between β1- and β2-ARs are the β1-AR selective antagonists metoprolol, bisoprolol, and nebivolol.[5] In contrast, β3-ARs are characterized by their relatively low affinity for propranolol,[41,55] by the selective β1-antagonist CGP 20712a,[42] or by their response to β3 selective agonists such as BRL 37344[42] or CL316243.[55] Two β-blocking agents in use or development, nebivolol and bucindolol, have β3-agonist activity that may contribute to their vasodilator properties or possibly to their myocardial effects.[5]

ALTERED β-ADRENERGIC RECEPTOR SIGNAL TRANSDUCTION IN THE FAILING HEART

As manifest in heart failure, chronic heightened adrenergic activation ultimately results in diminished β-AR-mediated signaling as a consequence of decreased in β1-AR gene expression (mRNA and protein expression),[58-61] uncoupling of both β1- and β2-ARs[62,63] secondary to receptor phosphorylation[64] from βARK1 (GRK2)[65] or other kinases, and to increases in the inhibitory G protein(Gαi) (**Fig. 6.4**).[66] In non-failing, adult human ventricles, β1-ARs constitute approximately 70% to 80% of all β-ARs. However, in individuals with heart failure the β1-AR is selectively downregulated, resulting in an ~60:40 ratio of β1- to β2-ARs.[60,67]

Phosphorylation of β-ARs occurs by the G-protein receptor kinase (GRK) family, specifically GRK2, which phosphorylates both β1- and β2 receptor subtypes in an agonist occupancy-dependent manner,[68] and GRK5,[69] a kinase of considerable importance linking β1-ARs to

epidermal growth factor receptor (EGFR) transactivation and cardioprotective effects,[70,71] but also to CaMKII signaling,[72] and β2-ARs to Src and MAP kinase (extracellular signal-regulated kinase [ERK]) signaling.[73] As initially described, β-ARs also can be phosphorylated and desensitized by other kinases including PKA and PKC.[74] Therefore in failing ventricular myocardium, both β1- and β2-receptor subtypes undergo desensitization, with β1-ARs exhibiting downregulation, and both β1- and β2-ARs uncoupling from PKA signaling. Similar results have been obtained in the in vivo setting with intravenous administration of dobutamine, demonstrating marked blunting of contractility in the failing human heart compared to no decrement in function with calcium infusion.[75]

The major consequence of β-AR downregulation and desensitization is that for a given level of adrenergic activation, less of the second messenger cAMP is produced. In turn, decreased formation of cAMP leads to diminished activation of PKA. However, decreased PKA activity does not necessarily translate into decreased phosphorylation of all putative PKA substrates. Related to the above, although PKA activity and PLB phosphorylation are decreased in heart failure,[76] cardiac RyR2s have been shown to be hyperphosphorylated.[77] The net phosphorylation "state" of the RyR and PLB, and thus their activities, is due, at least in part, to their being in separate subcellular A-kinase anchoring protein-scaffolded microdomains. In these discreet microdomains different PDEs control cAMP levels and PKA activation; phosphatase species and activities may also differ. Specifically, in the failing heart there is evidence for the downregulation of phosphatases PP1 and PP2A that are associated with RyR2, as well as to changes in PKA activity.[77,78] Alternatively, recent studies have shown that RyR2 can be phosphorylated by CaMKII,[79] inducing SR calcium leakiness and engendering arrhythmias, an effect that appears to be mediated by cardiac β1-ARs and the "exchange protein directly activated by cAMP-2," EPAC2.[80] Interestingly, a recent paper by Pereira and colleagues,[81] showed that the EPAC/CaMKII-mediated phosphorylation of RyR2 occurs through a pathway that includes AKT (also known as protein kinase B) and NOS1. The authors showed that increased cAMP levels activate EPAC, which in turn activates AKT resulting in NOS1 activation. NOS1 promotes S-nitrosylation of CaMKII resulting in phosphorylation of RyR2 and increased leakiness.

In contrast to the hyperphosphorylation of RyR2, PKA-mediated phosphorylation of PLB appears to be decreased in heart failure,[37] which is presumably due to reduced cAMP levels in the SERCA II-PLB microdomain and to the activation of the phosphatase PP1.[76] PP1 is regulated by protein phosphatase inhibitor I, PPI-1, a protein whose

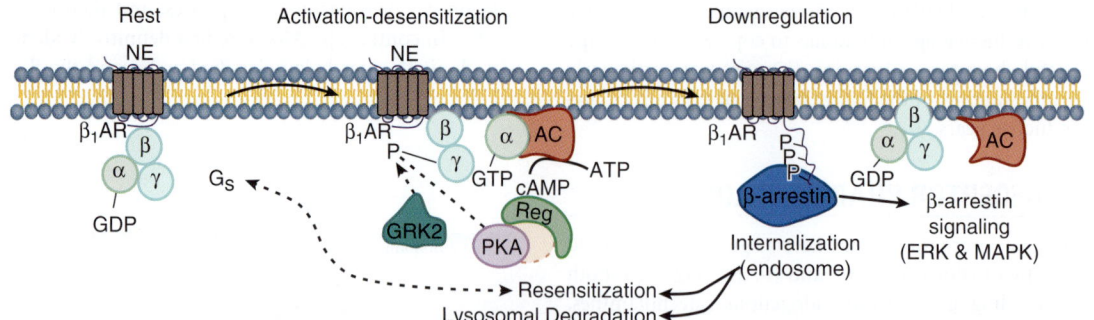

Fig. 6.4 Beta1-adrenergic receptor (β1AR) activation, desensitization, downregulation, and recycling. Prolonged β1AR activation causes recruitment of a G-protein receptor kinase (GRK2) that phosphorylates the receptor and favors recruitment of beta-arrestin (β-arrestin). β-arrestin promotes its own signaling cascades (e.g., via extracellular receptor and MAP kinase [ERK and MAPK]) as well as internalization of the β1AR into endosomes. From there, β1AR can either be degraded or recycled to the cell surface. NE, Norepinephrine (Modified from Bers DM. *Excitation-Contraction Coupling and Cardiac Contractile Force.* Dordrecht, Netherlands: Kluwer Academic; 2001).

abundance is itself downregulated in heart failure.[82] The reduced PLB phosphorylation results in a greater inhibition of SR Ca^{2+} ATPase (SERCA II), resulting in an impaired ability of the heart to both relax and contract.[83] In contrast, hyperphosphorylation of RyR2 results in defective channel function during excitation-contraction coupling.[84] Together, these changes result in decreased contractility in response to adrenergic stimulation and a propensity for developing arrhythmias. Unfortunately, however, the relationship between RyR2 phosphorylation state and its biological relevance is not as clear as might be desired, as articulated in a recent set of "controversies" articles.[85,86]

Substantial evidence from model systems points to significant differences between β_1- and β_2-ARs and their ability to stimulate apoptosis in cardiac myocytes[12] with stimulation of the β_1- but not the β_2-AR pathway resulting in an increased rate of cardiomyocyte apoptosis. Disruption of β_2-AR coupling to Gi by treatment with pertussis toxin can abrogate the potential protective, anti-apoptotic signaling pathways rendering the β_2-AR pro-apoptotic.[87] Chesley and colleagues,[88] have provided evidence to support the supposition that the anti-apoptotic effects of β_2-AR are mediated in part by the stimulation of the PI3K and the Akt-PK-D pathways.

In addition to the mechanisms described above, the pro-apoptotic effect of the β_1-AR pathway also may be due to increased CaMKII activity. Zhu and colleagues,[89] have shown that β_1-AR stimulation results in myocyte apoptosis, which is independent of PKA activation but is dependent on CaMKII, suggesting that β_1-AR stimulation may selectively result in CaMKII activation independently. These studies demonstrate that inhibition of CaMKII, LTCC phosphorylation, or buffering of intracellular Ca^{2+} results in an attenuation of β_1-AR mediated apoptosis; conversely, overexpression of CaMKIIδ_c induces apoptosis. In addition, Yoo and colleagues,[90] using transgenic mice with knockouts of β-AR subtypes, have demonstrated that post-infarct, isoproterenol-mediated increases in CaMKII signaling and apoptosis are dependent exclusively on the β_1-AR. However, recent data from Dewenter and colleagues[91] indicate that CaMKII signaling persists despite the use of β-blockers in both experimental and human heart failure, arguing for the development and use of selective CaMKII inhibitors in heart failure. This conclusion is supported by the findings of Kreusser and colleagues,[92] indicating that in a mouse transverse aortic constriction (TAC) model, double knockout of CaMKIIδ/γ progression of cardiac dysfunction and deposition of fibrosis is attenuated.

Excessive β_1-AR signaling also activates the fetal gene program (**see also Chapter 1**).[32,34] In this context, a change in MHC isoform expression favoring the low(er) ATPase activity β isoform would be expected to decrease contractile function, as would the downregulation in SERCA II, another adult gene that is considered part of the adult-fetal program. Although the signaling cascades responsible for this activation are complex, CaMKII appears to play a prominent role,[32] and the altered expression of so-called fetal and adult genes appears mediated by β_1- and not β_2-AR stimulation.[32,34] CaMKII activity is upregulated in the failing human heart,[93,94] suggesting that despite the desensitization that occurs in more proximal β_1-receptor signaling steps, adverse signaling through CaMKII may be maintained or even enhanced (**see also Chapter 1**).

As described above, CaMKII is involved in various pathologic processes in heart failure including apoptosis, arrhythmias and changes in gene expression. To gain a better understanding of the role of CaMKII in pathologic cardiac disease, knockout mouse models of CaMKII and a transgenic model overexpressing a CaMKII peptide inhibitor have been generated.[95,96] Mice expressing the inhibitory peptide are resistant to pathological changes related to β-AR stimulation, and do not exhibit decreases in fractional shortening, increases in heart/body weight or decreases in left ventricular internal diameter.[97] Different results are obtained in knockout mouse model studies. In response to TAC in 6-week-old animals, knockout of CaMKIIδ blunted fibrosis and reduced heart/body weight ratio, myocyte area, and pathologic changes in gene expression.[98] In an 8-week TAC model, CaMKIIδ downregulation did not prevent the development of pathologic hypertrophy, but blunted the transition to heart failure, including chamber dilation, ventricular dysfunction, lung edema, cardiac fibrosis, and apoptosis.[79] However, a 6-week-old CaMKII knockout mouse model of severe thoracic aortic banding showed improved contractility, increased myofilament sensitivity to Ca^{2+}, decreased apoptosis but increased fibrosis. However, no improvement in ejection fraction/fractional shortening was observed. The authors also showed that knockout of CaMKII in the setting of severe heart failure may be detrimental due to reduced efficiency of β-AR regulation of contraction and exacerbation of diastolic dysfunction.[96] These studies suggest that although CaMKII is likely to be primarily detrimental, it may also be important for β-AR regulation of contractile function in the failing heart.

In contrast to the general desensitization phenomena exhibited by β_1- and β_2-ARs in failing human ventricular myocardium, β_3-ARs exhibit upregulation.[99] Since the β_3-AR knockout mouse undergoes excessive remodeling in response to pressure overload,[100] increased expression of β_3-ARs in the failing human heart may be a salutary adaptive mechanism.

MOLECULAR BASIS OF β-ADRENERGIC RECEPTOR SIGNALING

Canonically, β_1- and the β_2-ARs couple to stimulatory G-proteins, Gs, which are composed of three subunits, an α-subunit, and a $\beta\gamma$-heterodimeric subunit, **Fig. 6.5**. Both the α and $\beta\gamma$ subunits are competent to signal independently Gαs is a member of the much larger class of G-protein α-subunits, of which there are ~20 subtypes. Their heterogeneity is a central basis of specificity for GPCR signaling, a subject reviewed in detail elsewhere.[101] Additional layers of signaling diversity are afforded by combinatorial permutations of various $\beta\gamma$-heterodimeric subunits (5 β-subtypes and 11 γ subtypes) with the various α-subunits.

As a result of agonist stimulation, G-protein α and $\beta\gamma$ subunits dissociate with the free αs-subunit acting to stimulate adenylate cyclases (AC), for which there are multiple isoforms.[102] In cardiac tissues, the most abundant isoforms are AC V and VI with the activities of each being feedback inhibited by increases in cytosolic calcium. In turn, adenylate cyclase stimulation increases production of cAMP that, in turn, binds to the regulatory subunits of PKA. Binding causes the dissociation of the regulatory and catalytic subunits of PKA, with the catalytic subunits proceeding to phosphorylate consensus serine (S) and threonine (T) residues on a broad spectrum of intracellular target proteins. In a number of tissues, including cardiac, PKA and its targets are in close approximation because of A-kinase anchoring proteins (AKAPs).[103] An association between the β_2-AR and AKAP79 has been described.[104] Additionally, there is recent clarity as to the scaffolding proteins that interact with β_1-ARs.[105,106] Thus, unique interactions between β_1- and β_2-ARs and specific AKAPs and/or other anchoring proteins support the "micro-domain" concept of receptor subtype-specific signaling, discussed in greater detail below.

Via the "canonical" Gαs/adenylyl cyclase pathway, β-AR stimulation results in the phosphorylation by PKA of a number of proteins including (LTCC, $CaV_{1.2}$)[107] and PLB, the primary modulator of the sarcoplasmic reticulum (SR)-associated ATP-dependent calcium pump, SERCA II, as well as modulatory proteins associated with regulation of the contractile apparatus, for example, troponin I (TnI).

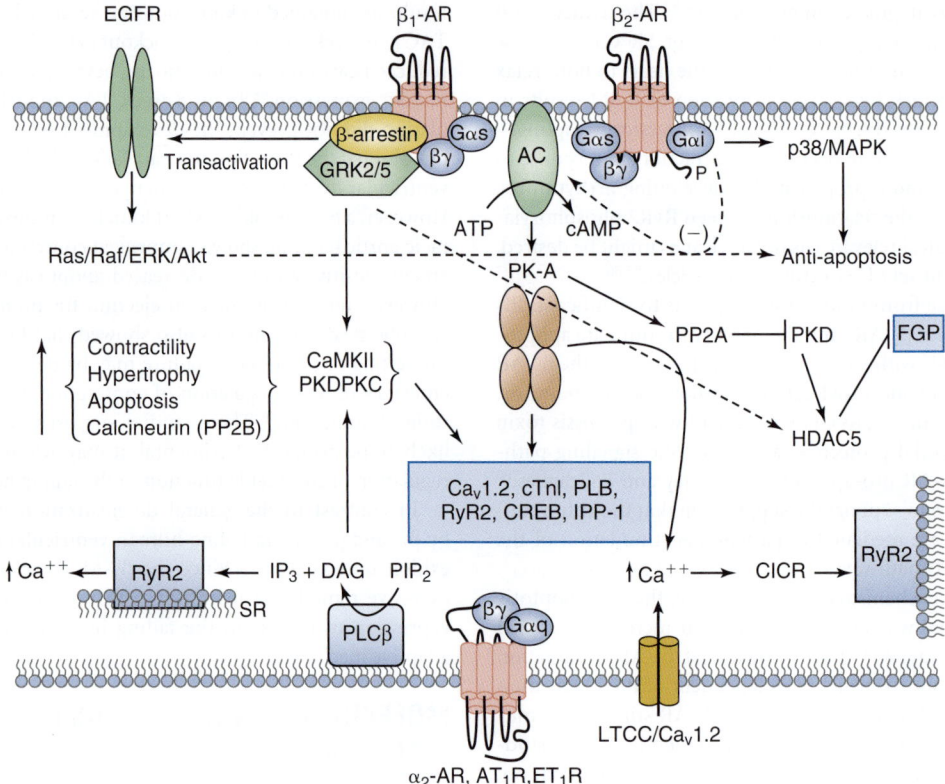

Fig. 6.5 Signal transduction pathways stimulated by β-ARs. Canonically, both *β₁- and β₂-AR* signal via the stimulatory G-protein, Γαs, to stimulate adenylyl cyclase *(AC)* activity increasing cAMP production and activating PKA. Downstream targets of PKA include L-type *Ca⁺⁺* channels, contractile proteins (e.g., TnI), and the regulator of sarcoplasmic reticulum calcium uptake, phospholamban *(PLB)*. Increased [Ca⁺⁺]i results in increased contractility and, if persistent, apoptosis. The β₁-AR activates at least two other pathways: *CaMKII* and the epidermal growth factor receptor *(EGFR)*. Increased CaMKII activity results in increased [Ca⁺⁺]i and calcineurin phosphatase activity, which activates pro-hypertrophic transcription factors causing the re-expression of the fetal gene program *(FGP)*; it also accelerates the rate of myocyte apoptosis. In contrast, β₁-AR-mediated stimulation of the EGFR is a cardio-protective, anti-apoptotic pathway. The β₂-AR can also couple to the inhibitory G-protein, Gi, resulting in a direct inhibition of AC activity as well as activation of pro-hypertrophic *MAPKs* and anti-apoptotic pathways. (Adapted from Port JD. Beta-adrenergic signaling: complexities and therapeutic relevance to heart failure. *Curr Signal Transduct Ther.* 2012;7:120–131.)

More directly, however, PKA phosphorylates β-ARs,[108] as well as other GPCRs, resulting in partial uncoupling and desensitization of receptors to further agonist stimulation. Changes in the phosphorylation state of calcium-handling proteins results in increased [Ca⁺⁺]i and enhanced rates of myocardial contraction and relaxation. However, the increase in intracellular calcium has a number of other effects beyond enhanced contractility, including the activation of a number of calcium-sensitive enzymes, for example, Ca⁺⁺/calmodulin and calcineurin (phosphatase PP2B).[109] On a more global level, changes in [Ca⁺⁺]i can result in profound changes in gene expression patterns.

It has been known for some time that β₁- and β₂-ARs differ in their efficiency of coupling to adenylate cyclase and to cAMP production, with the β₂-AR subtype being more efficiently coupled to cAMP production than is the β₁-AR.[59] In trabeculae isolated from the human heart, selective stimulation of contraction by either receptor pathway generally correlates well with receptor abundance.[58,62,63] However, the fact that the β₂-AR produces more cAMP per unit of stimulus does not necessarily translate into a greater inotropic potential for β₂-ARs. Rather, these data favor an argument that there is distinct intracellular compartmentalization of cAMP pools produced by β-ARs,[110] with the existence of discrete microdomains of high cAMP concentration

in cardiomyocytes. Specifically, in neonatal cardiomyocytes, high concentrations of cAMP are found in the proximity of T tubules and the junctional SR. An argument is also made that diffusion of cAMP outside of these microdomains is quickly curtailed by the action of PDEs. Support for this notion is the finding that there appears to be close coordination between agonist-stimulated recruitment of PDEs to the β₂-AR, a process facilitated by interaction with β-ARs, and the attenuation of signaling. Recent data indicate that the differential signaling and architecture of β₁- and β₂-ARs appears to be defined, in part, by a differential association with PDEs,[111] with PDE4 activity preferentially targeting cAMP produced by the β₁-AR, whereas cAMP produced by the β₂-AR being targeted by multiple subtypes of PDEs. Perhaps counterintuitive to the highly localized responses of β-ARs being dictated by scaffolding proteins is the recent study by Nikolaev and colleagues,[112] demonstrated in transgenic mice that isoproterenol-mediated increases in cAMP in cardiac tissues leads to "far-reaching" cAMP signals for the β₁-AR, whereas β₂-AR generated cAMP appears to remain locally confined. An excellent recent study detailing the compartmentalization of β-AR signaling, the interplay of PDEs, phosphatases, and subtype specific spaciotemporal patterning has recently been published by Xiang.[113]

A very recent study delineates further cAMP and β-AR compartmentalization. Interestingly, in murine models, β_2-ARs and cAMP demonstrate anatomical variation such that at the apex of the heart β_2-ARs uniquely modulate increased contractility.[114] This appears to be primarily due to variations in the size and organization of T-tubules and caveolae impacting microdomains.

It is clear that both the β_1-AR and the β_2-AR pathways couple to signaling pathways beyond the "traditional" Gαs/adenylyl cyclase pathway.[115] Perhaps the best example of this diversity of signaling is the finding that the β_2-AR can interact with the inhibitory G-protein, Gαi. This is of interest in the setting of CHF, for two reasons. As described earlier, increased circulating NE concentrations result in chronic activation of β-ARs. This, in turn, results in increased βARK activity and an increased phosphorylation state of β-ARs resulting ultimately in the uncoupling of the receptor from the stimulatory Gαs signaling pathway. It is this phosphorylated form of the β_2-AR that has an increased propensity to couple to the inhibitory Gαi pathway[116] and its downstream effectors, including inhibition of AC and activation of MAPKs. Amplifying this effect is the finding that the abundance of Gαi proteins is significantly elevated in the failing human heart.[117] Thus, the increased phosphorylation state of the β_2-AR and the increased abundance of Gαi protein both facilitate increased trafficking of β_2-AR signaling via Gαi-associated pathways. The ramifications of this are potentially significant, particularly in regard to protective, anti-apoptotic effects as well as to myocardial growth regulatory effects.

The β_1-AR, although thought to be less "promiscuous" than the β_2-AR in its ability to couple to pathways other than to Gαs, nonetheless does exhibit signaling via additional pathways, as noted above, to the CaMKII pathway. However, recent data from Wang and colleagues support the conclusion that the β_1-AR can indeed couple to Gαi, an effect uniquely promoted by the β-AR antagonist, carvedilol.[118] In fact, Gαi appears to be required for β_1-AR β-arrestin-biased signaling for both EGFR transactivation and for MAPK signaling. However, unlike β_2-AR Gαi-mediated ERK activation, carvedilol-induced β_1-AR/Gαi MAPK signaling does not appear to require Gβγ nor GRK/PKA receptor phosphorylation.[118] As noted above, current published evidence supports the finding that carvedilol's induction of β_1-AR/Gαi interaction is unique; it will be of future interest to determine whether or not nebivolol, also a β-arrestin-biased agonist,[119] has any requirement for Gαi.

At least in part, β_1-AR extra-Gαs coupling, much like that of the β_2-AR, appears to be facilitated by the specificity of the carboxy-terminus PDZ (PSD-95/Dlg/ZO-1) domain of the receptor peptide, a domain that drives the interaction with proteins containing specific PDZ recognition motifs. An excellent review on the general topic of regulation of β-AR signaling by scaffolding proteins has been published by Hall and Lefkowitz.[120] Examples of β_1-AR interacting proteins are PSD-95, MAGI-2, the endophilins (SH3p4/p8/p13), and CNrasGEF, all of which appear to have unique downstream roles. The association of the β_1-AR with PSD-95, which is a neuronal-associated protein, distinctly places the β_1-AR in the proximity of the synapse,[121] a location perhaps driven by adrenergic innervation. Here, PSD-95 appears to inhibit the internalization of the β_1-AR,[122] an effect that is modulated by the kinase GRK5. Conversely, interaction of the β_1-AR with endophilins appears to negatively modulate Γαs coupling and to promote β_1-AR internalization.[123] A more detailed picture of the β_1-AR SAP97-AKAP79/150 scaffold at its PSD-95/DLG/ZO1 motif has been demonstrated to be necessary for both PKA mediated phosphorylation of the β_1-AR as well as for receptor trafficking.[105,106] This is in contrast to the findings describing the association of the β_1-AR with CNrasGEF (PDZ-GEF1), an effector molecule that activates Ras, and thus growth pathways. In this case, the mechanism of Ras activation is rather unique given that it

appears to be via Gαs rather than the well-documented Gβγ signaling pathway.

Additional evidence detailing the importance of PDZ-mediated interactions has been described by Xiang and colleagues.[124] Specifically, mutation of the PDZ motif by disruption of the carboxy-terminus renders the β_1-AR significantly more sensitive to agonist-mediated cell surface downregulation. Further, deletion of C-terminal amino acids renders the β_1-AR more β_2-AR-like in that it becomes capable of interacting with Gi. Thus, even though the β_1-AR[122] and β_2-AR[125] both contain PDZ motifs, the interacting proteins that each couples to are unique and serve as an important basis of different regulatory and signaling properties. To expand this concept, the β_2-AR, has been shown to modulate signaling independent of its interactions with G-proteins. For example, the β_2-AR appears to couple to at least three other pathways: (1) NHERF, which in turn regulates the function of the Na^+/H^+ exchanger[126]; (2) to a non-PKA-dependent interaction with L-type calcium channels[31,115]; and (3) coupling to the phosphatidylinositol 3′-kinase pathway (PI3K), a pathway associated with the inhibition of apoptosis, and to the PI3K-PTEN pathway, which is relevant to the regulation of both myocardial contractility and cell size and shape.[127]

As alluded to above, β-AR stimulation results in the dissociation of the stimulatory G-protein, Gs, into α and βγ subunits, each of which are signaling entities. A major function of the βγ heterodimer is to recruit βARKs in proximity to the receptor. By virtue of the lipid-modified (isoprenylation) of the γ subunit, which promotes localization of the βγ subunit to the sarcolemmal membrane, the heterodimer is in position to orchestrate the co-localization of the β-AR with βARK. Protein/protein interaction of the βγ subunit with βARK occurs via a pleckstrin homology (PH) domain.[128] In this way agonist-dependent, βARK-mediated phosphorylation of β-ARs serves as an important mode of β-AR desensitization.[68] In addition to playing a scaffolding role, βγ subunits are also signaling molecules in their own right. Downstream targets of signaling include subsets of adenylyl cyclases, PI3K, K^+ channels, and Ras/Raf/MEK/MAPK pathway(s) (**see Fig. 6.5**).

Recently, significant attention has been paid to the specifics of β-AR localization and receptor trafficking. Differential targeting of β-AR subtypes to specific intracellular compartments has been described.[129] Of note is the apparent caveolar co-localization of the β_2-ARs with the inhibitory protein, Gαi, as well as with PKA subunits and with GRK2. What is now becoming clear is that the localization of the β_2-AR to the caveolar compartment is an essential component of its signaling capabilities.[130] In contrast, β_1-ARs, as well as a number of other proteins including Gαs, and ACs V and VI, are not specifically associated with caveolae; instead, these proteins have a more generalized distribution.

An important and newly emergent concept of β-AR signaling is that of the connection between β_1-AR signaling with the cardioprotective effects of the EGFR pathway. Work from Rockman and colleagues[70,131,132] has shown that GRK5/6 mediated phosphorylation of the β_1-AR targets the association of β-arrestin to the receptor, which, in addition to activating MAP kinases, facilitates the activation of matrix metalloproteinases causing the release of heparin-bound EGF, which then activates the EGFR. Activation of the EGFR leads to activation of Ras/Raf/ERK/Akt and subsequent anti-apoptotic, cardioprotective effects (**see Fig. 6.5**).

Recent evidence indicated that the differentiation of β_1- versus β_2-AR signaling also extends to the cardiac progenitor cells (CPCs) and their differentiation and survival. Interestingly, β-AR stimulation appears to promote the differentiation of CPCs via β_2-ARs. However, once these cells become committed to a myocyte lineage, they begin to express β_1-ARs. Counteracting that progression, continued β-AR stimulation via β_1-AR leads to a loss of CPCs.[133]

REGULATION OF β-ADRENERGIC RECEPTORS GENE EXPRESSION

Genes encoding β-ARs are regulated at virtually every level, including transcriptional, posttranscriptional/pretranslational, translational, and posttranslational. Much like proto-oncogenes and cytokines, β-ARs can profoundly affect a number of cellular functions affecting cell viability—thus the need for stringent, rapid, and redundant regulatory mechanisms. β-AR expression, at the levels of both mRNA and protein, is the result of a number of independently regulated processes.

At the level of transcriptional regulation, both positive and negative transcriptional regulatory elements exist within the 5′-untranslated regions (UTRs) of β-ARs. Cell culture model systems have provided evidence regarding the effects of a number of transcriptional regulatory pathways starting with the most obvious, that of the direct effects of β-AR stimulation. Increases in cAMP can lead to a transient upregulation of β-AR mRNA via a cAMP-responsive element (CRE)-mediated transcriptional effect. However, it is recognized that in heart failure, at least for the β_1-AR, mRNA and protein are unequivocally downregulated.[64] Therefore, CRE-mediated upregulatory effects are unlikely to be important in the chronic setting. Conversely, β-AR genes have the potential to be negatively regulated by the transcriptional suppressor, ICER (inducible cAMP early repressor). Evidence points to a role for ICER in a pathophysiological feedback loop with its upregulation causing a persistent downregulation of PDE3A—a finding associated with increased isoproterenol-mediated cardiomyocyte apoptosis.[134] However, others have not found a downregulation in PDE3 in the failing human heart.[135]

In the cardiac context, a number of other transcriptional regulators of β-AR genes are also known to be important. Most notably, transcriptional regulation of β-AR genes by glucocorticoid and thyroid hormone-responsive elements can have significant effects via their respective consensus DNA binding elements (e.g., glucocorticoid response elements [GREs] and thyroid hormone response elements [TREs]).[136,137] In general, glucocorticoids have been associated with causing an upregulation of β_2-ARs and a reciprocal downregulation of β_1-Ars,[136,138] whereas thyroid hormone has been uniformly associated with upregulation of β-AR expression.[139]

For β-ARs expressed in myocardial tissues, a concordant relationship between mRNA and protein appears to be well preserved.[60] Thus, mechanisms regulating β-AR mRNA abundance likely significantly impact β-AR protein expression. To this end, nucleic acid motifs, known as A + U-rich elements (AREs), found within the 3′UTRs of several β-ARs, are known to be the target for a number of mRNA binding proteins associate with changes in mRNA turnover. Previous evidence has confirmed a relationship between agonist-mediated stimulation of β-ARs, the production of cAMP, and the destabilization of β-AR mRNA resulting in reduced mRNA and ultimately protein abundance.[140] However, additional evidence points to the role of MAPK pathways as critical regulators of the stability of ARE-containing mRNAs, including those encoding β-ARs.[141] In particular, several proteins associated with mRNA changes in mRNA turnover have been demonstrated to bind to β-AR AREs. These include AUF1/hnRNP D, which is associated with increased mRNA turnover[142]; HuR, which is associated with the stabilization of numerous ARE-containing mRNAs[143]; KSRP, which increases turnover of ARE-containing mRNAs, drives muscle cell differentiation, and modulates Wnt/β-catenin and PI3K/AKT signaling[144]; and tristetraprolin (TTP), which is associated with turnover of tumor necrosis factor α (TNFα) mRNA.[145] How each of these proteins specifically affects β-AR mRNA turnover in the myocardial tissues remains to be explored.[146] However, given the evidence that the homozygous deletion of TTP in transgenic mice results in a dramatic upregulation of TNFα and a subsequent cardiomyopathy,[147] there is little doubt that these mechanisms are in play.

Other means of posttranscriptional regulation include modulation of translational efficiency that can be controlled by RNA-binding proteins and by microRNAs. From the perspective of RNA-binding proteins, both HuR and TIAR appear to modulate β-AR gene expression via their ability to interact with U-rich nucleotide sequences.[148] From the perspective of microRNAs, it is well documented that they change in expression secondary to heart failure[149-152] and increased β-AR signaling.[153] In turn, several microRNAs are candidates to modulate β-AR expression, with miR let-7 being directly shown to do so. Previously, Wang and colleagues,[154] demonstrated that overexpression of let-7 causes downregulation of the β-AR as well as an increased association of β_2-AR mRNA with the Ago2/RISC complex. More recently, Liggett and colleagues have demonstrated that prolonged exposure to β-agonist drives a cAMP/PKA-dependent CREB-mediated increased let-7f expression, and in turn, downregulated β_2-AR expression.[155] Given the preservation of let-7 binding sites in the β_1-AR 3′UTR, it would not be surprising if a similar regulatory pattern were seen.

MYOPATHIC POTENTIAL OF INDIVIDUAL COMPONENTS OF ADRENERGIC RECEPTOR PATHWAYS

The development and study of transgenic animal models has provided a wealth of information with regard to understanding the role of adrenergic receptor signaling in CHF. This section will summarize a few of the more relevant findings obtained from animal models containing cardiac-targeted overexpression or deletion of various components of adrenergic receptor pathways. The impact of these changes on the development or prevention of cardiomyopathy is discussed.

β_1- and β_2-Adrenergic Receptors

The idea that significant differences exist between β_1- and β_2-AR signaling in the heart has been reinforced by data from a number of transgenic mouse models. One of the more notable initial observations was that overexpression of each receptor subtype can result in strikingly different cardiac phenotypes. As originally reported by Milano and colleagues,[156] overexpression of the wild-type β_2-AR in mice, at relatively high abundance (~50- to 200-fold), was associated with increased basal AC activity, enhanced contractility, and elevated left ventricle (LV) function. Interestingly, no pathology was apparent in animals up to 4 months of age. In a longer-term study, Liggett and colleagues[157] reported comparable effects of increased β_2-AR on the myocardium (i.e., enhanced cardiac function from birth); however, this group also noted linear gene dose-dependence with regard to the development of cardiomyopathy. Animals expressing more than 60× the background β-AR concentration maintained their hyperdynamic state for more than 1 year without an apparent increase in mortality. In contrast, overexpression of the β_2-AR at ~100-fold resulted in progressive cardiac enlargement, the development of heart failure, and premature death occurring at close to 1 year of age. At ~350 times the level of wild-type expression, the β_2-AR produced a cardiomyopathy, resulting in premature death in 50% of animals as early as week 25.[157]

Compared to the extremely high levels of β_2-AR expression required to produce myopathic results, wild-type β_1-AR overexpression at relatively low abundance (~20- to 40-fold) can lead to markedly decreased contractility and LV function and increased hypertrophy and fibrosis, resulting in progressive myocardial failure and premature death.[158,159] The pathophysiological mechanism(s) responsible for the detrimental effects of β_1-AR overexpression in these animals are only partially understood. Chronic increases in PKA activity are likely to be a component of the pathology associated with β_1-AR overexpression, as overexpression of the catalytic subunit of PKA is, in its own right, cardiomyopathic.[160] However, in the failing heart, cAMP abundance, and therefore PKA activity, is generally decreased.[37] Thus, it is possible or perhaps even likely that β_1-AR-mediated CaMKII activity, which is increased in CHF, underlies the observed pathology. Indeed, in a study by Dockstader and colleagues,[153] where β_1-AR Arg or Gly389 polymorphic variants were overexpressed, bioinformatic analysis detected a strong signature for the CaMKII pathway activation in Arg389 animals.

Initial studies reported an increase in systolic function in young animals overexpressing the β_1-AR, with a progressive decline in LV function occurring with age.[158,159] Interestingly, this appears to occur prior to any structural alterations, such as fibrosis, which do not become apparent until at least 4 months, depending on level of expression. In this same study,[158] the mechanism of contractile dysfunction was found to involve impaired Ca^{2+} handling in cardiac myocytes, characterized by marked prolongation of intracellular Ca^{2+} transients. Subsequent examination of the expression levels of various SR proteins involved in Ca^{2+} release and uptake revealed a modest increase in the expression of SERCA II protein in animals at 2 months of age, and increased phosphorylation of PLB at Ser16, a critical regulatory site, was also detected. Collectively, these results indicate that impaired Ca^{2+} handling is likely another major causal factor in producing early contractile dysfunction in β_1-AR overexpressors, with these changes occurring prior to the appearance of interstitial fibrosis or other structural alterations.

α_1-Adrenergic Receptors

Both α_{1a} and α_{1b}-ARs are expressed at the protein level in human ventricular myocardium and neither one is downregulated in heart failure.[161] Transgenic animal models that overexpress each subtype have been described. Overexpression of the wild-type α_{1b}-AR results in a dilated cardiomyopathy.[162] In contrast, α1A transgenic cardiac overexpression produces an increase in contractility without hypertrophy.[163] Importantly, double knockout of both α_1 subtypes results in the acceleration of remodeling in response to pressure overload,[164] suggesting, on balance, that α_1-ARs play an adaptive role in maintenance of myocardial chamber integrity. Moreover, of the two subtypes, the α_{1a}-AR appears to be particularly devoid of myopathic potential and is contractility enhancing, at least in rodents, the inference being that selective agonists may have therapeutic potential.[161,163]

G-Proteins and Adenylate Cyclases

As described above, the G-proteins involved in adrenergic signaling are several, including Gs and Gi, which modulate AC activity, and Gq, which is linked to activation of PLC. Similar to that observed with the β-ARs, overexpression of each of these downstream signaling components results in a variety of cardiac phenotypes. Transgenic mice overexpressing wild-type Gαs have been described with this model, and are characterized by having a chronically increased heart rate, enhanced chronotropic and inotropic responses to agonist, altered β-AR density, and an increased frequency of cardiac arrhythmias.[165] Over time, myocardial performance in Gαs-overexpressing animals declines and LV dilatation is observed. Likewise, myocyte hypertrophy, apoptosis, and fibrosis become evident with age, and animals die prematurely. In addition, there is evidence that overexpression of Gαs is associated with an increase in L-type Ca^{2+} currents, an effect that appears to be independent of cAMP and AC activation. From these data, it has been suggested that Gαs may directly regulate the activity of L-type calcium channels. Interestingly, much like transgenic models of β-AR overexpression,[166] the pathophysiological changes observed with

Gαs overexpression can be prevented, and survival improved, through treatment with β-blockers.[167]

Transgenic mice that overexpress Gαq also exhibit a myopathic phenotype characterized by marked myocyte hypertrophy, increased expression of hypertrophy-related genes, and increased fibrosis, ultimately resulting in decreased myocardial contractility.[168] The mechanism of cardiomyopathy appears to involve, at least in part, cross-regulation to β-AR signaling pathways by Gαq or its downstream effectors.[169] Mice that overexpress Gαq exhibit decreased AC activity in response to the agonist, which is apparently due to impaired functional coupling of β-ARs to AC, since β-AR density is unchanged when compared to wild-type expression levels. In addition, β-AR stimulation of L-type Ca^{2+} channels is depressed in Gαq overexpressors, and expression levels of Gi are increased, as is PKC activity. In this model, the inhibition of Gαi unexpectedly caused sudden death, suggesting that the change in Gαi expression may be a compensatory mechanism to counteract other detrimental signaling caused by the Gq pathway.

Cardiac-targeted overexpression of a modified Gi-coupled receptor has been reported.[170] Mice that contain this modified receptor reportedly exhibited significant ventricular conduction delays, which can be attenuated by treatment with pertussis toxin, strongly suggesting a Gi-dependent mechanism. Moreover, these animals developed a pronounced dilated cardiomyopathy, resulting in death by 15 weeks of age. These results were the first to suggest a potential causal role for increased Gi signaling in the development and progression of heart failure,[170] and stand in distinction to the notion that the Gi pathway is simply protective, acting to abrogate the deleterious stimulatory effects of the Gαs pathway. In fact, overexpression of the carboxy-terminus of Gαi (GiCT), a peptide construct that inhibits Gi signaling, has been demonstrated to enhance apoptosis associated with ischemia.[171]

In contrast to the above, overexpression of more distal components of the Gs signaling pathways, specifically ACs V or VI, does not appear to cause any form of cardiomyopathy.[172] Agonist-stimulated AC activity is higher in this model, and basal and stimulated PKA activities are also increased; however, these effects translate into modestly enhanced inotropic, lusitropic, or chronotropic function. Further, no long-term histopathological sequelae or deleterious changes in cardiac function have been noted with AC overexpression.[172] Based on this profile, preliminary (Phase 2) gene therapy trials utilizing adenovirus-mediated gene transfer of adenylyl cyclases have occurred.[173] In this study, an adenovirus AC6 construct underwent intracoronary delivery in patients with an ejection fraction of less than 40%. It appears that AC6 delivery is both safe and efficacious in terms of increasing cardiac performance with larger follow-up trials likely being justified.

G-Protein Receptor Kinases

As described above, GRKs are central to modulating β-AR signaling and do so from a variety of perspectives. GRK-mediated phosphorylation of β-ARs desensitize and uncouple the receptors from their signaling pathways. They are the facilitators of receptor internalization and downregulation and, as mentioned earlier, in the case of GRK5, can affect cross-talk between canonical β-AR signaling pathways and other kinase pathways, including those of MAPKs and tyrosine kinases. Worth noting is the extensive work surrounding GRK2, which has been historically described as βARK2. Increased expression and/or activity of GRK2 has been implicated in progression of heart failure and post-myocardial infarction,[174] and the use of a GRK2 mini-peptide that acts as an inhibitor appears to be of potential therapeutic benefit.[174] The deleterious effects of GRK2 have been linked, in part, to PKA-mediated phosphorylation of the β_2-AR leading to Gi-biased signaling,[175] and to pro-death signaling via HSP90 mitochondrial targeting of GRK2.[176]

ADRENERGIC RECEPTOR POLYMORPHISMS AND THEIR IMPORTANCE IN HEART FAILURE NATURAL HISTORY OR THERAPEUTICS

Polymorphisms of many genes, including a number of components of adrenergic receptor signaling pathways and the renin-angiotensin-aldosterone system, have the potential to influence the progression of cardiovascular disease and/or response to individual therapeutic agents. Depending on the genetic variant and the end-point assessed, variable response may be either generalized to a class of agents (i.e., β-blockers) or delimited to an individual agent.[177]

In groundbreaking work performed by Liggett and collaborators, the effects of polymorphic variants of α- and β-ARs have been shown to have profound effects on receptor signaling and response to pharmacological agents, and potentially to clinical outcomes. For more detailed information on the subject, several reviews (e.g., references 178 and 179) of adrenergic receptor polymorphisms have been published. As with many genes, a number of haplotypes have been described.[180] Further, allele frequencies and combinations of complex haplotypes are not uniform across racial[26] or geographical populations.[178,180]

Of particular importance in heart failure, two major polymorphic loci have been identified for the human β1-AR gene: variations at nucleotides 145 and 1165 encode either a serine (Ser) or glycine (Gly) variant amino acid position 49 (Ser49Gly), or an arginine (Arg) or Gly variant at amino acid position 389 (Arg389Gly). Data indicate that the minor allele Gly49 variant is significantly more susceptible to agonist-induced downregulation than is the Ser49 variant,[181] even though the two variants do not appear to be different in terms of their ability to couple to stimulation of adenylyl cyclase and production of cAMP. In contrast, the 389 Arg and minor allele Gly variants of the β1-AR have completely different signal transduction properties.[182,183] The Arg389 variant of the human β1-AR is much more efficiently coupled to adenylyl cyclase stimulation than is the Gly389 variant,[183] with three to four times greater signal transduction capacity.[182] The Arg389 variant transduces greater inotropic effects in isolated preparations of both nonfailing and failing human hearts,[182] and has a greater portion of receptors exhibiting constitutive activity.[166,182,183] Perhaps most importantly, in transfected cells and human ventricular myocardial membranes, compared to Gly389 the Arg389 variant has a higher affinity for agonists,[183] including a ~fivefold greater fraction of receptors in a high-affinity, agonist-binding state for NE.[184] This high affinity for NE compared to Gly389, β2- and β3-ARs means that *the β1 389Arg AR is the norepinephrine receptor in the human heart.*

For NE binding[184] and inotropic stimulation[182] the Gly389 allele is dominant negative, so that myocardial preparations from heterozygotes and Gly homozygotes have similar attenuation of function properties. This means that the genotype frequencies in the general US population are evenly divided between Arg389 homozygous and Gly389 carriers (heterozygotes + Gly389 homozygotes). For historical reasons, the Gly389 variant has been considered to be the "wild-type" allele as it was first to be cloned[47]; however, its frequency in the Caucasian and African-American populations of ~0.27 and ~0.42, respectively,[182] establishes the Arg389 variant as the major allele. The human genome is unique in containing a substantial fraction of Gly389 alleles; all other genomes examined to date are 100% Arg389.[182]

As a follow-up to cell-based studies, transgenic mouse studies where the β1-AR Arg389Gly receptor variants have been overexpressed clearly demonstrate that Arg389 is markedly more pathologic.[153,166] Additionally, Arg389 mice are more pharmacologically responsive to β-blocker therapy[166]—a notion that fits with the increased function receptor variant being able to be suppressed to a greater degree.[182] Interestingly, overexpression of 389Arg or Gly β1-AR variants results

in different gene expression patterns for mRNA[153,166] and miRNA,[153] which, when examined temporally, appear to vary more quantitatively than qualitatively.[153]

Over the past several years, a number of clinical studies have attempted to associate clinical event and remodeling outcomes to patient β1-AR 389Arg/Gly genotype.[182,184-187] An example of a study reporting differential reverse remodeling efficacy for carvedilol in patients with β1-AR Arg389Gly variants was by Chen and colleagues.[188] However, a study by Metra and colleagues[186] could not confirm this result. Consistent with this finding, in a well-designed prospective clinical trial, Sehnert and colleagues[187] found no effect of β1-AR 389Arg/Gly variants on the primary endpoint of transplant-free survival for heart failure patients receiving either carvedilol or metoprolol. Improvement in reverse remodeling effected by metoprolol treatment in β1-AR 389Arg homozygotes but not Gly carriers was reported by Terra and colleagues,[189] but was not confirmed in another study of genotyped heart failure clinic patients.[190] For metoprolol's effects on clinical endpoints, in a pharmacogenetic substudy of the MERIT-HF trial, White and colleagues[191] reported that metoprolol CR/XL did not interact with the β1-AR Arg389Gly polymorphism for effects on the combined endpoint of mortality or heart failure hospitalization, which is in agreement with metoprolol data from Sehnert and colleagues.[187] From a statistical standpoint, the most robust data on the effects of the β1 Arg389Gly polymorphism on β-blocker clinical effects come from a large (*n* = 2460, 765 deaths) heart failure clinic population prospectively followed in a National Heart, Lung, and Blood Institute genomics study at two large heart failure referral centers.[185] β-blockers treatment occurred in 83%, 90% of whom received carvedilol or metoprolol. There was no evidence of any effect of the β1 Arg389Gly polymorphism on mortality in β-blocker-treated patients, where mortality was lower compared to untreated patients, but only in Caucasians.[185] In marked contrast to these clinical endpoint pharmacogenetic studies investigating the effects of carvedilol and metoprolol CR/XL,[187,191] Liggett and colleagues,[182] demonstrated an effect of β1-AR 389Arg/Gly variants on mortality and other endpoints for the investigational β-blocker/sympatholytic agent bucindolol, and that this relationship can be modified by the presence or absence of an α2C-AR insertion/deletion polymorphism.[184] Thus for clinical endpoints, differential therapeutic effects of β-blockers by β1-AR Arg389Gly polymorphism may be agent dependent. The basis for the β1-AR 389 polymorphism differential effects of bucindolol, but not carvedilol or metoprolol, may reside in the novel pharmacologic properties of bucindolol, which include promoting inactivation of constitutively active β1-AR 389Arg receptors[182] and NE lowering.[21,184] The Arg389 β1-AR variant's much higher affinity for NE compared to its Gly389 counterpart[184] means that NE lowering would have preferentially favorable effects in subjects who are β1389 Arg homozygotes.[184]

The effects of the β1-AR Arg389Gly polymorphism on the risk of developing heart failure and on disease progression also have been investigated. A study by Small and colleagues[54] investigated the potential synergism between β1-AR and α2c-AR polymorphisms and found a significantly increased risk of developing heart failure in African-American subjects, in β1389 Arg homozygotes who were also homozygous for the loss of function α2c-AR 322-325 deletion (Del) allele.[54] The β1-AR Arg389 allele did not appear to be a risk factor for developing heart failure in and of itself,[166] but its presence synergistically increased the risk associated with the α2c-AR Del allele.[184,192] The increased risk of developing heart failure in patients who are β1389 Arg and α2c Del combination homozygotes was driven by results in the African-American cohort,[54] who have a 10-fold higher allele frequency for the Del allele.[54,182] These results could not be confirmed in a European population[193] or in a large epidemiologic study in an African-American population.[194] The hypothesis for the synergistic risk of the $\beta_1$389Arg and α_{2c} Del homozygous genotype was that based on the loss of tonic inhibition of NE release in adrenergic nerves patients with α_{2c} Del prejunctional receptors would have an increase in adrenergic drive that would then signal through hyperfunctional $\beta_1$389Arg receptors.[54,166] However, in subjects with established CHF, the α_{2c} Del polymorphism is not associated with a statistically significant increase in systemic venous NE levels,[192] so this hypothesis may not be correct.

In the placebo arms of both the BEST[182] and MERIT-HF[191] DNA substudies that examined effects of the β_1-AR Arg389Gly polymorphism on clinical endpoints, there was no evidence of any differences between patients who were Arg homozygous and those who were Gly carriers. However, in the Cresci and colleagues two-center genomics study,[185] Caucasian patients untreated with β-blockers who were homozygous for $\beta_1$389 Arg had an improved survival compared to Gly389 patients. Thus, there are mixed reports for the β_1-AR Arg389Gly polymorphism affecting heart failure risk and disease progression, and larger, prospective studies are needed.

Recently evidence has emerged that the cardiac arrhythmias atrial fibrillation and ventricular tachycardia/fibrillation (VT/VF) may be even more sensitive than heart failure endpoints to differential pharmacologic intervention targeting β_1-AR Arg389 homozygotes versus 389Gly genotypes.[195,196] In a pharmacogenetic substudy of the BEST trial, bucindolol produced a 74% reduction in the risk of developing atrial fibrillation in patients with a β_1-AR Arg389Arg genotype versus no risk reduction in 389Gly genotypes.[195] A similar completely differentiated treatment effect was found for VT/VF.[196]

A number of polymorphisms also have been described for the human β_2-AR, the best characterized of which is the presence of either a threonine (Thr) or isoleucine (Ile) at amino acid position 164.[197] The allele frequency of the 164 Ile, minor allele is quite low (−5%), and only 1% to 5% of the population is heterozygous Thr/Ile. Remarkably, no homozygous Ile/Ile subjects have been identified, possibly because of the myocardial dysfunction and mortality associated with this loss of function polymorphism. Similar to the β_1-AR Arg389 variant, the Thr164 β_2-AR is much more efficiently coupled to adenylyl cyclase activation than is the Ile164 variant.[197] The presence of the Ile164 allele is associated with reduced exercise capacity[198] and reduced transplant-free survival.[199] In a transgenic mouse model system, overexpression of the human β_2-AR Ile164 leads to impaired cardiac function,[197] a finding that recapitulates the observation that this allele is associated with reduced exercise capacity and reduced survival in patients with heart failure.[198] Because of the extremely low Ile164allele frequency, no intervention studies have been reported for effects in Thr164Ile heterozygotes.

Kaye and colleagues[200] and Metra and colleagues[186] have reported that a polymorphism of the β_2-AR that affects agonist mediated downregulation, Gln27Glu, where the Glu allele confers resistance, is associated with a more favorable left ventricular ejection fraction (LVEF) response to carvedilol. In terms of effects on clinical endpoints, de Groote and colleagues[201] reported no effects on mortality in a modest-sized heart failure clinic population in 91% of those treated with β-blockers.

As described earlier, one of the major regulators of β-AR signaling are the GRKs. Interestingly, a Gln greater than Leu41 variant of GRK5 has been shown to be protective against heart failure–associated death or transplantation in an African-American population,[185,202] where the Leu allele is ~20 times more frequent than in Caucasian populations. The authors speculate that the increased agonist-mediated uncoupling of the β-AR by GRK5-Leu41 is, in essence, the equivalent of "genetic β-blockade."[179,202]

There would seem a high likelihood that beyond what has already been described, other polymorphic variants of adrenergic receptors, other GPCRs, and any number of downstream effectors will eventually be described. A significant question that remains to be addressed is whether or not the presence of specific polymorphisms, alone or in combination, are primary factors in the predisposition to, or in the rate of progression of, heart failure. The issue of whether β_1 Arg389Gly polymorphisms can alter the clinical response to bucindolol will be answered by prospective Phase 3 clinical trials.

NONCATECHOLAMINE LIGANDS THAT ACTIVATE MYOCARDIAL β-ADRENERGIC RECEPTORS, AND THEIR ROLE IN PRODUCING DILATED CARDIOMYOPATHIES

It doesn't require a biogenic amine to activate a GPCR; work spanning decades has demonstrated that auto-antibodies (AAbs) to the extracellular loops of GPCRs can bind to β_1-[203] and β_2-ARs,[204] and that the consequent signaling[205] can have adverse biologic effects on the myocardium and cardiac myocytes.[206] These AAbs act differently than catecholamine agonists, by activating the AR trough in a different motif.[207] From the standpoint of heart failure, there is no doubt that AAbs to the first and second extracellular loops of the human β_1-AR can produce a dilated cardiomyopathy,[206] and that removal of these AAbs by immunoadsorption[208] can improve myocardial function. Major questions remain as to the incidence of AAbs in dilated or ischemic cardiomyopathies, and their role in a general heart failure population. Some of these questions are being addressed by an ongoing Etiology, Titre-Course, and Survival (ETiCS) study that is being conducted in Europe.[209]

There are several approaches, beyond immunoadsorption, to deal with these AAbs, including the administration of decoy peptides[210] and aptamers that bind to the AAbs with high affinity.[206] Some of these approaches, coupled with a companion diagnostic, may make their way through clinical development over the next several years,[211] and if so will likely be incorporated into the heart failure armamentarium.

SUMMARY AND FUTURE DIRECTIONS

Adrenergic mechanisms are markedly altered in CHF and exert major effects on the natural history of the clinical syndrome. Adrenergic abnormalities can be classified into two major groups: those that produce a sustained increase in adrenergic drive and those that cause defects or qualitative shifts in β-AR signal transduction. Within each category there is the potential for benefit and harm, and successful therapeutic intervention involves interfering with the harmful components without compromising the beneficial aspects. A pharmacological concept evolving in this context is that of biased GPCR ligands,[212] and other approaches involving the use of β_1-selective antagonists in combination with a second agent to enhance beneficial adrenergic effects have been tested or are undergoing testing.[5]

It should be clear from the scope of this review that adrenergic receptor signaling is far more complex than our naïve supposition that the binding of catecholamines to receptors simply increases the abundance of the second messengers, cAMP and Ca^{++}, thereby affecting an increase in myocardial contractility and heart rate. Although the importance of these functions has not been diminished, adrenergic receptors are now recognized to be important effectors of any number of cellular processes important to cardiac myocyte biology. Undoubtedly, the diversity and complexity of these signaling paradigms will continue to unfold. It is hoped that an increased appreciation of these processes, as well as the recognition that genetic variation is important to both disease progression and to therapeutic response, will lead to advances in heart failure therapeutics.

KEY REFERENCES

2. Esler M, Kaye D, Lambert G, Esler D, Jennings G. Adrenergic nervous system in heart failure. *Am J Cardiol*. 1997;80(11A):7L–14L.

5. Bristow MR. Treatment of chronic heart failure with beta-adrenergic receptor antagonists: a convergence of receptor pharmacology and clinical cardiology. *Circ Res*. 2011;109(10):1176–1194. Epub 2011/10/29. doi: 10.1161/CIRCRESAHA.111.245092.

6. Packer M, Bristow MR, Cohn JN, et al. The effect of carvedilol on morbidity and mortality in patients with chronic heart failure. U.S. Carvedilol Heart Failure Study Group. *N Engl J Med*. 1996;334(21):1349–13455.

7. MERIT. Effect of metoprolol CR/XL in chronic heart failure: Metoprolol CR/XL Randomised Intervention Trial in Congestive Heart Failure (MERIT-HF) [see comments]. *Lancet*. 1999;353(9169):2001–2007.

8. Bucindolol Investigators. A trial of the beta-blocker bucindolol in patients with advanced chronic heart failure. *N Engl J Med*. 2001;344(22):1659–1667.

30. Cohn JN, Pfeffer MA, Rouleau J, et al. Adverse mortality effect of central sympathetic inhibition with sustained-release moxonidine in patients with heart failure (MOXCON). *Eur J Heart Fail*. 2003;5(5):659–667.

34. Lowes BD, Gilbert EM, Abraham WT, et al. Myocardial gene expression in dilated cardiomyopathy treated with beta-blocking agents. *N Engl J Med*. 2002;346(18):1357–1365.

58. Bristow MR, Ginsburg R, Umans V, et al. Beta 1- and beta 2-adrenergic -receptor subpopulations in nonfailing and failing human ventricular myocardium: coupling of both receptor subtypes to muscle contraction and selective beta 1-receptor down- regulation in heart failure. *Circ Res*. 1986;59(3):297–309.

75. Fowler MB, Laser JA, Hopkins GL, Minobe W, Bristow MR. Assessment of the beta-adrenergic receptor pathway in the intact failing human heart: progressive receptor down-regulation and subsensitivity to agonist response. *Circulation*. 1986;74(6):1290–1302.

150. Sucharov C, Bristow MR, Port JD. miRNA expression in the failing human heart: functional correlates. *J Mol Cell Cardiol*. 2008;45(2):185–192. doi: 10.1016/j.yjmcc.2008.04.014.

The full reference list for this chapter is available on ExpertConsult.

Role of Innate Immunity in Heart Failure

Douglas L. Mann

Although clinicians recognized the pathophysiological importance of inflammation in the heart as far back as 1669, the formal recognition that inflammatory mediators were activated in the setting of heart failure did not occur for another three centuries. Since the initial description of inflammatory cytokines in patients with heart failure in 1990,[1] there has been a growing interest in the role that these molecules play in regulating cardiac structure and function, particularly with regard to their potential role in disease progression in heart failure. This interest has expanded recently with the recognition that inflammatory mediators are part of a much larger, highly integrated biological system referred to as the innate immune system. In the present chapter we will summarize the recent growth of knowledge that has taken place in this field, with a particular emphasis on the pathophysiologic role that innate immunity plays in the progression of heart failure.

OVERVIEW OF INNATE IMMUNITY

The adult heart responds to tissue injury by synthesizing a series of proteins that promote homeostasis, either by activating mechanisms that facilitate tissue repair or, alternatively, by upregulating mechanisms that confer cytoprotective responses within the heart. The literature suggests that proinflammatory cytokines serve as the downstream "effectors" of the innate immune system by facilitating tissue repair within the heart. What has been less well understood, until recently, is how these myocardial innate immune responses are coordinated following tissue injury.

The relatively recent discovery that the innate immune system is activated by pattern recognition receptors (PRRs) that recognize conserved motifs on pathogens (so-called pathogen-associated molecular patterns [PAMPs]) has provided important new insights with respect to our understanding of the role of inflammation in health and disease (**Fig. 7.1**).[2] Typical examples of PAMPs include the lipopolysaccharides (LPS) of gram-negative organisms, the teichoic acids of gram-positive organisms, the glycolipids of mycobacterium, the zymosans of yeast, and the double-stranded RNAs of viruses. These PAMPs are unique to these pathogens, and in some cases are required for their virulence. Thus, one of the quintessential features of the innate immune system is that it serves as an "early warning system" that enables the host to accurately and rapidly discriminate self from non-self. PRRs are also activated by molecular patterns of endogenous host material that is released during cellular injury or death, so-called damage-associated molecular patterns (DAMPs).[3-5] DAMPs can be derived from dying or injured cells, damaged extracellular matrix proteins, or circulating oxidized proteins. Thus, molecular patterns released by damaged or dying cells are capable of eliciting inflammatory responses analogous to the immune response that is triggered by PAMPs. Importantly, PRRs are constitutively expressed on most cardiac cells, while adaptive immune receptors are not. The most important PRRs include Toll-like receptors (TLRs), NOD-like receptors (NLRs), RIG-I-like receptors (retinoic acid inducible), pentraxins, and C-type lectin receptors (CLRs). As will be discussed, the long-term consequences of sustained activation of innate immunity can lead to progressive left ventricle (LV) remodeling and LV dysfunction, thereby contributing to the pathogenesis of heart failure (**Table 7.1**).

EXPRESSION AND REGULATION OF PATTERN RECOGNITION RECEPTORS IN THE HEART

Toll Receptors

The toll receptor was originally discovered as a protein that was responsible for dorsoventral polarity in the fly. Subsequent studies demonstrated that the human homolog of the *Drosophila* toll protein was sufficient to activate NF-κB-dependent genes in mammalian cells.[6] At the time of this writing, 13 mammalian TLR paralogs have been identified, of which 10 functional TLRs have been identified in humans (functional TLRs 11–13 are only expressed in mice). TLRs 1 to 6 are expressed on the cell surface of mammalian cells, whereas TLR 3, 7, and 9 are expressed in intracellular compartments, primarily endosomes and the endoplasmic

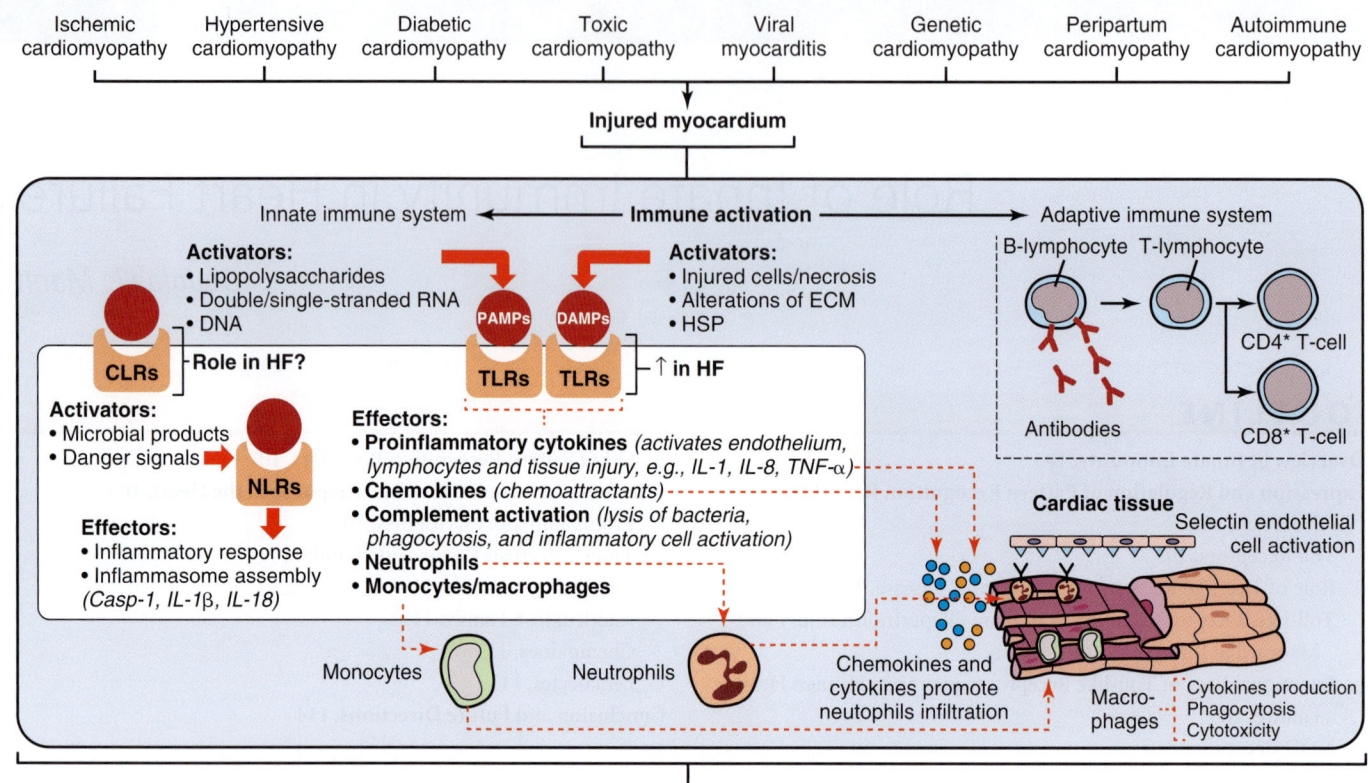

Fig. 7.1 Interaction between cardiac disease states and the various components of the innate immune system. *Casp-1*, Caspase-1; *CLR*, C-type lectin receptor; *DAMP*, danger-associated molecular pattern; *ECM*, extracellular matrix; *HF*, heart failure; *HSP*, heat-shock protein; *IL*, interleukin; *NLR*, NOD-like receptor; *PAMP*, pathogen-associated molecular pattern; *TLR*, Toll-like receptor; *TNF*, tumor necrosis factor. Modified from Frantz S, Falcao-Pires I, Balligand JL, et al. The innate immune system in chronic cardiomyopathy: a European Society of Cardiology [ESC] scientific statement from the Working Group on Myocardial Function of the ESC. *Eur J Heart Fail*. 2018;20(3):445–459.

TABLE 7.1 Effects of Inflammatory Mediators on Left Ventricular Remodeling

Alterations in the Biology of the Myocyte
- Myocyte hypertrophy
- Contractile abnormalities
- Fetal gene expression

Alteration in the Extracellular Matrix
- Matrix metalloproteinase activation
- Degradation of the matrix
- Fibrosis

Progressive Myocyte Loss
- Necrosis
- Apoptosis

reticulum, with the ligand-binding domains facing the lumen of the vesicle. TLR10 is the most recent member of the human TLR receptor family discovered; however, its function and direct ligand are still unknown. Humans also encode a TLR11 gene, but it contains several stop codons, and the protein is not expressed.

Messenger RNA (mRNA) for TLRs 1 to 10 have been identified in the human heart.[7] Of note, the relative expression levels of mRNA for TLRs 2, 3, and 4 is approximately 10-fold higher than TLRs 1, and 5 to 10.[7] Although expression levels of TLRs have not been identified in human myocytes, TLR2, 3, 4, and 6 mRNA have been identified in

cardiac myocytes from neonatal rats.[8] Although less is known regarding the regulation of TLR expression in heart failure, the experimental literature suggests that sustained activation of TLR signaling following cardiac injury is maladaptive and can lead to heart failure. Two studies have shown that TLR4 expression is increased in the hearts of patients with advanced heart failure.[9,10] Moreover, the pattern of TLR4 expression in cardiac myocytes differs in heart failure, in that there are focal areas of intense TLR4 staining in failing cardiac myocytes, in contrast to the diffuse pattern of TLR4 staining observed in nonfailing myocytes.[9]

As shown in **Fig. 7.2A**, the signaling pathway that is used by the TLR family of receptors is highly homologous to that of the interleukin-1 receptor (IL-1R) family (see below). TLRs are type 1 membrane-spanning receptors that have a leucine-rich repeat (LRR) extracellular motif and an intracellular signaling motif that is similar to IL-1. With the exception of TLR3, all TLRs interact with an adaptor protein termed MyD88 (myeloid differentiation factor 88) via their Toll interleukin receptor (TIR) domains (Fig. 7.2B). MyD88-dependent signaling through TLR2 and TLR4 requires an adaptor protein termed TIRAP (TIR domain-containing adaptor protein) to initiate signaling. When stimulated, MyD88 sequentially recruits IL-1 receptor associated kinases 4, 1, and 2 (IRAK4, IRAK1, and IRAK2) to the receptor complex. Phosphorylation of IRAK1 on serine/threonine residues by IRAK4 results in recruitment of tumor necrosis receptor-associated factor 6 (TRAF6) to the complex, which is responsible for early responses to TLR signaling. More recent studies have suggested an important role for phosphorylation of IRAK2 by IRAK4 in terms of

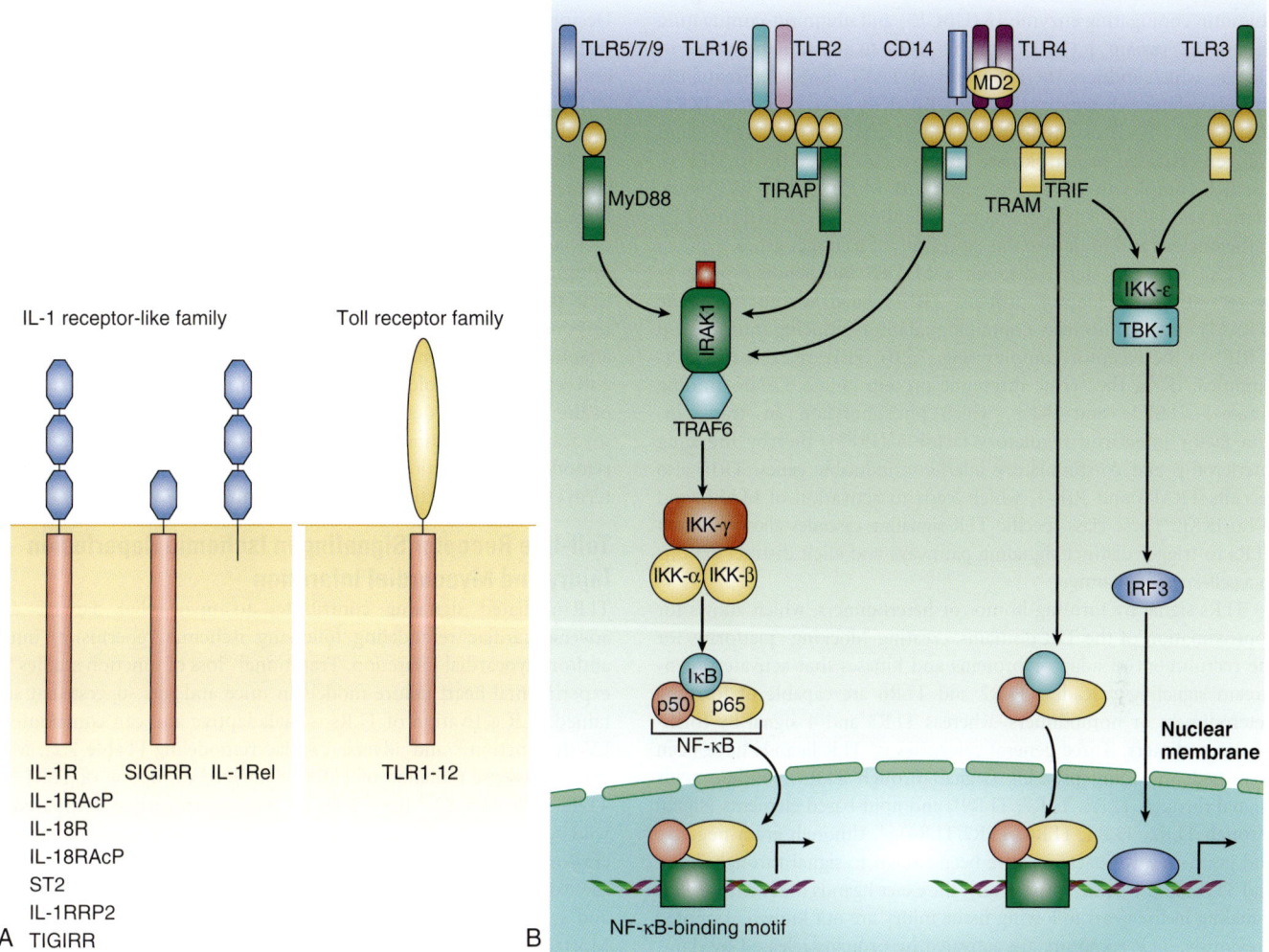

Fig. 7.2 Toll-like receptors (*TLRs*) structure and signaling. (A) *TLRs* and interleukin-1 *(IL-1)* receptors have a conserved cytoplasmic domain that is known as the Toll/IL-1 R domain. The TIR domain is characterized by the presence of three highly homologous regions (known as boxes 1, 2, and 3). Despite the similarity of the cytoplasmic domains of these molecules, their extracellular regions differ markedly: TLRs have tandem repeats of leucine-rich regions (known as leucine rich repeats, *LRR*), whereas IL-1 Rs have three immunoglobulin *(Ig)*-like domains. (B) Stimulation of TLRs triggers the association of MyD88, which in turn recruits IRAK4, thereby allowing the association of IRAK1. IRAK4 then induces the phosphorylation of IRAK1. TRAF6 is also recruited to the receptor complex, by associating with phosphorylated IRAK1. Phosphorylated IRAK1 and TRAF6 then dissociate from the receptor and form a complex with TAK1, TAB1, and TAB2 at the plasma membrane (not shown), which induces the phosphorylation of TAB2 and TAK1. IRAK1 is degraded at the plasma membrane, and the remaining complex (consisting of TRAF6, TAK1, TAB1, and TAB2) translocates to the cytosol, where it associates with the ubiquitin ligases UBC13 and UEV1A. This leads to the ubiquitination of TRAF6, which induces the activation of TAK1. TAK1, in turn, phosphorylates both MAP kinases and the IKK complex, which consists of IKK-α, IKK-β and IKK-γ (also known as IKK1, IKK2, and NEMO, respectively). The IKK complex then phosphorylates IκB, which leads to its ubiquitination and subsequent degradation. This allows to the nucleus and induce the expression of its target genes. The MyD88 dependent pathway is used by TLR1, TLR2, TLR4, TLR5, TLR6, TLR7, and TLR9. TIRAP, a second TIR-domain-containing adaptor protein, is involved in the MyD88-dependent signaling pathway through TLR2 and TLR4. In contrast, TLR3- and TLR4-mediated activation of interferon *(IFN)*-regulatory factor 3 *(IRF3)* and the induction of IFN-β occur in a MyD88-independent manner. As shown, a third TIR-domain-containing adaptor, TRIF, is essential for the MyD88-independent pathway through TLR3 and TLR4. TRAM, a fourth TIR-domain containing adaptor, is specific to the TLR4-mediated, MyD88-independent/TRIF-dependent pathway. TRIF mediates the activation of the noncanonical IKKs, IKK-ε, and TBK1, and MAP kinase. Note TLR3 is predominately located within endosomes (not illustrated). Modified from Akira S, Takeda K. Toll like receptor signaling. *Nat Rev Immunol.* 2004;7:499–511.

mediating late responses to TLR signaling.[11] Phosphorylated IRAK1 and TRAF6 dissociate from the receptor and form a complex at the plasma membrane with transforming growth factor-activated kinase 1 (TAK1), a mitogen-activated protein kinase kinase kinase, as well as TAK1-binding protein 1 (TAB1) and TAK1-binding proteins 2 or 3 (TAB2 or TAB3), resulting in the phosphorylation of TAB2/3 and TAK1. IRAK1 is degraded at the plasma membrane, and the remaining complex (consisting of TRAF6, TAK1, TAB1 and TAB2 or TAB3) translocates to the cytosol, where it associates with the ubiquitin ligases ubiquitin conjugating enzyme 13 (UBC13) and ubiquitin-conjugating enzyme E2 variant 1 (UEV1A). This leads to the ubiquitylation of TRAF6, which induces the activation of TAK1. TAK1 subsequently phosphorylates IκB kinase (IKK) α/IKKβ/IKKγ (also known as IKK1, IKK2, and NF-κB essential modulator [NEMO], respectively) and mitogen-activated protein kinase kinase 6 (MP2K6, MKK6, MEK6). The IKK complex then phosphorylates IκB, which leads to its ubiquitylation and subsequent degradation. This allows NF-κB to translocate to the nucleus and to induce the expression of its target genes.[12,13]

TLR4 also can signal through a MyD88 independent pathway by recruiting the adaptor proteins TRIF-related adaptor molecule (TRAM) and TIR-domain-containing adaptor-inducing interferon-β (TRIF) to the receptor complex (Fig. 7.2B). TRIF recruits the non-canonical IKKs, the serine-threonine-protein kinase TANK-binding kinase-1 (TBK1) and IKKε, which phosphorylate the transcription factor interferon regulatory factor 3 (IRF3), thereby inducing interferon-β and co-stimulatory interferon-inducible genes. TRIF also recruits TRAF6 and RIP-1, which leads to activation of MAPK and IKKα/IKKβ. These class-specific TLR signaling cascades allow different TLRs to trigger distinct signaling pathways and elicit distinct actions in a cell-specific manner.

TLRs signal by forming homo- or heterodimers, which allows for approximation of the TIR domains, creating "docking" platforms for the recruitment of adaptor proteins and kinases that activate downstream signaling cascades. TLR2 and TLR6 are capable of forming heterodimers or homodimers, whereas TLR3 and 4 signal by forming homodimers. Three general categories of TLR ligands have been identified, including proteins (signal through TLR5), nucleic acids (signal through TLR3, TLR7, TLR9), and lipid-based elements (signal through TLR2, TLR4, TLR6, TLR2/TLR6).[14] Although gram-negative and gram-positive bacteria have been shown to signal through TLR4 and TLR2 in the heart, respectively, the exact ligands that activate TLR signaling in the heart following tissue injury are not known. As noted previously, TLR receptors are activated by proteins released by damage-associated molecular patterns released by injured and/or dying cells, as well as by fragments of the extracellular matrix (see Fig. 7.1).[4,15]

Given the importance TLR signaling, it is not surprising that nature has evolved multiple pathways to negatively regulate TLR signaling. TLR-signaling pathways are negatively regulated by several molecules that are induced following stimulation of TLRs, including IL-1-receptor-associated kinase M IRAK-M,[16] suppressor of cytokine signaling 1 (SOCS1), and Src homology 2 domain-containing inositol 5-phosphatase 1 (SHIP-1) a phosphatase that hydrolyzes the 5′phosphate of PI-3,4-P2, which inhibits PI3 kinase-dependent TLR-MyD88 interactions and NF-kβ activation, and thus negatively regulates TLR signaling.[17] TRIM30α destabilizes the TAK1 complex by promoting the degradation of TAB2 and TAB3,[18] whereas myeloid differentiation primary-response protein 88 short (MyD88s), an alternatively spliced variant of MyD88, blocks the association of IRAK4 with MyD88. Sterile-alpha and Armadillo motif containing protein (SARM) is a novel adaptor protein that specifically blocks TRIF-dependent but not MyD88-dependent signaling.[19] TOLLIP (Toll interacting protein) is thought to maintain immune cells in a quiescent state and/or terminate TLR-mediated signaling, by interacting with the cytoplasmic TIR domains of TLR2 and TLR4 and suppressing IRAK1phosphorylation. Finally, the TIR (Toll/IL-1R)-domain-containing receptors single immunoglobulin IL-1 receptor related (SIGIRR) molecule and ST2 have also been shown to negatively regulate TLR signaling. Another highly conserved mechanism for regulating innate immunity is being revealed for microRNAs, so-called immuno-miRs, that regulate innate immune gene expression by preventing mRNA translation by promoting mRNA degradation.

Role of Toll-like Receptors in Myocardial Disease

Deciphering the role that the innate immune system plays in myocardial disease has been challenging, insofar as it has been difficult to reconcile two sets of conflicting observations, one of which suggests that TLR signaling is beneficial, and the other of which suggests that TLR signaling following ischemic injury is deleterious. Recent "reductionist" studies that have been performed ex vivo, or that have employed chimeric TLR-deficient mice that harbor wild-type bone marrow cells have allowed for a clearer understanding of the central (i.e., myocardial) and peripheral (i.e., bone marrow-derived) effects of the innate immune system following ischemic injury. The aggregate data suggest that short-term activation of TLR signaling confers cytoprotective responses within the heart, whereas longer-term TLR signaling is maladaptive and results in the upregulation of proinflammatory cytokines and cell adhesion molecules, which leads to activation and recruitment of the "peripheral" neutrophils, monocytes, and dendritic cells to the myocardium, resulting in increased cell death and adverse cardiac remodeling. The sections that follow will focus on the deleterious long-term effects of the activation of innate immunity in the heart.

Toll-like Receptor Signaling in Ischemia Reperfusion Injury and Myocardial Infarction

TLR-mediated signaling contributes to myocardial damage and adverse cardiac remodeling following ischemia reperfusion injury and/or myocardial infarction. Traditional "loss of function studies" in experimental heart failure models in mice and rats suggest that sustained TLR activation of TLRs is maladaptive and can contribute to LV dysfunction[20] and adverse cardiac remodeling (**Table 7.2**). Mice with a missense mutation of TLR4 or targeted disruption of TLR4,[21-23] TLR2,[24] or MyD88[25] have reduced infarct sizes when compared to wild-type controls. Moreover, mice pretreated with a TLR4 antagonist (Eritoran)[26] had reduced nuclear translocation of NF-κB, decreased the expression of proinflammatory cytokines (e.g., IL-1, IL-6, TNF), and smaller infarct sizes when compared to vehicle treated animals. Mortality and LV remodeling are reduced in mice with targeted disruption of TLR4 or TLR2.[24,27] Studies performed ex vivo in TLR2-deficient mice suggest that the LV dysfunction that supervenes following I/R is mediated through TLR2-TRAP-mediated upregulation of TNF.

Functional Role of Toll-like Receptor Signaling in Human Heart Failure

The experimental literature reviewed above suggests that sustained activation of TLR signaling following cardiac injury is maladaptive and can lead to a heart failure phenotype. Unfortunately, very little is known with respect to the role of the innate immune system in the failing human heart. To date, two studies have shown that TLR4 expression is increased in the hearts of patients with advanced heart failure.[9,10] Moreover, the pattern of TLR4 expression in cardiac myocytes in heart failure, in that there are focal areas of intense TLR4 staining in failing cardiac myocytes, in contrast to the diffuse pattern of TLR4 staining observed in nonfailing myocytes.[9] To further clarify the role of innate immunity in the failing heart, a recent study examined the expression profiles of 59 innate immune genes using gene arrays that were from explanted hearts from patients with ischemic cardiomyopathy (ICM), idiopathic dilated cardiomyopathy (DCM), and viral cardiomyopathy (VCM); gene arrays from nonfailing hearts were used as the appropriate controls.[28] This bioinformatic study showed that there were distinct gene expression profiles for innate immune genes in failing and nonfailing hearts, and that there were distinct gene expression profiles for innate immune genes in ICM and DCM hearts. Although these provisional studies suggest that the innate immune system is activated in human heart failure, it will be important to more

TABLE 7.2   **Toll-like Receptor Signaling Modulation of Myocardial Ischemia Reperfusion Injury and Cardiac Remodeling**

Mice	Infarct Models	Effects in Knockout Mice
TLR2 Signaling		
TLR2−/−	I/R (30′ I/60R′)[93]	Sizes, reduced neutrophil recruitment, reduced ROS and cytokines
TLR2−/−	Permanent coronary ligation[26]	Survival rate, attenuated remodeling, but same infarct sizes at 4 wk
TLR4 Signaling		
C57 BL/10 ScCr	I/R (60′ I/24 h R)[25]	Sizes, reduced MPO activity and complement 3 deposition
C3H/HeJ	I/R (60′ I/120′ R)[23]	Sizes, decreased cardiac expression of TNF, MCP-1, and ILs
C3H/HeJ	I/R (60′ I/24 h R)[24]	Sizes, but no gain in LV function
C3H/HeJ	I/R (30′ I/120′ R)[28]	Sizes, reduced pJNK, reduced cytokine expression
WT with eritoran	I/R (30′ I/120′ R)[28]	Sizes, reduced pJNK, reduced cytokine expression
C3H/HeJ	Permanent coronary ligation[94]	Remodeling, improved systolic function, reduced cytokine expression
C57 BL/10 ScCr	Permanent coronary ligation[29]	Function on day 6 after infarction, improved survival rate, reduced LV remodeling and apoptosis at 4 wk.
MyD88−/−	I/R (30′ I/24 h R)[27]	Sizes, improved LV function, and attenuated cytokine expression and neutrophil recruitment

MCP-1, Monocyte chemoattractant protein-1; *MPO*, myeloperoxidase; *MyD88*, myeloid differentiation primary-response gene 88; *pJNK*, phosphorylated JNK; *ROS*, reactive oxygen species; *TLR*, Toll-like receptor.
Modified from Chao W. Toll-like receptor signaling: a critical modulator of cell survival and ischemic injury in the heart. *Am J Physiol Heart Circ Physiol.* 2009;296:H1–H12; Topkara VK, Evans S, Zhang W, et al. Therapeutic targeting of innate immunity in the failing heart. *J Mol Cell Cardiol.* 2011;51:594–599.

precisely determine the expression levels of the different components of the innate immune system, as well as link activation of the innate immune system to the development and progression of heart failure.

NOD Receptors

NLRs have emerged as important PRR superfamily members in health and disease.[29] NLRs cooperate with TLRs in regulating inflammatory and cellular homeostatic responses. The canonical structure of the NLR consists of three domains, including a central NACHT (NOD nucleotide-binding domain) domain, which is common to all NLRs, and is responsible for ATP mediated oligomerization. As shown in **Fig. 7.3** the majority of NLRs contain C-terminal LRRs, which detect the presence of cognate ligands. The N-terminal domain is responsible for homotypic protein–protein interaction and consist of either a caspase recruitment domain (CARD), a pyrin domain (PYD), or an acidic transactivating domain or baculovirus inhibitor repeats (BIRs) domain.

Five subfamilies of NLRs can be distinguished based on their N-terminal effector domains, which impart unique functional characteristics to each NLR. The founding NLR members are NOD1 (NLRC1) and NOD2 (NLRC2), which are part of the larger NLRC subfamily (NLRC 1–5). NLRCs are characterized by the presence of a CARD domain that allows for direct interaction between members of this family and other CARD carrying adaptor proteins. NOD1 (NLRC1) and NOD2 (NLRC2) serve as important sensors of bacterial peptidoglycan (PGN) and are crucial for tissue homeostasis and host defense against bacterial pathogens (48). NLRs with an N-terminal acidic transactivation domain are termed NLRA (CIITA), and serve as transcriptional regulators of MHC class II antigen presentation (44). NLRB (NAIP) proteins have a BIR domain, and play important roles in host defense and cell survival. NLRX1 is the only described member of the NLRX subfamily that contains an N-terminal mitochondria-targeting sequence required for its trafficking to the mitochondrial membrane (Fig. 7.3A). Members of the PYD-containing NLRP subfamily (NLRP 1–14) are best known for their role in inducing the formation of the oligomeric inflammatory complex termed the "inflammasome." The inflammasome (Fig. 7.3B) is composed of an NLRP, the proinflammatory caspase-1, and the apoptosis-associated

speck-like protein (ASC). The ASC contains an N-terminal PYD and a C-terminal CARD, which enables it to bring caspase-1 and NLRPs into close proximity. Upon activation, NLRP3 recruits ASC and caspase-1, which is required for the cleavage and maturation of the inflammatory cytokines IL-1β and IL-18. More recently, a more complex model for NLRP3-inflammasome activation has been proposed where two adaptors, ASC and mitochondrial antiviral signaling (MAVS) protein, are required for optimal inflammasome triggering.[30]

The NLRP3 inflammasome has been shown to play an important role in the heart following tissue injury (Fig. 7.3B).[29] The NLRP3 and other important key components of the inflammasome are not constitutively expressed in cardiac myocytes, but can be upregulated in leukocytes and cardiac myocytes by proinflammatory cytokines and/or DAMPs or PAMPs. After the inflammasome is "primed," a second "trigger" is required for the activation of the NLRP3, which is largely, but not exclusively, dependent on the intracellular K+ concentration. As shown in Fig. 7.3B, lysosomal destabilization activates a signaling pathway that indirectly leads to increased membrane permeability and K+ efflux. Leakage of cathepsin B from lysosomes also has been shown to activate the inflammasome. Additional triggers include extracellular ATP binding to the P2X purinoreceptor 7 (P2X7), which triggers K+ efflux, leading to a conformational change in NLRP3 that allows for recruitment of ASC (Fig. 7.3B). The NLRP3 inflammasome is critically involved in the response to injury during acute myocardial infarction (AMI), and is responsible for the production of IL-1β and the ensuing systemic inflammatory response. Experimental studies in small and large animals show that NLRP3 inflammasome-targeted therapies might be a viable strategy for the reduction of infarct size and the prevention of heart failure following AMI (reviewed in reference [29]).

Other Pattern Recognition Receptors

The pentraxins, including pentraxin3 (PTX3), serum amyloid P (SAP), and C-reactive protein (CRP), are involved in innate immunity and inflammatory signaling in cardiovascular disease. Pentraxins are useful biomarkers for ischemic heart disease and heart failure. Elevated levels of CRP provide important prognostic information for a variety of clinical settings and have been used to identify patients with coronary artery disease who are more likely to have cardiac events. CLRs

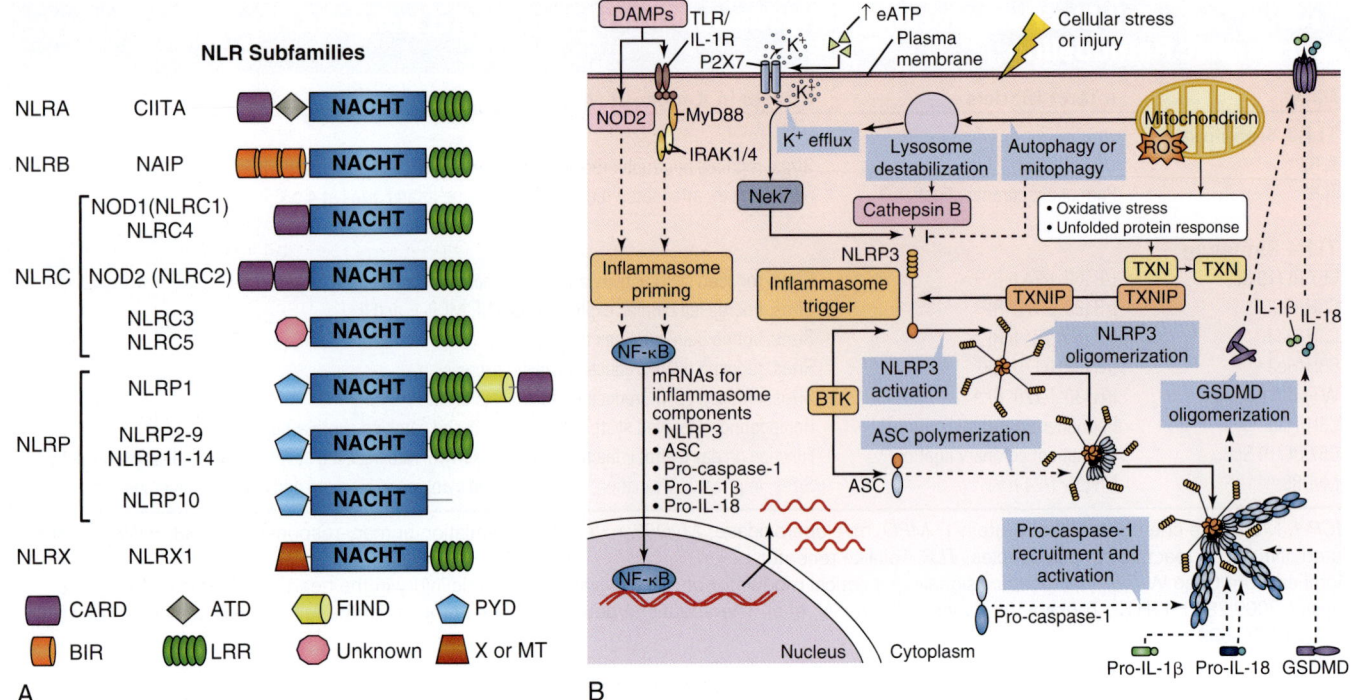

NLR Subfamilies

Fig. 7.3 (A) Schematic representation of individual nod-like receptor *(NLR)* domains. Human NLRs are sub-classified into five categories: NLRA, NLRB, NLRC, NLRP, and NLRX. All 22 human NLRs contain a central NACHT domain and a C-terminal ligand-sensing LRR domain, with the exception of NLRP10. The N-terminal domains ascribe functional properties to the NLRs; however, the function of some of the domains is still unclear. *ATD*, Acidic transactivation domain; *BIR*, baculoviral inhibition of apoptosis protein repeat domain; *CARD*, caspase association and recruitment domain; *FIIND*, function to find domain; *LRR*, leucine-rich repeats; *MT*, targets NLRX1 to the mitochondria; *PYD*, pyrin domain. (A, from Saxena M, Yeretssian G. NOD-Like Receptors: Master Regulators of Inflammation and Cancer. *Front Immunol.* 2014;5:327). (B) Pathways for formation of the NLRP3 inflammasome. The formation of the inflammasome in the heart requires two independent steps: priming and triggering. The priming signal is dependent on the activity of nuclear factor *(NF)*-κB through stimulation of the membrane Toll-like receptors *(TLRs)* and the downstream signaling mediated by myeloid differentiation primary response protein MyD88 and interleukin-1 *(IL-1)* receptor-associated kinases *(IRAKs)*. The TLRs sense extracellular threats through damage-associated molecular patterns *(DAMPs)* and prime the cells to respond to the potential injurious conditions by increasing the transcription and translation of inflammasome components and the associated cytokines (IL-1β and IL-18). These cytokines function in a paracrine fashion on the membrane cytokine receptor and converge on the same pathways to amplify the signal. A similar priming effect is mediated by nucleotide-binding oligomerization domain-containing protein 2 *(NOD2)*. The primary signal is necessary but insufficient to form the inflammasome in cardiomyocytes in the absence of the trigger signal. The activation of NACHT, LRR, and PYD domains-containing protein 3 *(NLRP3)* is mediated by extracellular and/or intracellular pathways. The increase in extracellular ATP *(eATP)* activates the P2X purinoreceptor 7 *(P2X7)* and leads to K+ efflux, a step that triggers NLRP3 activation. Lysosomal destabilization by indigestible material is another mechanism that leads to NLRP3 activation by leakage of the lysosomal enzyme cathepsin B and by induction of K+ efflux. The serine/threonine–protein kinase Nek7 senses the K+ efflux and binds NLRP3, allowing its activation. Thioredoxin-interacting protein *(TXNIP)* links oxidative stress and the unfolded protein response to NLRP3 activation. TXNIP is freed from thioredoxin *(TRX)* and binds NLRP3. The mitochondria also have an important role in producing reactive oxygen species *(ROS)*. Furthermore, ineffective clearance of mitochondrial debris by mitophagy contributes to lysosomal destabilization. By contrast, effective mitophagy and autophagy suppress the activation of NLRP3. The tyrosine–protein kinase BTK also binds NLRP3 and apoptosis-associated speck-like protein containing a CARD *(ASC)*, leading to inflammasome activation after ischemia. The active NLRP3 oligomerizes, forming a circular structure that functions as a platform for the polymerization of ASC into filaments, which in turn work as a central core from which caspase 1 filaments branch, forming a star-like structure. Active caspase 1 cleaves the inactive pro-IL-1β and pro-IL-18 into the active forms, IL-1β and IL-18. Gasdermin D *(GSDMD)* is an additional substrate of caspase 1 that oligomerizes upon cleavage and forms pores in the cell membrane with the N-terminal fragments, which allow the extracellular release of active IL-1β and IL-18. (B, modified from Toldo S, Abbate A. The NLRP3 inflammasome in acute myocardial infarction. *Nat Rev Cardiol.* 2018;15:203–214.)

are a family of proteins with one or more C-type lectin domains, which require calcium for binding. CLRs display a diverse range of functions, including innate immune response, cellular apoptosis, and cell–cell adhesion. Very little is known about the role of C-type lectins and cardiac function. RIG-I-like receptors (retinoic acid-inducible gene-I-like receptors [RLRs]) are cytosolic innate immune sensors that detect pathogenic RNA and trigger a systemic antiviral response. RLRs cooperate in signaling crosstalk networks with TLRs and activate the innate immunity, as well as modulate adaptive immune response. There are three RLRs: RIG-I, melanoma differentiation-associated gene 5 (MDA5), and laboratory of genetics and physiology 2 (LGP2). Overexpression of MDA5 in the heart has been shown to protect the heart from viral injury.

EFFECTORS OF THE INNATE IMMUNE RESPONSE IN THE HEART

Proinflammatory Cytokines

Cytokines are 15 to 30 KDa proteins that are secreted by cells in response to activation on the innate immune system. Whereas proinflammatory cytokines have traditionally been thought to be produced by the immune cells, it is now widely recognized that cytokines are expressed by a broad variety of nucleated cell types, including cardiac myocytes. Thus, from a conceptual standpoint, these molecules should be envisioned as proteins that are produced locally within the myocardium by "cardiocytes" (i.e., cells that reside within the myocardium), in response to one or more different forms of environmental stress. The section that follows will review the biological properties of the canonical proinflammatory cytokine families, including the tumor necrosis factor (TNF) super family (TNFSF), the IL-1 family (IL-1F), and the IL-6 family.

Tumor Necrosis Factor Superfamily

The TNF superfamily consists of 19 well-characterized ligands (TNFSF) and 34 TNF receptor superfamily (TNFRSF). Members of the TNF superfamily of ligands and receptors are expressed in a broad variety of cell types, including myocardial cells.[31] Without exception, all members of the TNF superfamily exhibit proinflammatory activity. Of note, recent studies have identified a potential role for TNFSF ligands/receptors in terms of mediating inflammatory responses in the heart, including TNF/TNFR1,TNFR2 (TNFSF2/TNFRSF1A, TNFRSF1B), FasL/Fas (TNFSF6/TNFRSF6), TWEAK (TNF-like weak inducer of apoptosis)/TWEAKR (TNFSF12/TNFRSF12),[32] and RANKL (Receptor activator of NF-kB ligand)/RANK (TNFSF11/TNFRSF11A).[33] Cardiac-restricted overexpression of FasL does not lead to a DCM[34] and will not be discussed further herein.

Tumor necrosis factor. TNF (TNFSF2), the prototypical member of the TNF superfamily, has a broad variety of pleiotropic biological capacities. Besides its cytostatic and cytotoxic effects on certain tumor cells, it influences growth, differentiation, and/or function of virtually every cell type investigated, including cardiac myocytes.[35] In most cell types studied TNF is initially synthesized as a nonglycosylated transmembrane protein of approximately 25 Kda. A 17 Kda fragment is proteolytically cleaved off the plasma membrane of the cell by a membrane-bound enzyme termed TACE (TNF-α convertase [ADAM17]) to produce the "secreted form," which circulates as a stable 51 Kda TNF homotrimer (**Fig. 7.4**). Clinical studies have shown that TNF mRNA and protein is expressed in failing human hearts but is not detectable in nonfailing hearts.[36]

TNF is initially expressed as a functional 26-kDa homotrimeric transmembrane that may be cleaved by a metalloproteinase termed TACE (see Fig. 7.4). Once TNF is cleaved, it is released into the circulation as 17-kDa protein that assembles as a functional 60-kDa homotrimer. The function of TNF is relayed by two structurally distinct receptors, termed TNF receptor 1 (TNFR1; TNFRSF1A, p55, CD120a) and TNF receptor 2 (TNFR2, TNFRSF1B, p75, CD120b). The TNFRs belong to the TNFRSF, a group of type I transmembrane glycoproteins that are characterized by a conserved homologous cysteine-rich domain in their extracellular region. Previous studies have identified the presence of both types of TNFRs in nonfailing[37] and

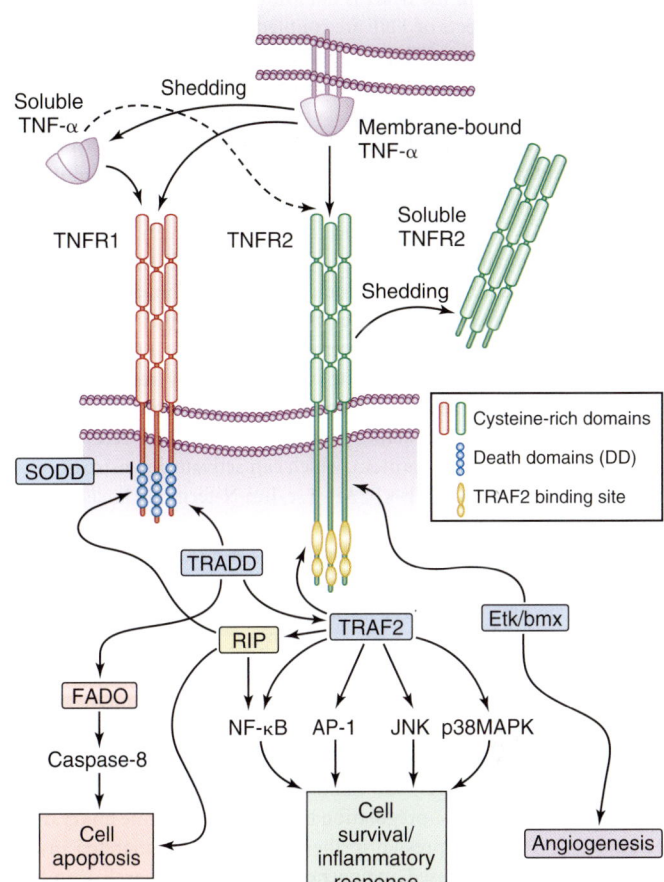

Fig. 7.4 Overview of tumor necrosis factor *(TNF)* signaling. TNF is initially expressed as a functional 26-kDa homotrimeric transmembrane that may be cleaved by a metalloproteinase termed TACE (TNFα-converting enzyme [ADAM-17]). Once TNF is cleaved, it is released into the circulation as 17-kDa protein that assembles as a functional 60-kDa homotrimer. The function of TNF is relayed by two structurally distinct receptors, termed TNF receptor 1 (TNFR1; TNFRSF1A, p55, CD120a) and TNF receptor 2 (*TNFR2*, TNFRSF1B, p75, CD120b). The TNFRs belong to the TNFR superfamily, a group of type I transmembrane glycoproteins that are characterized by a conserved homologous cysteine-rich domain in their extracellular region. Both TNFRs can be "shed" (cleaved) from the cell membrane, and are retained in the circulation as circulating "soluble" receptors (referred to as sTNFR1 and sTNFR2, respectively). Both of these soluble receptors retain their ability to bind ligand, as well as to inhibit the biological activities of TNF. The main structural difference between TNFR1 and TNFR2 is the presence of a death domain *(DD)* in the cytoplasmic domain of TNFR1. The binding of TNF allows TRADD (TNF receptor-associated death domain protein) to interact with the DD. TRADD is an essential partner of TNFR1 for signal transduction that recruits the downstream adapter molecule FADD (fas-associated death domain), which initiates the caspase pathway responsible for apoptotic cell death. TRADD can also interact directly with RIP (receptor interacting protein) and TRAF2 (TNF receptor-associated factor 2 protein), which can activate downstream signaling pathways, such as NF-κB, AP- 1, c-Jun N-terminal kinase stress kinases *(JNK)*, and p38MAPK. (From Ernandez T, Mayadas TN. Immunoregulatory role of TNFalpha in inflammatory kidney diseases. *Kidney Int.* 2009;76:262–276.)

failing human myocardium.[36] Both TNF receptor subtypes have been immunolocalized to the adult human cardiac myocyte, thus providing a potential basis for beginning to understand the signaling pathways that are utilized by TNF. Although the exact functional significance of

TNFR1 and TNFR2 in the heart is not known at present, the majority of the deleterious effects of TNF are coupled to activation of TNFR1,[38] whereas the activation of TNFR2 appears to exert protective effects in the heart. Both TNFRs can be shed (cleaved) from the cell membrane, and are retained in the circulation as circulating "soluble" ("s") receptors (referred to as sTNFR1 and sTNFR2, respectively). Both of these soluble receptors retain their ability to bind ligand and to inhibit the biological activities of TNF. The main structural difference between TNFR1 and TNFR2 is the presence of a death domain (DD) in the cytoplasmic domain of TNFR1. The binding of TNF allows TRADD (TNF receptor-associated death domain protein) to interact with the DD. TRADD is an essential partner of TNFR1 for signal transduction that recruits the downstream adapter molecule FADD (FAS-associated death domain), which initiates the caspase pathway responsible for apoptotic cell death (**see also Chapter 2**). TRADD can also interact directly with receptor interacting protein (RIP) and TNF receptor-associated factor 2 (TRAF2) protein, which can activate downstream signaling pathways, such as NF-κB, AP- 1, c-Jun N-terminal kinase stress kinases (JNK), and p38MAPK.

TNF-like weak inducer of apoptosis (TWEAK). TNF-like weak inducer of apoptosis (TWEAK, TNFSF12), a member of the TNFSF of ligands, is first synthesized as a type II transmembrane protein, which is cleaved from the membrane. TWEAK functions primarily as a soluble cytokine with diverse biological roles, including proinflammatory activity, angiogenesis, regulation of cell survival, and myoblast differentiation/proliferation.[39] TWEAK induces apoptosis indirectly through secondary activation of the TNF/TNFR1 pathway. The expression of TWEAK is relatively low in normal tissues, including the heart, but undergoes dramatic upregulation in the setting of tissue injury. For example, TWEAK is expressed in the border zone of infarcted myocardium, wherein increased angiogenesis is observed, as well as in the nonischemic myocardium remote from the infarct area.[39] Recent studies have suggested that sustained elevated circulating levels of TWEAK, induced via transgenic or adenoviral-mediated overexpression of soluble TWEAK, were sufficient to provoke LV dilation, LV fibrosis, LV dysfunction, and increased mortality in mice.[32] Moreover, circulating levels of TWEAK are elevated in patients with nonischemic cardiomyopathy compared to patients with ICM and/or normal controls.[32]

The receptor for TWEAK, TWEAKR (Fn14, TNFSFR12A), is the smallest member of the TNFR family. TWEAKR is a type 1 transmembrane protein (102 aa), which is expressed both constitutively and in an inducible manner in many tissues including the brain, kidney, liver and heart.[39] TWEAKR is highly upregulated in the border zone of the heart following left anterior descending artery ligation.[39] Both norepinephrine and angiotensin II also strongly upregulate TWEAKR in isolated neonatal cardiomyocytes.[39] TWEAKR contains sequence motifs within the cytoplasmic domain that promote aggregation of a family of adaptor proteins termed TRAF1, 2, and 3 (TNF receptor associated factor), which in turn activate intracellular signal transduction cascades, including nuclear factor-kappaB (NF-κB), the mitogen-activated protein kinases JNK, p38, and extracellular signal-regulated kinase (ERK).

Receptor activator of NF-kB ligand (RANK ligand). Osteoprotegerin (OPG [TNSFR11B]) and RANKL (TNFSF11) are two cytokines that have been classically associated with the regulation of bone remodeling. In bone, RANKL activates osteoclasts, and hence bone resorption, after binding to RANK. In contrast, OPG acts as a decoy receptor for RANKL, and thereby inhibits bone resorption. In experimental models of cardiac injury, OPG and RANKL are both increased in direct relation to the severity of heart failure and/or in relation to hemodynamic pressure overload.[33] Studies in rats postmyocardial infarction have revealed increased levels of mRNA for OPG, RANKL, and RANK within the ischemic zone, and increased protein

levels of OPG in the remote zone in fibroblasts and cardiac myocytes.[33] Studies in patients with heart failure have shown that OPG levels are increased in association with worsening New York Heart Association (NYHA) class, LV dysfunction, and elevated levels of B-type natriuretic peptide.[33] Heart failure patients also had increased levels of RANKL; however, increased levels were only observed in patients with NYHA class IV heart failure. Furthermore, there was increased RANK and RANKL immunoreactivity in cardiac myocytes, vascular smooth muscle cells, and endothelial cells in failing human hearts when compared to nonfailing human hearts. Viewed together, these findings suggest a potential role for the RANKL/RANK/OPG axis in heart failure; however, given that both RANKL and its cognate antagonist OPG are both elevated in experimental and clinical heart failure, the clinical significance of this axis remains unclear at present.

Interleukin-1 Family

Although the original IL-1 family (IL-1F) consisted of IL-1α (IL-1 F1) and IL-β (IL-1 F2), the IL-1 family has now expanded to include seven ligands with agonist activity (IL-1α and IL-1β, IL-18 (IL-1F4), IL-33 (IL-1F11), IL-36α (IL-1F6), IL-36β (IL-1F7), IL-36γ (IL-1F8), three receptor antagonists (IL-1Ra [IL-F3], IL-36Ra [IL-F5], IL-38 [IL-F10]), and an anti inflammatory cytokine (IL-37 [IL-10]). Members of the IL-1 receptor (IL-1R) family include six receptor chains forming four signaling receptor complexes, two decoy receptors (IL-1R2, IL-18BP), and two negative regulators (TIR8 or SIGIRR [IL-1R8], IL-1RAcPb).[40]

Interleukin-1α and Interleukin-1β. IL-1α (IL-F1) and IL-1β (IL-F2), which are encoded by separate genes, are the "founding" members of the IL-1 family of cytokines. Analogous to TNF, IL-1α and IL-β are responsible for controlling proinflammatory reactions following tissue injury. With the notable exception of IL-1Ra, each member of the IL-1 family is synthesized first as a precursor that does not have a clear signal peptide for processing or secretion. The immature form of IL-1β, pro-IL-1β, is synthesized within mammalian cells as a 31 kD precursor. Processing of IL-1β to a 17 kD "mature" form requires cleavage by IL-1-converting enzyme or by caspase-1, which is activated by the inflammasome, a multiprotein oligomer consisting of caspase 1, NLRP3, and ASC (see Fig. 7.3B). Once IL-1β is processed, the mature form is secreted rapidly from the cell. IL-1β is the main form of circulating IL-1. IL-1α is constitutively expressed as membrane-bound protein. For the most part, IL-1α remains intracellular or is retained on the cell membrane, and is therefore not detected in the circulation unless the cell dies and releases its intracellular content. Unlike IL-1α, the inactive or proform of IL-1β is only marginally active. IL-1α and IL-1β both bind to common receptors, which explains the similarity of effects of the two molecules. A third specific ligand, the IL-1 receptor antagonist (IL-1RA), binds the IL-1RI with similar specificity and affinity but does not activate the receptor and trigger downstream signaling, and thus acts as a competitive inhibitor.[41] Similar to TNF, IL-1β appears to synthesized within the myocardium in response to stressful environmental stimuli, and both IL-1β mRNA and protein have been detected in the hearts of patients with DCM.[29,42] Blocking the IL-1 pathway with Canakinumab, a human monoclonal antibody that blocks IL-1β activity, was shown to improve cardiovascular outcomes in patients with a prior myocardial infarction and an elevated CRP level (>2 mg/L), in the multicenter CANTOS (Canakinumab Anti-inflammatory Thrombosis Outcome Study) trial.[43]

IL-1α and IL-1β, which are encoded by separate genes, each independently bind the type I IL-1 receptor (IL-1R1). As shown in **Fig. 7.5**, the IL-1 receptor accessory protein (IL-1RAcP) is recruited to the type I IL-1 receptor and serves as a coreceptor that is required for signal transduction of IL-1/IL-1RI complexes. IL-1RAcP is required for activation of IL-1R1 by other IL-1 family members, especially IL-18 and IL-33. Whereas early work on the IL-1 receptor (IL-1R) suggested that there was a single receptor, subsequent cross-linking studies have suggested the presence of a low-affinity (80 kDa; IL-1RI) receptor and a higher-affinity receptor (68 kDa, IL-1RII), each coded for by a single gene product.[44] The type I receptor (IL-1RI) transduces a signal, whereas the type II receptor (IL-1RII) binds IL-1α and IL-1β but does not transduce a signal. Indeed, IL-1 RII acts as a sink for IL-1, and has been termed a "decoy" receptor. The extracellular domains of the IL receptors or "soluble" portions of the IL-1RI, IL-1RII, and sIL-1RAcP (termed sIL-1RI, sIL-1RII, and sIL-1RAcP, respectively) circulate in health and disease and function as natural "buffers" that are capable of binding to IL-lα, IL-1β, or to IL-1Ra.[45]

The IL-1 receptor/IL-1RAcP complex leads to recruitment of the adaptor protein MyD88 (myeloid differentiation primary response gene 88) to the Toll-IL-1 receptor (TIR) domain of both IL-1RI and IL-1RAcP, leading to phosphorylation of IRAK4, analogous to TLR signaling (Fig. 7.2A). IL-1, IL-1RI, IL-RAcP, MYD88, and IRAK4 form a stable IL-1–induced signaling module, which subsequently phosphorylates IRAK1 and IRAK2 (see Fig. 7.5). This is followed by the recruitment and oligomerization of TRAF6, which serves as a ubiquitin E3 ligase that, together with the ubiquitin E2 ligase complex, attaches K63-linked polyubiquitin chains to several IL-1-signaling intermediates, including IRAK1 and the adaptor proteins TAB2 and 3 and TAK1. Ubiquitination of TAK1 promotes its association with TRAF6 and with MEKK3 with the subsequent formation of at least two TAK1 and MEKK3 signaling complexes that activate the NF-κB, c-Jun N-terminal kinase (JNK), and p38 MAPK pathways.[41]

Interleukin-18. Interleukin 18 (IL-18, IL-1F4) is a relatively new member of the IL-1 superfamily.[46] Similar to IL-1β, IL-18 is synthesized as an inactive precursor and is cleaved to its active form by caspase-1. Although IL-18 was initially recognized for its ability to induce interferon-γ (IFN-γ) and its capacity to induce T-helper 1 (Th1) responses, IL-18 was subsequently found to play an important role in LPS-induced hepatotoxicity, which stimulated further study of the role of IL-18 in other settings. Relevant to the present discussion is the recent observation that IL-18 had been shown to be produced in the heart during ischemia reperfusion injury and endotoxemia.[47] Importantly, IL-18 activates NF-κB, which is a transcriptional regulator of many proinflammatory cytokines and cellular adhesion molecules in the heart. In vitro studies have shown that IL-18 increases the production of TNF and IL-1β in murine macrophages and human monocytes and induces the expression of ICAM-1 and VCAM-1 on endothelial cells and monocytes.[46] In vivo studies have shown specific blockade of IL-18 using IL-18 binding protein improves contractile function in human atrial tissue following ischemia reperfusion injury,[48] and lipopolysaccharide-induced LV dysfunction in experimental animals.[48]

The IL-18 receptor (IL-18R) is related to the IL-1 family of receptors, and is composed of a ligand-binding subunit, I-1Rrp1 and an accessory subunit, AcPL, both of which share sequence homology to the IL-1R family.[49] Moreover, the signal transduction pathways utilized by IL-1β and IL-18 are similar. In addition, there is a third receptor-like chain, the IL-18 binding protein (IL-18BP), that lacks a transmembrane domain and thus does not signal. IL-18BP is produced constitutively and is secreted, and thus acts as a potent inhibitor of IL-18 activity.

Interleukin 33. As noted above, IL-33 (IL-F11) belongs to the IL-1 superfamily. IL-33 was identified in a search for the ligand for the ST2 receptor (see below). IL-33 induces helper T cells, mast cells, eosinophils, and basophils to produce type 2 cytokines. The mode by which IL-33 exerts its effect has not been fully established, but it probably acts similarly to other members of the IL-1 family. That is, precursor IL-33 is cleaved by caspases and is then released into the interstitium

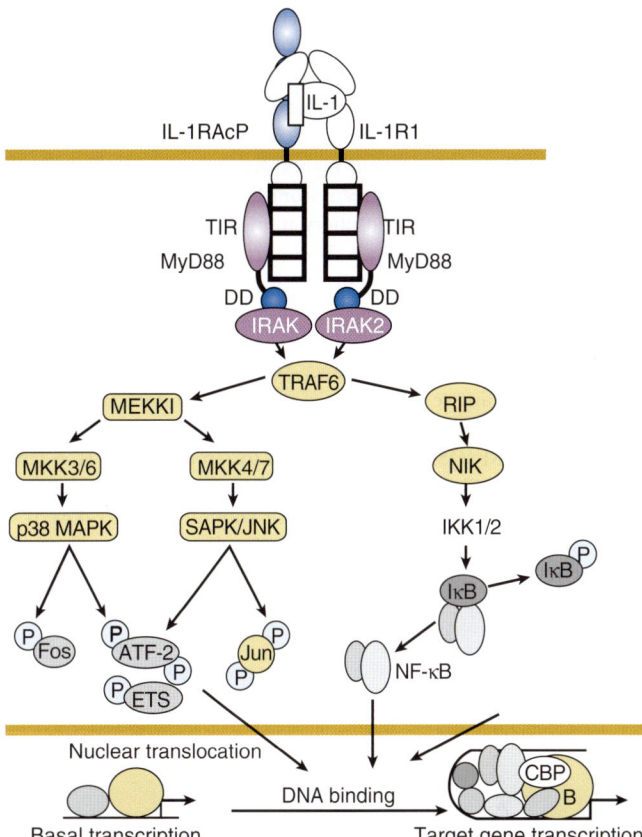

Fig. 7.5 Intracellular signaling pathways activated by interleukin-1 *(IL-1)*. Binding of IL-1 to the type I IL-1 receptor *(IL-1R1)* leads to the recruitment of the IL-1R accessory protein *(IL-1RAcP)*. The cytoplasmic Toll/IL-1 receptor *(TIR)* domains of the receptor recruit MyD88 via its TIR, and the MyD88 death domain *(DD)* recruits the IL-1 receptor–associated kinases *(IRAK and IRAK2)* to the receptor complex before being rapidly phosphorylated and degraded. The IRAKs mediate tumor necrosis factor receptor-associated factor 6 *(TRAF6)* oligomerization, initiating various protein kinase cascades, the major ones of which involve (1) the stress-activated protein kinases, p38 mitogen-activated protein kinase *(MAPK)*, and c-Jun N-terminal kinase *(JNK)*, which lead to the activation of activator protein-1 *(AP-1)* (c-Fos/c-Jun), activating transcription factor-2 *(ATF-2)*, and E Twenty-Six *(ETS)* factors, among other transcription factors; and (2) inhibitor of κB *(IκB)* kinases 1 and 2 *(IKK-1 and IKK-2)*, which lead to the activation of nuclear factor κB *(NFκB)*. (Modified from Firestein GS. Role of the chondrocyte in cartilage pathology. In: Firestein GS, et al., editors. *Kelley's Textbook of Rheumatology.* 8th ed. Philadelphia: Saunders; 2008:52–55.)

as an active cytokine, where it stimulates signaling in target cells.[50] In the heart IL-33 is produced by cardiac fibroblasts in response to biomechanical strain. In vitro studies have shown that IL-33 markedly antagonizes angiotensin II and phenylephrine-induced cardiomyocyte hypertrophy; moreover, recombinant IL-33 reduced hypertrophy and fibrosis and improved survival after pressure overload in mice.[51] Thus, IL-33 appears to activate a cardioprotective program in the heart.

ST2 is the cognate receptor for IL-33. There are four isoforms of ST2 (sST2 [soluble]), ST2L (membrane bound), ST2V, and ST2LV. The overall structure of ST2L is similar to the structure of the type I IL-1 receptors, which are comprised of an extracellular domain of three linked immunoglobulin-like motifs, a transmembrane segment and a TIR cytoplasmic domain. sST2 lacks a transmembrane and cytoplasmic domain contained within the structure of ST2L and includes a unique nine amino-acid C-terminal sequence.[50] Whereas ST2L is constitutively expressed primarily in hematopoietic cells, sST2 expression is largely inducible in a variety of cell types, including cells that reside in the heart. Interestingly, high baseline ST2 levels are a significant predictor of cardiovascular death and heart failure (**see also Chapter 33**) independently of baseline characteristics and NT-proBNP in patients with an ST-segment myocardial infarction.[52] The signaling pathways that are downstream from IL-33/ST2 signaling are still unclear but may include phosphorylation of ERK 1/2, p38 MAPK, JNKs, and activation of NF-κB. However, the relationship between ST2L and NF-κB activation is a matter of ongoing debate.[50]

Interleukin-6 Family

Based on their functional redundancy, structural similarity, and use of a common signaling receptor, IL-6, leukemia inhibitory factor (LIF), cardiotrophin-1 (CT-1), ciliary neurotrophic factor (CNTF), IL-11, and oncostatin M (OSM) are considered to represent the "IL-6 family" of cytokines (**Fig. 7.6A**). Inclusion in the IL-6 family is based on a helical cytokine structure and receptor subunit makeup. The IL-6 family of cytokines triggers downstream signaling pathways in multiple cell types, including cardiac myocytes, either through the homodimerization of the gp130 receptor or through the heterodimerization of

gp130 with a related transmembrane receptor (see Fig. 7.6A). All IL-6 type cytokines potentially activate signal transducer and activator of transcription 3 (STAT3), and to a lesser extent STAT1 through their common gp130 subunits. The specificity of cytokine signaling within the IL-6 family is determined by the composition of the cytoplasmic domains associated with the signal-competent receptor complex.[53] For example, IL-6 initiates formation of a signaling receptor complex by binding to an IL-6 receptor (IL-6R), which then heterodimerizes with gp130 to initiate IL-6 signaling. On the other hand, LIF, CT-1, and CNTF all transduce signaling events through heterodimerization of LIF receptors (LIFRβ) and gp130. The SOCS (also referred to as cytokine-inducible SH2 proteins [CIS]) are a family of specific negative regulatory feedback elements of JAK/STAT signaling (Fig. 7.6B). Expression of some SOCS family members is regulated transcriptionally by STATs, thereby acting as a negative feedback loop for JAK-STAT signaling. Both SOCS-1 and SOCS-3 interact with the kinase domain of various JAK proteins, thereby preventing STAT phosphorylation. Previous clinical studies showed that the plasma level of IL-6, CT-1, LIF, and gp130 are elevated in patients with advanced heart failure, and that high levels are associated with a poor prognosis for heart failure patients.[54,55]

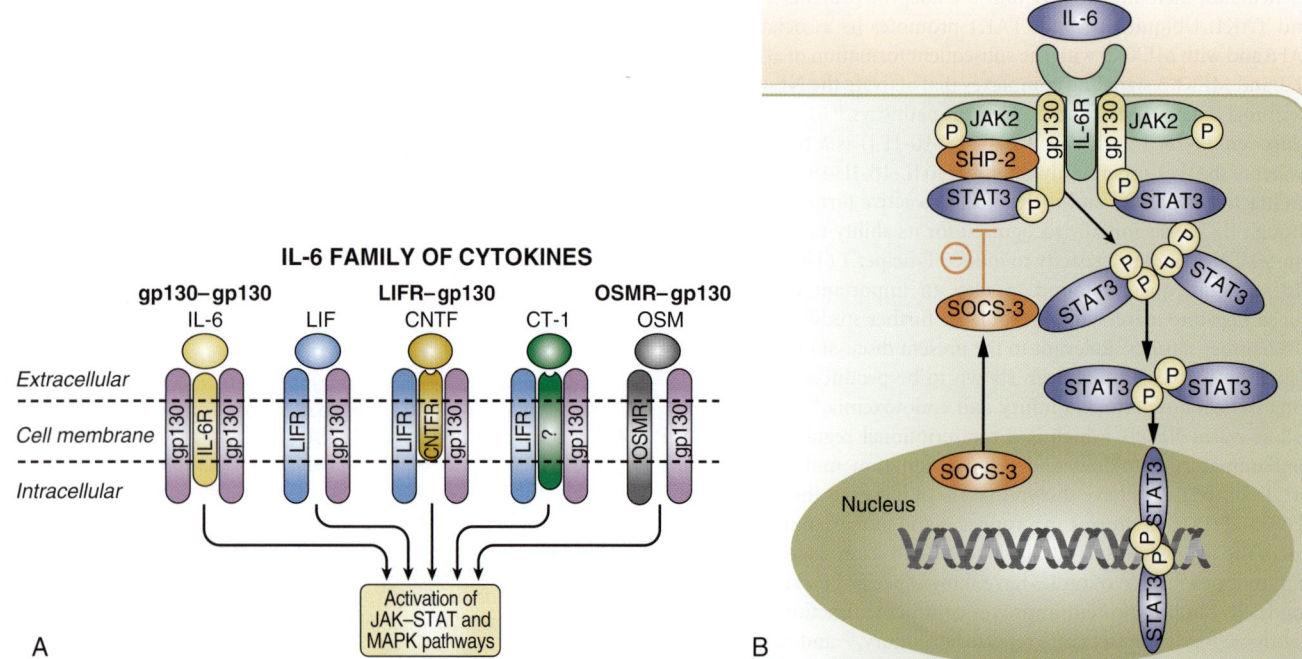

Fig. 7.6 Interleukin-6 *(IL-6)* family of cytokines. (A) Various combinations of receptor subunits and signaling pathways are used by different members of the IL-6 cytokine family. gp130 homodimers associate with specific IL receptors such as the IL-6 receptor *(IL-6R)* to mediate the actions of IL-6. Leukemia inhibitory factor *(LIF)* binds to heterodimers of LIF receptor *(LIFR)* and gp130. LIFR–gp130 heterodimers can also associate with other receptor subunits to bind ciliary neurotrophic factor *(CNTF)* and cardiotrophin 1 *(CT-1)*. The oncostatin M receptor *(OSMR)* forms heterodimers with gp130 to bind oncostatin M *(OSM)*. The signal-transducing subunit gp130 is found in all complexes and is responsible for the intracellular activation of the Janus-activated kinase–signal transducer and activator of transcription *(JAK/STAT)* and the mitogen-activated protein kinase *(MAPK)* pathways. (B) IL-6 stimulation induces the expression of a number of proinflammatory gene products via activation of the JAK/STAT, MAPK, and PI3K signaling cascades. Ligand binding of IL-6 to IL-6R induces dimerization of the gp130 receptor, which activates the associated JAK tyrosine kinases. The JAKs phosphorylate recruitment sites for the STAT proteins and the scaffold protein SHP2, which is linked to MAPK and PI3K signaling cascades. As shown, the suppressor of cytokine signaling *(SOCS)* proteins can negatively modulate gp130 mediated JAK-STAT signaling. (A, modified from Bauer S, Kerr BJ, Patterson PH. The neuropoietic cytokine family in development, plasticity, disease and injury. *Nat Rev Neurosci.* 2007;8:221–232. B, modified from Walters TD, Griffiths AM. Mechanisms of growth impairment in pediatric Crohn's disease. *Nat Rev Gastroenterol Hepatol.* 2009;6:513–523.)

Interleukin-6. Human IL-6 is produced as a 212-amino-acid precursor and is processed to a 184-amino-acid soluble form following cleavage of a signal sequence during secretion of the mature protein.[56] The mature protein is a 26-kDa glycoprotein[57] with a number of alternative N- and O-linked glycosylation sites. IL-6 can be detected in the circulation following Gram-negative bacterial infection or TNF infusion, as well as following myocardial stunning,[58] and appears to be secreted in direct response to TNF or IL-1, which are thought to induce IL-6 gene expression by activation of NF-kB.[56] Recently, IL-6 has been shown to exist in the circulation in "chaperoned" complexes of molecular mass 400 to 500, 150 to 200, and 25 to 35 kDa in association with binding proteins that can include soluble IL-6R, anti-IL-6 antibodies, and anti-sIL-6R antibodies, and others. Sustained high levels of different circulating IL-6 complexes are observed in cancer patients subjected to particular active anticancer immunotherapy regimens. However, "chaperoned" IL-6 complexes have not yet been reported in heart failure.[59] The human IL-6R is a glycoprotein with a molecular mass of 80 kDa. In contrast to the receptors for IL-1 and TNF, the cytoplasmic domain of IL-6 is not necessary for intracellular signaling to occur. Moreover, when bound to its receptor, IL-6 is known to associate with a second membrane glycoprotein with a molecular mass of 130 kDa (gp130). Thus, the current evidence suggests that the IL-6R system is composed of two functional chains: a 80 kDa IL-6 binding protein, termed IL-6R, and a 130 kDa "docking protein," termed gp130, which transmits the intracellular signal.[56] Importantly, IL-6Rs are expressed with low abundance in adult cardiac myocytes, whereas mice that are deficient in gp130 are embryonic lethal because their hearts do not develop.[60] In contrast, double transgenic mice that have been genetically engineered to overexpress both IL-6 and IL-6R develop substantial concentric hypertrophy.[61]

IL-6 signaling through IL-6 /gp130 receptor induces phosphorylation and activation of Janus kinase (JAK) proteins (Fig. 7.6B), which are constitutively associated with the cytoplasmic domains of the gp130 receptor. JAK proteins phosphorylate gp130, creating docking sites for STAT3 proteins via interaction through their SH2 domains. The STAT proteins are phosphorylated on specific tyrosine residues by the associated JAKs, thereby inducing the formation of parallel STAT dimers (Fig. 7.6B). The STAT dimers dissociate from the receptor and translocate into the nucleus, where they bind to specific DNA sequences and regulate the expression of target genes. Three major signaling pathways have been identified downstream from IL-6/gp130 mediated signaling: JAK-STAT signaling, mitogen-activated protein kinase (MAPK) signaling, and the PI3K/AKT signaling.[55] In the heart, STAT proteins regulate the expression of gene-encoding proteins involved in angiogenesis, inflammation, apoptosis, extracellular matrix composition, and cellular signaling.[62] The JAK-STAT pathway has been shown to be involved in ischemia/reperfusion injury, hypertrophy, and postpartum cardiomyopathy.[62,63] Moreover, the JAK-STAT pathway has also been reported to interfere with the renin-angiotensin system (RAS), which is involved in the pathophysiology and progression of hypertrophy and heart failure (**see Chapter 5**).

Leukemia Inhibitory Factor. LIF is a 181 amino acid glycoprotein that was originally identified as a cytokine that inhibited the proliferation of the murine myeloid leukemic cell line M1, and induced these cells to differentiate into macrophages. There are several forms of LIF; however, the best studied is a secreted and variably glycosylated protein (34–63 kDa) that varies depending on the cell type and context, ranging from proliferation and survival to differentiation and apoptosis. LIF signals, at least in part, through the transmembrane protein gp130 that heterodimerizes with the LIF receptor (LIFR) (Fig. 7.6A). The pleiotropic effects of LIF function may be due, at least in part, to

the integration of the different signaling pathways that can be induced once LIF is combined with its receptor gp130-LIFR.

Analogous to IL-6, LIF signals through JAK-STAT, MAPKs, and the PI3K/AKT pathways.[64] LIF-induced activation of the JAK/STAT pathway is linked to cardiac myocyte cell growth, whereas activation of the MAPK, PI(3)-kinase pathways, and the JAK/STAT pathways is linked to cytoprotection.[64] LIF has also been shown to contribute to homing of bone marrow–derived cardiac progenitors in a postinfarct model. The contribution of LIF signaling to contractile function is unclear, with studies suggesting that LIF induces the downregulation of the sarcoplasmic reticulum Ca2+ ATPase (SERCA) gene and protein expression, whereas others suggest LIF induces increased intracellular Ca2+ concentrations in cardiac myocytes secondary to increased L-type Ca2+ currents.[64] Whether LIF offers protection to the heart under chronic stress, such as hypertension-induced cardiac remodeling and heart failure, is not known.

Cardiotrophin-1. CT-1 is a 201 amino acid protein that was originally identified for its ability to induce a hypertrophic growth in neonatal cardiac myocytes.[65] Subsequent studies have shown that CT-1 is synthesized by cardiac myocytes and noncardiac myocytes in response to mechanical stress. Analogous to LIF, the signaling pathways downstream from CT-1 include the JAK/STAT pathway, the MAPK pathway, and the PI3K/AKT pathway.[66] The predominant actions of CT-1 include cytoprotection, cell hypertrophy, cell proliferation, and collagen synthesis. CT-1 exerts a dose-dependent decrease in blood pressure in rats, which is sensitive to nitric oxide synthase inhibition. Although the acute administration of CT-1 had no immediate effect of LV dP/d*t*, long-term exposure to CT-1 provoked contractile dysfunction in heart tissue engineered from rat cardiac myocytes. Peripheral circulating levels of CT-1 increase in relation to worsening NYHA functional class and correlate with LV mass index in patients with DCM. However, at the time of this writing it is unclear whether elevated levels of CT-1 are biological markers or biological mediators of worsening heart failure.

Chemokines

Chemokines are a distinct family of cytokines that regulate biological processes such as chemotaxis, collagen turnover, angiogenesis, and apoptosis. The chemokine superfamily is divided into four groups (CXC, CX3C, CC, and C) according to the relative positioning of the first two closely paired cysteines of their amino acid sequence. Chemokines exert their effects by interacting with G protein–linked transmembrane receptors, referred to as chemokine receptors, that are found on the surfaces of their target cells. A major role of chemokines is the recruitment and activation of specific subpopulations of leucocytes that play a pivotal role in the immune response and inflammation. While chemokine-dependent functions are essential for the control of infection, wound healing, and hematopoiesis, excessive chemokine activation may result in inappropriate inflammation leading to cell death and tissue damage. Studies have shown that circulating levels of CC chemokines are elevated in patients with ischemic and nonischemic heart failure, including macrophage chemoattractant protein-1 (MCP-1), macrophage inflammatory protein-1α (MIP-1α), and RANTES (regulated on activation normally T-cell expressed and secreted). The highest levels of these chemokines were noted in patients with NYHA class IV heart failure.[67] Given that these chemokines can attract inflammatory cells to the heart, they may contribute to disease progression in heart failure.

Leukocytes

Monocytes/macrophages and neutrophils are the most important cellular effectors of the innate immune system.[68] Although there has been considerable research on the role of leukocytes in the early phase of myocardial infarction and ischemia reperfusion injury,[69] as shown in

TABLE 7.3   Comparison of Acute Versus Chronic Effects of Components of the Innate Immune System After Experimental Myocardial Infarction

	<4 wk after MI	>4 wk after MI
Humoral Immune Response		
TNF	Decreased LV function	Chronic overexpression leads to Heart failure[34]
TLR	TLR 2$^{-/-}$ protected	Data lacking
	TLR 4$^{-/-}$ protected	Data lacking
Cellular Immune Response		
Neutrophils	Depletion maladaptive	Data lacking
Macrophages	Depletion maladaptive	Splenectomy protective
T-cells	T helper cell depletion maladaptive	Data lacking
B- cells	B cell depletion adaptive	Data lacking

LV, Left ventricle; MI, myocardial infarction; TLR, Toll-like receptor; TNF, tumor necrosis factor.
Modified from Frantz S, Falcao-Pires I, Balligand JL, et al. The innate immune system in chronic cardiomyopathy: a European Society of Cardiology (ESC) scientific statement from the Working Group on Myocardial Function of the ESC. Eur J Heart Fail. 2018;20(3):445–459.

TABLE 7.4   Deleterious Effects of Inflammatory Mediators in Heart Failure

Left ventricular dysfunction
Pulmonary edema in humans
Cardiomyopathy in humans
Reduced skeletal muscle blood flow
Endothelial dysfunction
Anorexia and cachexia
Receptor uncoupling from adenylate cyclase experimentally
Activation of the fetal gene program experimentally
Cardiac myocyte apoptosis experimentally

Table 7.3, there are very limited data on the role of monocytes/macrophages, neutrophils, T-cells, and B-cells in the chronic phase of cardiac injury. The extant literature suggests that a chronic proinflammatory response might be detrimental in heart failure; however, the role of specific leukocyte subsets in terms of mediating the chronic proinflammatory response has not been defined.

CONCLUSION AND FUTURE DIRECTIONS

In this chapter we have focused on the experimental evidence, which suggests that the activation of the innate immune system with the subsequent elaboration of inflammatory cytokines plays an important role in the progression of heart failure, by virtue of the deleterious effects that these molecules exert on the heart and the peripheral circulation. Indeed, pathophysiologically relevant concentrations of these molecules mimic many aspects of the so-called heart failure phenotype in experimental animals, including LV dysfunction, LV dilation, activation of fetal gene expression, cardiac myocyte hypertrophy, and cardiac myocyte apoptosis (**Table 7.4**). Thus, analogous to the proposed role for neurohormones, proinflammatory cytokines would appear to represent another distinct class of biologically active molecules that can contribute to heart failure progression. Nonetheless, the early attempts to translate this information to the bedside not only have been disappointing but also have, in many instances, led to worsening heart failure.[70] While one interpretation of these findings is that inflammatory mediators are not viable targets in heart failure, an alternative point of view is that we simply have not targeted proinflammatory mediators with agents that can be used safely in the context of heart failure, or alternatively, that targeting a single component of the inflammatory cascade is not sufficient in a disease as complex as heart failure. These statements notwithstanding,

the observed decrease in cardiovascular endpoints with Canakinumab in the CANTOS trial[43] demonstrated that inflammatory mediators can be targeted safely in heart disease. Although the CANTOS trial was not a heart failure trial per se, it provides an important proof of concept for targeting inflammation in heart failure in future studies. However, it bears emphasis that it may be necessary to use biomarkers to select heart failure patients who have ongoing inflammation despite optimal medical therapy. Indeed, a recent consensus statement from the Translation Research Committee of the Heart Failure Association of the European Society of Cardiology suggested that there may not be a common inflammatory pathway that characterizes all of the different forms of heart failure, and that going forward it will be important to design specific antiinflammatory approaches for different types and stages of heart failure, and to determine the specific inflammatory pathways that are activated in different forms of heart failure.[71]

KEY REFERENCES

1. Levine B, Kalman J, Mayer L, Fillit HM, Packer M. Elevated circulating levels of tumor necrosis factor in severe chronic heart failure. N Engl J Med. 1990;223:236–241.
3. Mann DL. Innate immunity and the failing heart: the cytokine hypothesis revisited. Circ Res. 2015;116:1254–1268.
9. Frantz S, Kobzik L, Kim YD, et al. Toll4 (TLR4) expression in cardiac myocytes in normal and failing myocardium. J Clin Invest. 1999;104:271–280.
12. Frantz S, Ertl G, Bauersachs J. Mechanisms of disease: Toll-like receptors in cardiovascular disease. Nat Clin Pract Cardiovasc Med. 2007;4:444–454.
35. Gulick TS, Chung MK, Pieper SJ, Lange LG, Schreiner GF. Interleukin 1 and tumor necrosis factor inhibit cardiac myocyte b-adrenergic responsiveness. Proc Natl Acad Sci U S A. 1989;86:6753–6757.
36. Torre-Amione G, Kapadia S, Lee J, et al. Tumor necrosis factor-a and tumor necrosis factor receptors in the failing human heart. Circulation. 1996;93:704–711.
43. Ridker PM, Everett BM, Thuren T, et al. Antiinflammatory therapy with canakinumab for atherosclerotic disease. N Engl J Med. 2017;377:1119–1131.
45. Dinarello CA. Biological basis for interleukin-1 in disease. Blood. 1996;87:2095–2147.
63. Hilfiker-Kleiner D, Kaminski K, Podewski E, et al. A cathepsin D-cleaved 16 kDa form of prolactin mediates postpartum cardiomyopathy. Cell. 2007;128:589–600.
70. Mann DL. Inflammatory mediators and the failing heart: past, present, and the foreseeable future. Circ Res. 2002;91:988–998.

The full reference list for this chapter is available on ExpertConsult.

Oxidative Stress in Heart Failure

Aaron L. Sverdlov, Doan T. M. Ngo, Wilson S. Colucci

OUTLINE

Oxidative stress is increased in heart failure (HF), and experimental studies suggest that this contributes to structural and functional changes in the heart that are central to both cardiac dysfunction and disease progression.

REACTIVE OXYGEN SPECIES AND ANTIOXIDANT SYSTEMS (FIG. 8.1)

Reactive Oxygen Species

Reactive oxygen species (ROS) are a by-product of aerobic metabolism, and so the highly metabolically active myocardium is rich in ROS (**see Chapter 17**). As in all tissues, ROS are handled in the myocardium by both soluble and enzymatic antioxidant systems. However, differences in subcellular and tissue compartmentalization of ROS, as well as levels of ROS, contribute to the downstream effects. It is now clear that ROS signaling pathways are complex and in many cases essential for normal signal transduction and cardiovascular physiology.[1] "Oxidative stress" occurs when the production of ROS exceeds the capacity of antioxidant defense systems. In general, ROS cascades begin with the formation of *superoxide anion (O_2^-)* by either enzymatic or nonenzymatic one-electron reduction of molecular oxygen. The unpaired electron in O_2^- is an unstable free radical that reacts with itself and other oxygen-containing species, and directly or indirectly with organic molecules—including lipids, nucleic acids, and

proteins—ultimately leading to regulation or disruption of cellular functions. All aerobic organisms, from bacteria to man, have evolved a complex antioxidant defense system of enzymatic and nonenzymatic components to defend against the unavoidable formation of ROS.[2] In parallel, there has been the evolution of specific ROS-generating systems that are used both in the immune system, where the toxicity of ROS is exploited to fight infectious organisms,[3] as well as in all cell types, where ROS act as signaling intermediates for the purpose of triggering specific intracellular processes.

Primary Antioxidant Systems

Primary antioxidant enzymes, defined here as those that directly interact with ROS, include superoxide dismutase (SOD), catalase, and other peroxidases. These enzymes work in parallel with nonenzymatic antioxidants to protect cells and tissues from ROS. The mitochondrial enzymes manganese superoxide dismutase (MnSOD) and glutathione peroxidase (GPx) appear to be the most important in controlling myocardial levels of O_2^- and H_2O_2. Approximately 70% of the SOD activity in the heart, and 90% of that in the cardiac myocyte, is attributable to *MnSOD (SOD2)*.[4] The remainder consists of *cytosolic Cu/ZnSOD (SOD1)*, with less than 1% contributed by *extracellular SOD (ECSOD, SOD3)*.[5] This is in contrast to other organs, where Cu/ZnSOD plays a greater role. The relative importance of MnSOD in the regulation of oxidative stress in the

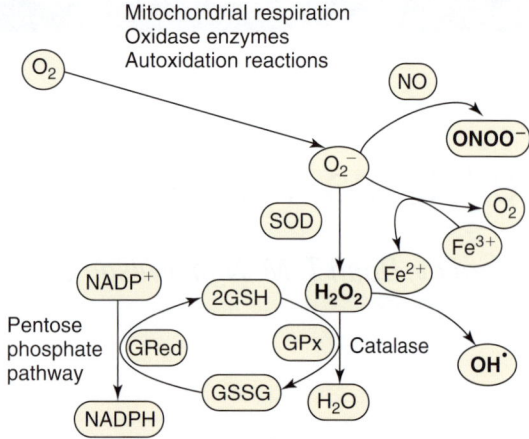

Fig. 8.1 Reactive Oxygen Species (ROS) and Antioxidant Enzyme Systems. Enzymatic or nonenzymatic formation of superoxide anion leads to the formation of other ROS *(shown in bold)*. Potentially toxic ROS are removed by the enzymes superoxide dismutase *(SOD)*, glutathione *(GSH)* peroxidase *(GPx)*, and catalase. The presence of Fe^{2+} or nitric oxide *(NO)* can allow the formation of hydroxyl radical *(OH•)* and peroxynitrite *(ONOO−)*, respectively. These latter reactions are favored when the activity of SOD is decreased. O_2^- can increase the formation of OH• by reducing Fe^{3+} to Fe^{2+}. Glutathione plays a central role in cellular antioxidant defenses not only as a reducing agent for the action of GPx, but also through direct reactions with ROS. Glutathione is recycled by the enzyme glutathione reductase, which requires NAD(P)H. Thus, indirectly, the pentose phosphate pathway, by supplying NAD(P)H, also plays an important role in antioxidant defenses.

myocardium is highlighted by the demonstration that mice deficient in MnSOD die soon after birth with dilated cardiomyopathy.[6] In contrast, mice deficient in CuZnSOD or ECSOD have no overt myocardial phenotype.[5] As the only SOD located in the mitochondria, MnSOD plays a critical role in the control of mitochondrial ROS generated during normal oxidative phosphorylation (see later discussion). The phenotype of the MnSOD knockout mouse therefore also underscores the importance of the mitochondria as a source of ROS in the myocardium.

H_2O_2, the product of SOD, is handled by catalase and/or one of several GPxs. *Catalase* is expressed in the cytosol, where it is located primarily in peroxisomes (pCAT) and in the mitochondria (mCAT). Catalase contains four porphyrin heme groups that interact with H_2O_2 to facilitate its decomposition to water and oxygen. Transgenic expression of either pCAT or mCAT exerts beneficial effects on cardiac structure and function in a variety of animal HF models,[7-9] suggesting that H_2O_2 is an important oxidant species in the failing heart. Compared with O_2^-, H_2O_2 is longer lasting and able to cross cellular membranes.

GPx are a family of selenium-containing enzymes that catalyze the removal of H_2O_2 through oxidation of reduced glutathione (GSH), which is recycled from oxidized glutathione (GSSG) by the nicotinamide adenine dinucleotide phosphate (NADPH)–dependent glutathione reductase (GRed). GPx-1 is encoded on the nuclear genome but localizes both to the cytosol and mitochondria.

Ancillary Antioxidant Mechanisms

Several enzymes and molecules play a supporting role in regulating oxidative stress and/or the effects of oxidants on targets. The activity of GPx requires stoichiometric quantities of *glutathione* (GSH), and therefore decreased levels of GSH inhibit the activity of GPx. GRed requires NAD(P)H as a reductant to recycle GSSG to GSH. Glutathione is also a direct scavenger of reactive oxygen and nitrogen species. Cells replenish GSH both by de novo GSH synthesis and through the action of glutathione reductase on GSSG. In this context, enzymes in the pentose phosphate pathway and glucose 6-phosphate dehydrogenase

(G6PD), the rate-limiting enzyme in this pathway, are ancillary antioxidant enzymes that are critical to cellular antioxidant defenses.[10] In mice, chronic GSH depletion causes worse LV function, fibrosis, and survival in response to pressure overload, and GSH supplementation ameliorates the phenotype.[11] Increased oxidative stress lowers the GSH/GSSG ratio, which may thus be used as a measure of myocardial oxidative stress.[12] Unlike the levels of lipid peroxidation products, which can reflect oxidative stress inside and/or outside of the cell, the GSH/GSSG ratio specifically measures intracellular oxidative stress. Other thiol-containing proteins, such as *metallothionein*, have significant antioxidant functions through direct scavenging of ROS and may play a role in the failing heart.[13] Overexpression of metallothionein suppresses mitochondrial oxidative stress, cardiac apoptosis, and the development of diabetic cardiomyopathy (**see also Chapter 17**).[14]

Several thiol-containing proteins modulate the effects of ROS. The *thioredoxin (Trx)* system consists of Trx reductase, Trx, peroxiredoxin, and NADPH (**Fig. 8.2**).[15] This system, like HO-1 and metallothionein, is induced by a variety of oxidative stresses, and Trx levels are increased in the myocardium[16] and blood[17] of patients with HF. Trx exerts an antioxidant effect by scavenging ROS, but also interacts directly with multiple cellular signal transduction pathways and activates HO-1 and Bcl-2.[18] *Thioredoxin-interacting protein (Txnip)* interacts with Trx via a disulfide bond, decreasing thioredoxin activity and thus increasing oxidative stress.[19]

The *glutaredoxin (Grx)* system is similar in organization and function to the Trx system, but has a much higher selectivity for cysteine thiols that are glutathiolated, and thus may play an important role in the regulation of protein function via glutathionylation.

The *peroxiredoxins* (Prx) are a family of antioxidant enzymes that reduce H_2O_2 and which may also interact with Trx and Grx, from which they accept electrons in order to be active. Although Prxs are abundant, their precise role in the heart remains to be determined.

Heme oxygenase-1 (HO-1) is induced by oxidative stress and serves a cytoprotective function through the breakdown of pro-oxidant heme into equimolar amounts of carbon monoxide, biliverdin/bilirubin, and free ferrous iron. Carbon monoxide and bilirubin exert direct cardioprotective effects via their respective anti inflammatory and antioxidant actions.[20,21]

Vitamin antioxidants play a role in the control of ROS cascades and the prevention of free radical chain reactions. Vitamin E (α-tocopherol) and vitamin C (ascorbic acid) prevent lipid peroxidation and membrane breakdown. α-Tocopherol is a fat-soluble vitamin that concentrates in cellular membranes. Through the aromatic ring head group, α-tocopherol is able to form a "stable" tocopheryl radical when it reacts with ROS and lipid peroxy radicals. Ascorbic acid reacts with tocopheryl radicals, thereby converting them back to tocopherol. Circulating and tissue levels of α-tocopherol have been used as measures of both antioxidant capacity and oxidative stress.[12]

MARKERS OF OXIDATIVE STRESS IN HUMAN HEART FAILURE

Oxidation products of several organic molecules, including lipids, proteins, and nucleic acids, have been used to assess oxidative stress in HF (**Table 8.1**). While these methods can individually be criticized for their relative lack of specificity, collectively the data support the conclusion that there is increased systemic and myocardial oxidative stress in patients with HF.

Lipid Oxidation Products

Lipid peroxidation products, such as *malondialdehyde* (MDA)[22] and *4-hydroxy-nonenal*,[23] are increased, and total thiol levels are decreased in patients with ischemic and nonischemic cardiomyopathy compared

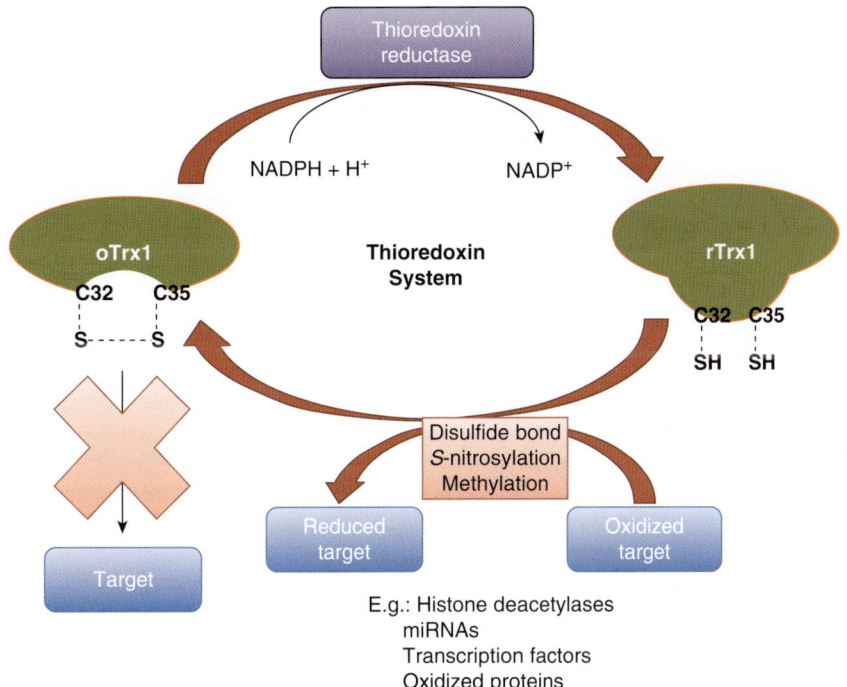

Fig. 8.2 Thioredoxin System. Reduced thioredoxin 1 *(rTrx1)* with free Cys32 *(C32)* and Cys35 *(C35)* can interact with and reduce oxidized target molecules having disulfide bonds. Although this reaction produces oxidized thioredoxin 1 *(oTrx1)* with an intramolecular disulfide linkage between Cys32 and Cys35, the oxidized Trx1 can be reduced again (recycled) by TrxR in the presence of the electron donor, NADPH. (From Nagarajan N, Oka S, Sadoshima J. Modulation of signaling mechanisms in the heart by thioredoxin 1. *Free Radic Biol Med.* 2017;109:125–131.)

with subjects without HF.[24] MDA is an independent predictor of death in patients with chronic HF.[22] *Exhaled pentane,* a volatile lipid peroxidation product, is increased in patients with HF.[25] The *8-isoprostanes* (8-iso-prostaglandin $F_{2\alpha}$) are a family of prostaglandin $F_{2\alpha}$ isomers formed by the peroxidation of arachidonic acid through a non-cyclo-oxygenase-mediated reaction catalyzed by free radicals.[26] In contrast to reactive aldehydes, lipid hydroperoxides, and conjugated dienes, 8-isoprostanes are more stable products of lipid peroxidation and thus may be a more useful indicator of oxidative stress.[27] 8-Isoprostanes measured in the pericardial fluid of patients with HF undergoing open heart surgery correlated with increasing New York Heart Association (NYHA) functional class.[28] Plasma and urinary isoprostanes correlate with the clinical severity of HF, antioxidant status, and blood B-type natriuretic peptide (BNP).[29] *Plasma oxidized LDL* (oxLDL), a marker of oxidative stress, is elevated in HF patients and predicts mortality and morbidity independent of conventional factors.[30,31]

Glycoprotein and DNA Products

Oxidation products of glycoproteins and nuclear DNA are increased in patients with HF. Serum *pentosidine,* an advanced glycation end product, is an independent risk factor for cardiac events in patients with HF.[32] Plasma *carbonyls* are increased in patients with more symptomatic HF, and associated with higher C-reactive protein (CRP) and BNP,[33] as well as progressive LV remodeling.[22] *8-Hydroxy-2-deoxyguanosine (8-OHdG),* formed when DNA is oxidatively damaged, is increased in myocardium of animals with cardiac hypertrophy[34] and tachycardia-induced cardiomyopathy,[35] and in both the serum and myocardium of patients with HF.[36] Plasma levels of 8.OHdG correlate with NYHA functional class, cardiac function, and several other biomarkers such as plasma BNP, tumor necrosis factor-α (TNF-α), and sCD40L, while urinary 8-OHdG levels correlate with symptoms and functional severity of HF.[36]

Other Oxidative Stress Markers

Uric acid, produced by the ubiquitous ROS-generating xanthine oxidase, is released from the failing human heart in inverse relation to LV ejection fraction.[37] Increased serum uric acid levels are associated with worse hemodynamic function and correlate with plasma NT-proBNP in patients with HF.[38] Uric acid was an independent predictor of mortality in the SENIORS trial, which included patients with both systolic and diastolic HF.[39] Uric acid is elevated in patients presenting with acute decompensated HF.[40] However, in high-risk HF patients with reduced ejection fraction and elevated uric acid levels, xanthine oxidase inhibition with allopurinol failed to improve clinical status, exercise capacity, quality of life, or left ventricular ejection fraction (LVEF).[41]

Biopyrrins are oxidized metabolites of bilirubin, which are increased in HF, probably secondary to hepatic dysfunction and/or increased HO-1 activity. Urinary biopyrrin levels are elevated and correlate with blood BNP and the severity of HF.[42]

Free thiols, which are a part of the antioxidant machinery, are oxidized in the presence of excess ROS, leading to depletion of their plasma levels. This phenomenon has been observed in patients with HF.[43]

Myeloperoxidase (MPO), a peroxidase enzyme abundant in granulocytes, is increased in the circulating blood of patients with HF and is an independent predictor of death, heart transplantation, or HF hospitalization.[44] Among patients with acutely decompensated HF, elevated MPO concentrations are associated with a higher 1-year mortality, even when adjusted for BNP levels.[45] MPO predicts the risk of developing HF in aging individuals.[46]

Ceruloplasmin, an acute-phase reactant and protein involved in cooper transport, has been shown to have ferroxidase I activity that is responsible for the conversion of reactive Fe^{2+} into Fe^{3+}, thereby preventing Fe^{2+} from participating in the generation of hydroxyl

TABLE 8.1 Studies of Oxidative Stress Markers in Human Heart Failure

Markers	Studies	Findings
MDA, Thiols, SOD, GPx	McMurray et al.[219]	Increased plasma MDA, decreased plasma thiols in patients with CAD and LV dysfunction
	Belch et al.[220]	Increased plasma MDA, decreased plasma thiols in patients with CHF; weak correlation between decreasing thiols and worsening LV function
	McMurray et al.[24]	Increased MDA, decreased plasma thiols in both CAD and non-CAD patients with HF
	Ghatak et al.[221]	Increased MDA, and reduced erythrocyte SOD and GPx activities in CHF; weak correlation with LV function; improved by vitamin E administration
	Radovanovic et al.[22]	Increased MDA in CHF; MDA predicted death
	Keith et al.[222]	Correlated oxidative stress with NYHA clinical class, as well as levels of soluble TNF receptor levels as marker of prognosis
	Mak et al.[23]	Plasma unsaturated aldehydes including 4-OH-nonenal were elevated in association with impaired LV contractile function in HF patients
	Polidori et al.[223]	Plasma MDA was higher in patients with severe CHF than those with moderate disease
	Campolo et al.[224]	Reduced cysteines and MDA were increased in CHF patients
MPO	Tang et al.[44]	MPO was associated with an increased likelihood of more advanced HF, and predictive of worse long-term clinical outcomes
	Tang et al.[46]	MPO predicted development of HF in aging subjects
	Reichlin et al.[45]	MPO predicted higher mortality in acute decompensated HF
8-Isoprostanes	Mallat et al.[28]	Pericardial 8-isoprostanes in patients undergoing open-heart surgery correlated with preoperative NYHA functional class
	Kameda et al.[225]	Pericardial 8-isoprostanes correlated with LV end-diastolic volume, and activities of MMP-2 and MMP-9 and gelatinolysis in CAD patients
	Polidori et al.[29]	Plasma F2 isoprostanes correlated with antioxidant status and NYHA class
	Nonaka-Sarukawa et al.[226]	Urinary 15-Ft-isoprostanes increased in proportion to the severity of CHF, and correlated with plasma BNP and serum IL-6
PON-1	Kim et al.[54]	PON-1 activity was reduced in HF
	Tang et al.[55]	Indirect measure of PON-1 activity independently predicted high risk of cardiac events in systolic HF
Glutathione S-transferase	Andrukhova et al.[51]	Serum levels of glutathione S-transferase are associated with EF and NYHA class
Breath pentane	Sobotka et al.[25]	Increased exhaled pentane in CHF compared with controls; pentane levels reduced by captopril therapy
Pentosidine	Koyama et al.[32]	Serum pentosidine was an independent risk factor for cardiac events in patients with HF
Plasma carbonyls	Amir et al.[33]	Serum oxidative stress levels increased with NYHA functional class and were associated with higher CRP and BNP
	Radovanovic et al.[22]	Increased plasma carbonyls in CHF; carbonyls correlated with echocardiographic remodeling indices
8-Hydroxy-2′-deoxyguanosine	Watanabe et al.[227]	Correlated with NYHA functional class, left atrial diameter, LV end-diastolic diameters, LV end-systolic diameters, and plasma BNP
	Kono et al.[228]	Increased in both the serum and myocardium of patients with HF; reduced with carvedilol therapy
	Pignatelli et al.[229]	Serum levels increased in CHF progressively from class I-II to class III-IV; correlated with TNF-α and sCD40L
	Kobayashi et al.[230]	Urinary levels correlated with symptoms and functional severity of HF
	Nagayoshi et al.[231]	Higher levels in CAD vs. non-CAD HF patients despite same NYHA class
Uric acid	Cicoira et al.[232]	Elevated serum uric acid levels correlated with parameters of diastolic dysfunction in HF
	Anker et al.[233]	Uric acid predicted mortality in patients with moderate to severe CHF
	Kojima et al.[234]	Correlated with Killip classification and mortality in patients with acute MI
	Sakai et al.[37]	Positive transcardiac gradient increased with the severity of HF, and inversely correlated with LV ejection fraction
	Kittleson et al.[38]	High uric acid was associated with increased cardiac filling pressure and reduced cardiac index; correlated with NT-proBNP
	Ioachimescu et al.[235]	An independent predictor of death in patients at high risk of cardiovascular disease
	Manzano et al.[39]	Independent predictor of mortality in the SENIORS trial patients with systolic and diastolic HF
	Bishu et al.[40]	Elevated levels in acute decompensated HF
Oxidized LDLs	Charach et al.[30]	Plasma levels predicted mortality and morbidity in HF patients
Phospholipid transfer protein	Chen et al.[56]	Higher levels associated with LV systolic function
Biopyrrins	Hokamaki et al.[42]	Urinary biopyrrin levels were elevated, and correlated with blood BNP and severity of HF
Ceruloplasmin	Dadu et al.[48]	Higher levels correlate with incident HF even after adjustment for other biomarkers
	Saunders et al.[49]	
Serum free thiols	Koning et al.[43]	Higher levels correlate with lower levels of NT-proBNP, decreased rehospitalization rate, and increased patient survival

CAD, Coronary artery disease; *CHF,* congestive heart failure; *EF,* ejection fraction; *GPx,* glutathione peroxidase; *HF,* heart failure; *LV,* left ventricular; *MDA,* malondialdehyde; *MPO,* myeloperoxidase; *NYHA,* New York Heart Association; *PON-1,* paraoxonase-1; *SOD,* superoxide dismutases.

radicals, GPx activity, and the ability to inhibit MPO.[47] Elevated plasma ceruloplasmin levels are associated with incident HF,[48] even after adjusting for other biomarkers, such as BNP, troponin, and CRP.[49] While ceruloplasmin, per se, was not associated with mortality in HF, low serum ferroxidase I activity, presumably as a result of ceruloplasmin nitration, was a predictor of HF mortality.[50]

Glutathione S-transferase P1 participates in the detoxification of ROS and maintenance of the cellular redox state, and is elevated in the plasma of patients with HF in proportion to systolic dysfunction and functional class.[51]

Thioredoxin 1 (Trx1), part of the thioredoxin antioxidant defense system described previously, decreases oxidative stress by reducing peroxiredoxin, which in turn reduces H_2O_2. Trx1 was shown to be an independent predictor of cardiac events survival in HF patients.[52]

Paraoxonase-1 (PON-1) is a high-density lipoprotein (HDL)-associated glycoprotein that contributes to the systemic antioxidant activities of HDL.[53] PON-1 is decreased in HF patients[54]; decreased serum arylesterase activity, a measure of diminished antioxidant properties of PON-1, predicts higher risk of long-term adverse cardiac events in patients with systolic HF.[55]

Phospholipid transfer protein (PLTP) modulates lipoprotein metabolism and plays a role in inflammation and oxidative stress. A higher PLTP activity is associated with depressed LV systolic function.[56]

MECHANISMS OF INCREASED OXIDATIVE STRESS IN HEART FAILURE (FIG. 8.3)

Increased oxidative stress may occur as a result of the increased generation of ROS, decreased clearance of ROS by various antioxidant systems, or both. Both mitochondria and several enzyme systems that generate O_2^- may produce pathophysiologic amounts of O_2^- in the failing heart.

Oxidases

The *NAD(P)H oxidase (NOX)* family consists of at least five transmembrane enzymes that mediate electron transfer from NAD(P)H to molecular oxygen to generate O_2^-. The NOX-2 isoform was first described in the neutrophil, where it is responsible for the oxidative burst, which produces large amounts of cytotoxic ROS. Other isoforms produce lower levels of ROS that can act as signaling intermediates.[57,58] NOX-2 and NOX-4 are the predominant isoforms in cardiac myocytes, and both have been implicated in mediating hypertrophy.[59,60] NOX-2 is located in the plasma membrane, whereas the localization of NOX-4 is less certain but appears to include the endoplasmic reticulum (ER) and/or mitochondrial membranes. NOX-2 mediates LV hypertrophy and failure in response to activation of the renin-angiotensin system,[58] but not in response to pressure overload.[61] NOX-4 also appears to contribute to oxidative stress and to be involved in mediating cardiac hypertrophy and failure in response to hemodynamic stress, though the data are conflicting.[62-64]

Xanthine oxidoreductase consists of two interconvertible forms, xanthine dehydrogenase and xanthine oxidase, both of which are involved in the conversion of hypoxanthine and xanthine to uric acid. The constitutive xanthine dehydrogenase uses NAD+ primarily as an electron acceptor, whereas the inducible xanthine oxidase transfers electrons to molecular oxygen, yielding ROS. In addition, xanthine oxidoreductase can generate O_2^- via NADH oxidase activity and produce NO via nitrate and nitrite reductase activities.[65] Thus activation of xanthine oxidoreductase may cause both oxidative and nitrosative stress. The expression of xanthine oxidase is increased in the hearts of

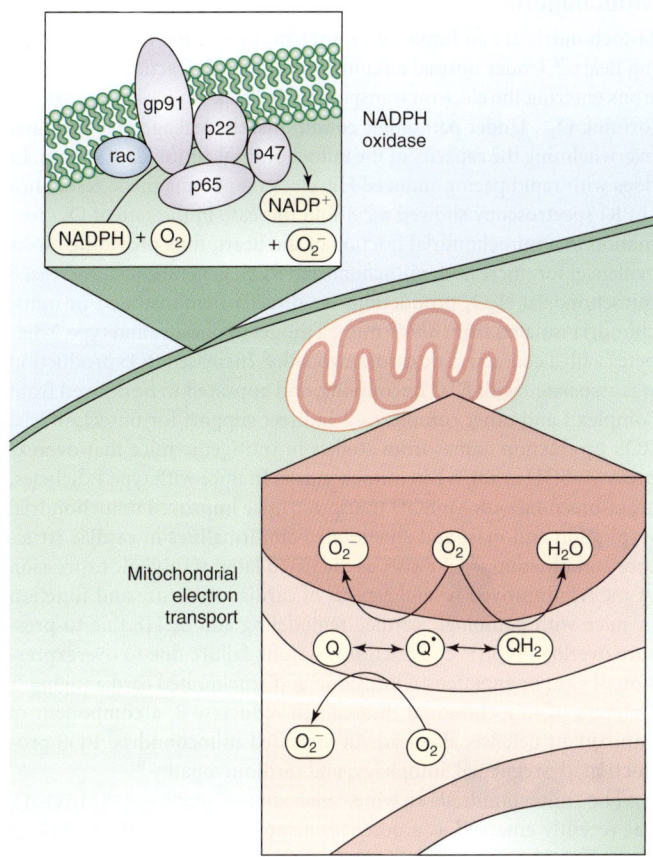

Fig. 8.3 NAD(P)H Oxidases and Mitochondria as Sources of Reactive Oxygen Species (ROS) in the Heart. An NAD(P)H oxidase is expressed in cardiac myocytes similar to that found in neutrophils and vascular cells. The oxidase is composed of at least five subunits, with two membrane proteins that comprise the oxidase activity and three cytoplasmic proteins that serve regulatory functions. The complex catalyzes the one-electron reduction of O_2 to O_2^-, with NADPH or NADH as a reducing cofactor. The mitochondrial electron transport chain creates a proton-motive force through the transfer of electrons from NADH dehydrogenase (complex I) and succinate dehydrogenase (complex II) to ubiquinone (Q), thereby forming reduced ubiquinone (QH_2). Partially reduced ubiquinone ($Q^.$) is a radical that can reduce O_2 to O_2^-. This oxygen "leakage" is a potentially large source of ROS, and has been implicated in the increased oxidative stress in HF (see text).

rats with HF[66,67] and patients with dilated cardiomyopathy.[68] In animal models of HF, xanthine oxidase inhibitors (e.g., allopurinol, oxypurinol, febuxostat) attenuate the production of ROS, improve cardiac function, decrease LV size, improve β-adrenergic receptor sensitivity, improve myocardial energetic coupling,[69,70] inhibit fetal gene expression, and improve Ca^{2+} handling.[71] In rats with pressure overload, the magnitude of improvement in cardiac function with oxypurinol is related to the initial level of xanthine oxidase activity.[72]

In patients with HF, allopurinol reduced plasma MDA, improved endothelium-dependent flow-mediated response,[73,74] reduced myocardial oxygen consumption, and improved myocardial efficiency.[68] In acute and short-term human studies, oxypurinol increased LV ejection fraction and reduced LV end-diastolic volume.[75] However, in a dedicated randomized controlled study of HF patients with elevated uric acid levels (EXACT-HF study), chronic allopurinol treatment failed to lead to an improvement in clinical status, exercise capacity, quality of life, or LVEF.[41]

Mitochondria

Mitochondria are an important source of myocardial ROS in the failing heart.[76] Under normal circumstances, a small fraction of the electrons entering the electron transport chain "leak" to molecular oxygen forming O_2^-. Under pathologic conditions, the leakage may increase, overwhelming the capacity of the mitochondrial antioxidant system. In dogs with rapid pacing-induced HF, electron paramagnetic resonance (EPR) spectroscopy showed a 2.8-fold increase in the rate of O_2^- formation in a mitochondrial fraction of the heart, thus providing direct evidence for increased mitochondrial ROS generation.[77] Increased mitochondrial H_2O_2 production was directly demonstrated in mitochondria isolated from *db/db* mice, a model of obesity, and type 2 diabetes with a characteristic cardiomyopathy. Increased ROS production was associated with ETC uncoupling, and appeared to be derived from complex I and other complexes.[78] Indirect support for mitochondrial ROS production comes from studies in transgenic mice that overexpress MnSOD or mCAT in mitochondria. In mice with type 1 diabetes, cross-breeding with MnSOD transgenic mice improved mitochondrial respiration and mass and ameliorated abnormalities in cardiac structure and function.[79] Likewise, as discussed later, transgenic expression of mCAT improved several aspects of cardiac structure and function in mice with pathologic cardiac remodeling and/or HF due to pressure overload (aortic constriction), systolic failure due to overexpression of Gαq or angiotensin infusion,[7] and ameliorated cardiac aging.[80] Deletion of mitochondrial thioredoxin reductase 2, a component of antioxidant defense, also leads in increased mitochondrial ROS production, dysregulated autophagy, and cardiomyopathy.[81]

The mitochondrial enzyme, *monoamine oxidase-A* (MAO-A), has recently emerged as a potent generator of ROS in the heart—in particular, H_2O_2. Cardiac MAO-A expression is increased in models of HF and cardiac aging.[82] Overexpression of MAO-A in the heart is associated with aging and HF, resulting in significant mitochondrial and lysosomal dysfunction and cardiac damage.[83] This is thought to be mediated by ROS-dependent inhibition of nuclear translocation of transcription factor-EB, a master regulator of autophagy and lysosome biogenesis.[84]

A pathologic role of mitochondrial ROS has also been confirmed in obesity-mediated cardiomyopathy. Wild-type mice fed a high-fat, high-sucrose diet develop a cardiomyopathy characterized by LV hypertrophy and diastolic dysfunction.[85] In this model, there is an increase in mitochondrial ROS production, particularly from complexes I and II, that precedes the development of obesity.[9,86,87] Importantly, overexpression of mCAT prevents both mitochondrial and nonmitochondrial abnormalities in this model and restores a near normal cardiac phenotype,[9] suggesting a major mechanistic role of mitochondrial ROS in the pathogenesis of obesity-mediated cardiomyopathy. Although these studies show that mitochondrial ROS is a key mediator of cardiac dysfunction, they do not absolutely establish the source of the ROS. For example, ROS from nonmitochondrial sources may cause mitochondrial dysfunction and may include ETC electron leakage, leading to further ROS generation (i.e., ROS-mediated ROS release).[88]

Nitric Oxide Synthase

Nitric oxide (NO) is a free radical that can modify the myocardial response to oxidative stress both directly and indirectly. NO is synthesized in the conversion of L-arginine to L-citrulline by a family of nitric oxide synthases (NOS). NO, a free radical gas, is buffered in the cell by reactions with glutathione, and reacts reversibly with sulfhydryl groups of proteins forming *S*-nitrosothiols that can alter protein function.[89] Through chemical reactions with ROS, NO can either *decrease* or *increase* the oxidative stress in a cell or tissue. Under normal circumstances, myocardial NO is produced at low levels by *endothelial NOS (eNOS or NOS3)*. NOS3, which is present in virtually all cell types in the myocardium, including myocytes, fibroblasts, and endothelial cells, is regulated by a calcium-sensitive interaction with calmodulin.[90] *Inducible nitric oxide synthase (NOS2)* is not regulated by Ca^{2+} and when induced is capable of producing high levels of NO. Though NOS2 is expressed minimally in the normal myocardium, it is induced by exposure to cytokines, hypoxia, and other stimuli in both myocytes and nonmyocytes, leading to a marked increase in the production of NO.[91] NOS2 can catalyze the formation of O_2^-,[92] particularly in the setting of arginine depletion, and may contribute directly to the formation of ROS.[93] The expression and activity of NOS2 are increased in the myocardium of patients with idiopathic and ischemic dilated cardiomyopathies.[94]

Low levels of NO, as are formed by NOS3, may decrease the level of oxidative stress by decreasing the production of O_2^- through inhibition of oxidative enzymes.[95] Through the activation of guanylate cyclase, NO can inhibit signaling and transcription factors that modify myocyte hypertrophic and apoptotic signaling.[96] Mice lacking NOS3 have worse ventricular function late after MI,[97] consistent with the notion that NOS3-derived NO is beneficial for the failing heart. Higher levels of NO increase oxidative stress by reacting with O_2^- to generate *peroxynitrite (ONOO$^-$)*, a free radical that is toxic and longer-lived than either NO or O_2^-.[98] ONOO$^-$ can react with many cell constituents, including tyrosine residues of susceptible proteins such as MnSOD, causing irreversible inactivation.[99] Based on the relative rate constants for the reaction of O_2^- with SOD versus NO, the formation of ONOO$^-$ is favored when the levels of O_2^- and/or NO are high or the level of SOD is low.

High concentrations of NO can have direct toxic effects on cardiac myocytes in vitro. The cytotoxic effect of cytokines on cardiac myocytes in culture is inhibited by the NOS inhibitor L-NMMA.[100] Cytokine-induced apoptosis can be prevented by either an inhibitor of NOS2 or an SOD-mimetic, thus implicating ONOO$^-$. In mice, late post-MI NOS2 expression is increased in the remote myocardium, and NOS2 knockout mice have less myocyte apoptosis, improved contractile function, and increased survival.[101] Likewise, in animal models of autoimmune and viral myocarditis, the amount of myocardial injury was reduced by aminoguanidine, an inhibitor of NOS2.[102] Treatment with aminoguanidine also decreased the amount of O_2^- anion formed, suggesting the presence of NOS2-dependent O_2^- production or the inactivation of MnSOD by ONOO$^-$.[103] The divergent effects of NO were revealed when mice with viral myocarditis were treated with L-NAME. A low dose improved survival, HF, and myocardial necrosis, whereas the highest dose worsened survival.[104] Similarly, stretch-induced myocyte apoptosis is inhibited by an NO donor.[105] Potential mechanisms for a protective effect of low NO levels include inhibition of enzymes in the programmed cell death pathway[96] and decreased mitochondrial ROS production.[95]

NOS can be *uncoupled* due to oxidation of the essential cofactor tetrahydrobiopterin,[106] leading to the generation of O_2^-. ROS production from uncoupled eNOS contributes to HF[107] and diastolic dysfunction,[108] and the cardiac phenotype is improved by supplementation with tetrahydrobiopterin. Uncoupling of NOS may be caused by ROS from other sources (e.g., mitochondria or other oxidases), thus providing a mechanism for amplification of ROS.

Decreased Antioxidant Activity

ROS are exquisitely regulated by a large number of interacting and, to some extent, redundant antioxidant systems. Impaired function of one or more of these antioxidant systems can lead to an increase in oxidative stress. In guinea pigs with pressure overload due to aortic banding, both SOD and GPx activity decreased during the progression to HF, in association with a decrease in the ratio of GSH/GSSG, indicating an increase in myocardial oxidative stress.[109] Similar changes in antioxidant capacity and oxidative stress occur in the rat heart late after myocardial infarction (MI).[12,110] Decreased antioxidant enzyme capacity and depletion of vitamin E occurred in a large animal model of volume overload–induced HF secondary to mitral regurgitation.[111] Two studies found no decrease in SOD or GPx activity in pathologic samples from explanted human hearts at the time of cardiac transplant,[112,113] whereas in another study, MnSOD activity was reduced in the failing human heart, apparently due to a posttranscriptional level mechanism because mRNA expression was not decreased.[114]

Sirtuins, a seven-member family of NAD^+-dependent histone deacetylases, have recently emerged as major regulators of multiple native antioxidant defense systems.[115] Sirt1, which is predominantly localized to the nucleus, can deacetylate and activate FoxO1 to upregulate expression of antioxidants, including MnSOD, catalase, and Trx1, as well as a number of antiapoptotic factors.[116] Deacetylation of p66Shc, a master regulator of ROS, by Sirt1 has been shown to be a key protective mechanism against diabetes-medicated vascular oxidative stress.[117] In addition to its ability to regulate redox stress, the activity of Sirt1 in turn can be redox regulated and decreased by oxidative posttranslational modifications (OPTM) including S-glutathiolation.[118–120] Similarly, Sirt3, another well-studied member of sirtuin family that is located in mitochondria, has been shown to block cardiac hypertrophy by decreasing ROS production via activation of FoxO3-dependent antioxidant systems, including MnSOD and catalase, as well as via suppression of Ras activation and inhibition of the MAPK-ERK and PI3K–Akt signaling pathways.[121] While Sirt5, Sirt6, and Sirt7 play protective roles against ROS-induced injury, their role in the heart is not well documented.[116]

Nonenzymatic Auto-Oxidation

Reactions involving several organic molecules may contribute to the formation of ROS in vivo. Oxidation of norepinephrine and epinephrine to *adrenochrome* and O_2^- has been proposed as a mechanism for myocardial injury in the presence of chronic adrenergic stimulation.[122] Thiol compounds, including cysteine and GSH, can auto-oxidize to form O_2^-, particularly in the presence of transition metals such as iron. The cardiotoxicity of *iron* overload is likely a combination of this plus Fenton chemistry to generate hydroxyl radicals. *Myoglobin* can autoxidize from oxymyoglobin to metmyoglobin with the release of O_2^-.[123]

OXIDATIVE STRESS AND ANTIOXIDANT THERAPY IN ANIMAL MODELS OF HEART FAILURE

Work in animal models has allowed greater insight regarding the sources and consequences of oxidative stress in HF. Studies have been performed in a variety of models of HF, with a range of antioxidant strategies.

Hemodynamic Overload

The aortic constriction model of HF occurs in two phases. In the initial days after constriction there is LV hypertrophy, whereas over the ensuing weeks there is progressive chamber dilation, wall thinning, and systolic failure. Several types of antioxidant intervention have been shown to ameliorate one or both phases of this model.

NAD(P)H Oxidase Transgenic Mice

The NOX-2 and NOX-4 isoforms of NAD(P)H oxidase are predominant in cardiac myocytes.[124] In mice, NOX-2 knockout prevented cardiac hypertrophy and fibrosis caused by chronic sub-pressor

infusion of angiotensin,[125] suggesting a role in the response to neurohormones. However, NOX-2 knockout did not inhibit the hypertrophic response to pressure overload with aortic constriction.[61,126] NOX-4 appears to modulate the hypertrophic response to pressure overload, although the exact role remains unclear. In one study, NOX-4 knockout mice did better after aortic constriction, and NOX-4 transgenic mice did worse.[62] NOX-4 overexpression was associated with increased mitochondrial ROS and worse mitochondrial function.[62] The latter was supported by another study where NOX-4 transgenic mice had significantly higher production of ROS, and manifested cardiac interstitial fibrosis.[64] In that study, the mechanism seemed to be related to the upregulation of cardiac fetal genes and activation of the Akt-mTOR and NFκB signaling pathways.[64] However, another group using a similar aortic constriction model found that NOX-4 knockout mice developed worse LV failure with aortic constriction, whereas NOX-4 overexpressing animals were protected.[63] These experiments illustrate the complexity of redox systems, which on the one hand can mediate pathophysiologic processes and on the other are essential to normal cellular and defense mechanisms. For example, knockout of both NOX-2 and NOX-4 exacerbated ischemia-reperfusion injury in the heart, suggesting that low-level ROS production by the NOX system is required for the activation of protective mechanisms.[127]

NOS3 Knockout and Tetrahydrobiopterin

Aortic constriction causes less LV hypertrophy and fibrosis in NOS3 knockout mice, suggesting that uncoupled NOS3 contributes to myocardial oxidative stress.[128] Likewise, treatment with oral tetrahydrobiopterin (BH4), a cofactor necessary for NOS coupling, recoupled NOS3, decreased oxidative stress, and decreased both LV hypertrophy and fibrosis.[129]

Thioredoxin and *N*-2-Mercaptopropionyl Glycine

N-2-mercaptopropionyl glycine (MPG) is a low-molecular-weight antioxidant analogue of glutathione, which scavenges H_2O_2. Administration of MPG to mice decreased markers of myocardial oxidative stress and myocardial hypertrophy 7 days after aortic constriction.[130] In transgenic mice, cardiac-specific overexpression of a dominant-negative Trx-1 worsened, and overexpression of wild-type Trx-1 ameliorated the response to aortic constriction.[34] Consistent with a protective effect of Trx-1, cardiomyocyte-specific knockout of Txnip, which inhibits Trx, protected from early, but not late, pressure overload–induced cardiac dysfunction.[131]

Peroxisomal Catalase

Left ventricular (LV) hypertrophy and failure associated with a generalized increase in myocardial oxidative stress and specific oxidative modifications of SERCA at cysteine 674 and tyrosine 294/5 due to ascending aortic constriction is ameliorated by myocyte-specific overexpression of pCAT.[132] Furthermore, SERCA cysteine modifications were also prevented. This is consistent with the ability of pCAT to reverse aging-associated myocardial dysfunction via decrease in cysteine OPTM.[133]

Vitamins E and C, and Resveratrol

In guinea pigs subjected to aortic banding, vitamin E (α-tocopherol) had no effect on LV hypertrophy early after banding, but at late time points prevented the transition to HF.[134] In the same model, vitamin C (ascorbic acid) administration to guinea pigs with aortic banding inhibited LVH.[135] Resveratrol, a naturally occurring polyphenol antioxidant present in grapes, decreased LV hypertrophy and improved diastolic relaxation early after aortic constriction in the rat model.[136]

Mitochondrial Antioxidants

Transgenic overexpression of mCAT[137] or administration of an anti-oxidant peptide targeted to mitochondria[138] exerts broad beneficial effects in mice with aortic constriction, resulting in less LV hypertrophy and progression to failure. The effects of mCAT were associated with correction of the mitochondrial proteome.[138] Euk-8 is a potent SOD-mimetic, catalase-mimetic, and free radical scavenger.[139] In mice with aortic constriction, Euk-8 decreased LV hypertrophy and progression to failure and improved survival.[140] Elamipretide, a cell-permeable and mitochondrial inner membrane-targeting peptide, is known to protect mitochondrial cristae structure, reduce oxidative stress and improve ATP synthesis.[141] Elamipretide has been shown to ameliorate LV hypertrophy/cardiac failure in a model of angiotensin II-induced cardiomyopathy[142] and pressure overload,[138] likely via a decrease in mitochondrial ROS generation.[141]

Heart Failure in Gαq-Transgenic Mice

The G protein Gαq mediates many of the effects of neurohormones and mechanical strain in cardiac myocytes, and its overexpression in mice leads to pathologic myocardial remodeling that progresses to a severe dilated cardiomyopathy.[143] Myocyte-specific overexpression of catalase that is expressed primarily in the peroxisomes (pCAT) had no effect on the early phenotype of LV dilation and contractile dysfunction at the time of weaning, but prevented the subsequent progression to HF.[8] A key mechanism for improvement in contractile function appeared to be prevention of OPTM of SERCA at cysteine 674.[144] In another study, overexpression of catalase targeted to the mitochondria (mCAT) prevented progressive adverse remodeling and failure.[7] In the same study, mCAT also alleviated adverse remodeling in response to chronic angiotensin infusion,[7] and the effects in both models were mimicked by an orally administered antioxidant peptide targeted to the mitochondria,[142] thus highlighting the importance of mitochondrial ROS and demonstrating the potential therapeutic utility of this approach.[145]

Anthracycline-Induced Cardiomyopathy (Fig. 8.4)

Anthracycline causes cardiotoxicity via several mechanisms including excess free radical production induced by the quinone group; modulation in topoisomerase 2β activity, leading to DNA strand breaks; alterations in the multidrug-resistant (MDR) efflux proteins, leading to higher levels of intracardiac levels of anthracycline; and decreased progenitor cell population.[146] The anthracyclines induce myocyte apoptosis and necrosis in a dose-dependent manner.[127] Both NOX-2 and mito-chondria-derived ROS have been implicated as potential mediators of these effects.[147,148] The apoptosis, but not necrosis, could be inhibited by the addition of the iron chelator dexrazoxane, which has shown promise clinically in the prevention of anthracycline cardiotoxicity.[149] These results implicate hydroxyl radicals formed via the Fenton reaction in anthracycline-induced apoptosis. Anthracycline cardiotoxicity can be acute, occurring within days, or chronic, developing over months or even years. Both acute and chronic doxorubicin (Dox) cardiac toxicity and oxidative stress in mice were improved by transgenic overexpression of a variety of antioxidant proteins including metallothionein,[150,151] pCAT,[152,153] sirtuin 3,[154] and thioredoxin.[15] In animal models of Dox-induced cardiomyopathy, vitamin C administration ameliorated both oxidative stress and Dox-induced cardiac dysfunction.[155]

MODELS OF DIASTOLIC DYSFUNCTION (SEE ALSO CHAPTER 11)

HF with preserved ejection fraction due to diastolic dysfunction is a major cause of HF in *metabolic heart disease (MHD)* and aging. MHD is associated with increased oxidant stress. For example, in diabetic *(db/db)* mice, a model of type 2 diabetes, there are increased levels of MDA and 4-hydroxynonenol (4HNE) in the myocardium, and increased H_2O_2 production by cardiac mitochondria.[78] Mice fed a diet high in fat and sucrose develop obesity, type 2 diabetes, and metabolic syndrome characterized by increased oxidative stress markers (e.g., HNE), mitochondrial ROS production, and decreased ATP synthesis in the heart in

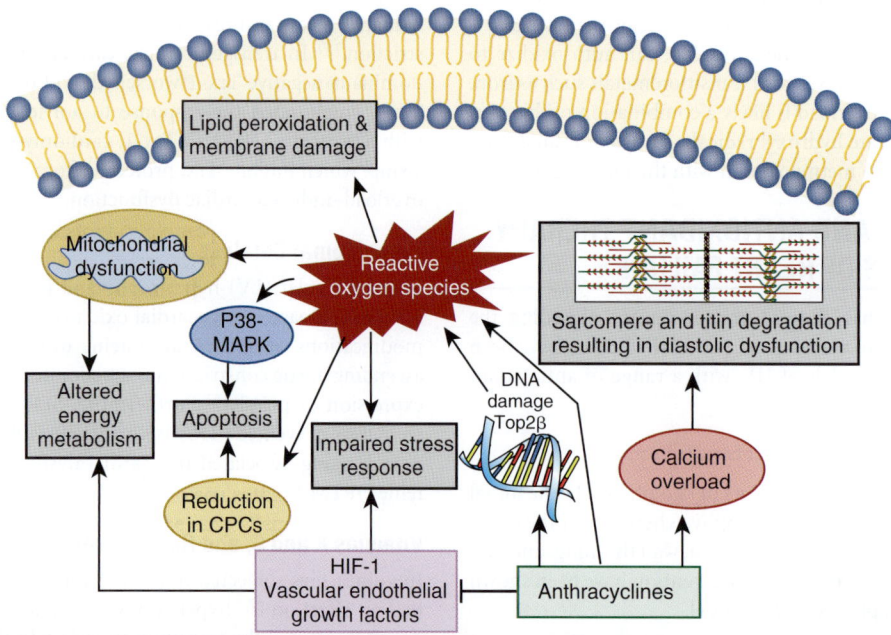

Fig. 8.4 Proposed Mechanisms of Anthracycline Cardiotoxicity. Using anthracyclines results in the generation of reactive oxygen species *(ROS)*, potentially via topoisomerase 2β inhibition, as well as calcium overload, reduction in cardiac progenitor cells (CPCs), and hypoxia-inducible factor (HIF) inhibition. *ER,* Endoplasmic reticulum. (From Ky B. Cardio-oncology. In: Zipes DP, Libby P, Bonow RO, Mann DL, Tomaselli GF, eds. *Braunwald's Heart Disease: A Textbook of Cardiovascular Medicine.* Philadelphia: Elsevier; 2019:1641–1650.)

association with LV fibrosis, hypertrophy, and diastolic dysfunction.[85,86] In these mice, treatment with *resveratrol*, a polyphenol with antioxidant properties, normalized the markers of oxidative stress and improved the cardiac structure and function.[85] Similarly, overexpression of mCAT in this model normalized mitochondrial ROS production, ATP synthesis, and respiration, as well as diastolic function, and significantly attenuated LV hypertrophy.[9] Likewise, transgenic overexpression of HO-1 ameliorated LV dysfunction, myofibril disarray, oxidative stress, inflammation, apoptosis, and autophagy in mice with diabetic cardiomyopathy.[156] *Vitamin E* supplement also improved LV function and decreased myocardial 8-isoprostanes and oxidized glutathione accumulation in rodents with diabetic cardiomyopathy.[157] In *aging mice*, transgenic overexpression of either pCAT[158] or mCAT[80] lessened LV hypertrophy and improved LV diastolic function. In addition, pCAT decreased the oxidation of SERCA[158] and mCAT decreased mitochondrial DNA mutations and improved mitochondrial biogenesis.[137] These studies emphasize the central role of oxidative stress in the aging heart.

Other Experimental Heart Failure Models

LV dilation and failure *late post-MI* are related to chronic hemodynamic overload. Although less studied than the aortic constriction model, late post-MI remodeling and failure appear to be ameliorated by antioxidants. The ROS scavenger DMTU prevented both pump dysfunction and chamber dilation in mice post-MI.[159] Probucol decreased the levels of myocardial oxidative stress, preserved myocardial systolic function, and improved animal survival.[160] In rabbits with *pacing-induced* cardiomyopathy, antioxidant vitamins decreased tissue oxidative stress and attenuated cardiac dysfunction.[35] Elamipretide, mitochondria-targeting peptide, improved LV systolic function, normalized plasma biomarkers, and reversed mitochondrial abnormalities in LV myocardium of dogs with advanced ischemic HF.[161]

HUMAN TRIALS OF ANTIOXIDANT THERAPIES

Antioxidant vitamins have not been successful in altering the outcomes in patients with HF in large randomized clinical trials.[162] The reasons for this could be numerous, including nonspecific nature of vitamins and/or their inability to reach the subcellular compartments, where their actions would have been beneficial. Other approaches have involved more targeted agents. Oxypurinol, an inhibitor of xanthine oxidase, did not improve outcomes in patients with moderate and severe HF.[163] The Q-SYMBIO trial[164] showed improvement in survival rates in patients with congestive heart failure (CHF) treated with coenzyme Q10; however, several limitations of the trial have been identified, and larger trials are necessary to confirm these results.[165] Another mitochondria-targeted antioxidant, elamipretide, in a small study resulted in favorable changes in LV volumes after a single-dose infusion.[166]

MECHANISMS OF ROS-MEDIATED LEFT VENTRICULAR REMODELING AND HEART FAILURE (FIG. 8.5)

Left Ventricular Remodeling (see also Chapter 12)

Several mechanisms contribute to myocardial remodeling, including myocyte hypertrophy, myocyte slippage, myocyte apoptosis, and/or alterations in the turnover and properties of the extracellular matrix (**see also Chapter 4**). The stimuli for remodeling include increased wall stress, inflammatory cytokines, and neurohormones such as catecholamines and angiotensin II. In vitro and in vivo studies have shown that ROS mediate many of the effects of remodeling stimuli, thereby playing an important role in pathologic remodeling.

Myocyte Hypertrophy

A number of stimuli implicated in mediating cardiac remodeling exert pro-hypertrophic actions in ROS-dependent manner.[57] In cardiac myocytes, in vitro partial inhibition of CuZnSOD[167] and exposure to low concentration of exogenous H_2O_2[168] caused myocyte hypertrophy that was inhibited by antioxidants. Likewise, low-amplitude mechanical strain of cardiac myocytes caused amplitude-dependent ROS formation and myocyte hypertrophy, and the hypertrophic effect was inhibited by an SOD-mimetic.[169] Similarly, myocyte hypertrophy stimulated by angiotensin II or TNF-α is mediated by ROS.[170] Myocyte production of angiotensin II and TNF-α has been implicated in the response to mechanical strain.[160] α-Adrenergic receptor stimulation also induces myocyte ROS formation and stimulates myocyte hypertrophy through ROS-dependent pathways.[171] The ROS-mediated hypertrophic effects of these stimuli act via Gαq, NAD(P)H oxidases, and activation of the ras/raf/MEK/ERK signaling cascade (see later discussion), including endothelin, α₁-adrenergic agonists, and mechanical strain.[159,171,172]

Myocyte Death

ROS-mediated *apoptosis and programmed necrosis* contribute to the myocardial failure.[173] In contrast to the growth effects of low levels of ROS generated by specific oxidases and acting via specific signaling systems, ROS-mediated myocyte cell death generally involves higher

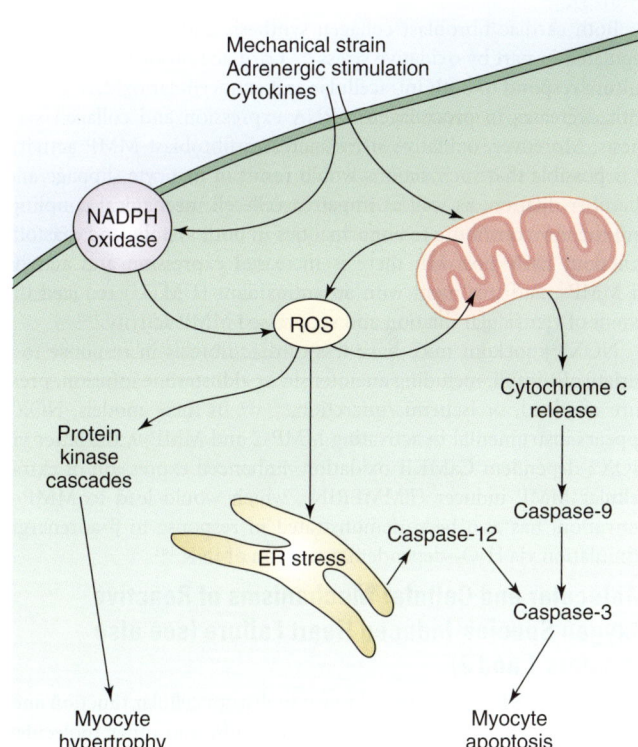

Fig. 8.5 Schematic Presentation of the Effects of Reactive Oxygen Species (ROS) on Myocyte Hypertrophy and Apoptosis. Through activation of kinase cascades such as mitogen-activated protein kinase (*MAPK*), ROS can induce myocyte hypertrophy. Mitochondrial ROS may be particularly prone to induce apoptosis by stimulating the mitochondrial release of cytochrome c, which is necessary for the activation of caspase cascades. When the ER is overwhelmed by the stress, caspase-12 is released and activates caspase-3 and the final programmed cell death pathway. *CPC,* Cardiac progenitor cell; *HIF,* hypoxia-inducible factor.

levels of ROS. For example, whereas partial inhibition of SOD causes myocyte hypertrophy, more complete inhibition causes apoptosis.[167] Low concentrations of exogenous H_2O_2 cause hypertrophy, whereas higher concentrations cause apoptosis.[168,174] In papillary muscle, mechanical strain induces ROS formation and myocyte apoptosis.[105] In cardiac myocytes, in vitro low-amplitude mechanical strain causes myocyte hypertrophy, whereas high-amplitude strain causes apoptosis that is inhibited by SOD-mimetic.[169] As discussed later, myocyte apoptosis may involve regulation of mitochondrial death pathways by the Bcl-2 family proteins. *Programmed necrosis,* which involves similar stimuli as apoptosis, albeit acting via distinct signaling pathways, has also been described in cardiomyocytes.[175]

Interstitial Fibrosis

As discussed in **Chapter 4**, one mechanism for ventricular chamber dilation is via alterations in the interstitial matrix of the myocardium. Individual ventricular myocytes are mechanically coupled to other cells via interstitial matrix proteins that connect to the sarcomere via integrins and intermediate filaments. Like intracellular proteins, there is a regular turnover of interstitial matrix proteins that is regulated by proteases and the protein synthetic machinery of the cardiac cells. Collagen is the major component of the interstitium that contributes to the structural integrity of the myocardium. Myocardial collagen content is regulated by the balance between synthesis and degradation, the latter primarily due to the action of matrix *metalloproteinases (MMPs).*[176]

Both cardiac fibroblast collagen synthesis and MMP activity are regulated in part by oxidative stress.[177] Cardiac fibroblasts in primary culture respond to both intracellular and extracellular oxidative stress with decreases in procollagen mRNA expression and collagen synthesis. Moreover, oxidative stress increases fibroblast MMP activity. It is possible that such actions would result in myocyte slippage and chamber dilation, as well as impaired cell-cell mechanical coupling, and thereby contribute to abnormalities in both systolic and diastolic function. Early post-MI, there is increased expression and activity of MMPs, and treatment with an antioxidant (DMTU) reduced the extent of ventricular dilation and suppressed MMP activity.[178]

NOX2 knockout mice have less cardiac fibrosis in response to a variety of stimuli, including angiotensin or aldosterone infusion, pressure overload, or ischemia/infarction.[179,180] In these models, NOX2 appears instrumental in activating MMP-2 and MMP-9, the latter via NOX2-dependent CaMKII oxidation. Enhanced expression of extracellular MMP inducer (EMMPRIN), which would lead to MMP-2 activation, has also been demonstrated in response to β-adrenergic stimulation via H_2O_2-dependent activation of JNK.[181]

Molecular and Cellular Mechanisms of Reactive Oxygen Species-Induced Heart Failure (see also Chapters 1 and 2)

Although ROS have long been known to disrupt cellular function and/or viability via damage to proteins and lipids, and other molecules, it is now recognized that ROS can regulate physiologic protein function by means of *OPTM*[182] (**Fig. 8.6**). Under normal conditions, low physiologic levels of ROS regulate homeostatic functions, a process called *redox signaling.* However, elevated levels of ROS that are present in the hypertrophied or failing heart have the ability to cause exaggerated signaling that promotes detrimental effects such as hypertrophy, apoptosis, and impaired calcium regulation. The consequences of OPTM likely relate to the specific amino acids modified and the type of modification. There are likely several protein targets of OPTM in various models of HF. For example, a reversible glutathiolation of C674 of SERCA causes activation in response to low levels of ROS,

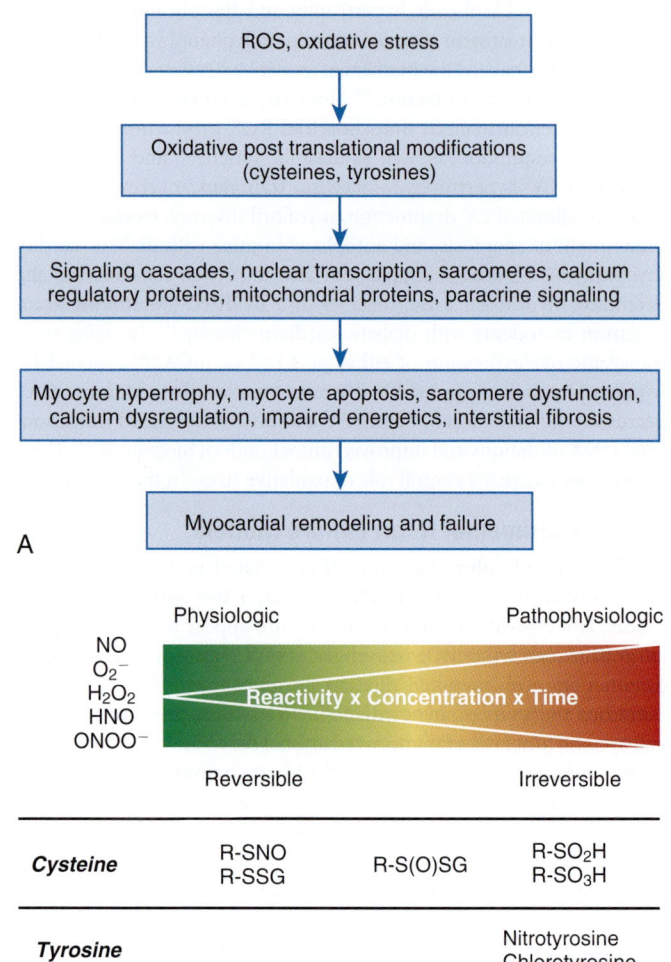

Fig. 8.6 Oxidative Stress in the Pathophysiology of Heart Failure. (A) Oxidative posttranslational modifications (OPTM) of proteins play a central role in transducing the effects of reactive oxygen species *(ROS)* in the myocardium. Increased ROS and oxidative stress lead to OPTM of reactive protein amino acids on key proteins involved in all aspects of cellular function, including intracellular signaling, sarcomere function, calcium regulation, mitochondrial energetics, and paracrine signaling to neighboring cells such as fibroblasts and endothelial cells. (B) OPTM exert a range of effects on protein function from physiologic to pathologic, depending on the target amino acid (e.g., cysteine, tyrosine) and the type (e.g., H_2O_2, $ONOO^-$), intensity (local concentration), and duration of oxidant exposure. In general, oxidant conditions of low intensity that occur under physiologic conditions cause reversible OPTM, such as glutathiolation (R-SSG) of a cysteine thiol. More intense oxidant levels that result from pathologic stimuli lead to irreversible OPTM, such as sulfonylation ($R-SO_3$) of a cysteine thiol. Reversible OPTM can be modulated by enzyme systems, such as thioredoxin and glutaredoxin, that reduce the OPTM, thereby reversing the effect and restoring normal homeostasis. In contrast, irreversible OPTM typically lead to a permanent decrease (or change) in protein function, are not subject to modulation, and may lead to degradation of the protein, resulting in a further loss of function. The continuous and dynamic nature of oxidant conditions, together with the ability for oxidants to be localized in their actions, allows for a broad spectrum of cellular effects that range from homeostatic to adaptive to maladaptive. Because ROS and protein OPTM are part of normal cellular homeostasis, treatment strategies that cause a global inhibition of ROS may have undesired effects.

whereas irreversible sulfonylation causes inactivation in response to higher levels of ROS.[183] Diet-induced obesity with resultant cardiomyopathy leads to widespread reversible cysteine OPTM in the heart, especially in mitochondrial proteins.[184] While some of those could be participating in redox signaling, reversible oxidation of C100 and C103 of mitochondrial complex II leads to decrease in its function, which likely contributes to impaired ATP synthesis and cardiac dysfunction observed in this model.[9]

Mitogen-Activated Protein Kinases

Many actions of ROS involve activation of one or more stress-responsive protein kinases in the mitogen-activated protein kinase (MAPK) superfamily, which include the *extracellular signal-regulated kinases (ERK),* the *p38.kinases,* and the *c-Jun N-terminal kinases (JNKs)* that mediate both translational and transcriptional events.[185] The effects of ROS on MAPK signaling appear to be concentration-dependent. Low levels of ROS activate ERK, leading to hypertrophic signaling, whereas higher levels activate the stress-kinases p38 and JNK that are coupled to apoptosis.[168] This pathway can be activated by hypertrophic stimuli such as α-adrenergic receptor stimulation[172] and mechanical strain,[169] leading to oxidation of specific cysteine thiols in Ras and subsequent downstream signaling via the Raf/MEK/ERK. Inhibition of ERK increases the apoptotic response to ROS, suggesting that ERK exerts a prosurvival effect.[174] Apoptosis may involve activation of JNK via ROS-mediated activation of apoptosis signal-regulating kinase 1 (ASK-1).[186-188] ROS-mediated apoptosis may also involve activation of CaMKII via oxidation of methionine residues,[189] leading to apoptosis via p38 kinase.[190]

Mitochondrial Signaling and Energetics (see also Chapter 17)

Mitochondria can be involved in ROS-mediated apoptosis in the heart through the release of cytochrome c from the intermembrane space (**see also Chapter 2**). Cytochrome c activates caspases 9 and 3, and may potentiate mitochondrial generation of ROS through effects on electron transport.[191] The process of cytochrome c release is modulated by the Bcl-2 family of proteins.[192] Proapoptotic members of the Bcl-2 family (Bax, Bad, and Bak) interact with the outer mitochondrial membrane and allow for cytochrome c release and dissipation of the membrane potential through what has been termed the *mitochondrial permeability pore transition.* Antiapoptotic members of the family (e.g., Bcl-2 and Bcl-xL) inhibit Bax-mediated cytochrome c release, caspase-3 activation, and the generation of ROS. In myocytes treated with direct addition of ROS, p53 activity increases in association with translocation of Bax and Bad from the cytosol to the mitochondrial fraction, leading to release of cytochrome c.[193] In contrast, extracellular ROS, and in particular O_2^-, may trigger apoptosis via changes in matrix/integrin interactions.[167]

In addition to being a source of ROS, mitochondria are a target for ROS. Mitochondrial DNA (mtDNA) is very susceptible to ROS damage, in part due to its limited repair activity and the substantial ROS production within the mitochondria in close proximity to mtDNA.[194] Since mtDNA number is a key determinant of gene expression, any reduction or damage to mtDNA may lead to impaired mitochondrial function. In failing myocardium, increased ROS generation was associated with a decrease in mtDNA number with evidence of DNA oxidative damage and impaired mitochondrial function because of decreased ETC activity.[195,196] High levels of oxidative damage to mtDNA can also activate mitochondrial apoptosis pathways.[194] In dogs with HF due to dyssynchronous pacing, mitochondrial ATP synthase activity is decreased in association with OPTM of the α-subunit of ATP synthase at cysteine 294.[197] In obesity-induced cardiomyopathy, decreased ATP synthesis, phosphocreatine content, free energy of

ATP hydrolysis, and impaired activity of ETC complexes were associated with OPTM of the mitochondrial ETC proteins.[9,86,198]

Endoplasmic Reticulum Stress Response

ROS may exert apoptotic effects via ER stress.[199] The ER is a multifunctional cellular organelle responsible for many cellular functions, including posttranslational processing of newly synthesized secretory and membrane proteins, maintenance of calcium homeostasis, and production and storage of macromolecules. A wide range of noxious stimuli, including ROS, hypoxia, ischemia, gene mutation, protein misfolding, and perturbed Ca^{2+} homeostasis, prompt an adaptive process known as the *unfolded protein response* (UPR) that couples the protein load to the folding capacity of the ER.[200] This process promotes the removal of the unfolded proteins to the ubiquitin proteasome for degradation in an attempt to restore cellular homeostasis.[201] If the capacity of UPR to remove unfolded proteins is insufficient, a maladaptive ER overload response (EOR) occurs that is associated with induction of C/EBP homologous protein (CHOP), cleavage of the ER-resident procaspase-12 to active caspase-12, and eventual programmed cell death through the activation of caspases 9 and 3. The UPR and EOR are activated in cardiac hypertrophy and failure.[201-203] Dilated cardiomyopathy occurs in transgenic mice overexpressing a mutant KDEL receptor for ER chaperones that sensitizes the cells to ER stress.[204] The UPR and EOR are activated in an autoimmune cardiomyopathy.[205]

ROS may mediate ER stress/apoptotic signaling via inhibition of antiapoptotic pathways, such as Akt and ARC (apoptosis repressor with caspase recruitment domain). For example, ROS-mediated Akt inactivation is associated with a decrease in prosurvival Bcl proteins[206]; ROS-mediated downregulation of ARC leads to sarcoplasmic reticulum (SR) calcium release with resultant caspase-3 cleavage and apoptosis.[207]

Calcium Handling

Myocytes isolated from the failing heart show markedly abnormal intracellular Ca^{2+} transients along with alterations in the expression and/or activity of Ca^{2+} handling proteins (**see also Chapters 1 and 2**). ROS can regulate the expression and/or activity of key calcium-regulating proteins.[208] The activity of *sarcoplasmic reticulum Ca^{2+}-ATPase (SERCA)* is decreased in the failing heart and appears to contribute to contractile dysfunction. ROS can decrease SERCA2 activity by decreasing protein expression[167] and by altering protein function due to OPTM.[183] Pathologic levels of ROS are associated with irreversible OPTM of SERCA cysteines and tyrosines that are known to inhibit activity. Sulfonylation of SERCA cysteine 674, which inhibits activity, is present in failing hearts due to transgenic Gαq overexpression,[144] aging,[158] and endotoxemia.[209] Transgenic expression of catalase prevented SERCA OPTM and impairment of calcium and myocyte function in the Gαq[144] and aging[158] mice.

ROS may activate the Na^+/Ca^{2+} exchanger,[210] leading to Ca^{2+} overload,[211] and has been implicated in the pathophysiology of myocardial failing.[212] ROS may also regulate the function of the SR *calcium release channel/ryanodine receptor 2 (RyR2)* and the *voltage-dependent Ca^{2+} channel.*[213,214] Oxidation of RyR2 prolongs opening of the channel, leading to increased calcium leaking out of the SR, causing SR calcium depletion and cytoplasmic overload.[215] In addition, oxidation of Ca^{2+} and calmodulin-dependent protein kinase II (CaMKII) leads to excessive enzyme activation, which in turn promotes cardiomyocyte death and HF.[216]

Impaired Energetics (see also Chapter 17)

In addition to profound effects on calcium regulation, oxidative stress has been shown to directly impair the cardiac mitochondrial ATP synthesis machinery. In dogs with HF due to dyssynchronous pacing, mitochondrial ATP synthase activity is decreased, in association with OPTM of the α-subunit of ATP synthase at cysteine 294.[197] In obesity-induced cardiomyopathy, decreased ATP synthesis, phosphocreatine content, free energy of ATP hydrolysis, and impaired activity of ETC complexes were associated with OPTM of the mitochondrial ETC proteins.[9,86,198]

SUMMARY AND FUTURE DIRECTIONS

Oxidative stress is elevated systemically and in the myocardium of patients with chronic myocardial failure. The cause of increased ROS in this setting is not completely understood, but appears multifactorial, including increased production of ROS because of increased metabolic activity, stimulated production by mechanical strain, neurohormonal activation, inflammatory cytokines, as well as decreased antioxidant activity. Based on in vitro and in vivo studies, it appears likely that increases in oxidative stress contribute to the ventricular remodeling and contractile dysfunction in the failing heart.

ROS exert many effects on myocardial structure and function. It is clear that oxidative stress can trigger a range of responses in myocytes in vitro, and that similar responses may occur in vivo in situations, leading to myocardial dysfunction. As in other tissues, oxidative stress can stimulate both the growth and death of cells. The mechanism by which various ROS activate cell signaling pathways remains an area of active investigation, and promises to offer new therapeutic targets for pharmacologic antioxidants. Our understanding of the precise mechanistic pathways and targets affected by oxidative stress in HF grows, but are yet to be reliably translated into human therapeutics.

There remain many unanswered questions about the role of oxidative stress in myocardial failure. In addition, the results of applying preclinical observations to develop therapeutic strategies for patients with HF have been disappointing. In developing therapeutic strategies targeted specifically at oxidative stress, we will need to understand in more detail (1) the relative contributions of decreased antioxidant activity versus increased formation of ROS; (2) the situations in which oxidative and/or nitrosative stress contribute to the pathogenesis of myocardial dysfunction in vivo; (3) the precise ROS involved; and (4) the optimal place in ROS cascades to intervene.

KEY REFERENCES

1. Brown DI, Griendling KK. Regulation of signal transduction by reactive oxygen species in the cardiovascular system. *Circ Res.* 2015;116:531–549.
7. Dai DF, Johnson SC, Villarin JJ, et al. Mitochondrial oxidative stress mediates angiotensin II-induced cardiac hypertrophy and Galphaq overexpression-induced heart failure. *Circ Res.* 2011;108:837–846.
9. Sverdlov AL, Elezaby A, Qin F, et al. Mitochondrial reactive oxygen species mediate cardiac structural, functional, and mitochondrial consequences of diet-induced metabolic heart disease. *J Am Heart Assoc.* 2016;5.
40. Bishu K, Deswal A, Chen HH, et al. Biomarkers in acutely decompensated heart failure with preserved or reduced ejection fraction. *Am Heart J.* 2012;164:763–770.e3.
58. Zhang M, Perino A, Ghigo A, Hirsch E, Shah AM. NADPH oxidases in heart failure: poachers or gamekeepers? *Antioxid Redox Signal.* 2013;18:1024–1041.
76. Brown DA, Perry JB, Allen ME, et al. Expert consensus document: mitochondrial function as a therapeutic target in heart failure. *Nat Rev Cardiol.* 2017;14:238–250.
107. Takimoto E, Kass DA. Role of oxidative stress in cardiac hypertrophy and remodeling. *Hypertension.* 2007;49:241–248.
165. Okonko DO, Shah AM. Heart failure: mitochondrial dysfunction and oxidative stress in CHF. *Nat Rev Cardiol.* 2015;12:6–8.
182. Kumar V, Calamaras TD, Haeussler D, et al. Cardiovascular redox and ox stress proteomics. *Antioxid Redox Signal.* 2012;17:1528–1559.
208. Wagner S, Rokita AG, Anderson ME, Maier LS. Redox regulation of sodium and calcium handling. *Antioxid Redox Signal.* 2013;18:1063–1077.

The full reference list for this chapter is available on ExpertConsult.

Natriuretic Peptides in Heart Failure: Pathophysiologic and Therapeutic Implications

Nina Dzhoyashvili, John C. Burnett

NATRIURETIC PEPTIDES: HISTORICAL BACKGROUND

The discovery of natriuretic peptides (NPs) changed the classical paradigm of the heart as solely a pump and developed the novel concept of the heart as an endocrine organ. The current and potential applications of NPs in clinical practice and medical research are endless. Currently, NPs remain the "gold standard" for the diagnosis and prognosis of heart failure (HF) and the evaluation of HF treatment efficacy. The NP story began in the 1950s when Gauer and his coworkers reported that distension of the left atrium after the expansion of an intra-atrial balloon resulted in a prompt diuresis linking this physiologic effect to the changes in circulating blood volume.[1] Concurrently, Kisch first described specific dense homogenous granules in atria using a new electron microscopy technique,[2] and Jamieson and Palade revealed the secretory nature of these granules.[3] Later, Poche found that the number of granules depends on water intake.[4] Indeed, Marie and colleagues confirmed that salt and water intake increases the numbers of granules in the atrial cardiomyocytes.[5] In cross-circulation experiments in canines, De Wardner described the humoral nature of a substance with natriuretic properties.[6] Although the presence of the "specific atrial granules" and their secretory phenotype were confirmed, the function of these storage granules remained a mystery.

In 1981 de Bold et al. performed the groundbreaking experiment that showed that the injection of atrial homogenates causes rapid renal sodium and water excretion and the reduction of blood pressure.[7] Interestingly, the manuscript describing for the first time natriuretic, diuretic, and vasodilatory properties of atrial natriuretic peptide (ANP) was initially rejected by the journal to which the study was submitted. Following this landmark study several individual groups purified, sequenced, and synthesized ANP.[8-11] Therefore ANP became the first peptide hormone isolated from the heart (**Fig. 9.1**). B-type NP (BNP), originally named brain-type natriuretic peptide, was first isolated from porcine brain tissues in 1988.[12] Further studies revealed that BNP is also synthesized by both atrial and ventricular cardiomyocytes and like ANP is responsive to mechanical stretch.[13,14] The discovery of ANP and BNP is considered a fundamental advance in the field of cardiovascular biology and has tremendously impacted HF treatment and diagnostics.

Urodilatin (URO) is a molecular form of ANP derived from the ANP prohormone proANP and processed in the kidney, resulting in a more renal-specific NP. C-type NP (CNP), a third peptide in NP family, was first extracted from porcine brain and then from endothelial cells.[15] CNP, like ANP, URO, and BNP, has a similar but distinct 17–amino acid disulfide bridge ring and is synthesized in vascular endothelium. Finally, the concept of the heart as an endocrine organ was importantly solidified by the landmark work of Murad's group, which identified 3′,5′-cyclic guanosine monophosphate (cGMP) as the second messenger of ANP, and seminal studies identified particulate guanylyl cyclase receptors (pGC-A and pGC-B) as the targets of ANP, URO, BNP, and CNP.[16,17]

The therapeutic effects of NPs have been widely applied in patients with acute decompensated heart failure (ADHF) (**see Chapter 36**). Synthetic ANP (Carperitide) and synthetic BNP (Nesiritide) have been approved in several countries for the treatment of HF. Carperitide was approved for the clinical management of ADHF in Japan in 1995. Nesiritide was considered as a first line therapeutic agent for ADHF. Initial clinical trials revealed that Nesiritide significantly led to beneficial hemodynamic and natriuretic effects, reduced pulmonary capillary wedge pressure, and increased cardiac output.[18,19] The Natrecor Study Group has also confirmed the beneficial hemodynamic effects of Nesiritide in patients with ADHF.[20] Moreover, Nesiritide was associated with significantly lower mortality than dobutamine in the PRECEDENT (Prospective, Randomized Evaluation of Cardiac Ectopy with Dobutamine or Natrecor Therapy) study,[21] caused a faster and greater improvement in pulmonary capillary wedge pressure compared with intravenous nitroglycerin.[22,23] Due to these results of the clinical trials, Nesiritide was approved for the treatment of ADHF in 2001 by the US Food and Drug Administration (FDA) and marketed under the trade name Natrecor.[24] However, meta-analysis of Natrecor clinical trials by Sackner-Bernstein raised concerns about Nesiritide-associated mortality and renal dysfunction in patients with ADHF.[25,26] These reports significantly contributed to a decline in both prescriptions and Nesiritide sales. The controversy between defenders of nesiritide, including its manufacturer, Johnson & Johnson, and their opponents was finally resolved by the Acute Study of Clinical Effectiveness of Nesiritide in Decompensated Heart Failure (ASCEND-HF) trial.[27] The trial included 7141 patients with ADHF who received continuous intravenous infusion of Nesiritide or placebo. Results showed that there were no significant differences in the

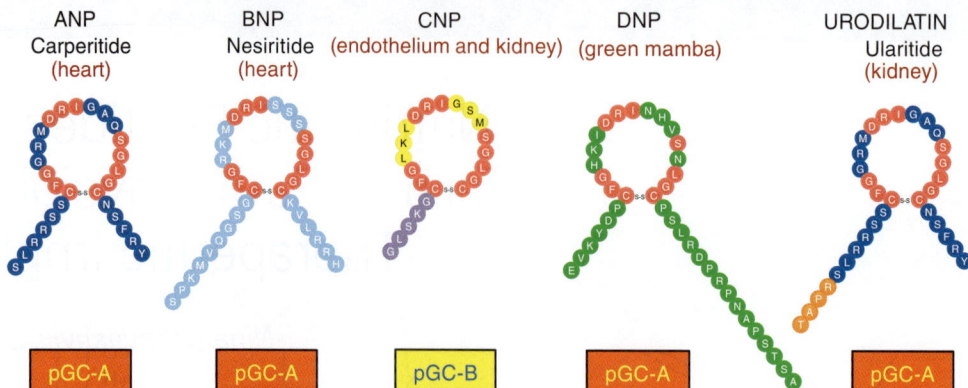

Fig. 9.1 Natriuretic peptides. Atrial natriuretic peptide *(ANP)*, B-type natriuretic peptide *(BNP)*, urodilatin, and *Dendroaspis* natriuretic peptide *(DNP)* bind to guanylyl cyclase A *(GC-A)*. C-type natriuretic peptide *(CNP)* binds to guanylyl cyclase B *(GC-B)*, ANP, BNP, CNP, and urodilatin are found in humans; DNP is found in the venom of the green mamba snake.

TABLE 9.1	General Characteristics of Natriuretic Peptides		
Characteristics	**ANP**	**BNP**	**CNP**
Gene	NPPA	NPPB	NPPC
Precursor	PreproANP (1–151)	PreproBNP (1–134)	PreproCNP (1–126)
Prohormone	ProANP (26–151)	ProBNP (27–134)	ProCNP (24–126)
Mature protein	NT-proANP (26–123)	NT-proBNP (27–102)	CNP-53 (74–126)
	ANP-28 (124–151)	BNP-32 (103–134)	CNP-22 (105–126)
Molecular weight of active peptide	3080.5	3464.05	CNP-53 (5801.7)
			CNP-22 (2197.63)
Clearance mechanisms	Neutral endopeptidase;	Neutral endopeptidase;	Neutral endopeptidase;
	NPR-C	NPR-C	NPR-C
Circulating half-life	3 min	20 min	3 min
Predominant tissue expression	Atrial cardiomyocytes	Ventricular cardiomyocytes	Vascular endothelium; Kidney

ANP, Atrial natriuretic peptide; *BNP*, B-type natriuretic peptide; *CNP*, C-type natriuretic peptide; *NPPA*, ANP gene; *NPPB*, BNP gene; *NPPC*, CNP gene; *NPR*, natriuretic peptide receptor.

incidence of death or renal injury. On the other side, the trial also showed no significant differences in the end point of dyspnea. In addition, standard doses of Nesiritide caused symptomatic and asymptomatic hypotension. Finally, Nesiritide was not recommended for routine treatment of ADHF. This information was important for further development of chimeric NP designs specifically for the treatment and prevention of HF.

GENERAL OVERVIEW OF NATRIURETIC PEPTIDE SYSTEM

The pharmacologic actions of NPs are based on interaction between specific molecular amino acid sequences in naturally occurring NPs and respective receptors (see Fig. 9.1 and **Table 9.1**). NPs all possess a similar but distinct 17–amino acid ring formed by an intramolecular disulfide bridge. This ring structure is essential for exerting biologic activity. ANP is synthesized and stored within atrial cardiomyocytes as a 151–amino acid preproANP peptide which is cleaved to generate 126–amino acid proANP. ANP is stored in atrial cardiomyocytes in granules as proANP.[28] Studies have established that the atrium is the major site of ANP synthesis in which the level of ANP mRNA expression is 100-fold higher than in the ventricles.[29] ANP is synthesized and stored within atrial cardiomyocytes as a 151–amino acid preproANP peptide which is cleaved to generate 126–amino acid proANP. When atrial myocytes are stretched, proANP is cleaved by corin, a myocardium-specific type II transmembrane protease, into the nonbiologically active N-terminus of pro-ANP and the biologically active C-terminal 28–amino acid ANP.[30] Corin is also involved in

BNP processing, which is initially synthesized as 134-amino acid preproBNP. After processing by corin or intracellular Golgi-localized protease furin, a low level of proBNP can be stored along with ANP in the atrial-specific granules.[31] In contrast to ANP, BNP is predominantly secreted by ventricular myocardium and is constitutively released. Both ANP and BNP are secreted in response to myocardial stretch induced by volume or hemodynamic overload.[32-34] Upon release into the circulation, proBNP is converted to a 76–amino acid inactive N-terminal fragment of proBNP and biologically active C-terminal 32–amino acid BNP.[35] The lack of ANP in genetically modified mice may lead to chronic hypertension, cardiac dilation, hypertrophy, fibrosis, and HF.[36] Mice lacking BNP do not develop cardiac hypertrophy or hypertension but display cardiac fibrosis that leads to ventricular stiffness, altered chamber compliance, and contractile dysfunction.[37] In the cardiovascular system, CNP can be produced in the myocardium but at low levels, and highly expressed in vascular endothelium. PreproCNP is a 126–amino acid peptide, which is cleaved by a signal peptidase to form 103–amino acid proCNP. The latter is cleaved by furin to produce the biologically active 22–amino acid CNP and a larger 53–amino acid inactive fragment.[38] Defects in CNP production lead to endothelial dysfunction, hypertension, atherogenesis, and aneurysm formation,[39] and reduced ability of CNP to activate pGC-B leads to hypertension, tachycardia, and impaired left ventricular systolic function.[40] Plasma CNP is also elevated in patients with HF, although its level is lower compared with ANP and BNP.[41-43] Due to increased expression levels of pGC-B in HF, CNP may exert cardioprotective action against myocardial injury.[44] Less information is known about the processing of URO.

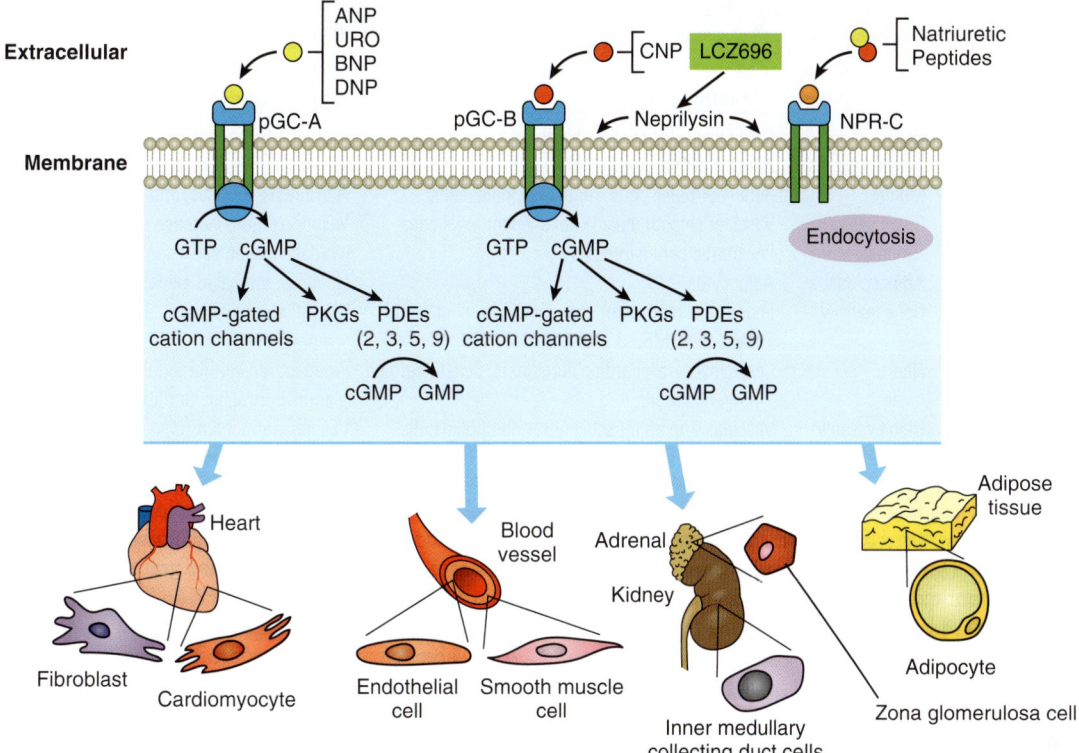

Fig. 9.2 Natriuretic peptide, receptor, and biologic targets: Particulate *(pGCA)* guanylyl cyclase signaling pathways. Natriuretic peptides bind to GC-A and/or GC-B (membrane-bound pGCs) and activate the signaling pathways of *(GC)* cyclic guanosine monophosphate *(cGMP)*. Once the intracellular concentration of cGMP increases, cGMP-gated cation channels, cGMP-dependent protein kinases, and phosphodiesterases generate important biologic responses in different tissues. *ANP,* Atrial natriuretic peptide; *BNP,* B-type natriuretic peptide; *CD-NP,* CD natriuretic peptide; *CNP,* C-type natriuretic peptide; *CU-NP,* CU natriuretic peptide; *DNP, Dendroaspis* natriuretic peptide; *GC-A,* particulate guanylyl cyclase A; *GC-B,* particulate guanylyl cyclase B; *GTP,* guanosine triphosphate; *NPR,* natriuretic peptide receptor; *PDEs,* phosphodiesterases; *PKGs,* cGMP-dependent protein kinases; *URO,* Urodilatin.

As introduced previously, NPs act via transmembrane GC-coupled receptors. The receptors pGC-A and pGC-B are composed of an extracellular domain, which binds endogenous ligands, a single transmembrane region, a kinase homology domain, and intracellular catalytic domain with GC activity (**Fig. 9.2**). The pGC-A receptor mediates the physiologic action of ANP and BNP by generating the intracellular secondary messenger cGMP, which acts on cGMP-dependent protein kinase, or protein kinase G (PKG), cGMP-gated ion channels, and cGMP-regulated phosphodiesterases (PDEs). Studies have established that pGC-A is mostly expressed in kidneys, vascular smooth muscle, endothelium, heart, and adrenals, as well as adipocytes. The pGC-B receptor is predominantly expressed in the brain, kidney, heart, lung, and bone.

NPR-C mediates the clearance of NPs through an internalization and degradation process.[45] NPR-C is expressed in several tissues, including kidneys, endothelium, heart, lungs, and adrenals.[46] Although NPR-C is mainly known as a receptor involving in NP clearance from the circulation by receptor-mediated endocytosis, key studies have reported NPR-C–mediated inhibition of endothelial and vascular smooth muscle cell (VSMC) proliferation. Moreover, NPR-C may be involved in modulating coronary endothelial cell permeability[47] and may be a target of CNP in modulating vascular tone.[39] In addition to proteolytic inactivation and NPR-C–mediated clearance, enzymatic pathways clear the NPs. Specifically, NPs can be cleaved by the zinc metalloprotease insulin-degrading enzyme[48] and by the membrane-bound zinc-dependent enzyme

neutral endopeptidase or neprilysin (NEP), which plays a critical role both in regulating NP levels and also serving as a therapeutic target.[49]

From a physiologic perspective, a growing concept is that the NP/pGC/cGMP system plays an important role in the long-term regulation of sodium and water balance and blood pressure homeostasis. An additional new role for the NP system is in metabolic regulation. In key genetic epidemiology studies, genetic variants of the ANP and BNP genes in which circulating ANP or BNP may be elevated, the phenotype is one of lower blood pressure, reduced risk for hypertension, and protection from obesity and metabolic syndrome.[50,51] From studies in genetically altered mice and physiologic and pharmacologic studies in animals and humans, the key biologic properties of NPs are summarized in **Table 9.2** and include inhibition of myocardial hypertrophy, organ fibrosis, maintenance of the endothelial barrier, vasorelaxation, natriuresis including an increase in glomerular filtration rate (GFR) and a decrease in proximal tubule reabsorption, suppression of aldosterone, and lipolysis.[52-54]

NATRIURETIC PEPTIDE SYSTEM IN HEART FAILURE: PATHOPHYSIOLOGY, DIAGNOSTICS, AND TREATMENT

HF in advanced stages is characterized by renal retention of sodium and water together with systemic and renal vasoconstriction and myocardial remodeling. The disease involves the prolonged activation of

TABLE 9.2   Natriuretic Peptide System Activation in Different Target Organs

Receptor	Ligand	Main Tissue Distribution	Specific Cells	Physiologic Actions
pGC-A	ANP, BNP	Heart	Cardiomyocytes cardiac fibroblasts,	Antiremodeling, antihypertrophy
		Adrenal glands	Adrenal glomerulosa cells	Inhibition of aldosterone synthesis and RAAS
		Kidney	Renal epithelial cells, renal mesangial cells	Natriuresis, diuresis, anti-inflammatory
		Blood vessels	Vascular smooth muscle cells, endothelial cells	Vasorelaxation, increase endothelial permeability
		Pancreas	Pancreatic beta islet cells	Increase insulin secretion
		Adipose tissue	Adipocytes	Lipolysis, fatty acid oxidation, WAT browning
		Bone marrow	Endothelial progenitor cells (EPCs), mesenchymal stem cells (MSCs)	Migration, proliferation, angiogenesis, tissue regeneration
pGC-B	CNP	Heart	Cardiomyocytes, cardiac fibroblasts, Sca-1+ cardiac progenitor cells	Proapoptotic, antiremodeling, antiproliferative, antihypertrophic, antifibrotic, myocardium regeneration
		Blood vessels	Vascular smooth muscle cells, endothelial cells	Vasorelaxation, antiremodeling
		Cartilage	Chondrocytes	Endochondral growth
		Nervous system	Stellate sympathetic neurons	Reduces cardiac sympathetic neurotransmission; suppresses food intake and regulate energy homeostasis
NPRC	ANP, BNP, CNP	All organs		Modulates NP biologic effects via natriuretic peptide clearance
		Heart	Cardiomyocytes and cardiac fibroblasts	Antiproliferative
		Kidney	Glomerular podocytes, glomerular mesangial cells, medullary interstitial cells	Regulate diuresis, natriuresis and blood volume
		Blood vessels	Vascular smooth cells, endothelial cells	Vasorelaxation, antiproliferative, antiremodeling
		Cartilage	Chondrocytes	Chondrocyte differentiation and bone growth

ANP, Atrial natriuretic peptide; *BNP*, B-type natriuretic peptide; *CNP*, C-type natriuretic peptide; *NPRC*, natriuretic peptide receptor-C; *pGC-A*, particulate guanylyl cyclase A; *RAAS*, renin-angiotensin-aldosterone system; *WAT*, white adipose tissue.

the sympathetic nervous system (SNS) (**see Chapters 6 and 13**) and renin-angiotensin-aldosterone system (RAAS) (**see Chapter 5**) that together contribute to the worsening of HF. The NP/pGC/cGMP system plays a counterregulatory role to all of these deleterious hallmarks of chronic HF.[55]

Although the NP system mediates beneficial actions in HF, especially in the early stages of HF, it is important to recognize that an "NP resistance" or "NP paradox" exists in which, despite elevation of circulating NPs in HF, there is overt HF with salt and water retention, activation of RAAS and SNS, and progressive myocardial failure and remodeling. This "resistance" or "paradox" in part is a result of abnormal molecular forms of circulating NPs, as well as increased activity of NEP and NPR-C, which may contribute to decreased efficacy of NPs. Importantly, reductions of NP convertases affect proNP processing and contribute to HF progression by reducing the processing of proNPs to biologically active NPs. Ichiki and colleagues found in a canine model of HF that the level of corin gene and protein expression decreased in HF.[56] Tripathi et al. showed in a mouse model of cardiomyopathy that cardiac corin gene expression was reduced in experimental HF and remained low during HF progression, whereas cardiac ANP and BNP gene expression and plasma levels increased only at the terminal stage of HF.[57] In human HF, Dong and colleagues confirmed that plasma corin levels were significantly reduced in HF.[58] Similarly, Ibebuogu and associates revealed that patients with HF have significantly low levels of plasma corin and higher levels of plasma uncleaved proANP.[59] This implies that impaired cleavage of proANP and reduced effectiveness of corin may contribute to the progression of HF. In addition, Zhou et al. suggested that low level of corin might be associated with higher risk of major adverse cardiovascular events, HF progression, and poor prognosis.[60] Interestingly, the authors also stated that plasma corin levels are significantly reduced in female patients. This

may indicate the presence of sex differences in the pathogenesis of HF as it relates to NPs. This study also suggested that the patients with higher corin-mediated processing of NP precursors might have better outcomes. It should also be noted that proBNP, also due to reduced processing by corin, is the predominant molecular form of immunoreactive BNP detected by clinical assays for BNP. Importantly, Huntley et al. recently tested the bioactivity of proBNP in activating the pGC-A receptor in human kidney cells. They reported that proBNP was markedly reduced in its potency to activate pGC-A and the second messenger cGMP.[61]

Additional mechanisms for impaired NP bioactivity in HF also include furin-mediated processing of NPs and NP glycosylation.[62] Nagai-Okatani and Minamino were the first who reported the mechanism of O-glycosylation of human proBNP. This study demonstrated that the upregulation of mucin-type O-glycosylation may contribute to the increase in sialylated O-glycan at Thr71, close to the processing site of proBNP, resulting in the inhibition of the binding of furin and the conversion of proBNP to bioactive BNP.[63]

It is now recognized that patients with HF may have higher concentration of circulating soluble NEP.[64] NEP is an integral type II, membrane-bound, zinc-dependent endopeptidase. NEP is found in high concentrations in kidneys and also in brain, lung, endothelial, and blood cells. NEP cleaves and degrades ANP, BNP, and CNP, as well as bradykinin, substance P, adrenomedullin, and vasoactive intestinal peptide.[65] The enzyme has an ectodomain, presenting the catalytic site, a transmembrane domain, and a short intracellular domain. NEP cleaves peptides with a molecular weight at 3000 Da or less and attacks peptides at the amino side of hydrophobic amino acids, with a preference for Phe or Leu, releasing di or tripeptides from the carboxy-terminus of peptides.[66] Thus enhanced NEP activity increases enzymatic clearance of the NPs, thus limiting their beneficial actions. From a biologic prospective, the clearance and degradation of NPs by NEP has led to the concept that the inhibition of NEP may enhance the activity of NPs and result in better regulation of sodium and water balance in HF. Previously, Martin and coworkers demonstrated that chronic oral administration of the NEP inhibitor (NEPi) Candoxatril prolongs the compensated phase of experimental early chronic HF. The treatment with NEPi led to enhanced renal actions of NPs, prevented sodium retention, and suppressed the activation of aldosterone.[67] However, the inhibition of NEP alone not only increases NP levels, but also raises the levels of circulating vasopressors, angiotensin II and endothelin I, that weaken the beneficial effect of the NPs. As a consequence, NEPi alone had little effect in patients with HF.[68] Therefore NEPi together with blockers of RAAS can potentially improve the treatment efficacy and prognosis of HF (see also Chapter 37).

Omapatrilat (OMA) was the first drug in this group that was extensively studied in several randomized clinical trials. Specifically, OMA was a single small molecule that could inhibit NEP but also angiotensin-converting enzyme (ACE), becoming a dual NEP/ACE inhibitor (NEPi/ACEi). Inhibition of Metalloprotease by Omapatrilat in a Randomized Exercise and Symptoms Study in Heart Failure (IMPRESS) showed an improved hemodynamic profile with OMA in patients with HF with reduced ejection fraction (HFrEF) when compared with ACEi, lisinopril, alone.[69] The Omapatrilat Versus Enalapril Randomized Trial of Utility in Reducing Events (OVERTURE) trial showed no significant difference between OMA and enalapril in reducing the primary end point of combined all-cause mortality and hospitalizations in patients with New York Heart Association (NYHA) class II to IV HF, although post hoc analysis revealed a strong signal for improvement with OMA. However, treatment with OMA caused a higher incidence of angioedema (0.8%) compared with the enalapril group (0.5%).[70]

Although both ACEi and angiotensin receptor blockers (ARBs) are considered first-line drugs in HF, ARBs do not inhibit the degradation of kinins, therefore reducing the risk of angioedema. It was considered logical to develop the next OMA-like drug based on the combination of ARBs and NEPi, a class that is now called ARNI. The novel drug Entresto (LCZ696), a combination of the ARB valsartan and the NEPi sacubitril, has been first compared with valsartan alone in the Prospective comparison of ARNI with ARB on Management of Heart Failure with Preserved Ejection Fraction (PARAMOUNT) trial in patients with HF with preserved ejection fraction (HFpEF) (see Chapter 39). The treatment with LCZ696 caused decreases in left atrial size and volume, as well as in more significant decline in N-terminal proBNP (NT-proBNP).[71] The Prospective Comparison of LCZ696 with ARB Global Outcome in HF with Preserved Ejection Fraction (PARAGON-HF) trial is currently underway and aims to evaluate the effect of LCZ696 compared with valsartan in the reduction of cardiovascular death and hospitalizations in patients with HFpEF. In the landmark study Prospective Comparison of ARNI with ACEI to Determine Impact on Global Mortality and Morbidity in Heart Failure (PARADIGM-HF) led by McMurray and associates in collaboration with scientists at Novartis, LCZ696 was compared with enalapril in patients with HFrEF. The study was stopped early because of significant reduction in HF hospitalization and a significant survival rate in the ARNI group (see Chapter 37). Although there was a nonsignificant trend for an increase for symptomatic hypotension and angioedema, this did not lead to serious cases or drug discontinuation.[72]

Although increased circulating NPs may have biologic significance as a compensatory mechanism in HF to oppose the deleterious RAAS and SNS pathways, plasma levels of BNP and NT-proBNP are powerful biomarkers for prognosis and risk stratification of HF, in addition to aiding in HF diagnosis.[73-75] The levels of BNP and NT-proBNP are strongly correlated to clinical status and survival rate of patients. Moreover, BNP and NT-proBNP may play a role in the medical management of HF both in guiding therapy and assessing the efficacy of therapy. This is discussed in greater detail in Chapter 33, which focuses on biomarkers and precision medicine.

The fact that the NP system counteracts the adverse effects of RAAS and other neurohumoral systems in HF as a key compensatory mechanism together with possible impaired bioavailability, as discussed previously, provides a powerful rationale for the development of NP-based HF therapy. Increasing the activity of NP or reducing their degradation may achieve a more favorable balance between RAAS/SNS and the NP system and therefore mediate beneficial actions on cardiorenal function and structure positively impacting outcomes, as was seen in the PARADIGM-HF trial.[72] Furthermore, the use of long-term NP therapy has also had positive outcomes in chronic HF. Specifically, Chen et al. reported that 8 weeks of twice-daily administration of subcutaneously administered BNP to patients with NYHA class III HF resulted in symptom improvement, reduced plasma renin activity, and improved myocardial structure and function with preservation of renal function.[76] Most recently, novel peptide-based NP therapies have emerged that go beyond the properties of the naturally occurring NPs and possess greater resistance to degradation by NEP. This is discussed next.

NOVEL DESIGNER NATRIURETIC PEPTIDES IN THE THERAPY OF HEART FAILURE

Advances in peptide engineering have resulted in the design, synthesis, and investigation of chimeric designer NPs.[77] It is increasingly recognized that peptide therapeutics permit a more targeted approaches through well-characterized receptors and molecular pathways, thus avoiding off-target actions associated with small molecules. Peptides also possess larger surface area than small molecules, which may optimize receptor activation. However, a limitation to peptide therapies is rapid degradation such as NEP, therefore limiting the bioavailability of peptides as compared with small molecules.

Breakthroughs in peptide engineering have accelerated peptide therapeutics in disease areas other than HF and include novel glucagon-like peptide (GLP)-1 receptor activators for diabetes; in human immunodeficiency virus (HIV), peptides target novel molecular markers; and more recently in cardiovascular (CV) disease we have seen the use of peptides such as seralaxin. Indeed, insights into peptide and receptor biology may result in peptide modifications resulting in innovative peptide analogues with enhanced activity and attractive properties.

Cenderitide is the most clinically advanced designer NP. Cenderitide (CD-NP) peptide fuses the 15–amino acid C-terminus of Dendroaspis natriuretic peptide (DNP), a pGC-A activator, isolated from the venom of the green mamba to the 22–amino acid human C-type NP, the latter a pGC-B activator (Fig. 9.3).[78] Thus Cenderitide is the only known NP that uniquely binds to both NP receptors (pGC-A and pGC-B) and consequently activates the second messenger cGMP through two separate and complementary receptor signaling pathways.[79] Moreover, Cenderitide is more resistant to NEP-mediated degradation due to the longer C-terminus.[80] A goal in the engineering of Cenderitide was to develop a less hypotensive NP as CNP/pGC-B has minimal action on blood pressure while lacking renal and RAAS-modulating action together with natriuretic and RAAS-suppressing actions of DNP/pGC-A activation. Such a dual receptor targeting property is also supported by the report by Ichiki et al. that myocardial production of CNP is reduced in human HF, whereas expression of pGC-B is preserved.[81] Thus such design and properties of Cenderitide may lead to enhanced cardiovascular and renal effects without causing profound

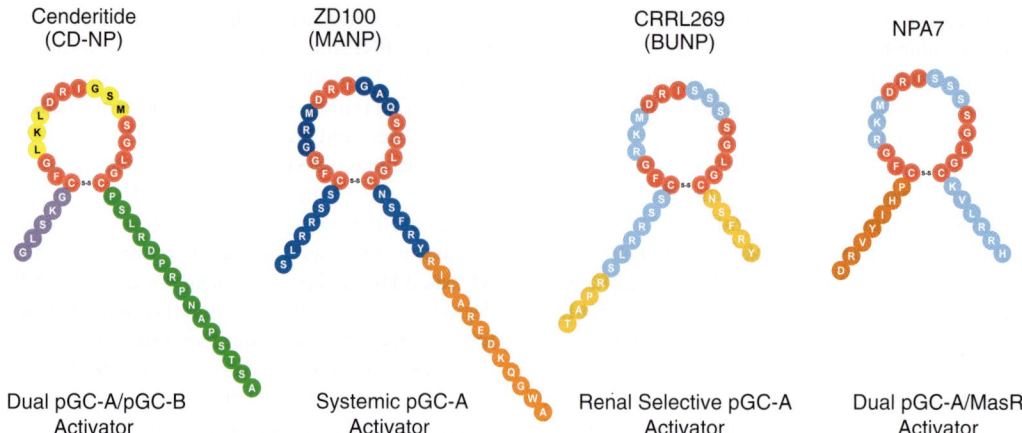

Fig. 9.3 Structures of designer natriuretic peptides *(NP)*: CD-NP (Cenderitide); MANP (ZD100); NPA7; CRRL269. *GC-A*, particulate guanylyl cyclase A; *GC-B*, particulate guanylyl cyclase B *MANP*, mutant atrial natriuretic peptide.

hypotension, which is the common side effect of recombinant ANP and BNP, because the avoidance of profound hypotension is the main concern in treating HF.[82] Importantly, Lee and associates demonstrated in healthy volunteers that Cenderitide activates cGMP, increases renal sodium excretion, and inhibits RAAS without clinically significant hypotension.[83] Kawakami et al. reported that, in a study of safety and tolerability, acute intravenous infusion of Cenderitide in subjects with stable HF and reduced EF was safe and well tolerated. Without hypotension, the drug also activated plasma and urinary cGMP.[84]

Although clinical studies of Cenderitide currently are focusing on HFpEF, Martin and colleagues reported the myocardial actions of chronic Cenderitide in an experimental model of early cardiac fibrosis and impaired diastolic function induced by unilateral nephrectomy to mimic mild chronic kidney disease (CKD).[85] Importantly, Cenderitide suppressed cardiac fibrosis and preserved diastolic function. The investigators suggested that such cardioprotective effect is related to pGC-A–mediated antiapoptotic and aldosterone-suppressing properties of Cenderitide. In addition and most importantly, pGC-B–mediated inhibition by Cenderitide of fibroblast proliferation may also contribute to the attenuation of cardiac fibrosis and remodeling, as supported by the direct antifibrotic actions of Cenderitide in human cardiac fibroblasts.[81]

Therefore human and animal studies demonstrate that Cenderitide is safe and improves cardiovascular and renal function without inducing significant levels of hypotension. Future clinical trials are needed to further assess the therapeutic effect of Cenderitide in patients with HF, including those with either HFrEF or HFpEF.

Mutant ANP (MANP) is a novel designer NP developed by fusing native 28–amino acid ANP to a unique 12–amino acid carboxyl terminal extension (see Fig. 9.3).[86] Similar to Cenderitide, MANP is highly resistant to degradation by NEP, in contrast to ANP, due to the unique 12–amino acid C-terminal extension.[87] MANP, like ANP, activates pGC-A. Thus MANP may be considered a biologically enhanced ANP-based analogue. Previously, McKie and colleagues reported that MANP exerts significantly greater plasma cGMP activation, higher diuretic and natriuretic activities, stronger GFR enhancing and RAAS inhibiting actions, better cardiac unloading, and larger blood pressure-lowering effects when compared with native ANP.[86] Thus MANP may improve cardiac function through enhancing cardiovascular and kidney function and promoting antihypertrophic, antifibrotic, and antiproliferative actions via direct actions on cardiomyocytes and fibroblasts and also via RAAS suppression. Together, these properties make MANP highly attractive in the treatment of HF. Indeed, in a

model of acute hypertensive HF, MANP compared with cGMP-activating drug nitroglycerine infusion was more cardiorenal protective and RAAS suppressing **(Fig. 9.4)**.[88] To date, the therapeutic potential of MANP in human HF remains unexplored, and further studies are warranted to better define the cardiorenal actions of MANP in HF.

We proposed a new first-in-class innovative cardiorenal protective NP, NPA7, which may be highly effective in the treatment of HF.[89] NPA7 uniquely targets pGC-A and Mas receptors that activate the NP/pGC-A/cGMP and ANG1-7/MasR/cAMP receptor pathways (see Fig. 9.3). The rationale to the design of NPA7 is that the simultaneous activation of two pathways may have synergistic actions resulting in greater antiinflammatory and antiapoptotic activities, stronger cardiorenal protective effects, and more significant inhibition of RAAS when compared with pGC-A or MasR activation alone. More recently, we showed that NPA7 in combination with furosemide showed renoprotective properties in a canine model of HF.[89] Experimental HF animals received NPA7 followed by furosemide infusion, or furosemide followed by NPA7, respectively. Hemodynamics, plasma Ang II, and plasma aldosterone were measured, and cardiorenal function was assessed. The results showed that NPA7 significantly decreased systemic vascular resistance and increased urinary flow and urinary sodium excretion. Although furosemide was natriuretic and diuretic, it significantly impaired renal hemodynamics and activated RAAS. Importantly, the combination of NPA7 with furosemide showed renal enhancing and synergistic natriuretic and diuretic efficacy while preserving GFR. In addition, interestingly, the optimal renal-enhancing action was observed with NPA7 pretreatment and less after furosemide pretreatment followed by NPA7 infusion. Furosemide is effective in providing symptomatic relief and remains the first-line therapy for HF patients with congestion. However, furosemide is associated with significant renal impairment, vasoconstriction, and RAAS activation. Therefore a strategy of pretreatment with NPA7 may enhance natriuresis and diuresis while preserving kidney function. Combination therapy including pretreatment with NPA7 may represent a novel cardiorenal protective strategy for the treatment of HF patients. Further studies are warranted to detail efficacy of NPA7 in HF.

CRRL269 (BUNP) is a novel renal-selective pGC-A–activating designer peptide, which has been recently engineered, synthesized, and investigated in vitro and in vivo with a goal of its potential as a peptide therapeutic for the cardiorenal syndrome (CRS) and acute kidney injury (AKI) (see Fig. 9.3).[90] BUNP integrates key amino acids (AAs) of BNP and urodilatin (URO). Because of such structure, BUNP possesses higher potency in terms of pGC-A activation and cGMP generation than

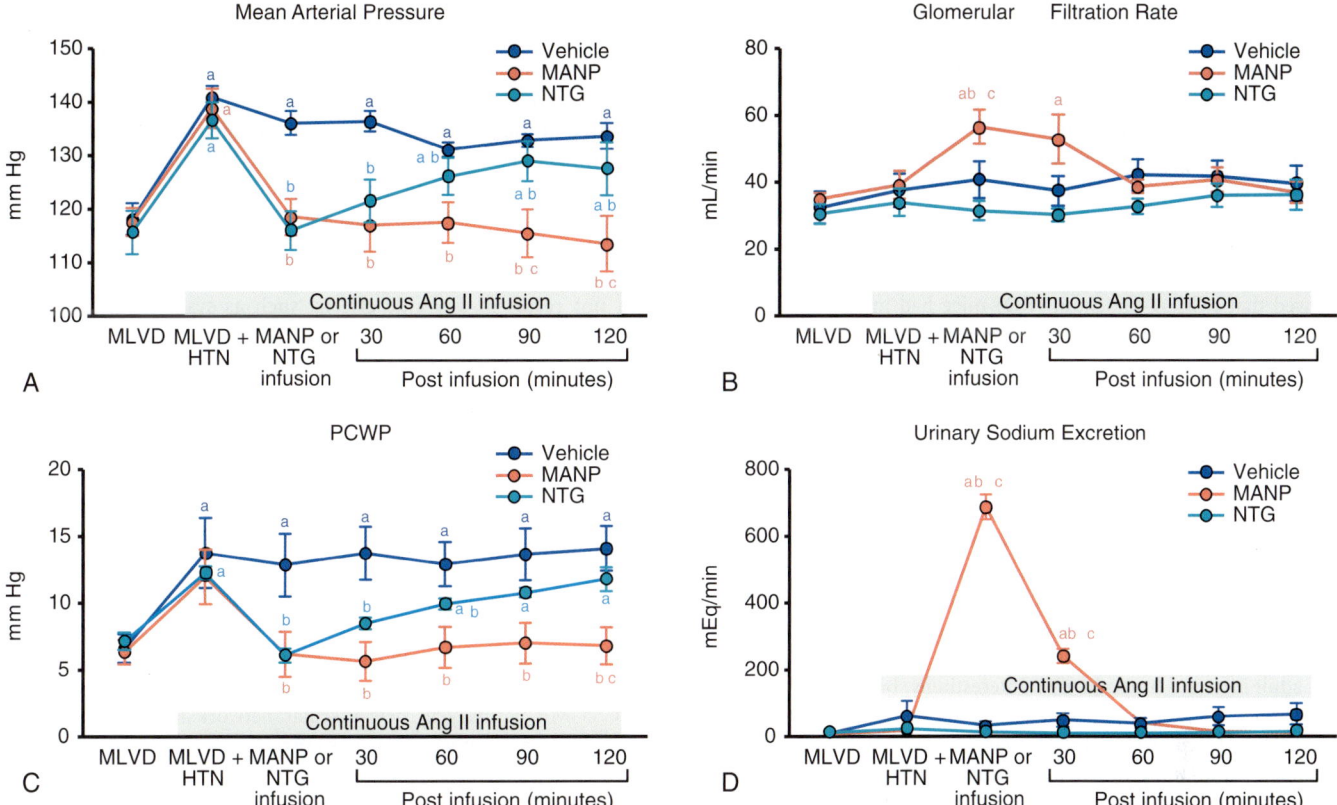

Fig. 9.4 Cardiorenal responses to mutant atrial natriuretic peptide *(MANP)* in experimental acute hypertensive heart failure: Cardiorenal actions of MANP, a pGC agonist, and NTG, an sGC activator, in experimental HF. MANP or NTG was administered in dogs with mild left ventricular dysfunction (MLVD) and MLVD + angiotensin II (Ang II)-induced hypertension (MLVD + HTN). The figure shows effects on (a) mean arterial blood pressure, (b) renal function, (c) mean pulmonary capillary wedge pressure *(PCWP)*, and (d) natriuresis at 30, 60, 90, and 120 minutes. [a]$P < .05$ versus MLVD and [b]$P < .05$ versus MLVD + HTN, 2-way ANOVA with pairwise comparison of individual timepoints within groups using the Tukey HSD method. [c]$P < .05$ for MANP versus vehicle at a specific time point, 2-way ANOVA with Bonferroni post tests. *HF*, Heart failure; *NTG*, nitroglycerin; *pGC*, particulate guanylyl cyclase; *sGC*, soluble guanylyl cyclase.

of BNP or URO. First, pGC-A activation and cGMP generation were examined after CRRL269 treatment of human embryonic kidney 293 (HEK293) cells overexpressing human pGC-A. Interestingly, CRRL269 at low concentrations generated significantly higher cGMP when compared with the same concentrations of ANP, BNP, or URO. At high peptide concentrations there was no significant difference between peptides in the level of cGMP. Importantly, these results were confirmed in kidney-specific cells such as human renal tubular and endothelial cells. In addition, CRRL269 produced a significant increase in urine flow and urinary sodium excretion, which was comparable with URO and even higher when compared with BNP. BNP was also more hypotensive than CRRL 269. Importantly, a clinical trial in ADHF reported that short-term treatment with URO (Ularitide) was not able to improve a clinical composite end point and reduce long-term cardiovascular mortality despite of favorable physiologic actions, which in part was attributable to URO-induced hypotension and reduction in renal perfusion pressure.[91] Taken together, CRRL269 exerts renoprotective properties in a dose-dependent manner, demonstrating enhanced natriuresis and diuresis and increased GFR with a lack of hypotension when compared with either BNP (nesiritide) or URO (Ularitide). These beneficial actions on renal function were also attributed to higher resistance to NEP degradation and RAAS suppression. These therapeutic benefits may provide a therapeutic advantage of CRRL269 in patients with HF and impaired renal function, and future studies are warranted to assess the cardiorenal actions of CRRL269 in HF.

ROLE OF NATRIURETIC PEPTIDES IN CARDIAC REGENERATION AND REPAIR

Conventional HF therapy fails to stimulate endogenous regenerative processes and remains insufficient to compensate for the loss of cardiomyocytes including loss of coronary vasculature. Regeneration is a complex and well-orchestrated process and includes several steps that involve the clearance of necrotic tissue, coordinated regulation of inflammation, extracellular matrix remodeling, and suppression of overactive fibrosis (**see Chapter 4**), with the formation of fully functional blood vessels and lymphatics. A new paradigm in cardiac regeneration has begun with the discovery that the adult heart has capacity for repair. Therefore stimulating regenerative capacity in situ with drugs may have therapeutic potential.

Stem cells used in cell therapies including bone marrow–derived mesenchymal stem cells (MSCs) or adipose tissue–derived stem cells may importantly secrete peptides with growth factor and cytokine-activating properties. These secreted factors act in a paracrine fashion and contribute to neovascularization, cytoprotection, and proliferation of endogenous cardiac progenitor cells (CPCs) and thus promote cardiac repair and regeneration.

NPs have been shown to reduce cardiomyocyte apoptosis and fibrosis and increase angiogenesis in damaged hearts. Several studies highlighted that NPs are involved in embryonic cardiac development. Abdelalim and coworkers reported that embryonic stem cells secrete high levels of BNP that regulate their proliferation.[92] Becker and colleagues demonstrated that ANP and BNP and their receptors are functionally overactive during early cardiac development and induce the proliferation of both embryonic and neonatal cardiomyocytes in a concentration-dependent manner.[93]

Cardiac regeneration following tissue injury shares many similarities with embryonic development. From this perspective, the role of pGC-A signaling in stem cell recruitment was reported by Mallela and colleagues.[94] Using a tumor model, they found that pGC-A colocalizes on endothelial progenitor cells (EPCs) and recruits MSCs. They also showed that pGC-A–knockout (KO) mice had impaired angiogenesis due to lack of stem cell recruitment. The role of the NP system in EPC attraction was also investigated by Shmilovich and colleagues.[95] They reported that BNP treatment leads to a significant increase in bone marrow EPC expressing Sca-1 and Flk-1. Similar results were found in the study in which Rignault-Clerc and associates found that BNP treatment of adult healthy or infarcted mice increased the number of Sca-1–positive cells expressing Nkx2.5 via the mechanism of pGC-A and PKG activation.[96] Bielmann and colleagues also suggested that BNP may play important role in cardiac regeneration in adults.[97] Several studies have described a new effect of NPs on CPCs. In agreement with Becker's study,[93] low doses of BNP stimulated CPC proliferation and differentiation into mature cardiomyocytes in neonatal and adult infarcted hearts in vivo. Interestingly, Bielmann showed different roles for NP receptors in cardiac regeneration. They reported that BNP-induced CPC proliferation in vitro was mediated via pGC-A, whereas BNP binding to pGC-B stimulated CPC differentiation into mature cardiomyocytes. Previously, Dickey et al. demonstrated that pGC-B is the predominant NP receptor in the failing mouse heart.[98] Therefore BNP might be the target during the design and development of NP-based drugs for cardiac tissue regeneration in BNP such as NPA7. In addition, CNP has been shown can stimulate Sca-1–positive cell proliferation via PKG and a PKG-independent mechanism, underscoring a potential for pGC-B as well in cardiac regeneration.

Along with the regulation of stem cell recruitment and damaged tissue replacement, NPs are involved in mechanisms of cardiac tissue remodeling. As both ANP and BNP are synthesized in the heart, their levels are closely associated with the stage of HF. In particular, ANP has a very important function in the inhibition of RAAS, endothelin synthesis, and SNS activity to inhibit these pathways. On the cellular level, ANP inhibits apoptosis and hypertrophy of cardiomyocytes and suppresses the proliferation cardiac fibroblasts and fibrosis. Because of these biologic actions, ANP prevents cardiac remodeling and improves LV function in patients after myocardial infarction (MI),[99] left ventricular aneurysm repair (LVR),[100] and experimental autoimmune myocarditis (EAM).[101] A similar role of BNP has been shown in patients with advanced HF and extensive cardiac scarring.[102] Considering the mechanisms of BNP-mediated actions on injured heart tissue, Tsuruda revealed that BNP is a regulator of extracellular matrix production via decreases in collagen synthesis and increases matrix metalloproteinases (MMPs).[103] In HF, the activation of the RAAS serves as a compensatory mechanism to maintain cardiac output, whereas Ang II is known to be an activator of transforming growth factor-β1 (TGF-β1) that causes cardiac fibrosis. Kapoun showed that BNP suppresses TGF- β1–mediated cardiac fibroblast proliferation and TGF-β1–related fibrotic genes.[104] Therefore the antiremodeling effects of BNP including the control of fibroblast proliferation, profibrotic gene expression, and the ECM degradation via a cGMP/PKG pathway provide the opportunity for an effective peptide treatment strategy of chronic HF.

The role of CNP in cardiac remodeling has been less investigated. Endothelial cells mainly secrete CNP as a paracrine factor producing local effects such as the inhibition of VSMC and migration via

the pGC-B/cGMP pathway. Several studies have shown that gene transfer of CNP can prevent coronary restenosis. Morishige and associates found that gene transfer of CNP can prevent coronary artery remodeling after balloon injury in pigs in vivo.[105] CNP was detected at the site of transfection in the media and the adventitia of coronary arteries, where the level of cGMP was also significantly higher compared with an untreated group. This indicates that CNP might be secreted by fibroblasts and VSMCs where CNP stimulates cGMP generation, which in turn inhibits VSMC transformation, fibrosis, and vascular remodeling. Importantly, CNP gene therapy did not result in any side effects, such as systemic hypotension, which can be considered as one of the advantages of CNP-based therapy. These in vivo and in vitro findings support a role of CNP as a regulator of myocardial structure via control of fibroblast and VSMC function and inhibition of vascular remodeling. It should be noted that Cenderitide coactivates both pGC-B (like CNP) and pGC-A (like ANP and BNP). Cenderitide is also able to modulate cardiac tissue structure due to the suppression of TGF-β1–mediated Col I production in cardiac fibroblasts. Thus Cenderitide possesses the strong antifibrotic action on cardiac fibroblasts and prevents ventricular remodeling. The modulating action of Cenderitide in regeneration has to date not been investigated.

Angiogenesis is an important component of tissue regeneration following tissue injury and organ failure. The importance of the NP/pGC/cGMP pathway in new vascular network formation has been confirmed in transgenic mice overexpressing BNP and after gene transfer of CNP in ischemic muscles.[106] Specifically, Yamahara and colleagues demonstrated that angiogenesis is significantly potentiated in cGKI-transgenic mice but reduced in cGK-KO mice, thus indicating that cGMP/cGMP-dependent protein kinase (cGK) pathway is critical for angiogenesis in vivo. Kook and coworkers previously revealed that ANP can support endothelial cell proliferation and migration.[107] This study also observed that the regenerative effect of ANP depends on concentrations and that low physiologic concentrations of ANP result in an increase of cGMP, cGK, Akt, and ERK1/2 activations. The proangiogenic potential of pGC-A has also been shown in several studies. As discussed in part previously, Mallela and associates showed that endothelial cells extracted from pGC-A-KO mice displayed decreased ability to form capillary-like structures in vitro.[94]

Angiogenesis, a critically important process in organ preservation, is closely linked to inflammation and stem/progenitor cell recruitment, as discussed previously. Indeed, pGC-A-KO aortic rings showed decreased endothelial sprouting and significant reduction in expression of CXC chemokine receptor type 4 (CXCR4) and CD31 after lipopolysaccharide (LPS) treatment, suggesting the importance of CD31-positive and CXCR4-positive progenitor cells in inflammation-induced angiogenesis. The important role of pGC-A in vascular regeneration was also shown by Kuhn and coworkers.[108] In particular, it was found that in mice with systemic or endothelial–restricted deletion of the pGC-A gene, vascularization in ischemic tissues is significantly suppressed. In addition to an antiangiogenic effect, the depletion of pGC-A receptor caused mild cardiac fibrosis and significant left ventricular diastolic dysfunction. Interestingly, Kuhn also found that the local depletion of pGC-A gene in VSMCs did not affect angiogenesis. However, VSMCs may affect angiogenesis via the CNP/pGC-B pathway. VSMCs and ECs have close contact within a blood vessel. Doi and coworkers found that CNP overexpression in VSMCs significantly enhanced endothelial cell proliferation.[109] CNP is commonly referred as an endothelium-derived factor that contributes to the regulation of vascular tone and arterial blood pressure. In VSMCs, CNP inhibits their growth and proliferation by the occupation of pGC-B. CNP appears to be a potent stimulator of a proangiogenic VSMC phenotype, which may be essential to accelerated reendothelization and vascular repair during injury-induced vascular remodeling. The role of the NPs and their receptor signaling pathway in cardiac and vascular regeneration, which is highly relevant to novel therapeutic of HF, remains an exciting area of future investigation and translation.

CONCLUSIONS AND FUTURE DIRECTIONS

The pioneering translational research of the role of the NPs in the pathophysiology of HF has laid down the rationale for their development as HF therapeutics, especially their use as chronic therapies. Specifically, preclinical data indicate that deficiencies of the NP system may contribute to the progression of HF. Furthermore, NPs play a crucial role in maintaining cardiovascular and renal homeostasis. An important therapeutic advantage of NPs as therapies is their cardiorenoprotective properties that allow them to be used for the treatment as well as prevention of HF progression. The identification of NP receptors and molecular signaling pathways for the endogenous NPs has resulted in the development of innovative designer NPs that possess higher resistance to enzymatic degradation and stronger therapeutic effects. Furthermore, synthetic strategies also allow for the chemical modification of peptide structures, including the replacement of natural amino acids and incorporation of nonnatural amino acids, and backbone modification that extend half-life and improve solubility and peptide stability, and other physical and pharmacologic properties.[78] It is clear that the heart is not merely a pump but rather a critically important endocrine organ whose physiology and pathophysiology has enormous relevance to the pathophysiology, diagnostics, and therapeutics of HF.

KEY REFERENCES

2. Kisch B. Electron microscopy of the atrium of the heart. I. Guinea pig. *Exp Med Surg*. 1956;14(2-3):99–112.
7. De Bold AR, Borenstein HB, Veress AT, et al. A rapid and potent natriuretic response to intravenous injection of atrial myocardial extract in rats. *Life Sci*. 1981;28:89–94.
12. Sudoh T, Kangawa K, Minamino N, et al. A new natriuretic peptide in porcine brain. *Nature*. 1988;332:78–81.
15. Sudoh T, Minamino N, Kangawa K, et al. C-type natriuretic peptide (CNP): a new member of natriuretic peptide family identified in porcine brain. *Biochem Biophys Res Comm*. 1990;168:863–870.
41. Burnett Jr JC, Kao PC, Hu DC, et al. Atrial natriuretic peptide elevation in congestive heart failure in the human. *Science*. 1986;231(4742):1145–1147.
72. McMurray JJ, Packer M, Desai AS, et al. Angiotensin-neprilysin inhibition versus enalapril in heart failure. *New Engl J Med*. 2014;371(11):993–1004.
74. Januzzi J, van Kimmenade R, Lainchbury J, et al. NT-proBNP testing for diagnosis and short-term prognosis in acute destabilized heart failure: an international pooled analysis of 1256 patients: the international collaborative of NT-proBNP study. *Eur Heart J*. 2006;27:330–337.
78. Lisy O, Huntley BK, McCormick DJ, et al. Design, synthesis, and actions of a novel chimeric natriuretic peptide: CD-NP. *J Am Coll Cardiol*. 2008;52(1):60–68.
86. McKie PM, Cataliotti A, Huntley BK, et al. A human atrial natriuretic peptide gene mutation reveals a novel peptide with enhanced blood pressure-lowering, renal-enhancing, and aldosterone-suppressing actions. *J Am Coll Cardiol*. 2009;54(11):1024–1032.
90. Chen Y, Harty GJ, Huntley BK, et al. CRRL269: a novel designer and renal enhancing pGC-A peptide activator. *Am J Physiol Regul Integr Comp Physiol*. 2018;314(3):R407–R414.

The full reference list for this chapter is available on ExpertConsult.

Systolic Dysfunction in Heart Failure

David A. Kass

Depressed systolic function is a core manifestation in nearly half of all patients with heart failure (HF). The underlying mechanisms are many and include defects in sarcomere function (**see Chapter 2**), abnormal excitation-contraction coupling and calcium homeostasis,[1] ion channel dysfunction (**see Chapter 1**), mitochondrial and metabolic abnormalities,[2,3] depressed cell survival signaling, enhanced autophagy and mitophagy,[4,5] abnormal proteostasis,[6] redox pathobiology (**see Chapter 8**),[7] inflammation (**see Chapter 7**),[8] signal transduction abnormalities,[9] and vascular insufficiency.[10] Systolic depression is also impacted by cross-talk between cells and signaling from the cardiac interstitium and muscle cells.[11-13] Lastly, there are external factors, such as abnormal venous (preload) and/or arterial (impedance) loads, pericardial constraints, neurological controls, and other factors, which can potently influence net systolic performance.

The most direct demonstration of systolic depression in heart muscle is obtained from isolated muscle or myocytes in which sarcomere function, calcium transients, and force are measured. Human data largely stem from explanted hearts from transplant recipients or myocardium removed at time of ventricular assist device implantation. Data from membrane skinned human myocytes obtained from heart biopsies are suitable for sarcomere function studies but not the analysis of intact cell behavior. The results of such studies are discussed in detail in **Chapter 2**. The inability to study intact myocytes from biopsies has proven to be a major limitation, as common forms of heart disease, including HF with a preserved ejection fraction (EF) and mutations of the dystrophin-sarcoglycan complex, are not treated with heart transplantation, and ideal animal models remain lacking. Thus, our understanding of human myocyte biology in these syndromes is sketchy at best.

Chamber systolic function is routinely assessed using strain-based measures, such as fractional shortening or EF, tissue Doppler measures, and simple pressure parameters such as the peak rate of pressure rise (dP/dt_{max}). These measures are not specific to underlying systolic dysfunction, nor are they capable of identifying the type of underlying defects. This is not just of academic concern as these ambiguities have undoubtedly contributed to the rather disappointing results of efforts to improve systolic function to date. EF is the most common measure used, yet it lacks both specificity and sensitivity to changes in underlying contractility.[14] Drugs dosed to enhance EF may risk overshooting a safety margin in the effort to provide a clear quantitative change. The current classification of HF based on EF (e.g., HF with a reduced or preserved EF) is historical and convenient but also arbitrary, and unfortunately it misses critical features of underlying systolic function. Even hearts with reduced EF can have markedly disparate myocardial properties; an infarcted heart could reflect loss of a region of the wall replaced by scar, whereas another heart could reflect diffuse cardiodepression.

Here, we review our current understanding of the various mechanisms underlying systolic depression in the failing heart, the relationship between properties determined by the muscle and dysfunction as assessed in the chamber level, how systolic function is best measured in the intact heart and its relation to loading conditions, cardiac-vascular interactions and their influence on systolic function in both left and right ventricles, and lastly newer translational efforts to treat systolic dysfunction.

CELLULAR AND MOLECULAR DETERMINANTS: A VIEW FROM 30,000 FEET

The greatest advances in understanding of HF over the past decade have come from the elucidation of its molecular-cellular determinants and their impact at the organ level. Most of this work comes from studies in mice with genetic manipulations, and is discussed in some detail in **Chapter 1**.

Systolic force generation starts at the level of the actin-myosin cross-bridge, which, in turn, is coupled via structural proteins to the surface membrane to transduce into net chamber contraction. Sarcomere proteins play a central role in systolic dysfunction revealed by HF causing mutations that depress molecular motors[15,16] and the myriad of post-translational modifications that alter their function.[17] Mouse models recapitulating sarcomere defects that induce dilated cardiomyopathy (DCM) exhibit reduced power generation and loss of function of the actin–myosin cross-bridge.[18] Mutations in titin are common, perhaps reflecting its enormous size, and are associated with DCM.[19,20] The most frequent mutations inducing hypertrophic cardiomyopathy are in myosin-binding protein C (MyBP-C), though they can also induce dilated

HF.[21,22] The phosphorylation of troponin I (TnI), tropomyosin, myosin light chain, MyBP-C, and titin also impacts contractility (see Chapter 2). Troponin I and -T phosphorylation[23] modulates myofilament calcium sensitivity, whereas MyBP-C phosphorylation is required for β-adrenergic stimulated contractility.[24,25] Both TnI and MyBP-C can also undergo proteolytic cleavage in the setting of ischemic injury, with the former resulting in a loss-of-function peptide,[26] and the latter in a poison peptide fragment[27]—both inducing DCM.

HF also entails disruption of intermediate filament proteins that structurally couple the sarcomere to the cell membrane. Loss of function mutations in muscle limb protein, plasma membrane sarcoglycan-dystrophin complex, focal adhesion complexes, including vinculin and metavinculin, and nuclear or mitochondrial membrane linking filaments, such as laminin, lamin, and desmin, are associated with DCM.[28,29]

Another major cause of systolic impairment are abnormalities of calcium homeostasis (see Chapters 1 and 2).[30,31] This involves ion channels at the plasma membrane and intracellular proteins and calcium storage systems such as the sacroplasmic reticulum (SR). Cycling of calcium via the SR is regulated by phospholamban (PLN) through its control of the SR calcium ATPase (SERCA), but other proteins are involved, including histidine-rich calcium-binding protein, HS-associated protein X-1 (HAX-1), and heat shock protein 20.[30] Posttranslational regulation PLN by phosphatase PP1c is controlled by inhibitor I-1, and reduced I-1 levels observed in failing hearts results in dephosphorylation of PLN and systolic depression.[32] Abnormal activation of protein kinase C α that inhibits I-1 has been proposed as a mechanism.[33] Hyperactive calcium release from the SR is common in failing hearts and particularly linked to excessive calcium-calmodulin activated kinase II phosphorylation of the ryanodine receptor.[34] Other modifications of calcium-handling proteins including oxidation,[35] nitrosylation,[36] and SUMOylation[37] also impair excitation-contraction coupling in the failing heart. Another set of non-voltage gated nonselective cation channels known as transient receptor potential channels can cause abnormal mechanosensing and prohypertrophic/fibrotic signaling.[38-40] Relevant species in the heart include TRPV2, TRPC1, TRPC3, and TRPC6.

Molecular signaling abnormalities are vast in the failing heart, and as an increasing number have been manipulated by genetic gain- and loss-of-function studies, their role in contractile failure has been revealed. Beyond specific genes and proteins, broad epigenetic transcriptional regulators such as BET-bromodomains (gene readers),[41] nonprotein coding messenger RNAs (mRNAs) including microRNA (miRNA),[42] long-non-coding RNA,[43] and circular RNAs[44] are also important. Lastly, the global biochemical milieu that the failing heart operates within has itself become a focus of attention. The presence of obesity, with diabetes and proinflammatory conditions, is changing the metabolic and signaling conditions in which even an otherwise "healthy" heart operates.[45] Changes in high-energy phosphate metabolism and fuel substrate utilization have a major impact on systolic function and reserve (see Chapter 17).[3,46-48]

Lastly, it is important to note that systolic dysfunction extends well beyond the myocyte, engaging the extracellular matrix, and the organ systems to which the heart is coupled. Studies suggest inadequate vasculogenesis to match demands of a hypertrophied ventricle contributes to dysfunction.[10] MiRNAs expressed only in fibroblasts can impair heart function,[49,50] while inversely, molecular signaling in the myocyte can potently impact interstitial fibrosis and inflammatory responses.[11,51] Inflammatory modulation and matrix remodeling—often associated with metalloproteinase stimulation—can also impact myocyte performance (see Chapter 4). Signaling from peripheral organs, such as the kidney, lung, and liver, are known to impact heart function. Thus therapy to improve systolic function should be viewed broadly and include factors extrinsic to the myocyte itself.

MEASURING SYSTOLIC FUNCTION: A PRIMER ON PRESSURE-VOLUME RELATIONS

EF is the most common index of contractile function though it lacks specificity and sensitivity. In fact, EF mostly reflects chamber dilation (end-diastolic volume) rather than contractility, since it is a ratio of stroke volume to end-diastolic volume, and the former is generally maintained until late-stage HF. Second, EF is sensitive to loading changes, notably afterload, but in dilated or hyperdynamic hearts, also to preload. From the 1960s to the 1990s, cardiovascular physiologists focused on developing more specific contractility measures based on various combinations of pressure, volume, or flow. By plotting simultaneous chamber pressure versus volume, Suga, Sagawa, and colleagues revealed how ventricular pressure-volume (PV) loops and relations provided a very powerful framework to dissect intrinsic cardiac contractile and diastolic properties from the loading systems to which the heart was coupled.[52] This framework has since become the primary method used to identify more precise properties of the intact heart and separate them from those mediated by loading.

The fundamental concept underlying PV depictions of heart contraction is that heart muscle acts like a spring with a time-varying stiffness constant. The spring constant at the level of a chamber is called elastance, and the time-varying elastance (elastance is the inverse of compliance), which is easily derived from simultaneous pressure and volume measurements of a ventricular chamber, shows stiffness transitioning from diastole to systole and back again (Fig 10.1A). This time-varying elastance waveform shape is remarkably conserved among mammals (see Fig. 10.1B),[53] among patients with various forms of heart disease or acute modifications.[54] It is also conserved among many gene-mutation models in mice.[55] An exception is in heart muscle lacking MyBP-C. This sarcomere protein imposes a restraint on cross-bridge cycling kinetics,[56,57] and is required for systolic elastance to be sustained once ejection starts.[55] A newly therapy for HF in clinical trials, omecamtiv mecarbil, invokes a mechanism to prolong the time to peak elastance (discussed more below), and so also changes this underlying shape.[58] Fig. 10.1C shows how this approach differs from a β-adrenergic receptor agonist (dobutamine).

Fig 10.2A displays typical human left ventricular (LV) PV data obtained at rest and during transient reduction of chamber preload volume. The loop furthest to the right shows the rest condition, and the labeling depicts end-diastole (point A), isovolumic contraction (point A-B), opening of the aortic valve (point B), ejection (point B-C), isovolumic relaxation (point C-D), opening of the mitral valve and initiation of diastolic filling (point D), and diastolic filling (point D-A). The loop width is stroke volume, the ratio of width to end-diastolic volume is EF, and the loop area is external (or stroke) work. When ventricular preload is rapidly reduced, both stroke volume and systolic pressure decline with each ensuing beat. This is the Frank–Starling relationship. Indeed, the same data can be used to generate typical Frank–Starling curves by plotting end-diastolic pressure for each beat versus the respective stroke volume (or cardiac output). The loops also reveal the ventricular end-systolic elastance (Ees), the slope of the end-systolic PV relationship formed by the upper-left corners of each loop. This corner point (end-systole) is determined as the time of peak elastance (Pressure/[Volume-V_o]); where V_o is the chamber end-systolic volume at zero pressure. The collection of points from multiple cardiac cycles at varying loads forms the end-systolic PV relationship (ESPVR). The position and slope of this relation define systolic function. An important feature of the ESPVR is its relative insensitivity to changes in vascular loading. As shown, it is generated over a range of preload, and its linearity (often but not always

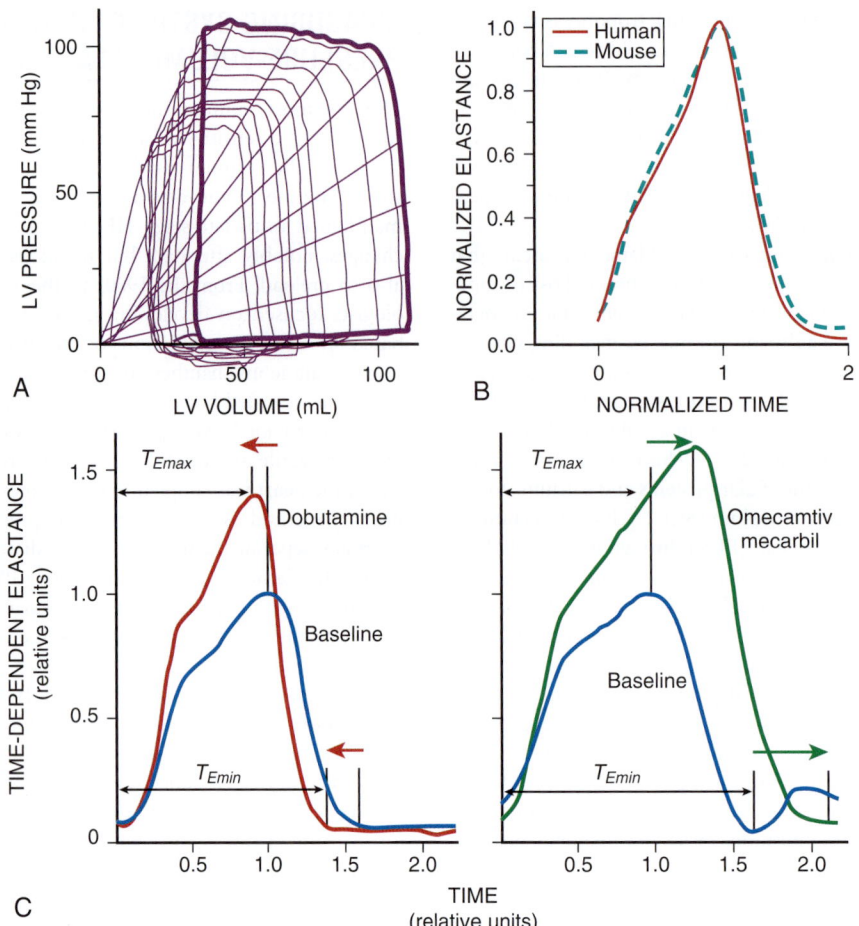

Fig. 10.1 Time-varying elastance in the human heart. (A) Generation of time-varying elastance from multiple cardiac cycles. Linear spokes represent isochrones (connecting points on each loop at the same time), and their slope reflects the instantaneous chamber stiffness or elastance achieved at that point in the cycle [Elastance = Pressure/(Volume–Vo)]. The time-varying elastance is the change in this slope throughout the heartbeat (E[t]). (B) E(t) curves shown normalized to both peak amplitude and time to peak amplitude from the average of greater than 50 human subjects with varying cardiac diseases and from mice. There is remarkable consistency across species in the shape of the waveform, supporting a highly conserved behavior. (C) Time-varying elastance curves in experimental model of heart failure in response to two different types of inotropic stimulation. On the left is the response to the β-adrenergic receptor agonist dobutamine, which increases both the magnitude of elastance rise and rate of rise and hastens subsequent decay (e.g., both contraction/relaxation kinetics are faster). The kinetic changes are related to targets of protein kinase A phosphorylation induced by the agonist. On the right is the response to the myosin activator omecamtiv mecarbil. A similar augmentation of peak elastance is achieved, but in this case, the myofilament response to calcium increases without any PKA stimulation. There is prolongation of contraction, delay in reaching peak elastance, and no acceleration of relaxation. *LV*, Left ventricle. (From Malik FI, Hartman JJ, Elias KA, et al. Cardiac myosin activation: a potential therapeutic approach for systolic heart failure. *Science.* 2011;331:1439–1443.)

the case) indicates that the slope (Ees) is preload insensitive. The ESPVR is also fairly afterload insensitive, although this is not absolute. The behavior observed in the heart is also found in single cardiac myocytes, in this case plotting sarcomere length versus tension **Fig. 10.2B**.[59] As in the whole heart, myocyte end-systolic stiffness is fairly insensitive to the load applied to the cell.

PV analysis facilitates the assessment of acute changes in contractility. This is shown by clinical example in **Fig. 10.2C** in a patient before and after receiving the calcium channel blocker verapamil by intravenous injection.[60] The decline in contractility is depicted by the reduced Ees. As verapamil is also a vasodilator, EF did not decline, and indeed for a long time the impact of this commonly used clinical drug on contractility was underappreciated because of this. In acute settings, changes in Ees can be unambiguously

interpreted as altered contractility. However, contractility changes may manifest by shifting the entire relationship upward and leftward with or without a slope change, and this also should be interpreted as a rise in contractile performance. It is the position and not solely the slope of the relation with such acute changes that is important. Ees is also impacted by ventricular geometric changes independent of underlying muscle properties, so alterations with chronic disease are not as directly equitable with contractility change. For example, with dilated HF, PV relations shift to rightward and Ees often declines. The right shift reflects chronic chamber dilation, while the slope, can decline due to dilation per se, but also due to depressed contractility. An example of this behavior is shown in **Fig. 10.2D** from a mouse model.[61] There are geometric formulas that estimate myofibrillar stress and strain from

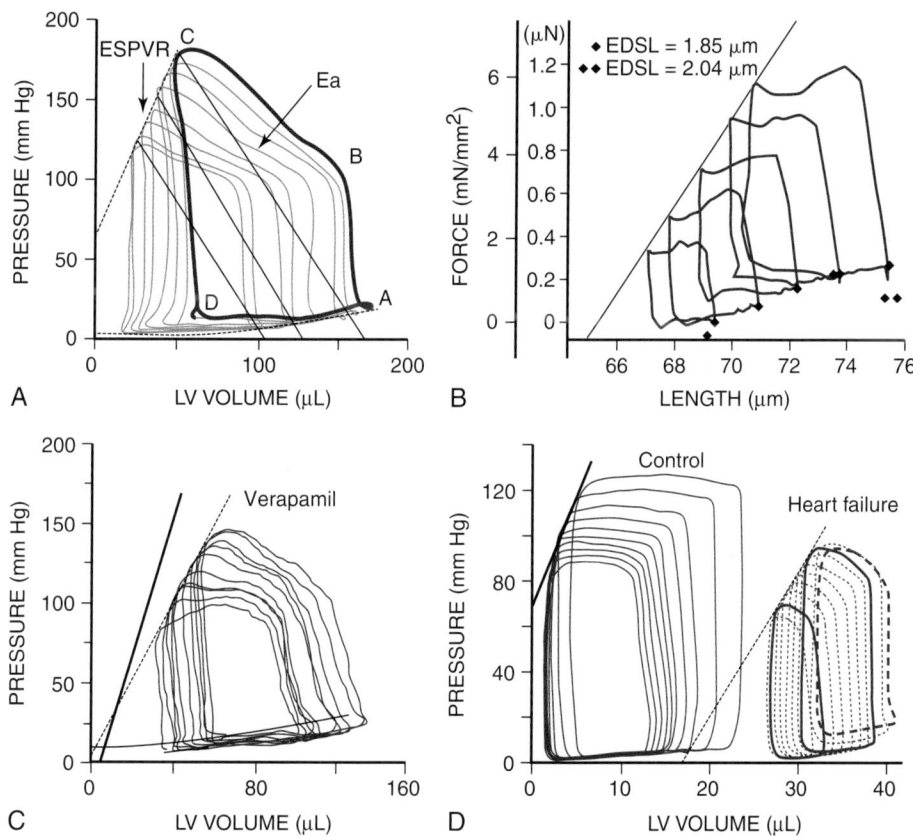

Fig. 10.2 Pressure-volume *(PV)* analysis of cardiac function. (A) Resting *(dark solid loop)* PV loop and multiple cycles derived by varying preload volume in human subjects. Each loop cycle moves counterclockwise in time as preload volume was reduced in this subject; *(A)* end diastole, *(B)* ejection onset, *(C)* end systole, *(D)* onset of diastolic filling. The upper left corners of the set of loops define the end-systolic PV relation *(ESPVR)*, a valuable measure of chamber systolic function, with slope end-systolic elastance *(Ees)*. The group of diagonal lines drawn within several of the beats denotes the arterial load, indexed by their slope (ignoring the negative direction), which is the effective arterial elastance *(Ea)*; Ea, end-systolic pressure/stroke volume. Ea is similar for each beat despite the decline in preload, a reflection of the fact that the arterial afterload or impedance load is little altered by preload in this range. Ea is a useful measure of ventricular afterload, and the ratio of Ees/Ea is a useful measure of ventricular–vascular interaction. (B) Similar types of data but obtained from a single cardiac myocyte, with force and sarcomere length measured and controlled to generate "loops." As in the intact heart, there is a time-varying stiffening of the myocyte, and a linear end-systolic force-length dependence. Thus, this behavior is intrinsic to the cardiac myocyte. (C) Prototypical response of ESPVR to a change in contractile state. Data shown are due to acute intravenous verapamil injection in a human subject.[65] (D) Example of ventricular remodeling and cardiac systolic depression with sustained cardiac failure. Data in this example were generated using a mouse model of heart failure (MKK3 overexpression). *EDSL,* End-diastolic sarcomere length; *LV,* left ventricle. (*B,* from Iribe G, Helmes M, Kohl P. Force-length relations in isolated intact cardiomyocytes subjected to dynamic changes in mechanical load. *Am J Physiol Heart Circ Physiol.* 2007;292:H1487–H1497.)

pressure-dimension data,[62] and these can provide a more chamber-geometry independent index of muscle stiffness.

Fig. 10.2A displays another key feature of PV loops, their simultaneous depiction of total vascular afterload. The diagonal line connecting the lower right to upper left is known as the *effective arterial elastance* (Ea),[63,64] and it incorporates both mean resistance and pulsatile vascular loading imposed on the heart during systole. Ea is calculated from the ratio of end-systolic pressure/stroke volume. It is not synonymous with vascular stiffness; its value is actually most influenced by mean arterial resistance and heart rate (Ea = ESP/SV ≈ R × HR). We do not typically think of HR as an "afterload" but, for any given arterial resistance, a pure rise in HR increases the systemic blood pressure as cardiac output increases. The net effective systolic afterload imposed on the heart is thus greater. However, unlike arterial blood pressure, Ea is minimally altered if only cardiac preload is changed

(note how in Fig. 10.2A, diagonal lines from beats with different preloads remain parallel; e.g., Ea is the same). Clinical use of Ea and Ees to assess heart-vascular interaction have shown changes with aging, disease, and drugs, and as a marker of cardiovascular risk.[65-67] Such analysis also has been extended to the right ventricle (RV) in patients with pulmonary hypertension.[68]

There are some caveats to the ESPVR and its mathematical analysis. First, while the relation is often linear over a constrained range of physiological loading, its overall shape is more often nonlinear, and concaves downward. This is a particularly common observation in small mammals, such as mice, and it should be considered when linear fits are used. There are methods to parameterize the relation independent of a model-fit that can circumvent this problem.[69] Ees is also impacted by noncontractile properties such as chamber geometry, hypertrophy, and interstitial fibrosis, inflammation, and edema. Ees rises with aging in conjunction with arterial stiffening,[66,70] though this more likely reflects changes in passive than systolic-developed stiffness.[70] Cardiac hypertrophy also manifests by a rise in ventricular Ees.[71,72] This can reflect hypercontractility, but similar behavior is found in hearts with gene mutations inducing hypertrophy with depressed sarcomere function,[73] as the hypertrophy can still stiffen muscle in the absence of abnormally enhanced contraction.

BEAT-TO-BEAT REGULATION OF SYSTOLIC FUNCTION

There are three primary mechanisms that regulate beat-to-beat systolic performance of cardiac muscle. They involve the dependence of systolic force on (a) sarcomere length at the onset of contraction, (b) tension imposed during contraction, and (c) beat frequency. In the intact heart, these components translate to the impact of chamber end-diastolic volume (preload), systemic vascular impedance or wall stress (afterload), and heart rate on cardiac systolic function.

Acute Stretch—The Frank-Starling Effect

With an abrupt length increase, cardiac myocytes and muscle display an immediate rise in force without corresponding changes in intracellular calcium. This is the essence of the behavior shown by the multiple loops at varying preload in Fig. 10.2A. This response was first attributed to changes in actin-myosin filament overlap, but the marked steepness of the relation between force and sarcomere length, and its variability with contractile states, led to abandoning this hypothesis.[74]

In 1982, Hibberd and Jewell[75] revealed a left shift of the steady-state force-Ca^{2+} relationship with increasing length, both at submaximal and maximal calcium activation, establishing length-dependent Ca^{2+} activation as a central mechanism. However, the underlying mechanism for this has remained uncertain. One theory is that muscle lengthening reduced interfilament spacing between actin and myosin (i.e., stretch in one direction, compressed spacing in the orthogonal direction), favoring cross-bridge formation.[76] The most recent work supports a critical role of titin in potentiating the recruitment of rested-to-ready strongly bound cross-bridges.[77] Stretch extends the I-band region of titin, a protein that spans the entire sarcomere and binds both actin, myosin, and myosin binding protein C (MyBP-C).[78,79] As titin is obliquely oriented to the sarcomere axis and attaches to both myosin and MyBP-C, it imposes a passive strain to alter the geometry of the thick-filament proteins. This favors the population of more force-generating cross-bridges. The magnitude of this effect rises with systolic activation, recruiting more such cross-bridges.[80]

Effect of Systolic Load—The Anrep Effect

The Anrep or slow force response (SFR) is observed in muscle exposed to an abrupt increase in systolic load. Unlike the Frank-Starling response that is immediate and occurs without a change in myocyte intracellular Ca^{2+}, the SFR evolves over several minutes and is coupled to increased Ca^{2+}. It can be measured by a rise in elastance (or ESPVR left shift) or increase in muscle force.[81-83] The precise source of calcium and its controlling mediators remain the subject of investigation. One culprit are members of stretch-activated channels (SACs) that augment intracellular Ca^{2+} (or Na^+) and thus contraction, with TRP channel members playing a role. As previously mentioned, cardiac muscle expresses various stretch-responsive TRP channels, including TRPC1, TRPC3, TRPC6, and TRPV1, and they play a role in acute and chronic responses to afterload increase. Seo and colleagues[84] first reported that the SFR is depressed in myocytes lacking TRPC6 (but not TRPC3). Moreover, they found the SFR is potently suppressed by activation of threonine/serine cGMP-stimulated kinase (PKG). This effect required the presence of TRPC6 that can be phosphorylated by PKG to block

conductance (Fig. 10.3A, B). Intriguingly, the SFR is greatly increased in myocytes from a mouse model of Duchenne muscular dystrophy (e.g., lacking dystrophin and utrophin),[84] and this is consistent with hyperactive TRPC6 mechano-responses. TRPC6 is activated by diacylglycerol coupled to $G_{q/11}$ protein coupled receptors, such as the angiotensin type 1 receptor. This receptor is itself mechano-sensitive[85] and could thereby contribute to the Anrep response.

Another explanation for the SFR attributes Ca^{2+} entry to reverse mode Na^+-Ca^{2+} exchange (NCX) triggered by a rise in intracellular Na^{2+}.[86] This model starts with stretch activation of a Gq-receptor, the endothelin type-A receptor coupled to AT1 ligand-independent activation, that in turn stimulates PI3K and Akt.[83] The cascade involves transactivation of epidermal growth factor receptor (EGFR) to stimulate ERK phosphorylation[87] and activate the surface membrane Na^+/H^+ exchanger to elevate intracellular sodium. Na^+ is then exchanged for Ca^{2+} by the NCX, leading to the rise in force. How this mechanism would be blocked by PKG remains unclear.

The relevance of the SFR in the intact heart and to HF relates to its role in maintaining cardiac output when the heart confronts a rise in afterload stress. For example, a rise in systemic resistance is countered by an increase in cardiac contractility so that stroke volume (and in turn cardiac output) are maintained. This process, termed *homeometric autoregulation* in the 1950s by Stanley Sarnoff, would be particularly important in a failing heart that displays a greater decline in ejected volume at higher afterload.

Effect of Heart Rate

Systolic function of cardiac muscle is also influenced by beat frequency. This occurs within a single cycle and is the consequence of altered myocyte Ca^{2+} entry (more depolarizations/minute of the L-type Ca^{2+} channel and thus greater net Ca^{2+} entry) and increased cycling of Ca^{2+} into and out of the SR.[88] The latter not only is intrinsic to SR calcium handling kinetics but also is controlled by rate responsiveness of Ca^{2+}-calmodulin dependent kinase II.[89] In humans, raising heart rate alone from 70 to 150 per minute increases LV contractility by 100%, and similar ranges are observed in large mammals.[90,91] Mice, who operate at ~500 per minute at rest, display a much smaller change in contractility from heart rate increase.[92] Assessing how heart rate impacts contractility requires measures insensitive to loading (e.g., Ees), as chamber filling and effective afterload both vary with heart rate (inversely and directly, respectively). Importantly, contractility dependence on heart rate is markedly blunted in dilated and hypertrophic heart disease as a primary manifestation of depressed SR calcium handling (see Chapters 1 and 2).[93,94] Fig. 10.3C shows this phenomenon in an intact canine model of dilated HF. Increasing heart rate augments contractility (indexed by Ees) in the normal heart, but this is depressed in a dilated failing heart. Costimulation with a β-adrenergic agonist (dobutamine) further enhances HR-augmentation of contractility, since PKA-dependent phosphorylation of the L-type Ca^{2+} channel and PLN (among other proteins) themselves elevate intracellular Ca^{2+}. The failing heart has both depressed β-adrenergic signaling and SR function, so this combined augmentation is depressed. Failure of the force-frequency dependence is important with exertion when both sympathetic and chronotropic stimulation normally occurs.

INTEGRATIVE MEASURES OF SYSTOLIC FUNCTION

There are many other measures of systolic chamber function that are commonly used to index contractile function. These can be divided into measures of early isovolumic contraction (e.g., dP/dt_max, isovolumic contraction time); early-mid ejection phase (e.g., maximal ventricular power, flow acceleration, peak strain velocities, peak velocity

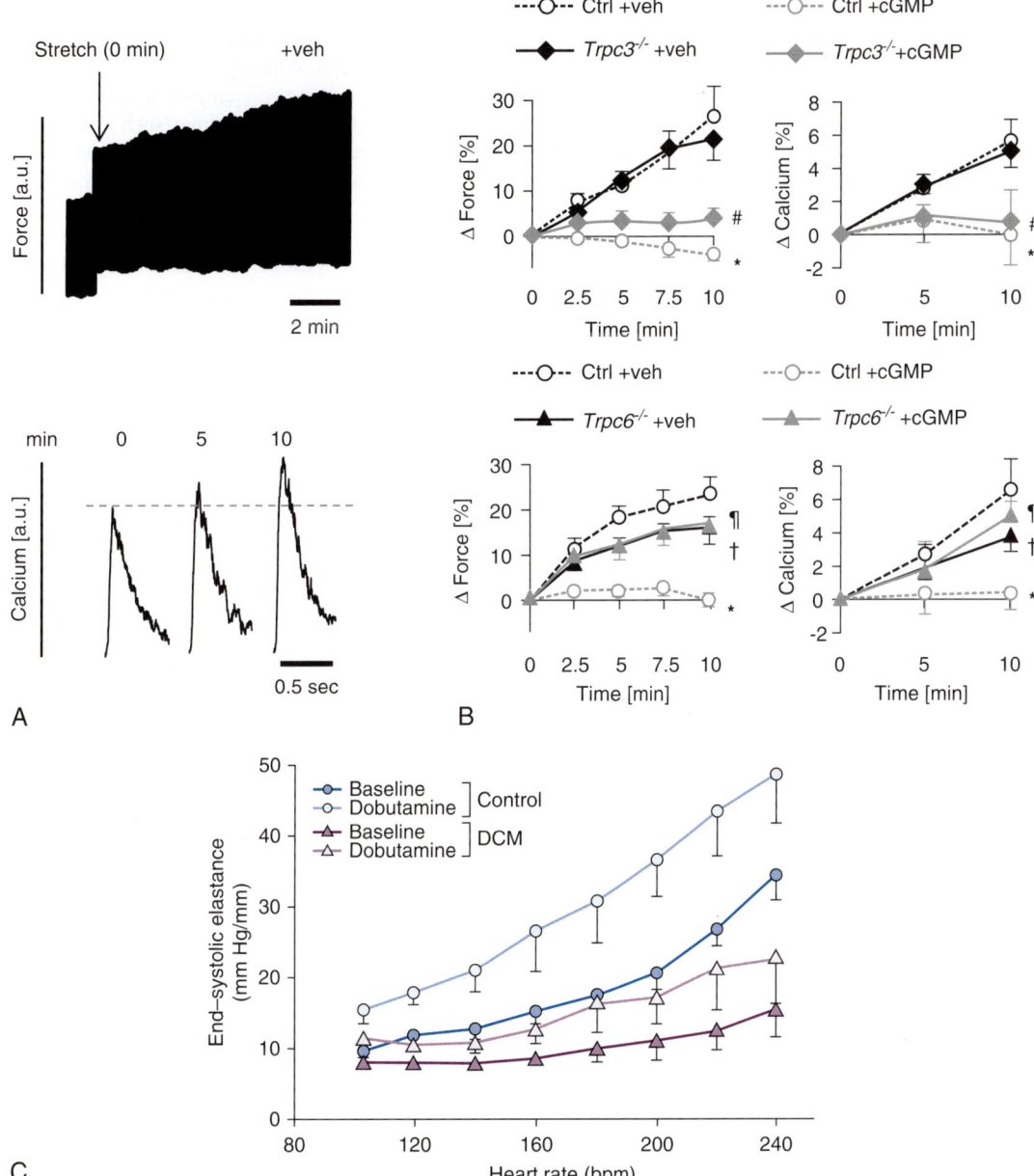

Fig. 10.3 (A) Demonstration of the Anrep phenomenon, also known as slow force response or stress-stimulated contractility. Shown are data from isolated papillary muscle contracting isometrically before and after an abrupt increase in length. The initial rise in peak and developed force at time 0 reflects the Frank–Starling effect, and there is no change in peak calcium (dashed line in lower tracing reflects steady-state peak prior to the stretch). However, over the ensuing 10 minutes, there is a gradual rise in developed and peak force and peak calcium, which reflects the Anrep effect. (B) Relation between change in developed force or peak calcium and time following a rise in systolic stress. Data were derived from experiments as shown in panel A. Muscle lacking TRPC6 (but not TRPC3) show a decline in the load-stimulated contractility rise (in both force and calcium). When muscle was incubated with cGMP to stimulate PKG, this dependence is largely eliminated so long as TRPC6 is expressed. In the absence of TRPC6 (e.g., in TRPC6$^{-/-}$ muscle), cGMP has no impact on the relation. (C) Force-frequency dependence in intact heart from conscious dog with and without cardiac failure *(DCM)*. The relation is generated in the intact heart, so frequency is presented as heart rate (HR), and contractile force indexed by end-systolic elastance to reduce the potential impact of load-dependent changes. The relation is depressed in cardiac failure. Furthermore, there is an augmentation in the HR-dependent rise in elastance, with concomitant β-adrenergic stimulation provided by dobutamine. This is consistent with an interaction between enhanced calcium transients that are stimulated by the dobutamine and increased intracellular calcium cycling due to higher beat frequency. The interaction of the two mechanisms is also depressed somewhat in cardiac failure. Data are shown as the relative percent increase from resting heart rate. *DCM*, Dilated cardiomyopathy. (A and B, adapted from Seo K, Rainer PP, Lee DI, et al. Hyperactive adverse mechanical stress responses in dystrophic heart are coupled to transient receptor potential canonical 6 and blocked by cGMP-protein kinase G modulation. *Circ Res.* 2014;114:823–832; and C, adapted from Senzaki H, Isoda T, Paolocci N, Ekelund U, Hare JM, Kass DA. Improved mechanoenergetics and cardiac rest and reserve function of in vivo failing heart by calcium sensitizer EMD-57033. *Circulation.* 2000;101:1040–1048.)

of shortening-stress dependence); and late systolic parameters (e.g., stroke work-derived indexes, Ees). To an extent, each of these is influenced by intrinsic systolic properties of the heart muscle, its integration into the chamber, and the loading system to which the heart is coupled. There really is no precise measure of "contractility"—a term that is itself more conceptual rather than physical. Furthermore, not all measures of chamber function index the identical behavior, and there can be discrepancies among these measurements. This is particularly true in mouse models where genetic engineering can decouple components of systolic contraction from one another.

Chamber systole begins with isovolumetric contraction, and is most often quantified by the maximal rate of pressure (or force) development. The peak first derivative of pressure (dP/dt_{max}) is one of the most common measures of chamber systolic function, largely due to its simplicity and ease of determination (just need pressure). It is also arguably the least directly relevant to net ejection performance by the heart, as it occurs before the aortic valve opens. dP/dt_{max} is typically depressed in cardiomyopathy, and its absolute level found in human HF is remarkably consistent, being near 1000 mm Hg/sec (normal being near 1600–1800 mm Hg/sec). It remains a very commonly used parameter in mouse studies. A major caveat to dP/dt_{max} is its strong preload dependence. In mice, a change of as little as 2 to 3 microliters of end-diastolic volume (10% decline) can markedly alter dP/dt_{max} (**Fig. 10.4A**).[53] This dependence is minimized by regressing dP/ systolic

dt_{max} from multiple beats at varying end-diastolic volumes versus EDV from the same cycles. While this approach is rarely used clinically due to its complexity, it is easily employed experimentally.[95] dP/dt_{max} is also influenced by internal loading (such as reflected by intermediate filaments, microtubules, and titin), the extracellular matrix (i.e., edema, inflammation, collagen dysregulation), the phosphorylation state of MyBP-C, sarcomere cross-bridge properties (e.g., cooperativity upon activation), and the dynamic coordination of contraction by different portions of the cardiac chamber wall. The latter is rendered abnormal in the presence of conduction delays, such as a left bundle branch block (LBBB), and the resulting discoordination depresses dP/dt_{max} even without any primary change in contractile function of the myocytes. When one side of the heart contracts early while the opposite side remains in diastole, pressure force is dissipated by stretching the still-relaxed wall, and the rate of pressure rise is slowed. Acute increases in dP/dt_{max} associated with biventricular stimulation of a dyssynchronous failing heart occur within a single beat, and similarly do not indicate a change in underlying contractile function, but rather chamber-level consequences of improved coordination of wall contraction.[96]

Early-to-mid systolic parameters reflect times when shortening velocity (e.g., wall motion correlated to peak flow from the heart) and flow is maximal. Peak velocity of chamber shortening varies inversely with wall stress, and this hyperbolic relation has been used

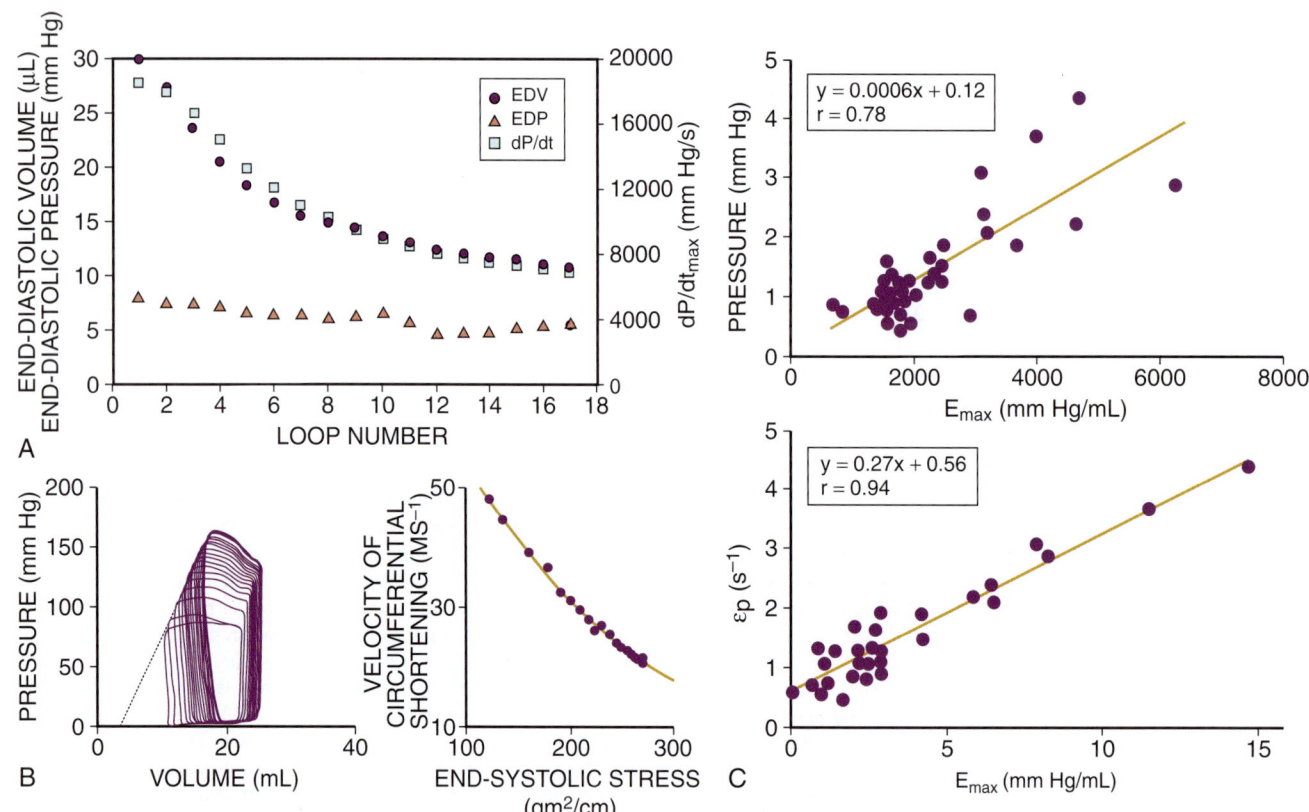

Fig. 10.4 Indices of contractility in the intact heart. (A) Preload dependence of dP/dt_{max} in a mouse. Data are derived from a series of cycles at varying preload; beat 0 is at high preload, beat 17 at low preload. Although there is negligible change in end-diastolic pressure for these cycles, preload volume *(EDV)* declines in direct correlation with dP/dt_{max}. This dramatically shows the marked preload-dependence of dP/dt_{max}, particularly in this species. (B) Generation of velocity of shortening-stress relations from pressure-volume data at varying afterloads. (C) Correlation of myocardial systolic strain rate (εp; *y*-axis) or chamber dP/dt_{max} to maximal end-systolic elastance (E_{max}). As determined here, Emax is the same thing as Ees. Both εp and dP/dt_{max} are commonly used to index contractility. (From Greenberg NL, Firstenberg MS, Castro PL, et al. Doppler-derived myocardial systolic strain rate is a strong index of left ventricular contractility. *Circulation.* 2002;105:99–105.)

as a measure of contractility (**see Fig. 10.4B**). Noninvasive image-based measures include tissue Doppler peak systolic velocity (**see Chapter 32**), or load-incorporating variants, such as maximal ventricular power (needs to be adjusted for preload volume), or the circumferential shortening velocity adjusted for wall stress. Maximal power is the peak product of ventricular pressure and outflow, and can be derived noninvasively from Doppler flow imaging and cuff/tonometry-derived blood pressure data.[97,98] Maximal power is then adjusted for chamber end-diastolic volume to derive a parameter with little load dependence.[98,99] The latter is not the case if afterload changes are marked, as may apply to the right heart in severe pulmonary hypertension.[100] This index displays far more marked sensitivity to contractile function than does the EF, and can be measured during exercise stress procedures.[101]

Tissue Doppler imaging has given rise to strain and strain-rate analysis.[102] These approaches essentially quantify myocardial wall motion—as obtained from magnetic resonance imaging. Actual regional stresses remain unknown, yet these also influence measured strains and strain rates. Nonetheless, strain rate has been found to correlate with dP/dt_{max} and indices derived from end-systolic PV relations (**see Fig. 10.4C**), and clearly is prominently influenced by chamber systolic function. In genetic models of hypertrophic cardiomyopathy, tissue Doppler has been used to define early abnormalities of chamber function that precede the evolution of cardiac hypertrophy. Tissue Doppler has been widely employed to index contractile discoordination in patients with cardiac failure and conduction delay.[103]

The most commonly used late-systolic parameter is EF—the chamber translation of fractional shortening. EF is easy to measure, its value is independent of calibration errors of absolute volume assessment (i.e., it is dimensionless), it is only moderately sensitive to inotropic changes, and it is not very sensitive to pure alterations in cardiac filling volume (preload), and inversely dependent on afterload and heart rate. In human heart disease, EF mostly reflects the presence of chamber dilation/remodeling since the numerator (stroke volume) is relative preserved in many forms of heart disease until very late stage decline, whereas the denominator (EDV) can increase markedly. It is unfortunate in this regard that we continue to categorize HF by EF, including the nomenclature of HF with a reduced or preserved, and mid-range EF,[104] insofar as these categories do not imply meaningful differences in underlying myocardial pathophysiology, molecular mechanisms, or necessarily what type of intervention is likely to be most successful.

While the Frank-Starling curve remains an important element of systolic analysis, its utility is limited by strong afterload and heart rate dependencies, and ambiguities associated with the use of end-diastolic filling pressure to index preload. An alternative approach, developed over 50 years ago, was to assess relations between cardiac stroke work and preload (preload-recruitable stroke work), with the latter indexed by end-diastolic volume rather than pressure.[105] Stroke work (area of a PV loop) is less afterload dependent than stroke volume, as it incorporates pressure as well, and the stroke work–end-diastolic volume (SW-EDV) relation is both linear and minimally influenced by chamber load, while still reflecting systolic function. It has a distinct advantage among all the systolic function indexes in that its units are of force (the volume terms drop out from numerator and denominator). This makes it more chamber-size independent, and values of the slope of the relation lie between 75 and 90 mm Hg in normal hearts from mouse and rat up through to dog, pig, and human. As with Ees, methods to assess preload recruitable stroke work (PRSW) from single-beat data using noninvasive analysis have been reported.[106,107]

IMPACT OF PERICARDIAL LOADING ON SYSTOLIC FUNCTION

The pericardium surrounds all chambers of the heart and has the capacity to alter transmural wall stress and the relation between diastolic distending pressures and volumes. This results in an important impact on the apparent Frank-Starling relation.[108] For example, pericardial constraining forces are largely responsible for the apparent descending limb of the Frank-Starling relation in dilated failing hearts. This fall in force at high preload was classically attributed to the overstretch of the sarcomere with a loss of thick and thin filament overlap. However, this is not possible in cardiac muscle due to the complex collagen weave that surrounds each cell in the myocardial syncytium, as well as cytoskeletal membrane proteins within the myocyte. Rather, Tyberg and colleagues revealed that high preload can result in a decline in transmural pressure (not absolute chamber pressure) due to constraining forces provided by the pericardium.[109,110] In patients with DCM, increased end-diastolic pressures may not be associated with elevated transmural pressure due to higher pericardial pressure. This is not the result of fluid pressure in the pericardial space, but from the membrane itself, which does not over stretch as the heart dilates. When preload is reduced, the pericardial pressure declines, so that transmural distending pressures can actually rise, filling the heart with more blood even as the apparent intracavity diastolic pressure is declining. Plots of cardiac output (CO) versus end-diastollic pressure (EDP) appear biphasic, rising at lower EDP and falling at higher EDP, whereas the same data plot as CO versus EDV is upward linear.[109,110]

VENTRICULAR–ARTERIAL INTERACTION

The interaction of the heart and arterial system into which it ejects critically determines cardiac output, EF, stroke work, mechanical efficiency, systolic pressure, and many other key integrated properties. Depending upon the matching of heart to vessel, these variables can be either optimized or not. This interaction also explains differences in cardiac output and systolic blood pressure responses to changes in arterial or venous dilation or inotropy between normal, hypertrophied, and failing hearts.

Among the more successful methods to assess ventricular-vascular coupling is the one derived from the PV framework, employing Ees to index the systolic heart property, and Ea to index the arterial load.[111] As noted in Fig. 10.2A, E_a is the ratio of end-systolic pressure to stroke volume and its value is dominated by mean arterial resistance and heart rate. It is also influenced by phasic (reactive) loading properties of the arterial system; that is, properties due to wall compliance, wave reflections, inertance, etc. Coupling is then expressed by a ratio of E_a to the ESPVR slope (E_a/E_{es} or E_{es}/E_a) (**Fig. 10.5A**).

When the E_a/E_{es} ratio is near 1.0, the transfer of energy or stroke work from heart to arterial system is near optimal, and the heart operates at near optimal cardiac efficiency.[112,113] In normal individuals, this ratio is near 0.8, and this is maintained during exercise,[114] with concomitant rises in both Ees and Ea. This behavior is conserved across mammals, and may relate to an evolutionary process designed to maintain the lowest cardiac/body size ratio.[115]

In hearts with depressed contractility, work and power output are far from optimal, as they fall with higher vascular loading (greater Ea) and myocardial depression (lower Ees). Asanoi and colleagues[116] first reported coupling ratios in patients with normal, moderate, and severely depressed LV function, finding ratios >3 (**see Fig. 10.5B**) in DCM.

The interaction of Ees and Ea provides a useful means of understanding and/or predicting the response of a given heart to a particular

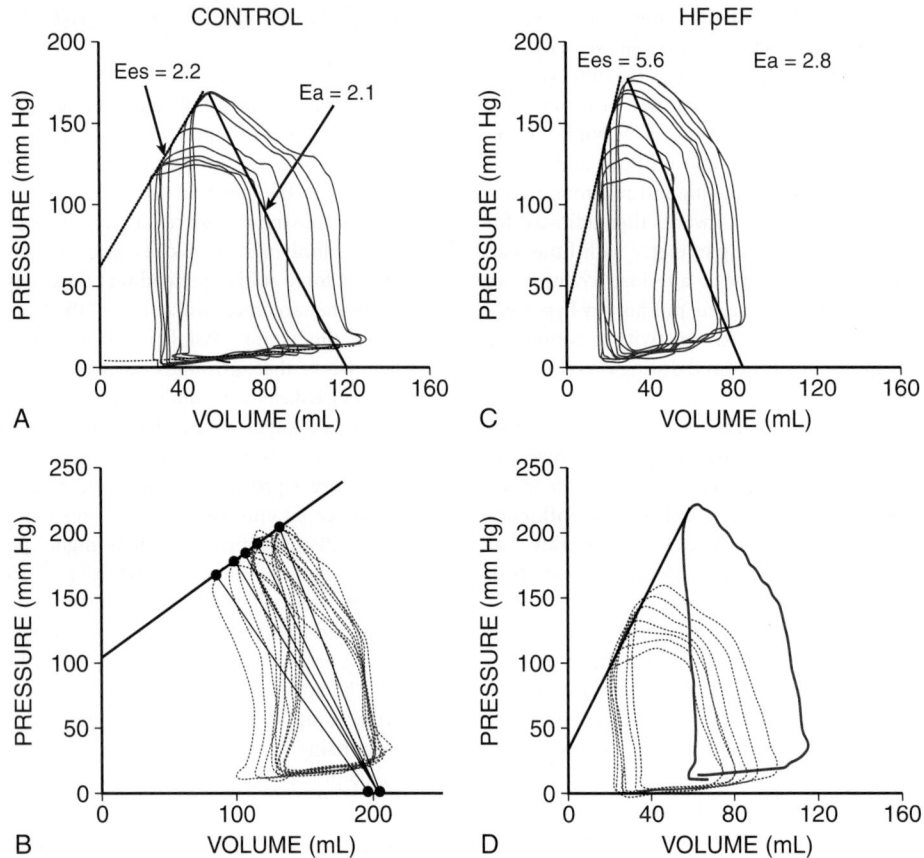

Fig. 10.5 Ventricular-arterial coupling. (A) Resting human pressure–volume (PV) relations showing normal matching between end-systolic elastance *(Ees)* and arterial elastance *(Ea)*. This matching results in optimized cardiac function and efficiency. (B) In contrast, the failing heart displays a reduced Ees (depressed systolic function) and elevated Ea (higher afterload), yielding a decline in chamber power output and metabolic efficiency. (C) Subject with congestive heart failure and preserved ejection fraction *(EF)*. In such patients, Ees appears elevated over age/pressure-matched controls and is accompanied by a further rise in Ea because of reduced vascular distensibility. (D) This pathophysiology can explain marked increases in blood pressure and cardiac workload with exertion. Shown here is an example subject during an isometric hand exercise, with the resting PV loops *(dotted lines)* and stress-response loop as *solid lines*. *HFpEF*, Heart failure with preserved ejection fraction. (From Kawaguchi M, Hay I, Fetics B, et al. Combined ventricular systolic and arterial stiffening in patients with heart failure and preserved EF: implications for systolic and diastolic reserve limitations. *Circulation* 2003;107:714–720.)

therapeutic intervention. A little algebra helps clarify how this works.[117] From the definition of $E_{es} = P_{es}/(V_{es}-V_o) = P_{es}(V_{ed}-SV-V_o)$, where Pes, Ves are end-systolic pressure and volume, Ved is end-diastolic volume, SV is stroke volume, and Vo is the zero-pressure intercept of the ESPVR, and for Ea=Pes/SV, one can write:

$$E_{es} \times (V_{ed} - SV - Vo) = E_a \times SV$$

Solving for SV yields:

$$SV = E_{es} \times (V_{ed} - Vo) / (E_a + E_{es}) = (V_{ed} - Vo) / ([E_a/E_{es}] + 1)$$

What Equation 10.2 indicates is that if you have a depressed contractility (low Ees), then the changes in Ea more potently alter the Ea/Ees ratio, and thereby have a greater impact on stroke volume. In a patient with a high Ees (as with hypertrophic heart disease), the Ea/Ees ratio will be less altered by changes in Ea, and similarly stroke volume (SV) will remain unaltered despite vascular afterload changes. An example of the former is shown in Fig. 10.5C in a DCM patient with high systemic resistance who was then administered a bolus of intravenous nitroglycerin. The resulting beat-to-beat decline in arterial resistance resulted in an increase in PV loop width (stroke volume) by nearly 50%, improving cardiac output. Combined increases in Ees and Ea also influence the pressures developed by the heart in response to changes in chamber filling and arterial load. Increased ventricular systolic stiffening means that even small increases or decreases in preload will amplify into marked changes in systolic pressure. This may contribute to the increased diuretic and orthostatic sensitivity in the elderly. Reduced Ees in DCM predicts minimal systolic pressure change despite unloading.

Adverse ventricular-arterial interaction plays an important role in a subgroup of HF patients with preserved EF (HFpEF).[118] While defined more or less arbitrarily as having an EF >50%, this does not mean that either the heart or its vascular load are normal. Indeed, studies found a higher Ees coupled to a higher Ea, predicting greater energy costs to increasing cardiac output, and correlating with depressed exertional capacity. Tandem increases in Ees and Ea are also observed with normal aging,[70] with women developing both properties at a faster rate than men.[66] This may contribute to a prevalence of HFpEF in older women.[72]

Fig. 10.5D shows an example of a patient with HF and preserved EF, demonstrating the greatly increased stiffening of the ventricle during systole, and increased vascular stiffening. EF may appear normal in such individuals, but this does not necessarily mean that systolic function is normal and the problem resides solely with diastolic abnormalities. Increased chamber systolic stiffening and its impact on ventricular-arterial interaction may play an important pathophysiologic role in symptom lability, and in hypertension and dysfunction during stress as shown in Fig. 10.5D when the same patient performed an isometric hand-grip to increased arterial resistance. Importantly, increased Ees at rest in HFpEF patients does not necessarily mean that the hearts have normal contractile reserve. Indeed, studies have found various measures of load-independent systolic function: Ees, PRSW, and Power$_{max}$-Index fail to increase normally in these patients when stimulated by supine exercise.[119]

PULMONARY HYPERTENSION AND SYSTOLIC FUNCTION OF THE RIGHT VENTRICLE

The disease that imposes the most profoundly abnormal vascular load on a ventricle is pulmonary hypertension. Unlike the systemic circulation where resistance is constrained to a maximum of ~2× normal, pulmonary artery resistance often rises five to six times over normal. Moreover, the distribution of resistance and capacitive vessels between the systemic and pulmonary circulations are quite different, and this has major implications for restoring optimized ventricular-vascular interaction for the two sides of the circulation. For the arterial circulation, the proximal thoracic aorta is the primary source of arterial compliance[120] and is geographically distinct from the more distal resistance arterioles. However, in the lung, compliance is distributed in the periphery, primarily in the same vessels that provide resistance.[121] This property results in a rather tight inverse relation between total pulmonary vascular compliance (the major factor controlling pulsatile RV loading) and resistance, which does not occur in the systemic circulation.[122] **Fig. 10.6A** depicts this interdependence derived from >1000 patients with varying levels of pulmonary vascular disease. An implication of this interdependence is that in patients with high levels of pulmonary vascular resistance (positioned on the lower right of the hyperbola), compliance is also very low, so pulsatile RV loading is high. This load is itself a trigger for pathological stress and hypertrophic remodeling for the RV. The normal pulmonary vasculature operates near the bend of this hyperbola, and during exercise, a decline in resistance in the lung is accompanied by increased compliance as the data shift further to the left and upward. This does not occur in patients with pulmonary artery hypertension (PAH), who start at the lower right on this curve, and despite shifting somewhat leftward with exercise, still have abnormal pulsatile load and high resistance.

Another factor that comes into play regarding pulmonary afterload and its impact on the RV is that the afterload is affected by the venous downstream pressure; for example, mean left atrial pressure. This provides a back-pressure for the forward-pressure/flow wave generated by the RV during contraction, and the effect is to enhance systolic wave reflection in the pulmonary arterial circuit essentially increasing the pulsatile RV afterload.[122] This is demonstrated in Fig. 10.6B, where patients with or without an elevated pulmonary capillary wedge pressure (PCWP) are shown in the same pulmonary resistance versus compliance plot. For any given resistance, the total pulmonary vascular compliance is reduced (greater pulsatile load impact) if the PCWP is elevated. This provides coupling of LV diastolic pressure elevation as often occurs with systolic HF and greater RV pulsatile loading. Thus, from the standpoint of ventricular-vascular coupling of the RV and pulmonary vasculature, changes in left heart filling pressures play an important role. Indeed, pulmonary vascular compliance has been identified as an independent risk factor for worse clinical outcome in

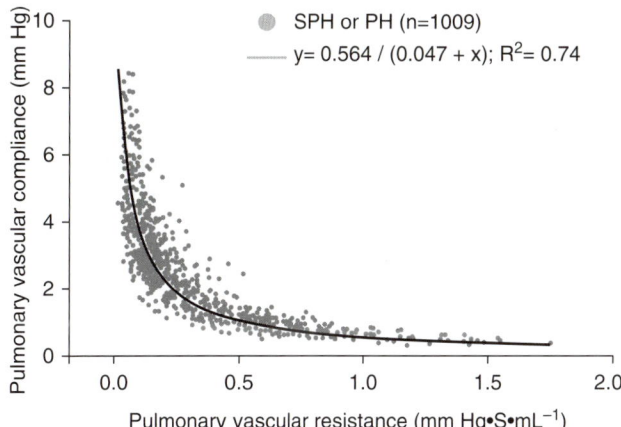

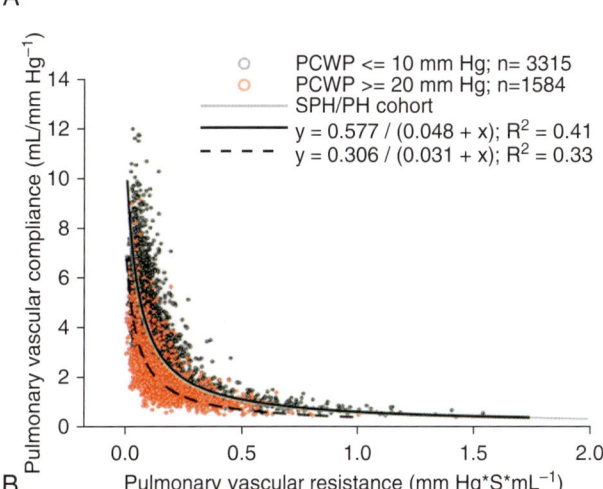

Fig. 10.6 (A) Inverse relation between pulmonary vascular resistance and total pulmonary vascular compliance. There is a hyperbolic relation between these variables, reflecting the shared anatomical sources for both behaviors in pulmonary vessels, which is in the periphery of the lung. These data were from >1000 patients undergoing right heart catheterization. (B) Similar relations are shown for patients with a reduced pulmonary capillary wedge pressure *(PCWP)* versus those with elevated pressure. The latter group *(red symbols)* displays a lower level of pulmonary vascular compliance for any given resistance, essentially shifting the hyperbolic relationship downward. This links abnormal diastolic pressures of the left heart with increased pulsatile pulmonary vascular and thus right heart loading in heart failure syndromes. *SPH/PH;* Suspected or previously confirmed pulmonary hypertension in patients presenting for right heart catheterization. (Data from Tedford RJ, Hassoun PM, Mathai SC, et al. Pulmonary capillary wedge pressure augments right ventricular pulsatile loading. *Circulation.* 2012;125:289–297.)

patients with HF.[123] They may both relate to the impact they have on RV load and maladaptation.

In the face of pathological pulmonary vascular loading, the RV must compensate and does so by increasing mass and Ees in an attempt to restore ventricular-vascular coupling. This puts an enormous stress on the RV, yet remarkably many ventricles appear up to the task. However, an example where this does not occur is PAH associated with systemic sclerosis (SSc-PAH). Patients with SSc-PAH display higher mortality than those with other forms of PAH.[124] Early theories laid the blame on a stiffer pulmonary vascular system imposing greater pulsatile loading on the RV. In a study of SSc-PAH patients, we demonstrated that this is not the case.[68] Rather, PV analysis of the RV in these patients identified rest and reserve-stimulated systolic failure in striking contrast to patients with idiopathic PAH (IPAH), (**Fig. 10.7A, B**).[68] Interestingly, this contractile depression was not identified by conventional measures of RV function based on image-derived indexes. Abnormal vascular load undoubtedly played a role in the ambiguity of convention measures but not PV indexes. RV contractility also does not increase during supine exercise in SSc-PAH, but does in IPAH. This depresses ventricular-vascular coupling in the SSc-PAH group.[125] Further study has revealed abnormalities of the sarcomere to explain disparate RV contractile function in SSc-PAH versus IPAH, with the former having very depressed maximal Ca^{2+}-activated myocyte tension (see Fig. 10.7C).[126] This maximal tension measured in isolated human myocytes from endocardial biopsies is inversely correlated with the extent to which in vivo LV dilate during exercise to compensate for their lack of inotropic reserve (see Fig. 10.7D). These findings have shifted the focus of attention from PAH to RV systolic failure due to a sarcomere defect, in SSc-PAH patients. They also demonstrate that underlying myocardial disease may be difficult to detect by standard measures, and are likely more prevalent than we have suspected.

TREATING SYSTOLIC DYSFUNCTION

Despite a defining role in HF for many patients, the amelioration of systolic dysfunction by pharmacotherapy has proven to be a difficult task (**see Chapter 37**). Only a few decades ago, the main treatment was digitalis, although its impact on contractility was quite modest. Current use of digitalis as an inotrope is very limited. Rather, methods largely rely on cyclic adenosine monophosphate (cAMP) generation by stimulation of the β-adrenergic pathway (e.g., dobutamine) or inhibiting cAMP-targeting phosphodiesterase type 3 (e.g., milrinone). Both ultimately stimulate contraction by cAMP-dependent activation of protein kinase A, enhancing calcium cycling, myofilament function, and other proteins critical to force generation and relaxation. Central to their effects are a rise in intracellular calcium, and while useful, chronic stimulation has been detrimental,[127] stymying efforts with these approaches.

The development of genetically engineered mice revealed that stimulating various downstream components of the β-adrenergic pathway surprisingly improves HF outcome. Several of these have been targeted in clinical trials using small molecules or gene transfer approaches. An example is the inhibition of β-receptor kinase GRK-2, which normally phosphorylates the β-receptor to suppress signaling and stimulate receptor internalization and desensitization (**see Chapter 6**). Mutant versions of GRK-2 that lack this kinase activity have been successful in ameliorating various models of HF and myocardial infarction in rodents and large mammals.[128,129] Preclinical large animal studies using paroxetine, an antidepressant that also stimulates GRK-2, proved beneficial in a model of myocardial infarction.[130] Another approach is to target adenylate cyclase (AC). While blockade of AC type 5 is associated with reduced HF,[131] upregulation of AC type 6 may improve contraction more safely.[132] This was recently tested in a phase II trial of 42 patients with DCM, with AC-6 delivered by adenovirus-mediated gene transfer. While no change in exercise capacity was observed, there was a small but significant improvement in dP/dt_{max} without arrhythmia.[133] Further studies are under consideration. Still another approach used gene therapy to enhance expression of SERCA2a. While initially promising, clinical end points for efficacy were not met in the subsequent multicenter trial.[134] These data suggest that how and where in the cell cAMP is being generated is critical, that this signaling is very compartmentalized, and the effects differ accordingly.

Several pharmaceuticals now being developed for HF have effects on the sarcomere, and have highlighted the use of peak ventricular

elastance as a core systolic index. These agents augment myofilament response to calcium, and broadly referred to as *calcium sensitizers*, or *sarcomere enhancers*. They can function by interacting with troponin, tropomyosin, myosin ATPase, or other proteins. There are several theoretical advantages of such agents. First, by bypassing the adrenergic system and directly targeting the myofilaments, these drugs are equally effective in failing as in normal hearts. An example of this behavior is shown in **Fig. 10.8A**. In this canine model of HF,[135] the dobutamine-stimulated contraction is markedly depressed compared with the normal control response, whereas the response to the sensitizer, EMD-57033, which is thought to target the myosin head to enhance actin attachment, is similar in both conditions. A second feature is that they can enhance contraction without requiring the ATP needed when this is accomplished by the cAMP-dependent pathway. The extent of energy savings depends on their mechanism of action, and so far no completely "free lunch" effect has been identified. Third, they impact later phases of systolic function, such as the duration of systole, but do not accelerate early contraction as a β-agonist does. An example (see Fig. 10.2B) is with the myosin ATPase activator, omecamtiv mecarbil,[58,136] which prolongs systole and time to peak elastance, compared to dobutamine, which shortens this time period. Omecamtiv mecarbil[58] is currently being studied in HF with a reduced EF, in the phase III Registrational Study With Omecamtiv Mecarbil/AMG 423 to Treat Chronic HF With Reduced EF(GALACTIC-HF; NCT02929329).

Finally, increasing calcium sensitivity means that the impact on systolic function will itself vary with the stimulation of calcium by other means. At rest, calcium activation is reduced, so the impact on rest contractility of the sensitizer is commensurately less. However, with exercise, there are the catecholamine and heart rate–triggered changes that, even while depressed, can still enhance the calcium trigger and thus increase the inotropic effect from the sensitizer. This is demonstrated in a dog study of levosimendan (see Fig. 10.8B).[137] Improved systolic function with the drug was modest at rest but much more marked in animals doing treadmill exercise. (Levosimendan is currently approved for acute therapy of HF in Europe but not in the United States.)

Another approach to increasing contractility is with nitroxyl, or HNO. This is the protonated form of nitric oxide; the molecule does not dissociate as with an acid, but rather interacts with negative charged cysteine residues (thiolates) on selective proteins, which, in turn, modify heart function.[138-140] The reaction is reversibly controlled by the redox state, in that enhancing reducing conditions can block it. HNO was first reported to enhance systolic function in the intact canine heart model of HF, and later cellular mechanisms for this effect have been revealed. These include demonstration of direct enhancement of SR calcium uptake and release,[141] which appears due to its formation of a disulfide between cysteines in the intramembrane region of PLN.[142] HNO also targets the myofilaments with disulfide bonds to link actin and tropomyosin, and on the myosin heavy chain and myosin light chain-1.[140] Novel HNO donors have been developed and tested in humans and are currently being evaluated in the phase IIb STANDUP AHF clinical trial (Evaluate the Safety and Efficacy of 48-Hour Infusions of HNO [Nitroxyl] Donor in Hospitalized Patients With HF [NCT03016325]).

SYSTOLIC EFFECTS OF DYSSYNCHRONY AND RESYNCHRONIZATION (SEE ALSO CHAPTER 38)

It has long been recognized that discoordinate cardiac contraction itself reduces the systolic performance of the chamber, and recent developments in therapies to resynchronize contraction have shown this to be a valuable target for HF treatment. Conduction disease at or above the

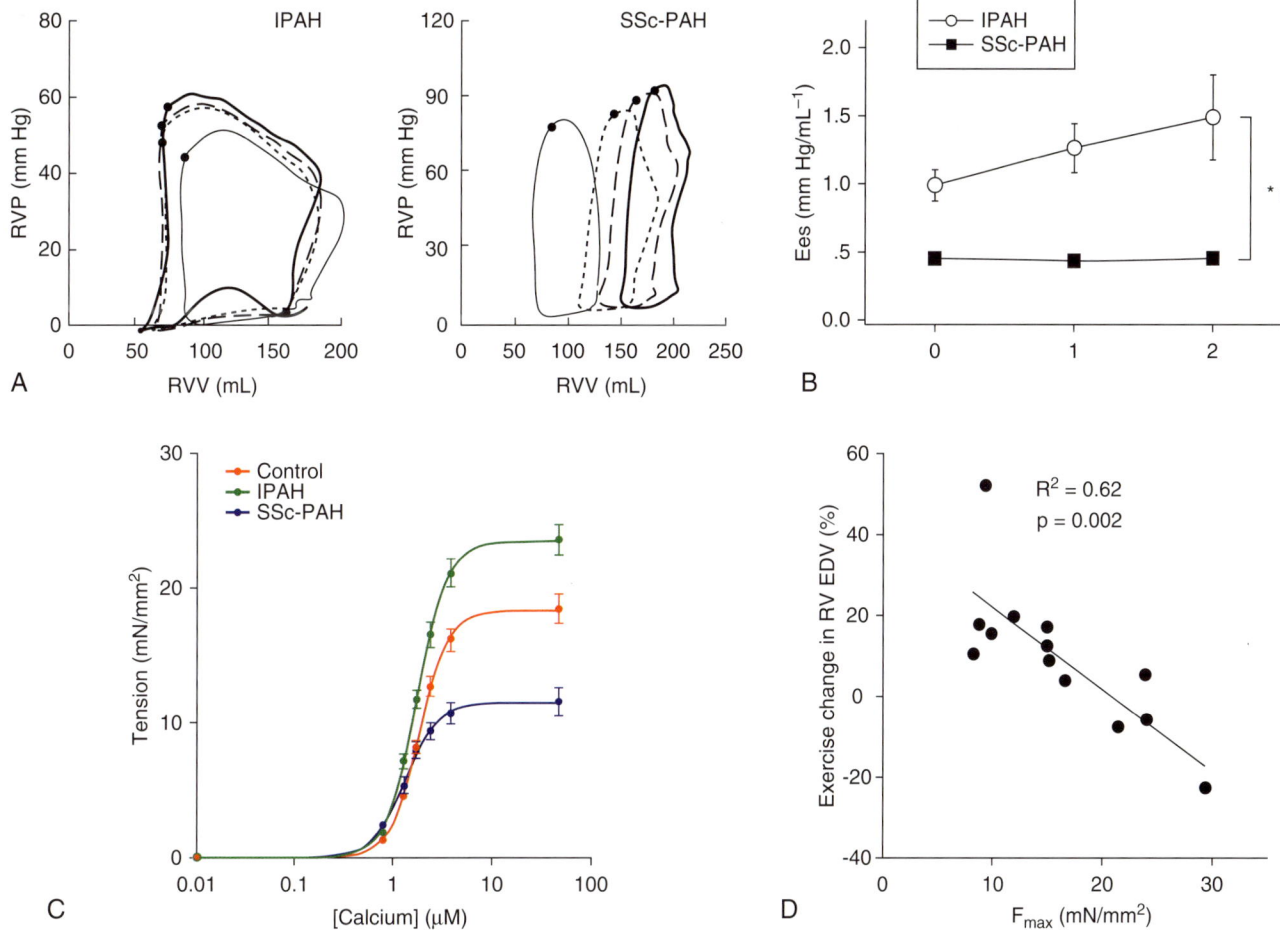

Fig. 10.7 (A) Example pressure-volume (PV) loops from patients with pulmonary artery hypertension *(PAH)* due to idiopathic disease *(IPAH)* or systemic sclerosis *(SSc-PAH)* at rest and during matched stages of supine bicycle exercise. __ Baseline; - - - Exercise Stage 1; __ __ __ Exercise Stage 2; **bold** _ Exercise Stage 3. The IPAH subject demonstrates a rise in contractility (upper corners of PV loops shift up to the left with each stage), whereas the SSc-PAH subject does not, but rather displays cardiac dilation. The use of the Frank–Starling mechanism is a way to offset the lack of contractile reserve in the SSc-PAH patient. (B) Summary results for right ventricular contractility *(Ees)* in both patient groups at rest and with exercise shows this disparity. (C) Steady-state force-calcium dependence measured in isolated right ventricle myocytes obtained from patients with either IPAH or SSc-PAH. The former shows increased function with higher maximal calcium activated force as compared to controls, while the SSc-PAH cells display the opposite, with reduced function. (D) Myocyte maximal calcium activated force inversely relates to the extent of right ventricular end-diastolic volume change during supine exercise measured in the same patient from which the right ventricular biopsy was obtained. *EDV,* End-diastolic volume; *RVP,* right ventricular pressure; *RVV,* right ventricular volume. (Data from Hsu S, Houston BA, Tampakakis E, et al. Right ventricular functional reserve in pulmonary arterial hypertension. *Circulation.* 2016;133:2413–2422.)

atrioventricular (AV) node affects chronotropic competence and effective preload (and left atrial pressure). Both short and excessively long AV delays reduce net LV filling.[143,144] Infranodal conduction delay—commonly LBBB pattern—induces discoordinate contraction.[145-147] DCM hearts, with an LBBB, display early activation of the septal wall with lateral prestretch, followed by markedly delayed lateral contraction with late systolic septal stretch toward the RV. Cardiac discoordination induced by LBBB or RV-ventricular pacing depresses systolic function, increasing the end-systolic volumes at a given pressure (rightward shift of the ESPVR), prolongs isovolumic relaxation,[148] and has been coupled to widening of the QRS complex.[149] The energetic cost of contraction can increase relative to effective ejection, because the early activated myocardium largely serves to increase preload on the lateral free wall, leaving the late activated wall to contract at higher stress while wasting work by stretching the more pliable early activated territory.[150,151]

These mechanical effects of discoordinate contraction were the impetus for studies performed over a decade ago in which right ventricular preexcitation was used to treat patients with hypertrophic cardiomyopathy.[152] In such patients, the institution of RV-apex pacing increased end-systolic volumes, reduced dP/dt$_{max}$ and other parameters of systolic function, and importantly in this instance, resulted in a decline in hyperdynamic ejection and thus cavity obliteration. Importantly, this effect did not depend on the presence of asymmetric hypertrophy, but was equally, if not more, effective in individuals with concentric left ventricular hypertrophy (LVH) associated with symptoms of cardiac failure.[153] **Fig. 10.9A** shows time tracings of apical segmental volume in a patient with hypertrophic cardiomyopathy subjected to acute RV apical pacing. Whereas the original data show normal timing of systolic ejection and filling, pacing results in premature contraction of the region, and later restretch (volume increase) during what is still systole. This results in residual systolic volume

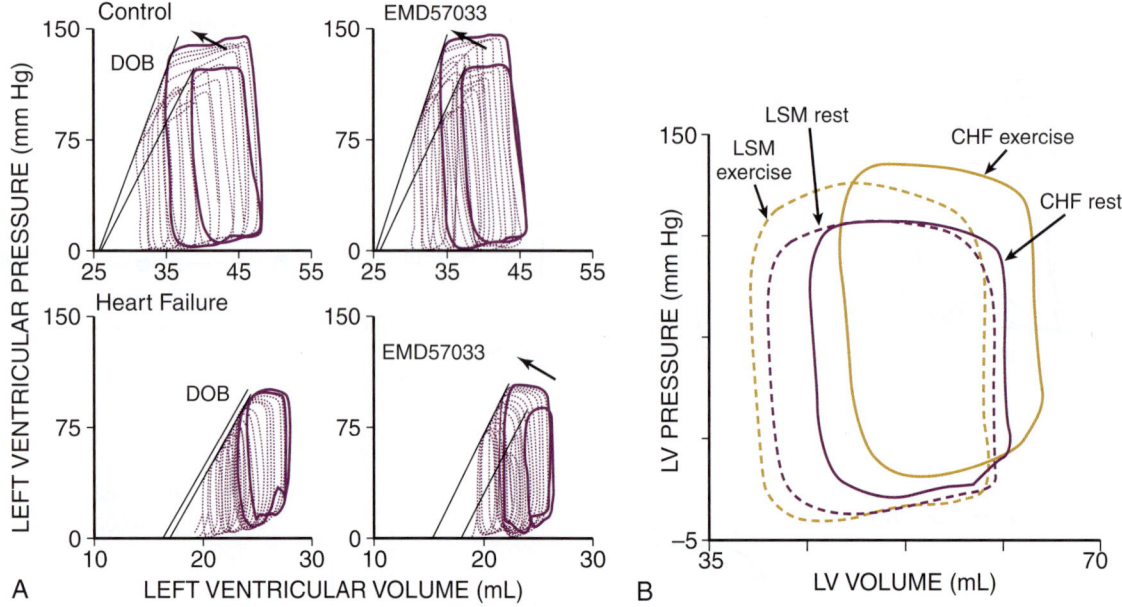

Fig. 10.8 (A) Influence of dobutamine *(DOB)* versus a calcium sensitizer (EMD-57033) on contractile reserve in normal versus failing hearts. In thez control hearts *(upper panels)*, both drugs stimulate contractility almost identically, reflected by the leftward shift and slope increase in the end-systolic pressure-volume relation. However, in failing hearts *(lower panels)*, the response to dobutamine is markedly depressed, whereas the contractile response to the sensitizer is maintained, consistent with its more distal site of action, directly on the myofilaments. (B) Enhanced effectiveness from a calcium sensitizer on systolic function during exercise in a canine model of heart failure. The improvement in function reflected by the left shift of the PV loop and increase in its width (stroke volume) is modest in the heart when at rest, but potentiated during exercise. *CHF,* Congestive heart failure; *LSM,* levosimendan (acute intravenous) treated CHF. (A, from Senzaki H, Isoda T, Paolocci N, et al. Improved mechanoenergetics and cardiac rest and reserve function of in vivo failing heart by calcium sensitizer EMD-57033. *Circulation.* 2000;101:1040–1048. B, from Tachibana H, Cheng HJ, Ukai T, et al. Levosimendan improves LV systolic and diastolic performance at rest and during exercise after heart failure. *Am J Physiol Heart Circ Physiol.* 2005;288:H914–H922.)

that is not ejected, so the end-systolic PV relation shifts rightward (see Fig. 10.9B).[71] Though therapeutic generation of ventricular dyssynchrony in patients with septal hypertrophy proved less effective,[154,155] a small single-center trial in patients with concentric LVH and cavity obliteration found benefits from reducing systolic contraction in these patients. Larger controlled trials still need to be done.

The opposite approach—resynchronizing the LV in individuals with DCM and underlying basal discoordination because of LBBB—has been far more successful (**see Chapter 38**). Biventricular pacing or univentricular pacing of the LV lateral free wall can recoordinate contraction and is associated with systolic improvement.[96,156,157] Cardiac resynchronization effects manifest abruptly (i.e., rise in dP/dt$_{max}$, arterial pressure, Fig 10.9C), occurring within one beat, and reflect increased systolic flow. When displayed as ventricular PV loops, the resynchronization effect can be observed as a widening of the loop (enhanced stroke volume), decline in end-systolic wall stress (left shift of end-systolic PV point), and increased cardiac work (see Fig. 10.9D). Importantly, the latter is not accompanied by increases in energy consumption, but it can occur with a net decline in energy consumption.[156] Studies have not demonstrated major effects on diastolic function to date, although there is evidence of reverse cardiac remodeling associated with this therapy.

These initial studies established an improvement in systolic function at the chamber level, although, as with acute dyssynchrony, this was likely because of the coordination of contraction and was not a primary improvement in myocardial contractility. However, chronic cardiac resynchronization therapy (CRT) treatment enhances rest and

systolic reserve function, demonstrated by exercise capacity and the response to increases in heart rate. This has been coupled to upregulation in myocardial gene expression of β_1-receptors, PLN, and SERCA2a, among other genes.[158,159] Animal models of dyssynchronous HF and CRT revealed improved resting myocyte function and adrenergic reserve (**Fig. 10.9E**).[160,161] Cells were obtained from hearts with a LBBB and subjected to 6 weeks of rapid pacing, which induces DCM, but with CRT, pacing was switched from atrial to bi-ventricular for the latter 3 weeks. The mechanisms included reversal of abnormalities of calcium cycling regulation and improved adrenergic signaling cascades, with suppressed inhibitory G proteins, upregulation of β_1-receptor-coupled signaling and AC activation, and upregulation of regulator of G-protein signaling: RGS2 and RGS3. Another mechanism by which CRT improves systolic function is by enhancing myofilament-calcium sensitivity. As observed in a canine model, this involves the reactivation of glycogen synthase kinase 3-β, enhancing phosphorylation of several proteins that localize to the Z-disk and M-band.[162] Thus chronic CRT does enhance systolic function by mechanisms that involve more than chamber-level mechanics. Other studies have revealed potent influences on mitochondrial ATP synthesis,[163] ion channels involved with repolarization and arrhythmia,[164,165] and other features.[166]

A somewhat surprising discovery that has evolved from work on CRT pathobiology was that temporarily exposing a synchronous failing heart to a period of dyssynchrony (e.g., 6 hours at night) followed by resynchronization during the remainder of the day improved cardiac function as well.[167] The effects of pacemaker-induced transient asynchrony (PITA)

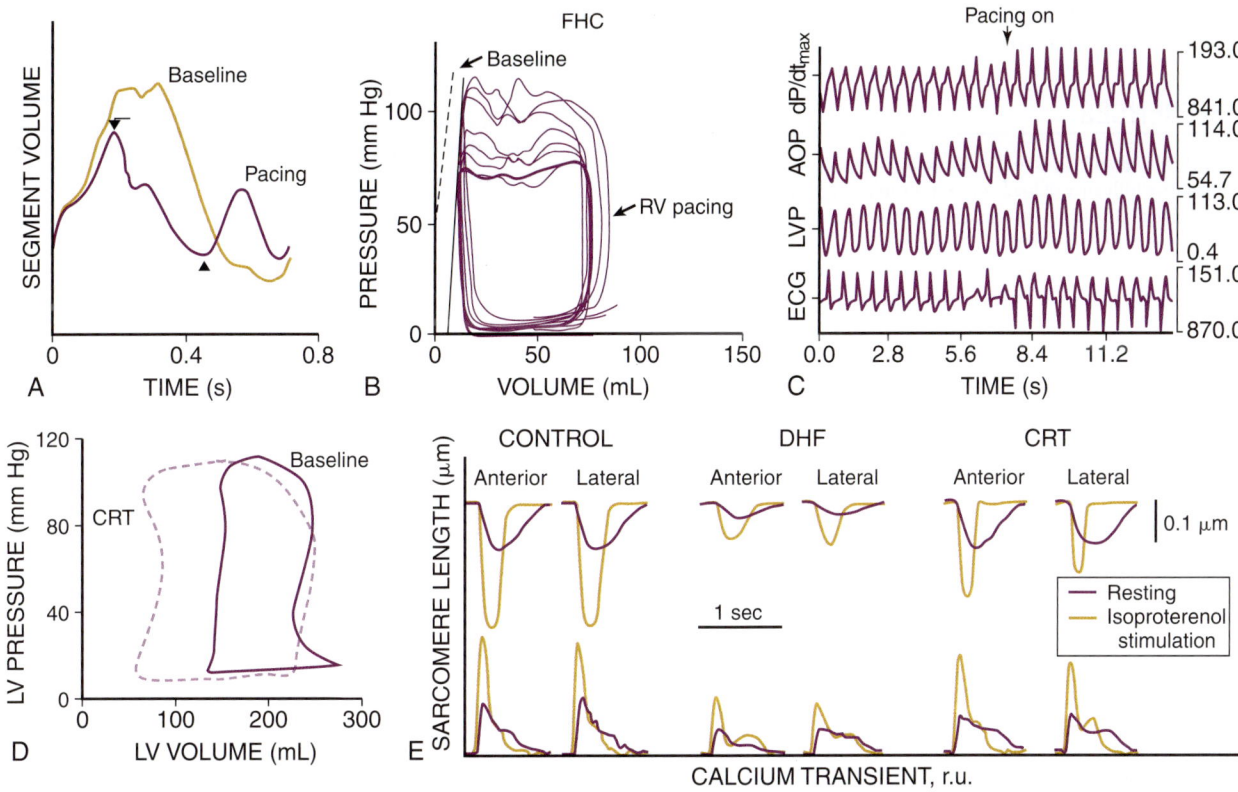

Fig. 10.9 Impact of ventricular discoordination and resynchronization on chamber systolic function. (A) Dyssynchrony generated by right ventricle *(RV)* apex pacing in the human ventricle, with local pressure-apical volume loops displayed. The resting condition *(baseline)* shows normal timing of systolic ejection. With early stimulation of this region, shortening occurs at low pressure but is converted to stretch later in systole as the rest of the heart contracts. (B) Global pressure–volume relations during RV apex pacing are compared with sinus controls *(dashed end-systolic PV relationship [ESPVRs])*. Dyssynchrony results in an increase in end-systolic volume, a rightward shift of the ESPVR, and thus a decline in effective systolic function. (C) Resynchronization in human dilated cardiomyopathy (DCM) patient with left bundle branch block (LBBB). Acute biventricular stimulation enhances dP/dt_max, aortic pressure *(AOP)* and the pulse magnitude, and peak left ventricle pressure *(LVP)* as shown after the *arrow*. This effect is near immediate. (D) Example of pressure-volume loops with resynchronization *(dashed line)* showing enhanced function, increased loop width, and left shift of end-systolic point *(upper left corner)*. This is opposite to the effect in panel B when dyssynchrony was induced by RV-apex pacing. (E) Myocyte contraction and calcium transients at rest and after adrenergic stimulation. Cells are isolated from hearts with normal function, dyssynchronous heart failure *(DHF)*, or resynchronized heart failure *(CRT)*. DHF cells display markedly depressed rest function and calcium transients, and their responsiveness to isoproterenol (ISO) stimulation is depressed. CRT cells display improvements in both rest and ISO responses for both shortening and calcium transients. These changes are observed in cells obtained throughout the heart, specifically from both early- and late-activated regions. *FHC,* Familial hypertrophic cardiomyopathy. (B, from Pak PH, Maughan WL, Baughman KL, et al. Mechanism of acute mechanical benefit from VDD pacing in hypertrophied heart: similarity of responses in hypertrophic cardiomyopathy and hypertensive heart disease. *Circulation.* 1998;98:242–248, 1998.)

in dogs with dilated HF and no dyssynchrony were analogous to those observed with CRT, in that β-adrenergic responsiveness, receptor signaling, and myofilament function improved and chamber size declined. However, the underlying molecular mechanisms appear somewhat different. The concept borrows from a form of conditioning, where exposure to a potentially pathological stress for a defined period of time results in a biological response that improves the heart once the stress is removed. This has the potential to provide a pacemaker-based systolic enhancement therapy in HF patients without dyssynchrony, and future trials are planned.

SUMMARY

Although central to many forms of HF, systolic dysfunction has been historically difficult to accurately diagnose and to therapeutically

target. Development of newer imaging tools and methods to utilize PV relation-based analytics is helping. While a conclusion that improving systolic function was a "fool's errand," as the heart would ultimately capitulate under the increased demands imposed by increased contractility, results with CRT provided optimism that it depended more on how this was accomplished. Methods to impact cAMP signaling in different compartments than those obtained from adrenergic stimulation or PDE3 inhibition are showing promise. Newer agents to modulate myofilament function may provide first-in-class sarcomere activators that safely ameliorate systolic depression. Insights from CRT have now led to the notion of using dyssynchrony as a drug, with temporary exposure and reversal serving as a potential systolic therapy. Thus, after nearly 20 years of relative inactivity, there are many new efforts in process that may well alter our approach to systolic failure. As they evolve, the assessment of systolic function and its response to therapy will undoubtedly regain importance to HF physicians and researchers.

KEY REFERENCES

14. Kass DA, Maughan WL, Guo ZM, Kono A, Sunagawa K, Sagawa K. Comparative influence of load versus inotropic states on indexes of ventrricular contractility: experimental and theoretical analysis based on pressure-volume relationships. *Circulation*. 1987;76:1422–1436.
63. Kelly RP, Ting CT, Yang TM, et al. Effective arterial elastance as index of arterial vascular load in humans. *Circulation*. 1992;86:513–521.
72. Kawaguchi M, Hay I, Fetics B, Kass DA. Combined ventricular systolic and arterial stiffening in patients with heart failure and preserved ejection fraction: implications for systolic and diastolic reserve limitations. *Circulation*. 2003;107:714–720.
84. Seo K, Rainer PP, Lee DI, et al. Hyperactive adverse mechanical stress responses in dystrophic heart are coupled to transient receptor potential canonical 6 and blocked by cGMP-Protein kinase G modulation. *Circ Res*. 2014;114:823–832.
96. Kass DA, Chen CH, Curry C, et al. Improved left ventricular mechanics from acute VDD pacing in patients with dilated cardiomyopathy and ventricular conduction delay. *Circulation*. 1999;99:1567–1573.
108. Dauterman K, Pak PH, Nussbacher A, Arie S, Liu CP, Kass DA. Contribution of external forces to left ventricle diastolic pressure: implications for the Clinical Use of the Frank-Starling Law. *Annals Int Med*. 1995;122:737–742.
125. Hsu S, Houston BA, Tampakakis E, et al. Right ventricular functional reserve in pulmonary arterial hypertension. *Circulation*. 2016;133:2413–2422.
167. Kirk JA, Chakir K, Lee KH, et al. Pacemaker-induced transient asynchrony suppresses heart failure progression. *Sci Transl Med*. 2015;7:319ra207.
113. Sunagawa K, Maughan WL, Sagawa K. Optimal arterial resistance for the maximal stroke work studied in isolated canine left ventricle. *CircRes*. 1985;56:586–586.
162. Kirk JA, Holewinski RJ, Kooij V, et al. Cardiac resynchronization sensitizes the sarcomere to calcium by reactivating GSK-3beta. *J Clin Invest*. 2014;124:129–138.

The full reference list for this chapter is available on ExpertConsult.

Alterations in Ventricular Function: Diastolic Heart Failure

Loek van Heerebeek, Walter J. Paulus

Heart failure (HF) with preserved ejection fraction (EF; HFpEF) currently accounts for greater than 50% of all HF cases, and its prevalence relative to HF with reduced EF (HFrEF) continues to rise at a rate of 1% per year (**see also Chapter 39**).[1] By 2020, the prevalence of HFpEF is projected to exceed 8% of people older than 65 years of age, and the relative prevalences of HFpEF and HFrEF are predicted to be 69% and 31%, respectively, turning HFpEF into the most prevalent HF phenotype.[1] Outcomes in patients with HFpEF and HFrEF are equally poor, with 5-year mortality rates up to 75% in both HF phenotypes.[2] In contrast to HFrEF, modern HF pharmacotherapy did not improve outcome in HFpEF, which is related to incomplete understanding of HFpEF pathophysiology, patient heterogeneity, suboptimal trial designs, and lack of insight into primary pathophysiologic processes.[3] Patients with HFpEF are frequently elderly females, and patients have a high prevalence of noncardiac comorbidities, which independently adversely affect myocardial structural and functional remodeling.[4] Furthermore, although diastolic left ventricular (LV) dysfunction represents the dominant abnormality in HFpEF, numerous ancillary mechanisms are frequently present, which also negatively affects cardiovascular reserve.[3] Over the past decade, clinical and translational research has led to improved insight into HFpEF pathophysiology and the importance of comorbidities and patient heterogeneity. Recently, a new paradigm for HFpEF has been proposed, which suggests that comorbidities drive myocardial dysfunction and remodeling in HFpEF through coronary microvascular inflammation.[4] In the conceptual framework of HFpEF treatment, emphasis may need to shift from a "one-size-fits-all" strategy to an individualized approach based on phenotypic patient characterization and diagnostic and pathophysiologic stratification of myocardial disease processes. This chapter describes these novel insights from a pathophysiologic standpoint.

PHYSIOLOGY OF DIASTOLIC FILLING AND COMPLIANCE

Normal diastolic function allows adequate filling of the heart without an excessive increase in diastolic filling pressure both at rest and with exercise. LV relaxation starts at end-systole, and LV pressure falls rapidly when the LV expands, creating a left atrial (LA)-to-LV pressure gradient when LV diastolic pressure drops below LA pressure (**Fig. 11.1**A).[5] This accelerates blood out of the LA and produces rapid early diastolic LV filling, with the LA-to-LV pressure gradient being considered a measure of LV suction.[5] Following filling of the LV, the pressure gradient from the LA to the LV apex decreases and then transiently reverses. The reversed mitral valve pressure gradient decelerates and then stops the rapid flow of blood into the LV in diastole. During the midportion of diastole (diastasis), the LA and LV pressures equilibrate and mitral flow nearly ceases. Late in diastole, atrial contraction produces a second LA-to-LV pressure gradient that again propels blood into the LV (see Fig. 11.1A). After atrial systole, as the LA relaxes, its pressure decreases below LV pressure, causing the mitral valve to begin closing.[5]

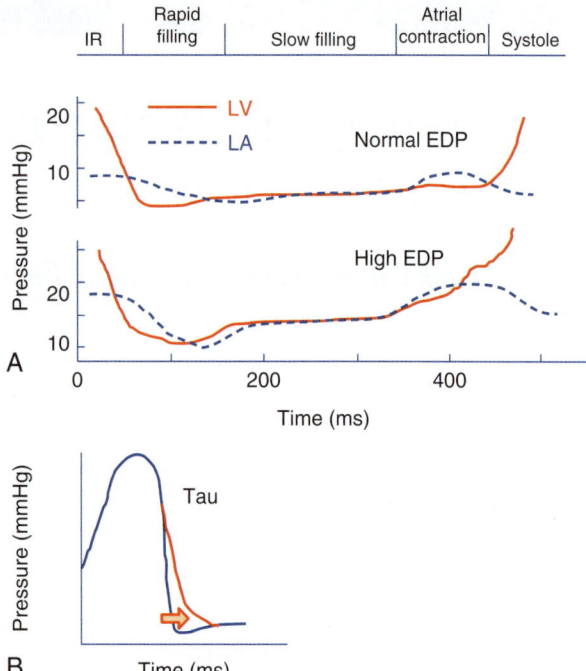

Fig. 11.1 (A) The four phases of diastole are marked in relation to pressure recordings from the left atrium *(LA)* and left ventricle *(LV)*. The first pressure crossover corresponds to the end of isovolumic relaxation *(IR)* and mitral valve opening. In the first phase, LA pressure exceeds LV pressure, accelerating mitral flow. Peak early diastolic mitral valve blood flow velocity approximately corresponds to the second crossover. Thereafter LV pressure exceeds LA pressure, decelerating mitral flow. These two phases correspond to rapid filling. This is followed by slow filling, with almost no pressure differences. During atrial contraction, LA pressure again exceeds LV pressure with late diastolic filling from LA contraction. (B) Time constant of isovolumic relaxation (Tau) indicates the rate of LV pressure fall. Tau becomes shorter when LV pressure fall accelerates and longer when LV pressure fall slows. *EDP*, End-diastolic pressure.

DIASTOLIC DYSFUNCTION

Normally, early diastole is responsible for the majority of ventricular filling, but with disturbed myocardial relaxation the rate of early diastolic LV pressure decline is reduced, which increases the time to reach minimal LV diastolic pressure and augments the importance of the contribution of atrial contraction for diastolic filling.[5] As LA pressure increases, early diastolic filling becomes more dominant despite impaired myocardial relaxation. Early filling is initiated by increased LA pressure, which pushes the blood into the LV, instead of the negative LV diastolic pressure, which pulls the blood from the LA by suction (see Fig. 11.1A). As diastolic function worsens, LA pressure is elevated and myocardial relaxation is impaired at rest, as evident from prolongation of the time constant of isovolumic relaxation (see Fig. 11.1B). Most of diastolic LV filling now occurs during early diastole, and LA contraction may not be sufficient. In this situation, LA contraction pushes blood back into the pulmonary veins, especially if pulmonary venous diastolic forward flow is already completed at the time of atrial contraction.[5] The term diastolic dysfunction indicates an abnormality of diastolic distensibility, filling, or relaxation of the LV, regardless of whether the EF is normal or abnormal and regardless of whether the patient is symptomatic or asymptomatic. After adjustment for established HF risk factors, asymptomatic antecedent LV diastolic dysfunction was associated with incident HF in individuals recruited in the Framingham Heart Study.[6] Thus diastolic dysfunction refers to abnormal mechanical (diastolic) properties of the ventricle and is present in virtually all patients with HF. The term HFpEF refers to a clinical syndrome characterized by symptoms or signs of HF, preserved LVEF, and diastolic LV dysfunction.[7]

INVASIVE MEASUREMENT OF DIASTOLIC FUNCTION: RELAXATION AND CHAMBER STIFFNESS

Evidence of abnormal LV relaxation, filling, diastolic distensibility, and diastolic stiffness can be acquired invasively during cardiac catheterization.[7] Ventricular pressure fall is the hemodynamic manifestation of myocardial relaxation, and the rate of global LV myocardial relaxation is reflected by the exponential course of isovolumic LV pressure fall (see Fig. 11.1B). Isovolumic relaxation can be quantitated by calculating the peak instantaneous rate of LV pressure decline, peak (−)dP/dt, and the time constant of isovolumic LV pressure decline, tau (τ) (see Fig. 11.1B).[7] Tau is inversely related to the rate of LV pressure fall, becoming shorter when LV pressure fall accelerates and longer when LV pressure fall slows, such that τ greater than 48 milliseconds represents evidence for delayed relaxation.[7] Another invasive approach that can be used to determine LV chamber stiffness and compliance is through measurement of LV pressure volume loops with the use of high-fidelity LV conductance catheters, which simultaneously measure LV pressure and LV volume (**Fig. 11.2**A).[8] By changing preload (e.g., transient inferior vena caval occlusion) or afterload (e.g., administration of phenylephrine), a family of loops is obtained (see Fig. 11.2B). The end-diastolic pressure-volume relationship (EDPVR), constructed by connecting the end-diastolic pressure-volume points of each loop, is nonlinear and defines the passive physical properties of the chamber with the myocardium in its most relaxed state. The end-systolic pressure-volume relationship (ESPVR), constructed by connecting the end-systolic pressure-volume points of each loop, defines a reasonably linear relationship that characterizes properties of the chamber with the myocardium in a state of maximal activation at a given contractile state (see Fig. 11.2B).[8] An important difference between HFrEF and HFpEF patients resides in these pressure-volume loops, with HFrEF being characterized by decreased contractility and downward and rightward displacement of the LV ESPVR (see Fig. 11.2C), whereas HFpEF is characterized by preserved global contractility but impaired LV relaxation, elevated filling pressures, and increased stiffness with an upward and leftward shift of the LV EDPVR, representing raised LV end-diastolic pressure at any given LV end-diastolic volume (see Fig. 11.2C).[8] This steep LV EDPVR in patients with HFpEF seems the most important determinant for impaired exercise tolerance, with deficient early diastolic LV recoil, blunted LV lusitropic or chronotropic response, vasodilator incompetence, and deranged ventriculovascular coupling serving contributory roles.[9] Elevated LV filling pressures constitute the hallmark of diastolic LV dysfunction, and filling pressures are considered elevated when the mean pulmonary capillary wedge pressure (PCWP) is greater than 12 mm Hg or when the LVEDP is greater than 16 mm Hg.[7]

NONINVASIVE MEASUREMENT OF DIASTOLIC FUNCTION: ECHOCARDIOGRAPHY

Echocardiography provides assessment of cardiac structural and functional remodeling and is most commonly used to assess LV diastolic (dys)function. Tissue Doppler (TD) echocardiography of early diastolic mitral annular movement, designated as e′ or E′ velocity, provides a noninvasive estimate of myocardial relaxation.[5] The ratio of peak early Doppler mitral valve flow velocity (E) divided by e′ (E/e′ ratio) provides a noninvasive assessment of diastolic LV filling pressure. Because E depends on LA driving pressure, LV relaxation kinetics, and age and because e′ depends mostly on LV relaxation kinetics and age, in the E/e′ ratio, effects of LV relaxation kinetics and age are eliminated, and the ratio becomes a measure of LA driving pressure or LV filling pressure. With a value of E/e′ greater than 15, LV filling pressures are elevated, and this is considered diagnostic evidence for diastolic LV dysfunction. In contrast, when *E/e′* ratio is less than 8, LV filling

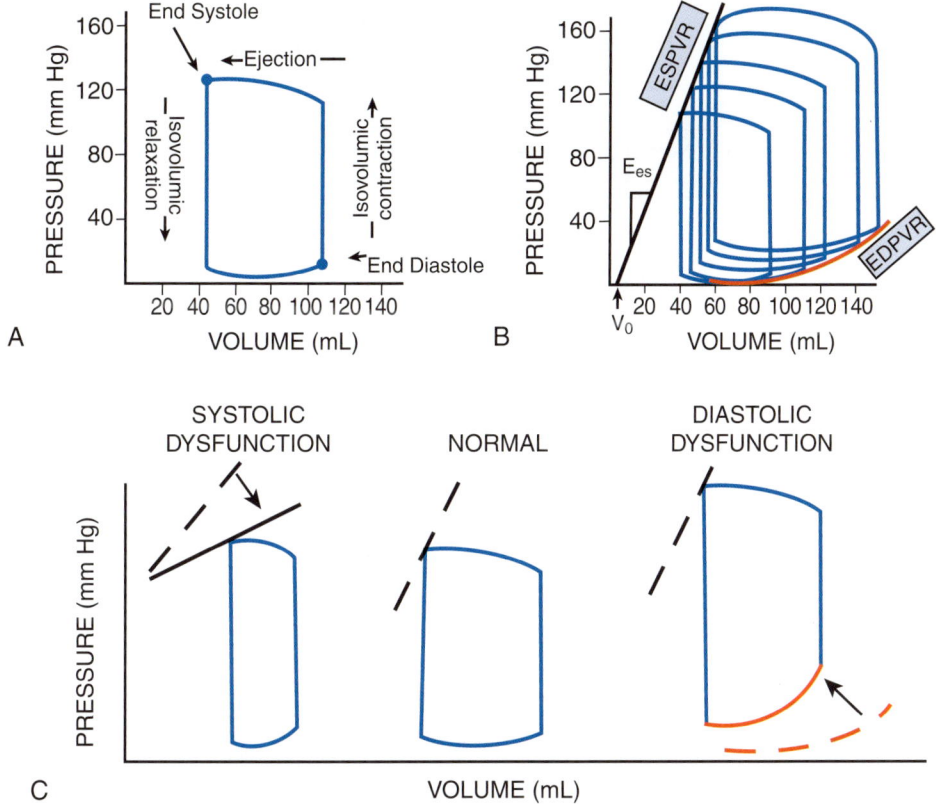

Fig. 11.2 (A) The four phases of the cardiac cycle are displayed on the pressure-volume loop, which is constructed by plotting instantaneous pressure versus volume. This loop repeats with each cardiac cycle and shows how the heart transitions from its end-diastolic state to the end-systolic state and back. (B) With a constant contractile state and afterload, a progressive reduction in ventricular filling pressure causes the loops to shift toward lower volumes at both end systole and end diastole. When the resulting end-systolic pressure-volume points are connected, a reasonably linear end-systolic pressure-volume relationship *(ESPVR)* is obtained. The linear ESPVR is characterized by a slope *(E$_{es}$)* and a volume axis intercept *(V$_0$)*. In contrast, the diastolic pressure-volume points define a nonlinear end-diastolic pressure-volume relationship *(EDPVR)*. (C) In systolic dysfunction, contractility is depressed and the ESPVR is displaced downward and to the right; there is diminished capacity to eject blood into a high-pressure aorta. In diastolic dysfunction, chamber stiffness is increased and the EDPVR is displaced up and to the left; there is diminished capacity to fill at low diastolic pressures. The LVEF is low in systolic dysfunction and normal in diastolic dysfunction. *LVEF,* Left ventricular ejection fraction.

pressures are low, and this is considered diagnostic evidence of absence of HFpEF. An *E/e′* ratio ranging from 8 to 15 is considered suggestive but nondiagnostic evidence of diastolic LV dysfunction and needs to be implemented with additional echocardiographic measurements or evidence of elevated biomarkers to confirm the diagnosis of HFpEF.[7]

Estimation of Left Ventricle Filling Pressures

In contrast to earlier studies, which demonstrated close correlation of the E/e′ ratio with LV filling pressures, recent studies combining right heart catheterization and echocardiography demonstrated that E/e′ did not reliably track changes in left-sided filling pressures at rest and during alterations in loading conditions,[10] whereas in some patients, elevated filling pressure is observed only during exercise.[11] Therefore normal filling pressure at rest does not exclude clinically significant diastolic dysfunction or HFpEF. In addition, presence of structural LV and/or LA remodeling is suggestive for diastolic LV dysfunction.

Left Ventricle Hypertrophy

LV geometry can be described based on the LV mass (hypertrophy) and the relative wall thickness (RWT), which describes the relationship between wall thickness and cavity size (concentricity). LV hypertrophy can occur in the context of increased RWT (concentric hypertrophy) or normal to reduced RWT (eccentric hypertrophy).

Increased concentricity can also occur in the absence of frank hypertrophy (concentric remodeling). LV concentric remodeling and/or hypertrophy was present in 59% to 77% of HFpEF patients included in the Treatment of Preserved Cardiac Function Heart Failure With an Aldosterone Antagonist (TOPCAT)[12] and Irbesartan in HFpEF (I-PRESERVE)[13] trials with concentric LV remodeling and/or hypertrophy being related to increased mortality and HF hospitalization.[14]

Left Atrial Dysfunction

LA volume is strongly associated with severity of diastolic LV dysfunction, independent of LVEF, age, gender, and cardiovascular risk score, and patients with HFpEF frequently demonstrate both increased LA volume and impaired LA function, which are independently associated with worse outcome.[15,16] The principal role of the LA is to modulate LV filling and cardiovascular performance by functioning as a reservoir for pulmonary venous return during ventricular systole, a conduit for pulmonary venous return during early ventricular diastole, and a booster pump that augments ventricular filling during late ventricular diastole.[15,16] In the I-PRESERVE and TOPCAT echocardiographic substudies, 65% of HFpEF patients had LA dilatation.[14,17] In HFpEF patients enrolled in TOPCAT, lower peak LA strain was associated with older age, higher prevalence of atrial fibrillation and LV hypertrophy, worse LV systolic and diastolic function, and higher risk of HF hospitalization.[15]

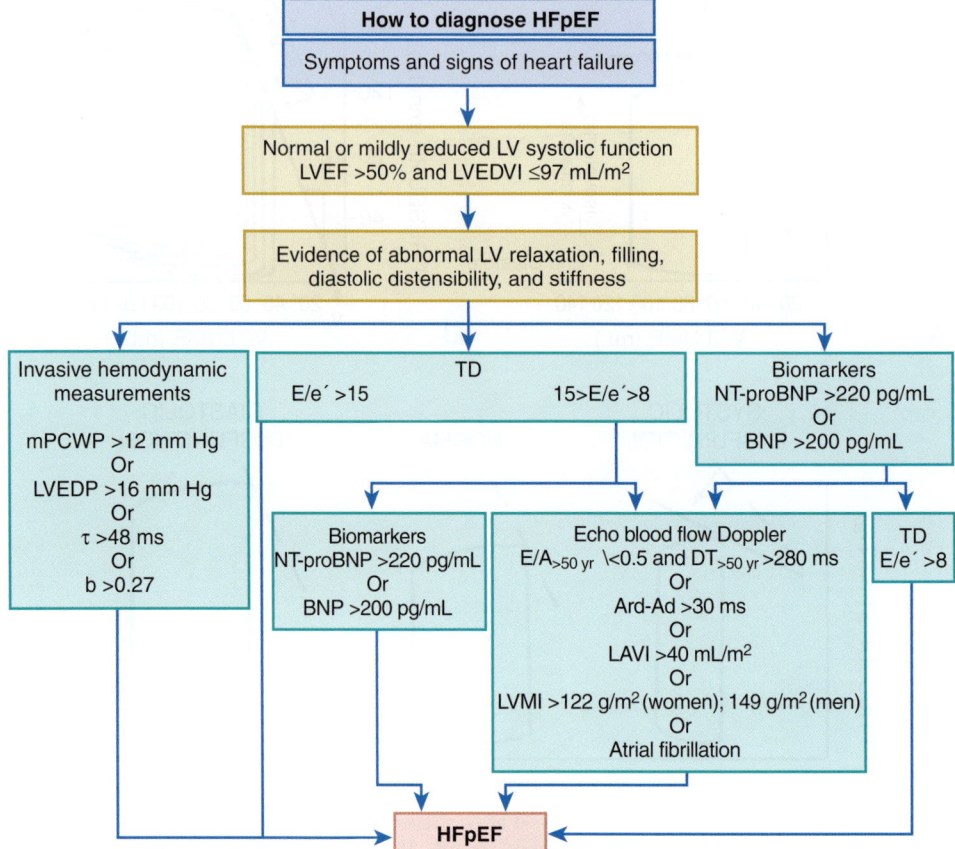

Fig. 11.3 Diagnostic Flowchart on "How to Diagnose HFpEF." *τ*, Time constant of left ventricular relaxation; *Ad*, duration of mitral valve trial wave flow. *Ard*, duration of reverse pulmonary vein atrial systole flow; *b*, constant of left ventricular chamber stiffness; *BNP*, B-type natriuretic peptide; *DT*, deceleration time; *e′*, velocity of mitral annulus early diastolic motion; *E*, early mitral valve flow velocity; *E/A*, ratio of early (E) to late (A) mitral valve flow velocity; *HFpEF*, heart failure with preserved ejection fraction; *LAVI*, left atrial volume index; *LV*, Left ventricle; *LVEDP*, left ventricular end-diastolic pressure; *LVEDVI*, left ventricular end-diastolic volume index; *LVEF*, left ventricular ejection fraction; *LVMI*, left ventricular mass index; *mPCWP*, mean pulmonary capillary wedge pressure; *NT-proBNP*, N-terminal proBNP; *TD*, tissue Doppler.

NATRIURETIC PEPTIDES (SEE ALSO CHAPTERS 9 AND 33)

Natriuretic peptides (NPs) represent the third modality that can be used in the diagnosis of HFpEF.[7] Atrial natriuretic peptide (ANP) and B-type natriuretic peptide (BNP) are produced by atrial and ventricular myocardium in response to an increase of atrial or ventricular diastolic stretch due to volume or pressure overload, and their secretion results in natriuresis, vasodilation, and improved LV relaxation. Cardiac myocytes produce proBNP, which is subsequently cleaved in the blood into N-terminal (NT)-proBNP and BNP.[18] NP levels are lower in HFpEF than in HFrEF, which is usually attributed to lower LV diastolic wall stress in HFpEF because of concentric LV remodeling.[1,19] Recently, a cushioning effect of epicardial fat was also suggested to contribute to the low NP levels in HFpEF as it dampens LV distension in diastole.[20] The latter finding explains why low NT-proBNP plasma levels are frequently observed in HFpEF patients suffering from obesity, a highly prevalent comorbidity and important contributor to HFpEF.[4] Indeed, patients with invasively proven HFpEF frequently even have low or even normal NP levels.[21] A recent study, which used combined rest and exercise PCWP measurements to diagnose HFpEF, reported a median value of 406 pg/ml with 18% of patients having a normal plasma NT-proBNP level (<125 pg/mL).[21] In early-stage HFpEF, increase of LV filling pressures, which triggers NP release, can be limited to conditions of physical exercise with normal or near-normal filling pressures at rest.[21] Low NP

expression was confirmed in LV myocardial biopsies of HFpEF patients, who had four times lower myocardial proBNP$_{108}$ content than HFrEF patients.[22] Therefore, when used for diagnostic purposes, NPs do not provide diagnostic standalone evidence of HFpEF and always need to be implemented with other noninvasive investigations.[7] Despite low levels of NPs in HFpEF, NPs remain an indicator of disease severity in HFpEF as they predicted prognosis in several HFpEF outcome trials. In the Coordinating Study Evaluating Outcomes of Advising and Counseling in Heart Failure (COACH) trial, BNP levels were lower in HFpEF than in HFrEF, but, for a similar elevation in BNP, prognosis was equally poor in both conditions.[19] In the I-PRESERVE trial, baseline log transformed NT-proBNP was the strongest predictor of all three outcomes.[23]

DIAGNOSIS OF HEART FAILURE WITH PRESERVED EJECTION FRACTION

According to current recommendations, three obligatory conditions need to be satisfied for the diagnosis of HFpEF: (1) presence of signs or symptoms of congestive HF; (2) presence of preserved LV systolic function, defined as LVEF greater than 50% and LV end-diastolic volume index (LVEDVI) less than 97 mL/m²; and (3) evidence of diastolic LV dysfunction determined either by invasive measurements or by echocardiography alone or by echocardiography in conjunction with biomarkers (**Fig. 11.3**).[7] Decompensated patients with HFpEF typically display overt congestion on physical examination and chest

	Clinical Variable	Values	Points
H₂	Heavy	Body mass index > 30 kg/m²	2
	Hypertensive	2 or more antihypertensive medicines	1
F	Atrial fibrillation	Paroxysmal or persistent	3
P	Pulmonary hypertension	Doppler echocardiographic estimated pulmonary artery systolic pressure >35 mm Hg	
E	Elder	Age > 60 years	1
F	Filling pressure	Echocardiographic E/e′ >9	1
	H₂FPEF score		Sum (0–9)

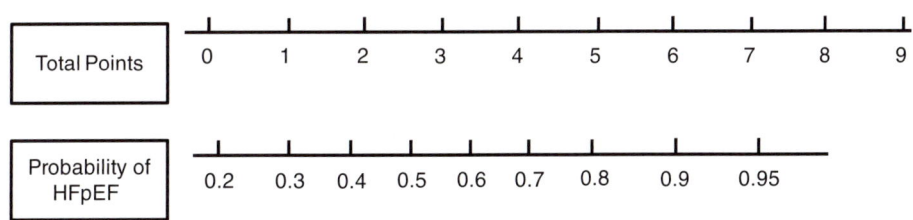

Fig. 11.4 Description of the H₂FPEF score and point allocations for each clinical characteristic *(top box)*, with associated probability of having heart failure with preserved ejection fraction *(HFpEF)* based upon the total score as estimated from the model *(lower box)*.

radiography, and in this setting the diagnosis is straightforward. However, compensated, euvolemic patients presenting with exertional dyspnea in the absence of overt clinical, radiographic, or biomarker evidence of congestion present a greater diagnostic challenge. The reference standard to diagnose HFpEF in these patients is by right heart catheterization followed by invasive exercise testing if resting intracardiac pressures are normal.[21] Because of its invasive nature, technical complexity, and cost, this test is impractical for routine evaluation but is more logically reserved for situations in which diagnosis remains uncertain after less invasive test results are equivocal.[21] To make this determination, the probability of disease must first be estimated, allowing clinicians to decide whether disease is likely present or absent, or intermediate, when more definitive testing is required. A recent study evaluated clinical data from consecutive patients for whom the diagnosis of HFpEF or a noncardiac etiology of dyspnea was ascertained conclusively by invasive exercise testing to develop a scoring system that can be used in the diagnostic evaluation of HFpEF.[24] HFpEF patients were identified by elevated PCWP at rest (≥15 mm Hg) or during exercise (≥25 mm Hg).[11,21] Logistic regression was performed to evaluate the ability of clinical findings to discriminate cases from controls, and a scoring system was developed and validated in a separate test cohort. Obesity, atrial fibrillation, age greater than 60 years, treatment with two or more antihypertensives, echocardiographic E/e′ ratio greater than 9, and echocardiographic pulmonary artery systolic pressure greater than 35 mm Hg were selected as the final set of predictive variables. A weighted score based on these six variables was used to create a composite score (H₂FPEF score) ranging from 0 to 9 (**Fig. 11.4**).[24] The odds of HFpEF doubled for each 1-unit score increase (odds ratio [OR] 1.98 1.74–2.30], $P < .0001$) with an area under the curve (AUC) of 0.841 ($P < .0001$) (see Fig. 11.4). By establishing the probability of disease, the H₂FPEF score may be used to effectively rule out disease among patients with low scores (e.g., 0 or 1), establish the diagnosis with reasonably high confidence at higher scores (e.g., 6–9), and identify patients for whom additional testing is needed with intermediate scores (e.g., 2–5) (see Fig. 11.4).[24]

HEART FAILURE WITH PRESERVED EJECTION FRACTION: HIGH DIASTOLIC LEFT VENTRICLE STIFFNESS

In the absence of endocardial or pericardial disease, high diastolic LV stiffness results from increased myocardial stiffness, which is regulated by the extracellular matrix (ECM) and the cardiomyocytes (**Fig. 11.5**).[4]

Regulation of Diastolic Stiffness by the Extracellular Matrix

The ECM contributes to passive stiffness in diastole and prevents overstretch, myocyte slippage, and tissue deformation during ventricular filling, and components of the ECM also serve as modulators of growth and tissue differentiation (**see also Chapter 4**).[25] The ECM is composed of fibrillary proteins (such as collagen and elastin), nonfibrillary proteins (such as aminoglycans, fibronectin, laminin), and bioactive proteins (such as transforming growth factor-β [TGF-β], matrix metalloproteinases [MMPs], tissue inhibitors of matrix metalloproteinases [TIMPs], and matricellular proteins).[25] Collagen importantly determines ECM-based stiffness, through regulation of its total amount, expression of collagen type I, and degree of collagen cross-linking, which are increased and linked to diastolic LV dysfunction[26] and outcome[27] in patients with HFpEF. Diffuse interstitial myocardial fibrosis, assessed by magnetic resonance imaging–derived T1 mapping, was recently shown to predict invasively measured LV stiffness in patients with HFpEF.[28] Collagen metabolism requires sequential, highly orchestrated and regulated steps: (1) procollagen synthesis and secretion, (2) procollagen postsynthetic processing, (3) collagen posttranslational modification, and (4) collagen degradation (**Fig. 11.6**). Each of these steps is altered in HFpEF, contributes either individually or in aggregate to LV diastolic dysfunction, is mirrored in plasma biomarkers, and serves as a unique treatment target.[29] In HFpEF, fibroblasts are presumed to convert to myofibroblasts because of exposure to TGF-β as a result of monocyte/macrophage myocardial

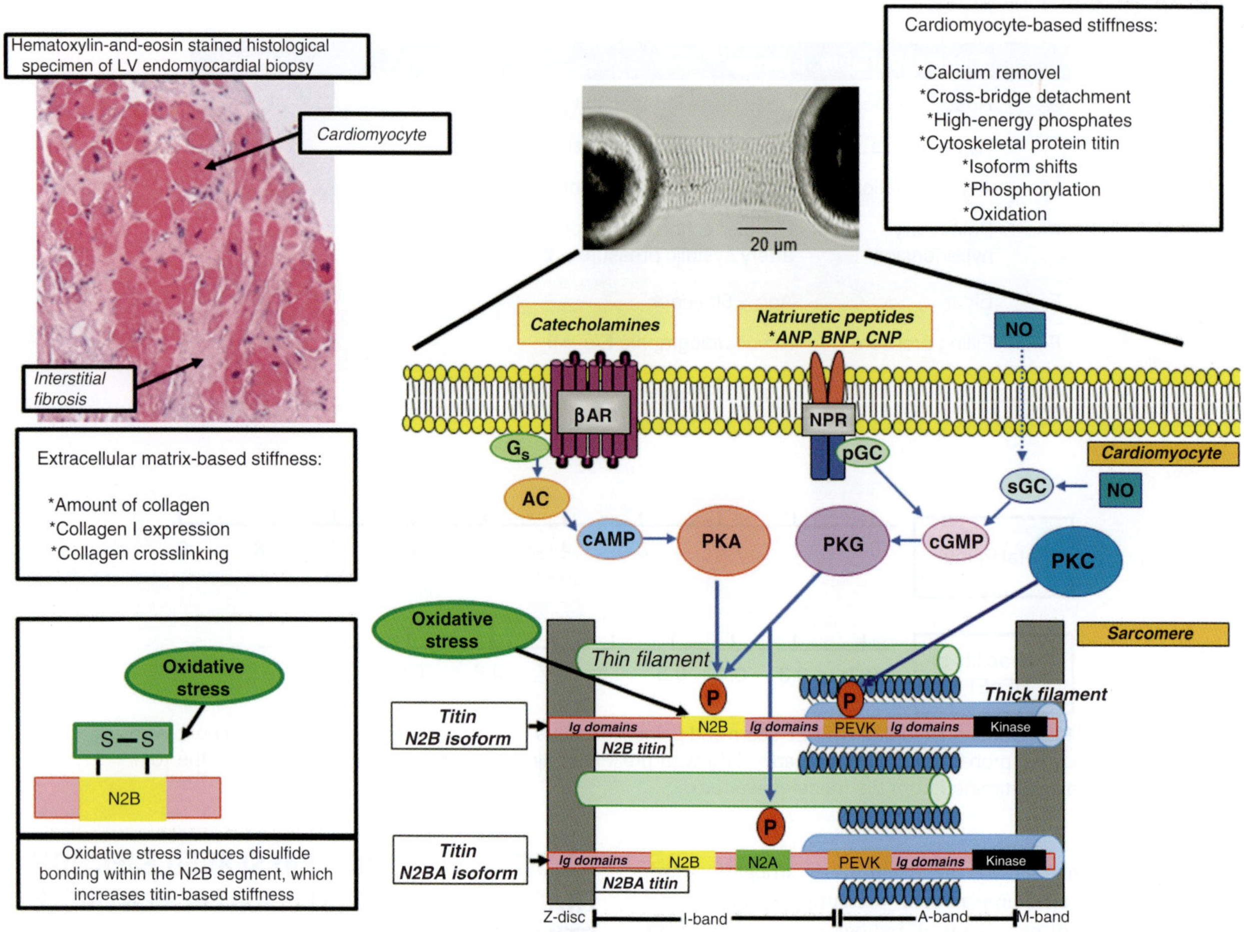

Hematoxylin-and-eosin stained histological specimen of LV endomyocardial biopsy

Cardiomyocyte

Interstitial fibrosis

Cardiomyocyte-based stiffness:

*Calcium removel
*Cross-bridge detachment
*High-energy phosphates
*Cytoskeletal protein titin
  *Isoform shifts
  *Phosphorylation
  *Oxidation

20 μm

Catecholamines

Natriuretic peptides
*ANP, BNP, CNP

NO

βAR

NPR

Gs

pGC

Cardiomyocyte

sGC

NO

Extracellular matrix-based stiffness:

*Amount of collagen
*Collagen I expression
*Collagen crosslinking

AC

cAMP

PKA

PKG

cGMP

PKC

Oxidative stress

Oxidative stress

S—S

N2B

Oxidative stress induces disulfide bonding within the N2B segment, which increases titin-based stiffness

Sarcomere

Thin filament

Thick filament

Titin N2B isoform

P

P

Ig domains   N2B   Ig domains   PEVK   Ig domains   Kinase

N2B titin

Titin N2BA isoform

P

Ig domains   N2B   N2A   PEVK   Ig domains   Kinase

N2BA titin

Z-disc   I-band   A-band   M-band

Fig. 11.5 Extracellular Matrix and Cardiomyocytes Determine Myocardial Stiffness. Extracellular matrix–based stiffness is predominantly regulated by collagen. Cardiomyocyte-based stiffness is predominantly regulated by the giant elastic sarcomeric protein titin (see text). Cardiomyocyte signaling pathways involved in regulating cardiac titin stiffness. Titin-based stiffness can be modulated by reversible phosphorylation of the N2B segment by both PKA and PKG. Activation of PKA results from stimulation by signaling through the β-adrenergic pathway, which is coupled to the second messenger cAMP. Activation of PKG results from stimulation by the second messenger cGMP. Generation of cGMP results from either activation of sGC by NO or from activation of pGC by NPs. PKC mediated phosphorylation of the PEVK segment of titin increases cardiomyocyte stiffness. Oxidative stress–mediated formation of disulfide bonds in the N2B segment of titin increases cardiomyocyte stiffness. *Circled Ps* indicate phosphorylatable sites. βAR, β-Adrenergic receptor; *AC*, adenylyl cyclase; *Ang II*, angiotensin II; *ANP*, atrial natriuretic peptide; *BNP*, brain-type natriuretic peptide; *CaMKII*, Ca^{2+}/calmodulin-dependent protein kinase II; *cAMP*, cyclic adenosine monophosphate; *cGMP*, cyclic guanosine monophosphate; *CNP*, C-type natriuretic peptide; *ERK2*, extracellular signal–regulated kinase-2; *ET-1*, endothelin-1; *G*, G-stimulatory protein; *GPCR*, G protein–coupled receptor; *Ig's*, immunoglobulin domains; *LV*, left ventricle; *MEK1/2*, MAPK/ERK kinase-1 and -2; *NO*, nitric oxide; *NPR*, natriuretic peptide receptor; *PDE5*, phosphodiesterase type 5; *PDE5*, phosphodiesterase type 5; *PEVK*, unique sequence rich in proline, glutamic acid, valine, and lysine; *pGC*, particulate guanylate cyclase; *PKC*, Ca^{2+}-dependent protein kinase C; *Raf*, rat fibrosarcoma protein; *Ras*, rat sarcoma protein; *sGC*, soluble guanylate cyclase.

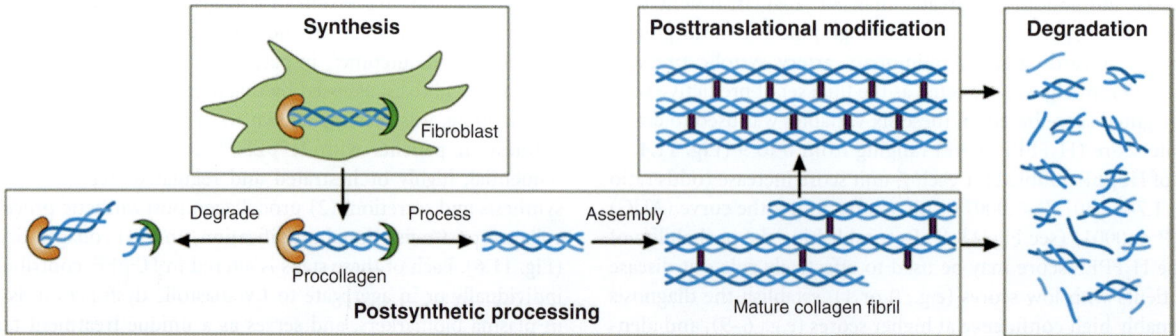

Synthesis

Fibroblast

Posttranslational modification

Degradation

Degrade   Process   Assembly

Procollagen

Postsynthetic processing

Mature collagen fibril

Fig. 11.6 Collagen metabolism involves sequential steps consisting of procollagen synthesis, procollagen processing to collagen fibrils, posttranslational modification of collagen fibrils, and collagen degradation.

TABLE 11.1   Unequal Structural, Functional, and Ultrastructural Left Ventricle Characteristics in HFpEF and HFrEf

	HFpEF	HFrEF
LV structure/function		
End-diastolic volume	↔	↑
End-systolic volume	↔	↑
Wall thickness	↑	↔
Mass	↑	↑
Mass/volume ratio	↑	↓
Remodeling	Concentric	Eccentric
Ejection fraction	↔	↓
Stroke work	↔	↓
End-systolic elastance	↔	↓
End-diastolic stiffness	↑	↓
LV ultrastructure		
Myocyte diameter	↑	↔
Myocyte length	↔	↑
Myocyte remodeling	Concentric	Eccentric
Fibrosis	Interstitial/reactive	Focal/replacement

HFpEF, Heart failure with preserved ejection fraction; *HFrEF*, heart failure with reduced ejection fraction.

infiltration, whereas matrix degradation is decreased because of altered expression of MMPs and upregulation of TIMPs.[30] Distinct expression profiles of MMPs and TIMPs also correspond to differences in ECM geometry, composition, and homeostatic mechanisms in HFpEF versus HFrEF. HFpEF is more often associated with interstitial, reactive fibrosis and HFrEF with focal, replacement fibrosis (Table 11.1).[8] As recently shown in LV biopsies, increased diastolic LV stiffness in hypertensive HFpEF patients was caused by both the ECM and elevated intrinsic cardiomyocyte stiffness.[31]

Regulation of Myocardial Stiffness by the Cardiomyocyte (see also Chapters 1, 2 and 9)

High intrinsic cardiomyocyte stiffness importantly contributes to high diastolic LV stiffness in HFpEF.[22,31] Cardiomyocyte stiffness is mainly determined by the elastic sarcomeric protein titin, which functions as a bidirectional spring, responsible for early diastolic recoil and late diastolic distensibility (see Fig. 11.5).[32] Titin spans a half sarcomere running from the Z disc to the M band with an elastic spring element in the I band of the sarcomere.[32] Titin-based cardiomyocyte stiffness results from dynamic changes in expression of stiff (N2B) and compliant (N2BA) isoforms and from posttranslational modifications including titin isoform phosphorylation and oxidative changes of the N2B segment.[32] Phosphorylation of the N2B segment decreases titin-based myofilament stiffness. Kinases known to phosphorylate the N2B segment include extracellular signal regulated kinase-1/2 (ERK1/2), cAMP-dependent protein kinase A (PKA), cGMP-dependent protein kinase (PKG), and calcium/calmodulin-dependent kinase II (CaMKII). In contrast, phosphorylation of the PEVK-region increases titin-based myofilament stiffness, mediated by phosphorylation by Ca^{2+}-dependent protein kinase C (PKCα) (see Fig. 11.5).[32] Hypophosphorylation of the N2B segment and hyperphosphorylation of PEVK can act complementary to elevate passive tension (e.g., in end-stage HF) and are important to fine-tune passive myocardial stiffness and diastolic function in the heart.

Cardiomyocyte stiffness was higher in patients with HFpEF than in patients with HFrEF or aortic stenosis (AS) and correlated with reduced myocardial concentration of the pivotal second messenger cGMP and

lower activity of its effector kinase PKG in HFpEF than in HFrEF or AS (**Fig. 11.7**).[22] The generation of the second messenger molecule cGMP results from activation of soluble guanylate cyclase (sGC) by nitric oxide (NO) and from activation of particulate GC (pGC) by NPs (**Fig. 11.8**).[33] Once generated, cGMP activates PKG, allowing PKG-mediated phosphorylation of a vast number of target proteins, exerting a wide range of downstream effects such as enhanced reuptake of calcium (Ca^{2+}) into the sarcoplasmic reticulum (SR), inhibition of Ca^{2+} influx, suppression of hypertrophic signaling through inhibition of G protein–coupled receptors and the transient receptor potential canonical channel; inhibition of ischemia-reperfusion injury through phosphorylation of the ATP-sensitive potassium channel; and stimulation of LV relaxation and LV distensibility by phosphorylation of troponin I and the stiff titin N2B segment (see Fig. 11.8).[33] In addition to posttranslational modifications of titin consisting of lack or excess phosphorylation at specific sites along the titin molecule, altered diastolic stiffness was recently suggested to also originate from titin being damaged by oxidative or physical stress.[34,35] Using single-molecule atomic force microscopy force-extension measurements on recombinant immunoglobulin (Ig) domain polyprotein constructs, it was shown that the human titin N2-B-unique sequence (N2-B[us]) contains up to three disulfide bridges under oxidizing conditions, leading to increased titin-based cardiomyocyte stiffness.[34] In addition, mechanical unfolding of titin Ig domains exposes buried cysteine residues, which then can be S-glutathionylated. S-glutathionylation of cryptic cysteines greatly decreases the mechanical stability of the parent Ig domain, as well as its ability to fold. Both effects favor a more extensible state of titin.[35] Recently, it was demonstrated that the family of small heat shock proteins (sHSPs), including HSP27 and αB-crystallin, provide myofilamentary protection upon cardiomyocyte harmful insults.[36-38] Typically, sHSPs are upregulated under diverse stress situations, and their overexpression protects cells from oxidative stress, energy depletion, and other unfavorable conditions.[36] In the heart, αB-crystallin and HSP27 are induced during ischemic injury, heat stress, or end-stage failure.[36,37] In response to potentially harmful insults, the myocyte sHSPs, including αB-crystallin and HSP27, preferentially translocate from the cytosol to the myofibrils, where they bind to the sarcomeric Z disc and/or I band (**Fig. 11.9**).[37] Previous exposure of cardiomyocytes to stretch and low pH caused a rise of cardiomyocyte stiffness and was indeed suppressed by HSP27 and αB-crystalline.[37] Sarcomere stretch unfolds titin domains, exposing concealed hydrophobic sites, leading to aggregation of titin Ig domains, which results in loss of function and increased cardiomyocyte stiffness.[37] Interestingly, HSP27 and αB-crystallin provided protection against titin aggregation, with lowering of cardiomyocyte stiffness.[37] Administration of αB-crystallin also reversed the combined effects of prestretch and acidic pH on the diastolic passive tension ($F_{passive}$)—sarcomere length (SL) relation in cardiomyocytes isolated from LV tissue samples of patients with dilated cardiomyopathy (DCM) or AS (**Fig. 11.10**).[38] In AS and DCM cardiomyocytes, αB-crystallin lowered diastolic stiffness well below baseline values, as previously reported after administration of PKA or PKG.[22,39] This supports overlapping effects of titin phosphorylation and stretch-induced titin aggregation possibly because of preexisting stretch-induced titin aggregation obstructing phosphorylation at sites that specifically increase titin elasticity. This finding has important therapeutic implications because it implies limited efficacy of drugs that increase PKA or PKG activity for treatment of diastolic LV dysfunction related to high cardiomyocyte stiffness and could relate to the failure of dobutamine to improve diastolic LV dysfunction[40] and of phosphodiesterase (PDE) 5 inhibitors to improve exercise tolerance or hemodynamics in HFPEF.[41,42] In addition, upregulation and subsarcolemmal localization of αB-crystallin was observed in AS and DCM

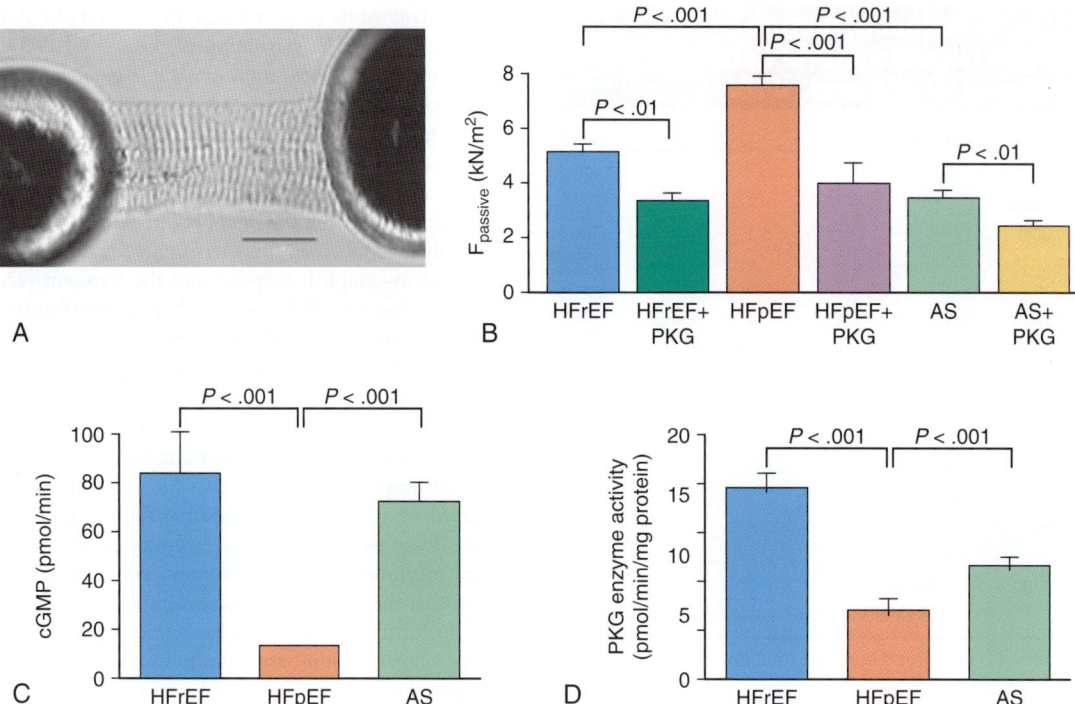

Fig. 11.7 (A) Single permeabilized cardiomyocyte mounted between force transducer and piezoelectric motor. (B) Higher cardiomyocyte passive tension in heart failure with preserved ejection fraction *(HFpEF)* than in heart failure with reduced ejection fraction *(HFrEF)* and aortic stenosis *(AS)*. After in vitro administration of cGMP-dependent protein kinase *(PKG)* there was a larger decrement in cardiomyocyte passive tension in HFpEF than in HFrEF and AS. (C) Lower myocardial cGMP concentration in HFpEF than in HFrEF or in AS. (D) Lower myocardial PKG activity in HFpEF than in HFrEF or in AS. *cGMP*, cyclic guanosine monophosphate.

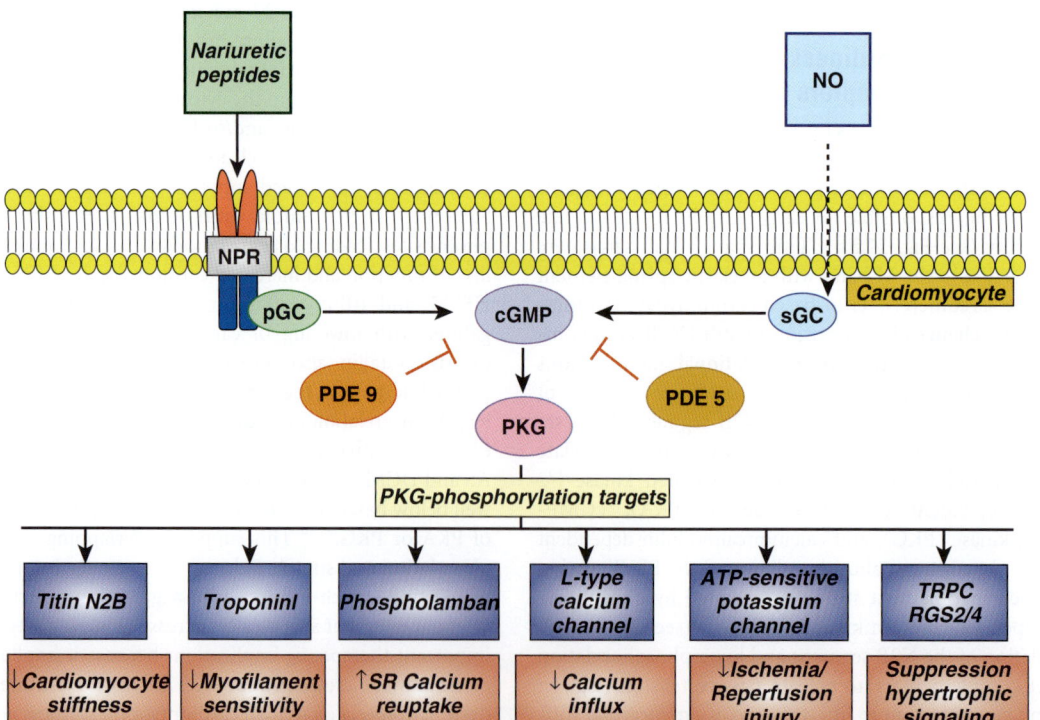

Fig. 11.8 Myocardial cGMP-PKG Signaling. See text for details. *cGMP*, cyclic guanosine monophosphate; *PDE5*, phosphodiesterase type 5; *pGC*, particulate guanylate cyclase; *PKG*, cGMP-dependent protein kinase; *NO*, nitric oxide; *NPR*, natriuretic peptide receptor; *sGC*, soluble guanylate cyclase; *SR*, sarcoplasmic reticulum.

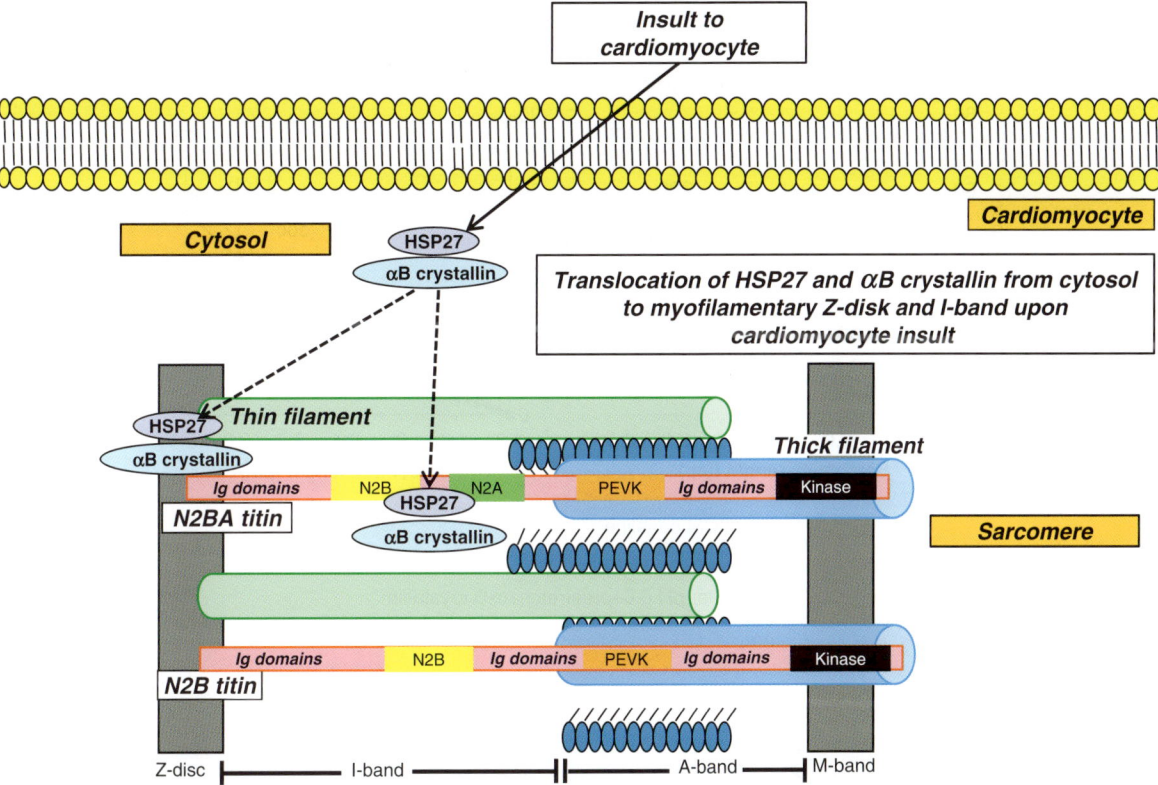

Fig. 11.9 Protective Actions of Heat Shock Proteins. See text for details. *αB*-crystallin, alpha B-crystallin; *HSP27*, heat shock protein 27; *Ig*, immunoglobulin domains; *PEVK*, unique sequence rich in proline, glutamic acid, valine, and lysine.

cardiomyocytes.[38] Because of the close vicinity of capillaries (*white arrows* in **Fig. 11.11**), the localization of αB-crystallin in subsarcolemmal aggresomes was consistent with signals from the microvascular endothelium being involved in their formation. The subsarcolemmal localization also suggested that endogenous αB-crystallin was diverted from the sarcomeres and therefore failed to exert its protective action on titin distensibility, which was, however, restored after administration of exogenous αB-crystallin. The latter finding supports future therapeutic efforts to raise concentration of αB-crystallin in failing myocardium through direct administration of αB-crystallin, through administration of αB-crystallin analogues or through administration of HSP-inducing drugs such as geranylgeranylacetone or NYK9354.

The downregulation of myocardial cGMP-PKG signaling seen in HFpEF was related to reduced myocardial BNP expression and increased microvascular inflammation and oxidative stress, which impair both the NP-cGMP and NO-cGMP axes (**Fig. 11.12**).[22] Reduced myocardial BNP expression in HFpEF could have resulted from a number of factors, including concomitant obesity and insulin resistance (IR), which are known to lower myocardial BNP expression and concentric LV remodeling/hypertrophy, which lowers both systolic and diastolic LV wall stress.[43] Reduced myocardial BNP expression in HFpEF could result from concentric LV remodeling/hypertrophy and obesity-mediated clearance and impaired production. In addition, increased expression of PDE type 9 breaks down cGMP specifically generated through the NP-pGC axis (see Fig. 11.8).[44] Impaired NO-cGMP signaling could result from the increased inflammation and oxidative stress observed in HFpEF, which was inferred from the high prevalence of comorbidities such as hypertension, obesity, type 2 diabetes mellitus (T2DM), chronic obstructive pulmonary disease (COPD), anemia, and renal dysfunction.[1,4,22] In addition, HFpEF patients are generally older and more often female, suggesting that older age and gender-specific characteristics may contribute to HFpEF pathophysiology.[1,4,22]

COMORBIDITIES IN HEART FAILURE WITH PRESERVED EJECTION FRACTION (SEE ALSO CHAPTER 39)

Increased Age

Half of all HF diagnoses and 90% of all HF deaths occur in patients older than 70 years, and HF incidence doubles with each decade of life.[45] Aging is associated with increased LV wall thickness, myocardial collagen deposition, cardiomyocyte hypertrophy, arterial stiffening, and with disturbed diastolic calcium handling, β-adrenergic signaling, and mitochondrial and endothelial dysfunction, which impair LV relaxation and early filling.[45] Ventricular systolic and diastolic stiffness increase in tandem with normal aging, particularly in women, even as arterial stiffness decreased or remains stable.[46]

Female Gender

Women more frequently have concentric LV remodeling, higher EF, increased systolic and diastolic LV stiffness, and higher pulsatile arterial loading with increased age-dependent vascular stiffening compared with men.[46,47] Estrogens exert several cardiovascular protective effects, including inhibition of RAAS activation and myocardial fibrosis, stimulation of NO bioavailability and mitochondrial biogenesis, and regulation of cardiomyocyte calcium handling.[48]

Chronic Obstructive Pulmonary Disease

Reduced forced expiratory volume in 1 second in COPD independently predicts incident HF, which was attributed to the low-grade systemic inflammation present in COPD.[49] COPD is both a premorbid identifier of HFpEF[50] and a contributor to HFpEF mortality.[51] In a

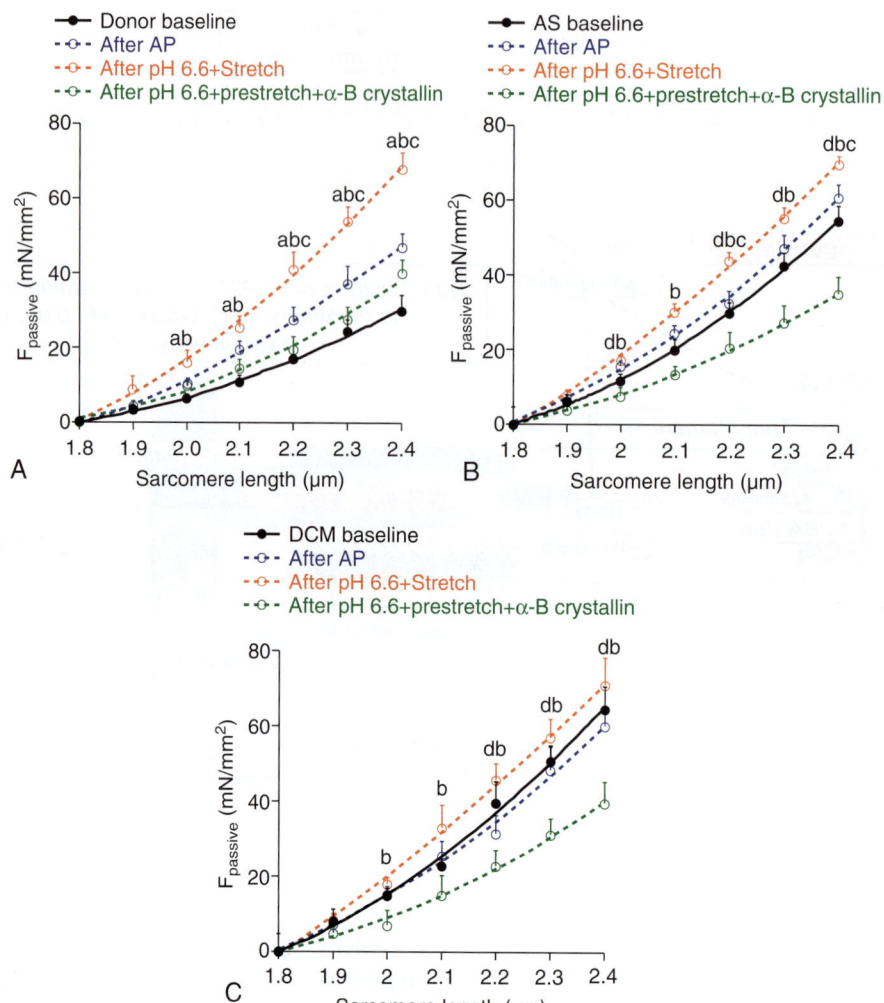

Fig. 11.10 Passive in Single Myocytes. (A) In donor cardiomyocytes, $F_{passive}$ significantly increased after administration of alkaline phosphatase *(AP)* and increased further after performing a prestretch in an acidic environment. After in vitro administration of αB-crystallin, $F_{passive}$ fell to a position slightly lower than after AP. (B) In aortic stenosis (AS) cardiomyocytes, no significant change in $F_{passive}$ was observed after incubation with AP. After the prestretch in pH 6.6, $F_{passive}$ increased significantly compared with baseline, but in vitro treatment with αB-crystallin lowered $F_{passive}$ to a level significantly lower than baseline. (C) In dilated cardiomyopathy (DCM) cardiomyocytes, incubation with AP had no effect on $F_{passive}$, but performing a prestretch in an acidic environment significantly increased passive stiffness. After in vitro treatment with αB-crystallin, $F_{passive}$ fell to a level significantly below baseline. [a]$P < .05$ AP versus baseline; [b]$P < .05$ pH 6.6+prestretch versus AP; [c]$P < .05$ αB-crystallin versus pH 6.6+prestretch; [d]$P < .05$ αB-crystallin versus baseline.

population-based study, greater severity of COPD was linearly related to impaired LV filling, reduced stroke volume, and lower cardiac output without changes in LVEF.[52]

Anemia

HFpEF patients demonstrate a high prevalence of anemia, which is associated with increased risk of HF hospitalization and overall mortality.[53,54] Inflammation importantly contributes to anemia in HF,[55] through impaired production of erythropoietin and causing bone marrow dysfunction.[56] In HF with or without anemia, iron deficiency contributes to immune responses and oxidative stress.[57]

Renal Dysfunction

Chronic kidney disease is present in approximately 30% to 40% of HF patients and is an important predictor of mortality.[58] HF and chronic renal failure frequently coexist, which can be related to common risk factors, such as hypertension, diabetes, and atherosclerosis, but also

to common pathogenic mechanisms such as neurohumoral activation, inflammation, and oxidative stress.[59] Impaired renal function was recently also identified as a risk factor for developing HFpEF.[60] HFpEF and renal dysfunction are mutually promoting.[59] HFpEF promotes renal dysfunction by (1) an elevated central venous pressure, which results from pulmonary hypertension and right ventricular (RV) dysfunction; (2) inability to increase cardiac output following arterial vasodilation because of chronotropic incompetence and fixed LV stroke volume[61]; (3) systemic inflammation, endothelial dysfunction, and low NO bioavailability, which reduces renal blood flow[62,63] and sodium excretion.[64] Renal dysfunction promotes HFpEF by worsening systemic inflammation, endothelial dysfunction, and NO bioavailability, in part, because of renal-specific mediators, such as high levels of fibroblast growth factor 23, phosphorus, parathyroid hormone, or uremic toxins, and low levels of vitamin D or erythropoietin.[59] Endothelial inflammatory activation is associated with microalbuminuria, which was recently shown to be associated with LV diastolic

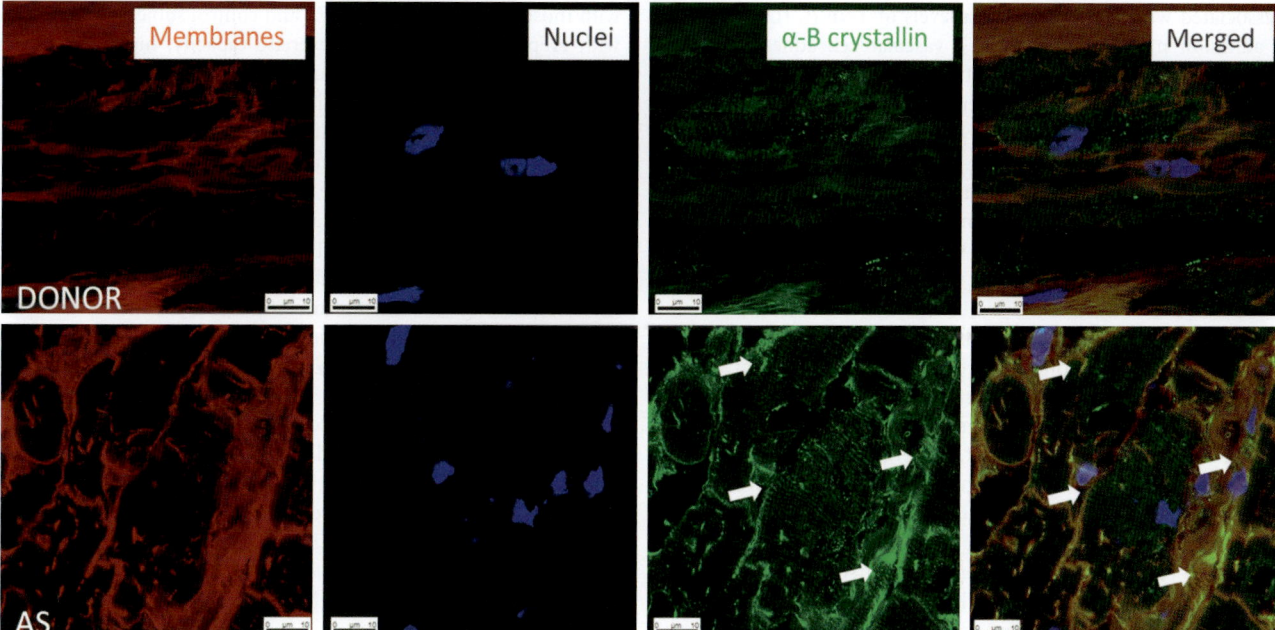

Fig. 11.11 Confocal Laser Microscopy for αB-Crystallin in Donor and Aortic Stenosis (AS). Confocal laser microscopic images were obtained from left ventricular (LV) myocardium of donor and AS patients with immunohistochemical visualization of cell membranes (A), nuclei (B), and αB-crystallin (C). In myocardium of AS patients, intensity of αB-crystallin expression (C) was higher than in donor with visualization in the merged images (D) of subsarcolemmal aggresomes especially in the vicinity of capillaries (white arrows).

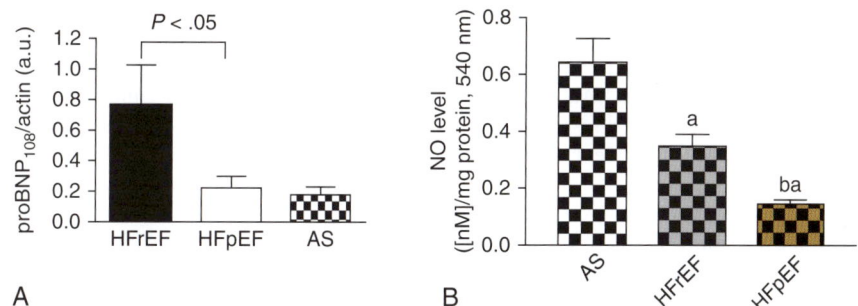

Fig. 11.12 (A) Myocardial proBNP$_{108}$ expression, assessed by Western blot analysis and normalized for actin, is lower in heart failure with preserved ejection fraction (HFpEF) than in heart failure with reduced ejection fraction (HFrEF) and similar in HFpEF and aortic stenosis (AS). Representative Western blot lanes showing myocardial proBNP$_{108}$ and actin expression. (B) Myocardial nitrite/nitrate concentrations were lower in HFpEF than in AS and HFrEF patients and lower in HFrEF than in AS patients. [a]$P < .05$ HFpEF versus AS; [b]$P < .05$ HFpEF versus HFrEF, [a]$P < .05$ HFrEF versus AS.

dysfunction[65] and to predict incident HFpEF.[60] Limited tolerability of systemic vasodilation and impaired sodium excretion are of therapeutic importance.[66] Impaired sodium excretion implies the arterial pressure–natriuresis relationship to be shifted to the right. Under these conditions, a fall in arterial pressure because of systemic vasodilation without cardiac output increase is especially deleterious because it leads to additional sodium retention and extracellular volume expansion, which wipes out any direct beneficial effect of vasodilation on LV filling pressures.[66] HFpEF in the presence of renal dysfunction recently emerged as a distinct phenotype with more LV hypertrophy, a larger LV systolic functional deficit, impaired LA mechanics, RV dysfunction, and poor prognosis.[67,68] The latter relates to exaggerated reactive pulmonary hypertension and RV dysfunction. Because of RV dysfunction, renal venous congestion importantly contributes to renal dysfunction in HFpEF.

Hypertension

Arterial hypertension is highly prevalent in HFpEF (approximately 60%–88%).[1,69] Adverse cardiovascular effects of hypertension include LV hypertrophy, myocardial fibrosis, elevated arterial stiffness, and systemic inflammation.[70] The importance of overload is unclear because, in a concentrically remodeled LV with normal EF, a favorable late-systolic Laplace relation protects LV myocardium from loading increments provoked by large reflected arterial pressure waves. However, in the presence of a minor LV shortening deficit, hypertensive HFpEF patients may develop late-peaking systolic LV wall stress. This may explain the favorable effects in HFpEF patients of the sodium-restricted Dietary Approaches to Stop Hypertension (DASH) diet, which improves ventricular-arterial coupling.[71] Inflammation, oxidative stress, and endothelial dysfunction are importantly involved in hypertension.[72] Endothelial dysfunction in hypertensive patients was associated with increased plasma levels of TNF-α, IL6, intercellular adhesion molecule 1 (ICAM-1), vascular cell adhesion molecule 1 (VCAM-1), E-selectin, C-reactive protein (CRP), and the von Willebrand factor, which is a marker of endothelial activation.[73] In salt-sensitive hypertension, high salt intake leads to systemic oxidative stress[74] possibly because of renal production of proinflammatory cytokines. Arterial hypertension can affect myocardial remodeling and dysfunction in HFpEF through myocardial overload or systemic inflammation.[75]

Metabolic Risk Factors

HFpEF patients demonstrate a high prevalence of metabolic risk factors including metabolic syndrome, overweight/obesity, and T2DM.[1,69,76] Obesity and T2DM are strongly related to IR and the metabolic syndrome (a constellation of cardiovascular risk factors, including obesity, hypertension, IR, hyperglycemia, dyslipidemia, microalbuminuria, and hypercoagulability).[77,78] The prevalence of these metabolic risk factors is expected to reach pandemic proportions in the next few decades,[77] and these metabolic risk factors have all been prospectively identified as precursors of incident HF and are independently associated with early development of diastolic LV dysfunction.[79,80] The frequent clustering of these metabolic risk factors causes synergistic adverse myocardial effects including myocardial hypertrophy and fibrosis,[80] reduced myocardial energetic reserve,[81] impaired myocardial relaxation,[80-82] increased diastolic LV and cardiomyocyte stiffness,[83] myocardial and systemic inflammation, oxidative stress, and endothelial dysfunction,[84,85] which importantly contribute to myocardial dysfunction and remodeling and result in downregulation of NO-cGMP-PKG signaling.[86] Diabetes mellitus increases titin-based cardiomyocyte stiffness in LV samples from HFpEF[83] and AS patients.[84] Insulin modulates titin isoform composition in a phosphoinositide 3 kinase (PI3K)/Akt pathway–dependent manner[87] and insulin modulates titin phosphorylation properties via ERK1/2-, PKG- and PKCα-dependent phosphorylation.[88] Administration of insulin to cultured cardiomyocytes activated the PI3K/AKT/eNOS signaling cascade and increased PKG-dependent titin N2-Bus phosphorylation.[88] Furthermore, insulin induced titin N2-B(us) phosphorylation, presumably mediated by ERK1/2. These findings suggest that reduced cGMP pool and ERK1/2 activity observed in diabetic hearts are linked to insulin deficiency and impaired insulin signaling.

Obesity has reached epidemic proportions worldwide and is a common finding in patients with HFpEF.[89] Obesity has many deleterious effects on the cardiovascular system, mediated by changes in volume status, cardiac loading, energy substrate use, tissue metabolism, and systemic inflammation, which are believed to promote disease progression.[20,90] A detailed characterization of cardiovascular structure, function, and reserve capacity was performed in obese subjects with HFpEF (body mass index [BMI] ≥ 35 kg/m^2) compared with nonobese HFpEF (BMI < 30 kg/m^2) and control subjects without HF.[20] Compared with both subjects with nonobese HFpEF and control subjects, subjects with obese HFpEF displayed increased plasma volume, more concentric LV remodeling, greater RV dilatation, more RV dysfunction, increased epicardial fat thickness, and greater total epicardial heart volume, despite lower NT-proBNP levels. PCWP was correlated with body mass and plasma volume in obese HFpEF but not in nonobese HFpEF. The increase in heart volumes in obese HFpEF was associated with greater pericardial restraint and heightened ventricular interdependence, reflected by increased ratio of right- to left-sided heart filling pressures, higher pulmonary venous pressure relative to LV transmural pressure, and greater LV eccentricity index. Interdependence was enhanced as pulmonary artery pressure load increased. Compared

with those with nonobese HFpEF and control subjects, obese patients with HFpEF displayed worse exercise capacity, higher biventricular filling pressures with exercise, and depressed pulmonary artery vasodilator reserve.[20] Recently, a trial of 20-week caloric restriction diet was feasible and appeared safe in older, obese HFpEF patients, and it significantly improved symptoms, peak oxygen consumption (VO$_2$) and quality-of-life scores.[91] The combination of weight loss diet with endurance exercise training was additive and produced a large (2.5 mL/kg/min) increase in peak VO$_2$. The increase in peak VO$_2$ was strongly correlated with reduced body fat mass, increased percent lean body mass, higher thigh muscle/intermuscular fat ratio, and lower biomarkers of inflammation, all of which support the hypothesis that overweight/obesity contributes to exercise intolerance in HFpEF through systemic inflammation.[91]

Therefore highly prevalent comorbidities in HFpEF patients share systemic inflammation and endothelial dysfunction as common and unifying factors, and inflammation and endothelial dysfunction have been unequivocally demonstrated to play an important pathophysiologic role in patients with HFpEF.

INFLAMMATION AND ENDOTHELIAL DYSFUNCTION

Myocardial inflammation importantly contributes to ECM changes and diastolic dysfunction in HFpEF (**Fig. 11.13**).[30,85] In an endomyocardial biopsy study, when compared with controls, HFpEF patients had increased inflammatory cell TGF-β expression, and both myocardial collagen and the quantity of inflammatory cells correlated with diastolic LV dysfunction.[30] In addition, LV endomyocardial biopsies showed microvascular endothelial activation, increased expression of endothelial adhesion molecules, high oxidative stress, uncoupling of endothelial NO synthase, and low myocardial NO levels in HFpEF patients.[35] Recent studies demonstrated a high prevalence of endothelial dysfunction in HFpEF patients, which was related to reduced exercise capacity[92] and worse outcome.[93] Microvascular endothelial inflammation is also associated with myocardial capillary rarefaction, which has been demonstrated in HFpEF myocardium.[94] In an autopsy study, cardiac structural and ultrastructural characteristics were compared between patients with premortem diagnosis of HFpEF and age-appropriate control subjects who died from noncardiac causes and had no prior HF.[94] HFpEF patients had heavier hearts, more severe coronary artery disease (CAD), more extensive LV fibrosis, and lower myocardial capillary density. Lower myocardial capillary density in HFpEF was observed regardless of the severity of epicardial coronary disease.[94] In both control and HFpEF subjects, the severity of myocardial fibrosis was inversely associated with myocardial vascular density. Group differences in LV fibrosis were attenuated after adjustment for myocardial vascular density, suggesting that reduced myocardial vascular density contributes to myocardial fibrosis. Heart weight, fibrosis, and myocardial capillary density were similar in HFpEF patients with CAD versus without CAD.[94]

THE NEW PARADIGM FOR HEART FAILURE WITH PRESERVED EJECTION FRACTION

Recently, a novel paradigm of HFpEF was published, which proposes that comorbidities (and especially obesity) drive structural and functional remodeling in HFpEF through induction of systemic inflammation.[4] Systemic inflammation leads to coronary microvascular endothelial inflammation and dysfunction. This affects LV diastolic dysfunction through macrophage infiltration, which stimulates TGF-β mediated transformation of fibroblasts into myofibroblasts, resulting

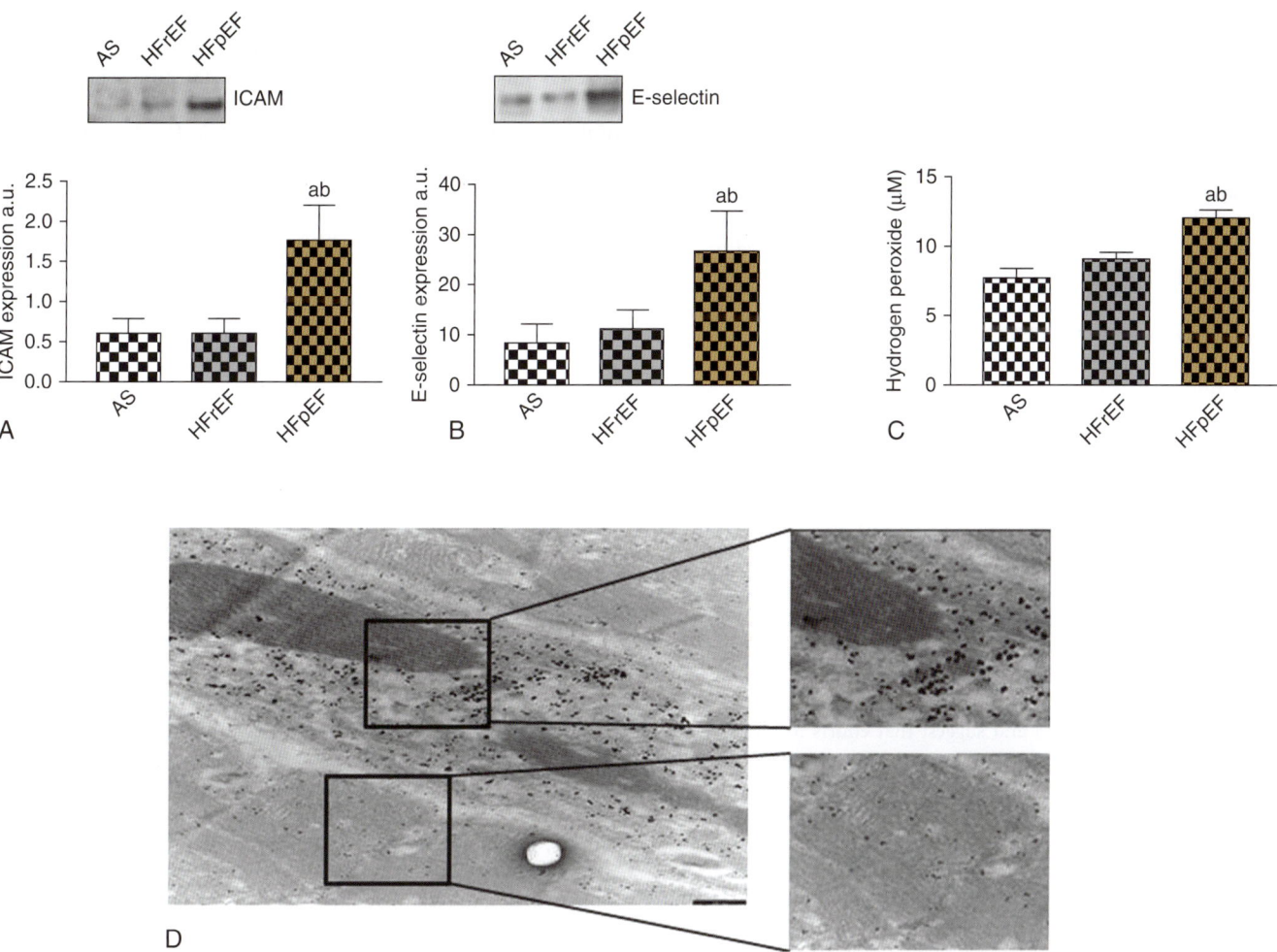

Fig. 11.13 (A) Intercellular adhesion molecule 1 *(ICAM-1)* expression was higher in heart failure with preserved ejection fraction *(HFpEF)* than in aortic stenosis *(AS;* [a]*P* < .05 vs. AS) and heart failure with reduced ejection fraction *(HFrEF;* [b]*P* < .05 vs. HFrEF). (B) E-selectin levels were higher in HFpEF than in HFrEF and AS ([a]*P* < .05 vs. AS) and HFrEF ([b]*P* < .05 vs. HFrEF). (C) Myocardial hydrogen peroxide concentrations were higher in HFpEF than in AS and HFrEF ([a]*P* < .05 vs. AS; [b]*P* < .05 vs. HFrEF). (D) Immunogold-labeled electron microscopy showed myocardial localization of 3-nitrotyrosine.

in myocardial interstitial fibrosis and through altered paracrine signaling to cardiomyocytes. Because of the proinflammatory state, coronary microvascular endothelial cells produce reactive oxygen species, which limits NO bioavailability for adjacent cardiomyocytes. Limited NO bioavailability decreases sGC activity, thereby lowering cGMP generation, leading to reduced PKG activity. Reduced cardiomyocyte cGMP-PKG signaling augments cardiomyocyte stiffness through hypophosphorylation of titin and increases cardiomyocyte hypertrophy because of impaired PKG-mediated antihypertrophic activity.[4]

HEART FAILURE WITH PRESERVED EJECTION FRACTION: A SYSTEMIC DISORDER

Strong support for an extramyocardial origin of HFpEF came from parabiosis experiments in which hearts of young animals acquired HFpEF-like features when exposed to blood from old animals and vice versa, because hearts of old animals reversed HFpEF-like features when exposed to blood of young animals.[95] The extramyocardial origin of HFpEF differs from the intramyocardial origin of HFrEF, where remodeling is driven by cardiomyocyte cell death because of ischemia, infection, or toxicity.[4] Distinct origins of HFpEF and HFrEF are mirrored by unequal LV structural and ultrastructural remodeling (see

Table 11.1).[4] Biomarker profiles in HFpEF and HFrEF are consistent with the distinct origins of both HF phenotypes because they show lower markers of myocardial injury (high-sensitivity troponin T) or of myocardial stress (NT-proBNP) in HFpEF.[96,97] Lower high-sensitivity troponin T is explained by less cardiomyocyte damage as a result of limited upregulation in HFpEF myocardium of nicotinamide adenine dinucleotide phosphate oxidase 2 evident in infiltrating macrophages or endothelial cells but not in cardiomyocytes.[85] Lower NT-proBNP is explained by concentric LV remodeling/hypertrophy in HFpEF in contrast to eccentric remodeling/hypertrophy in HFrEF[18] and by obesity,[20] which is highly prevalent in HFpEF patients. In HFpEF, chronic systemic inflammation affects not only the myocardium but also other organs such as lungs, skeletal muscles, and kidneys.[4] Although HFpEF patients may stop exercising because of a rapid and brisk rise in LV filling pressures, in a substantial subset of patients effort tolerance is limited by inappropriate pulmonary vasoconstriction (as shown by the development of pulmonary hypertension) or by inadequate peripheral skeletal muscle vasodilation, perfusion, and oxygen use (as shown by the absence of the widening of the arteriovenous oxygen difference which usually accompanies exercise).[98,99] Systemic inflammation also affects the renal microcirculation and the ability of the kidneys to excrete a sodium load. Inability to excrete a sodium load contributes to the progressive volume expansion observed during transition from chronic compensated to acute decompensated HFpEF[8] and explains the efficacy of diuretics because they restore the pressure-natriuresis relationship. HFpEF represents a complex and heterogeneous clinical syndrome, in which multiple cardiac and vascular abnormalities, cardiovascular risk factors, and overlapping extracardiac comorbidities may be present in various combinations.[3,4,100-102] HFpEF is difficult to define, as illustrated by various diagnostic classifications and inclusion criteria of clinical trials.[3] These factors contributed to heterogeneity of HFpEF patients recruited into trials and registries. In the past, no consensus was present on the optimal cutoff value of LVEF, and different cutoffs have been used across classifications and trials ranging from LVEF≥40% to greater than 50%.[3] Although diastolic LV dysfunction represents the dominant abnormality in HFpEF, ancillary mechanisms were also found to contribute, such as systolic LV dysfunction,[103] ventricular-vascular stiffening,[104] impaired systemic vasodilatory reserve,[92,105] chronotropic incompetence,[92] pulmonary hypertension,[106,107] RV dysfunction,[108,109] chronotropic incompetence,[92,110,111] skeletal muscle dysfunction,[112,113] microvascular capillary rarefaction,[114] CAD,[115,116] and atrial fibrillation.[117-119] Prevalent atrial fibrillation in HFpEF goes along with a more advanced stage of cardiac remodeling evident from a larger LA and uniformly carries a worse prognosis.[117-119] Prevalent atrial fibrillation was shown to be associated with incident HFpEF and prevalent HFpEF with incident atrial fibrillation.[120] These interactions suggest atrial fibrillation to beget HFpEF and vice versa and suggest that efforts to restore sinus rhythm could be included in a HFpEF treatment strategy.

HETEROGENEITY IN HEART FAILURE WITH PRESERVED EJECTION FRACTION

The underlying phenotypic heterogeneity is likely far greater in HFpEF than in HFrEF and may be an important reason for the failure of HFpEF clinical trials.[8-11] Despite the diversity of the HFpEF syndrome, the treatment strategy thus far has focused on a "one-size-fits-all" approach that has worked relatively well for chronic HFrEF. However, virtually all clinical syndromes benefit from more tailored, personalized therapy, and this may also be true of HFpEF. Indeed, presence of subtle systolic LV dysfunction, endothelial dysfunction, pulmonary hypertension, and RV dysfunction are all carrying prognostic implications and probably identify distinct subgroups of HFpEF patients. In a recent study, phenomapping analysis using statistical learning algorithms, demonstrated that HFpEF patients recruited according to uniform diagnostic criteria could be divided into three main distinct subgroups, which differed markedly in clinical characteristics, cardiac structure and function, invasive hemodynamics, and outcome, despite similar end-systolic and end-diastolic elastances on LV pressure-volume analysis.[102] In addition, a latent class analysis study demonstrated six distinct subgroups of HFpEF patients enrolled in the I-PRESERVE and CHARM-PRESERVED (Clinical study of candesartan in patients with heart failure and preserved left ventricular systolic function) trials with significant differences in event-free survival. The two subgroups with the worst event-free survival in both studies were characterized by a high prevalence of obesity, hyperlipidemia, diabetes mellitus, anemia, and renal insufficiency and by female predominance, advanced age, lower BMI, and high rates of atrial fibrillation, valvular disease, renal insufficiency, and anemia.[121]

Pathophysiologic Stratification in Heart Failure With Preserved Ejection Fraction

Clinical and translational studies demonstrated varying degrees of ventricular and cardiomyocyte hypertrophy, interstitial fibrosis, and capillary rarefaction,[4,94] which implies distinct and possibly

evolutionary stages of myocardial disease progression. Although neurohumoral inhibition did not improve primary end points in the large HFpEF trials, many of them reached statistical significance for secondary end points, subgroups, or post hoc analyses.[122,123] Because of these findings, the involvement of RAAS in HFpEF appears more subtle than in HFrEF, probably requiring upfront identification of subgroups of HFpEF patients rather than a "one-fits-all strategy." Such a stratification approach with identification of myocardial structural and functional abnormalities in the individual HFpEF patient could be highly relevant for determination of potential therapeutic responsiveness and selection of appropriate treatment strategies. For instance, the efficacy of RAAS inhibitors to improve adverse myocardial remodeling is likely very different in HFpEF patients with minor, modest, or severe stages of myocardial hypertrophy, fibrosis, and capillary rarefaction (**Fig. 11.14**). Presence of atrial fibrillation is likely to emerge as an indicator of an advanced stage of myocardial disease in HFpEF. A recent subgroup analysis of HFpEF patients recruited in the RELAX trial indeed showed presence of atrial fibrillation to be indicative of long-standing HFpEF.[117] In this study, HFpEF patients with atrial fibrillation were older than those in sinus rhythm but had similar symptom severity, comorbidities, and renal function. Despite comparable LV size and mass, AF was associated with worse systolic (lower EF, stroke volume, and cardiac index) and diastolic (shorter deceleration time and larger LA) function compared with sinus rhythm. Patients with AF had higher pulmonary arterial systolic pressure (PASP) and increased NT-proBNP, aldosterone, endothelin-1, troponin I, and C-telopeptide for type I collagen levels, suggesting more severe neurohumoral activation, myocyte necrosis, and fibrosis.[117] In summary, understanding the phenotypic heterogeneity of HFpEF, which includes the etiologic and pathophysiologic heterogeneity of the syndrome, may allow more targeted and successful HFpEF clinical trials and result in patient-tailored therapeutic strategies.

SUMMARY AND FUTURE DIRECTIONS

HFpEF represents a complex disorder with a heterogeneous constellation of comorbidities, underlying pathogenic mechanisms, and lack of effective treatment and poses a formidable challenge for clinicians and translational researchers. Over the past decade, significant progress has been made in understanding HFpEF pathophysiology and recognizing the importance of comorbidities and disease heterogeneity. However, numerous issues regarding underlying pathophysiologic mechanisms remain unresolved. For instance, patients with substantial diastolic dysfunction with or without structural heart disease in the setting of hypertensive heart disease may behave differently from those with chronotropic incompetence or from those with normal blood pressure but inflammatory activation in the setting of metabolic risk factors. In addition, pathogenic mechanisms may vary in the course of HFpEF disease trajectory and could therefore differentially influence structural and functional myocardial dysfunction at different time courses of the disease. Furthermore, the additive role of preexisting or newly developing noncardiac comorbidities on structural and functional remodeling in HFpEF is incompletely understood. Therefore improved subclassification of HFpEF patients, increased procurement of HFpEF myocardial tissue (e.g., through LV endomyocardial biopsy procurement), and improvement in experimental HFpEF models are important future goals in enhancing our understanding of HFpEF pathophysiology. Stimulation of crosstalk and formation of collaborative networks between translational researchers and clinicians is of great interest to enhance insight into structural and functional cardiovascular dysfunction in the setting of coexisting variable pathogenic mechanisms and comorbidities in HFpEF patients. Importantly, the conceptual framework of HFpEF treatment may need to shift from a "one-fits-all" strategy to an individualized approach based on phenotypic patient characterization

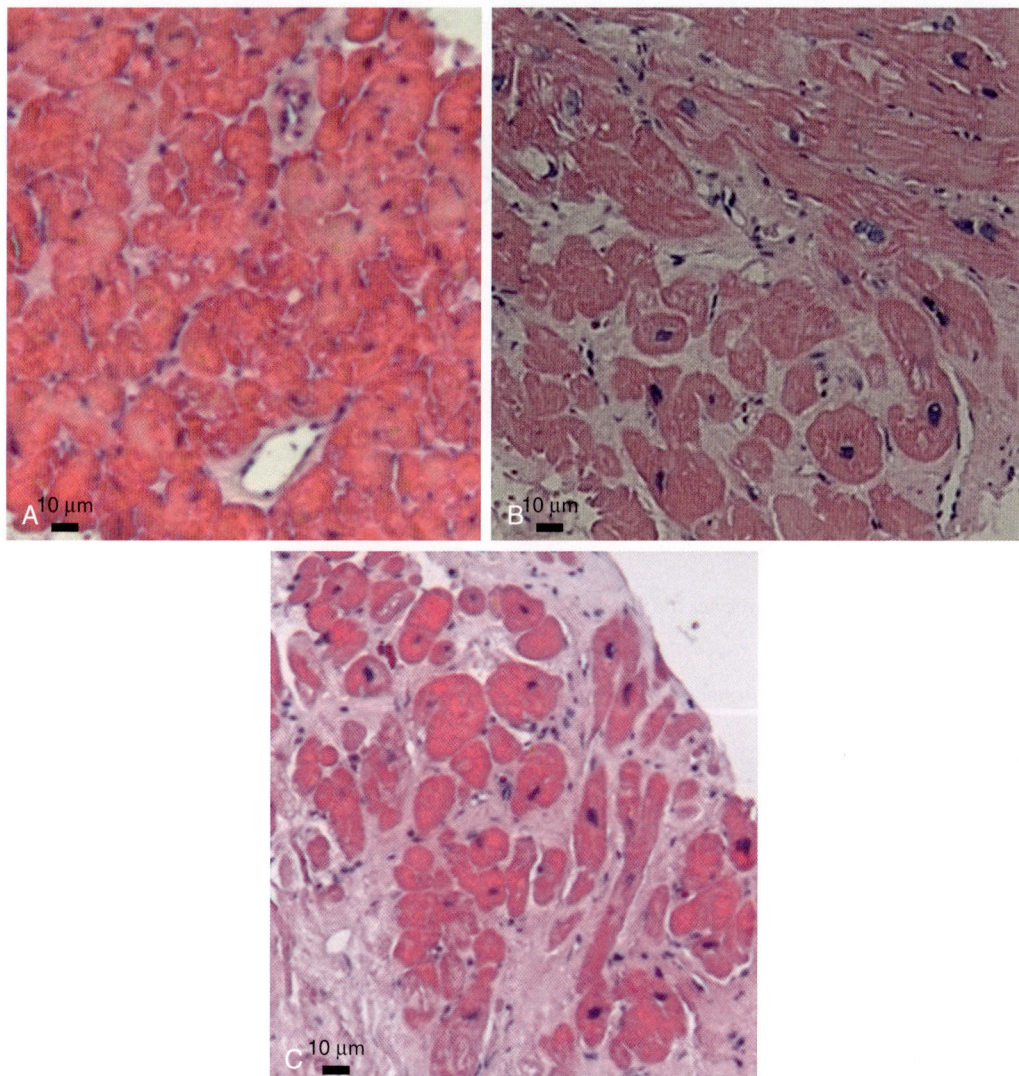

Fig. 11.14 Distinct Stages of Structural Myocardial Disease in Heart Failure With Preserved Ejection Fraction *(HFpEF)*. (A–C), Histologic images of LV myocardium from HFpEF patients, demonstrating minor (A), moderate (B), and severe (C) interstitial fibrosis.

and diagnostic and pathophysiologic stratification of myocardial disease processes. This could ultimately provide an inroad for improved identification of specific treatment targets and enhance development of "personalized therapy" for HFpEF patients.

ACKNOWLEDGMENT

Supported by grants from CVON (Cardioavasculair Onderzoek Nederland), Dutch Heart Foundation, The Hague (RECONNECT, EARLY HFPEF).

KEY REFERENCES

4. Shah SJ, Kitzman DW, Borlaug BA, et al. Phenotype–specific treatment of heart failure with preserved ejection fraction: a multi–organ roadmap. *Circulation.* 2016;134(1):73–90.
20. Obokata M, Reddy YN, Pislaru SV, et al. Evidence supporting the existence of a distinct obese phenotype of heart failure with preserved ejection fraction. *Circulation.* 2017;136(1):6–19.
22. van Heerebeek L, Hamdani N, Falcão-Pires I, et al. Low myocardial protein kinase G activity in heart failure with preserved ejection fraction. *Circulation.* 2012;126(7):830–839.
24. Reddy YN, Carter RE, Obokata M, et al. A simple, evidence based approach to help guide diagnosis of heart failure with preserved ejection fraction. *Circulation.* 2018;138:870–889.
32. Linke WA, Hamdani N. Gigantic business: titin properties and function through thick and thin. *Circ Res.* 2014;114(6):1052–1068.
38. Franssen C, Kole J, Musters R, et al. αB Crystallin reverses high diastolic stiffness of failing human cardiomyocytes. *Circ Heart Fail.* 2017;10(3):e003626.
85. Franssen C, Chen S, Unger A, et al. Myocardial microvascular inflammatory endothelial activation in heart failure with preserved ejection fraction. *JACC Heart Fail.* 2016;4(4):312–324.
94. Mohammed SF, Hussain S, Mirzoyev SA, et al. Coronary microvascular rarefaction and myocardial fibrosis in heart failure with preserved ejection fraction. *Circulation.* 2015;131(6):550–559.
102. Shah SJ, Katz DH, Selvaraj S, et al. Phenomapping for novel classification of heart failure with preserved ejection fraction. *Circulation.* 2015;131:269–279.
104. Borlaug BA. Mechanisms of exercise intolerance in heart failure with preserved ejection fraction. *Circ J.* 2014;78(1):20–32.

The full reference list for this chapter is available on ExpertConsult.

Alterations in Ventricular Structure: Role of Left Ventricular Remodeling and Reverse Remodeling in Heart Failure

Luigi Adamo, Douglas L. Mann

One of the major conceptual advances in the field of heart failure (HF) has been the recognition that HF progresses because of the structural changes that occur in the heart in response to hemodynamic, neurohormonal, epigenetic and genetic factors. Although the complex changes that occur in the heart during left ventricular (LV) remodeling have traditionally been described in anatomic terms, the process of LV remodeling arises secondary to changes in biology of the cardiac myocyte, histological changes resulting from changes in the volume of myocyte and nonmyocyte components of the myocardium, as well as macroscopic changes in the geometry and architecture of the LV chamber (**Table 12.1**). Clinical studies have shown that resolution of the cardiac injury that led to myocardial dysfunction and/or the implementation of medical and device therapies that reduce HF morbidity and mortality, results in a reversal of LV remodeling, which is characterized anatomically by a return in LV volume and mass toward normal values, as well as a shift in the LV end-diastolic pressure-volume relationship (EDPVR) to the left. These salutary changes represent the summation of a series of integrated biologic changes in cardiac myocyte size and function, as well as modifications in LV structure and organization. For want of better terminology, these changes have been referred to collectively as *reverse remodeling*.[1,2] A small subset of patients experience sufficient reverse remodeling to regain a normal ejection fraction (EF) in a process that has been referred to as *myocardial recovery*.[3] The rate of normalization in left ventricular ejection fraction (LVEF) depends on the underlying etiology of the cardiomyopathy.[4] Moreover, there is growing body of evidence that suggests that, even among patients who experience a complete normalization in LVEF, there is tremendous heterogeneity and that a significant proportion will have recurrent LV dysfunction and recurrent HF events.[5,6] The importance of understanding the biology of LV remodeling, reverse LV remodeling,

and the subtleties of myocardial recovery is that it may lead to the identification of novel therapeutic targets for treating/reversing HF. In the chapter that follows, we will discuss the changes that occur during the process of LV dilation in HF with a reduced EF. The remodeling that occurs in HF with a preserved EF is discussed in **Chapter 11**.

LEFT VENTRICULAR REMODELING

The term *left ventricular (LV) remodeling* describes the changes in mass, volume, shape, and composition observed in the LV in response to mechanical stimulation and systemic neurohormonal activation.[7,8] Conceptually, these changes can be envisioned as occurring within the cardiac myocyte, in the histological structure of the myocardium, and within the LV chamber.

Alterations in the Biology of the Cardiac Myocyte

The changes that occur in the biology of the failing cardiac myocyte include (1) cell hypertrophy (**see Chapter 2**); (2) reactivation of fetal genes; (3) β-adrenergic desensitization (**see Chapter 6**); (4) loss of myofibrils and progressive disarray of the cytoskeleton; (5) changes in excitation-contraction coupling leading to alterations in the contractile properties of the myocyte (**see Chapter 2**); and (6) modifications of myocyte metabolism (**see Chapter 17**). Collectively these changes lead to decreased shortening and delayed relaxation of the failing cardiac myocyte.

Two basic patterns of cardiac hypertrophy occur in response to hemodynamic overload (**Fig. 12.1**). In pressure overload hypertrophy (e.g., with aortic stenosis or hypertension), the increase in systolic wall leads to the addition of sarcomeres in parallel, an increase in myocyte cross-sectional area, and increased LV wall thickening. This

TABLE 12.1 Overview of Left Ventricular Remodeling

Alterations in Myocyte Biology

Hypertrophy
Reactivation of fetal genes
• adrenergic desensitization
Loss in myofibrils and progressive disarray of the cytoskeleton
Changes in excitation contraction coupling
Modifications of myocyte metabolism

Myocardial Changes

Myocyte loss
• Necrosis
• Apoptosis
• Autophagy
Alterations in extracellular matrix
• Matrix degradation
• Myocardial fibrosis
Alteration in the microvasculature

Alterations in Left Ventricular Chamber Geometry

Left ventricular (LV) dilation
Increased LV sphericity
LV wall thinning
Mitral valve incompetence

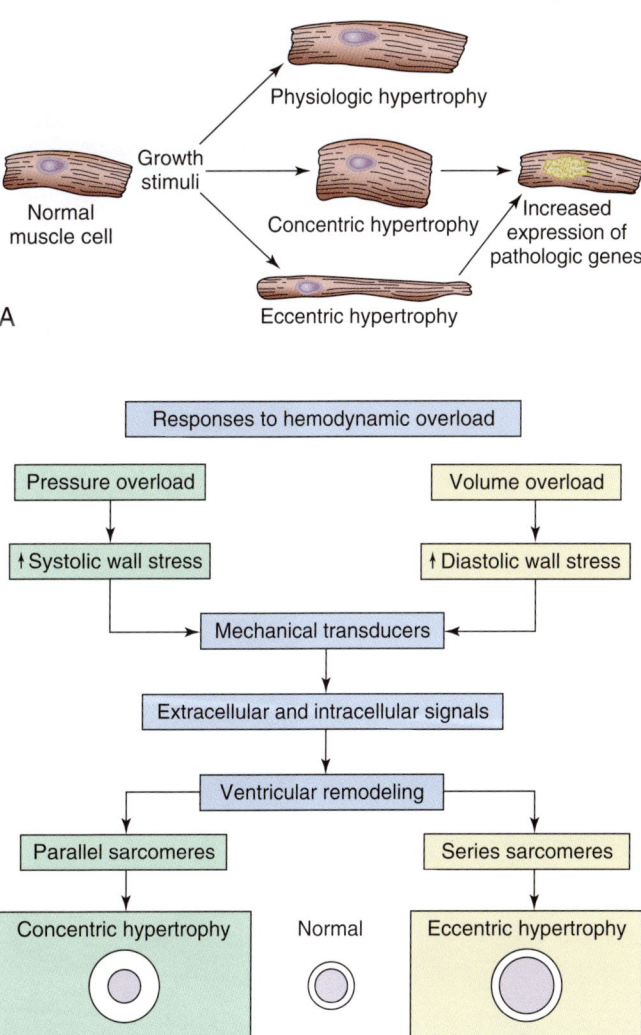

A

B

Fig. 12.1 Patterns of cardiac myocyte hypertrophy. (A) Morphology of cardiac myocytes in response to hemodynamic pressure and volume overloading. Phenotypically distinct changes in the morphology of myocyte occur in response to the type of hemodynamic overload that is superimposed. When the overload is predominantly due to an increase in pressure, the increase in systolic wall stress leads to the parallel addition of sarcomeres and widening of the cardiac myocytes. When the overload is predominantly due to an increase in ventricular volume, the increase in diastolic wall stress leads to the series addition of sarcomeres, and thus lengthening of cardiac myocytes. (B) The pattern of cardiac remodeling that occurs in response to hemodynamic overloading depends on the nature of the inciting stimulus. When the overload is predominantly due to an increase in pressure (e.g., with systemic hypertension or aortic stenosis), the increase in systolic wall stress leads to the parallel addition of sarcomeres and widening of the cardiac myocytes, resulting in concentric cardiac hypertrophy. When the overload is predominantly due to an increase in ventricular volume, the increase in diastolic wall stress leads to the series addition of sarcomeres, lengthening of cardiac myocytes, and left ventricular (LV) dilation, which is referred to as eccentric chamber hypertrophy. (Modified from Hunter JJ, Chien KR. Signaling pathways for cardiac hypertrophy and failure. *N Engl J Med.* 1999; 341:1276; Colucci WS, editor. *Heart Failure: Cardiac Function and Dysfunction*, 2nd ed. Philadelphia: Current Medicine; 1999:4.2; and Mann DL. Pathophysiology of heart failure. In: Libby PL, Bonow RO, Mann DL, et al., editors. *Braunwald's Heart Disease*, 8th ed. Philadelphia: Saunders; 2004:541–560.)

pattern of remodeling has been referred to as *concentric hypertrophy* (see Fig. 12.1A) and has been linked with alterations in calcium/calmodulin-dependent protein kinase II-dependent signaling.[9] In contrast, in volume overload hypertrophy (e.g., with aortic and mitral regurgitation), increased diastolic wall stress leads to an increase in myocyte length with the addition of sarcomeres in series, thereby engendering increased LV dilation. This pattern of remodeling has been referred to as *eccentric hypertrophy* (so named because of the position of the heart in the chest) or a *dilated phenotype* (see Fig. 12.1A) and has been linked with Akt activation.[9] Patients with HF classically present with a dilated LV with or without LV thinning. The myocytes from these failing ventricles have an elongated appearance that is characteristic of myocytes obtained from hearts subjected to chronic volume overload. Cardiac myocyte hypertrophy leads to reactivation of portfolios of genes that are normally not expressed postnatally. The reactivation of these fetal genes, the so-called fetal gene program, is also accompanied by decreased expression of a number of genes that are normally expressed in the adult heart including the gene for the β1 adrenergic receptor with resulting β-adrenergic desensitization (**see Chapter 6**). As will be discussed below, activation of the fetal gene program may contribute to the contractile dysfunction that develops in the failing myocyte in many other ways. The stimuli for the genetic reprogramming of the myocyte include mechanical stretch/strain of the myocyte, neurohormones (e.g., NE, angiotensin II), inflammatory cytokines (e.g., tumor necrosis factor [TNF], interleukin-6 [IL-6]), other peptides and growth factors (e.g., ET), and reactive oxygen species (e.g., superoxide, NO). These stimuli occur both locally within the myocardium, where they exert autocrine/paracrine effects, as well as systemically where they exert endocrine effects.

The early stage of cardiac myocyte hypertrophy is characterized morphologically by increases in the number of myofibrils and mitochondria, as well as enlargement of mitochondria and nuclei (**Fig. 12.2**). At this stage the cardiac myocytes are larger than normal

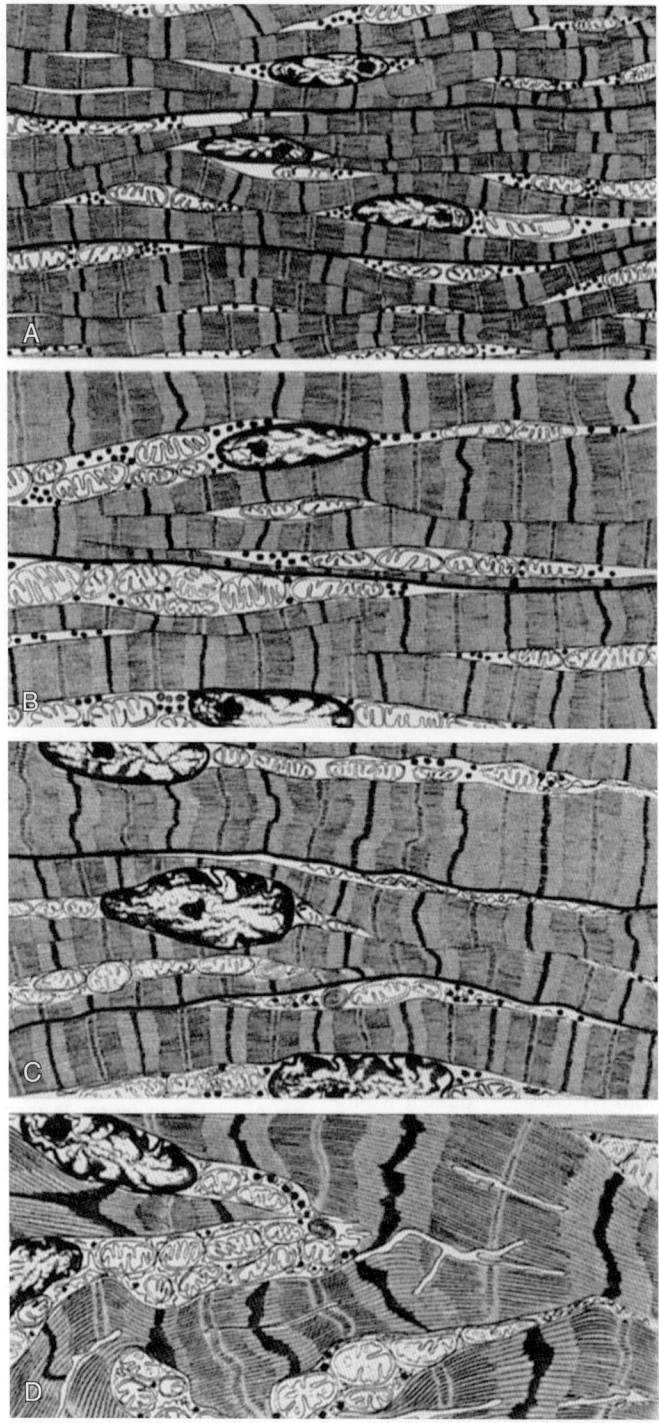

Fig. 12.2 The early stage of cardiac hypertrophy (A) is characterized morphologically by increases in the number of myofibrils and mitochondria and enlargement of mitochondria and nuclei. Muscle cells are larger than normal, but cellular organization is largely preserved. At a more advanced stage of hypertrophy (B) preferential increases in the size or number of specific organelles, such as mitochondria, along with irregular addition of new contractile elements in localized areas of the cell, result in subtle abnormalities of cellular organization and contour. Adjacent cells may vary in their degree of enlargement. Cells subjected to long-standing hypertrophy (C) show more obvious disruptions in cellular organization, such as markedly enlarged nuclei with highly lobulated membranes, which displace adjacent myofibrils and cause breakdown of normal Z-band registration. The early preferential increase in mitochondria is supplanted by a predominance (by volume) of myofibrils. The late stage of hypertrophy (D) is characterized by loss of contractile elements with marked disruption of Z bands, severe disruption of the normal parallel arrangement of the sarcomeres, deposition of fibrous tissue, and dilation and increased tortuosity of T tubules. (From Ferrans VJ. Morphology of the heart in hypertrophy. *Hosp Pract.* 1983;18:69.)

and have preserved cellular organization. As hypertrophy continues, there is an increase in the number of mitochondria, as well as the addition of new contractile elements in localized areas of the cell. Cells subjected to long-standing hypertrophy show more obvious disruptions in cellular organization, such as markedly enlarged nuclei with highly lobulated membranes, accompanied by the displacement of adjacent myofibrils with loss of the normal registration of the Z bands. The late stage of hypertrophy is characterized by loss of contractile elements (myocytolysis) with marked disruption of Z bands, severe disruption of the normal parallel arrangement of the sarcomeres, accompanied by dilation and increased tortuosity of T tubules.

Failing human cardiac myocytes also undergo a number of other important changes expected to lead to a progressive loss of contractile function, including decreased α-myosin heavy chain gene expression with a concomitant increase in β-myosin heavy chain expression.[10] The cytoskeleton of the myocyte consists of actin, the intermediate filament desmin, the sarcomeric protein titin, and α- and β-tubulin that form microtubules by polymerization. Vinculin, talin, dystrophin, and spectrin represent a separate group of membrane-associated proteins. The failing myocyte shows alterations in cytoskeletal proteins,[11] and in numerous experimental models cytoskeletal and/or membrane-associated proteins have been implicated in the pathogenesis of HF. This is accompanied by alterations in excitation-contraction coupling that have been closely linked to myocardial contractile dysfunction (**see Chapter 2**). These changes include modification in the abundance of critical Ca^{2+} regulatory proteins including sarcoplasmic endoreticular Ca^{2+} ATPase (SERCA), ryanodine receptor (RyR), L-type calcium channel (LTCC), and sarcolemmal Na^+/Ca^{2+} exchanger (NCX). Furthermore, several lines of evidence suggest that the failing myocyte experiences metabolic changes, which leads to impaired efficiency of myocardial energetics (**see Chapter 17**). When the contractile performance of isolated failing human myocytes was examined under very simple experimental conditions, investigators found that there is an approximately 50% decrease in cell shortening in failing human cardiac myocytes when compared with nonfailing human myocytes.[12]

Alterations in the Myocardium

The alterations that occur in failing myocardium may be categorized broadly into those that occur within the cardiac myocyte compartment, those that occur in the volume and composition of the extracellular matrix (ECM), as well as changes in the myocardial microvasculature. With respect to the changes that occur in the cardiac myocyte component of the myocardium, there is increasing evidence to suggest that progressive myocyte loss may contribute to the development of LV dysfunction and LV remodeling. Necrotic and apoptotic cell death are discussed in **Chapter 2**. Whereas the distinction between necrosis and apoptosis is obvious in certain circumstances, the dividing line between these two conditions is often less clear in the failing heart. And indeed, similar mechanisms can operate in both types of cell death. Thus instead of the existence of distinct types of cell death in HF, there is likely a continuum of cell death responses that contribute to progressive myocyte loss and disease progression.

Changes within the ECM constitute the second important myocardial adaptation that occurs during cardiac remodeling and include changes in overall collagen content, changes in the relative contents of different collagen subtypes, changes in collagen cross-linking, and modifications of the connections between cells and the ECM via integrins. Studies in failing human myocardium have shown that there is a quantitative increase in collagen I, III, VI, and IV; fibronectin; laminin; and vimentin, and athat the ratio of type I collagen to type III collagen is decreased in patients with ischemic cardiomyopathy.

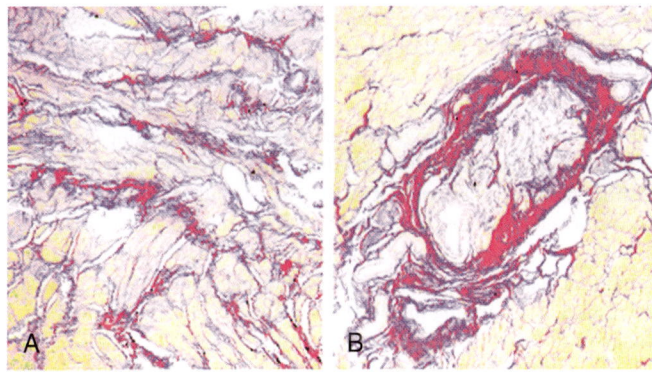

Fig. 12.3 **Myocardial fibrosis.** Histologic section of a human myocardial biopsy specimen showing (A) interstitial and (B) perivascular fibrosis using picrosirius red staining. (Modified from Lopez B, Gonzales A, Varo N, et al. Biochemical assessment of myocardial fibrosis in hypertensive heart disease. *Hypertension.* 2001;38:1222.)

Moreover, clinical studies suggest that there is a progressive loss of cross-linking of collagen in the failing heart, as well as loss of connectivity of the collagen network with individual myocytes, which would be expected to result in profound alterations in LV structure and function. Further, loss of cross-linking of the fibrillar collagen has been associated with progressive LV dilation following myocardial injury. The accumulation of collagen can occur on a "reactive" basis around intramural coronary arteries and arterioles (perivascular fibrosis) or in the interstitial space (interstitial fibrosis), and does not require myocyte cell death (**Fig. 12.3**). Alternatively, collagen accumulation can occur as a result of microscopic scarring (replacement fibrosis) that develops in response to cardiac myocyte cell necrosis. This scarring or "replacement fibrosis" is an adaptation to the loss of parenchyma and is therefore critical to preserve the structural integrity of the heart. The increased fibrous tissue would be expected to lead to increased myocardial stiffness, which would presumably result in decreased myocardial shortening for a given degree of afterload. In addition, myocardial fibrosis may provide the structural substrate for atrial and ventricular arrhythmias, thus potentially contributing to sudden death. Although the full complement of molecules responsible for fibroblast activation is not known, many of the classical neurohormones (e.g., angiotensin II, aldosterone) and cytokines (ET, transforming growth factor-β [TGF-β], cardiotrophin-1) that are expressed in HF are sufficient to provoke fibroblast activation. And indeed, the use of angiotensin-converting enzyme (ACE) inhibitors, β-blockers, and aldosterone receptor antagonists has been associated with a decrease in myocardial fibrosis in experimental HF models.[13]

Although the fibrillar collagen matrix was initially considered to form a relatively static complex, it is now recognized that these structural proteins can undergo rapid turnover. As discussed in **Chapter 4**, one of the more exciting developments with respect to understanding the pathogenesis of cardiac remodeling has been the discovery that a family of collagenolytic enzymes, collectively referred to as *matrix metalloproteinases (MMPs),* are activated within the failing myocardium. Conceptually, disruption of the ECM would be expected to lead to LV dilation and wall thinning as a result of mural realignment (slippage) of myocyte bundles and/or individual myocytes within the LV wall, as well as LV dysfunction as a result of dyssynchronous contraction of the LV. Although the precise biochemical triggers that are responsible for activation of MMPs are not known, it bears emphasis that TNF, as well as other cytokines and peptide growth factors that are expressed within the failing myocardium, is capable of activating MMPs. However, the biology of matrix remodeling in HF is likely to be much more complex than the simple presence or absence of MMP activation. In fact, degradation of the matrix is also controlled by glycoproteins termed *tissue inhibitors of matrix metalloproteinases (TIMPs)*, which are capable of regulating the activation of MMPs by binding to and preventing these enzymes from degrading the collagen matrix of the heart. The TIMP family presently consists of four distinct members, known as TIMP-1, -2, -3, and -4, each of which is constitutively expressed in the heart by fibroblasts, as well as myocytes. TIMPs-1, -2, -3, and -4 are secreted proteins that act as the natural inhibitors of active forms of all MMPs, although the efficiency of MMP inhibition varies among the different members. The existing literature suggests that MMP activation can lead to progressive LV dilation, whereas TIMP expression favors progressive myocardial fibrosis (**see Chapter 4**).

The histologic modifications of the failing myocardium are not limited to the ECM but also involve significant changes in the relationship between cardiac myocytes and their blood supply. In fact, although cardiac growth and angiogenesis are tightly coordinated during development and physiologic cardiac growth,[14] following hemodynamic overload and/or cardiac injury it is easy to observe a mismatch between cardiac myocyte growth and blood supply that may lead to contractile dysfunction and cell death. This has been especially well documented in patients with dilated cardiomyopathy that have a reduced myocardial capillary density.[15,16] Thus impaired capillary growth may contribute to the development and/or progression of HF.

Changes in Left Ventricular Geometry

The changes that occur in the biology of the cardiac myocyte and the myocardium (cardiac myocytes and ECM) lead to progressive LV dilation and increased sphericity of the ventricle. The increase in LV end-diastolic volume, along with LV wall thinning that can occur in some settings, sets the stage for progressive functional *ventricular-afterload mismatch* that contributes further to a decrease in stroke volume. Moreover, the high end-diastolic wall stress might be expected to lead to (1) hypoperfusion of the subendocardium, with resultant ischemia and worsening of LV function; (2) increased oxidative stress with resultant activation of families of genes that are sensitive to free radical generation (e.g., TNF and interleukin-1β); and (3) sustained expression of stretch-activated genes (angiotensin II, endothelin, and TNF) and/or stretch activation of hypertrophic signaling pathways. Increasing LV dilatation and sphericity also result in tethering of the papillary muscles, resulting in incompetence of the mitral valve and the development of "functional mitral regurgitation." Whereas the amount of functional mitral regurgitation was once thought to be mild, the advent of noninvasive imaging modalities has shown that functional mitral regurgitation is clinically significant. Apart from the more obvious problem of loss of forward blood flow, mitral regurgitation presents yet a second problem to the heart insofar as the mitral regurgitation results in further hemodynamic overloading of the ventricle. Taken together, the mechanical burdens that are engendered by LV remodeling might be expected to lead to decreased forward cardiac output, increased LV dilation (stretch), and increased hemodynamic overloading, any or all of which are sufficient to contribute to disease progression independently of the neurohormonal status of the patient. Moreover, the aforementioned changes in LV structure and function might be expected to make the cardiovascular system less responsive to normal homeostatic control mechanisms, such as increased adrenergic drive. Thus alterations in the remodeled ventricle may foster a self-amplifying situation in which worsening neurohormonal activation occurs in response to the inability of the remodeled LV to respond appropriately to these compensatory mechanisms. Moreover, at some point in time it is predictable that the aggregate end-organ changes that occur within the cardiomyopathic ventricle may progress to the point that no amount of neurohormonal stimulation can maintain cardiovascular homeostasis, at which point HF may progress independent of the neurohormonal statues of the patient.

Clinical Studies Linking Left Ventricular Remodeling With Untoward Patient Outcomes

Natural history studies have shown that progressive LV remodeling is directly related to future deterioration in LV performance and a less favorable clinical course in patients with HF.[17-19] White and colleagues[20] were among the first to demonstrate that LV volume had greater predictive value for survival postinfarction than did LVEF. These authors measured LV volumes, LVEF, and severity of coronary arterial occlusions and stenosis at 1 to 2 months after a first or recurrent myocardial infarction. Survivors were followed for a mean of 78 months (range 15–165 months). There were 101 cardiac deaths, of which 71 (70%) were sudden (instantaneous or found dead). Multivariate analysis with log rank testing and the Cox proportional hazards model showed that end-systolic volume had greater predictive value for survival than did end-diastolic volume or EF. Interestingly, the severity of coronary occlusions and stenosis showed additional prediction of only borderline significance. Similar findings were reported by St. John Sutton and associates,[21] who studied LV enlargement after myocardial infarction in an echocardiographic sub-study of the Survival and Ventricular Enlargement (SAVE) Trial in which patients were randomized to placebo or captopril after an acute myocardial infarction. These investigators found that, irrespective of treatment assignment, baseline LV systolic area and the percent change in LV area were strong predictors of cardiovascular mortality and adverse cardiovascular events. At 1 year, LV end-diastolic and end-systolic areas were significantly larger in the placebo than in the captopril group. Moreover, approximately 25% of the patients who survived 1 year experienced a major adverse cardiovascular event. Relevant to the present discussion, patients who experienced an adverse cardiovascular outcome had a greater than threefold increase in LV cavity size than did patients with an uncomplicated course. In a prospective study of 36 patients with dilated cardiomyopathy, Douglas and associates used two-dimensional echocardiography to study the functional consequences of changes in LV size and shape.[18] In this study, nonsurvivors died an average of 11 months after initiation of the study, whereas survivors were followed up for an average of 52 months (range 40–76 months). Survivors had a smaller LV end-diastolic short-axis dimension when compared with nonsurvivors. Moreover, the ratio of short- to long-axis end-diastolic dimensions was more spherical in those with poorer survival (ratio 0.76 vs. 0.68, $P < .02$). More recently, Vasan and colleagues studied the impact of changes in LV size on mortality in subjects that were followed in the Framingham study.[19] They examined the relation of the LV end-diastolic and end-systolic internal dimensions, as measured by M-mode echocardiography, to the risk of HF in subjects who had not sustained a myocardial infarction and who were free of HF at the time of enrollment. Data were analyzed using a sex-stratified proportional-hazards regression to assess the association between baseline LV internal dimensions and the subsequent risk of HF, after adjusting for age, blood pressure, hypertension treatment, body mass index, diabetes, valve disease, and interim myocardial infarction. HF was diagnosed based on Framingham criteria (two major, or one major and two minor criteria).[22] These investigators found that during an 11-year follow-up period, HF developed in approximately 1.6% of the subjects. The risk-factor-adjusted hazard ratio for congestive HF was 1.47 (95% confidence interval, 1.25–1.73) for each increment of 1 standard deviation in LV end-diastolic dimension (height indexed). Similar results were obtained using LV end-systolic dimension

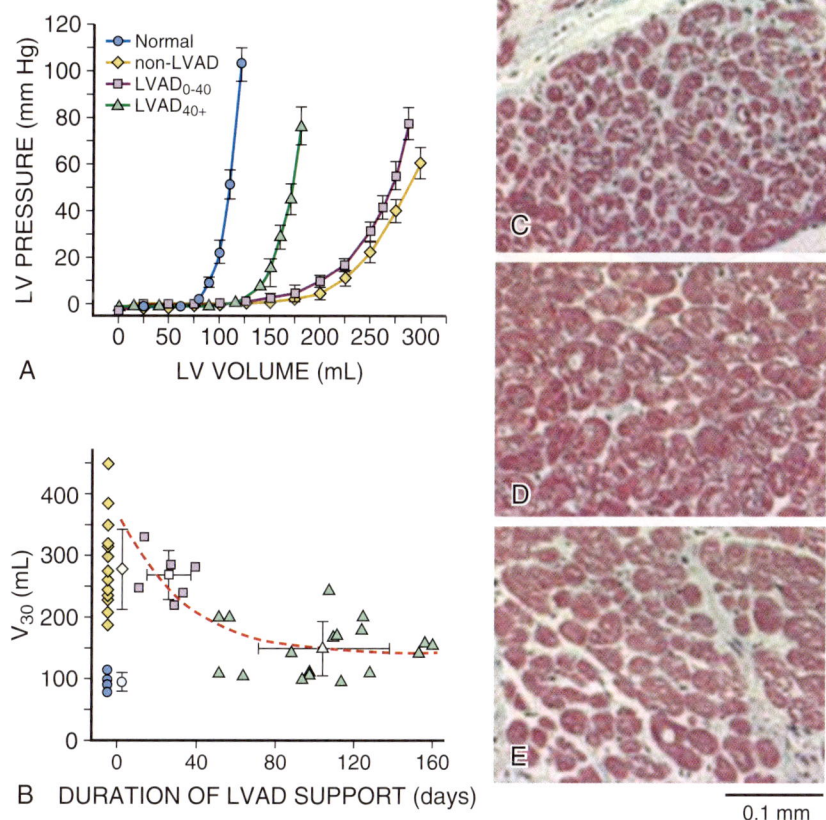

Fig. 12.4 The ventricular end-diastolic pressure-volume relationship, which is initially shifted far rightward in heart failure (HF), shifts, over time, back toward normal. (A) Average end-diastolic pressure volume relationships from normal human hearts, from failing hearts not supported with LVAD, hearts supported with an LVAD for less than 40 days, and hearts supported with in LVAD for more than 40 days. (B) Heart size, indexed by V30, the volume required to achieve an end-diastolic pressure of 30 mm Hg as a function of duration of LVAD support from individual hearts (see insert for symbol key). Also shown are values from normal and failing hearts not supported by LVAD. Underlying the reduction in heart size is regression of cellular hypertrophy. (C) Cross-section of normal human myocardium. (D) In chronic heart failure, the myocytes are markedly hypertrophic. (E) After LVAD support, LV myocardial hypertrophy regresses (individual myocyte cross-sectional area reduced). Increased interstitial fibrosis is also noted. All myocardial samples used for C to E were fixed in an unloaded state. *LV,* Left ventricle; *LVAD,* left ventricular assist device. (From Madigan JD, Barbone A, Choudhri AF, et al. Time course of reverse remodeling of the left ventricle during support with a left ventricular assist device. *J Thorac Cardiovasc Surg.* 2001;121:902–908.)

(hazard ratio = 1.43; 95% confidence interval, 1.24–1.65). Vasan and colleagues concluded that an increase in LV internal dimension is a risk factor for congestive HF in men and women who have not had a myocardial infarction. Thus, both the increased LV size and LV sphericity are predictive of untoward outcomes in HF patients with ischemic and dilated cardiomyopathy.

REVERSE LEFT VENTRICULAR REMODELING

The term *reverse remodeling* was first used to describe the leftward shift in the LV end-diastolic pressure-volume curve of the failing heart following hemodynamic unloading with a ventricular assist device (**Fig. 12.4**) or a myocardial wrap with latissimus dorsi muscle.[1,2] An important feature of the decrease in LV size with reverse remodeling was that the change in LV geometry persisted even if the inciting therapy was abruptly stopped, suggesting that the change in properties reflected intrinsic biologic changes in the LV chamber as opposed to changes in LV volume that occur simply in response to a decrease in LV filling pressure. **Fig. 12.5** shows that reverse LV remodeling has been observed in a wide variety of clinical settings, even when the HF is

quite severe, including viral myocarditis, postpartum cardiomyopathy, or after removal of a cytotoxic agent. A recurring observation in all these clinical studies is that reverse remodeling is associated with an improvement in the clinical manifestations and outcomes in HF, raising the interesting possibility that reverse remodeling is linked mechanistically to the observed improved HF outcomes. Remarkably, this observation held true also when studying patients with the same EF. Patients with mid-range EF (40%–50%) who had entered this category after experiencing reverse remodeling and improvement in LVEF were in fact found to have better outcomes than patients who had mid-range EF but had not experienced reverse remodeling.[23] As illustrated in Fig. 12.5, three major causes of dilated cardiomyopathy are associated with spontaneous recovery of LV function and reverse LV remodeling, including abnormal energetics, inflammation, and toxic insults. The greatest degree of recovery and/or normalization of LV function was observed in cardiomyopathies associated with abnormal energetics, whereas the cardiomyopathies associated with the least degree of recovery and/or normalization of LV function occurred with myocarditis and postpartum cardiomyopathy. There is also extensive clinical trial–based evidence supporting the potential for reverse remodeling

increase in EF after 4 months of therapy. In a dog model of HF induced by intracoronary microembolization, therapy with a cardiac support device resulted in a return in β-MHC, α-MHC, ANP, and BNP toward values observed in sham-operated animals.[47] Taken together, these data suggest that both drug and device therapies contribute to reversal of the fetal gene program that has been associated with abnormal contractile function of the cardiac myocyte. However, what is not clear from the extant literature is which of the above changes is/are necessary and/or essential for myocardial recovery.

As noted above, one of the signatures of advancing HF is a reduction in β₁-adrenergic receptor (β-AR) density, isoproterenol-mediated adenylate cyclase stimulation, and isoproterenol-stimulated muscle contraction.[48] β-AR desensitization can be reversed with pharmacologic and device therapies that have been shown to improve patient outcomes. In a sub-study of an MDC (metoprolol in dilated cardiomyopathy) trial, treatment with selective β₁-blocker metoprolol resulted in significantly increased total β-receptor density in the heart. Interestingly, carvedilol had no effect on β-adrenergic receptor (β-AR) density despite the fact that it was associated with a marked improvement in myocardial function and a reduction in cardiac adrenergic activity.[49] In a randomized, double-blind, placebo-controlled study, the use of the ACE inhibitor lisinopril resulted in a significant increase in myocardial β-AR density in a subset of HF patients with high baseline cardiac adrenergic activity.[50] Normalization of reduced β-adrenergic receptor density and enhanced inotropic responsiveness to isoproterenol have been demonstrated consistently in LVAD-supported failing hearts.[51-53] The enhanced β-adrenergic responsiveness with LVAD support was associated with a decrease in GRK2 protein levels and total GRK activity, but no significant change in GRK5 protein and mRNA levels. Similar findings have been observed following CRT therapy. After 4 months of CRT, β₁-adrenergic receptor expression was significantly upregulated at the transcriptional level in HF patients.[54] Treatment with a cardiac support device resulted in increased inotropic responsiveness in a canine model of HF.[55]

Mechanical unloading with LVAD support results in restoration of cytoskeletal organization. Vatta and colleagues reported that there was loss of the N-terminal region of dystrophin (which links to the sarcomere through actin) in patients with both ischemic and dilated cardiomyopathy, and that mechanical unloading resulted in increased N-terminal dystrophin expression.[56] The change in the level of expression of dystrophin was comparable in the RV and the LV after mechanical unloading; however, a greater degree of normalization was achieved in patients treated with pulsatile-flow LVADs than among those treated with continuous-flow LVADs.[57] Mechanical support with an LVAD has been reported to increase immunostaining for major sarcomeric proteins, including actin, troponin C, troponin T, tropomyosin, and titin, with a small nonsignificant decrease in myosin,[58] along with changes in the intracellular distribution of desmin, vinculin, and tubulin and an increase in desmin protein content, with no change in the content or distribution of α-actinin.[59] Interestingly, in one small study, there was a specific pattern of changes in mRNA expression levels for both sarcomeric and nonsarcomeric cytoskeletal proteins in the myocardium (increased β-actin, α-tropomyosin, α₁-actinin, α-filamin A, with decreased troponin T3, α₂-actinin, and vinculin) in patients who were bridged to recovery when compared with HF patients who were not supported, suggesting that alterations in cytoskeletal structure might play an important role in and serve as a marker of myocardial recovery (see later discussion).[60] Studies in canine models have shown that treatment with CRT can be associated with a normalization in the deposition of α-actinin.[61]

Collectively, the above genomic and proteomic changes would be expected to lead to functional improvements in the failing cardiac myocyte. And indeed, there is a significant increase in contractility (maximal calcium-saturated force generation) in cardiac myocytes isolated from hearts that have undergone LVAD support, when compared with myocytes isolated before LVAD support.[62]

As discussed in **Chapter 2**, changes in the abundance of critical Ca²⁺ regulatory proteins, including SERCA, ryanodine receptor (RyR), L-type calcium channel (LTCC), and sarcolemmal Na⁺/Ca²⁺ exchanger (NCX), likely play an important role in the contractile dysfunction of the failing cardiac myocyte. In a transgenic mouse model of HF overexpressing tropomodulin, treatment with β-blockers resulted in normalization of SERCA and NCX protein levels and LTCC density and function.[63] RyR phosphorylation was unchanged by treatment with β-blockers in this transgenic model. Clinical studies have shown that treatment with β-blockers results in increased myocardial SERCA mRNA and protein content (see Fig. 12.6),[39,64] a trend toward a decrease in myocardial PLB and NCX protein content,[64] and reduced PKA-mediated hyperphosphorylation of RyR.[65] Similarly, administration of ACE inhibitors or ARBs in a post-MI rat model of HF significantly attenuates the reduction in myocardial SERCA, RYR, and PLB mRNA and protein levels.[66,67] Mechanical unloading with LVAD support has provided the clearest insight into the importance of changes in excitation-contraction coupling during myocardial recovery. As summarized in **Fig. 12.7**, the return of contractile function in failing hearts following LVAD-induced unloading is associated with altered gene expression of key Ca²⁺ regulatory proteins, including NCX, SERCA2a, and RyR, and changes in calcium cycling.[68,69] Moreover, protein kinase A-mediated hyperphosphorylation of RyR was restored to normal in failing hearts following LVAD support.[70] Nonetheless, the significance of some of the reported changes in gene expression is uncertain, insofar as only SERCA2 protein levels increased, whereas protein levels of the RYR and NCX were unchanged following LVAD support. Cardiac resynchronization therapy significantly increased mRNA expression for SERCA2a, RyR, and SERCA/NCX mRNA in HF patients.[55] Importantly, improvement in SERCA expression occurred only in patients who clinically responded to CRT.[46] Although treatment with a cardiac support device did not result in changes in SERCA2a and phospholamban expression, treatment with a cardiac support device resulted in increased SERC2A-mediated Ca⁺² uptake in an experimental model.[71]

A number of authors have investigated the effect of medical and device therapies on myocardial metabolisms. While data is limited, the available evidence shows that medical and device therapies that lead to reverse remodeling improve myocardial metabolic efficiency. Treatment with β-adrenergic blockers was shown to decrease fatty acid uptake and overall myocardial oxygen consumption in the face of an increase in LV performance.[72] CRT was shown to increase cardiac performance without significant changes in myocardial oxygen consumption, therefore increasing myocardial efficiency.[73] A study of paired human myocardial tissue from 31 advanced HF patients at LVAD implant and at heart transplant showed that LVAD-induced mechanical unloading of the failing human heart induced upregulation of glycolysis without a parallel increase in pyruvate utilization for mitochondrial oxidation. The observed pyruvate mitochondrial oxidation mismatch suggests that there was persistent mitochondrial dysfunction, despite hemodynamic unloading of the heart (**Fig. 12.8**).[74]

Reversal of Alterations in the Myocardium

In addition to the salutary changes in the biology of the adult cardiac myocyte that occur during reverse remodeling, there are a number of important histological changes that also occur within the myocardium, including a reduction in cell loss, changes in the microvascular structure, and changes in the volume and composition of the ECM.

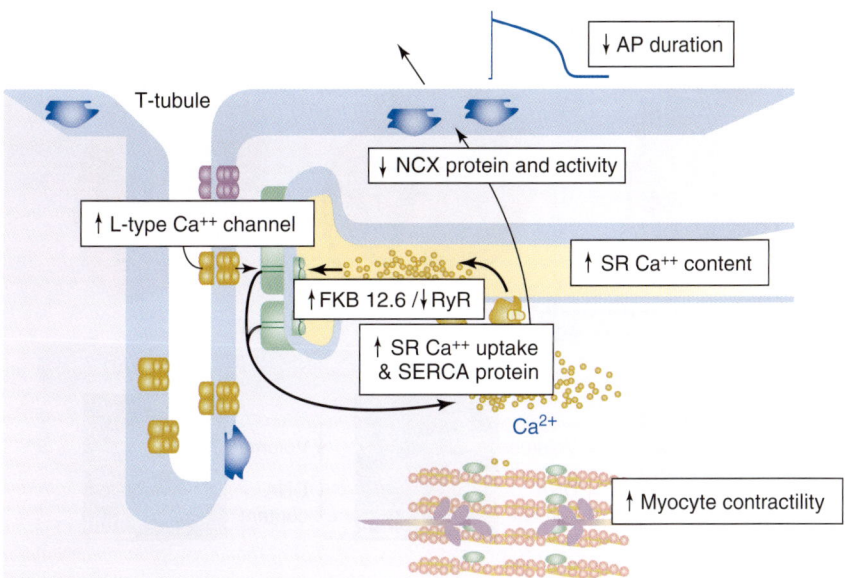

Fig. 12.7 Summary of changes in excitation-contraction coupling in cardiac myocytes from hearts that have been supported with a left ventricular assist device (LVAD). As shown, there is an increase in the inward Ca^{2+} current through the L-type Ca^{2+} channel, a decrease in the levels and activity of the sodium-calcium exchanger *(NCX)*, increased Ca^{2+} content of the sarcoplasmic reticulum *(SR)*, decreased activity of the ryanodine receptor *(RyR)*, and decreases in FKB 12.6 levels (a regulatory protein that prevents Ca^{2+} release from the RyR). Collectively, these changes would be expected to lead to improved myocyte contractility. (Key: The arrows indicate increases [↑] or decreases [↓] in various parameters.) *SERCA*, Sarcoplasmic endoreticular Ca^{2+} ATPase. (Modified from Soppa GK, Barton PJ, Terracciano CM, et al. Left ventricular assist device-induced molecular changes in the failing myocardium. *Curr Opin Cardiol.* 2008;23:206–218.)

While there is no evidence that medical and device therapies reverse the cardiomyocyte loss characteristic of the failing heart, there is evidence that chronic therapy with β blockers reduces HF associated apoptosis in canine models of HF.[75]

As noted above, both the amount and the organization of the fibrillar collagen are important determinants of myocardial structure and function in the failing heart. β-blockade with metoprolol significantly decreased replacement fibrosis in a dog model of HF.[76] Consistent with this finding, treating patients with dilated cardiomyopathy with β-blockers for 4 months resulted in decreased myocardial collagen types I and III mRNA expression in paired myocardial RV biopsy samples.[77] Experimental studies suggest that ACE inhibitors reduce collagen deposition in the failing myocardium in various models of HF, and this salutary effect is mediated, at least in part, by kinins.[78,79] Similarly, treatment of patients with ischemic cardiomyopathy with captopril resulted in decreased total collagen content, decreased collagen type III levels, and normalization of the collagen type I:III ratio, when compared with untreated HF patients.[80] Angiotensin receptor type I (AT_1) blockers also reduce myocardial collagen content in experimental HF models; however, this decrease was not attenuated by blockade of the bradykinin B_2-receptor, suggesting that antagonism of the renin angiotensin system alone is sufficient to reverse myocardial fibrosis.[79] Treatment with eplerenone in a dog model of HF significantly attenuated LV collage volume fraction by reducing both interstitial and replacement fibrosis[81] and normalized mRNA and protein expression of MMPs 1, 2, and 9, but had no effect on mRNA levels of TIMP-1 and -2.[82]

Mechanical circulatory support with LVADs also leads to important changes in the ECM and myocardial fibrillar content and organization. There are conflicting reports on the effect of LVAD support on LV myocardial collagen content, with several reports showing increased myocardial collagen content relative to levels observed in failing hearts

that have not been supported with LVADs,[83-87] whereas other reports suggest that the collagen volume fraction decreases.[88,89] Although the reason(s) for this discrepancy is not known, it may be related to differences in HF etiology, differences in the degree of inotropic and/or pharmacologic support, and the duration of LVAD support. Of note, one report suggests that longer duration of LVAD support results in increased myocardial collagen volume fraction in a time-dependent manner (**Fig. 12.9**).[29] Another potential explanation is that collagen content decreased in LVAD-supported patients taking ACE inhibitors and increased in patients not taking ACE inhibitors.[90]

The biologic basis for these changes is suggested by two studies that show that LVAD support resulted in decreased levels of MMP 1 and 9 and increased expression of TIMP-1 and -2, resulting in decreased MMP-1/TIMP-1 ratio (favoring collagen accumulation) and an increase in the ratio of insoluble to total soluble collagen (a measure of collagen cross-linking).[84,90] Moreover, these changes were amplified by concomitant therapy with ACE inhibitors during the period of LVAD support.[91] Serial myocardial biopsies from HF patients revealed a significant reduction in the collagen volume fraction following CRT,[33,92] with a significant decrease in MMP-9 levels in the group of patients who underwent reverse remodeling (i.e., "responders").[93]

Experimental studies suggest that myocardial capillary density is restored toward normal values following treatment with pharmacologic therapies that have been shown to improve patient outcomes in HF.[76,79,81] Moreover, some of these same therapies also lead to improved myocardial blood flow in patients with HF.[94-96] Whether the improved myocardial blood flow is related to increased angiogenesis, altered hemodynamic loading conditions, or both is not known. Analysis of changes in gene expression before and after LVAD support revealed significant alterations in genes that are involved in the regulation of vascular networks, including upregulation of Sprouty-1 and downregulation of neurophilin (VEGF receptor), stromal derived

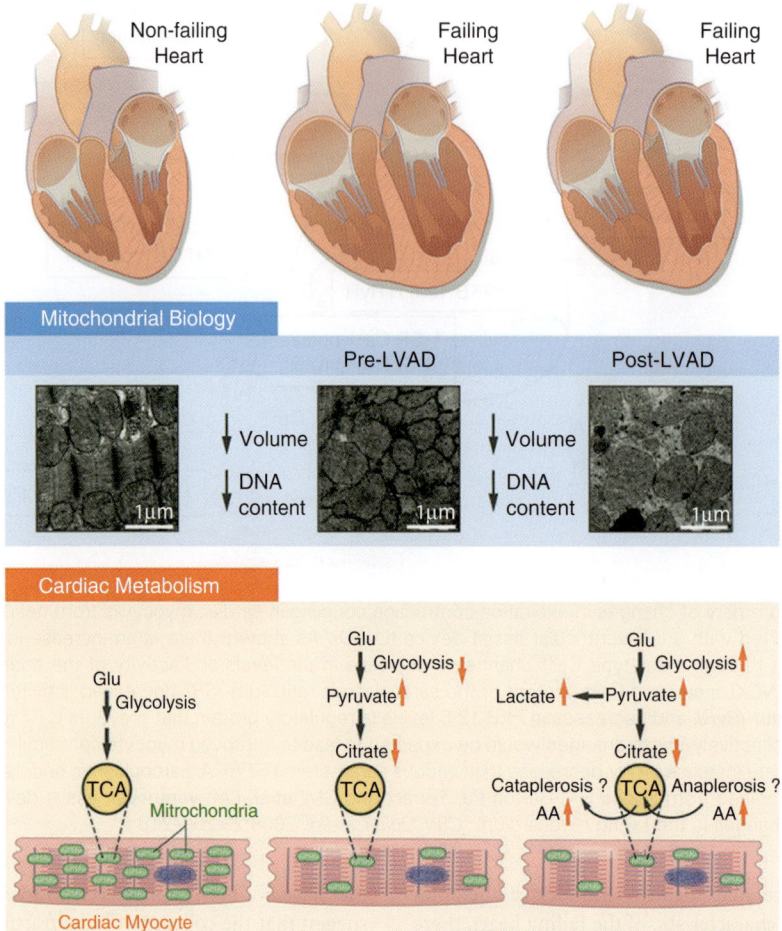

Fig. 12.8 Metabolic reverse remodeling induced by treatment with a left ventricular assist device *(LVAD)*. The failing heart is characterized by a reduction in the volume and number of mitochondria. This is associated with a depression of both glycolysis and the tricarboxylic acid *(TCA)* cycle and an accumulation of Pyruvate. In a heart supported with LVAD, there is an increase in glycolysis without a corresponding increase activity of the TAC cycle that is associated with an accumulation of lactate. The role that the replenishment (anapleirosis) and depletion (catapleirosis) of intermediates of the TCA cycle play in this process remains unknown. (From Diakos NA, Navankasattusas S, Abel DE, et al. Evidence of glycolysis up-regulation and pyruvate mitochondrial oxidation mismatch during mechanical unloading of the failing human heart: implications for cardiac reloading and conditioning. *JACC Basic Transl Sci.* 2016;1(6):432–444.)

factor-1, FGF9, and endomucin[97] Sprouty-1 was immunolocalized to the microvasculature, and the upregulation of Sprouty-1 in endothelial cells was associated with a decrease in VEGF-induced endothelial proliferation, which suggests that Sprouty-1 may serve as an intrinsic mediator of cardiac remodeling by regulating angiogenesis.[97] Studies in HF patients who underwent CRT revealed increased myocardial capillary density and an improvement in the distribution pattern of myocardial blood flow.[92,98]

Reversal of Changes in Left Ventricular Geometry

As noted previously, clinical studies with ACE inhibitors, β-blockers, aldosterone antagonists, LVADs, and CRT have shown that these treatment modalities lead to a return of cardiac myocyte biology toward normal and to changes in the ECM that favor increased structural integrity of the heart and reverse remodeling. In the following section, we will review the literature that shows that drugs and devices that favorably impact clinical outcomes are accompanied by reverse LV remodeling as measured by reduction in LV volume, reduction in LV sphericity, normalization of LV wall thickness, and reduction in MV incompetence. These different domains of LV remodeling

have not always been studied in detail in each study, but they have all been shown to be associated, to some extent, with normalization of LV volume and EF. As illustrated in **Fig. 12.10A**, treatment with ACE inhibitors prevented worsening LV remodeling but did not lead to reverse remodeling in a substudy of SOLVD,[99] whereas treatment with β-blockers resulted in decreased LV end-diastolic volumes when compared with the placebo (diuretics and ACE inhibitors) in a substudy of the ANZ (Australia New Zealand) trial (see Fig. 12.10B).[100] In an echocardiographic substudy of the Val-HeFT (Valsartan in HF) trial, treatment with valsartan added to an ACE inhibitor and/or β-blocker significantly resulted in decreased LV internal diastolic diameter (LVIDd)/body surface area from 4 months to greater than 24 months (see Fig. 12.10C).[101] Similarly, the addition of spironolactone to candesartan resulted in a significant decrease in LV volume index at 1 year when compared with candesartan alone (see Fig. 12.10D).[102]

Device therapies also lead to a reduction in the ventricular volume. Although pulsatile-flow devices provide a greater degree of ventricular unloading than continuous-flow devices,[103] the continuous-flow LVADs appear to be as effective as pulsatile-flow LVADs with regard to the degree of LV reverse remodeling (see Fig. 12.10E).[103,104] In the

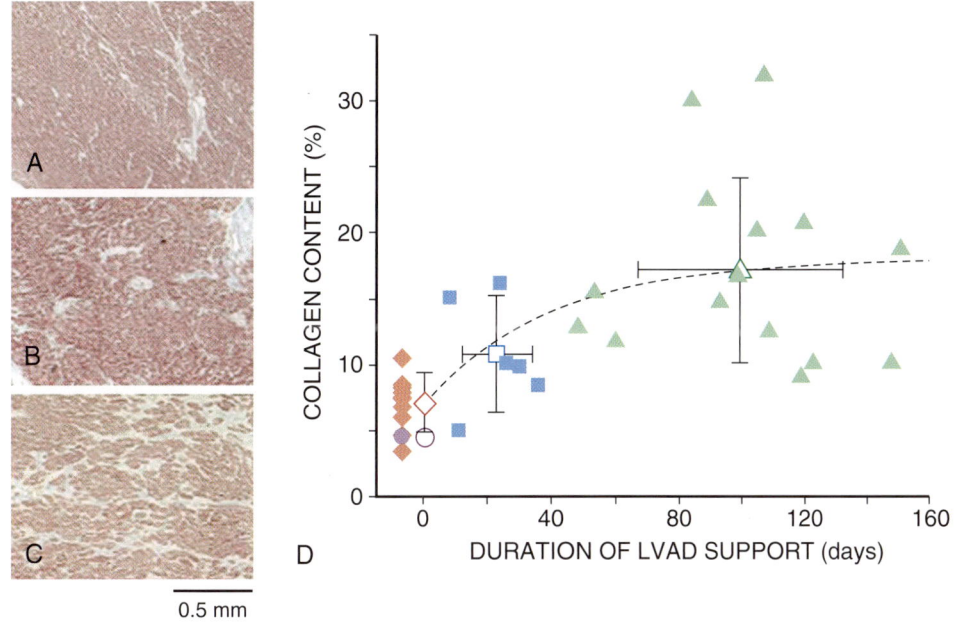

Fig. 12.9 Effect of the duration of LVAD support on myocardial collagen content. Trichrome-stained sections of LV free wall demonstrating relative myocardial collagen content for (A) normal (B) non-LVAD, and (C) LVAD$_{40+day}$ groups. (D) Relative myocardial collagen content versus duration of LVAD support (*squares,* LVAD$_{0-40\ days}$; *triangles,* LVAD$_{40+days}$; *diamonds,* non-LVAD; *circles,* normal). (Modified from Madigan JD, Barbone A, Choudhri AF, et al. Time course of reverse remodeling of the left ventricle during support with a left ventricular assist device. *J Thorac Cardiovasc Surg.* 2001;121:902–908.)

MIRACLE (Multicenter In-Synch Randomized Clinical Evaluation) trial, CRT led to improvements in LVEF, mitral regurgitant area, and LV end-diastolic diameter at 6 months in patients with moderate to severe HF and prolonged QRS (**see Chapter 38**).[105] Similar findings have been reported in the MUSTIC (MUltisite STimulation in Cardiomyopathy) and CARE-HF (Cardiac Resynchronization in Heart Failure) studies, which employed a longer follow-up period (**see also Chapter 38**).[106,107] CRT was also shown to induce a normalization of LV shape in one of the few studies that specifically investigated changes in the LV "sphericity index" in response to therapy.[108]

In addition to the drugs and devices discussed above, a variety of surgical techniques to reverse the maladaptive ventricular remodeling in patients with HF have been explored. As discussed in **Chapter 19**, myocardial revascularization should be considered in patients with evidence of myocardial viability and depressed LV dysfunction.

MYOCARDIAL REMISSION AND MYOCARDIAL RECOVERY

Clinical studies have shown that reverse LV remodeling with normalization of LV structure and function is associated with stabilization of the clinical syndrome of HF. This group of patients are often referred to as having "HF with recovered EF."[109] However, among patients who experience normalization of the LVEF , a significant proportion remain at increased risk of future HF, whereas a smaller percentage remain free from HF events.[5] Based on the disparate clinical outcomes of reverse remodeling, it has been suggested that the term *myocardial recovery* should be used to describe the rare normalization of the molecular, cellular, myocardial, and LV geometric changes that are associated with freedom from future HF events, whereas the term *myocardial remission* should be used to refer to the normalization of the molecular, cellular, myocardial, and LV geometric changes that provoke cardiac remodeling that are insufficient to

prevent the recurrence of HF in the face of normal and/or perturbed hemodynamic loading conditions.[110] Although the biologic differences between myocardial recovery and myocardial remission are not known, it bears emphasis that, as described above, in most instances, reverse LV remodeling normalization of the HF phenotype does not lead to a "normal" heart (**Fig. 12.11A**). First, gene expression profiling studies have shown that only approximately 5% of genes that are dysregulated in failing hearts revert back to normal following LVAD support, despite typical morphologic and functional responses to LVAD support.[41,44,111] Second, although maximal calcium-saturated force generation is improved in myocytes following LVAD support, force generation is still less than in myocytes from nonfailing controls, despite reversal of cardiac myocyte hypertrophy.[36] Third, as noted previously, the majority of studies that have examined changes in the ECM following LVAD have suggested that the ECM does not revert to normal on its own and can actually be characterized by increased myocardial fibrosis. Moreover, our current understanding of changes in the ECM during LVAD support have focused on ECM content and not on the more fundamental issues of its three-dimensional organization or with the interactions between the collagen matrix and the resident cardiac myocytes, which are likely to be critically important. Fourth, although the LV EDPVRs of LVAD-supported hearts are shifted leftward, and overlap those found in nonfailing ventricles, the ratio of LV wall thickness-to-LV wall radius does not return to normal despite normalization of LV chamber geometry.[112] Rather, this ratio remains elevated at nearly twice the normal ratio. This has important implications for LV function, insofar as LV wall stress depends critically on this ratio (Laplace's Law). Given that end-diastolic wall stress represents the load on the cardiac myocyte at the onset of systole, the observation that the LV wall thickness-to-LV wall radius ratio is not normalized despite the normalization of LV global chamber properties, suggests that the cardiac myocytes in reverse-remodeled ventricles are still exposed to increased physiologic

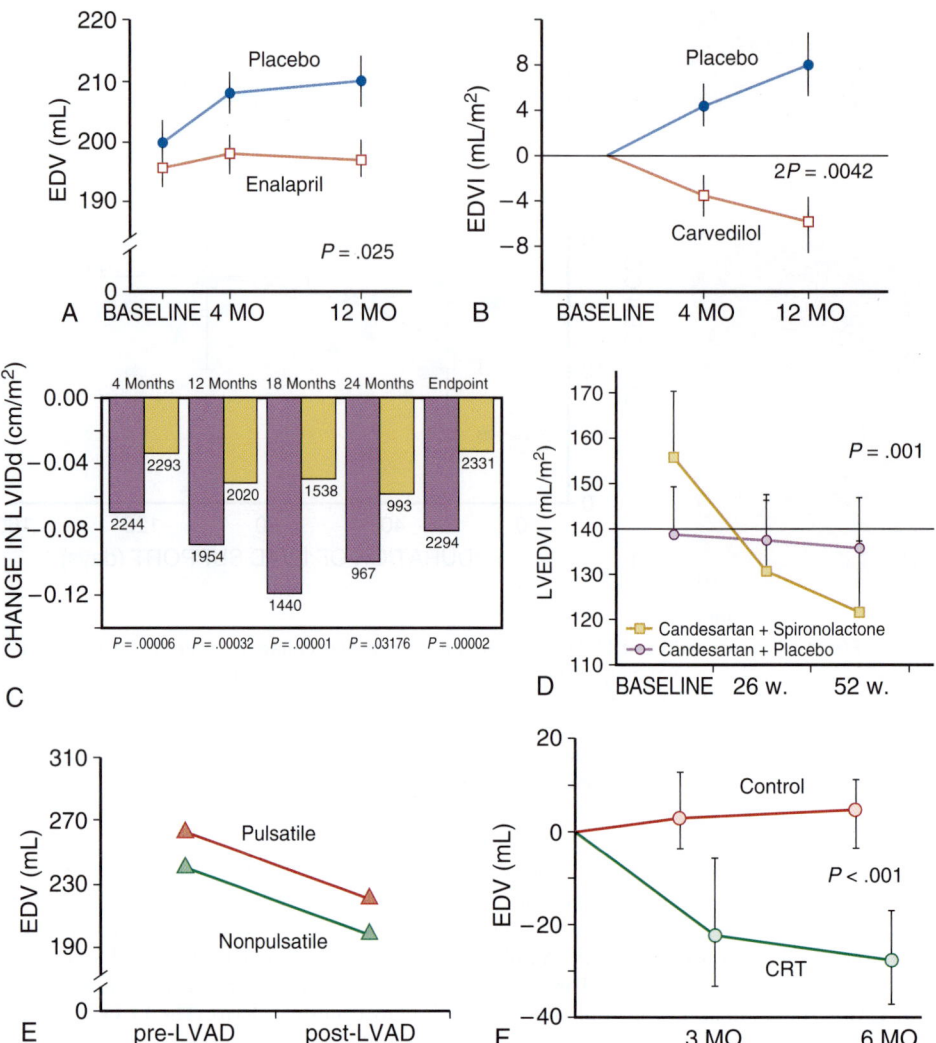

Fig. 12.10 Reverse cardiac remodeling following pharmacologic and device therapies in patients with heart failure. (A) Changes in LV end-diastolic volume (LVEDV) in the placebo and enalapril-treated patients in SOLVD compared to the placebo. (B) Changes in LV volume index from baseline during the 12-month follow-up period in the ANZ trial compared to the placebo. (C) Changes in LV end-diastolic dimension in patients treated with valsartan added to an ACE inhibitor and/or β-blocker significantly resulted in decreased LV internal diastolic diameter (normalized to body surface area [BSA]). (D) Changes in LV volume index in patients treated with spironolactone and candesartan compared to candesartan alone. (E) Changes in LVEDV in pulsatile versus continuous flow LVADs. (F), Change in LVEDV at 3 and 6 months after CRT compared to the control group in the MIRACLE trial. *ACE,* Angiotensin-converting enzyme; *EDV,* end-diastolic volume; *LVAD,* left ventricular assist device. (A to F, modified, respectively, from Greenberg B, Quinones MA, Koilpillai C, et al. Effects of long-term enalapril therapy on cardiac structure and function in patients with left ventricular dysfunction. Results of the SOLVD echocardiography substudy. *Circulation.* 1995;91:2573–2581; Doughty RN, Whalley GA, Gamble G, et al. Left ventricular remodeling with carvedilol in patients with congestive heart failure due to ischemic heart disease. *J Am Coll Cardiol.* 1998;29:1060–1066,; Wong M, Staszewsky L, Latini R, et al. Valsartan benefits left ventricular structure and function in heart failure: Val-HeFT echocardiographic study. *J Am Coll Cardio.* 2002;40:970–975; Chan AK, Sanderson JE, Wang T, et al. Aldosterone receptor antagonism induces reverse remodeling when added to angiotensin receptor blockade in chronic heart failure. *J Am Coll Cardiol.* 2007;50:591–596; Klotz S, Deng MC, Stypmann J, et al. Left ventricular pressure and volume unloading during pulsatile versus nonpulsatile left ventricular assist device support. *Ann Thorac Surg.* 2004;77:143–149; and St John Sutton MG, Plappert T, Abraham WT, et al. Effect of cardiac resynchronization therapy on left ventricular size and function in chronic heart failure. *Circulation.* 2003;107:1985–1990.)

stresses. Whether this represents loss of functioning cardiac myocytes or failure of the three-dimensional organization of the ECM to revert to normal is unknown. Fifth, in a single-center retrospective cohort study, an analysis of the left ventricular global longitudinal strain (GLS) among patients with fully recovered LVEF showed that most

patients with normalized LVEF have a subnormal GLS and that GLS correlates with the likelihood of maintaining a normal LVEF during follow-up.[6] Thus, normalization of the HF phenotype during reverse LV remodeling typically does not signify that the cellular/molecular biology and physiology of these hearts actually becomes normal,

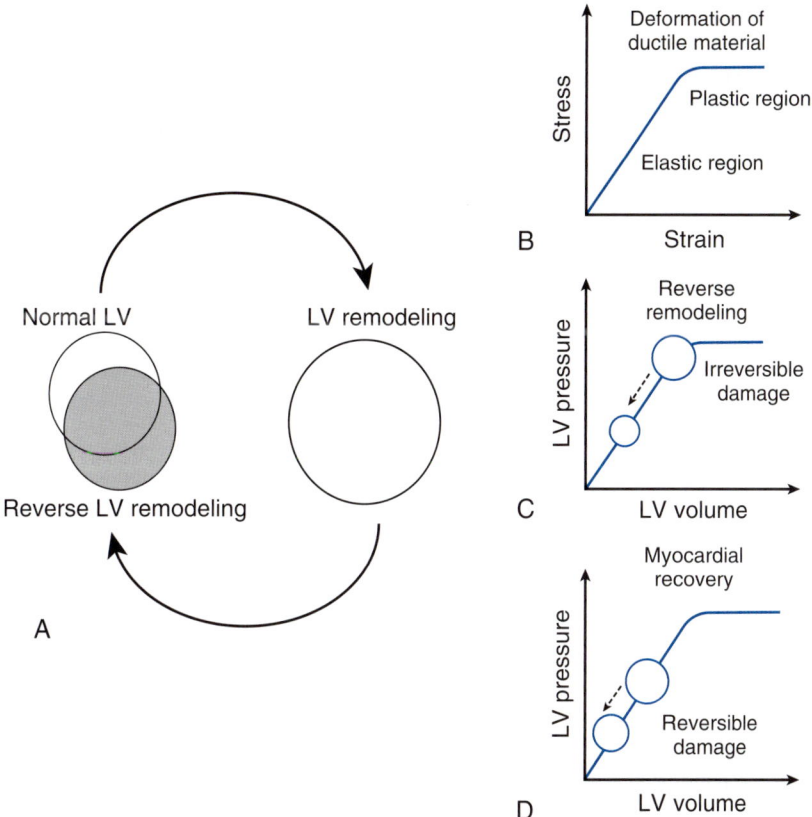

Fig. 12.11 Myocardial recovery and remission. (A) Proposed hypothetical model suggesting that reverse LV remodeling represents the summation of complex interactions between multiple biological networks that adopt a novel less pathological configuration, which only partly overlaps with the configuration present in naïve hearts (B) Diagram of a stress-strain curve of a ductile material, illustrating the relationship between an applied force (stress) and deformation (strain). Deformation can lead to reversible changes in a material (elastic deformation) if the properties of the material are not changed, but marked deformation can lead to irreversible changes (plastic deformation). (C) Hypothetical model of reverse remodeling in a heart that has undergone irreversible damage (plastic deformation). (D) Hypothetical model of reverse remodeling with recovery in a heart that has undergone reversible damage (elastic deformation). *LV,* Left ventricle. (A, modified from Weinheimer CJ, Kovacs A, Evans S, et al. Load-dependent changes in left ventricular structure and function in a pathophysiologically relevant murine model of reversible heart failure. *Circ Heart Fail.* 2018;11(5):e004351; Mann DL, Barger PM, Burkhoff D. Myocardial recovery: myth, magic or molecular target? *J Amer Coll Cardiol.* 2012;60:2465–2472.)

which may explain why reverse remodeling does not invariably lead to freedom from future HF events.

Although the potential biological differences between myocardial recovery and myocardial remission are not known, there are parallels in mechanical engineering science that may help to illuminate potential important differences and frame future mechanistic discussions. In mechanics, deformation of a material refers to the change in the shape or size of an object due to an applied force. Fig. 12.11B shows a representative stress versus strain diagram of a material that is exposed to an increased load. With increasing stress, there is an increase in the length of the material, up until the point when no further changes in length are possible without the material breaking. Importantly, if the material returns to its original state when the load is removed, this is referred to as *elastic deformation*. In contrast, if during the application of stress the mechanical properties of the material are changed irreversibly, such that the object will return only part way to its original shape when the stress is removed, this is referred to as *plastic deformation*. It is sometimes the case that elastic deformation occurs under a certain level of stress and plastic deformation occurs when that stress level is exceeded. Regardless, the important distinction is whether or not the material returns to its original state when the stress is removed. Although precise parallels between cardiac remodeling in HF and the deformation of solid materials following loading are not appropriate, there could be a parallel between reverse remodeling and plastic deformation, inasmuch as the reverse remodeled heart does not revert completely to normal after cessation of hemodynamic overloading (see Fig. 12.11C). Although speculative, it is possible that myocardial recovery is more analogous to elastic deformation in that the recovered heart reverts back to normal after hemodynamic overloading is removed (see Fig. 12.11D). Thus, myocardial remission represents a reversal of the HF phenotype that occurs in hearts that have undergone irreversible damage, whereas myocardial recovery represents a reversal of the HF phenotype that occurs in hearts that have undergone reversible damage. Although the biological motifs that separate reversible (elastic) from irreversible (plastic) changes in the heart are not known, it is likely that the progressive loss of cardiac myocytes and the progressive erosion of the native 3-dimensional organization of the ECM surrounding the cardiac myocytes will be critical determinants that distinguish between reverse remodeling and myocardial recovery. This model is consistent with the observation that the great majority of clinical examples of myocardial recovery in the literature occur after transient injury (e.g., viral infection, inflammation, toxic injury) rather than longer-standing and/or permanent injury (e.g., myocardial infarction, genetic abnormalities), and, therefore, the ability of the heart to "recover" to a state as close as possible to its original state is related to the nature of the inciting injury and the extent of underlying myocardial damage that occurs during the resolution of cardiac injury.

SUMMARY AND FUTURE DIRECTIONS

As discussed herein, the failing heart undergoes a number of maladaptive changes in LV structure and function that contribute to disease progression in the clinical syndrome of HF. Numerous clinical and epidemiologic studies have also suggested that HF is potentially reversible and that the heart is capable of undergoing favorable reversal of the changes in LV structure and function that are associated with stabilization of the clinical syndrome of HF. Although the various components of reverse remodeling have been carefully studied and annotated, it is presently unclear exactly how these changes contribute to restoration of normal LV structure and function. That is, we simply do not understand what the essential biologic "drivers" of myocardial recovery are, nor do we understand how they are coordinated. More importantly, we do not understand why reverse LV remodeling is sometimes associated with freedom from recurrent HF events (i.e., myocardial recovery) but much more often is associated with recurrence of HF events at a future point in time.[5,109] Epidemiological data suggests that the likelihood of experiencing reverse remodeling depends on the type and extent of damage that cause LV remodeling, and, therefore, the myocardium might be described as an object that, when exposed to a load, can undergo a reversible (elastic) deformation, but, when the load exceeds a certain threshold, experiences an irreversible (plastic) deformation. In line with this conceptual framework, data from animal models suggests that the reverse remodeled heart is characterized by a persistence of dysregulated gene networks.[113,114] Thus reverse LV remodeling of the heart represents a "less or nonpathologic state" that is comprised of dysregulated gene networks that are either partially or completely normalized and of persistently dysregulated gene networks that assume a different biological set point. The observation that gene networks undergo hysteretic expression[111,115] is consistent with the well-recognized observation that most soft tissues exhibit hysteresis when mechanically loaded and unloaded, indicating that although the biological properties of the stretched tissue return toward the normal unstressed state, they do not return to their original state.[116] While this model explains the epidemiological data indicating that patients with recovered LVEF almost univocally remain at increased risk of future cardiovascular events, the molecular and mechanistic basis of the difference between reverse remodeled and naïve hearts remain largely unknown. As more and more therapies to foster reverse remodeling are becoming available and our ability to interrogate the biology of the myocardium is improving, it is likely that the learning curve will remain steep for the foreseeable future.

KEY REFERENCES

1. Kass DA, Baughman KL, Pak PH, et al. Reverse remodeling from cardiomyoplasty in human heart failure. External constraint versus active assist *Circulation*. 1995;91:2314–2318.
2. Levin HR, Oz MC, Chen JM, Packer M, Rose EA, Burkhoff D. Reversal of chronic ventricular dilation in patients with end-stage cardiomyopathy by prolonged mechanical unloading. *Circulation*. 1995;91:2717–2720.
5. Merlo M, Stolfo D, Anzini M, et al. Persistent recovery of normal left ventricular function and dimension in idiopathic dilated cardiomyopathy during long-term follow-up: does real healing exist? *J Am Heart Assoc*. 2015;4:e001504.
6. Adamo L, Perry A, Novak E, Makan M, Lindman BR, Mann DL. Abnormal global longitudinal strain predicts future deterioration of left ventricular function in heart failure patients with a recovered left ventricular ejection fraction. *Circ Heart Fail*. 2017;10.
8. Cohn JN, Ferrari R, Sharpe N. Cardiac remodeling—concepts and clinical implications: a consensus paper from an international forum on cardiac remodeling. Behalf of an International Forum on Cardiac Remodeling *J Am Coll Cardiol*. 2000;35:569–582.
18. Douglas PS, Morrow R, Ioli A, Reicheck N. Left ventricular shape, afterload, and survival in idiopathic dilated cardiomyopathy. *J Am Coll Cardiol*. 1989;13:311–315.
20. White HD, Norris RM, Brown MA, Brandt PW, Whitlock RM, Wild CJ. Left ventricular end-systolic volume as the major determinant of survival after recovery from myocardial infarction. *Circulation*. 1987;76:44–51.
109. Basuray A, French B, Ky B, et al. Heart failure with recovered ejection fraction: clinical description, biomarkers, and outcomes. *Circulation*. 2014;129:2380–2387.
110. Mann DL, Barger PM, Burkhoff D. Myocardial recovery: myth, magic or molecular target? *J Amer Coll Cardiol*. 2012;60:2465–2472.
111. Margulies KB, Matiwala S, Cornejo C, Olsen H, Craven WA, Bednarik D. Mixed messages: transcription patterns in failing and recovering human myocardium. *Circ Res*. 2005;96:592–599.

The full reference list for this chapter is available on ExpertConsult.

Alterations in the Sympathetic and Parasympathetic Nervous Systems in Heart Failure

John S. Floras

Despite substantive advances in medical and device therapy of heart failure, symptom burden and rates of hospitalization and death remain high. Increased plasma norepinephrine (NE) concentration, its rate of appearance in coronary sinus efflux, and diminished tonic and reflex heart rate modulation were among the first characteristics of heart failure with reduced ejection fraction (HFrEF) that were shown to identify individuals at particular risk of premature death.[1,2] This chapter, which focuses on the autonomic disturbances of heart failure, will review mechanisms responsible for between-patient variation in their magnitude and the relevance of altered sympathetic and vagal regulation of the heart and circulation to the pathophysiology and management of this condition.[1-5] The autonomic phenotype of heart failure patients with preserved ejection fraction (HFpEF) is less well characterized (**see also Chapters 11** and **39**),[6] but extant knowledge will be summarized. Reference to animal models will be limited to concepts as yet unstudied in humans. Disturbances of autonomic thermoregulatory mechanisms in heart failure[7] will not be discussed.

ASSESSMENT OF HUMAN SYMPATHETIC AND PARASYMPATHETIC NERVOUS SYSTEM ACTIVITY

A range of distinct yet complementary invasive and noninvasive methods are available for this purpose (**see also Chapter 42**). Their application has yielded important insights into mechanisms of autonomic dysregulation in heart failure but, as highlighted in **Table 13.1**, each has specific shortcomings as well as utility. None, thus far, has an established role in clinical practice.

Catecholamines

Venous plasma NE concentrations, acquired at rest, reflect primarily neurotransmitter release from upstream forearm skeletal muscle and provide little insight into the magnitude and duration of other sympathetic nerve or adrenal responses to emotional stimuli or exercise. Moreover, the effect of heart failure or its therapies on neurotransmitter release cannot be deduced definitively solely from changes in

TABLE 13.1   Methods to Assess Human Autonomic Cardiovascular Regulation

	Vagal	Sympathetic	Comment	Research Utility	Clinical Utility
Heart rate (HR) at rest	Yes	Yes		+	++
HR response to Valsalva maneuver	Yes	Yes		+	+
HRV: time domain	Yes	If with BP	Quantitation of spontaneous blood pressure (BP) → HR relationship to estimate arterial baroreflex regulation of sinoatrial deceleration (vagal) or acceleration (sympathetic)	++	+++
HRV: frequency domain	Yes	Yes	High-frequency spectral power reflects vagal HR modulation; spectral power at lower frequencies primarily sympathetic HR modulation; Concurrent BP → HR spectral power transfer function to estimate arterial baroreflex regulation of HR	++	+
HR responses to drug stimuli	Yes	Yes	Arterial baroreceptor stimulation by phenylephrine elicits immediate vagal response; unloading by vasodilators elicits reflex sympathetic response	+++	++
HR response to mechanical stimuli	Yes	Yes	Responses to lower body negative or positive pressure primarily sympathetic; to negative or positive neck pressure primarily vagal	++	?
Blood pressure (BP) variability	?	?	Time or frequency domain measures not specific to autonomic regulation; Principal utility when evaluated in conjunction with HRV spectrum	?	?
Arterial/venous norepinephrine (NE)	No	Yes	Global nonspecific index	+	++
Urinary NE excretion	No	Yes	Global nonspecific index	+	++
NE spillover to plasma	No	Yes	Total body or organ-specific (heart, kidney, limb muscle, brain) data	+++	+
Sympathetic nerve recordings	No	Yes	Multi-unit or single-unit efferent muscle sympathetic nerve activity (MSNA); Sympathetic reflex response to baroreceptor, chemoreceptor, muscle mechanoreflex and metaboreflex, and other reflex simulation or inhibition can be estimated in time domain; Concurrent BP → MSNA spectral power transfer function estimates arterial baroreflex efferent sympathetic regulation in frequency domain	+++	+
Sympathetic nerve imaging	No	Yes	Nuclear tracers or PET ligands to assess principally cardiac sympathetic innervation and NE uptake	++	++

HRV, Heart rate variability.

plasma catecholamine concentrations. The majority of NE released from sympathetic vesicles is subject to neuronal or extraneuronal uptake; only a small fraction either acts on postjunctional adrenoceptors or appears in plasma. Low cardiac output reduces neuronal and extraneuronal clearance, causing plasma NE concentrations to rise.[8]

The isotopic method addresses such limitations but at increased complexity and cost. Total body NE spillover into plasma is determined from the dilution of tritium-labeled NE during its steady-state infusion in tracer concentrations. If venous effluent from an organ, such as the heart, kidney, or brain, is collected simultaneously with an arterial sample, the difference in tritium-labeled NE between vein and artery can be used to calculate its local extraction (Extr) by neuronal and extraneuronal transport mechanisms. Organ-specific NE spillover (NES) can then be determined by the equation:

$$NES = [(NE_v - NE_a) + (NE_a \times Extr)] \times PF$$

with NE_a and NE_v representing arterial and venous concentrations of unlabeled NE and PF plasma flow. Neuronal NE re-uptake and storage can be estimated by calculating spillover of tritium-labeled dihydroxyphenylglycol (DHPG), an intraneuronal metabolite.[8]

Microneurography

Multifiber or single-unit recordings from postganglionic nerves supplying muscular or cutaneous vascular beds capture the dynamic nature of sympathetic nerve firing and illustrate its reflex control (**Fig. 13.1**).[9-12] Skin sympathetic nerve activity is not modulated by input from high- or low-pressure baroreceptor reflexes. It responds preferentially to alerting stimuli or cold with burst firing

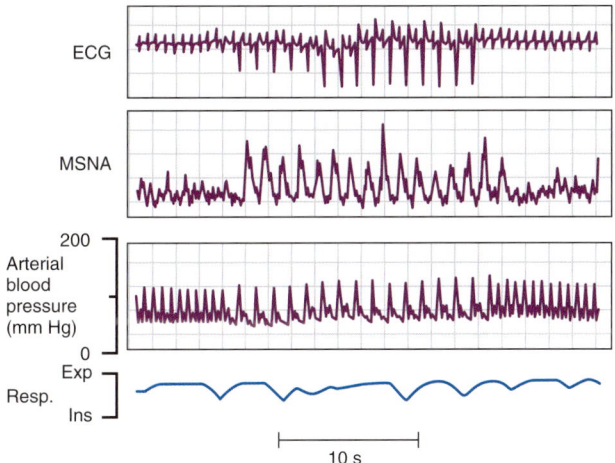

Fig. 13.1 The electrocardiogram *(ECG)*, mean voltage neurogram for *(MSNA)*, blood pressure, and respiratory excursions in a young man with end-stage heart failure due to dilated cardiomyopathy. Paroxysms of ventricular bigeminy result in a doubling of the blood pressure cycle length, a longer diastolic period, and lower diastolic blood pressure. These changes are registered immediately by the arterial baroreceptors and result in a corresponding increase in the duration of the sympathetic burst and a marked increase in burst amplitude. These are reversed with the restoration of sinus rhythm. (Courtesy John S. Floras, MD.)

occurrence independent of the cardiac cycle, whereas sympathetic discharge directed at skeletal muscle resistance vessels is entrained by input from arterial and cardiopulmonary mechanoreceptors. Muscle sympathetic nerve activity (MSNA) exhibits distinctive pulse-synchronicity, with multiunit bursts appearing 1.1 to 1.3 seconds after the preceding R wave of the electrocardiogram. In healthy subjects, MSNA is activated by reductions in diastolic or cardiac filling pressure, exercise, hypoxia, hypercapnia, and arousal from sleep, and is inhibited by lung inflation. In healthy resting individuals, the magnitude of MSNA correlates with both renal and cardiac NE spillover. Isometric exercise elicits proportionately similar increases in MSNA and cardiac norepinephrine spillover (CNES). In HFrEF, however, such concordance is lost.[13]

Arterial Baroreflex Sensitivity

Because cardiac cycle length responds more rapidly to the release and metabolism of acetylcholine than of NE, the normally brisk sinus node response to an acute perturbation in blood pressure is mediated primarily by arterial baroreceptor reflex-mediated vagal activation or withdrawal. One method of determining the strength, or gain, of reflex vagal heart rate regulation is to quantify the bradycardic response to a bolus of a vasoconstrictor drug, such as phenylephrine, or the tachycardic response to nitroprusside- or nitroglycerin-induced hypotension. Longer ("steady state") infusions of these vasoactive agents elicit competing sympathetic influence. The use of such drugs for this purpose has several limitations. Nitrate donors affect sino-atrial discharge directly. By causing sustained vasoconstriction or dilation, these drugs mechanically distort baroreceptor nerve endings. Their action is nonspecific, affecting also mechanoreceptors situated in the atria and pulmonary vasculature. Heart rate responses to carotid sinus baroreceptor stimulation by neck suction or unloading by neck pressure have been studied, but aortic arch baroreceptors will elicit counter-regulatory reflex responses to any arterial pressure changes these maneuvers induce.

Algorithms have been developed to track spontaneous fluctuations in blood pressure and heart rate from continuous noninvasive

or invasive recordings, and to identify, within such time periods, brief sequences with concordant changes in systolic blood pressure and the subsequent R-R intervals (inverse of heart rate).

Common to such methods is the construction of regression equations relating changes in output (pulse interval; in milliseconds) to changes in input (systolic blood pressure; mm Hg from antecedent cardiac cycles. The slope of this estimates the gain of the arterial baroreflex control of heart rate. Values obtained by this spontaneous sequence method are qualitatively similar to those derived using vasoactive drugs.

Reflex regulation of central sympathetic outflow can be evaluated similarly by relating changes in MSNA to changes in arterial pressure during graded infusions of pressors and vasodilators, or by constructing, under resting drug-free conditions, regression equations relating spontaneous changes in MSNA to preceding diastolic blood pressures.[14] By their nature, such methods cannot establish if any reduction in the arterial baroreflex gain of either heart rate or sympathetic nerve firing accrues from conduit artery inelasticity, diminished neural transduction of baroreceptor stretch, central neuroplastic adaptation, or efferent nerve dysfunction.

Heart Rate Variability

The half-life of acetylcholine is too brief and its actions too local to permit assay. Instead, tonic vagal heart rate modulation is estimated indirectly, most often and best validated by determining beat-to-beat variation either within the time domain (e.g., the standard deviation of all nonectopic pulse intervals occurring within a specified period) or within the frequency domain, using spectral analysis. A complimentary method, termed heart rate turbulence analysis, evaluates beat-to-beat variations in heart rate that follow a premature ventricular complex. Algorithms commonly employed to derive heart rate power spectra include Fast Fourier Transformation, autoregression, and coarse-graining spectral analysis (CGSA). The complexity of the heart rate variation is such that a range of additional analytic methods, both linear and nonlinear, have been proposed to characterize the information contained more fully, but few have been adopted broadly for research, clinical, or prognostic purposes.[15]

Because atropine abolishes high-frequency (0.15–0.5 Hz) spectral power, oscillations in heart rate within this band have been attributed to parasympathetic activity, with respiration as its primary rhythmic stimulus. Conversely, because maneuvers known to increase central sympathetic outflow, such as standing, tilt, and exercise, increase low-frequency (0.05–0.15 Hz) spectral power, whereas decreases are observed during sleep or after β-blockade or central sympatholysis with clonidine, heart rate fluctuations within these frequencies initially were considered specific representations of sympathetic neural modulation. However, parasympathetic oscillatory input also influences power spectral frequencies below 0.15 Hz. For this reason, a (contentious) ratio between low- and high-frequency power has been proposed as an estimate of "sympathovagal balance."

Oscillatory autonomic contributions to heart rate variability are superimposed on a broadband nonharmonic fractal signal, most prominent between 0.00003 and 0.1 Hz (i.e., at very low and low frequencies). Using CGSA, this nonharmonic power can be quantified by plotting the log of spectral power as a function of the log of frequency (l/f$^\beta$ plot) then extracted, yielding more precise estimates of residual harmonic contributions to low- and high-frequency (0.15–0.50 Hz) power. For this reason, CGSA becomes particularly useful when evaluating autonomic contributions to heart rate variability in patients with heart failure, whose harmonic spectral power is both concentrated within the very low- and low-frequency ranges and are markedly diminished relative to the nonharmonic signal.

Frequency domain analysis should be appreciated primarily for the insight it allows into mechanisms responsible for short- and long-term heart rate oscillations and for its prognostic value in populations with cardiovascular disease. At best, it provides an estimate of the extent to which parasympathetic and cardiac sympathetic discharge and neurotransmitter release modulate heart rate within these specific frequency bands, but not of the intensity of such neural discharge or the magnitude of sympathetic outflow directed elsewhere, for example, to the ventricle, kidney, or regional vascular beds.

Cross-Spectral Analysis

Algorithms used to derive power spectra for heart rate can also be applied to blood pressure, respiratory signals, and MSNA. Cross-spectral analysis between two such variables can establish their coherence, the influence of input on output, and the phase delay between these signals. For example, the gain of the transfer function between systolic blood pressure (input) and pulse interval (output) oscillations within the low- or high-frequency regions (α coefficient) estimates arterial baroreceptor reflex control of heart rate (although agreement with values obtained using vasoactive drug methods is poor), and the gain of the transfer function between blood pressure (input) and MSNA (output) estimates arterial baroreflex modulation of central sympathetic outflow.

Tracer Imaging With Catecholamine Analogues

Nuclear iodine-123 metaiodobenzylguanidine (^{123}I-MIBG) or ^{11}C-metahydroxyephredrine (^{11}C-HED) positron emission tomographic (PET) imaging infer the integrity and homogeneity of cardiac sympathetic innervation and NE transport and indirectly, by calculating tracer uptake and washout, an approximation of its neural release.[16-18] PET imaging provides superior spatial resolution.[18] PET tracer analogues of β-adreno-, muscarinic, and nicotinic receptors are being evaluated for potential clinical application.[18]

SYMPATHETIC ACTIVATION AND PARASYMPATHETIC WITHDRAWAL IN HUMAN HEART FAILURE (SEE ALSO CHAPTERS 6 AND 42)

Heart Failure With Reduced Systolic Function

The onset of HFrEF is characterized by a cardiac-specific autonomic "signature," with the loss of tonic and reflex vagal heart rate modulation and selective increase in cardiac NE spillover; total body or renal NE spillover and MSNA are not elevated.[1,2,8] Indeed, in many patients with asymptomatic or mild to moderate symptomatic HFrEF, plasma NE concentrations and sympathetic nerve firing rates are similar to those of age-matched healthy subjects (**Figs. 13.2** and **13.3**).[1,8,13,19]

Sympathetic Activation

Relative to the unaffected population, cohort-mean plasma NE concentration increases as asymptomatic HFrEF progresses to overt congestion. In more advanced HFrEF, heightened adrenal sympathetic nerve activity stimulates medullary epinephrine and NE release into plasma.[1,8]

In health, approximately 25% of total body NE spillover arises from the kidney and about 2% from the heart.[8] In patients with left ventricular dysfunction and congestion, studied before the advent of contemporary therapies, calculated NE clearance was one-third lower, and total body NE spillover double that of control subjects. Approximately 60% of this increase resulted from a 5- to 20-fold elevation in cardiac and a 2- to 3-fold greater renal NE spillover into plasma. Mental stress and cycling exercise elicit further increases in cardiac neurotransmitter

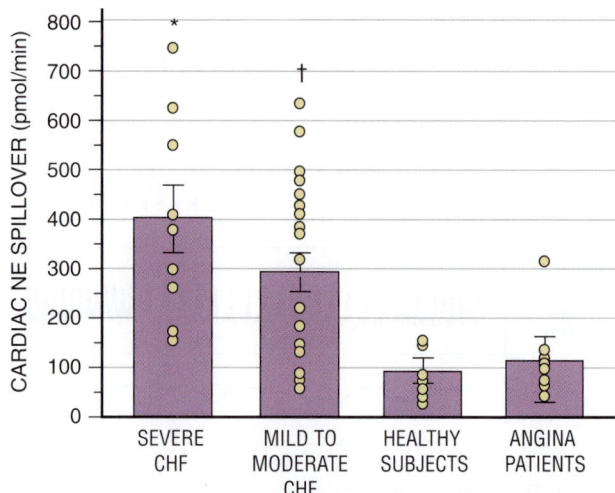

Fig. 13.2 Individual and mean ± SEM values for cardiac norepinephrine *(NE)* spillover in patients with mild-to-moderate and severe chronic heart failure *(CHF)*, healthy subjects, and patients with stable angina pectoris. *Statistically significant difference (*P* < .05) between severe CHF and both control groups. †Statistically significant difference (*P* < .05) between mild-to-moderate CHF and both healthy subjects and angina patients. (From Rundqvist B, Elam M, Bergmann-Sverrisdottir Y, Eisenhofer G, Friberg P. Increased cardiac adrenergic drive precedes generalized sympathetic activation in human heart failure. *Circulation.* 95;169–175, with permission from the American Heart Association.)

release, indicating preservation of myocardial adrenergic reserve.[8] Preferential activation of cardiac sympathetic nerve traffic also is evident in the paced-ovine HFrEF model.[20]

Microneurographic recordings provided definitive evidence that the majority of this increase in total body NE spillover can be attributed to greater central sympathetic outflow rather than altered neurotransmitter reuptake or clearance.[1,2,8] Single-unit recordings from patients with HFrEF in sinus rhythm display both higher firing probability and recruitment of previously silent efferent neurons, but no increase in the proportion of cardiac cycles associated with multiple discharges; whereas those who develop atrial fibrillation exhibit a significantly greater incidence of multiple firing, which would evoke more NE release and consequently greater vasoconstriction. In contrast, sympathetic discharge to skin is not increased.[1,2,10,12]

There is little or no correlation, in patients with HFrEF, between left ventricular ejection fraction (LVEF) and MSNA burst incidence. Indeed, if oxygen uptake at maximum exercise capacity (peak VO$_2$) is relatively preserved, resting MSNA can remain within the range of age-matched control subjects, despite profound left ventricular systolic dysfunction. However, their sympathoneural response to exercise is exaggerated (**Fig. 13.4**).[19]

In the frequency domain, heart failure and age-matched control subjects display similar total MSNA power, harmonic power, nonharmonic power between 0 and 0.5 Hz, and spectral density within the very low (0–0.05 Hz) and high (0.15–0.5 Hz) frequency bands. However, low-frequency oscillations in the mean voltage neurogram are diminished markedly or absent, despite near-maximal sympathetic burst incidence, indicating loss of central or reflex modulation of efferent sympathetic traffic proportional to heart failure severity.[21]

Parasympathetic Withdrawal

Responses to infusions of both phenylephrine and sodium nitroprusside (expressed either as msec/mm Hg or as beats/min/mm Hg) and to carotid sinus baroreceptor stimulation by neck suction diminish in

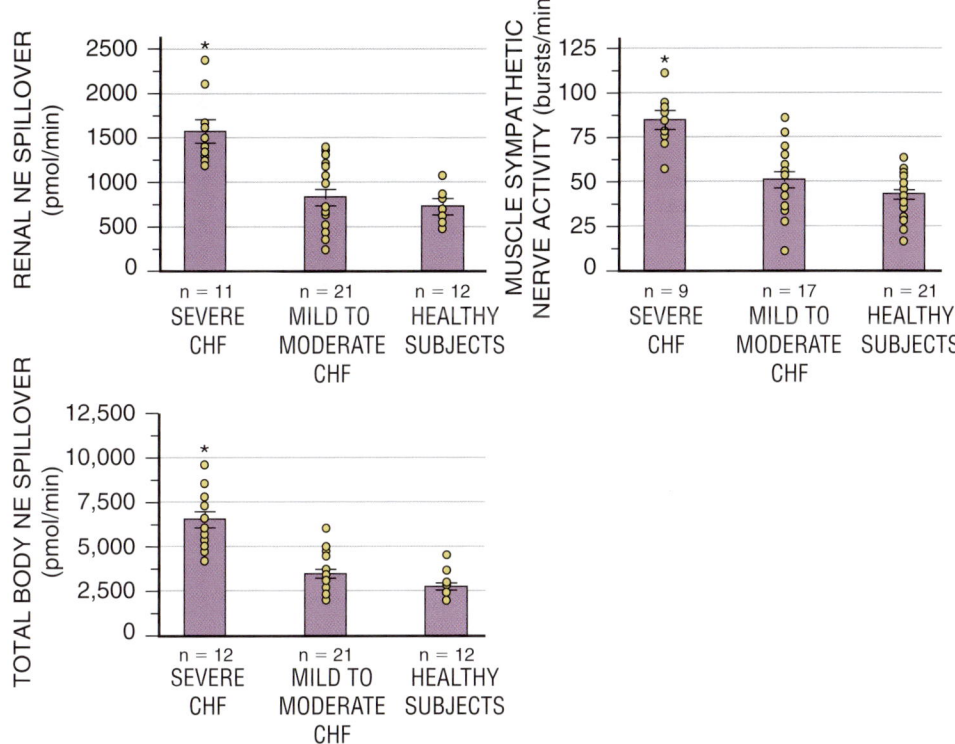

Fig. 13.3 Individual and mean ± SEM values for renal and total body norepinephrine *(NE)* spillover and muscle sympathetic nerve activity in the groups defined in the legend of **Fig. 13.2**. *Statistically significant difference (P < .05) between severe chronic heart failure *(CHF)* and both healthy subjects and mild-to-moderate CHF. (From Rundqvist B, Elam M, Bergmann-Sverrisdottir Y, Eisenhofer G, Friberg P. Increased cardiac adrenergic drive precedes generalized sympathetic activation in human heart failure. *Circulation.* 95;169–175:1997, with permission from the American Heart Association.)

proportion to the resting heart rate, the left ventricular systolic dysfunction, the New York Heart Association (NYHA) functional symptom class, mitral regurgitation severity, blood urea nitrogen, and the standard deviation of all normal-to-normal pulse intervals (SDNN), a time domain index of tonic vagal heart rate modulation.[1,2]

In NYHA Class II patients, the low-frequency component of the heart rate power spectrum predominates, but as heart failure progresses, saturation or downregulation of cardiac postjunctional β-adrenoceptors and impairment of postsynaptic β-adrenoreceptor signal transduction decreases sinoatrial responsiveness to neurally released NE. There is less variation in the heart rate. Low-frequency spectral power is attenuated more often than augmented and relates inversely rather than directly to both the discharge frequency of muscle sympathetic nerves or the cardiac NE spillover.[1,22]

Heart Failure With Preserved Ejection Fraction (see also Chapters 11 and 39)

Our understanding of this phenotype would benefit from more extensive and rigorous investigation. To date, HFpEF cohort sizes have been small, the definitions of HFpEF inconsistent (some conflate hypertension plus impaired relaxation with HFpEF), the quality of studies published often have been suboptimal, and few have considered the confounding excitatory influences of age and left ventricular hypertrophy, with blunted stimulation of inhibitory ventricular afferents, on sympathetic activity.[6] Although long-standing hypertension is a well-recognized risk factor for HFpEF and itself is often accompanied by chronic sympathetic excitation, no prospective studies have as yet determined whether such long-term autonomic imbalance increases the risk of incident HFrEF.

In the Studies of Left Ventricular Dysfunction (SOLVD) registry, mean plasma NE concentrations of patients with pulmonary congestion and LVEF greater than 45% were not increased. In general, heart rate variability is diminished, the sympathetic nervous system appears less activated than in patients with HFrEF, and cardiac NE transport function, as assessed using ^{123}I-MIBG imaging, not as defective.[6] A series of 15 patients with restrictive cardiomyopathy due to endomyocardial fibrosis and a LVEF greater than 50 who were studied at least 6 months after endocardial resection surgery described increases in MSNA burst frequency and incidence, sympathetic contributions to heart rate variation, and decreases in indices of tonic and reflex vagal heart rate modulation that were comparable to those observed concurrently in a matched cohort of patients with dilated cardiomyopathy.[23] The recent discovery of an excitatory reflex engaged by high atrial pressure *(vide infra)*[10] identifies a potential causal mechanism that could elicit sympathoexcitation in both HFrEF and HFpEF.

CLINICAL CONSEQUENCES OF AUTONOMIC IMBALANCE

Cardiac

Fractional shortening is diminished in mice with defective vesicular acetylcholine transport; deficient neurotransmitter release is accompanied by more extensive fibrosis in response to exogenous angiotensin II.[24] The impact of impaired vagal tone in human heart failure on heart rate modulation, inflammatory pathways, the regulation of left ventricular performance, and the progression of HFrEF have been reviewed in detail.[1-5]

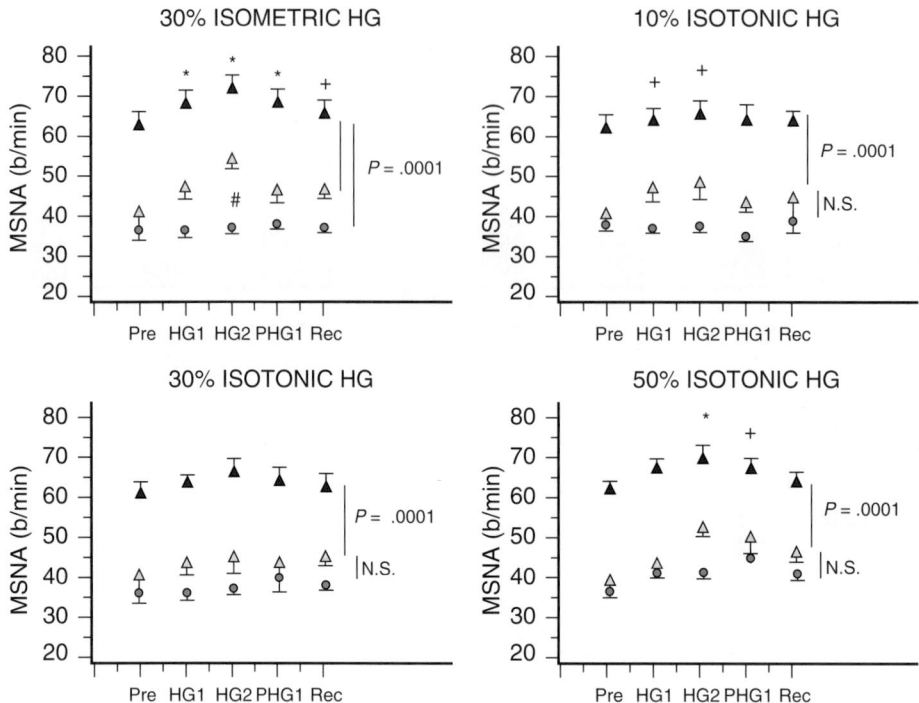

Fig. 13.4 Muscle sympathetic nerve activity *(MSNA)* response to handgrip *(HG)* exercise in participants with heart failure and reduced left ventricular ejection fraction (LVEF) whose peak oxygen uptake (VO$_{2peak}$) was less than 56% predicted (▲, n = 8; mean LVEF 18%) or VO$_{2peak}$ was >56% predicted (△, n = 6; mean LVEF 20%) and in healthy age-matched control subjects (●, n = 10). Stated *P* values refer to the significance level of the main effect of group; *P < .05 vs. pre-HG in both heart failure groups; +P < .05 vs. pre-HG in VO$_{2peak}$ greater than 56% predicted only; #P < .05 vs. VO$_{2peak}$ greater than 56% predicted compared with normal subjects. *N.S.,* Not significant. (From Notarius CF, Atchison DJ, Floras JS. Impact of heart failure and exercise capacity on sympathetic response to handgrip exercise. *Am J Physiol Heart Circ Physiol.* 2001;280:H969–H976.)

The combination of early vagal withdrawal plus a selective increase in cardiac NE spillover constitute adaptive autonomic responses, which are engaged to maintain peripheral tissue perfusion in the face of compromised ventricular performance. However, once congestion becomes manifest, the heart is subject to the greatest proportional increase in regional NE spillover, and thus, the failing heart is the organ exposed for the longest duration to the greatest magnitude of sympathetic activation. The direct adverse myocardial consequences of such intense cardiac adrenergic drive, which are reviewed in **Chapters 6** and **10,** include: an increase in heart rate; induction of myocyte necrosis and apoptosis; fibrosis; decreased β$_1$-adrenergic receptor density; diminished β$_1$-adrenoceptor responsiveness to catecholamines and altered β$_1$-adrenergic receptor signal transduction with upregulation of G-protein-coupled receptor kinase 2; defective calcium regulation by the sarcoplasmic reticulum; induction of proinflammatory cytokine expression; greater oxidative stress; increased muscarinic M2 receptor expression; destruction of sympathetic nerve terminals; and depletion of myocardial NE content—all of which contribute to the relentless progression of cardiac dysfunction.[5,25,26] Nonuniform NE depletion and sympathetic denervation disturb the temporal coordination of right and left ventricular contraction and relaxation and alter the dispersion of refractoriness, leading to ventricular dyssynergy and promoting arrhythmogenesis.[17,27] In human experiments, muscarinic stimulation was found to exert a negative lusitropic effect and to antagonize the effect of beta-adrenergic stimulation in patients with HFrEF.[28]

Peripheral

Sympathetically mediated constriction of capacitance and resistance vessels increases both preload and afterload; diminished conduit artery compliance impairs ventricular-vascular coupling. Stimulation of renal sympathetic nerves activates the renin-angiotensin-aldosterone axis (**see also Chapter 15**), promotes tubular absorption of sodium and water, increases renal vascular resistance, and blunts the renal responsiveness to atrial natriuretic peptide. Angiotensin II–mediated efferent arteriolar vasoconstriction and atrial natriuretic peptide–mediated afferent arteriolar vasodilation strive to maintain glomerular filtration in the face of renal hypoperfusion.

Exercise

Exercise constrained by dyspnea or fatigue is a common heart failure symptom indicative of decreased oxygen delivery (central) or utilization (peripheral). Limiting central mechanisms include heart failure–associated reductions in ventilation, diffusion, chronotropic competence, and cardiac output. Also, β$_2$-adrenoceptor polymorphisms associated with impaired exercise performance have been identified. Proposed peripheral limiting mechanisms include sarcopenia, impaired mitochondrial respiration, and diminished oxygen transport due to augmented neurogenic vasoconstriction. In heart failure patients (but not in healthy age-matched controls) maximal oxygen uptake (peak VO$_2$) during exercise correlates inversely to resting MSNA but not cardiac NE spillover.

In recent experiments, fibular MSNA was recorded continuously while subjects performed contralateral one-leg cycling without and against resistance. In contrast to healthy controls, whose burst incidence fell, exercise increased MSNA in those with HFrEF; overall there was a significant inverse relationship between the maximum MSNA elicited by one-leg exercise and subjects' peak VO$_2$ (**Fig. 13.5**).[11,29] Sympathetically mediated reductions in blood flow below levels required to meet local metabolic demands during exercise

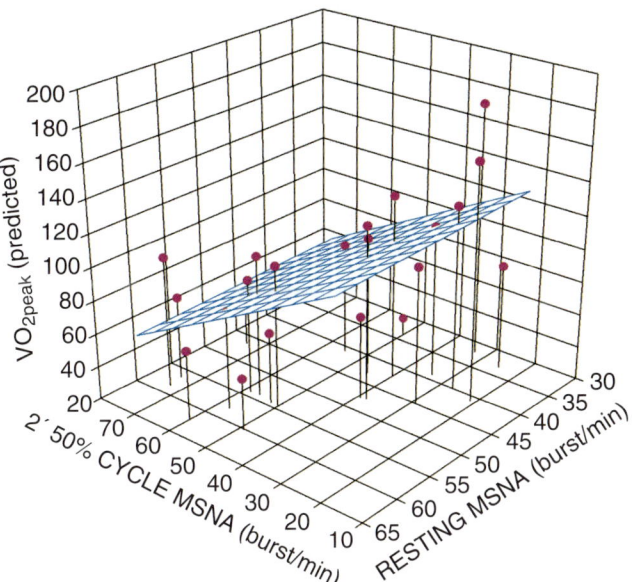

Fig. 13.5 Relationship between peak oxygen uptake (VO$_{2peak}$) and muscle sympathetic nerve activity (*MSNA*) burst frequency at rest and 2 minutes into one-leg cycling (contralateral limb) at 50% of VO$_{2peak}$ in a cohort with and without HFrEF. The three-dimensional graph shows individual data points and regression plane. The slope relating VO$_{2peak}$ to exercise-induced MSNA is significant ($P = .03$) and remains so when adjusted for baseline MSNA; the slope relating VO$_{2peak}$ to resting MSNA is not ($P = .93$). (From Notarius CF, Millar PJ, Murai H, Morris BL, Floras JS. Inverse relationship between muscle sympathetic activity during exercise and peak oxygen uptake in subjects with and without heart failure. *J Am Coll Cardiol.* 2014;63:605–606, with permission from the American College of Cardiology Foundation.)

could attenuate endothelium-mediated vasodilatation and stimulate metaboreceptor afferents in skeletal muscle. Consequent reflexive increases in central sympathetic outflow could further diminish exercise capacity.

Mortality

Before widespread clinical adoption of angiotensin-converting enzyme inhibitors and β-adrenoceptor antagonists, the prognostic weight of a single resting plasma NE concentration was superior to that of heart rate, plasma renin activity, serum sodium or stroke index; if this exceeded 800 pg/mL, life expectancy was less than 1 year. In the pre β-blocker era, survival of transplant candidates was inversely proportional to cardiac NE spillover.[30] In those treated chronically with β-adrenoceptor antagonists, renal has proven superior to cardiac NE spillover for the prediction of death or transplantation.[31] However, cardiac NE content can also predict the mode of death: in a cohort of 116 patients (mean LVEF, 19%), followed on average for 18 months, the risk of sudden death was two- to threefold greater if estimated cardiac NE stores and cardiac NE spillover exceeded median values. By contrast, individuals with depleted myocardial NE stores and high cardiac NE spillover (reflecting chronically increased neurotransmitter turnover and reduced reuptake and storage) had a two- to fourfold greater risk of death from progressive pump failure.[32]

Each of MSNA, diminished baroreflex sensitivity, loss of heart rate variability, abnormal heart rate turbulence, and augmented chemosensitivity to both hypoxia and hypercapnia have been linked to premature death, whether due to progressive myocardial failure or arrhythmia. An attenuated reflex heart rate response to phenylephrine has similar

prognostic implications in patients treated or not treated with beta-adrenoceptor antagonists. Loss of both complexity in the heart rate signal, as estimated by nonharmonic power-law regression parameters, and low-frequency harmonic power, appears to be the most sensitive frequency domain predictors of sudden death.[1,2,5] Abnormal ^{11}C-HED or ^{123}I-MIBG uptake by ventricular sympathetic nerves can also identify HFrEF patients at increased risk of sudden cardiac arrest or premature death (**Fig. 13.6**).[16,17,33]

MECHANISMS DISTURBING AUTONOMIC EQUILIBRIUM

Alterations in the neurogenic control of the circulation stimulated by the onset and progression of heart failure can arise from one or more regulatory components, such as those participating in the generation and conveyance of inhibitory and excitatory input to brainstem vasomotor neurons, the cortical modulation of central nervous system integration and catecholamine turnover, or the determination of release and receptor responsiveness to neurotransmitters (**Fig. 13.7**).[1,2]

Afferent Influences

In healthy resting subjects, the reflex effect of sympathoinhibitory input from carotid sinus and aortic arch "arterial high-pressure" and the cardiopulmonary "low-pressure" mechanoreceptors outweighs any excitatory contributions from arterial chemoreceptors, muscle mechanoreceptors or metaboreceptors, or renal afferent nerves. The efferent vagal component of the baroreceptor heart rate reflex is also subject to arterial baroreceptor afferent input. Consequently, healthy resting individuals display low sympathetic nerve firing and high heart rate variability. Reflex vagal and sympathoneural responses to acute perturbations in blood pressure are brisk.

Arterial Baroreceptor Reflexes

Arterial baroreceptor nerve discharge is activated by the pressure wave of systole and diminishes or falls silent during diastole. Systolic stimulation of baroreceptor discharge increases parasympathetic and decreases efferent sympathetic outflow reflexively. When arterial pressure falls below mechanoreceptor stimulation threshold, release of baroreceptor restraint on sympathetic motor neurons permits efferent sympathetic fiber discharge.

Because arterial baroreceptor modulation of heart rate is diminished in patients with HFrEF and baroreceptor afferent nerve discharge is less responsive to changes in local distending pressure in experimental models of ventricular systolic dysfunction, it had been concluded that the arterial baroreflex regulation of vagal and sympathetic outflow in human HFrEF are impaired in parallel. However, assessment of the baroreceptor–heart rate reflex in humans relies upon the indirect estimation of sinoatrial responsiveness to two distinct and differentially regulated autonomic inputs. In experimental canine heart failure, it is impaired vagal ganglionic neurotransmission that diminishes parasympathetic responsiveness to baroreceptor stimulation; sinoatrial acetylcholinesterase is reduced, and muscarinic receptors are upregulated. By contrast, cardiac-specific sympathetic neural modulation is attenuated by downregulation or desensitization of β-adrenoceptors[26] rendering the sinoatrial node less responsive to reflexively elicited changes in neurally released NE. In patients with HFrEF the variability and complexity of heart rate are attenuated, but the variability of blood pressure is similar to that of age-matched healthy subjects.[1]

In patients with HFrEF, reports of significant inverse relationships between stroke work index and MSNA and between cardiac output and cardiac NE spillover suggest the arterial baroreflex regulation of

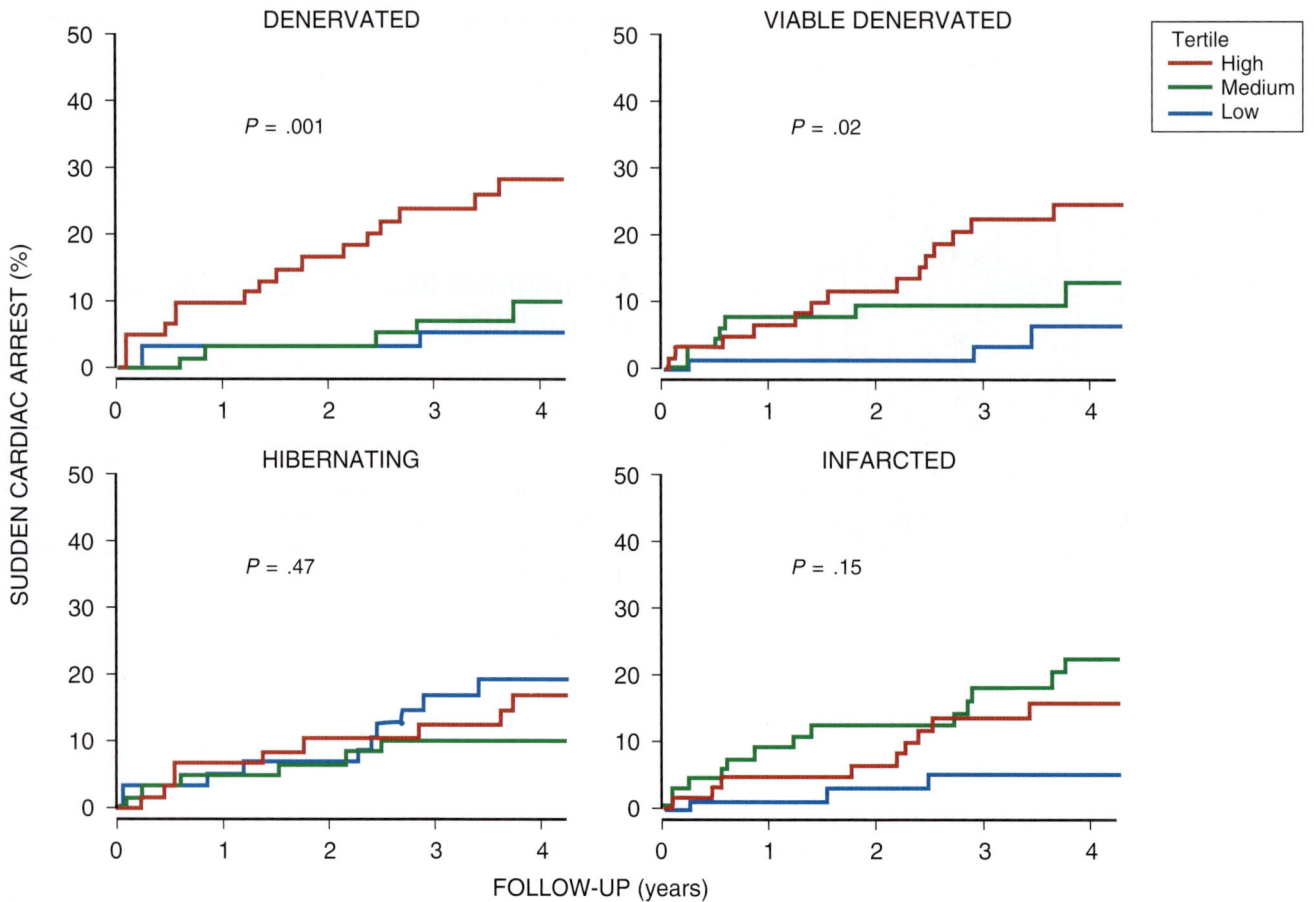

Fig. 13.6 Kaplan-Meier curves over a median follow-up of 4.1 years demonstrating that myocardial sympathetic denervation (both total volume of denervated myocardium, as well as viable denervated myocardium, *upper panels*) quantified using ^{11}C-HED positron emission tomographic imaging can identify heart failure with reduced ejection fraction patients with ischemic cardiomyopathy at high, medium, and low risk of sudden cardiac death. By contrast, neither hibernating myocardium nor total infarct volume *(lower panels)* identified risk significantly. (From Fallavollita J, Heavey BM, Luisi AJ, et al. Regional myocardial sympathetic denervation predicts the risk of sudden cardiac arrest in ischemic cardiomyopathy. *J Am Coll Cardiol.* 2014;63:141–149, with permission from the American College of Cardiology Foundation.)

efferent sympathetic discharge responds appropriately to the altered hemodynamics of heart failure. Two challenges to any interpretation of experiments in HFrEF involving vasoactive drugs are: (1) muscle sympathetic burst firing is pulse synchronous, with an incidence (i.e., bursts/100 cardiac cycles) approaching 100%; and (2) heart rate responses to arterial baroreceptor perturbation by phenylephrine or nitroprusside are markedly attenuated. Consequently, there is little opportunity, arithmetically, to modify a cardiac frequency–dependent multiunit representation of sympathetic nerve firing. If the reported effect of these drug interventions on MSNA burst frequency is re-expressed relative to cardiac frequency (or as changes in absolute units, rather than as a percentage of baseline values), then the gain of the arterial baroreflex regulation of MSNA is not appreciably impaired.[1]

Several lines of evidence, obtained using different approaches and summarized in **Table 13.2**, reveal relatively intact arterial baroreflex modulation of efferent sympathetic outflow in human heart failure. An instructive illustration is the rapidity with which MSNA responds to the initiation and termination of ventricular bigeminy (see Fig. 13.1). Further evidence for preserved arterial baroreflex function is provided by experimental heart failure models. Brandle et al.,[34] who found no differences in the time course of changes in hemodynamics and plasma NE concentrations during the development of heart failure in dogs with and without sinoaortic baroreceptor denervation, concluded that impairment of the arterial baroreflex

could not be responsible for sustaining the increase in sympathetic outflow observed in this experimental model. In sheep, cardiac sympathetic nerve activity (CSNA), recorded directly, was significantly increased and the baroreceptor regulation of heart rate was profoundly impaired, but the arterial baroreflex control of both CSNA and renal sympathetic nerve traffic did not differ from that of control animals.[35]

Human cardiac and renal efferent responses to arterial baroreceptor unloading are dissimilar. In one study, nitroprusside-induced hypotension (to offload low- as well as high-pressure mechanoreceptors) elicited, as anticipated, an 85% increase in renal NE spillover in healthy control subjects, but no net change in heart failure subjects (albeit from a nearly threefold higher baseline).[36] In a subsequent experiment, a hypotensive dose of nitroglycerin lowered renal NE spillover in individuals with systolic dysfunction but not in healthy control subjects.[37] These data point to the emergence, in HFrEF, of an important inhibitory effect of cardiopulmonary baroreceptor unloading on the arterial baroreflex regulation of renal NE spillover.

Cardiopulmonary Reflexes

In healthy subjects, reflexes arising from afferent nerve endings situated in the heart and pulmonary veins elicit sympathoinhibition and forearm vasodilation when stimulated by increases in cardiac filling pressure or volume, or by inotropic force. Conversely, phlebotomy or

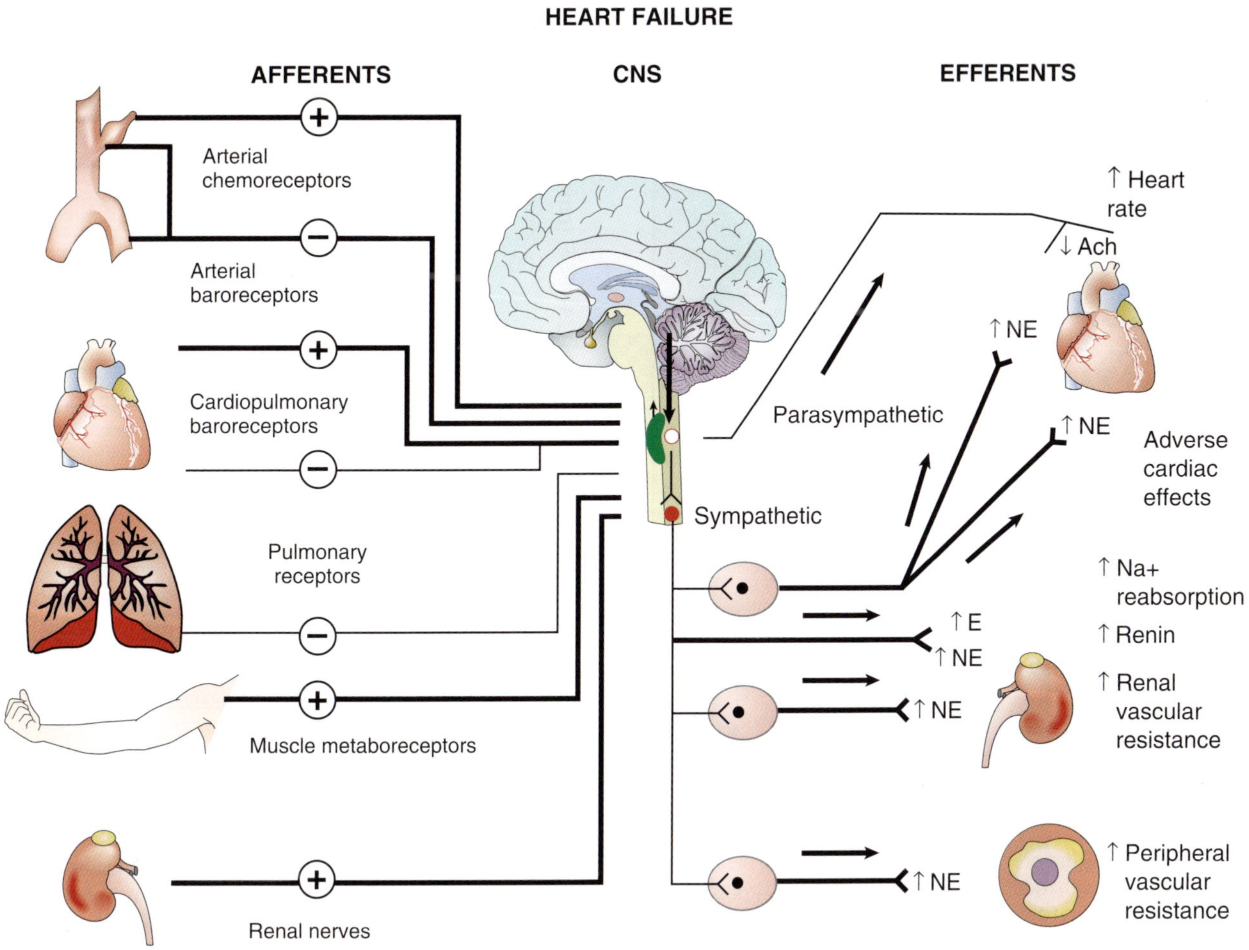

HEART FAILURE

Fig. 13.7 Mechanisms participating in the autonomic disturbances of heart failure with reduced ejection fraction. Input from arterial and cardiac mechanoreceptor and chemoreceptor, arterial chemoreceptor, pulmonary stretch receptor, muscle metaboreceptor and mechanoreceptor, and renal afferent nerves converge to modulate sympathetic outflow about a centrally mediated set-point increase, involving an angiotensin II-AT$_1$ receptor-NADPH-superoxide pathway. As systolic function deteriorates, input effecting sympathoinhibition (−) by stimulating ventricular and a population of atrial mechanoreceptor afferent nerves decreases *(thin line)*, whereas inhibitory modulation of efferent sympathetic nerve traffic by arterial baroreceptors *(thick line)* is preserved. Efferent vagal heart rate responses to arterial baroreflex perturbations are attenuated *(thin line)*. Excitatory (+) afferent input arises from a normally quiescent atrial reflex, activated by increases in cardiac filling pressures; chemically sensitive ventricular afferent nerve endings, triggered by ischemia; augmented sympathoexcitatory input from arterial chemoreceptors; exercising skeletal muscle in heart failure; and renal afferent nerves *(thick lines)*. The central set point for sympathetic outflow *(arrow pointing down)* is raised further by central chemoreceptor stimulation, by sleep apnea, and by obesity. Efferent mechanisms for increased NE spillover include prejunctional facilitation of its release and impaired NE uptake. The time course through which these mechanisms are engaged differs between individuals. Relatively asymptomatic systolic dysfunction is characterized by a selective increase in cardiac NE release and a reduction in tonic and reflex vagal heart rate modulation. As heart failure advances, there is a generalized increase in sympathetic nerve traffic to the heart, adrenal, kidney, skeletal muscle, and other vascular beds *(thick arrow shafts, thick lines)*. *Ach*, Acetylcholine; *CNS*, central nervous system; *E*, epinephrine; *Na+*, sodium; *NADPH*, nicotinamide adenine dinucleotide phosphate; *NE*, norepinephrine. (Reproduced with permission of the author. Copyright 2016 John Floras. All rights reserved.)

nonhypotensive lower body negative pressure (LBNP) provoke sympathoexcitation. After observing similar gains in the arterial baroreflex control of MSNA in healthy and HFrEF subjects, but in the latter attenuated responses to stimuli that increased or decreased cardiac filling pressure without affecting systemic blood pressure, Dibner-Dunlap and colleagues[38] concluded that the cardiopulmonary, rather than the arterial, baroreflex was impaired in human heart failure (see Fig. 13.7). Subsequently, nonhypotensive LBNP was shown to significantly increase total body NE spillover in control subjects with normal LVEF but not in individuals with impaired ventricular systolic

function.[39] In a more recent study, low-dose nitroglycerin selectively reduced pulmonary artery pressures, yet did not alter renal NE spillover in either HFrEF or healthy subjects.[37]

However, such selective impairment of inhibitory cardiopulmonary reflex responses does not explain the direct correlations seen, in more advanced heart failure, between MSNA and pulmonary artery or capillary wedge pressure, nor accounts for the selective augmentation in cardiac NE spillover in mild to moderate heart failure, which is apparent before any concomitant increase in total body or renal NE spillover or in MSNA.[13] Those observations suggest that a second,

TABLE 13.2 Evidence for Preserved Arterial Baroreflex Modulation of Sympathetic Activity in Human Heart Failure

Concept	Observation
MSNA pulse synchronicity lost after sinoaortic baroreceptor denervation	Pulse synchronicity preserved, even in end-stage HF
Pause with decay in DBP after premature beat increases reflexively MSNA burst amplitude, duration, and area; rise in DBP after postextrasystolic beat inhibits MSNA	Extrasystolic augmentation of MSNA amplitude, duration and area and postextrasystolic suppression replicated in HF; duration or suppression proportional to magnitude of diastolic overshoot
MSNA bursts track previous DBP with 1.2–1.3 s lag	Synchronization of sympathetic neural alternans with pulsus alternans
Frequency domain estimate of arterial BR gain derived by cross-spectral analysis with BP oscillations as stimulus and MSNA oscillations as response	Transfer function gain in HF and healthy subjects similar across all frequency bands; calculated gain highest in high-frequency range
Arterial BR unloading with SNP elicits reflex increase in TNES	Similar reflex increase in TNES in HF and healthy subjects
LV pacing in HF increases DBP	Acute inverse DBP–MSNA relationship immediately from RV to LV pacing
Muller maneuver increases acutely intrathoracic aortic and LV transmural pressures	MSNA inhibited similarly in HF and control subjects

BP, Blood pressure; *BR*, baroreceptor reflex; *DBP*, diastolic blood pressure; *HF*, heart failure with reduced ejection fraction; *LV*, left ventricular; *MSNA*, muscle sympathetic nerve activity; *RV*, right ventricular; *SNP*, sodium nitroprusside; *TNES*, total body norepinephrine spillover.

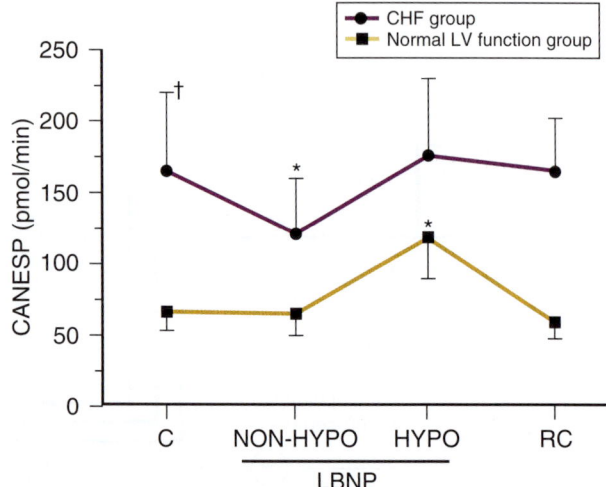

Fig. 13.8 Cardiac norepinephrine spillover (*CANESP*) responses to non-hypotensive and hypotensive (*HYPO*) lower body negative pressure (*LBNP*). *Upper line*: HFrEF group (*CHF*). *Lower line*: normal left ventricular (*LV*) function group. *C*, Control; *HFrEF*, heart failure with reduced ejection fraction; *RC*, recovery. *P < .05 vs. normal LV function group at control state. (Data from Azevedo ER, Newton GE, Floras JS, Parker JD. Reducing cardiac filling pressure lowers cardiac norepinephrine spillover in patients with chronic heart failure. *Circulation*. 2000;101:2053–2059.)

independent and cardiac-specific sympathoexcitatory reflex, responsive to pathological increases in cardiopulmonary blood volume or pressure, may become operative in human heart failure. Indeed, in dogs with pacing-induced congestion, Wang and Zucker documented sensitization of cardiac sympathetic afferents responsive to chemical stimulation; this reflex was potentiated by acute volume expansion.[40]

Several observations in individuals with HFrEF support the concept of activation, by increased filling pressure, of a cardiac-specific sympathoexcitatory reflex. These include detection of a positive relationship between pulmonary capillary wedge pressure and cardiac NE spillover and reductions in cardiac NE spillover when atrial, pulmonary, and systemic arterial pressures are reduced concomitantly by sodium nitroprusside infusion,[41] or when positive airway pressure is applied acutely to reduce atrial and pulmonary venous transmural pressure (consequent reductions in intrathoracic aortic and left ventricular transmural pressure should increase sympathetic outflow reflexively). Importantly, nonhypotensive LBNP, applied to reduce selectively cardiac filling and pulmonary pressures, decreases cardiac NE spillover in HFrEF, but not in control subjects with normal left ventricular systolic function (**Fig. 13.8**).[39] Conversely, increasing the intensity of LBNP to induce systemic hypotension elicits a significant increase in cardiac NE spillover in control subjects only (see Fig. 13.8).[39] The most plausible interpretation of these findings is that a physiological increase in cardiac NE spillover evoked reflexively by the unloading of high- and low-pressure mechanoreceptors when both atrial and systemic blood pressures are reduced is countered, in HFrEF, by concurrent withdrawal of a second stimulus arising from myelinated mechanoreceptor afferents, situated within the venous–atrial

junctions that reflexively and selectively excite cardiac adrenergic drive when distended (see Fig. 13.7).

In some with HFrEF, LBNP elicits forearm vasodilation rather than vasoconstriction, and saline infusion induces a paradoxical (i.e., an effect opposite to that in control subjects) increase in forearm vascular resistance. These observations suggest that when stimulated acutely, the ensuing reflex sympathoexcitation may target skeletal muscle as well as the ventricle. When interpreting multiunit MSNA responses, prior investigators had assumed that all single-unit discharge incorporated within the envelope discharged uniformly in response to reductions in cardiac filling pressure. Recent experiments documenting single-unit sympathetic firing proved this hypothesis incorrect.[10] In humans with HFrEF there is, relative to controls, a proportionately greater subpopulation of single-muscle sympathetic fibers that respond to lower body positive pressure paradoxically, with increased discharge.[10] Thus, the multiunit MSNA preparation in this setting summates discharge from single units exhibiting directionally opposite responses to increased cardiac filling pressure. The excitatory reflex likely is elicited by the stretch of atrial unmyelinated afferent nerve endings, whereas the generally more dominant inhibitory response arises from stimulation, by increased pressure, volume, and inotropy, of atrial and ventricular myelinated afferents. Should a subpopulation of sympathetic units innervating the kidney also increase firing, in parallel, in response to intracardiac pressure or volume, and augment renal sodium retention, that effect would result in further stimulation of these cardiopulmonary afferents, which could then amplify efferent discharge via this positive feedback loop.

A pressor reflex, stimulated by a selective increase in pulmonary artery pressure and accompanied by increased renal sympathetic nerve firing, has been identified in dogs with normal ventricular function.[42] With secondary pulmonary hypertension so prevalent in the heart failure population, this discovery adds to the list of potential sympathoinhibitory benefits of lowering cardiopulmonary pressure and blood volume in HFrEF.

Chronic atrial fibrillation in heart failure is accompanied by an increase at rest, relative to sinus rhythm, in the single-unit MSNA

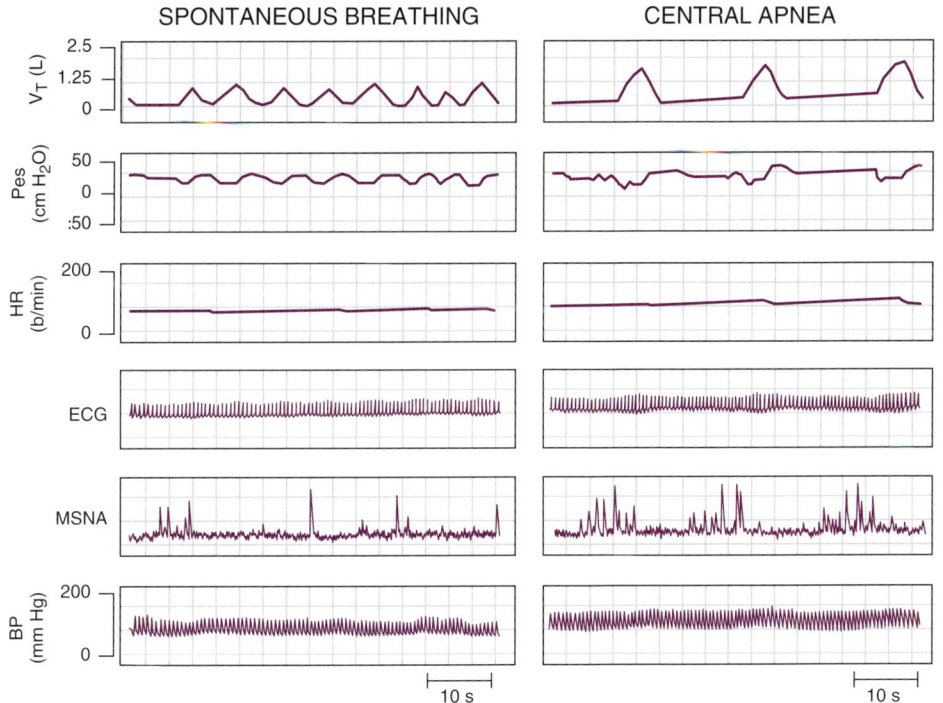

Fig. 13.9 Tidal volume *(V$_T$)*, esophageal pressure *(Pes)*, heart rate *(HR)*, the electrocardiogram *(ECG)*, muscle sympathetic nerve activity *(MSNA)*, and blood pressure *(BP)* in a young man with dilated cardiomyopathy who within a few minutes oscillates, while awake, between a normal breathing pattern and one of spontaneous central apnea. Note the marked activation of central sympathetic outflow and increased BP during apnea. (Courtesy John S. Floras, MD.)

firing frequency and the incidence of multiple firing of single-units within each cardiac cycle (inversely proportional to the diastolic pressure nadir, which varies according to cycle length), but not multiunit MSNA burst frequency[43] or cardiac NE spillover. The increase in cardiac NE ordinarily elicited by head-up tilt is attenuated.[44]

In summary, a large body of evidence indicates that the higher sympathetic nerve firing or NE release rates, which are evident in the majority of patients with HFrEF, represents the integration of a least three mechanoreflex-mediated responses, with the principal sources of excitation originating in mechanoreceptors situated within the heart and pulmonary vessels (see Fig. 13.7). In some patients with HFrEF, such adaptation may fully account for the prevailing level of sympathetic activity at rest but not during activity. In most patients, however, the contribution of nonbaroreflex mediated excitatory reflexes or central resetting of sympathetic outflow also should be considered.

Nonbaroreflex Mechanisms

In HFrEF patients, age, hypertension, metabolic syndrome, anemia, obesity, and uremia have been shown to independently increase multiunit MSNA.[1,2]

Pulmonary Stretch Reflexes. The distension of pulmonary stretch receptors by inspiration inhibits reflexively sympathetic outflow. In healthy subjects, breathing frequency correlates positively with MSNA burst frequency, and reflex sympathoneural responses to hypoxia and hypercapnia. This influence of breathing pattern on oscillations in sympathetic discharge is preserved in heart failure patients,[45] in whom decreased tidal volume, high respiratory frequency,[46] and brief periods of apnea elicit marked increases in MSNA (**Fig. 13.9**). With heart failure, greater lung inflation is required to inhibit MSNA completely.[45] Rapidly adapting airway vagal sensory receptors, responding to inflation and deflation, are also stimulated by increases

in left atrial pressure and extravascular pulmonary fluid volume; by triggering hyperpnea, this reflex pathway, in turn, can initiate cycles of Cheyne–Stokes respiration (CSR).

Peripheral Chemoreceptor Reflexes. The contribution of arterial chemoreceptors to sympathetic activation in experimental models of HFrEF has been reviewed in detail by Schultz and associates.[47] Reduction in carotid blood flow and increases in the plasma concentrations of chemoreceptor-stimulating metabolites augment reflex ventilatory and sympathetic responsiveness to hypoxia.[3,48] In two studies, inhalation of 100% O$_2$ to suppress peripheral chemoreceptor input had no effect on group mean values for MSNA; other investigators report an augmented peripheral chemoreceptor response to hypoxia in ~40% of patients with medically treated HFrEF. The latter finding likely signals the presence of comorbidities, such as sleep apnea, anemia, or chronic kidney disease.[2]

Peripheral chemoreceptor sensitization affects several adverse autonomic disturbances. These include higher plasma NE and epinephrine concentrations; further impairment of the arterial baroreflex control of heart rate; augmented very-low-frequency heart rate and blood pressure spectral power; loss of low-frequency heart rate variability; the development of periodic oscillations in breathing at very low frequency both during sleep and in the awake state; enhanced ventilatory responses to exercise; a higher likelihood of developing nonsustained ventricular tachycardia; and attenuation of the arterial baroreflex regulation of MSNA.[2] With respect to the latter, Despas and colleagues reported that in a subset of heart failure patients exhibiting increased peripheral chemosensitivity, MSNA at rest was elevated, and the slope of the relationship between spontaneous changes in diastolic blood pressure and MSNA was attenuated; inhalation of 100% oxygen was restored both to values recorded in heart failure patients with normal chemoreceptor responsiveness.[14] Carotid chemoreceptor reflex-induced sympathetic activation in heart failure may assume greater importance during exercise than in the resting state.[49]

Myocardial Ischemia and Infarction.

When evaluated 6 months after uncomplicated myocardial infarction, patients with relatively preserved LVEF (mean 52%) had significantly higher MSNA burst incidence than did either matched patients with stable coronary artery disease but without prior necrosis or control subjects.[50] In a cohort of well-matched treated patients with chronic ischemic or nonischemic dilated cardiomyopathy, MSNA was significantly higher and peak VO_2 was significantly lower in those with ischemic pathogenesis.[51]

There are several mechanisms by which myocardial ischemia or prior infarction could stimulate sympathetic outflow acutely or chronically, independent of ventricular systolic dysfunction per se. Acutely, both anterior and inferoposterior wall ischemia elicit sympathoexcitation by stimulating cardiac sympathetic afferent nerves; this reflex is blocked by stellectomy. If ischemia were to impair pump function, causing a drop in arterial pressure, the resultant unloading of sinoaortic baroreceptors should elicit a further, reflexive increase in sympathetic outflow. Vagal afferents arising from inferoposterior ventricular segments normally evoke a depressor response; infarction can sever this reflex.

Excitatory Reflexes Arising From Skeletal Muscle.

Several stimuli arising from skeletal muscle elevate sympathetic outflow reflexively to a greater extent in patients with HFrEF than in otherwise healthy individuals (see Fig. 13.7). These include: (1) increases in muscle venous pressure; (2) the muscle mechanoreflex, which can be elicited by passive stretch; and (3) the muscle metaboreflex, which arises primarily from type IV sensory fibers and is activated by exercise metabolites at a lower workload in individuals with HFrEF than in age-matched healthy control subjects.[1,2,19]

Isometric exercise (handgrip, at 30% of maximum voluntary contraction) elicits a greater efferent neural response in heart failure by increasing the probability that a single MSNA unit will fire within each cardiac cycle.[52] The multiunit MSNA response to exercise and to postexercise skeletal muscle ischemia is more prominent in heart failure patients with low peak predicted VO_2 than in those with peak VO_2 greater than 56% of predicted, independent of LVEF (see Fig. 13.4).[19] In contrast to healthy middle-aged subjects in whom MSNA burst incidence in the contralateral leg falls, when patients with HFrEF perform dynamic exercise (one-leg cycling) contralateral MSNA, the burst incidence increases.[11] The responsible mechanisms and functional consequences of such sympathoexcitation have yet to be determined.

Excitatory Reflexes Arising From the Kidney.

Renal afferent nerves discharge in response to increased intrarenal pressure or hypoperfusion-induced ischemia. Stimulation of chemically sensitive nerve endings by bradykinin, adenosine, urea, or acidosis elicits reflex firing of ipsilateral and contralateral renal and systemic sympathetic nerves. This chemoreflex becomes evident in HFrEF patients with chronic kidney disease[53] or elevated right atrial pressure.[54] When administered to patients with HFrEF and renal insufficiency, 100% oxygen reduced sympathetic nerve firing and augmented the relationship between diastolic blood pressure and MSNA, revealing an important and qualitatively opposite influence of chronic kidney disease on arterial chemoreceptor and baroreceptor reflexes.[55,56]

Sleep-Related Breathing Disorders.

Sympathetic outflow, heart rate, stroke volume, and systemic vascular resistance all diminish during normal non–rapid eye movement (non-REM) sleep. Blood pressure typically falls 20% to 25% from average waking levels. Arterial baroreflex vagal control of the heart rate is augmented. Paroxysms of sympathetic discharge provoking surges in heart rate and blood pressure occur during REM sleep, but in general REM comprises only 15% of sleep time. Systolic dysfunction itself is associated with briefer sleep duration and interrupted sleep,[57] resulting in a greater 24-hour adrenergic burden, even in the absence of sleep apnea.

In the contemporary era of drug and device therapy, approximately 50% of patients with chronic symptomatic HFrEF or HFpEF will have obstructive or central sleep apnea (CSA).[58] Each pause in breathing elicits profound increases in MSNA by deactivating pulmonary stretch receptors and by stimulating peripheral and central chemoreceptors via hypoxia and hypercapnia. Such sympathetic excitation is independent of, and in addition to, any reflex responses to mechanoreceptor unloading resulting from pump failure or systemic hypotension in heart failure. Inspiratory efforts against a collapsed upper airway, as occurs in obstructive sleep apnea (OSA), will generate extreme negative swings in intrathoracic pressure (i.e., an abrupt increase in left ventricular afterload). Because impaired systolic performance is accompanied by increased sensitivity to afterload, in those with HFrEF obstruction provokes an acute fall in stroke volume and diastolic blood pressure. This unloading of arterial baroreceptors then elicits a reflex increase in MSNA. The magnitude of sympathetic excitation is greater in individuals with HFrEF than in those with normal left ventricular systolic function, who are better able to maintain systemic blood pressure when confronted by increased afterload. Arousal from sleep, which terminates an apneic event, is accompanied by a further surge in central sympathetic outflow, a rise in blood pressure often exceeding waking levels, and a decrease in the vagal contribution to heart rate variability. In severely affected patients, these cycles of apnea and arousal recur repeatedly over the course of each night. Moreover, the aftereffects of apnea during sleep include sustained increases in MSNA during wakefulness.[58] In community-dwelling men, severe OSA has been shown to increase the 10-year risk of incident heart failure by 58%.[59] The recurrent cycles during sleep of increased afterload, reduced oxygen saturation, and sympathetic excitation, followed after awakening by sustained upward resetting of central sympathetic outflow, are the mechanisms most likely responsible for this progression.

In patients with HFrEF and sleep apnea, the failing ventricle and peripheral circulation are exposed to a greater adrenergic burden than necessary for circulatory homeostasis. From a sampling of 60 patients with HFrEF receiving evidence-based therapies, of whom 43 had an apnea-hypopnea index (AHI) of 15 events/hour or more, Spaak et al. identified significantly higher MSNA during wakefulness in those with coexisting sleep apnea; in those without, MSNA was similar to that documented in age-matched control subjects (**Fig. 13.10**).[60] In patients with HFrEF and predominantly OSA, MSNA was increased by 11 bursts/100 heartbeats; when OSA was abolished in a subset of such patients, by 1 month of continuous positive airway pressure (CPAP), MSNA fell by 12 bursts/100 heartbeats.[60,61] Such data provide important evidence in human heart failure for convergence, on central sympathetic neurons, of input from two independent sympathoexcitatory influences (heart failure, and sleep apnea) that interact to increase MSNA; because the independent contribution of sleep apnea is approximately 50% of that observed in individuals without OSA, such summation likely occurs through a process of mutual inhibition (**Fig. 13.11**). This additional OSA-mediated sympathoexcitation has adverse consequences: the rates of defibrillator discharge are greater and survival is shorter in patients with HFrEF and untreated OSA. Those with ischemic cardiomyopathy are at particular risk.[58]

Over the course of their sleep, some patients transit from predominantly obstructive apnea to mainly central events. This precession is accompanied by prolongation of circulation time and a reduction in PCO_2 below the threshold for central apnea. These observations suggest that these repetitive increases in left ventricular afterload during airway obstructions cause systolic function to deteriorate over the

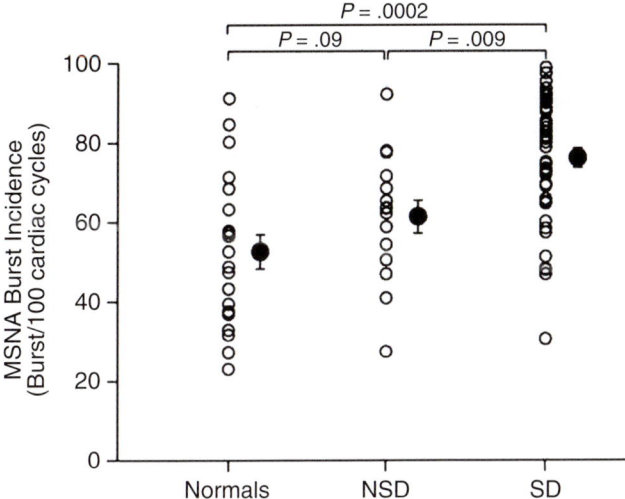

Fig. 13.10 Scattergrams and means ± standard errors for muscle sympathetic burst incidence (bursts/100 cardiac cycles) in treated heart failure with reduced ejection fraction (HFrEF) patients with *(SD)* and with no sleep related breathing disorders *(NSD)*, as compared with age-matched healthy laboratory controls. Note that MSNA in treated HFrEF patients without sleep apnea is not significantly greater than that of healthy subjects, whereas the coexistence of sleep apnea with heart failure is accompanied by significantly higher MSNA (*P* = .005). *MSNA,* Muscle sympathetic nerve activity. (From Floras JS. Sympathetic nervous system activation in human heart failure. Clinical implications of an updated model. *J Am Coll Cardiol.* 2009;54:375–385, with permission of the American College of Cardiology Foundation.)

course of the night, increasing venous return and pulmonary congestion. This, in turn, will stimulate hyperventilation followed by hypocapnia, initiating cycles of CSA with CSR.[58]

Compared with heart failure patients matched for LVEF and other clinical characteristics, but without sleep-related breathing disorders, those with CSA have higher nocturnal urinary NE excretion, and increased plasma NE concentrations while awake. The magnitude of such activation is proportional to the frequency of arousal from sleep and the degree of apnea-related hypopnea. MSNA during wakefulness is also greater in heart failure patients with CSA than in those without.[60] Mansfield and colleagues[62] reported higher rates of cardiac and total body NE spillover in heart failure patients with CSA than in those without CSA or with OSA, and attributed such differences to greater hemodynamic decompensation in those with CSA. The cardiac washout rate of ^{123}I-MIBG also has been shown to be greater in heart failure patients with central apnea than in those with OSA or without a sleep-related breathing disorder.[63]

Central Integration and Interactions

Information arising from arterial baroreceptor and chemoreceptor inputs is integrated within the nucleus tractus solitarius, which regulates—via projection to the caudal then rostral ventrolateral medullae (VLM)—discharge of sympathetic preganglionic neurons in the intermediolateral cell column of the spinal cord. Adjacent respiratory centers, suprabulbar subcortical regions, and a cortical autonomic network all interact with brainstem motoneurons to reset the magnitude of central sympathetic outflow to modulate such discharge during both wakefulness and sleep.[64]

Experimental Heart Failure Models

Zucker's group has documented the central augmentation of cardiac sympathetic afferent reflex regulation of renal sympathetic nerve

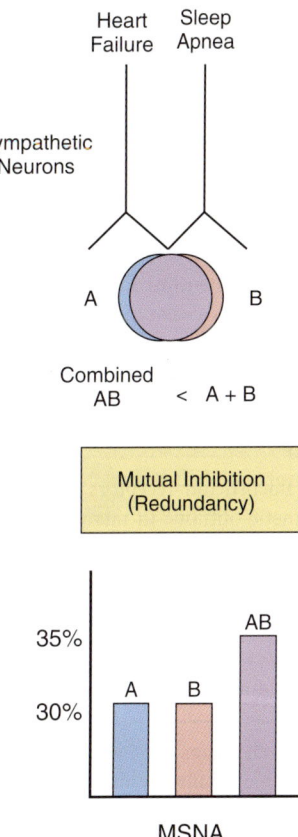

Fig. 13.11 Convergence of afferent input from two sets of reflexes (in this example, heart failure and sleep apnea) eliciting directionally similar (in this example, excitatory) effects on muscle sympathetic nerve activity *(MSNA)* may summate and interact centrally through mutual inhibition (redundancy), simple additive summation, or mutual facilitation. The difference in MSNA recorded during wakefulness in heart failure patients with and without obstructive sleep apnea *(OSA)*[60] is eliminated when OSA is abolished.[61] Improvements in left ventricular ejection fraction and congestion with treatment[58] should diminish MSNA concurrently and independently. Taken together, these observations are consistent with the concept that these two sympathoexcitatory stimuli interact centrally through an overlapping (i.e., redundant) process of mutual inhibition.

activity, which arises from increases in brain angiotensin II, decreases in local synthesis of neuronal NO (which exerts sympathoinhibitory actions at several sites), the generation of reactive oxygen species, the activation of rho kinase, and consequent changes in neural excitability via modulation of ion channel function. In their experience, it is increased central enhancement of cardiac reflex gain, rather than loss of arterial baroreceptor input, that increases the set-point for sympathetic outflow in heart failure.[65,66]

Exogenous angiotensin II inhibits vagal discharge, induces inflammation, increases central sympathetic outflow, and interacts with the arterial baroreflex at several sites within and outside the blood-brain barrier. In dogs without heart failure, the hypotensive response to chronic carotid baroreceptor stimulation is attenuated if angiotensin II is infused concurrently.[67] The cardiac sympathetic afferent reflex in dogs is potentiated by chronic central infusion of angiotensin II; in rats with chronic heart failure this reflex can be normalized by central administration of antisense oligodeoxynucleotides to AT₁ receptor mRNA. In contrast, in the ovine paced heart failure model, cardiac activity, but not renal sympathetic nerve activity, was significantly increased relative to healthy controls; only the former was attenuated by acute intracerebroventricular infusion of losartan.[20] Sympathetically mediated increases in renal renin release in heart failure could thereby generate a positive feedback loop, further amplifying nerve firing through these central actions of angiotensin II.

In a rat model of HFrEF, an increase in renal sympathetic outflow and resetting of its regulation by the arterial baroreceptor reflex could be reversed by intracerebroventricular infusion of Fab fragments (to inhibit ouabain-like activity), inhibitors of angiotensin II AT_1 receptor function or an angiotensin-converting enzyme inhibitor; such sympathetic excitation was absent in transgenic rats deficient in brain angiotensinogen. In a rabbit heart failure model, sympathoexcitation resulted from increased rostral VLM angiotensin AT_1 receptor and NAD(P)H oxidase subunit gene expression with consequent upregulation of superoxide production.[68] This pathway appears modifiable by lipophilic statins.[69]

Central mineralocorticoid receptors also participate in the regulation of sympathetic outflow. In rats with experimental heart failure, intracerebroventricular infusion of spironolactone reduced renal sympathetic nerve firing and augmented its arterial baroreflex regulation. Aldosterone of adrenal origin is capable of stimulating the brain renin-angiotensin system by increasing paraventricular (hypothalamic) nucleus angiotensin AT_1 receptor mRNA, protein, and NAD(P)H oxidase subunit gene expression and, concurrently, plasma NE concentrations.

Determining mechanisms by which immune and inflammatory mechanisms initiate centrally mediated sympathoexcitation has become a focus of intense research. There is now compelling evidence for a bidirectional relationship between the adaptive and innate immune system and the sympathetic nervous system, with central neural angiotensin II at its crux.[70,71] There is, in parallel, extensive literature concerning reflex vagal control of immunity.[72] Such interactions are likely to induce similar adrenergic and vagal disturbances in HFrEF.[2] Infarction induces neural and myocardial inflammation,[73] and a central cytokine-mediated pathway in experimental heart failure has been shown to activate the sympathetic nervous and renin-angiotensin systems.[74,75] The latter processes can be attenuated by antiinflammatory cytokines, TNF-α receptor 1 knockdown, mineralocorticoid receptor blockade, or ablation of the forebrain subfornical organ, which lacks a blood-brain barrier.[76,77]

Clinical Studies

By measuring NE appearance rates in the internal jugular vein, along with those of its lipophilic metabolites, 3-methoxy-4-hydroxyphenylglycol (MHPG) and 3,4-DHPG, Esler's group has demonstrated significant increases in human heart failure in internal jugular spillover of MHPG, DHPG, epinephrine, and of the serotonin metabolite, 5-HIAA, plus a significant positive correlation between brain NE turnover and cardiac NE spillover. Selective sampling of venous effluent from cortical and subcortical regions detected fourfold higher suprabulbar subcortical turnover of NE in treated heart failure patients than in control subjects. Cortical NE turnover tended to be lower. Furthermore, there was a significant positive correlation between subcortical NE turnover and total body NE spillover in the HFrEF group, an observation consistent with these authors' hypothesis that activation of noradrenergic neurons projecting rostrally from the brain stem mediates sympathetic excitation in heart failure.[78] Because of their participation in arousal, vigilance, and circulatory control in the rat, brain NE-containing nuclei in the locus coeruleus have received particular attention. Chronic sleep disruption in heart failure (even in the absence of nocturnal breathing disorders)[57] may establish a state of heightened arousal, increasing adrenergic drive as a consequence.[58] In patients with both HFrEF and OSA there is an inverse relationship between MSNA and a subjective measure of daytime sleepiness.[79]

As heart failure advances, ventilatory responses to central chemoreceptor stimulation by hypercapnia are augmented[80,81] and within-breath sympathoinhibition is attenuated.[80] Increased central chemoreflex responsiveness to CO_2 facilitates the cyclical breathing oscillations characteristic of CSA; apneas act, in turn, to further stimulate central sympathetic outflow, with exaggerated sympathoexcitation[80] and carryover of high MSNA into the awake state.[60] Di Vanna and colleagues[81] described, in HFrEF patients with Class II to III symptoms, increased MSNA responses to hypercapnic (central) and well as hypoxic (peripheral) chemoreflex stimulation. In series comprising 60 consecutive patients with Class I to III HFrEF (mean LVEF 31%), 47% exhibited increased sensitivity to hypercapnia. Extension of this cohort to 110 consecutive patients, followed for a mean of 29 months, reported a 4-year survival of only 49% in those with increased sensitivity to both hypoxia and hypercapnia, compared with 100% in those with normal chemosensitivity.[82]

Efferent Mechanisms
Ganglionic Neurotransmission

The principal defect in the parasympathetic modulation of heart rate in experimental heart failure appears to lie at the level of vagal ganglionic neurotransmission.[83] Conversely, by stimulating sympathetic ganglionic and adrenomedullary neurotransmission, increases in angiotensin II in heart failure could augment NE and epinephrine release.

Prejunctional Mechanisms and Efferent Sympathovagal Interactions

In the hamster model of dilated cardiomyopathy, early increases in cardiac NE turnover, tyrosine hydroxylase and dopamine beta-hydroxylase activity and cardiac dopamine stores are followed by the depletion of myocardial NE content and the destruction of sympathetic nerve terminals.[26] In a rabbit model of pacing induced heart failure, ventricular systolic dysfunction and an increase in plasma NE were followed by a reduction in cardiac NE uptake and transporter density, and a subsequent decrease in myocardial beta-receptor density, with gradual normalization after pacing ended.[84]

In human HFrEF, NE spillover into the coronary sinus is increased disproportionately to its neuronal release, implying a contributory role for reduced efficiency of NE uptake by cardiac sympathetic nerve endings in the selective increase in cardiac NE spillover observed at the onset of this condition.[85] Consistent with this concept, Rundqvist and associates[13] calculated the fractional extraction of NE to be 87% in healthy controls, but only 60% in patients with HFrEF. Radioligand binding experiments in ventricles derived from patients with Class II to IV HFrEF detected a decrease in NE uptake-1 carrier density of up to 30%.[86]

Release of NE from sympathetic nerve endings and the discharge of acetylcholine from vagal nerves also can be augmented or suppressed by endogenous or exogenously administered agonists, acting on a wide variety of prejunctional receptors. NE release can be facilitated if prejunctional $β_2$-adrenoceptors are stimulated by its endogenous agonist, epinephrine. In advanced heart failure, circulating epinephrine may be transported into sympathetic nerve terminals, incorporated into vesicles along with NE, and released as a cotransmitter, exerting a local prejunctional sympathofacilitatory action.[8] In contrast, $α_2$-adrenoceptors inhibit NE release. Observations in human heart failure suggest regional selectivity, with left ventricular but not forearm $α_2$-adrenoceptors retaining this inhibitory capacity.[1]

Polymorphisms of prejunctional adrenergic receptors might contribute to interindividual variation in NE release. In a retrospective genetic-association study, Small et al.[87] detected a 6-fold increase in the risk of developing heart failure in African-American subjects homozygous for the hypofunctioning prejunctional α_{2C} Del322-325 polymorphism, and a 10-fold increase in those who were also homozygous for the hyperfunctional postjunctional β_1Arg329 receptor. The latter demonstrates greater affinity, in vivo, for adenylyl cyclase, and an augmented generation of contractile force in right ventricular trabeculae of nonfailing and failing hearts exposed to isoproterenol. These authors proposed that heart failure risk accrued from a synergistic enhancement of two adrenergic signal transduction pathways. However, this specific publication did not report heart rate. Subsequently, Kaye and associates,[88] in a cohort of patients with severe heart failure, detected no relationship between the α_{2C} Del322-325 or $\beta2$-adrenoceptor polymorphisms and the rate of cardiac NE release. Curiously, the relationship between NE release and heart rate was steeper in β_2-adrenoceptor Arg 16 homozygotes, implying greater postjunctional responsiveness.

Muscarinic M_2 receptors on adrenergic nerve endings also attenuate NE release when stimulated by acetylcholine. In subjects with impaired left ventricular systolic function and increased cardiac adrenergic drive, intracoronary infusion of acetylcholine decreased cardiac NE spillover, an effect not seen in control subjects with normal left ventricular systolic function. Receptor blockade with atropine had no effect in the heart failure group, but did have increased cardiac NE spillover in control subjects.[89] Conversely, increased NE release from sympathetic nerve endings inhibits acetylcholine release by stimulating prejunctional α_1-adrenoceptors on vagal nerve endings.[90]

Neuregulin-1 signaling has been identified as an important antiadrenergic pathway, requiring eNOS-mediated muscarinic receptor activation. Neuregulin-1 expression initially increases then decreases as heart failure progresses.[91] In advanced HFrEF, other sympathetic neurotransmitters, such as neuropeptide Y (NPY), also may exert a vagolytic action by inhibiting acetylcholine release. In experimental preparations, prejunctional AT_1 receptors have been shown to facilitate neural and adrenal release of catecholamines when stimulated by angiotensin II; however, this action has not been discerned in human HFrEF.[92]

Chronic exposure to either sympathomimetic circulating β_1-adrenoceptor activating antibodies, present in some patients with dilated cardiomyopathy, or negatively inotropic β_2-adreno- and M_2 muscarinic acetylcholine receptor antibodies can impair ventricular systolic performance.[93]

THERAPEUTIC IMPLICATIONS (SEE ALSO CHAPTERS 37 AND 42)

Parenteral positive inotropic agents were among the earliest therapies for heart failure. Acutely, dobutamine infusion causes a significant reduction in cardiac NE spillover, an effect attributed to reductions in cardiac filling pressures, and activation of ventricular mechanoreceptors.[94] However, the application of isotope dilution methodology to heart failure patients disproved the concept that the failing heart required inotropic support to compensate for sympathetic denervation, and in several trials chronic administration of sympathomimetics increased mortality. Use of these agents is now restricted to short-term palliative strategies.

The translational consequence of the large body of experimental and clinical work reviewed in this chapter has been a surge in the number of investigator- and industry-initiated investigations of therapies targeting one or more elements of the autonomic disequilibrium of heart failure.[1-4] Such initiatives are predicated upon four hypotheses: (1) in most patients, the magnitude of sympathetic activation exceeds that required to maintain cardiovascular homeostasis; (2) the

adrenergic and parasympathetic disturbances of HFrEF are reversible; (3) identification of patient-specific mechanisms engendering excess sympathetic drive affords the opportunity to institute targeted individualized interventions adjunctive to evidence-based drug and device therapies; and (4) pharmacological, lifestyle, or device interventions that attenuate sympathoexcitation or augment vagal tone will improve symptoms and prognosis.

Pharmacological Interventions

Several contemporary heart failure therapies counter (directly or indirectly) the adverse effects of excessive cardiac and sympathetic activity or augment vagal tone, or both, yielding improved symptoms or prognosis. Landmark placebo-controlled trials, involving carvedilol, bisoprolol and metoprolol, demonstrating the symptom, hemodynamic, and mortality benefits of long-term β_1- and nonselective β-blockade for patients with heart failure due to depressed left ventricular systolic function (**see Chapter 37**) earned these agents a Class I indication in contemporary HFrEF guidelines. In a trial involving participants aged $\geq$ 70 years selected on the basis of heart failure symptoms and signs, regardless of ejection fraction, nebivolol, a β_1-adrenoceptor antagonist and β_3-agonist, also reduced the composite primary outcome comprising all-cause mortality or cardiovascular hospital admission.[95]

Neither carvedilol nor metoprolol reduces MSNA.[96] Rather, these and other β-adrenoreceptor antagonists address the earliest autonomic disturbances identified in HFrEF by shielding the heart from the adverse consequences of excessive NE, by attenuating β_1-mediated stimulation of renin, and by augmenting tonic and reflex heart rate modulation while preserving homeostatic oscillations in MSNA.[97] Carvedilol, unlike metoprolol, decreases total body and cardiac NE spillover by ~30%, presumably due to the blockade of sympathetic prejunctional β_2-adrenoceptors that facilitate neural NE release.[96] Importantly, β-adrenoceptor blockade does not protect the heart, kidney, or periphery from α-adrenoceptor mediated vasoconstriction or renal sodium retention (carvedilol's peripheral α-blocking actions diminish over time),[98] or from vasoconstriction caused by greater corelease with NE in heart failure of neurotransmitters such as ATP or NPY.

When given intravenously, 0.1 mg clonidine, an α_2-adrenoceptor and imidazoline I_1 receptor agonist, lowered arterial NE concentrations, cardiac NE spillover, and left ventricular +dP/dt by 47%, 58%, and 15%, respectively.[99] Administered for 2 months via transdermal patch, 0.1 mg of daily clonidine reduced muscle sympathetic burst frequency by 26% and plasma NE concentrations by 47%.[100] As yet, no long-term outcome trial has tested this agent.

Autonomic balance may also be improved pharmacologically, as an ancillary property of existing therapies, through sensitizing baroreceptor afferents (digitalis); relief of congestion, unloading of sympathoexcitatory atrial afferents, and partial attenuation of sleep-related breathing disorders (diuretics); elevating endogenous natriuretic peptide concentrations (by injection, infusion, or neutral endopeptidase inhibition); countering central and peripheral sympathoexcitatory and vagolytic effects of angiotensin AT_1 receptor stimulation (angiotensin converting enzyme inhibitors or angiotensin receptor antagonists); or by blocking mineralocorticoid receptors.[1-3] Although none of these drug-based strategies in isolation restores autonomic equilibrium in HFrEF, several prolong survival or reduce hospitalizations.

In both hypertension and HFpEF, centrally mediated sympathoexcitation can be countered by chronic administration of lipophilic statins.[69,101] Efferent vagal tone can be augmented by centrally acting acetylcholinesterase inhibitors, such as donazepil.[3] The limited available data suggest that ivabradine increases time-domain indices of heart rate variability in concert with pulse interval. Additional pharmacological strategies exhibiting therapeutic potential include peripheral chemoreflex desensitization (caffeine; dopamine), peripheral acetylcholinesterase inhibition (pyridostigmine), inflammasome modulation and the combination of β_2-adrenoceptor or β_3-adrenoceptor agonism with β_1-adrenoceptor blockade.[1-3,5,102,103] Digitoxin, which has both vagotonic and antiinflammatory properties, is being evaluated in a large prospective European HFrEF trial.[3]

Abnormalities identified by cardiac imaging, such as the ^{123}I-MIBG heart/mediastinum uptake ratio or defect score (signs, in individuals with HFrEF, of increased risk for malignant ventricular arrhythmias and premature cardiac death),[16,27] improve with chronic β-adrenoceptor blockade and, in patients with HFpEF, with the angiotensin II AT_1 receptor antagonist, candesartan.[18]

Whereas several such pharmacological modulators of the autonomic nervous system improve clinical outcome, sympatholytic interventions appear harmful. In both a pilot study[104] and a large-scale mortality trial,[105] there was an excess of deaths in those allocated moxonidine, a centrally acting I_1-agonist. When the β-adrenoceptor antagonist bucindolol was tested in HFrEF, there was an increase in mortality accompanied by a marked fall in plasma NE concentration.[106] Of note, prerandomization NE concentrations were not elevated in many moxonidine trial participants, and skipping doses may have caused intense rebound surges in NE, heart rate, blood pressure, and ventricular ectopic frequency.[104] Whether bucindolol diminished neural NE release, increased NE clearance, or attenuated sympathetic outflow cannot be established from plasma concentrations alone. The hypothesis that targeting directly central sympathetic outflow will improve prognosis is unlikely to be affirmed until a definitive and practical screening biomarker for sympathetic activation becomes available for routine research and clinical use.

Nonpharmacological Interventions

Patients with HFrEF whose autonomic profile places them at high risk may be offered adjunctive personalized interventions targeting their individually specific sympathoexcitatory or vagoparvic disturbances. The attractiveness of device over drug therapies for this purpose is that such interventions can be designed to target specific pathways, can be programmed to apply timed or constant stimulation, are less likely to be cause systemic adverse effects, and do not depend upon patient adherence for efficacy.[2-5,58,107]

Cardiac Resynchronization Therapy (see also Chapter 38)

In short-term uncontrolled trials, biventricular pacing, which was programmed to narrow temporal and spatial dispersion of left ventricular contraction, lowered mean MSNA by ~30%[108] and augmented tonic and reflex vagal heart rate modulation.[109] In one experiment, acute conversion from synchronous to nonsynchronous pacing increased MSNA by 25%.[110] Whether such responses can be sustained with time has yet to be determined by any randomized, controlled trial.

In a prospective study in which 45 consecutive patients were restudied 6 months after receiving cardiac resynchronization–defibrillator devices, improvement in group mean time domain indices of vagal heart rate modulation and ^{123}I-MIBG estimates of cardiac sympathetic nerve terminal function were noted. However, in a substantial minority, biventricular pacing did not affect ^{123}I-MIBG kinetics, and plasma concentration of nerve growth factor, a sympathetic neurotrophin, was unchanged.[111] The prevalence of obstructive and CSA is unaffected by biventricular pacing; in a cohort of 472 patients screened 6 months after cardiac resynchronization–defibrillator implantation, in 80%, the AHI exceeded 5 events/hr and in 64% was greater than 15 events/hr.[112] In the canine paced model, cardiac resynchronization

therapy was shown to augment cholinergic as well as adrenergic signaling.[25]

Cardiac Sympathetic Denervation

The sympathoinhibitory, vagotonic, and antiischemic consequences of left-sided cardiac sympathetic denervation have been exploited as management of refractory ventricular arrhythmia. With increased cardiac NE spillover and vagal withdrawal being the initial autonomic HFrEF phenotype, with deepening autonomic disturbances accompanying its progression and increasing mortality risk, and with ventricular arrhythmias being the principal cause of sudden cardiac death, there is a sound rationale to extend its application to heart failure. A feasibility and safety trial randomized 30 patients with HFrEF and NYHA Class II or III symptoms to left cervico–thoracic sympathetic blockade by videothorascopic clipping under general anesthesia in addition to continued optimal medical therapy. There were no adverse surgical effects in the 10 participants who proceeded safely through surgery. After 6 months, LVEF, 6 minutes' walking distance, symptoms were significantly improved; other study endpoints were not changed.[113] A randomized safety and feasibility pilot study of surgical removal of the lower half of the left stellate ganglion (T1) and thoracic ganglia (T2–T4), in anticipation of a larger phase III efficacy trial, is currently under way.[114]

Carotid Baroreceptor Stimulation (see also Chapter 42)

The demonstration of preserved arterial baroreflex modulation of sympathetic outflow in human HFrEF established a compelling physiological rationale to investigate, in this condition, the autonomic, hemodynamic, and clinical impact of electrical activation of afferent nerves arising from the carotid sinus. Importantly, such stimulation occurs distal to the mechanoreceptor, bypassing any local impairment of signal transduction that might be present. In dogs with experimental chronic heart failure, carotid baroreceptor activation lowered plasma NE and angiotensin II concentrations and improved survival relative to unstimulated control animals.[115]

Recent technical advances permit surgical envelopment of the carotid sinus by electrodes connected to an implanted pulse generator, achieving durable responses to bi- or unilateral stimulation.[3] In a seven-patient HFrEF cohort followed for 43 months, chronic baroreceptor afferent stimulation was accompanied by sustained reduction in MSNA and modest improvements in its reflex control and in LVEF without any corresponding reductions in either blood pressure or heart rate.[116] In a subsequent trial involving 146 patients with HFrEF (LVEF ≤35%) reporting NYHA Class III symptoms who were randomly allocated "baroreceptor activation therapy," 6 months of stimulation lowered N-terminal pro-BNP (NT-proBNP) concentration and improved 6-minute walk distance, quality of life, and functional class rank. In the cohort as a whole, stimulation did not affect LVEF, but an increase was detected in those who were not being treated concurrently with cardiac resynchronization.[117,118] Whether patients or their clinicians would accept such surgery in practice in the absence of positive long-term outcome data has yet to be established.

Carotid Body Denervation

In both rabbit and rat models of experimental heart failure, denervation of the carotid body improved autonomic cardiovascular modulation, the density of arrhythmia, and the AHI.[119,120] When ablation was performed 2 weeks after coronary artery ligation, there was relative preservation of ventricular structure and function; survival improved by ~90%.[119] A review of the experimental and clinical literature stimulated Paton and colleagues to propose targeting the carotid body of HFrEF patients with increased chemosensitivity to attenuate both sympathoexcitation and sleep-disordered breathing.[121] In a series of 10 men with HFrEF (mean LVEF 27%) who underwent either bilateral (6) or right-sided (4) carotid body resection, surgery improved ventilator responses to peripheral chemoreflex stimulation and exercise capacity but reduced MSNA by only 8% and had adverse effects on O_2 saturation during sleep. Subsequently, two subjects died.[122] An alternate, catheter-based ultrasound approach also has been tested in humans. With such limited safety and efficacy data thus far, the future progress of such an investigation is difficult to predict.

Diet

Benefits of sodium restriction may extend beyond relief of congestion. In a multivariable analysis of patients with HFrEF who underwent polysomnography and whose sodium intake was estimated by detailed validated food records, a significant positive correlation was noted between sodium intake and the AHI.[123]

Exercise Training

A systematic review of several small studies reports beneficial neuromodulatory effects of chronic exercise training in HFrEF—reductions in resting MSNA and its reflex modulation and increases in vagal components of heart rate variability both at rest and during recovery from exercise and a fall in total body NE spillover—but few subjects have been studied thus far. The six studies reporting MSNA were all conducted at the same institution, and the durability of these responses is unknown.[124] Experimental mechanisms by which exercise training has been shown to repair autonomic equilibrium include mitigation of central neural oxidative stress and angiotensin AT_1 receptor upregulation, normalization of altered nitric oxide metabolism and GABA- and glutamate-mediated cardiovascular neurotransmission, diminution of peripheral chemosensitivity, reduction of renal sympathetic nerve-mediated sodium and water retention, and generalized improvement in baroreceptor and chemoreceptor reflex regulation of the heart and circulation.[124,125] Four months of exercise training reduced the AHI and the MSNA of HFrEF patients with OSA. It also reduced the MSNA of those with CSA but had no effect on their AHI.[126] Clinical Trial NCT03111017 is testing the hypotheses in patients with HFpEF, aged ≥ 60 years, that 16 weeks of exercise training will lower MSNA and that such a reduction will correlate with improved exercise capacity.

Positive Airway Pressure

Conventional pharmacological or device management of HFrEF has no appreciable impact on the presence or severity of OSA. By contrast, nocturnal nasal CPAP immediately abolishes upper airway obstruction and four of its sympathoexcitatory consequences: apnea, hypoxia, hypercapnia, and arousal from sleep. In patients with HFrEF and OSA, CPAP reduces nocturnal blood pressure and heart rate and increases arterial baroreflex modulation of the heart rate. Thus, the sympathoinhibitory and vagotonic effects of CPAP during sleep alone may be sufficient to benefit heart failure patients with coexisting OSA. By reducing, when present, right ventricular constraint on left ventricular filling, positive airway pressure acutely increases stroke volume and cardiac output; this, in turn, could reduce central sympathetic outflow reflexively.[58]

Removal of these nocturnal mechanical, chemical, and adrenergic insults with treatment should restore autonomic equilibrium, in theory, and permit the recovery of ventricular systolic function. Indeed, in a randomized trial of 1-month duration involving HFrEF patients with OSA (with a similar proportion of ischemic and dilated cardiomyopathy), nightly use of CPAP abolished apnea; improved left ventricular structure and ejection fraction and the arterial baroreflex regulation of heart rate and heart rate variability; lowered systolic blood pressure,

heart rate, and MSNA during wakefulness; and reduced ventricular ectopy during sleep.[2,58,61] A second, 3-month trial, enrolling patients with milder OSA (AHI > 5 events/hr) and LVEF less than 55% also observed, with treatment, a significant increase in the latter and a reduction in urinary NE excretion.[127] In a third trial lasting 6 to 8 weeks, CPAP improved ^{11}C-hydroxyephedrine retention, a probe of presynaptic cardiac sympathetic nerve function, and in those with an AHI of greater than 20 events/hr it augmented myocardial efficiency.[128]

In a 3-month randomized trial involving heart failure patients with CSA, the nightly application of CPAP suppressed the AHI and reduced nocturnal urinary NE by 41% to values similar to those obtained in clinically matched heart failure patients without CSA. CPAP also reduced plasma NE during wakefulness by 22%.[2,58] In an event-driven trial involving 258 heart failure patients with CSA, a mean of 2 years of CPAP treatment did not improve transplant-free survival overall, but this intervention only reduced the AHI from 40 to 20 events/hr.[129] In a post hoc efficacy analysis, CPAP improved transplant-free survival of those patients in whom the AHI was suppressed below 15 apneic or hypopneic events/hr; that is, the threshold for recruitment into this trial.[130]

Adaptive servo-ventilation (ASV) provides both end-expiratory pressure support to abolish obstructive apnea and either minute volume (mv)- or peak flow (pf)-triggered ventilation to effectively suppress CSR. Thus, ASV has the potential to mitigate or reverse central adaptations to chronic intermittent hypoxia, hypercapnia, and arousal, which result in daytime as well as nighttime sympathetic activation and vagal inhibition. Results of observational studies involving HFrEF patients with CSA have been encouraging, with ASV reducing plasma NE concentrations and arrhythmic events and improving cardiac ^{123}I-MIBG kinetics and survival.[131,132] However, in an event-driven trial involving 1325 participants with symptomatic HFrEF (LVEF ≤ 45%) and an AHI greater than 15 with predominantly (≥ 50%) CSA and a central AHI ≥ 10 who were randomly allocated to mv-ASV and followed for a mean of 2.6 years, there were no between-group differences with respect to the primary endpoint, a composite that included death from any cause, cardiac transplantation, LV assist device implantation, resuscitation after sudden cardiac death, appropriate defibrillator discharge, or unplanned admission for worsening HF, or most secondary endpoints, such as symptoms, NT-pro-BNP or inflammatory markers. Catecholamines were not measured. Hazard ratios for two secondary endpoints, all-cause (1.28; 95% CI, 1.06–1.55; $P = .01$) and cardiovascular mortality (1.34; 9% CI 1.09–1.65; $P = .006$), were increased in those allocated mv-ASV.[133] These findings have generated considerable discussion concerning cause, reproducibility, and generalizability of these findings, which may be specific to the device algorithm, the magnitude of pressure support applied, and the characteristics of patients enrolled, resulting in admonition against the clinical application of mv-ASV to treat CSA-CSR outside of well-monitored clinical trials.[58]

A nonrandomized observational study involving OSA subjects with HFrEF suggested that abolition of apneas by CPAP improved survival.[134] The hypothesis that treating, with pf-ASV, HFrEF patients who either have OSA but are not sleepy, or CSA, will reduce a composite primary endpoint comprising death, cardiac transplantation, left ventricular assist device implantation, and cardiovascular hospitalization is currently being tested in a multinational trial (ADVENT-HF; NCT01128816).

Renal Denervation (see also Chapter 42)

Efferent renal sympathetic nerves, predominantly unmyelinated fibers with catecholamine-containing terminals innervating proximal and distal tubules, exhibit pulse-synchronous firing that is modulated by arterial and atrial baroreceptor reflex input, breathing, muscle contraction, and other stimuli. They are intimately involved in the pathophysiology of heart failure: when renal nerves are stimulated, they increase, proportional to discharge frequency, renin release (β_1-mediated), renal tubular sodium and water reabsorption (α_1-mediated), and renal vascular resistance (α_1-mediated).[135] Indeed, in the contemporary β-blocker, renal NE spillover has been identified as a potent marker of risk of future death or transplantation.[31]

A randomized controlled trial of heart failure patients requiring high doses of furosemide for clinical stability highlighted the restraint imposed by these efferents on both natriuresis and diuresis.[136] In experimental models, renal denervation, which severs both efferent nerves and afferent nerves (the latter comprised of subpopulations engaged selectively by mechanical or chemical stimuli), attenuated pathological sodium and water retention, lowered blood pressure,[135] improved filling pressures and LVEF, and increased the threshold for induction of atrial and ventricular arrhythmias.[3]

Several nonsurgical means of renal denervation have been developed.[3] The greatest cumulative clinical experience, thus far, has been with percutaneous single-electrode catheter-based delivery of radiofrequency energy into renal arteries and their distal branches. As proof of principle, renal NE spillover was assessed in 10 patients with drug-resistant hypertension before and 15 to 30 days after this procedure. Renal NE spillover fell, on average, by 47%.[137] Uncontrolled series, with 6 months of follow-up, reported reductions in total peripheral resistance (by 19%, on average),[138] MSNA, and inflammatory markers.[139] In a rat model, denervation inhibited renal neprilysin activity.[140] However, the largest sham-controlled blinded trial of renal denervation for drug-resistant hypertension did not discern a significant effect on systolic blood pressure at 6 months.[141] Several factors, including incomplete understanding of human renal neuroanatomy when this trial was designed,[3] have been advanced to explain this neutral finding.

A pilot study of seven patients, with 6-month follow-up, reported that denervation could be performed safely in HFrEF without causing hypotension or increasing creatinine.[142] This was confirmed in a randomized trial involving 60 patients who were found to have lower NT-proBNP and systolic blood pressure and improved LVEF and symptom class when restudied 6 months after radiofrequency ablation.[143] A single-center, randomized, open-controlled trial involving 25 patients with HFpEF was stopped early due to difficulties with recruitment. Renal denervation had no impact on quality of life indices, exercise capacity, cardiac structure and function, glomerular filtration, or macro- or micro-vascular biomarkers.[144] Several research consortia are now investigating, in greater depth, the therapeutic potential of multielectrode and also nonradiofrequency-based denervation technologies for patients with either HFrEF (who are not hypotensive) or HFpEF.[3]

Spinal Cord Stimulation (see also Chapter 42)

Offered initially to assist in the management of chronic pain or refractory angina, midthoracic cord stimulation also modulates autonomic tone via engaging spinal projections to higher regulatory centers. In experimental heart failure and postinfarction preparations, spinal cord stimulation increased LVEF and decreased plasma NE and NT-proBNP concentrations, the incidence of spontaneous ventricular arrhythmias, and the inducibility of atrial fibrillation.[4] A nonrandomized human safety and efficacy study evaluated the effects of 6 months of continuous T1–T3 stimulation at 90% to 110% of the paresthesia threshold. NYHA Class, quality of life measures, left ventricular dilatation, LVEF, and peak VO$_2$ all improved.[4] However, in a subsequent randomized trial of 66 patients with LVEF less than 35% (NCT01112579),

12 hours of daily T2–T4 stimulation using a different technology and algorithm had no impact on the primary outcome of LV end-systolic volume index, or on any secondary study endpoint, including cardiac ^{123}I-MIBG kinetics.[145] It is still uncertain whether these findings relate to the particular stimulation protocol applied or represent conceptual failure.

Vagal Nerve Stimulation (see also Chapter 42)

In animal models of HFrEF, chronic cervical vagal nerve stimulation has been shown to reduce sympathetic outflow, improve efferent parasympathetic tone, restore autonomic balance, reverse adverse ventricular remodeling, and prolong survival. Vagal stimulation also affords the opportunity to test the concept that human immune system function in HFrEF can be influenced beneficially by modulating by the autonomic nervous system.[2,3]

A clinical multicenter open-label study involving a small series of HFrEF subjects reported, after 1 year of stimulation, an increase in LVEF from 21% to 34%, a 9 beats/min lower heart rate, and augmented vagal heart rate modulation, and a substantial number of serious adverse effects, including two judged to be procedurally related and three deaths.[146] Three subsequent randomized trials, evaluating different stimulation sites, frequencies, currents, and duty cycles, were unable to establish definitive evidence of therapeutic benefit with respect to primary clinical or surrogate endpoints.[147-149] Two of these reported material procedure–related complications.[148,149] The largest such trial, INcrease Of VAgal TonE in CHF (INNOVATE-HF), which was designed to determine the impact of chronic vagal pacing on a primary combined endpoint of all-cause mortality and first heart failure hospitalization, was stopped on the basis of futility after randomizing 707 patients according to a 3:2 intervention:control ratio. Secondary analyses did report improved symptoms and walking distance.[147] A more rigorous appreciation of the anatomy and function of neural networks engaged by vagal stimulation, elucidation of the optimal stimulation site and protocol, and avoidance of device-related complications, all appear necessary for this strategy to advance.[3] Moreover, there may be limited potential for such stimulation to modify heart rate or its tonic variation if the principal defect in the parasympathetic modulation of heart rate is deficient vagal ganglionic neurotransmission.[83,150]

SUMMARY AND FUTURE DIRECTIONS

The last three decades have witnessed a major transformation in our conception of how neural dysregulation of the heart and circulation arises in heart failure then drives its progression. Mechanisms and processes responsible for the autonomic phenotype of heart failure are more nuanced and patient-specific than initially envisaged. Impaired tonic and reflex vagal modulation of heart rate is a virtually universal accompaniment of left ventricular systolic dysfunction, but such individuals can differ considerably with respect to the magnitude, extent, and mechanisms of their sympathetic activation. Although the set point for central sympathetic outflow is increased in the majority, in a substantial minority of patients with asymptomatic or symptomatic left ventricular systolic dysfunction plasma NE concentrations, MSNA, and total body NE spillover fall within the ranges exhibited by healthy individuals of similar age and sex. Since sympathetic activation is not a universal characteristic of treated left ventricular systolic dysfunction, patients exhibiting little or no adrenergic activation are unlikely to gain appreciable clinical benefit from adding sympathoinhibitory interventions.

Current evidence in humans permits five conclusions with respect to mechanoreceptor reflex regulation of heart rate and sympathetic nervous system activity in human HFrEF (see Fig. 13.7): (1) the arterial baroreceptor reflex regulation of heart rate by the vagus nerve is impaired; (2) the arterial baroreflex regulation of MSNA remains rapidly responsive to changes in diastolic blood pressure; (3) pulmonary mechanoreceptor-mediated inhibition of sympathetic outflow is preserved; (4) the sympathoinhibitory cardiopulmonary reflex control of MSNA is attenuated; and (5) elevated cardiac filling pressures stimulate a normally quiescent sympathoexcitatory reflex, resulting in increased cardiac NE spillover and discharge rate of a subpopulation of efferent muscle sympathetic fibers.[1,2,10] As elevated atrial pressures are common to HFrEF and HFpEF, the latter mechanism could elicit an increase in efferent sympathetic nerve activity in both phenotypes.

From this perspective, the heterogeneity and time course of organ-specific sympathetic activation and parasympathetic withdrawal in HFrEF can be considered appropriate to individual hemodynamic profiles, as summarized in **Table 13.3**. Patients will progress from asymptomatic to end-stage HFrEF via different pathways and at different rates. In some, the initial insult may be a sudden drop in cardiac output and blood pressure, which will reflexively activate the sympathetic nervous and renin-angiotensin systems and decrease vagal tone to achieve a state of relative compensation. If, on the other hand, relatively normal stroke volume and blood pressure can be maintained by increases in left ventricular end-diastolic volume, rather than cardiac filling pressure, such patients would be less likely to manifest evidence, at rest, for hemodynamically mediated sympathetic activation. As myocardial contractile performance deteriorates, heart rate will rise through arterial baroreflex-mediated vagal withdrawal and sympathetic activation to maintain cardiac output and systemic arterial pressure. Over time, unloading of arterial baroreceptors by a decline in systolic or pulse pressure will elicit further diminution of cardiac vagal modulation, generalized neurohumoral activation (resulting from reflex increases in sympathetic outflow to the heart, kidney, and skeletal muscle), and loss of low-frequency MSNA spectral modulation, due to impaired neuroeffector transduction. By removing the inhibitory or restraining effect of lung inflation on central sympathetic outflow, pulmonary congestion, altered lung mechanics, and increased work of breathing will cause a further step-up in nerve traffic; indeed, it is those patients with short, shallow breaths who display the highest values for MSNA.[46] Other sympathoexcitatory comorbidities that elevate the setpoint for central sympathetic outflow or neurotransmitter release above levels required to maintain hemodynamic stability may be present, but vary considerably in potency between patients.[1,2]

For heart failure with reduced systolic function, it is now evident that several therapies that modulate sympathetic and vagal outflow or antagonize the postjunctional actions of neurally released and circulating catecholamines also decrease morbidity and prolong survival (**Table 13.4**). There are three important hypotheses for future investigation: (1) whether there is a causal relationship between such autonomic modulation and improved outcomes; (2) whether patients with heart failure but preserved systolic function exhibit similar alterations in sympathetic and parasympathetic function by these several baroreflex and nonbaroreflex mediated mechanisms; and (3) whether a robust and scalable biomarker for sympathetic activation in heart failure can be identified, validated, and commercialized.

A range of additional sympathomodulatory strategies, acting upon autonomic afferents, or within central sites of cardiovascular autonomic regulation, or upon elements of the efferent sympathetic nervous system, are currently within the preclinical or clinical stages of investigation (see Table 13.4). Equipoise persists as to whether there is specific benefit to treating either OSA or CSA when present in HFrEF; thus far there are few data concerning targeted treatment of sleep apnea in patients with HFpEF.[58] Autonomic modulation via implanted devices, such as carotid baroreceptor and vagal nerve stimulators, cardiac resynchronization therapies, or renal nerve or carotid body ablative interventions, has attracted worldwide interest and considerable intellectual and financial resources[3-5,107]; however, thus far, the yield on these investments has been low.[3] Under investigation is the novel strategy of optogenetic modulation of sympathetic activity, whether directed at the heart or other vascular beds.[151]

TABLE 13.3 Time Course and Heterogeneity of Autonomic Disturbances in Human Heart Failure

Abnormality	Autonomic Consequence
Acute heart failure with pulmonary congestion and hypotension	Generalized activation of sympathetic and renin-angiotensin-aldosterone systems; parasympathetic withdrawal
Chronic increase in left atrial pressure	Activation of cardiac sympathetic afferents causing reflex increase in efferent cardiac SNA
	Decrease in tonic +/– reflex vagal HR modulation
	Decreased prejunctional muscarinic receptor-mediated inhibition of NE release
Chronic increase in left ventricular end-diastolic pressure and volume	Reflex inhibition of sympathetic outflow to kidneys, skeletal muscle, and other systemic vascular beds
Chronic exposure to increased cardiac SNA	Impaired cardiac β-mediated signal transduction
	Increased prejunctional α_1-mediated inhibition of Ach release
Chronic reduction in stroke volume and systemic blood pressure	Impaired arterial baroreflex regulation of HR
	Reflex sympathetic activation resulting from intact and responsive arterial baroreflex regulation of muscle SNA, total body NE spillover, +/– cardiac NE spillover, +/– renal NE spillover
Pulmonary congestion	Decreased inhibition of central sympathetic outflow by pulmonary stretch reflexes stimulated by lung inflation
	Decreased respiratory sinus arrhythmia (vagal)
	Increased muscle SNA
	Decreased tonic and reflex vagal HR modulation
Chemoreceptor and muscle metaboreceptor activation	Increased muscle SNA and decreased vagal HR modulation during sleep
Co-existing sleep apnea	Increased daytime plasma NE

Ach, Acetylcholine; *HR*, heart rate; *NE*, norepinephrine; *SNA*, sympathetic nerve activity.

TABLE 13.4 Sympathetic Activation in Heart Failure: Therapeutic Opportunities

Afferent Neural Modulation
Cardiac resynchronization therapy
Carotid baroreceptor reflex activation
Carotid chemoreceptor reflex attenuation
Exercise
Renal denervation
Unloading of cardiopulmonary sympathoexcitatory afferents
Vagal nerve stimulation

Central Neural Action
Central acetylcholinesterase inhibition
Centrally acting adrenergic agonists, antagonists, antioxidants, and immune-modulators
Exercise training
Treating sleep apnea

Efferent Modulation
Adrenergic receptor blockade
Augmented norepinephrine uptake
Augmented vagal neurotransmission
Peripherally acting acetylcholinesterase inhibition
Prejunctional inhibition of norepinephrine release
Renal denervation
Spinal cord stimulation
Vagal nerve stimulation

This breadth of therapeutic opportunity holds great promise for patients with heart failure with both impaired and preserved systolic function with marked sympathetic excitation and vagal withdrawal, despite adherence to current evidence-based drug and device therapy, as they are still at high residual risk for increased morbidity, hospitalization, malign arrhythmias, and premature mortality. That autonomic disequilibrium is fundamental to the pathogenesis, progression, and prognosis of heart failure has been recognized since the early 1980s, but our understanding of the mechanisms responsible, and our translation of this knowledge into new therapies, continues to evolve. Proving the efficacy of β-adrenergic therapy for large cohorts of patients with impaired systolic function should not be considered the end of this chapter of heart failure research and innovative therapy, but its beginning.

KEY REFERENCES

2. Floras JS, Ponikowski P. The sympathetic/parasympathetic imbalance in heart failure with reduced ejection fraction. *Eur Heart J.* 2015;36:1974–1982.
3. van Bilsen M, Patel HC, Bauersachs J, et al. The autonomic nervous system as a therapeutic target in heart failure: a scientific position statement from the Translational Research Committee of the Heart Failure Association of the European Society of Cardiology. *Eur J Heart Fail.* 2017;19:1361–1378.
4. Chatterjee NA, Singh JP. Novel interventional therapies to modulate the autonomic tone in heart failure. *J Am Coll Cardiol HF.* 2015;3:786–802.
5. Florea VG, Cohn JN. The autonomic nervous system and heart failure. *Circ Res.* 2014;114:1815–1826.
6. Verloop WL, Beeftink MM, Santema BTBPJ, Cramer MJ, Doevendans PA, Voskuil M. A systematic review concerning the relation berween the sympathetic nervous system and heart failure with preserved left ventricular ejection fraction. *PLoS One.* 2015;10(2):e0117332.
10. Millar PJ, Murai H, Floras JS. Paradoxical muscle sympathetic reflex activation in human heart failure. *Circ.* 2015;131:459–468.
11. Notarius CF, Millar PJ, Murai H, et al. Divergent muscle sympathetic responses to dynamic leg exercise in heart failure and age-matched healthy subjects. *J Physiol.* 2015;593:715–722.
17. Fallavollita JA, Heavey BM, Luisi AJ, et al. Regional myocardial sympathetic denervation predicts the risk of sudden cardiac arrest in ischemic cardiomyopathy. *J Am Coll Cardiol.* 2014;63:141–149.
26. Lymperopoulos A, Rengo G, Koch WJ. Adrenergic nervous system in heart failure: pathophysiology and therapy. *Circ Res.* 2013;113:739–753.
58. Floras JS. Sleep apnea and cardiovascular risk: an enigmatic risk factor. *Circ Res.* 2018;122:1741–1764.

The full reference list for this chapter is available on ExpertConsult.

Alterations in the Peripheral Circulation in Heart Failure

Eduard Shantsila, Ahsan A. Khan, Gregory Y. H. Lip

OUTLINE

The complex pathology of heart failure (HF) can be attributed, at least in part, to important changes that occur in the peripheral circulation. As cardiac output declines, systemic perfusion pressure is maintained predominantly by peripheral vasoconstriction and sodium retention, both of which can be attributed to complex interactions among the autonomic nervous system (**see also Chapter 13**), neurohormonal mechanisms, and the kidney (**see also Chapter 15**). These homeostatic mechanisms tend to preserve circulation to the brain and heart while decreasing blood flow to the skin, skeletal muscles, splanchnic organs, and kidneys. Impaired circulation of skeletal muscle with a diminished oxygen supply is a major contributor to exercise intolerance and fatigue, a common and sometimes debilitating symptom in patients with HF.[1-3] The sympathetic nervous system is activated very early in the disease process (**see also Chapter 13**), whereas the renin-angiotensin system is usually activated when clinical symptoms develop (**see also Chapter 5**). Vasopressin is released mainly in very advanced stages of chronic HF when systemic perfusion is already threatened. Furthermore, chronic severe HF is associated with an increased endothelial release of locally acting vasoconstricting factors such as endothelin.

These endogenous vasoconstricting factors are counterbalanced in part by endogenous vasodilators.[4-6] In normal individuals, natriuretic peptides attenuate the release of norepinephrine, renin, and vasopressin, as well as their actions on peripheral blood vessels and within the kidneys. In addition, the continuous release of endothelium-derived relaxing factor (nitric oxide) from the endothelium normally counteracts the vasoconstricting factors. In fact, the continuous basal release of nitric oxide keeps the peripheral vasculature in a dilated state. However, in patients with HF, the effects of circulating and locally active vasodilators are attenuated. The release of atrial natriuretic peptide (ANP) is blunted in chronic HF, and the effects of both ANP and B-type natriuretic peptide (BNP) lose their ability to suppress the release of renin or dilate peripheral blood vessels (**see also Chapter 9**). In addition, the vascular availability of nitric oxide is severely diminished in patients with chronic HF.[7] Thus diminished vasodilator forces leave the actions of vasoconstrictors unopposed. It is important to note that the interaction of the sympathetic and renin-angiotensin system even amplifies their vasoconstricting effects. Increased sympathetic activity increases the release of renin and vice versa, and angiotensin enhances the release of both norepinephrine and vasopressin.

PATHOPHYSIOLOGIC INSIGHTS

One of the important insights that has emerged from studies on the peripheral circulation in HF is that endothelial dysfunction plays a significant role in the pathogenesis, symptomatic status, and prognosis in HF. It contributes to the impaired coronary and systemic perfusion and reduced exercise capacity in patients with HF.[8] The endothelium is a monolayer of cells that cover the luminal side of the heart and all blood vessels, from the aorta to the capillaries. Historically, the endothelium was considered a relatively inert "border" between the blood and surrounding tissues. However, over the past two decades the endothelial cells, building blocks of the endothelium, were found to exert an extremely diverse range of activities implicated in cardiovascular biology and pathology. Indeed, the endothelium regulates vasomotor function, hemostatic status, angiogenesis, the balance of prooxidant and antioxidant, and proinflammatory and antiinflammatory processes.[9] Adjacent endothelial cells can exhibit differential signaling to modulate functional properties of specialized cardiomyocytes (e.g., "pacemaker cells").[10] All these activities are highly relevant to the clinical status of the patients with compromised cardiac function, who are vulnerable to even minor shifts in hemodynamic and homeostatic state.[1-3] Of note, the vast majority of research data in HF have focused on HF with impaired systolic function with previously limited information available on HF with preserved ejection fraction (HFpEF). However, evidence for the role of endothelial dysfunction in HFpEF is growing (**see also Chapter 11**).[11] For example, Lee and colleagues showed that patients with HFpEF have impaired macrovascular and microvascular functions as compared with age- and sex-matched controls.[12] Cardiac endothelial dysfunction plays a key role in HFpEF leading to cardiomyocyte dysfunction, unfavorable left ventricular (LV) concentric remodeling and resulting diastolic dysfunction.[13]

Although the term *endothelial dysfunction* is used throughout the chapter, there is a continuum from endothelial *activation* to endothelial "dysfunction" and endothelial "damage."[4,5] Endothelial *activation* usually refers to a physiologic response to various stimuli (including inflammatory cytokines), such as bleeding and infection, aiming to preserve homeostatic stability of the host (protective changes). Endothelial "activation" may involve increased expression and shedding of some surface adhesion molecules, release of von Willebrand factor, and fibrinolytic factors. A crucial aspect of "activation" is that it is reversible upon cessation of the activating agent(s). In contrast, endothelial *dysfunction* refers to the situations of sustained excessive (e.g., increased reactive oxygen species [ROS] production) or depressed (e.g., impaired vasodilation) endothelial performance. Given that endothelial "dysfunction" could follow chronic "activation" (e.g., by prolonged and inappropriate activation by inflammatory cytokines), there is clear overlap between the two states. In terms of blood flow control, a major pathologic feature of endothelial dysfunction (in the context of cardiovascular disorders) is a functional deficiency of endothelial nitric oxide synthase (eNOS). This results in the reduced bioavailability of nitric oxide and excessive formation of ROS within the vascular wall and leads to endothelial dysfunction.[8] Dysfunction may be reversible, whereas endothelial *damage* refers to the extreme degree of endothelial dysfunction characterized by premature apoptosis/death of endothelial cells. Increased shedding of the circulating endothelial cells and high plasma concentrations of von Willebrand factor are considered markers of endothelial damage. Such damage is unlikely to be reversible.[4]

Although the endothelium serves as a critical regulator of different aspects of vascular biology, such as hemostasis and inflammation, its ability to produce nitric oxide is pivotal for the different endothelial-dependent functions related to the development and progression of HF. In addition to the regulation of the hemodynamics, nitric oxide acts as a potent modulator of myocardial oxygen consumption in the failing heart.[6,7] The reduced availability of nitric oxide in HF stems either from its reduced production by eNOS or accelerated nitric oxide degradation by ROS (**Fig. 14.1**). Downregulation of constitutively expressed eNOS by the endothelium is a characteristic feature of endothelial dysfunction that can be related to LV impairment.[14] Paradoxically, the chronic production of nitric oxide by inducible nitric oxide synthase (iNOS) in HF exerts detrimental effects on ventricular contractility and circulatory function.[15] However, direct evidence for a pathogenic role of iNOS in human HF remains limited. Treatment with NOS inhibitors has no effect on the contraction of the failing heart or β-adrenoceptor sensitivity of ventricular myocytes.[16,17]

Mice lacking eNOS have abnormal cardiac nitric oxide production, impaired myocardial glucose uptake, and pathologic concentric LV remodeling, whereas eNOS overexpression reduced severity of HF.[18-20] Targeted overexpression of the eNOS gene within the vascular endothelium in mice has attenuated cardiac and pulmonary dysfunction and led to dramatic improvement in survival during severe HF.[20] On the other hand, Scherrer-Crosbie et al. have demonstrated that eNOS-deficient mice have increased end-diastolic diameter and end-diastolic volume and depressed contractility, fractional shortening, and survival when compared with wild-type mice after 4 weeks of coronary artery ligation.[21] Interestingly, the capillary density was lower in postinfarction eNOS-deficient mice compared with wild-type animals, indicating a role for nitric oxide in postinfarction capillary preservation.[21] Reduced eNOS activity leads to the hypertrophic growth of cardiomyocytes in vitro and eNOS deficiency in mice was associated with impaired myocardial angiogenesis.[22,23] Although eNOS mRNA is reduced in LV

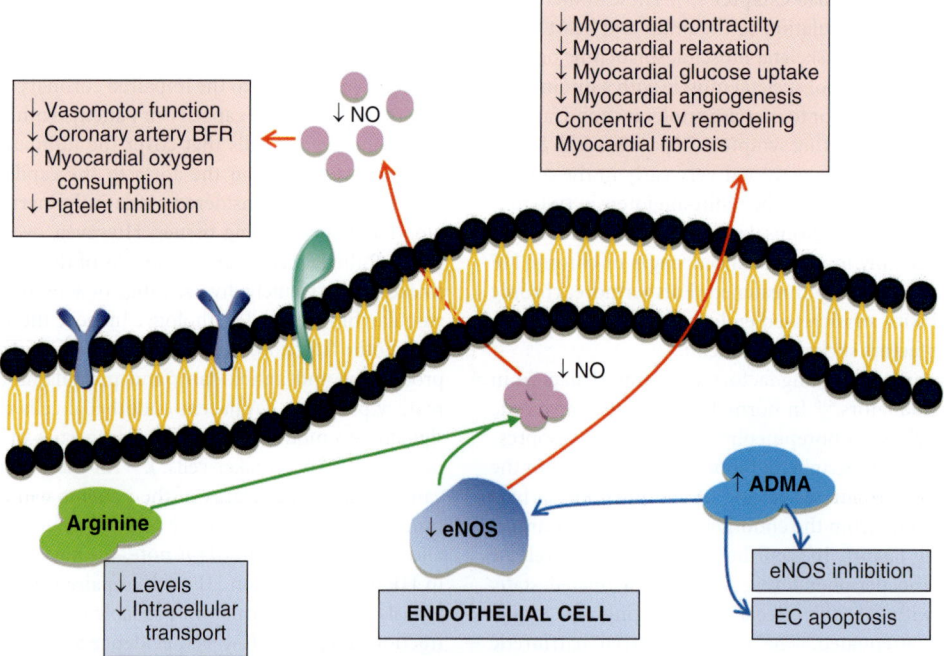

Fig. 14.1 Mechanisms and effects of vasomotor endothelial function in heart failure. Vasomotor endothelial dysfunction is featured by reduced *endothelial nitric oxide synthase (eNOS)* expression and nitric oxide *(NO)* production. It can also be contributed by diminished arginine availability and its impaired intracellular function, as well as upregulation of the endogenous eNOS inhibitor, asymmetric dimethylarginine *(ADMA)*. In heart failure, these abnormalities lead to the reduced coronary blood flow reserve, increased myocardial oxygen consumption, impaired cardiac function, angiogenesis, enhanced cardiac remodeling, and fibrosis. *BFR*, Blood flow reserve; *EC*, Endothelial cell; *LV*, left ventricular.

tissue of patients with end-stage HF, iNOS mRNA is upregulated and associates with impaired myocardial relaxation.[16] iNOS is located primarily and invariably in the endothelium and smooth muscle cells of the myocardial vasculature, and its expression is associated with the condition of HF per se rather than related to HF etiology.[24] Patients with advanced HF have increased circulating levels of proinflammatory cytokines.[25,26] Several studies have shown that proinflammatory cytokines such as interleukin-1β (IL-1β), tumor necrosis factor-α (TNF-α), and interferon-γ (IFN-γ) stimulate nitric oxide synthesis in cardiac myocytes by inducing iNOS expression.[27-29] Nitric oxide induced by cytokines leads to sustained reduced myocardial contractility and negative chronotropic effects on cardiac myocytes.[30]

An excess in ROS causes endothelial dysfunction by accelerating nitric oxide inactivation (**see also Chapter 8**). The family of multisubunit nicotinamide adenine dinucleotide phosphate (NADPH) oxidases is a major contributor to the increase in superoxide anion production and oxidative stress is upregulated in HF.[31] Depression of the endothelial function and eNOS activity may directly lead to increased ROS release, thus maintaining a vicious circle of oxidative stress. In a rat model of diastolic HF, the increase in cardiac eNOS expression by the eNOS enhancer, AVE3085 (which is an activator of eNOS transcription), is accompanied by the reduction in NADPH oxidase, as well as attenuation of cardiac hypertrophy, fibrosis, and diastolic dysfunction.[32]

Antioxidant capacity is also diminished in HF. In animal experiments, activity of different superoxide dismutase (SOD) isoforms is present in the failing myocardium and gene transfer of extracellular SOD significantly improves endothelial function.[33-35] Increased xanthine-oxidase and reduced extracellular SOD activity is closely associated with increased vascular oxidative stress in HF patients, indicating increased oxidative burden and loss of vascular oxidative balance as possible contributors to endothelial dysfunction in HF.[36]

There are in vivo and in vitro data for impaired arginine (eNOS substrate) transport in human HF.[37] This is mediated by the biochemical system y+ carrier, which is principally represented by the CAT-1 transporter.[38] The arginine uptake and mitochondrial expression of the CAT-1 arginine transporter are significantly reduced in HF.[38] Williams and colleagues have shown that higher mitochondrial L-arginine availability achieved by transfection of a mitochondrially targeted CAT-1 significantly improved cardiomyocyte response to mitochondrial stresses, reduced oxidative stress, and improving survival.[38] In addition, circulating levels of asymmetric dimethylarginine (ADMA; an endogenous inhibitor of eNOS and circulating proinflammatory cytokines) are increased in HF, further contributing to endothelial dysfunction and accelerated apoptosis of endothelial cells.[39] In patients with ischemic chronic HF elevated plasma, ADMA levels tend to be related to higher New York Heart Association (NYHA) functional classes, increased N-terminal (NT)-proBNP levels, and worse clinical outcomes.[40] A strong correlation has been demonstrated between eNOS downregulation and endothelial apoptosis.[41] Of some interest, the β-blocker carvedilol suppresses the caspase cascade and excessive human umbilical vein endothelial cell apoptosis induced by the serum from HF patients or addition of TNF-α.[42]

Inflammatory changes are common in patients with HF, with numerous studies reporting high concentrations of cytokines (e.g., TNF-α and IL-6) and C-reactive protein (CRP) (**see also Chapter 7**).[25,43-46] These biomarkers strongly correlate with HF severity and are strong and independent predictors of mortality.[43-47] In animal models, inflammation is not an innocent bystander but is rather an active participant in HF development and progression.[48] A dysfunctional endothelium also facilitates a proinflammatory status in HF by release of inflammatory factors, such as pentraxin 3 (**see also Chapter 33**). Endothelial activation of nuclear factor-κB, a key proinflammatory

transcriptional factor, is more prominent in patients with severe HF undergoing heart transplantation.[49] Of note, pentraxin 3 levels independently predict cardiac death or HF-related rehospitalization.[50] Despite the strong evidence of a detrimental impact of inflammation in HF outcome, data on specific biologic therapies against TNF-α (i.e., using etanercept and infliximab) have been generally disappointing (**see also Chapter 7**).[51,52]

Endothelial Dysfunction in Clinical Heart Failure

Direct evidence of involvement of the endothelial dysfunction in the genesis of hemodynamic abnormalities in HF derives from data on infusion of NG-monomethyl-L-arginine (L-NMMA), an inhibitor of nitric oxide production, to volunteers with HF.[53] Administration of L-NMMA increases median pulmonary and systemic vascular resistances and arterial pressures, characteristic features of the HF syndrome. Numerous studies have demonstrated peripheral endothelium-dependent vasomotor abnormalities in HF assessed by brachial artery flow-mediated dilation (FMD) or forearm blood flow changes in response to acetylcholine.[54-56] However, many such studies show weak, if any, correlations between these measures of endothelial dysfunction and clinical parameters of HF severity, cardiac contractility, or wedge pressure.[56-58]

Although the presence of endothelial dysfunction has been uniformly reported in ischemic HF, the evidence is less robust in the case of nonischemic cardiomyopathy. Some data show no evidence of endothelial dysfunction in HF, whereas some reports show a lesser degree of endothelial abnormalities and other data suggest similar abnormalities in ischemic and nonischemic cardiomyopathy.[54,59-61] Both endothelial-dependent and endothelial-independent vasodilation have demonstrated HF secondary to valvular heart disease.[62] Although endothelial dysfunction is a feature of HF of any etiology, multiple cardiovascular risk factors and comorbidities that are common in patients with ischemic HF (e.g., diabetes, systemic atherosclerosis) can contribute to systemic endothelial impairment per se. In contrast, patients with nonischemic HF tend to have more localized endothelial dysfunction limited to the cardiac vasculature. The evidence supporting this concept will be discussed later.

Endothelial Dysfunction of the Coronary Circulation in Heart Failure

Evidence of endothelial dysfunction of coronary arteries is uniformly present in patients with HF of any etiology.[63] Coronary artery endothelial dysfunction appears to play a particular role in nonischemic cardiomyopathy. As opposed to ischemic HF, in which atherosclerosis often affects multiple vascular sites, pathogenic processes in many forms of nonischemic cardiomyopathy are predominantly confined to the heart itself. Under these circumstances, prominent coronary endothelial dysfunction may be seen without any signs of peripheral artery endothelial dysfunction present. In some patients with nonischemic HF, impairment of endothelial function may occur and be attributable to the unmatched circulatory demand related to the failing heart. Of note, in patients with nonischemic LV dysfunction, significant impairment of the endothelial function is evident despite normal epicardial coronary arteries.[64] Profound coronary endothelial dysfunction seen in patients with acute-onset dilated cardiomyopathy suggests early involvement of the endothelium in the pathogenic process.[65]

In ischemic HF, coronary endothelial impairment parallels systemic endothelial dysfunction and involves both resistance and conductance vessels. However, coronary endothelial dysfunction in ischemic HF can vary substantially in its severity, possibly reflecting individual pathologic features of the disease (e.g., inflammatory activity).[66] Pathophysiologic significance of dysfunctional coronary endothelium in ischemic cardiomyopathy is supported by the link between the degree of depression of the coronary blood flow reserve (an index of coronary endothelial dysfunction), magnitude of unfavorable cardiac geometry, and rise in BNP levels.[67,68]

Activity of the coronary endothelium affects both systolic and diastolic cardiac function. Vasomotor capacity of the coronary arteries is predictive of subsequent improvement in LV contractility.[65] The status of coronary endothelium is also independently linked to the impaired cardiac relaxation in patients with preserved systolic function.[69] In addition, in patients with ischemic heart disease, coronary endothelial dysfunction predicts progression of the myocardial diastolic dysfunction.[70] The details of molecular mechanisms that link endothelial dysfunction and abnormalities in cardiac contractility and relaxation are still to be understood; however, the altered balance between the generation of nitric oxide and the elimination of nitric oxide in the heart has been shown to be important with respect to the transition from cardiac hypertrophy to HF in experimental animals.[71] Both activity and expression of the normal eNOS in cardiac tissue are reduced, whereas potentially detrimental iNOS is increased in failing human hearts.[71,72] A direct mutual relationship between the coronary endothelial perturbations and pathogenesis of cardiac dysfunction in humans is difficult to establish, and to some extent coronary endothelial dysfunction could still be secondary to the other cardiac pathologic processes.

Systemic Nature of Endothelial Dysfunction in Heart Failure

As was mentioned previously, in most patients with HF, endothelial dysfunction is not confined to a single arterial bed but rather shows a systemic pattern of distribution with peripheral arteries, such as the brachial or radial artery being affected in parallel with the heart vessels. The systemic nature of the endothelial abnormalities spreads beyond the arterial tree itself. Accumulating evidence shows the endothelial dysfunction in systolic HF also involves the venous and capillary endothelium. Endothelium-dependent venodilation is impaired in chronic HF but particularly so in the acute decompensated phase of the disease.[73] Improvement in vasomotor venous function in patients with decompensated systolic HF is accompanied by increase in exercise tolerance.[73] Animal experiments showed inflammatory activation of the venous endothelial cells secondary to vascular stress and peripheral blood flow congestion typical of HF.[74] However, knowledge of clinical significance of the venous endothelial function in this disorder is limited, and evidence of any independent role of venous endothelial abnormalities in the pathogenesis and prognosis in HF is lacking. It is likely that the bulk of venous endothelial abnormalities may be a consequence rather than a course of HF.[75] Similar to arterial endothelial arterial dysfunction, changes in activity of the venous endothelium appear to vary depending on HF etiology, with no venous endothelial dysfunction evident in patients with chronic nonischemic HF even when the arterial endothelial dysfunction is present.[76]

Resting exhaled nitric oxide, a marker of pulmonary endothelial nitric oxide production, is increased in HF, potentially indicating preserved endothelial function of the pulmonary vessels.[77] Although one may speculate about the possibility that enhanced nitric oxide production may play a role in counterbalancing systemic endothelial dysfunction, this hypothesis seems unlikely. It is not clear whether this increased nitric oxide generation is mediated by eNOS associated with normal endothelial function or iNOS associated with uncontrolled nitric oxide release under conditions of abnormal systemic homeostasis (e.g., in sepsis) and responsible for excessive oxidative stress. The fact that patients with HF have reduced ability to increase nitric oxide release by pulmonary arteries during exercise despite enhanced resting nitric oxide production points toward the presence of endothelial dysfunction in the pulmonary vascular system. The presence of systemic

endothelial dysfunction in HF is also supported by studies that have demonstrated a defective endothelium-dependent dilatory response of the microvascular bed.[78,79] Microvascular endothelial dysfunction, together with reduced capillary density seen in systolic HF, may significantly contribute to the chronic hypoxia of peripheral tissues, symptoms of fatigue, and poor exercise tolerance.[80]

Chronic dysfunction in the endothelium in HF contributes to the remodeling of peripheral arteries, resulting in the hypertrophy and reduced elastic properties.[81,82] Impaired endothelium-dependent vasodilation correlates with the vascular wall hypertrophy and abnormalities of the local arterial elastic characteristics, such as distensibility and compliance.[82,83] This systemic nature of endothelial dysfunction seen in HF reflects the concept of the endothelium as a single unique organ. Nevertheless, this approach also acknowledges significant diversity in phenotype and function of endothelial cells located within different segments of the vascular tree. Further research is still required to provide a holistic view on systemic versus local endothelial disarrangements in the pathophysiology of HF.

ENDOTHELIAL DYSFUNCTION AND CLINICAL OUTCOMES IN HEART FAILURE

Evidence of clinical significance of vasomotor endothelial dysfunction in patients with HF is provided by several prospective outcome studies (**Table 14.1**). All these studies consistently demonstrate an independent relationship between the degree of endothelial dysfunction and the risk of negative outcome. This relationship was true across a population of patients ranging from mild HF (NYHA class I) with relatively preserved cardiac contractility to those with advanced disease (NYHA class IV) with severely depressed LV function.[84,85] Systemic levels of the natural eNOS inhibitor, ADMA, which are elevated in systolic HF, independently predict a reduced effective renal plasma flow.[86] This potentially makes endothelial dysfunction partly responsible for the progressive deterioration of renal function seen in many patients with HF.

Although the severity of vasomotor endothelial dysfunction may vary among patients with ischemic or nonischemic cause of HF, the predictive power of endothelial dysfunction on prognosis does not depend on the HF etiology. Once developed, endothelial dysfunction bears similarly high risk of unfavorable events in both ischemic and nonischemic HF. Moreover, endothelial dysfunction of coronary arteries in patients after cardiac transplantation also independently predicts the risk of future cardiovascular events and death.[87] Endothelial dysfunction may be also accountable for some cases of suboptimal response to cardiac resynchronization therapy. The association of clinical improvement after cardiac resynchronization therapy and magnitude of endothelium-dependent vasodilation is independent from the factors commonly used to select patients for treatment, such as QRS complex duration, LV ejection fraction, or degree of LV dyssynchrony.[88] Improvement in exercise tolerance after cardiac resynchronization therapy is accompanied by improvements in endothelial vasodilatory capacity, although a causative relationship between the changes cannot be established.[88] Recently, endothelial dysfunction has been shown to be of prognostic significance in patients with HFpEF.[89,90] However, the clinical significance of the endothelial dysfunction in HF is somewhat limited by relatively small populations of the studied patients, as well as the short- to middle-term duration of follow-up.

Circulating Markers of Endothelial Dysfunction in Heart Failure

The impairment of endothelial function in HF is not limited to vasomotor capacity but apparently affects all the diverse aspects of the endothelial activity, including proinflammatory activation of endothelial cells

TABLE 14.1 Endothelial Dysfunction and Clinical Outcomes in Heart Failure

Study	Study Population	NYHA / Ejection Fraction	Measure of Endothelial Function	Follow-up Duration	Outcome	Results[a]
Shechter et al.[85]	82 (100% IHF)	IV/22 ± 3	FMD	14 months	Death	HR (median FMD) 2.04; 95% CI 1.09–5.1, $P = .03$
de Berrazueta et al.[175]	242 (38% IHF)	I–IV/36 ± 13	FBF in response to ACH (VOP)	5 years	Composite of death, heart attack, angina, stroke, NYHA class IV, or hospitalization due to HF	HR [Exp(B)] 0.67; SE 0.18, $P = .01$
Heitzer et al.[84]	289 (56% IHF)	I/41 ± 7	FBF in response to ACH (VOP)	4.8 years	Composite of death from cardiac causes, hospitalization due to HF, heart transplantation	HR 0.96; 95% CI 0.94–0.98, $P = .007$
Katz et al.[176]	149 (33% IHF)	II–III/25 ± 1	FMD	28 months	Death or urgent transplantation	HR (1% decrease in FMD) 1.20; 95% CI 1.03–1.45, $P = .027$
Katz et al.[176]	110 (56% IHF)	II–III/25 ± 1	Exhaled NO production	13 months	Death or urgent transplantation	HR 1.31; 95% CI 1.01–1.69, $P = .04$
Fischer et al.[177]	67 (64% IHF)	II–III/47 ± 10	FMD	46 months	Composite of cardiac death, hospitalization due to HF, or heart transplantation	HR [Exp(B)] 0.665; SE 0.18, $P = .01$
Kübrich et al.[87]	185 heart transplant recipients (32% IHF)	75 ± 10	Coronary vasomotor function	60 months	Composite of death, progressive HF, myocardial infarction, percutaneous or surgical coronary revascularization	RR 1.97; CI 1.1–3.6, $P = .028$

[a]For all, endothelial function was an independent predictor of outcome.
ACH, Acetylcholine; *CI*, confidence interval; *FBF*, forearm blood flow; *FMD*, flow-mediated dilation; *HF*, heart failure; *HR*, hazard ratio; *IHF*, ischemic heart failure; *NO*, nitric oxide; *NYHA*, New York Heart Association; *RR*, relative risk; *SE*, standard error; *VOP*, venous occlusion plethysmography.

and failure of the antioxidant defense system (**Fig. 14.2**). Among multiple regulatory proteins produced by the endothelium, several have emerged as useful blood markers of endothelial activation or damage. In respect to the HF, increased levels of plasma markers of endothelial activation (e.g., E-selectin) and damage (e.g., von Willebrand factor) are commonly seen (**Table 14.2**). However, most of these studies compared data obtained from patients with HF with those from healthy individuals. Consequently, it is difficult to differentiate precisely the scale to which the endothelial changes are attributable to the HF per se or to comorbidities and risk factors (such as hypercholesterolemia), which are often seen in patients with HF and known to be associated with endothelial perturbation. The influence of comorbidities and risk factors on endothelial function may partly explain why levels of von Willebrand factor and E-selectin do not always correlate with measures of HF severity, such as LV ejection fraction, BNP, HF functional status, or exercise tolerance.[91,92] This viewpoint is also supported by lack of significant differences in parameters of plasma markers of endothelial activation and damage between patients with acute decompensated and chronic HF. Furthermore, increased concentrations of E-selectin and von Willebrand factor in HF were reported in patients with concomitant diabetes but not in diabetes-free patients.[93]

Counts of circulating endothelial cells, another index of endothelial damage, are increased to similar degree in subjects with acute and chronic HF and correlate with other measures of endothelial damage/dysfunction (e.g., levels of von Willebrand factor and E-selectin and FMD).[55,94] In relation to clinical parameters, circulating endothelial cell counts parallel plasma levels of BNP but not LV contractility or HF functional class.[55,94]

Endothelin-1 is a very powerful vasoconstrictor, and overproduction is related to the pathogenesis of various cardiovascular diseases.[95] Although produced by endothelial cells, the role of blood endothelin-1

levels—a marker of endothelial dysfunction—has significant limitations. First, its generation is not exclusive to the endothelium, and it is also produced by vascular smooth muscle cells.[95] Second, this regulatory protein predominantly acts in a paracrine manner being released toward the location of the vascular smooth muscles rather than to the arterial lumen. Nevertheless, endothelin-1 overexpression is implicated in endothelial dysfunction, and its plasma levels correlate with degree of impairment of the endothelium-mediated vasodilation.[96] Plasma endothelin-1 levels are increased in HF patients and inhibit endothelial activity by stimulation of ADMA production, at least in experimental HF.[97,98] Consequently, increased endothelin-1 activity in HF represents one of the mechanisms responsible for endothelial dysfunction. In experimental work, pharmacologic inhibition of the endothelin-1 pathway significantly improved vasomotor endothelial function.[99] In addition, in patients with HF, vasomotor endothelial function improved following administration of small doses of an endothelin A receptor blocker.[100] However, endothelin receptor blockers failed to demonstrate any significant clinical benefits in randomized clinical trials conducted on patients with HF.[101]

PROTHROMBOTIC TRANSFORMATION OF THE ENDOTHELIUM IN HEART FAILURE

Chronic HF is an independent and major risk factor for venous thromboembolism (VTE) and confers a considerable prothrombotic risk in both inpatient and outpatient settings.[102-104] The annual incidence of VTE is 1.7% to 2.7% in HF compared with approximately 0.1% in the general population.[105] The frequency of PE in patients with HF ranges from 0.9% to 39% and deep vein thrombosis (DVT) varies from 10% to 59%.[106] Three large, well-designed, double-blinded, placebo-controlled studies of hospitalized medical patients at risk of VTE showed

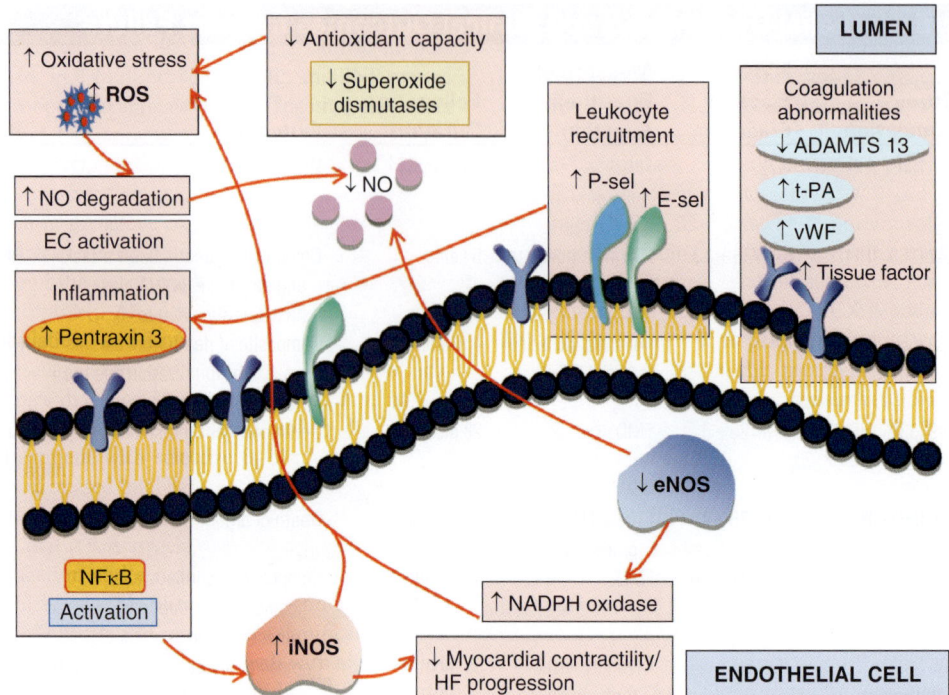

Fig. 14.2 Diversity of endothelium-related abnormalities in HF. Endothelial dysfunction in HF parallels enhanced oxidative stress, which contributes to accelerated nitric oxide *(NO)* degradation, and proinflammatory activation of endothelial cells *(ECs)*. Activated endothelium produces different inflammatory molecules, such as pentraxin, and also attracts inflammatory cells (leukocytes) in the vascular wall, thus completing the vicious circle on proinflammatory changes. In addition, dysfunctional endothelium shifts toward a prothrombotic phenotype, associated with increased production of von Willebrand factor, tissue factor, tissue type plasminogen activator *(t-PA)*, and reduced expression of ADAMTS 13. *eNOS,* Endothelial NO synthase; *E-sel,* soluble E-selectin; *HF,* heart failure; *iNOS,* inducible NO synthase; *NFκB,* nuclear factor-κB; *P-sel,* soluble P-selectin; *ROS,* reactive oxygen species.

that 25% to 50% of these admissions were due to HF.[107-109] Although the genesis of prothrombotic risk in HF is multifactorial and includes low cardiac output, dilation of cardiac chambers, and stasis of blood in peripheral vascular beds, endothelial damage/dysfunction is considered an important contributor to this process.[101]

The prominent antithrombotic characteristics of healthy endothelial cells are changed dramatically in the dysfunctional endothelium.[101] For example, the abundance of inflammatory cytokines in HF triggers endothelial expression of tissue factor, a trigger of the extrinsic coagulation cascade.[110] Active endothelial production of tissue factor results in downstream activation of factor Xa and leads to cleavage of prothrombin to form thrombin. In acute HF, high tissue factor levels are significantly correlated with inflammatory markers and are highly increased in those who died during the follow-up period.[111] In addition, tissue factor is a significant predictor of poor prognosis in chronic HF.[112]

Platelet abnormalities in observed HF are also partly attributable to endothelial impairment.[113] A dysfunctional endothelium triggers expression of platelet-activating factor, which facilitates platelet adhesion to endothelial cells and upregulates production of von Willebrand factor.[114] Dysfunctional endothelial cells release large amounts of von Willebrand factor, further promoting platelet activation and adhesion. Activity of ADAMTS13, a key von Willebrand factor–cleaving protease pivotal in the pathogenesis of prothrombotic thrombogenic purpura and hemolytic thrombogenic syndrome, is decreased in HF, being negatively correlated with BNP levels, NYHA class, and endothelial dysfunction.[115] In addition, high levels of the tissue type plasmin activator antigen (tPA), predominantly produced by endothelial cells, are independently predictive of a poor prognosis in HF.[116]

TREATMENT OF ENDOTHELIAL DYSFUNCTION IN HEART FAILURE

Pharmaceutical Agents and Endothelial Function

Given the general acceptance of the importance of endothelial dysfunction in the pathogenesis and outcome of HF, the endothelium became a target for various therapeutic interventions. Activation of the renin-angiotensin-aldosterone axis seen in HF negatively affects function of endothelial cells and disturbs nitric oxide downstream signaling (**Fig. 14.3**).[117] Favorable effects of angiotensin-converting enzyme (ACE) inhibitors on the endothelium in HF are achieved via different mechanisms, including reduction in production of vasoconstrictor prostanoids, upregulation of eNOS, and inhibition of endothelial cell apoptosis (**see also Chapter 37**).[118-120] The clinical effectiveness of inhibitors of the renin-angiotensin-aldosterone system, such as ACE inhibitors or spironolactone, in HF appears to be partly attributable to their beneficial effects on the vascular endothelium.

All published studies uniformly show improvement in endothelium-dependent vasomotor capacity and reduction in the blood levels of von Willebrand factor using neurohormonal antagonists in HF (**Table 14.3**). Several studies, including the African American Heart Failure Trial (A-HeFT), have demonstrated that improvement in morbidity, mortality, and functional status in HF treated by ACE inhibitors was linked to the improvement in endothelial function.[121,122] The capacity of various ACE inhibitors to restore endothelial function may differ significantly, and the prescription of higher treatment doses may be required.[123,124] However, the relative impact of the endothelial effects in the overall benefit of such therapy is unclear, and there is little

TABLE 14.2 Plasma Markers of Endothelial Function in Heart Failure

Study	Study population	EF, % (Inclusion Criteria/Actual)	Etiology	Controls	Marker	Results
Kistorp et al.[93]	195 CHF with diabetes	≤45/30 ± 8 in diabetic group, 30 ± 8 in nondiabetic group	74% IHF in diabetic group, 51% IHF in nondiabetic group	116 healthy	E-selectin	↑ diabetes group ↔ in nondiabetic
	147 CHF without diabetes				vWF	↑ diabetes group ↔ in nondiabetic
Chong et al.[94]	35 with AHF	≤40/30 (21–33) in AHF, 30 (29–33) in CHF	63% IHF in AHF group, 83% IHF in CHF group	32 healthy	E-selectin	↑ in AHF and CHF ↔ AHF vs. CHF
	40 with CHF				vWF	↑ in AHF and CHF ↔ AHF vs. CHF
					sTM	↑ in AHF and CHF ↑ AHF vs. CHF
Vila et al.[178]	59 CHF	Not specified	Not specified	59 healthy	vWF	↑
					thrombospondin-1	↓
Chong et al.[92]	137 CHF	≤45/30 (25–35)	61% IHF	106 healthy	E-selectin	↔
					vWF	↔
Chong et al.[94]	30 with AHF	≤40/30 (22–32) in AHF group, 30 (29–34) in CHF	70% IHF in AHF group, 80% IHF in CHF group	20 healthy	E-selectin	↑ in AHF and CHF ↔ AHF vs. CHF
	30 with CHF				vWF	↑ in AHF and CHF ↔ AHF vs. CHF
					CECs	↑ in AHF and CHF ↔ AHF vs. CHF
Leyva et al.[179]	39 CHF	Not specified/22 ± 12 in IHF, 26 ± 16 in DCM	59% IHF	16 healthy	E-selectin	↑ (↔ IHF vs. DCM)
Chong et al.[55]	30 CHF	<40/31 (29–35)	77% IHF	20 healthy	vWF	↑
					sTM	↔
					CECs	↑

↑, Increased; ↓, decreased; ↔, no changes; *AHF*, acute heart failure; *CECs*, circulating endothelial cells; *CHF*, chronic heart failure; *DCM*, dilated cardiomyopathy; *EF*, ejection fraction; *IHF*, ischemic heart failure; *sTM*, soluble thrombomodulin; *vWF*, von Willebrand factor.

evidence to justify the preference of particular ACE inhibitors based on their endothelial effects.

The majority of reported trials showed that treatment with statins improves endothelial function in HF regardless of its cause (**Table 14.4**). The exact mechanisms of the pleiotropic properties of statins on endothelium are not clear but appear to be independent of their cholesterol-lowering effects.[125,126] The statins enhance coronary nitric oxide generation in pacing-induced HF and improve endothelial function in normolipidemic patients with HF.[127-130] The cholesterol-independent nature of endothelial responses to statins is further supported by lack of any endothelial effects of ezetimibe, despite similar cholesterol-lowering capacity.[131] Furthermore, statins reduce circulating levels of the adhesion molecules intercellular adhesion molecule 1 (ICAM-1) and E-selectin, which are markers of endothelial dysfunction.[132] Statins also inhibit platelet and leucocyte adhesion and improve endothelial function.[132] It is not clear if statins have any direct specific effect on the endothelial cells to increase their production of nitric oxide. Systemic effects of statins are more likely to be implicated. Antioxidant properties of the statins were also proposed to play a role, but direct mechanistic links between the two processes are difficult to prove, leaving room for debate.[133-135] In the context of lack of evidence from randomized clinical trials to support beneficial effects of statins on outcomes in HF, endothelial dysfunction alone cannot constitute an indication for initiation of statin therapy. Obviously, many patients with HF will still receive statins because of background ischemic heart disease. A number of other medications, such as sildenafil, allopurinol, etanercept, and growth hormone, have shown favorable effects on endothelial dysfunction in HF; the clinical utility of such effects remains ambiguous

until results of appropriately designed randomized trials are available (see Table 14.3).

Nutritional Supplements and Endothelial Function in Heart Failure

L-Arginine serves as a substrate for eNOS to produce nitric oxide, and an insufficient supply of the amino acid is suggested to contribute to the development of endothelial dysfunction. In addition, L-arginine supplementation reduces concentrations of endogenous nitric oxide inhibitor ADMA, known to be elevated in HF.[39] In animals with low L-arginine levels, supplementation with a low, but not high, dose of the amino acid ameliorated endothelial dysfunction. Similar results were obtained on patients with HF. Although smaller doses of L-arginine (e.g., 8 g daily) improved endothelial function, such effects were absent in individuals receiving a higher (20 g daily) dose.[136,137] Small to moderate doses of L-arginine significantly improved exercise capacity over a 6-week treatment period in a single placebo-controlled trial study performed in patients with HF.[138] However, longer-term effects of L-arginine supplementation and its impact on clinical outcomes in HF remain unclear. Furthermore, administration of higher L-arginine doses in HF was complicated by elevation in urea and aspartate transaminase levels.[137] Accordingly, currently available evidence does not justify routine use of L-arginine supplements in HF.

A similar situation occurs with some other nutritional supplements with favorable effects on endothelial dysfunction in HF. For example, vitamin C intake can increase endothelium-dependent vasodilatory capacity, and it inhibits endothelial cell apoptosis in congestive HF (see Table 14.3).[139] Despite these predominantly short-term benefits, there

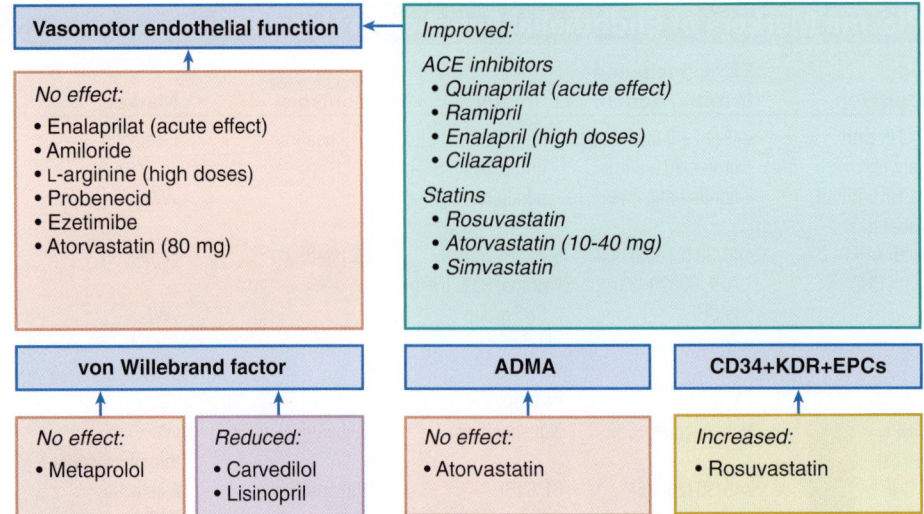

Fig. 14.3 Effects of therapeutic interventions on characteristics of endothelial function in patients with systolic heart failure. *ACE,* Angiotensin-converting enzyme; *ADMA,* asymmetric dimethylarginine; *EPCs,* endothelial progenitor cells.

is no robust evidence for routine supplementation of the diet of HF patients with antioxidant vitamins. Recently, flavanol-rich chocolate improved endothelial function in chronic HF, and its inclusion in a diet may be a suitable option.[140]

Exercise and Endothelial Function in Heart Failure

Regular moderate physical activity has become a crucial part of the healthy lifestyle recommended for patients with HF. Regular physical training in individuals with systolic LV impairment improves HF-related symptoms, exercise capacity, and quality of life and predicts a better prognosis.[141] Ultimately, cumulative analysis of the literature indicates some capacity of regular physical training to delay progression of the disease.[142] The pathophysiologic mechanisms of exercise-mediated benefits in HF are numerous and include inhibition of excessive neurohormonal activation, amelioration of inflammatory responses and oxidative burden, improvement of cardiovascular hemodynamics, and reduction of peripheral vascular resistance.[142] Vascular endothelium plays a prominent role in those processes.

Endothelial cells are capable of sensing vascular flow as changes in sheer stress. The endothelium responds to increases in luminal sheer stress by enhanced production of nitric oxide followed by relaxation of vascular wall smooth muscles and vasodilation. This process represents the essence of vasomotor function of the endothelium, and it is commonly assessed as arterial flow–mediated dilation. Physical activity provides a direct physiologic stimulus, and gentle (but regular) stimulation of the endothelium increases its nitric oxide synthase expression, accelerates L-arginine transport, and increases basal nitric oxide release.[143-147] In addition, physical training enhances the generation of proangiogenic factors, such as vascular endothelial growth factor (VEGF) and mobilization of endothelial progenitor cells, with presumable effect of development/remodeling of the vascular tree.[148,149]

Studies involving regular aerobic exercise in both ischemic and nonischemic systolic HF have consistently yielded beneficial effects on systemic endothelial function (**Table 14.5**). In contrast, static exercise confined to isolated muscle groups, such as handgrip training, has limited if any effect on systemic endothelial function.[150] The intensity and modality of the physical activity can influence resulting changes in the endothelial performance. Bouts of high-intensity exercise can lead to acute release of inflammatory cytokines and oxidative stress and thus have a detrimental effect on endothelial function.[151,152]

However, the endothelium does benefit from regular moderate aerobic exercise. Under these conditions, better vasomotor endothelial capacity is reflected by improvement in cardiac contractility and reverse LV remodeling.[153]

GENETIC PREDISPOSITION TO ENDOTHELIAL DYSFUNCTION IN HEART FAILURE

In the Genetic Risk Assessment of Heart Failure (GRAHF) substudy of the A-HeFT, the eNOS genotype differed between white and black patients with HF (**Fig. 14.4**).[154] In black patients the -786T allele was associated with lower LV ejection fraction.[154] The prevalence of allele Glu298 was significantly higher in HF patients, and the Glu298Glu genotype was associated with an increased prevalence of hypertension.[155] In addition, HF patients homozygous for eNOS promoter polymorphism (thymidine to cytosine transition [T(-786)C]) were found to have a more advanced cardiac autonomic imbalance (i.e., abnormal heart rate variability).[156] In the GRAHF study, the Glu298Asp polymorphism was associated with reduced effectiveness of fixed-dose combination of isosorbide dinitrate and hydralazine, which improved only the composite score of survival, hospitalization, and quality of life in Glu298Glu allele carriers.[154] In addition, poorer event-free survival was confirmed in HF patients with Asp298 variant of eNOS, particularly in those with nonischemic HF.[157]

ENDOTHELIAL PROGENITORS AND ANGIOGENIC FACTORS IN HEART FAILURE

Conflicting reports have been published on the numbers of circulating CD34+ hematopoietic progenitors, with some studies observing reduction or no change in their levels irrespective of HF etiology.[158] HF severity rather than its cause appears to be the main factor affecting levels of CD34+ cells. Indeed, CD34+ cells have been shown to be increased in mild HF and are depressed in severe HF, when compared with HF-free controls.[159] Other studies confirm a significant inverse correlation between CD34+, CD133+, CD34+/CD133+, and NYHA functional class, as well as their progressive reduction from NYHA class I-II to NYHA class III HF independent of cause.[160,161]

It is likely that a reduction in CD34+ cell levels is secondary to HF rather than an element of HF pathogenesis itself and is likely to

TABLE 14.3 Clinical Studies on the Effects of Pharmaceutical Agents and Nutritional Supplements on Endothelial Function in Heart Failure

Author	Study	Number of HF Patients	EF, %	Treatment[a]	Duration	Results
Boman et al.[180]	R, DB, controlled	267 (53% IHF)	25 ± 7	Carvedilol 25 mg bd or metoprolol 50 mg bd	1 year	↓vWF by carvedilol ↔vWF by metoprolol
Hornig et al.[123]	R, PC	40 (34% IHF)	≈25	Quinaprilat, enalaprilat, IA	Acute effects	↑FMD by quinaprilat ↔FMD by enalaprilat
Hryniewicz et al.[181]	R, PC, DB	64 (52% IHF)	25 ± 1	Ramipril 10 mg or sildenafil 50 mg or combination	Acute effects 1–4 hr	↑FMD (with all 3 treatments)
Drakos et al.[124]	NR	11		Enalapril 10–30 mg bd	4–8 weeks	↑FMD with higher doses
Tavli et al.[182]	NR	30 (100% IHF)	25 ± 5	Cilazapril 5 mg	3 days	↑FMD
Gibbs et al.[183]	NR	40 (80% IHF)	30	Lisinopril 10 mg od, or BB (bisoprolol 5 mg or carvedilol 25 mg od)	6 months	↓vWF
Poelzl et al.[122]	NR	33 (40% IHF)	≈24	Optimized dose of various ACEI and BB	3 months	↑FMD in responders defined by improvement in functional capacity
Farquharson et al.[184]	R, DB, PC, crossover	10 (100% IHF)	31 ± 6	Spironolactone 50 mg daily	1 month	↑FBF in response to ACH (VOP)
Macdonald et al.[185]	R, DB, PC, crossover	43 (67% IHF)	<25	Spironolactone 12.5–50 mg daily	3 months	↑FBF in response to ACH (VOP)
Abiose et al.[186]	NR	20	24 ± 9	Spironolactone	8 weeks	↑FMD
Farquharson et al.[187]	R, PC, DB	10 (100% IHF)	20 ± 8	Amiloride 5 mg od	1 month	↔FBF in response to ACH (VOP)
Belardinelli et al.[188]	R, PC, DB	51 (100% IHF)	33 ± 5	Trimetazidine 20 mg tid	4 weeks	↑RA response to ACH (US)
Ito et al.[189]	NR	12 NIHF	34	Vitamin C 1 g, IV	Acute effects	↔FMD
Hornig et al.[190]	PC	15 (20% IHF)	21	Vitamin C 0.25 g, IA; 1 g bd, oral	Acute effects 4 weeks	↑FMD
Ellis et al.[191]	R, PC, DB, crossover	10		Vitamin C 2 g, IV	Acute effects	↑FMD
Ellis et al.[192]	PC	40 NIHF	<35	Vitamin C 2 g, IV; 2 g bd, oral	Acute effects 1 month	↑FMD
Erbs et al.[193]	NR	18 (50% IHF)	25 ± 4	Vitamin C 0.5 g, IA	Acute effects	↑RA response to ACH (US)
George et al.[194]	R, PC, DB	30		Allopurinol 300 od or bd	4 weeks	↑FBF in response to ACH (VOP) (more with 300 mg bd)
Doehner et al.[195]	DB, PC, crossover	14 (79% IHF)	≈23	Allopurinol 300 mg od	1 week	↑FMD
Hambrecht et al.[136]	R	40 (40% IHF)	19 ± 3	L-arginine 8 g daily	4 weeks	↑FBF in response to ACH (VOP)
Hirooka et al.[196]	NR	20 NIHF	≈43	L-arginine 50 mg, IA	Acute effects	↑FBF in response to RH (VOP)
Chin-Dusting et al.[137]	R, PC, DB	20 (60% IHF)	21	L-arginine 20 g daily	4 weeks	↔FBF in response to ACH (VOP)
Paul et al.[197]	R, PC, DB	22 (100% IHF)	27 ± 7	Methyltetrahydrofolate, IV	Acute effects	↔PWA (salbutamol-mediated changes AI) ↓ADMA
Napoli et al.[198]	R, DB, PC	16 (31% IHF)	<40	Growth hormone (4 IU, SC every other day)	3 months	↑FBF in response to ACH (VOP)
Fichtlscherer et al.[199]	Controlled	18 (50% IHF)	25 ± 1	Etanercept 25 mg, SC, single dose	7 days	↑FBF in response to ACH (VOP)
Fuentes et al.[200]	R, PC, DB	22 (41% IHF)		800 mg magnesium oxide bd	3 months	↑small artery elasticity index
George et al.[194]	R, PC, DB	26		Probenecid 1 g daily	4 weeks	↔FBF in response to ACH (VOP)
Patel et al.[201]	NR	19 (100% IHF)	27 ± 2	Dobutamine 3 μg/kg/min, IV	72 hr	↑FMD for ≥2 weeks
Freimark et al.[202]	Controlled	20 (100% IHF)		Dobutamine, 3.5 μg/kg/min, IV, 5 hr twice a week	4 months	↑FMD

TABLE 14.3   Clinical Studies on the Effects of Pharmaceutical Agents and Nutritional Supplements on Endothelial Function in Heart Failure—cont'd

Author	Study	Number of HF Patients	EF, %	Treatment[a]	Duration	Results
Schwarz et al.[203]	R, PC	31 NIHF	19 ± 7	GTN 10^{-9} mol/L, IA	20 min or 12 hr	↑FBF in response to ACH (VOP)
Guazzi et al.[204]	DB, PC	16 (63% IHF)	≤45	Sildenafil 50 mg	Acute effects	↑FMD

[a]Oral administration unless indicated otherwise.

ACEI, Angiotensin-converting enzyme inhibitor; *ACH,* acetylcholine; *ADMA,* asymmetric dimethylarginine; *AI,* augmentation index; *BB,* beta-blocker; *bd,* twice daily; *DB,* double blind; *EF,* ejection fraction; *FBF,* forearm blood flow; *FMD,* flow-mediated dilation; *GTN,* glyceryl trinitrate; *HF,* heart failure; *IA,* intra-arterial; *IHF,* ischemic heart failure; *IU,* international units; *IV,* intravenous; *NIHF,* nonischemic heart failure; *NR,* nonrandomized; *od,* once daily; *PC,* placebo controlled; *PWA,* pulse wave analysis; *R,* randomized; *RA,* radial artery; *RH,* reactive hyperemia; *SC,* subcutaneously; *VOP,* venous occlusion plethysmography; *vWF,* von Willebrand factor.

TABLE 14.4   Clinical Studies on Statins and Endothelial Function in Heart Failure

Author	Study	Number of HF Patients	Mean EF, %	Treatment[a]	Duration	Results
Erbs et al.[134]	R, PC	42 (27% IHF)	30 ± 1	Rosuvastatin 40 mg od	12 weeks	↑FMD ↑CD34/KDR + EPCs
Gounari et al.[131]	R, DB, crossover	22 (100% IHF)	30 ± 1	Rosuvastatin 10 mg od or ezetimibe 20 mg od	4 weeks	↑FMD with rosuvastatin ↔FMD with ezetimibe
Bleske et al.[126]	R, PC, DB	15 NIHF	25 ± 9	Atorvastatin 80mg	12 weeks	↔FMD
Strey et al.[205]	R, DB, PC, crossover	23 NIHF	30 ± 8	Atorvastatin 40 mg od	6 weeks	↑FMD ↓endothelin-1
Young et al.[133]	R, PC, DB	24 (17% IHF)	31 ± 8	Atorvastatin 40 mg od	6 weeks	↑FMD ↔ADMA
Castro et al.[206]	R, PC	38	27 ± 12	Atorvastatin 20 mg od	8 weeks	↑FMD
Strey et al.[130]	R, PC, crossover	240 NIHF	<40	Atorvastatin 40 mg od	6 weeks	↑FBF in response to ACH (VOP)
Tousoulis et al.[129]	R, controlled	38 (66% IHF), cholesterol levels <220 mg/dL	≤35	Atorvastatin 10 mg od	4 weeks	↑FBF in response to RH
Tousoulis et al.[207]	R, controlled	38 (100% IHF)	≈25	Atorvastatin 10 mg od or atorvastatin 10 mg od plus vitamin E 400 IU/day	4 weeks	↑FBF in response to RH in both treatment groups, but more in atorvastatin alone group
Tousoulis et al.[208]	R, DB, crossover	22 (100% IHF)		Atorvastatin 10 mg od Atorvastatin 40 mg od	4 weeks	↑FMD with 40 mg od only
Landmesser et al.[135]	R	20 (33% IHF)	23	Simvastatin 10 mg od or ezetimibe 10 mg od	4 weeks	↑RA FMD ↑EPC ("early" EPC colonies) (for both with simvastatin but not ezetimibe)

[a]Oral administration unless indicated otherwise.

ACH, Acetylcholine; *ADMA,* asymmetric dimethylarginine; *DB,* double blind; *EF,* ejection fraction; *EPC,* endothelial progenitor cell; *FBF,* forearm blood flow; *FMD,* flow-mediated dilation; *HF,* heart failure; *IHF,* ischemic heart failure; *IU,* international units; *KDR,* kinase insert domain receptor; *NIHF,* nonischemic heart failure; *od,* once daily; *PC,* placebo controlled; *R,* randomized; *RA,* radial artery; *RH,* reactive hyperemia; *VOP,* venous occlusion plethysmography.

reflect bone marrow depression and anemia common in severe HF. These hypotheses are supported by observations that implantation of ventricular assist devices was associated with a transient increase in CD34+ cells in parallel with a reduction in BNP levels.[162] In addition, CD34+ cell numbers in HF are not affected by physical exercise testing, and transcoronary transplantation of CD34+ cells into patients with a history of an anterior myocardial infarction did not have any effect on endothelial function.[163,164] Numbers of "early" endothelial progenitor cells counted in culture are reduced in HF, being inversely related to NYHA class but not to VEGF, NT-proBNP, or CRP levels.[161,165] Migratory activity of such "early endothelial progenitor cells" is significantly impaired in HF (particularly of ischemic etiology), correlates with endothelial dysfunction, and can be normalized by physical exercise.[158,163] Functional impairment of circulating progenitors in HF is

TABLE 14.5 Exercise and Endothelial Function in Heart Failure

Author	Study Design	HF (n)	Mean EF, %	Exercise Program	Duration	Results
Wisloff et al.[153]	R, controlled	27 (100% IHF)	29	Treadmill: (i) Aerobic interval training: four 4-min intervals at 90%–95% PHR, with 3 min active pauses (walking at 50%–70% PHR) (ii) Moderate continuous training (walked at 70%–75% PHR for 47 minutes)—3 tpw	12 weeks	↑FMD (more with aerobic interval training than moderate continuous training)
Miche et al.[150]	NR	42 (77% IHF)	23	Weekly, cycle ergometer training (3 times), a 6-min walk (twice) and muscle strength training (twice)	4 weeks	↔FMD (irrespective of the presence of diabetes)
Sarto et al.[149]	NR	22 (64% IHF)	31	Cycle ergometer (55 min)—3 tpw	8 weeks	↑CD34+/KDR+ EPC ↑EC-CFU
Bank et al.[209]	NR	7	23	Handgrip exercise (30 min)—4 tpw	4-6 weeks	↔FBF in response to ACH (↑ in healthy controls)
Parnell et al.[144]	Controlled	21 (30% IHF)	22	Walking, light hand weights, and cycling (50%–60% of maximal HR) plus home-based program—3 tpw	8 weeks	↑L-arginine transport ↑FBF in response to ACH
Kobayashi et al.[210]	R, controlled	28 (46% IHF)	31	Cycle ergometer training (in two 15 min sessions per day)—2–3 tpw	3 months	↑FMD in tibial arteries ↔FMD in brachial arteries
Linke et al.[211]	R, controlled	22 (45% IHF)	25	Cycle ergometer (6 times a day for 10 min, at 70% peak oxygen consumption)	4 weeks	↑RAD in response to ACH
Hornig et al.[212]	NR	12	21	Handgrip training (70% of the maximal workload for 30 min)—daily	4 weeks	↑RAD in response to ACH
Hambrecht et al.[145]	R, controlled	20 (35% IHF)	24	Cycle ergometer (6 times daily for 10 min at 70% PHR)—first 3 weeks, followed by twice daily (40 min in total)—5 tpw	6 months	↑Femoral artery blood flow in response to ACH ↑Basal endothelial NO formation

ACH, Acetylcholine; *EC-CFU*, endothelial cell colony-forming units; *EF*, ejection fraction; *EPC*, endothelial progenitor cells; *FBF*, forearm blood flow; *FMD*, flow-mediated dilation; *HF*, heart failure; *HR*, heart rate; *IHF*, ischemic heart failure; *KDR*, kinase insert domain receptor; *NO*, nitric oxide; *NR*, nonrandomized; *PHR*, peak heart rate; *R*, randomized; *RAD*, radial artery dilation; *tpw*, times per week.

also supported by increased numbers of late apoptotic progenitors, particularly in severe HF, which correlated inversely with ejection fraction and positively with NYHA class.[166] In 107 patients with chronic HF, "early endothelial progenitor cells" were independent predictors of all-cause mortality.[165] In addition, NT-proBNP dose dependently increased the numbers and proliferative and functional capacity of human "early endothelial progenitor cells" in vitro.[167] Systemic BNP administration to mice led to a significant increase in bone marrow Sca-1/Flk-1+ endothelial progenitors and improvement in blood flow and capillary density in the ischemic limbs.[167]

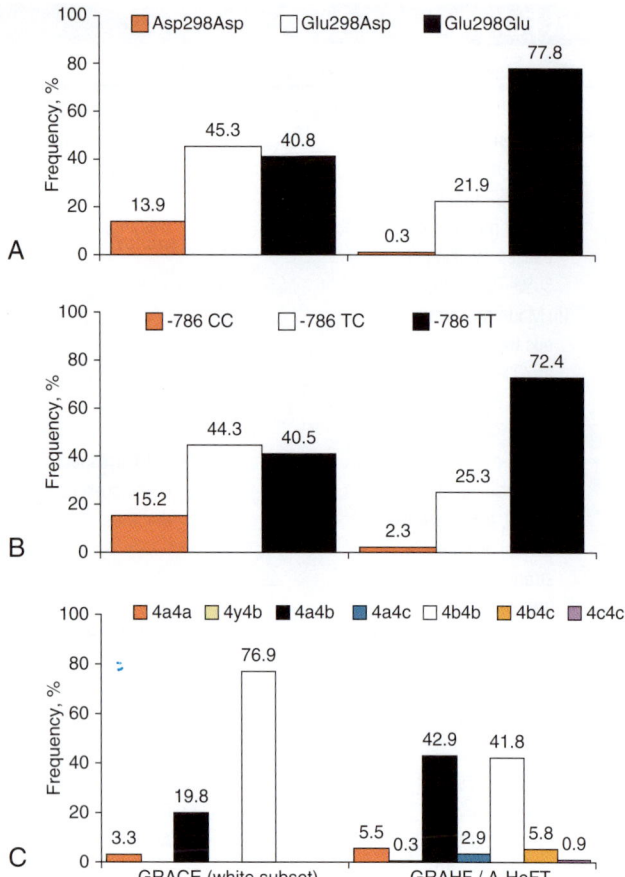

Fig. 14.4 Racial differences in NOS3 alleles: genotype frequencies for the NOS3 polymorphisms in the white heart failure cohort in Genetic Risk Assessment of Cardiac Events (GRACE) and the African-American heart failure cohort from Genetic Risk Assessment of Heart Failure (GRAHF). (A) Exon 7 Glu298Asp: prevalence of the Glu298 allele is significantly higher (*P* < .001) in GRAHF. (B) e786 T/C promoter: prevalence of the e786 T allele in significantly higher (*P* < .001) in GRAHF. (C) Intron 4 27 base-pair variable number repeat: 4y 5 2 repeats, 4a 5 4 repeats, 4b 5 5 repeats, 4c 5 6 repeats; prevalence of the 4a, y, and c alleles is significantly higher in GRAHF (*P* < .001).

CD34+KDR+ cells seem to be only significantly reduced in patients with very severe HF.[161,163] Indeed, numbers of CD34+KDR+ cells in HF are unaffected by physical exercise or implantation of ventricular assist devices.[162,163] In one randomized study, 3 months' treatment with high doses of rosuvastatin increased CD34+KDR+ cells and their integrative capacity, which paralleled a significant improvement of FMD and ejection fraction.[134]

Cell transplantation for myocardial regeneration has been shown to have beneficial effects on cardiac function after myocardial infarction (**see also Chapters 3 and 41**). In a study of patients with ischemic cardiomyopathy (ejection fraction <22%), transplantation of autologous bone marrow CD133+ cells improved functional status from NYHA class III-IV to I-II in all participants, and the approach was feasible and safe.[168] In addition, another study involving the implantation of CD133+ cells in the infarcted zone in seven candidates for cardiac

transplantation was associated with NYHA improvement, reduced NT-pro-BNP levels and risk of sudden death, and a significant increase in ejection fraction by 24 months after treatment.[169] However, the last study was small and lacked a control group, and two of the seven patients died during the period of the observation; thus larger controlled trials are essential to draw any robust conclusion on such therapies in HF.

Abnormal levels of angiogenic factors such as angiopoietin-2 and VEGF have been reported in HF patients.[170] VEGF levels are reduced in congestive HF but upregulated in acute HF.[171,172] VEGF did not independently predict outcome in chronic HF, and a pathophysiologic role of angiogenic factors in human HF is unclear.[112] However, VEGF treatment reduces myocardial apoptosis, promotes capillary growth, and preserves myocardial contractility and prolonged survival in animal studies.[173,174] In summary, the biologic and pathologic roles of altered production of angiogenic factors are still not entirely clear. They may reflect a degree of compensatory angiogenesis in patients with ischemic HF, but it is more plausible that these changes reflect an ongoing process of vascular remodeling in response to the hemodynamic changes. The potential of these pathways as therapeutic targets is still to be determined.

CONCLUSIONS AND FUTURE DIRECTIONS

Endothelial dysfunction is common in patients with systolic HF and is implicated in the pathophysiology of the disease, symptomatic status, and outcome. Endothelial abnormalities in HF are complex and involve apparently all aspects of the activity of the endothelial cells, including their vasomotor, hemostatic, antioxidant, and inflammation-related functions. There is substantial variability in the pattern of endothelial dysfunction among patients with systolic HF depending on its cause. In patients with ischemic cardiomyopathy, systemic endothelial dysfunction is typically seen within coronary and peripheral arteries, as well as the microvascular bed. In contrast, patients with nonischemic cardiomyopathy show more localized dysfunction of cardiac arteries, which may be present with or without systemic vascular involvement.

There are several pharmaceutical agents and nutritional components with suggested beneficial effects on endothelial function. However, any prognostic benefits of these agents need to have robust evidence from randomized clinical trials before their clinical implementation. At present, none of the existing agents is recommended for use in HF solely based on their endothelial properties. Improvement of endothelial function by regular aerobic physical exercise contributes to overall success of the physical training in HF. However, isolated bouts of extreme physical activity in sedentary patients may have a negative impact on the endothelium by triggering oxidative and inflammatory responses and should be avoided.

Importantly the prognostic significance of endothelial dysfunction in HF has not yet translated effectively to the clinical setting, primarily because of the significant methodologic limitations of its assessment. Indeed, the methods commonly used for research purposes lack standardization, tend to be operator dependent, and are sometimes invasive. Increasingly better understanding of molecular mechanisms of endothelial dysfunction in HF will help to identify new targets for future treatments aimed at restoring endothelial function and improved patient outcomes.

KEY REFERENCES

5. Blann AD, Woywodt A, Bertolini F, Bull TM, Buyon JP, Clancy RM, et al. Circulating endothelial cells. Biomarker of vascular disease. *Thromb Haemost*. 2005;93(2):228–235.

30. Ikeda U, Shimada K. Nitric oxide and cardiac failure. *Clin Cardiol*. 1997;20(10):837–841.

40. Hsu CP, Lin SJ, Chung MY, Lu TM. Asymmetric dimethylarginine predicts clinical outcomes in ischemic chronic heart failure. *Atherosclerosis*. 2012;225(2):504–510.

62. Nakamura M, Yoshida H, Arakawa N, Mizunuma Y, Makita S, Hiramori K. Endothelium-dependent vasodilatation is not selectively impaired in patients with chronic heart failure secondary to valvular heart disease and congenital heart disease. *Eur Heart J*. 1996;17(12):1875–1881.

70. Ma LN, Zhao SP, Gao M, Zhou QC, Fan P. Endothelial dysfunction associated with left ventricular diastolic dysfunction in patients with coronary heart disease. *Int J Cardiol*. 2000;72(3):275–279.

94. Chong AY, Lip GY, Freestone B, Blann AD. Increased circulating endothelial cells in acute heart failure: comparison with von Willebrand factor and soluble E-selectin. *Eur J Heart Fail*. 2006;8(2):167–172.

104. Howell MD, Geraci JM, Knowlton AA. Congestive heart failure and outpatient risk of venous thromboembolism: a retrospective, case-control study. *J Clin Epidemiol*. 2001;54(8):810–816.

128. Landmesser U, Engberding N, Bahlmann FH, Schaefer A, Wiencke A, Heineke A, et al. Statin-induced improvement of endothelial progenitor cell mobilization, myocardial neovascularization, left ventricular function, and survival after experimental myocardial infarction requires endothelial nitric oxide synthase. *Circulation*. 2004;110(14):1933–1939.

145. Hambrecht R, Fiehn E, Weigl C, Gielen S, Hamann C, Kaiser R, et al. Regular physical exercise corrects endothelial dysfunction and improves exercise capacity in patients with chronic heart failure. *Circulation*. 1998;98(24):2709–2715.

163. Van Craenenbroeck EM, Beckers PJ, Possemiers NM, Wuyts K, Frederix G, Hoymans VY, et al. Exercise acutely reverses dysfunction of circulating angiogenic cells in chronic heart failure. *Eur Heart J*. 2010;31(15):1924–1934.

The full reference list for this chapter is available on ExpertConsult.

Alterations in Kidney Function Associated With Heart Failure

Tamar S. Polonsky, George L. Bakris

Control of circulating blood volume is a tightly regulated physiological process and is critical for maintaining cardiovascular homeostasis. Under normal homeostatic conditions, there is extensive cross-talk between the kidney and the heart (the "cardiorenal axis") that is essential for regulation of salt and water homeostasis. However, as will be discussed here, in the setting of heart failure (HF), the normal mechanisms that control sodium and water balance become dysregulated secondary to the activation of neurohormonal pathways that lead to increased sympathetic activity (**see Chapter 13**) and increased activation of the renin-angiotensin system, with a resultant increase in peripheral vasoconstriction and sodium and water reabsorption.[1]

As discussed in **Chapter 13**, a decline in cardiac function results in a change in the "effective" arterial blood volume of the peripheral circulation, which can lead to a decrease in kidney function. For example, among 156,743 US veterans with HF and an estimated glomerular filtration rate (eGFR) ≥60 mL/min/1.73m^2, adults with HF had a 2.12-, 2.06-, and 2.13-fold higher multivariable-adjusted risk of incident chronic kidney disease (CKD), composite of CKD or mortality, and rapid eGFR decline, respectively.[2] The kidney acts as both a bystander and a contributor to several maladaptive processes, to maintain organ perfusion. However, reduced kidney function as a consequence of reduced cardiac output and reduced kidney blood flow is only one component of the complex cardiorenal interaction.[3] Substantial evidence also supports the role of additional pathways, such as neurohormonal mechanisms (**see Chapters 5**, **6**, and **13**) and venous congestion, in the deterioration of kidney and cardiac function.[4]

EPIDEMIOLOGY OF CHRONIC KIDNEY DISEASE AND THE IMPACT ON HEART FAILURE

Kidney dysfunction is commonly seen in both stable patients and those with acute decompensated heart failure (ADHF). Ezekowitz and colleagues demonstrated that almost 40% of outpatients with both coronary artery disease and HF have Stage 3 or higher CKD, defined as an eGFR less than 60 mL/min/1.73m^2.[5] The prevalence of Stage 3 or higher CKD was as high as 64% among patients admitted for ADHF.[6]

The presence of CKD is one of the most important prognostic factors for patients with HF, regardless of whether the ejection fraction (EF) is preserved or reduced (**Fig. 15.1**).[7] In a prospective cohort of 754 adults referred to an outpatient HF clinic, a 1% increase in 1-year mortality was seen for every 1 mL/min decrease in creatinine clearance.[8] In an observational study of 24,331 adults with HF, Smith and colleagues found a graded association of eGFR with hospitalization for HF, all-cause hospitalization, and mortality. The association was similar between patients with preserved (n = 14,579) and reduced (n = 9762) EF. Importantly, patients with CKD experienced the same reduction in mortality from treatment with angiotensin-converting enzyme inhibitors and beta-blockers as did patients with normal kidney function, although they were less likely to receive the medications.[8]

The presence of CKD is also associated with poor short-term outcomes. Data from the Acute Decompensated HF National Registry (ADHERE) showed that in-hospital mortality increased from 1.9% among patients with normal kidney function to 7.6% and 6.5% among patients with baseline CKD and kidney failure, respectively.[6] While GFR remained a significant predictor of mortality after adjusting for confounders, the blood urea nitrogen (BUN) level remained the single best predictor. Other investigators have confirmed the usefulness of BUN as a marker of increased risk.[9] In the Acute and Chronic Therapeutic Impact of a Vasopressin Antagonist in Chronic Heart Failure (ACTIV in CHF trial), patients with a baseline BUN greater than 40 mg/dL experienced an event rate of 30%, whereas patients whose baseline BUN less than 18 mg/dL had an event rate of 8.6%.[10] It is likely that, in the acute setting, BUN is a marker of neurohormonal activation, which leads to constriction of the afferent arteriole, secretion of vasopressin, and enhanced reabsorption of sodium, water, and urea. These pathways will be discussed in more detail as follows.

WORSENING KIDNEY FUNCTION AND PROGNOSIS

Worsening kidney function (WKF) among patients admitted with ADHF is often defined as an increase in creatinine ≥0.3 mg/dL. As many as one-third of patients may experience WKF, which typically occurs in the first 3 to 4 days of admission, but has also been shown

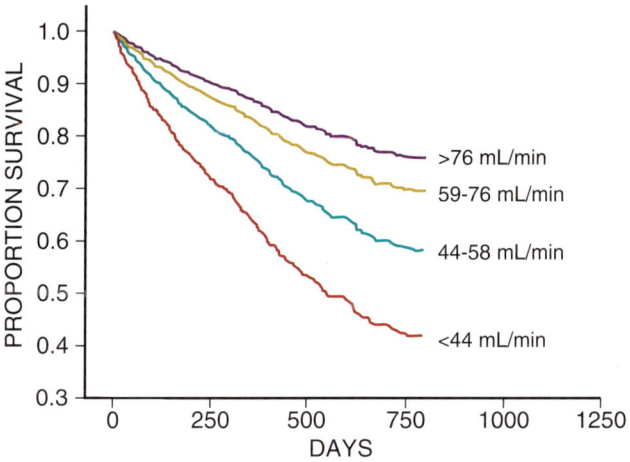

Fig. 15.1 Proportional relationship of calculated glomerular filtration rate (using the Cockcroft-Gault equation) with mortality in Cox-adjusted survival analysis. Patients had heart failure (New York Heart Association Class III or IV, left ventricular ejection fraction <35%) and were enrolled in the Second Perspective Randomized study of Ibopamine on Mortality and Efficacy (PRIME-II) trial, which investigated the oral dopamine agonist ibopamine. (From Boerrigter G, Costello-Boerrigter L, Burnett JC. Alterations in renal function in heart failure. In: Mann DM, ed. *Heart Failure: A Companion to Braunwald's Heart Disease.* 2nd ed. Philadelphia: Saunders; 2011:292; and modified from Hillege HL, Girbes AR, de Kam PJ, et al. Renal function, neurohormonal activation, and survival in patients with chronic heart failure. *Circulation.* 2000;102:203–210.)

to occur in the week after hospital discharge.[11] In the Prospective Trial of Intravenous Milrinone for Exacerbations of Chronic Heart Failure (OPTIME-CHF), 12% of participants experienced a greater than 25% decrease in eGFR and 39% experienced a greater than 25% increase in BUN.[12] In a meta-analysis of eight randomized controlled trials of renin-angiotensin-aldosterone system (RAAS) inhibitors in stable outpatients (6 HFrEF, 1 HFpEF and 1 that included both populations), the incidence of WKF was slightly higher in HFrEF compared with HFpEF (12% vs. 7%). Risk factors for WKF include baseline creatinine greater than 1.5 mg/dL, diabetes, and pulmonary edema.[13]

While earlier studies suggested that WKF portended a worse prognosis, more recent analyses suggest that the association of WKF with prognosis is highly dependent on the clinical context.[14] For example, in a study of 599 adults admitted to the hospital with ADHF, the development of WKF was associated with 1-year mortality only in patients who also had signs on physical exam of congestion at the time of hospital discharge.[15] In a study of 1232 adults admitted for ADHF, Salah and colleagues compared the relative contribution of a decrease in N-terminal-pro-B-type natriuretic peptide (NT-pro-BNP) and WKF to prognosis.[16] The authors found that WKF was not associated with 180-day mortality or readmission to the hospital for CVD among patients who had at least a 30% reduction in their NT-pro-BNP. In addition, the change in NT-pro-BNP did not predict development of severe WKF (defined as an absolute increase in serum creatinine ≥0.5 mg/dL), suggesting that severe WKF is multifactorial, and not simply explained by overly aggressive diuresis. Ibrahim and colleagues also evaluated the relative importance of NT-pro-BNP versus WKF in a randomized controlled trial of biomarker-guided HF therapy for patients with class II-IV HF with reduced ejection fraction (HFrEF).[17] The authors found that adults who achieved NT-pro-BNP levels less than 1000 pg/mL were on higher doses of RAAS inhibitors, regardless of WKF. Further, patients with WKF but an NT-pro-BNP less than 1000 pg/mL experienced significantly fewer events at 1 year (worsening

HF, hospitalization for HF or CVD death) compared with patients with no WKF but an NT-pro-BNP greater than 1000 pg/mL. Paradoxically, in the Diuretic Optimization Strategies Evaluation (DOSE) trial, a prospective multicenter trial investigating strategies of loop diuretic administration, increases in serum creatinine were associated with a lower risk for death, emergency room visits within 60 days, or rehospitalization (hazard ratio [HR] = 0.81 per 0.3 mg/dL increase, 95% CI 0.67–0.98, P = .026). Moreover, compared with those with stable kidney function, there was a strong association between improved kidney function (n = 28) and the composite endpoint (HR = 2.52, 95% CI = 1.57–4.03, P < .001). Taken together, available data suggest that for both acute and chronic management of HFrEF, it is important to prioritize decongestion and the use of evidence-based therapy, such as RAAS inhibitors, even with modest degrees of WKF.

There are few studies comparing the risk of WKF in patients with HFpEF versus HFrEF. In a meta-analysis of eight RCTs of RAAS inhibitors versus placebo (6 HFrEF, 1 HFpEF, 1 both), adults with HFrEF who were randomized to RAAS inhibitors and had WKF experienced higher rates of HF hospitalization, compared with patients who experienced no WKF (RR, 1.19 [1.08–1.31]; P < .001). However, the risk associated with WKF in patients allocated to placebo was larger (RR, 1.48 [1.35–1.62]; P < .001), and significantly different from patients randomized to RAAS inhibitors with WKF (P for interaction = .005). Adults with HFpEF who were taking RAAS inhibitors also experienced a higher risk of hospitalization if they developed WKF compared with those without WKF (RR 1.78, 95% CI 1.43–2.21). However, unlike adults with HFrEF, WKF for those on placebo did not confer an increased risk of hospitalization. While is it possible that the pathophysiology of WKF differs between HFrEF and HFpEF, it is likely that the use of RAAS inhibitors simply unmasked greater disease severity.[18]

PATHOPHYSIOLOGY OF CHRONIC KIDNEY DISEASE IN HEART FAILURE

The homeostatic relationship between the heart and kidneys with respect to maintenance of body fluid homeostasis has been appreciated for centuries. Indeed, Sir William Withering noted that patients with "dropsical" conditions, characterized by the swelling of soft tissues due to the accumulation of excess water, often experienced a brisk diuresis following the administration of foxglove.[19] In the early phases of HF, the ratio of the glomerular filtration rate to kidney blood flow (referred to as the filtration fraction) is maintained, and can even be increased. This is largely due to vasoconstrictor peptides, such as arginine vasopressin (AVP), angiotensin II, and norepinephrine (NE), which help maintain GFR by maintaining blood pressure and constricting the efferent arteriole resulting in increased intraglomerular capillary pressure (**Fig. 15.2**). The remainder of the chapter will review some of the normal physiology that controls salt and water homeostasis, and some of the cardio-kidney pathways activated and contributed to a failing heart in clinical HF.

PERIPHERAL VOLUME SENSORS

Baroreceptors and Mechanoreceptors

Numerous pressure receptors (baroreceptors, mechanoreceptors) are located in critical areas in the circulatory tree—the carotid sinus, aortic arch, afferent glomerular arterioles in the kidney, and the superior and inferior vena cava.[20-22] The receptors detect alterations in pressure and stretch of the vessel wall. In volume-depleted states, where stretch is decreased, there is a subsequent loss of tonic inhibition by the parasympathetic nervous system, which results in reflex increase sympathetic neural tone (**Fig. 15.3**). The baroreceptors of the carotid body

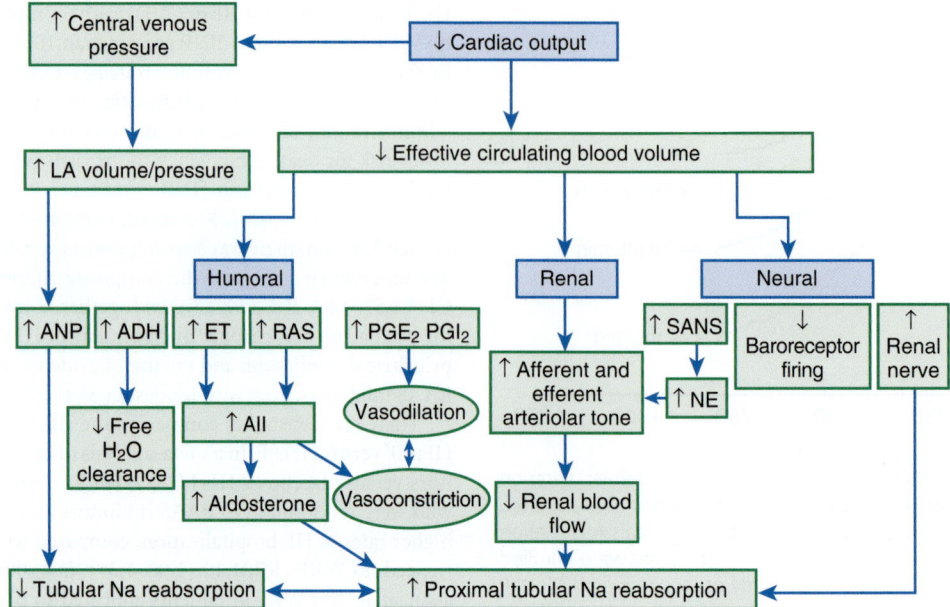

Fig. 15.2 Intraglomerular changes in heart failure (HF). Glomerular function is regulated by glomerular hydrostatic pressure, which is controlled by arterial blood pressure and segmental vascular resistances at the level of pre- and postglomerular vessels (i.e., afferent and efferent arterioles). In the early phases of HF, the ratio of the glomerular filtration rate to renal blood flow (i.e., the filtration fraction) is maintained largely because of vasoconstrictor peptides such as arginine vasopressin, angiotensin II, and norepinephrine *(NE)* that help maintain the glomerular filtration rate by maintaining blood pressure and constricting of the efferent arteriole, resulting in increased intraglomerular capillary pressure. *ADH,* Antidiuretic hormone; *AII,* angiotensin II; *ANP,* atrial natriuretic peptide; *ET,* endothelin; *LA,* left atrial; *PGE₂,* prostaglandin E₂; *PGI₂,* prostaglandin I₂; *RAS,* renin-angiotensin system; *SANS,* sympathetic autonomic nervous system.

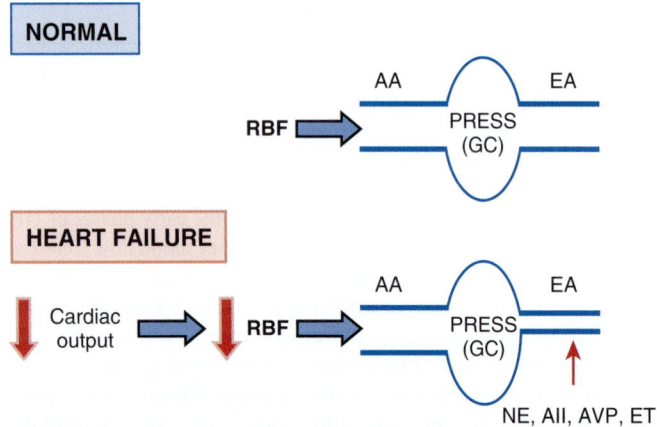

Fig. 15.3 Overview of the neurohormonal, hemodynamic, and neural changes impacting renal function in heart failure. *AA,* Afferent arteriole; *AII,* angiotensin II; *AVP,* arginine vasopressin; *EA,* afferent arteriole; *ET,* endothelin; *NE,* norepinephrine; *PRESS (GC),* pressure in the glomerular capsule; *RBF,* renal blood flow.

and aortic arch contribute to the antinatriuretic response observed in HF patients. Studies have demonstrated a reduction in urinary output and sodium excretion following volume expansion in the presence of carotid sinus excitation, despite a constant arterial pressures.[23,24]

The atria also possess baroreceptors of two types: (1) type A, located primarily at the entrance of the pulmonary veins, which discharge at the onset of systole and are not affected by volume; and (2) type B, which demonstrate increased activity with atrial filling and increase atrial size.[25,26] The neuronal inputs of the cardiac atria and

the carotid body are transmitted to the medulla and hypothalamus through cranial nerves IX and X.[20] Atrial transmural pressure has a significant influence on kidney function.[27] Experiments in dogs show that decreased atrial wall distension culminated in decreased sodium excretion and urine flow rate by the kidney.[25] In addition, the normal diuretic response to volume expansion was attenuated when atrial wall distension was limited. Other studies examine the interaction between the carotid body and neuronal control of sodium homeostasis. For example, infusion of hypertonic saline increased neural activity along the tracts, leading to the hypothalamus and medulla.[26] Conversely, increased left atrial stretch decreased activity of these neural tracts, and with a resultant increase in the urinary flow rate and sodium excretion.[25] Plasma levels of atrial natriuretic peptide (ANP) were increased, while AVP and aldosterone levels were decreased.[28] The atria and ventricles have their own baroreceptors that stimulate secretion of ANP and brain natriuretic peptide (BNP) in response to atrial or ventricular distension. ANP release can stimulate up to a 10-fold increase in sodium excretion.[27] ANP and BNP will be discussed in more detail as follows.

The Juxtaglomerular Apparatus

The juxtaglomerular apparatus of the kidney serves as a intrarenal baroreceptor that is composed of four basic elements: the terminal portion of the afferent arteriole, the macula densa (a segment of the distal tubule), the extraglomerular mesangial region, and the efferent arteriole at the glomerulus (summarized in **Fig. 15.4**).[29] Because of its location in the nephron, it is highly sensitive to changes in volume as induced by various diuretic classes, and thus it is sensitive to changes in kidney perfusion pressure. The juxtaglomerular apparatus is also known to be adrenergically innervated, and has β-1 adrenoreceptors.

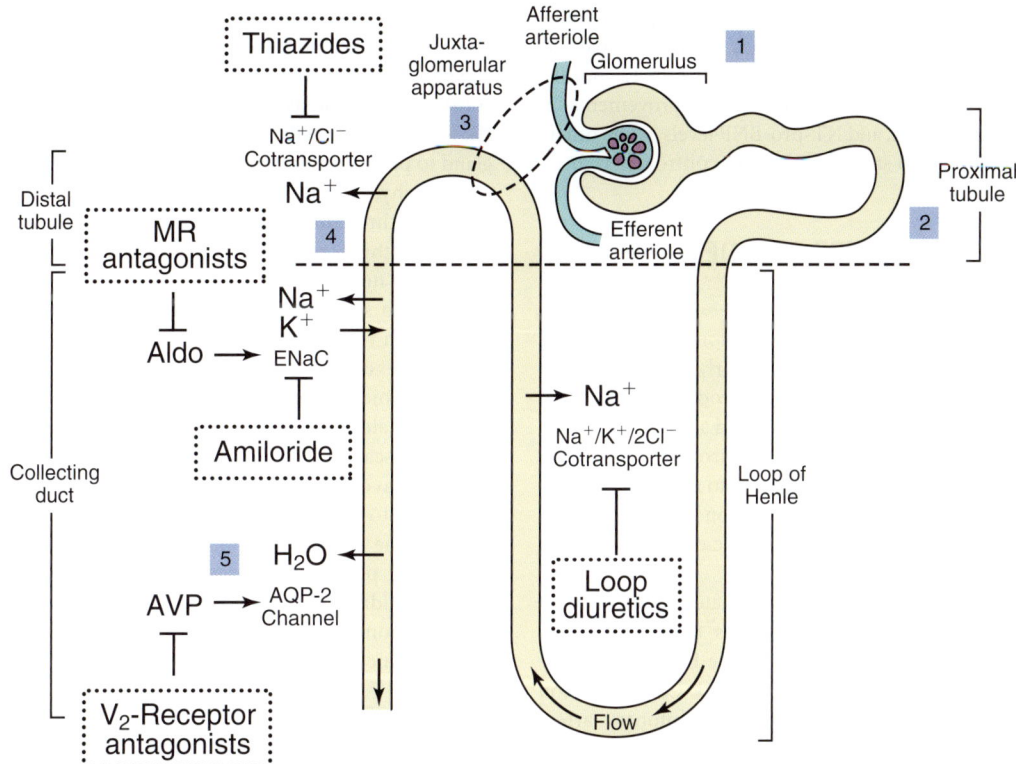

Fig. 15.4 Schematic of a single nephron with major sites of action of some conventional diuretics and the natriuretic peptides. The juxtaglomerular apparatus, located at the junction of the afferent arteriole and the distal tubule, contains renin-secreting cells. Natriuretic peptides have diverse renal actions: they can (1) increase glomerular filtration, (2) oppose proximal reabsorption of sodium by opposing angiotensin II and the sympathetic nervous system, (3) inhibit tubuloglomerular feedback and the secretion of renin, (4) inhibit sodium reabsorption in the distal tubule, and (5) promote free water excretion by opposing arginine vasopressin. *Aldo,* Aldosterone; *AQP-2,* aquaporin 2 water channel; *AVP,* arginine vasopressin; *ENaC,* epithelial sodium channel; *MR,* mineralocorticoid; *V2-Receptor,* vasopressin 2 receptor. (From Boerrigter G, Costello-Boerrigter L, Burnett JC. Alterations in renal function in heart failure. In: Mann DM, ed. *Heart Failure: A Companion to Braunwald's Heart Disease.* 2nd ed. Philadelphia: Saunders; 2011:292.)

TABLE 15.1 Factors That Inhibit or Stimulate the Renin-Angiotensin-Aldosterone System

Inhibit Activity	Stimulate Activity
Arginine vasopressin	Activation of renal sympathetic nerves
Angiotensin II	Catecholamines
Salt loading	Hypotension
β-adrenoceptor antagonists	Baroreceptor stimulation
Potassium	Hypoperfusion
Adenosine	Prostaglandin E and I series
Hypocalcemia	Upright posture
Hyperkalemia	Hypovolemia

Sympathetic stimulation or decreases in volume or perfusion pressure can all stimulate the juxtaglomerular apparatus response to release renin into the afferent arteriole. Renin then converts angiotensinogen, which is formed in the liver, to angiotensin I (**see also Chapter 5**). Angiotensin-converting enzyme converts angiotensin I to angiotensin II, which is a potent vasoconstrictor and stimulates secretion of aldosterone from the adrenal cortex. Other factors that stimulate the renin-angiotensin-aldosterone system are noted in **Table 15.1**. Most beta-blockers used clinically can cause adverse hemodynamic alterations in the kidney, including a decline in kidney blood flow and a

GFR, and a reduction of renin release with a subsequent antinatriuretic response, most prominently with upright posture.[30] However, neither nebivolol nor carvedilol appears to have adverse effects on renal hemodynamics.[31,32]

RENAL SYMPATHETIC NERVES

Renal sympathetic nerve activity has been found to be intimately related to body fluid homeostasis. Immunofluorescent electron microscopic and histochemical studies have demonstrated kidney nerves in the afferent and efferent arterioles, proximal and distal tubules, ascending limb of the loop of Henle, and the juxtaglomerular apparatus.[33] Dopaminergic receptors have also been found in the tubules and kidney nerves.[34] Increased kidney sympathetic activity leads to a decrease in kidney blood flow and a reduction in urinary sodium excretion. These effects are mediated, in part, by α1-adrenoreceptors.[34,35] Renal sympathetic activity is also modulated by salt intake. Low-salt diets increase and high-salt diets decrease nerve activity.[33] Increased kidney sympathetic nerve activity has been documented in states of volume (salt) depletion, and contributes to the associated elevation of plasma renin activity, reduction in kidney blood flow, and the subsequent antinatriuretic state.[36]

Given the importance of sympathetic activity in HF, there is interest in applying kidney denervation to this population.[37-40] Catheter-based kidney denervation involves catheterization of the femoral artery, and then applying radiofrequency energy circumferentially to the endothelium of the distal kidney artery. Pilot studies of up to 60 participants have not shown any adverse safety events over 6 to 12 months follow-up. Some studies have shown significant improvements in ejection fraction, 6-minute walk, and NT-pro-BNP levels, while others have shown neutral effects. No studies with sham controls have been reported.[41-44]

CENTRAL VENOUS PRESSURE AS A DETERMINANT OF KIDNEY FUNCTION

Early animal models have confirmed the association between central venous pressure (CVP) and kidney function. As early as 1931, Winton used a canine model to demonstrate that urine production decreased substantially at venous pressures of 20 mm Hg, and almost completely stopped at pressures greater than 25 mm Hg.[45] Chronic thoracic vena cava obstruction has been used as a model in dogs to study the association of elevated pressures in HF with kidney function.[46] Hemodynamic changes in the dogs included a decrease in cardiac output, GFR, and kidney plasma flow.

Studies in patients with heart failure demonstrate that an elevated CVP identifies those patients who will progress to develop WKF based on cardiac hemodynamic parameters. In the Evaluation Study of Congestive Heart Failure and Pulmonary Artery Catheterization Effectiveness (ESCAPE) trial—a comparison of pulmonary artery catheter-guided treatment for acute HF versus clinical assessment—there was no correlation between pulmonary capillary wedge pressure (PCWP), cardiac index (CI), or systemic vascular resistance with baseline kidney function.[47] Right atrial pressure was the only hemodynamic measure that was significantly associated with baseline kidney function. In a retrospective analysis of more than 2500 adults who underwent a right heart catheterization, Damman and colleagues found that, above a CVP of 6 mm Hg, there was a progressive decline in kidney function.[48] In a study of 145 patients hospitalized for ADHF, Mullens and colleagues found that the mean baseline CVP in patients who developed WKF was significantly higher than those who did not develop WKF (18 ± 7 mm Hg vs. 12 ± 6 mm Hg, $P < .001$).[49] Interestingly, the mean CI was higher in those who developed WKF compared with those who did not (2.0 ± 0.8 vs. 1.8 ± 0.4 L/min/m^2, $P = .008$), again challenging the notion that CKD in HF is primarily secondary to poor forward flow.[50]

Research on the association of venous congestion and CKD has also extended to studies of intra-abdominal pressure (IAP). For example, among 40 consecutive patients admitted with ADHF, 60% had an elevated IAP, defined as ≥ 8 mm Hg.[51] Of note, none of the patients complained of abdominal symptoms on admission or during therapy. Overall, mean arterial pressure, CVP, PCWP, and CI were comparable between those with and without an elevated IAP. However, those with an elevated IAP had a higher baseline creatinine (2.3 ± 1.0 mg/dL vs.1.5 ± 0.8 mg/dL, $P < .009$) and at follow-up (1.8 ± 0.8 mg/dL vs. 1.3 ± 0.9 mg/dL, $P < .04$). Among the patients with elevated IAP at baseline, improvement in kidney function was associated with an improvement in IAP, and not any other hemodynamic measurements.

NEUROHORMONAL REGULATION OF KIDNEY FUNCTION

The Renin-Angiotensin-Aldosterone System

The renin-angiotensin-aldosterone system plays a central role in the maladaptive response of sodium and water reabsorption as HF progresses (see also Chapter 5). Table 15.1 lists the factors that stimulate the renin-angiotensin-aldosterone system. Elevated renin secretion occurs early in the course of HF.[52] As noted previously, circulating levels of renin enzymatically cleave angiotensinogen, which results in the generation of angiotensin I (Ang I), and is converted to a potent vasoconstrictor, angiotensin II. Angiotensin II is later converted to Ang III, which then directly stimulates the zona glomerulosa of the adrenal gland to produce aldosterone.

The physiological effects of Ang II are many and varied. These include stimulation of central neural centers associated with increased thirst mechanisms, as well as a heightened activity of ganglionic nerves, via its effects on the autonomic nervous system. Ang II also serves to increase aldosterone synthesis, thus increasing sodium reabsorption by the kidney, which ultimately may raise arterial pressure and worsen sodium retention, if present. However, normal subjects usually exhibit an escape from the salt-retaining effects of aldosterone within a 3-day period.[53,54] Conversely, in HF, this escape phenomenon is not achieved.[55] In addition, these patients have elevated plasma aldosterone levels, which might be secondary to poor hepatic clearance.[56] In spite of this fact, spironolactone, the aldosterone antagonist, does not consistently affect sodium or potassium excretion in patients with congestive HF.[57] Thus, as kidney perfusion declines in concert with decreased cardiac function, loop diuretics are the only effective agents that may be used to achieve a diuresis.

Catecholamines

Catecholamines play a vital role in HF. Studies have shown that intrarenal blood flow is reduced when the effective circulating volume is reduced and sympathetic tone is increased. Studies by Chidsey and colleagues documented very high plasma NE levels in patients with HF.[58] More importantly, elevated plasma NE levels correlate with activation of the sympathetic nervous system, as well as mortality in this patient population.[59] Enhanced sympathetic tone contributes to sodium avidity in several ways. Increased sympathetic nervous system activity secondary to withdrawal of parasympathetic tone by the baroreceptors leads to direct enhancement of proximal tubule sodium reabsorption in the proximal tubule and the loop of Henle.[33] Post-glomerular capillary pressure falls and oncotic pressure rises, further enhancing proximal tubular reabsorption.

The contribution of dopamine to improvement of cardiac function and maintenance of kidney hemodynamics has received much attention. Dopamine affects kidney hemodynamics by vasodilation of afferent and efferent arterioles and intralobular arteries enhancing kidney blood flow without increase in glomerular filtration.[60] Dopamine inhibits proximal tubule reabsorption of sodium related in part to attenuation of aldosterone secretion.[61] However, despite the theoretical benefits of dopamine, its use in a randomized trial of low-dose dopamine versus placebo among adults hospitalized with ADHF and an eGFR 15.60 mL/min/1.73m^2 did not enhance decongestion or improve kidney function (see also Chapter 36).[62]

Natriuretic Peptides (see also Chapter 9)

The natriuretic peptides help counteract many of the maladaptive pathways in HF, making them attractive therapeutic agents. Two structurally related proteins—BNP, ANP—have been found in the heart. C-type natriuretic peptide (CNP) is a related peptide that is secreted mainly by the vascular endothelium. The peptides are discussed extensively in Chapter 9.

Myocardial stretch is the stimulus for BNP and ANP secretion. ANP and BNP have several favorable biologic properties.[63] The primary functions in the kidney are summarized in Table 15.2. ANP and BNP have been shown to block sympathetic nervous activity in the cardiovascular system and in the kidney.[64,65] Both bind to

TABLE 15.2 Effects of Natriuretic Peptides on the Kidney

Decrease	Increase
Arterial pressure	Glomerular filtration rate
Angiotensin II (inhibits action)	Renal blood flow (transient)
Vasopressin (inhibits action)	Sodium excretion
Renin secretion	Tubular flow rate
Aldosterone secretion	Potassium excretion (minimal)
	Calcium, phosphate, and magnesium excretion

natriuretic peptide receptors (NPR-A) on target cells, leading to the production of cyclic guanosine monophosphate, which then mediates many of the physiologic effects. The greatest concentration of receptors in the kidney is found in the glomerulus and medulla.[66] ANP and BNP increase glomerular filtration and prevent sodium reabsorption. The increase in glomerular filtration rate versus the relatively blunted effect on kidney blood flow implies that ANP dilates the afferent arteriole of the nephron while constricting the efferent arteriole, promoting natriuresis.[67] This is discussed more extensively in **Chapter 9**.

Patients with kidney disease require special consideration when measuring BNP or NT-proBNP levels, because stage 3 or higher CKD is associated with higher concentrations of both hormones (**see also Chapter 33**).[68] Investigators have therefore sought to determine whether the elevation simply represents decreased clearance of the natriuretic peptides or increased secretion because of cardiac disease. In a study of 103 non-dialysis-dependent adults with CKD, plasma BNP level was greater in those with CKD compared with hypertensive controls (28 ± 4 pg/mL vs. 162 ± 21 pg/mL), suggesting that the increase in natriuretic peptide levels was secondary to impaired renal function.[69] Interestingly, however, 2-D echo derived measures of volume overload were independent predictors of BNP levels, even after controlling for kidney function.

Those with kidney disease required higher cutoffs of NT proBNP for the diagnosis of HF, compared with patients with normal kidney function (**see also Chapter 33**).[70] Among patients with a GFR less than 60 mL/min/1.73m^2, a cut point of 1200 pg/mL provided a sensitivity of 89% and specificity of 72%. Even after adjustment for multiple confounders, including kidney function, NT-proBNP remained a significant predictor of mortality. In a meta-analysis including 4287 patients, the area under the curve (AUC) for the diagnosis of ADHF using NT-proBNP ranged from 0.66 to 0.89 with a median cut-point of 1980 pg/mL for adults with an eGFR less than 60 mL/min/1.73m^2; the AUC ranged from 0.72 to 0.95 with a cut-point of 450 pg/mL in patients with eGFR greater than 60 mL/min/1.73 m^2.[71]

Neprilysin is the primary enzyme responsible for degradation of the natriuretic peptides, and is most abundant in the proximal kidney tubular cells (**see also Chapter 9**).[72] Neprilysin inhibition (NEPi) results in potent natriuresis and vasodilation; in the kidney, this vasodilatory effect reduces intraglomerular pressure and proteinuria.[72] Evidence for the outcome benefit of a neprilysin inhibitor comes from the results of the Prospective comparison of ARNi with ACEi to Determine Impact on Global Mortality and morbidity in Heart Failure trial (PARADIGM-HF) study (**see also Chapter 37**),[73] which showed a striking improvement in cardiovascular outcomes with fixed dose sacubitril (and ARNi) and valsartan (an ARB). It is interesting to note that in PARADIGM-HF, fewer patients with sacubitril/

valsartan compared with enalapril experienced a creatinine greater than 2.5 mg/dL (3.3% vs. 4.5%, $P < .007$) or a potassium greater than 6.0 mmol/L (4.3% vs. 5.6%, $P < .007$). The increase in albumin excretion seen with valsartan/sacubitril may represent a direct effect on the glomerulus. Prior studies demonstrated an increased intracapillary pressure and concomitant relaxation of mesangial cells, with a secondary increase in glomerular filtering surface area and subsequent loss of protein.[74]

Arginine Vasopressin

AVP, also known as antidiuretic hormone (ADH), is a peptide hormone, which is derived from a prehormone precursor that is synthesized in the hypothalamus. It is then transported and stored in the posterior part of the pituitary gland and is released in response to multiple mechanisms associated with volume depletion and increased osmolality. In the kidney, AVP facilitates urinary concentration primarily by modulating the passage of water and urea from the collecting ducts into the medullary interstitium.[75,76] In advanced HF, AVP contributes to development of hyponatremia and maintenance of glomerular capillary pressure.[76] Of note, AVP does not have a role in edema formation in most other pathophysiologic circumstances. There are multiple mechanisms responsible for AVP release in HF. Baroreceptors, parasympathetic stimuli, and intracardiac receptors have been implicated in the control of AVP release in animal studies.[77,78] As HF advances, baroreceptor dysfunction results in increased sympathetic tone and unopposed secretion of vasopressin. This, coupled with the intense thirst produced by Ang II, yields a scenario that culminates in hyponatremia, which predicts increased mortality in patients with HF.

In the cardiovascular system, vasopressin (as the name suggests) increases systemic and peripheral vascular resistance. While this property has made it useful in the treatment of vasodilatory shock, the physiological effects of AVP have a potentially detrimental hemodynamic effect in the setting of HF.[79] Oral vasopressin V2 receptor antagonist tolvaptan has been evaluated in patients with HF, and even though it did improve hyponatremia, there was no effect on long-term morbidity and mortality in this patient population (**see also Chapter 36**).[80] Moreover, in the multicenter, open-label, randomized Kanagawa Aquaresis Investigators Trial of Tolvaptan on HF Patients with Renal Impairment (K-STAR), tolvaptan added to furosemide resulted in a greater diuretic effect than increasing the dose of furosemide, even in normonatremia patients with CHF complicated by CKD stages G3b-5.[81]

Prostaglandins

The intrarenal prostaglandin system has been implicated in the regulation of kidney hemodynamics and kidney sodium excretion in HF. Plasma levels of prostaglandins (e.g., PGE2 and prostacyclin) are elevated in patients with HF, especially in those patients with hyponatremia.[82,83] With the exception of PGF2 and thromboxane, the kidney prostaglandins are all vasodilators. In addition, they alter sodium reabsorption at both thick ascending loop of Henle and the cortical collecting tubule.[84] These actions counteract, at least in part, other hemodynamically active peptides, such as AVP, Ang II, and NE.[85] The importance of prostaglandins as modulators of kidney function in patients with HF is exemplified by Dzau and colleagues.[82] In this study, patients with severe HF had PGI2 and PGE2 metabolite levels 3 to 10 times above levels found in normal subjects. The subset of patients with hyponatremia challenged with prostaglandin synthetase inhibitor, indomethacin, had significant decreases in CI, along with elevation of PCWP and systemic vascular resistance.

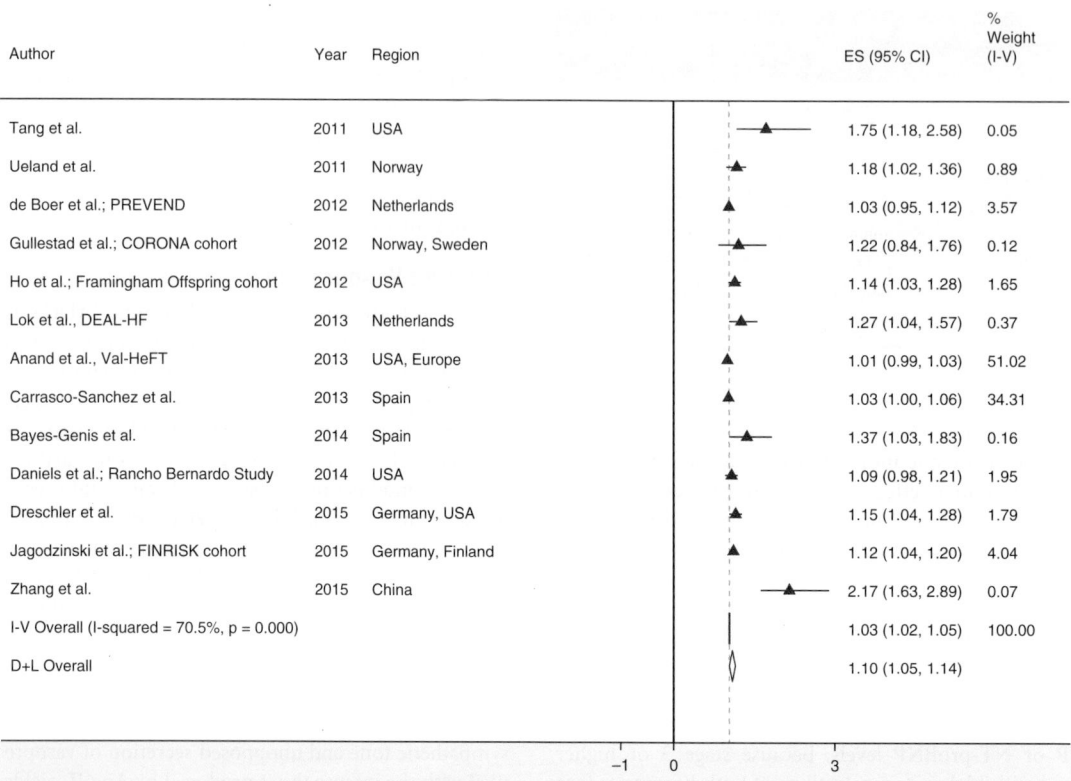

Author	Year	Region		ES (95% CI)	% Weight (I-V)
Tang et al.	2011	USA		1.75 (1.18, 2.58)	0.05
Ueland et al.	2011	Norway		1.18 (1.02, 1.36)	0.89
de Boer et al.; PREVEND	2012	Netherlands		1.03 (0.95, 1.12)	3.57
Gullestad et al.; CORONA cohort	2012	Norway, Sweden		1.22 (0.84, 1.76)	0.12
Ho et al.; Framingham Offspring cohort	2012	USA		1.14 (1.03, 1.28)	1.65
Lok et al., DEAL-HF	2013	Netherlands		1.27 (1.04, 1.57)	0.37
Anand et al., Val-HeFT	2013	USA, Europe		1.01 (0.99, 1.03)	51.02
Carrasco-Sanchez et al.	2013	Spain		1.03 (1.00, 1.06)	34.31
Bayes-Genis et al.	2014	Spain		1.37 (1.03, 1.83)	0.16
Daniels et al.; Rancho Bernardo Study	2014	USA		1.09 (0.98, 1.21)	1.95
Dreschler et al.	2015	Germany, USA		1.15 (1.04, 1.28)	1.79
Jagodzinski et al.; FINRISK cohort	2015	Germany, Finland		1.12 (1.04, 1.20)	4.04
Zhang et al.	2015	China		2.17 (1.63, 2.89)	0.07
I-V Overall (I-squared = 70.5%, p = 0.000)				1.03 (1.02, 1.05)	100.00
D+L Overall				1.10 (1.05, 1.14)	

Fig. 15.5 Meta-analysis of the predictive value of galectin-3 on heart failure development and all-cause mortality. Data are corrected for changes in nt-proBNP. D + L, ¼ DerSimonian-Laird model; ES, ¼ effect estimate. (From Imran TF, Shin HJ, Mathenge N, et al. Meta-analysis of the usefulness of plasma Galectin-3 to predict the risk of mortality in patients with heart failure and in the general population. *Am J Cardiol.* 2017;119:57-64.)

BIOMARKERS OF KIDNEY DYSFUNCTION

There have been numerous studies evaluating various biomarkers on cardiovascular outcomes and kidney disease progression in people with both HF and CKD (**see also Chapter 33**). Few biomarkers are predictive of both CKD progression and worsening HF; however, galectin-3 has been shown predictive in both settings.

Galectin-3 was prospectively analyzed utilizing data from 9148 Atherosclerosis Risk in Communities (ARIC) Study participants with measured plasma galectin-3 levels over different time periods.[86] One group was evaluated without presence of CKD or HF. Another group of 1983 CKD cases were followed for a median time of 16 years. A significant, graded, positive association between galectin-3 and incident CKD was noted. The association remained significant after adjustment for eGFR, urine albumin-to-creatinine, ratio, troponin T, and N-terminal pro- BNP. This relationship between galectin-3 levels and CKD progression was also seen in the Framingham cohort.[87]

A meta-analysis evaluating galectin-3 as a biomarker of myocardial fibrosis, inflammation, and CVD mortality as well as incident HF found a strong positive relationship. The meta-analysis reviewed 32,350 participants (323,090 person-years of follow-up) with a mean age of 57 years, 47.2% of whom were women. They were followed for a median of 5 years (**Fig. 15.5**). The results support the concept that elevated plasma galectin-3 is associated with a higher risk of all-cause mortality, CVD mortality, and HF.

Taken together, galectin-3 and nt-ProBNP, previously shown to be predictive of poor outcomes in HF and CKD, will hopefully be useful in the future to manage such patients earlier and improve prognosis.

SUMMARY AND FUTURE DIRECTIONS

The importance of the kidney in HF has been recognized for more than a century. As discussed herein, the kidney maintains sodium balance by regulating intravascular volume. Under physiologic conditions, the control of sodium homeostasis by the kidney is regulated by hormones synthesized and released by the heart, which act upon the glomerulus and the tubular epithelium to enhance natriuresis and suppress sodium-retaining factors such as aldosterone. However, in HF, the cardiorenal axis becomes perturbed leading to an inappropriate volume expansion of the vascular and extravascular space. Thus far, our enhanced understanding of physiologic and pathophysiologic, biochemical, and mechanical mechanisms in which this cardiorenal axis interacts in the maintenance of sodium homeostasis has provided important diagnostic and novel therapeutic opportunities that may ultimately delay the progression of HF.

KEY REFERENCES

4. Lazich I, Bakris GL. Renal hemodynamic changes in heart failure. In: BAKRIS GL, ed. *The Kidney in Heart Failure*. New York: Springer Science+Business Media; 2012:27–38.

11. Blair JE, Pang PS, Schrier RW, et al. Investigators E. Changes in renal function during hospitalization and soon after discharge in patients admitted for worsening heart failure in the placebo group of the EVEREST trial. *Eur Heart J.* 2011;32:2563–2572.

14. Damman K, Valente MA, Voors AA, O'Connor CM, van Veldhuisen DJ, Hillege HL. Renal impairment, worsening renal function, and outcome in patients with heart failure: an updated meta-analysis. *Eur Heart J.* 2014;35:455–469.

16. Salah K, Kok WE, Eurlings LW, Bettencourt P, Pimenta JM, Metra M, et al. Competing risk of cardiac status and renal function during hospitalization for acute decompensated heart failure. *JACC Heart Fail.* 2015;3:751–761.

17. Ibrahim NE, Gaggin HK, Rabideau DJ, Gandhi PU, Mallick A, Januzzi Jr JL. Worsening renal function during management for chronic heart failure with reduced ejection fraction: results from the Pro-BNP Outpatient Tailored Chronic Heart Failure Therapy (PROTECT) study. *J Card Fail.* 2017;23:121–130.

43. Patel HC, Rosen SD, Hayward C. Renal denervation in heart failure with preserved ejection fraction (RDT-PEF): a randomized controlled trial. *Eur J Heart Fail.* 2016;18:703–712.

55. Weber KT. Aldosterone in congestive heart failure. *N Engl J Med.* 2001;345:1689–1697.

71. Schaub JA, Coca SG, Moledina DG, Gentry M, Testani JM, Parikh CR. Amino-terminal pro-B-type natriuretic peptide for diagnosis and prognosis in patients with renal dysfunction: a systematic review and meta-analysis. *JACC Heart Fail.* 2015;3:977–989.

73. McMurray JJ, Packer M, Desai AS, Investigators PH. Committees. Angiotensin-neprilysin inhibition versus enalapril in heart failure. *N Engl J Med.* 2014;371:993–1004.

81. Tominaga N, Kida K, Inomata T. Effects of tolvaptan addition to furosemide in normo- and hyponatremia patients with heart failure and chronic kidney disease stages G3b-5: a subanalysis of the K-STAR study. *Am J Nephrol.* 2017;46:417–426.

The full reference list for this chapter is available on ExpertConsult.

Alterations in Skeletal Muscle in Heart Failure

P. Christian Schulze, Michael J. Toth

The syndrome of heart failure (HF) is characterized by adaptations in numerous physiologic systems that contribute to disease symptomology and progression. The cardinal symptom of HF, exercise intolerance, which manifests as dyspnea and skeletal muscle fatigue, has long been attributed to cardiac insufficiency. However, research over the past three decades has conclusively demonstrated a role for adaptations in the skeletal musculature in these symptoms. The overall goal of this chapter is to summarize the skeletal muscle adaptations to HF identified in clinical studies and model systems. When possible, we extend the description of these adaptations to the cellular and molecular levels. We present this evidence with a focus on describing how skeletal muscle adaptations contribute to diminished skeletal muscle and whole body physiological functional capacity, which, in turn, would contribute to exercise intolerance.

SKELETAL MUSCLE ADAPTATIONS IN HEART FAILURE

Dyspnea and fatigue, resulting in diminished exercise tolerance, are among the main factors contributing to decreased social and physical functioning and quality of life of HF patients.[1] There has long been evidence that measures of cardiac function, such as ejection fraction and cardiac output, only poorly correlate with a patient's capacity to exercise, suggesting the involvement of factors other than cardiac insufficiency. Furthermore, many studies of the effects of exercise in patients with HF have failed to demonstrate improvements in cardiac output, stroke volume, or ejection fraction, despite showing gains in exercise capacity and peak oxygen uptake (VO_2).[2] The lack of a close correlation between central hemodynamics and exercise tolerance has led to investigations into alterations in peripheral skeletal muscle. As will be discussed later, the view that alterations in skeletal muscle metabolism, structure, mass, and function play a rate-limiting role in the functional capacity in patients with HF is now broadly accepted. **Fig. 16.1** provides

a broad hypothetical framework for how factors related to the syndrome of HF (disease-related effectors) diminish skeletal muscle functional capacity (functional phenotypes) and promote exercise intolerance (fatigue and dyspnea) via their effects on skeletal muscle structure and function (skeletal muscle adaptations). To date, most studies have evaluated skeletal muscle adaptations in patients with HF with reduced ejection fraction (HFrEF). As knowledge has grown regarding the syndrome of HF with preserved ejection fraction (HFpEF), work has begun to accumulate on the skeletal muscle phenotype in these patients (**see also Chapters 11** and **39**). Although still limited in number, studies show comparable changes in skeletal muscle metabolism, structure, and function in patients with HFpEF as seen in patients with HFrEF.[3-5] Nonetheless, the majority of work has focused on patients with HFrEF, and we will refer to those studies throughout the text as simply "HF," unless adaptations are specified as being evaluated in HFpEF patients.

The myopathy associated with HF affects both cardiac and skeletal muscle and encompasses alterations in structure and function. Regarding skeletal muscle, the classical model of the myopathy of HF includes a loss of muscle size, strength, and oxidative capacity. More specifically, HF patients experience skeletal muscle atrophy secondary to muscle fiber atrophy, and this loss of muscle quantity may account for a large proportion of the reduction in peak VO_2.[6] Patients also experience muscle weakness,[6] which is due in part to muscle atrophy, but there are also unique effects of the disease to reduce intrinsic skeletal muscle contractile function.[7] Finally, patients exhibit abnormal skeletal muscle metabolism, with a shift toward glycolytic pathways, changes in mitochondrial function[8,9] and structure,[10] and decreased oxidative enzyme activity.[8] This is due in part to a shift from fatigue-resistant, oxidative type I fibers toward oxidative, type II fibers.[11] Altogether, these abnormalities in skeletal muscle structure, function, and cell viability are intimately linked to each other and contribute to the abnormal exercise response, enhanced fatigability, and progressive symptom complex of patients with HF.

Disease-related effectors

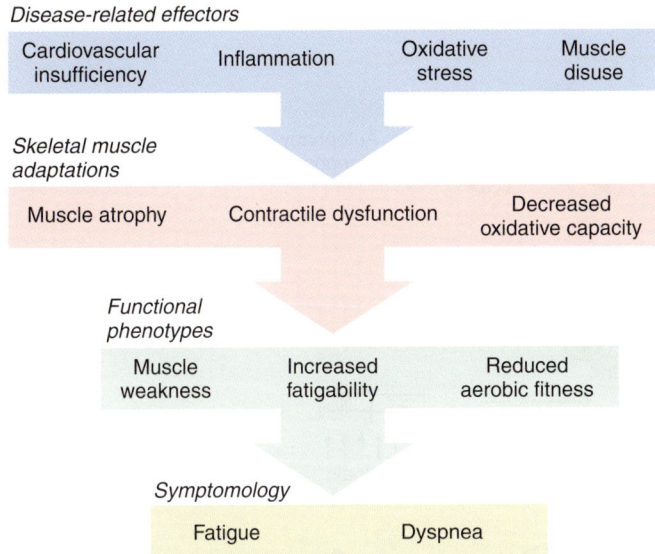

Fig. 16.1 Broad hypothetical framework for how factors related to heart failure syndrome (disease-related effectors) diminish skeletal muscle functional capacity (functional phenotypes) and promote exercise intolerance (fatigue and dyspnea) via their effects on skeletal muscle structure and function (skeletal muscle adaptations).

SKELETAL MUSCLE ATROPHY

HF patients develop generalized muscle atrophy. Calf muscle volume, assessed by magnetic resonance imaging, revealed reduced muscle volume in patients with HF and significant water and/or fat infiltration.[12] Muscle atrophy develops in patients with severe HF compared with age- and gender-matched controls.[13] However, some studies report normal muscle mass in patients with HF.[14] This disparity may relate to the patients studied, because muscle atrophy may develop secondary to weight loss or inactivity in a subset of the HF population.[15] However, HF patients generally experience some degree of muscle atrophy during the course of the disease.

The mechanisms that mediate skeletal muscle wasting and atrophy have been studied in patients with HF and animal models of cardiac dysfunction. Muscle atrophy occurs during periods of negative muscle protein imbalance, which are due to decreased protein synthesis, increased protein degradation, or both. There is controversy on the impact of clinical status and disease exacerbations on muscle atrophy in HF. The majority of studies have shown no defects in either muscle protein synthesis or breakdown in clinically stable HF patients.[15] It is possible that muscle atrophy initiation and progression is directly linked to episodes of disease exacerbation and hospitalization, which are accompanied by bed rest, malnutrition, and other factors that may incite atrophy. Unfortunately, no studies have examined patients during acute disease exacerbation to test this postulate or determine what metabolic defects might account for muscle atrophy, although one study has evaluated patients shortly after hospitalization and found evidence for enhance muscle protein breakdown.[16]

Skeletal muscle atrophy contributes to exercise intolerance in HF patients. Strong correlations have been found between muscle mass and peak VO_2.[6] Moreover, in contrast to nondiseased individuals, in patients with severe HF, the addition of upper arm exercise significantly increases peak VO_2, suggesting the importance of skeletal muscle mass in determining peak VO_2 in patients with HF.[17] Thus there is ample evidence supporting a role for muscle atrophy in promoting exercise intolerance. We will now consider the mechanisms underlying this loss of skeletal muscle.

Skeletal Muscle Protein Synthesis and Reduced Anabolic Hormones/Effectors

Skeletal muscle protein synthesis is controlled by mechanoresponsive pathways and paracrine growth factor signaling loops, such as the local insulin-like growth factor-1 (IGF-1) system, but also responds to systemic stimuli, including growth hormone (GH), systemic IGF-1, anabolic steroids, and others. The GH/IGF-1 axis plays a key role in skeletal muscle growth and differentiation. Low systemic IGF-1 levels have been associated with a reduced leg muscle cross-sectional area (CSA) and total muscle strength in HF patients.[18] Catabolic syndromes, such as chronic inflammation, sepsis, or cancer, show an altered state of the GH/IGF-1 axis, most probably due to a peripheral IGF-1 deficiency because of an impaired IGF-1 response to GH but also abnormal intrahepatic responses to GH.[19] This has been attributed, in part, to increased serum levels and the local expression of proinflammatory cytokines, such as interleukin-1β (IL-1β) and tumor necrosis factor-α (TNF-α).

In humans with advanced HF and animal models of ischemic cardiomyopathy, reduced local expression of IGF-1 was detected in skeletal muscle compared with controls, accompanied by an increased expression of the IGF-1 receptor in the presence of normal serum levels of IGF-1.[18,20] The serum concentration of the proinflammatory cytokines IL-1β and IL-6 were not found to be significantly changed, whereas TNF-α showed a trend toward higher levels in HF. Notably, the local expression of both IL-1β and TNF-α is increased in chronic HF[20,21] and can be reduced by aerobic exercise training.[21] Furthermore, a decreased single muscle fiber CSA in HF has been linked to local expression of IL-1β and impaired expression levels of expression of IGF-1 in skeletal muscle.[20] These results suggest that, despite normal serum levels of IGF-1 and proinflammatory cytokines, the local expression of IGF-I is substantially reduced in HF, indicating a reduction in local anabolic stimuli. Because decreased IGF-1 levels and a reduced muscle fiber CSA correlate with increased levels of IL-1β, these results point toward a cytokine-mediated local catabolic process that is mediated, in part, through reductions in anabolic hormone expression.

Local expression of IGF-1 in skeletal muscle is mainly regulated by two different mechanisms. The first is GH receptor–dependent,[22] a mechanism which, at least in part, is impaired in HF-induced weight loss due to a peripheral GH resistance.[23] In addition, skeletal muscle IGF-1 expression is modulated in response to alterations in muscle use, and the expression of IGF-1 increases significantly in response to work-overload and passive stretch.[24] In contrast, TNF-α and other cytokines may decrease skeletal muscle expression of IGF-1.[25,26]

In addition to its classical role to enhance protein synthesis, IGF-1 has antiapoptotic effects in various tissues, protecting against cytokine-mediated apoptosis.[27] These findings suggest that IGF-1 may regulate cell survival by modulating both proapoptotic and antiapoptotic stimuli. Thus the increased rate of skeletal muscle apoptosis in HF[28] may be explained by a decline in local IGF-1 expression. This is suggested by preclinical models, where stimulation of IGF-1 production via GH administration reduces atrophy via reductions in apoptosis.[29]

In male HF patients, deficiencies in circulating total testosterone, dehydroepiandrosterone (DHEA), and IGF-1 are common and correlate with a poor prognosis.[30] Testosterone maintains skeletal muscle mass by increasing fractional muscle protein synthesis. In addition, testosterone appears to stimulate IGF-1 expression, but the exact molecular pathways are incompletely understood. At supraphysiologic doses, testosterone appears to act through androgen receptor–independent mechanisms. In HF patients, serum levels of free testosterone and DHEA are decreased, and this decrease correlates with HF severity. Perhaps most importantly, replacement of testosterone improves exercise capacity, muscle strength, and metabolic function.[31]

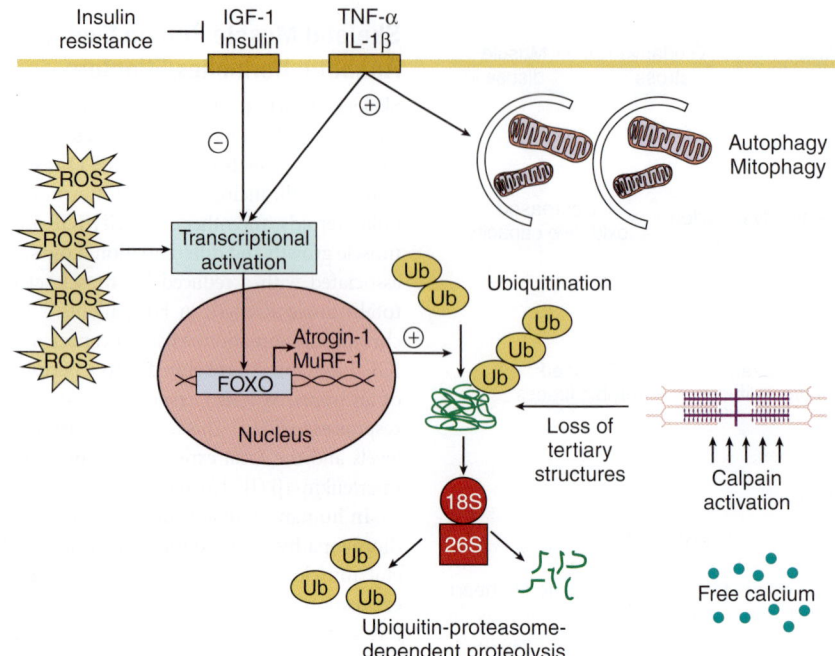

Fig. 16.2 Regulation of muscle atrophy occurs through several highly conserved pathways of proteolytic changes in skeletal muscle. These are identical for various disease states, as well as disuse and immobilization. The main proteolytic pathway in skeletal muscle is the adenosine triphosphate (ATP)–dependent degradation of proteins through ubiquitination and action of the *26S* proteasome. This pathway is transcriptionally regulated through FOXO transcription factors and expression of atrogenes, such as *MURF-1* and atrogin-1. Activation of calcium-dependent calpains occurs due to increased levels of intracellular calcium released from the sarcoplasmic reticulum. Calpains are primarily responsible for destruction of tertiary structure and subsequent exposure of proteolytic cleavage sites. Finally, lysosomal protein degradation, or autophagy, is a highly regulated process that contributes to the destruction of cellular organelles. All these pathways likely contribute to skeletal muscle atrophy in advanced heart failure. *IGF-1*, Insulin-like growth factor-1; *IL-1β*, interleukin-1β; *ROS*, reactive oxygen species; *TNF-α*, tumor necrosis factor-α.

Finally, insulin resistance is a hallmark of advanced HF. This metabolic abnormality is more pronounced during acute decompensated HF and improves upon cardiac recompensation.[32] Moreover, improved cardiac output through left ventricular assist device placement results in reduced insulin resistance and improved glucose homeostasis in advanced HF.[33] The effects of insulin to promote skeletal muscle anabolism occur during the daily cycle of feeding and fasting, where it serves to promote postprandial anabolism by reducing skeletal muscle protein breakdown. Studies have suggested that HF patients experience impaired suppression of insulin's effects to reduce protein breakdown in response to meal-associated stimuli and that this impaired response was related to the circulating IL-6 level.[34] Thus tissue insulin sensitivity, possibly secondary to immune activation, may contribute to skeletal muscle atrophy.

Skeletal Muscle Protein Breakdown and Increased Catabolic Hormones/Effectors

HF is a catabolic state, with increased levels of various catabolic hormones.[35] Several authors have suggested a role for myostatin in muscle atrophy in patients with advanced HF.[36] Myostatin is a local and circulating factor secreted from skeletal muscle with antianabolic and antihypertrophic actions. In fact, such a mechanism may be operable in patients, because circulating levels of myostatin,[37] and other transforming growth factor (TGF) receptor ligands, such as activin,[38] are increased in HF patients. Whatever might be the proximal hormonal/circulating effector, local skeletal muscle protein breakdown is mediated by several cellular systems that include lysosomal proteases, the adenosine triphosphate (ATP)–dependent ubiquitin-proteasome system, and the Ca^{2+}-dependent calpain

system (**Fig. 16.2**). Specifically the ubiquitin–proteasome system has been implicated in the enhanced protein breakdown of atrophying skeletal muscle in a number of disease models,[39] including chronic HF.[40] Of particular interest is a group of ubiquitin-conjugating enzymes (E3-ligases) that target proteins for degradation by the proteasome. Through transcriptional screening, two E3-ligases, atrogin-1 (also called MFbx-1) and MURF-1 (muscle ring finger protein-1), have been identified to be highly induced in processes of muscular atrophy of different origin. Gomes and colleagues reported the identification and initial description of an increased expression of atrogin-1 (also called MAFbx-1), a muscle-specific E3-ligase, following starvation.[41] Through a comparable analysis of genes regulated in atrophying muscle caused by different mechanisms, Bodine and colleagues identified the same gene (here called MAFbx-1) and, additionally, MURF-1, another E3-ligase.[42] Through adenovirally mediated overexpression of these genes, their catabolic effects were demonstrated. Furthermore, animals with targeted deletion of MAFbx-1 or MURF-1 exhibit less muscular atrophy in response to denervation and hind limb suspension.[41]

Increased atrogin-1 has been reported in other animal models of muscular atrophy induced by immobilization, denervation, hind limb suspension,[42] starvation,[41] and sepsis.[43] The induction of atrogin-1 expression prior to muscle weight loss in starvation suggests that the activation of this gene is involved in the development and progression of muscle protein loss.[41] In support of this possibility, overexpression of atrogin-1 in C_2C_{12} myotubes induced atrophy in vitro, whereas muscular atrophy following denervation was prevented in animals with targeted deletion of atrogin-1.[42] Intriguingly, infusion of the proinflammatory cytokine IL-1β induces the expression of atrogin-1[42] and TNF-α increases the ubiquitin-conjugating capacity in myocytes,[44] findings that again support the hypothesis of cytokines as putative mediators of muscular atrophy. Prior studies have shown transcriptional activation of E3 ligases in muscle of animals with left ventricular dysfunction[40] and humans with advanced HF,[45] whereas other reports did not show these changes.[46] This might relate to the type of muscle injury and severity of HF.[16] However, the exact mechanisms underlying the transcriptional activation of atrogin-1 by IL-1β remain to be elucidated.

Activation of the renin-angiotensin system results in vasoconstriction and elevated skeletal muscle concentration of angiotensin II (Ang II), which increases local oxidative stress, increases muscle proteolysis, and lowers skeletal muscle concentration of IGF-1. These mechanisms may accelerate protein degradation while decreasing protein synthesis. Loss of skeletal muscle mass contributes to muscle reflex alterations in HF.[47] In normal subjects, muscle reflex activation helps to raise blood pressure and thereby maintain muscle perfusion during muscle acidosis. In HF, muscle reflex activation occurs at the onset of exercise, resulting in vasoconstriction and limited skeletal muscle perfusion.

SKELETAL MUSCLE CONTRACTILE DYSFUNCTION

Skeletal muscle contractile dysfunction has received relatively minimal attention as a precipitant of functional limitations in the clinical syndrome of HF. Despite this lack of attention, data suggest that HF is associated with marked reductions in skeletal muscle contractility. Skeletal muscle atrophy contributes to this diminished contractile function, but there is evidence for diminished function per unit muscle size (i.e., intrinsic contractile dysfunction). Studies under both static (isometric) and dynamic (isokinetic) conditions suggest intrinsic contractile deficits in HF patients on the order of 15% to 25%.[6,34] This reduction is greater in cachectic versus noncachectic patients[48] and is not corrected by cardiac transplantation,[49] although ventricular assist device implantation has been shown to mitigate upper extremity weakness.[50] Of note, studies show that these decrements in muscle function persist when patients are compared with controls who are matched for habitual physical activity level,[51] arguing that decreased contractility is not a consequence of muscle disuse. Moreover, reduced contractility is not related to impairments in central motor drive or neural transmission.[6,51] Thus there is compelling evidence that HF alters the intrinsic contractile properties of skeletal muscle and that the resulting muscle weakness contributes to exercise intolerance.[6]

Myofilament Contractile Adaptations

Alterations in skeletal muscle contractile function in HF may relate to changes in myofilament protein expression, their function, or both. Regarding the former, adult human skeletal muscle is composed of three fiber types, characterized primarily by the type of myosin isoform expressed. **Table 16.1** details the structural and functional features of these types of muscle fibers. In general, most skeletal muscles contain a mixture of these fiber types, with myosin heavy chain (MHC) I and IIA being predominant and with very few fibers that express only the fastest MHC isoform (MHC IIX). This differs from rodents, which express a fourth fiber type MHC IIB that is faster and less oxidative than all the other fiber types. There are other contractile proteins whose expression varies by fiber types, but the functional character of each fiber is largely dictated by the type of myosin expressed.

Myofilament Protein Expression

One of the most often cited, skeletal muscle adaption to HF is the shift in fiber type toward a more fast-twitch, glycolytic phenotype, which is reflected by a change in expression of MHC toward a more fast-twitch

TABLE 16.1 Structural and Functional Features of Muscle Fibers

Fiber Type	HUMAN FIBER TYPES			LOW-ORDER MAMMALS
	Type I (Red)	Type IIA (Red)	Type IIX (White)	Type IIB (White)
Contraction time	Slow	Moderate fast	Fast	Very fast
Oxidative capacity	High	High	Intermediate	Low
Mitochondrial density	High	High	Medium	Low
Glycolytic capacity	Low	High	High	High
Resistance to fatigue	High	Fairly high	Intermediate	Low
Major storage fuel	Triglycerides	Creatine phosphate, glycogen	Creatine phosphate, glycogen	Creatine phosphate, glycogen
Capillary density	High	Intermediate	Low	Low

isoform (IIA or IIX). The loss of slow-twitch, oxidative fibers has been demonstrated in animal models[52] and humans[11] and has long been held as a mechanism underlying the reduction in aerobic fitness.[11] More recent studies have confirmed that this adaptation is also apparent in HFpEF patients.[5] However, this switch toward a fast-twitch phenotype is apparent upon muscle disuse, raising the possibility that it may be a by-product of the physical inactivity that accompanies the HF syndrome. Early work that compared MHC expression between HF patients, healthy controls, and stroke patients confined to bed rest for more than 1 year as "inactive" controls argued against this notion.[11] Whether patients who undergo muscle disuse secondary to loss of central neural activation represent the degree of activity restriction that occurs with HF,[53] which is arguably more modest than being bedridden, is questionable. In fact, studies that have carefully matched HF patients to controls for fitness/activity level have observed no effect of HF to alter MHC isoform expression/fiber type.[46,54]

Discordance between studies finding/not finding a shift in fiber type/MHC expression with HF may be explained by the advent of the use of angiotensin-converting enzyme inhibitors (ACEi) and angiotensin receptor blockers, as that these agents reverse the shift in fiber type back toward a more slow-twitch phenotype.[55] However, more recent studies in human patients have observed this fiber type switch in patients taking an ACEi.[56] In fact, studies conducted by the same laboratory in separate cohorts of human patients taking these medications have both observed and not observed changes in muscle fiber type,[46,56] with the only difference between the two cohorts being the activity status of controls. This further highlights the potential modulating role of physical activity on fiber type characteristics in the HF population. Building on this notion, and considering that a similar switch in fiber type from a slow- to a fast-twitch phenotype is emblematic of muscle disuse, the effects of these medications might reflect their ability to improve symptomology and, in turn, increase physical activity in patients.

In addition to alterations in the expression of specific isoforms of MHC, recent studies have found evidence for a select reduction in the expression of myosin relative to other contractile proteins on the order of 15% to 20% (**Fig. 16.3**).[46,56] Mechanical assessments that reflect cross-bridge number

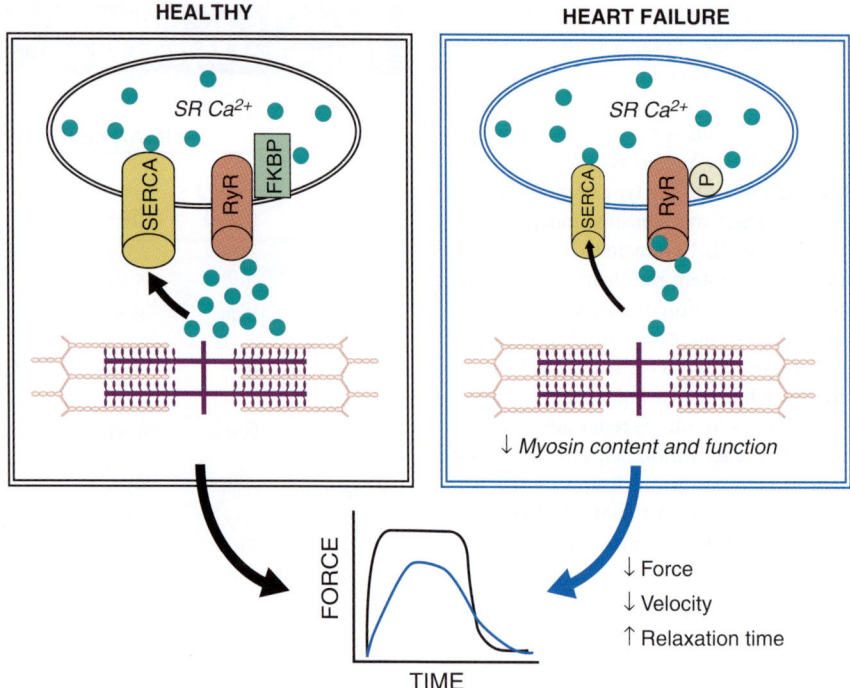

Fig. 16.3 Effects of heart failure (HF) to decrease skeletal muscle contractile function. HF impairs intracellular Ca²⁺ release, thereby diminishing activation of myofilament proteins and lessening contractile force (lower plateau of the force tracing). In addition, HF reduces myosin protein expression and myosin-actin cross-bridge function, which likely has the net effect of reducing contractile velocity (ascending limb of the force tracing). In addition, evidence suggests that HF increases relaxation time (descending limb of the force tracing), possibly secondary to reduced Ca²⁺ reuptake into the sarcoplasmic reticulum (SR). Collectively, these adaptations likely reduce contractile force, velocity and, in turn, power output, leading to a reduced capacity for physical work. In addition, adaptations in myofilament function and Ca²⁺ dynamics may contribute to increased fatiguability of skeletal muscle. *FKBP,* FK506 binding protein; *RyR,* ryanodine receptor; *SERCA,* sarcoplasmic reticulum Ca²⁺ ATPase.

were similarly reduced,[46] suggesting that these results are not attributable to variation in biochemical extraction of myosin. Moreover, these reductions are similar in magnitude with what has been observed in animal models[52] and have been shown to related to functional decrements.[56] Importantly, this loss was not related to muscle disuse, as suggested by some studies,[57] because patients were matched to controls for physical activity level.[46] Similar patterns of myosin loss have been shown in other clinical conditions (e.g., chronic obstructive pulmonary disease [COPD], critical care myopathy [58,59]), suggesting this may be a common contractile protein adaptation related to some aspect of acute/chronic disease.

Myofilament Protein Function

Several lines of evidence suggest that skeletal muscle contractile protein function is impaired in HF patients, but the exact nature of this effect is in dispute. We will first consider the effect of HF on myofilament protein function. Preclinical models have generally shown minimal effects of HF on peripheral skeletal muscle myofilament protein function, as assessed in chemically skinned single muscle fibers.[60] In contrast, studies in clinical patients have shown profound reductions (~30%–50%) in single muscle fiber contractile force per unit fiber CSA (i.e., tension).[61] Together with clinical studies showing relationships between whole muscle strength and circulating cytokines in HF patients[62] and similar magnitude reductions in muscle tension with acute and chronic cytokine administration,[63] these results have led to the notion that the immune activation that accompanies HF contributes to exercise intolerance, in part, through impairment of muscle contractile function. However, recent studies that more carefully

matched HF patients to controls for age and physical activity status have found no reduction in tension in single muscle fibers from HF patients.[7] Conflicting results among studies of human muscle fibers may relate to the fact that prior studies have used control populations that differ in age from patients by greater than 10 years, and no account was taken for the physical activity status of groups.[61] Here again, when the physical inactivity of HF patients is taken into consideration, the impact of the HF syndrome is lessened.

Despite the absence of an effect on contractile protein force production, HF does alter other aspects of contractile protein function; specifically, the kinetics of the myosin–actin cross-bridge interaction were slowed in HF patients compared with age- and activity-matched controls.[7] Such alterations in the myosin–actin cross-bridge function, although potentially beneficial in maintaining muscle fiber force generating capacity,[7] can have detrimental consequences. A slowing of cross-bridge kinetics would presumably slow contractile velocity,[64] which could, in turn, reduce muscle power output. Indeed, there is some evidence from preclinical models for reduced contractile velocity with HF.[65] A reduction in the contractile velocity of muscle would contribute to an overall reduction in muscle power output.[51] Thus some proportion of the reduced work capacity of skeletal muscle in HF patients, which would directly influence performance during a peak exercise test, may relate to deceased contractile velocity secondary to impaired cross-bridge function (see Fig. 16.3). Indeed, drugs that enhance myofilament protein function improve muscle contractility and power output and, in turn, increase exercise performance.[66]

Excitation-Contraction Coupling Adaptations

Although alterations in myofilament protein function may explain diminished contractile velocity and, in turn, power production, they do not appear to explain reduced force production (i.e., muscle strength). This may be explained, instead, by impaired excitation-contraction coupling (ECC). More specifically, diminished calcium (Ca^{2+}) release from the sarcoplasmic reticulum leads to decreased myofilament activation and, in turn, force production (see Fig. 16.3). In addition, impaired ECC function may partially underlie the fatigue that HF patients report on exertion. In the next section, we review evidence that HF alters the ECC system. Because most of the components of the ECC system intrinsic to skeletal muscle cannot be assessed in humans, this discussion primarily relies on data from animal models.

Most of the research in this field has focused on Ca^{2+} release and reuptake from the sarcoplasmic reticulum. Early work in the rat coronary artery ligation model of HF showed that reduced skeletal muscle (extensor digitorum longus; fast-twitch muscle) tension was accompanied by decreased intracellular Ca^{2+} release.[67] In addition, HF animals were associated with accelerated fatigue rates, as assessed by the decrease in tension following repeated tetanic contractions. Other studies have further suggested that Ca^{2+} uptake may also be impaired in HF, based on diminished expression of the sarcoplasmic reticulum Ca^{2+} ATPase (SERCA).[68,69] These seminal results stimulated research in this area because such decrements in Ca^{2+} release and reuptake could underlie greater fatiguability in skeletal muscle in HF.

Studies that included slow- (soleus) and fast-twitch muscles/isolated muscle fibers of rats using the same coronary artery ligation model of HF showed conflicting results. Under nonfatigued conditions, there were no decrements in contractile strength with HF, although there was evidence for slowed relaxation times.[70] Interestingly, contrary to the previously mentioned reports of a loss of SERCA protein expression, this study found no effect of HF on SERCA expression, despite the presence of its resultant physiological phenotype (i.e., slowed relaxation). Moreover, there were no prominent differences between HF and control animals during fatiguing contractions in tension development or intracellular Ca^{2+} levels,[70] although force relaxation was markedly slowed in the slow-twitch soleus muscle. Follow-up studies by this same group, where contractile properties of the soleus muscle were assessed in situ using a protocol that more closely simulated submaximal contractile activity, observed a reduced relaxation rate in HF animals, which was also accompanied by increased fatigability.[71] Subsequent studies in isolated single muscle fibers have further suggested that increased fatigability in HF animals was not associated with impaired Ca^{2+} release.[72] Instead, the authors assert that impairments in myofilament protein function may develop with fatiguing contraction to produce the reduction in tension. This could potentially be explained by reduced cross-bridge kinetics detailed previously,[7] because maneuvers that increase the rate of cross-bridge cycling reduce skeletal muscle fatigue.

More recent studies, also conducted in the rat coronary ligation model of HF, have further supported impaired sarcoplasmic reticulum (SR) Ca^{2+} release. Ward and colleagues[73] showed a transient reduction in the intracellular Ca^{2+} in HF animals. Ca^{2+} sparks, which are spontaneous, localized Ca^{2+} release events that play an important role in dictating aggregate intracellular Ca^{2+} release, have smaller amplitude, slower temporal kinetics, and greater spatial spread. In these same studies, the sarcoplasmic reticulum Ca^{2+} release channel, the ryanodine receptor, was hyperphosphorylated and had less associated FKBP12 (also known as calstabin). Further work showed that protein kinase A–mediated phosphorylation of the ryanodine receptor causes dissociation of FKBP12, which normally functions to inhibit the channel.[74] This conspiration of changes in ryanodine receptor biochemistry is associated with a "leaky" channel phenotype that has been found in

cardiomyocytes in models of HF and is thought to contribute to disease progression.[75] This is significant because it links the well-known heightened sympathetic nervous system activity in the HF syndrome to the skeletal muscle contractile phenotype. In fact, this leaky channel phenotype may be important for exercise intolerance in HF because it has been suggested to contribute to fatigue in humans.[76]

Whether similar alterations in intracellular Ca^{2+} dynamics are present in humans with HF is unknown. Using isolated sarcoplasmic reticulum vesicles, recent studies have found no alterations in Ca^{2+} release, uptake, or leak in patients compared with controls.[77] In addition, contrary to animal models, some studies have suggested an upregulation of Ca^{2+} uptake in patients with HF compared with controls,[78] although some studies suggest downregulation of the expression of these proteins.[79] Thus the balance of available evidence, although quite small, suggests that the phenotype of ECC in human HF may not be adequately reflected in available animal models. This could be due to the fact that measurements in human samples are necessarily different than in animal models. Alternatively, discordant results may be explained by the fact that patients are treated with pharmacologic agents that counteract some of the pathologic Ca^{2+} regulatory alterations (e.g., beta-blockers may prevent ryanodine receptor hyperphosphorylation and the resulting calcium release abnormalities). Further work is required to clearly define the ECC phenotype in human HF to determine its contribution to reduced skeletal muscle contractile strength.

DECREASED OXIDATIVE CAPACITY AND METABOLISM

Exercise intolerance, defined subjectively as dyspnea and fatigue upon exertion and clinically as a reduced peak oxygen uptake during an incremental exercise test, is the cardinal symptom of chronic HF. Although this decrement was originally attributed to cardiac insufficiency, work over the past three decades has led to an appreciation of noncardiac, or peripheral, adaptations to the HF syndrome that contribute to exercise intolerance.[80] The relative importance of skeletal muscle versus vascular versus neural adaptations that may explain reduced functional capacity in HF patients has been debated, and the exact admixture of pathophysiologic adaptations contributing to exertional intolerance is likely variable among patients. Instead of offering a resolution to these arguments, we will describe what is known about how HF affects skeletal muscle specifically, with a concentration on what is known about the unique effect of the syndrome of HF. We focus our efforts mostly on those adaptations confined to skeletal muscle, because **Chapter 14** provides an in-depth discussion of skeletal muscle vascular adaptations.

Mitochondrial Adaptations

Much of the early work in this field used phosphorus magnetic resonance spectroscopy (MRS), coupled with isolated limb exercise, to noninvasively monitor inorganic phosphate, phosphocreatine, and ATP levels and cellular pH in skeletal muscle to assess oxidative metabolism. Early studies from a number of laboratories throughout the 1980s and 1990s showed that HF was characterized by intrinsic deficits in skeletal muscle oxidative capacity that yield disproportionately greater increases in inorganic phosphate and reductions in pH for a given exercise load (**Fig. 16.4**). Importantly, these abnormalities were shown to be independent of blood flow,[9] muscle atrophy,[12] and fiber type adaptations,[8] suggesting an intrinsic deficit in oxidative metabolism. At approximately the same time, ultrastructural studies of skeletal muscle tissue from HF patients showed evidence of significant mitochondrial rarefaction,[10] providing a potential subcellular mechanism underlying the aforementioned metabolic derangements identified by

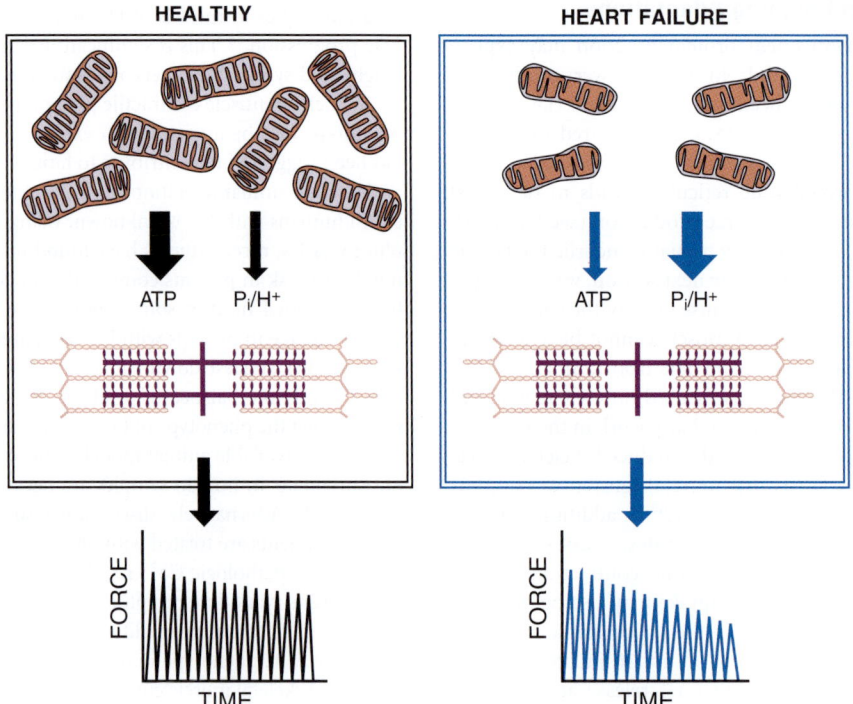

Fig. 16.4 Effects of heart failure (HF) to impair oxidative capacity and hasten muscle fatigue in skeletal muscle. HF contributes to both structural and functional impairment of skeletal muscle oxidative capacity. HF contributes to quantitative and function changes in mitochondria, including mitochondrial loss, disrupted ultrastructure (decreased cristae), and reduced capacity for oxidative adenosine triphosphate (ATP) production. This leads to increased inorganic phosphate levels (Pi), greater acidity, and suboptimal ATP provision during exercise. Increased Pi, reduced pH, and decreased ATP availability would conspire to impair myofilament contractile function. Collectively, these alterations lead to more rapid muscle fatigue during repetitive muscular activity, as indicated by a more rapid reduction in force production (bottom force tracings). Such a reduction in skeletal muscle oxidative capacity would contribute to decreased tissue oxygen use and, in turn, reduced whole body peak oxygen consumption.

MRS. Early studies showing reduced activity of a variety of oxidative enzymes in HF patients[8] further suggested impaired energy metabolism. More recently, studies have identified similar adaptations in patients with HFpEF.[81] Collectively, these results implicate impaired oxidative metabolism, and mitochondrial structure/function in particular, in the symptomology of HF. Along with the fiber type alterations discussed previously, these energetic abnormalities have become a hallmark of the skeletal muscle myopathy of HF. In addition, impaired skeletal muscle oxidative metabolism in HF has served as evidence to support the recommendation of aerobic exercise training as an intervention to alleviate exercise intolerance in HF, considering that the primary effect of such exercise to improve aerobic fitness in cardiac populations likely derives from its effects on skeletal muscle oxidative capacity.[82]

Recent studies have also highlighted the role of metabolic signaling through peroxisome proliferator-activated receptor δ (PPAR) δ signaling. Administration of a pharmacologic agonist of PPARδ increased skeletal muscle oleic acid oxidation in mice with HF compared with placebo treatment.[83] PPARδ stimulation increased oxidative gene expression, improved running endurance, and preserved fatty acid oxidation, suggesting that drugs that modify metabolic function might correct skeletal muscle dysfunction in HF.

However, a considerable body of research has raised doubts about whether HF per se alters skeletal muscle oxidative capacity generally or mitochondrial content or function specifically. Using MRS, Chati and colleagues[84] found no group differences in ATP, inorganic phosphate, or pH during exercise when HF patients were compared with sedentary

controls who were recruited to match patients for their low level of physical activity. In contrast, they found that trained control subjects (>14 hr/wk of physical training) showed slower ATP depletion, inorganic phosphate accumulation, and acidification than HF patients or sedentary controls. In another study, which used saponin-skinned muscle fibers, Mettauer and coworkers[54] observed no effect of HF on oxidative metabolism in patients versus sedentary controls (peak VO₂ < 110% of predicted), whereas lower oxidative rates were found in both of these groups compared with active controls (peak VO₂ > 110% of predicted). Finally, Williams and colleagues,[85] working with isolated mitochondria, showed no differences in ATP production rates between HF patients and sedentary controls (no specification for the designation of "sedentary" was provided). Thus, when studying muscle oxidative function using a variety of techniques, from isolated mitochondria to in vivo, these data suggest that a large proportion of the effect of HF on skeletal muscle oxidative capacity may be explained by the chronic physical inactivity that characterizes these patients, rather than the disease process itself. This conclusion should be tempered by the fact that studies have shown defects in oxidative metabolism in forearm muscles, which should not be impacted by muscle disuse,[9] arguing for some contribution from the disease.

Similar questions arise regarding the potential involvement of muscle disuse in the mitochondrial rarefaction observed in HF patients.[10] More recent studies that have matched HF patients and controls for physical activity level did not observe a reduction in mitochondrial content.[86] In fact, the early studies of Drexler and colleagues emphasized that mitochondrial loss is only apparent in patients with later-stage

HF, where one might expect more pronounced reductions in physical activity. Arguing against muscle disuse as the precipitant for mitochondrial loss, a recent study has shown mitochondrial rarefaction in HF patients compared with sedentary controls.[87] Thus there is still ambiguity as to whether there is a unique effect of HF on mitochondrial content/morphology. However, from the preceding discussion, it should be apparent that any mitochondrial structural abnormalities that might be present have minimal effects on overall mitochondrial function when the effects of physical inactivity are taken into account.

Another consideration that should be factored into this discussion is the effect of medications. Many of the early studies establishing an effect of HF on skeletal muscle oxidative capacity and mitochondrial biology were performed prior to the widespread use of vasodilator therapy. This point is noteworthy because some studies in preclinical models of ischemic cardiomyopathy (coronary artery ligation model) have shown that initiation of an ACEi following coronary infarct can mitigate impaired mitochondrial function related to HF.[88] Thus one reason for the failure of more recent studies to observe an effect of HF on skeletal muscle oxidative capacity may relate to the evolution of HF therapies. Indeed, Drexler and colleagues[10] noted that mitochondrial loss could be largely corrected in patients with treatment that led to sufficient functional improvements. Whether these medications have a unique effect to modulate skeletal muscle oxidative function, or instead derive their benefits from effects on nonmuscle systems that indirectly improve muscle function via reduced disease burden and/or increased physical activity, is not apparent. Arguing against the former, studies in preclinical models suggest that ACEi does not modulate skeletal muscle oxidative capacity through alterations in mitochondrial function.[89] Whatever the mechanism, there are clearly effects of HF medications on skeletal muscle oxidative capacity that should be considered when discerning which factors incite decreased aerobic capacity in these patients.

Interventions to improve skeletal muscle oxidative function in HF patients have substantial benefits. HF is characterized by reduced habitual physical activity[53] and acute periods of profound muscle disuse during hospitalization, both of which diminish overall oxidative capacity. Thus aerobic exercise training remains attractive as a means to improve overall functional capacity in HF patients. In fact, some degree of exercise training may be required to remediate the "detraining effects" that the disease imposes on skeletal muscle, as studies have shown that skeletal muscle energetic abnormalities persist after correction of cardiac insufficiency via transplantation.[90] There is substantial evidence that mitochondrial biology and skeletal muscle oxidative capacity can be improved with aerobic training,[91,92] and that such improvements can be elicited with relatively low-intensity exercise (40% of peak oxygen uptake;[93]). Thus rehabilitation programs that use aerobic exercise training remain an attractive adjunct to classical HF therapeutics to improve functional capacity and quality of life.

Fiber Type Adaptations

Decreased oxidative capacity in HF patients may be a function of disease-related fiber type shifts toward a more fast-twitch, glycolytic phenotype. As addressed previously, these alterations in fiber type, as reflected by alterations in the expression of MHC protein, are largely related to muscle disuse, rather than a unique effect of the disease process. Regardless of the inciting factor, and beyond its role in dictating skeletal muscle oxidative capacity, fiber type composition plays an important role in determining overall functional capacity, as assessed by peak oxygen consumption.[94] More specifically, lower slow-twitch fiber content is associated with exercise intolerance. In this light, interventions to counter the switch towards a fast-twitch fiber type, such as aerobic exercise, would clearly be beneficial in maintaining and/or improving functional capacity. Indeed, the effect of aerobic training to shift muscle

fiber type composition towards a more slow-twitch phenotype in HF patients is well founded.[95] In addition to exercise training, certain HF medications may exert similar beneficial effects on muscle fiber composition. As noted previously, studies in patients [55] have shown that antagonism of angiotensin II via ACEi or angiotensin receptor blockers shifts skeletal muscle fiber composition towards a more slow-twitch phenotype. Commensurate with these shifts in fiber type was an increase in peak aerobic capacity. This provides a potential cellular-level explanation for how medications may alter muscle oxidative capacity and, furthermore, raises the intriguing possibility that one of the cornerstone therapies for HF may derive some of its beneficial effects, at least in part, from improvements in skeletal muscle abnormalities.

Vascular Adaptations (see also Chapter 14)

Impaired peripheral vascular flow dynamics are only partially explained by reduced cardiac output, and abnormal tissue perfusion through impaired microcirculation constitutes another important disturbance of vascular flow dynamics in HF. This is particularly important in HF because vascular flow dynamics relate to intrinsic properties of skeletal muscle affecting exercise performance. In oxidative muscle, capillary density is higher in comparison with more glycolytic muscle types. This relates directly to endurance function and exercise performance. Of note, exercise training in normal cohorts, as well as in HF subjects, increases not only muscle function but also skeletal muscle capillary density, which suggests that improved peripheral microcirculatory flow dynamics are linked to improved oxidative function.

Capillary density measured as the ratio of capillaries per muscle fiber shows a consistent reduction in the skeletal muscle of HF patients compared with controls.[10,85,96] This has been linked to reduced exercise tolerance.[96] However, this relation has been difficult to reproduce in the continuum of clinical stages of patients with HF, suggesting that certain degrees of structural and functional derangements in skeletal muscle are necessary to develop a persistent and significant vascular phenotype. Metabolic changes relating to differences in oxygen use and ability to extract oxygen from the peripheral circulation, as what might be expected with reduced mitochondria content and function described previously, might in fact be required to promote changes in capillary density. In this context, intrinsic skeletal muscle adaptations may feed back to the vasculature to provoke maladaptive changes.

EFFECTORS OF SKELETAL MUSCLE ADAPTATIONS

Hypoperfusion

Reduced cardiac output and decreased capillary density of skeletal muscle are directly linked.[96] Although cardiac output at rest is only minimally impaired in HF, most changes occur during exercise during a state of increased oxygen demand of the working skeletal muscle. Therefore the imbalance of oxygen and energy supply to skeletal muscle is in particular impaired during exercise and physical work. Although this corresponds to the clinical symptoms of advanced HF, it does not fully explain the underlying mechanisms. Several studies have suggested that impaired cardiac output and pulsatility in advanced HF lead to reduced shear stress in the vascular endothelium and therefore to a reduction in shear-released nitric oxide,[97] one of the strongest vasodilators. Furthermore, the chronic activation of the renin-angiotensin-aldosterone system and a hyperadrenergic state in advanced HF favors a vasoconstriction of the peripheral vasculature. With that, peripheral hypoperfusion, both at rest and particularly during exercise, is worsened. In turn, the beneficial effects of peripheral vasodilator therapy on improving cardiac output and peripheral perfusion are explained by this phenomenon.

Reduced capillary density, progressive vasodilation, and impaired oxidative metabolism are linked by the molecular response to chronic hypoperfusion and low-grade ischemia. Several studies have confirmed that both in the myocardium and in skeletal muscle, ischemia and ischemia/reperfusion result in a switch toward a more glycolytic metabolism.[98] This is, in part, explained by the ability of the cell to produce ATP, even in the absence of oxygen through glycolysis. In contrast, oxidative metabolism requires a sufficient oxygen supply. Although fatty acid oxidation seems to be particularly affected, all other substrates for oxidative metabolism, including glucose, amino acids, and lactate, require oxygen-dependent metabolic steps as part of mitochondrial generation of ATP. Therefore the increased glycolytic capacity of skeletal muscle in advanced HF might be a direct reflection of impaired tissue oxygenation in combination with other pathomechanisms discussed in this section.

Inflammation

Although increased levels of circulating cytokines such as TNF-α, IL-6, and IL-1β in chronic disease states are a well-established finding, an increased local expression of proinflammatory cytokines, and their potential role in mechanisms leading to muscular atrophy, has only recently attracted more attention.[18,20,21] Circulating cytokine levels do not reflect tissue levels and their potential activity due to unknown autocrine/paracrine effects, in contrast to the typical endocrine action of circulating hormones/metabolites. Moreover, tissue-specific expression further complicates the analysis of their exact action. It is possible that enhanced local expression of proinflammatory cytokines precedes an increase in circulating levels and therefore represents a more sensitive indicator of local skeletal muscle abnormalities in HF.

One possible mechanism leading to an increased local expression of proinflammatory cytokines might be found in an enhanced activation of the transcription factor NF-κB. This transcription factor regulates the expression of proinflammatory cytokines (e.g., TNF-α and IL-1β).[99] Moreover, both cytokines and angiotensin II[100] trigger their local expression by a receptor-mediated activation of NF-κB. The activation of NF-κB occurs in chronic muscle diseases and has been implicated in reduced maturation and regeneration of skeletal muscle.[101] Furthermore, NF-κB regulates the expression of the inducible isoform of the nitric oxide synthase (iNOS), which is overexpressed in skeletal muscle in HF patients[102] and may lead to muscle atrophy[103] and contractile dysfunction.[104]

Oxidative Stress

Increased oxidant activity can lead to detrimental effects on skeletal muscle structure and function and evolves under conditions where the generation of reactive oxygen/nitrogen species (ROS/RNS) exceeds the capacity of antioxidant systems. Several lines of evidence suggest that HF is accompanied by increased oxidative stress in skeletal muscle, with potential significance for skeletal muscle structure and function.

Studies have shown increased oxidative modification of proteins, lipids, and DNA in animal models[105,106] and humans.[102,107] However, whether this is due to increased generation of ROS/RNS or diminished antioxidant activity is uncertain. Studies have shown increased generation of ROS[108] and expression NOS[102,106] and reduced expression of decreased expression of antioxidant systems.[106] However, the proximal factor contributing to these precipitants of increased oxidative stress in skeletal muscle in HF is unclear. Numerous investigators have suggested that this relates to increased immune activation,[104] and recent studies in animal models have implicated a potential role for increased angiotensin II,[109] but substantiation of any of these mechanisms in humans is lacking.

Elevated skeletal muscle oxidative stress may contribute to both muscle atrophy and dysfunction. Studies have shown that enhanced oxidative stress contributes to muscle atrophy.[110] In fact, recent studies have suggested that increased antioxidant expression secondary

to genetic manipulation in animal models of HF may prevent muscle atrophy.[111,112] Oxidative modification of proteins important for muscle contraction (e.g., ECC proteins, myofilament proteins)[104] or oxidative metabolism (mitochondrial proteins, creatine kinase) could impair skeletal muscle strength or endurance, leading to exercise intolerance. Indeed, studies in human HF have shown that increased oxidative modification of myofilament proteins is related to reduced exercise capacity.[107] Interestingly, studies in animal models have shown that β-blockers can reduce oxidative protein modifications in HF.[113] Moreover, if angiotensin II contributes to increased skeletal muscle oxidative stress in HF,[109] ACEi and angiotensin receptor blockers may further diminish oxidant activity. This may explain at least part of the effects of these two drugs to alleviate HF symptomology. In addition, recent studies have shown that aerobic exercise training can increase antioxidant systems and reduce oxidative protein modification,[114] which may, in part, mediate the beneficial effects of exercise training on exercise tolerance.

Muscle Disuse

Weight-bearing activity is significantly curtailed in HF patients,[53] which may relate to psychological barriers to performing certain activities.[115] Thus one could argue that a large proportion of the skeletal muscle myopathy of HF actually represents physical inactivity/deconditioning that accompanies the syndrome,[116] rather than a unique effect of the disease. This may seem like an unnecessary distinction because it is axiomatic that individuals with HF are less active than their healthy counterparts, with physical inactivity frequently being both a cause and a consequence of their underlying heart disease. However, defining which specific skeletal muscle adaptations are directly attributable to the disease process or its sequelae is important for understanding which may be amenable to exercise countermeasures. More specifically, defining which aspect of the skeletal muscle pathology of HF is due to muscle disuse could also help to define the modality that would be most effective at remediating that defect because much is known about how different training paradigms impact various facets of skeletal muscle biology (e.g., resistance exercise training might be more effective at correcting contractile deficits, whereas aerobic exercise training would be more effective at correcting mitochondrial adaptations/oxidative deficiencies).

It is necessary to distinguish between acute and chronic muscle disuse because the magnitude and character of disuse is likely to differ. Acute disuse likely occurs during hospitalization due to acute disease exacerbation or health decline due to other comorbidities. Hospitalization for acute HF is accompanied by bed rest, which is known to lead to dramatic alterations in skeletal muscle. However, with treatment and reambulation, many of these acute adaptations may remediate. Indeed, even some of the most profound adaptations in skeletal muscle, such as mitochondrial rarefaction, can be largely corrected with successful treatment and reambulation.[10] This is again a necessary distinction because most of the seminal work in this field did not clarify the clinical state of the patients studied or their proximity to hospitalization. Thus it is unclear to what extent many of the hallmark muscle adaptations to HF represent transient adaptations to factors associated with hospitalization, such as profound muscle disuse, and which are truly attributable to the underlying disease. In contrast, chronic disuse in HF patients represents a drop in normal daily activities on the order of approximately 50%.[53] To what extent such a drop in habitual activity might contribute to the skeletal muscle adaptations observed in HF is unclear, but even short periods of this magnitude of inactivity can affect skeletal muscle in older adults.[117] Thus many of the skeletal muscle adaptations observed in HF patients are likely the result of either acute or chronic reductions in muscle use, rather than any unique effect of the disease process.[116]

CONTRIBUTION OF SKELETAL MUSCLE ADAPTATIONS TO SYMPTOMOLOGY

How do skeletal muscle adaptations contribute to the major symptoms of exercise limitation in HF patients: dyspnea and muscle fatigue? As the previous discussion of potential precipitating factors should reveal, the skeletal muscle adaptations occurring in any one individual patient are likely to be complex and unique. Thus there is no simple answer to this question, because it will likely be highly variable among patients, as well as within patients throughout the course of the disease. However, some generalizations are possible.

In acute HF, much of the symptomology likely occurs secondary to circulatory congestion and cardiac insufficiency. However, there are accompanying alterations in skeletal muscle size and function, characterized by muscle atrophy, contractile dysfunction, and reduced oxidative capacity, which may further lessen exercise tolerance, because all of these adaptations would reduce overall physiologic functional capacity. In other words, any given physical activity would require a greater relative percentage of an individual's physiologic capacity and, accordingly, be more likely to provoke dyspnea and fatigue. Aside from this simple lowering of physiologic capacity, muscle adaptations may contribute to symptomology in ways that have been classically assigned to cardiac contractile dysfunction/circulatory congestion. For instance, increased metabolite generation owing to impaired oxidative capacity, together with enhanced sensory nerve activation (either by mechanoreceptor or metaboreceptor hypersensitivity) in skeletal muscle, may increase vasoconstriction and ventilatory drive,[118] which would contribute to muscle fatigue and dyspnea. The precipitating factor for increased sensory nerve stimulation (e.g., metabolic dysfunction in skeletal muscle leading to enhanced metabolite generation and/or effects of acute HF on sensory neurons) is not known, but it is clear that these adaptations in skeletal muscle likely figure into the symptomology of acute HF.

In chronic HF, the contribution of these skeletal muscle adaptations to symptomology is primarily through their capacity to limit physiologic capacity. For instance, reduced oxidative capacity, owing to reduced mitochondrial content and function, as well as fiber type switching toward a more glycolytic phenotype, contribute to dyspnea and fatigue directly. In the case of the former, metabolic derangements leading to excessive metabolite production (e.g., increased acidity) increase ventilatory drive by activating sensory afferents.[119] Regarding the latter, excessive metabolite generation, such as increased intracellular phosphate levels,[9] decreases myofilament force production,[120] which is the primary physiologic marker of muscular fatigue. These adaptations, and others, such as muscle atrophy and weakness, would also contribute to the subjective sensation of fatigue by reducing the overall physiologic capacity and would cause patients to perceive any activity as more demanding. Thus, as can be gleaned from this discussion, there are a large number of possible combinations of skeletal muscle adaptations that can contribute to dyspnea and fatigue in the context of either acute or chronic HF.

SUMMARY AND FUTURE DIRECTIONS

HF is characterized by marked adaptations in skeletal muscle quantity and functionality that contribute to the primary symptoms of fatigue and dyspnea. Many of these adaptations likely result from skeletal muscle disuse that accompanies the syndrome of HF, but heightened inflammation, oxidative stress, and hypoperfusion probably also contribute (**Fig. 16.5**). Accordingly, exercise training appears to be an

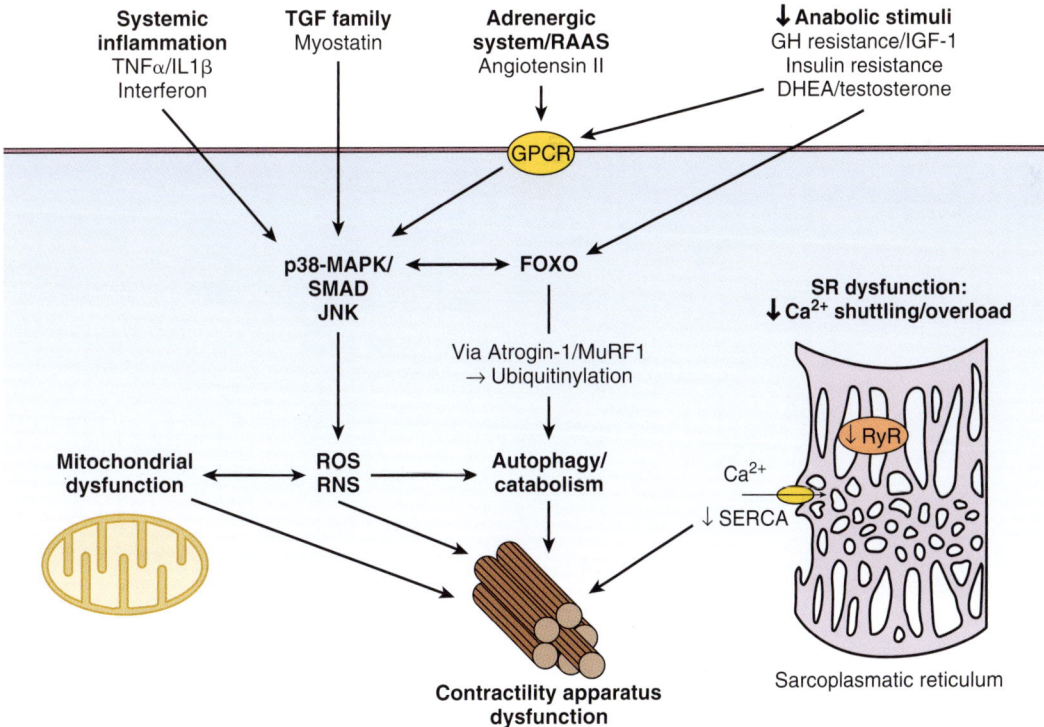

Fig. 16.5 Summary of pathophysiologic mechanisms impairing skeletal muscle function in heart failure. *DHEA*, Dehydroepiandrosterone; *GH*, growth hormone; *IGF-1*, insulin-like growth factor-1; *IL-1β*, interleukin-1β; *JNK*, c-Jun N-terminal kinase; *RAAS*, renin-angiotensin-aldosterone system; *RNS*, reactive nitrogen species; *ROS*, reactive oxygen species; *SERCA*, sarcoplasmic reticulum Ca²⁺ ATPase; *SR*, sarcoplasmic reticulum; *TGF*, transforming growth factor; *TNF-α*, tumor necrosis factor-α. From Kennel PJ, Mancini DM, Schulze PC. Skeletal muscle changes in chronic cardiac disease and failure. *Compr Physiol.* 2015;5(4):1947–1969.

effective countermeasure for many of these skeletal muscle adaptations and should be considered as a standard treatment in suitable patients. Various standard HF medications may also counteract some of the skeletal muscle adaptations, raising the intriguing possibility that at least some portion of their clinical benefit derives from their ability to influence skeletal muscle structure and function, either directly or indirectly. Taken together, this evidence solidifies a role for skeletal muscle adaptations in the symptomology of HF.

KEY REFERENCES

1. Downing J, Balady GJ. The role of exercise training in heart failure. *J Am Coll Cardiol.* 2011;58:561–569.
5. Kitzman DW, Nicklas B, Kraus WE, et al. Skeletal muscle abnormalities and exercise intolerance in older patients with heart failure and preserved ejection fraction. *Am J Physiol Heart Circ Physiol.* 2014;306:H1364–H1370.
23. Anker SD, Volterrani M, Pflaum CD, et al. Acquired growth hormone resistance in patients with chronic heart failure: implications for therapy with growth hormone. *J Am Coll Cardiol.* 2001;38:443–452.
36. Heineke J, Auger-Messier M, Xu J, et al. Genetic deletion of myostatin from the heart prevents skeletal muscle atrophy in heart failure. *Circulation.* 2010;121:419–425.

45. Gielen S, Sandri M, Kozarez I, et al. Exercise training attenuates MuRF-1 expression in the skeletal uscle of patients with chronic heart failure independent of age. *Circulation.* 2012;125:2716–2727.
46. Miller MS, VanBuren P, LeWinter MM, et al. Mechanisms underlying skeletal muscle weakness in human heart failure: alterations in single fiber myosin protein content and function. *Circ Heart Fail.* 2009;2:700–706.
54. Mettauer B, Zoll J, Sanchez H, et al. Oxidative capacity of skeletal muscle in heart failure patients versus sedentary or active controls subjects. *J Am Coll Cardiol.* 2001;38:947–954.
76. Bellinger AM, Reiken S, Dura M, et al. Remodeling of ryanodine receptor complex causes "leaky" channels: a molecular mechanism for decreased exercise capacity. *Proc Natl Acad Sci.* 2008;105:2198–2202.
109. Inoue N, Kinugawa S, Suga T, et al. Angiotensin II-induced reduction in exercise capacity is associated with increased oxidative stress in skeletal muscle. *Am J Physiol.* 2012;302:H1202–H1210.
116. Rehn TA, Munkvik M, Lunde PK, Sjaastad I, Sejersted OM. Intrinsic skeletal muscle alterations in chronic heart failure patients: a disease-specific myopathy or a result of deconditioning? *Heart Fail Rev.* 2011;17:421–436.

The full reference list for this chapter is available on ExpertConsult.

Alterations in Cardiac Metabolism in Heart Failure

Heiko Bugger, Adam R. Wende, E. Dale Abel

OUTLINE

OVERVIEW OF CARDIAC METABOLISM

Hallmarks and Regulation of Cardiac Energy Metabolism

Cardiac energy metabolism is essential to maintain cardiac pump function. To enable the heart to beat 100,000 times a day for a lifetime, the heart exhibits a highly regulated and efficient system for adenosine triphosphate (ATP) regeneration, generating up to 6 kg of ATP every day, which is 15- to 20-fold its own weight. Thus the heart is one of the most metabolically active organs, and its prolific capacity for generating energy is underscored by the very high density of mitochondria and their unique patterns of distribution relative to areas of high energy utilization such as sarcomeres (the contractile unit) and the sarcolemma where significant changes in ionic flux occurs.[1] Under physiologic conditions, the heart generates more than 95% of its ATP by oxidative metabolism of energy substrates; 60% to 70% of ATP arises from the oxidation of fatty acids (FAs), and 30% to 40% from the oxidation of glucose and other substrates such as lactate, amino acids, and ketone bodies, depending on their availability in the circulation.[2] Utilization of FAs for ATP regeneration initially requires FA uptake into the cardiomyocyte via fatty acid transporters such as CD36 and the fatty acid transporters (FATP, family of proteins). Following esterification to acyl CoA by acyl-CoA synthetase, they are imported into mitochondria by transient coupling to carnitine via the carnitine palmitoyltransferase (CPT) system. Once imported into mitochondria, acyl Coenzyme A (CoA) is oxidized in the β-oxidation spiral to yield acetyl CoA and flavin adenine dinucleotide (FADH). Utilization of glucose requires sarcolemmal glucose uptake via the classical insulin-responsive glucose transporter 4 (GLUT4) and the constitutive glucose transporter (GLUT1).[3] Recent evidence suggests that some glucose might enter the heart via the sodium-glucose transporter (SGLT1).[4] However, GLUT4, which shuttles to the cell surface with cardiomyocyte contraction, likely accounts for the bulk of myocardial glucose uptake. Upon entering the heart, most of the glucose is

metabolized via glycolysis to yield ATP, reduced nicotinamide adenine dinucleotide (NADH), and pyruvate. Additional metabolic branches of glycolysis such as the hexosamine biosynthetic pathway (HBP) or the pentose phosphate pathway (PPP) yield metabolites that play an important role in signal transduction, oxidation-reduction REDOX regulation, and nucleic acid synthesis. Pyruvate is imported into mitochondria via the mitochondrial pyruvate transporter and decarboxylated by pyruvate dehydrogenase (PDH) to acetyl CoA. Acetyl CoA derived from metabolic precursors such as glucose, FAs, and others (e.g., ketones) enters the (tricarboxylic acid) TCA cycle. Oxidation of acetyl CoA in the TCA cycle generates NADH and FADH, which donate electrons to the electron transport chain (ETC), which pumps protons into the mitochondrial intermembrane space to generate the proton-motive force that is dissipated via ATP synthase to ultimately regenerate ATP from adenosine diphosphate (ADP) by the process of oxidative phosphorylation (OXPHOS) (**Fig. 17.1**).

Several modes of regulation adapt cardiac energetics to acute or chronic changes in energy demand. Long-term regulation of cardiac energy metabolism is usually governed by changes in gene expression. For example, transcriptional regulators that regulate genes that encode mitochondrial enzymes of mitochondrial OXPHOS can be induced or repressed by various stimuli that correlate with changes in cardiac substrate metabolism. These transcriptional regulators include nuclear receptors that regulate genes that encode fatty acid oxidation (FAO) enzymes such as peroxisome proliferator activated (PPAR)α, PPARβ/δ, and estrogen related receptor (ERR)α, transcription factors that increase OXPHOS gene expression (transcription factor A of mitochondria [TFAM], nuclear respiratory factors [NRFs], ERRα), and transcriptional coactivators that regulate both the expression of FAO and OXPHOS genes (PPAR gamma coactivator [PGC]-1α, PGC-1β) (**Table 17.1**).[5] Thus conditions of FA excess such as obesity and diabetes are associated with increased expression of transcriptional regulators of FAO, whereas heart failure (HF), which is associated with

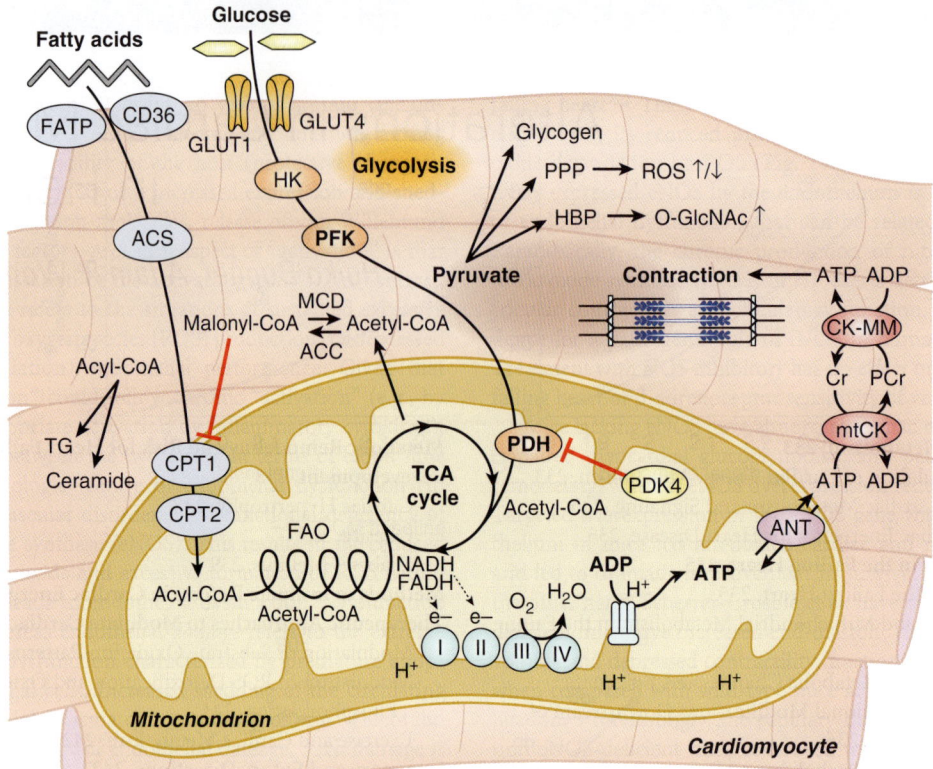

Fig. 17.1 Simplified overview of myocardial energy substrate utilization and regulatory mechanisms in the normal heart. Fatty acids (FA) enter the heart via transporters such as CD36 and fatty acid transport proteins (FATP) and are converted to FA-acyl-CoA by the enzyme family acyl CoA synthetase (ACS). These acyl CoA enter the mitochondria via carnitine palmitoyl transferases (CPT) and are oxidized within mitochondria for ATP regeneration. Alternatively, they are used for the synthesis of triglycerides or ceramides. Mitochondrial uptake and subsequent oxidation of acyl CoA are regulated by intracellular levels of malonyl CoA, the steady state levels of which are governed by activities of malonyl CoA decarboxylase (MCD) and acetyl CoA decarboxylase (ACC). Glycolysis, which is regulated by multiple enzymes, including hexokinase (HK) and phosphofructokinase (PFK), generates pyruvate. Pyruvate is imported into the mitochondria via the inner mitochondrial membrane pyruvate carrier and is oxidized by pyruvate dehydrogenase (PDH) for ATP regeneration. PDH activity may be inhibited by increased levels and activity of pyruvate dehydrogenase kinase (PDK4). Alternatively, glycolytic intermediates may be used to increase glycogen storage or to increase flux into the pentose phosphate pathway (PPP) or to catalyze the hexosamine biosynthetic pathway (HBP). ATP generated from intramitochondrial substrate oxidation is delivered to myofibrils by the phosphocreatine shuttle to maintain cardiac contraction.

TABLE 17.1	**Regulators of Myocardial Energy Metabolism**	
Molecule	**Predominant Functions in Heart**	**Mechanism of Action**
PPARα	Increase FAO gene expression	Transcription factor
PGC-1α, PGC-1β	Increase FAO and OXPHOS gene expression, increase mitochondrial biogenesis, ROS detoxification	Transcriptional coactivator
ERRα	Increase FAO and OXPHOS gene expression	Transcription factor
TFAm	mtDNA replication, OXPHOS gene expression	Transcription factor
NRF1	OXPHOS gene expression	Transcription factor
AMPK	Increase FA uptake and oxidation, increase glucose uptake, increase glycolysis, inhibit anabolic pathways	Protein kinase
SIRT1, SIRT3, SIRT5	Increase FA and glucose oxidation, increase mitochondrial function, ROS detoxification	Deacylase

FA, Fatty acid; *mtDNA*, mitochondrial DNA.

decreased mitochondrial energetics capacity is associated with repression of PGC-1α. Mechanisms that acutely regulate short-term changes in energetics include signaling pathways that drive regulatory pathways via posttranslational mechanisms. One of the best-studied pathways is adenosine monophosphate-activated protein kinase (AMPK) activation, which drives catabolic pathways and inhibits anabolic pathways

by phosphorylation of specific metabolic enzymes that regulate glycolysis, glycogen synthesis, and FAO. A second pathway is protein deacetylation of a broad variety of metabolic enzymes, including FAO enzymes, TCA cycle enzymes, PDH, OXPHOS subunits, and the F_OF_1-ATPase by a family of NAD+-dependent deacylases called sirtuins,[6] which links cardiac metabolic capacity with nutrient sensing via NAD+.

Allosteric regulation of metabolic enzymes represents another important mechanism for the short-term regulation of cardiac metabolism. This is classically exemplified by the "Randle cycle," whereby increased FA utilization inhibits glucose utilization via increased generation of citrate, which inhibits glycolysis, and the reverse Randle cycle, whereby increased malonyl CoA that may occur when glucose utilization is increased in turn allosterically inhibits CPT1 and mitochondrial FA utilization. Cardiac energy metabolism is also acutely regulated by various stress hormones (e.g., catecholamines), cytokines, insulin signaling, changes in workload, or concentrations of metabolic substrates.

Crosstalk Between Cardiac Metabolism and Signaling

Although the main function of myocardial energy substrate metabolism is to generate ATP, metabolic intermediates also serve as signaling molecules. Both glycolysis and mitochondrial energy metabolism generate and consume NADH and thereby participate in the regulation of the NAD^+/NADH ratio, which can be considered an indicator of the cellular energy charge. Accordingly, this ratio increases during energy demand and decreases under conditions of sufficient ATP supply, which in turn regulates the activity of sirtuins, which not only regulate energetics but also cellular senescence, growth, mitochondrial biogenesis, and reactive oxygen species (ROS), among other mechanisms (see also Chapter 8).[7] In addition to entering glycolysis, glucose may also enter other pathways such as the PPP and the HBP. Flux through the HBP generates glucosamine that increases O-GlcNAcylation of many proteins that regulate diverse cellular functions. These include proteins, the modification of which modulates transcription factor activity, epigenetic regulation, cellular Ca^{2+} homeostasis, cell growth, cell survival, oxidative stress, and mitochondrial function.[8] Flux through the PPP regulates the generation of NADPH, which, as a substrate for NADPH oxidases, serves an important generator of cytosolic ROS. PPP intermediates also maintain the levels of reduced glutathione. Thus PPP flux participates importantly in the regulation of cellular REDOX. The redox state of cells plays important roles in multiple cellular signaling pathways, including oxidative modification of regulatory proteins that includes targets such as phosphatases, protein kinases (A, D, and G), cytokines, mitogen-activated protein kinases, or insulin signaling.[9,10] In this regard, the activity (i.e., forward or reverse mode) of the mitochondrial nicotinamide nucleotide transhydrogenase (NNT), which transfers electrons between NAD(H) and NADP(H) to balance ATP production and antioxidant capacity, is dependent on metabolic demand and cardiac workload.[11] Another metabolite affecting intracellular signaling is citrate, the conversion of which to acetyl CoA by ATP-citrate lyase may contribute to direct enzyme acetylation by cytosolic acetyltransferases, as well as to nuclear histone acetylation and subsequent epigenetic regulation of gene expression.[12] The examples discussed here are not exhaustive because many additional metabolites, such as succinate, are being identified and may regulate signaling pathways within the heart under basal conditions or in response to stressors such as ischemia/reperfusion.[13]

Significance of Cardiac Energetics for Heart Disease

Impaired cardiac metabolism and energy depletion are well recognized to contribute to cardiac dysfunction and reduced efficiency in terms of energy transfer to contractile work (see also Chapter 2). These changes, which contribute to many cardiac pathologies by impairing ATP-dependent intracellular processes such as myofilament contraction and maintenance of ion homeostasis, have been described in prevalent disorders such as myocardial ischemia reperfusion injury, diabetes-related cardiac dysfunction, cardiac hypertrophy, and HF.[2] In ischemia reperfusion, ATP regeneration is impaired due to limited oxygen and substrate supply and to persistent impairment in OXPHOS and

mitochondrial integrity. In cardiac hypertrophy, substrate preference may shift toward a relative increase in glucose utilization, accompanied by early defects in mitochondrial function, whereas in HF, overall mitochondrial oxidative metabolism can be impaired. In diabetes, increased FAO and impaired glucose utilization are associated with impaired mitochondrial ATP generation, mitochondrial uncoupling, and impaired cardiac efficiency that may be characterized by increased myocardial oxygen consumption.

Recent work has revealed important sex differences in cardiac metabolism in healthy subjects and in individuals with cardiac dysfunction or high-risk conditions such as diabetes. Myocardial oxygen consumption (MVO_2) and myocardial FA utilization (MFAU) are higher in healthy females relative to males[14] and may be related to estrogen.[15] These differences persisted in individuals with type 2 diabetes (T2D)[16] and in those with HF with preserved ejection fraction (HFpEF) (see also Chapters 11 and 39).[17] Myocardial blood flow (MBF) rates were higher in women with HFpEF, and MBF was correlated with better event-free survival. Despite lower rates of MFAU, diabetic men exhibited greater impairment in diastolic relaxation. In a study of normal, obese, and T2D subjects, diabetes and obesity reduced glucose utilization, but sex also had a powerful effect on glucose utilization, with levels of glucose utilization being lower in females. Because glucose uptake and metabolism rates were relatively low in nonobese women, they were not markedly different from those in obese and T2DM women. Thus the potentially detrimental effects of obesity and diabetes on myocardial glucose metabolism appear to be more pronounced in men than women.[18]

The relevance of altered myocardial metabolism for disease development and progression is underpinned by a number of clinical trials that investigated the effects of specific metabolic interventions, in particular in HF. Some of these trials have yielded promising results despite small patient numbers, including improvements in ejection fraction (EF), HF symptoms, and HF hospitalization, although data from large randomized controlled clinical trials investigating hard clinical end points are lacking to date.[19] Finally, a number of metabolic cardiomyopathies have been described in which a single mutation or enzyme deficiency may lead to cardiac failure, likely due to impairment in cardiac energetics, further emphasizing the direct relationship between myocardial energy metabolism and HF development. These defects include systemic carnitine deficiency, malonyl carboxylase deficiency, deficiency of FAO enzymes, and inherited mutations in mitochondrial (mtDNA).[20] This chapter will review mechanisms, diagnostic approaches, and potential therapeutic strategies related to metabolic dysfunction in the failing heart.

METABOLIC DYSFUNCTION IN THE FAILING HEART

Energy Depletion in the Failing Heart

Continuous cardiac pump function requires the regeneration of large amounts of ATP. Energy depletion is a well-established characteristic of HF irrespective of its etiology. When directly examined, energy deprivation in failing human hearts is characterized by a reduction in the phosphocreatine (PCr)/ATP ratio.[21] The PCr shuttle transfers ATP from mitochondria to myofilaments and transfers ADP back to the mitochondria for rephosphorylation. PCr receives its phosphate group from ATP by the creatine kinase reaction, which favors ATP synthesis over PCr synthesis by approximately 100-fold. Thus, when ATP demand outweighs ATP availability, the PCr/ATP ratio declines first and represents a sensitive and powerful index of the energetic state of the heart. In HF patients, PCr/ATP was found to be reduced, and the magnitude of this reduction correlates with New York Heart Association (NYHA) functional class, systolic and diastolic function, and mortality.[22,23] In addition, mitochondrial respiratory capacity and rates of ATP synthesis are markedly decreased in HF patients, both in ischemic and nonischemic dilated cardiomyopathy.[24,25] An unresolved question remains as to whether impaired cardiac energetics are cause or consequence of HF. There is a large body of evidence particularly from animal studies that support a causal role, between energy depletion and the pathophysiology of HF. However, cardiac mitochondria isolated from failing hearts at the time of left ventricular assist device (LVAD) implantation might not reveal intrinsic defects, and metabolomics analysis reveals improved mitochondrial metabolism after ventricular unloading, suggesting that some degree of mitochondrial plasticity might exist in failing hearts.[26,27] It is also noteworthy that animal studies that directly seek to increase mitochondrial biogenesis in HF models might not necessarily improve ventricular function in the face of ongoing hemodynamic stress.[28] Thus it is likely that the mitochondrial changes associated with HF might reflect both an adaptive response and a direct contributor to ventricular dysfunction.

Substrate Utilization and Mitochondrial Metabolism in the Failing Heart

The metabolic alterations related to impaired cardiac energetics in HF are manifold. Although studies of substrate utilization in HF have yielded conflicting results, most studies show a decrease in FAO, which is most pronounced in the advanced stages of the disease.[29,30] In parallel, a relative increase in glucose utilization (glycolysis and glucose oxidation) is frequently observed during the evolution of pathologic cardiac hypertrophy and early in HF. However, glucose oxidation is invariably markedly reduced in the later stages of the disease (**Fig. 17.2**). Although the report of conflicting results may be related to differences in the etiology and stages of HF, the adaptive or maladaptive character of preferential glucose oxidation remains a subject of debate. Support for a beneficial role of increased glucose utilization comes from interventional studies suggesting that inducing a relative increase in glucose utilization could be beneficial, as will be discussed further later. HF-associated changes in substrate preference may be related to decreased PPARα signaling, resulting in reduced expression of FAO genes, and decreased signaling of PGC-1 coactivators that may downregulate both expression of FAO and OXPHOS genes.[5] The mechanisms for increased glucose utilization remain incompletely understood. Increased glucose uptake and glycolysis may be related to increased GLUT1 expression and activation of AMPK. In addition, chronic or intermittent tissue hypoxia may increase hypoxia-inducible factor 1-α (HIF1α) levels, which may also increase glycolysis. Reduced FA capacity might also increase glucose utilization via the Randle phenomenon. Reduced glucose oxidation when it develops has been primarily attributed to reduced PDH activity or mitochondrial pyruvate uptake.[2,31] The imbalance between the coupling of (increased) glycolysis to (reduced) glucose oxidation contributes to lactate accumulation and intracellular acidosis. Activation of the sodium hydrogen exchange and other mechanisms in turn lead to Na^+ and Ca^{2+} overload, which places an additional energetic burden on the cardiomyocyte. The ATP requirements for restoring ion homeostasis, in addition to the ongoing need for myofilament contraction, further exacerbate impaired cardiac contractility and efficiency.[32]

Although most studies have focused on glucose and FA metabolism, recent studies in humans and animal models have revealed that the failing heart increases ketone body utilization.[33,34] Increased ketone body utilization by the failing heart could reflect an adaptation that maintains cardiac contractile function in the face of significant restriction in substrate availability from other sources. Whether or not increasing ketone body utilization by pharmacologic, dietary, or other means in the context of HF will improve cardiac function is not known

but is an area of active investigation. HF is also associated with the increased de novo synthesis and accumulation of the lipid derivative ceramide, which has been proposed to be mechanistically linked to ventricular dysfunction.[35] In vitro studies have linked ceramide accumulation to cell death and mitochondrial dysfunction in cultured cardiomyocytes.[36] Finally, recent studies have suggested that HF is also associated with impaired catabolism of branched-chained amino acids (BCAAs). In animal models with genetic impairment in BCAA metabolism, HF ensues.[37] The clinical utility or modulating BCAA metabolism in humans with HF remains to be determined. However, clinical trials have now been initiated in which hypoalbuminemic patients with HF have been treated with BCAA supplementation.[38]

In the advanced stages of HF, the general impairment in oxidative capacity is due in part to defective ETC and F_OF_1-ATPase activity (see Fig. 17.2). Reduced expression of nuclear- and mitochondria-encoded subunits of the ETC and F_OF_1-ATPase, oxidative damage of mitochondrial proteins, lipids, and DNA, impaired activity and formation of OXPHOS complexes and respiratory supercomplexes, reduced TCA cycle enzyme activities, posttranslational protein modification (e.g., hyperacetylation, phosphorylation), increased proteolysis, decreased NNT activity, defects in mitochondrial dynamics, increased mitophagy and apoptosis, and cardiolipin remodeling are some, but not all of the mechanisms, that have been associated with impaired mitochondrial respiration and ATP synthesis in the failing heart.[39,40] Decreased activity of sirtuin 1, 3, 5, 6, and 7 may contribute to HF due to overall slowing of oxidative metabolism by decreasing the removal of specific protein acetylations from a broad variety of energy metabolic enzymes (PDH, FAO enzymes, TCA cycle enzymes, OXPHOS subunits, F_OF_1-ATPase) leading to changes in their activity. Finally, increased mitochondrial oxidative stress resulting from inhibition of ROS detoxification represents another important mechanism that contributes to impaired mitochondrial bioenergetics in the failing heart.[7,41]

Novel Concepts Linking Metabolic Changes and Epigenetic Changes and Posttranslational Modifications Downstream of Metabolic Intermediates

As discussed earlier, an important consequence of altered metabolic function in the failing heart is energy or ATP depletion. However, it is now becoming widely accepted that the intermediates of metabolic pathways act as signaling molecules to alter protein function and gene expression. Two areas of research where disruption of cardiac metabolism has become linked to mechanisms of HF include studies of posttranslational modifications (PTMs) and more specifically the recently expanding area of epigenetics.[42,43] In fact, these areas have received so much attention that entire issues of journals have been dedicated to the role of PTMs in heart metabolism.[44] It is also important to note that these two areas are not completely separate, because many of the PTMs that occur on contractile and metabolic proteins also contribute to epigenetics (e.g., acetylation, methylation, O-GlcNAcylation). Briefly, epigenetics includes regulation of gene expression by PTM of histones, modification of DNA (i.e., methylation and hydroxymethylation), and posttranscriptional regulation by noncoding RNAs (i.e., microRNAs [miRNAs] and long noncoding RNA [lncRNA]). Although many of the initial studies concerning epigenetics were focused on inherited changes impacting gene expression, recent work has shown that acquired alterations in epigenetic marks contribute both to disease susceptibility and progression.[45,46] These observations place metabolism at the nexus of causality and consequence of epigenetic alterations; and unraveling these interactions has resulted in a number of novel insights.

Many risk factors associated with HF (e.g., obesity and diabetes) lead to excessive or dysregulated nutrient utilization that alters the

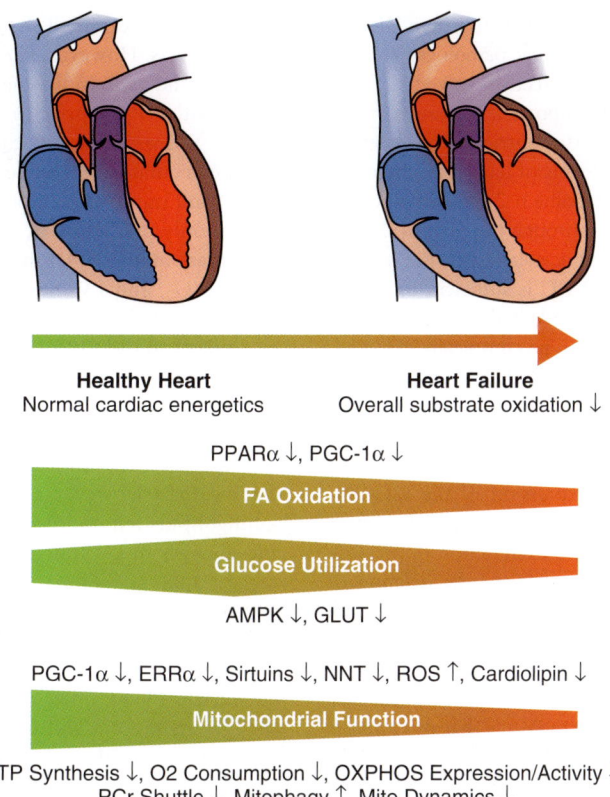

Fig. 17.2 Changes in cardiac energetics during heart failure development. During HF development, fatty acid (FA) oxidation may progressively decline, which is accompanied by an increase in glucose oxidation during the stages of hypertrophy and early heart failure. In advanced heart failure, impaired oxidation of both FA and glucose exacerbate cardiac energy depletion, which is compounded by multiple additional mitochondrial defects that progressively develop during HF progression.

concentrations of substrates or allosteric regulators that control mediators of PTMs such as histone or lysine acetyl transferases (KATs), histone or lysine deacetylases (KDACs), methyltransferases, and O-GlcNac transferase (OGT). In addition, impaired mitochondrial function that accompanies HF also independently regulates metabolites (e.g., NAD$^+$, acetyl-CoA) that may further impact the regulation of these enzymes. For example, in human end-stage HF there is an elevation in acetyl CoA levels that correlates with increased acetylation of mitochondrial proteins.[34,47] Because these modifications alter mitochondrial oxidative function, they exacerbate and perpetuate the link between energy starvation and PTMs that may both contribute to the progression of HF. Very recent evidence found that in HF there is an elevation of the miRNA, miR-195, which in turn decreases levels of the mitochondrial deacetylase sirtuin 3 (SIRT3), leading to enhanced mitochondrial protein acetylation, that ultimately contributes to mitochondrial dysfunction by dysregulating ATP synthase and PDH complex.[48] Importantly, loss of SIRT3 activity by genetic ablation in mice was sufficient to induce mitochondrial and contractile dysfunction.[49] In theory, this would further alter the acetyl CoA pool, leading to additional modulation of protein acetylation. These studies, along with numerous others on SIRT1 and SIRT6 and the extensive literature on protein acetylation, have made this an enticing area of potential therapeutic intervention,[50] including regulation by a number of naturally occurring phytochemicals (e.g., resveratrol, curcumin).[51]

Although less well studied, the serine and threonine O-linked addition of β-N-acetyl-glucosamine (O-GlcNAcylation) has emerged as an important albeit controversial factor in HF.[52] Some of the early limitations in studies of protein O-GlcNAcylation resulted from

technical hurdles in measuring site-specific modifications, many of which have recently been overcome.[53] Unlike many PTMs, the addition or removal of which are generally mediated by numerous enzymes, O-GlcNAcylation addition and removal is regulated by single gene products, namely OGT and O-GlcNAcase (OGA), respectively. This has led to the speculation that the primary form of regulation of this pathway is the rate of flux through multiple metabolic pathways such as glucose, amino acids, FA, and nucleotide metabolism leading to accumulation of N-acetyl glucosamine or its precursors.[54] More recently, subcellular redistribution of OGT and OGA has also been postulated to govern the regulation of protein O-GlcNAcylation.[55]

Increased protein O-GlcNAcylation has been described in samples obtained from failing human or rodent hearts[56] and correlates with decreased cardiac mitochondrial oxidative function, particularly in the context of diabetes.[57] In contrast, in the context of ischemia, increased O-GlcNAcylation is associated with protection against cardiac injury,[58] by inhibiting calcium overload and reactive oxygen species generation[59] or by increasing cardiac stem cell survival.[60] Interestingly, O-GlcNAcylation might not mediate cardiac hypertrophy induction in mouse models, because inducible cardiomyocyte ablation of OGT in the context of transverse aortic constriction exacerbated LV remodeling despite reduced protein O-GlcNAcylation.[61] Similar to other PTMs, miRNAs also regulate O-GlcNAcylation pathways. miR-539, which negatively regulates OGA expression, is increased in HF, leading to increased protein O-GlcNAcylation, representing an additional potential avenue for future therapeutic regulation.[62] More work is needed to understand the nuanced physiology of O-GlcNAcylation in the adaptive responses of the heart to stress and how disruption of cardiac metabolism in HF may perturb O-GlcNAcylation and contribute to cardiac pathology.[63]

Additional metabolites that might not be directly involved in classical substrate oxidation are also emerging as important mediators of epigenetic modifications that could contribute to ventricular remodeling. Specifically, in HF associated with some forms of leukemia, there is a resultant increase in levels of the oncometabolite D-2-hydroxyglutarate (D2-HG), which leads to both altered flux through the citric acid cycle as well as altered histone methylation and acetylation in the heart.[64] Furthermore, the authors showed that D2-HG is sufficient to impair cardiac performance and reduce ATP levels.[64] Whether similar mechanisms exist in other forms of HF remains to be completely explored. As discussed elsewhere in this chapter, human HF is associated with increased ketone body utilization,[33,34] which may alter tissue levels of D-β-hydroxybutyrate (BHB). These observations raise interesting mechanistic links between substrate metabolism and adverse cardiac remodeling. Cardiomyocyte-specific overexpression of the rate-limiting enzyme in BHB oxidation, D-β-hydroxybutyrate dehydrogenase I (BDH1), attenuates cardiac remodeling and dysfunction in pressure overload–induced HF,[65] whereas cardiomyocyte-specific deletion of a related enzyme, succinyl-CoA:3-oxoacid CoA transferase (SCOT), exacerbates contractile dysfunction in the context of pressure overload–induced HF.[66] Although some of this is likely explained by changes in metabolic substrate flux to ATP generations, a number of studies have also identified that BHB is a critical signaling molecule that also impacts epigenetic pathways.[67]

This section has not provided an exhaustive review of the role of PTMs in HF. Additional PTMs likely play important roles in normal physiology, and their disruption in HF progression is potentially linked causally to altered cardiac metabolism in HF and in turn to the pathophysiology of LV remodeling. For example, methylation,[68] palmitoylation,[69] small ubiquitin-like modifier mediated modifications (SUMOylation),[70] succinylation,[71] and others have all been linked to regulating cellular pathways that are directly linked to cardiac dysfunction. For example, we are only beginning to appreciate the scope of epigenetic modifications that may be mediated by changes in metabolic flux, which could contribute to dysregulated gene expression in the context of HF. Novel modifications are now being increasingly identified, such as DNA hydroxymethylation,[72] occurring in combination with the previously discussed PTMs on histones,[73] as well as splice variants in the histones themselves.[74] These modifications could all be changing in HF in complex ways and in response to comorbidities that are associated with disease progression. It is probable that systems biology approaches will be required to elucidate these complexities.

Crosstalk Between Cardiac Metabolism and Systemic Metabolism

Most studies that have examined the relationship between cardiac metabolism and HF in humans have focused on HF with reduced EF. However, HFpEF represents a major and growing clinical problem (see also Chapter 39). Risk factors for HFpEF cluster with those that are associated with the metabolic syndrome such as obesity, insulin resistance, and T2D. Changes in cardiac metabolism that are associated with obesity have been reviewed extensively elsewhere.[75] In summary, obesity is associated with increased myocardial FA utilization, decreased glucose oxidation, increased myocardial oxygen consumption, decreased cardiac efficiency, and myocardial steatosis. These changes have also been associated with or mechanistically linked in some animal models with increased myocardial fibrosis and inflammation. Given the heterogeneity of comorbidities associated with HFpEF, relatively few studies have

systematically examined changes in cardiac substrate metabolism in these subjects. However, Peterson and colleagues have conducted a series of studies in individuals with obesity and the metabolic syndrome with HFpEF prior to and after bariatric surgery. Weight loss surgery was associated with improvement in systemic metabolic parameters that paralleled regression of left ventricular hypertrophy (LVH) and improvement of diastolic relaxation. In the initial studies, the only predictors of improved LV relaxation were decreased body mass index (BMI), improved insulin resistance, reduction in total MVO_2, and LV mass. The relationship between total MVO_2 and LV relaxation was independent of BMI. However, changes in FA utilization did not predict an improvement in LV relaxation.[76] In a follow-up study by the same group, bariatric surgery in obese women with HFpEF led to improved symptom index, regression of LVH, and improved diastolic function, which occurred in parallel with improvement in hepatic steatosis but with no change in cardiac steatosis. However, although circulating levels of ceramide and sphingolipids fell, there was no correlation between these changes and changes in LV function.[77] Taken together, these observations suggest that systemic (noncardiac changes) might play a more important role in the pathophysiology of HFpEF than changes in cardiac metabolism per se. Potential candidate mechanisms include changes in skeletal muscle insulin sensitivity, increased skeletal muscle blood flow, decreased peripheral vascular resistance, changes in the circulating concentrations of adipokines such as adiponectin, or other novel metabolic regulators such as fibroblast growth factor-21 (FGF-21).[78] These findings, which are consistent with clinical observations that interventions such as exercise, which might improve symptoms in HFpEF, might mediate its beneficial effects by addressing pathophysiologic mechanisms in the periphery as opposed to the heart.

Recent studies in animals have also suggested that changes in cardiac muscle per se might have profound effects on systemic metabolic homeostasis. HF is associated with increased circulating concentrations of natriuretic peptides. Studies by the Collins' group suggest that these peptides may activate natriuretic peptide signaling pathways in brown adipose tissue that may activate the thermogenic program of brown adipocytes to increase energy expenditure.[79] Although decreased natriuretic receptor signaling in adipose tissue has been associated with insulin resistance in subjects without HF, the relationship between this pathway and energy expenditure in HF patients remains to be determined. It will be interesting to determine, for example, if aberrant activation of thermogenesis by increased concentrations of natriuretic peptides could contribute to cardiac cachexia. Other intriguing reports in animal models have shown that manipulation of specific molecular pathways in the heart, such as the transcriptional regulator MED13, might modulate systemic glucose metabolism and insulin sensitivity via a miRNA miR-208a that is secreted from the heart.[80]

METABOLIC REMODELING AND RISK FOR HEART FAILURE DEVELOPMENT

Cardiac Hypertrophy

LVH is an independent risk factor for HF development and increases mortality by more than twofold.[81] Pressure overload due to hypertension and aortic stenosis, and postinfarction remodeling are the most frequent causes of human LVH. Although LVH is in principle an adaptive response, this process becomes maladaptive if left untreated and may progress to cardiac dysfunction and failure. However, despite its importance, the transition from hypertrophy to HF in humans is incompletely understood. The most consistent data on energy metabolism in hypertrophied hearts are available from animals subjected to chronic pressure overload, such as surgically mediated transverse aortic constriction or spontaneously hypertensive rats. In these models, most studies report an early decrease in FAO, which is likely the consequence of decreased PPARα and also decreased PGC-1 signaling, which leads to decreased expression of CPT1 and FAO enzymes.[82] In parallel, glucose uptake and glycolysis rates increase, while glucose oxidation may decrease and thereby impair the coupling of glycolysis to glucose oxidation. This uncoupling increases lactate production and may cause myocardial acidosis, which may contribute to contractile dysfunction.[83] The substrate switch toward a relative increase in glucose utilization during hypertrophy is considered a reprogramming of energy metabolism to a "fetal" pattern of energy substrate metabolism and may be beneficial for cardiac energetics because glucose may represent a more "oxygen-efficient" energy substrate, in addition to other mechanisms. Increased glucose utilization during hypertrophy may result from activation of AMPK, which increases glucose uptake and stimulates glycolysis by increasing GLUT4 trafficking to the sarcolemma and by activation of phosphofructokinase. AMPK activation results from increased AMP levels, probably indicating myocardial energy starvation that is already present during the stage of compensated hypertrophy. Indeed, in animal models and in human cardiac hypertrophy, the PCr/ATP ratio is decreased, although ATP levels remain unaltered. However, after transition to HF, the PCr/ATP ratio further declines, accompanied by a relevant decrease in myocardial ATP content.[25] In addition to altered substrate oxidation, downstream defects within mitochondria such as impaired mitochondrial respiratory capacity, ATP synthesis and OXPHOS activities have been observed during hypertrophy, a phenotype which becomes even worse after transition into cardiac failure.[40] Although it remains a subject of debate whether a myocardial energy deficit represents the cause or consequence of hypertrophy and HF, studies in transgenic mice with increased glucose uptake or increased AMPK activity show a normalization of the PCr/ATP ratio and attenuation of HF development. These observations support the concept that energy starvation may already occur in hypertrophy or that biochemically evident but functionally as yet insignificant alterations in cardiac energy metabolism occur in hypertrophied hearts, aggravation of which following or during transition to HF ultimately contributes to cardiac dysfunction and increased risk of HF.[84] It is likely that beneficial effects of some manipulations to increase myocardial energy utilization are more likely to succeed if flux through the entire metabolic pathway is enhanced and the coupling of substrate utilization to oxidation is optimized.

Obesity

Epidemiologic data reveal a consistent association between obesity and HF.[85] The mechanisms linking obesity and HF are multifactorial and include increased incidence of coronary atherosclerosis, hypertension, sleep apnea and pulmonary hypertension, and volume overload. Moreover, obesity increases the risk for insulin resistance and T2D, which might also independently contribute to HF risk. Many studies in humans and animal models have also identified intrinsic changes within the heart in the context of obesity that could contribute to the increased risk of HF. These changes have been extensively reviewed[75,86] and will be summarized briefly. Obesity is associated with increased myocardial FA utilization. Increased use of FA as a metabolic substrate increases myocardial oxygen consumption and reduces cardiac efficiency. Increased myocardial lipid uptake is also associated with myocardial storage of triglycerides (myocardial steatosis). Although the mechanisms linking myocardial steatosis and HF are incompletely understood, it is believed that the accumulation of lipid in the heart promotes "lipotoxicity" probably on the basis of the generation of lipid metabolites that activate signaling pathways that contribute to cellular

dysfunction such as impaired autophagy or cell death. The increase in FA utilization in obesity is associated with reduced glucose uptake and oxidation, which could potentially increase the risk of myocardial injury in the context of ischemia when the dependence of metabolism on glycolysis is increased.

Studies in humans and animals with obesity have suggested that mitochondrial energy metabolism might also become impaired. Early changes that have been noted in animals with diet-induced or genetic obesity include evidence of mitochondrial uncoupling that could be related to the induction or activation of uncoupling proteins such as uncoupling protein 3 (UCP3).[87-89] Increased mitochondrial ROS generation has been shown to increase the activation of UCP3 and other mitochondrial proteins such as the adenine nucleotide translocase.[88] Activation of mitochondrial uncoupling increases mitochondrial proton leak and oxygen consumption, which has been postulated to contribute to increased rates of myocardial oxygen consumption and reduced cardiac efficiency. Obesity leads to generalized insulin resistance and hyperinsulinemia. Studies in humans and animals suggest that, in contrast to skeletal muscle in which insulin resistance is associated with reduced activation of insulin signaling intermediates, in the heart, insulin signaling might actually be increased. Insulin is known to be a potent growth factor in the heart, and hyperinsulinemic activation of insulin signaling might contribute to LVH.[90] In some animal models, protracted high-fat feeding may lead to spontaneous ventricular dysfunction that is associated with altered signaling via forkhead transcription factors, which is a downstream mediator of insulin signaling.[91] Animal studies have also suggested a crosstalk between myocardial insulin signaling and adrenergic signaling pathways that promote myocardial fibrosis.[92,93] Obesity and insulin resistance might also contribute to myocardial pathology by increasing inflammatory signaling.[94]

Diabetes Mellitus

Diabetes mellitus increases the risk of HF. The burden of HF in diabetes is largely borne by individuals with T2D, which accounts for greater than 95% of all diabetes. Epidemiologic studies reveal clear evidence of subclinical myocardial injury, as evidenced by troponin leak, in individuals with no clinical evidence of HF but who have diabetes or are at high risk for developing T2D.[95] In addition, many asymptomatic patients with T2D exhibit evidence of impaired diastolic relaxation that can be detected by echocardiography, particularly when coupled with speckle tracking.[96] The increased risk of HF in diabetes has been termed diabetic cardiomyopathy. Mechanisms for diabetic cardiomyopathy have been extensively reviewed.[97,98] There is overlap between the mechanisms described previously linking HF and obesity and those that link diabetes and HF. However, it is very likely that given additional systemic metabolic abnormalities such as hyperglycemia and elevated circulating concentrations of FA and inflammatory cytokines, the myocardial maladaptations in diabetes are more severe than those described in obesity. For example, diabetes mellitus is invariably associated with impaired mitochondrial OXPHOS capacity that exacerbates mitochondrial energetic impairment and mitochondrial uncoupling. In addition, oxidative stress is likely to be more severe in diabetes relative to individuals who are obese. Hyperglycemia also activates signaling mechanisms described elsewhere in this chapter, such as those that are downstream of the hexosamine biosynthetic signaling pathway. Other pathways linked to glucotoxicity include accumulation of advanced glycation end products, which have been implicated in the pathogenesis of diabetes-associated myocardial fibrosis.[99] Impaired excitation-contraction (E-C) coupling secondary to impaired function of the sarcoplasmic reticulum (SR) has also been described. It is noteworthy that simply normalizing blood glucose might not be sufficient to mitigate the risk of HF in diabetes. Indeed, many therapeutic glucose-lowering agents have been suggested to increase the risk of HF hospitalizations, whereas others do not.[100] Thus a consideration of cardiovascular outcomes has now become an important facet in the approval of new glucose-lowering agents and an important consideration in the choice of agent when treating individuals at high risk for cardiovascular complications. Recent trials have revealed a reproducible effect of a relatively new class of antidiabetic agents, SGLT2 inhibitors, in reducing not only cardiovascular mortality but also the prevalence of HF and hospitalization for HF.[100] Although there has been much speculation regarding the mechanisms for the cardioprotection such as increasing circulating ketones, volume contraction, and blood pressure lowering, the basis for the beneficial impact of SGLT2 inhibitors on HF and cardiovascular (CV) mortality is not understood.

METHODS TO EVALUATE DEFECTS IN CARDIAC ENERGETICS

Many approaches have been used for estimating rates of cardiac substrate utilization and metabolism. The underlying principles and methods for measuring cardiac metabolism were recently summarized in great detail in a scientific statement from the American Heart Association.[101] This section will briefly review approaches that have been adapted for studies in humans and their clinical utility. Cardiac metabolism can be evaluated by measuring the arteriovenous (AV) differences in oxygen and endogenous or isotopically labeled substrates by sampling the coronary sinus (venous) and the aortic root (arterial). In cases where cardiac tissue is being obtained such as following implantation of an LVAD, preinfusion of heavy labeled substrates will lead to isotopic enrichment of metabolite pools that can be determined in the myocardial tissue sample obtained. Analyses of these samples using mass spectrometry–based metabolomics approaches have the potential to provide novel insights regarding myocardial substrate flux and substrate utilization.[102] These invasive approaches, although powerful, have limited utility for routine clinical use.

The most widely used approach in human studies to provide important insights into the physiology and pathophysiology of cardiac metabolism is positron emission tomography (PET) following labeled fluorodeoxyglucose (FDG) or ^{11}C-labeled palmitate. FDG-PET is now the clinical standard for detecting viable myocardium and has been used to describe changes in cardiac glucose metabolism in various pathophysiologic states such as exercise, cardiac hypertrophy, HF, obesity, and diabetes. PET tracers have also been used to determine MBF and oxygen consumption rates to estimate myocardial efficiency.[101]

Proton (^{1}H) magnetic resonance spectroscopy (MRS) has been adapted for measuring intramyocellular triglyceride. These studies have demonstrated, for example, that myocardial lipid content is increased in the hearts of subjects with the diabetes, obesity, and the metabolic syndrome and the impact of dietary interventions on these changes.[103,104] Moreover, by linking metabolite determinations with measures of cardiac contractile function, correlations between indices of LV relaxation and myocardial lipid content, for example, have been described in individuals with diabetes.[105,106] Phosphorous ^{31}P MRS has been used for decades to determine levels and flux of high-energy phosphates within the heart, including flux through creatine kinase. Landmark studies using this approach demonstrated depletion of the phosphocreatine pool in the failing heart and changes in these ratios in various pathophysiologic states such as diabetes and following specific dietary interventions.[107-111] ^{13}C MRS has been used in experimental studies in animal models to track metabolic fluxes in the heart through diverse pathways such as glycolysis, and the TCA cycle. The low sensitivity of ^{13}C has limited clinical utility. However, hyperpolarized ^{13}C approaches, although still in development, hold the promise of using this approach to determine carbon flux in the intact human heart.[101]

Metabolomics profiling describes the use of mass spectrometry to measure the absolute or relative concentrations of small organic biomolecules. Targeted metabolomics measures known metabolites, using existing standards, and nontargeted metabolomics describes an unbiased approach that has the potential to profile a wide range of novel circulating metabolites. Based on the predication that metabolites generated within the myocardium might enter the circulation, some groups are now seeking to identify metabolomics signatures that may characterize clinical or subclinical cardiac injury as occurs following ischemia or in high-risk conditions such as diabetes mellitus.[112-114] For example, in patients with aortic stenosis undergoing transaortic valvular replacement, circulating concentrations of long-chain acyl carnitines correlated with indices of adverse LV remodeling and were normalized following valve replacement.[115] These observations suggest that relief of pressure overload was associated with enhanced and complete mitochondrial FAO in the heart or periphery in parallel with increased insulin sensitivity. When parallel analyses are conducted where tissues are available, powerful insights can be gained by comparing circulating metabolomics patterns with those in cardiac tissue. The integration of these data sets with genomic and transcriptional analyses provides important inputs for network analyses, which are likely to yield new insights into the regulation of myocardial substrate utilization and metabolism in health and disease.

THERAPEUTIC APPROACHES TO MODULATE CARDIAC ENERGETICS

Despite clinical improvement and positive effects on morbidity and mortality in the face of an expanding armamentarium of new drugs in recent decades, the long-term prognosis for HF patients remains poor. The increasing and promising evidence for (and recognition of) a role of myocardial metabolic dysfunction and energy depletion in etiology, pathophysiology, and progression of HF has fostered the concept of targeting cardiac energy metabolism as a novel therapeutic strategy. The term metabolic modulation describes all intervention strategies that alter patterns of myocardial substrate utilization and maintain or restore sufficient regeneration of ATP to ultimately counteract myocardial metabolic dysfunction with the goal of reversing energy depletion. The as yet limited but growing evidence from clinical trials investigating the effect of myocardial metabolic modulation in HF will be summarized next.

Modulation of Substrate Oxidation Patterns

Inhibition of FAO is the most intensively investigated intervention in the context of metabolic modulation (**Fig. 17.3**). Inhibition of CPT1, a key regulatory enzyme of FA import into mitochondria, results in decreased FAO and a reciprocal increase in glucose oxidation via activation of PDH. Additional beneficial effects may arise from reduction of accumulated lipid peroxides within mitochondria, and by rebalancing of carbon and nucleotide phosphate fluxes secondary to increased lactate and amino acid uptake. In rats, treatment with the irreversible CPT1 inhibitor etomoxir improved LV function and prevented LV dilation.[116] In a human trial, treatment of 10 HF patients with etomoxir once daily in addition to standard medical therapy for 3 months improved LV EF and cardiac output during exercise compared with pretreatment values.[117] Unfortunately, a further placebo-controlled trial had to be stopped prematurely due to few cases of hepatotoxicity, although a trend toward increased exercise capacity in

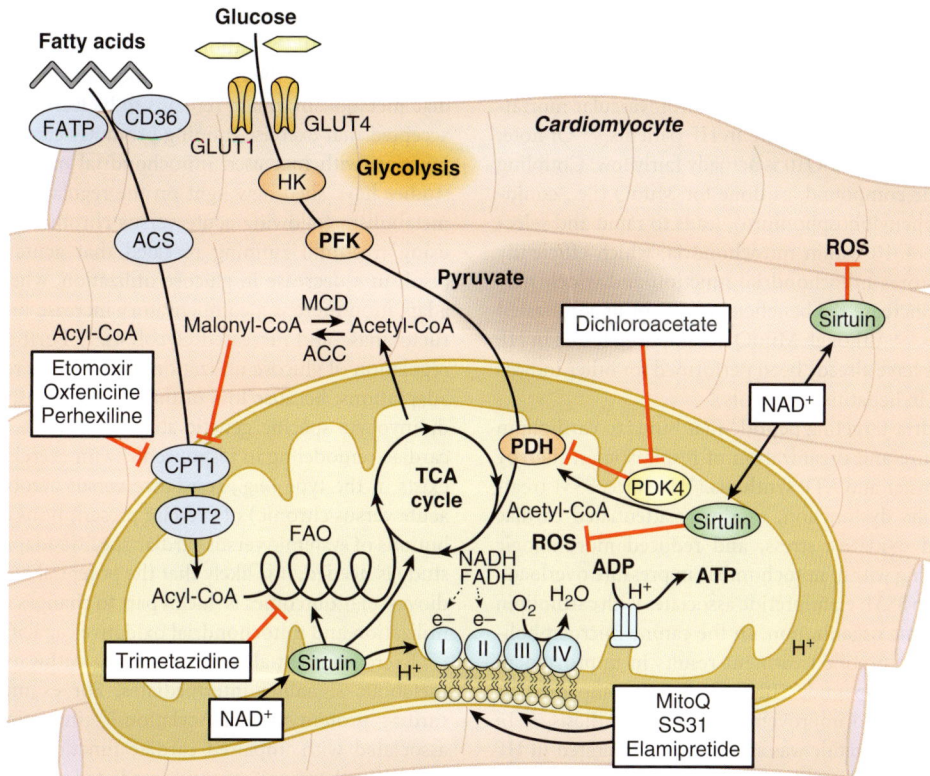

Fig. 17.3 Overview of pharmacologic interventions available to modulate myocardial energy metabolism in HF. A relative increase in glucose utilization may be achieved by inhibiting acyl CoA uptake into mitochondria. Strategies to achieve this include inhibition of CPT-1 using etomoxir, oxfenicine, or perhexiline or by predominant inhibition of enzymes of the beta oxidation spiral using trimetazidine. A similar switch in substrate utilization may be achieved by inhibition of PDK4 by dichloroacetate, which results in disinhibition of PDH. Optimization of respirasome organization by SS31 or elamipretide, and normalization of mitochondrial CoQ levels by MitoQ treatment improve electron transport and ATP synthesis in the respiratory chain. Activation of intramitochondrial and extramitochondrial sirtuins by exogenous NAD+ supplementation may result in global activation of catabolic pathways that increase ATP synthesis while limiting detrimental ROS production.

etomoxir-treated HF patients was observed, despite the small number of patients that could be analyzed.[118] Caution is warranted in end-stage HF in which substrate utilization is globally repressed. Indeed, following acute FAO inhibition in patients with advanced HF, outcomes were actually worsened.[119,120] Oxfenicine, another irreversible CPT1 inhibitor, delayed the development of cardiac dysfunction and remodeling in the canine pacing-induced HF model; however, clinical trials in HF patients using oxfenicine are lacking.[119] In contrast, several clinical trials exist for perhexiline, a potent and reversible CPT1 inhibitor. In HF patients, perhexiline treatment improved EF, peak exercise oxygen consumption, NYHA class, and PCr/ATP ratio.[121] However, it should be noted that mechanisms in addition to or besides CPT1 inhibition may contribute to these beneficial effects, such as inhibition of NADPH oxidase 2 (NOX2), reduced expression of thioredoxin-interacting protein (TXNIP), activation of Krüppel-like factor 14, and inhibition of mechanistic target of rapamycin (mTOR).[122] Trimetazidine also induces a switch from FAO toward glucose utilization but only partially inhibits FAO by inhibition of long-chain 3-ketoacyl-CoA thiolase and only weakly inhibits CPT1. This agent has been used clinically in some parts of the world as an antianginal, and as such, data from numerous clinical trials are generally available. Treatment of patients with HF improves NYHA functional class, increases EF, and decreases LV end-systolic volume.[123,124] In a meta-analysis, trimetazidine treatment was found to reduce HF hospitalizations, to improve NYHA class, to improve EF, and to

ameliorate LV remodeling and was generally well tolerated, with only minor side effects.[125] Another mechanism to inhibit FAO with potentially promising beneficial therapeutic effects in HF is inhibition of malonyl CoA decarboxylase, which inhibits CPT1 by increasing malonyl CoA levels, which has been shown to improve EF in preclinical HF studies.[126] Instead of reciprocal activation of glucose oxidation via inhibition of FAO, direct activation of glucose oxidation using dichloroacetate was shown to improve LV function, to reduce myocardial oxygen consumption, and to improve LV mechanical efficiency after short-term treatment in HF patients.[32] Unfortunately, the clinical use of this specific substance is complicated due to dose-dependent severe peripheral neuropathy. In contrast to the therapeutic concept of FAO inhibition, a number of studies have demonstrated beneficial effects of increasing FA utilization in animal models of HF using genetic engineering (e.g., deletion of acetyl CoA decarboxylase) or by treatment with PPARα agonists; however, no clinical trials to date have tested PPARα agonist treatment as a specific metabolic therapy in HF.

Modulation of ROS Detoxification and Oxidative Phosphorylation

Defects in electron transport, OXPHOS, and increased mitochondrial oxidative stress are believed to contribute to impaired cardiac energetics in HF. Because coenzyme Q10 (CoQ10) is a component of the ETC and also exerts radical scavenging capacity, it represents an essential cofactor for mitochondrial functional integrity. Levels of CoQ10 tend to decline with age, and significant positive correlation exists between HF severity and severity of CoQ10 deficiency.[127] In a recent randomized controlled trial, CoQ10 therapy in addition to standard therapy over 2 years was shown to be safe and to reduce cardiovascular mortality and hospital admission for heart failure in HF patients.[128] Of note, mitochondrial accumulation of CoQ10 is actually fairly low. Coupling of CoQ10 to a lipophilic compound, as done for MitoQ (i.e., conjugation of CoQ10 to triphenylphosphonium), leads to rapid and selective accumulation of CoQ10 within mitochondria, which efficiently detoxifies ROS and restores mitochondrial function and which may be expected to further increase the beneficial effects of unconjugated CoQ10 treatment in HF.[129] Although MitoQ has not been tested in HF patients, human studies have already been performed for other indications (e.g., liver disease in hepatitis C patients).

SS31 is a mitochondria-targeting peptide that binds to cardiolipin and protects the structure and organization of respirasomes, thereby optimizing electron transfer and ATP synthesis.[130] In mice, SS31 treatment normalized systolic dysfunction, markedly attenuated cardiac remodeling, attenuated oxidative stress, and reduced morphologic and proteomic remodeling within mitochondria in pressure overload–induced HF.[131] Similar to SS31, elamipretide associates with cardiolipin and maintains respirasome organization. In the canine microembolization model of HF, elamipretide treatment results in improvement of EF and brain natriuretic peptide (BNP) levels, accompanied by decreased ROS generation and improvement in ATP synthesis.[132] In a phase 2 clinical trial, elamipretide was safe and well tolerated in HF patients.[133] Future clinical studies will reveal whether this class of metabolic modulators will improve clinical end points in HF patients.

NAD$^+$ is an important acceptor for reducing equivalents generated by the TCA cycle and plays an important role in the regulation of electron transfer and OXPHOS. Recent studies in animal models have suggested that NAD$^+$ depletion, or increased NAD$^+$ catabolism, may contribute to impaired myocardial energetics in the failing heart.[134] Repletion of the NAD$^+$ pool with precursors such as nicotinamide riboside (NR) have been shown to improve left ventricular function in animal models of HF.[135] NR (a member of the vitamin B family) is widely available and has been shown in pilot human studies to be well absorbed and to increase cellular pools of NAD$^+$. Sirtuins are NAD$^+$-dependent enzymes that regulate numerous fundamental functions within cells, including oxidative substrate metabolism, and ROS production and detoxification. Sirt1, Sirt3, Sirt5, Sirt6, and Sirt7 have been shown to either accelerate the development of HF in animal studies when absent or to attenuate HF severity when overexpressed.[7,41] SIRT1 can increase mitochondrial biogenesis, increase FAO, and decrease oxidative stress. SIRT3 and SIRT5 may increase the activity of a large number of energy metabolic enzymes (TCA cycle, FAO, PDH, ETC) and detoxify ROS. The adverse effect of the reduction in NAD$^+$/NADH ratios, described in animal models and humans with HF, could be due in part to reduced activity of Sirtuins. Thus increasing NAD$^+$ bioavailability, including exogenous NAD$^+$ supplementation leading to sirtuin activation, attenuates myocardial ischemia reperfusion injury, the development of pathologic hypertrophy, and contractile dysfunction in HF models, in concert with improvements in substrate oxidation, mitochondrial function, and oxidative stress.[134] Exogenous NAD$^+$ supplementation may thus be a promising future target to boost cardiac energetics, and clinical trials investigating safety, bioavailability, and effect on cardiometabolic functions have already been initiated.

Exercise and Cardiac Metabolism

In addition to pharmacologic regulation of metabolic pathways, lifestyle modifications also represent potential avenues that may alter disease progression. Exercise remains a powerful approach to alter myocardial metabolic capacity that may modulate the susceptibility to or course of HF.[136] Although decades of research have advanced our understanding of the molecular mechanisms linking exercise and cardiac metabolism, much remains to be learned. For example, it is well accepted that exercise training promotes cardiac hypertrophy in conjunction with increased mitochondrial oxidative capacity.[137] Recent studies have shed new light on the regulation of myocardial glucose metabolism following acute versus chronic exercise. Studies in mice using treadmill running revealed that acute responses to exercise result in a decrease in glucose utilization, whereas following exercise adaptation there is a compensatory increase in myocardial phosphofructokinase and increased glycolysis.[138] Furthermore, it appears that regulation of glucose utilization in exercise is required for physiologic adaptations, because loss of the glucose transporter GLUT4, via cardiomyocyte specific genetic ablation in mice, resulted in pathologic cardiac remodeling in response to swim exercise training.[139] Diversity exists in the type (e.g., resistance versus aerobic) and duration (e.g., acute versus chronic) of exercise prescriptions and the relative contributions of systemic versus cardiac specific adaptations. Although more study is needed, it is likely that the potential benefit of exercise in cardiovascular outcomes is due in part to changes in myocardial substrate utilization and mitochondrial oxidative capacity.

Exercise might also alter signaling pathways that are mediated by metabolic signaling intermediates. For example, exercise decreases cardiac protein O-GlcNAcylation,[140] induction of which has been associated with impaired cardiac function in the context of diabetes.[141] Furthermore, exercise-mediated reduction in diabetic heart O-GlcNAcylation is associated with elevated acetyltransferase activity,[142] which might contribute to global patterns of protein acetylation further underscoring the close relationship between exercise, metabolism, PTMs, and cardiac function. HF is associated with lower levels of an N-terminal proteolytically derived fragment of histone deacetylase 4 (HDAC4-NT) and exercise increases HDAC4-NT levels, which correlated with maintenance of cardiac performance.[143] One proposed mechanism of action was via altering gene expression that regulated HBP flux and protein O-GlcNAcylation of the calcium sensor stromal interaction molecule 1 (STIM1). Interestingly, the role of O-GlcNAcylation and STIM1 was previously suggested to alter susceptibility to HF in diabetes.[144] However, the relative paucity of studies evaluating the direct effect of heart metabolism in response to exercise in HF patients underscores the need for future studies that will extend beyond analyses of systemic adaptations.

SUMMARY AND FUTURE DIRECTIONS

Cardiac contractile performance is inextricably linked with the profound capability of the heart to efficiently generate high-energy phosphates via the metabolism of diverse fuels. The high content of mitochondria relative to other organs underscores the importance of substrate oxidation and metabolism to the maintenance of cardiac performance. Although much work has focused on the mechanisms regulating substrate fluxes, substrate preference, and mitochondrial capacity, recent studies have begun to reveal the critical role of metabolites as signaling intermediates. In addition to regulating metabolite flux, energy generation, and energy utilization, these signaling pathways likely regulate other cellular functions within the cardiomyocyte and other cardiac cells. These pathways may modulate the cardiac adaptations to hemodynamic stress, including those that may lead to myocardial injury. Future research seeking to further elucidate these pathways and to determine the extent to which they can be therapeutically manipulated may lead to novel approaches for cardioprotection and the treatment of HF.

KEY REFERENCES

1. Doenst T, Nguyen TD, Abel ED. Cardiac metabolism in heart failure: implications beyond ATP production. *Circ Res*. 2013;113(6):709–724.
2. Stanley WC, Recchia FA, Lopaschuk GD. Myocardial substrate metabolism in the normal and failing heart. *Physiol Rev*. 2005;85(3):1093–1129.
32. Lopaschuk GD. Metabolic modulators in heart disease: past, present, and future. *Can J Cardiol*. 2017;33(7):838–849.
43. Wende AR. Post-translational modifications of the cardiac proteome in diabetes and heart failure. *Proteomics Clin Appl*. 2016;10(1):25–38.
64. Karlstaedt A, Zhang X, Vitrac H, et al. Oncometabolite d-2-hydroxyglutarate impairs α-ketoglutarate dehydrogenase and contractile function in rodent heart. *Proc Natl Acad Sci*. 2016;113(37):10436–10441.
75. Abel ED, Litwin SE, Sweeney G. Cardiac remodeling in obesity. *Physiol Rev*. 2008;88(2):389–419.
82. Abel ED, Doenst T. Mitochondrial adaptations to physiological vs. pathological cardiac hypertrophy. *Cardiovasc Res*. 2011;90(2):234–242.
90. Riehle C, Abel ED. Insulin signaling and heart failure. *Circ Res*. 2016;118(7):1151–1169. 2016.
97. Boudina S, Abel ED. Diabetic cardiomyopathy revisited. *Circulation*. 2007;115(25):3213–3223.
101. Taegtmeyer H, Young ME, Lopaschuk GD, et al. Assessing cardiac metabolism: a scientific statement from the American Heart Association. *Circ Res*. 2016;118(10):1659–1701.

The full reference list for this chapter is available on ExpertConsult.

18

Epidemiology of Heart Failure

Andreas P. Kalogeropoulos, Lampros Papadimitriou, Javed Butler

Improved outcomes of acute cardiac conditions, population aging, increasing prevalence of lifestyle risk factors, and advances in heart failure (HF) therapeutics all have led to an increasing prevalence of HF. Because of these trends, HF has become a public health priority in developed countries and a major noncommunicable syndrome in developing regions. In the United States, the population prevalence of HF among adults, currently estimated at 2.5%, is projected to increase to approximately 3.0% by year 2030. HF has a high lifetime incidence and unfavorable prognosis, especially after hospitalization. At age 45, lifetime risks for HF in the United States range from 20% to 46%, depending on gender and race.[1] Despite decreasing mortality trends,[2,3] the average 1-year mortality after a hospitalization for HF ranges between 30% and 35%, depending on demographic characteristics,[2-5] with wide regional variation.[6] Five-year survival after HF diagnosis in population studies does not exceed 50% in most systems, regardless of setting (outpatient vs. inpatient),[3,7-10] and is as low as 25% in older inpatients regardless of left ventricular ejection fraction (EF).[9] These survival rates are lower compared with several forms of cancer.[10] HF also significantly affects quality of life.[11] Beyond the impact on quantity and quality of life, HF adds substantially to the cost of health care systems.

PATIENT CHARACTERISTICS

Demographic Distribution

HF is a disease of older adults. In a recent population-based report from the United Kingdom, mean age at diagnosis was 76.7±12.6 years.[12] A similar median age (76–77 years) at HF diagnosis was reported for inpatients in Denmark, with most patients diagnosed between age 66 and 85.[13] In Canada, although patients diagnosed in specialty clinics were slightly younger (median, 69 years) compared with general clinic outpatients (72 years), and those diagnosed in the emergency department (75 years) were younger compared with inpatients (77 years), the majority of cases in the population were diagnosed between ages 57 and 84.[14]

Men and women are equally affected by HF. However, age at onset and type of HF affect sex predominance.[15,16] In the United Kingdom, women accounted for 49.0% of new HF cases.[12] A similar 1:1 sex ratio for new cases has been reported in the United States around the world.[8,15,17] However, although higher rates of coronary artery disease in men lead to male preponderance in younger patients, susceptibility to diastolic dysfunction leads to a higher proportion of women affected by HF at older ages. Men are more likely to develop HF with reduced EF (HFrEF), whereas women are more prone to HF with preserved EF (HFpEF).[16,18] In the United Kingdom, age at diagnosis in men was 74±13 years versus 79±12 years in women.[12] A similar difference has been reported in Sweden.[8] Finally, in large studies, HF appears to affect all races equally.[1,19,20]

Comorbidities (see also Chapter 48)

As a disease of older adults, HF is rarely encountered in isolation. More than 80% of patients have ≥2 concomitant chronic conditions, and most have ≥3.[12,21,22] The most common are hypertension, ischemic heart disease, diabetes mellitus, cerebral and peripheral vascular disease, atrial fibrillation, chronic kidney disease, chronic obstructive lung disease, anemia, and depression. As average age at HF diagnosis increases over time,[12] the number of comorbidities and medications in patients with HF increases as well.[12,13,23] In the United Kingdom, the number of comorbidities in patients with HF increased from 3.4±1.9 in 2002 to 5.4±2.5 in 2014, and the percentage of patients with ≥3 additional conditions increased from 68% to 87%.[12] In the US National Health and Nutrition Examination Survey (NHANES), the average number of prescription medications in patients with HF increased from 4.1 in 1988–1994 to 6.4 in 2003–2008.[23] Overall, there is a shift from a model where HF was mainly a consequence of coronary artery disease with male preponderance toward a disease of older adults equally affecting both sexes and accompanied by a complex medical profile.[24] Among the 493 older adults (age 70–79 years at inception) who developed HF in the Health, Aging, and Body Composition Study,[25] 36.8% had no prior coronary artery disease.

PREVALENCE AND INCIDENCE

Estimates and Trends

Most contemporary national health care databases in developed countries indicate that the age-standardized incidence of HF at the population level is declining,[7,12–14] and that age-standardized prevalence of HF is increasing only slightly, the latter being probably the result of advances in HF therapeutics. However, because of population aging, the crude incidence remains high and the crude prevalence and number of patients with HF keeps increasing. Estimates vary according to the methods and definitions used. The population incidence of HF is currently estimated between 200 and 400 cases annually per 100,000 individuals in most developed countries, and the crude prevalence ranges between 1% and 3%. **Table 18.1** summarizes the population prevalence of HF in health care databases around the world.

In a comprehensive epidemiologic study from the United Kingdom,[12] the population-based incidence of HF in 2014 was 332/100,000 person-years, a 7% decline from 2002; the decline was similar for men and women. Despite this decline, crude incidence increased by 2% and the number of new HF cases increased by 12% between 2002 and 2014, largely due to an increase in population size and age.[12] In the same study, although the age- and sex-standardized prevalence of HF increased only slightly from 1.5% to 1.6%, the number of patients with HF increased by 23% over the same period.[12]

Similar trends have been reported in North America and continental Europe. In a study of 2.3 million Medicare beneficiaries (age ≥65), although incident HF declined by 32% between 2004 and 2013, prevalence increased from 16.2% to 17.2%.[26] In Olmsted County, Minnesota, the adjusted incidence of HF declined from 316/100,000 in 2000 to 219/100,000 in 2010.[7] The decline was greater for HFrEF than for HFpEF. In Ontario, Canada, HF incidence decreased by 32.7% between 1997 and 2007 (from 455 to 306/100,000 person-years), with a comparable decrease in both inpatient and outpatient settings.[27] In Sweden, despite a relative decline in incidence by 24% between 2006 and 2010 (average, 380 cases per 100,000 person years), the prevalence of HF remained unchanged.[8] In Germany, the age- and sex-standardized incidence of HF in 2006 was 270/100,000 person years.[28] In Italy, the incidence of hospitalized new HF cases in Lombardy decreased between 2005 and 2012 (from 362 to 313/100,000 adults), but with an increasing proportion of patients aged ≥85 years.[29] However, in a study of in-hospital new HF cases in Denmark between 1995 and 2012, although HF incidence declined overall and in older persons (>50 years), there was an increasing trend in younger (≤50 years) persons.[13]

TABLE 18.1 Population Prevalence of HF in Registries and Surveys Across the World

Country	Population Sample	Study Period	Ascertainment of Heart Failure Cases	Total (%)	Men (%)	Women (%)
Germany[28]	6.3 million	2006	Primary or secondary hospital diagnosis or confirmed outpatient diagnosis of HF (ICD-10 codes I50, I11.0, I13.0, I13.2, I97.1) between 2004 and 2006	1.7	1.8	1.6
Australia[90]	8707 subjects	2008–2009	National study of general practice activity, random sample, physician-provided information on chronic conditions	1.5[a]		
Sweden[8]	2.1 million	2010	Primary or secondary diagnosis of HF (ICD-10 code I50) in primary care (2003–2010), secondary care (1997–2010), or during hospitalization (1997–2010)	2.2[a]	2.2	2.2
Spain[15]	7.5 million	2012	Hospital diagnosis of HF (ICD-9-CM codes 402.X1, 404.X1, 404.X3, 428.X) or outpatient diagnosis followed by loop diuretic prescription between 2011 and 2012	1.2 (among age >15)		
United States[91]	5761 respondents	2013–2014	NHANES, multistage probability sampling, self-reported HF[a]	1.9[a]	1.8	2.0
United Kingdom[12]	4.0 million	2002–2014	ICD-10 codes (I50.X, I42.0, I42.9, I11.0, I13.0, I13.2, I25.5) for in-hospital and NHS Read codes for primary care diagnosis of HF in any diagnostic position	1.6	1.8	1.2
South Korea[32]	1.4 million	2014	Adult patients with any outpatient or inpatient services with a primary or secondary diagnosis of HF (ICD-10 codes I50.X, I11.0, I13.0, I13.2, I42.0, I42.5, I25.5) in 2014	1.2 (among age >18)		

[a]Estimated prevalence in the national population.
HF, Heart failure; *ICD-9-CM*, International Classification of Diseases, Ninth Revision, Clinical Modification; *ICD-10*, International Classification of Diseases, Version 10; *NHANES*, US National Health and Nutrition Examination Survey; *NHS*, National Health Service.

Impact of Demographics and Socioeconomic Status

Age

Age is a major contributor to development of HF, and therefore the incidence and prevalence of HF is considerably higher among middle-aged or older adults. In a meta-analysis of community-based studies, the median prevalence of HF among persons age ≥60 was 11.8% (4.7%–13.3%).[30] The effect of age on HF prevalence is demonstrated in the NHANES data (**Fig. 18.1**). Among Danish adults, the annual incidence of new in-hospital HF diagnosis in 2012 was <0.01% in ages 18 to 35 but >1% in ages >74 (**Fig. 18.2**).[13] In the United States, the annualized incidence of HF ranges between 1% and 2% among older adults (age ≥65), depending on age group and race.[4,25]

Sex

Age-standardized incidence and prevalence of HF is higher in men,[8,12,28,31] but more women develop HF later in life, therefore contributing almost equally to new HF cases, and therefore the crude prevalence is either only slightly higher in men or comparable between men and women.[8,12,28,31,32] In the United Kingdom, although the age-standardized incidence was higher in men than in women (incidence rate ratio 1.52, 95% CI 1.50–1.54), the total number of incident cases was only 9% higher in men because of the greater number of women in the older age groups.[12] In the Atherosclerosis Risk in Communities cohort, incidence of HF was higher in men versus women for both blacks and whites and across age groups, but these differences diminished in the >75 age group.[4] In Denmark, men had a higher incidence rate than women overall, except in the >74 age group.[13] In Germany, the age-standardized incidence rate of HF was 230/100,000 person-years in women and 310 in men, with the sex gradient diminishing with age.[28]

Race

Although lifetime risk for HF appears to be comparable or even higher in Caucasian versus African American patients,[1] the latter are more vulnerable to HF at a younger age and more susceptible to the effects of hypertension.[4,33] However, these differences tend to diminish with advancing age.[19,34] In the Health, Aging and Body Composition Study (70–79 years old at inception), there was no race interaction with blood pressure for incident HF.[34] In the Multi-Ethnic Study of Atherosclerosis (MESA), the incidence of HFpEF for patients 70±9 years old at baseline was similar across all races and ethnicities.[19]

Socioeconomic Status

Socioeconomic status is a key determinant of HF risk. In the United Kingdom, among persons of the same age and sex, those in the most deprived socioeconomic quintile were more likely to experience HF (incidence rate ratio 1.61, 95% CI 1.58–1.64) than their affluent counterparts, and this was more pronounced in the younger age groups.[12] Patients from the most deprived quintile were about 3.5 years younger at diagnosis versus those from the least deprived (74.5±13 years vs. 78±12 years).[12] In a study of 27,000 relatively young (age, 55.5±10.4 years), low-income white and black men and women in the United States who were receiving Centers for Medicare and Medicaid Services in years 2002–2009, HF incidence was 328 cases per 100,000 person-years, considerably higher for age compared with other cohorts, with little variation across race or sex.[20]

Lifetime Risk of Heart Failure

In a project that pooled more than 700,000 person-years of follow-up in the United States (85% white, 15% black), lifetime risk for HF at age 45 was estimated at 30% to 42% in white men, 20% to 29% in black men, 32% to 39% in white women, and 24% to 46% in black women.[1] Lifetime risk for HF was higher with higher blood pressure and body mass index (BMI) at all ages.[1] Women are more likely to develop HF as the first manifestation of cardiovascular disease.[35]

Prevalence of Preclinical (Stage A and B) Heart Failure

As with most chronic diseases, HF is a progressive condition amenable to early preventive interventions (**see also Chapter 35**). To emphasize this concept, the American Heart Association and the American College of Cardiology have proposed a scheme that classifies HF into four stages. Stage A indicates the presence of risk factors but no clinical or subclinical disease. Stage B refers to asymptomatic cardiac structural or functional abnormalities usually detectable by cardiac imaging (i.e., subclinical disease). Stage C refers to stable symptomatic HF, whereas Stage D is used to indicate advanced symptomatic HF that is refractory to pharmacotherapy.

Because of the need for systematic imaging to detect subclinical disease, limited data exist on the population prevalence of HF stages. In the Atherosclerosis Risk in Communities (ARIC) study,[17] among 6,118 participants age 67 to 91 years, 52% were categorized as Stage A and 30% as Stage B in the 2011–13 visit. In the Framingham study,[36] among 6770 participants (54% women) with a mean age of 51, the prevalence of Stage A and B was 36.5% and 24.2%, respectively. The prevalence of Stage B increased

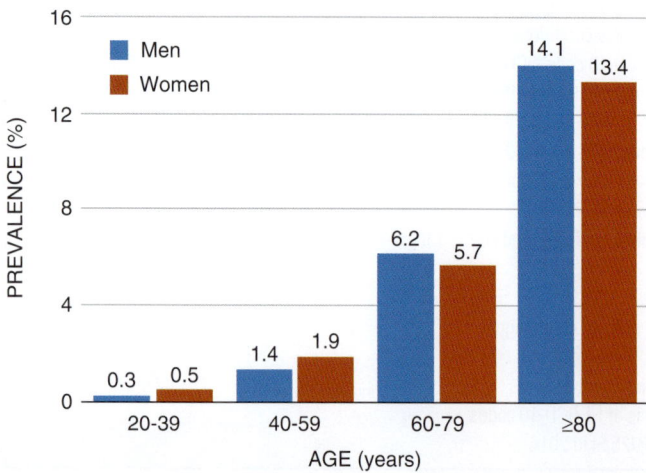

Fig. 18.1 Prevalence of heart failure by gender and age in the United States. From US National Health and Nutrition Examination Survey, 2011–2014.

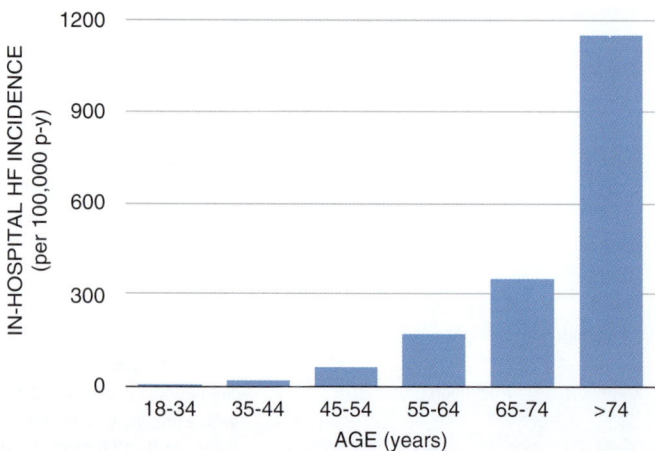

Fig. 18.2 Incidence of in-hospital heart failure diagnosis among adults in Denmark, 2012. Data from Christiansen MN, Køber L, Weeke P, et al. Age-specific trends in incidence, mortality, and comorbidities of heart failure in Denmark, 1995 to 2012. *Circulation*. 2017;135:1214–1223.

steadily with age, from 17.6% in the ≤54 age group to 42.9% in the ≥75 age group (**Fig. 18.3**). Compared with healthy participants, mortality was two-fold higher among participants with Stage B HF after a mean of 7 years.[36]

MAJOR CONTRIBUTORS TO HEART FAILURE

Heart Failure After Acute Coronary Syndromes (see also Chapter 19)

Coronary artery disease is a major driver of HF. Previous longitudinal studies have shown that reductions in short- and long-term mortality after acute myocardial infarction (AMI) in the past decades have been translated into increasing rates of HF. In recent registries, post-AMI HF is declining, as a result of increasing use of early interventional strategies. However, HF continues to be a major problem in patients recovering from AMI or acute coronary syndrome (ACS). Estimates of HF after AMI vary as a result of varying definitions of both AMI and post-AMI HF.

Among Medicare beneficiaries (age ≥65) in the United States, rates for HF within 1 year after AMI declined modestly from 16.1% in 1998 to 14.2% in 2010.[37] Similar trends, albeit at lower absolute HF rates due to a more stringent definition, have been reported for Australia.[38] Among 25,000 patients without HF admitted for a first ACS in Alberta, Canada, between 2002 and 2008, HF during index admission occurred in 13.6% of patients with ST-elevation AMI, 14.8% of those with non-ST-elevation AMI, and 5.2% of those with unstable angina.[39]

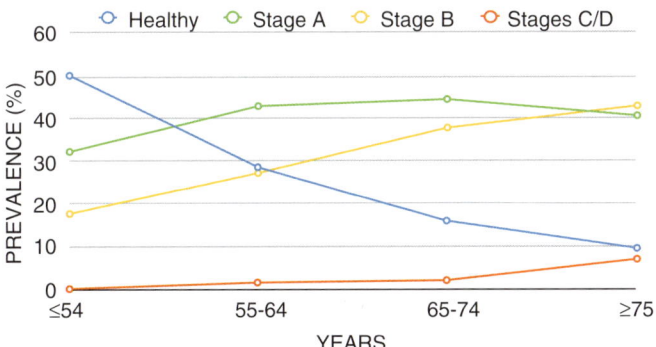

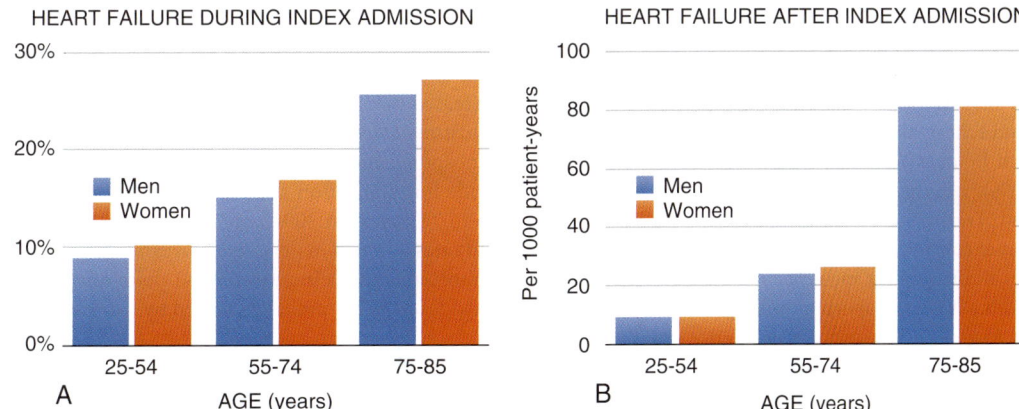

Fig. 18.3 Prevalence of heart failure stages in the Framingham Heart Study, Massachusetts. Data from Xanthakis V, Enserro DM, Larson MG, et al. Prevalence, neurohormonal correlates, and prognosis of heart failure stages in the community. *JACC Heart Fail.* 2016;4:808–815.

Incident HF rates at 1 year were 23.4%, 25.4%, and 16.0%, respectively, indicating that HF continues to be a common complication of AMI. Revascularization was associated with 18% lower risk for HF after the index admission.[39] In a Swedish national registry, primary percutaneous coronary intervention increased from 6.0% to 91.5% between 1996 and 2008, accompanied by a decrease in the incidence of HF (defined as presence of crackles or the use of IV diuretics or inotropes) during index hospitalization from 46% to 28%.[40] The decrease was more pronounced for ST-segment elevation AMI. Notably, reduction in post-AMI HF rates has been reported for HFrEF but not HFpEF.[41] In a comprehensive study from Norway, 18.7% of patients developed new HF during index admission for a first AMI between 2001 and 2009, depending on age (**Fig. 18.4A**).[42] Among patients discharged without HF, 12.6% were admitted or died because of HF after a median of 3.2 years. The annual incidence of HF was 3.1% in men and 4.6% in women (*P* < .01) (see Fig. 18.4B). Risk for HF was highest during the first 6 months of follow-up.[42]

Hypertension (see also Chapter 25)

Along with coronary artery disease, hypertension has the highest population-attributable risk for HF. In the Health ABC Study (age 70–79 at inception), there was a continuous direct association between systolic blood pressure (SBP) and HF risk for levels of SBP as low as <115 mm Hg.[34] The 10-year incidence of HF with SBP <120, 120 to 139, 140 to 159, and ≥160 mm Hg at baseline was 5.9%, 10.5%, 14.8%, and 22.8%, respectively, and more than half of cases occurred in individuals with SBP <140 mm Hg.[34] The impact of SBP control on HF risk was impressively demonstrated in the landmark Systolic Blood Pressure Intervention Trial (SPRINT), which compared intensive (<120 mm Hg) with conventional (<140 mm Hg) target SBP; intensive SBP target reduced risk of HF by 37% (HR 0.63; 95% CI, 0.46–0.85; *P* = .003) consistently across all subgroups.[43]

Older adults and black patients with hypertension are especially vulnerable to HF. In the Second Australian National Blood Pressure Study (ANBP2), which compared an angiotensin-converting inhibitor-based versus a thiazide diuretic-based regimen in hypertensive patients aged 65–84 years, the incidence of HF was 0.63% per year; 0.79% in men and 0.48% in women over a median of 10.8 years, without difference between arms.[44] The 5-year incidence of HF was 3.0% in hypertensive patients aged 55 to 80 without HF assigned to either losartan- or atenolol-based treatment in the Losartan Intervention For Endpoint reduction in hypertension (LIFE) trial; however, the incidence was higher among black versus nonblack patients (7.0 vs. 3.1%).[33]

Fig. 18.4 Heart failure after first acute myocardial infarction (A) during index admission and (B) post index admission in Norway, 2001–2009. Data from Sulo G, Igland J, Nygård O, et al. Prognostic impact of in-hospital and postdischarge heart failure in patients with acute myocardial infarction: a nationwide analysis using data from the Cardiovascular Disease in Norway [CVDNOR] project. *J Am Heart Assoc.* 2016;5:e002667.

Diabetes (see also Chapter 48)

Several studies have highlighted the impact of increasingly prevalent metabolic risk factors, including diabetes, glucose intolerance, and insulin resistance on HF risk. Glycemic control appears to be directly associated with HF risk.[45] In the Swedish National Diabetes Registry, among patients with type 1 diabetes (age, 39±13 years; 45% women), the incidence of new hospitalized HF was 340 events per 100,000 patient-years and increased monotonically with hemoglobin A1c (HbA1c), with a range of 140 to 520 events per 100,000 patient-years between patients in the lowest (<6.5%) and highest (≥10.5%) categories of HbA1c.[46] In the same registry, poor glycemic control (HbA1c >7%) was associated with increased risk of hospitalization for new HF in type 2 diabetes (age, 66±12 years; 45% women); the annualized incidence increased significantly, from 1.38% for patients with HbA1c <6.0% to 2.58% for patients with HbA1c ≥10.0%.[47] Risk was higher for men, older patients, and longer diabetes duration. However, in a study that modeled HbA1c as a time-updated variable in ~8700 individuals with type 2 diabetes, both HbA1c <6% (HR 1.60; 95% CI, 1.38–1.86) and HbA1c >10% (HR 1.80; 95% CI, 1.60–2.16) were associated with risk of HF, pointing to a U-shaped relationship between HbA1c and HF precipitation.[48]

Obesity

Obesity and associate metabolic derangements are important drivers of HF from a public health perspective. In the Cardiovascular Lifetime Risk Pooling Project, lifetime risk for HF was higher with higher body mass index (BMI) at all ages in both blacks and whites, and did not diminish substantially with advancing index age.[1] In the MESA prospective cohort, a multicenter observational cohort study following 6814 subjects (mean age 62±10 years; 47% men), BMI has been identified as an independent predictor of HF with 40% higher risk for every 5 kg/m^2 higher BMI (HR 1.40; 95% CI 1.10–1.80).[49] However, the increased risk for HF with obesity may be largely mediated by obesity-related conditions. In the MESA study, the associations of BMI and waist circumference with incident HF became nonsignificant after adjusting for obesity-related conditions (hypertension, dysglycemia, hypercholesterolemia, left ventricular hypertrophy, kidney disease, and inflammation).[50]

Atrial Fibrillation (see also Chapter 38)

Atrial fibrillation (AF) is common among patients with HF and worsens prognosis. Conversely, AF confers increased risk for HF, especially HFpEF. In the Framingham Heart Study, among 1,737 individuals with new AF (mean age, 75±12 years; 48% women), more than one-third (37%) had HF. Conversely, among 1166 individuals with new HF (mean age, 79±11 years; 53% women), more than half (57%) had AF. Prevalent AF was more strongly associated with incident HFpEF versus HFrEF.[51] In Olmsted County, Minnesota, among approximately 3,500 patients with new AF (age 71±15 years, 45.5% women), a substantial excess risk of HF was observed after AF diagnosis, with a standardized morbidity ratio of 9.60, 2.13, and 1.70 at 90 days, 1 year, and 3 years, respectively.[52] Among patients with EF data, 61% had HFpEF (EF ≥50%) and 39% had HFrEF (EF <50%).[52] In the community-based Outcomes Registry for Better Informed Treatment of Atrial Fibrillation (ORBIT-AF), among ~6500 outpatients with AF in the United States (median age 74 years, 43.6% female) annualized HF incidence was 1.58% over a 2-year follow-up period, with a higher proportion of HFpEF versus HFrEF.[53] Of note, in contrast to general HF cases, the incidence of HF after AF does not seem to be declining in recent years.[52,54]

Renal Disease

Renal impairment is common in HF and portends a worse prognosis. Conversely, HF commonly follows renal dysfunction. In a study of ~10,000 men (mean age, 67 years), an estimated glomerular filtration rate (eGFR) <60 mL/min per 1.73 m^2 was associated with a twofold risk of HF compared with eGFR ≥60 mL/min per 1.73 m^2 after a median of 10 years.[55] Even moderate renal impairment, despite the absence of diabetes and hypertension, was associated with a higher risk of HF. A similar increase in HF risk was observed in three community cohorts in the United States, pooling data from ~14,500 participants (age, 63±12 years; 59% women; 44% black), where chronic kidney disease (CKD—defined as <60 mL/min per 1.73 m^2) was present in 10% of participants.[56] Annualized incidence of HF was 2.20% among those with versus 0.62% without CKD. Risk for HF was higher in blacks and Hispanics.[56] Besides CKD, acute kidney injury also carries HF risk. In a cohort of 300,000 hospitalized US veterans without HF, a 0.3-mg/dL or 50% increase in serum creatinine from baseline to peak hospital value was associated with 23% increased 2-year risk for HF.[57] Of note, in a cohort of more than 3500 patients with CKD, cystatin C-based eGFR and albuminuria predicted risk for HF better than creatinine-based eGFR; anemia, insulin resistance, inflammation, and poor glycemic control were additional risk factors.[58]

HOSPITALIZED HEART FAILURE (SEE ALSO CHAPTER 36)

Trends in Hospitalization Rates

Hospitalization for decompensated (or "acute") HF has become the epicenter of intensive research (and debate), both from a therapeutic and a health care perspective. Hospitalization represents a turning point in the natural history of HF, with a striking increase in adverse outcomes afterwards. Many therapies have been evaluated for acute HF, but none has been shown to improve outcomes. The pathophysiologic mechanisms that lead to increased mortality and morbidity after hospitalization for HF are still uncertain. Hospitalization rates and trends vary widely across health care systems, as financial and administrative incentives are different. Recent reports from the United States and other countries report a decrease in hospitalizations for HF. However, these trends are not consistent across health care systems, and the total burden of HF hospitalizations remains high, secondary to population aging and increasing HF prevalence.

In the United States, annual hospitalization rates for HF as a primary diagnosis among adults ≥18 years declined from 553/100,000 people in 2001–2005 to 489/100,000 in 2006–2019 and 416 in 2010–2014.[59] However, the rates for HF as a secondary diagnosis remained stable at ~1400 admissions per 100,000 people annually.[59] In France, the overall age-standardized rate of primary HF hospitalizations was 250/100,000 people in 2012, with only a small change from 2002.[60] Of note, although the age-standardized rate was higher in men (320 vs. 200/100,000 people), the crude rate was comparable between men and women. In Germany, primary HF-related hospitalizations increased by 65.4% between 2000 and 2013, and by 28.4% after age adjustment (from 261 to 335/100,000), and HF was the leading cause of hospitalizations and in-hospital deaths in 2013.[61] In Murcia, Spain, crude hospitalization rates for a primary diagnosis of HF increased by 76.7% between 2003 and 2013, from 128 to 226/100,000 people, and rates doubled in persons ≥75 years.[62] Importantly, the Elixhauser comorbidity index increased by ~1 point during the study period and episodes, with >6 points increased by twofold.[62]

Length of Stay

Length of stay is highly system dependent. In the large Acute Study of Clinical Effectiveness of Nesiritide in Decompensated Heart Failure (ASCEND-HF) trial, mean length of stay ranged from 4.9 to 14.6 days across 27 countries.[63] In a nationally representative sample of primary HF hospitalizations in the United States, mean length of stay declined from 6.1 days in 1996 to 5.3 in 2009.[64] However, despite attempts to shorten length of stay worldwide, the burden of HF on hospitals has proven difficult to curb. In Germany, the absolute number of HF-related hospital days increased by 22% from 2000 to 2013, despite a 26% decrease in the average length of stay (from 14.3 to 10.6 days).[61] Also, data from registries and clinical trials indicate that there is a trade-off between length of stay and short-term readmission rates in patients admitted for HF.[63]

Effect of Heart Failure Hospitalization on Outcomes

Hospitalization has a dramatic impact on HF outcomes, especially mortality, that is evident in both short- and long-term studies. In the Italian HF registry, 1-year mortality was 24% among patients admitted for HF (19.2% for de novo HF and 27.7% for worsening HF) and 5.9% in outpatients.[65] In the European Society of Cardiology Heart Failure Long-Term (ESC-HF-LT) registry, all-cause 1-year mortality rate was 23.6% for inpatient versus 6.4% for outpatient enrollees. The corresponding composite endpoint of mortality or HF hospitalization within 1 year was 36.0% and 14.5% for inpatients and outpatients, respectively.[66] Among Medicare beneficiaries with new-onset HF between 2004 and 2013 in the United States, unadjusted 1-year mortality was 31.9% and 13.5% for HF diagnosed as inpatient and outpatient, respectively.[26] In the CHARM clinical trial program, which enrolled ~7600 patients with New York Heart Association class II to IV HF, rates of cardiovascular mortality and HF hospitalization were more than 50% higher among patients with previous HF hospitalization (71% of patients) over a median follow-up of 3 years.[67] The magnitude of increased risk was similar in patients with HFrEF or HFpEF, and varied inversely with the time interval between hospitalization and enrollment.

HEART FAILURE WITH REDUCED, MIDRANGE, AND PRESERVED EJECTION FRACTION

The majority of HF cases result from abnormalities in LV myocardial function. However, the spectrum of the underlying LV functional abnormalities is wide, ranging from normal LV size and preserved EF but predominant LV diastolic dysfunction to severe LV dilatation and markedly reduced EF. In fact, abnormalities of both systolic and diastolic LV function have been described in most HF patients, irrespective of EF. Despite the varying cutoffs used to define preserved EF, ranging from >40% to ≥55%, EF is still considered important in the classification of HF because of distinct patient demographics, comorbid conditions, prognosis, and response to therapies. Recently the European Society of Cardiology guidelines introduced the term HF with midrange EF (HFmrEF) to describe patients with borderline EF (41%–50%).[68] However, the distribution of EF among HF patients is highly dependent on the data source.

Distribution of Ejection Fraction in HF Registries and Cohorts

Most studies point toward an increasing proportion of HFpEF relative to HFrEF cases in recent years as a result of population aging. Among 894 Framingham Study participants with new-onset HF (mean age 75, 52% women), HFpEF increased (EF ≥50%: 41.0% in 1985 to 1994 vs. 56.2% in 2005 to 2014) and HFrEF decreased (EF <40%: 44.1% vs. 31.06%) over time, while HFmrEF remained unchanged (EF 40% to <50%: 14.9% vs. 12.8%).[69] In contrast to community studies and unselected cohorts, HFpEF is usually less frequent in specialty registries and trials (**Table 18.2**). Nevertheless, between 15% to 25% of patients are classified as HFmrEF in most studies.

Patient Characteristics According to Ejection Fraction

There is an age and sex distribution gradient across EF categories. Among ~12,000 patients with new HF diagnosis from four centers in the United States, the mean age of patients with HFrEF was 69.1 years versus 71.6 in HFmrEF and 74.7 in HFpEF; the percentage of women was 32.6%, 38.4%, and 57.1%, respectively.[24] Those with a history of coronary artery bypass surgery, mitral or aortic valvular disease, atrial fibrillation or flutter, or a diagnosis of hypertension were more likely to have HFpEF, as were those with a diverse range of noncardiac comorbid conditions, including lung disease, liver disease, depression, and dementia. Patients with a history of AMI were more likely to have HFrEF.[24] In the ESC-HF-LT registry, outpatients with HFrEF were younger (64 years vs. 69), more commonly male (78% vs. 52%), ischemic (49% vs. 24%), and with left bundle branch block (24% vs. 9%), but less likely to have hypertension (56% vs. 67%) or atrial fibrillation (18% vs. 32%), compared with HFpEF. Patients with HFmrEF resembled HFrEF in terms of age, sex, and ischemic etiology but had less left ventricular and atrial dilation.[18]

OUTCOMES

Despite advances in HF therapy in the past 20 years, HF-related mortality and rehospitalization rates at the population level have proven difficult to curb, secondary to (1) increasing patient age and comorbidity burden[12]; (2) diminishing returns of newer treatments as neurohormonal blockade effects reach a plateau; (3) negative results of trials with pharmaceuticals targeting non-neurohormonal pathways; (4) lack of effective treatments for patients hospitalized for HF; and (5) lack of effective treatments for patients with HFpEF. On the positive side, HF mortality appears to be decreasing in long-term trends analyses for both outpatients and inpatients, albeit at different rates for various subgroups. Currently, 1-year mortality for outpatients with HF in observational studies in developed countries ranges between 5% and 10%[18,65,66]; however, it is considerably higher (between 10% and 20%)

TABLE 18.2 Distribution of Ejection Fraction in Recent Heart Failure Registries and Cohorts

Region	HFrEF	HFmrEF	HFpEF	Midrange EF Definition	Setting	Study Design	Age (Years)	Female (%)
Europe, Turkey, Israel, Egypt[18]	60	24	16	40%–50%	Outpatient	Registry	64.8±13.3	28.2
Switzerland, Germany[92]	65	17	18	40%–49%	Outpatient	Clinical Trial	76.6±7.7	36.9
Sweden[93]	56	21	23	40%–49%	Mixed	Registry	74±12	29–55
Europe, Latin America, Australia[94]	52	25	23	40%–49%	Inpatient	Registry	28.3% >75 years	36.2
Spain[95]	41	16	43	40%–49%	Inpatient	Registry	71.8±12.1	37.7
United States[9]	46	8	46	41%–49%	Inpatient	Registry	80 (74–86)	54.0

EF, Ejection fraction; *HFmrEF,* heart failure with midrange ejection fraction; *HFpEF,* heart failure with preserved ejection fraction; *HFrEF,* heart failure with reduced ejection fraction in national registries,[27] developing regions,[6] and older adults.[26] For hospitalized patients, 1-year mortality is generally >20% and exceeds 30% in several national registries.[3,26-28,65,66,70] Readmission rates remain high, with >20% of patients in the United States readmitted within 30 days[70-72] and between one-half and two-thirds readmitted within 1 year.[70,73,74] Of note, concerted efforts to reduce readmissions in the United Stated have been associated with unfavorable mortality trends,[73] highlighting the challenges of improving outcomes in an ever-aging and medically complex HF population.

Outcomes in Outpatients
Mortality

In contrast to hospitalized patients, data for ambulatory patients with HF are less abundant. In the ESC-HF-LT registry, mortality at 1 year was 8.8% among ~5500 outpatients with HFrEF (EF ≤40%, age 64±13 years, 21.6% women), 7.6% among ~2200 patients with borderline or midrange EF (EF 40%-50%, age 64±14 years, 31.5% women), and 6.3% among ~1,500 patients with HFpEF (EF >50%, age 69±14 years, 47.9% women) (**Fig. 18.5**).[18] In a retrospective cohort receiving care in an academic center in the United States, mortality was 5.7%, 11.1%, and 16.3% at 1, 2, and 3 years, respectively, among 1350 patients with HFrEF (EF ≤40%, median age 63, 34.3% women).[75] The corresponding mortality rates for the 466 patients with HFpEF (EF >40%, median age 72, 56.9% women) in the same cohort were 4.0%, 7.8%, and 13.2%.

Mortality is higher in national registries, which encompass older and sicker patients. Among 11,600 patients with HFrEF in the US IMPROVE HF registry (EF ≤35%, median age 71 years), mortality at 2 years was 22.1%.[76] In a Veterans Affairs cohort of 6600 ambulatory men with HFrEF (EF <50%, age 70±10 years), 2-year mortality was 25.5% versus 19.8% among the ~2800 patients with HFpEF (EF ≥50%, age 71±10 years), P < .001 for the difference.[77] Importantly, mortality was affected by the number of comorbid conditions in both HFrEF and HFpEF patients. On a positive note, mortality in outpatients appears to be declining in the past two decades. In a study using administrative data from Ontario, Canada, 1-year risk-adjusted mortality decreased from 17.7% in 1997 to 16.2% in 2007 (P = .02).[27]

Quality of care, especially adherence to evidence-based practices, critically affects outcomes in HFrEF. In IMPROVE HF, each 10% improvement in a composite care metric was associated with a 13% lower odds of 24-month mortality (adjusted odds ratio, 0.87; 95% CI, 0.84–0.90).[76] In the international, quality improvement–oriented QUALIFY registry, mortality at 6 months was generally below 7% among outpatients with HFrEF but was highly dependent on adherence to guideline recommended practices.[78]

Hospitalization and Composite Outcomes

In the ESC-HF-LT registry, 31.9% of ambulatory patients with HFrEF were hospitalized within 1 year, and approximately half of the admissions (14.6% of patients) were for HF (see Fig. 18.5). By 1 year, all-cause hospitalization rates were lower for patients with HFpEF and those with HF and midrange EF (HFmrEF); also, the rate of HF hospitalizations was lower for HFpEF and HFmrEF versus HFrEF patients (see Fig. 18.5). The 1-year composite of death or HF hospitalization, commonly used in clinical trials, occurred in 21.2%, 15.0%, and 14.6% for patients with HFrEF, HFmrEF, and HFpEF, respectively.[18] Similar rates for this composite (20.0% and 12.7% for HFrEF and HFpEF, respectively, at 1 year) were reported by a cohort in the United States.[75]

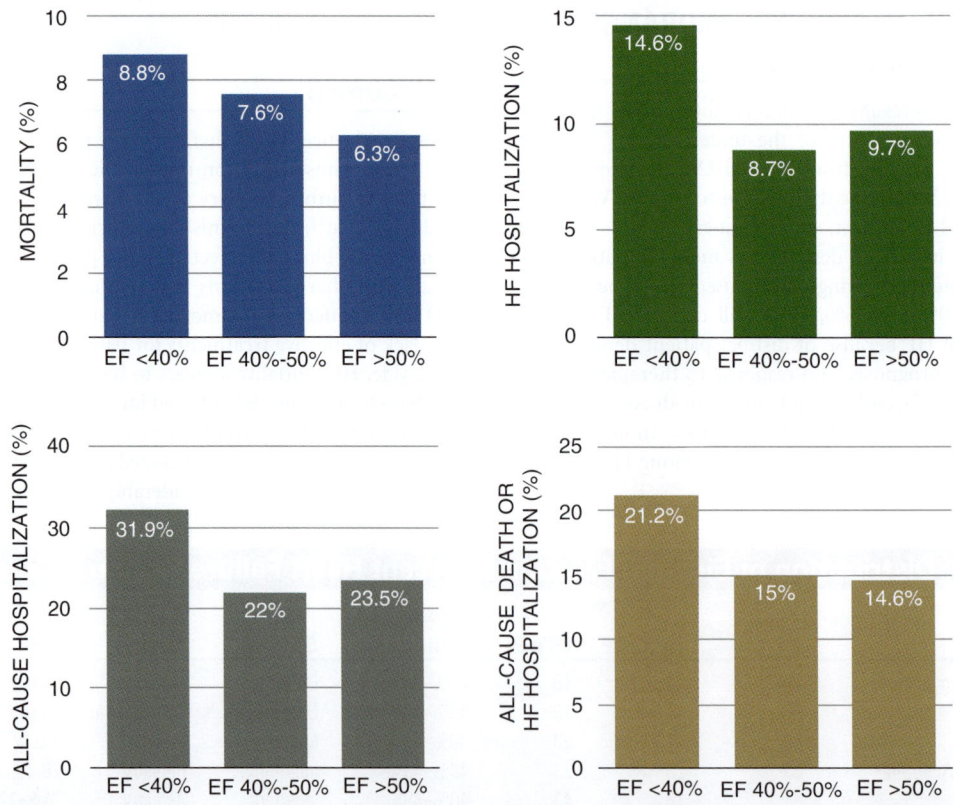

Fig. 18.5 Outcomes at 1 year in outpatients with heart failure in the ESC Heart Failure Long-Term Registry. *EF,* Ejection fraction; *HF,* heart failure. Data from Chioncel O, Lainscak M, Seferovic M, et al. Epidemiology and one-year outcomes in patients with chronic heart failure and preserved, mid-range and reduced ejection fraction: an analysis of the ESC Heart Failure Long-Term Registry. *Eur J Heart Fail.* 2017;19:1574–1585.

Progression to Stage D Heart Failure

Over time, a proportion of patients with ambulatory (Stage C) HF will develop advanced symptoms, usually defined as New York Heart Association functional class IIIB to IV, refractory to optimal therapy, therefore reaching advanced (Stage D—also referred to as "refractory" or "end-stage") HF. In a study of 964 outpatients in the United States with baseline EF ≤40%, the 3-year progression to Stage D HF was 12.2% (annualized rate: 4.5%).[79] By 3 years, 25.1% of patients had either progressed to Stage D or died (annualized rate: 9.2%). Progression was faster in blacks, nonischemic HF, and those in worse functional class. Lower EF and blood pressure, renal and hepatic dysfunction, and chronic lung disease were additional risk factors.[79]

Long-Term Outcomes

Limited data exist on long-term outcomes among ambulatory HF patients. Among ~23,500 patients with HF in England who were seen in primary care and had no HF hospitalization record (median age 79, 51.3% women), 5-year survival was 43.9% compared with 88.1% in the age- and sex-matched general population.[80] In a primary care cohort in Scotland, 5-year survival among ~10,300 men with HF (mean age at diagnosis, 70.5±12.2 years) and ~9100 women with HF (mean age at diagnosis, 76.4±15.5 years) was 55.8% and 49.5%, respectively, and was comparable to or worse than several forms of cancer.[10]

Outcomes in Outpatients With Improved or Recovered Ejection Fraction

Patients who initially present with HFrEF but subsequently demonstrate improved or recovered EF (HFrecEF) have a distinct clinical course and, as a rule, better outcomes than patients with persistent HFpEF or HFrEF. In a single-center outpatient cohort from the United States, preserved (>40%) EF at inception was present in 37.7% of 2166 outpatients.[75] Of these, more than 40% had previously reduced (≤40%) EF. Mortality significantly decelerated among patients with HFrecEF after 1 year. Age- and sex-adjusted 3-year mortality was 16.3%, 13.2%, and 4.8% in patients with HFrEF, HFpEF, and HFrecEF, respectively. Compared with HFpEF or HFrEF, patients with HFrecEF had fewer all-cause and HF-related hospitalizations.[75] In a Spanish cohort of more than 1000 referral outpatients, 1 in 4 HFrEF patients showed recovery of EF from <45% to ≥45% within 1 year.[81] Patients with HFrecEF had lower all-cause, cardiovascular, and HF-related mortality as well as sudden-death rates and experienced fewer hospitalizations.[81]

Prognosis of Hospitalized Heart Failure

The focus of health care systems on reducing the cost of HF has led to a wealth of outcomes data on patients hospitalized with acute HF. However, despite intensive quality-of-care initiatives in recent years, outcomes after a HF hospitalization, especially readmissions, have been remarkably resistant to change. Although in-hospital and 30-day mortality have been decreasing over the past decades, the pressure to reduce length of stay has led to a trade-off between days spent in the hospital and 30-day readmissions.[63,82] More recently, the introduction of financial penalties in the United States as part of a program to reduce readmissions after an admission for HF has been associated with increased 30-day and 1-year mortality.[73] **Table 18.3** summarizes recent evidence on short- and long-term mortality estimates after hospitalization for HF.

Short-Term Outcomes

Overall, in-hospital mortality rates are currently below 10% in developed countries. In the United States, in-hospital mortality among patients admitted with a primary diagnosis of HF declined from 4.5% in 2001 to 2.9% in 2014, although the decline has slowed in recent years and regional variation is considerable.[59,83] In Italy, in-hospital mortality remained unchanged at 9.4% in Lombardy between 2000 and 2012; this estimate included patients (13%) with HF as secondary diagnosis, who have higher mortality rates.[29] In the same study, mortality decreased among patients <75 years old; however, the percentage of older patients increased in the same period.[29] Similar in-hospital mortality (9.3%) has been reported for years 2000–2013 in Germany.[61] In a younger cohort (age, 59±15 years) from seven Gulf countries in 2012, mortality was 6.3%.[84] Of note, length of stay (and therefore time at risk) is considerably shorter in the United States compared with Europe or Asia, and this may partially explain the lower in-hospital mortality.[59,61,84]

Because 30-day outcomes after an admission for HF have become a hospital performance metric and, more recently, a financial incentive, most data on 30-day mortality and readmissions come from the United States. Despite improvements in 30-day mortality, the 30-day readmission metric has proven remarkably resistant to quality improvement initiatives. In several studies, 30-day mortality and readmissions have divergent secular trends. In 416 US hospitals participating in the Get With the Guidelines—Heart Failure (GWTG-HF) registry, the 30-day risk-adjusted readmission rate among Medicare beneficiaries declined from 20.0% in 2006–2010 to 18.4% in 2012–2014.[73] However, 30-day risk-adjusted mortality increased from 7.2% to 8.6% during the same period, and 1-year readmission and mortality rates followed a similar pattern, raising concerns about unintended consequences of the readmission reduction program. Short-term readmission rates vary widely in other systems. In ASCEND-HF, the mean country-level all-cause 30-day readmission rate ranged from 2.5% to 25.0%, and countries with longer length of stay had significantly lower readmission rates.[63]

Long-Term Outcomes

Admission for HF is accompanied by high mortality in the following months. In the Efficacy of Vasopressin Antagonism in Heart Failure Outcome Study with Tolvaptan (EVEREST) trial, mortality decreased immediately after discharge, reached a low at 90 days, and increased steadily thereafter.[85] Despite a decrease over the past few decades, 1-year mortality after hospitalization for HF remains high and exceeds 30% in several systems (see Table 18.3). In recent reports, 1-year mortality appears to have reached a plateau.

In Denmark, 1-year mortality after hospitalization for HF declined from 45% to 33% between 1983–1987 and 2008–2012, with slower decline in recent years.[3] The slowing decline of 1-year mortality in recent years has been reported by studies from Australia (2005–2014, 1-year mortality 32%)[86] and Canada (33.8% in 2007).[27] In the ESC-HF-LT registry (age, 69±13; 37.4% women), 1-year mortality was 23.6%, and varied from 21.6% to 36.5% across countries.[66]

Hospitalization for HF is associated with poor long-term survival, especially in older adults, and limited life expectancy compared with the general age- and sex-matched population. Among patients age ≥65 admitted for HF between 2005 and 2009 in hospitals participating in the GWTG-HF program (median age, 80; 54% female), median survival was 2.1 years.[9] In adjusted analyses, 5-year mortality was similar in patients with HFrEF (75.3%), HFmrEF (75.7%), and HFpEF (75.7%), and median survival was considerably shorter for age compared with the general population.[9] In England, 5-year mortality among patients who survived 3 months after the diagnosis of HF (median age, 80; women 50%) was 78.3% for those not receiving primary care and 56.1% for those receiving primary care, compared with 11.9% in an age- and sex-matched population.[80]

TABLE 18.3 Mortality Rates After Hospitalization for Heart Failure

	Source	Mortality Estimates	Notes
In-hospital			
United States	National Inpatient Sample[59]	4.5% (2001) to 2.9% (2014)	ICD-9-CM codes, primary diagnosis
	GWTG-HF[96]	HFpEF: 3.32% (2005) to 2.35% (2010)	Quality improvement initiative
		HFrEF: 3.03% (2005) to 2.83% (2010)	
		HFmrEF: 2.69% (2005) to 2.88% (2010)	
Italy	Lombardy region, administrative data[29]	• 9.4% without temporal trend (2000–2012)	ICD-9-CM codes
		• Acute HF episodes: 9.1%	
		• Cardiomyopathies without acute HF: 5.6%	
		• With HF as secondary diagnosis: 15.9%	
Germany	German Federal Health Monitoring System[61]	14.8% (2000) to 9.3% (2013)	ICD10-GM codes, primary diagnosis
France	French National Hospitalization Database[60]	7.8% (2012)	ICD-10 codes, primary diagnosis
Gulf Area	Gulf Acute HF Registry[97]	6.5% (2012)	Mean age, 59±15 years
Sub-Saharan Africa	Survey[98]	4.2% (2007–2010)	Mean age, 52±18 years
30-day			
United States	Medicare enrollees from the GWTG-HF program[73]	7.2% (2006– 2010)	Risk-adjusted estimates
		8.6% (2012–2014)	
International	ALARM-HF Registry[94]	9.4% (2006–2007)	Patients with documented EF
1-year			
USA	Medicare enrollees from the GWTG-HF program[73]	31.3% (2006–2010); 36.3% (2012–2014)	Risk-adjusted estimates
Europe	Multicenter registry[66]	23.6% (2011–2013)	Prospective study, only consenting patients included
International	INTER-CHF cohort[6]	30.6% (unadjusted)	Middle- or low-income countries
Italy	Italian Network Registry[65]	24.0% (2007–2009)	Prospective study, only consenting patients included
		De novo HF: 19.2%	
		Worsening HF: 27.7%	
Gulf Area	Gulf Acute HF Registry[97]	20.2% (2012)	Mean age, 59±15 years
Germany	Administrative data[28]	23% (2006)	Primary diagnosis, new cases only
Denmark	Registry[3]	34.6% (2003–2007)	ICD codes, primary or secondary diagnosis, new cases only
		32.7% (2008–2012)	
Canada	Administrative data[27]	35.7% (1997) to 33.8% (2008)	ICD codes
5-year			
USA	GWTG-HF[9]	HFrEF: 75.3%, HFpEF: 75.7%	Quality improvement initiative
		HFmrEF: 75.7%	
Denmark	Registry[3]	64.1% (2003–2007)	ICD codes, primary or secondary diagnosis, new cases only
		61.3% (2008–2012)	

ALARM-HF, Acute Heart Failure Global Registry of Standard Treatment; *EF,* ejection fraction; *GWTG-HF,* Get With the Guidelines—Heart Failure; *HF,* heart failure; *HFmrEF,* heart failure with midrange ejection fraction; *HFpEF,* heart failure with preserved ejection fraction; *HFrEF,* heart failure with reduced ejection fraction; *ICD-9-CM,* International Classification of Diseases, 9th Revision, Clinical Modification; *ICD-10-GM,* International Classification of Diseases, 10th revision, German Modification; *INTER-CHF,* International Congestive Heart Failure Study.

Long-term post-HF admission mortality is highly dependent on age, with 1-year rates approaching 50% in the oldest old (**Fig. 18.6**).[29,87] Most studies indicate that postadmission mortality is similar in men and women.[3] However, mortality seems to differ across race. In the GWTG-HF registry, 1-year mortality was significantly lower among black patients (29.5%) compared with whites (37.8%), Asians or Pacific Islanders (35.1%), and Hispanics (32.2%).[70] Hospitalization for decompensated chronic HF carries higher risk compared with hospitalization for de novo HF.[65] Finally, patients with HFrEF have slightly higher 1-year mortality compared with HFmrEF and HFpEF, but these differences appear to be related to patient characteristics.[88]

Outcomes After Post-AMI Heart Failure (see also Chapter 19)

Post-AMI HF outcomes have proven difficult to improve, especially among older adults, and development of HF still portends a significantly worse prognosis among AMI survivors. Most registries report a twofold increase in mortality with HF. In the United States, the 1-year post-AMI incidence of HF declined slightly between 1998 and 2010, but 1-year mortality after HF was steadily >40%.[37] In Sweden, despite a marked decrease in post-AMI HF incidence and mortality between 1996 and 2008, 1-year mortality was still twofold higher with HF and still >30% in 2008.[40] Similar trends and relative risks have been reported from Australia and Norway.[38,89]

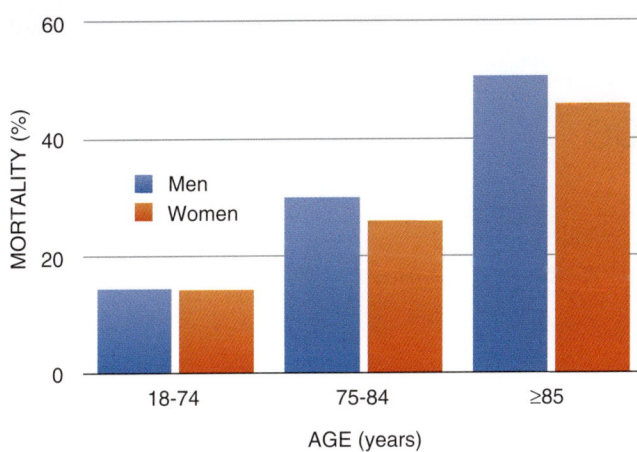

Fig. 18.6 Mortality at 1 year in patients hospitalized for heart failure in Lombardy, Italy, 2005–2012. Data from Frigerio M, Mazzali C, Paganoni AM, et al. Trends in heart failure hospitalizations, patient characteristics, in-hospital and 1-year mortality: a population study, from 2000 to 2012 in Lombardy. *Int J Cardiol.* 2017;236:310–314.

KEY REFERENCES

9. Shah KS, Xu H, Matsouaka RA, et al. Heart failure with preserved, borderline, and reduced ejection fraction: 5-year outcomes. *J Am Coll Cardiol.* 2017;(17):39761; pii: S0735-1097.
12. Conrad N, Judge A, Tran J, et al. Temporal trends and patterns in heart failure incidence: a population-based study of 4 million individuals. *Lancet.* 2018;391:572–580.
16. Brouwers FP, de Boer RA, van der Harst P, et al. Incidence and epidemiology of new onset heart failure with preserved vs. reduced ejection fraction in a community-based cohort: 11-year follow-up of PREVEND. *Eur Heart J.* 2013;34:1424–1431.
18. Chioncel O, Lainscak M, Seferovic PM, et al. Epidemiology and one-year outcomes in patients with chronic heart failure and preserved, mid-range and reduced ejection fraction: an analysis of the ESC Heart Failure Long-Term Registry. *Eur J Heart Fail.* 2017;19:1574–1585.
36. Xanthakis V, Enserro DM, Larson MG, et al. Prevalence, neurohormonal correlates, and prognosis of heart failure stages in the community. *JACC Heart Fail.* 2016;4:808–815.
40. Desta L, Jernberg T, Löfman I, et al. Incidence, temporal trends, and prognostic impact of heart failure complicating acute myocardial infarction. The SWEDEHEART Registry (Swedish Web-System for Enhancement and Development of Evidence-Based Care in Heart Disease Evaluated According to Recommended Therapies): a study of 199,851 patients admitted with index acute myocardial infarctions, 1996 to 2008. *JACC Heart Fail.* 2015;3:234–242.
63. Eapen ZJ, Reed SD, Li Y, et al. Do countries or hospitals with longer hospital stays for acute heart failure have lower readmission rates? Findings from ASCEND-HF. *Circ Heart Fail.* 2013;6:727–732.
73. Gupta A, Allen LA, Bhatt DL, et al. Association of the hospital readmissions reduction program implementation with readmission and mortality outcomes in heart failure. *JAMA Cardiol.* 2018;3:44–53.
75. Kalogeropoulos AP, Fonarow GC, Georgiopoulou V, et al. Characteristics and outcomes of adult outpatients with heart failure and improved or recovered ejection fraction. *JAMA Cardiol.* 2016;1:510–518.
79. Kalogeropoulos AP, Samman-Tahhan A, Hedley JS, et al. Progression to stage d heart failure among outpatients with stage c heart failure and reduced ejection fraction. *JACC Heart Fail.* 2017;5:528–537.

The full reference list for this chapter is available on ExpertConsult.

Heart Failure as a Consequence of Ischemic Heart Disease

G. Michael Felker, Douglas L. Mann, James D. Flaherty, Robert O. Bonow

Despite significant progress in the prevention and treatment of cardiovascular disease over the past 30 years, national statistics indicate that the incidence and prevalence of heart failure (HF) continue to rise.[1] This has occurred during a time period in which death rates from coronary artery disease (CAD) and stroke have declined. HF and CAD are both age-related conditions (the prevalence of HF is 1% between the ages of 50 and 59 years, but 10% above the age of 75 years).[2] The increased survival after myocardial infarction (MI) and advances in medical and device therapies (e.g., β-blockers and implantable cardioverter-defibrillators [ICDs]) for the prevention of sudden cardiac death (SCD) have increased the pool of patients with both CAD and HF.[3-5]

PREVALENCE OF CORONARY ARTERY DISEASE IN HEART FAILURE

CAD has emerged as a dominant causal factor in HF (**see also Chapter 18**). Survivors of acute MI, even when not complicated by HF, have a relatively high incidence of subsequent HF hospitalization.[6] This is due not only to the initial ventricular insult caused by the MI but also the progressive nature of CAD (**Fig. 19.1**). The Framingham Heart Study suggests that the factors contributing to HF are changing, as evidenced by a decrease in valvular heart disease and left ventricular (LV) hypertrophy but an increase in MI as a risk factor from 1950 to 1998.[3] In this analysis, the odds of a prior MI as a cause of HF increased by 26% per decade in men and 48% per decade in women. In contrast, hypertension as a cause of HF decreased by 13% per decade in men and 25% in women, and valvular heart disease as a cause of HF decreased by 24% per decade in men and 17% in women.

In the Studies of Left Ventricular Dysfunction (SOLVD) registry, which enrolled 6273 patients, CAD was determined as the underlying cause of chronic HF in approximately 70% of patients, whereas hypertension was invoked as the primary cause in only 7% of cases.[7]

Of note, there was a history of hypertension in 43% of patients. There were striking racial differences observed in this registry. HF was considered due to CAD in 73% of white patients but only 36% of African-American patients (**see also Chapter 40**).

Pooling data from 26 multicenter trials of chronic HF since 1986, with greater than 43,000 patients, revealed that 62% carried a diagnosis of CAD (**Table 19.1**).[8-33] This number may actually underestimate the true prevalence of CAD in this population because in clinical practice and in most studies there is no systemic assessment of coronary artery anatomy. In addition, most of these trials excluded patients with a recent MI, angina, or objective evidence of active ischemia. In a study of 136 patients (<75 years old) hospitalized with de novo HF, a review of the clinical, angiographic, and myocardial perfusion imaging data was used to determine that CAD was the primary cause in greater than 50% of cases.[34] In this study alone, two-thirds of all patients who underwent angiography had obstructive CAD (defined as >50% luminal stenosis), although CAD was not considered the primary causal factor in all cases. In a recent analysis of a large US acute HF registry, myocardial ischemia was found to be a leading precipitating factor for hospitalization.[35]

PROGNOSTIC SIGNIFICANCE OF CORONARY ARTERY DISEASE IN HEART FAILURE

The presence of CAD in patients with HF has been shown to be independently associated with a worsened long-term outcome in numerous studies.[36] Atherosclerosis is an important contributing cause of death in HF patients through a variety of mechanisms, including SCD, progressive ventricular failure, MI, renal failure, and stroke. In patients with HF, the long-term prognosis is directly related to the angiographic extent and severity of CAD.[37,38] This has been demonstrated both in HF patients with LV systolic dysfunction and in those with preserved systolic function.[39]

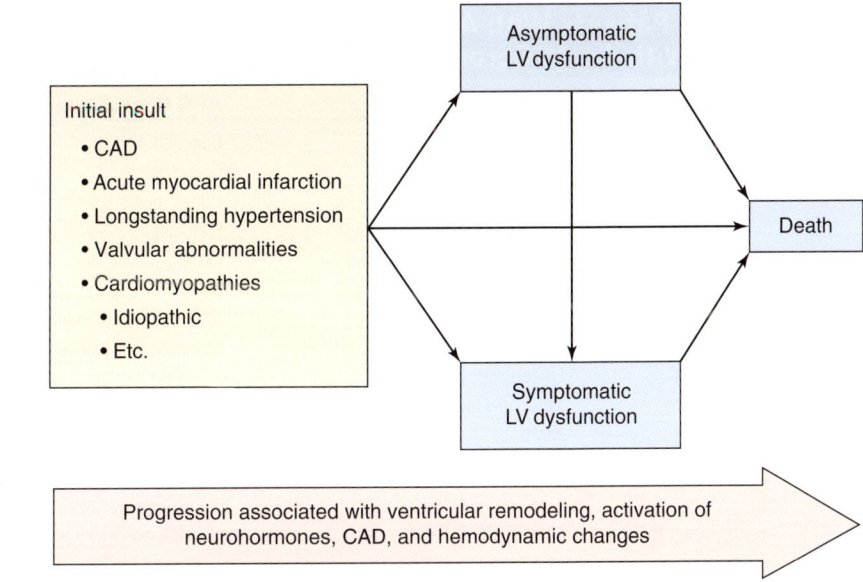

Fig. 19.1 Coronary artery disease *(CAD)* contributes to left ventricular *(LV)* dysfunction not only during an initial insult (e.g., myocardial infarction) but throughout its progression. In addition, progression of chronic heart failure is associated with ventricular remodeling, activation of neurohormones, and hemodynamic changes.

TABLE 19.1 Prevalence of Coronary Artery Disease in 26 Multicenter Chronic Heart Failure Trials Reported by the *New England Journal of Medicine* Since 1986			
Trial	**Year**	**N**	**CAD**
VHEFT-1	1986	642	282
CONSENSUS	1987	253	146
Milrinone	1989	230	115
PROMISE	1991	1088	590
SOLVD-T	1991	2569	1828
VHEFT-2	1991	804	427
SOVLD-P	1992	4228	3518
RADIANCE	1993	178	107
Vesnarinone	1993	477	249
STAT-CHF	1995	674	481
Carvedilol	1996	1094	521
PRAISE	1996	1153	732
DIG	1997	6800	4793
VEST	1998	3833	2236
RALES	1999	1663	907
DIAMOND	1999	1518	1017
Nesiritide	2000	127	58
COPERNICUS	2001	2289	1534
BEST	2001	2708	1587
Val-HeFT	2001	5010	2880
MIRACLE	2002	453	108
COMPANION	2004	1520	842
SCD-HeFT	2005	2521	1310
CARE-HF	2005	813	309
RethinQ	2007	172	90
Dronedarone	2008	627	407
Total		**43,444**	**27,074**

CAD was documented to be present in nearly 65% of patients.
CAD, Coronary artery disease.

Recent data suggest that the mechanism of SCD may differ between ischemic and nonischemic HF, with acute coronary events representing the major cause of SCD in patients with CAD.[40,41] In the Assessment of Treatment with Lisinopril and Survival (ATLAS) study, 54% of patients with chronic HF and CAD who died suddenly had autopsy evidence of acute MI.[40] In another autopsy study of 180 patients with known ischemic cardiomyopathy, acute MI was responsible for 57% of the deaths.[41] This study revealed that before autopsy data were available, many deaths as a result of acute MI in patients with HF were misclassified as caused by progressive HF or arrhythmias. In another study of patients with HF and left ventricular systolic dysfunction (LVSD) 25% of repeat hospitalizations were attributed to acute coronary syndrome (ACS).[42] However, approximately 10% of patients with a history of HF who were subsequently hospitalized for ACS were originally classified as having a nonischemic cause. These findings further emphasize the importance of accurately assessing for the presence of CAD in patients with HF.

PATHOPHYSIOLOGY OF ACUTE HEART FAILURE IN PATIENTS WITH CORONARY ARTERY DISEASE

Underlying Coronary Artery Disease

Patients hospitalized with acute HF differ from patients with chronic ambulatory HF with respect to prognosis and early management (**see also Chapter 36**).[43] Patients with CAD who develop acute HF do so with either an ACS or a non-ACS presentation. Although the majority of such patients do not have ACS, there is considerable overlap in these two presentations with respect to clinical characteristics (**Table 19.2**) and potential therapies (**Table 19.3**). However, the approach to the patient with ACS has become more standardized in clinical practice guidelines compared with the acute HF patient with a non-ACS presentation. Myocardial injury is common in both, but in ACS patients it is usually the principal cause of HF, whereas in non-ACS patients myocardial injury may be the result of worsening HF. In these latter patients, cardiac troponin levels are frequently elevated in patients with acute HF, representing myocardial injury (**see also Chapter 33**). In the era of high-sensitivity troponin assays, the values of troponin in AHF

TABLE 19.2 **Characteristics of Patients With Acute Heart Failure Syndrome and Coronary Artery Disease Versus Patients With Acute Coronary Syndrome Complicated by Heart Failure**

	AHFS and CAD	ACS Complicated by HF
Dyspnea	Common	Common
Chest discomfort	Uncommon	Common
Prior HF	Common	Uncommon
BNP/N-terminal pro-BNP	Elevated	Elevated
Troponin	Normal or elevated[a]	Usually elevated
Left ventricular systolic function	Normal or depressed	Normal or depressed
Diagnostic testing for CAD[b] (ischemia/viability/angiography)	Uncommon	Standard (per guidelines)
Myocardial revascularization	Uncommon[b]	Standard (per guidelines)
Secondary prevention for CAD	Underused	Standard (per guidelines)
In-hospital mortality	Relatively low	Relatively high
Early after-discharge death or rehospitalization	High	High

[a]Typically low-level elevation.
[b]During index hospitalization.
ACS, Acute coronary syndrome; *AHFS*, acute heart failure syndrome; *BNP*, B-type natriuretic peptide; *CAD*, coronary artery disease; *HF*, heart failure.

TABLE 19.3 **Therapies for Acute Heart Failure Syndrome and Coronary Artery Disease Versus Acute Coronary Syndrome Complicated by Heart Failure**

	AHFS and CAD	ACS Complicated by HF
Immediate Therapies		
Nitrates	Yes	Yes
Antiplatelet agents	Yes	Yes
Anticoagulation	No	Yes
Inotropes	Avoid if possible	Avoid if possible
Statins	Yes	Yes
Renin-Angiotensin System Modulation		
ACE-I or ARB	Yes	Yes
Aldosterone blockade (if LVSD)	Yes	Yes
β-blockers	Yes	Yes
Early angiography/revascularization	Yes[a]	Yes[a]

[a]If jeopardized myocardium present (ischemia or viability).
ACE-I, Angiotensin-converting enzyme inhibitor; *ACS*, Acute coronary syndrome; *AHFS*, acute heart failure syndrome; *ARB*, angiotensin receptor blocker; *CAD*, coronary artery disease; *HF*, heart failure; *LVSD*, left ventricular systolic dysfunction.
From Flaherty JD, Bax JJ, De Luca L, et al. Acute heart failure syndromes in patients with coronary artery disease early assessment and treatment. *J Am Coll Cardiol.* 53:254–263, 2009.

patients often surpass the acute MI threshold (i.e., the 99th upper reference limit [URL]) and may demonstrate a typical rise and fall.[44] Such events have been classified as "acute myocardial injury" rather than type II myocardial infraction in the new fourth universal definition of MI, although this is primarily a semantic distinction.[45] Regardless, these acute elevations of troponin in HF are a marker of worse outcomes.[46-51]

In acute HF, a high LV diastolic pressure can result in subendocardial ischemia (even in the absence of epicardial coronary disease). Experimental evidence suggests that troponin release is correlated with both LV loading conditions and microvascular dysfunction. Excessive neurohormonal activation can exacerbate ischemia via increased cardiac contractility and reduced coronary perfusion because of endothelial dysfunction. In addition, patients with acute HF and CAD often have hibernating or stunned myocardium.[52] Together, all of these factors may result in myocardial injury.

Low systemic blood pressure combined with elevated LV diastolic pressure reduces coronary perfusion, and in this setting, the autoregulation between coronary artery perfusion pressure and coronary vasoactive tone may be lost or impaired in patients with obstructive epicardial CAD. This may contribute to myocardial injury (as reflected by cardiac enzyme elevation) and worse outcomes. This may help to explain why patients with acute HF and underlying CAD have a worse outcome than those without CAD and have improved outcomes if they have a history of myocardial revascularization.[50,53]

Acute Coronary Syndromes

Approximately 10% to 20% of patients with ACS have concomitant acute HF, and approximately 10% of ACS patients develop HF in-hospital.[54-59] In the EuroHeart Survey II on HF, 42% of all de novo HF cases were due to ACS.[60] Patients with ACS and ST-segment elevation typically have a high degree of myocardial injury. ACS patients with HF but without ST-segment elevation also have significant cardiac enzyme elevation but a smaller degree of injury.[49] The short-term risk of adverse outcomes in ACS patients with HF is directly proportional to the level of troponin elevation.[61] Most of these patients do not have a history of HF or LVSD.[54,56]

Patients with ACS complicated by HF have markedly increased short- and long-term mortality rates compared with ACS patients without HF.[54-56,61-69] ACS patients who develop HF after the initial presentation have even higher mortality rates.[55,59] The prognosis of ACS complicated by HF is directly related to the Killip class.[55,57,59] Compared with Killip class I patients, patients with an ACS in Killip class II or III HF are four times more likely to die in-hospital.[56,59] The risk goes up to 10-fold for patients with cardiogenic shock (Killip class IV). Among ACS patients who recover from transient HF, the majority develop recurrent HF.[6]

PATHOPHYSIOLOGY OF CHRONIC HEART FAILURE IN PATIENTS WITH CORONARY ARTERY DISEASE AND REDUCED EJECTION FRACTION

HF in the setting of CAD is a heterogeneous condition with several possible factors contributing to clinical manifestations of HF and LVSD and/or diastolic dysfunction. First and foremost, the sequelae of MI, with loss of functioning myocytes, development of myocardial

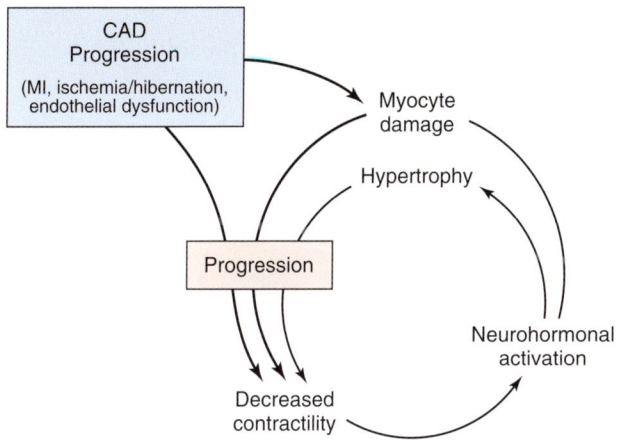

Fig. 19.2 Progression of coronary artery disease *(CAD)* leads to decreased contractility, which stimulates neurohormonal activation of chamber remodeling, hypertrophy, and myocyte damage. *MI,* Myocardial infarction. (Adapted from Gheorghiade M, Bonow RO. Chronic heart failure in the United States: a manifestation of coronary artery disease. *Circulation.* 1998;97[3]:282–289.)

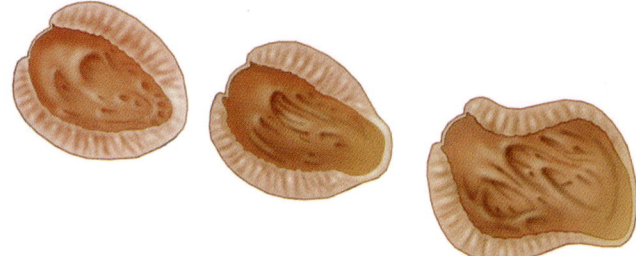

Fig. 19.3 Remodeling of Left Ventricle After ST-Elevation Myocardial Infarction (STEMI). *Left,* Apical STEMI (white zone of left ventricle). Over time, the infarct zone elongates and thins. Progressive remodeling of the left ventricle occurs *(center* and *right),* ultimately converting the left ventricle from an oval shape to a spherical shape. Pharmacologic and catheter-based reperfusion strategies for STEMI have a favorable impact on this process by minimizing the extent of myocardial necrosis *(left)* through prompt restoration of flow in the epicardial infarct vessel. (Modified from McMurray JJV, Pfeffer MA, eds. *Heart Failure Updates,* London: Martin, 2003.)

fibrosis, and subsequent LV remodeling, result in chamber dilation and neurohormonal activation that lead to progressive deterioration of the remaining viable myocardium.[70] This is a well-recognized clinical process that can be ameliorated after acute MI by the use of angiotensin-converting enzyme (ACE) inhibitor therapy, beat-blocking agents, mineralocorticoid receptors, and myocardial revascularization.[71-74] Second,[75] the majority of patients surviving MI have significant atherosclerotic disease in coronary arteries other than the infarct-related artery.[76] Thus superimposed on the LV with irreversibly damaged myocardium, there is often a considerable degree of jeopardized myocardium served by a stenotic coronary artery either within the infarct zone or remote from the infarcted tissue. This may result in myocardial ischemia/hibernation, contributing to LV dysfunction and the risk of recurrent MI producing further deterioration in LV function or SCD. Finally, endothelial dysfunction, a characteristic feature of atherosclerotic CAD, may also contribute importantly and independently to the progression of LV dysfunction (**Fig. 19.2**).[77]

Left Ventricular Remodeling (see also Chapter 12)

LV remodeling is the process by which the LV's size, shape, and function are altered in response to acute injury and/or hemodynamic overload. As reviewed in detail in **Chapter 12**, LV remodeling occurs secondary to mechanical, neurohormonal, and genetic factors (**Fig. 19.3**).[70] The severe loss of myocardial cells after acute MI results in an abrupt increase in loading conditions that induces a unique pattern of remodeling involving the infarct zone, the infarct border zone, and the remote noninfarcted myocardium.[70] Myocyte necrosis initiates a process of reparative changes, which consist of dilation, hypertrophy, and the formation of a collagen scar. Other factors may influence this process, including the location and transmurality of the infarct, the extent of myocardial stunning beyond the initial infarction, infarct-related artery patency, and local trophic factors.[70] Postinfarction remodeling has been arbitrarily divided into an early phase (within 72 hours) and a late phase (beyond 72 hours). In patients with transmural MI, the early phase involves expansion of the infarct, with thinning and bulging that may result in ventricular rupture, aneurysm, mitral insufficiency, and ventricular tachyarrhythmias. Late remodeling involves the LV globally and is associated morphologically with dilation, hypertrophy, and myocyte hypertrophy (see Fig. 19.3).[70] Importantly, LV remodeling creates a de novo

mechanical burden for the heart and can integrated processes contribute independently to the progression of HF.[78]

Myocardial Ischemia

Under basal conditions, episodes of reversible myocardial ischemia caused by a severe coronary artery stenosis superimposed on the LV with depressed systolic function may produce transient worsening of LV function. This exacerbates dyspnea on exertion and fatigue. In many patients, these HF symptoms, stimulated by exercise, represent an anginal equivalent that may occur in the absence of chest pain.

Transient LV dysfunction can aggravate symptoms during stress or spontaneous ischemia in patients with CAD and HF. Ischemia can also produce a rapid and massive increase in the concentration of all three endogenous catecholamines (norepinephrine, epinephrine, dopamine) in the myocardial interstitium, which is mediated by inhibition of neuronal reuptake mechanisms.[79] High myocardial catecholamine concentration may have a deleterious effect on cardiac myocytes.[80-82]

Ischemia may also lead to myocyte apoptosis, which may result in progression of LV dysfunction without a clear ischemic event.[83] This situation also indicates that ischemia from a chronic stenosis can produce substantial myocyte loss in the absence of significant necrosis or fibrosis. Ischemia may also cause an increase in endothelin production that may have a negative effect on LV function.[84] Aggressive medical and surgical interventions designed to ameliorate ischemia appear to have a substantial impact on limiting apoptosis.

Hibernation/Stunning

Episodes of transient myocardial ischemia may cause prolonged LVSD that persists after the ischemic insult itself has resolved. This process is termed *stunning,* which is similar to more severe and protracted myocardial stunning that results from coronary occlusion and reperfusion (**Fig. 19.4A**).[85] Recurrent episodes of myocardial ischemia that produce repetitive myocardial stunning may contribute to overall LV dysfunction and HF symptoms.

Another important mechanism for systolic dysfunction with additive effects on LV performance is myocardial hibernation. Once considered a process in which myocardial contraction is downregulated in response to chronic reduction in myocardial blood supply,[86-88] the current evidence supports the hypothesis that persistent contractile dysfunction in patients with chronic CAD represents a process of

CONSEQUENCES OF ACUTE ISCHEMIA

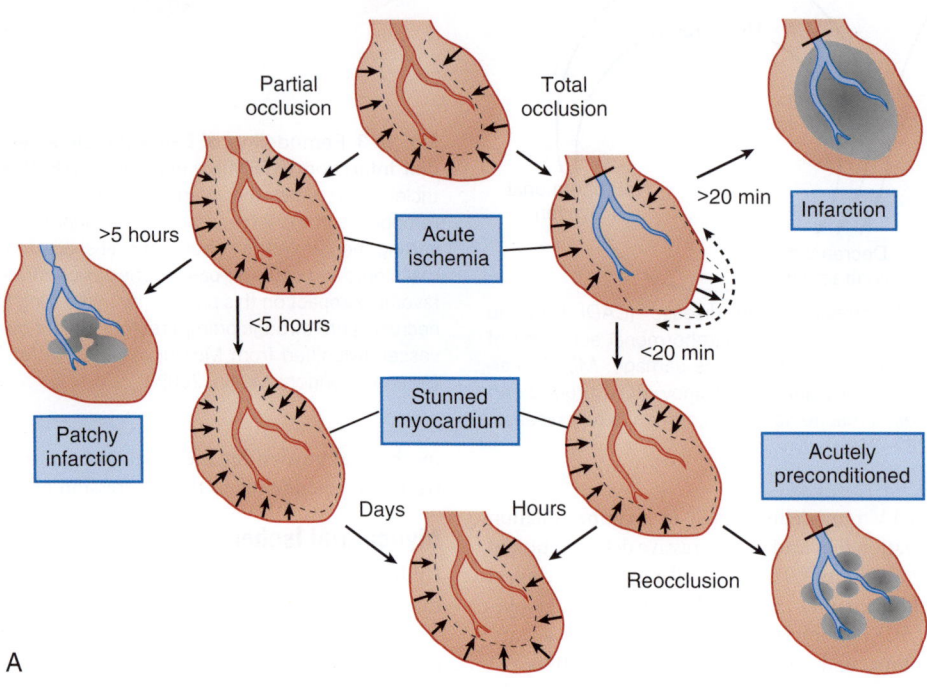

Partial occlusion

Total occlusion

Acute ischemia

>20 min

Infarction

>5 hours

Patchy infarction

<5 hours

<20 min

Stunned myocardium

Acutely preconditioned

Days

Hours

Reocclusion

A

CONSEQUENCES OF CHRONIC REPETITIVE ISCHEMIA

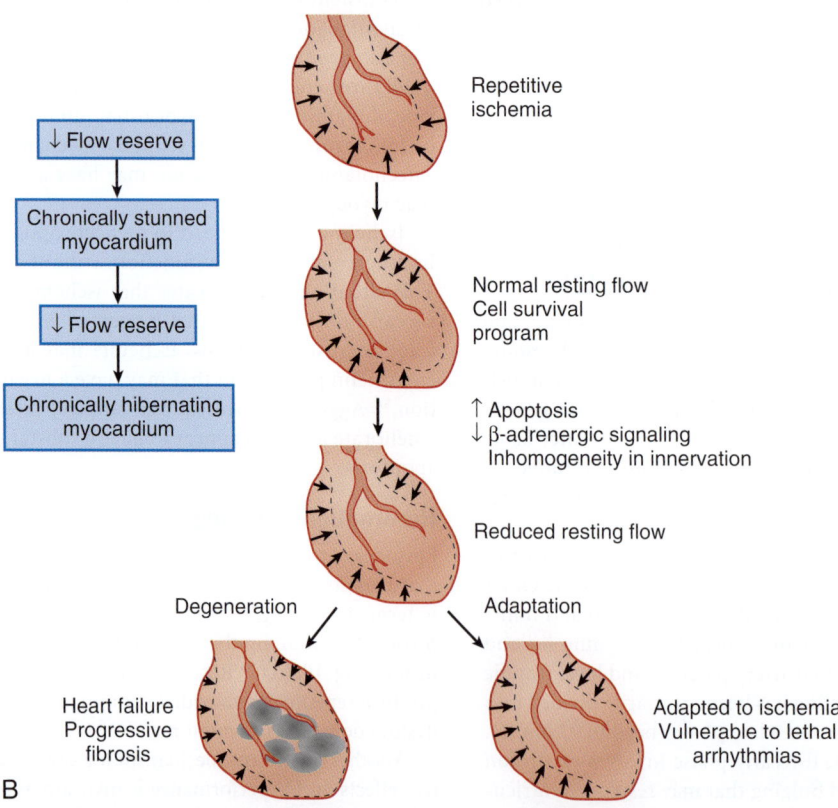

Repetitive ischemia

↓ Flow reserve

Chronically stunned myocardium

↓ Flow reserve

Chronically hibernating myocardium

Normal resting flow
Cell survival program

↑ Apoptosis
↓ β-adrenergic signaling
  Inhomogeneity in innervation

Reduced resting flow

Degeneration

Adaptation

Heart failure
Progressive fibrosis

Adapted to ischemia
Vulnerable to lethal arrhythmias

B

Fig. 19.4 Effects of Ischemia on Left Ventricular Function and Irreversible Injury. The ventriculograms illustrate contractile dysfunction (*dashed lines* and *arrows*). (A) Consequences of acute ischemia. A brief total occlusion *(right)* or a prolonged partial occlusion (caused by an acute high-grade stenosis, *left*) leads to acute contractile dysfunction proportional to the reduction in blood flow. Irreversible injury begins after 20 minutes following a total occlusion but is delayed for up to 5 hours following a partial occlusion (or with significant collaterals) caused by short-term hibernation. When reperfusion is established before the onset of irreversible injury, stunned myocardium develops and the time required for recovery of function is proportional to the duration and severity of ischemia. With prolonged ischemia, stunning in viable myocardium coexists with subendocardial infarction and accounts for reversible dysfunction. Brief episodes of ischemia preceding prolonged ischemia elicits protection against infarction (acute preconditioning). (B) Effects of chronic repetitive ischemia on function distal to a stenosis. As stenosis severity increases, coronary flow reserve decreases and the frequency of reversible ischemia increases. Reversible repetitive ischemia initially leads to chronic preconditioning against infarction and stunning (not shown). Subsequently, there is a gradual progression from contractile dysfunction with normal resting flow (chronically stunned myocardium) to contractile dysfunction with depressed resting flow (hibernating myocardium). This transition is related to the physiologic significance of a coronary stenosis and can occur in a time period as short as 1 week or develop chronically in the absence of severe angina. The cellular response during the progression to chronic hibernating myocardium is variable, with some patients exhibiting successful adaptation with little cell death and fibrosis and others developing degenerative changes difficult to distinguish from subendocardial infarction. (From Canty JM. Coronary blood flow and myocardial ischemia. In: Libby P, Bonow RO, Mann DL, et al, eds. *Braunwald's Heart Disease*. Philadelphia, PA: Saunders, 2008.)

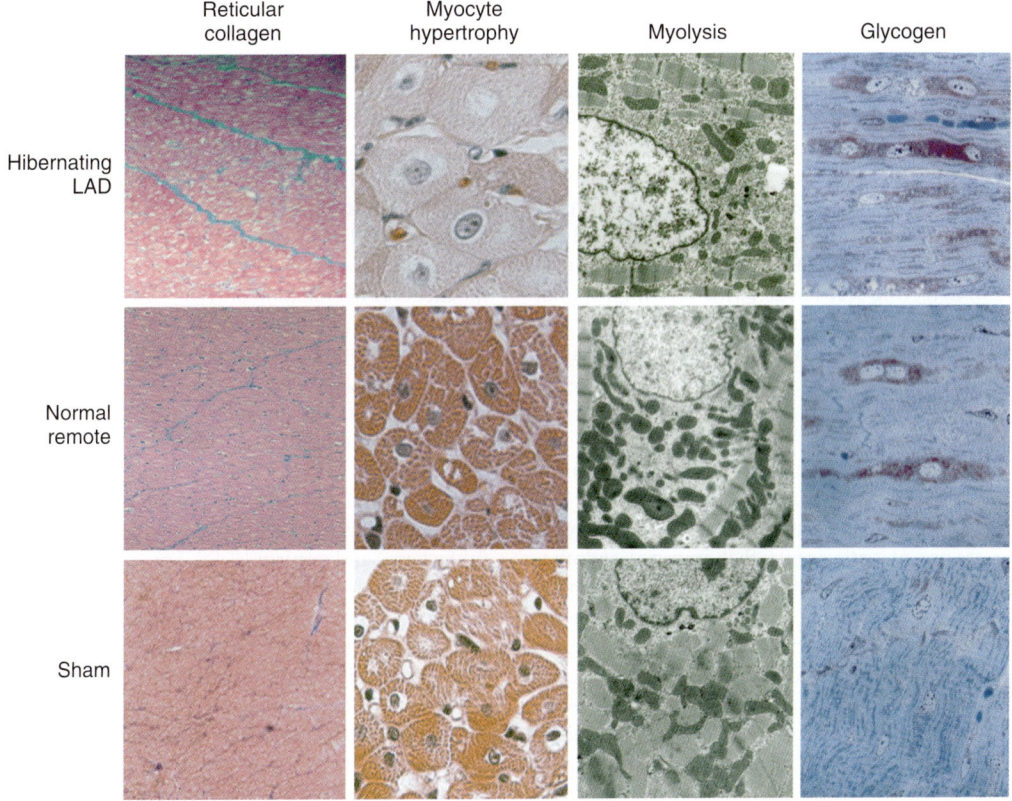

Fig. 19.5 Myocyte Cellular Changes in Hibernating Myocardium. The increased myocyte loss results in compensatory myocyte cellular hypertrophy in hibernating myocardium. Although reticular collagen is regionally increased (approximately 2%), there is no evidence of infarction. The electron microscopic characteristics of hibernating myocardium demonstrate myofibrillar loss, an increased number of small mitochondria, and increased glycogen content. Although these are markedly different from normal myocardium (sham), biopsies of normal remote, nonischemic segments show similar morphologic changes, indicating that these structural abnormalities are not directly related to ischemia nor are they the cause of regional contractile dysfunction. *LAD,* Left anterior descending artery. (From Canty JM Jr, Fallavollita JA. Hibernating myocardium. *J Nucl Cardiol*. 2005;12[1]:104–119.)

programmed disassembly of contractile elements following repeated episodes of reversible ischemia (see Fig. 19.4B).[89-93] Thus rather than a "protective" mechanism, hibernation represents a disadvantageous process that, left uncorrected, may lead to apoptosis and myocyte loss, replacement fibrosis, graded and reciprocal changes in alpha- and beat-adrenergic receptor density, progressive LVSD, and the risk of ventricular arrhythmias (**Fig. 19.5**). This process may affect a substantial number of HF patients. Among patients with HF, CAD, and LVSD, approximately 50% have evidence of viable but dysfunctional myocardium.[94-96]

Diagnosis

Hibernating myocardium should be suspected in all patients with CAD and chronic LV dysfunction of any degree, regional and global.[96] Up to 50% of patients with CAD and chronic LV dysfunction have significant areas of dysfunctional but viable myocardium.[97] Hibernating myocardium can be determined with the use of imaging techniques that detect myocardial contractile reserve, preserved metabolic activity, or cell membrane integrity within the region of dysfunctional myocardium.[74,98-101] Intact perfusion, cell membrane integrity, and intact mitochondria can be evaluated with single-photon emission tomography using thallium 201–and/or technetium 99m–labeled traces. Preserved glucose metabolism can be assessed by positron emission tomography using F18-fluorodeoxyglucose. Contractile reserve can be unmasked by infusion of low-dose dobutamine during echocardiography. The use of these techniques has been associated with improved survival in patients with chronic HF and significant viability who underwent myocardial revascularization.[98-102]

Cardiac magnetic resonance imaging is also an established technique to assess myocardial viability and the potential for recovery of LV function.[103-105] Resting cine MRI can be used to assess LV end-diastolic wall thickness. An end-diastolic wall thickness less than 5 to 6 mm is a marker of transmural MI and virtually excludes the presence of viable myocardium. In dysfunctional myocardium with preserved end-diastolic wall thickness (6 mm), detection of contractile reserve during low-dose dobutamine infusion confirms the presence of viable myocardium. Gadolinium-based contrast agents have been used to detect nonviable myocardium because these agents accumulate selectively in areas of scar tissue.[103,104] It should be noted that this technique is extremely sensitive in detecting scar tissue (with very high spatial resolution), but the absence of scar tissue does not permit discrimination between normal tissue and hibernating or stunned myocardium.

Clinical Implications

The presence of viable but dysfunctional myocardium can be used to predict a favorable response to myocardial revascularization and pharmacologic therapy.[102,106,107] The restoration of blood flow with revascularization or treatment with agents that improve endothelial function and blood flow, such as statins and beat-blockers, may improve contractility in a hibernating area.[106-109] In contrast, agents such as dobutamine and milrinone, especially at high doses, may precipitate myocardial necrosis and are associated with worse long-term outcomes in patients with CAD and HF.[110-113] Hibernating myocardium is associated with global alterations in LV volume and shape, not just impairment of underperfused segments.[100] This explains why myocardial revascularization of hibernating territories can promote reverse remodeling globally.[114]

However, the clinical importance of routine viability testing remains controversial based on the results of the viability testing in the Surgical Treatment for Ischemic Heart Failure (STICH) trial, described in more detail later.

Endothelial Dysfunction

Available data suggest that the coronary endothelium plays an important role not only in the control of blood flow and vascular patency but also in the physiologic modulation of myocardial structure and function.[115] Thus endothelial dysfunction, an inherent component of the pathophysiology of atherosclerotic CAD, may directly affect ventricular function.[116]

Endothelial Vasodilators

The endothelial release of nitric oxide relaxes vascular smooth muscle cells in association with activation of guanylyl cyclase and increased levels of cyclic glucose monophosphate. NO is the most potent endogenous vasodilator and is responsible for the maintenance of vasovascular tone. NO also inhibits smooth muscle cell proliferation and migration, leukocyte adhesion, and platelet aggregation.[117,118]

Endothelial Vasoconstrictors

The major endothelin-derived vasoconstrictive substances include angiotensin II and endothelin. Angiotensin II is a potent vasoconstrictor that also exerts a variety of effects on vascular structure and function.[119] Studies of angiotensin II indicate the involvement of the renin-angiotensin system in many aspects of vascular homeostasis. Angiotensin II increases the production of plasminogen activator inhibitor type 1, the primary endogenous inhibitor of tissue plasminogen activator, and promotes vascular growth in addition to stimulating the production of other growth factors.[120] Angiotensin II also enhances platelet aggregation, sensitizes the platelets to the effects of direct platelet agonists, and stimulates the production of endothelin.[121] Endothelin is the most potent endogenous vasoconstrictor yet identified and promotes proliferation of smooth muscle cells and secretion of extracellular matrix, which contribute to the formation of atherosclerotic plaque.[122]

Disordered endothelial function in patients with CAD stimulates vasoconstriction, smooth muscle migration and proliferation, increased lipid deposition in the vessel wall, and possibly coronary thrombosis. This promotes myocardial ischemia, which may further contribute directly or indirectly to the progression of LV dysfunction.[116,123-125] The release of endothelin is also increased in failing myocardium.[126] Angiotensin II contributes to the release of endothelin and the excessive degradation of NO.[124] Taken together, these observations make a case for an interplay between the failing myocardium and the coronary endothelium that potentiates the progression of both CAD and LV dysfunction.

Properties of the normal endothelium serve to relax vascular tone and inhibit smooth muscle growth, platelet aggregation, and leukocyte adhesion. Many drugs that reduce mortality and reinfarction in patients with CAD have the potential to improve endothelial function, including lipid-lowering agents, ACE inhibitors, nonselective β-blockers, and aspirin.[127-130] For example, marked reduction of serum cholesterol is associated with a rapid recovery of endothelial function, improvement of myocardial perfusion, and reduction of myocardial ischemia.[131-137] An improvement in tissue perfusion is an important goal in patients with HF in terms of both the peripheral and the coronary circulation.

In summary, endothelial dysfunction may further reduce blood flow, promote progression of coronary atherosclerosis, and have direct negative effects on the myocardial cells and the interstitium.[138,139]

Clinical Manifestations

Reinfarction. Patients with HF and CAD are at increased risk for reinfarction. In clinical trials, the rate of infarction or reinfarction is relatively low, with a fatal MI rate of 3%.[140] However, in one study, more than half of patients with HF and CAD who died suddenly had autopsy evidence of an acute ischemic event (e.g., coronary clot, recent infarct),[40] suggesting that the number of patients with plaque rupture is not accounted for in clinical trials.

Sudden Cardiac Death. The risk of SCD after MI has significantly declined in recent years.[141] However, the occurrence of HF post-MI is associated with a markedly increased risk of SCD.[141] In several clinical HF trials, SCD accounted for 20% to 60% of deaths, depending on the severity of HF.[142] In the Metoprolol CR/XL Randomised Intervention Trial in Congestive Heart Failure (MERIT-HF), 64% of patients in New York Heart Association (NYHA) class II who subsequently died had SCD compared with 59% of patients in class III and 33% of patients

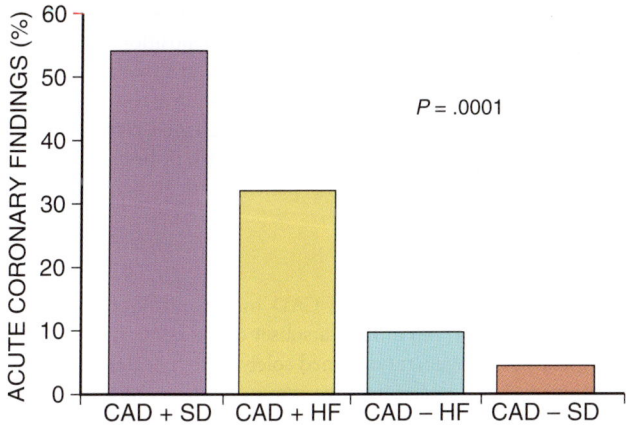

Fig. 19.6 Relation of acute coronary findings to mode of death and presence of coronary artery disease in the Assessment of Treatment with Lisinopril and Survival (ATLAS) trial. Patients with sudden cardiac death had the highest prevalence of acute coronary findings. +, Presence of CAD; –, absence of CAD. *CAD,* Coronary artery disease; *HF,* heart failure; *SD,* standard deviation. (From Uretsky BF, Thygesen K, Armstrong PW, et al. Acute coronary findings at autopsy in heart failure patients with sudden death: results from the assessment of treatment with lisinopril and survival [ATLAS] trial. *Circulation.* 2000;102[6]:611–616.)

in class IV.[143] Several factors have been implicated in the high rate of SCD in patients with HF. These include subendocardial ischemia, ventricular hypertrophy, stretching of myocytes, a high sympathetic tone, abnormal baroreceptor responsiveness lowering the threshold for a malignant arrhythmia, potassium and magnesium depletion, and coronary artery emboli from atrial or LV thrombi.[142] However, CAD probably contributes directly to SCD.[142] Patients with CAD and systolic HF have dilated hearts, large regions of myocardial scar, and obstructive epicardial coronary stenosis. CAD and its major structural consequences (i.e., plaque rupture, thrombosis, and infarction) constitute the most common structural basis of SCD.[144,145]

Uretsky and colleagues reported the relative importance of an acute coronary event as a trigger for SCD in patients with HF who were studied in the ATLAS trial, which included 3164 patients with moderate to severe systolic HF.[40] There were 1383 deaths (43.7%) during the follow-up period of 3 to 5 years. An autopsy was performed in only 188 patients, and the postmortem data were available in only 171 patients (12.4% of the total patients who died). Patients who died in this study were older and had both more symptoms and a higher prevalence of CAD than the surviving patients. The patients who died and did not undergo autopsy were similar to those who died and were subjected to autopsy. Acute coronary findings were observed in 54% of the patients with significant CAD who died suddenly (**Fig. 19.6**). The ATLAS study was the first to demonstrate that recent coronary events are frequently unrecognized in patients with moderate to advanced HF symptoms who die suddenly, especially in patients with CAD.

Other studies have documented a high frequency of plaque rupture or coronary thrombosis in patients with CAD who suffered SCD.[144,146] However, it should be noted that these studies reported a much higher incidence of ruptured plaque, ranging from 57% to 81%, than the ATLAS autopsy study.[40,144,146] However, the prevalence of clinical acute coronary findings in the same series ranged from 21% to 41%, which was similar to the ATLAS study.[40] Because the autopsy findings reported in ATLAS were based on routine clinical examinations, it is unlikely that the examinations involved the degree of detail necessary to observe ruptured plaque and small thrombi. Therefore it is possible that the rate of acute coronary events may have been even higher than reported. This study underlines the importance of strategies to prevent

and treat acute coronary events to successfully prevent SCD in patients with HF. For example, in the ATLAS trial, two-thirds of patients had CAD but only 40% of this group was taking aspirin.[40]

Among patients with HF who receive an ICD for the primary prevention of SCD, those who receive shocks have a markedly increased short-term risk of death compared with those who do not receive shocks. This risk may be much higher in patients with CAD.[147,148] A recent analysis of the Sudden Cardiac Death in Heart Failure Trial (SCD-HeFT) revealed that patients with HF due to CAD who received an appropriate ICD shock had a threefold increased risk of mortality compared with patients with HF and a nonischemic cause who received an appropriate ICD shock. This suggests that among patients with HF, those with CAD can develop fundamental alterations in the underlying arrhythmic substrate that predisposes them to SCD.

CORONARY ARTERY DISEASE AND DIASTOLIC HEART FAILURE (SEE ALSO CHAPTER 39)

The vast majority of HF trials conducted over the past 30 years have studied patients with LVSD. However, HF with relatively preserved systolic function is present in approximately half of all patients hospitalized with HF.[149-156] Among patients with HF and preserved systolic function, approximately 60% have documented CAD.[153] Over the past two decades, the relative proportion of patients with HF and preserved systolic function has risen steadily relative to those with LVSD.[150] Patients with HF and preserved systolic function tend to be older than those with HF and LVSD. Thus the relative rise in this category of HF is reflective of an aging population. This rise has also corresponded to increased rates of CAD, hypertension, diabetes, and atrial fibrillation in this population. Among patients hospitalized with HF, the early and long-term risk of death is similar for patients with preserved systolic function and LVSD.[151,154-156] However, patients with HF and preserved systolic function are more likely to die from other cardiac comorbidities, including CAD, rather than progressive HF when compared with patients with HF and LVSD.[157,158]

When systolic function is preserved, it is assumed that the majority of these patients have HF signs and symptoms on the basis of abnormal LV diastolic function.[159] A variety of factors predispose to abnormalities in diastolic functional behavior of the LV and lead to elevating filling pressures, impaired forward output, or both, despite normal systolic function.[160] Myocardial ischemia is one of the leading factors. Pulmonary congestion can be caused by reversible episodes of ischemia, which impair LV relaxation and increase LV filling pressure.[161]

The prognosis in patients with HF and preserved systolic function in the presence of CAD may be directly related to the angiographic burden of CAD. Data from the Duke experience demonstrated that patients with HF and preserved systolic function have a worse 5-year survival if they have left main or three-vessel CAD versus those with one- to two-vessel CAD.[42] Similarly, according to the Coronary Artery Surgery Study (CASS) registry, the 6-year survival rate of patients with normal ejection fraction and HF symptoms was 92% in patients with no CAD, 83% in patients with one- or two-vessel CAD, and 68% in patients with three-vessel disease.[162]

There is a need for reappraisal on whether systolic function is truly normal at the time when HF symptoms are present in patients diagnosed with HF and "normal" systolic function. The majority of studies of this syndrome did not report the timing of the evaluation demonstrating normal systolic function relative to the episodes of HF itself.[163] In other studies, the evaluation was performed days to weeks after the episode.[164] Transient ischemia may cause regional systolic dysfunction, which in many patients was severe and extensive enough to cause a brief but profound reduction in global LV function.[164] The pathophysiologic changes in regional and global systolic function form the basis for exercise radionuclide ventriculography and exercise echocardiography as diagnostic tests for myocardial ischemia due to CAD. It may be that many patients with apparently normal systolic function and HF caused by CAD do not have isolated diastolic dysfunction but instead have transient systolic and diastolic dysfunction at the time when myocardial ischemia induces HF symptoms.

DIABETES, HEART FAILURE, AND CORONARY ARTERY DISEASE (SEE ALSO CHAPTER 48)

In terms of cardiovascular risk, a diagnosis of diabetes is comparable to a diagnosis of CAD.[165,165] The prevalence of documented CAD in diabetic patients has been shown to be as high as 55%, compared with 2% to 4% for the general population.[167] Diabetic patients with a history of MI have a markedly worse prognosis than individuals with only one of these conditions.[165,166] A significant number of patients with HF have diabetes: 23% in the CONSENSUS (Cooperative North Scandinavian Enalapril Survival Study) trial, 25% in SOLVD (Studies of Left Ventricular Dysfunction), 20% in V-HeFT (Vasodilator Heart Failure Trial), 20% in ATLAS (Assessment of Treatment with Lisinopril and Survival), 27% in RESOLVD (Randomized Evaluation of Left Ventricular Dysfunction), 42% in the OPTIMIZE-HF (Organized Program To Initiate Lifesaving Treatment in Hospitalized Patients With Heart Failure) registry, and 44% in the ADHERE (Acute Decompensated Heart Failure National Registry).[9,11,40,168-171] Diabetes is an independent risk factor for the development of HF.[172-174] In the Framingham Heart Study, the relative risk for developing HF in diabetic patients was 3.8 for men and 5.5 for women, respectively, compared with nondiabetic patients.[174] The risk of developing HF in diabetic patients has been directly related to glycemic control.[175,176] In the United Kingdom Prospective Diabetic Study (UKPDS), for each 1% increase in glycosylated hemoglobin level, the risk of HF rose by 12%.[176]

The presence of diabetes in patients with HF is associated with substantially higher mortality rates.[177-186] Several studies suggest that the increased risk in diabetic patients with HF compared with nondiabetic patients with HF is limited to individuals with concomitant CAD.[183-186] Diabetic patients with CAD also have worse outcomes following myocardial revascularization.[187] Derangements associated with diabetes, including hyperglycemia, insulin resistance, dyslipidemia, inflammation, and thrombosis, contribute to the development of hypertension, endothelial cell dysfunction, accelerated atherogenesis, and coronary thrombosis.[187,188] In addition, diabetic patients exhibit more complex and diffuse anatomic patterns of CAD, including more lipid-rich plaques and intracoronary thrombi but less compensatory vascular remodeling.[187,189-191]

Diabetes directly contributes to HF in patients with LVSD, diastolic dysfunction, or both.[192,193] The increased mortality in patients with HF in the presence of diabetes has been observed in patients with either LVSD or preserved systolic function.[179] Ventricular dysfunction in patients with HF and diabetes has been termed *diabetic cardiomyopathy* and is the result of the complex interplay between the sympathetic nervous system and the renin-angiotensin-aldosterone system (RAAS), increased levels of circulation cytokines, alterations in heart rate variability, and increased oxidative stress.[194] Chronic hyperglycemia leads to the glycation of collagen and elevated serum levels of advanced glycation end products, which results in increased myocardial stiffness.[195] Pathologically, this cardiomyopathy is characterized by myocyte atrophy, interstitial fibrosis, increased periodic acid–Schiff (PAS)-positive material, intramyocardial microangiopathy, and

depletion of myocardial catecholamines.[196] In diabetic patients with HF and LVSD, myocardial fibrosis and the deposition of advanced glycation end products predominate, whereas in those with HF and preserved systolic function, increased cardiomyocyte resting tension is a more important mechanism.[193] There is increased recognition that therapies for diabetes may interact with the risk of both incident HF and the risk of disease progression in patients with known HF (**see also Chapters 17 and 48**).

Therapeutic Options

Recognition that progression of CAD may contribute importantly to progression of HF, in at least a subset of patients, shifts the focus from medical management designed solely to reduce neurohormonal activation and alleviate congestive symptoms to a strategy designed to use aggressive secondary prevention measures. Those efforts to slow the progression of CAD include attention to reducing the risk of acute coronary events by plaque stabilization, reducing ischemia, and enhancing endothelial function. It is noteworthy that the classes of drugs that have shown conclusively to improve survival in HF—ACE inhibitors, angiotensin receptor blockers (ARBs), β-blockers, and aldosterone antagonists (**see also Chapter 37**)—address those factors. The beneficial effects of these drugs may relate as much to their vascular protective effects as to their neurohormonal blocking effects. Patients hospitalized with HF are frequently undertreated for CAD. For example, ACS patients with acute HF are less likely to receive antiplatelet agents, β-blockers, ACE inhibitors, or statins than ACS patients without HF.[42,47,48,155,197] In addition to pharmacologic therapy, myocardial revascularization, surgical therapy, and cardiac device therapy may play an important role in the treatment of patients with HF in the setting of CAD.

Immediate Management of the Hospitalized Patient

The immediate management of acute HF usually occurs in the emergency department (**see also Chapter 36**).[198] There is considerable overlap in the presentation and management of acute HF patients with CAD and ACS versus CAD and non-ACS (see Tables 19.2 and 19.3). In patients with underlying CAD who are not hypotensive, nitrates may provide a rapid reduction of myocardial ischemia and improve coronary perfusion. In patients with severe pulmonary edema, the combination of high-dose nitrates and low-dose diuretics (vs. low-dose nitrates and high-dose diuretics) led to significantly decreased rates of mechanical ventilation and MI.[199] In a large acute HF registry, the use of intravenous nitroglycerin or nesiritide was associated with lower in-hospital mortality compared with treatment with dobutamine or milrinone.[200] However, compared with intravenous nesiritide in acute HF patients, of whom greater than 60% had documented CAD, intravenous nitroglycerin has been associated with less deterioration of renal function and a trend toward less mortality at 30 days.[201-202]

Inotropes may be particularly harmful when used in HF patients with CAD. Experimentally, the use of dobutamine in a model of HF with hibernating myocardium led to increased myocardial necrosis.[203] Hospitalized HF patients with troponin elevation have significantly higher in-hospital mortality when inotropes are used.[51] In the Outcomes of a Prospective Trial of Intravenous Milrinone for Exacerbations of Chronic Heart Failure (OPTIME-CHF) trial, use of the phosphodiesterase inhibitor milrinone in patients with CAD was associated with increased postdischarge mortality compared with a placebo.[112] In general, a decrease in coronary perfusion as a result of a decrease in blood pressure and/or an increase in heart rate resulting from inotropes with vasodilator properties, or inotropes used in conjunction with vasodilators, may be particularly deleterious in HF patients with CAD.[113,204] In a recent series of 112 inotrope-dependent patients with stage D HF patients not eligible for transplantation, there was no difference in the adjusted mortality rate observed between those treated with milrinone and those treated with dobutamine.[205]

Long-Term Therapies for the Heart Failure Patient With Coronary Artery Disease

Renin-angiotensin-aldosterone system modulators. The RAAS regulates sodium balance, fluid volume, and blood pressure, which has a profound impact on HF and CAD (**see also Chapter 5**).[206] The use of ACE inhibitors or ARBs is strongly indicated in HF patients with LVSD and is also indicated for the secondary prevention of cardiovascular events in all patients with CAD.[207-209]

Endothelial dysfunction plays a fundamental role in many forms of cardiovascular disease and is the final common pathway through which most cardiovascular risk factors contribute to inflammation and atherosclerosis. Angiotensin II is a powerful vasoconstrictor and also stimulates smooth muscle cells (hyperplasia), fibroblast proliferation, collagen deposition, inflammation, and thrombosis. All these maladaptations can be mitigated by the use of ACE inhibitors or ARBs.[128,206,210] In the SOLVD and the SAVE (Survival and Ventricular Enlargement) trials, the ACE inhibitors enalapril and captopril not only reduced overall mortality in patients with CAD but also reduced the rate of nonfatal MI and unstable angina.[211,212] In the SAVE trial, a 25% decrease in MI with captopril occurred despite the selection criteria, which excluded patients with residual ischemia who were considered at great risk of reinfarction.[212] The reduction of acute ischemic events would not have been anticipated only on the basis of the hemodynamic or neurohormonal effects of ACE inhibitors. Moreover, in the SOLVD trial, the reduction of unstable angina and MI with enalapril was not evident until more than 6 months after randomization.[211] This suggests that the beneficial effects of enalapril on ischemic events was not due to an immediate effect related to a primary or secondary reduction in LV afterload.

The addition of eplerenone, an aldosterone antagonist, to optimal medical therapy in ACS patients with acute HF and LVSD significantly reduced death and rehospitalization in the Eplerenone Post-Acute Myocardial Infarction Heart Failure Efficacy and Survival Study (EPHESUS) trial (**Fig. 19.7**).[105] The reduction in death corresponded with a decrease in SCD, which may be due to the inhibition of myocardial fibrosis.[213]

β-blockers. β-Blockers are effective for the reduction of death and rehospitalization in patients with HF and CAD.[99] The continuation or predischarge initiation of β-blockers in patients hospitalized with HF is associated with improved medication adherence and an early survival advantage.[214-216] Patients with viable but dysfunctional myocardium derive greater improvement in LV function and remodeling from β-blocker therapy than those without viability.[97,114]

The improvement in survival with β-blockers in the MERIT-HF and CIBIS II (Cardiovascular Insufficiency Bisoprolol Study II) trials was more pronounced in patients with HF and documented CAD than in patients with a presumed nonischemic cause.[142,217] However, improvement in survival was slightly more pronounced in patients with presumed nonischemic HF and mild to moderate HF studied in the US Carvedilol trials and in patients with severe HF patients studied in the Carvedilol Prospective Randomized Cumulative Survival (COPERNICUS) trial.[18,19] These differential effects were minor because the reduction in mortality in each of these four trials was less than 30% and there was a nonsignificant difference in mortality benefit between ischemic and nonischemic patients.[218] In MERIT-HF, mortality was slightly higher in diabetic patients with HF who were treated with metoprolol succinate than in nondiabetic patients with HF, and carvedilol showed similar reductions for

diabetic and nondiabetic patients in both the US Carvedilol trials and COPERNICUS. The benefit of carvedilol in CAD patients was later confirmed in post-MI patients in the Carvedilol Post-Infarct Survival Control in LV Dysfunction (CAPRICORN) study.[219] In this study of 1959 post-MI patients with a left ventricular ejection fraction (LVEF) of 40% or less, the addition of carvedilol to ACE inhibitor therapy led to a 20% relative reduction in all-cause mortality at a mean follow-up of 1.3 years (**Fig. 19.8**).[219] The differences observed with β-blockers in outcomes based on the presence of CAD in HF patients may be due to cause-related differences in pathophysiologic derangements on the β-adrenergic signal transduction pathway.[220] This may also relate to the more severe symptoms of patients enrolled in COPERNICUS, differences in β_1-selectivity versus β_1-nonselectivity, or other pharmacologic differences between β-blocking agents, such as α-blockade, antioxidant effect, and lipophilicity.[221]

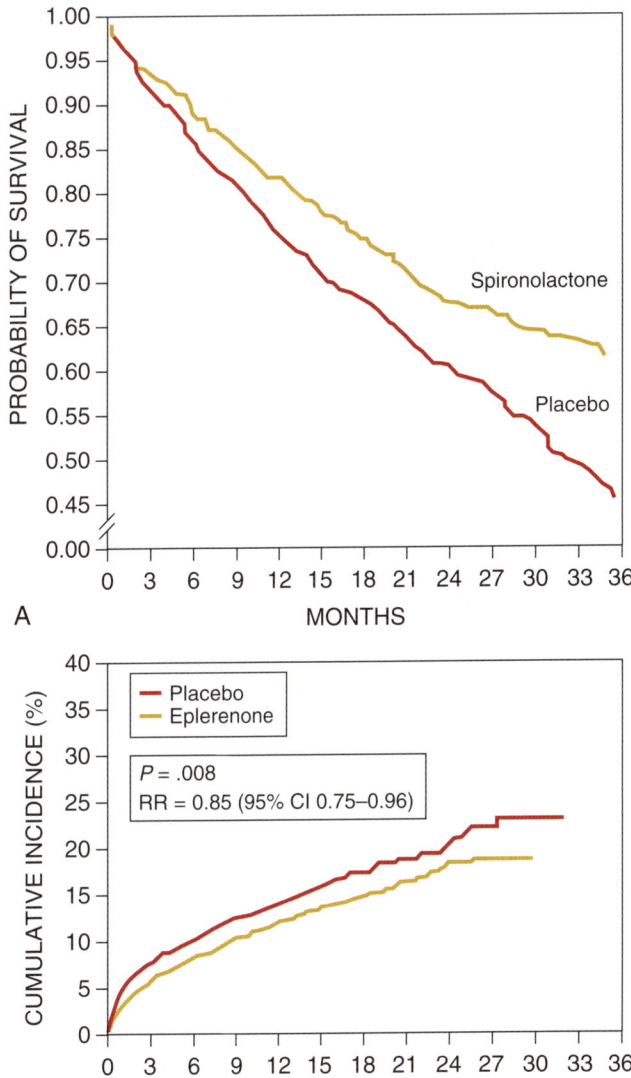

Fig. 19.7 (A and B) Trials testing aldosterone antagonists. *RR,* Relative risk. (Modified from Pitt B, Zannad F, Remme WJ, et al. The effect of spironolactone on morbidity and mortality in patients with severe heart failure. Randomized aldactone evaluation study investigators. *N Engl J Med.* 1999;341[10]:709–717; Pitt B, Remme W, Zannad F, et al. Eplerenone, a selective aldosterone blocker, in patients with left ventricular dysfunction after myocardial infarction. *N Engl J Med.* 2003;348[14]:1309–1321.)

Lipid-lowering agents. Statin therapy is strongly recommended in patients with CAD.[222] The benefits of statins may be caused by plaque stabilization and improvements in endothelial function. The Cholesterol and Recurrent Events (CARE) trial, which demonstrated beneficial effects of pravastatin in patients with mild elevation of serum cholesterol after MI, prospectively randomized a subset of patients with an ejection fraction between 25% and 40%[223]; these patients had similar characteristics to those entered into post-MI ACE inhibitor trials, such as SAVE.[224] Pravastatin significantly decreased cardiac events in this subgroup. Similarly, in the Scandinavian Simvastatin Survival Study (4S), simvastatin decreased the development of HF symptoms after MI; among patients who experienced HF, simvastatin decreased mortality from 32% to 25%.[225] Furthermore, in patients with either stable CAD or ACS, the use of high-dose statin therapy is associated with a decreased risk for HF hospitalization compared with low-dose statin therapy.[226-227]

Dyslipidemia is associated with an increased risk for the development of HF that is independent of its association with MI.[228] This risk has been further linked to individual lipoprotein components, notably the apoB/apoA-1 ratio and triglyceride levels.[229]

In unselected HF patients, the use of statins is associated with lower mortality, including the elderly and patients with preserved systolic function.[230-232] However, the Controlled Rosuvastatin Multinational Trial in Heart Failure (CORONA) showed that rosuvastatin therapy in older patients (60 years or older) with chronic HF and LVSD did not lead to a decrease in all-cause death (**Fig. 19.9A**), although there was a reduction in HF hospitalizations.[233] There was also a trend toward fewer coronary events in the patients treated with rosuvastatin. In the Gruppo Italiano per lo Studio della Sopravvivenza nell'Insufficienza Cardiaca Heart Failure (GISSI-HF) trial, the use of rosuvastatin in patients with chronic HF (mean age 68 years, 90% with LVSD, 40% ischemic cause) did not decrease mortality or cardiovascular hospitalization at 4 years (see Fig. 19.9B).[234] These data suggest that statin

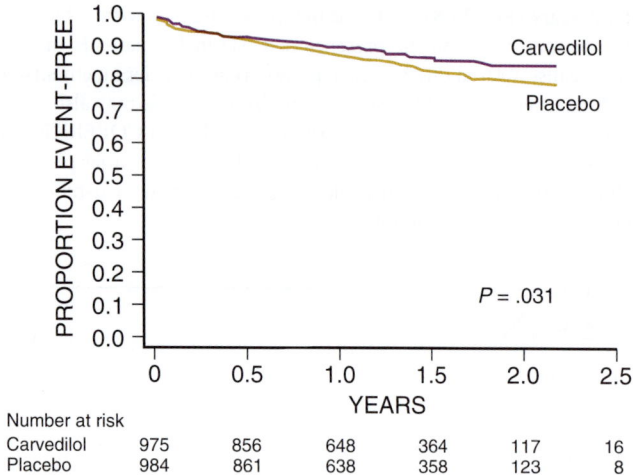

Fig. 19.8 Effect of carvedilol on morbidity and mortality in patient with left ventricular dysfunction after acute myocardial infarction in the CAPRICORN study. (From Dargie HJ. Effect of carvedilol on outcome after myocardial infarction in patients with left ventricular dysfunction: the CAPRICORN randomized trial. *Lancet.* 2001;357[9266]:1385–1390.)

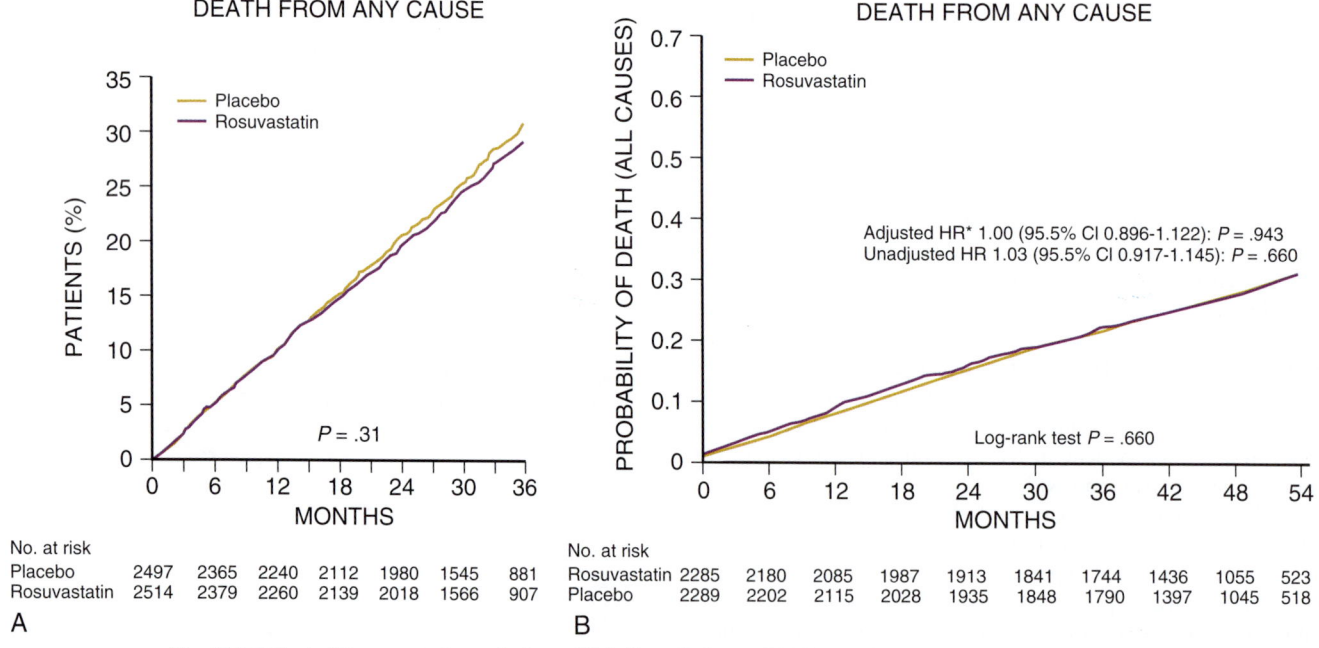

Fig. 19.9 Effect of Rosuvastatin on Patients With Heart Failure. (A) Effects of rosuvastatin on all-cause death in older patients (60 years of age) with chronic HF and LVSD in the CORONA study. (B) Effects of rosuvastatin on all-cause death in patients with chronic HF with depressed and preserved systolic function in the GISSI-HF trial. [a]Estimates were calculated with a Cox proportional hazards model, with adjustments for admission to hospital for heart failure in the previous year, previous pacemaker, sex, diabetes, pathologic Q waves, and angiotensin receptor blockers. *CI,* Confidence interval; *CORONA,* Controlled Rosuvastatin Multinational Trial in Heart Failure; *GISSI-HF,* Gruppo Italiano per lo Studio della Sopravvivenza nell'Insufficienza Cardiaca Heart Failure; *HF,* heart failure; *HR,* heart rate; *LVSD,* left ventricular systolic dysfunction. (Modified from Kjekshus J, Apetrei E, Barrios V, et al. Rosuvastatin in older patients with systolic heart failure. *N Engl J Med.* 2007;357[22]:2248–2261; Tavazzi L, Maggioni AP, Marchioli R, et al. Effect of rosuvastatin in patients with chronic heart failure (the GISSI-HF trial): a randomised, double-blind, placebo-controlled trial. *Lancet.* 2008;372[9645]:1231–1239.)

therapy may be important for the prevention of HF and ischemic events in patients with CAD but may be unable to impact mortality in patients with chronic HF and LVSD.

Fish consumption and dietary supplementation with n-3 polyunsaturated fatty acids (PUFAs) in individuals with and without established CAD is associated with reduced cardiovascular mortality.[173,235,236] In a separate GISSI-HF trial, the use of n-3 PUFA in patients with chronic HF (mean age, 67 years; 90% with LVSD; 50% ischemic cause) led to a 2% absolute risk reduction in mortality (27% vs. 29% at 4 years, P = .041) and a similar reduction in cardiovascular hospitalization.[237] It is suspected that n-3 PUFA may exert their beneficial effect via the reduction of arrhythmic events and not ischemic events. Because the use of ICD therapy in this trial was low (7%), the impact of this therapy on patients with chronic HF and LVSD with appropriate indications for ICD therapy is unclear.

Antiplatelet and anticoagulation therapy.
The use of antiplatelet therapy (i.e., aspirin or clopidogrel) is strongly indicated in the presence of CAD for the secondary prevention of cardiovascular events.[238] Dual antiplatelet therapy, clopidogrel added to aspirin, has been shown to be beneficial in ACS patients for the prevention of recurrent ischemic events and was associated with an 18% reduction in subsequent HF.[239] There is experimental evidence that aspirin inhibits the acute arterial and venous vasodilator response to ACE inhibitors in patients with chronic HF.[240] However, there is no prospective evidence that this potential interaction is clinically relevant. Nevertheless, it may be prudent to limit the combination of aspirin and ACE inhibitor therapy in HF patients to those with established CAD.

LVSD is independently associated with an increased risk of ischemic stroke.[241] The use of oral anticoagulation is strongly indicated in HF patients with atrial fibrillation and patients with confirmed or suspected LV thrombus. However, to date, there is a lack of evidence that the use of oral anticoagulation in HF patients without atrial fibrillation has a beneficial effect on cardiovascular events, including embolic stroke.[242,243]

Myocardial revascularization.
The role of surgical management of HF patients with stable CAD has been an area of uncertainty. The three major randomized clinical trials that have compared coronary artery bypass graft (CABG) surgery with medical management, the Veterans Administration Cooperative Study, the European Coronary Surgery Study, and the CASS, all excluded patients with HF or severe LVSD. Historically, registries and databases have been used to inform decision making for patients with ischemic cardiomyopathy. For example, a report from the Duke database compared CABG surgery versus medical therapy over a 25-year period. Medical therapy was used in 1052 patients and CABG in 339.[72] Unadjusted and adjusted survival (Cox proportional-hazards model) strongly favored CABG after 30 days and at 10 years. This analysis included all groups by extent of CAD and by different subgroups (**Fig. 19.10**). Adjusted overall survival at 1 year, 5 years, and 10 years was 83% versus 74%; 61% versus 37%; and 42% versus 13%, respectively, for CABG versus medical therapy (all P < .0001). Other similar analyses in patients with chronic systolic HF and CAD appear to corroborate a protective effect for CABG.[244]

It has been hypothesized that revascularization may improve outcomes in patients with HF and dysfunctional but viable myocardium. In a meta-analysis of greater than 3000 patients with LVSD, revascularization was associated with markedly decreased yearly mortality (3.2% vs. 16.0%, P < .0001) if viability was present.[102] In patients without hibernating myocardium, revascularization did not improve survival. A different retrospective observational study examined the role of myocardial revascularization in approximately 4000 patients with chronic HF.[245] At 1 year, patients who underwent revascularization had substantially reduced mortality (11.8% vs. 21.6%; hazard ratio [HR], 0.52; 95% confidence interval [CI] 0.47–0.58). The survival curves continued to diverge through 7 years of follow-up.

In 2002 the National Institutes of Health initiated funding for the STICH trial. The STICH trial was a prospective randomized study that enrolled more than 2200 patients at approximately 100 centers.

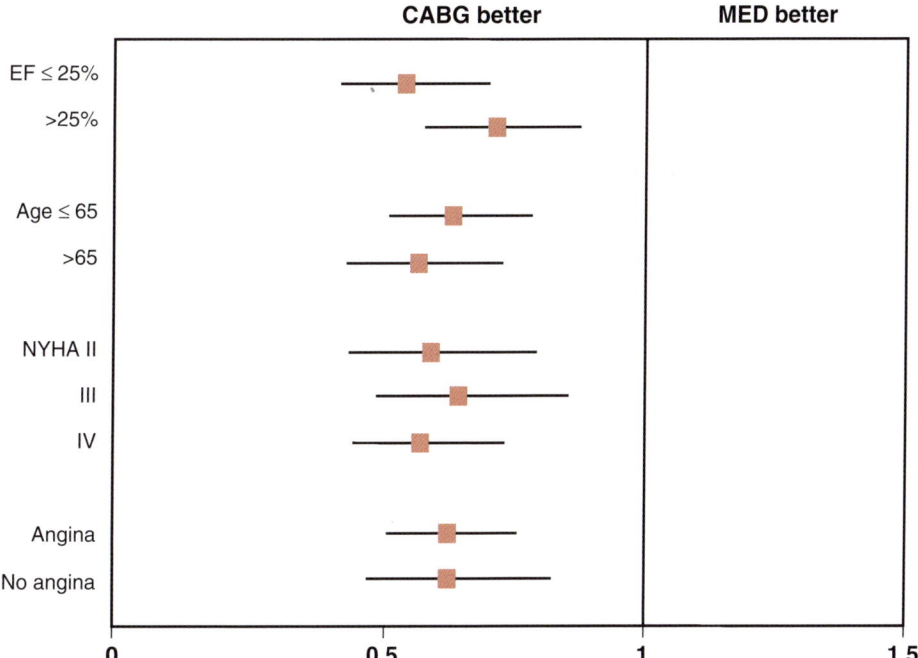

Fig. 19.10 Subgroup analysis of coronary artery revascularization versus medical therapy in patients with heart failure. Hazard ratios (95% confidence interval) for mortality for a number of baseline characteristics all favored CABG. *CABG*, Coronary artery bypass grafting; *EF*, ejection fraction; *MED*, medical therapy; *NYHA*, New York Heart Association. (Modified from O'Connor CM, Velazquez EJ, Gardner LH, et al. Comparison of coronary artery bypass grafting versus medical therapy on long-term outcome in patients with ischemic cardiomyopathy [a 25-year experience from the Duke Cardiovascular Disease Databank]. *Am J Cardiol.* 2002;90[2]:101–107.)

Patients with CAD and LVSD amenable to CABG were randomized to combinations of three different treatment strategies: CABG, surgical ventricular reconstruction (SVR), and intensive medical therapy. The trial was designed to address two primary hypotheses: (1) CABG combined with medical therapy improves long-term survival when compared with medical therapy alone, and (2) SVR provides an additional long-term survival benefit when combined with CABG and medical therapy.

The results of the second arm of the study were published first.[246] One thousand patients were randomized to CABG alone (499) or CABG with SVR (modified Dor procedure) (501). SVR reduced the end-systolic volume index by 19%, as compared with a reduction of 6% with CABG alone. Cardiac symptoms and exercise tolerance improved from baseline to a similar degree in the two study groups. However, there was no significant difference in a composite of death from any cause and hospitalization for cardiac causes, which was the primary outcome of the trial (**Fig. 19.11**). The results from hypothesis 2 of the STICH trial may indicate that a stricter definition of what constitutes an LV aneurysm may need to be applied in future studies of SVR if this procedure is to maintain clinical relevance. Post hoc analyses of the SVR group from STICH suggest a benefit from SVR in patients with smaller preoperative and/or postoperative LV volumes.[247,248] There are also reports of more refined SVR techniques that may achieve better long-term clinical results.[249]

This first arm (hypothesis 1) of the STICH trial randomized 1212 patients with an LVEF of 35% or less and CAD amenable to CABG to medical therapy alone or medical therapy plus CABG. The results of a large subset of patients who underwent myocardial viability testing were reported simultaneously.[250] Overall, there was no survival advantage conferred by CABG over medical therapy alone during the follow-up period in the intention-to-treat analysis (**Fig. 19.12A**). However, in a prespecified analysis, patients who underwent CABG had significantly less death from cardiovascular causes (see **Fig. 19.12B**). This reduction in cardiovascular death after CABG has been attributed to a decrease in SCD and fatal pump failure events.[251] Nine percent of patients were assigned to but did not undergo CABG, whereas 17% of patients assigned to medical therapy alone crossed over to CABG in the follow-up period. In an as-treated analysis, the hazard ratio for patients who either randomized to CABG or who crossed over to CABG during the first year of follow-up was 0.70 (95% CI 0.58–0.84, $P < .001$) compared with those who did not undergo CABG.[252] These initial conclusions from STICH have been reassessed in light of the findings of the extended follow up of the STICH trial, STICHES (discussed more later). The presence of myocardial viability, demonstrated by single-photon emission computed tomography (SPECT) and/or dobutamine echocardiography, in the STICH trial was associated with improved survival. However, this association was not statistically significant after adjustment for other baseline variables (see Fig. 19.12C). Furthermore, there was no significant interaction between the presence of viable myocardium and the assigned treatment with respect to mortality, suggesting a limited role for viability testing in treatment selection. Patients with myocardial viability did have a significantly reduced risk for a composite of death or hospitalization (HF 0.59, 95% CI 0.47–0.74), a relationship that remained significant on multivariate analysis ($P = .003$). Overall, this subgroup had more comorbidities and a lower mean LVEF than patients who did not undergo viability testing, implying that it may not be appropriate to extrapolate the results to the entire study population. Also left unanswered is the role of emerging techniques to assess myocardial viability, in particular delayed-enhancement cardiovascular magnetic resonance (CMR) imaging. CMR may have a more powerful role in defining the burden of myocardial scar, which has recently been shown to be indirectly associated with improvement in contractility after revascularization.[253]

Long-term follow-up of the STICH trial: STICHES. In any treatment comparison of surgical therapy versus medical therapy, interpretation of the results must acknowledge that surgery involves upfront risk (for perioperative morbidity and mortality) in the hopes of longer-term benefits. This logic suggested the need for longer-term follow-up of the STICH trial to better characterize longer-term risks and benefits.[254] In this light, the STICH investigators conducted extended follow-up, out to a median follow-up duration of 9.8 years from randomization. In this extended analysis, the primary end point (death from any cause) occurred in 359 of 610 patients in the CABG group and 398 of 602 in the medical therapy group (HR = 0.82, $P = .02$). Similarly, CABG improved the secondary end points of cardiovascular death (HR = 0.79, $P = .006$) and the composite of death or HF hospitalization (HR = 0.81, $P = .002$) (**Fig. 19.13**). Taken as a whole, these data broadly support the long-term benefits of CABG in appropriate patients who meet the criteria of the STICH study.

STICH largely applies to the outpatient setting because 95% of those who underwent CABG did so on an elective basis. Studies have shown that outcomes in patients with HF in the setting of an ACS are improved by a strategy of early myocardial revascularization.[255] This includes patients with and without ST-segment elevation and those in cardiogenic shock.[256] Despite this, patients with ACS complicated by HF are less likely to undergo revascularization than ACS patients without HF.[6,255] Non-ACS patients hospitalized with acute HF have improved early survival if they have a history of myocardial revascularization, although this a retrospective finding.[49,53] This relationship has been observed in acute HF patients with LVSD or preserved systolic function. These data generate the hypothesis that early revascularization will be beneficial in acute HF patients with ischemia due to CAD. A management strategy for the acute HF failure based on the presence, extent, and severity of CAD could help identify appropriate candidates for optimal medical therapy for CAD and, when indicated, myocardial revascularization (**Fig. 19.14**). The performance of in-hospital angiography in patients with acute HF and CAD is associated with an increased use of aspirin, statins, β-blockers, ACE inhibitors, and myocardial revascularization and improved postdischarge outcomes.[257]

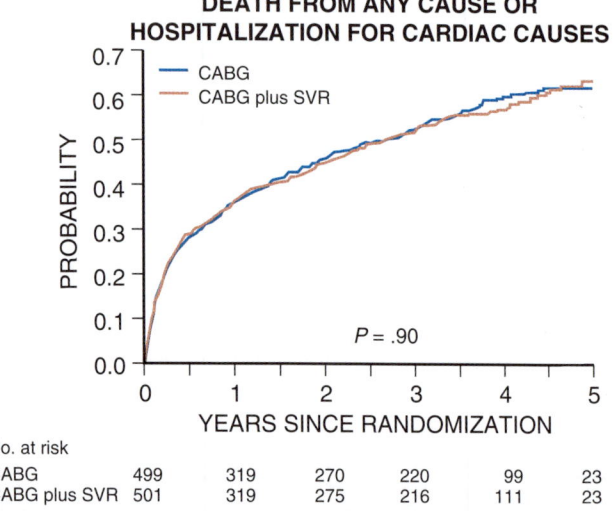

DEATH FROM ANY CAUSE OR HOSPITALIZATION FOR CARDIAC CAUSES

— CABG
— CABG plus SVR

$P = .90$

YEARS SINCE RANDOMIZATION

No. at risk

CABG	499	319	270	220	99	23
CABG plus SVR	501	319	275	216	111	23

Fig. 19.11 Effect of coronary artery bypass surgery with or without surgical ventricular reconstruction on all-cause death and hospitalization for cardiac causes in the Surgical Treatment for Ischemic Heart Failure trial. *CABG*, Coronary artery bypass graft; *SVR*, surgical ventricular reconstruction. (Modified from Jones RH, Velazquez EJ, Michler RE, et al. Coronary bypass surgery with or without surgical ventricular reconstruction. *N Engl J Med.* 2009;360[17]:1705–1717.)

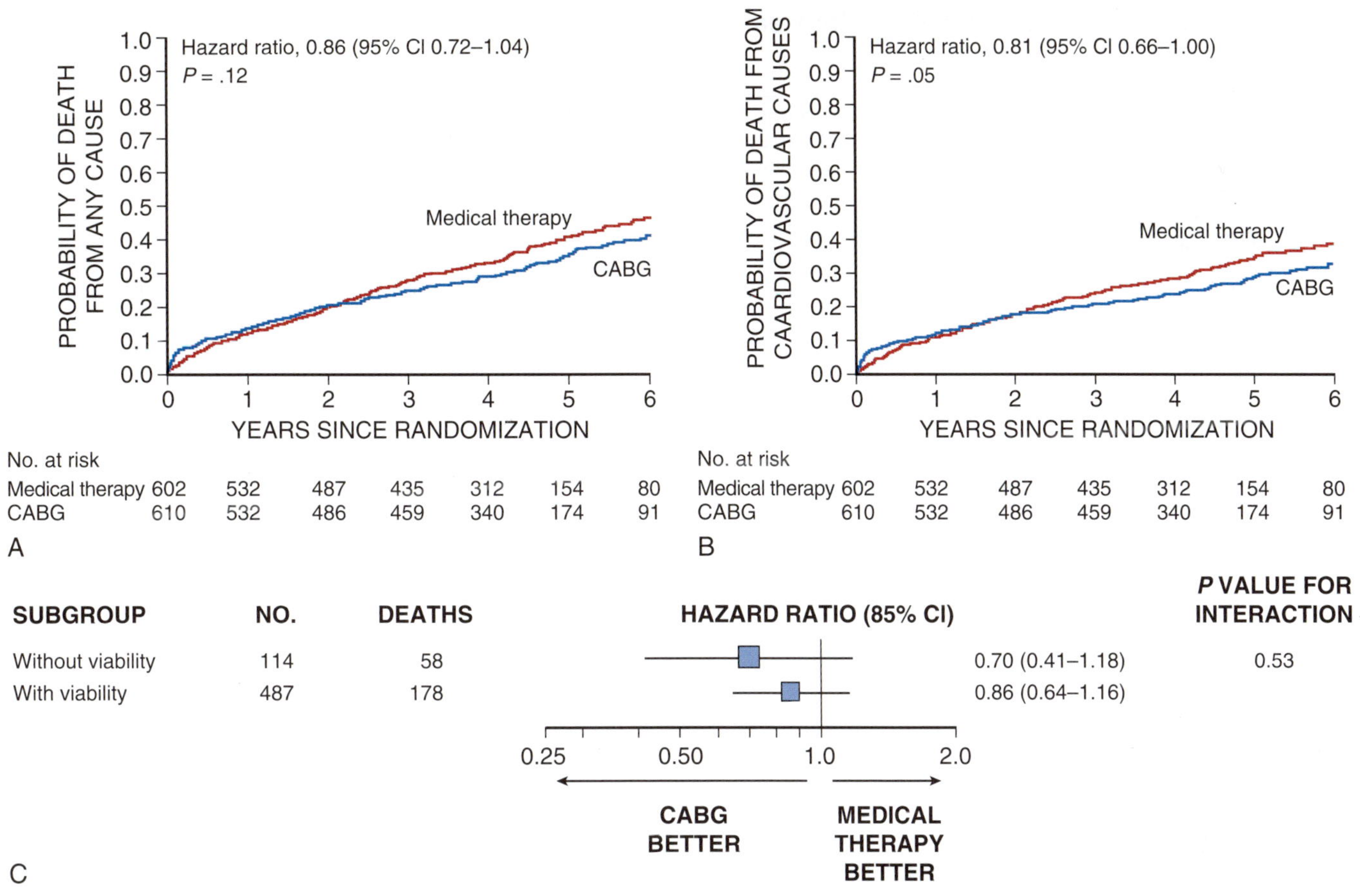

Hazard ratio, 0.86 (95% CI 0.72–1.04)
P = .12
PROBABILITY OF DEATH FROM ANY CAUSE
1.0
0.9
0.8
0.7
0.6
0.5
0.4
0.3
0.2
0.1
0.0
Medical therapy
CABG
0 1 2 3 4 5 6
YEARS SINCE RANDOMIZATION
No. at risk
Medical therapy 602 532 487 435 312 154 80
CABG 610 532 486 459 340 174 91
A
Hazard ratio, 0.81 (95% CI 0.66–1.00)
P = .05
PROBABILITY OF DEATH FROM CAARDIOVASCULAR CAUSES
1.0
0.9
0.8
0.7
0.6
0.5
0.4
0.3
0.2
0.1
0.0
Medical therapy
CABG
0 1 2 3 4 5 6
YEARS SINCE RANDOMIZATION
No. at risk
Medical therapy 602 532 487 435 312 154 80
CABG 610 532 486 459 340 174 91
B
SUBGROUP
NO.
DEATHS
HAZARD RATIO (85% CI)
P VALUE FOR INTERACTION
Without viability 114 58 0.70 (0.41–1.18) 0.53
With viability 487 178 0.86 (0.64–1.16)
0.25
0.50
1.0
2.0
CABG BETTER
MEDICAL THERAPY BETTER
C

Fig. 19.12 Influence of coronary artery bypass graft *(CABG)* on mortality compared with medical therapy alone in the surgical treatment for ischemic heart failure (STICH) trial. (A) Per the intention-to-treat analysis, there was not a significant impact of CABG on mortality. (B) CABG was associated with a decreased risk of death from cardiovascular causes. (C) After control for baseline variables, there was no significant interaction between viability status and treatment assignment with respect to mortality. (Modified from Velazquez EJ, Lee KL, Deja MA, et al for the STICH Investigators. Coronary artery bypass surgery in patients with left ventricular dysfunction. *N Engl J Med*. 2011;1364[17]:1601–1616; Bonow RO, Maurer G, Lee KL, et al. for the STICH Investigators. Myocardial viability and survival in ischemic left ventricular dysfunction. *N Engl J Med*. 2011;364[17]:1617–1625.)

100%
90%
80%
70%
60%
50%
40%
30%
20%
10%
0%
All cause death
CV death
Death or CV hosp
Death or HF hosp
Death or any hosp
Death or revasc
Death or nonfatal MI
Death or nonfatal stroke
CABG
Medical

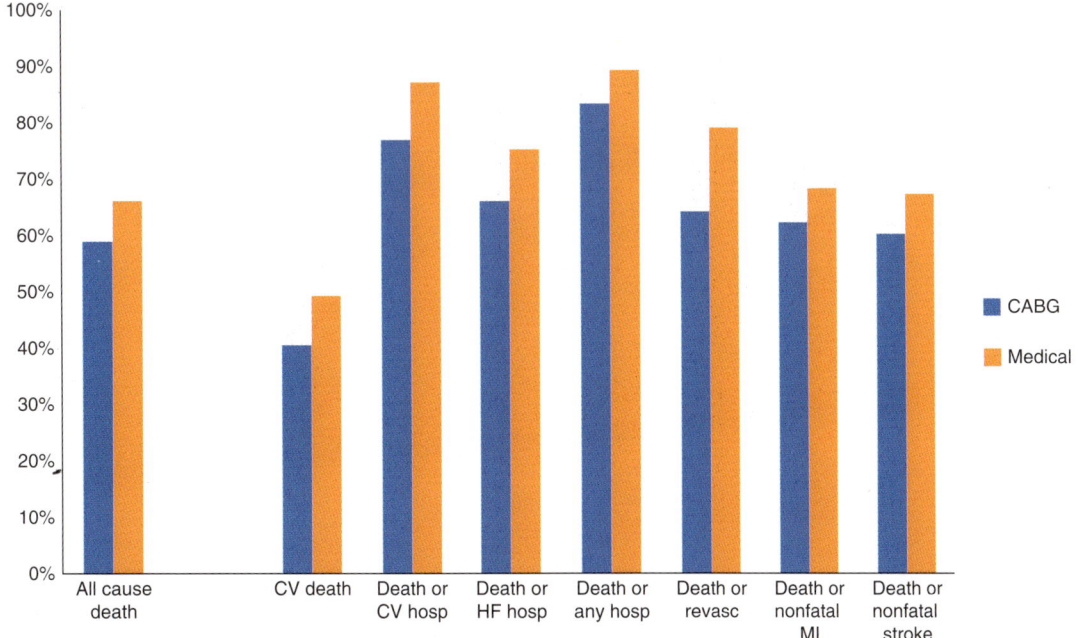

Fig. 19.13 Primary and secondary endpoints from long term follow up of the STICH study. *CABG*, Coronary artery bypass surgery; *CV*, cardiovascular; *HF*, heart failure, *MI*, myocardial infarction. (Data from Velazquez EJ, Lee KL, Jones RH, et al. Coronary-artery bypass surgery in patients with ischemic cardiomyopathy. *N Engl J Med*. 2016;374:1511–1520.)

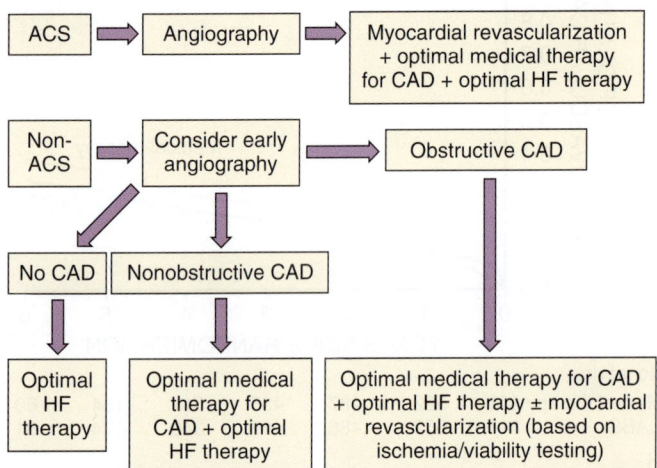

Fig. 19.14 A proposed algorithm for the management of acute heart failure patients on the basis of presence, extent, and severity of CAD. [a]For those patients with remote or no history of coronary angiography. *ACS*, Acute coronary syndrome; *CAD*, coronary artery disease; *HF*, heart failure. (From Flaherty JD, Bax JJ, De Luca L, et al. Acute heart failure syndromes in patients with coronary artery disease early assessment and treatment. *J Am Coll Cardiol.* 2009;53[3]:254–263.)

CONCLUSIONS

The progression of LV dysfunction, worsening of HF, and death in many patients with CAD may be related to the progressive nature of CAD, in addition to the neurohormonal mechanisms that exacerbate myocardial dysfunction. This progression does not require a discrete coronary event such as an acute MI. Myocardial ischemia or hibernation (or both) may contribute to symptoms of HF. In addition, myocardial hibernation appears to be an unstable process that may progress with time to myocyte loss, apoptosis, and replacement fibrosis, leading to more LV dysfunction. As previously noted, endothelial dysfunction may also lead to progression of myocardial dysfunction. Measures specifically target reduction in the risk of subacute ischemic events and improvement in outcomes.

KEY REFERENCES

37. Felker GM, Shaw LK, O'Connor CM. A standardized definition of ischemic cardiomyopathy for use in clinical research. *Circulation.* 2002;39:210–218.
40. Uretsky BF, Thygesen K, Armstrong PW, et al. Acute coronary findings at autopsy in heart failure patients with sudden death: results from the assessment of treatment with lisinopril and survival (ATLAS) trial. *Circulation.* 2000;102:611–616.
45. Thygesen K, Alpert JS, Jaffe AS, et al. Fourth universal definition of myocardial infarction (2018). *J Am Coll Cardiol.* 2018. [in press].
70. Sutton St John, Sharpe N. Left ventricular remodeling after myocardial infarction: pathophysiology and therapy. *Circulation.* 2000;101:2981–2988.
72. O'Connor CM, Velazquez EJ, Gardner LH, et al. Comparison of coronary artery bypass grafting versus medical therapy on long-term outcome in patients with ischemic cardiomyopathy (a 25-year experience from the Duke cardiovascular disease databank). *Am J Cardiol.* 2002;90:101–107.
75. Pitt B, Remme W, Zannad F, et al. Eplerenone, a selective aldosterone blocker, in patients with left ventricular dysfunction after myocardial infarction. *N Engl J Med.* 2003;348:1309–1321.
187. Flaherty JD, Davidson CJ. Diabetes and coronary revascularization. *JAMA.* 2005;293:1501–1508.
250. Bonow RO, Maurer G, Lee KL, et al. STICH Trial Investigators: myocardial viability and survival in ischemic left ventricular dysfunction. *N Engl J Med.* 2011;364:1617–1625.
252. Velazquez EJ, Lee KL, Deja MA, et al. Coronary-artery bypass surgery in patients with left ventricular dysfunction. *N Engl J Med.* 2011;364:1607–1616.
254. Velazquez EJ, Lee KL, Jones RH, et al. Coronary-artery bypass surgery in patients with ischemic cardiomyopathy. *New Engl J Med.* 2016;374:1511–1520.

The full reference list for this chapter is available on ExpertConsult.

Heart Failure as a Consequence of Dilated Cardiomyopathy

Biykem Bozkurt

OUTLINE

DEFINITION

The term *dilated cardiomyopathy* (DCM) refers to a spectrum of heterogeneous myocardial disorders (**Table 20.1**) that are characterized by ventricular dilation and depressed myocardial contractility in the absence of abnormal loading conditions (such as hypertension or valvular disease) or ischemic heart disease sufficient to cause global systolic impairment.[1] Such a definition with emphasis on anatomic description has been challenging, as there could be heterogeneity of expression of the same disease with different phenotypes, or a phenotype may progress from one to another during clinical course (e.g., hypertrophic or infiltrative cardiomyopathies may progress to a dilated form).[2] Although DCM is recognized as a final common pathway for a myriad of cardiac disorders that either damage the heart muscle or, alternatively, disrupt the ability of the myocardium to generate force and subsequently cause chamber dilation, this anatomical characterization fails to emphasize etiology. From a pathologic standpoint, the term DCM is traditionally used to designate an idiopathic or unknown process, but the morphological categorization should not undermine the necessity of search for an etiology and a specific diagnosis. It is likely that the term "dilated cardiomyopathy" will gradually be replaced with specific diagnoses underlining the etiology.

Recent proposed classifications, such as MOGE(S), describe (**Fig. 20.1**) the morphofunctional phenotype (M), organ involvement (O), genetic inheritance pattern (G), etiological annotation (E) including genetic defect or underlying disease/substrate, and the functional status (S) of the disease using both the American College of Cardiology/American Heart Association stage and New York Heart Association (NYHA) functional class. This approach does not dichotomize the classification as dilated versus hypertrophic cardiomyopathies; recognizes the flexibility of potential transitions between morphofunctional types; defines involvement of different cardiac structures and extra cardiac organs; emphasizes etiology such as genetic causes, progression of symptomatology, and functional status; and provides more precision for diagnosis and prognosis.[3]

In clinical practice and multicenter trials, heart failure has often been categorized into ischemic and nonischemic cardiomyopathy, and the term DCM has been interchangeably used with nonischemic cardiomyopathy. Though this approach may be practical, it is overly simplistic and fails to recognize that the term "nonischemic cardiomyopathy" may include cardiomyopathies due to volume or pressure overload—such as hypertension or valvular heart disease—that are not conventionally accepted under the definition of DCM, and also fails to recognize specific etiologies of DCM.

TABLE 20.1 Etiologies of Dilated Cardiomyopathy

Idiopathic
  Idiopathic dilated cardiomyopathy
Familial (hereditary)
  Autosomal dominant
  X-chromosomal
  Polymorphism
  Other
Toxic
  Ethanol
  Cocaine and other cardiotoxic illicit drugs
  Adriamycin, trastuzumab, and other cardiotoxic chemotherapy
  Catecholamine excess
  Phenothiazines, antidepressants
  Cobalt
  Carbon monoxide
  Lead
  Lithium
  Cyclophosphamide
  Amphetamine
  Pseudoephedrine/ephedrine
Inflammatory: Infectious etiology
  Viral (coxsackie virus, parvovirus, adenovirus, echovirus, influenza virus, HIV)
  Spirochete (leptospirosis, syphilis)
  Protozoal (Chagas disease, toxoplasmosis, trichinosis)
Inflammatory: Noninfectious etiology
  Collagen vascular disease (scleroderma, lupus erythematosus, dermatomyositis, rheumatoid arthritis, sarcoidosis)
  Kawasaki
  Hypersensitivity myocarditis
Miscellaneous acquired cardiomyopathy
  Postpartum cardiomyopathy
  Obesity
Metabolic/nutritional
  Thiamine
  Kwashiorkor Pellagra
  Scurvy
  Selenium deficiency
  Carnitine deficiency
Endocrine
  Diabetes mellitus
  Acromegaly
  Thyrotoxicosis
  Myxedema
  Uremia
  Cushing disease
  Pheochromocytoma
Electrolyte imbalance
  Hypophosphatemia
  Hypocalcemia
Physiologic agents
  Tachycardia
  Heat stroke
  Hypothermia
  Radiation
Autoimmune disorders
Infiltrative cardiomyopathies (DCM usually after progression from restrictive cardiomyopathy, in end-stage)
  Cardiac amyloidosis
  Hemochromatosis
Stress/catecholamine induced cardiomyopathy

DCM, Dilated cardiomyopathy; *HIV,* human immunodeficiency virus.

EPIDEMIOLOGY OF DILATED CARDIOMYOPATHY

Due to challenges and changes in approaches to definition and diagnosis, geographical, environmental, and genetic variation, the reported incidence of DCM varies in publications. In Western populations, the annual incidence of DCM is about 5 to 8 cases per 100,000 of the population.[2,4] The prevalence is considerably higher in underdeveloped and tropical countries due to various infectious and environmental factors.[5] As populations go through epidemiological, socioeconomic transitions, health care modifications, and changes in exposure to cardiotoxic agents, the prevalence of DCM will continue to change. Changes in patterns of drug and substance abuse, development of chemotherapy and biological agents with cardiotoxicity, the development of obesity, new metabolic and dietary trends globally, and the success in treatment of protozoal diseases in Latin America will continue to play a dynamic role in the epidemiology of DCM. The true incidence may be underestimated also due to underreporting or underdetection of asymptomatic cases of DCM.

In most multicenter, randomized trials in heart failure, approximately 30% to 40% of the enrolled patients have nonischemic DCM. According to the Acute Decompensated Heart Failure National Registry (ADHERE), 47% of the patients admitted to the hospital with heart failure have nonischemic cardiomyopathy, but the true incidence of DCM is unknown.[6]

Compared with whites, blacks have almost a threefold increase in risk for developing DCM, not explained solely by differences in hypertension, cigarette smoking, alcohol use, or socioeconomic factors.[7] Moreover, the risk of mortality is almost twofold higher among blacks compared with age-matched whites with DCM. While the reasons for these differences are not exactly known, potential explanations include differences in genetic predisposition, etiology, risk factors, comorbidities, lack of access to medical care, and differences in response to therapy.

Epidemiological data suggesting sex-related differences in the occurrence and prognosis of DCM are conflicting and confounded by differing etiologies and underrepresentation of women in clinical trials, though the "true" incidence of DCM in women independent of hypertension is not well known. In some studies, women with idiopathic DCM had more advanced heart failure (HF) and a trend toward worse survival compared with men.[8]

NATURAL HISTORY OF DILATED CARDIOMYOPATHY

DCM represents a heterogeneous spectrum of myocardial disorders that may each progress at different rates.[9] Furthermore, diagnosis may be delayed as the onset may be insidious, particularly in the case of familial and/or idiopathic dilated cardiomyopathies. Approximately 4% to 13% of the patients with DCM will present with asymptomatic left ventricular dysfunction and left ventricular dilatation. Once symptomatic, prognosis is relatively poor, with 25% mortality at 1 year and 50% mortality at 5 years (**Fig. 20.2**).[10] The cause of death appears to be primarily pump failure in approximately 70%, whereas sudden cardiac death accounts for approximately 30% of all deaths. The existing clinical studies suggest that patients with idiopathic DCM have a lower total mortality than ischemic cardiomyopathy.[11] The absence of a rigorous definition of DCM in many studies may account for this discrepancy and make interpretation of the results difficult. Further studies targeting specific etiologies of heart failure could be particularly important to achieve benefit above and beyond conventional treatment strategies that target heart failure as a single disease entity.

Since addition of guideline directed therapies, prognosis may be more favorable, perhaps reflecting earlier diagnosis and better treatment.[12] Approximately 25% of DCM patients with the recent onset of symptoms of heart failure will improve spontaneously.[13]

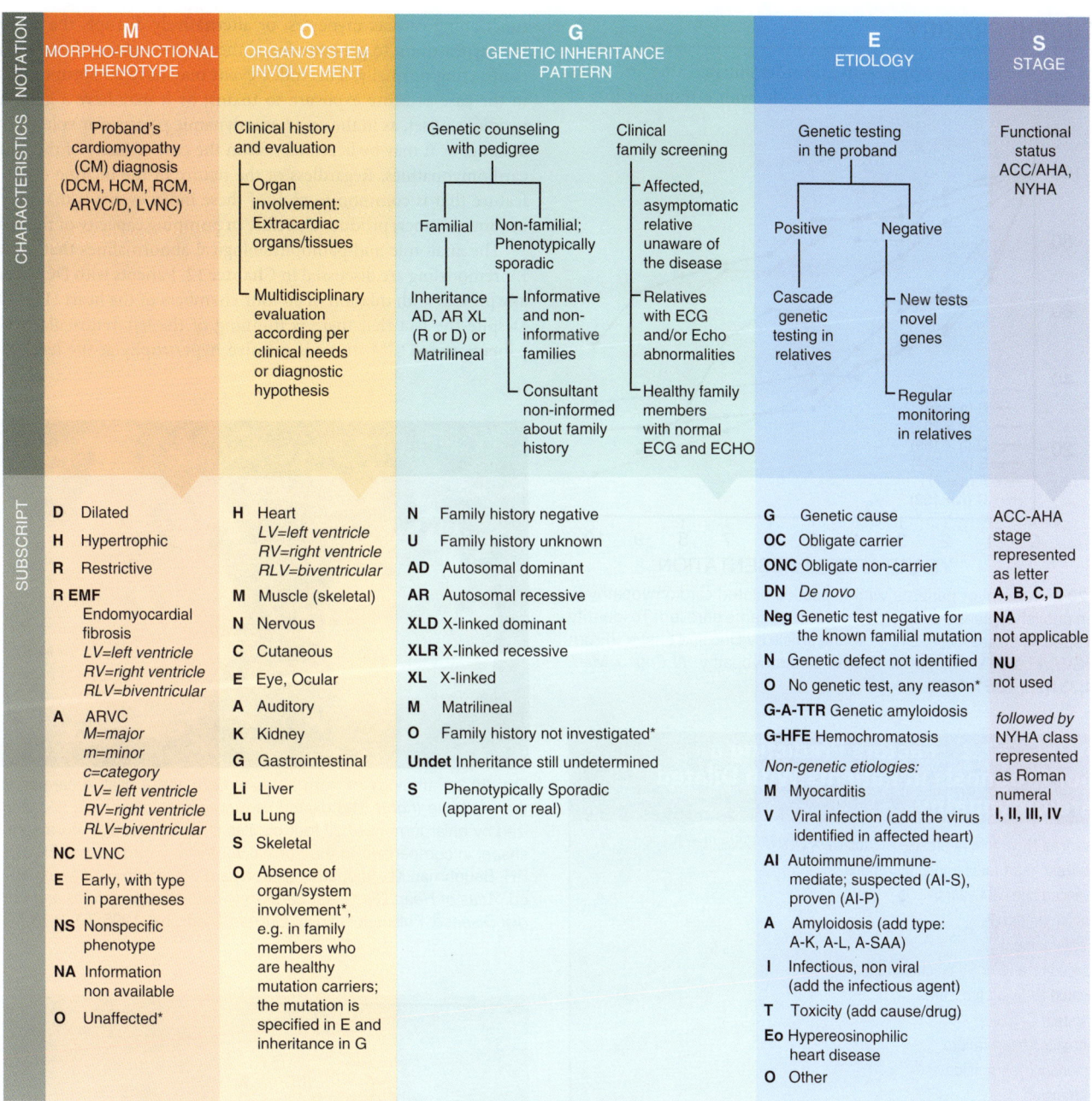

Fig. 20.1 Classification of cardiomyopathy according to MOGE(S) nosology. M, Morphofunctional phenotype; O, organ involvement; G, genetic inheritance pattern; E, etiology. (Annotation provides the description of the specific disease gene and mutation, as well as a description of nongenetic etiology). S, symptoms and functional status according to ACC/AHA staging and NYHA Class. A color code assigned to each variant can provide information about the potential role of the identified variant: affects function or probably affects function (red); variant of unknown significance (VUS) (yellow); and probably does not affect function (or probably no functional effect) or does not affect function (no functional effect) (green). DCM, Dilated cardiomyopathy. (From Arbustini E, Narula N, Tavazzi L, et al. The MOGE[S] classification of cardiomyopathy for clinicians. *J Am Coll Cardiol.* 2014;64[3]:304–318.)

This statement notwithstanding, patients with longer duration of symptoms and/or with severe clinical decompensation and advanced disease generally have less chance of recovery.[13]

As shown in **Table 20.2**, there are a number of other parameters that predict a poor prognosis in patients with DCM, including biventricular enlargement, reduced left and right ventricular ejection fraction, persistent S_3 gallop, right-sided heart failure, elevated left ventricular (LV) filling pressures, moderate to severe mitral regurgitation, pulmonary hypertension, ECG findings of left bundle branch block, recurrent ventricular tachycardia, renal and hepatic dysfunction, elevated levels of natriuretic peptides, persistently elevated cardiac troponin levels, peak oxygen consumption less than 10 to 12 mL/kg/min, serum sodium less than 137 mmol/L, advanced NYHA class, and age over 64 years.

PATHOPHYSIOLOGY

DCM may be viewed as a progressive disorder initiated after an "index event" that either damages the heart muscle, with a resultant loss of

functioning cardiac myocytes, or alternatively disrupts the ability of the myocardium to generate force, thereby preventing the heart from contracting normally. This index event may have an abrupt onset, as in the case of acute exposure to toxins; or it may have a gradual or insidious onset, as in the case hemodynamic pressure or volume overloading; or it may be hereditary, as in the case of many of the familial cardiomyopathies. Regardless of the nature of the inciting event, the feature that is common to each of these index events is that they all, in some manner, produce a decline in pumping capacity of the heart.

The anatomic and pathophysiological abnormalities that occur in LV remodeling are discussed in **Chapter 12**. Patients with DCM generally present with dilation of all four chambers of the heart (**Fig. 20.3**). Despite the fact that there is thinning of the left ventricular wall in patients with DCM, there is massive hypertrophy at the level of the

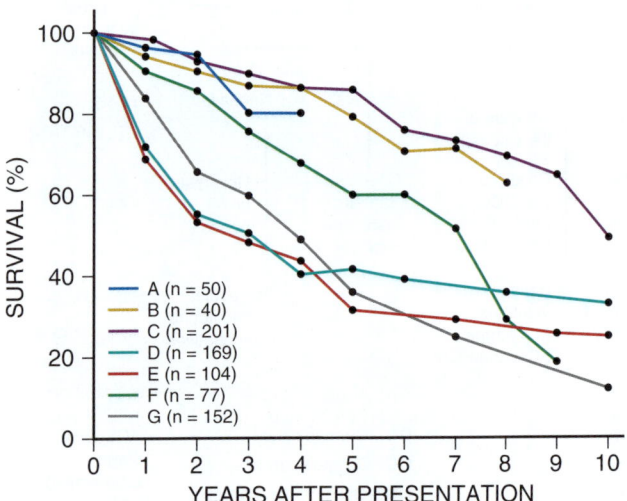

Fig. 20.2 Survival of patients with idiopathic dilated cardiomyopathy in seven published series (A–G). *n*, number of patients enrolled. To identify each specific series, please refer to the article by Dec and Fuster. (From Dec GW, Fuster V. Idiopathic dilated cardiomyopathy. *N Engl J Med.* 1994;331[23]:1564–1575.)

TABLE 20.2 Factors Predicting a Poor Prognosis in Patients With Dilated Cardiomyopathy

Advanced New York Heart Association class (NYHA Class III or IV)
Recurrent heart failure hospitalizations
Advanced age (>64 years)
LV enlargement
RV enlargement
Reduced LV and/or RV ejection fraction
Elevated LV filling pressures
Persistent S_3 gallop
Right-sided heart failure
Pulmonary hypertension
Hypotension
Moderate-severe mitral regurgitation
ECG findings of LBBB, persistent tachycardia, wide QRS
Recurrent ventricular tachycardia
Reduced heart rate variability
Late potentials of QRS in signal average ECG
Myocytolysis on endomyocardial biopsy
Elevated levels of natriuretic peptides (NT-proBNP or BNP)
Elevated levels of proinflammatory cytokines and other inflammatory biomarkers
Elevated cardiac injury markers; serum cardiac troponin T, troponin I levels
Peak oxygen consumption <10–12 mL/kg/min
Reduced contractile response
Serum sodium <137 mmol/L
Impaired kidney function (elevated creatinine, reduced EGFR)
Impaired liver function (elevated transaminases, elevated bilirubin)

BNP, Brain natriuretic peptide; *ECG,* electrocardiogram; *EGFR,* estimated glomerular filtraiton rate; *LBBB,* left bundle branch block; *LV,* left ventricular; *NT-proBNP,* N-terminal pro-brain natriuretic peptide; *RV,* right ventricular.

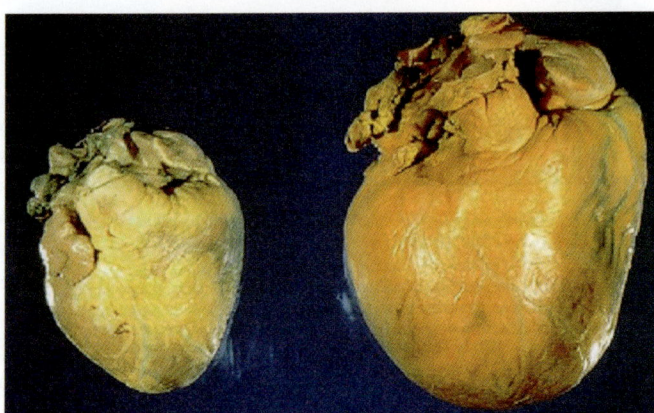

Fig. 20.3 Pathology of normal heart *(left)* and a dilated cardiomyopathic ventricle *(right)*. The dilated cardiomyopathic ventricle is characterized by enlargement of all four cardiac chambers, and a more spherical shape, in comparison to the normal ventricle. (From Kasper EK, Hruban RH, Baughman KL. Idiopathic dilated cardiomyopathy. In: Abelman WH, ed. *Atlas of Heart Diseases: Cardiomyopathies, Myocarditis and Pericardial Disease*. Philadelphia, PA: Current Medicine; 1995:3.1–3.18.)

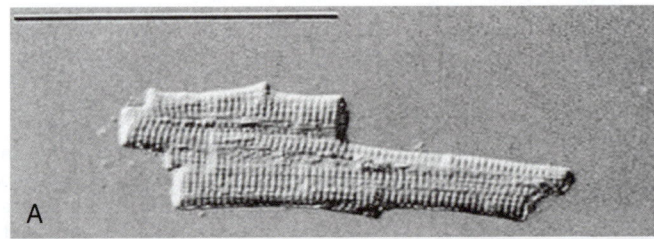
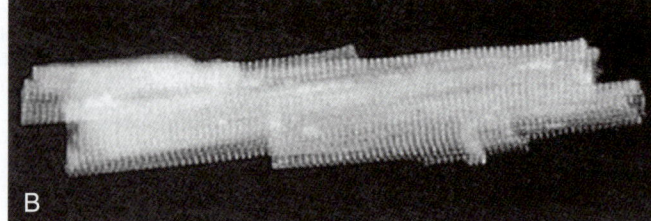

Fig. 20.4 Cardiac myocyte structure *(A)* in normal myocardium and in dilated cardiomyopathy *(B)*. Cardiac myocytes isolated from myocardium from patients with dilated cardiomyopathy have an elongated shaped as the result of the sarcomeres being formed in series. (From Gerdes AM, Kellerman SE, Moore JA, et al. Structural remodelling of cardiac myocytes in patients with ischemic cardiomyopathy. *Circulation.* 1992;86[2]:426–430.)

intact heart, as well as at the level of the cardiac myocyte, which has a characteristic elongated appearance that is observed in myocytes obtained from hearts subjected to chronic volume overload (**Fig. 20.4**). The coronary arteries are usually normal in DCM, although it should be emphasized the end-stage "ischemic cardiomyopathies" (**see also Chapter 19**) may also present with a dilated phenotype. The cardiac valves are anatomically normal; however, there is usually left ventricular dilation, global hypokinesis (**Fig. 20.5**), tricuspid and mitral annular dilatation due to cavity enlargement, distortion of subvalvular apparatus, and stretching of the papillary muscles giving rise to valvular regurgitation. Intracavitary thrombi are common usually in the ventricular apex (**Fig. 20.6**).

DIAGNOSTIC STRATEGIES IN DILATED CARDIOMYOPATHY

Patients with DCM should undergo appropriate diagnostic evaluation for specific etiology with an aim toward individualized and targeted management strategies according to etiology. A common diagnostic and management approach for patients with heart failure with reduced ejection fraction (HFrEF) may be appropriate for most, but further

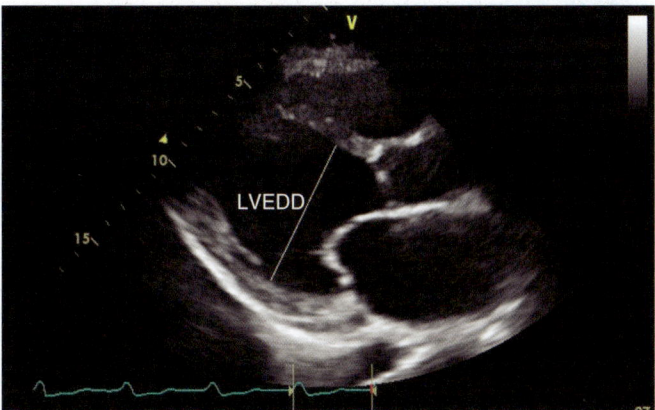

Fig. 20.5 Left ventricular dilatation in dilated cardiomyopathy by transthoracic echocardiography. In this parasternal long-axis image, the LV dimension is measured at the level of the mitral leaflet tips *(white line)*. The LV is severely dilated in this example with a dimension of 7 cm. (Image courtesy Harris Health System, Houston, TX.)

diagnostic and treatment strategies should target specific etiologies in patients with DCM. A diagnostic algorithm approach for evaluation of a patient with DCM is summarized in **Fig. 20.7**.

GENERAL MANAGEMENT STRATEGIES OF DILATED CARDIOMYOPATHY

Patients with DCM should be treated according to guideline-directed management and treatment (GDMT) strategies for patients with HFrEF, as most treatment strategies for HFrEF are appropriate for patients with DCM (**see Chapter 37**).[14,15] In addition, however, when a specific treatment strategy is available or preferred for a specific etiology, that specific management strategy should be considered first, and/or in addition to GDMT for HFrEF.[2]

In most large-scale clinical trials in HFrEF, DCM has not been captured as a specific etiology, and subgroups for etiology have been usually divided into two general groups: ischemic or nonischemic. The differential treatment benefit seen in nonischemic patients compared with patients with ischemic cardiomyopathy that has been observed in several earlier randomized clinical trials such as with digoxin[16] or amiodarone[17] suggested that there may be therapeutic differences between ischemic and nonischemic heart failure. Contrarily, earlier reports of survival benefit with β-blockers[18] or amlodipine[19] in patients with nonischemic but not ischemic cardiomyopathy have not been reproduced in subsequent large-scale randomized trials, in which the benefit was similar in both the ischemic and nonischemic heart failure patients. Currently, it is accepted that guideline-directed medical and device therapies, including implantable cardioverter defibrillator (ICD) and cardiac resynchronization therapy (CRT) for HF, are beneficial in both in ischemic and nonischemic HF patients, including DCM. Thus it is appropriate to achieve optimization of therapies according to the general guidelines for HFrEF patients, and specific management strategies for specific etiologies of DCM should be considered when appropriate.[2]

MYOCARDIAL DISEASES PRESENTING AS DILATED CARDIOMYOPATHY

The most common causes of DCM are genetic, idiopathic, toxic, inflammatory, infectious, or metabolic. However, it should be recognized that

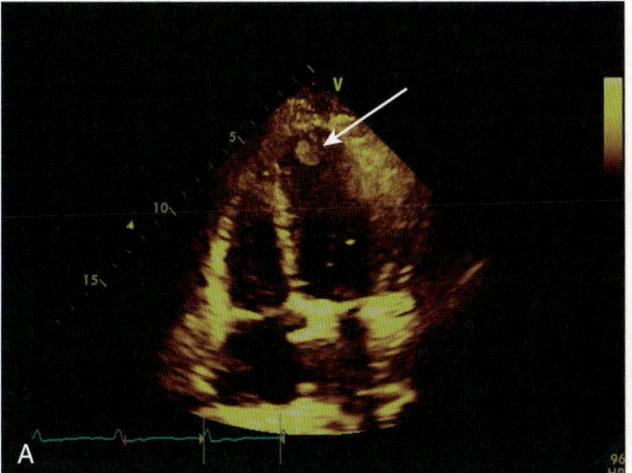
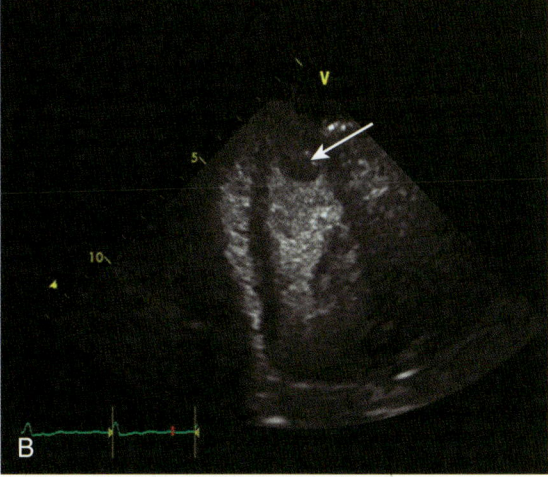

Fig. 20.6 Left ventricular apical thrombus in a patient with dilated cardiomyopathy. Apical 4 chamber view without (A) and with perfluorocarbon contrast (B) demonstrating a circular mass in the LV apex consistent with thrombus *(arrows)*. (Images courtesy Harris Health System, Houston, TX.)

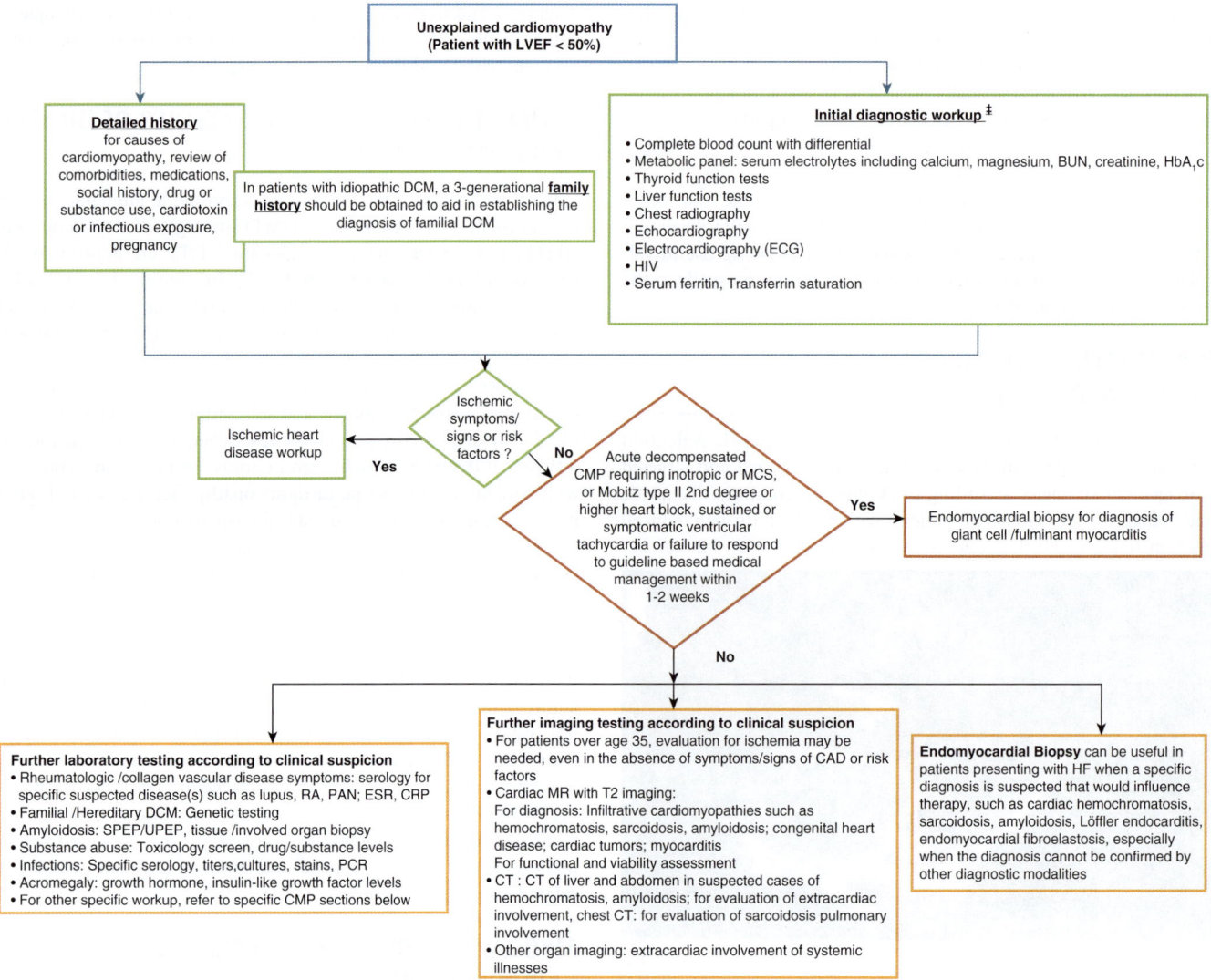

Fig. 20.7 Diagnostic Algorithm for Dilated Cardiomyopathies. These diagnostic tests are part of routine workup of initial evaluation of a HF patient according to most recent ACCF/AHA Guideline for the Management of Heart Failure. *CAD,* Coronary artery disease; *CMP,* cardiomyopathy; *CT,* computerized tomography; *MR,* magnetic resonance; *PAN,* polyarthritis nodosa; *PCR,* polymerase chain reaction; *RA,* rheumatoid arthritis; *SLE,* systemic lupus erythematosus; *SPEP,* serum protein electrophoresis; *UPEP,* urine protein electrophoresis. (Reprinted with permission. From Bozkurt B, Colvin M, Cook J, et al. Current diagnostic and treatment strategies for specific dilated cardiomyopathies: a scientific statement from the American Heart Association. *Circulation.* 2016;134(23):e579–e646; and Yancy CW, Jessup M, Bozkurt B, et al. 2013 ACCF/AHA guideline for the management of heart failure: a report of the American College of Cardiology Foundation/American Heart Association Task Force on practice guidelines. *Circulation.* 2013;128[16]:e240–e327. ©2016 American Heart Association, Inc.)

the exact prevalence of the various forms of DCM will vary based on the demographics of the patient population and the ability to identify a specific etiology. In the section that follows, we will review that various specific etiologies that lead to the development of DCM.

Idiopathic Dilated Cardiomyopathy

Although the term idiopathic DCM has become synonymous with that of DCM in some heart failure parlance, the term "idiopathic" was originally intended to characterize the subset of DCM patients in whom no known etiological cause for ventricular dilation and depressed myocardial contractility was apparent. However, with increasing sophistication in diagnostic testing, clinicians have become aware that most cases of so-called idiopathic DCM may occur as the result of inherited and/or spontaneous mutations of genes that regulate cardiac structure and/or function (**see also Chapter 24**), such

as the genes for cytoskeletal proteins, or in some cases a consequence of undiagnosed hypertension, autoimmune diseases, toxins (such as cardiotoxic chemotherapy, alcohol, or illicit drugs), or viral myocarditis. Nonetheless, in the context of the present chapter, we use the terminology of idiopathic DCM to refer to those patients with DCM whose etiological cause remains unknown. It is likely that the proportion of patients with idiopathic DCM will diminish with increased sophistication in detection of genetic cardiomyopathies and other specific cardiomyopathies.

Familial/Genetic Cardiomyopathies

There is growing evidence that many cases of previously diagnosed "idiopathic" dilated cardiomyopathies have a genetic basis. It is estimated that at least 30% of DCM cases are familial or genetic. Such causes, including noncompaction cardiomyopathies; dystrophin, titin-related, or other sarcomere, cytoskeleton, nuclear lamina–related genetic cardiomyopathies; X-linked cardiomyopathies; muscular dystrophy–associated cardiomyopathies; other familial dilated cardiomyopathies; and arrhythmogenic right ventricular cardiomyopathies, are discussed in detail in **Chapter 24**.

Cardiomyopathy Due to Cardiotoxins
Alcoholic Cardiomyopathy

Alcoholism is an important cause of DCM.[20] The clinical diagnosis of alcoholic cardiomyopathy is suspected when biventricular dysfunction and dilation are noted in an individual with a long and heavy alcohol abuse history, in the absence of other known causes for myocardial disease. Alcoholic cardiomyopathy most commonly occurs in men 30 to 55 years of age who have been heavy consumers of alcohol for more than 10 years.[20] Women represent approximately 14% of the alcoholic cardiomyopathy cases, but may develop cardiomyopathy with a less total lifetime exposure to alcohol compared with men.[20] Mortality rates due to alcoholic cardiomyopathy are greater in men compared with women, and in blacks compared with white.[20] Even before the clinically overt symptoms of heart failure, left ventricular systolic dysfunction and atrial fibrillation are common. The point at which these abnormalities appear during the course of an individual's lifetime of drinking, such that the abnormalities can be called a DCM, is not well established and is highly individualized.

The risk of developing alcoholic cardiomyopathy appears to be related to both the amount and duration alcohol intake. In general, alcoholic patients consuming greater than 90 g of alcohol a day (approximately seven to eight standard drinks per day) for more than 5 years are at risk for the development of asymptomatic alcoholic cardiomyopathy. On the other hand, mild to moderate alcohol consumption has been reported to be protective against development of heart failure in the general population.[21,22] These paradoxical findings (i.e., alcohol may be protective against development of heart failure in certain populations when used in moderation, but detrimental in others, especially when used in excess over longer periods of time) suggest that duration of exposure and individual genetic susceptibility play an important role in pathogenesis. Persistent DCM develops in only a small percentage of chronic drinkers, and the role of genetic predisposition, or the presence of synergistic cardiovascular factors such hypertension or arrhythmias in the development of alcohol-related cardiomyopathy, are not clear at the present time.

Studies in experimental animals have demonstrated that both acute and chronic ethanol administration impairs cardiac contractility. Alcohol results in acute as well as chronic depression of myocardial contractility, even when ingested by normal individuals in quantities consumed during social drinking.[23] Compensatory mechanisms such as vasodilation or sympathetic stimulation may mask the direct acute myocardial depressant effects of alcohol.

Despite the known deleterious effects of alcohol, it has been difficult to produce heart failure in animal models in which ethanol has been administered. Thus the direct causal relationship between alcohol consumption and the development of cardiomyopathy has not been rigorously demonstrated in experimental models, despite the long-recognized clinical relationship between alcohol consumption and the development of DCM. Potential mechanisms invoked to explain the depressed myocardial function include the direct toxic effects of alcohol on striated muscle (most alcoholics have manifestations of skeletal myopathy and cardiomyopathy); shifts in the relative expression of the α-myosin heavy chain to β-MHC; alterations in cellular calcium, magnesium, or phosphate homeostasis; and formation of fatty acid ethyl esters impairing mitochondrial oxidative phosphorylation.[20] In acute ethanol toxicity, free radical damage and/or ischemia may occur,

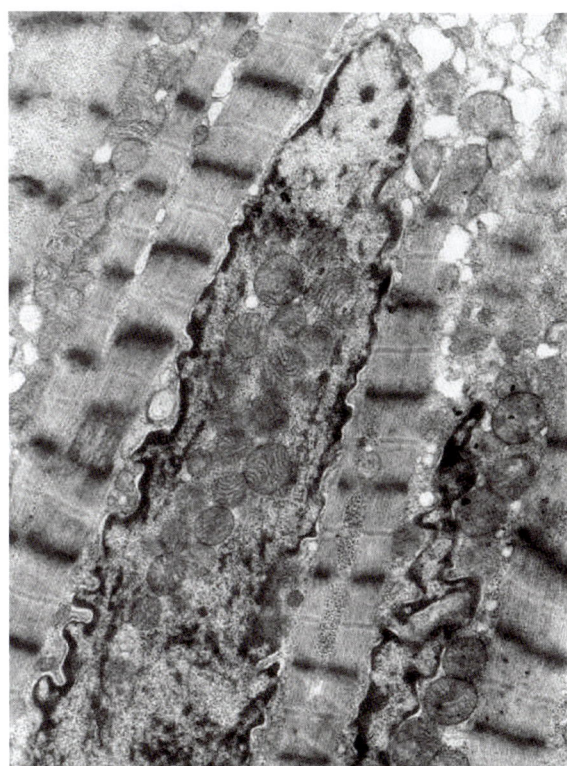

Fig. 20.8 Electron microscopy of cardiomyocytes of patients with alcoholic cardiomyopathy revealing the presence of nuclei with mitochondria accumulated in their core, associated with chromatin displacement to periphery of the nucleus. (From Bakeeva LE, Skulachev VP, Sudarikova YV, Tsyplenkova VG. Mitochondria enter the nucleus [one further problem in chronic alcoholism]. *Biochemistry [Mosc]*. 2001;66[12]:1335–1341.)

possibly due to increased xanthine oxidase activity or β-adrenergic stimulation, respectively. Both autopsy and endomyocardial biopsy specimens from alcoholic cardiomyopathy patients reveal marked mitochondrial swelling, fragmentation of cristae, swelling of endoplasmic reticulum, entrance of mitochondria into the nucleus potentially promoting attack of mitochondria by nuclear proteins and the attack of nuclear DNA by proteins of the mitochondrial intermembrane space, and cytoskeletal disorganization and destruction of myofibrils (**Fig. 20.8**).[24] Several studies suggest that heavy drinking alters both lymphocyte and granulocyte production and function, raising the possibility that myocardial damage may occur secondary to inflammatory and autoimmune mechanisms comparable to those observed in myocarditis. The point at which the changes in mitochondrial, sarcoplasmic reticulum, contractile protein, and calcium homeostasis culminate in intrinsic cell dysfunction is not completely understood. Application of insulin-like growth factor (IGF)-1 has been reported to attenuate the apoptotic effects of ethanol in primary neonatal myocyte cell cultures.[20]

Genetic traits such as multiple point mutations in the mitochondrial DNA have been reported to influence the occurrence, pathogenesis, and progression of alcoholic cardiomyopathy, which may explain interindividual variations in the sensitivity of the myocardium to alcohol-induced myocardial damage.[25] In addition, nutritional deficiencies, such as thiamine deficiency, may play an additive role to the direct myocardial damage of ethanol. Thus the cardiomyopathy that develops following chronic alcohol consumption appears to be multifactorial in origin.

The management of patients with alcohol cardiomyopathy begins with total abstinence from alcohol, in addition to the conventional management of heart failure. There are currently no studies of specific pharmacotherapies in patients with alcoholic cardiomyopathy other than the standard therapy of heart failure; however, there are numerous reports that detail the reversibility of depressed left ventricular dysfunction after the cessation of drinking.[26] Many heart failure programs limit alcoholic beverage consumption to no more than one or two alcoholic beverage servings daily for all patients with left ventricular dysfunction, regardless of the etiology.[14] Even if the depressed left ventricular function does not normalize completely, the symptoms and signs of congestive heart failure improve after abstinence.[26] However, the overall prognosis remains poor, with a mortality of 40% to 50% within 3 to 6 years, if the patient is not abstinent.[20] Survival is significantly lower for patients who continue to drink compared with patients with idiopathic DCM or alcoholic cardiomyopathy patients who abstain.[20]

Cocaine Cardiomyopathy

Long-term abuse of cocaine, a drug that causes postsynaptic norepinephrine reuptake blockade, can result in DCM, even without presence of coronary artery disease, vasculitis, or regional myocardial injury. This has been termed as "cocaine related cardiomyopathy" and likely reflects the direct toxicity of the cocaine on the myocardium. In patients with cocaine abuse, depressed LV function has been reported in 4% to 18% of the screened patients without heart failure symptoms.[27-29]

Electrocardiogram may reveal increased QRS voltage, early repolarization, ischemic or nonspecific ST-T changes, or pathologic Q waves. Episodes of ST elevation may be seen during Holter monitoring. Echocardiogram usually reveals left ventricular hypertrophy, depressed left ventricular ejection fraction, and dilation. Segmental wall motion abnormalities usually suggest myocardial injury; however, approximately 18% to 20% of patients with cocaine abuse manifest global hypokinesia. Cardiac catheterization in these patients may reveal normal coronaries or mild coronary artery disease not significant enough to explain the extent of myocardial dysfunction. Accelerated coronary atherosclerosis, coronary vasculitis, coronary spasm, or coronary thrombosis can also be seen in cocaine-related heart disease.

Cocaine may produce left ventricular dysfunction through its direct toxic effects on the myocardium, by provoking coronary arterial spasm (and hence myocardial ischemia), and by causing increased release of catecholamines, which may be directly toxic to cardiac myocytes. These effects will decrease myocardial oxygen supply and may increase demand if heart rate and blood pressure rise. The vasoactive effects of cocaine are further complicated with enhanced platelet aggregation, anticardiolipin antibody formation, and endothelial release of potent vasoconstrictors such as endothelin-1. Up regulation of tissue plasminogen activator inhibitors, increased platelet aggregation, and decreased fibrinolysis by cocaine predispose to coronary thrombosis and/or microvascular disease.[27] Myocarditis with inflammatory lymphocyte and eosinophils has also been reported, raising the possibility of hypersensitivity myocarditis due to cocaine or associated contaminants. Scattered foci of myocyte necrosis, contraction band necrosis, and foci of myocyte fibrosis have been reported in patients with cocaine abuse. In addition, experimental studies and clinical case reports suggest that cocaine may cause lethal arrhythmias. Cocaine prolongs repolarization by a depressant effect on potassium current and may generate early after depolarizations.[27]

Other than abstinence, very little is known about the treatment of cocaine-induced cardiac dysfunction. Indeed, there are case reports of reversibility of cardiac function after cessation of drug use. In patients who develop cardiomyopathy, the traditional therapy for LV dysfunction is appropriate. Given that some of the toxicity of cocaine is

caused by catecholamine excess and/or myocardial ischemia, the use of β-adrenergic blocking agents appeared to be a logical treatment, both in terms of preventing further disease progression, as well as for treating the ventricular arrhythmias that are prone to develop in this setting. Two decades ago, the treatment of cocaine-induced cardiovascular effects favored the use of β-blockers, especially propranolol. As the clinical use of propranolol increased, reports of accentuation of cocaine-induced hypertension and myocardial ischemia began to surface, blaming the unopposed alpha effects of the β-blockers. Although these reports were isolated, the routine use of propranolol and subsequently all β-blockers were considered relatively contraindicated in treating cocaine-induced cardiovascular emergencies. The end result is that an entire generation of potent and selective β-adrenergic blocking agents have been overlooked, both for acute and chronic treatment of cocaine-related cardiac disease, due to the possibility of "unopposed alpha effects." The focus of treatment shifted from the cardiovascular effects to combating central nervous stimulation. As a result, benzodiazepines have been the drug of choice in treating the cerebrovascular and subsequent systemic hyperadrenergic complications of cocaine, and nitroprusside or phentolamine being advocated for peripheral vasodilatory effects. It is now becoming apparent that treatment of cardiovascular effects of cocaine should involve a multifactorial approach to combat both central nervous system and peripheral vasospastic effects of cocaine. An observational study demonstrated that β-blocker treatment did not result in any a major adverse cardiovascular in patients with HFrEF, and there were no significant differences in HF readmissions or mortality rates compared with β-blocker treatment in HFrEF patients with and without cocaine use.[30] Within HF patients with cocaine use, mortality rates were not significantly different between patients treated with non-cardioselective versus cardioselective β-blockers.[30] According to the AHA Scientific Statement on Current Diagnostic and Treatment Strategies for Specific Dilated Cardiomyopathies,[2] it is considered reasonable to treat patients with cocaine-related cardiomyopathy who have demonstrated abstinence for more than 6 months with standard therapy for LV dysfunction including β-blockers. In patients at risk for relapse for cocaine abuse, a nonselective β-blocker treatment with α_1, β_1, β_2 receptor antagonism is reasonable because of potential protection against the unopposed alpha agonism effects of cocaine with β_1-receptor antagonist treatment alone.[2] It should also be noted that β-blockers are not recommended to be used in the acute setting of cocaine-related acute coronary syndrome.

Cardiomyopathy Related to Other Stimulant Drugs

Especially among adult patients, crystal amphetamine and methamphetamine abuse have been associated with reports of myocardial infarction, pulmonary edema, and cardiomyopathy cases.[31] Methamphetamine users have an almost fourfold increased risk of developing cardiomyopathy compared with nonusers.[32,33] Methamphetamine-associated cardiomyopathy may be reversible with appropriate medical therapy and cessation of use. By some reports, late gadolinium enhancement cardiovascular MR has been helpful to identify the magnitude of fibrosis and likelihood of recovery in methamphetamine-associated cardiomyopathy cases.[34] Although rare, misuse or overdose of drugs used for attention-deficit/ hyperactivity disorder (ADHD) such as methylphenidate, dextroamphetamine, and dextroamphetamine-amphetamine have been associated with myocardial infarction, cardiomyopathy, and sudden death in case reports.[35]

Over the past decade, novel or atypical drugs have emerged and have been associated with cardiovascular toxicity. Cardiostimulant drugs such as ecstasy (3,4-methylenedioxy-N-methylamphetamine [MDMA]);[36] "bath salts" containing synthetic cathinones such as mephedrone methylenedioxypyrovalerone, which have

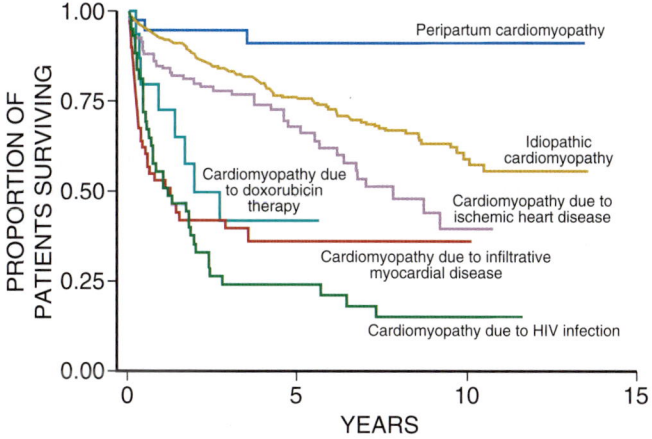

Fig. 20.9 Survival according to different etiologies of dilated cardiomyopathy. In a cohort of patients who underwent endomyocardial biopsy as part of an evaluation for heart failure due to unexplained cardiomyopathy, when compared with the patients with idiopathic cardiomyopathy, survival was significantly better in patients with peripartum cardiomyopathy and significantly worse among the patients with cardiomyopathy due to infiltrative myocardial disease, human immunodeficiency virus (HIV) infection, therapy with doxorubicin, and ischemic heart disease. (From Felker GM, Thompson RE, Hare JM, et al. Underlying causes and long-term survival in patients with initially unexplained cardiomyopathy. *N Engl J Med*. 2000;342[15]:1077–1084.)

amphetamine/cocaine-like properties;[37] and khat chewing, which contains cathinone,[38] have cardiotoxic effects and have been implicated in cases of myocardial infarction, arrhythmia, cardiac arrest, and cardiomyopathy.[2] Synthetic cannabinoids have been reported to result in acute congestive heart failure from myocardial stunning, respiratory failure, and death.[39]

Chemotherapy (See Also Chapter 46)

Cardiotoxicity is a well-known side effect of several cytotoxic drugs, especially of the anthracyclines, and can lead to long-term morbidity. Anthracyclines, such as doxorubicin and daunorubicin, produce cardiac toxicity possibly by increasing oxygen free radical generation, platelet activating factor, prostaglandins, histamine, calcium and C-13 hydroxy metabolites, or by interfering with sarcolemmal sodium potassium pump and mitochondrial electron transport chain. Formation of oxygen free radicals that are generated by iron-catalyzed pathways appears to be the most important pathway in the pathogenesis of anthracycline-induced cardiomyopathy, as it has been noted that iron-chelating agents that prevent generation of oxygen free radicals, such as dexrazoxane, are cardio-protective.[2] The prognosis of anthracycline induced cardiomyopathy relates to the time course of treatment and preexisting additional risk factors for myocardial injury such as radiation, coexisting coronary artery disease, and preexisting cardiac dysfunction. Prior XRT to the heart/mediastinum also increases the risk of doxorubicin-induced cardiomyopathy.[2] In general, patients with anthracycline-induced cardiomyopathy have a worse survival than that seen with idiopathic DCM (**Fig. 20.9**). Other chemotherapeutic agents in cancer associated with cardiac toxicity complication are the monoclonal antibody trastuzumab (herceptin), high-dose cyclophosphamide, taxoids, mitomycin-C, 5-fluorouracil, certain antivascular endothelial growth factor (VEGF) inhibitors and proteasome inhibitors, such as bortezomib and carfilzomib, and interferons.[2] In contrast to anthracycline-induced cardiac toxicity, trastuzumab-related cardiac dysfunction does not appear to increase with cumulative dose or to be associated with ultrastructural changes in the myocardium, and is

generally reversible. This topic is discussed in further detail in **Chapter 46**.

Other Myocardial Toxins

In addition to the classic toxins described previously, as shown in Table 20.1, there are a number of other toxic agents that may lead to left ventricular dysfunction and heart failure, including cobalt, phenothiazines, clozapine, antidepressants, carbon monoxide, lead, lithium, methysergide, pseudoephedrine, ephedrine, cobalt, anabolic steroids, hydroxychloroquine, and catecholamines.[2] One such agent, ephedra, which has been used for the purposes of athletic performance enhancement and weight loss, has been linked to a high rate of serious adverse outcomes, including left ventricular systolic dysfunction, development of heart failure, and cardiac deaths ultimately resulting in a ban of this agent by the US Food and Drug Administration (FDA). High doses of decongestants, such as pseudoephedrine or ephedrine, have also been implicated in cardiotoxicity and are recommended not to be overused.[2]

INFLAMMATION-INDUCED CARDIOMYOPATHY

There is increasing evidence that inflammation and/or inflammatory processes may contribute to the overall pathogenesis of DCM (**see also Chapter 7**). Moreover, there is evidence that biological properties of inflammatory mediators, such as proinflammatory cytokines, are also sufficient to produce a dilated cardiac phenotype.[40] As discussed later, both infectious and noninfectious inflammatory processes may lead to the development of DCM. Although a great many infections and noninfectious processes may impact the myocardium, and may transiently lead to systolic dysfunction and congestive symptomatology, the great majority of these infections and noninfectious processes do not lead to the development of DCM. Therefore, in the section that follows, we will focus primarily on those disease states that are considered to lead to DCM.

Infectious Causes

There are a number of infectious diseases that can lead to DCM, including viral myocarditis (**see Chapter 28**), Chagas disease (**see Chapter 28**), and acquired immunodeficiency syndrome (AIDS), which will be discussed in detail in the following sections.

Acquired Immunodeficiency Syndrome

Several investigators have reported that there is an association between AIDS and DCM. Reviews and studies published before the introduction of highly active antiretroviral therapy regimens have correlated the incidence and course of human immunodeficiency virus (HIV) infection with development of DCM in both children and adults. In a long-term echocardiographic follow-up by Barbaro and coworkers,[41] 8% of initially asymptomatic HIV positive patients were diagnosed with DCM and advanced heart failure during 5 years follow-up. The mean annual incidence rate of heart failure was 15.9 cases per 1000 HIV-infected patients. The extent of immunodeficiency of the patients, as assessed by the CD4 count, influenced the incidence of DCM; specifically, there was a higher incidence among patients with a CD4 count of less than 400 cells per cubic millimeter.

It has been demonstrated that targeted myocardial expression of HIV transactivator in transgenic mice results in cardiomyopathy and mitochondrial damage,[42] emphasizing the role of the HIV infection itself in AIDS cardiomyopathy. The role of HIV type 1 infection of cardiac myocytes in the development of DCM in HIV has not been fully characterized. Even though human myocardial cells are not known to express CD4 cells, an autopsy series of persons dying from acquired immunodeficiency syndrome–related illnesses demonstrates

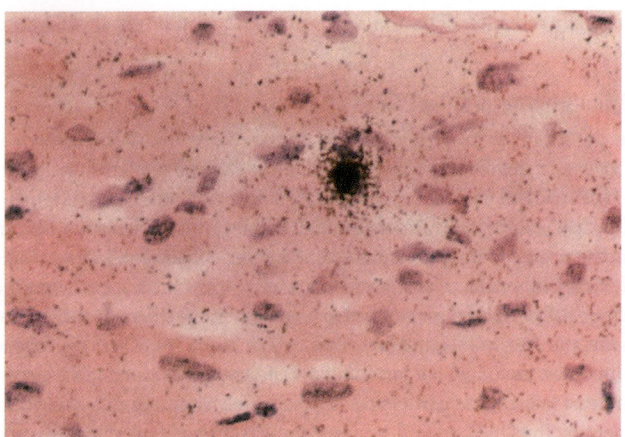

Fig. 20.10 In situ hybridization of human immunodeficiency virus (HIV) RNA probe in a section of myocardial tissue obtained at autopsy from acquired immunodeficiency syndrome patients. Using sulfur-35-labeled ribonucleic acid probes, HIV nucleic acid sequences were detected in cardiac tissue sections. The black grains in the emulsion overlying a presumed cardiac myocyte indicate positive hybridization with HIV nucleic acid sequences (counterstained with hematoxylin and eosin, ×335). (From Grody WW, Cheng L, Lewis W. Infection of the heart by the human immunodeficiency virus. *Am J Cardiol.* 1990;66[2]:203–206.)

histological evidence of myocarditis in approximately 50% of the patients.[43] By in situ hybridization techniques, HIV nucleic acid sequences were detected in cardiac tissue sections in 27% of the patients who died of AIDS (**Fig. 20.10**).[44] Symptomatic heart failure is seen in approximately half of these patients with myocardial involvement. Other than treatment for HIV with antiretroviral therapy, the treatment of heart failure in patients with symptomatic HIV cardiomyopathy is the same as the conventional treatment for patients with HFrEF. The prognosis of HIV cardiomyopathy remains poor, with a more than 50% mortality rate in 2 to 3 years (see Fig. 20.9).[45]

Noninfectious Causes
Hypersensitivity Myocarditis

Hypersensitivity to a variety of agents may result in allergic reactions that involve the myocardium, characterized by peripheral eosinophilia, and a perivascular infiltration of the myocardium by eosinophils, lymphocytes, and histiocytes. These infiltrates may be occasionally associated with necrosis. A variety of drugs, most commonly the sulfonamides, penicillins, methyldopa, and other agents such as dobutamine, amphotericin B, streptomycin, phenytoin, isoniazid, tetanus toxoid, hydrochlorothiazide, and chlorthalidone have been reported to cause allergic hypersensitivity myocarditis. Most patients are not clinically ill but may die suddenly, presumably secondary to an arrhythmia. Hypersensitivity myocarditis is recognized only rarely clinically, but may be sufficient to produce global and/or regional myocardial dysfunction detected by noninvasive methods. This entity is often first diagnosed on postmortem examination, and occasionally on endomyocardial biopsy.[46]

Systemic Lupus Erythematosus

Although a number of cardiac abnormalities can be present in patients with systemic lupus erythematosus (SLE), in a small percentage of patients, DCM can be present. Global left ventricular dysfunction has been reported in approximately 5% of patients with SLE, and correlates with disease activity. However, myocardial involvement is frequently found at autopsy or at endomyocardial biopsy and is less easily detected clinically. The myocardial lesions are characterized by

an increase in interstitial connective tissue and myocardial scarring. Recent studies suggest that depolarization abnormalities on signal average EKG accompanied with echocardiographic evidence of abnormal left ventricular filling may reflect the presence of myocardial fibrosis and could be a marker of subclinical myocardial involvement in SLE patients.[47] Cardiac involvement may manifest itself by conduction system abnormalities such as complete atrioventricular heart block. Especially neonatal lupus is characterized by congenital heart block, as well as cardiomyopathy, cutaneous lupus lesions, hepatobiliary disease, and thrombocytopenia. Abnormal levels of serum cTnT and cTnI can be associated with increased disease activity, including in those with a normal C, and may have a role in screening for cardiac involvement.[48] However, it should be noted that these patients may have falsely elevated levels due to assay detection with antibody formation.

Scleroderma

The development of DCM is rare in patients with scleroderma. A recent echocardiographic study showed that although there was no difference in LV dimensions or fractional shortening in patients with scleroderma, there was indication of systolic impairment in the majority of patients.[49] A distinctive focal myocardial lesion ranging from contraction band necrosis to replacement fibrosis without morphologic abnormalities of the coronary arteries is noted in approximately half of the patients with scleroderma. This is postulated to be due to intermittent vascular spasm with intramyocardial Raynaud phenomenon. Thus progressive systemic sclerosis can lead to conduction abnormalities, arrhythmias, heart failure, angina pectoris with normal coronary arteries, myocardial fibrosis, pericarditis, and sudden death. Late contrast enhancement with gadolinium may be used to characterize patchy fibrosis and myocardial edema interspersed with normal myocardium in scleroderma. Cardiac involvement in systemic sclerosis portends an ominous prognosis, and is probably most directly related to the extent of myocardial fibrosis.[2]

Rheumatoid Arthritis

Cardiac involvement in rheumatoid arthritis generally results from the development of myocarditis and/or pericarditis. However, rarely development of DCM can be seen in these patients. In a retrospective study of 172 patients with juvenile rheumatoid arthritis, symptomatic cardiac involvement occurred in 7.6% of patients, including pericarditis, perimyocarditis, and myocarditis. Both myocarditis and pericarditis are regarded as poor prognostic factors in rheumatoid arthritis.[50] Myocardial involvement in rheumatoid arthritis is thought to be secondary to disturbances in the microcirculation secondary to microvasculitis, and can occur in the absence of any clinical symptoms of ECG changes.[2]

Sarcoidosis

Cardiac sarcoidosis is most commonly recognized in patients with systemic or other manifestations of sarcoidosis, and cardiac involvement may occur in isolation and go undetected. Cardiac sarcoidosis may present as asymptomatic LV dysfunction, symptomatic heart failure, atrioventricular block, atrial or ventricular arrhythmia, and sudden cardiac death. Although untested in clinical trials, early use of high-dose steroid therapy may halt or reverse cardiac damage.[51] Cardiac magnetic resonance imaging and/or positron emission tomography imaging with fluorodeoxyglucose imaging can be useful to diagnose cardiac sarcoidosis and/or follow response to therapy.[2] Cardiac involvement is patchy with granulomas and fibrosis, and endomyocardial biopsy may demonstrate myocardial granulomas characterized by clusters of mononuclear cells and giant cells. In the setting of ventricular tachyarrhythmia, patients may require placement of an implantable cardioverter-defibrillator for primary prevention of sudden cardiac death. Though most present with restrictive cardiomyopathy features with mildly depressed or preserved left ventricular ejection fraction (LVEF), elevated filling pressures, enlarged atria, and restrictive filling pattern by echocardiography, in advanced stages, the cardiac features may progress to DCM. Endomyocardial biopsy can be useful to confirm cardiac sarcoidosis when pathology yields evidence of noncaseating granulomas, but absence does not rule out the possibility of cardiac sarcoidosis.

Patients with cardiac sarcoidosis are usually treated with corticosteroids. Other immunosuppressive therapies (e.g., methotrexate, azathioprine, mycophenolate mofetil, cyclophosphamide, pentoxifylline, and thalidomide) can be used in patients who cannot tolerate corticosteroids, or in patients who continue to worsen clinically despite corticosteroid treatment. Ventricular arrhythmia, advanced degree atrioventricular block, and progressive decline in LV function are ominous signs. In addition to consideration for ICD, referral for cardiac transplantation and/or MCS should be made for patients with advanced HF in the absence of significant extracardiac burden of sarcoid disease.[2]

Peripartum Cardiomyopathy

Peripartum cardiomyopathy (PPCM) is a disease of unknown cause in which severe left ventricular dysfunction occurs during the last trimester of pregnancy or the early puerperium in the absence of an identifiable cause for the cardiac failure other than pregnancy. In the past, the diagnosis of this entity was made on clinical grounds; however, modern echocardiographic techniques have allowed more accurate diagnoses by excluding cases of diseases that mimic the clinical symptoms and signs of heart failure. The former historical diagnostic restriction of the time frame to last month of pregnancy or first 5 months postpartum for diagnosis has been challenged by observations that almost 20% of the patients developed symptoms of heart failure and were diagnosed with PPCM earlier than the last gestational month.[52] Hence, a more contemporary definition of PPCM is a cardiomyopathy presenting with HF secondary to left ventricular dysfunction toward the end of pregnancy or in the months following delivery, where no other cause of heart failure is found.[53]

The incidence varies geographically. Based on available literature, the incidence of PPCM appears to be 1 in 1000 in South Africa, 1 in 300 in Haiti,[53] and 1 in 2200 to 4000 in the United States.[54] Risk factors for PPCM include advanced maternal age, multiparity, obesity, black race, twinning, pregnancy induced hypertension, preeclampsia, and long-term tocolysis. In a population study using the National Hospital Discharge Survey to evaluate incidence of PPCM in the United States in more than 51 million live births, there was a trend toward increased incidence of PPCM from 1990 to 2002. Between 1990 and 1993, the incidence of PPCM was 1 in 4350 live births and increased to 1 in 2229 live births between 2000 and 2002.[2]

Although its etiology remains unknown, most theories have focused on the hemodynamic, inflammatory, oxidative, and immunologic stresses of pregnancy and genetic susceptibility. An immune pathogenesis is supported by the findings of lymphocytic myocarditis on myocardial biopsy; high titers of auto-antibodies against selected cardiac tissue proteins in a majority of women with PPCM; fetal microchimerism (fetal cells in maternal blood) in some patients with PPCM; and the fact that multiparity or previous exposure to fetal antigens are significant risk factors.[55] More recent studies have suggested that a defective antioxidant cascade may play a role, specifically implicating the activation of prolactin-cleaving protease cathepsin D and production of proapoptotic derivatives of prolactin with potentially detrimental cardiovascular actions in the pathophysiology.[56] This concept was supported by the observation that in mice, treatment with bromocriptine, an inhibitor of prolactin secretion, prevented the development of PPCM.[56] Regarding genetic etiology, familial clustering of PPCM in certain cases have suggested that a subset of PPCM may be a part of the spectrum of familial DCM, presenting in the peripartum period. Recent studies suggest that PPCM may share genetic mutations similar to idiopathic DCM. In a recent study, the distribution of truncating variants in a large series of women with PPCM was found to be remarkably similar to those found in patients with idiopathic DCM. Two-thirds of identified truncating variants were in *TTN*, which encodes the sarcomere protein titin.[57]

The prognosis of PPCM is related to the recovery of ventricular function. In contrast to patients with idiopathic DCM, significant improvement in myocardial function is seen in more than 50% of patients in the first 6 months after presentation (see Fig. 20.9).[55] However, for those patients who do not recover to normal or near normal function, the prognosis is similar to other forms of DCM. Cardiomegaly that persists for more than 4 to 6 months after diagnosis indicates a poor prognosis. In a contemporary multicenter IPAC (Investigations of Pregnancy Associated Cardiomyopathy) prospective cohort study, 100 North American women with PPCM were followed for 1 year postpartum;[58] 88% were receiving β-blockers and 81% ACE inhibitors or angiotensin receptor blockers. Most women recovered; however, 13% had major events or persistent severe cardiomyopathy. Black women had more LV dysfunction at presentation and at 6 and 12 months postpartum. Severe LV dysfunction and greater remodeling at study entry were associated with less recovery. No subjects with both a baseline LVEF less than 0.30 and a left ventricular end-diastolic diameter (LVEDD) ≥6.0 cm recovered by 1 year postpartum, whereas 91% with both a baseline LVEF ≥0.30 and an LVEDD less than 6.0 cm recovered(**Fig. 20.11**).[58] The mortality of PPCM has been reported to be lower than that of other forms of cardiomyopathies. In the United States, the mortality after diagnosis of PPCM has ranged from 0% to less than 10% in contemporary analyses.[2] Heart transplantation is performed in 5% to 10% of patients with PPCM.[2] In South Africa and Haiti, mortality related to PPCM appears to be significantly higher than in the United States, up to 15% to 28% at 2 years.[2]

Diagnosis is based on the clinical presentation of congestive heart failure and objective evidence of left ventricular systolic dysfunction. Symptoms may mimic those encountered in a normal pregnancy, which may contribute to delayed or missed diagnosis impacting outcomes. Electrocardiogram findings may be nonspecific. Sinus tachycardia, atrial fibrillation, atrial flutter, and ventricular tachycardia have been reported. Among patients with LVEF greater than 30% at diagnosis, restoration of normal LVEF is more likely. Echocardiography is most commonly used to evaluate suspected PPCM, and may demonstrate moderate-to-severe left ventricular systolic dysfunction, left ventricular dilatation, four-chamber enlargement, mitral and tricuspid regurgitation, biatrial enlargement, elevated pulmonary pressures, and right ventricular (RV) enlargement. The left ventricle may not always be dilated; however, an initial left ventricular end-systolic diameter of ≤5.5 cm has been shown to predict recovery of left ventricle function. LV thrombus has been found on initial echocardiography in 10% to 17% of patients, and PPCM is associated with an increased incidence of thromboembolism compared with DCM from other etiologies. Other imaging modalities such as cardiac magnetic resonance imaging (MRI) do not show any specific pattern in PPCM to help differentiate from other causes of cardiomyopathy, although it can give a more accurate measurement of chamber volumes and ventricular function than echocardiography. Cardiac MRI has been evaluated in several small studies and case reports, and is a reasonable choice as the imaging modality for patients suspected of PPCM. The use of gadolinium during a cardiac

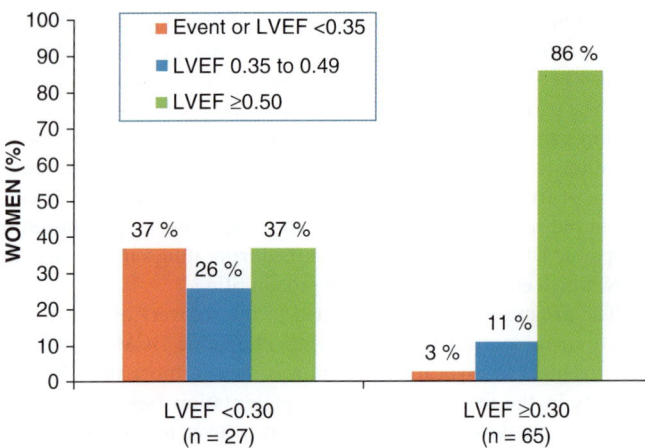

Fig. 20.11 Final status based on the initial LVEF of patients with peripartum cardiomyopathy. Comparison of status at the end of the study based on the initial LVEF. *Red column*, percentage of women with no recovery (event or final LVEF <0.35); *blue column*, percentage of women with partial recovery (final LVEF 0.35–0.49); *green column*, percentage of women with complete recovery (LVEF ≥0.50). Recovery was evident in 86% of women with a baseline LVEF ≥0.30, compared with 37% of those with an LVEF less than 0.30, p <0.001. *LVEF*, Left ventricular ejection fraction. (Modified from McNamara DM, Elkayam U, Alharethi R, et al. Clinical outcomes for peripartum cardiomyopathy in North America: results of the IPAC Study (Investigations of Pregnancy-Associated Cardiomyopathy). *J Am Coll Cardiol.* 2015;66[8]:905–914.)

MRI is not recommended during pregnancy. Natriuretic peptide levels (brain natriuretic peptide [BNP] or NT-proBNP) are usually elevated. Measuring cardiac troponin may be considered, as it has moderate predictive ability for ventricular recovery, and levels inversely correlate with LV function recovery at follow-up.[59] Markers of inflammation such as C-reactive protein, interferon–γ, and Fas/apolipoprotein-1 are usually elevated in patients with PPCM, but their role in diagnosis or prognosis is uncertain at this time.

For management of PPCM, a multidisciplinary approach involving a cardiologist, obstetrician, intensivist, anesthesiologist, and pediatrician is essential and should be engaged as early as possible. Pregnant women with PPCM should be referred to a center with experience with this condition for multidisciplinary care, with close monitoring before, during, and after delivery. Initial management is similar to that of other forms of nonischemic cardiomyopathy and includes oxygen, fluid restriction, loop-diuretics and/or other diuretics, nitrates, and hydralazine (safe to use during pregnancy), especially for hypertension. Angiotensin-converting enzyme inhibitors should be avoided in the second and third trimesters but are safe to use postpartum. For patients with PPCM, β-blockers can be used, although with caution, with monitoring of fetal heart rate and growth. β-blockers can be used when not contraindicated during pregnancy, and they can be used postpartum. During pregnancy, β-1 selective agents are preferred because β-2 receptor blockade may have an antitocolytic effect. Diuretics should be used when appropriate to treat volume overload, yet should be used sparingly to avoid reductions in fetal blood flow. Inotropic agents can be used in patients with signs of low cardiac output or with persistent congestion, despite diuretics/afterload-reducing agents. Anticoagulation is recommended in patients with PPCM, as these patients have a high incidence of LV thrombus, especially patients with an LVEF less than 35%. Heparin (unfractionated and low-molecular-weight) is favored in pregnancy since, unlike warfarin, it does not cross the placenta. Warfarin should be avoided, as it is teratogenic in early pregnancy and has a risk of causing fetal cerebral

hemorrhage in the second and third trimesters. Prompt delivery is recommended for patients with PPCM who are unstable. Vaginal delivery is preferred for patients with PPCM. Delivery through cesarean section should be reserved for patients with PPCM who are critically ill or for other obstetric indications. Earlier delivery may not be required if the mother and fetus are stable.

After delivery, PPCM should be treated according to current guidelines for heart failure. Implantable defibrillators and advances in medical therapy have significantly reduced the risk of sudden death, and all-cause mortality rates. It may be reasonable to wait for 6 months or longer of optimal medical therapy in patients with PPCM to allow for possible myocardial recovery when considering the timing of cardiac device placement such as ICD or CRT. For those patients who remain refractory to conventional pharmacologic therapy, cardiac transplantation and mechanical circulatory support are viable options.

Other treatment strategies summarized in the following paragraph remain investigational. A single nonrandomized study suggested that immunosuppression may benefit women with biopsy-proven myocarditis.[60] The Myocarditis Treatment Trial, however, did not show any benefit of immunosuppressive medications,[61] and given the risks of immunosuppressive therapy, they are currently not widely utilized. Similarly, the use of intravenous immunoglobulin was associated with an increase in LVEF in a retrospective study,[62] but the placebo controlled IMAC trial (Controlled Trial of Intravenous Immune Globulin in Recent-Onset Dilated Cardiomyopathy) failed to show a significant improvement with immune globulin treatment of adult patients with recent-onset cardiomyopathy; thus intravenous immunoglobulin (IVIG) is not routinely used in PPCM. With recognition of the potential detrimental role of the prolactin cascade, small studies have studied prolactin blockade with bromocriptine and reported improvement in LVEF and NYHA functional class.[63] In a more recent multicenter study, 63 patients with PPCM were randomized to 1 week versus 8 weeks of bromocriptine therapy postpartum, and there were no significant differences between the short- or long-term therapy, but there was no control arm without bromocriptine.[64] The generalizability of these studies are unclear, given the small sample sizes, lack of a control arm with placebo in the most recent study, the higher than expected mortality rate in the standard care group in the former study, and differences in PPCM characteristics in patients in Africa as compared with those elsewhere. Further studies aimed at clearly establishing the efficacy and safety of bromocriptine are needed before it can be recommended for the treatment of PPCM. Similarly, in a single center small study, pentoxifylline, an antiinflammatory agent, was associated with better LVEF, NYHA class, and survival.[65] The promising role of pentoxifylline in PPCM remains experimental until it is validated by a larger scale, placebo-controlled, randomized clinical trials. Breast-feeding is controversial, and conflicting data exist. While in general breast-feeding can be continued in stable patients, it is not recommended for women who are decompensated and critically ill. The risk and benefits of breast-feeding for mother and child need to be balanced carefully.[2]

PPCM is associated with a high risk of recurrence in subsequent pregnancies both in patients who have recovery of LV function and in those with persistent LV dysfunction. Patients with PPCM who recover their LV function have a lesser chance of recurrence compared with those with persistent LV dysfunction. The increased deterioration of LV function in subsequent pregnancy in patients with persistent LV dysfunction leads to a worse prognosis (20%–30% mortality in subsequent pregnancy), whereas patients with a full recovery of LV function have negligible mortality in subsequent pregnancies. Appropriate counseling regarding subsequent pregnancies and contraception is important, and women with LVEF of less than 25% at diagnosis of

PPCM or persistent LV dysfunction should be advised against a subsequent pregnancy. Every subsequent pregnancy in women with PPCM should be managed in high-risk perinatal centers, as subsequent pregnancies are associated with a high risk of recurrence despite recovered LV function. Even in the setting of normalized ventricular function, women with a history of PPCM should be counseled that a subsequent pregnancy carries a 20% risk of recurrent HF and LV dysfunction. Dobutamine stress testing has been recommended in women with apparent recovery of LV function who are considering a pregnancy in order to assess contractile reserve and further risk-stratify the potential for recurrence, but this has not been prospectively validated.[2]

Autoimmune Mechanisms

There has been increasing evidence suggesting that abnormalities in cellular and humoral immunity may contribute to the overall pathogenesis of DCM. Circulating auto-antibodies to a variety of cardiac antigens including G-protein linked receptors (such as those to β_1-adrenoreceptors and muscarinic receptors), mitochondrial antigens, adenosine diphosphate, adenosine triphosphate carrier proteins, and cardiac myosin heavy chain have been identified in patients with DCM. In this regard, it is interesting to note that immunization with certain cardiac muscle (but not skeletal) antigens such as α-myosin heavy chain can result in the development of a dilated cardiac phenotype in certain susceptible strains of mice. Moreover, a meta-analysis has shown that there is increased expression of the antigens of genes located at the major histocompatibility complex (MHC) on chromosome 6, which is the locus that is responsible for regulating immune responses. This study showed that HLA Class II antigens such as DR4 or DQw4 were present in 63% of the patients with cardiomyopathy as compared with 26% in the control subjects.[66] Features that support an autoimmune etiology in patients who present with myocarditis and DCM include familial aggregation, a weak association with HLA-DR4 haplotype, abnormal expression of HLA class II antigens in cardiac tissue, and detection of organ- and disease-specific cardiac auto-antibodies by immunofluorescence and immunoabsorption techniques. Nonetheless, a precise interpretation of these findings has been complicated by the knowledge that low titers of autoantibodies, which can be part of the normal immunologic repertoire, are not always pathogenic. For example, tissue injury secondary to ischemia or infection may lead to autoantibody production because of alterations of self-antigens or exposure of antigens that are normally sequestered from the immune system. In such situations, the generation of autoantibodies is the result, and not the cause, of the tissue injury. Furthermore, observations about autoimmune responses are generally made in patients with established disease; accordingly, any inferences regarding cause and effect are, invariably, indirect and circumstantial.

ENDOCRINE AND METABOLIC CAUSES OF CARDIOMYOPATHY (SEE ALSO CHAPTER 17)

Obesity

Obesity cardiomyopathy is defined as congestive heart failure due entirely or predominantly to obesity. Heart failure in the markedly obese usually develops over a long period of time, and can be directly related to the duration of obesity. Initially the dyspnea and edema in these patients is simply related to alterations in left ventricular compliance and diastolic heart failure, with resultant elevated filling pressures. However, with chronicity, some of these patients will develop significant left ventricular hypertrophy and increased left ventricular mass, and some subsequently develop DCM. Although the precise reasons for obesity-related heart failure are not known, it is thought that the excessive adipose accumulation results in increase in circulating

blood volume and subsequently a persistent increase in cardiac output, cardiac work, and systemic blood pressure, which ultimately leads to myocardial failure. Furthermore, there is increased prevalence of hypertension and coronary artery disease in obese patients, which may also contribute to the development of DCM in these patients. Cardiac myocyte injury by lipotoxicity has been implicated as a potential mechanism, especially in individuals with metabolic syndrome and insulin resistance. Cardiac lipotoxicity is hypothesized to arise from an imbalance between fatty acid uptake and utilization, leading to the inappropriate accumulation of free fatty acids and neutral lipids within cardiomyocytes. This lipid overload causes cellular dysfunction, cell death, and eventual organ dysfunction.[67] Obesity-related hypoventilation and sleep apnea may also contribute to the pathophysiology. A study examining the relation between obesity and heart failure in participants in the Framingham Heart Study[68] reported that after adjustment for established risk factors, there was an increase in the risk of heart failure of 5% for men and 7% for women for each increment of 1 in body-mass index. When compared with subjects with a normal body-mass index, obese subjects had a doubling of the risk of heart failure. Obesity alone was estimated to account for 11% of cases of heart failure in men and 14% of those in women.[68] Given the high prevalence of obesity in the last decade, strategies to promote optimal body weight may reduce the population burden of heart failure. In addition to its recognized risk for development of heart failure, intuitively, one would anticipate that obesity would adversely affect the outcome of patients with established heart failure. Interestingly, however, there is a recognized paradox with obesity and heart failure: in patients with established heart failure, obesity is associated with better clinical outcomes (**Fig. 20.12**).[69] This paradox, though not clearly understood, may partly be due to comparison of individuals in noncatabolic state with ability to gain weight with individuals who are lean or cachectic due to advanced heart failure; selective survival of different subtypes of obese individuals; earlier detection or misdiagnosis of heart failure in obese patients due to increased prevalence of dyspnea and edema; differences in etiology of heart failure in obese (hypertension, diabetes) versus nonobese (coronary artery disease); and the endocrine/paracrine role of the adipose tissue, which may also participate in metabolic turnover or rapid degradation of certain chemokines and neurohormones, including natriuretic peptides. Ongoing studies will provide more insight into the obesity paradox in heart failure.

Although there are anecdotal reports regarding symptomatic improvement following weight reduction in obesity induced heart failure, large-scale clinical trials on the role of weight loss in heart failure patients with obesity have not yet been performed.[70,71] The safety and efficacy of weight loss drugs such as orlistat, sibutramine, lorcaserin, or phentermine-topiramate have not been tested in large-scale trials in cardiac patients. There has been concern against use of sibutramine in heart failure due to reports of development of cardiomyopathy, and this medication is contraindicated in heart failure.[72] In small scale pilot studies, orlistat appeared to be tolerated and effective in weight loss in heart failure patients with obesity, but ongoing investigations are underway regarding its hepatic safety profile.[73] The safety of lorcaserin, an agonist of the 5-hydroxytryptamine (5-HT, or serotonin) receptor 5-HT2C, in patients with heart failure, is unknown; the initial FDA-approval includes a provision mandating postmarketing studies to assess for adverse cardiovascular effects. The Food and Drug Administration's approval of phentermine-topiramate combination is indicated for use in adults with a body mass index (BMI) greater than 30 kg/m² and at least one weight-related condition such as hypertension, type 2 diabetes, or dyslipidemia, but again safety or efficacy in heart failure is unknown. Similarly, there are no large-scale studies on safety or efficacy of weight loss with lifestyle modification with diet or exercise in obese heart failure

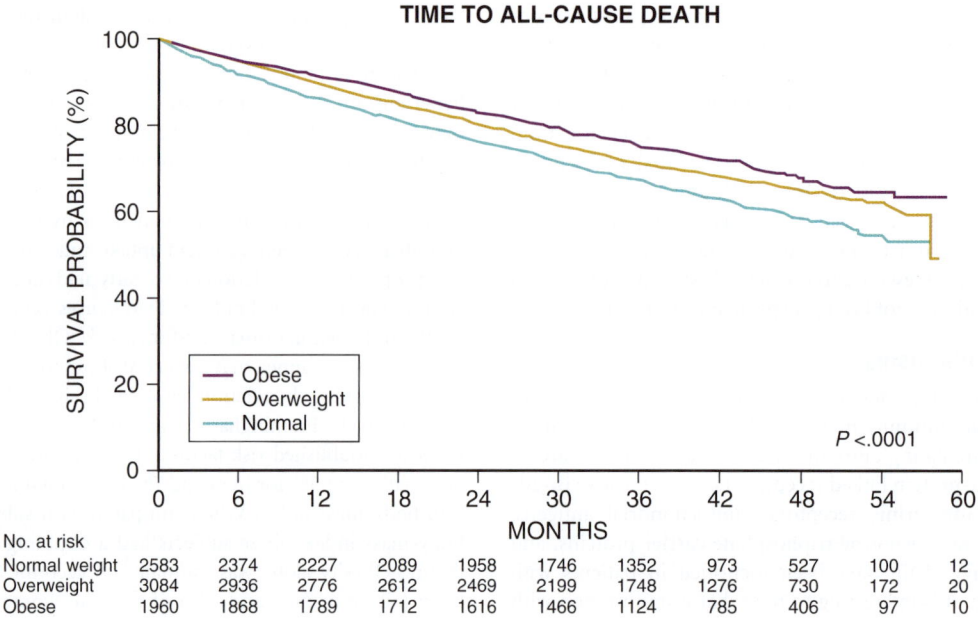

Fig. 20.12 Kaplan-Meier survival curves by body mass index in the obese, overweight, and normal-weight groups in patients with heart failure. The number of patients at risk for death at each 6-month interval is shown below the figure. (From Bozkurt B, Deswal A. Obesity as a prognostic factor in chronic symptomatic heart failure. *Am Heart J.* 2005;150[6]:1233–1239.)

patients. Since the prevalence of obesity is increasing in the general, as well as in the heart failure population, examination of obesity and prevention and treatment options will be critical in heart failure patients.

Ephedra, which has been used for the purposes of athletic performance enhancement and weight loss, has been linked to a high rate of serious adverse outcomes, including left ventricular systolic dysfunction, development of heart failure, and cardiac deaths, ultimately resulting in a ban of this agent by the FDA.

Obesity surgery, or bariatric surgery, is recommended for class 2 obesity or above (BMI ≥35 kg/m²), and possibly in individuals with BMI 30 to 34.9 kg/m² when associated with comorbid conditions such as diabetes, sleep apnea, or systemic hypertension. Although severe heart failure or systolic dysfunction is considered a general contraindication to bariatric surgery, there are a few studies that have investigated its safety and efficacy in obese patients with HF,[71,74] with improvement in LVEF and NYHA functional class. Clearly, further prospective studies are needed to better define which patients can be safely referred for bariatric surgery, optimal surgical techniques, as well as effects on long-term outcomes.

Diabetic Cardiomyopathy

Since its first description in 1972, a considerable amount of experimental, pathological, epidemiological, and clinical data have accumulated to support the existence of "diabetic cardiomyopathy." So far, a large body of literature suggests that the occurrence of diabetic cardiomyopathy is an independent phenomenon from macro-angiographic changes in coronary arteries and hypertension. Diabetes is now well recognized as an independent risk factor for the development of heart failure, despite correcting for age, hypertension, obesity, hypercholesterolemia, and coronary artery disease. This subject is covered in further detail in **Chapter 17**.

Hyperthyroidism

Hyperthyroidism has been implicated in causing DCM; however, in view of the increased cardiac contractile function of patients with hyperthyroidism, the development of heart failure is unexpected

and raises the question of whether there truly is a direct causal association between hyperthyroidism and cardiomyopathy. Patients with hyperthyroidism may occasionally have exertional dyspnea or other symptoms and signs of heart failure. Many of these clinical manifestations may be attributed to the direct effects of thyroid hormone on cardiovascular hemodynamics. In most patients with hyperthyroidism, cardiac output is high, and the subnormal response to exercise may be the result of an inability to increase heart rate maximally or to lower vascular resistance further, as normally occurs with exercise. The term "high-output failure" is not appropriate for all cases of cardiomyopathy related to hyperthyroidism, because the ability of the heart to maintain increased cardiac output at rest and with exercise is usually preserved.[75] Occasional patients with severe, long-standing hyperthyroidism have poor cardiac contractility, low cardiac output, and symptoms and signs of heart failure, including a third heart sound and pulmonary congestion. This complex of findings most commonly occurs with persistent sinus tachycardia or atrial fibrillation, and is the result of so-called tachycardia-related heart failure. In older patients with heart disease, the increased workload that results from hyperthyroidism may further impair cardiac function and thus result in DCM. The presence of ischemic or hypertensive heart disease may compromise the ability of the myocardium to respond to the metabolic demands of hyperthyroidism. Histological examination usually reveals a nonspecific pattern, including foci of lymphocytic and eosinophilic infiltration, fibrosis, fatty infiltration, and myofibril hypertrophy. Although enhanced adrenergic activity contributes to the hyperdynamic state in hyperthyroidism, β-adrenergic blockade does not fully return the heart rate or contractility to normal, which may suggest a primary cardiac effect of thyroid hormone with contributory effects of catecholamines.[75]

Hypothyroidism

Abnormalities in cardiac systolic and diastolic performance have been reported both in experimental and clinical studies of hypothyroidism; however, the classic findings of myxedema do not usually indicate cardiomyopathy. The most common signs are bradycardia, mild hypertension, a narrowed pulse pressure, and attenuated activity on the precordial examination. Pericardial effusions and nonpitting edema (myxedema) can occur in patients with severe, long-standing hypothyroidism. The low cardiac output is caused by bradycardia, a decrease in ventricular filling, and a decrease in cardiac contractility. Systemic vascular resistance may increase by as much as 50%, and diastolic relaxation and filling are slowed.[75] However, heart failure is rare, because the cardiac output is usually sufficient to meet the lowered demand for peripheral oxygen delivery. Positron-emission tomographic studies of oxygen consumption in patients with hypothyroidism have revealed that myocardial work efficiency is lower than in normal subjects. From 10% to 25% of patients have diastolic hypertension, which, combined with the increase in vascular resistance, raises cardiac afterload and cardiac work.[75] Abnormal systolic force may improve with thyroid hormone replacement but does not return to normal levels, suggesting the possibility of persistent myocardial dysfunction. Thyroid hormone replacement should be initiated at low doses and titrated slowly, as left ventricular failure may be precipitated. Interestingly, patients with heart failure also have low serum tri-iodothyronine concentrations, and the decrease is proportional to the degree of heart failure. Whether such changes in thyroid hormone metabolism contribute to further impairment of cardiovascular function in patients with heart failure is not known.[75]

Acromegaly and Growth Hormone Deficiency

Impaired cardiovascular function has recently been demonstrated to potentially reduce life expectancy both in growth hormone deficiency and excess. Experimental and clinical studies have supported the evidence that growth hormone and IGF-I are implicated in cardiac development.[76] In most patients with acromegaly, a specific cardiomyopathy, characterized by myocardial hypertrophy with interstitial fibrosis, lympho-mononuclear infiltration, and areas of monocyte necrosis, results in biventricular concentric hypertrophy.[76] Myocardial dysfunction is a major cause of morbidity and mortality in acromegaly, and appears to be related to both the severity and duration of growth hormone excess. Some reports indicate that the treatment of acromegaly might improve cardiac function in the short term, but the long-term prognosis is questionable. Reduction of the LV mass, leading to a consequent improvement of diastolic filling, has been reported after short- and long-term treatment with octreotide.[76]

In contrast, patients with childhood or adulthood-onset growth hormone deficiency may suffer both from structural cardiac abnormalities, such as narrowing of cardiac walls, and functional impairment, which combine to reduce diastolic filling and impair left ventricular response to peak exercise. In addition, growth hormone deficiency patients may have an increase in vascular intima-media thickness and a higher occurrence of atheromatous plaques that can further aggravate the hemodynamic conditions and contribute to increased cardiovascular and cerebrovascular risk. Several studies have suggested that the cardiovascular abnormalities can be partially reversed by suppressing growth hormone and IGF-I levels in acromegaly or after growth hormone replacement therapy in growth hormone deficiency patients.[76] Receptors for both growth hormone and IGF-I are expressed by cardiac myocytes; therefore, growth hormone may act directly on the heart or via the induction of local or systemic IGF-1, while IGF-1 may act by endocrine, paracrine, or autocrine mechanisms. Experimental studies suggested that growth hormone and IGF-1 have stimulatory effects on myocardial contractility, possibly mediated by changes in intracellular

calcium handling. Thus, much attention has been focused on the ability of growth hormone to increase cardiac mass, suggesting its possible use in the treatment of chronic heart failure. Initial studies demonstrated that treatment with growth hormone may result in improvement in hemodynamic and clinical status of patients with heart failure; however, two randomized, placebo-controlled studies did not show any significant growth hormone-mediated improvement in cardiac performance in patients with DCM, despite significant increases in IGF-1.[77]

NUTRITIONAL CAUSES OF CARDIOMYOPATHY

Thiamine Deficiency

Thiamine serves as a cofactor for several enzymes involved primarily in the carbohydrate catabolism and is found in high concentrations in the heart, skeletal muscle, liver, kidneys, and brain. The most common cause of thiamine deficiency in Western countries is chronic alcoholism and anorexia nervosa; AIDS and pregnancy can account for other rare causes of thiamine deficiency. A state of severe depletion can develop in patients on a strict thiamine-deficient diet in approximately 18 to 21 days. Prolonged and large doses of diuretic use can be associated with thiamine deficiency, especially in patients hospitalized with HF.

The major manifestations of thiamine deficiency in humans involve the cardiovascular (wet beriberi) and nervous (dry beriberi, or neuropathy, and/or Wernicke-Korsakoff syndrome) systems. The cardiovascular signs and symptoms include dyspnea, fatigue, leg edema, and palpitations. Tachycardia is common, and there are usually increased jugular venous pressure and warm extremities. Biventricular heart failure is present, and the circulation is usually hyperkinetic. Ultimately circulatory collapse, metabolic acidosis, or shock can develop, at which time the disease has advanced from chronic beriberi to fulminating beriberi heart failure (Shoshin beriberi). Severe lactic acidemia in the presence of a high cardiac output and extremely low oxygen consumption are the classic features of acute fulminant cardiovascular beriberi, which, if unrecognized and untreated, can lead to high cardiac output failure and death. Treatment for Beriberi should consist of administration of thiamine, along with other conventional treatment of circulatory support and heart failure. The main cause is diet being very low in thiamine, and more common in regions where diet includes predominantly white rice or processed food without grain ingredients. Studies on the effects of B-vitamin supplementation in patients with HF are currently lacking.

Carnitine Deficiency

L-carnitine and its derivative, propionyl-L-carnitine, are organic amines necessary for oxidation of fatty acids, the deficiency of which may be associated with a syndrome of progressive skeletal myopathy and lipid vacuoles on muscle biopsy. They have also been shown to reduce intracellular accumulation of toxic metabolites during ischemia, demonstrate protective effect on muscle metabolism injuries, inhibit caspases, and decrease the levels of TNF-α and sphingosine, as well as reduce apoptosis of skeletal muscles cells, and thus have been implied in the treatment of congestive heart failure. Genetic causes of carnitine deficiency are associated with cardiomyopathy, and L-carnitine deficiency has been documented in the failing heart. Several metabolic genes, including the muscle carnitine palmitoyl transferase-1, the key enzyme for the transport of long-chain acyl-coenzyme A (acyl-CoA) compounds into mitochondria, are downregulated in the failing human heart.[78] Inhibitors of carnitine palmitoyl-transferase I (CPT I), such as etomoxir, have been developed as agents for treating diabetes mellitus. Despite initial promising preclinical and phase II clinical results, a double-blind randomized multicenter clinical trial with etomoxir in heart failure was stopped prematurely, because unacceptably high liver transaminase levels were detected in four patients taking etomoxir.[79]

Selenium Deficiency

Selenium deficiency is associated with cardiomyopathy and congestive heart failure in geographic areas where dietary selenium intake is low.[80] This has been named as the Keshan disease, due to the geographical prevalence of a specific form of DCM in northeast China, in which the soil has a low selenium content. Chronic selenium deficiency may also occur in individuals with malabsorption and long-term selenium-deficient parenteral nutrition. Selenium deficiency is implicated in causing cardiomyopathy as a result of the depletion of selenium-associated antioxidant enzymes, selenoenzymes, which protect cell membranes from damage by free radicals. The cardiomyopathy is manifested by insidious onset of congestive heart failure or a complication of sudden death or thromboembolic phenomena. The heart shows biventricular enlargement and histologically exhibit edema, mitochondrial swelling, hypercontraction bands, widespread myocytolysis, and extensive fibrosis.[80]

HEMATOLOGIC CAUSES OF CARDIOMYOPATHY

Cardiomyopathy Due to Iron Overload: Hemochromatosis and Thalassemia

Iron-overload cardiomyopathy manifests itself as systolic or diastolic dysfunction secondary to increased deposition of iron in the heart, and occurs with common genetic disorders such as primary hemochromatosis and beta-thalassemia major.

Hereditary hemochromatosis is an inherited disorder of iron metabolism and is the most common hereditary disease of northern Europeans, with a prevalence of approximately 5 per 1000. It is an autosomal recessive disorder of iron metabolism characterized by increased iron absorption and deposition in the liver, pancreas, heart, joints, and pituitary gland. Without treatment, death may occur from cirrhosis, primary liver cancer, diabetes, or cardiomyopathy. In 1996, HFE, the gene for hereditary hemochromatosis, was mapped on the short arm of chromosome 6.[81] Two mutations, C282Y and H63D, have been implicated in hereditary hemochromatosis. The H63D mutation is significantly increased in patients with DCM.[81] HFE is considered as a candidate gene for population-based genetic testing for diagnosis and detection of hemochromatosis. The complications of hemochromatosis can be devastating, but its clinical management is simple and effective if the disease is identified early in its progression.

Although the exact mechanism of iron-induced heart failure remains to be elucidated, the toxicity of iron in biological systems is attributed to its ability to catalyze the generation of oxygen-free radicals. It has been shown that chronic iron-overload results in dose-dependent increases in myocardial iron burden, decreases in the protective antioxidant enzyme activity, increased free-radical production, and increased mortality.[82] These findings suggest that the mechanism of iron-induced heart dysfunction involves, at least in part, free radical-mediated processes. Myocardial iron deposition is most prominent in and around contractile elements and less common in the conduction system, in contrast to sarcoidosis and amyloidosis, in which the pathologic process commonly involves the conduction system.[82] The mechanism by which iron produces cellular dysfunction is not yet clear, as fibrosis may not be prominent. This also implies that the disease process is reversible if the tissue iron concentration can be controlled. Myocardial iron deposits do not occur until other organs such as liver, pancreas, and connective tissues are saturated with iron. Thus the extracardiac manifestations are present before the cardiomyopathy develops.[82]

Iron overload can occur either as a result of inappropriate excess iron absorption, as in the case of hemochromatosis or thalassemia major, or due to multiple transfusions. The most important manifestations of heart disease in hemochromatosis are congestive heart failure and cardiac arrhythmia. During the initial phases of the cardiomyopathy, the hemodynamic profile represents a restrictive pattern. As the severity of cardiomyopathy advances, DCM with biventricular enlargement and heart failure ensue. The spectrum of arrhythmia ranges from minor abnormalities on the electrocardiogram to supraventricular arrhythmia, atrioventricular conduction block, and ventricular tachyarrhythmia, presumably due to myocardial dysfunction and iron deposition in the conduction system and atrioventricular node. The ECG most commonly shows decreased voltage and nonspecific ST and T wave changes; Q waves are uncommon. Among patients with beta-thalassemia major, biventricular DCM remains the leading cause of mortality. In some patients, a restrictive type of left ventricular cardiomyopathy or pulmonary hypertension is noted. The clinical course, although variable and occasionally fulminant, is more benign in recent than in older series.

The diagnosis of hemochromatosis is suggested by elevated serum ferritin and increased ratio of iron to total iron binding capacity (TIBC). Serum transferrin saturation (serum iron/TIBC of >45% and elevated serum ferritin >200 μg/L in men or >150 μg/L in women) supports the diagnosis.[2] If hereditary hemochromatosis is suspected, especially with a known family history, testing for the HFE genotype should be performed. The most definitive test for calculation of iron stores in the body is by measurement of iron concentration by liver biopsy. Magnetic resonance imaging can also be very useful to identify the iron laden organs and cardiac involvement. Though not required to demonstrate cardiac involvement in every case, endomyocardial biopsy can be useful in the assessment of cardiac iron deposition. The echocardiogram usually reveals increased systolic and diastolic ventricular dimensions, and reduced left ventricular ejection fraction.

Before phlebotomy and chelation therapy, survival among patients with hemochromatosis and heart failure was less than 20% in 5 years. The actuarial survival rates of the individuals who are homozygous for the C282Y mutation of the hemochromatosis gene C282Y have been reported to be 95%, 93%, and 66%, respectively, at 5, 10, and 20 years.[83] Similarly, in patients with thalassemia major, cardiac failure is one of the most frequent causes of death. Chelation therapy, including newer forms of oral chelators, such as deferoxamine, and phlebotomy have dramatically improved the outcome of hemochromatosis. Similarly, chelation therapy has improved prognosis in beta-thalassemia major both by reducing the incidence of heart failure and by reversing cardiomyopathy. It is important to start therapy early, as treatment may prevent or reverse cardiac involvement. Early diagnosis and treatment by phlebotomy before tissue damage has occurred is essential, because life span seems to be normal in treated patients but markedly shortened in those who are not. In addition, genetic counseling with evaluation of first-degree relatives is mandatory.[82] New imaging modalities, especially magnetic resonance imaging, is expected to improve early diagnosis and risk stratification for treatment. By increasing the proportion of patients on optimal chelation, survival in patients with hemochromatosis or beta-thalassemia may further improve.

HEMODYNAMIC AND STRESS-INDUCED CARDIOMYOPATHY

Tachycardia-Induced Dilated Cardiomyopathy

Tachycardia-induced cardiomyopathy is a reversible cause of HF characterized by LV myocardial dysfunction caused by increased ventricular rate. The concept that incessant or chronic tachycardia can lead to reversible LV dysfunction is supported both by animal models of chronic pacing as well as human studies documenting improvement in ventricular function with tachycardia rate or rhythm control. Sustained rapid pacing in experimental animal models can produce severe biventricular systolic dysfunction. In humans, descriptions of reversal of cardiomyopathy with rate or rhythm control of incessant or chronic tachycardias have been reported with atrial tachycardias, accessory pathway reciprocating tachycardias, atrioventricular node reentry, and atrial fibrillation with rapid ventricular responses.[84] Tachycardia-mediated cardiomyopathy is characterized by LV dilatation without hypertrophy; however, during the recovery phase, hypertrophy and persistent diastolic dysfunction occur, suggesting irreversible structural changes despite apparent recovery. Tachycardia as the causative factor of cardiomyopathy is implied by the presence of tachyarrhythmia in the presence of and preceding LV dysfunction, and restoration of hemodynamic and myocardial derangements following elimination of the tachyarrhythmia. Although there are data suggesting that a heart rate greater than 100 beats/min may lead to cardiomyopathy, the heart rate at which cardiomyopathy occurs is not well defined, and may differ according to underlying genetic, hemodynamic, rhythm, and compensatory differences. Regardless, clinicians should be aware that controlling the arrhythmia may result in improvement and even complete normalization of systolic function.[84] Catheter ablation may be required and is often curative. Tachycardia-induced cardiomyopathy may be a more common mechanism of LV dysfunction than recognized, and aggressive treatment of the arrhythmia should be considered.

Premature Ventricular Contractions and Cardiomyopathy

Increased burden of premature ventricular contractions (PVCs) and, similarly, sustained bigeminy or trigeminy in a structurally otherwise normal heart have been associated with the development of cardiomyopathy in certain patients. Improvement and/or resolution of cardiomyopathy has also been reported after elimination or suppression of PVCs, raising the question of a possible PVC-induced cardiomyopathy.[85] Frequently patients may present after the onset of ventricular dysfunction, thus determining whether PVCs are causative or a result of the cardiomyopathy is challenging. The proposed mechanisms underlying PVC-induced cardiomyopathy include ventricular dyssynchrony and increased myocardial oxygen demand. This is supported by evidence that left bundle branch block (LBBB) creates dyssynchrony that can impair diastolic function and worsen mitral regurgitation. PVC burden is related to cardiomyopathy; PVC burden ≥20% is independently associated with cardiomyopathy.[86] The RV outflow tract was the most common origin of PVCs, present in 52%. Radiofrequency ablation has been reported to result in normalization of LVEF, and those patients who did not respond to radiofrequency ablation had progression of cardiomyopathy.[86] PVC-induced cardiomyopathy should be suspected as an etiology of cardiomyopathy in young and otherwise healthy asymptomatic patients without a cardiac history or family history of cardiomyopathy, with greater than 10,000 to greater than 20,000 PVCs per 24 hours, with presence of outflow tract or fascicular morphology, and especially if the patient has an improvement of LV function with PVC suppression and has recovery of LV function with ablation.[2]

Stress-Induced Cardiomyopathy

Stress cardiomyopathy is characterized by acute, usually reversible LV dysfunction in the absence of significant CAD, usually triggered by acute emotional or physical stress.[87] This phenomenon was initially identified by a distinctive pattern of "apical ballooning," first described in Japan as Takotsubo, and often affected postmenopausal women.[88] A majority of patients have a clinical presentation similar to that of acute coronary syndrome and may have transiently elevated cardiac enzymes such as cardiac troponin. Though apical ballooning is seen in most, other diverse ventricular contraction patterns have been defined by cardiovascular magnetic resonance imaging or by echocardiography (Fig. 20.13).[88] In the majority, left ventricular function usually returns to normal rapidly, although delayed recovery over 2 months has been described.[89] Despite reversal to normal cardiac function in most, studies have demonstrated that both short-term mortality and long-term mortality are higher than previously recognized.[88] Resolution of LV dysfunction occurs usually within a week. Right and/or left ventricular thrombi have been described and are usually associated with embolic events underlining the importance of anticoagulation in these patients.

Diagnostic criteria have been proposed for apical ballooning syndrome, which usually require the following criteria to be met: (1) transient hypokinesis, akinesis, or dyskinesis of the LV mid segments with or without apical involvement; the regional wall motion abnormalities extending beyond a single epicardial vascular distribution, where a stressful trigger is often but not always present; (2) absence of obstructive coronary disease or angiographic evidence of acute plaque rupture; (3) new electrocardiographic abnormalities (ST-segment elevation and/or T-wave inversion) or modest elevation in cardiac troponin; and (4) absence of pheochromocytoma or myocarditis.[2]

Despite extensive research, the cause and pathogenesis of stress cardiomyopathy remain incompletely understood. Different emotional or psychological stressors have been identified to precede the onset. Both circulating epinephrine and norepinephrine released from adrenal medullary chromaffin cells and norepinephrine released locally from sympathetic nerve terminals are significantly increased in the acute phase of Takotsubo cardiomyopathy implicated in direct catecholamine toxicity, adrenoceptor-mediated damage, epicardial and microvascular coronary vasoconstriction and/or spasm, and increased cardiac workload, to myocardial damage, which has a functional counterpart of transient apical left ventricular ballooning.[90] The relative preponderance among postmenopausal women suggests that estrogen deprivation may play a facilitating role, probably mediated by endothelial dysfunction.[90]

Though usually benign and rapidly reversible, clinical spectrum can be heterogeneous with about one-third either male, less than 50 years of age, without a stress trigger, or with in-hospital death, nonfatal recurrence, embolic stroke, or delayed normalization of ejection fraction, underlining the importance of follow-up in these patients. Management needs to be individualized with elimination of psychosocial and cardiac stressors, and initiation of standard guideline directed medical therapy.

SUMMARY AND FUTURE DIRECTIONS

As noted at the outset, the dilated cardiomyopathies constitute one of the largest groups of myopathic disorders that are responsible for

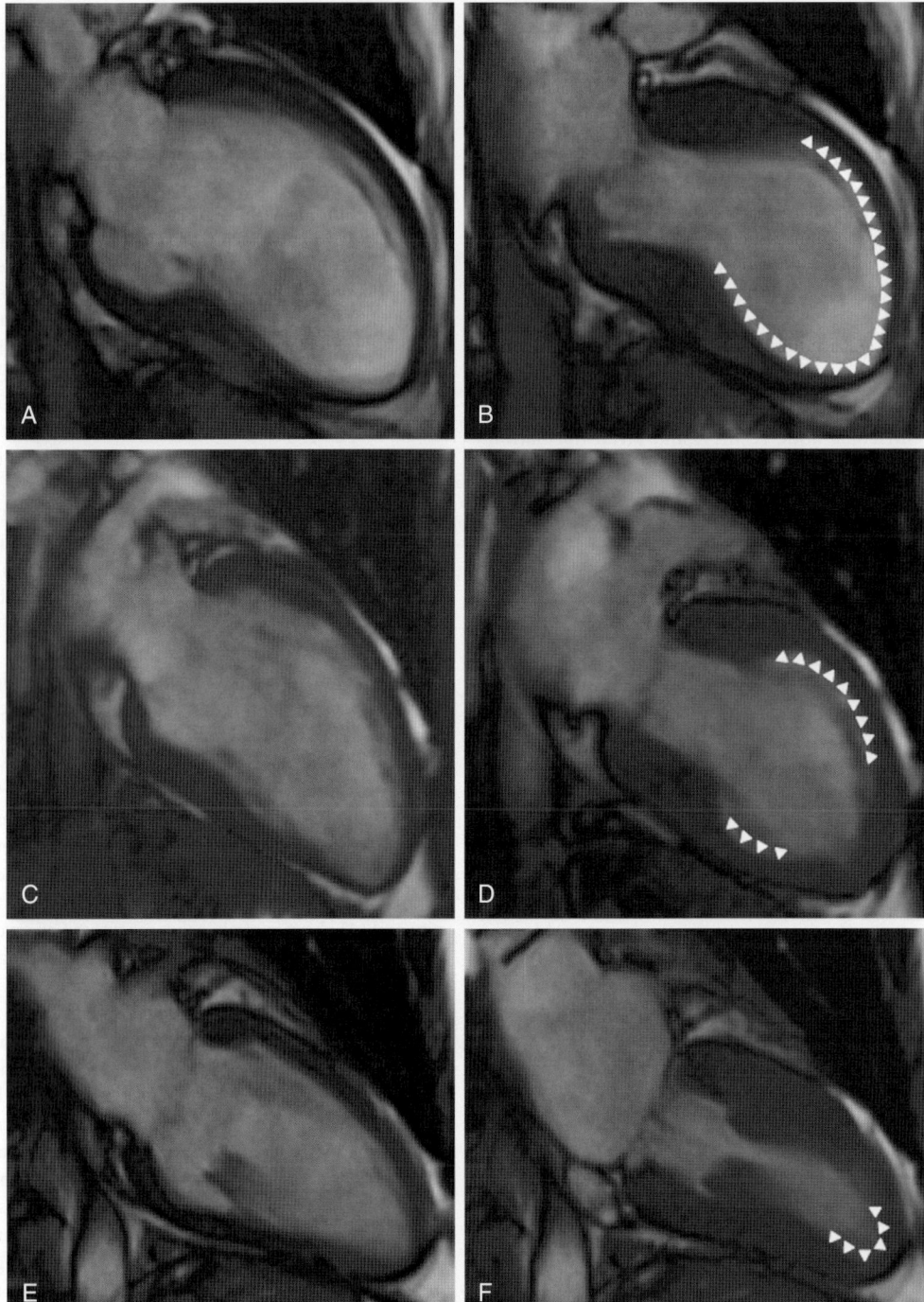

Fig. 20.13 Diversity of left ventricular contraction patterns in stress cardiomyopathy, as demonstrated by cardiac magnetic resonance imaging in vertical long-axis view (A, C, and E) diastole; (B, D, and F) systole. Three types are depicted: (A and B) most common pattern of mid and apical left ventricular (LV) akinesia: Takotsubo type *(arrowheads)*; (C and D) mid-LV akinesia *(arrowheads)* with sparing of apical region; and (E, F) apical LV contraction abnormality only *(arrowheads)*. (From Sharkey SW, Windenburg DC, Lesser, JR, et al. Natural history and expansive clinical profile of stress [tako-tsubo] cardiomyopathy. *J Am Coll Cardiol.* 55[4]:333–341, 2010.)

TABLE 20.3 Specific Treatment Approaches to Dilated Cardiomyopathies

Etiology for DCM	Specific Treatment
Alcoholic	Abstinence
Cocaine, illicit drugs	Abstinence
Collagen vascular disease	
SLE, RA, sarcoidosis	Steroids, cytotoxic or immunomodulating agents
Scleroderma	Steroids, Ca channel blockers for Raynaud
Kawasaki disease	IV Immunoglobulin
Viral myocarditis	Prednisone and immunosuppressant therapy or transplant for fulminant course
Chagas disease	Benznidazole, nifurtimox
HIV/AIDS	Highly active retroviral therapy, increase CD4 count
Nutritional deficiency	
Thiamine, selenium, or carnitine deficiency)	Replacement
Hyperthyroidism/hypothyroidism	Achieve euthyroid state
Uremia	Dialysis
Pheochromocytoma	Removal of tumor
Tachycardia induced	Ablation, maintenance of sinus rhythm
Stress-induced cardiomyopathy	Management of psychosocial stress
Peripartum cardiomyopathy	Multidisciplinary high-risk pregnancy management, avoid subsequent pregnancy if LV function does not normalize
Chemotherapy-induced cardiomyopathy	Reduce dose or discontinue, avoid cardiotoxic other chemotherapy combinations and XRT, initiate early standard treatment for heart failure
Genetic	Genetic counseling, prenatal diagnosis, new experimental treatment modalities with gene editing, RNA silencing or RNA interference

AIDS, Acquired immunodeficiency syndrome; *DCM,* dilated cardiomyopathy; *HIV,* human immunodeficiency virus; *IV,* intravenous; *LV,* left ventricle; *RA,* rheumatoid arthritis; *SLE,* systemic lupus erythematosus; *XRT,* radiation therapy.

systolic heart failure. Recent advances have allowed for the identification of specific genetic, metabolic, infectious, inflammatory, toxin-induced, nutritional, autoimmune, endocrine, nutritional, and hematological causes for DCM. Although the current treatment strategies for the DCM are similar to those for ischemic cardiomyopathy (**see Chapters 37 and 38**), as illustrated in **Table 20.3**, there are also a number of "etiology specific" treatment strategies that clinicians should be consider when treating patients with DCM. While many of these strategies have not been tested in randomized clinical trials, they provide a useful basis for individualizing the care of patients with various etiologies of DCM. Further, the observation that reverse remodeling and recovery of left ventricular function are almost exclusively observed in patients with DCM (**see also Chapter 12**) raises the intriguing possibility that etiology specific treatment strategies in DCM may be more beneficial beyond the generic treatment of HFrEF.

KEY REFERENCES

2. Bozkurt B, Colvin M, Cook J, et al. Current diagnostic and treatment strategies for specific dilated cardiomyopathies: a scientific statement from the American Heart Association. *Circulation.* 2016;134(23):e579–e646.
3. Arbustini E, Narula N, Tavazzi L, et al. The MOGE(S) classification of cardiomyopathy for clinicians. *J Am Coll Cardiol.* 2014;64(3):304–318.
9. Felker GM, Thompson RE, Hare JM, et al. Underlying causes and long-term survival in patients with initially unexplained cardiomyopathy. *N Engl J Med.* 2000;342(15):1077–1084.
10. Dec GW, Fuster V. Idiopathic dilated cardiomyopathy. *N Engl J Med.* 1994;331(23):1564–1575.
12. Sugrue DD, Rodeheffer RJ, Codd MB, Ballard DJ, Fuster V, Gersh BJ. The clinical course of idiopathic dilated cardiomyopathy. A population-based stud. *Ann Intern Med.* 1992;117(2):117–123.
14. Yancy CW, Jessup M, Bozkurt B, et al. 2013 ACCF/AHA guideline for the management of heart failure: a report of the American College of Cardiology Foundation/American Heart Association Task Force on Practice Guidelines. *Circulation.* 2013;128(16):e240–e327.
15. Yancy CW, Jessup M, Bozkurt B, et al. 2017 ACC/AHA/HFSA focused update of the 2013 ACCF/AHA guideline for the management of heart failure: a report of the American College of Cardiology/American Heart Association Task Force on Clinical Practice Guidelines and the Heart Failure Society of America. *Circulation.* 2017;136(6):e137–e161.
55. Elkayam U, Tummala PP, Rao K, et al. Maternal and fetal outcomes of subsequent pregnancies in women with peripartum cardiomyopathy. *N Engl J Med.* 2001;344(21):1567–1571.
87. Maron BJ, Towbin JA, Thiene G, et al. Contemporary definitions and classification of the cardiomyopathies: an American Heart Association scientific statement from the Council on Clinical Cardiology, Heart Failure and Transplantation Committee; quality of care and outcomes research and functional genomics and translational biology interdisciplinary working groups; and Council on Epidemiology and Prevention. *Circulation.* 2006;113(14):1807–1816.
90. Pelliccia F, Kaski JC, Crea F, Camici PG. Pathophysiology of takotsubo syndrome. *Circulation.* 2017;135(24):2426–2441.

The full reference list for this chapter is available on ExpertConsult.

Restrictive and Infiltrative Cardiomyopathies and Arrhythmogenic Right Ventricular Dysplasia/Cardiomyopathy

Joshua M. Hare

Restrictive cardiomyopathy is the least prevalent of cardiomyopathies relative to dilated (**see Chapter 20**) and hypertrophic forms (**see Chapter 23**) of heart muscle diseases.[1] All forms of cardiomyopathy are diseases of heart muscle that result from a myriad of insults, such as genetic defects (**see Chapter 24**), cardiac myocyte injury, or infiltration of myocardial tissues.[2,3] Thus cardiomyopathies result from insults to both cellular elements of the heart, notably the cardiac myocyte, and processes that are external to cells, such as deposition of abnormal substances into the extracellular matrix. Disorders that lead to the abnormal deposition of noncompliant materials in the myocardium preferentially lead to the restrictive cardiomyopathy phenotype,[4] the prototypic causes being deposition of excessive fibrosis and amyloid proteins (**see Chapter 22**).[5] Cardiomyopathies are traditionally defined on the basis of structural and functional phenotypes, notably dilated (characterized primarily by an enlarged ventricular chamber and reduced cardiac performance),[6] hypertrophic (characterized primarily by thickened, hypertrophic ventricular walls and enhanced cardiac performance), and restrictive (characterized primarily by thickened, stiff ventricular walls that impede diastolic filling of the ventricle; cardiac systolic performance is typically close to normal).[4] A fourth, and increasingly appreciated, structural and functional phenotype is a cardiomyopathy that primarily involves the right ventricle—arrhythmogenic right ventricular dysplasia/cardiomyopathy (ARVD/C). This chapter will review restrictive/infiltrative cardiomyopathies and ARVD/C.

RESTRICTIVE AND INFILTRATIVE CARDIOMYOPATHY

Relative to the dilated (**see Chapter 20**) and hypertrophic (**see Chapter 23**) cardiomyopathies, restrictive cardiomyopathy occurs with lower frequency in the developed world. Specific forms of restrictive cardiomyopathy, such as endomyocardial disease (EMD) (**Table 21.1**), are important causes of morbidity and mortality common in specific geographic locales, especially in underdeveloped countries.[7-9] The pathophysiologic feature that defines restrictive cardiomyopathy is the increase in stiffness of the ventricular walls, which causes heart failure because of impaired diastolic filling of the ventricle (**see also Chapters 11, 23, and 39**).[10] In early stages of the syndrome, systolic function may be normal, although deterioration in systolic function is usually observed as the disease progresses.[4]

Restrictive cardiomyopathy must be distinguished from constrictive pericarditis, which is also characterized by normal or nearly normal

TABLE 21.1 Classification of Types of Restrictive Cardiomyopathy According to Cause

Myocardial

Noninfiltrative
Idiopathic cardiomyopathy[a]
Familial cardiomyopathy
Hypertrophic cardiomyopathy
Scleroderma
Pseudoxanthoma elasticum
Diabetic cardiomyopathy

Infiltrative
Amyloidosis[a]
Sarcoidosis[a]
Gaucher disease
Hurler disease
Fatty infiltration

Storage Disease
Hemochromatosis
Fabry disease
Glycogen storage disease

Endomyocardial
Endomyocardial fibrosis[a]
Hypereosinophilic syndrome
Carcinoid heart disease
Metastatic cancers
Radiation[a]
Toxic effects of anthracycline[a]
Drugs causing fibrous endocarditis (serotonin, methysergide, ergotamine, mercurial agents, busulfan)

[a]These conditions are more likely than the others to be encountered in clinical practice.
From Kushwaha SS, Fallon JT, Fuster V. Restrictive cardiomyopathy. *N Engl J Med* 1997;336:267–276; Hare JM. The dilated and restrictive cardiomyopathies. In: Bonow RL, et al., eds. *Braunwald's Heart Disease*. 9th ed. Philadelphia: Elsevier; 2011:1561–1581.

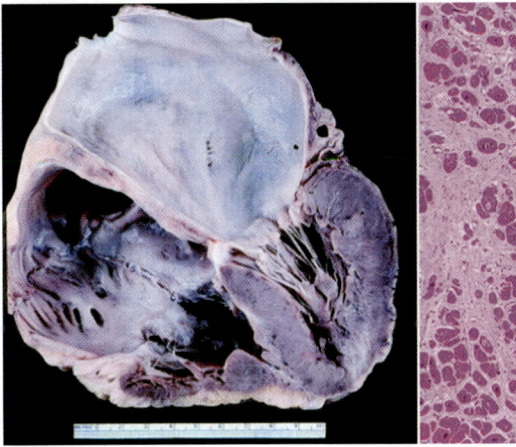

Fig. 21.1 Pathology of idiopathic restrictive cardiomyopathy in a 63-year-old woman. *Left,* Gross cardiac specimen shown in four-chamber format, demonstrating prominent biatrial enlargement, with normal size ventricles. *Right,* Light microscopy showing marked interstitial fibrosis *(light pink areas).* Hematoxylin and eosin; magnification 120×. Modified from Ammash NM, Seward JB, Bailey KR, Edwards WD, Tajik AJ. Clinical profile and outcome of idiopathic restrictive cardiomyopathy. *Circulation.* 2000;101:2490; Hare JM. The dilated and restrictive cardiomyopathies. In: Bonow RL, Mann D, Zipes D, Libby P, ed. *Braunwald's Heart Disease.* 9th ed. Philadelphia: Elsevier; 2011:1561–1581.

Clinical Evaluation

Cardiac Catheterization and Endomyocardial Biopsy

Restrictive Cardiomyopathy Versus Constrictive Pericarditis. A classic diagnostic challenge is to differentiate restrictive cardiomyopathy from constrictive pericarditis, which manifests with similar clinical and hemodynamic features. Cardiac catheterization is a key step in this evaluation (**see also Chapter 31**). Although there is equalization of diastolic pressures in constrictive pericarditis (pressures differ by no more than 5 mm Hg), they may vary to a greater extent in restrictive cardiomyopathy. Pulmonary hypertension is worse in restrictive cardiomyopathy, with systolic pulmonary pressures often exceeding 50 mm Hg. In constrictive pericarditis, the plateau of right ventricular diastolic pressure is usually at least one-third of peak systolic pressure; in restrictive cardiomyopathy, this is most often lower. Hemodynamically both conditions have a rapid early diastolic pressure decline followed by a rapid rise and plateau in early diastole, the so-called square root sign. The atrial pressure tracing manifests either a classic square root pattern or an M or W waveform when the *x* descent is also rapid. Both *a* and *v* waves are prominent and frequently have the same amplitude. Right- and left-sided atrial filling pressures are elevated, although in the case of restrictive cardiomyopathy the left ventricular filling pressure typically is 5 mm Hg or more than the right ventricular diastolic pressure. This difference may be accentuated by the Valsalva maneuver, exercise, or a fluid challenge.

Endomyocardial biopsy can also be valuable in the evaluation of these patients to exclude an infiltrative process or cardiomyopathic-appearing myocytes and received a class IIa recommendation in the guidelines.[16] A normal-appearing biopsy supports the diagnosis of a pericardial process. Surgical exploration is needed far less often, given the availability of biopsy and imaging technology (see later discussion).[17]

Prognosis

Restrictive cardiomyopathy carries a variable prognosis dependent on the cause (**Fig. 21.2**). Most often, especially in the case of amyloidosis,

systolic function but abnormal ventricular filling.[4] Differentiation[11] of these two conditions represents a classic diagnostic challenge and is one of significant clinical importance because pericardial constriction may be treated successfully with pericardiectomy.[12]

Approximately 50% of cases of restrictive cardiomyopathy result from specific clinical disorders, whereas the remainder represent an idiopathic process. The most common specific cause of restrictive cardiomyopathy is infiltration caused by amyloidosis—there are both acquired and genetic causes of amyloid (**see Chapter 22**).[13] Although there are other specific pathologic presentations associated with restrictive cardiomyopathy, their precise etiology often remains obscure. Like dilated cardiomyopathy (DCM), there are inflammatory and genetic factors important in the cause of restrictive cardiomyopathy. Recently, mutations in the troponin T *(TNNT2),* troponin I *(TNNI3),* α-actin *(ACTC),* and β-myosin heavy chain *(MYH7)* genes coding for these sarcomere subunits have been mapped as causes of restrictive cardiomyopathy.[2,3,14] The identification of specific infiltrative processes may have prognostic and therapeutic implications.[15] The abnormal diastolic properties of the ventricle are attributable to myocardial fibrosis, infiltration, or scarring of the endomyocardial surface. Myocyte hypertrophy is common, particularly in idiopathic restrictive cardiomyopathy (**Fig. 21.1**).

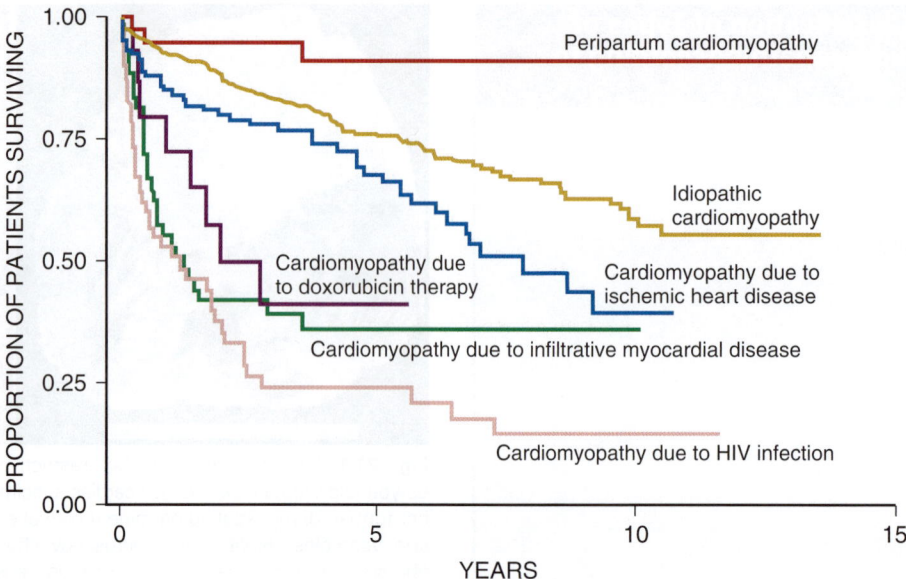

Fig. 21.2 Adjusted Kaplan-Meier estimates of survival among patients with infiltrative cardiomyopathies. Survival of patients with idiopathic cardiomyopathy is shown for comparison. Modified from Felker GM, Thompson RE, Hare JM, et al. Underlying causes and long-term survival in patients with initially unexplained cardiomyopathy. *N Engl J Med.* 2000;342:1077; Hare JM. The dilated and restrictive cardiomyopathies. In: Bonow RL, et al., eds. *Braunwald's Heart Disease.* 9th ed, Philadelphia: Elsevier; 2011:1561–1581.

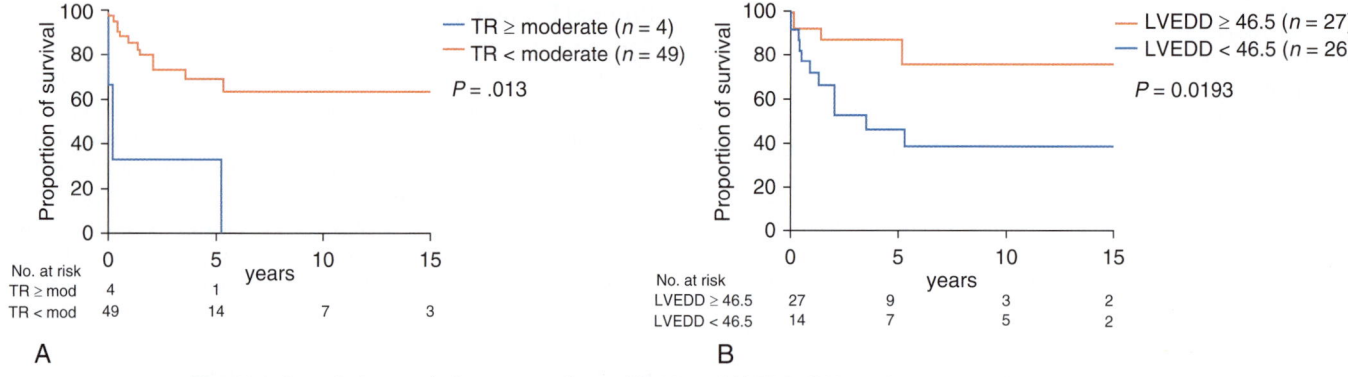

Fig. 21.3 Cumulative survival rate according to TR (A) and LVEDD (B) in patients with idiopathic restrictive cardiomyopathy. *LVEDD,* Left ventricular end-diastolic diameter; *TR,* tricuspid regurgitation. Modified from Hong JA, Kim MS, Cho MS, et al. Clinical features of idiopathic restrictive cardiomyopathy: a retrospective multicenter cohort study over 2 decades. *Medicine [Baltimore].* 2017;96:e7886.

it is invariably progressive with an accelerated mortality.[18] Hong and colleagues recently reported in a series of patients ($n = 53$) with idiopathic restrictive cardiomyopathy that 5-year survival was 64% and that predictors of mortality were tricuspid regurgitation and smaller left ventricular (LV) chamber size[4] (**Fig. 21.3**). There is no specific therapy for the idiopathic form of restrictive cardiomyopathy, but intensive fluid and supportive management is required to maintain a patient with a reasonable quality of life. There are ongoing aggressive attempts to devise therapies for secondary forms of restrictive cardiomyopathy tailored to the cause (e.g., iron removal in hemochromatosis or enzyme replacement therapy in Fabry disease).

Clinical Manifestations

Patients with restrictive cardiomyopathy frequently present with exercise intolerance that results from an impaired ability to augment cardiac output during increasing heart rate because of the restriction of diastolic filling. Other notable symptoms are weakness, dyspnea, and edema. Exertional chest pain is reported by some but not all patients. With advancing disease, profound edema occurs that includes peripheral edema, hepatomegaly, ascites, and anasarca. These patients represent the most difficult volume management because of the balance between volume status and hypotension that can result during diuresis because of reduced preload filling of the ventricles. Physical examination is notable for an elevated jugular venous pulse, often with the Kussmaul sign, and a rising jugular pressure during inspiration (because of the restriction to filling). Both S_3 and S_4 gallops are common and the apical pulse is palpable (in contrast to constrictive pericarditis). Patients with restrictive cardiomyopathy are highly prone to developing atrial fibrillation.[4]

Laboratory Studies

Computed tomography and magnetic resonance imaging (MRI) are valuable for differentiating constrictive and restrictive disease.[17] A thickened pericardium supports the diagnosis of pericardial constriction. Other ancillary tests also may be helpful. For example, chest roentgenography may detect pericardial calcification. The electrocardiogram (ECG) may disclose atrial fibrillation. Echocardiography should be routinely performed in patients suspected of restrictive cardiomyopathy or constriction and may reveal biatrial dilation and increasing wall thickness associated with myocardial infiltration, as well as alterations in the appearance of the myocardium (e.g., speckling). Doppler echocardiography supplemented with tissue Doppler reveals evidence of myocardial relaxation with increased early left ventricular filling velocity, decreased atrial filling velocity, and decreased isovolumetric relaxation time. The latter findings are additionally useful for the discrimination from constrictive disease.[4,19] Brain naturetic peptide (BNP) levels may be used to discriminate between restrictive cardiomyopathy and constrictive disease, with concentrations approximately five times greater in the former compared with the latter.[20]

INHERITED AND ACQUIRED INFILTRATIVE DISORDERS CAUSING RESTRICTIVE CARDIOMYOPATHY

The heritable metabolic disorders resulting from the myocardial accumulation or infiltration of abnormal metabolic products represent an important cause of restrictive cardiomyopathy. These disorders produce classic restrictive cardiomyopathy with diastolic impairment and variable degrees of systolic dysfunction. The heritable metabolic disorders include Fabry disease, Gaucher disease, the glycogenoses, and the mucopolysaccharidoses. Early diagnosis is increasingly important because of the availability, in some cases, of effective enzyme replacement therapy.

Fabry Disease

Fabry disease, or *angiokeratoma corporis diffusum universale*, is an X-linked recessive disorder that results in deficiency of the lysosomal enzyme α-galactosidase A, and the resultant accumulation of glycosphingolipids (most notably globotriaosylceramide) in lysosomes.[21,22] The major clinical features result from the accumulation of glycolipid substrate in the endothelium. More than 160 different mutations are described that have a varying impact, ranging from the absence of α-galactosidase activity to an attenuated level of activity of this enzyme. Patients with absent α-galactosidase activity exhibit widespread systemic manifestations with prominent kidney and cutaneous manifestations, whereas those with an attenuated level of enzyme activity have atypical variants of Fabry disease that may cause isolated myocardial disease. Histologic evaluation of the heart demonstrates diffuse involvement of the myocardium, vascular endothelium, conduction system, and valves—most notably the mitral valve.

Cardiac Findings

Patients with Fabry disease often experience angina pectoris and myocardial infarction caused by the accumulation of lipid species in the coronary endothelium, although epicardial coronary arteries are angiographically normal. The ventricular walls are thickened and have mildly diminished diastolic compliance with normal systolic function. Mild mitral regurgitation may be present. Diastolic abnormalities detected by Doppler echocardiography may be one of the earlier manifestations preceding cardiac hypertrophy, although cardiac MRI may be the preferred diagnostic method.[23] Males almost always present with symptomatic cardiovascular involvement, whereas female carriers may be completely asymptomatic or have only minimal symptoms.[24] Other common features of the disorder include systemic hypertension, congestive heart

failure, and mitral valve prolapse. Echocardiography demonstrates increased ventricular wall thickness, which may mimic hypertrophic cardiomyopathy.[21] Although echocardiography may not be sufficient to do so, cardiac MRI may be able to differentiate Fabry disease from other infiltrative processes such as amyloidosis.[25,26] The surface ECG may reveal a short PR interval, atrioventricular block, and ST segment and T wave abnormalities. The endomyocardial biopsy and low plasma α-galactosidase A activity offer a definitive diagnosis, which has therapeutic implications because enzyme replacement therapy for Fabry disease is safe and effective[27]; moreover heart biopsy may be used to monitor response to therapy.[28] Administration of recombinant α-galactosidase A can ameliorate the stores of globotriaosylceramide from the heart and other tissues, leading to symptomatic, clinical, and echocardiographic improvement (**Fig. 21.4**).[27,28] Although enzyme reduction therapy is the mainstay of treatment, substrate reduction therapy (upstream inhibition of glycosphingolipids biosynthesis) and gene therapy are also being evaluated.

Gaucher Disease

Gaucher disease results from a heritable deficiency of β-glucosidase, which leads to an accumulation of cerebrosides in diffuse organs including spleen, liver, bone marrow, lymph nodes, brain, and heart. Cardiac disease manifests as a stiffened ventricle caused by reduced chamber compliance, leading to impaired cardiac performance. Other manifestations include left ventricular failure and enlargement, hemorrhagic pericardial effusion, and sclerotic, calcified left-sided valves. Gaucher disease is responsive to enzyme replacement therapy or, in more extreme cases, hepatic transplantation; both therapies contribute to reducing tissue infiltration by cerebrosides and can lead to varying degrees of clinical improvement.[29]

Hemochromatosis

Hemochromatosis results from excessive deposition of iron in a variety of parenchymal tissues, notably the heart, liver, gonads, and pancreas. The classic pentad is a symptom complex of heart failure, cirrhosis, impotence, diabetes, and arthritis. The most frequent form of hemochromatosis is inherited as an autosomal recessive disorder that arises from a mutation in the *HFE* gene, which codes for a transmembrane protein that is responsible for regulating iron uptake in the intestine and liver. Hemochromatosis may also arise from ineffective erythropoiesis secondary to a defect in hemoglobin synthesis, as well as from chronic liver disease, or may be acquired as a result of chronic and excessive oral or parenteral intake of iron or blood transfusions.[30]

Iron deposition in the heart is almost always accompanied by varying degrees of infiltration of the liver, spleen, pancreas, and bone marrow, although the degrees of different organ system involvement may not parallel each other. Cardiac involvement produces a mixed pattern of systolic and diastolic dysfunction that is often accompanied by arrhythmias. The severity of hemochromatosis is less, and age of onset is later in women because of the menstrual loss of iron. Cardiac toxicity results directly from the free iron moiety, in addition to adverse effects of tissue infiltration. Death results most frequently from cirrhosis and hepatocellular carcinoma, whereas cardiac mortality accounts for an additional one-third of the mortality and is particularly important in the group of male patients who present at relatively younger ages.

Pathology

Grossly the hearts are dilated, and ventricular walls are thickened. Iron deposits locate preferentially in the myocyte sarcoplasmic reticulum, more frequently in ventricular versus atrial cardiomyocytes.

BASELINE **POST-TREATMENT**

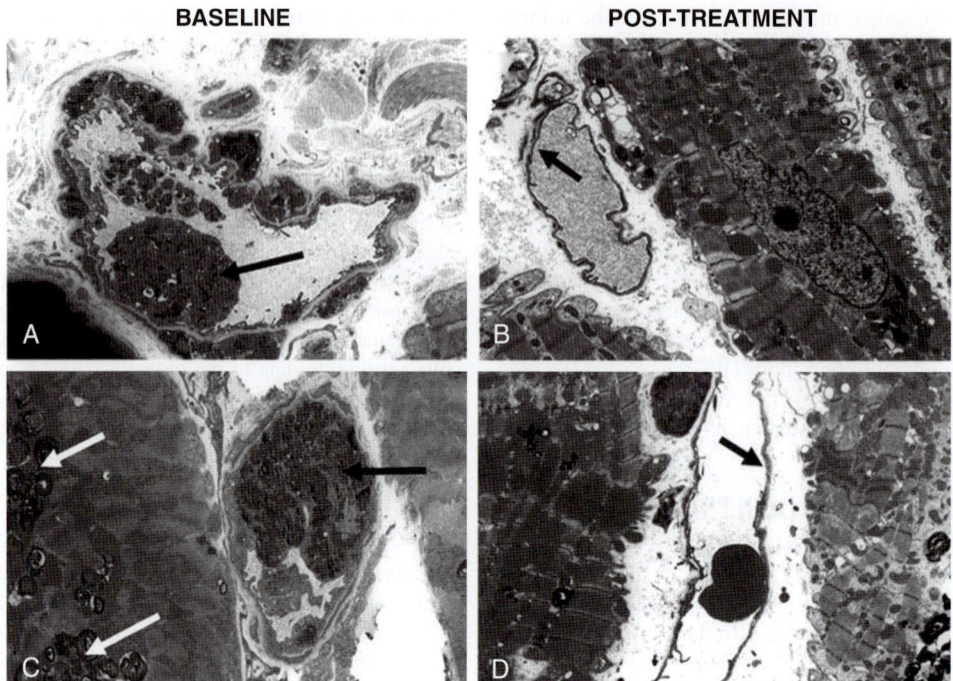

Fig. 21.4 Electron microscopy demonstrates clearance of globotriaosylceramide from cardiac capillaries. (A and C) The substrate accumulates in the endothelial cells of the cardiac capillaries and protrudes into the capillary lumen. (B and D) By 12 months after treatment, the substrate has been cleared from the endothelium. From Thurberg BL, Fallon JT, Mitchell R, et al. Cardiac microvascular pathology in Fabry disease: evaluation of endomyocardial biopsies before and after enzyme replacement therapy. *Circulation.* 2009;119:2561–2567.

Frequently, the conduction system is involved, and loss of myocytes with fibrosis is often present. The degree of iron deposition correlates with the extent of myocardial dysfunction.

Clinical Manifestations

Symptoms at presentation vary widely, and some patients are asymptomatic, although evidence exists for myocardial involvement. Echocardiography reveals increased left ventricular wall thickness, ventricular dilation, and ventricular dysfunction. Both computed tomography and MRI are useful to detect early subclinical myocardial involvement at a time when therapy is most effective.[31] ECG manifestations occur with advancing cardiac involvement and include ST segment and T wave abnormalities, and supraventricular arrhythmias.

Clinical and echocardiographic features usually are diagnostic, and endomyocardial biopsy is confirmatory but because of false negativity cannot definitively rule out the diagnosis. Evaluation of iron metabolism may aid in the diagnosis. Plasma iron levels are elevated, total iron-binding capacity is low or normal, and serum ferritin, urinary iron, liver iron, and especially saturation of transferrin are markedly elevated. Management should include repeated phlebotomies and/or treatment with chelating agents such as desferrioxamine. For advanced disease, cardiac transplantation carries acceptable 5- and 10-year survival rates, and combined liver and heart transplantation is described.[32,33]

Glycogen Storage Disease

Patients with type II, III, IV, and V glycogen storage diseases may have cardiac involvement. However, survival to adulthood is rare, with the exception of patients with type III disease (glycogen debranching enzyme deficiency). The most typical cardiac involvement is left ventricular hypertrophy, with electrocardiographic and echocardiographic findings, often with the absence of symptoms. A subset of patients may present with overt cardiac dysfunction, arrhythmias, and presentation of a DCM.

Inflammatory Causes of Infiltrative Cardiomyopathy (see also Chapter 20)

Sarcoidosis

Sarcoidosis is a systemic inflammatory condition characterized by the formation of noncaseating granulomas, most commonly involving the lungs, reticuloendothelial system, and skin. Sarcoid has been reported to involve essentially all tissues, including the heart, which is recognized in 20% to 30% of autopsies of affected patients. Cardiac impairment may also arise secondary to pulmonary sarcoidosis, in which case extensive pulmonary fibrosis leads to advancing right-sided heart failure. The main clinical manifestations of sarcoid heart disease result from infiltration of the conduction system and myocardium, producing heart block, malignant arrhythmias, heart failure, and sudden cardiac death. Patients with cardiac sarcoidosis may also present with a restrictive cardiomyopathy caused by increased ventricular chamber stiffness.[34]

Pathology. Noncaseating granulomas surrounded by multinucleated giant cells are the diagnostic feature of the disorder and are found in multiple organs. In the heart they infiltrate the myocardium and lead to the formation of fibrotic scars. The condition must be separated from two other inflammatory conditions of the heart—chronic active myocarditis and giant cell myocarditis (**see Chapter 28**). Giant cell myocarditis, which is characterized by diffuse giant cell inflammation in the absence of discrete granulomas, has a much more fulminant course than cardiac sarcoid (**Fig. 21.5**).[16,35] In sarcoidosis, the granulomas may

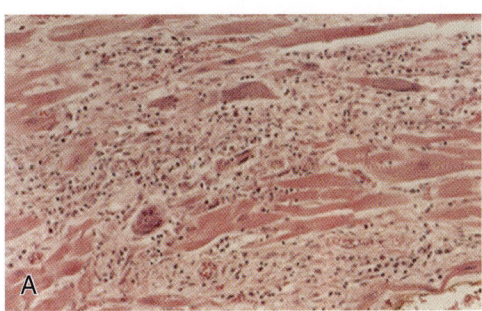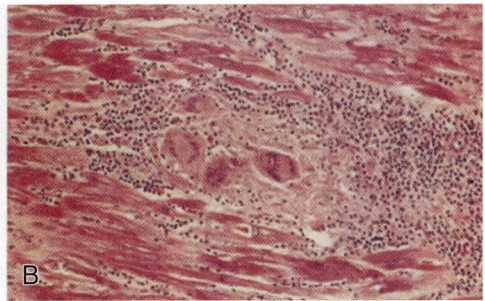

Fig. 21.5 Sarcoid versus giant cell myocarditis. Giant cell myocarditis (A) is characterized by lymphocytic infiltration, myocyte necrosis, and giant cells. Sarcoidosis (B) is characterized by the presence of true noncaseating granulomas. From Hare JM. Etiologic basis of congestive heart failure. In: Colucci WS, ed. *Atlas of Heart Failure.* 5th ed. Philadelphia: Current Medicine LLC; 2008.

involve discrete areas of the ventricular walls in a patchy fashion, increasing the likelihood of a false-negative endomyocardial biopsy result. Granulomas are most commonly observed in the interventricular septum and left ventricular free wall, and patients with conduction system disease typically have involvement of the basal portion of the interventricular septum. Left ventricular aneurysm formation may occur with extensive transmural free wall involvement. In terms of the coronary anatomy, the large conductance vessels are usually spared, but small coronary artery branches may be involved.

Clinical Manifestations. The clinical manifestations result from infiltration of the conduction system and myocardium. The most devastating presentation is that of sudden death caused by malignant ventricular arrhythmia. Patients may also present with heart block, congestive heart failure, and syncope. Both atrial and ventricular arrhythmias are common.[36] Patients may be asymptomatic despite significant cardiac involvement. Heart failure may result from direct myocardial involvement or cor pulmonale as a result of extensive pulmonary fibrosis. Survival may range from months to years, with the presence of a positive endomyocardial biopsy heralding a grave outcome.[37] An excellent long-term outcome may be achieved with aggressive immunosuppression. Isolated cardiac sarcoid has been reported.

The initial detection of cardiac sarcoidosis often results from the presence of bilateral hilar lymphadenopathy on chest roentgenogram in individuals with clinical or ECG findings suggesting myocardial disease. Endomyocardial biopsy should be performed if available because of the importance of positive findings, but it has a high false-negative rate.[16,37] Advanced cytogenetic analysis of biopsy samples may distinctly show a high number of CD209+ dendritic cells and CD68+ macrophages and less likely CD163+ M2 macrophages (nonischemic cardiomyopathy controls). Multiple imaging modalities assist in assessing diagnosis and prognosis. Echocardiography may demonstrate either global or regional left ventricular dysfunction and rarely may reveal aneurysm formation. Echocardiography is also valuable to evaluate right ventricular hypertrophy and to estimate pulmonary artery systolic pressures. Cardiac MRI is emerging as a highly sensitive and specific test (**Fig. 21.6**).[38] Other modalities include myocardial nuclear imaging with thallium 201, technetium 99m, which can reveal segmental perfusion defects because of granulomatous inflammation, and (^{18}F)-fluorodeoxyglucose positron emission tomography (**Fig. 21.7**), which can reveal focal uptake consistent with sarcoid. Uptake of technetium pyrophosphate, gallium, or labeled antimyosin antibody may also contribute to making the diagnosis.

The physical examination may show evidence of extracardiac sarcoid or may be totally normal. An apical systolic murmur as a result of mitral regurgitation is frequently present, often arising from cardiac chamber dilation as opposed to direct papillary muscle infiltration. Murmurs of tricuspid regurgitation, pulmonic regurgitation, and right-sided third heart sounds suggest pulmonary hypertension and cor pulmonale. Both S_3 and S_4 are frequently appreciated.

Electrocardiography typically demonstrates nonspecific findings suggestive of myocardial involvement, with T wave abnormalities commonly present. The ECG is highly valuable to assess the degree of conduction system involvement in terms of intraventricular delays and atrioventricular block. Q waves may be present indicating severe and extensive myocardial replacement and fibrosis. Typical findings on echocardiography include left ventricular dilation with global or regional hypokinesis, right-sided enlargement and hypertrophy, possible left ventricular aneurysm formation, and not infrequently, pericardial effusion. Occasionally, increased echogenicity suggests an infiltrative process.

Management. Sarcoidosis is generally treated with immunosuppression, which can be highly effective.[16,34] Conduction disturbance, arrhythmias, and myocardial dysfunction may all respond to corticosteroids. Steroids effectively halt the progression of inflammation, and some studies suggest that therapy may offer improved survival. Other drugs that may be of benefit in sarcoidosis and are steroids sparing include hydroxychloroquine, methotrexate, azathioprine, leflunomide, mycophenolate mofetil, and cyclophosphamide. Infliximab or adalimumab for tumor necrosis factor-α inhibition and rituximab against the CD20 antigen on the surface of B lymphocytes have also been used for steroid-resistant refractory cases. It is important to distinguish cardiac sarcoidosis from giant cell myocarditis (**see Chapter 28**), a much more aggressive disorder that requires intensive immunosuppression and frequently mechanical support or heart transplantation. Although antiarrhythmic therapy is often ineffective for controlling malignant arrhythmias, implantable cardioverter defibrillator (ICD) therapy is appropriate for patients at risk for sudden cardiac death. Catheter ablation is indicated for patients with ventricular arrhythmias refractory to immunosuppressive and antiarrhythmic therapy. Implantation of a permanent pacemaker is often required in the case of conduction system disease. Advanced heart failure therapies in the form of left ventricular assist device (LVAD) implantation or heart or heart-lung transplantation should be considered in the case of intractable heart failure, although recurrence of sarcoid may occur in the grafted organ.

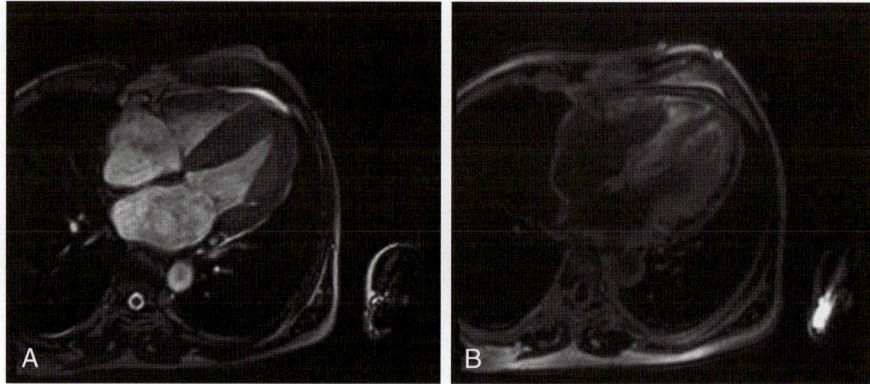

Fig. 21.6 Cardiac magnetic resonance imaging of patient with cardiac sarcoidosis. (A) Early gadolinium phase. Note the thickened heart walls. (B) Diffuse late gadolinium enhancement of the myocardium. From Muchtar E, Blauwet LA, Gertz MA. Restrictive cardiomyopathy: genetics, pathogenesis, clinical manifestations, diagnosis, and therapy. *Circ Res.* 2017;121:819–837.

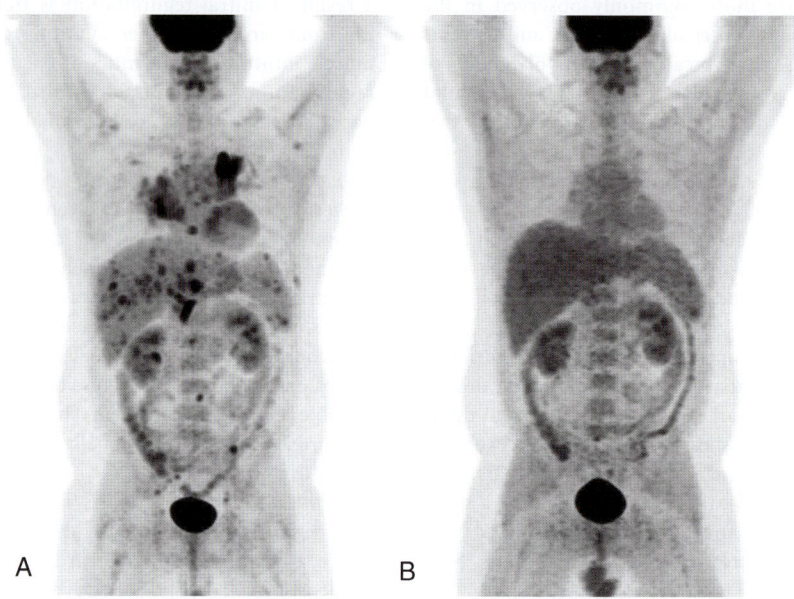

A   B

Fig. 21.7 Fluorodeoxyglucose (FDG)–positron emission tomography/computed tomography imaging in a patient with cardiac and extracardiac sarcoidosis (maximum intensity projection). (A) Multiple focal sites of increased FDG activity in the heart, peribronchovascular, portocaval, periportal, mesenteric, pelvic and inguinal lymph nodes, liver, spleen, and bones can be noted. (B) After 6 months of immunosuppression, no focal hypermetabolic lesions are detected. From Muchtar E, Blauwet LA, Gertz MA. Restrictive cardiomyopathy: genetics, pathogenesis, clinical manifestations, diagnosis, and therapy. *Circ Res.* 2017;121:819–837.

Endomyocardial Disease

Definition and Pathogenesis

A common form of restrictive cardiomyopathy found in a geographic location close to the equator is known as endomyocardial disease. EMD is common in equatorial Africa and manifests less frequently in South America, Asia, and nontropical countries, including the United States. Two variants are described that, despite similar phenotypes, are likely unique processes, both manifesting as aggressive endocardial scarring obliterating the ventricular apices and subvalvular regions. Endomyocardial fibrosis (EMF) or Davies disease is the first variant and occurs primarily in tropical regions, and the second, Löffler endocarditis parietalis fibroplastica, or the hypereosinophilic syndrome, is encountered in more temperate zones. Although the pathologic appearance of these two disorders is similar, there are sufficient differences between them, suggesting that they indeed are two distinct entities. Löffler endocarditis is more aggressive and rapidly progresses, affects mainly males, and is associated with hypereosinophilia, thromboemboli, and systemic arteritis; EMF occurs in a younger distribution, affects young children, and is only variably associated with eosinophilia.

Differences Between Löffler Endocarditis and Endomyocardial Fibrosis

Overlap between Löffler endocarditis and EMF is suggested by the observation that both diseases are attributable to the direct toxic effects of eosinophils in the myocardium. It is suggested that hypereosinophilia (regardless of cause) produces the first phase of EMD, which is characterized by necrosis, intense myocarditis, and arteritis (i.e., Löffler endocarditis). This phase lasts for a period of months and is then followed by a thrombotic stage a year following the initial presentation, in which a nonspecific thickening of the myocardium with a layer of thrombus replaces the inflammatory portion of the myocardium. In the late phase, final healing is achieved by the formation of fibrosis, at which point the clinical features of EMF are present. Most of the support for this three-stage pathophysiology, namely necrotic, thrombotic, and fibrotic, comes from autopsy studies. Nonetheless, definitive evidence that each patient passes sequentially through these stages is lacking.

Role of Eosinophils

The mechanisms by which eosinophils participate in the development of cardiac disease is not completely understood. These cells have the capacity to directly infiltrate tissues or release factors that may exert toxicity. The observation that patients with Löffler endocarditis have degranulated eosinophils in their peripheral blood supports the idea that these granules contain cardiotoxic substances capable of causing the necrotic phase of EMD, which leads to the thrombotic and fibrotic phases once the eosinophilia resolves. It is conceivable that this effect may occur only in temperate zones of the world, because the link between eosinophilia and EMF is less clear (although parasitic diseases have increased incidence), suggesting that in tropical countries EMF may result from a different mechanism. Factors implicated include elevated cerium levels, high vitamin D, serotonin toxicity, hypomagnesemia, and ingestion of a cyanogenic glycoside, linamarin (found in the cassava tuber).

Löffler Endocarditis: The Hypereosinophilic Syndrome

In temperate climates, EMD is closely associated with significant hypereosinophilia, which can have several different causes. Hypereosinophilia associated with Löffler endocarditis usually is characterized by eosinophil counts exceeding $1500/mm^3$ for at least 6 months. Most patients with this degree of hypereosinophilia will have cardiac involvement. The eosinophilia may be secondary to leukemia, reactive disorders such as parasite infection, allergies, granulomatous syndromes, hypersensitivity, or neoplastic disorders. In addition, patients with Churg-Strauss syndrome, characterized by asthma or allergic rhinitis and a necrotizing vasculitis, often have cardiac involvement.[39]

Pathology. Hypereosinophilic syndrome involves several organ systems beyond the heart, including the lungs, brain, and bone marrow. Both chambers of the heart are involved and manifest with endocardial thickening of the inflow regions and ventricular apices. Histologically there are variable degrees of eosinophilic myocarditis of the myocardium and subendocardium, thrombosis and inflammation of small intramural coronary vessels, mural thrombosis containing eosinophils, and endocardial fibrotic thickening several millimeters thick.

Clinical Manifestations. Patients with hypereosinophilic syndrome exhibit weight loss, fever, cough, rash, and congestive heart failure. Early in the course of cardiac involvement, patients may be asymptomatic, but with progression in excess of 50%, patients will have overt congestive heart failure and/or cardiomegaly. Murmurs of mitral regurgitation are common. Systemic emboli occur frequently—resulting in neurologic and renal sequelae. Death results from heart failure associated with renal, hepatic, or pulmonary involvement. Sudden cardiac death and syndromes mimicking acute myocardial infarction are described.

Laboratory Examination. Chest roentgenography may demonstrate an enlarged cardiac silhouette accompanied by evidence of pulmonary congestion or less frequently pulmonary infiltrates. Changes on the *ECG* are nonspecific and include ST segment and T wave abnormalities. Atrial fibrillation and conduction defects, most notably right bundle branch block, are often noted. The echocardiogram often shows regional thickening of the posterobasal portion of the left ventricular wall, with substantial impairment in the motion of the posterior leaflet of the mitral valve. The apex may be obliterated by thrombus. The atria are often dilated, and there is Doppler ultrasound evidence of atrioventricular regurgitation. As is typical for restrictive cardiomyopathy, systolic function is often normal. Hemodynamic measurements support a restrictive cardiomyopathic appearance with abnormal diastolic filling, secondary to the dense endocardial scarring and reduced size of the ventricular cavity from the organized thrombus. Regurgitation through atrioventricular valves results from involvement of their respective supporting structures. *Cardiac catheterization* reveals markedly elevated ventricular filling pressures, and there may be evidence of tricuspid or mitral regurgitation. A characteristic feature on *angiocardiography* is largely preserved systolic function with obliteration of the apex of the ventricles. *Endomyocardial biopsy* can provide diagnostic confirmation but is not always positive.

Management. There is a role for both medical and surgical therapy in improving quality and quantity of life in patients with Löffler endocarditis. There is evidence that both corticosteroids and cytotoxic drugs such as hydroxyurea may have an important favorable effect on survival. In refractory patients, treatment with interferon may offer a valuable adjunctive therapy. Routine supportive cardiac therapy with diuretics, neurohormonal blockade, and anticoagulation as indicated are appropriate for management of these patients. Surgical therapy consisting of endocardiectomy and valve replacement or repair appears to provide significant symptomatic palliation once the fibrotic stage of the disease manifests.

Endomyocardial Fibrosis

EMF is a disorder found typically in tropical and subtropical Africa, notably in Uganda, Nigeria, and Mozambique, and as such is a major cause of morbidity and mortality, accounting for 25% of cases of congestive heart failure and death in equatorial Africa.[7,40-42] A recent population-based study in rural Mozambique revealed a prevalence of the disorder, affecting 19.8% of the population.[7] In the latter study, only 48 of 211 patients were symptomatic at the time of detection, and familial occurrence was high.

The disease is increasingly recognized in other tropical and subtropical regions within 15 degrees of the equator including India, Brazil, Colombia, and Sri Lanka.[6] Importantly, it is also recognized in the Middle East, particularly Saudi Arabia.[41] Cardiac dysfunction occurs because of fibrous lesions that affect the inflow of the right and/or left ventricles (LVs) and that may also involve the atrioventricular valves, thereby producing regurgitant lesions. EMF has increased incidence among the Rwanda tribe of Uganda and in individuals of low socioeconomic status.[8] It has a slight male preponderance, is most common in children[42] and young adults,[7] but has been described in individuals into the sixth decade of life. Although most cases occur in black individuals, there are occasional presentations in white subjects residing in temperate climates. There are rare reports of EMF in individuals who have not resided in tropical areas.

Pathology

EMF affects both the right and left ventricles in approximately 50% of patients, purely the left in 40%, and the right ventricle alone in the remaining 10%.[9,41] The typical gross appearance is that of a normal to slightly enlarged heart. The right atrium may be dilated in

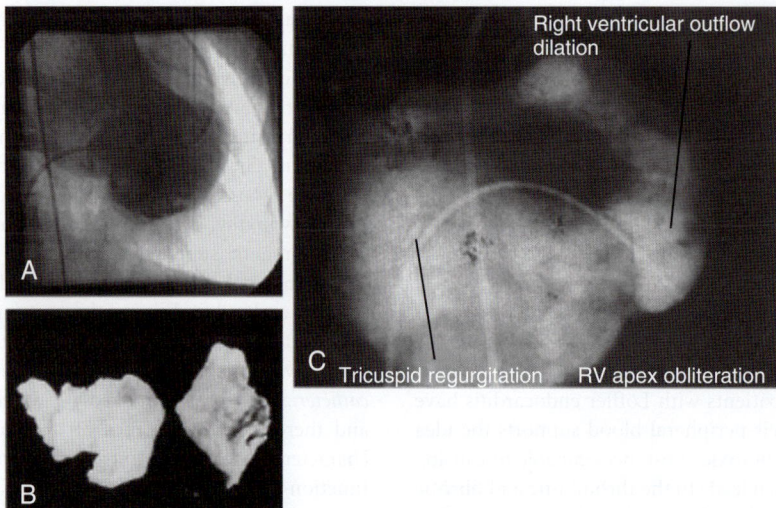

Fig. 21.8 Right- and left-sided endomyocardial fibrosis (EMF). (A) Left-sided EMF is characterized by apical obliteration, patchy filling defects, and severe mitral regurgitation. (B) The management of EMF often requires surgical excision of the endocardial fibrosis. Depicted are pieces of excised endocardial fibrosis. (C) Right ventricular (RV) angiogram of a patient with RV EMF showing right ventricular outflow tract dilation, RV apex obliteration, and tricuspid regurgitation. [A and B] From Joshi R, Abraham S, Kumar AS. New approach for complete endocardiectomy in left ventricular endomyocardial fibrosis. *J Thorac Cardiovasc Surg.* 2003;125:40–42; [C] from Seth S, Thatai D, Sharma S, et al. Clinico-pathological evaluation of restrictive cardiomyopathy (endomyocardial fibrosis and idiopathic restrictive cardiomyopathy) in India. *Eur J Heart Fail.* 2004;6:723–729; Hare JM. The dilated and restrictive cardiomyopathies. In: Bonow RL, et al., eds. *Braunwald's Heart Disease.* 9th ed. Philadelphia: Elsevier; 2011:1561–1581.

proportion to the severity of right ventricular involvement. There is often a pericardial effusion, which may be large. The right-sided heart border may be indented because of apical scarring. The hallmark feature of the disorder is fibrotic obliteration of the apex of the affected ventricle(s) (**Fig. 21.8**). The fibrosis involves the papillary muscles and chordae tendineae, leading to atrioventricular valve distortion and regurgitation. In the left ventricle, the fibrosis extends from the apex to the posterior mitral valve leaflet, usually sparing the anterior mitral leaflet and the ventricular outflow tract. Endocardial calcific deposits can be present, involving diffuse areas of the ventricle. The fibrotic tissue often creates a nidus for thrombus formation, which can be extensive. Atrial thrombi also occur. The process usually does not involve the epicardium, and the coronary artery obstruction is distinctly uncommon.

Histologic Findings

EMF is clearly apparent histologically, presenting as a thick layer of collagen overlying loosely arranged connective tissue.[41] In addition, there are fibrous and granular septations extending into the underlying myocardial tissue. Myocyte hypertrophy is common.[9] Although cellular infiltration is uncommon, interstitial edema is frequently present. Fibroelastosis that is found in the ventricular outflow tracts beneath the semilunar valves often represents a secondary process caused by local trauma. Examination of intramural coronary arteries may show involvement with medial degeneration, the deposition of fibrin, and fibrosis.

Clinical Manifestations

The symptomatic status of patients at presentation relates to which ventricles are involved. Ascites out of proportion to the pedal edema is hallmark of the disease. Pulmonary congestion signals left-sided involvement, whereas predominantly right-sided disease may

mimic restrictive cardiomyopathy and/or constrictive pericarditis. Atrioventricular valve regurgitation is common. The disease may be heralded by an acute febrile illness or may be simply insidious. EMF is a relentless and progressive process, although the time course of decline may vary considerably, with some patients appearing to have periods of stability. Modes of death include progressive heart failure, infection, infarction, sudden cardiac death, and complications of surgery. Atrial fibrillation and ascites are reported to be poor prognostic indicators.[43,44]

Right Ventricular Endomyocardial Fibrosis

In pure or predominant right ventricular involvement, the right ventricular apex is characterized by fibrous obliteration, which may extend to involve the supporting structures of the tricuspid valve, with ensuing tricuspid regurgitation. Patients exhibit an elevated jugular venous pressure, a prominent *v* wave with rapid *y* descent, and a right-sided S_3 gallop. There is prominent hepatomegaly with a pulsatile liver, ascites, splenomegaly, and peripheral edema, but pulmonary congestion is typically absent because of the lack of left-sided involvement. In this regard, pulmonary artery and pulmonary capillary wedge pressures are normal. A large pericardial effusion is often present. The right atrium may be enormously dilated. The *ECG* often has findings consistent with right-sided enlargement, especially a qR pattern in lead V_1, and supraventricular arrhythmias are common. The chest roentgenogram often demonstrates obvious right atrial prominence, a pericardial effusion, and calcification in the walls of the right and, less frequently, the left ventricle. Echocardiography demonstrates thickening of the right ventricle with obliteration of the apex, a dilated atrium, hyperechoic endocardial surfaces, and abnormal septal motion in patients with tricuspid regurgitation. On angiography, the right ventricular apex is typically not visualized because of fibrous obliteration; tricuspid regurgitation, right atrial enlargement, and filling defects in the right atrium caused by thrombi may be present.

Left Ventricular Endomyocardial Fibrosis

In cases of predominant left-sided disease, fibrosis involves the ventricular apex and often the chordae tendineae or the posterior mitral valve leaflet producing mitral regurgitation. The associated murmur may be late systolic, characteristic of a papillary muscle dysfunction murmur, or may be pansystolic. Findings of pulmonary hypertension may be prominent, and an S_3 protodiastolic gallop is frequently present. The ECG usually shows ST segment and T wave abnormalities, low-voltage QRS complexes if a pericardial effusion is present, or left ventricular hypertrophy. Left atrial abnormality is often noted. As with right-sided involvement, atrial fibrillation is often present and portends a poor prognosis. Echocardiography reveals increased endocardial echoreflectivity, preserved systolic function, apical obliteration, an enlarged atrium, pericardial effusion of varying size, and Doppler ultrasound evidence of mitral regurgitation. Pulmonary hypertension is typically observed during cardiac catheterization, as well as left atrial hypertension and a reduced cardiac index. Left ventriculography shows mitral regurgitation, and ventricular filling defects caused by intracavitary thrombi may be present. Coronary arteriography usually excludes obstructive epicardial vessel stenoses.

Biventricular Endomyocardial Fibrosis

Biventricular EMF is more common than either isolated right- or left-sided disease. The typical clinical presentation of EMF resembles right ventricular EMF; however, a murmur of mitral regurgitation is indicative of left-sided involvement. Unless left ventricular involvement is extensive, severe pulmonary hypertension is absent and the right-sided findings are the predominant mode of presentation. Approximately 15% of patients will experience systemic embolization, and only 2% will have infective endocarditis.

Diagnosis. Detection of EMF in individuals from the appropriate geographic area requires typical clinical and laboratory findings, as well as angiography. Eosinophilia is variably present and may result from parasitic infection.[8] Endomyocardial biopsy is diagnostic, but false-positives can occur because of the patchy nature of the disease. Insofar as myocardial biopsy may be complicated by systemic emboli, left-sided myocardial biopsy is contraindicated.

Management. The medical management of EMF remains challenging. One-third to one-half of patients with advanced disease die within 2 years, whereas those who are less symptomatic fare better. The development of atrial fibrillation is a poor prognostic indicator, although symptomatic relief can be achieved with rate control.[43] Heart failure is difficult to control, and diuretics are effective only in early stages of disease, losing efficacy with advanced ascites. Once EMF progresses to severe endocardial fibrosis, surgical resection with atrioventricular valve replacement on affected sides is the treatment of choice.[45-49] Surgical therapy consisting of endocardiectomy and valve replacement or repair usually results in hemodynamic improvement with reductions in ventricular filling pressure, increased cardiac output, and normalized angiographic appearance. Operative mortality is quite high, between 15% and 25%, and may be lower if valve replacement is not necessary.[46] Fibrosis may recur, although there are case reports of excellent long-term survival.[47-49]

Endocardial Fibroelastosis

Endocardial fibroelastosis (EFE) is a disorder of fetuses and infants of unclear cause that is characterized by deposition of collagen and elastin leading to ventricular hypertrophy and diffuse endocardial thickening.

Causes are not completely understood, and there are reports of associations with viral infections (especially mumps), metabolic disorders, autoimmune disease, and congenital left-sided obstructive lesions. Two recent reports implicate mitochondrial disorders and placental insufficiency.[50,51] Like DCM, EFE usually progresses to severe congestive heart failure and subsequent death. The echocardiographic finding of a highly reflective endocardial surface of the ventricular myocardium suggests EFE.

NEOPLASTIC INFILTRATIVE CARDIOMYOPATHY— CARCINOID HEART DISEASE

Carcinoid syndrome results from the metastasis of carcinoid tumors from the gut to the heart.[52] The symptoms include marked cutaneous flushing, diarrhea, bronchoconstriction, and endocardial plaques composed of a unique type of fibrous tissue. The symptom complex is caused in large part by the release of serotonin and other circulating substances secreted by the tumor. Essentially all patients experience diarrhea and flushing, 50% have cardiac lesions detected echocardiographically, and approximately 25% of the patients have severe right-sided involvement.

Carcinoid tumors originate largely from the gut, with 60% to 90% being found in the small bowel and appendix, and the remainder arising from other regions of the gastrointestinal tract or the bronchi. Carcinoid tumors arising in the ileum pose the greatest risk of metastasis, most likely affecting regional lymph nodes and the liver. Carcinoid tumors arising in the liver affect the heart. The severity of the cardiac lesions is related to the circulating concentrations of serotonin and 5-hydroxyindoleacetic acid (its primary metabolite), which are produced primarily by carcinoid tumors in the liver. The observation that the right side of the heart is preferentially affected in carcinoid syndrome reflects inactivation of the circulating toxic substances in the lung; the 5% to 10% of individuals presenting with left-sided lesions are likely to have right-to-left shunts or tumor involvement of the lungs.

Pathology

The characteristic lesions are fibrous plaques involving locations "downstream" of the tricuspid and pulmonic valves, the endocardium, and the intima of the venae cavae, pulmonary artery, and coronary sinus. Both stenotic and regurgitant valvular lesions result from fibrotic distortion originating in plaques.[52] The plaque material appears as a layer of fibrous tissue composed of smooth muscle cells, collagen, and mucopolysaccharides overlying the endocardium and, in some cases, extending into the underlying regions. Interestingly, identical pathology results from exposure to the anorectic drugs fenfluramine and dexfenfluramine. Occasionally there is actual metastasis of the tumor to one or both of the ventricles.

Clinical Manifestations

Cardiac murmurs indicating right-sided valve involvement are widely appreciated. A systolic murmur of tricuspid regurgitation along the left sternal border is almost always present, and pulmonic valve murmurs of either stenosis or regurgitation may also be present. The chest roentgenogram may be either normal or may show cardiac enlargement and pleural effusions or nodules. The pulmonary artery trunk is most often not enlarged, and poststenotic dilation is also absent, differentiating pulmonic involvement from congenital pulmonic stenosis. Although there are no specific changes on the ECG diagnostic of carcinoid heart disease, it is not uncommon to encounter right atrial enlargement without other findings of right ventricular hypertrophy, nonspecific ST segment and T wave abnormalities, and sinus tachycardia. Patients with advanced disease are likely to have low QRS voltage. Echocardiography often reveals tricuspid or pulmonary valve thickening and enlargement of the right atrium and ventricle; a minority of patients may have a small pericardial effusion. Cardiac MRI may offer additional value in evaluating the right side of the heart that may be difficult to image with echocardiography.[53]

Management

For mild congestive heart failure, standard therapy with diuretics and neurohormonal antagonists is appropriate. Both somatostatin analogues and chemotherapy can lead to improved symptoms and possibly enhanced survival, but neither is effective at ameliorating progressive cardiac disease in patients with carcinoid syndrome. A key element of management is relief of stenotic lesions of the tricuspid and pulmonary valves. This may be achieved with either balloon valvuloplasty or surgery, both of which can achieve symptomatic relief. Operative mortality is traditionally high, but it has improved significantly in experienced centers.[52]

ARRHYTHMOGENIC RIGHT VENTRICULAR DYSPLASIA/CARDIOMYOPATHY

ARVD/C, first described in 1977 by Fontaine and coworkers, is a genetic form of cardiomyopathy characterized prototypically by fibrofatty infiltration of the right ventricle (**Figs. 21.9** and **21.10**). ARVD/C accounts for 20% of cases of sudden cardiac death, and, importantly, the prevalence of this condition is higher among young athletes dying suddenly.[54,55]

Presenting Symptoms and Natural History

Patients typically present between the teenage years to their 40s, with only 10% falling outside of this age range. The natural history of the disorder is characterized by four phases—a concealed phase in which patients are asymptomatic, a phase characterized by an overt clinical manifestation of an electrical system disturbance, progression to signs and symptoms of right ventricular failure, and finally frank biventricular congestive heart failure. Accordingly, presenting symptoms range from palpitations to syncope and sudden cardiac death. A majority of patients who subsequently experience sudden cardiac death have a history of syncope, which thus represents an important prognostic event.[55] Progression to heart failure occurs in the minority of patients but is the predominant mode of death in individuals who are protected from sudden cardiac death by ICD implantation. The risk factors that increase the probability of ventricular arrhythmias include a reduced left ventricular ejection fraction (LVEF), a positive electrophysiologic study (EPS), and an individual who exercises for more than 6 hours per week.[56,57]

Pathology

Characteristically, a heart affected with ARVD/C exhibits fatty or fibrofatty replacement of the myocardium predominantly affecting the right ventricle. Rarely the process extends to the LVs.

Genetics

Several genes and gene loci are associated with ARVD/C, and both autosomal dominant and recessive modes of inheritance are described. Most but not all genes encode for desmosomal proteins.[58] Implicated genes include desmoplakin, junctional plakoglobin (JUP), the cardiac ryanodine receptor, plakophilin-2 (PKP2), and transforming growth factor-b3. JUP mutations are causally implicated in Naxos disease, a

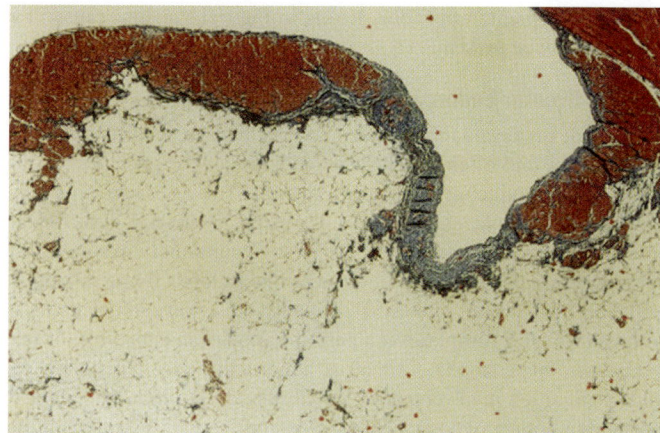

Fig. 21.9 Arrhythmogenic right ventricular dysplasia/cardiomyopathy (ARVD/C). Histologic appearance of ARVD/C showing fibrosis, adipose infiltration, and myocardial thinning. Modified from Hare JM. The etiologic basis of congestive heart failure. In: Colucci WS, ed. *Atlas of Heart Failure.* Philadelphia: Current Medicine LLC; 2008:29–56; Hare JM. The dilated and restrictive cardiomyopathies. In: Bonow RL, et al., eds. *Braunwald's Heart Disease.* 9th ed. Philadelphia: Elsevier; 2011:1561–1581.

syndrome characterized by ARVD/C, wooly hair, and palmoplantar keratoderma. Individuals with mutations in PKP2 present at younger ages and are more likely to have malignant arrhythmias.[54] This finding suggests the prognostic importance of genetic testing for ARVD/C. In addition, immunohistochemical detection of plakoglobin is proposed to be of value in diagnosis.[58]

Diagnosis

A task force has set diagnostic criteria to aid in the study and characterization of ARVD/C. The diagnostic criteria involve features obtained from imaging, ECG, signal-averaged ECG, and histologic criteria, as well as a positive family history and a history of arrhythmias.[59] Early diagnosis of ARVD/C remains challenging. Although endomyocardial biopsy may offer valuable diagnostic information, cardiac MRI is emerging as a more definitive diagnostic tool.[60] The main limitation of endomyocardial biopsy is a high false-negative rate because of sampling error and the fact that the right ventricle septum may lack the characteristic histologic changes; however, immunohistochemical detection of plakoglobin may enhance the value of tissue diagnosis.[58] Tandri and colleagues have reported that characterization of the ventricular wall morphology with delayed enhancement gadolinium MRI correlated well with histologic findings, as well as with inducibility of ventricular tachycardia during electrophysiologic testing.[60]

Management

Patients diagnosed with ARVD/C should receive an ICD. Antiarrhythmic therapy is appropriate before ICD insertion and, in some cases, after in patients who have recurrent ICD firings. Use of an ICD can have an enormous clinical impact in reducing the major cause of mortality in affected individuals. It is also recommended that patients receive neurohormonal blockade with angiotensin-converting enzyme inhibitors and β-adrenoreceptor antagonists. In individuals progressing to overt heart failure, management involves the same principles for the treatment of other forms of cardiomyopathy. Consideration of heart transplantation is indicated for patients with overt biventricular failure.

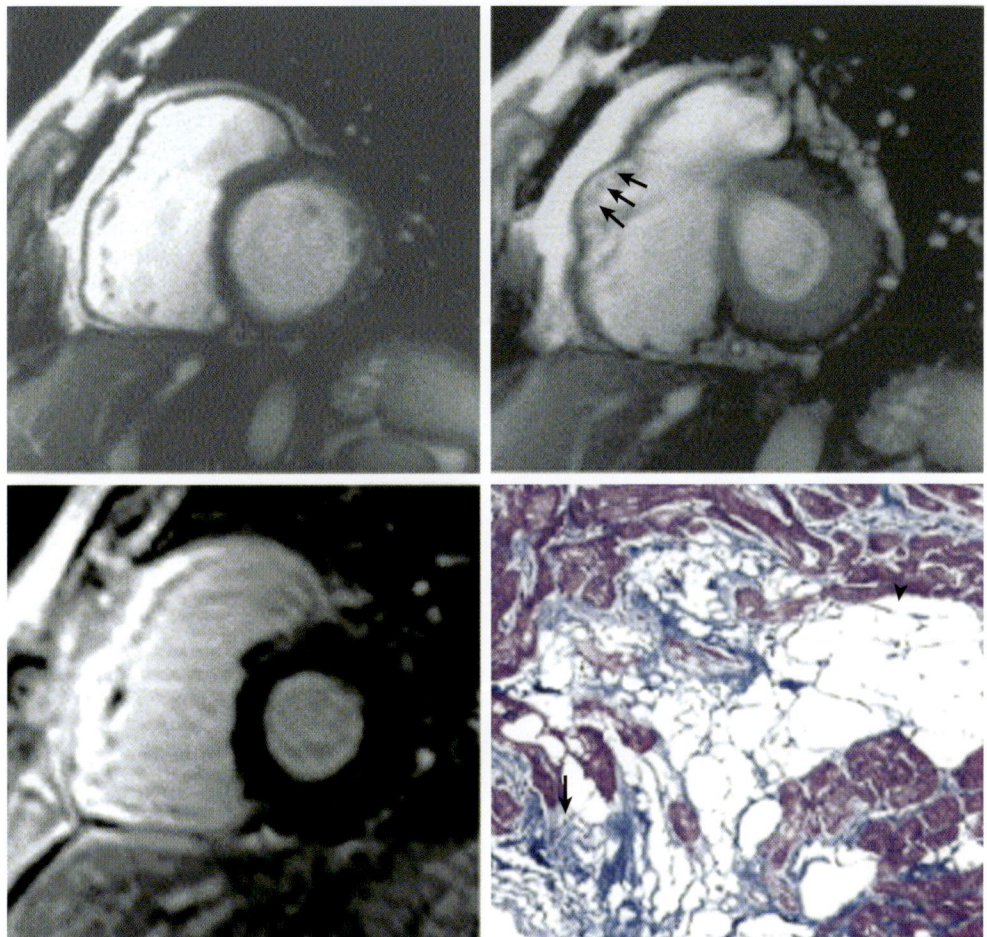

Fig. 21.10 Arrhythmogenic right ventricular dysplasia/cardiomyopathy (ARVD/C). The *top left* and *right* panels represent the end-diastolic and end-systolic frames of a short-axis cine magnetic resonance image (MRI) showing an area of dyskinesia on right ventricular (RV) free wall characterizing a focal ventricular aneurysm *(arrows)*. The *bottom left* panel displays the delayed-enhanced MRI with increased signal intensity within the RV myocardium *(arrows)* at the location of RV aneurysms. The *bottom right* panel shows the corresponding endomyocardial biopsy. Trichrome stain of the right ventricle at high magnification shows marked replacement of the ventricular muscle by adipose tissue. The adipose tissue cells *(arrowhead)* are irregular in size and infiltrate the ventricular muscle. There is also abundant replacement fibrosis *(arrow)*. There is no evidence of inflammation. Modified from Tandri H, Saranathan M, Rodriguez ER, et al. Noninvasive detection of myocardial fibrosis in arrhythmogenic right ventricular cardiomyopathy using delayed-enhancement magnetic resonance imaging. *J Am Coll Cardiol* 2005;45:98–103; Hare JM. The dilated and restrictive cardiomyopathies. In: Bonow RL, et al. eds. *Braunwald's Heart Disease*. 9th ed. Philadelphia: Elsevier; 2011:1561–1581.

SUMMARY AND FUTURE PERSPECTIVES

Our current understanding of processes leading to restrictive cardiomyopathy remains incomplete, as evidenced by the large percentage of patients who are assigned as having idiopathic disease. The strong genetic basis of restrictive cardiomyopathies and ARVD/C, coupled with high throughput technologies, will allow for the possibility of widespread genetic testing of affected individuals and their family members, as well as studies that correlate genotype with prognosis and treatment outcome. Genetic testing will also facilitate understanding of which patients have a genetic cause of their disease as opposed to a genetic predisposition to an environmental insult. In addition to genetics, measurement of expressed genes (transcriptomics), microRNA

abnormalities, and proteins (proteomics) has the potential to aid in understanding cause, prognosis, and individualized responses to therapy (precision medicine). A key example of the latter is the attempt to identify patients with a viral cause of cardiomyopathy and treat those patients with appropriate antiviral therapy on the one hand and those without viral infection with immunosuppressive therapy on the other hand. The most recent advance with significant future implications is the observation that the body, including the bone marrow and the heart, possesses reservoirs of endogenous stem cells regulated in stem cell niches—the discovery of these cells and their niches offers new insights into the causes of restrictive cardiomyopathy and may in the future provide a new therapeutic avenue.

KEY REFERENCES

2. Gallego-Delgado M, Delgado JF, Brossa-Loidi V, et al. Idiopathic restrictive cardiomyopathy is primarily a genetic disease. *J Am Coll Cardiol.* 2016;67:3021–3023.

3. Kostareva A, Kiselev A, Gudkova A, et al. Genetic spectrum of idiopathic restrictive cardiomyopathy uncovered by next-generation sequencing. *PloS one.* 2016;11:e0163362.

4. Hong JA, Kim MS, Cho MS, et al. Clinical features of idiopathic restrictive cardiomyopathy: a retrospective multicenter cohort study over 2 decades. *Medicine (Baltimore).* 2017;96:e7886.

12. Hemmati P, Greason KL, Schaff HV. Contemporary techniques of pericardiectomy for pericardial disease. *Cardiol Clin.* 2017;35:559–566.

17. Rammos A, Meladinis V, Vovas G, Patsouras D. Restrictive cardiomyopathies: the importance of noninvasive cardiac imaging modalities in diagnosis and treatment-a systematic review. *Radiol Res Pract.* 2017;2017:2874902.

23. Hazari H, Belenkie I, Kryski A, et al. Comparison of cardiac magnetic resonance imaging and echocardiography in assessment of left ventricular hypertrophy in fabry disease. *Can J Cardiol.* 2018;34:1041–1047.

40. Gallagher J, McDonald K, Ledwidge M, Watson CJ. Heart failure in sub-saharan Africa. *Card Fail Rev.* 2018;4:21–24.

56. Maupain C, Badenco N, Pousset F, et al. Risk stratification in arrhythmogenic right ventricular cardiomyopathy/dysplasia without an implantable cardioverter-defibrillator. *JACC Clin Electrophysiol.* 2018;4:757–768.

57. Wang W, James CA, Calkins H. Diagnostic and therapeutic strategies for arrhythmogenic right ventricular dysplasia/cardiomyopathy patient. *Europace.* 2018. https://doi.org/10.1093/europace/euy063.

The full reference list for this chapter is available on ExpertConsult.

Cardiac Amyloidosis

Adam Castaño, Mathew S. Maurer

Amyloidosis is a deposition disease in which proteins with unstable structures misfold and aggregate into amyloid fibrils, which deposit in the heart, kidneys, liver, peripheral nerves, gastrointestinal tract, lungs, and soft tissues. Amyloid fibrils are insoluble nonbranching structures 7 nm to 10 nm wide and of variable length that are resistant to proteolysis. Under normal light microscopy when stained with Congo red, amyloid deposits display a hyaline pink appearance and under polarized light, change to a characteristic apple-green birefringence.[1] When viewed by electron microscopy, amyloid fibrils appear as needle-like filamentous bundles with a unique cross β-pleated sheet configuration.

Cardiac amyloidosis (CA) is an increasingly recognized cause of heart failure (HF). Among the thirty proteins known to form amyloid fibrils that deposit in the extracellular space leading to disruption of tissue architecture and organ dysfunction, cardiologists predominantly encounter amyloidosis caused by three proteins that infiltrate the heart: (1) immunoglobulin light chain (AL) and transthyretin (ATTR) amyloidosis due to (2) a mutation (hATTR, also known as hereditary or familial amyloid cardiomyopathy) or (3) wild-type (wtATTR, also known as senile or age-related CA). In developing nations, secondary amyloid A (AA) is more prevalent due to chronic infections and inflammatory conditions. Uncommon variants also known to affect the heart or aorta include atrial natriuretic peptide (ANP), apolipoprotein A1 (AApoA1), fibrinogen (Afib), gelsolin (Agel), and lactadherin amyloid (**Table 22.1**).

EPIDEMIOLOGY

Light-chain cardiac amyloidosis (AL-CA) is a rare condition with an estimated incidence of 10 cases per million individuals and thus ~3000 new diagnoses per year in the United States.[2] Among new cases, 30% to 50% present with symptomatic cardiac involvement. AL amyloid is caused by plasma cell dyscrasia, which spans the spectrum from monoclonal gammopathy of undetermined significance (MGUS) to AL and multiple myeloma. Approximately 10% to 15% of patients with AL amyloidosis meet criteria for multiple myeloma.[3]

Emerging data suggest that transthyretin cardiac amyloidosis (ATTR-CA) is not uncommon, especially due to wtATTR, which will become the most commonly diagnosed form of CA. Evidence suggests it is underdiagnosed as a cause of common cardiovascular conditions in older adults, including heart failure with a preserved ejection fraction (HFpEF) and aortic stenosis (AS), and is commonly seen in subjects with degenerative orthopedic conditions such as lumbar spinal stenosis, biceps tendon rupture, and bilateral carpal tunnel syndrome. Among patients with HFpEF over 75 years of age at autopsy, 32% have amyloid deposits, compared with 8% in those less than 75 years of age.[4] In hospitalized patients with HFpEF who underwent nuclear scintigraphy, 13% had wtATTR-CA.[5] Similarly, nuclear scintigraphy in patients undergoing transcatheter aortic valve replacement (TAVR) for severe calcific AS revealed a prevalence of 16% overall and 22% among men.[6] In patients undergoing surgery for degenerative lumbar spinal stenosis, almost all had amyloid in surgical specimens of the ligamentum flavum, and transthyretin (TTR) was identified immunohistochemically as the causative protein in one-third of resected tissues.[7] Among patients with wtATTR-CA, biceps tendon rupture has been observed in 33% of patients, occurring in the dominant arm in 95% and bilaterally in 24% of patients.[8]

TABLE 22.1   Types of Cardiac Amyloid

Amyloid Type	Amyloidogenic Protein	Extent of Cardiac Involvement
AL	Immunoglobulin light chain of κ or λ subtype	Frequent and severe cardiac involvement
ATTR	Transthyretin	
hATTR (*familial*)	Mutant transthyretin	Severe with particular mutations (Val122Ile, Thr60Ala, Ile68Leu, Leu11Met)
wtATTR (*senile*)	Wild-type transthyretin	Frequent and severe cardiac involvement is typical
AA	Serum amyloid A protein	Usually involves kidney first causing nephrotic syndrome; severe cardiac involvement can occur
Afib	Mutant fibrinogen	Cardiac autonomic dysfunction can occur
AGel	Gelsolin	Cardiac involvement possible
Apo A1	Mutant apolipoprotein A1	Severe cardiac involvement can occur
ANP	Atrial natriuretic peptide	Atrial involvement may occur

AA, Reactive systemic amyloidosis (amyloid A protein); *AGel,* hereditary gelsolin amyloidosis; *Afib,* hereditary fibrinogen amyloidosis; *AL,* light chain amyloidosis; *ANP,* atrial natriuretic peptide; *Apo A1,* mutant apolipoprotein A1 molecules; *ATTR,* transthyretin amyloidosis; *hATTR,* hereditary transthyretin amyloidosis; *TTR,* transthyretin; *wtATTR,* wild-type transthyretin amyloidosis.

TABLE 22.2   Phenotypic Comparison of Most Common Types of Cardiac Amyloidosis in North America

Clinical Characteristic	AL	wtATTR	ATTR Val122Ile	ATTR Thr60Ala
Median age, years	55	75	70	60
Sex	Equal	>90% male reported to date	Male predominant	Equal
Ethnic background	None	White	African-American or Afro-Caribbean	Irish
Peripheral neuropathy	+++	+	+	+++
Frequency of neuropathy	++	+	+	++

Mutations in the *TTR* gene, which are inherited in an autosomal dominant fashion, can also lead to ATTR-CA (**see also Chapter 24**). Over 120 mutations have been described, of which some have varying phenotypes and are endemic to specific geographic regions. For example, the Val122Ile or Leu111Met mutations lead to a predominant cardiomyopathy, while Val30Met causes a predominant neuropathy, also known as familial amyloidotic polyneuropathy (FAP), and Glu89Gln and Thr60Ala lead to a mixed cardiomyopathy/neuropathy (**Table 22.2**). Among mutations in the USA, Val122Ile is the most common.[9] Val122Ile affects almost exclusively individuals of African or Afro-Caribbean descent with a population prevalence of 3.4% and is under-recognized as a cause of HF.[10,11] Another common mutation, Thr60Ala, is the most common variant in the UK with an estimated population prevalence of 1% in northwest Ireland. The prevalence and penetrance of Val30Met, which is endemic to Portugal, Sweden, Japan, and Brazil, varies widely with region and age of onset. The disease prevalence is 1 in 100,000 individuals in nonendemic areas such as the United States, compared with 1 in 538 individuals affected in endemic areas of Portugal. Penetrance can also vary geographically with 22% at age 60 years in Sweden, compared with 80% at 50 years in Portugal.[12] Patients with early-onset disease manifest with peripheral neuropathy, while those with late-onset disease typically present with a concomitant cardiomyopathy.

NATURAL HISTORY

In AL-CA, the presence and extent of cardiac involvement is the major determinant of survival. Without successful treatment, patients who present with AL-CA and symptomatic HF have a median survival of 6 months.[13] The efficacy of chemotherapy targeting the underlying plasma cell clone is the next most important determinant of survival.[14] Overall survival has improved with advances in therapy for plasma cell

dyscrasias but still remains low at ~42% at 4 years.[15] Despite a hematologic response, survival is dependent on underlying cardiac function, and patients may die of progressive HF or sudden cardiac death (SCD). Pulseless electrical activity and electromechanical dissociation are often the cause of SCD, although ventricular tachyarrhythmias, bradycardia, and thromboembolism are not uncommon sequelae.

Original reports suggested that the median survival of patients with wtATTR-CA was greater than 5 years, but contemporary studies demonstrate worse outcomes with a median survival of 3.5 years from initial evaluation.[16-18] This discrepancy stems largely from the difficulty in determining the precise time of disease onset. Initial clinical manifestations of TTR amyloid deposition may include bilateral carpal tunnel syndrome, which is present in ~70% of individuals an average 5 to 7 years before the start of cardiac manifestations.[19] Other early signs of amyloid deposition include atrial arrhythmias and progressive effort intolerance, which are difficult to definitively attribute to amyloidosis given these occur commonly in older adults. In an early longitudinal multicenter investigation, the Transthyretin Amyloid Cardiac Study (TRACS), which studied advanced patients, mortality with ATTR-CA was high and was worse in patients with hATTR Val22Ile compared to wtATTR.[16] Common causes of death included HF, SCD, and sepsis. These data have been corroborated by the Transthyretin Amyloidosis Outcome Survey (THAOS), which reported significantly worse age-adjusted survival from time of enrollment over 3 years in patients with hATTR-CA Val122Ile compared to wtATTR-CA (HR 1.947, P = .013).[9,20] A single-center study demonstrated significantly worse overall and age-adjusted survival from time of diagnosis in patients with hATTR-CA Val122Ile compared with wtATTR-CA (median survival 47 months vs. 59 months, P = .01), with survival diverging well after 24 months from diagnosis.[21]

Physiologic derangements in ATTR-CA include a reduction in chamber capacitance, decline in contractility, and increase in arterial elastance, which lead to progressive left ventricular (LV) dysfunction. Blood pressure falls due to a reduction in cardiac output and heart rate increases to compensate for a reduced forward stroke volume. Among patients with wtATTR-CA, a positive troponin T, presence of a pacemaker, and New York Heart Association (NYHA) class IV symptoms were associated with a worse outcome.[22] Clinical assessments at 6-month increments in the TRACS study in patients with advanced disease demonstrated marked disease progression: mean 6-minute hall walk declined 26 m, N-terminal pro-B-type natriuretic peptide (NT-proBNP) increased 1816 pg/mL, and left ventricular ejection fraction (LVEF) fell 3%. In advanced ATTR-CA, cardiac cachexia ensues, which may be mediated by right HF, liver congestion, and altered bowel flora.

CLINICAL FEATURES

Misdiagnosis and Obstacles to Early Diagnosis

CA is often misdiagnosed for other causes of left ventricular hypertrophy (LVH) such as hypertrophic cardiomyopathy (HCM), hypertensive cardiomyopathy, and HFpEF. Neuropathy in patients with FAP is often mistaken for chronic inflammatory demyelinating polyneuropathy (CIDP). Consequent delays in diagnosis have detrimental consequences for patients. A survey in 533 participants with AL amyloidosis, 37% of whom had cardiac involvement, revealed that the average time from initial symptoms to diagnosis was 2 years.[23] Nearly one-third of patients reported visiting more than five physicians before receiving a diagnosis of amyloidosis, while only 8% received the diagnosis after visiting one physician. Despite seeing cardiologists more frequently than hematologists and nephrologists, cardiologists only made the diagnosis in 19% of cases. Similarly, approximately 50% of patients with ATTR-CA receive a diagnosis within 6 months, typically by a cardiologist.

CA is a "great mimicker," and the diagnosis is delayed due to both physician and disease-related factors.[24] A multidisciplinary amyloid team of cardiologists, neurologists, nephrologists, and hematologists is optimal for diagnosis and management, but such teams are rare and isolated to a few academic medical centers. The late presentation of AL-CA and the absence of disease-modifying treatments for ATTR-CA have also led physicians to express nihilism about prognosis and management options. An important disease-specific cause of diagnostic uncertainty is the heterogeneous phenotype of CA, which ranges from an isolated cardiomyopathy to systemic involvement with minimal cardiac involvement. Phenotypic variability within inherited ATTR is also influenced by genetic heterogeneity, geography, endemic region of origin, age, sex of the proband and transmitting parent, as well as amyloid fibril composition. The traditional requirement of histopathologic evidence of amyloid infiltration in involved tissues also delays diagnosis, as expertise in endomyocardial biopsy and amyloid-specific histopathologic techniques is typically restricted to specialty centers.[25]

Raising Clinical Suspicion for Cardiac Amyloidosis

A heightened clinical suspicion for CA is the key step in avoiding misdiagnosis and delayed diagnosis. The presence of noncardiac signs such macroglossia and periorbital purpura, while specific, are present only in a minority of cases of AL-CA and absent in ATTR-CA. A patient with unexplained LVH or restrictive cardiomyopathy should immediately prompt consideration of CA. Additional red flags may include a history of carpal tunnel syndrome in ATTR (especially bilateral with a history of repeated carpal tunnel surgeries), atraumatic rupture of the biceps tendon, a history of total knee or hip arthroplasty,[26] surgeries for degenerative lumbar spinal stenosis, unexplained neuropathic pain, and orthostatic hypotension. In addition, a diagnosis of "hypertensive cardiomyopathy" in a patient with normal or low blood pressure or "HCM" in a patient aged 60 years or older should raise clinical suspicion for CA.

Diagnosis

When CA is suspected, the diagnosis must be systematic and directed toward defining the specific amyloid subtype and assessing the burden of amyloid infiltration in the myocardium and other organs.

Electrocardiography

Low QRS voltage on electrocardiography (ECG) is touted as a classic and pathognomonic sign specific to CA but occurs as a late phase phenomenon associated with poor prognosis. In contemporary series, the prevalence of low voltage is relatively low and varies with CA subtype, ranging from 20% in ATTR to 60% in AL.[27] The absence of low QRS voltage therefore should not preclude the diagnosis of CA, particularly in patients with ATTR-CA in whom 30% present with LVH or left bundle branch block (LBBB). The hallmark ECG feature of CA is a disproportionately low QRS voltage to LV mass ratio.[28] A pseudo-infarct pattern, defined as pathologic Q waves in at least two contiguous leads without obstructive coronary artery disease, is present in up to 70% of cases and is more sensitive for CA than low voltage. Patients with CA may also develop progressive conduction disease such that AV block in an older patient with increased LV wall thickness should raise suspicion for CA.

Laboratory Testing

To date, no blood test exists to detect TTR oligomers to diagnose ATTR-CA. In AL-CA, however, quantification of serum free light chains (FLCs) and identification of an abnormal monoclonal band on immunofixation of serum and/or urine have a combined sensitivity of 99% for identifying AL-CA. However, up to 5% of the population over 65 years of age has MGUS, and therefore an abnormal ratio of kappa (κ) to lambda (λ) FLCs alone is not specific for AL amyloidosis.[41] An abnormal κ/λ ratio in elderly patients who in fact have ATTR-CA with concurrent MGUS can lead to misdiagnosis of AL-CA in up to 10% of cases (even at referral centers).[29] Interpretation of FLC concentrations must also take into account renal function, as FLCs are filtered by the glomeruli. Renal dysfunction can lead to increased serum FLC concentrations and affects κ and λ light chains differently. Therefore making a diagnosis of AL-CA is more challenging in patients with chronic kidney disease, and a wider reference range for a normal κ/λ ratio has been proposed in this population.[30]

Natriuretic peptides tend to be markedly elevated in CA, typically out of proportion to LV systolic function.[31] In AL-CA, circulating light chains are directly toxic to cardiomyocytes by modulating p38 mitogen-activated protein kinase and subsequent downstream upregulation of NT-proBNP expression.[32] Direct injection of light chains from subjects with AL amyloidosis into zebrafish results in impaired cardiac function, pericardial edema, and increased cell death with eventual 100% mortality relative to light chain control samples isolated from patients with multiple myeloma.[33] Therefore for the same degree of hemodynamic derangement, plasma NT-proBNP levels are higher in patients with AL compared with ATTR-CA. Amyloid infiltration can also trigger cardiomyocyte apoptotic pathways with subsequent elevation in serum troponin levels, which can lead to false diagnoses of an acute coronary syndrome. Consequently, in patients with unexplained new-onset HF, measurement of serum FLCs, NT-proBNP, and troponin may raise the suspicion of AL-CA. These tests are especially important in patients with a preexisting clonal plasma cell dyscrasia such as MGUS or smoldering myeloma, or in patients with unexplained increased LV wall thickness.

Cardiac Imaging (see also Chapter 32)

In clinical practice, transthoracic echocardiography, speckle tracking strain echocardiography, and cardiac magnetic resonance (CMR) often raise suspicion for CA (**Fig. 22.1**), while bone radiotracer scintigraphy can be diagnostic of ATTR-CA. As these modalities are complementary to one another, the focus should be to define the specific diagnostic goal and selecting the corresponding imaging test.[34]

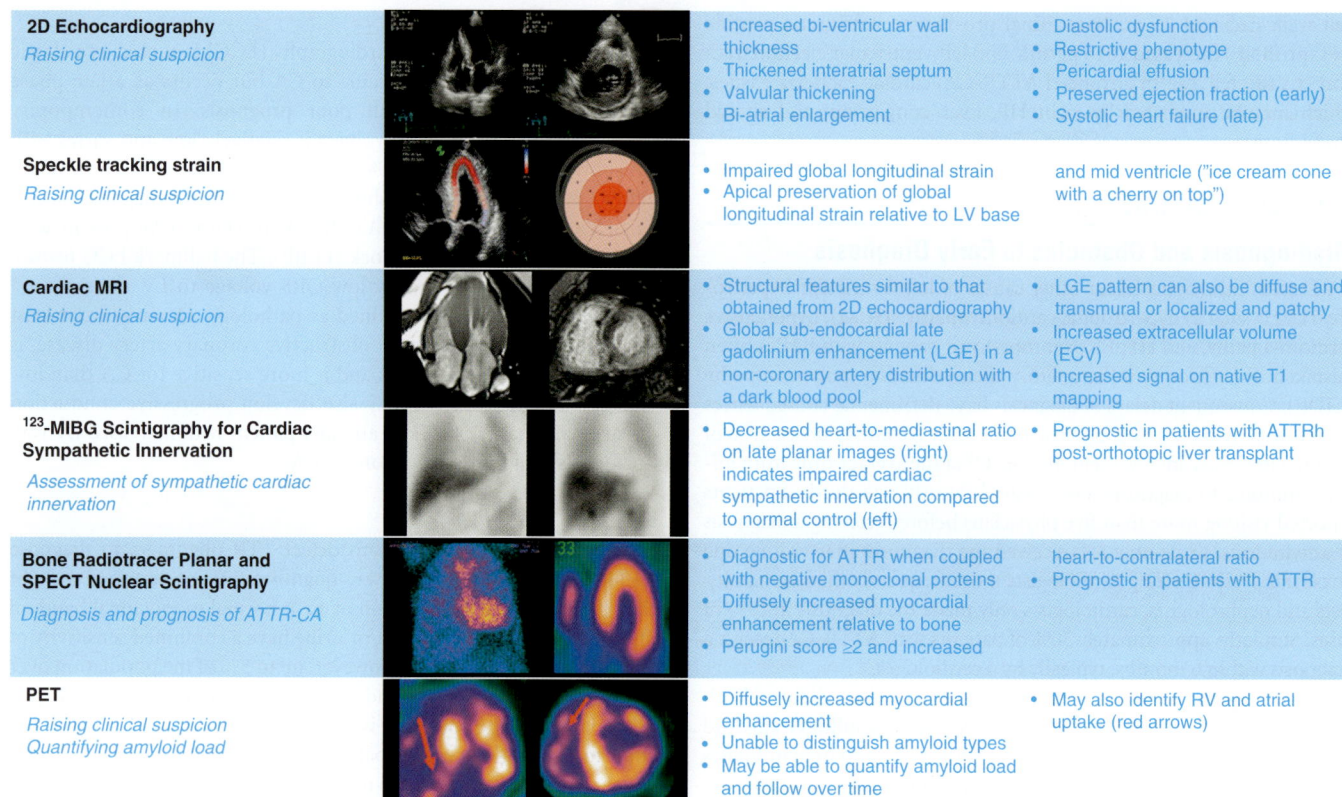

2D Echocardiography *Raising clinical suspicion*	• Increased bi-ventricular wall thickness • Thickened interatrial septum • Valvular thickening • Bi-atrial enlargement	• Diastolic dysfunction • Restrictive phenotype • Pericardial effusion • Preserved ejection fraction (early) • Systolic heart failure (late)
Speckle tracking strain *Raising clinical suspicion*	• Impaired global longitudinal strain • Apical preservation of global longitudinal strain relative to LV base	and mid ventricle ("ice cream cone with a cherry on top")
Cardiac MRI *Raising clinical suspicion*	• Structural features similar to that obtained from 2D echocardiography • Global sub-endocardial late gadolinium enhancement (LGE) in a non-coronary artery distribution with a dark blood pool	• LGE pattern can also be diffuse and transmural or localized and patchy • Increased extracellular volume (ECV) • Increased signal on native T1 mapping
¹²³-MIBG Scintigraphy for Cardiac Sympathetic Innervation *Assessment of sympathetic cardiac innervation*	• Decreased heart-to-mediastinal ratio on late planar images (right) indicating impaired cardiac sympathetic innervation compared to normal control (left)	• Prognostic in patients with ATTRh post-orthotopic liver transplant
Bone Radiotracer Planar and SPECT Nuclear Scintigraphy *Diagnosis and prognosis of ATTR-CA*	• Diagnostic for ATTR when coupled with negative monoclonal proteins • Diffusely increased myocardial enhancement relative to bone • Perugini score ≥2 and increased	heart-to-contralateral ratio • Prognostic in patients with ATTR
PET *Raising clinical suspicion* *Quantifying amyloid load*	• Diffusely increased myocardial enhancement • Unable to distinguish amyloid types • May be able to quantify amyloid load and follow over time	• May also identify RV and atrial uptake (red arrows)

Fig. 22.1 Role of cardiac imaging modalities for diagnosis and management of cardiac amyloidosis. *LV,* Left ventricle; *RV,* right ventricle. (¹²³-MIBG Scintigraphy courtesy Riemer Slart, MD, PhD. Cardiac MRI courtesy Steven Wolff, MD, PhD.)

Transthoracic Echocardiography. Echocardiographic features of CA are nonspecific, but in clinical context are highly suggestive of CA. In advanced disease, predominant abnormalities include symmetric thickening of the LV (though asymmetric hypertrophy is common), thickening of the right ventricular (RV) free wall, and a small pericardial effusion. Classically, thickening of the atrioventricular valves and interatrial septum and a "speckled" myocardium also occur, although "speckling" is less reliable with harmonic imaging. Amyloidosis is the archetype of LV diastolic dysfunction, with stages of diastolic impairment paralleling progressive disease. Impaired LV relaxation occurs in early CA, which progresses to restrictive pathophysiology. Analogous progression in RV diastolic dysfunction is reflected in Doppler signals of the RV inflow, superior vena cava, and hepatic vein flow velocities. CA also leads to impaired systolic performance, which precedes the onset of HF. In parametric polar maps of the LV, relative apical sparing of global longitudinal strain (LS) represents an important diagnostic clue for CA relative to other causes of LVH.[35] While differentiating AL from ATTR-CA by echocardiography is not possible, on average, patients with AL-CA tend to have more restrictive diastolic dysfunction and patients with ATTR-CA tend to have greater LV wall thickness.

Cardiac MRI. Structural information derived from CMR is similar to that acquired from echocardiography, but the opportunity to interrogate tissue composition with gadolinium-based contrast agents in CMR has led to an increase in the diagnosis of CA.[36] Gadolinium is a purely extracellular agent, which does not enter intact cardiomyocytes. Global subendocardial late gadolinium enhancement (LGE) in a noncoronary artery distribution is pathognomonic for CA, but LGE can also be diffuse and transmural or focal and patchy. T1 mapping, in which a quantitative signal from the myocardium is

measured before or after contrast administration, has shown increased precontrast T1 signal in patients with CA compared with HCM or healthy controls.[37] Pre- and postcontrast T1 data can also be used to calculate extracellular volume (ECV), a measurement of interstitial expansion, which is significantly elevated in patients with CA due to interstitial amyloid deposition.[38] Native T1 mapping does not require administration of contrast and is therefore safe in patients with renal impairment. Contemporary CMR enables assessment of amyloid burden via direct measurement of ECV, edema via measurement of native T1, and myocyte response via measurement of intracellular volume. Limitations to T1 mapping include nonstandardized reference ranges with different software platforms and limited availability. While CMR is safe, painless, and requires no radiation, its use is limited in patients with CA who have implanted ferromagnetic hardware or cannot tolerate lying immobile for the duration of the exam due to comorbidities such as spinal stenosis or HF. Protocols requiring the use of contrast may also be contraindicated in patients with renal impairment. Therefore in clinical practice, CMR may raise clinical suspicion of CA but is not diagnostic. Advanced CMR techniques provide insights into the pathophysiological processes underlying CA and monitoring of disease progression and response to therapy.

Myocardial Radiotracer Scintigraphy. Nuclear cardiac scintigraphy using technetium-labeled bone radiotracer has demonstrated high diagnostic accuracy in multiple studies. Radiotracers include technetium-3,3-diphosphono-1,2-propanodicarboxylic (^{99m}Tc-DPD), technetium-pyrophosphate (^{99m}Tc-PYP), and technetium-hydroxymethylene diphosphonate (^{99m}Tc-HMDP). A revival in nuclear cardiac scintigraphy for CA occurred when ^{99m}Tc-DPD planar scintigraphy demonstrated high sensitivity and specificity for differentiating ATTR-CA from other causes of LVH using a semiquantitative visual score (range 0–3 with score

0 = absent cardiac uptake, normal bone uptake; 1 = mild cardiac uptake inferior to bone uptake; 2 = moderate cardiac uptake with attenuated bone uptake; 3 = strong cardiac uptake with mild/absent bone uptake) and a quantitative heart-to-whole body (H/WB) ratio.[39] Like ^{99m}Tc-DPD, ^{99m}Tc-PYP in North America, using a quantitative heart-to-contralateral (H/CL) ratio, and ^{99m}Tc-HMDP in Europe using a quantitative heart-to-skull (H/S) ratio, exhibited high diagnostic accuracy for differentiating ATTR-CA from AL-CA and nonamyloid HFpEF.[40-42]

An international multicenter collaboration in 857 patients with CA who underwent either ^{99m}Tc-DPD, ^{99m}Tc-PYP, or ^{99m}Tc-HMDP planar radiotracer scintigraphy showed that grade 2 or 3 myocardial uptake was 100% specific for the diagnosis of ATTR-CA *in patients with no evidence of an abnormal monoclonal protein*.[43] The presence of a monoclonal protein was defined as an abnormal FLC ratio (<0.26 or >1.65) on serum Freelite assay or presence of a monoclonal protein on immunofluorescence of serum or urine. These data led to an international consensus that in select patients without evidence of an abnormal monoclonal protein, a positive radiotracer nuclear scan can diagnose ATTR-CA without the need for a biopsy. Planar nuclear scintigraphy is therefore an accurate and feasible imaging modality that may spare select elderly patients the need for invasive biopsy. These scans are faster than CMR, though they do require a supine position and minimal radiation exposure. A standardized protocol using ^{99m}Tc-PYP demonstrated the feasibility of a faster incubation period, less radiation exposure compared to other protocols, and shorter imaging time.[44] The molecular mechanism by which ^{99m}Tc-based bone radiotracers selectively bind to ATTR amyloid fibrils in the myocardium is unknown, but it has been suggested that the preferential binding may be a result of higher calcium content relative to other fibril types. Bone tracers can also detect early ATTR cardiac infiltration in asymptomatic allele carriers before echocardiographic or biomarker changes occur.[45]

Cardiac Positron Emission Tomography. Positron emission tomography (PET) radiotracers have also demonstrated high affinity for amyloid fibrils. Several radiotracers studied in small patient cohorts include ^{11}C-Pittsburgh compound B (PIB), and the [18]fluorine-labeled (^{18}F) compounds, ^{18}F-florbetapir, ^{18}F-florbetaben, and ^{18}F-sodium fluoride (NaF). Intense myocardial uptake of ^{11}C-PIB, ^{18}F-florbetapir, and ^{18}F-florbetaben in patients with CA (irrespective of AL and ATTR subtype) occurs with no uptake in amyloid negative controls.[46-48] A limitation of ^{11}C-PIB is its short radioactive half-life of 20 minutes, which restricts its use to centers with a nearby cyclotron and radiopharmacy infrastructure, while ^{18}F-florbetapir and ^{18}F-florbetaben have longer half-lives of 110 minutes allowing for widespread distribution to PET centers without a cyclotron. While these tracers may have potential for evaluating for CA, they do not differentiate between CA subtypes. Increased myocardial uptake of ^{18}F-NaF, which also has a half-life of 110 minutes, occurred in small cohorts of patients with ATTR-CA but not in AL or nonamyloid controls, suggesting specificity for ATTR.[49]

Tissue Biopsy and Confirmation of the Causative Precursor Protein

The diagnostic accuracy of a noncardiac biopsy is dependent on amyloid type and the source of examined tissue (**Table 22.3**). The yield of a noncardiac biopsy from the abdominal fat pad is higher in patients with AL compared with ATTR. In AL-CA, the yield of an abdominal fat pad biopsy can be as high as 84% while it is lower in hATTR-CA at 45% and in wtATTR-CA at 15%.[50] Therefore while the abdominal fat pad is a preferred initial site for harvesting tissue in subjects with AL-CA, a negative result is not sufficient to exclude the diagnosis, and in the

TABLE 22.3	**Clinical Misconceptions About Cardiac Amyloid**
Misconception	**Clinical Reality**
Cardiac amyloid is rare	• Cardiac amyloid is increasingly recognized and current epidemiology suggests ATTR-CA it is not an unusual cause of HF
A negative fat pad biopsy rules out the diagnosis of amyloid	• Fat pad biopsy has a low sensitivity for amyloid, especially for TTR amyloidosis • Tissue biopsy is required for the diagnosis of AL amyloid • Biopsy of the involved organ coupled with mass spectrometry is the gold standard for diagnosis • However, in patients without evidence of an abnormal monoclonal protein, a positive bone radiotracer scan using 99mTc-PYP, DPD, and/or HMDP may supplement the need for tissue biopsy
Low-voltage on an electrocardiography is an early diagnosis marker of CA	• Low voltage on ECG has a low sensitivity (<50%) for identifying CA and is a late phase phenomenon associated with adverse outcomes • Low voltage-to-mass ratio and pseudo infarcts are more sensitive electrocardiographic metrics of cardiac amyloid
Lack of disease-modifying treatment renders accurate diagnosis merely an academic exercise	• AL cardiac amyloid, if identified early, can be managed effectively with plasma cell therapy and is associated with excellent outcomes • Multiple disease-modifying therapies for ATTR-CA are in late phase clinical trials • Clinical implications of accurate diagnosis include modification of HF therapy, genetic counseling, and referral to an amyloid center for consideration of liver or heart transplantation, or inclusion in a clinical trial

AL, Light chain amyloidosis; *ATTR-CA,* transthyretin cardiac amyloidosis; *CA,* cardiac amyloidosis; *DPD,* diphospho-1,2-propanedicarbonacid; *ECG,* electrocardiogram; *HF,* heart failure; *HMDP,* hydroxymethylene diphosphonate ; *99mTc-PYP,* technetium 99m pyrophosphate; *TTR,* transthyretin.

context of high clinical suspicion, an endomyocardial biopsy should be pursued. Biopsy specimens also delineate the amyloidogenic precursor protein. Immunohistochemistry is the most widespread method of tissue typing and is commonly performed on formalin-fixed, paraffin-embedded sections for κ, λ, TTR, and serum amyloid A protein. A common pitfall is false-positive immunostaining for TTR in CA, which is confounded by the frequent lack of staining for immunoglobulin light chains. Mass spectrometry–based proteomic analysis is considered the gold standard for fibril typing and can frequently identify a mutant TTR genotype, although genetic sequencing is the gold standard for identifying TTR mutations.[51]

Genetic Analysis

Sequencing the *TTR* gene is recommended in all cases of ATTR-CA in conjunction with genetic counseling. Inherited hATTR-CA is indistinguishable from acquired wtATTR-CA based on clinical grounds or cardiac imaging. In addition, a family history indicating an autosomal dominant inheritance pattern is often absent due to incomplete and late disease penetrance. Though rare, the possibility of non-ATTR mutations including gelsolin, apolipoprotein A1, A2, and fibrinogen should be evaluated if these precursor proteins are found to cause CA and/or in the presence of a strong family history and a normal *TTR* gene sequence.[52]

CLINICAL MANAGEMENT

Biomarker Staging Systems

Laboratory testing plays an important role in clinical management using well-established prognostic models in AL amyloidosis. Current staging systems for AL-CA rely on the concentration of circulating FLCs and serum levels of NT-proBNP and cardiac troponin T (**Fig. 22.2**). These three biomarkers constitute the Mayo Clinic staging system, considered the most powerful prognostic tool in patients with AL-CA.[53] Patients are assigned a point for each of the following: difference between κ and λ FLC ≥18 mg/dL, cardiac troponin T ≥0.025 ng/mL, and NT-proBNP ≥1800 pg/mL, creating stages I to IV corresponding to scores of zero to three points, respectively. Median overall survival from diagnosis for stages I, II, III, and IV disease was 94.1, 40.3, 14, and 5.8 months, respectively (*P* < .001). Patients with marked elevations in both NT-proBNP and cardiac troponin have a particularly poor prognosis. An NT-proBNP >8500 pg/mL combined with a systolic blood pressure <100 mm Hg further stratifies patients within stage III with especially high mortality (stage IIIB). NT-proBNP is also a biomarker of disease progression and response to therapy. After treatment, a change in NT-proBNP level is a surrogate for survival with a decrease associated with improvement and an increase with worse overall survival.[14] Thus therapy can lead to meaningful increases in survival if it results in a reduction of light chains accompanied by a cardiac response, defined as a decline in NT-proBNP of >30% and >300 ng/L (assuming a baseline level ≥650 ng/L).[54]

Cardiac biomarkers may also be useful prognostic markers in patients with ATTR-CA. The Mayo Clinic developed a staging system in patients with wtATTR-CA using thresholds of troponin T (0.05 ng/mL) and NT-proBNP (3000 pg/mL) to designate stages I to III corresponding to both values below cutoff, one above, and both above, respectively. Overall survival rate over 4 years was 57%, 42%, and 18%, respectively (*P* < .001).[55] Another staging system stratified patients with ATTR-CA into three disease stages at baseline contingent on cut points of NT-proBNP >3000 ng/L and estimated glomerular filtration rate (eGFR) <45 mL/min. Stage I was defined as NT-proBNP ≤3000 ng/L and eGFR ≥45 mL/min, stage II if either NT-proBNP or eGFR crossed the cut point, and stage III if both crossed cut point. Median survival for stages I, II, and III disease was 69.2, 46.7, and 24.1 months, respectively (*P* < .0001).[56]

Prognostication from Advanced Cardiac Imaging

Several cardiac imaging parameters are also prognostic in CA. The myocardial contraction fraction (MCF), defined as the ratio of stroke volume to myocardial volume, has demonstrated superiority to LVEF in predicting survival.[57] Impaired global LS and the degree of apical sparing on speckle-strain echocardiography is also prognostic in CA and is associated with death or heart transplant.[58] The CMR-specific parameters, transmural LGE, native T1 mapping, and ECV, are also prognostic in patients with CA independent of biomarkers.[59,60] Planar cardiac nuclear scintigraphy in patients with ATTR-CA has also demonstrated prognostic utility using techniques to quantify myocardial retention such as H/WB ratio with ^{99m}Tc-DPD,[61] H/S ratio with ^{99m}Tc-HMDP,[62] and the H/CL ratio with ^{99m}Tc-PYP (see section on Myocardial Radiotracer Scintigraphy).[40]

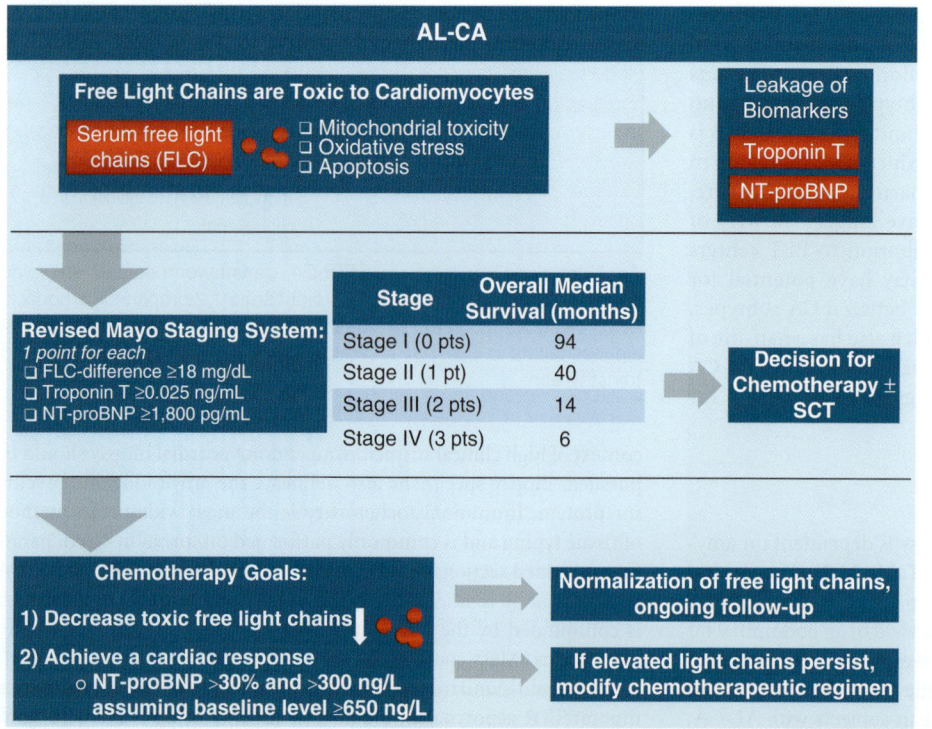

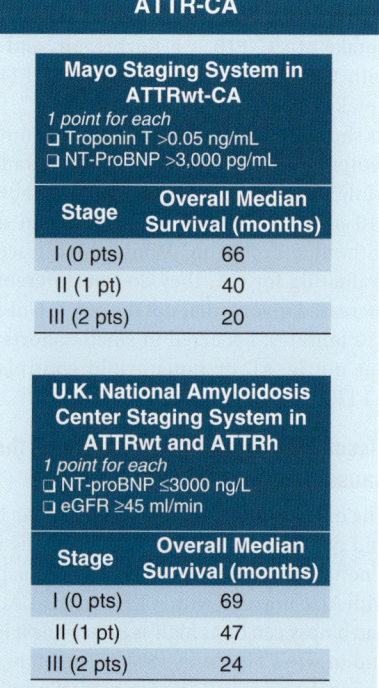

Fig. 22.2 Biomarkers for prognostication of disease and monitoring response to therapy in cardiac amyloidosis.

Supportive Nondisease-Modifying Therapies

The general principles underlying nondisease-modifying therapy for CA include symptom management, maintenance of euvolemia, avoidance of polypharmacy (particularly in elderly patients), avoidance of medications that may cause symptomatic hypotension, and consideration of pacemaker therapy for symptomatic conduction disturbances.

Diuretics

Patients with CA are often in a sodium-avid state and volume overloaded. Maintaining euvolemia is challenging given their load lability and risk of hypotension. Patients should be educated about the importance of dietary sodium restriction. Judicious use of bioavailable loop diuretics and aldosterone antagonists is required with frequent dose adjustments to address changes in volume status that may result from concomitant chemotherapies for AL amyloidosis, such as steroids. Diuretic resistance may develop in patients with advanced cardiomyopathy, mediated by high central venous pressures and a low stroke volume (type 2 cardiorenal syndrome) or in patients with AL with concomitant renal amyloid (type 5 cardiorenal syndrome). As clinical disease progresses and blood pressure falls, midodrine may be useful.

Drug Intolerances in Advanced CA

Intolerance to standard HF medications including angiotensin-converting enzyme inhibitors (ACEi), angiotensin receptor blockers (ARBs), and beta-blockers (BBs) is common in patients with cardiac amyloid. Such agents exacerbate symptomatic hypotension in the setting of concomitant autonomic dysfunction or by lowering heart rate and reducing cardiac output. Concerns have been raised that they may worsen outcomes, and thus they should be used with caution and, if employed, at low dosages.[63]

Calcium Channel Blockers and Digoxin

Calcium channel blockers (CCBs) are a relative contraindication in CA as they can worsen HF and lead to high degree heart block.[64] The affinity of TTR amyloid fibrils for various bone-seeking radiotracers is thought to be calcium related, which may suggest a potential mechanism for increased binding of CCBs to amyloid fibrils promoting hyperphysiologic effects. Nondihydropyridine CCBs (e.g., verapamil) should be avoided in patients with CA and concurrent hypertension and should not be used for rate control in those with atrial fibrillation (AF).

Patients with CA may also display high sensitivity to digoxin, which may cause abrupt cardiac rhythm disturbances or sudden death. An in vitro study demonstrated that isolated amyloid fibrils bind digoxin with high affinity with the majority of fibrils binding after only 15 minutes.[65] Caution with digoxin administration is generally recommended, but the adverse effects of digoxin do not appear to be as severe as with nondihydropyridine CCBs.[66]

Atrial Fibrillation, Thromboembolic Complications, and Anticoagulation

The overall prevalence of AF in ATTR-CA in the THAOS registry was 62.8% in wtATTR and 51.9% in hATTR Val122Ile.[9] While the presence of AF is not associated with survival in this population, it is associated with incident HF and thromboembolism.[67] In CA, blood stasis from AF compounded by endomyocardial damage and endothelial dysfunction from amyloid deposition are thought to lead to hypercoagulability and intracardiac thrombosis. In examined autopsy specimens, cases with AL compared with ATTR demonstrated a higher frequency of intracardiac thrombosis (51% vs. 16%, $P < .0001$) and fatal embolic events (26% vs. 8%, $P < .03$), while nonamyloid controls displayed none.[68] In multivariate analysis, AL subtype and LV diastolic dysfunction were independently associated

with thromboembolism (odds ratio [OR] 8.4, 95% confidence interval [CI] 1.8–51.2 and OR 12.2, 95% CI 2.7–72.7, respectively). A study employing transthoracic and transesophageal echocardiography in 156 patients with CA found intracardiac thrombi were present in 35% of patients with AL and 18% with ATTR ($P = .02$).[69] In multivariate analysis, LV diastolic dysfunction and low left atrial appendage emptying velocity, in addition to AF, were independently associated with intracardiac thrombosis. Thus a combination of systolic and diastolic ventricular dysfunction and chronic amyloid infiltration in the atria lead to atrial mechanical dysfunction, atrial enlargement, and blood stasis.[70] Atrial mechanical dissociation may also explain why some patients with CA develop atrial thrombosis even when in normal sinus rhythm.

In CA, risk assessment for thrombosis and subsequent decision for anticoagulation should not be based upon the CHA_2DS_2-VASc score alone.[71] The decision to administer anticoagulation should reflect a comprehensive clinical assessment of high-risk features specific to patients with CA. In addition to AF, the following are risk factors for thromboembolism: advanced LV diastolic dysfunction, low left atrial appendage emptying velocity, elevated heart rate, increased RV wall thickness (reflecting more advanced amyloid deposition with poor RV diastolic function and stasis), and AL versus TTR subtype. Anticoagulation may be considered in patients with AL amyloid even in normal sinus rhythm if they have low atrial velocities on Doppler of the mitral inflow. Novel oral anticoagulants have been used for thromboembolic risk reduction, but no studies to date have compared them head to head with warfarin in patients with CA.[67]

Permanent Pacemaker Implantation

Cardiac autonomic dysfunction and progressive conduction disease are common in CA, particularly due to hATTR Val30Met.[72] Over 50% of patients with hATTR Val30Met have abnormal 24-hour ECG recordings, highlighting the importance of cardiac monitoring. Permanent pacemaker (PPM) implantation has been required in 25% of patients with hATTR Val30Met, 36% Val122Ile, and 43% wtATTR-CA for high-degree conduction block, symptomatic bradycardia, and AF with a slow ventricular response.[73] Prophylactic PPM implantation in patients with hATTR Val30Met with conduction disturbances has been reported,[74] but retrospective analyses have not demonstrated PPM implantation to be associated with a mortality benefit. In fact, the presence of a PPM at baseline has been associated with worse survival in wtATTR-CA likely related to severity of disease and not to permanent pacing.[22] In patients with CA, adherence with class I guideline recommendations for PPM implantation is recommended.[75] Biventricular pacing may also play a role by mitigating ventricular dyssynchrony and subsequent reductions in stroke volume resulting from chronic RV pacing. Since patients with CA often become PPM dependent, a biventricular pacer may reduce symptoms, although additional research is required.

Implantable Cardioverter Defibrillators

The role of implantable cardioverter-defibrillator (ICD) therapy is controversial. Previously, prognosis in AL-CA with HF at presentation has been dismal (median survival <1 year), which directly conflicted with practice guidelines recommending ICD placement for primary prevention of SCD in patients with a reasonable life expectancy of greater than 1 year.[76] Thus ICDs are not typically implanted in patients with advanced AL-CA. Because SCD in patients with CA is often attributed to electromechanical dissociation rather than to a tachyarrhythmia argues further against the role of ICD implantation in this population.[77] However, with advances in the treatment of AL-CA, ICD therapy may be indicated for a subset of patients, such as those with syncope, nonsustained ventricular tachycardia (NSVT), or sustained VT.[78,79] A careful risk/benefit analysis may reveal those patients with CA who would specifically benefit from an ICD: i.e., unexplained syncope, a high burden of NSVT or sustained VT, and patients listed for organ transplantation.

Organ Transplantation

Liver Transplantation for hATTR With Predominant Neuropathic Mutations. The majority of TTR protein (95%) is produced by the liver. Orthotopic liver transplantation (OLT) replaces amyloidogenic mutant TTR with wild-type TTR and theoretically arrests amyloid formation. In contemporary practice, OLTs are performed as a preventative measure before the development of painful lower extremity sensorimotor neuropathy in patients with hATTR, most commonly due to Val30Met.[80] Survival after OLT in patients with early-onset hATTR Val30Met is ~73% at 10 years and lower on average in hATTR due to other neuropathic mutations. The long disease latency of CA also enables the practice of "domino liver transplantation" where the otherwise well-functioning hATTR Val30Met liver is transplanted into a different recipient. After OLT in patients with hATTR, there is still a risk of progressive CA or polyneuropathy as normal wild-type TTR from the transplanted liver can build up on already deposited mutant TTR present at the time of transplantation.[81] Thus after OLT, routine cardiac and neurologic evaluation should be implemented.

Orthotopic Heart and Combined Heart/Liver Transplantation. Combined orthotopic heart transplantation (OHT) and OLT may be considered in patients with mutations that result in advanced CA with a mixed neuropathic phenotype to eliminate the mutant precursor protein and prevent progression of neuropathy. Many amyloid centers perform isolated OHT for patients with hATTR that cause a predominant cardiac phenotype (e.g., Val122Ile). OHT has been controversial in patients with CA due to early data demonstrating lower survival compared with nonamyloid OHT recipients. At many centers, CA is a contraindication to OHT due to advanced age (especially in wtATTR) and comorbid conditions (**Table 22.4**). In the modern era, however, enhanced chemotherapy regimens for advanced AL-CA and better patient selection have led to comparable 5-year survival to nonamyloid OHT for both AL and ATTR subtypes.[82]

Disease-Targeted Therapies for AL-CA
Chemotherapy and Stem Cell Transplantation

The cornerstone of therapy for AL-CA is reducing clonal light-chain–producing plasma cells with chemotherapy. Arresting amyloid production reverses disease progression, preserves organ function, and enhances survival. Reducing FLC levels by at least 50% (ideally >90%) over a sustained period improves survival. In patients with adequate cardiac reserve, high-dose chemotherapy coupled with autologous stem cell transplant (ASCT) can be a definitive therapy.[83] Treatment of AL amyloidosis with high-dose melphalan plus ASCT, however, does not improve survival compared with standard-dose melphalan plus dexamethasone, although peritransplant mortality was 25%, emphasizing the importance of proper patient selection.[84] Immune modulators like thalidomide, lenalidomide, and pomalidomide, which are well tolerated in patients with multiple myeloma, can cause worsening HF in patients with AL amyloidosis. The proteasome inhibitor, bortezomib, effectively targets clonal plasma cells in a majority of patients and reduces circulating amyloidogenic monoclonal protein, although it can also worsen peripheral neuropathy. Daratumumab, a monoclonal antibody targeting the CD38-receptor and indicated for the treatment of patients with relapsed multiple myeloma, produced a rapid and profound hematologic response without unexpected toxicity in patients with heavily pretreated AL amyloidosis.[85]

TABLE 22.4   ISHLT Recommendations for Screening of Noncardiac Organs in Patients with AL Amyloid Prior to Consideration of OHT

Organ System	Screening Tests
Pulmonary	• Pulmonary function testing including arterial oximetry and diffusion capacity • CXR and CT to assess for interstitial disease, effusion • Thoracentesis may be necessary to differentiate amyloidosis from HF
Gastrointestinal	• Nutritional assessment including prealbumin, albumin • Assessment for bleeding by esophagogastroduodenoscopy, colonoscopy • Assessment of amyloid deposition on random biopsy • Assessment of intestinal motility with gastric-emptying studies
Hepatic	• Serum alkaline phosphatase and bilirubin *Alkaline phosphatase >1.5 above upper limit or normal in the absence of congestion should trigger a liver biopsy to assess for portal and parenchymal amyloid deposition*
Renal	• Measured creatinine clearance of eGFR and 24-hour urinary protein excretion *An eGFR or measured creatinine clearance <50 mL/min/1.73 m2 in the absence of decompensated HF or urinary protein excretion >0.5 g/24 hours should prompt renal biopsy to assess renal amyloid burden*
Coagulation	• Factor X and thrombin time *Patients with severe factor X functional deficiency (<25%) have <50% survival after autologous stem cell transplantation*

CXR, Chest x-ray; *eGFR*, estimated glomerular filtration rate; *HF*, Heart failure; ISHLT, International Society for Heart and Lung Transplantation; *OHT*, orthotopic heart transplantation.
Adapted from Mehra MR, Canter CE, Hannan MM, et al. The 2016 International Society for Heart Lung Transplantation listing criteria for heart transplantation: a 10-year update. *J Heart Lung Transplant.* 2016;35(1):1–23.

Disease-Modifying Therapeutic Opportunities for ATTR-CA

Given that no Food and Drug Administration (FDA)–approved drugs are currently available for treatment of ATTR-CA, medications that prevent and reverse TTR-mediated organ toxicity are currently under investigation (**Fig. 22.3**).

Silencers of TTR Gene Expression

RNA interference (RNAi) has emerged as an endogenous cellular mechanism for controlling gene expression. Small interfering RNAs (siRNAs) delivered to hepatocytes in formulations of lipid nanoparticles knock down target gene expression by triggering enzymatic degradation of messenger RNA (mRNA) in a sequence-specific manner. Systemic delivery of the siRNA compound, patisiran, targets a conserved sequence in the 3′ untranslated region of *TTR*, thereby specifically knocking down both mutant and wild-type *TTR* gene expression. The phase 3 study (APOLLO trial) in patients with hATTR with polyneuropathy (>50% of whom had cardiac

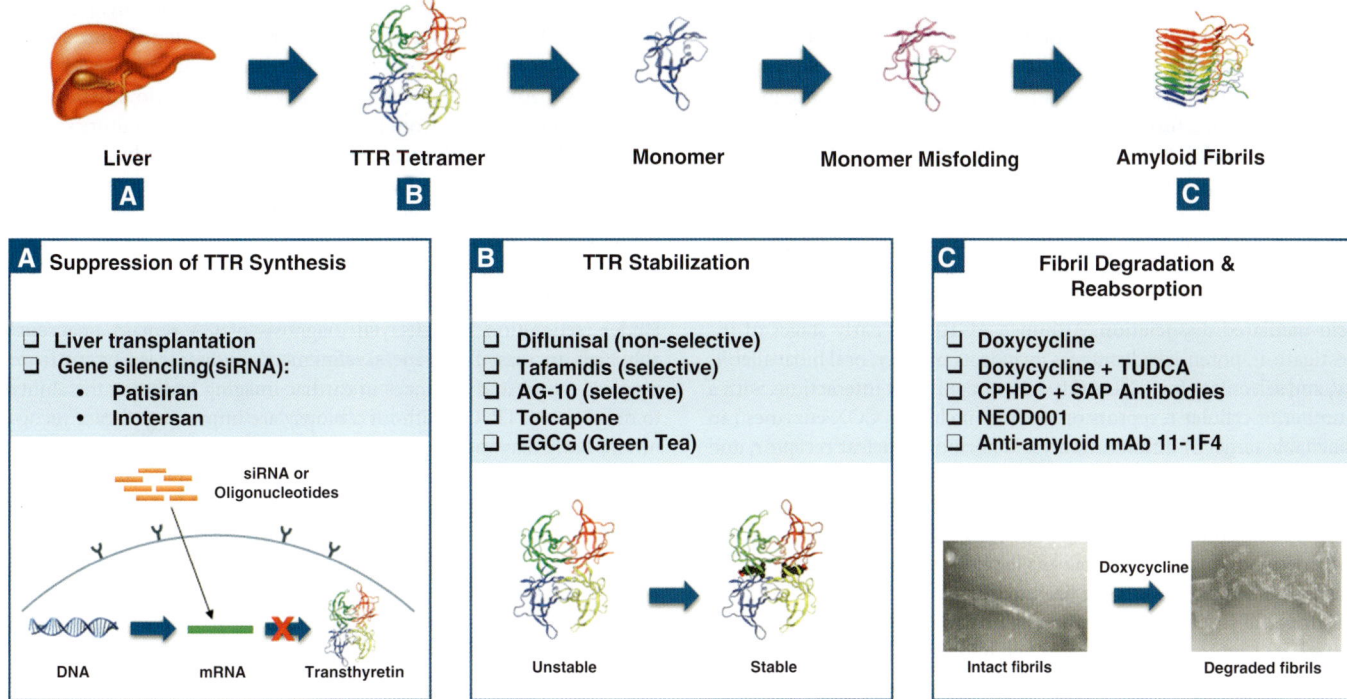

Liver **TTR Tetramer** **Monomer** **Monomer Misfolding** **Amyloid Fibrils**

A Suppression of TTR Synthesis

- ❑ Liver transplantation
- ❑ Gene silencling(siRNA):
  - Patisiran
  - Inotersan

siRNA or Oligonucleotides

DNA   mRNA   Transthyretin

B TTR Stabilization

- ❑ Diflunisal (non-selective)
- ❑ Tafamidis (selective)
- ❑ AG-10 (selective)
- ❑ Tolcapone
- ❑ EGCG (Green Tea)

Unstable   Stable

C Fibril Degradation & Reabsorption

- ❑ Doxycycline
- ❑ Doxycycline + TUDCA
- ❑ CPHPC + SAP Antibodies
- ❑ NEOD001
- ❑ Anti-amyloid mAb 11-1F4

Doxycycline

Intact fibrils   Degraded fibrils

Fig. 22.3 TTR disease modifying opportunities. *CPHPC,* (R)-1-[6-[(R)-2-carboxy-pyrrolidin-1-yl]-6-oxo-hexanoyl]pyrrolidine-2-carboxylic acid; *SAP,* serum amyloid P component; *siRNA,* small interfering RNAs; *TUDCA,* tauroursodeoxycholic acid.

involvement) showed that patisiran compared with placebo resulted in significant improvements in modified neuropathy impairment score (mNIS+7) at 18 months and secondary exploratory outcomes including Norfolk quality of life (QOL), 10-minute walk test, and modified body mass index (mBMI).[86] In a cardiac subgroup with wall thickness >13 mm, patisiran resulted in significant improvements in NT-proBNP, LV wall thickness, global LS, and gait speed compared to placebo. The ability of patisiran to lower mutant and wild-type TTR protein levels may provide a major advantage over OLT, which affects production of only mutant protein.

Antisense oligonucleotides (ASOs) also inhibit hepatic expression of TTR. ASOs are short synthetic RNAs that bind and inhibit translation of target mRNA, thereby suppressing wild type and mutant TTR. In a phase two-three randomized trial in patients with FAP, the ASO, inotersen, showed improvements in mNIS+7 score and the Norfolk QOL scale compared to placebo. Both approaches to TTR silencing (siRNA and ASO) have therapeutic potential in TTR-CA.

TTR Stabilization

As TTR tetramer dissociation is a rate-limiting step in the cascade of amyloid fibril formation, oral treatments have been studied with the aim to stabilize TTR tetramers.[87]

Diflunisal. Diflunisal, a nonsteroidal antiinflammatory drug (NSAID), binds and stabilizes TTR.[88] In a randomized, double-blind study in patients with FAP, diflunisal 250 mg bid significantly reduced neurologic impairment and preserved QOL at 2 years compared to placebo as demonstrated by the NIS+7 score and SF-36 QOL scale, respectively.[89] Diflunisal was well tolerated with no difference in serious adverse effects compared to placebo. Adverse events occurred in four patients and included gastrointestinal bleeding and congestive HF, known complications of chronic cyclooxygenase (COX) enzyme inhibition. Long-term safety and efficacy of diflunisal lasted beyond 2 years of treatment.[90] The efficacy in ATTR-CA is not well defined, but

an uncontrolled series from one center suggests a survival benefit.[91] The main advantages of diflunisal are that it is inexpensive, orally administered, and widely available.

Tafamidis. Tafamidis is a novel compound that binds to the thyroxine-binding site of the TTR tetramer and inhibits its dissociation into monomers, thereby blocking the rate-limiting step in the TTR amyloidogenesis cascade. Results from a clinical trial in the efficacy-evaluable population of patients with very early FAP Val30Met favored tafamidis 20 mg qd over placebo with respect to both co-primary endpoints, neuropathy impairment score of the lower limb (NIS-LL), and total QOL (TQOL).[92] TTR was stabilized in 98% of patients on tafamidis and 0% of placebo, and treatment was well tolerated. The 12-month open-label extension study in patients who earlier received blinded tafamidis or placebo showed that patients who continued on tafamidis had stable change rates in NIS-LL and total quality of life (TQOL) score, while in patients who switched from placebo, the monthly rate of change in NIS-LL and TQOL declined. Patients treated with tafamidis for 30 months had 55.9% greater preservation of neurologic function compared to patients who initiated tafamidis later. Adverse events were similar between groups and did not lead to any drug discontinuations. Tafamidis is now approved by the European Medicines Agency for treatment of stage 1 FAP and is currently available in Europe and Japan. With respect to ATTR-CA, the phase 3 clinical trial (ATTR-ACT [Transthyretin Amyloidosis Cardiomyopathy Clinical Trial]) in patients with hATTR and wtATTR, comparing tafamidis 20 or 80 mg qd with placebo, met its primary endpoint of reduction in the combination of all-cause mortality and frequency of cardiovascular-related hospitalizations at 30 months. An indication for use in ATTR-CA is expected.[92a]

EGCG (Green Tea). Epigallocatechin-3-gallate (EGCG), the most abundant catechin in green tea, inhibits amyloid fibril formation from a diverse array of substrate proteins including TTR.[93] A study in patients with wtATTR-CA showed that 600 mg po daily for at least

12 months resulted in a significant decrease in LV myocardial mass by 6% by CMR, while no change occurred in LVEF, LV wall thickness, and mitral annular plane systolic excursion.[94] These observations suggest that EGCG stabilizes and potentially inhibits the progression of CA, warranting further study.

Other Stabilizers in Early Phase Investigation. In a high-throughput screen for TTR ligands, the compound AG10 stabilized wild-type TTR and TTR Val122Ile in vitro.[95] AG10 prevents the dissociation of TTR Val122Ile in serum obtained from patients with ATTR-CA and protects human cardiomyocytes from amyloid toxicity. In human serum, AG10 also stabilizes wild-type TTR against acid-mediated dissociation. Although AG10 is in early stages of investigation, potential advantages include its potency, oral bioavailability, and selectivity for TTR. AG10 has no significant interactions with a number of cellular receptors or enzymes including COX enzymes (an inevitable target of diflunisal), thyroid hormone nuclear receptor, and a number of cytochrome P450 isozymes.

Tolcapone is an orally administered catechol-*O*-methyltransferase (COMT) inhibitor currently approved by the FDA as an adjunctive therapy to levodopa and carbidopa for the treatment of patients with Parkinson disease. It has since been repurposed as a potent TTR aggregation inhibitor, as it binds specifically to TTR in human plasma, stabilizes wild-type and mutant TTR, and inhibits amyloid cytotoxicity.[96] Safety and efficacy studies of AG10 and tolcapone are needed.

Fibril Degradation and Reabsorption

In addition to reducing the production of amyloid precursor protein, removal of already deposited amyloid is an area of active investigation.

Doxycycline and Combination Doxycycline + Tauroursodeoxycholic Acid. The tetracycline antibiotic, doxycycline, disrupts TTR fibrils in vitro. In a phase two open-label study in patients with ATTR, doxycycline 100 mg bid + tauroursodeoxycholic acid (TUDCA) 250 mg tid, a potent antiapoptotic and antioxidant biliary acid, showed an acceptable safety profile and no clinical progression of cardiac or neuropathic involvement over 1 year.[97]

Anti-SAP and Anti-TTR Antibodies. Serum amyloid P component (SAP) is a nonfibrillar glycoprotein present in all human amyloid deposits. In mice with amyloid deposits containing human SAP, antihuman SAP antibodies triggered a macrophage-mediated giant cell reaction that removed massive visceral amyloid deposits without adverse effects. An open-label phase one trial in patients with systemic amyloidosis demonstrated that the drug, (R)-1-[6-[(R)-2-carboxy-pyrrolidin-1-yl]-6-oxo-hexanoyl]pyrrolidine-2-carboxylic acid (CPHPC), efficiently depleted SAP from the plasma and allowed targeting of SAP in amyloid deposits by a humanized monoclonal IgG1 anti-SAP antibody.[98] At 6 weeks, treatment resulted in improvements in hepatic amyloid load, liver function tests, and liver stiffness. Infusion reactions but no serious adverse events occurred in some initial recipients of larger doses of antibody. Recently, the sponsor of this approach halted its development, given an unfavorable risk benefit profile.

Monoclonal antibodies targeted against monomeric amyloidogenic forms of TTR (anti-TTR mAb) have been developed and shown in vitro to induce antibody-dependent phagocytic uptake of TTR aggregates.[99] Anti-TTR mAbs specifically bind to amyloid deposits in cardiac samples derived from patients with hATTR-CA. Future studies need to delineate the pharmacokinetics of anti-TTR mAbs in different target tissues, efficacy in animal models, and therapeutic potential in patients with ATTR amyloidosis.

FUTURE PERSPECTIVES

Under-recognition and delayed diagnosis of CA remain unacceptably high. Increased awareness, refinements in disease subtyping from biopsied tissue, and advances in cardiac imaging including the ability to diagnose ATTR-CA without a biopsy are improving disease recognition. Early diagnosis is more important than ever before; new treatments for AL-CA are allowing for effective long-term management and emerging treatments for ATTR-CA based on a biological understanding of the disease are in late phase trials.

KEY REFERENCES

5. Gonzalez-Lopez E, Gallego-Delgado M, Guzzo-Merello G, et al. Wild-type transthyretin amyloidosis as a cause of heart failure with preserved ejection fraction. *Eur Heart J*. 2015;36(38):2585–2594.
6. Castano A, Narotsky DL, Hamid N, et al. Unveiling transthyretin cardiac amyloidosis and its predictors among elderly patients with severe aortic stenosis undergoing transcatheter aortic valve replacement. *Eur Heart J*. 2017;38(38):2879–2887.
9. Maurer MS, Hanna M, Grogan M, et al. Genotype and phenotype of transthyretin cardiac amyloidosis: THAOS (Transthyretin Amyloid Outcome Survey). *J Am Coll Cardiol*. 2016;68(2):161–172.
10. Quarta CC, Buxbaum JN, Shah AM, et al. The amyloidogenic V122I transthyretin variant in elderly black Americans. *N Engl J Med*. 2015;372(1):21–29.
18. Rapezzi C, Merlini G, Quarta CC, et al. Systemic cardiac amyloidoses: disease profiles and clinical courses of the 3 main types. *Circulation*. 2009;120(13):1203–1212.
43. Gillmore JD, Maurer MS, Falk RH, et al. Nonbiopsy diagnosis of cardiac transthyretin amyloidosis. *Circulation*. 2016;133(24):2404–2412.
53. Kumar S, Dispenzieri A, Lacy MQ, et al. Revised prognostic staging system for light chain amyloidosis incorporating cardiac biomarkers and serum free light chain measurements. *J Clin Oncol*. 2012;30(9):989–995.
84. Jaccard A, Moreau P, Leblond V, et al. High-dose melphalan versus melphalan plus dexamethasone for AL amyloidosis. *N Engl J Med*. 2007;357(11):1083–1093.
92. Coelho T, Maia LF, Martins da Silva A, et al. Tafamidis for transthyretin familial amyloid polyneuropathy: a randomized, controlled trial. *Neurology*. 2012;79(8):785–792.
95. Penchala SC, Connelly S, Wang Y, et al. AG10 inhibits amyloidogenesis and cellular toxicity of the familial amyloid cardiomyopathy-associated V122I transthyretin. *Proc Natl Acad Sci U S A*. 2013;110(24):9992–99927.

The full reference list for this chapter is available on ExpertConsult.

Heart Failure as a Consequence of Hypertrophic Cardiomyopathy

Ali J. Marian

OVERVIEW

Henri Liouville, a French pathologist, described the first case of hypertrophic cardiomyopathy (HCM) in 1869.[1] The patient was an elderly woman with symptoms of heart failure, a ventricular wall thickness of 3.5 to 4 cm and left ventricular outflow tract (LVOT) obstruction.[1] Dr. Liouville described the LVOT obstruction as "Rétrécissement cardiaque sous aortique," which literally translates to subaortic cardiac.[1] Since this initial description, there has been considerable interest in the unusual clinical and pathological manifestations of HCM.

Alexander Schmincke described diffuse muscular "hyperplasia" at the LVOT and pointed out the vicious cycle of left ventricular hypertrophy and outflow tract obstruction, perpetuating each other.[2] Robert L. Levy and William C. Von Glahn described HCM as "Cardiac Hypertrophy of Unknown Etiology in Young Adults" in 1933.[3] William Evans reported the familial nature of "idiopathic cardiomegaly" in 1949 and constructed the first documented pedigree of a family with HCM.[4] Donald Teare also noted the familial nature of HCM in a young adult patient with severe cardiac hypertrophy.[5] J.A.P. Paré and colleagues described the autosomal dominant mode of inheritance of HCM in a large French-Canadian family, whose genetic mutation was identified by Christine Seidman and colleagues three decades later.[6,7]

Lord Russell Brock in England and Andrew Glenn Morrow and Eugene Braunwald in the United States recognized the dynamic nature of LVOT obstruction in HCM and concluded that the obstruction was due to "systolic narrowing of the LVOT resulting from massive muscular hypertrophy."[8-10] Dr. Braunwald and colleagues coined the term "idiopathic hypertrophic subaortic stenosis."[11] They also described the unique hemodynamic feature known as the Brockenbrough phenomenon and characterized left ventricular diastolic dysfunction as a major feature of HCM, independent of LVOT obstruction.[12] These observations led Dr. Morrow and colleagues to introduce trans-aortic surgical myectomy in the 1960s, which is known as the Morrow operation. [13]

Advances in echocardiographic imaging led to the next phase of discoveries in HCM and the description of asymmetric septal hypertrophy (ASH) and the assessment of LVOT obstruction by Doppler imaging.[14-16] Echocardiography soon emerged as the most commonly used imaging tool in diagnosing HCM, the assessment of its severity, the detection of diastolic dysfunction, and the estimation of the LVOT gradient. Likewise, tissue Doppler and spectral imaging modalities provided valuable information on regional myocardial contraction and relaxation abnormalities as well as diastolic function.[17-20] These imaging modalities also offer utilities in the preclinical and early identification of family members who carry the causal mutations for HCM.[18,19]

The seminal discovery of the first causal mutation in familial HCM by Drs. Christine and Jon Seidman in 1990 ushered in the era of molecular genetics.[7] The discovery, which was made in the original French-Canadian family described by Paré 30 years earlier, shifted the paradigm of HCM from being an "obscure" disease to primarily a genetic disease of sarcomere and sarcomere-associated proteins. The genetic discoveries brought forth the routine applications of genetic testing in the diagnosis and management of patients with HCM.

Ulrich Sigwart introduced alcohol septal ablation for the reduction of LVOT obstruction in three patients who reported marked and rapid improvement in their symptoms.[21] The technique commonly known as percutaneous alcohol septal ablation has become an alternative modality to Morrow's procedure for the treatment of selected symptomatic HCM patients with LVOT obstruction who are refractory to medical therapy.

Progress in diagnosis and management of patients with HCM has continued unabated. Notable among the recent progresses is the use of defibrillators (implantable cardioverter-defibrillator, [ICD]) in prevention of sudden cardiac death (SCD) in HCM as an effective intervention, particularly in the secondary prevention of SCD.[22,23] In recent years a number of randomized clinical trials, albeit small-scale initial phase II and III studies, with new pharmacological agents have been initiated and are expected to pave the way for larger-scale efficacy studies. The findings could expand our pharmacopeia beyond the β blockers, which were established by Dr. Braunwald and colleagues, as the cornerstone of medical therapy for HCM more than half a century ago.[24] Finally, development of new patient-specific and genetic-based therapies are being developed, which might fulfill the goal of tailoring the treatment to the individual patient.

DEFINITION

HCM could be defined as a genetic disease of cardiac myocytes that grossly manifests with cardiac hypertrophy; often asymmetric, and a nondilated left ventricle with a preserved or increased ejection fraction (**Fig. 23.1**).[25] Thus, by definition, cardiac hypertrophy caused by loading conditions is excluded. Cardiac hypertrophy is commonly concentric but occasionally involves a specific left ventricular wall or apex. It is asymmetric with a predominant involvement of the interventricular septum in about quarter of the cases.

EPIDEMIOLOGY

HCM is a relatively common disease with an estimated prevalence of 1:500 (0.16% to 0.29%) in the world population.[26-29] Population frequency of HCM might be higher than that estimated based on the expression of cardiac hypertrophy with a wall thickness of 15 mm or greater, as expression of hypertrophy is age-dependent and often absent in the young individuals. It is estimated that approximately 50% of those with the underlying causal HCM mutations develop HCM by the third decade of life, ~75% by the fifth decade of life, and 95% by 50 years of age.[30,31] Because of the age-dependent penetrance of HCM mutations, HCM is more prevalent in the older populations, estimated at 0.29% (44/15,137) in the 60-year-old individuals who have had an echocardiogram.[27]

In the clinical diagnosis of HCM, phenocopy conditions should be considered, which might be present in 5% to 10% of those with the clinical diagnosis of HCM, particularly the children.[32-34] In addition, the presence of concomitant conditions leading to increased load, such systemic arterial hypertension, could complicate the clinical diagnosis, hence estimating the true prevalence of HCM.

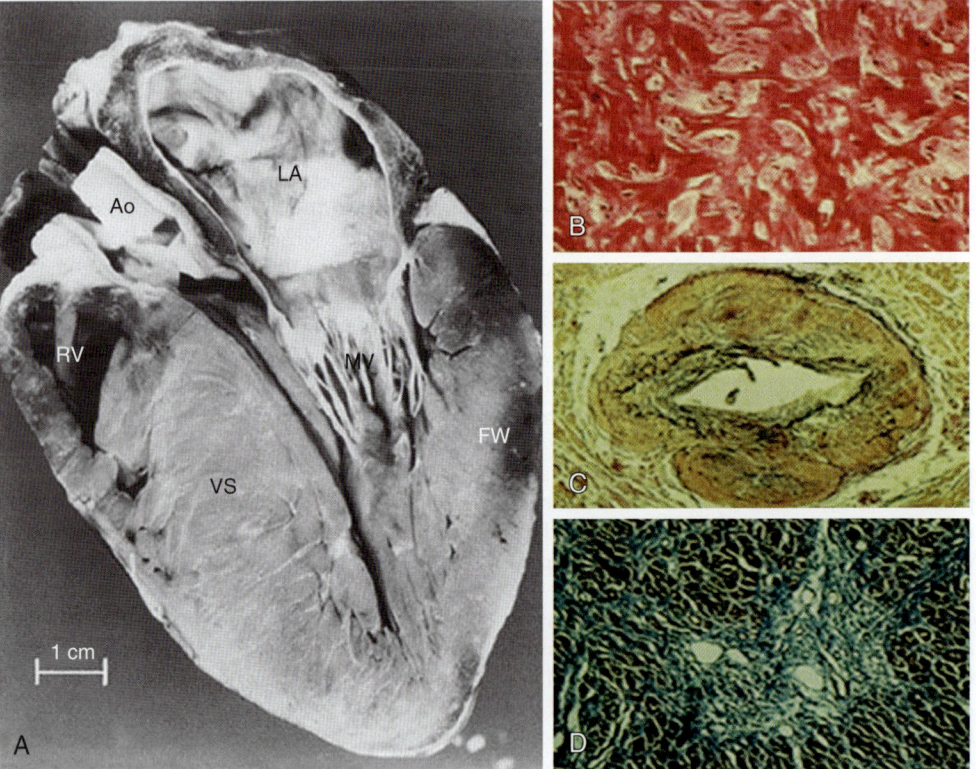

Fig. 23.1 Gross morphology and histopathology of hypertrophic cardiomyopathy (HCM). (A) Gross heart specimen shown in a cross-sectional plane similar to that of the echocardiographic (parasternal) long axis; pattern of left ventricle (LV) hypertrophy is asymmetric, disproportionately involving the ventricular septum (VS), which typically bulges into the left ventricular outflow tract. (B) Histopathology characteristic of LV in HCM with septal myocardium showing markedly disordered architecture with adjacent hypertrophied cardiac muscle cells arranged at perpendicular and oblique angles. (C) Intramural coronary artery with narrowed lumen and thickened wall, due primarily to medial (M) hypertrophy; (D) Scar in ventricular septum, representing repair process following clinically silent ischemia and myocyte death. *Ao,* Aorta; *FW,* free wall of left ventricle; *LA,* left atrium; *MV,* mitral valve; *RV,* right ventricle. (From Maron BJ. Sudden death in hypertrophic cardiomyopathy. *J Cardiovasc Transl Res.* 2009;2(4):368–380. Reproduced with permission of Springer.)

A genetic-based diagnosis might facilitate the accurate diagnosis of HCM in such cases (**see also Chapter 24**).

MOLECULAR GENETIC BASIS OF HYPERTROPHIC CARDIOMYOPATHY

HCM, a classic single gene disorder, is a familial disease in approximately two-thirds of cases and with an autosomal dominant pattern of inheritance.[35] HCM with an autosomal recessive or an X-linked mode of inheritance is rare.[36,37] The latter typically raises the possibility of a phenocopy condition, such as Fabry disease.[38]

Pioneering studies by Christine and Jon Seidman have led to the discovery of the first causal gene for HCM, namely the *MYH7* gene, which encodes sarcomere protein β-myosin heavy chain (MYH7), in the French-Canadian family that was originally described by Paré.[7] Subsequently, additional causal genes, including *MYBPC3*, *TNNT2*, *TPM1*, and *TNNI3*, which encode myosin-binding protein C proteins, cardiac troponin T, α-tropomyosin, and cardiac troponin I, respectively ,were mapped and identified.[39-42] Given that the well-established causal gene for HCM encodes sarcomere proteins, HCM is considered primarily a disease of sarcomere protein (**Fig. 23.2**).[39] Since the initial discoveries, over a dozen causal genes encoding sarcomere proteins and sarcomere-associated proteins, and thousands of mutations for HCM have been identified (**Table 23.1**).

The list of established causal genes for HCM includes *ACTC1* (cardiac α-actin), *MYL2* (myosin light chain 2), *MYL3* (myosin light chain 3), and *CSRP3* (muscle LIM protein).[43-45] In addition, *TTN* (titin), *TCAP* (telethonin), *MYOZ2* (myozenin 2), *TRIM63* (ubiquitin E3 ligase tripartite motif protein 63 or MuRF1), and *FHL1* (four and a half LIM domain 1) also are likely causal genes for HCM.[46-53] Finally, mutations in *TNNC1* (cardiac troponin C), *MYH6* (myosin heavy chain or α-myosin heavy chain), *PLN* (phospholamban), *CAV3* (caveolin 3), *ALPK3* (α kinase 3), and *JPH2* (junctophilin 2) have been associated with HCM.[54-59]

It is evident that HCM is a genetically heterogeneous disease. *MYH7* and *MYBPC3* are the two most common causal genes and together are responsible for approximately half of the familial HCM.[60-63] *TNNT2*, *TNNI3*, and *TPM1* are relatively uncommon causes of HCM and collectively are responsible for less than 10% of the HCM cases.[39,42,62,63] The remainder of the causal genes are even less common. Overall, the known causal genes account for about two-thirds of the HCM cases.

The majority of the causal mutations are missense mutations. Premature truncating mutations are rare with the exception of *MYBPC3* mutations, which are often insertion/deletion and frameshift mutations, leading to premature truncation of the encoded protein.[60,62,63] The frameshift mutations are often transcribed into unstable mRNAs, which are targeted for degradation by the nonsense-mediated decay (NMD). Similarly, whenever a premature truncated protein is expressed it is typically degraded by the ubiquitin proteasome system (UPS), leading to haploinsufficiency. Rare deletion mutations in *MYH7*, *TNNT2*, and others also have been reported.[64,65]

Population frequency of a specific HCM mutation is low and most mutations are either rare or private mutations. A notable exception is the p.Arg502Trp mutation in *MYBPC3*, which has been reported to occur in ~2.4% of HCM patients.[66] Likewise, the p.Val762Asp mutation in the *MYBPC3* gene has been reported in 3.9% of the Japanese population.[67] A few hot spots for mutation also have been reported.[68-70] Moreover, mutations do not exhibit an aggregation in a specific domain of the encoded protein, with the exception of mutations in *MYH7*, which show a predilection toward the globular head and hinge region of the protein, albeit mutations in the rod domain of *MYH7*, which have also have been described.[64,65,71] Finally, *MYH7* and *MYBPC3* are the two most common causal genes in apical HCM.[72,73]

The causal gene in approximately one-third of HCM remains unknown. The so-called missing causal genes typically pertain to the sporadic cases, where establishing the causality of the genetic variants unambiguously is exceedingly challenging if not impossible.[74] This

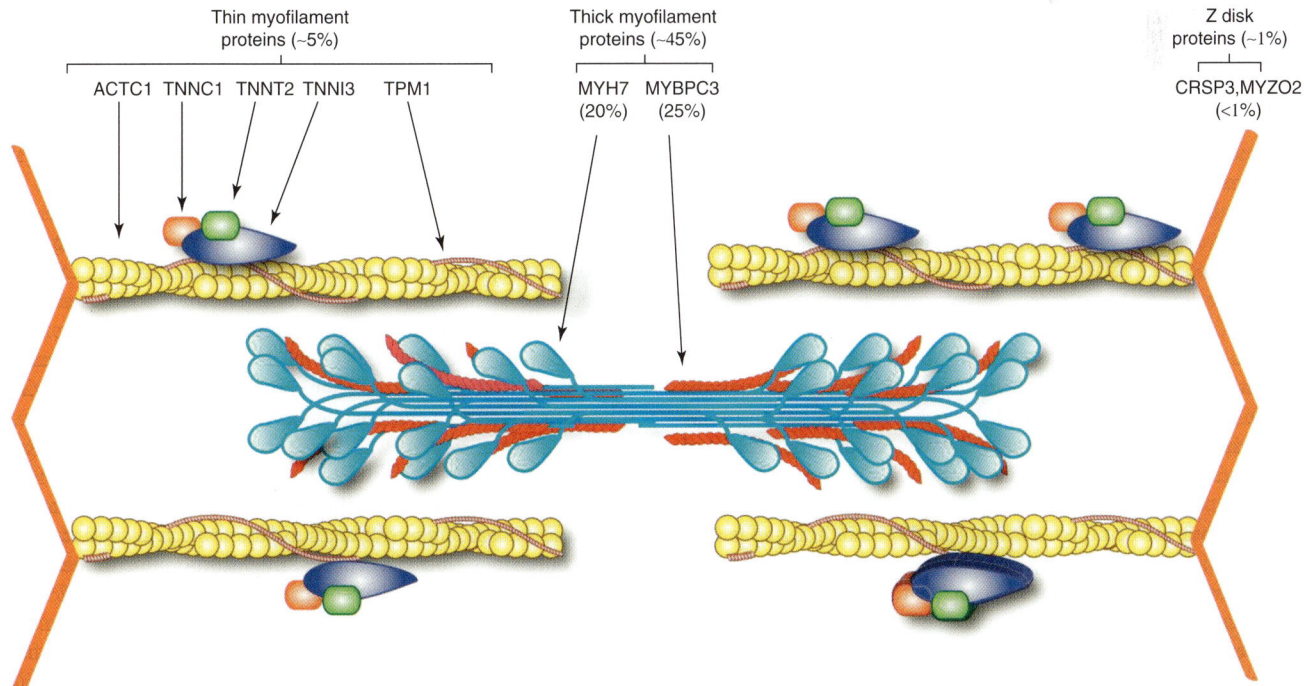

Fig. 23.2 The vast majority of clinically diagnosed hypertrophic cardiomyopathy (HCM) is caused by mutations in sarcomere proteins. Sarcomeres are comprised of thick and thin filaments and the Z disc. Therefore, HCM is primarily a disease of sarcomere proteins.

TABLE 23.1 Causal Genes for Hypertrophic Cardiomyopathy

Gene	Protein	Function
Causal Genes for HCM (strong evidence for causality)		
MYH7	β-Myosin heavy chain	ATPase activity, force generation
MYBPC3	Myosin binding protein-C	Cardiac contraction
TNNT2	Cardiac troponin T	Regulator of actomyosin interaction
TNNI3	Cardiac troponin I	Inhibitor of actomyosin interaction
TPM1	α-tropomyosin	Places the troponin complex on cardiac actin
ACTC1	Cardiac α-actin	Actomyosin interaction
MYL2	Regulatory myosin light chain	MYH7 binding protein
MYL3	Essential myosin light chain	MYH7 binding protein
CSRP3	Cysteine and glycine-rich protein 3	Muscle LIM protein (MLP), a Z disk protein
Causal Genes for HCM (moderate level evidence for causality)		
FHL1	Four-and-a-half LIM domains 1	Muscle development and hypertrophy
MYOZ2	Myozenin 2 (calsarcin 1)	Z disk protein
PLN	Phospholamban	Regulator of sarcoplasmic reticulum calcium
TCAP	Tcap (Telethonin)	Titin capping protein
TRIM63	Muscle ring finger protein 1	E3 ligase of proteasome ubiquitin system
TTN	Titin	Sarcomere function
Genes Associated with HCM (causality not definitive)		
ACTN2	Actinin, α-2	Z disk protein
ANKRD1	Ankyrin repeat domain 1	A negative regulator of cardiac genes
CASQ2	Calsequestrin 2	Calcium binding protein
CAV3	Caveolin 3	A caveolae protein
JPH2	Junctophilin2	Intracellular calcium signaling
LDB3	Lim domain binding 3	Z disk protein
MYH6	Myosin heavy chain α	Sarcomere protein expressed at low levels in the adult human heart
MYLK2	Myosin light chain kinase 2	Phosphorylate MYL2
NEXN	Nexilin	Z disc protein
TNNC1	Cardiac troponin C	Calcium sensitive regulator of myofilament function
VCL	Vinculin	Z disk protein

HCM, Hypertrophic cardiomyopathy.

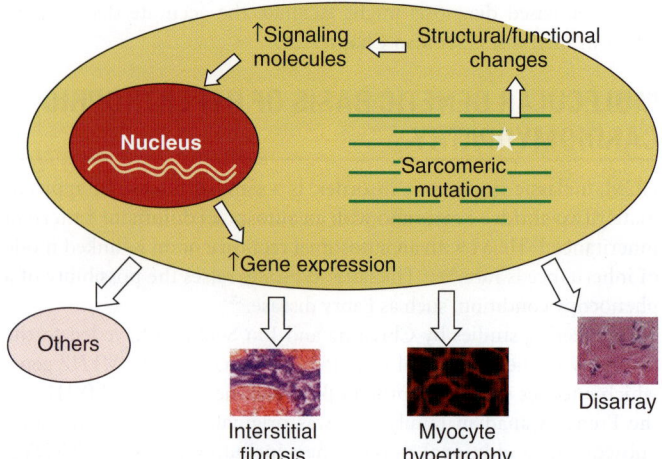

Fig. 23.3 (HCM), Pathogenesis of hypertrophic cardiomyopathy simplified into three stages of initial structural and functional defects followed by activation of signaling molecules, which lead to secondary gene expression leading to the HCM phenotype.

is in contrast to large families where the causal genes and mutations could be unambiguously identified through cosegregation and linkage analysis. The difficulty in identifying the "missing causal genes" in the sporadic cases, is in part intrinsic to genetic diversity of the humans, as each genome comprises about 4 million genetic variants, including about 11,000 nonsynonymous, and several thousand pathogenic variants.[75,76] In addition, the majority of the genetic variants is rare and population-specific, which makes it challenging to identify the responsible causal variant in a sporadic case. In addition, genetic variants exert a gradient of effect sizes, ranging from large and disease causing to clinically negligible.[77-79] Those with large effect sizes are expected to exhibit a high penetrance, cause familial disease where the variant cosegregates with inheritance of the phenotype. In contrast, variants with moderate effect sizes exhibit incomplete or low

penetrance in a familial setting and are often found in sporadic cases. Therefore, unambiguous ascertainment of genetic causality in such situations is difficult.

Finally, a subset of HCM, estimated to be about 5%, is caused by compound mutations in the same gene or two different genes.[63,67,80-85] Double mutations seem to be associated with a more pronounced phenotype.[67,80-83] Likewise, a small subset of HCM might be caused by multiple pathogenic variants, and hence, might be oligogenic in nature.[86]

PATHOGENESIS

The mechanistic molecular pathways connecting the causal mutations to the ensuing clinical and phenotypic features of HCM are diverse (**Fig. 23.3**). The mechanistic events could be sequentially categorized into three groups, based on the proximity of the genetic mutations, as follows:

- Proximal effects of the causal mutations, namely transcription and translation of the mutant proteins;
- Effects of the mutations on sarcomere structure and function, such as assembly and ATPase activity;
- Molecular pathways that are activated in response to structural and functional defects in the myofilaments/sarcomeres and link the mutations to the phenotypic features, such as trophic and mitotic factors.

Each set of the mechanistic categories entail a diverse array of events, likely reflecting the underpinning biological effects of the involved codon and protein. The mechanisms are likely to differ for HCM caused by mutations in genes other than those coding for the sarcomere proteins, including phenocopy conditions.

Effects of the Mutations on Transcription and Translation

Proximal defects are defined as the direct and most proximal effect of the mutations on gene transcription, translation, integrity, and stability of the encoded transcripts and proteins, and incorporation of the encoded proteins into sarcomeres. In keeping with the diversity of the genes and mutations involved, the proximal phenotypes are also diverse.

HCM mutations are mostly heterozygous missense mutations, which are typically translated into proteins, each encompassing a change in a single amino acid. However, a change in the nucleotide sequence could affect the efficiency of transcription as well as the translation of the encoded mRNA into the corresponding protein.[87-89] The suboptimal codon usage often leads to an allelic imbalance, which is often compensated for by the wild type allele. Thus, the majority of the missense mutations do not significantly affect, or only modestly affect, the expression levels of the corresponding proteins.[87,88] However, it seems that there is considerable variability in the transcript levels of mutant alleles among myocytes and in different regions of the myocardium, which might also influence the phenotypic expression of HCM.[88]

A fraction of HCM mutation is stop codon or insertion/deletion mutations that lead to premature truncation of the transcripts and the encoded proteins. The truncated transcripts and proteins are subject to several transcriptional and translational surveillance and quality control programs that target the prematurely truncated transcripts and proteins for degradation. Notable among them is the NMD pathway, which targets transcripts containing premature termination codon by releasing the elongation factors from the template and recruitment of the decay-inducing complex. Similarly, the prematurely truncated proteins are unstable and subjected to unfolded protein response and decay by UPS.[90-93]

In scenarios where the causal mutation leads to a gain- or loss-of-stop codon or results in a frame shift, expression of the mutant protein is reduced, and the net effect is reduced expression level of the involved protein and even haplo-insufficiency. This seems to be the predominant mechanism for mutations in the *MYBPC3*, which predominantly lead to premature truncation of the protein.[63,94]

Effects of Mutations on Sarcomere Assembly and Function

The majority of the mutant proteins carrying the causal mutations are stably expressed and incorporate into sarcomeres and myofibrils. However, the mutation by altering the three-dimensional (3-D) structure of corresponding protein could affect protein-protein interactions and reduce incorporation of the mutant protein into sarcomeres.[95] There is variability in the incorporation of the mutant proteins into sarcomere, which is expected to affect function of the assembled sarcomeres in cardiac myocytes.[89]

In interpreting the results of functional data, it is important to consider the differences in the sarcomere protein composition between mice and humans. While the mouse predominantly expresses α-myosin heavy chain or MYH6 (>95%) in the heart, the β-myosin heavy chain or MYH7 is the predominant myosin isoform in the human heart, comprising >90% of the total myosin heavy chain.[96-98] Differences in the MYH protein composition is relevant to functional studies of HCM mutations, as MYH6 and MYH7 show four- to six-fold differences in ATPase activities and actomyosin kinetics.[96,99-101]

Mutations impart a diverse array of functional defects by affecting various components of the actomyosin complex, including calcium sensitivity of the troponin complex, ATPase activity of myosin heavy chain, and generation of the force of contraction upon displacement of the actin filament by myosin heavy chain globular head. Under physiological conditions, the thin actin filament is released from the actomyosin complex upon binding of ATP to the globular head of the myosin. In the presence of HCM mutations, the sensitivity of this complex in releasing actin, upon binding of ATP to myosin globular head, is reduced. Consequently, in any given moment during a cardiac cycle, a higher number of myosin and actin are in a bound state than in a dissociated state, compared to the physiological condition. This is expected to affect both the systolic and diastolic phases of cardiac cycle. Consequently, the maximal tension development per each unit of the ATP is hydrolyzed, and hence, myocardial efficiency of force generation, is lower in HCM compared to the physiological state.[102-105] The effects of the mutations on the dissociation of actin and myosin upon

ATP binding, and hence, myocardial energetic efficiency, are variable leading to different degrees of functional impairment. For example, mutations in *MYH7* reduce myofibrillar ATPase activity more than those in the *MYBPC3*, resulting in a higher energy cost of tension generation for the *MYH7* rather than the *MYBPC3* mutations.[102,103] These functional alterations, such as reduced myocardial energetic efficiency, precede cardiac hypertrophy, as the impairment is also observed in the prehypertrophic stage in individuals who carry HCM mutations.[103] The increased energy cost of tension generation also correlates with the reduced ratio of cardiac phosphocreatine to ATP in the human hearts in HCM.[106] Experimental data in a transgenic rabbit model of HCM, which has a cardiac myosin isoform composition closely resembling that in the human heart, show reduced calcium sensitivity of the myofibrils ATPase activity early and prior to the development of cardiac hypertrophy.[105] Calcium sensitivity of maximum force generation also seems to vary among myocytes, which might be secondary to a variation in the expression levels of the mutant transcript.[88] Finally, different regions of the myocardium show differences in the expression levels and functions, suggesting a mosaic molecular and functional effect in HCM.[107]

The effects of mutations in thin filament proteins such as TNNT2 on sarcomere function seem to differ from mutations in the thick filaments, such as MYH7. Accordingly, mutations in the thick filament proteins enhance calcium sensitivity of force generation and ATPase activity of the myofilaments, as opposed to the effects of mutations in the thick filaments, which were discussed earlier.[108-111] The effects also precede the development of cardiac hypertrophy in the murine models.[112]

Molecular Pathways Liking the Initial Defects to the Phenotype

Defects in gene expression, sarcomere structure, and myocyte function, imparted by the HCM mutations, lead to activation of expression of large cadre of molecules, including the stress-responsive signaling pathways in the heart (see Fig. 23.3).[113] These dysregulated pathways mediate induction of cardiac hypertrophy, fibrosis, morphological, and functional phenotypes in HCM. As would be expected, the nature of the dysregulated transcriptional and signaling pathways are diverse and vary according to the biological functions of the proteins involved and the nature of the mutations. Among the dysregulated pathways in HCM are the calcineurin, mitogen activated protein kinases, and the transforming growth factor β pathways.[52,114-121] In addition, the noncoding RNA and epigenetic factors are also implicated.[122,123] The dysregulated pathways collectively lead to the induction of cardiac hypertrophy, interstitial fibrosis, and other morphological, histological, and functional features of HCM (see Fig. 23.3).

Determinants of the Clinical Phenotype of Hypertrophic Cardiomyopathy

The clinical phenotypes of HCM are secondary events resulting from complex and stochastic interactions of a number of dysregulated pathways and the environmental factors (**Fig. 23.4**). Consequently, a large number of factors contribute to the pathogenesis of clinical manifestations of HCM. Naturally, the causal mutations have the largest impact on the expression of the clinical phenotype; however, they are not the sole determinants, as the genetic background or the modifier genes and the additional pathogenic variants, the epigenetic factors, the noncoding RNAs, the posttranslational protein modifications, and the environmental factors all contribute to phenotypic expression of the disease (see Fig. 23.4). Nevertheless, despite the large effect size of the causal mutations, there is no clear genotype-phenotype correlation in HCM, and phenotypic expression of the disease is largely similar between *MYH7* and *MYBPC3*, which are the two most common causal genes in HCM.[124,125] The multiplicity of the phenotypic determinants along with their complex and stochastic interactions contribute to variability in the phenotypic expression of HCM (**Fig. 23.5**).[124,126,127]

The classic HCM is a single gene disorder with an autosomal dominant mode of inheritance. However, small families and probands have been described where multiple pathogenic variants seem to contribute to the pathogenesis of HCM.[80-82,85,86] Thus, in a sense, a subset of HCM might be digenic and oligogenic in etiology.[86] The presence of multiple pathogenic variants is associated with a more severe phenotype, including severe cardiac hypertrophy and outflow tract obstruction.[80-82,85,86]

Several modifier genetic variants and loci have been implicated as determinants of severity of the phenotype.[128-133] Notable among them

is an insertion/deletion variant in the angiotensin-1-converting enzyme 1 gene (*ACE*), which is associated with variation in the plasma levels of ACE.[134] The variant has been associated with the severity of cardiac hypertrophy as well as the risk of SCD in patients with HCM.[129-131] In a mouse model of HCM the *Fhl1* gene, encoding 4.5 LIM domains protein 1 is implicated as a possible modifier of cardiac hypertrophy and function.[135]

Among the external factors, loading conditions, including systemic arterial hypertension, are expected to influence phenotypic expression of HCM, including severity of cardiac hypertrophy. The so-called hypertensive hypertrophic cardiomyopathy of the elderly might represent a condition wherein the concomitant presence of systemic arterial hypertension influences expression of sarcomere protein mutations or pathogenic variants in the sarcomere genes. Likewise, isometric exercises would be expected to enhance expression of cardiac hypertrophy in those who carry the HCM mutations or pathogenic variants in genes encoding sarcomere proteins.

There is considerable phenotypic overlap for the phenotypic expression of mutations in genes known to cause cardiomyopathies. The causal gene for HCM might also cause other forms of cardiomyopathies, particularly dilated cardiomyopathy (DCM), which phenotypically contrasts HCM.[136-139] This is well illustrated for *TNNT2* and *MYH7*, which are known to cause either HCM or DCM.[7,140] Differences in the phenotypic expression of the mutations in a given gene might reflect the effects of the mutations on interactions of the mutant protein with other proteins, as well as calcium sensitivity of the myofilaments.[108,141-146] Mutations enhancing Ca^{+2} sensitivity of the myofibrillar force generation and ATPase activity could lead to HCM, whereas those reducing these functions lead to DCM.[108,141-148]

PHENOTYPIC FEATURES OF HYPERTROPHIC CARDIOMYOPATHY

Cardiac hypertrophy, the quintessential phenotypic feature of clinical HCM, develops primarily because of myocyte hypertrophy, and to

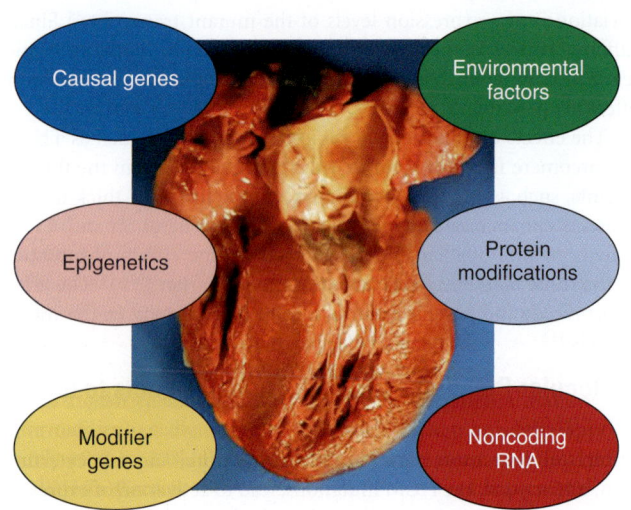

Fig. 23.4 Major expected determinants of clinical phenotype in patients with hypertrophic cardiomyopathy.

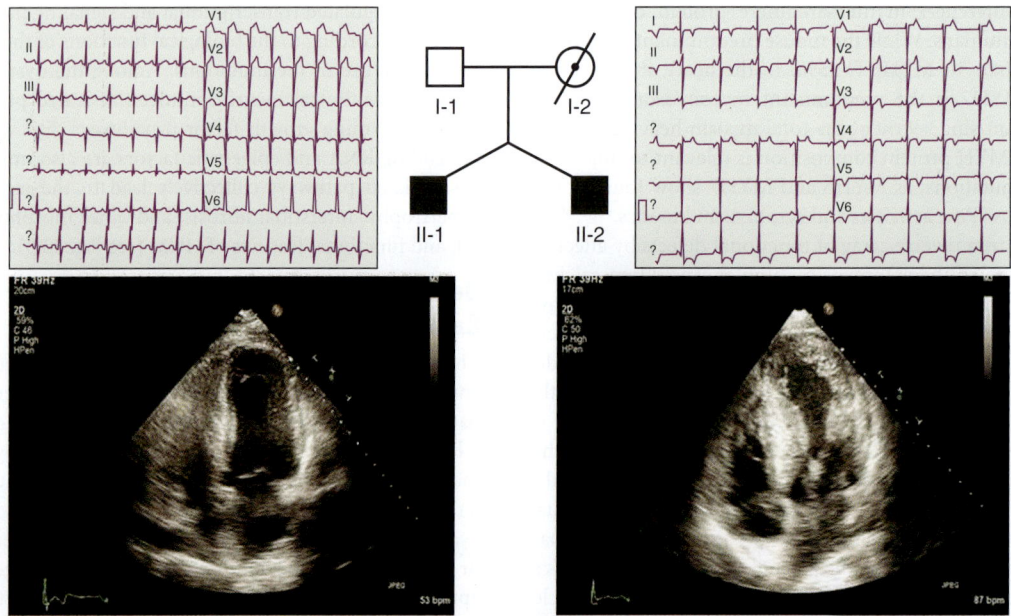

Fig. 23.5 Phenotypic variability. A truncated pedigree shows twin brothers with hypertrophic cardiomyopathy caused by the S48P mutation in *MYOZ2*. There is significant variability in the degree of cardiac hypertrophy on 12-lead electrocardiography (ECG) and echocardiograms between the two brothers.

some extent because of increased extracellular matrix volume. HCM is clinically diagnosed based on the detection of cardiac hypertrophy by a diagnostic modality, such as echocardiography. Cardiac hypertrophy is commonly defined as an end diastolic wall thickness of 13 mm or greater on an echocardiogram. In HCM, cardiac hypertrophy occurs in the absence of external loading conditions or is disproportionate to the external factors, and in the absence of other secondary causes, such as storage diseases. A left ventricular wall thickness of 15 mm or greater has been advocated as a more accurate indicator of hypertrophy in HCM, and it confers a greater specificity at the expense of reduced sensitivity in detecting HCM. Given that body size is a major determinant of cardiac size and wall thickness, a Z-score, reflecting deviation from an age- and sex-matched population average, is used in children to define cardiac hypertrophy.

Cardiac hypertrophy is commonly concentric, and in about a quarter of the cases it is asymmetric, predominantly involving the interventricular septum. Cardiac apex is occasionally the predominant site of involvement, which leads to the diagnosis of apical HCM. Such patients exhibit the characteristic deep T wave inversion in the precordial leads. Rarely, the other left ventricular wall or only the right ventricle is involved—the latter manifesting with right ventricular outflow tract obstruction.[149]

Cardiac hypertrophy, in the absence of a secondary cause, is the quintessential clinical diagnostic criterion for HCM. However, cardiac hypertrophy is the common response of the heart to a variety of stress, including increased loading conditions, such as systemic arterial hypertension. HCM is diagnosed when cardiac hypertrophy is judged to be disproportionate to the increased load. HCM might also be present concomitantly with systemic arterial hypertension, rendering the clinical diagnosis challenging. Phenotypic features, including ASH, increased left ventricular ejection fraction, a small left ventricular cavity size, and the presence of LVOT obstruction, would suggest the diagnosis of HCM in those with hypertension.

The distinction between physiological hypertrophy observed in professional athletes and pathological hypertrophy of HCM also could be challenging.[150] Again, characteristics described above, including the presence of a small left ventricular cavity size and LVOT obstruction, would indicate HCM, as athletes typically exhibit cardiac hypertrophy with an enlarged left ventricle.[150,151] Other features, including pathological Q waves, conduction defects, reduced tissue Doppler velocities, and reduced strain, would favor the diagnosis of HCM.[150-154]

Phenocopy conditions, such as glycogen storage diseases, lysosomal storage diseases, mitochondrial diseases, triplet repeat syndromes, and others, mimic HCM. The distinction is typically difficult, despite differences in the pathogenesis of HCM and its phenocopy conditions, such as Fabry disease.[38] Typically, a very high or low QRS voltage and presence of a delta wave on an electrocardiography (ECG) in a male patient with severe cardiac hypertrophy, as well as involvement of other organs, would hint at the possibility of a phenocopy condition. Genetic testing could lead to differentiation of HCM and its phenocopy conditions, although the yield of genetic testing is not high.

The pathological hallmark of HCM is myocyte disarray, which is defined as loss of normal parallel alignment of cardiac myocytes because of haphazardly oriented deformed myocytes that are enlarged and have pleiotropic nuclei (Fig. 23.6).[155] Disarray typically involves more than 10% of the myocardium and is typically present in conjunctions with hypertrophy and fibrosis.[155,156] Severe myocyte disarray has been associated with increased risk of SCD in patients with HCM.[157]

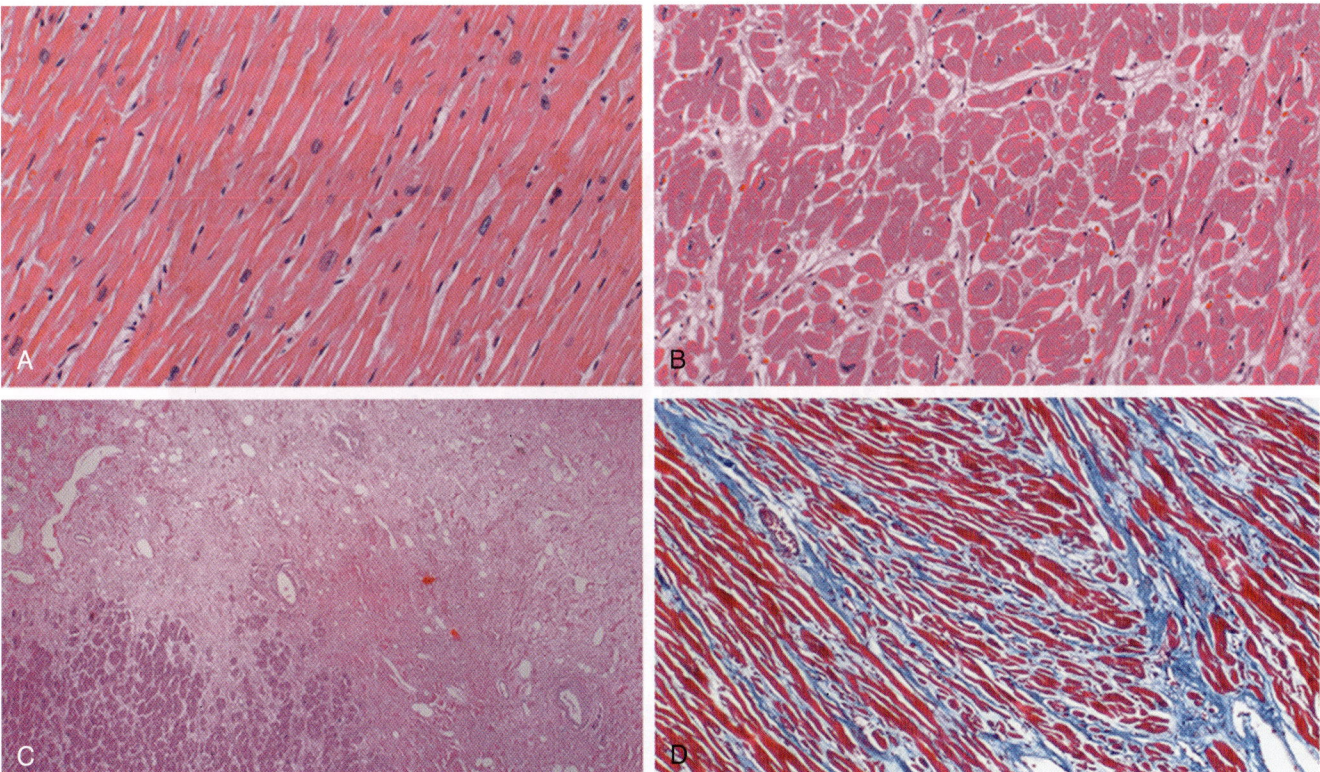

Fig. 23.6 Histological features of hypertrophic cardiomyopathy (HCM): (A) Hematoxylin and eosin (H&E)–stained thin myocardial section from a normal heart. (B) H&E-stained thin myocardial sections from a patient with HCM showing poorly organized myocytes and increased interstitial space. (C) Thin myocardial section from a patient with HCM showing a necrotic area bordering myocytes. (D) Masson trichrome-stained thin myocardial section from a patient with HCM showing increased interstitial fibrosis.

Another important histological feature of HCM is interstitial fibrosis, which is associated with an increased risk of cardiac arrhythmias, heart failure, and SCD (see Fig. 23.6).[158-160] Modern imaging techniques have enabled the detection and quantification of myocyte disarray and interstitial fibrosis without the need for an endomyocardial biopsy. Late gadolinium enhancement (LGE), detected and quantified by cardiac magnetic resonance (CMR) imaging, as a marker for extracellular volume fraction and interstitial fibrosis, is associated with the occurrence of cardiac arrhythmias and the risk of SCD in HCM.[159-162] Likewise, collagen cleavage products are useful biomarkers for the presence of interstitial fibrosis in HCM.[163-165] Other potential biomarkers for cardiac hypertrophy, cell death, and fibrosis, are cytokines, cardiac troponin T, and microRNAs.[166-171]

CLINICAL MANIFESTATIONS

The majority of patients with HCM are asymptomatic or minimally symptomatic, even though they typically exhibit reduced exercise tolerance. The common symptoms include palpitations, chest pain, and shortness of breath. The major clinical issues in patients with HCM include the management of cardiac arrhythmias and the risk of SCD; the management of heart failure, typically due to diastolic dysfunction; and the management of LVOT obstruction.

Chest Pain

Patients with HCM frequently experience chest pain, particularly the young individuals. It is commonly exercise induced, but otherwise does not follow the characteristics of angina pectoris of coronary origin. Chest pain presumably occurs because of a mismatch between the oxygen demand of hypertrophic myocardium and an inadequate supply partly because of increased intramural coronary vasculopathy, marked by thickening of arterial media, and a relatively reduced capillary density, leading to myocardial ischemia and even necrosis (see Fig. 23.6).[172] However, in older patients, concomitant coronary artery disease might be present. For those with no obstructive coronary artery disease, treatment with β-blockers and nondihydropyridine calcium channel blockers is effective in alleviating symptoms.

Heart Failure

Heart failure symptoms in patients with HCM are commonly due to diastolic dysfunction (**see also Chapter 11**) with an elevated left ventricular end diastolic pressure but a normal or increased left ventricular ejection fraction. Therefore, it is heart failure with preserved ejection fraction (HFpEF). Although the left ventricular ejection fraction is preserved, myocardial function, both systolic and more markedly diastolic, is impaired, as detected by modern imaging techniques such as tissue Doppler imaging, 3-D speckle tracking echocardiography, and CMR (**Fig. 23.7**).[19,173,174] Consequently, diastolic dysfunction is the major cause of heart failure in patients with HCM, and is a major prognosticator.[175] Symptom-wise, exercise intolerance and reduced cardiopulmonary capacity are the common early symptoms. Often, patients modify their lifestyle to cope with the symptoms. Therefore, detailed history taking is necessary to uncover the exercise intolerance. Exercise intolerance is often associated with findings of fluid retention such as peripheral edema. Exertional dyspnea is often progressive, and if untreated leads to the classic symptoms of fluid retention, such as orthopnea and paroxysmal nocturnal dyspnea, as well as peripheral edema. The symptoms are first responsive to medical treatment including the judicious use of diuretics. The use of diuretics is particularly concerning in those with an LVOT obstruction, as excess diuresis could induce hypovolemia, hypotension, and syncope.

The main risk factors for heart failure in patients with HCM include LVOT obstruction, severe cardiac hypertrophy, extensive interstitial fibrosis, and atrial fibrillation. LVOT in approximately one-third of the patients, and is a major contributor to elevated left ventricular end diastolic pressure and HFpEF.[176,177] LVOT obstruction results from cardiac hypertrophy, particularly asymmetric septal hypertrophy, which narrows the outflow tract, and a small left ventricle cavity size,

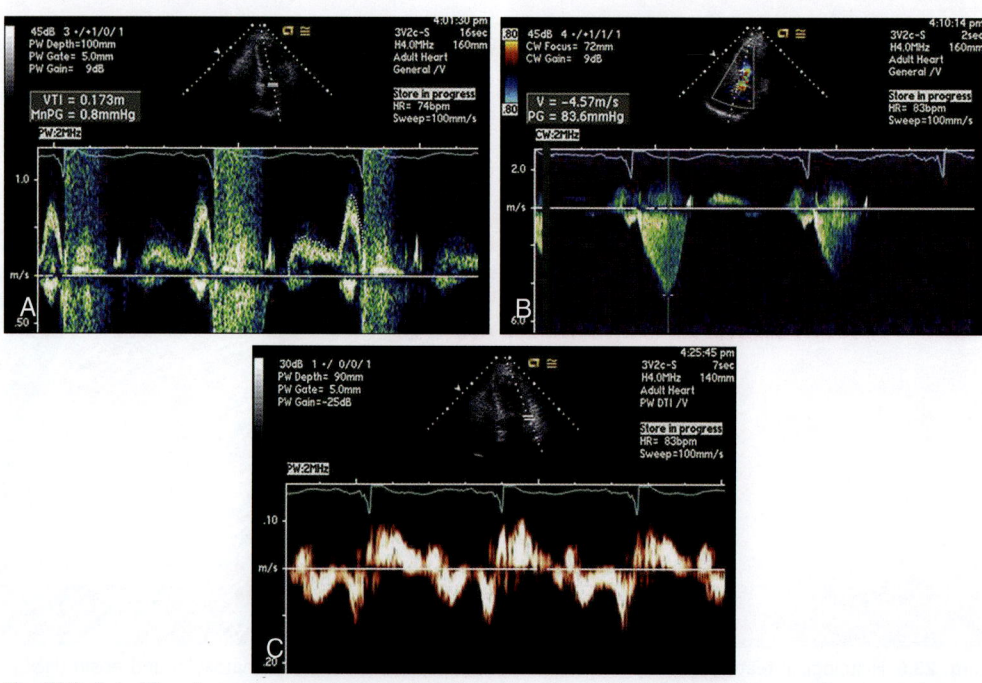

Fig. 23.7 Echo/Doppler evaluation of cardiac function in a patient with HCM and severe outflow tract obstruction. (A) Mitral inflow velocities showing diastolic dysfunction evidenced by decreased E and increased A velocities. (B) Doppler measurement of left ventricular outflow tract gradient, which is about 80 mmHg. (C) Reduced systolic and early diastolic velocities, which are early markers for HCM.

collectively leading to a Venturi effect and displacement of the anterior leaflet of the mitral valve toward septum during systole (systolic anterior motion) and obstruction of blood flow at the LVOT (see Fig. 23.6). Resting LVOT obstruction, defined a pressure gradient of >30 mm Hg, is present in approximately one-quarter of HCM patients, but is inducible with exercise in more than half of the patients.[178,179] As initially described by Sir Russell Brock and Dr. Braunwald, the obstruction is dynamic and varies with changes in contractility, stroke volume, and afterload.[8-11,180] It is an important contributor to the progression of cardiac hypertrophy and the risk of heart failure.[176,178]

Atrial fibrillation is also common and found in about one-quarter of patients with HCM. A new onset of atrial fibrillation is not well tolerated and often leads to heart failure.[181] Diastolic dysfunction infrequently progresses to refractory heart failure requiring heart transplantation. In addition, a small subset of patients with HCM, estimated to be about 5%, develop global systolic dysfunction with chamber dilatation and evolve into DCM, leading to heart failure with reduced ejection fraction.[136]

Ventricular Arrhythmias and Sudden Cardiac Death

SCD is the often the first manifestation of HCM, particularly in the young, but is fortunately infrequent, with an incidence of 0.5% to 2% per year in the overall HCM population.[182-184] Nonetheless, HCM is the most common cause of SCD in young competitive athletes, which is often tragic and occurs in the absence of prior symptoms.[185-187] However, minor symptoms might be present, which often are not pursued. Syncope is a major risk factor for SCD in patients with HCM.[183,188] It commonly occurs because of ventricular tachycardia and less commonly because of orthostatic hypotension resulting from hypovolemia, LVOT obstruction, and autonomic dysfunction.[183,188-190] SCD in HCM is typically because of ventricular tachycardia/fibrillation. Therefore, symptoms of palpitations, presyncope, and syncope necessitate additional investigation for cardiac arrhythmias, typically by long periods of telemetric rhythm monitoring.

Sustained ventricular tachycardia and repetitive nonsustained ventricular tachycardia, the latter particularly when associated with lightheadedness or presyncope, are major risk factors for SCD and necessitate implantation of an ICD.[188,189] A family history of SCD, reflective of the underpinning causal mutation and the genetic background, is also an important risk factor for SCD.[188,189] However, given the presence of considerable variability in the phenotypic expression of HCM, additional findings would be needed, besides a family history of SCD, to implant an ICD. However, there is no uniform opinion on the indications for an ICD implantation. Severe cardiac hypertrophy and extensive interstitial fibrosis are also associated with an increased risk of SCD in HCM.[161,188,191]

Supraventricular Arrhythmias

Atrial fibrillation/flutter and paroxysmal atrial tachycardia are the common forms of supraventricular tachycardias in HCM. The annual incidence of atrial fibrillation is about 3% per year.[181] Overall, about one-quarter of patients with HCM experience atrial fibrillation, which is often not well tolerated and is associated with adverse clinical outcomes.[181,192] The rapid heart rate, leading to a shortened diastolic phase, and the loss of atrial contraction in the presence of impaired left ventricular relaxation and compliance, lead to elevated left ventricular filling pressure and symptoms of heart failure. Likewise, reduced stroke volume could lead to hypotension and symptoms of lightheadedness, presyncope, and syncope. A preexcitation pattern on an electrocardiogram is detected in approximately 5% of patients with HCM, which might lead to AV nodal reciprocating arrhythmias. The preexcitation pattern is more common in patients with a phenocopy condition, such as glycogen storage diseases.[193]

Cardioversion is the treatment of choice for symptomatic new onset atrial fibrillation, followed by medical therapy to prevent recurrence. Recurrent and paroxysmal atrial fibrillation are treated with antiarrhythmic drugs. Atrial fibrillation increases the risk of thromboembolism. The annual incidence of thromboembolism in HCM is estimated to be about 4%.[181] Given the increased risk, stroke patients with atrial fibrillation require long-term anticoagulation.

Prognosis

Patients with HCM exhibit a spectrum of clinical course, ranging from SCD at a young age to a normal life expectancy. All things considered, HCM is a relatively benign disease, particularly in those without an LVOT obstruction who have a very low rate of complications.[177,192] The presence of LVOT obstruction increases the risk of heart failure, and in its absence, only about 10% of patients experience heart failure symptoms over the course of 6.5 years.[177] Overall, approximately two-thirds of patients with HCM do not have increased morbidity and experience a normal life expectancy.[192]

As mentioned, HCM is a relatively benign disease despite the risk of SCD. The annual mortality of garden variety adult patients with HCM is estimated at less than 1%.[194-196] This is also the case for patients with apical HCM, who exhibit a 15-year survival probability of approximately 95%.[192]

MANAGEMENT OF PATIENTS WITH HYPERTROPHIC CARDIOMYOPATHY

Genetic Testing

Genetic testing has become part of the routine evaluation of patients with HCM, particularly in the familial setting, where its impact is the largest. In this setting, genetic testing provides the opportunity to establish the causality of the pathogenic variant, which is typically identified by whole exome sequencing, upon cosegregation analysis. Likewise, it leads to identification of the mutation carriers prior to and independent of expression of the clinical phenotype. The latter group often is referred to genotype^Pos/phenotype^Neg individuals, but are best described as mutation carriers, which is the conventional nomenclature. Identification of the mutation carriers could provide the opportunity to intervene early to prevent and attenuate the evolving phenotype or slow its progression.[197] In addition, it leads to frequent evaluation and assessment, leading to early detection of HCM and interventions to reduce the risk of SCD.

Genetic testing in individuals who exhibit the clinical phenotype could offer insights into the molecular pathogenesis of HCM and enables the distinction between HCM causes by sarcomere protein mutations and the phenocopy conditions. The distinction is not inconsequential as treatment of the phenocopy conditions differ, as in the case of Fabry disease, where enzyme replacement therapy is available as a specific therapy.[198] The impact of genetic testing in genotype–phenotype correlation and assessing the severity of the disease or prognostication is less clear with the exception of double or multiple pathogenic variants, which are typically associated with a more pronounced phenotype.[67,80-83,86]

The main issue in genetic testing, typically performed by whole exome sequencing, is interpretation of the findings, as each exome contains a large number of pathogenic variants, including in the genes implicated in HCM. Consequently, the challenge is to discern the true pathogenic or causal variant from the rest. Identification of the true pathogenic variants is particularly challenging in sporadic cases and in small families. Therefore, unambiguous designation of causality of variants identified by genetic testing in an individual or in small families is almost impossible. The difficulty has become more evident in large-scale sequencing experiments, which show that approximately 5% to 10% of the general population carries one or two rare pathogenic variants in genes encoding sarcomere proteins.[199,200] Therefore, designation of all pathogenic variants in genes known to cause HCM would lead to a considerable overcall.[199,201]

The main disappointment in genetic testing is failure to identify the causal variant. Unfortunately, this is not uncommon as the yield of genetic testing by whole exome sequencing in HCM seems to be less than 50%.[202] The shortcoming is, in part, because of the imperfectness of the whole exome sequencing, which is often used for genetic testing, as well as difficulty in assigning the pathogenic or causal variant in a single individual or small families.

Management of Risk of Sudden Cardiac Death in Hypertrophic Cardiomyopathy

SCD, although not common, is often a tragic event. The incidence of SCD in HCM is between 0.5% and 2%.[182-184] The victims are typically young and often asymptomatic individuals who develop ventricular tachycardia/fibrillation during physical activity and competitive sports. HCM is the most common discernible cause of SCD in young competitive athletes.[22,187]

Several risk factors for SCD have been identified, including a history of syncope due to cardiac arrhythmias, runs of sustained and repetitive nonsustained ventricular tachycardia, a strong family history of SCD, and severe cardiac hypertrophy. While extended cardiac rhythm monitoring is valuable in detecting cardiac arrhythmias, and hence, evaluating the risk if SCD, the role of electrophysiological studies, tilt table testing, and exercise testing in the risk stratification for SCD have not been well established. Similarly, cardiopulmonary exercise testing, and exercise echocardiography could provide data on predicting cardiovascular events but their role in predicting the risk of SCD is unclear.[203-205] Likewise, LVOT obstruction is associated with an increased risk of heart failure but is not considered a major risk factor for SCD. Surgical septal myectomy in those with LVOT obstruction is associated with a reduced risk of SCD.[206]

HCM patients at an increased risk of SCD benefit from implantation of an ICD, which has been shown to be effective in detecting ventricular arrhythmias and intervening to terminate ventricular tachycardia and preventing SCD.[22,23,207,208] Every year 3% to 15% of adult patients with an ICD experience a proper ICD discharge.[22,23,207,208] The rate of proper ICD discharge is higher in adult patients who have experienced prior ventricular arrhythmias and in children.[22,23,207,208] Although the indication for an ICD implantation as a secondary prevention (i.e., in those with a prior event) is clear, an indication for the primary prevention of SCD is less clear, and is debatable. None of the known risk factors alone offer sufficient predictive value to justify implantation of an ICD. However, observational data suggest that the rate of ICD discharge does not differ among patients with one or multiple risk factors.[22] Retrospective data analysis shows that extreme cardiac hypertrophy is the most common risk factor in patients who receive an ICD implantation for the primary prevention of SCD and experience a proper ICD discharge.[23] The common practice is to implant an ICD in the primary prevention of SCD in patients who (1) experience sustained or repetitive nonsustained ventricular tachycardia; (2) experience syncope due to arrhythmias; (3) have severe cardiac hypertrophy; and (4) have a strong family history of SCD. However, a recent study reported that patients who had a maximum wall thickness of 35 mm or greater did not have an increased risk of SCD.[209] Other risk factors, such as extent of myocardial interstitial fibrosis, detected as LGE on CMR, are also considered in the evaluation for an ICD implantation.[23,159-161,210,211]

Management of Patients with Left Ventricular Outflow Tract Obstruction

LVOT obstruction at rest (a pressure gradient between left ventricle and the outflow tract of >30 mmHg) is present in approximately one-quarter of HCM patients. However, LVOT obstruction is inducible in about two-thirds of the patients with HCM (latent LVOT obstruction). A characteristic of LVOT gradient is its dynamic nature and variability. It changes to with maneuvers that affect loading conditions and left ventricular contractility. Often, the Valsalva maneuver or amyl nitrate is used to induce LVOT obstruction. It is best assessed noninvasively by Doppler imaging and invasively by cardiac catheterization and pull-back pressure recording.

LVOT obstruction is a risk factor for heart failure, hypotension, and syncope.[176] Symptomatic LVOT obstruction requires aggressive therapy, which is initially pharmacological intervention and more effectively septal myectomy, whether surgical or through alcohol ablation. Pharmacological treatment of LVOT obstruction comprises the use of β blockers, disopyramide, to a lesser extent, L-type calcium channel blockers. β blockers are the cornerstone of therapy and have been since the initial report by a group led by Dr. Braunwald in 1964.[24] The negative inotropic and parasympathetic agent disopyramide is commonly used in combination with a β blocker, the latter to attenuate its effects on increasing the heart rate. The combination has been shown to improve symptoms and reduce the LVOT gradient in about two-thirds of the patients.[212] Patients who do not tolerate β blockers or disopyramide, or remain symptomatic despite medical therapy, are treated with a nondihydropyridine class of calcium channel blockers. Dihydropyridines are avoided as they increase the risk of hypotension and syncope. Diuretics are used when there is evidence of fluid retention, but often at low doses to avoid the risk of volume depletion, hypotension, and syncope.

Surgical septal myectomy, which is referred to as the Morrow procedure, and alcohol septal ablation are highly effective in alleviating symptoms and reducing the LVOT obstruction. Both approaches are equally effective. The choice of the approach to septal myectomy depends on specific patient conditions. For example, surgical septal myectomy is the approach of choice in patients with concomitant coronary artery disease and in those who are at an increased risk of SCD.[206] However, alcohol septal ablation might be preferable in patients with comorbid conditions and when the surgical risk is high.

Management of Cardiac Arrhythmias

The typical arrhythmias in patients with HCM that require therapy are sustained and repetitive nonsustained ventricular tachycardia, atrial fibrillation, and other forms of supraventricular tachycardias. The most commonly used drugs are β-blockers, sotalol, amiodarone, and dronedarone. Flecainide is used for the treatment of ventricular and supraventricular arrhythmias typically in a subset of patients who already have an ICD implanted. It is not often used in those with an ICD implantation because of the concern about its proarrhythmic effects. The risk of atrial fibrillation is about 3% to 4% per year and approximately one-quarter of patients with HCM have atrial fibrillation.[181] New-onset atrial fibrillation is often not well tolerated, and such patients are typically converted to sinus rhythm upon electric or chemical cardioversion. Patients with chronic atrial fibrillation are treated with antiarrhythmic drugs as in atrial fibrillation due to other cardiovascular diseases. Because of the risk of thromboembolic stroke, which is estimated at about 4% per year, patients with chronic atrial fibrillation should be treated with oral anticoagulants.[181] Patients that do not respond to medical therapy are evaluated for radiofrequency catheter ablation, which is effective in the treatment of supraventricular arrhythmias and, to a lesser extent, in the treatment of ventricular arrhythmias.[213]

Experimental Therapies

Experimental therapies in HCM could be categorized into those who are addressing the secondary phenotypes, such as cardiac hypertrophy and fibrosis, and those who are designed to target the underlying molecular defect(s). In the first category, a number of pharmacological intervention studies have been conducted in animal models of HCM, targeting the renin–angiotensin–aldosterone system, oxidative stress, and selected signaling pathways with 3-hydroxy-3-methylglutaryl-coenzyme A (HMG-CoA) reductase inhibitors (statins).[118-120,214-216] These studies have shown remarkable effects in animal models of HCM but by and large their beneficial findings have not been extended to human patients with HCM, or at most the benefits have been modest.[217-221] A pilot placebo-controlled clinical trial that randomized 42 patients (HALT-HCM) showed no beneficial effects of N-acetylcysteine in regression and established hypertrophy and fibrosis in HCM (NCT01537926).[222] Likewise, diltiazem has been used to treat HCM mutation carries, which has shown only a modest benefit in early left ventricular remodeling, particularly in those with *MYBPC3* mutations.[197]

Understanding the underpinning mechanisms responsible for HCM has enabled development of specific therapies. The focus has been on myosin ATPase activity targeted by MYK-461, which is a small molecule inhibitor of myosin ATPase activity. It has been tested in a mouse model of HCM and has shown beneficial effects on the development of cardiac hypertrophy, myocyte disarray, and fibrosis.[223] Mavacamten (MYK-461) is an orally administered small molecule designed to reduce left ventricular contractility by allosterically modulating the function of cardiac myosin, thereby attenuating obstruction on HCM. The Food and Drug Administration (FDA) granted Orphan Drug Designation for mavacamten for the treatment of symptomatic obstructive HCM (HOCM) in 2016. Mavacamten is currently being evaluated in the PIONEER-HCM trial (NCT02842242), which is a Phase 2 open-label single-arm study to evaluate the safety, tolerability, and efficacy of MYK-461 in patients with symptomatic HOCM. The primary endpoint of the PIONEER trial is the level of reduction in the postexercise LVOT gradient over 12 weeks of drug treatment. Preliminary results from this trial showed statistically significant improvements in reductions to the LVOT gradient and peak VO2, as well as clinically meaningful improvements in the New York Heart Association functional class.

Likewise, an RNAi-based approach has been used to selectively target the mutant *Mhy6* allele in a mouse model, which exerted a modest effect on cardiac hypertrophy and fibrosis.[224] Other approaches that have been tested include exon skipping, inclusion, or trans-splicing, and AAV9-mediated gene targeting in mouse models of HCM.[225-227]

There are a number of ongoing clinical trials in human patients with HCM. A recent study (LIBERTY-HCM) tested the effects of eleclazine, a late sodium channel blocker, on exercise capacity (MVO2) and quality of life in patients with HCM (NCT02291237). The study was terminated prematurely because of a concern about the increased risk of ventricular arrhythmias associated with its use in patients with long QT syndrome.

SUMMARY AND FUTURE DIRECTIONS

The increased understanding of the diagnosis, clinical profile, and natural history of HCM has led to significant advances in management. Nonetheless, future investigative efforts will be necessary, including the development of even more precise risk stratification strategies to reliably identify patients at an unacceptably high risk for SCD deserving of consideration for ICD therapy. Recent experimental data in animal models of HCM have raised the potential utility of new pharmacologic and nonpharmacologic interventions in prevention and regression of cardiac phenotype, and the possibility of reducing the risk of cardiac arrhythmias. Large-scale randomized, clinical studies are ongoing to test the potential utility of such new interventions in reversing, attenuating, and/or preventing cardiac phenotype, as well as improving symptoms in HCM.

KEY REFERENCES

1. Braunwald E, Ebert PA. Hemodynamic alterations in idiopathic hypertrophic subaortic stenosis induced by sympathomimetic drugs. *Am J Cardiol.* 1962;10:489–495.
2. Morrow AG, Lambrew CT, Braunwald E. Idiopathic hypertrophic subaortic stenosis. II. Operative treatment and the results of pre- and postoperative hemodynamic evaluations. *Circulation.* 1964;30(suppl 4):120–151. SUPPL-51.
3. Sigwart U. Non-surgical myocardial reduction for hypertrophic obstructive cardiomyopathy. *Lancet.* 1995;346:211–214.
4. Geisterfer-Lowrance AA, Kass S, Tanigawa G, et al. A molecular basis for familial hypertrophic cardiomyopathy: a beta cardiac myosin heavy chain gene missense mutation. *Cell.* 1990;62:999–1006.
5. Thierfelder L, Watkins H, MacRae C, et al. Alpha-tropomyosin and cardiac troponin t mutations cause familial hypertrophic cardiomyopathy: a disease of the sarcomere. *Cell.* 1994;77:701–712.
6. Maron BJ, Gardin JM, Flack JM, et al. Prevalence of hypertrophic cardiomyopathy in a general population of young adults. Echocardiographic analysis of 4111 subjects in the CARDIA study. Coronary artery risk development in (young) adults. *Circulation.* 1995;92:785–789.
7. Maron BJ, Shirani J, Poliac LC, et al. Sudden death in young competitive athletes. Clinical, demographic, and pathological profiles. *JAMA.* 1996;276:199–204.
8. Maron BJ, Shen WK, Link MS, et al. Efficacy of implantable cardioverter-defibrillators for the prevention of sudden death in patients with hypertrophic cardiomyopathy. *N Engl J Med.* 2000;342:365–373.
9. Arad M, Maron BJ, Gorham JM, et al. Glycogen storage diseases presenting as hypertrophic cardiomyopathy. *N Engl J Med.* 2005;352:362–372.
10. Braunwald E, Lambrew CT, Rockoff SD, et al. Idiopathic hypertrophic subaortic stenosis. I. A description of the disease based upon an analysis of 64 patients. *Circulation.* 1964;30(suppl 4):3–119. SUPPL-119.

The full reference list for this chapter is available on ExpertConsult.

Heart Failure as a Consequence of Genetic Cardiomyopathy

Daniel P. Judge

The genetic contributions to heart failure are numerous and remarkably heterogeneous, extending from the monogenic forms of cardiomyopathy to more common polygenic diseases, such as hypertension, coronary atherosclerosis, and myocardial infarction. For monogenic diseases, the responsible mutations are rare but carry a very high pathogenic burden. Polygenic conditions typically include DNA variants that are common in healthy populations, imparting only a small pathogenic effect. For all of these conditions, both genetic factors and environmental stimuli likely work in synergy to cause cardiovascular disease. This chapter will focus on the monogenic disorders, such as familial dilated, hypertrophic, restrictive, and arrhythmogenic forms of cardiomyopathy, and their progression to heart failure.

In considering the genetic aspects of heart failure, one should contemplate not only the underlying cause of a familial form of cardiomyopathy, but also the pattern of familial segregation, or, more specifically, consider who else in the family is at risk of developing heart failure.[1] One should also recognize syndromic features of disorders that include familial cardiomyopathy. Genetic testing is an important aspect of the evaluation for familial cardiomyopathy, and it should be preceded by genetic counseling by a trained counselor. From a research perspective, improved understanding of the genetic basis for familial forms of cardiomyopathy should help to develop better treatments.

The following clinical scenario highlights many of these aspects. A 22-year-old man was referred for genetic evaluation due to his family history of dilated cardiomyopathy (DCM) and sudden cardiac death. He was healthy as a child and young adult, training for a triathlon without cardiac limitations or symptoms. His family history is shown in the pedigree in **Fig. 24.1**. His paternal grandfather died suddenly in his early 50s. No autopsy was performed, and his death was attributed to a "heart attack." Later, a paternal uncle had sudden cardiac death in his early 40s. This time an autopsy was performed, showing nonspecific features of DCM, without significant coronary atherosclerosis or inflammatory heart disease. Echocardiograms were performed for the surviving three siblings of this deceased individual, and two had asymptomatic DCM. The youngest in this generation progressed to end-stage heart failure, and he underwent cardiac transplantation. The father of the proband received an implanted cardioverter-defibrillator (ICD), and had multiple appropriate shocks for ventricular tachycardia despite his ejection fraction (EF) of 45%. Three years ago, the proband's echocardiogram showed left ventricular (LV) diameter 5.4 cm, EF 55%, and now his echocardiogram shows his LV diameter is 5.7 cm, and his EF is 50%. His electrocardiogram (ECG) is normal.

Several questions arise at this point: (1) Are the LV enlargement and mildly reduced EF due to his exercise or to early features of a genetic cardiomyopathy? (2) What is his risk of sudden cardiac death? (3) Should he continue to exercise? (4) Which asymptomatic family members carry the same genetic predisposition to DCM and sudden cardiac death? Recognition of a clear genetic cause will help to answer these questions. The male-to-male transmission excludes X-linked disorders, and the pattern is most consistent with autosomal dominant inheritance. This means that each child of an affected individual carries a 50% chance of inheriting the genetic predisposition. Notably, a mutation in *LMNA* encoding the nuclear envelope protein lamin A/C, could cause this condition. *LMNA* mutations are associated with high rates of sudden death and systemic manifestations.[2] Such a mutation may influence decisions about ICD placement and arrhythmia risk in the proband and family members.[3]

After genetic counseling, clinical genetic testing was performed in the proband's father using a panel of genes in which mutations cause DCM. His has a heterozygous substitution of a highly conserved arginine with a histidine at codon 636 in exon 9 of *RBM20*, encoding RNA Binding Motif Protein 20 (**Fig. 24.2**). This mutation was also present in the proband's affected paternal uncle, and absent in his paternal grandmother (probably present in his affected paternal grandfather). It has been published as a pathogenic mutation.[4] His targeted genetic testing

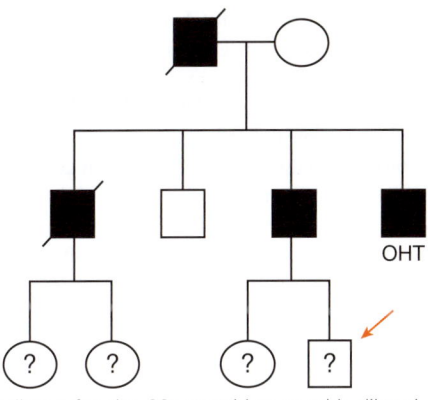

Fig. 24.1 Pedigree for the 22-year-old man with dilated cardiomyopathy. The proband is highlighted with a *red arrow*. *Circles* represent females, and *squares* represent males; *shading* indicates those with dilated cardiomyopathy or sudden cardiac death. A diagonal line through a square or circle indicates an individual who is deceased. OHT refers to orthotopic heart transplant.

RBM20 p.Arg636His

Human	MFREADRYGPERPRSRSPVSRSLSPRSHTPS
Macaque	LFREADRYGPERPRSRSPVSRSLSPRSHTPS
Gorilla	MFREADRYGPERPRSRSPVSRSLSPRSHTPS
Pig	MFREADRYGPERPRSRSPLHLLQFFPQPPGP
Cow	MFREAERYAPERPRSRSPVSRSLSPRSHTPS
Horse	MFREADRYGPERPRSRSPVSRSLSPSSSHSP
Chicken	LLREADSRYGTERPRSRSPISRSLSPRSHTPS
Rat	MLREADRYGPERPRSRSPMSRSLSPRSHSPP
Mouse	MLREADRYGPERPRSRSPMSRSLSPRSHSPP
Xenopus	MFRDTDRYRNERARSRSPVSRSLSPRSHTPS
Cave Fish	EMQEMDRYLPERARSRSPISRSLSPRSHSPS

Fig. 24.2 Conservation of the mutated amino acid. Arginine (Arg or R) at codon 636 is highly conserved among different species. Amino acids are shown with their single-letter abbreviations, and the position of the mutation is highlighted with *red text*. Substitution of this position with a histidine (His or H) disrupts an arginine/serine-rich domain, which is required for nuclear retention of the encoded protein.

shows that he also has this mutation. As such, his mild LV dilation and dysfunction are likely early features of genetic DCM. His sister and each of his paternal first cousins in **Fig. 24.1** also have this mutation, establishing their predisposition to DCM and sudden cardiac death.

CLINICAL PRESENTATIONS

People with familial forms of cardiomyopathy typically do not have overt symptoms until they have advanced dysfunction with very low cardiac output fairly late in the course of their disease. When cardiac function abruptly declines, as with acute ischemic or inflammatory injury to the heart, the sudden elevation of ventricular filling pressures usually causes prominent symptoms. With gradual loss of ventricular systolic function, physiological compensation due to neurohormonal activation causes progressive dilation of the heart and initial preservation of the stroke volume. Yet this same process of neurohormonal activation eventually becomes pathological, contributing to greater LV dilation and loss of systolic function.

The prevalence of familial DCM is often underestimated.[5] Though sometimes considered rare, careful assessment of the first-degree relatives of individuals with otherwise unexplained DCM for the same

condition has repeatedly shown 20% to 35% with familial DCM.[5,6] One study considered family members with LV enlargement greater than 112% of the size predicted on the basis of body surface area and normal systolic function as affected, and they reported a prevalence of familial DCM of 48% in a cohort that was previously considered to be idiopathic.[7] With this in mind, the American College of Cardiology/American Heart Association/American Society of Echocardiography (ACC/AHA/ASE) guidelines for the use of echocardiography provide a Class I recommendation for evaluation of first-degree relatives (parents, siblings, and children) of people with unexplained DCM.[8]

The genetic forms of cardiomyopathy are typically categorized based on the appearance of the heart. Because of pioneering research identifying its genetic basis, hypertrophic cardiomyopathy (HCM) is now usually well recognized as a familial condition (**see also Chapter 23**).[9] In contrast, nonischemic DCM can be caused by numerous other factors (**see also Chapter 20**).[10] Accordingly, familial DCM is less well recognized when it occurs. Incomplete pedigrees, age-dependent onset of symptoms, de novo mutations, recessive inheritance, and low penetrance are all factors contributing to failed recognition of familial forms of cardiomyopathy.[1] The phrase "heart attack" is a commonly used lay term that infers coronary thrombosis or occlusion, but it may otherwise refer to arrhythmic sudden death in the context of familial cardiomyopathy. Thus when discussing family history with individuals with idiopathic cardiomyopathy, it is important to clarify whether "heart attack" or sudden death occurred in the context of known coronary disease or extensive coronary atherosclerotic risk factors. If an autopsy was performed, it should be able to discern ischemic and nonischemic forms of heart failure. Familial cardiomyopathy also includes restrictive cardiomyopathy (RCM), which may overlap with DCM or HCM in some families and may be missed without careful imaging (**see also Chapter 21**).

The most easily recognized pattern of inheritance is autosomal dominant, but autosomal recessive, X-linked, and matrilinear (mitochondrial) patterns also occur. In X-linked forms of cardiomyopathy, female carriers may manifest the condition (X-linked dominant), though typically later and less severely than affected men. A familial trait like cardiomyopathy does not need to affect a large number of people in the family. In fact, recessive, X-linked, or de novo dominant forms of cardiomyopathy can appear without clear antecedent family history to alert healthcare providers to its underlying basis. Simply the presence of a single similarly affected family member allows for the diagnosis of familial cardiomyopathy.[11] A family history of early and unexplained sudden death, typically below the age of 35 years, may also be considered as a criterion for the diagnosis of familial cardiomyopathy.[11] In families with a single affected individual, the term "genetic cardiomyopathy" may be preferable to familial cardiomyopathy.

FINDINGS THAT INDICATE A GENETIC FORM OF CARDIOMYOPATHY

The main diagnostic tool in establishing the diagnosis of familial cardiomyopathy is ascertainment of a comprehensive family history. American College of Cardiology Foundation (ACCF)/AHA guidelines recommend review of at least three generations of family history.[12] This is best determined with a pedigree, in which each individual is represented by a circle (female) or square (male), with designation of phenotypic features by shading part or all of the circle or square. Rather than open-ended questions inquiring whether a family history of cardiomyopathy exists, health details for each person in the family should be reviewed, with particular attention to cardiovascular manifestations.

Although assessment of the family history and phenotypic characterization of family members who are at risk of inheriting the same genetic disorder is the best way to recognize inherited forms

TABLE 24.1   Noncardiac Findings Suggesting a Genetic Form of Cardiomyopathy

Organ	Manifestation	Consider
HEENT	Dysmorphic appearance	Chromosomal abnormality, *LMNA* mutation
	Blindness or unexplained loss of vision	Mitochondrial disorder
	Deafness or premature presbycusis	Mitochondrial disorder, *EYA4* mutation
	Unexplained corneal keratopathy	Fabry disease
	Retinopathy	Danon disease
Adipose	Lipodystrophy	*LMNA* mutation
Skin	Angiokeratomas	Fabry disease
	Palmoplantar kerato-dermas	Naxos, Carvajal, ARVC
	Hypohidrosis	Fabry disease
Central nervous system	Developmental delay	Chromosomal disorder
		Danon disease
		Mitochondrial disorder
		Presenilin mutation
Peripheral nervous system	Peripheral neuropathy	Fabry disease
		TTR amyloidosis
Skeletal muscle	Reduced strength, tone, or bulk	Cardio-skeletal myopathy
	Pseudohypertrophy	Cardio-skeletal myopathy
	Unexplained elevation of serum creatine kinase	Cardio-skeletal myopathy

ARVC, Arrhythmogenic right ventricular cardiomyopathy; *HEENT,* head eyes, ears, nose, and throat.

of cardiomyopathy, some additional features may help to make this diagnosis on initial presentation (**Table 24.1**). Because the heart and skeletal muscles both contain several of the same protein components, an individual with concomitant heart failure and skeletal myopathy usually has a monogenic condition to explain both findings, with rare systemic inflammatory exceptions. The manifestations of skeletal myopathy may be subtle, consisting of asymptomatic elevation of the serum creatine kinase level or abnormalities in muscle bulk (pseudohypertrophy or muscle hypotrophy). There is poor correlation between the severity of cardiac dysfunction and skeletal muscle weakness.

Mitochondrial disorders typically include cardiomyopathy, in addition to skeletal myopathy, blindness or loss of vision, early hearing loss, developmental delay, seizures, and/or short stature. Elevation of the resting lactic acid level in blood without hypoperfusion also suggests a mitochondrial disorder, and should prompt further evaluation for systemic manifestations. There are several forms of glycogen- and lysosomal-storage diseases with cardiac manifestations. These are usually recessive or X-linked disorders with loss-of-function mutations in enzymes, and they result in excessive production and deposition of intermediate metabolites.

Fabry Disease

Mutations in *GLA*, encoding alpha-galactosidase A, cause X-linked Fabry disease (or Anderson-Fabry disease).[13] Johannes Fabry in Germany and William Anderson in England simultaneously first reported this condition in 1898. The constellation of HCM, renal dysfunction, peripheral neuropathy, hypohydrosis, and angiokeratomas of the skin should raise concern for Fabry disease, but it can also occur with isolated cardiac involvement.[14] Corneal opacity (keratopathy) also occurs in Fabry disease, and it may be indistinguishable from amiodarone-induced corneal disease.

The age of onset for Fabry disease depends on gender and the type of mutation. Males with complete absence of alpha-galactosidase A enzyme activity typically have their initial symptoms during late childhood.[13] Males who have partial enzyme activity often present later in life with HCM, and often without systemic features. Clinical manifestations in women with a heterozygous *GLA* mutation range from asymptomatic to the full spectrum seen in affected men.[13] Since the responsible gene is on the X chromosome, male-to-male transmission of HCM in a family makes Fabry-associated HCM unlikely, unless Klinefelter syndrome (chromosome XXY) is present.

A clinical suspicion of Fabry disease can be confirmed by measurement of serum alpha-galactosidase A enzyme activity or by *GLA* genetic testing. Because women may have skewed inactivation of the X chromosome in different tissues, their serum alpha-galactosidase A enzyme activity may be normal in blood but deficient in the heart. Accordingly, blood enzyme activity is less reliable in women than in men, who have only a single copy of this gene. In one study, 90 probands with HCM underwent genetic analysis; 31/90 (34%) had sarcomere mutations, and 3/90 (3%) had *GLA* mutations.[15] None of these individuals had systemic features of Fabry disease. The inclusion of this gene in large panels for genetic evaluation of cardiomyopathies should help to increase recognition of Fabry disease, and particularly with isolated cardiac involvement.

Perhaps because of its position on the X chromosome and correlation with serum enzyme activity analysis in men, careful studies have identified less obvious mutations occurring deep in the introns of *GLA*.[16] Although complete loss of function of the enzyme usually causes the full spectrum of Fabry disease, partial loss may have cardiac- or renal-limited manifestations. For instance, the IVS4+919G>A was found to cause greater than 90% decrease in enzyme activity with later onset, cardiac-limited Fabry due to creation of abnormally spliced mRNA.[17] Although it was previously considered to be a very rare condition, newborn screening for Fabry has expanded in Asia, demonstrating that 0.13% of infants in Taiwan carry this mutation, presumably half of whom are male.[16]

The availability of replacement enzyme infusions for Fabry disease should lead to consideration of this condition in anyone with unexplained HCM. Most clinical panels for genetic testing for HCM include *GLA*. Alternatively, if an X-linked pattern of inheritance is not excluded with familial segregation of HCM, then a serum alpha-galactosidase A activity level may be useful for screening, particularly in men as compared to women with HCM. One study showed that treatment of affected individuals with recombinant human alpha-galactosidase A slowed progression to a composite endpoint, including cardiac, renal, and cerebrovascular complications or death, when compared to placebo.[18] The development of recombinant alpha-galactosidase A for the treatment of Fabry disease highlights the possibility of similar targeted therapy for related enzyme deficiencies.

Danon Disease

Danon and colleagues reported another X-linked glycogen storage disease with cardiomyopathy.[19] Phenotypic manifestations include cardiac hypertrophy with loss of systolic function, skeletal myopathy, developmental delay, and retinopathy. Loss-of-function mutations in *LAMP2*, encoding a lysosome-associated membrane protein, cause this condition, although enzyme replacement therapy is not currently available.[20]

One report highlighted the rapid progression and early mortality in a very small cohort of children (6 males and 1 female, age 7–17 years) with *LAMP2* mutations.[21] Four died from heart failure, one died from ventricular fibrillation refractory to defibrillator shocks, and one underwent cardiac transplantation with mean age of 21 years for these endpoints.[21] In a much larger cohort of 82 individuals with Danon disease from 36 separate families, in addition to 63 previously reported cases (145 people with this condition), another group more comprehensively characterized the natural history of this rare disorder.[22] In this report, the average ages of first symptom, cardiac transplantation, and death were 12.1, 17.9, and 19.0 years in men, and 27.9, 33.7, and 34.6 years in women, respectively. Cardiac transplantation appropriately addresses heart failure when it progresses to advanced stages, but progressive disease in other organ systems will occur in that context.

Familial Cardiac Amyloidosis

Cardiac amyloidosis may be suspected when there is discordance between imaging studies showing concentric ventricular hypertrophy and electrocardiograms demonstrating low ECG voltage (**see also Chapter 22**).[23] Mutations in *TTR*, encoding transthyretin, are the most common cause of inherited cardiac amyloidosis. Transthyretin is a carrier protein in the blood, binding to thyroid hormone and retinol binding protein. Mutations occur throughout the encoded protein, after cleavage of a 20-amino acid N-terminal signal peptide. In contrast with Human Genome Organisation (HUGO) nomenclature rules, the traditional numbering of mutations in this gene corresponds to the mature protein rather than the pro-protein. Accordingly, a clinical laboratory report may indicate that a mutation is p.Val50Met, then designating it by its more commonly recognized enumeration, Val30Met. Approximately 3.4% of African Americans carry one mutation (Val122Ile or p.Val142Ile by HUGO nomenclature) in heterozygosity or homozygosity, and its presence is associated with a higher frequency of heart failure after age 70 years.[24] The high prevalence of this allele among individuals with black African ancestry and the concomitantly high prevalence of heart failure with preserved EF (HFpEF) suggest that many older patients with black African ancestry and HFpEF may have unrecognized transthyretin cardiac amyloidosis. In one intriguing study looking at 650 self-identified black participants in the BEST (Beta-Blocker Evaluation in Survival) trial with NYHA (New York Heart Association) class III-IV heart failure, the prevalence of the Val122Ile mutation for those less than age 60 was 3.5%, whereas for those 60 years and older, the prevalence of this TTR mutation was 10%.[25] For other less common mutations in TTR, the likelihood of developing cardiac amyloid and the age at which it may develop should be tailored to the specific mutation.

Although far less common, other familial forms of amyloid can occur due to mutations in genes encoding apolipoprotein A-I (*APOA1*), apolipoprotein A-II (*APOA2*), gelsolin (*GSN*), fibrinogen A (*FGA*), and lysozyme (*LYZ*). Although these forms of familial amyloidosis do not typically involve the heart, systemic deposition of amyloid occurs in later stages and sometimes leads to cardiac dysfunction, which is similar to other forms of cardiac amyloidosis.

Arrhythmogenic Right Ventricular Cardiomyopathy

Arrhythmogenic right ventricular cardiomyopathy (ARVC) is genetic disorder characterized by right ventricular fibrofatty scar and prominent ventricular arrhythmias (**see also Chapter 21**).[26] Because of the uncommon presence of fat in the mid-wall of the RV, this condition was initially called arrhythmogenic right ventricular dysplasia (ARVD). However, "dysplasia" typically refers to malignancy or abnormal proliferation, which is not present in patients with this condition. Accordingly, the preferred term evolved to ARVC or ARVD/C.

Similar pathological changes and arrhythmia also occur in the left ventricle, leading to the eponym arrhythmogenic left ventricular cardiomyopathy (ALVC) and the broader category for both conditions— arrhythmogenic cardiomyopathy (ACM). Although the term ACM encompasses both conditions, detailed criteria have been used for the diagnosis of ARVC, and emerging recommendations classify ARVC as a subtype of ACM.

In one US study of 100 affected individuals, the median age at presentation was 26 years, with the initial diagnosis occurring postmortem in 31%.[27] The original description of this condition and subsequent diagnostic criteria focused on cardiomyopathies that predominantly (or exclusively) involved the RV.[28,29] Now, overlap with LV involvement is expanding the diagnosis to include all forms of ACM.[30] Naxos disease and Carvajal syndrome are two similar recessive disorders that also involve palmoplantar keratoderma and wooly hair. Noncardiac involvement in ARVC is quite rare, though subtle keratoderma or wooly hair may be present if carefully investigated.

The most frequent manifestation of ARVC is ventricular tachyarrhythmia, and once the condition is recognized with institution of appropriate antiarrhythmic therapies, the next priority for management becomes recognition and treatment of heart failure. One study identified at least one sign or symptom of heart failure in nearly half of all patients with ARVC.[31] Many individuals with ARVC have a long history of prominent aerobic exertion. In retrospective investigation, the amount of exercise, particularly after the diagnosis of ACM, directly correlates with the likelihood of further arrhythmia and development of heart failure.[32]

Approximately 50% of individuals with ARVC have a mutation in a component of the cardiac desmosome.[33] Immunohistochemical analysis for plakoglobin is consistently reduced and mislocalized in ARVC hearts, in contrast with HCM, DCM, ischemic cardiomyopathy, and control hearts.[34] Notably, cardiac sarcoid is commonly on the differential diagnosis for ARVC, and reduced plakoglobin immunoreactivity is quite similar in sarcoid as in ARVC.[35] Extending beyond the desmosome, mutations contributing to ARVC also occur in several other genes (**Table 24.2**).

Left Ventricular Noncompaction Cardiomyopathy

Left ventricular noncompaction cardiomyopathy (LVNC), which is also known as LV hypertrabeculation, has been described as a "new form of heart failure," but this likely reflects improved imaging technologies that have increased its recognition.[36] Early reports of this condition describe marked sinusoids in the ventricles with associated cardiac dysfunction and arrhythmias. LVNC is frequently associated with other cardiac malformations, with craniofacial abnormalities, and with concomitant skeletal myopathy.[37] Because of high resolution cardiac imaging, such as cardiac MRI and improved echocardiography, defined criteria have been developed.[38] Briefly summarized, the noncompacted endocardial layer has to be thicker than the compacted epicardial layer, with a ratio of noncompacted/compacted ≥2, with prominent and excessive trabeculations, and deep recesses filled with blood from the ventricular cavity. The incidence of thromboembolic complications appears higher in LVNC than in other forms of cardiomyopathy.[38]

LVNC often occurs in a familial pattern, and it is also associated with Barth syndrome, a rare X-linked disorder caused by loss-of-function mutations in tafazzin, encoded by *TAZ*. However, increased sensitivity of all forms of cardiac imaging, including echocardiography, cardiac computed tomography (CT), and cardiac magnetic resonance (CMR) has increased recognition of this diagnosis. For instance, in the Multi-Ethnic Study of Atherosclerosis (MESA), focal LVNC was observed in at least one LV myocardial segment in 43% of participants

TABLE 24.2 Genes With Mutations Known to Cause Cardiomyopathy

Encoded Protein's Cellular Location/Function	Gene	DCM	HCM	RCM	ARVC
Sarcomere/myofilament or Z-disc	ACTC	+	+	−	−
	ACTN2	+	+	−	−
	ANKRD1	+	+	−	−
	CSRP3	+	+	+	−
	MYBPC3	+	+	−	−
	MYH6	+	+	−	−
	MYH7	+	+	+	−
	MYL2	−	+	−	−
	MYL3	−	+	−	−
	MYLK2	−	+	−	−
	MYOZ2	+	+	−	−
	MYPN	+	+	+	−
	NEBL	+	−	−	−
	NEXN	+	+	−	−
	TCAP	+	+	−	−
	TNNC1	+	+	−	−
	TNNT2	+	+	+	−
	TNNI3	+	+	+	−
	TPM1	+	+	−	−
	TTN	+	+	−	+
Cytoskeleton	DES	+	−	+	+
	DMD	+	−	−	−
	DTNA	+	−	−	−
	FKTN	+	−	−	−
	FLNC	+	+	+	+
	LDB3	+	+	−	−
	OBSCN	+	+	−	−
	PDLIM3	+	−	−	−
	SGCD	+	−	−	−
	VCL	+	+	−	−
Calcium regulation	CAV3	+	−	−	−
	CALR3	−	+	−	−
	JPH2	−	+	−	−
	PLN	+	−	−	+
	PSEN1	+	−	−	−
	PSEN2	+	−	−	−
	RYR2	−	−	−	+
Nuclear envelope	EMD	+	−	−	−
	ILK	+	−	−	−
	LAMA4	+	−	−	−
	LAP2	+	−	−	−
	LMNA	+	+	+	+
	TMEM43	+	−	−	+
Ion channel	ABCC9	+	−	−	−
	SCN5A	+	−	−	+
Transcription factor or regulator of transcription	EYA4	+	−	−	−
	GATA4	+	−	−	−
	GATAD1	+	−	−	−
	NKX2-5	+	−	−	−
	PRDM16	−	−	−	−
	RAF1	+	+	−	−
	RBM20	+	−	−	−
Desmosome and associated cell junction	CDH2	−	−	−	+
	CTNNA3	−	−	−	+
	DSC2	−	−	−	+
	DSG2	+	−	−	+
	DSP	+	−	−	+
	JUP	−	−	−	+
	PKP2	−	−	−	+

TABLE 24.2 Genes With Mutations Known to Cause Cardiomyopathy—cont'd					
Encoded Protein's Cellular Location/ Function	**Gene**	**DCM**	**HCM**	**RCM**	**ARVC**
Mitochondria	*ANT1*	+	+	–	–
	FKRP	+	–	–	–
	FXN	–	+	+	–
	ND1	+	+	–	–
	tRNA	+	+	+	–
	TAZ	–	+	–	–
Storage disease	*GAA*	–	+	–	–
	GLA	–	+	–	–
	LAMP2	–	+	–	–
	PRKAG2	–	+	–	–
	TTR	–	+	+	–
Chaperone	*BAG3*	+	–	+	–
	CRYAB	+	–	+	–

ARVC, Arrhythmogenic right ventricular cardiomyopathy; *DCM,* dilated cardiomyopathy; *HCM,* hypertrophic cardiomyopathy; *RCM,* restrictive cardiomyopathy.

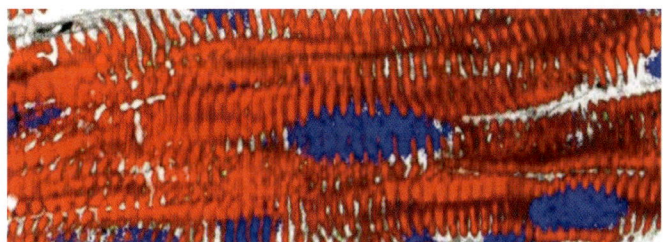

Fig. 24.3 The cardiac sarcomere. The cardiac sarcomeres make up myofibrils, which are highlighted in this image with immunostaining for cardiac troponin T *(red),* a component of the sarcomeres. Nuclei are stained with DAPI *(blue),* and wheat germ agglutinin *(white)* binds to the plasma membrane to demonstrate cell boundaries.

without known heart disease or hypertension, and LVNC was present in two segments in 6% of this cohort.[39] These findings were replicated by CMR in a population study performed in the UK, where 14.8% of individuals met at least one criterion for LVNC, and 4.4% had more extensive hypertrabeculation.[40] LVNC may be more prevalent among individuals of African ancestry, and one study showed that 8.1% of highly trained athletes carry this phenotype. Accordingly, some consider LVNC to be a distinct trait, like mitral valve prolapse (MVP), which can be found in families with and without cardiomyopathy.[41]

GENETIC CAUSES OF CARDIOMYOPATHY

Because of overlap among the etiologies of these phenotypes, including dilated, hypertrophic, restrictive, and right ventricular, the next section will be subdivided by etiology rather than specific cardiac morphologies. A list of genes with mutations known to cause cardiomyopathy in humans is shown in **Table 24.2.**

Sarcomere Mutations

The cardiac sarcomere is the primary subunit in myocytes used for generation of force (**Fig. 24.3**). Mutation in a gene encoding any component of the sarcomere can cause cardiomyopathy. Phenotypic manifestations related to sarcomere mutations include DCM, HCM, RCM, and there is also a report of *MYH7* mutation mimicking ARVC.[9,42-44] Oddly, prediction of the morphological consequence for the left ventricle by any particular sarcomere mutation is not currently feasible,

although phenotypes remain consistent for each individual mutation. Most missense substitutions in sarcomere genes are predicted to cause loss of function, though gain-of-function mutations would cause heterogeneity among individual subcellular units, and this could cause disease. In addition to mediating both contraction and relaxation of the heart, additional functions of the sarcomere and its network of associated proteins include integration, regulation, and coordination of cardiac signaling, sensation, and response to reactive oxygen species within the heart, and modulation of ubiquitination and autophagy.[45] With such central roles in cardiac function and homeostasis, it is not surprising that sarcomere dysfunction causes heart failure.

TTN encodes titin, the largest human protein. Spanning the entire sarcomere, it serves as a scaffold, contributing to myocyte elasticity. Truncating mutations in this gene are remarkably frequent among people with DCM.[46] However, not all exons in this large gene are spliced into cardiac transcripts. Accordingly, one must look closely at the location of the mutation and the expression of the encoded exon where the mutation occurs to decide if it is playing a role in a patient with DCM. The background rate of truncations in this gene is approximately 3%, with one study showing that 1% of patients with HCM and another sarcomere mutation also have truncating mutations in *TTN.*[46] This appears to contribute to several other forms of DCM, such as peripartum or Adriamycin-induced cardiomyopathy.[47,48]

Clinical Implications

Pathogenic heterozygous mutations tend to be sufficient to cause disease, and the presence of more than one mutation tends to worsen its severity within families. The diversity of phenotypes associated with sarcomere mutations limits the applicability of generalizations regarding sarcomere mutations. Among patients with HCM and mutations in *TNNT2* or *TNNI3,* encoding cardiac troponin T and cardiac troponin I, respectively, the likelihood of arrhythmia appears to be greater than that predicted by LV wall thickness. Regarding mutations in *TPM1,* encoding alpha-tropomyosin, one group has reported a wide range of onset and severity within families sharing the same mutation.[49] Because of the long history of investigation of genes encoding most elements of the cardiac sarcomere, clinical laboratories typically have a large number of variants from which to ascertain the likelihood of pathogenicity, and this increases the feasibility of using sarcomere mutation analysis among patients with all types of inherited cardiomyopathy.

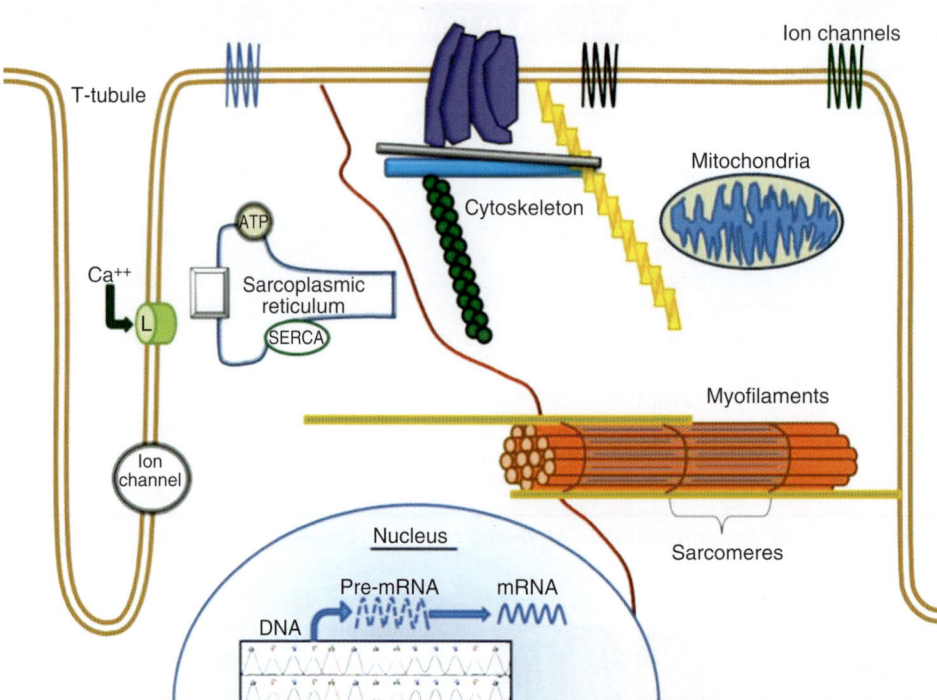

Fig. 24.4 Diagram of a cardiomyocyte. Mutations can occur in the genes encoding elements of the cardiac sarcomere and adjacent structures that make up myofilaments, the cytoskeletal proteins, those involved with calcium uptake into and release from the sarcoplasmic reticulum, the nuclear envelope, the cardiac ion channels, factors involved with DNA transcription into pre-mRNA and its splicing into mRNA, desmosomes, the mitochondria, or proteins that function as chaperones involved with cell stress. *ATP*, Adenosine triphosphatase; *SERCA*, sarcoendoplasmic reticulum Ca2+-ATPase.

Cytoskeletal Mutations

The cardiac cytoskeleton includes a large number of proteins that are responsible for the transmission of force, which is generated by the contractile elements of the sarcomere (**Fig. 24.4**). Dystrophin was the first cytoskeletal element that was recognized with mutations in association with DCM, among patients with Duchenne and Becker muscular dystrophies.[50] Subsequently, dystrophin gene mutations were identified in patients with X-linked DCM,[51] which suggested that other forms of familial DCM could be inherited through mutations affecting the cytoskeletal complex. Broadly interpreted, the cardiac cytoskeleton includes sarcoglycans, other associated glycoproteins, the basal lamina, and the intermediate filaments that link the sarcomeric Z-discs to the sarcolemma cell membrane. If the mutated gene encoding a cytoskeletal element is exclusively or predominantly expressed in the heart, then the phenotype should be isolated DCM. If the mutated cytoskeletal element is also present in skeletal muscle, then skeletal muscle weakness may also be present. More examples of genes encoding cytoskeletal elements that can be mutated in cardiomyopathy are listed in **Table 24.2**.

Clinical Implications

As in the example regarding dystrophin, many cytoskeletal proteins are present in both heart and skeletal muscle. Certain myofibrillar proteins, like desmin, are much more abundant in heart than skeletal muscle, and the range of severity in skeletal muscle dysfunction is quite large.[52] Among the cytoskeletal components with mutations resulting in cardiomyopathy, desmin is one in which arrhythmia can be a prominent feature, and recognition of a definite mutation in this gene should prompt earlier consideration for an ICD among affected individuals.

Mutations Altering Calcium Handling

Calcium is one of the most important cations for the relationship between electrical activation and mechanical function of cardiomyocytes, and it is intricately regulated (**see Fig. 24.4**). Accordingly, disruption or mutation of any of the regulatory components can result in either electrical or mechanical cardiac disease. When the mutation results primarily in mechanical dysfunction, it is also likely that arrhythmia is also a consequence. For instance, *PLN* encoding phospholamban is a gene in which mutations cause several forms of cardiomyopathy, and arrhythmia is prominent in this setting.[53] Phospholamban is a negative regulator of the sarcoplasmic reticulum calcium-adenosine triphosphatase (ATPase), and loss-of-function mutations might be predicted to cause improved cardiac function. However, the disruption of excitation-contraction coupling instead causes DCM or ARVC.[53,54] Mutations in the cardiac ryanodine receptor (encoded by *RYR2*) typically cause catecholaminergic polymorphic ventricular tachycardia without structural heart disease, although at least one report ties mutations in this gene to ARVC.[55]

Clinical Implications

Because of the intricate connection between calcium handling and arrhythmia, people with a mutation that alters cardiomyocyte calcium regulation should be evaluated closely for arrhythmia, regardless of their EF or severity of structural heart disease. Although there is not typically skeletal muscle disease with alterations in the cardiac calcium regulatory genes, one report highlights the possibility of overlap between DCM and Alzheimer dementia due to *PSEN1* or *PSEN2* mutations.[56]

Nuclear Envelope Mutations

Present in every nucleated cell, the nuclear envelope has emerged as far more than a passive structural membrane to encapsulate the nuclear contents. Several reports help to identify the role of the nuclear envelope components in the organization of chromatin, regulation of signaling and gene expression, nuclear-cytoplasmic transport, cell division, and aging.[57] Mutations in genes encoding elements of the nuclear envelope have a broad range of phenotypes, prominently including DCM, cardiac conduction disease, and heart failure.[58] Systemic manifestations include skeletal myopathy (limb girdle muscular dystrophy type 1b and Emery Dreifuss muscular dystrophy), partial lipodystrophy, premature aging, Charcot-Marie-Tooth disease, malignancy, and mandibuloacral dysplasia.[59]

LMNA is the most frequent nuclear envelope gene with mutations causing cardiovascular disease.[58] *LMNA* encodes two isoforms, lamin A and lamin C (sometimes called lamin A/C), and mutations in this gene cause dysmorphic nuclei (**Fig. 24.5**). People with *LMNA* mutations have higher rates of sudden death and worse cumulative survival than those with DCM without *LMNA* mutations.[2,60] Although the mechanisms for development of cardiac disease due to alterations of the nuclear envelope are not well known, a recent report demonstrated a role for lamin A/C and emerin in regulating nuclear translocation and downstream signaling of a mechanosensitive transcription factor, megakaryoblastic leukemia 1 (MKL1), which is important in cardiovascular development and function.[61]

Clinical Implications

Phenotypic features among patients with DCM that suggest a possible nuclear envelope mutation include unexplained elevation of creatine kinase, muscle weakness, cardiac conduction disease, frequent ventricular arrhythmias, or a family history of early sudden death. Recognition of a gene mutation that predisposes to life-threatening arrhythmia should prompt earlier use of implantable cardioverter-defibrillators.[3]

Ion Channel Mutations

Cardiac ion channel (**see Fig. 24.4**) mutations are most commonly recognized to cause inherited disorders of arrhythmia, such as Long QT Syndrome and, Brugada Syndrome.[62] Chronic tachycardia or cardiac arrest in that setting can cause a secondary form of structural cardiomyopathy, and rarely, mutations in ion-channel genes can cause a primary form of cardiomyopathy. Phospholamban is a regulator of the sarcoendoplasmic reticulum Ca2+-ATPase (SERCA2a) channel, and mutations have been reported in several different forms of cardiomyopathy, though somewhat surprisingly, heterozygous loss-of-function mutations in the SERCA2a gene do not cause impairment in cardiac performance.[63] Following a hypothesis that mutations in another regulator of myocyte calcium flux, the regulatory sulfonylurea receptor 2a subunit of the cardiac K_{ATP} channel encoded by *ABCC9*, could cause cardiomyopathy, investigators evaluated 323 individuals with unexplained DCM for mutations in this gene.[64] They identified two probands with functional alterations, establishing that cardiac ion-channel mutations can rarely cause DCM. Similarly, *SCN5A* encodes the Na$_V$1.5 cardiac sodium channel, and mutations in this gene cause type 3 Long QT and Brugada syndromes, as well as atrial fibrillation.[65,66] Investigation of a large family segregating DCM with prominent arrhythmia (atrial fibrillation, impaired automaticity, and conduction delay) led to linkage to chromosome 3p, and subsequently to a missense mutation in *SCN5A*.[67] These investigators subsequently looked for mutations in this gene among a cohort of 156 unrelated probands with DCM and identified that 4 (2.5%) also had a mutation in *SCN5A*.[67] Mutations in this gene are also associated with ARVC.[68]

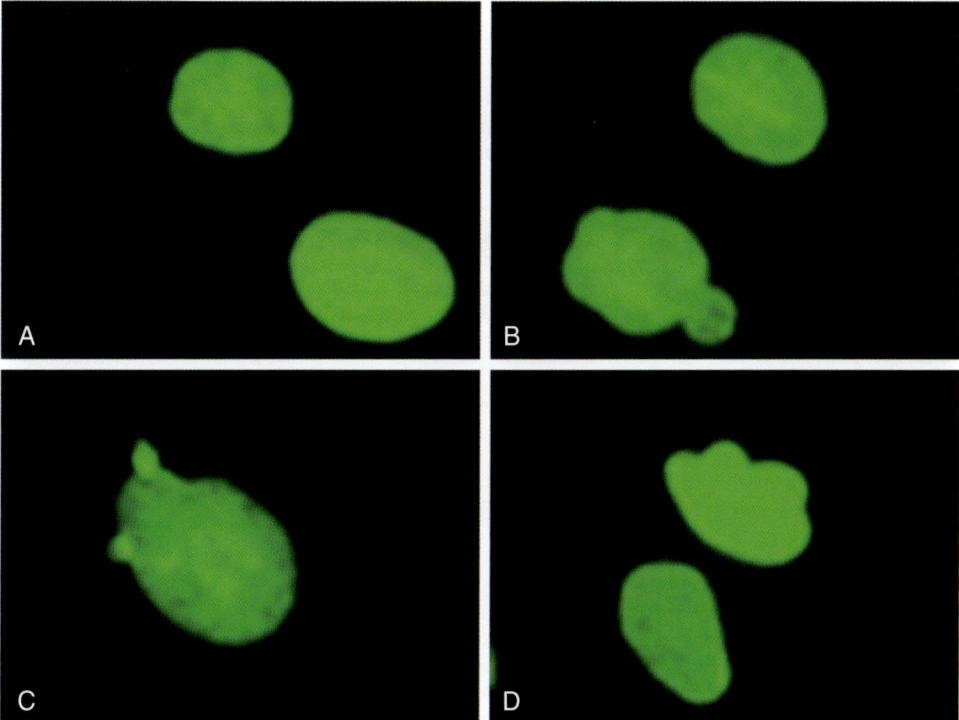

Fig. 24.5 Dysmorphic nuclei due to a LMNA mutation. Immunohistochemical staining for lamin A. Normal nuclei are shown in panel A, with dysmorphic nuclei in panels B, C, and D. The heterozygous *LMNA* mutation is p.Asp300Gly, and it causes cardiomyopathy with accelerated cardiovascular aging. From Kane MS, Lindsay ME, Judge DP, et al. LMNA-associated cardiocutaneous progeria: an inherited autosomal dominant premature aging syndrome with late onset. *Am J Med Genet A*. 2013;161:1599–1611.

Clinical Implications

Recognition of a mutation in *SCN5A* should prompt greater scrutiny for arrhythmia due to its association with Long QT and Brugada Syndromes, as well as atrial fibrillation. Importantly, certain drugs can prolong the QT interval, and they should be avoided among individuals with a mutation in an ion channel.

Transcription and Splicing Factor Mutations

Cardiac transcription factor mutations typically cause congenital malformations of the heart, though cardiomyopathy can also occur. For instance, *NKX2-5* mutations cause congenital cardiac malformations and cardiomyopathy.[69] Using a positional cloning approach in a large family segregating DCM with sensorineural hearing loss, investigators found linkage to chromosome 6q23–q24, and subsequently identified mutations in *EYA4*, encoding eyes-absent-4, a transcription factor.[70] In addition, mutations in *RBM20*, encoding a ribonucleic acid binding protein that regulates titin splicing, cause familial DCM with prominent arrhythmia.[71]

Clinical Implications

When mutations in a transcription factor gene that is associated with congenital malformations are identified, careful assessment for subtle or overt cardiac malformations should be performed in the proband and relatives who are at risk of inheriting the mutation. *RBM20* mutations, in particular, are associated with high rates of sudden cardiac death.

Desmosome Mutations

Desmosomes form cell junctions, and alterations in their components are associated with both cardiomyopathy and dermatologic disorders. Homozygous mutations in *JUP*, encoding junction plakoglobin, cause a recessive form of ARVC, wooly hair, and palmoplantar keratoderma called Naxos syndrome.[72]

Similarly, recessive mutations in *DSP*, encoding desmoplakin, cause a related disorder called Carvajal syndrome.[73] Since both desmoplakin and plakoglobin are components of the cardiac desmosomes, investigation next turned to mutations in other components in arrhythmogenic forms of cardiomyopathy or ARVC. The most prevalent gene with mutations underlying this phenotype is *PKP2*, encoding plakophilin-2.[74] Other gene mutations are noted in **Table 24.2** and shown schematically in **Fig. 24.6**. The phenotypes that result from desmosome mutations include right-, left-, and bi-ventricular cardiomyopathy, typically with frequent episodes of ventricular arrhythmia. In the most recently published criteria for ACM, the presence of a clearly pathogenic desmosome gene mutation helps to meet criteria.

There are several possible mechanisms whereby mutations in a component of the cardiac desmosome cause cardiomyopathy.[26] A simple structural model predicts that loss of cell adherence leads to apoptosis and scarring within the ventricle, particularly at sites with the greatest stress in response to exercise. A landmark publication demonstrated that disruption of the desmosome complex causes plakoglobin to accumulate in the nucleus, where it competes with beta-catenin for its downstream activation, thereby decreasing canonical Wnt/beta-catenin signaling.[75] This is also associated with abnormal cytoplasmic localization of glycogen synthase kinase-3-beta (GSK3β), and inhibition of GSK3β activates canonical Wnt signaling to improve the cardiomyopathy in mice with targeted desmosome mutations.[76] Loss of desmosomes may disrupt other cell junction complexes, and it also affects the sodium channel complex, which contributes to arrhythmia.[77] In another line of investigation, induced cardiomyocytes derived from patients with desmosome mutations helped to identify an important role for abnormal activation of the peroxisome proliferator-activated receptor gamma (PPARγ) pathway in this condition.[78]

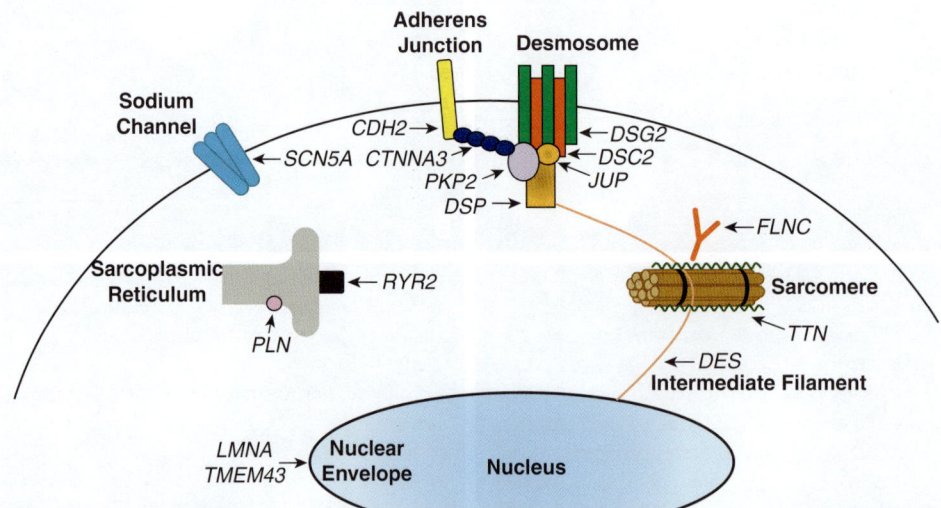

Fig. 24.6 Subcellular components in which mutations cause arrhythmogenic right ventricular cardiomyopathy (ARVC). Mutations in these proteins cause arrhythmogenic forms of cardiomyopathy. The cardiac desmosome is composed of transmembrane cadherins (desmocollins and desmogleins), armadillo proteins (plakoglobin and plakophilins), and plakins, such as desmoplakin. The adherens junction is another cell junction complex, composed of N-cadherin (encoded by *CDH2*), linked to the desmosome by alpha-T-catenin (*CTNNA3*). *SCN5A* encodes Na$_V$1.5, the major component of the sodium channel complex in cardiomyocytes. Two genes encoding elements of the nuclear envelope, *LMNA* and *TMEM43*, have been associated with ARVC, as have the genes encoding filamin C, desmin, titin, and two components of the sarcoplasmic reticulum (*PLN* and *RYR2*).

Clinical Implications

A few important factors should be taken into account for patients with desmosome gene mutations. First, penetrance of mutations in these genes seems lower, with one study showing that only 31% of first-degree relatives of probands with ARVC and a *PKP2* mutation also met diagnostic criteria, with wide intrafamilial variability among mutation carriers.[79] Another study showed that rare missense variation in these genes is commonly seen in control populations.[80] In the setting of a clear pathogenic mutation with cardiomyopathy, careful assessment for arrhythmia should be performed on a regular basis, particularly in those who do not yet have an ICD. Among patients with ARVC, a history of extensive athletic activity is common, and in a retrospective analysis, exercise increases age-related penetrance and risk of arrhythmia in desmosome mutation carriers.[81] Accordingly, clinicians should consider advising their patients who harbor desmosome gene mutations to decrease their aerobic exercise. Related investigation shows that restriction of exercise to the American Heart Association's minimum recommended level does not increase risk of ARVC disease progression.[82]

Mitochondrial Mutations

Heart muscle requires high levels of energy to maintain its constant requirement for delivering oxygen throughout the body. Production of energy relies heavily on mitochondria (**see Fig. 24.4**), and dysfunction of the mitochondria contributes to heart failure. In the setting of heart failure, there is a shift in the substrate for mitochondrial function, with a decline in fatty acid oxidation and a proportional increase in the oxidation of glucose in advanced phases.[83] Mitochondrial mutations that cause inherited forms of cardiomyopathy may occur with an isolated cardiac phenotype, but more often these mutations have multifaceted manifestations, including the involvement of many other tissues in which mitochondrial function is important for producing energy. Additional phenotypes that may be found in mitochondrial disorders include skeletal muscle disease, blindness, premature hearing loss, diabetes, encephalopathy, and seizures.[84] They may occur due to nuclear DNA mutations encoding components of the mitochondria, or in the approximately 16,600 nucleotides that comprise the mitochondrial DNA (mtDNA). If due to mtDNA mutation, then transmission to the next generation can only occur through female carriers. Differences in disease severity or age at presentation may be due to heteroplasmy or variation in the percentage of the mtDNA in which the mutation occurs. If the mtDNA mutation is homoplasmic, then the entire content of the mtDNA is mutant.

Mitochondrial disorders can cause HCM or DCM, sometimes occurring with concomitant LV noncompaction (hypertrabeculation), with or without systemic manifestations.[85,86] When cardiomyopathy occurs in isolation, it can be difficult to recognize a mitochondrial etiology without molecular genetic testing. Cardiomyopathy in Friedreich ataxia usually begins with concentric (nonobstructive) LV hypertrophy, with eventual loss of systolic function. The hypertrophy appears to be caused by a combination of fibrosis and marked proliferation of mitochondria with an associated loss of contractile elements.[87] Barth syndrome, another mitochondrial disorder, is an X-linked mitochondrial condition in which males typically present in infancy or childhood with DCM or LV noncompaction, associated with skeletal myopathy and neutropenia.[88]

Many treatment trials of mitochondrial forms of cardiomyopathy have focused on antioxidants. In addition to generating adenosine triphosphate (ATP), the mitochondria produce reactive oxygen species, such as superoxide and hydrogen peroxide, and mitochondrial dysfunction increases electron leakage from the mitochondrial transport chain.[89] To date, clinical trials for antioxidants, such as coenzyme Q10 and idebenone, have been not been convincing and these strategies remain experimental.[90]

Clinical Implications

Recognition of a mitochondrial form of cardiomyopathy is clinically important for several reasons. First, systemic manifestations should be assessed in organs in which mitochondrial production of energy is prominent, such as skeletal muscles, vision, and hearing. Once a nuclear versus mtDNA mutation is recognized, there will likely be important implications for risk assessment in family members. Although antioxidant treatments have greater appeal for mitochondrial disorders than in other forms of heart failure, a clear benefit from treatment with these medications is not yet known.

GENETIC TESTING

Research investigating the genetic basis of cardiomyopathy over the past twenty years has been remarkably successful. Traditional linkage studies initially facilitated the recognition of several genes in which mutations cause different forms of cardiomyopathy, and candidate-based studies, exome analysis, and whole genome association techniques have subsequently elucidated many other genes involved with these conditions. Improvements in the costs and efficiency of technologies applied to DNA sequencing have helped to bring genetic testing from the research benches to clinical applications. Today, the clinical use of genetic testing is gaining greater recognition for its value. Determination of a responsible gene mutation can help to support the clinical diagnosis, to identify individuals who are at risk of syndromic or extra-cardiac manifestations, to recognize those within the family who are at highest risk of developing cardiomyopathy, and for family planning.

Several different sets of guidelines for the clinical use of genetic testing for inherited cardiac disease have been published.[3,91-93] In this context, some common themes have emerged, such as recommendations for genetic counseling in conjunction with genetic testing, usually by masters'-trained counselors. A typical genetic counseling evaluation would include assessment of the pedigree, including the pattern of inheritance and determination of those who are at risk of cardiomyopathy.[94] Discussion of genetic testing should include the testing options that are available, the possible outcomes of these tests including uncertain or unexpected results, communication of results to family members, and the costs of such testing. Most physicians are not trained in helping patients deal with issues such as guilt arising from passing on a genetic predisposition to cardiomyopathy to their children.

Some experts recommend targeted analysis of the top few genes in which mutations occur, in an effort to minimize unnecessary genetic sequencing and to lower costs. This approach also simplifies the process and decreases the likelihood of finding nonpathogenic variation in genes that are included in larger sequencing panels. Others recommend larger panels since the costs are declining and the additional data may help to determine other genetic factors contributing to a disorder like cardiomyopathy in which there is reduced penetrance. One should decide between these two approaches based on availability and costs, as well as the feasibility of discerning pathogenicity of multiple variants based on co-segregation within the family if there are several individuals with cardiomyopathy and DNA available for testing. Whole exome and whole genome sequencing have become much more feasible over the past few years, though arguably these approaches are not more likely to identify pathogenic variants explaining cardiomyopathy than large panels, which typically include all genes in which mutations are known to cause cardiomyopathy. Filtering of the exome or genome results parallels the assessment of known genes in a large panel.

Looking to the future, the costs of DNA sequencing are rapidly declining, and we are learning the extent and potential pathogenicity of human genetic variation through large web-based platforms.[95] Because genotypes do not change, assessment of DNA sequence may soon become a standard aspect of primary care. For now, the use of genetic analysis is best if handled through highly specialized centers with expertise and familiarity with these topics.

KEY REFERENCES

1. Judge DP. Use of genetics in the clinical evaluation of cardiomyopathy. *JAMA.* 2009;302:2471–2476.
5. Michels VV, et al. The frequency of familial dilated cardiomyopathy in a series of patients with idiopathic dilated cardiomyopathy. *N Engl J Med.* 1992;326:77–82.
24. Quarta CC, et al. The amyloidogenic V122I transthyretin variant in elderly black Americans. *N Engl J Med.* 2015;372:21–29.
31. Gilotra NA, et al. Heart failure is common and under-recognized in patients with arrhythmogenic right ventricular cardiomyopathy/dysplasia. *Circ Heart Fail.* 2017;10 pii: e003819.
40. Weir-McCall JR, et al. Left ventricular noncompaction: anatomical phenotype or distinct cardiomyopathy? *J Am Coll Cardiol.* 2016;68:2157–2165.
43. Kamisago M, et al. Mutations in sarcomere protein genes as a cause of dilated cardiomyopathy. *N Engl J Med.* 2000;343:1688–1696.
46. Herman DS, et al. Truncations of titin causing dilated cardiomyopathy. *N Engl J Med.* 2012;366:619–628.
47. Ware JS, et al. Shared genetic predisposition in peripartum and dilated cardiomyopathies. *N Engl J Med.* 2016;374:233–241.
58. Fatkin D, et al. Missense mutations in the rod domain of the lamin A/C gene as causes of dilated cardiomyopathy and conduction-system disease. *N Engl J Med.* 1999;341:1715–1724.
93. Hershberger RE, et al. Genetic evaluation of cardiomyopathy—a Heart Failure Society of America practice guideline. *J Card Fail.* 2018;24:281–302.

The full reference list for this chapter is available on ExpertConsult.

Heart Failure as a Consequence of Hypertension

Florian Rader, Ronald G. Victor

INTRODUCTION: DEFINITION AND IMPACT

Hypertension (HTN) affects over 1 billion people worldwide and is the most prevalent risk factor for the development of heart failure.[1-4] Despite some improvements in the treatment and control of HTN,[5] the societal burden of hypertensive heart disease in an aging population has increased and heart failure—one major manifestation of hypertensive heart disease—continues to be the most frequent hospital admission diagnosis in the United States.[6,7] The term "hypertensive heart disease" encompasses a spectrum ranging from clinically silent structural remodeling, such as left ventricular hypertrophy (LVH), to the development of clinical symptoms—often decades later—such as heart failure. **Fig. 25.1** is a diagram of the progression and cardiovascular complications of hypertensive heart disease.

The human heart is a highly adaptive organ that responds to pressure overload by recruiting contractile elements in order to maintain normal left ventricular (LV) systolic wall stress; this includes myocyte hypertrophy with increased relative wall thickness (RWT), or concentric LVH.[8] Although LVH can precede the clinical diagnosis of HTN,[9] it is thought of as the inciting event in the development of hypertensive heart disease. Complex neurohumoral stimulation accompanies chronic HTN and eventually leads to cardiomyocyte dysfunction, pathologic increases in cardiac extracellular matrix (i.e., fibrosis), and disturbance of the intramyocardial microvasculature. LV diastolic dysfunction, left atrial enlargement, and atrial arrhythmias are early clinical signs of hypertensive heart disease. The development of ischemic events as a result of HTN is a common but not obligatory intermediate disease stage that can accelerate the progression of hypertensive heart disease.[10-12] Finally, increases in LV dimensions, worsening of systolic performance, and ventricular arrhythmias indicate severe or end-stage disease.[13,14]

LVH is a potent cardiovascular risk factor independent of the degree of blood pressure (BP) elevation or other comorbidities and correlates with biomarkers.[15-18] Regression of LVH with medical treatment, even in advanced stages of hypertensive heart disease, improves prognosis and thus may be an important therapeutic target.[19,20]

This chapter provides an overview of the diagnosis, epidemiology, molecular mechanisms, and treatment of hypertensive heart disease.

LEFT VENTRICULAR HYPERTROPHY

Epidemiology

As already described, LVH is a compensatory mechanism aimed at adapting to higher demands for LV work, including pressure load. The threshold between adaptive (healthy) and maladaptive (pathologic) hypertrophy is not clearly defined; this makes the estimation of pathologic LVH on a population level difficult. In the Multi-Ethnic Study of Atherosclerosis (MESA), comprising middle-aged and older men and women without a diagnosis of cardiovascular disease but with HTN, 11% of the participants met criteria for LVH by cardiac magnetic resonance imaging (MRI).[21] In the Dallas Heart Study, which included both hypertensive and normotensive persons ages 30 to 67 years, the overall prevalence of LVH by cardiac MRI was 9.4%, but it was higher in participants with elevated systolic BP.[22] These prevalence rates are among the most reliable estimates for the general adult population because they stem from population-based samples subjected to cardiac MRI for the detection of LVH. In contrast, estimates of LVH prevalence among hypertensive individuals vary markedly between studies depending on the testing modality used (e.g., electrocardiography [ECG] vs. echocardiography vs. cardiac MRI), the LVH diagnostic criteria employed, and, importantly, the demographics and comorbidity

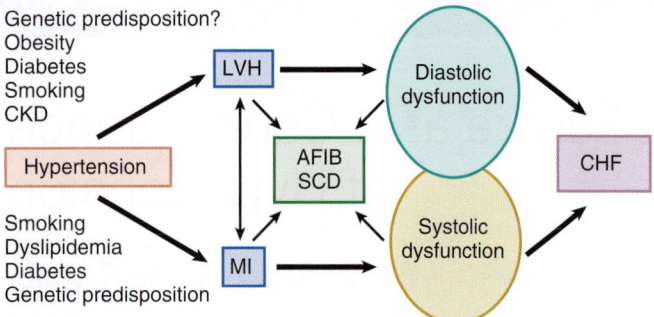

Genetic predisposition?
Obesity
Diabetes
Smoking
CKD

Smoking
Dyslipidemia
Diabetes
Genetic predisposition

Fig. 25.1 Risk factors and the progression of hypertensive heart disease and its complications. *AFIB*, Atrial fibrillation; *CHF*, congestive heart failure; *CKD*, chronic kidney disease; *LVH*, left ventricular hypertrophy; *MI*, myocardial infarction; *SCD*, sudden cardiac death.

profile of the study population. In a pooled analysis of studies using ECG as the diagnostic test, the reported prevalence of LVH ranged from 0.6% to 40% (average 24% in men and 16% in women).[23] Another pooled analysis of studies utilizing echocardiography for the detection of LVH showed less variable prevalence estimates, ranging from 36% to 41% among patients with HTN.[24]

Ethnic differences: In most population-based studies, non-Hispanic (NH) black individuals had a much greater prevalence of LVH than their NH white counterparts.[22,25,26] Specifically, in the Hypertension Genetic Epidemiology Network Study (HyperGEN),[27] middle-aged black adults with HTN had 2.5-fold greater odds for LVH by echocardiography even after adjustment for cardiovascular risk factors and body surface area (BSA). In the Dallas Heart Study, young and middle-aged black adults, including both normotensive and hypertensive individuals, had 1.8-fold greater odds of LVH by cardiac MRI after adjustment for systolic BP, body mass, age, gender, history of diabetes, and socioeconomic status.[22] The cause of this much greater propensity for LVH in blacks is unknown but could be related to the earlier onset,[28,29] less nocturnal dipping,[30-32] and greater severity of HTN.[5] However, the fact that the greater odds for LVH in blacks increased to 2.3-fold in the subgroup of hypertensive persons and that the prevalence of LVH was increased in blacks only if they were either in the prehypertensive or hypertensive range of systolic BP suggests a genetic predisposition of blacks to develop LVH in response to pressure overload, as discussed later (see section titled Genetic Factors in LVH). MESA compared left ventricular mass index (LVMI) with BSA between NH whites, NH blacks, and Hispanics of Mexican, Caribbean, and South/Central American origin. HTN was much more common in NH blacks than in all other groups. However, LVH (defined as >95th percentile of cumulative distribution separately for men and women) was more common in all Hispanic subgroups than in NH whites but was as frequently observed in Hispanics as in NH blacks.[33] Similarly, an increased prevalence of LVH in Hispanics and NH blacks compared with NH whites has also been observed in individuals with chronic kidney disease (CKD).[34] The Northern Manhattan Study—comprising a triethnic community cohort of NH white, NH black, and Hispanic participants—found that both Hispanics and blacks had worse echocardiography-derived LV diastolic indices than whites. However, these differences were not related to LV mass or HTN but rather to cardiovascular comorbidities and socioeconomic factors.[35] A comparison of Asian and white cohorts demonstrated a higher prevalence of ECG-determined LVH and worse LVH-related cardiovascular events in the former group.[36]

Gender differences: In general men have a greater LVMI as related to BSA than women. Therefore different threshold values have been established for the diagnosis of LVH in men and women. Using these different thresholds for the diagnosis of LVH, men tend to have a greater incidence of LVH even after adjustment for other characteristics thought of as risk factors for LVH.[22,27,37]

Risk factors for LVH: Besides the aforementioned demographic determinants of LVH, many other clinical risk factors have been identified. Not surprisingly, BP tracks LV mass in a linear fashion. However, single office BP measurements are only weakly associated with LV mass (**Fig. 25.2**),[38] whereas 24-hour ambulatory BP—a better measure of hemodynamic LV burden—is much more closely related to LV mass.[39] Another explanation for the weak correlation of BP measurements and LV mass are nonhemodynamic (i.e., neurohumoral) stimuli to myocardial muscle growth; these are discussed in the next section of this chapter. Epidemiologic studies have identified the following risk factors for LVH: In the MESA study of adults without clinical cardiovascular disease, LV mass was independently associated with current smoking and diabetes. More recently, even impaired glucose tolerance in nondiabetics was found to be a risk factor for LVH after adjustment for obesity.[40,41] Sleep-disordered breathing, even without symptoms of daytime sleepiness, has also been identified as a determinant of greater LV mass,[42,43] which is likely related to a greater prevalence of nocturnal HTN and sympathetic nerve activation[44] in these individuals.[45] Closely linked with sleep apnea is body mass index and subscapular skin fold thickness, which were associated with greater LV mass in the Coronary Artery Risk Development in Young Adults (CARDIA) study and in MESA.[46,47] CKD is closely linked with LVH, even when renal function is only mildly abnormal.[48] Inflammatory markers such as high-sensitivity C-reactive protein (hs-CRP) and interleukin 6 (IL-6) are determinants of LVH in CKD and thus may hint at the involved mechanisms.[49] The combination of black race and CKD is associated with a staggering LVH prevalence of 70% in this population.[50]

Pathophysiologic Mechanisms

Macroscopically LVH is an increase in myocardial muscle mass. However, on a cellular level, this greater muscle mass consists not only of increases in myocyte protein and the recruitment of contractile elements; other cell types—such as fibroblasts, vascular smooth muscle cells, and endothelial cells—also undergo changes that contribute to an altered extracellular matrix (i.e., the connective tissue) (**see also Chapter 4**). **Fig. 25.3** depicts the complex interplay between mechanical (hemodynamic) and neurohumoral stress and key pathways for stimulating hypertrophic gene expression.[51] The inability of the myocardial microvasculature to keep up with myocyte growth is a key aspect of the genesis hypertensive heart disease (see also **Fig. 25.2**). Although our understanding of the underlying mechanisms remains incomplete, decades of research have identified several molecular mechanisms, as reviewed by Cacciapuoti,[52] and genetic factors that influence the development of hypertensive heart disease.

Importance of hemodynamic burden: As mentioned earlier, the correlation between office/clinic BP measurement and LV mass is less than perfect.[53] There are several explanations for this finding: (1) Office BP is not a reliable surrogate for hemodynamic burden—24-hour ambulatory BP correlates much better.[39] (2) Neither office nor 24-hour ambulatory BP monitoring provides information on lifetime hemodynamic burden—on the onset and progression of HTN. (3) Neurohumoral stimulation linked to the development of LVH may differ between hypertensive individuals. (4) A genetic propensity for LVH may exists in some and be absent in other hypertensive patients. Racial/ethnic differences in the probability of developing LVH strongly suggest (but do not prove) a genetic component and are discussed separately.

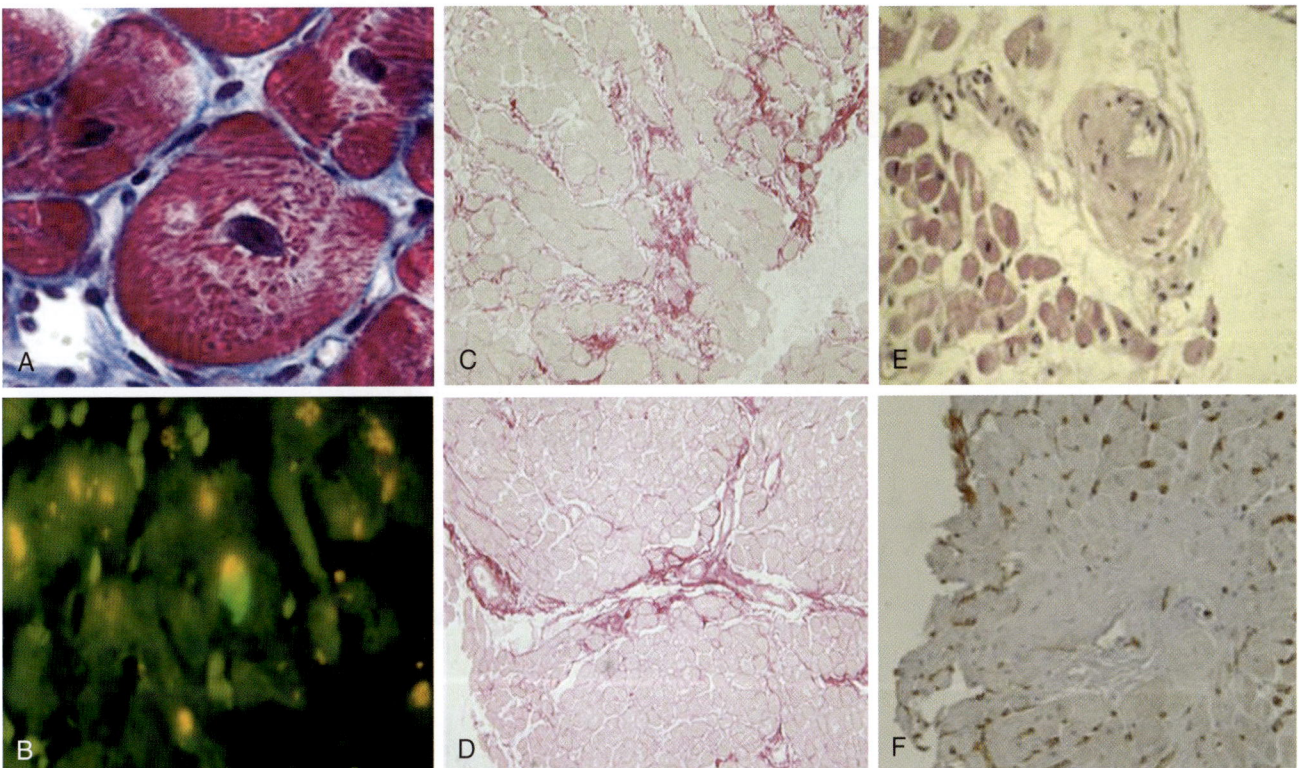

Fig. 25.2 The Hypertensive Myocardium. Histologic findings in left ventricular hypertrophy: cardiomyocyte hypertrophy (A), apoptosis (B), which among other mechanisms leads to interstitial (C), and perivascular fibrosis (D), arteriole remodeling (E), and capillary rarefaction (F), all of which perpetuate myocardial fibrosis. (From Moreno MU, Eiros R, Gavira JJ, et al. The hypertensive myocardium: from microscopic lesions to clinical complications and outcomes. *Med Clin North Am.* 2017;101[1]:43–52.)

Molecular Mechanisms

a. *The Renin-Angiotensin-Aldosterone System* (**see also Chapter 5**): Local release of angiotensin II causes the activation of G protein and rho protein, increasing protein synthesis in myocardial cells, and collagen synthesis in fibroblasts.[54-57] Overexpression of angiotensin II in transgenic mice causes pressure-independent LVH.[58] Angiotensin II may also stimulate the release of paracrine endothelin-1 from fibroblasts.[59] Clinical evidence for the importance of renin stimulation and angiotensin II in the development of LVH comes from the fact that angiotensin receptor blockers (ARBs) and angiotensin-converting enzyme (ACE) inhibitors are the most effective medical therapies used to reduce LVH in hypertensive individuals.[60]

b. *Aldosterone:* As described earlier, the renin-angiotensin-aldosterone system is important in the genesis of LVH. However, medical treatment with ACE inhibitors or ARBs does not protect against the effects of circulating aldosterone (i.e., aldosterone escape).[61] Cardiomyocytes express mineralocorticoid receptors.[62] Aldosterone itself has been shown to cause vascular[63] and cardiac inflammation,[64] myocardial fibrosis,[65] and cardiac hypertrophy.[66] In a hypertensive model of endothelial dysfunction, eplerenone prevented cardiac inflammation and fibrosis.[67] The nonselective aldosterone antagonist spironolactone and the selective aldosterone antagonist eplerenone provide clear clinical benefit in patients with systolic heart failure[68,69] and less clear benefit in patients with diastolic heart failure.[70,71] These agents decrease LVH as efficiently as an ACE-inhibitor and even more efficiently if given in combination with an ACE inhibitor.[72] These data strongly suggest that aldosterone is directly involved in the development of hypertensive heart disease. The interplay between hyperaldosteronism, LVH, and atrial fibrillation has been comprehensively reviewed by Saccia and colleagues.[73]

c. *Endothelin-1:* Endothelin has been shown to induce hypertrophy in animal models, and this phenotype can be suppressed by a pharmacologic endothelin-1 receptor blocker.[59,74,75] Direct evidence of endothelin-1 from human studies is lacking. As mentioned previously, there is an interplay between angiotensin II and endothelin-1.[59]

d. *Heat-Shock Proteins:* This is a group of intracellular proteins that become more abundant in cells exposed to thermal or other forms of stress; they regulate nuclear transcription factors. One of these is factor NF-κ-B, which was increased in a pressure-overload model in the rat and can be suppressed by either gene therapy with a viral vector or an antioxidant substance. As a result, the hypertrophic response to pressure overload was markedly attenuated in treated animals.[76] Furthermore, in mice with cardiomyocyte-restricted expression of an NF-κ-B superrepressor gene, both angiotensin II and isoproterenol induced

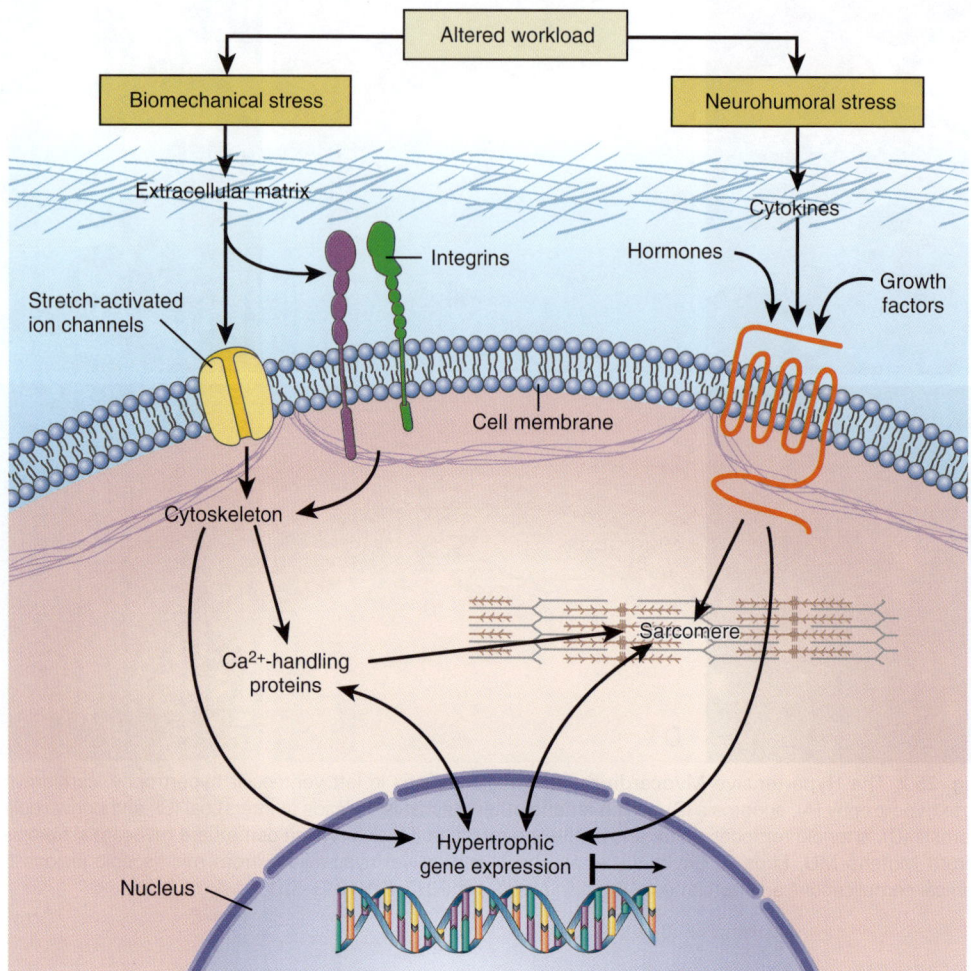

Fig. 25.3 Hemodynamic and Neurohumoral Stimuli and Pathways Leading to Myocyte Hypertrophy. Both mechanical and neurohumoral stress in hypertension stimulates local release of paracrine substances, which signal hypertrophic gene expression and sarcomeric hypertrophy. (From Hill JA, Olson EN. Cardiac plasticity. *N Engl J Med*. 2008;358:1370–1380.)

a hypertrophic response and the expression of hypertrophic markers, such as β-myosin heavy chain and natriuretic peptides, was reduced.[77] The proteasome-inhibitor PS-519, which is known to suppress NF-κ-B, prevented isoproterenol-induced LVH when given before and during isoproterenol infusion and caused regression of LVH in those animals, which already had isoproterenol-induced LVH.[78]

e. *G proteins:* Many substances involved in the hypertrophic response to pressure and stress—including phenylephrine, angiotensin II, and endothelin-1—bind to myocyte membrane receptors that activate G protein and small subforms of G proteins (i.e., Rho proteins). These proteins regulate transcription and have been shown to be involved in phenylephrine-induced LVH.[79] In addition, in transgenic mice that overexpress the carboxyl-terminal peptide of the G protein and thus inhibit normal G-protein activation, the slope of the hypertrophic response to increased LV pressure overload from transverse aortic banding was less steep.[80]

f. *Calcineurin:* Calcineurin is a calcium-dependent phosphatase; it dephosphorylates cytosolic factors, enabling them to translocate to the nucleus to activate transcription. Transgenic mice that overexpress calcineurin or its transcription factor targets develop cardiac hypertrophy and failure. This phenotype can be suppressed with pharmacologic calcineurin inhibition.[81]

Genetic Determinants of Left Ventricular Hypertrophy

In the Framingham Heart Study it was estimated that heritability of LVMI was between 0.24 and 0.32 in patients without known cardiac disease and a low risk-factor profile.[82] A much higher estimated heritability of 0.59 was found in a study of 182 monozygotic and 194 dizygotic twins. In addition, clinical observations have found a large variability of LV mass in patients with similar office BP and exceedingly high rates of LVH in certain race/ethnic populations.[22,27] This suggest a genetic predisposition for the development of LVH in response to pressure overload. Indeed, some genes associated with LVH have been identified: (1) *Corin* is the enzyme responsible for processing the preforms of atrial and brain natriuretic peptide (ANP and BNP), which are protective against LVH. Corin knockout mice develop HTN and cardiac hypertrophy.[82] Mutations of the corin I555(P568) gene were exclusive to African Americans in multiethnic samples with an allelic prevalence of 6% to 12%.[83] The association of this mutation with an increased prevalence of HTN and LVH in African Americans has been demonstrated in three independent population-based samples.[83] (2) *Protein C* overexpression causes progressive LVH and diastolic dysfunction in animals. (3) The bradykinin-2 receptor gene polymorphism, specifically the 9-bp receptor gene deletion, is associated with greater LV mass in subjects undergoing physical training.[84] (4) ACE gene polymorphism is also associated with both greater tissue and plasma ACE levels and a greater probability for LVH.[85,86]

CLASSIFICATION AND DIAGNOSIS OF HYPERTENSIVE HEART DISEASE

Hypertensive heart disease is classified using a combination of structural and functional criteria. Two distinct entities are excluded from these classifications and therefore not discussed in this section: (1) physiologic hypertrophy, as seen in pregnant women or athletes, which leads to moderate adaptive increases of LV internal dimensions and LV muscle mass but with normal RWT (0.32–0.42)[87] and normal Doppler-derived LV filling parameters, and (2) genetic or acquired hypertrophic cardiomyopathies in which pressure-independent LV wall thickening due to sarcomere-protein mutations occurs, as is seen in familial hypertrophic cardiomyopathy or with protein/glycolipid deposits as seen in amyloidosis or Fabry disease.

Clinical Presentation/Functional Classes

The onset of symptomatic heart failure and especially hospitalization for heart failure is an important indicator of poor outcomes and a high mortality rate, both in heart failure with preserved ejection fraction (HFpEF) and heart failure with reduced ejection fraction (HFrEF). Therefore the following consideration of symptoms in the classification of hypertensive heart disease is extremely important.[88]
- **Class I:** Subclinical diastolic dysfunction without LVH: Asymptomatic patients with abnormal LV relaxation/stiffness by Doppler echocardiography, a common finding in individuals above 65 years of age.[89]
- **Class II:** LVH
  - **IIA:** With normal or mildly abnormal functional capacity (New York Heart Association class I)
  - **IIB:** With abnormal functional capacity (New York Heart Association class II or greater)
- **Class III:** HFpEF—clinical signs and symptoms of cardiac decompensation (i.e., dyspnea, pulmonary edema) from increased left atrial pressure
- **Class IV:** HFrEF

Anatomic Classification of Left Ventricular Hypertrophy

The anatomic classification proposed by Ganau and colleagues (1992)[38] is based on echocardiographic measurements of LV geometry and muscle mass. LV geometry is determined by RWT calculated as doubling the width of the LV inferolateral wall and divided by the LV end-diastolic internal diameter in end-diastole. A RWT ≥0.44 is diagnostic of concentric LVH, whereas an RWT less than 0.44 with increased LV mass is indicative of eccentric remodeling. This category can be further distinguished from physiologic hypertrophy, which is characterized by mild increases of LV mass and an RWT between 0.32 and 0.44.[87] LV mass is best calculated according to the modified Simpson rule and most commonly indexed to

BSA.[90] **Fig. 25.4** depicts the four anatomic classes of LV mass and geometry.
- **Class I:** Normal LV
- **Class II:** Concentric remodeling without hypertrophy
- **Class III:** Concentric LVH
- **Class IV:** Eccentric LVH

Diagnostic Criteria for Left Ventricular Hypertrophy

LVH, the increase in LV myocardial mass beyond defined cutoffs, can be diagnosed by ECG, echocardiography, or cardiac MRI. Although cardiac MRI is the most accurate and precise method for determining LV mass, the preferred method is echocardiography because it is more widely available than cardiac MRI while also providing greater sensitivity than ECG.[91] ECG is a reasonable cost-conscious alternative to the more expensive testing modalities, especially in the asymptomatic hypertensive patient with a low index of suspicion for hypertensive heart disease in whom echocardiography is not necessarily indicated.[92] A clear limitation to the usefulness of screening for LVH irrespective of the testing modality is the fact that awareness of the presence or absence of LVH typically has little impact on physician behavior in the treatment of HTN.[93]

Electrocardiogram

Among the many published ECG-criteria for the diagnosis of LVH shown in **Table 25.1**, the Cornell criteria appear to be both reasonably sensitive and highly prognostic for cardiovascular events.[94] The sensitivity can be improved by using several ECG criteria in conjunction (i.e., Romhilt-Estes score, Perugia criteria). It is important to recognize that the sensitivity and specificity of ECG for the diagnosis of LVH depends on the severity of LVH in the study populations.

Echocardiography (see also Chapter 32)

Echocardiography is the preferred testing modality for the diagnosis of LVH. The use of calculated LV mass index provides both greater sensitivity and specificity for the diagnosis of LVH than linear measurements of the LV septum or posterior wall.[95] Of note, three-dimensional (3D) echocardiography may be as accurate and reproducible as cardiac MRI—the current gold standard for detecting LVH—but it is not widely used in clinical practice.[96,97] To determine LVH, LV mass is calculated using the following formula:

$$\text{Left ventricular mass} = 0.8 \times \left(1.04 \times \left[(\text{LVIDd} + \text{PWTd} + \text{SWTd})^3 - (\text{LVIDd})^3\right]\right) + 0.6\,g$$

and indexed to BSA; the latter is calculated according to Du Bois or Mosteller.[90,98] LVIDd indicates LV internal diameter in diastole; PWTd, posterior wall thickness in diastole; SWTd, septal wall thickness in diastole; and LVIDd, LV internal diameter in diastole. The severity of LVH is graded by LVMI, as shown in **Table 25.2**.

Computed Tomography

Computer tomography (CT) has excellent spatial resolution and can assess LV mass in 3D without geometric assumptions. However, poor temporal resolution, associated radiation, and less well-established normal values make CT the least utilized modality in assessing LVH.[99]

Cardiac Magnetic Resonance Imaging

Estimation of LV mass by two-dimensional (2D) echocardiography is based on linear measurements with the assumption that the LV is geometrically a prolate ellipsoid of revolution, which is often inaccurate. In contrast, cardiac MRI permits the estimation of LV mass by direct 3D tracing without any geometric assumptions. As a result, cardiac

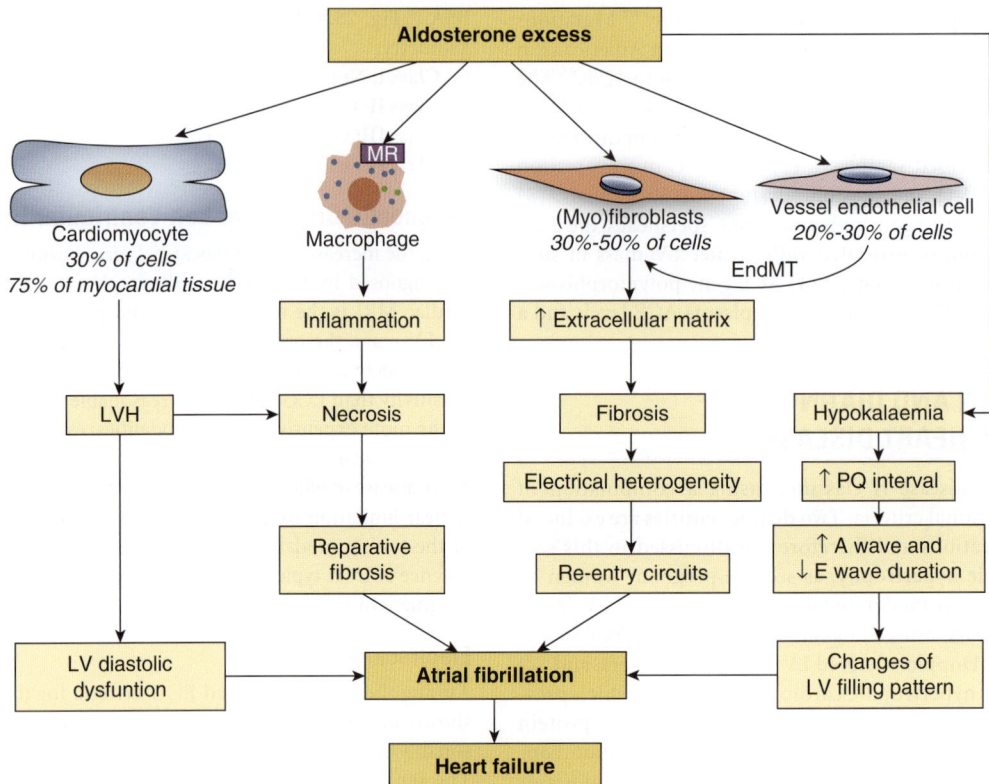

Fig. 25.4 Mechanisms by Which Aldosterone Excess Favors the Onset of Atrial Fibrillation. Aldosterone is one known stimulant for left ventricular hypertrophy. In addition, stimulation of inflammatory cascades and fibroblasts leads to additional myocardial thickening via necrosis and reparative and direct fibrosis, all of which lead to the clinical phenotypes of hypertensive heart disease. *LV*, Left ventricle; *LVH*, left ventricular hypertrophy. (From Seccia TM, Caroccia B, Adler GK, et al. Arterial hypertension, atrial fibrillation, and hyperaldosteronism: the triple trouble. *Hypertension.* 2017;69:545–550.)

MRI has been shown to be twice as precise as 2D echocardiography in determining LV mass with a 93% lower interstudy variability; it is therefore considered the gold standard.[100,101] However, higher cost, less availability, and poorer tolerability continue to limit its broad use as screening test for LVH in hypertensive patients.

COMPLICATIONS OF HYPERTENSIVE HEART DISEASE

Heart Failure With Preserved Ejection Fraction (see also Chapter 39)

HTN is the most prevalent cause of heart failure.[1] LV remodeling in response to pressure overload and neurohumoral stimulation causes structural geometric changes in the LV, and this process is initially adaptive. Later in the course of hypertensive heart disease, however, evidence of LV decompensation becomes evident. And diastolic dysfunction—abnormal LV relaxation and filling—typically occurs much earlier than systolic dysfunction.[102,103]

Diastolic function is determined noninvasively by echocardiography. The diastolic phase of the cardiac cycle consists of four distinct components: (1) *isovolumic relaxation*—which starts at closure of the aortic valve and ends with opening of the mitral valve; (2) passive filling of the LV—after opening of the mitral valve, rapid filling of the LV propelled by the pressure gradient between left atrium and the LV (i.e., pulsed Doppler-derived E-wave); (3) *diastasis*—when the pressure gradient between the LV and the left atrium approaches zero, flow across the mitral valve is equal to pulmonary vein inflow, which is limited by LV pressure

and compliance; and (4) *atrial contraction*—or pulsed Doppler-derived A-wave. Qualitative and quantitative evaluation of these four diastolic measures by Doppler echocardiography is essential to determine diastolic function and to estimate LV filling pressures noninvasively. Other echocardiographic surrogates of diastolic function are left atrial enlargement, a prevalent feature of hypertensive heart disease[104]; pulmonary vein flow pattern; and pulmonary arterial pressure. A detailed description of the evaluation of LV diastology is beyond the scope of this chapter. **Fig. 25.5** summarizes echocardiography-derived grading of diastolic dysfunction utilizing Doppler-derived measurement of the early and late mitral inflow and pulmonary vein patterns, tissue Doppler-derived atrioventricular annulus velocities, and color Doppler–derived mitral inflow propagation velocity.[105] Strain and strain rate can be assessed with echocardiography or MRI; these promise to be useful determinants of both the diastolic and systolic function of the LV. The association of some common measures of diastolic function with incident cardiovascular events, including heart failure, has been well established.[106-108]

HFpEF is a major public health concern. Some 43% of patients admitted for heart failure have normal left ventricular ejection fraction (LVEF).[109] HFpEF is linked to older age, female gender, diabetes, obesity, CKD, HTN, and coronary artery disease (CAD)[110]; thus, with an aging population, hospital admissions for heart failure, especially HFpEF, are increasing.[111] Even after adjustment for other cardiovascular risk factors, which are common in patients with HFpEF, this common form of heart failure is associated with a marked increase in all-cause mortality.[105,111] Although the clinical benefit of several medical and device-based therapies has been established in the treatment of systolic heart failure, HFpEF remains a therapeutic challenge. After

TABLE 25.1 Definition, Sensitivity, and Specificity of Some ECG Criteria for Left Ventricular Hypertrophy

ECG Criteria	Diagnostic Cutoff	Sensitivity	Specificity
R in aVL	≥1.1 mV	11	97
Sokolow-Lyon voltage[210] S in V$_1$ + R in V$_5$ or V$_6$	≥3.5 mV	13	93
Cornell voltage[211] S in V$_3$ + R in aVL	>2.8 mV (men) >2.0 mV (women)	19	97

Romhilt-Estes score[212]
Components:
1. Any of these:
    R or S in limb leads ≥20;
    S in V1 or V2 ≥30;
    R in V5 or V6 ≥30
2. ST-T vector opposite to QRS with digitalis
    ST-T vector opposite to QRS without digitalis
3. Left atrial enlargement in V1
4. Left axis deviation
5. QRS duration ≥0.09 sec
6. Intrinsicoid deflection in V5 or V6 >0.05sec
	total of ≥5 points
	3 points
	1 point
	3 points
	3 points
	2 points
	1 point
	1 point
		16	96

Perugia criteria[213] Components: 1. S in V$_3$ + R in aVL 2. LV strain (ST-T vector opposite to QRS) 3. Romhilt-Estes score	≥1 of the following criteria >2.4 mV (men) >2.0 mV (women) present ≥5 points	36	90

ECG, Electrocardiogram; *LV,* left ventricle.

TABLE 25.2 Severity of Left Ventricular Hypertrophy by Echocardiogram-Derived Left Ventricular Mass Indexed by Body Surface Area

Severity	LVMI in Men, g/m^2	LVMI in Women, g/m^2
Mild LVH	103–116	89–100
Moderate LVH	117–130	101–112
Severe LVH	≥131	≥113

LVH, Left ventricular hypertrophy; *LVMI,* left ventricular mass index. From Lang RM, Bierig M, Devereux RB, et al. American Society of Echocardiography's Guidelines and Standards Committee, European Association of Echocardiography. Recommendations for chamber quantification: a report from the American Society of Echocardiography's Guidelines and Standards Committee and the Chamber Quantification Writing Group, developed in conjunction with the European Association of Echocardiography, a branch of the European Society of Cardiology. *J Am Soc Echocardiogr.* 2005;18:1440–1463.

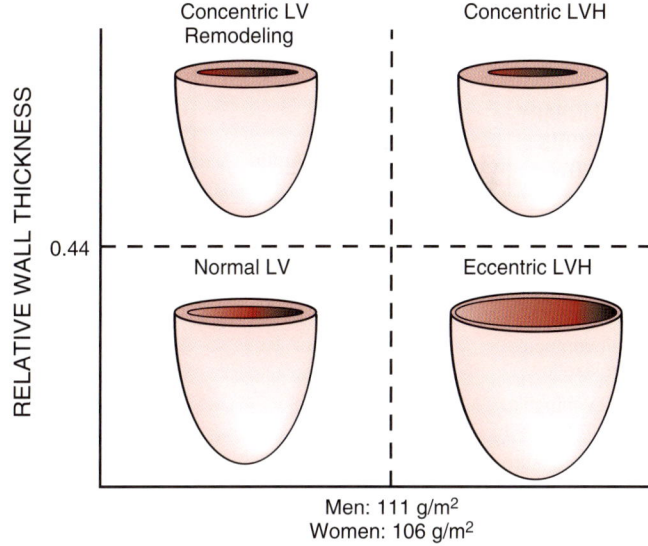

Fig. 25.5 Anatomic Classification of Hypertensive Heart Disease. Pressure overload of the left ventricle initiates concentric remodeling as a compensatory mechanism, followed by a frank increase in left ventricular mass above cutoff values for left ventricular hypertrophy. Left ventricular dilation with increased left ventricular mass occurs at a stage of decompensation. *LV,* Left ventricle; *LVH,* left ventricular hypertrophy. (Adapted from Ganau A, Devereux, Roman MJ, et al. Patterns of left ventricular hypertrophy and geometric remodeling in essential hypertension. *J Am Coll Cardiol.* 1992;19[7]:1550–1558.)

several randomized trials, no specific therapy has been identified that definitively alters the course of this disease and provides a mortality benefit for these patients.[112] Targeting the renin-angiotensin-aldosterone system has shown benefits in terms of LVH reduction [113-115] and improvements in diastolic function.[116-118] However, four large outcome trials studying the effects of the angiotensin blockers candesartan[119] and irbesartan,[120] the ACE-inhibitor perindopril,[121] and the aldosterone antagonist spironolactone[70] found that none of them showed a reduction in mortality rates in the active treatment arms. Nonetheless, spironolactone showed a reduction in heart failure hospitalizations, especially in North American study participants.[71] An echocardiographic substudy of this trial showed that more than a third of study participants had both normal systolic and diastolic function

(Fig. 25.6).[122] This finding suggests that current indicators of LV systolic and diastolic function are inadequate to diagnose cardiac dysfunction in a large portion of patients admitted for heart failure.

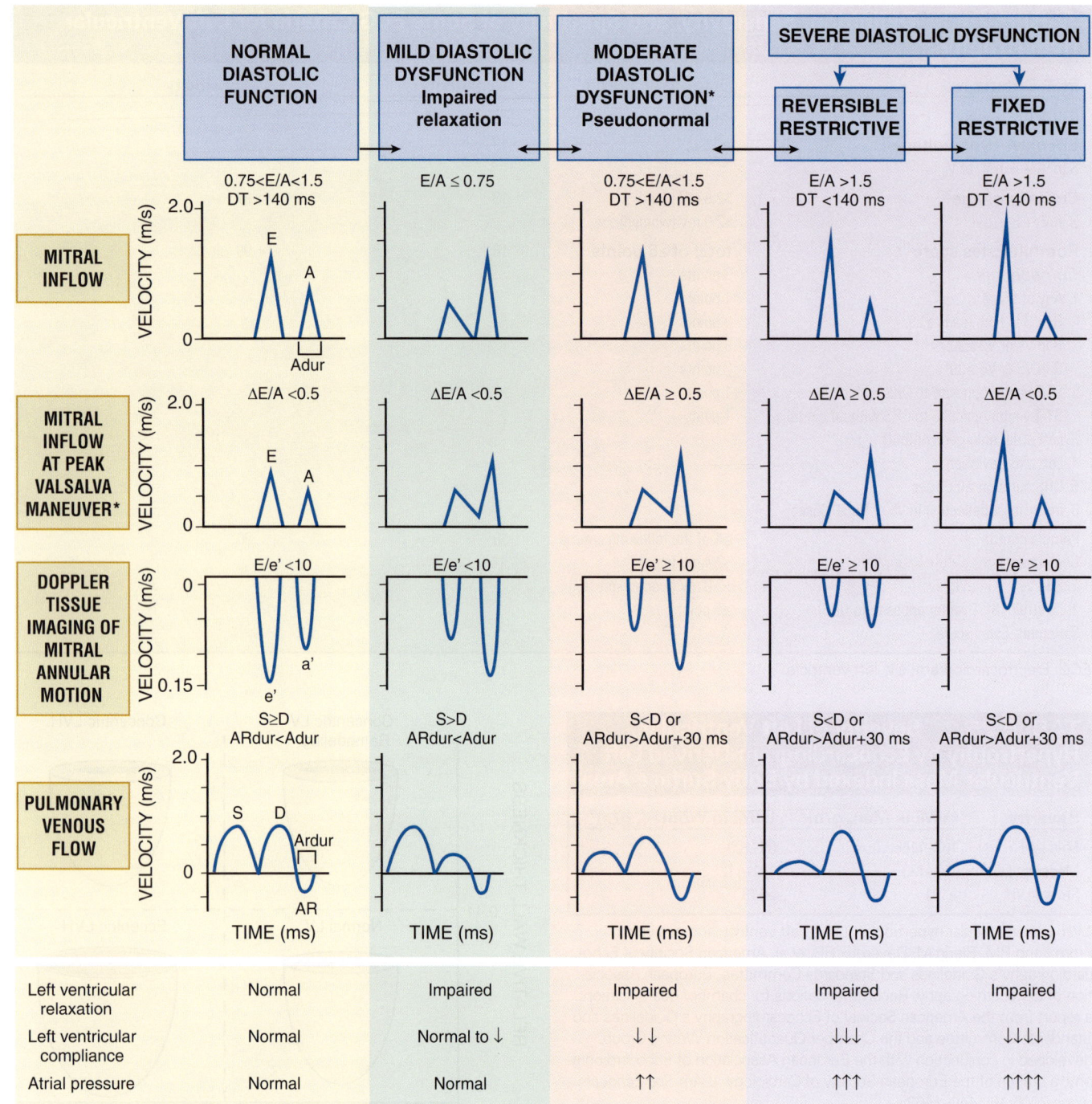

Fig. 25.6 Classification of diastolic function by Doppler/tissue Doppler echocardiography and correlating left ventricular and left atrial abnormalities. *A*, Late mitral inflow velocity during atrial contraction; *AR*, pulmonary vein flow reversal during atrial contraction; *ARdur* and *Adur*, duration of AR or A; *D*, diastolic component of pulmonary vein flow; *DT*, early mitral inflow deceleration time; *E*, early mitral inflow velocity; *e'*, early annular velocity by tissue Doppler; *S*, systolic component of pulmonary vein flow. (From Redfield MM, Jacobson SJ, Burnett JC, et al. Burden of systolic and diastolic ventricular dysfunction in the community: appreciating the scope of the heart failure epidemic. *JAMA.* 2003;289[2]:194–202.)

Systolic Heart Failure

Although LVEF has been shown to be an insensitive measure of systolic function, it is the most commonly used parameter for describing cardiac function in clinical practice. It is most commonly assessed with measurements of end-diastolic and end-systolic volume from 2D echocardiography. 3D echocardiography or cardiac MRI are considered the gold standard in the estimation of LVEF.[96,97,100,101] More sensitive indices of systolic function are global longitudinal strain, radial strain, circumferential strain, and LV torsion by speckle-tracking echocardiography, but these modalities are not yet widely used.[123-126] Decreased LVEF is an important predictor of mortality in ischemic and nonischemic cardiomyopathy, with major implications for medical treatment and the prevention of sudden cardiac death.[127,128] Although hospital admission for HFpEF is most common among white women, black males have the highest proportion of hospitalization for HFrEF.[109]

A link between LVH and systolic function was found in the population-based Cardiovascular Health Study.[129] Increased LVMI in relation to BSA was a strong predictor of depressed LV function after an average of 4.9 years of follow-up independent of age, baseline BP, diabetes, CAD, and Q-waves or atrial fibrillation on baseline ECG. This finding suggests that LVH is a direct or indirect—via ischemic events—predecessor of systolic deterioration in hypertensive heart disease. In patients with LVH, even minimal increases in natriuretic peptides and cardiac troponin may identify malignant subgroups with a high risk for progression to systolic heart failure and cardiovascular death.[130] The treatment of systolic heart failure—including medical therapies, device-based therapies, and the prevention of sudden cardiac death—is beyond the scope of this chapter and is described in other pertinent chapters of this book. It should be noted here, however, that a reduction of LVH with medical therapy also improves systolic LV function.[131,132]

Myocardial Ischemia

Convincing evidence exists that both HTN and LVH are potent risk factors for coronary heart disease. In the Framingham Heart Study, LVH was an important determinant of CAD in older participants.[133] Similarly, in the CARDIA study, LV mass by echocardiography was independently associated with coronary calcium in young adults.[134] Thus HTN, especially when accompanied by LVH, appears to cause progressive coronary plaque buildup to the point where the disease leads to cardiovascular events. Furthermore, LVH is associated not only with stable CAD from progressive arterial narrowing but also with increases in the risk of acute coronary plaque rupure.[135] In addition to macrovascular ischemia from epicardial CAD, microvascular ischemia is a hallmark of LVH and leads to cardiac complications. As a consequence, in hypertrophied hearts suffering ST-elevation myocardial infractions, the resulting infarct size is larger, the postinfarction LVEF is lower, and the risk of death and heart failure is more than doubled.[136] Therapeutic implications of microvascular blood flow disturbances are discussed in the last section of this chapter (Treatment Targets and the J-Curve Debate). Microvascular angina in the absence of obstructive epicardial CAD is now an established clinical entity and seems to be more common in women.[137,138] From a mechanistic point of view, both microvascular and macrovascular ischemia are key factors in the development of hypertensive heart disease and both perpetuate its progression.[11]

Atrial Fibrillation (see also Chapter 38)

Atrial fibrillation is the most common supraventricular arrhythmia, with a prevalence ranging from 0.1% in individuals younger than 55 years to 10% in octogenarians; moreover, the prevalence estimates are higher in Europe than in the United States.[139,140] As in the case of hypertensive heart disease and diastolic dysfunction, atrial fibrillation is closely linked to older age, HTN, obesity, and diabetes. HTN is the most prevalent modifiable risk factor for atrial fibrillation on a population level.[141,142] The severity of diastolic dysfunction,[143,144] as well as the degree of left atrial enlargement,[143,145] both correlate with the rate of incident atrial fibrillation. Increased left atrial pressure load from chronic HTN and diastolic dysfunction causes similar changes in the atrial myocardium as previously described in the ventricular myocardium in the development of LVH (see section titled Pathophysiologic Mechanism). Myocyte hypertrophy, interstitial fibrosis, cell loss, and changes in structural and electrophysiologic properties can lead to zones of conduction slowing and microreentrant circuits (i.e., "rotors") that perpetuate atrial fibrillation.[146-149] In animal models, pressure overload from aortic banding, angiotensin II infusion, and 5/6 nephrectomy—a model of CKD—all caused left atrial fibrosis and increased atrial fibrillation inducibility.[150] Oxidative stress and inflammation appear to be centrally involved, because pharmacologic antioxidants suppressed both left atrial fibrosis and atrial fibrillation inducibility in these animal models.[150] Important clinical sequelae of atrial fibrillation are thromboembolism and worsening heart failure, both from loss of atrial systole in preload-dependent stiff LV and from deterioration of systolic function from persistently elevated heart rates (i.e., tachycardia-mediated cardiomyopathy).[151] Higher BP was associated with an increased risk of stroke and thromboembolism in the ARISTOTLE (Apixaban for Reduction in Stroke and Other Thromboembolic Events in Atrial Fibrillation) trial.[152] Atrial fibrillation has also been associated with an increased risk of mortality independently of presence or absence of hypertensive heart disease.[153,154] In addition, new-onset atrial fibrillation increases the risk of sudden cardiac death in patient with LVH.[155] Therefore the prevention of atrial fibrillation could conceivably improve outcomes in hypertensive heart disease. This question has been asked in one large observational study[156] and two post hoc analyses of randomized studies.[157,158] In these studies, subjects who received an ARB had a significant (19%-37%) relative risk reduction for new-onset atrial fibrillation compared with control subjects. In contrast, in a large randomized trial for the prevention of recurrent (not new-onset) atrial fibrillation as the primary outcome, assignment to the ARB valsartan was ineffective.[159]

Sudden Cardiac Death

Patients with LVH have a greater incidence of ventricular premature beats and ventricular tachycardia[160-162] irrespective of the etiology of LVH.[163] Sudden cardiac death, which is most frequently caused by sustained ventricular tachyarrhythmias, is among the leading causes of death worldwide[164,165] and has been linked to LVH in large epidemiologic studies and registries.[12,13,16,133,166] In the Framingham Heart Study there was a 1.45-fold increase in sudden cardiac death risk for every 50 g increase in LV mass.[13] Although the mechanisms are not well understood, the arrhythmogenic substrate for sudden cardiac death may be subendocardial ischemia, interstitial fibrosis, increased sympathetic tone, increased tissue catecholamine levels, repolarization delay (i.e., prolongation of the QT interval), increased incidence of early afterdepolarizations, and a genetic predisposition of channelopathies in patients with LVH.[14,167] Interestingly, in a population-based study of sudden cardiac death victims, LVH by ECG and LVH by echocardiography showed little overlap and were, in terms of risk prediction, nearly distinct entities.[168] Because of the strong association between LVH and sudden cardiac death, the former may be a viable treatment target to prevent the latter. Indeed, regression of LVH decreased the incidence of sudden cardiac death in two large studies.[9,169] In the Losartan Intervention for Endpoint reduction in hypertension (LIFE) study, sudden cardiac death occurred at similar rates in both the atenolol and losartan treatment arms. However, absence of on-treatment LVH by Cornell voltage-duration product criteria on ECG was associated with a 66% risk reduction for incident sudden cardiac death even after adjustment for demographic and clinical characteristics. Given these and other encouraging results, it has been speculated that LVH could increase accuracy in the prediction of sudden cardiac death and thus make the implantation of implantable cardioverter defibrillators more cost-effective.[14]

All-Cause Mortality

LVH is a potent cardiovascular risk factor independent of the degree of BP elevation or other comorbidities.[15-17] In the Framingham Heart Study, adults above 40 years of age without apparent cardiovascular disease underwent echocardiography for the determination of LV mass. During a mean follow-up of 4 years, the relative risk for all-cause mortality for each 50 g increase in LV mass increased by 49% in men (adjusted relative risk [aRR] 1.49, confidence interval [CI] 1.14–1.94) and doubled in women (aRR 2.01, CI 1.44–2.81).[16] In patients who are treated for HTN, LVH carries a much greater risk for cardiovascular death. In an observational study of 280 patients with essential HTN, after a mean follow-up period of over 10 years, cardiovascular death occurred in 14% of individuals with LVH compared with 0.5% of individuals without LVH ($P < .0001$).[17] Conversely, in the LIFE study, absence of in-treatment LVH was associated with a markedly reduced risk for all-cause mortality (multivariable adjusted hazard ratio 0.36, CI 0.23–0.59, $P < .001$) (**Fig. 25.7**).[19] LV mass by echocardiography (not ECG) and age—not gender or BP—were the only independent predictors of cardiovascular events. Across the range of LV geometry, concentric LVH was associated with the greatest risk. Interestingly, an obesity paradox appears to exist for the association of LVH with all-cause mortality in women. In a large retrospective study of over 26,000 women with normal systolic LV function who underwent echocardiography in a major academic center, abnormal LV geometry was more common in obese than in nonobese individuals (**Fig. 25.8**). Although LVH—concentric more so than eccentric hypertrophy—was associated with increased all-cause mortality in both obese and nonobese individuals, this increase in mortality was much less dramatic in obese than in nonobese women .[170]

TREATMENT

General Considerations and Regression of Left Ventricular Hypertrophy

Although lifestyle-modifications and medical treatment are associated with both regression of LVH and improvements in cardiovascular outcomes in hypertensive heart disease, prevention of maladaptive LVH is arguably the most effective approach to reducing cardiovascular complications in chronic HTN. Especially in high-risk groups with a propensity for developing LVH—such as African Americans and to a lesser degree Hispanics[22,27,33]—early detection and aggressive treatment is key.[171] Once a diagnosis of LVH has been made, the cardiovascular prognosis is less favorable as compared with that of hypertensive persons without LVH (see also Fig. 25.7).[19] However, the temporal changes in LV mass while a patient is on antihypertensive medical therapy predict the incidence of cardiovascular events; therefore LVH itself is an important treatment target. Weight loss[172] (and bariatric surgery),[173] dietary salt restriction,[174,175] and treatment of obstructive sleep apnea with continuous positive airway pressure[176] are potential nonpharmacologic approaches for LVH regression and improvement in LV diastolic function, all of which are associated with only modest reductions of BP—the most important determinant of LVH regression. Although BP reduction is essential, there appear to be some differences independent of BP reduction between antihypertensive drug classes. Although some meta-analyses suggest that ACE inhibitors are more effective in reducing LV mass,[177,178] a more recent meta-analysis suggests the possible superiority of ARBs in reducing LV mass compared with other drug classes.[179] In another analysis[60] of 146 treatment arms of 80 double-blind, randomized controlled trials—after adjustment for treatment duration and change in BP—ARBs reduced LV mass on average by 13% (95% CI 8%–18%), calcium channel blockers by 11% (95% CI 9%–13%), ACE inhibitors by

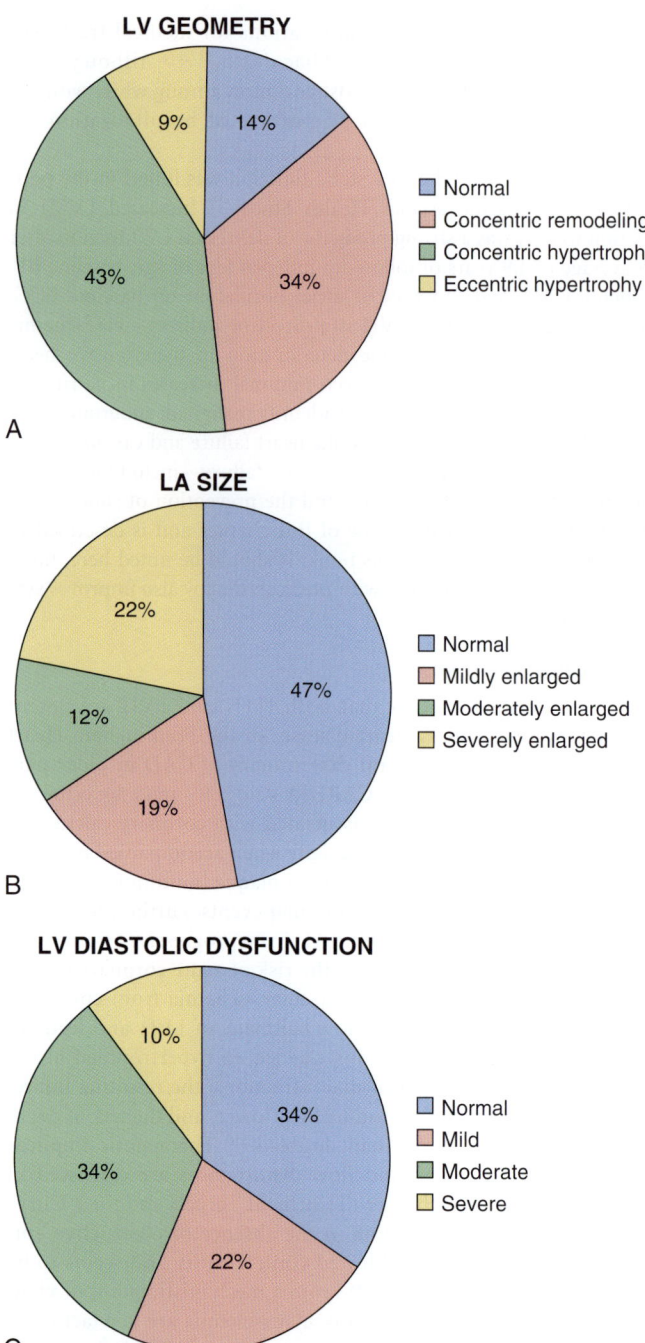

Fig. 25.7 Distribution of left ventricular (LV) geometry (A), left atrial (LA) size (B), and diastolic function (C) in patients with heart failure with preserved ejection fraction (HEFpEF) in the Treatment of Preserved Cardiac Function Heart Failure With an Aldosterone Antagonist trial. Panel A indicates that almost half of the HEFpEF patients did not meet the criteria for left ventricular hypertrophy, and panel C indicates that over one-third of HEFpEF patients had normal diastolic function by Doppler-echocardiography. (From Shah AM, Shah SJ, Anand IS, et al. Cardiac structure and function in heart failure with preserved ejection fraction: baseline findings from the echocardiographic study of the Treatment of Preserved Cardiac Function Heart Failure with an Aldosterone Antagonist trial. *Circ Heart Fail.* 2014;7:104–115.)

10% (95% CI 8%–12%), diuretics by 8% (95% CI 5%–10%), and beta blockers by 6% (95% CI 3%-8%). When drug classes were statistically compared regarding their effect on the reduction of LV mass, ARBs,

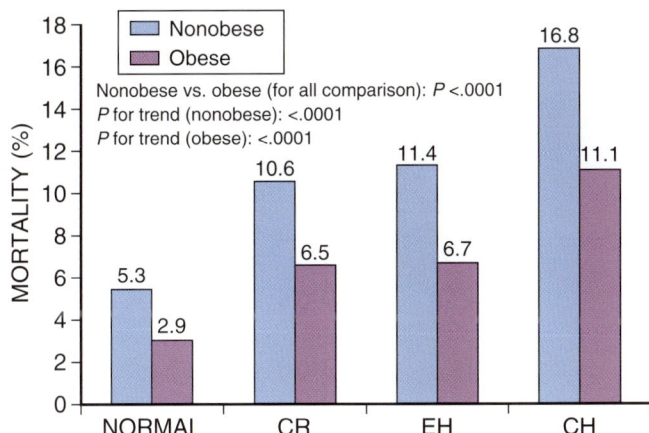

Fig. 25.8 Left ventricular geometry and risk of death among obese and nonobese women—another obesity paradox. Eccentric and especially concentric left ventricular hypertrophy is associated with increased mortality risk in both obese and nonobese women. However, the gradient is much steeper in nonobese women. *CH*, Concentric hypertrophy; *CR*, concentric remodeling; *EH*, eccentric hypertrophy. (From Patel DA, Lavie CJ, Artham SM, et al. Effects of left ventricular geometry and obesity on mortality in women with normal ejection fraction. *Am J Cardiol.* 2014;113[5]:877–880.)

ACE inhibitors, and calcium channel blockers were found to be more effective than beta blockers. In other studies, the direct renin inhibitor aliskirin[115] has been shown to reduce LV mass, whereas vasodilators (such as hydralazine and minoxidil), alpha blockers, and central sympatholytics (such as clonidine) may have no effect on LV mass.[180] A possible explanation for the lack of LV mass reduction with vasodilators may be reflex sympathetic activation[181]; in the case of central sympatholytics, their short half-life and rebound HTN may be explanatory.[182] However, the mechanisms leading to differential effects of the aforementioned drug classes are not well established. What has been established is that regression of LVH on treatment reduces cardiovascular events, including sudden death, myocardial infarction (MI), congestive heart failure, and stroke.[9,183-187] More recent data from the Systolic Blood Pressure Intervention (SPRINT) trial demonstrate that more intensive BP lowering reduced new ECG-diagnosed LVH and led to more LVH regression.[188] However, despite the normalization of BP, LVH does not always regress, suggesting that some of the changes in the development of LVH are irreversible and that LV pressure overload is not the only hypertrophic stimulus in some patients. Whether or not LVH regresses has important prognostic implications, especially for incident stroke. Patients who never had LVH and those whose LVH regressed while on treatment appear to have a similar risk for stroke, whereas patients whose LVH did not regress or those who developed LVH on treatment were at much higher risk for a cerebrovascular event (**Fig. 25.9**).[187] It should be briefly noted here that catheter-based renal denervation, which may or may not reliably lower BP,[189,190] has also been reported to reduce LV mass.[191] In addition, the reduction of renal dysfunction—such as microalbuminuria—may go hand in hand with LVH regression.[192]

Treatment Targets and the J-Curve Debate

As discussed in the previous section, it has been well established that the lowering of BP with medications in patient with HTN prevents future complications from hypertensive heart disease. What is less clear is the BP threshold for the initiation of antihypertensive therapy or the treatment target for lowering BP, which provides the most benefit in the prevention of cardiovascular events. A BP of 140/90 mm Hg is

a reasonable threshold/target recommended for most patients in HTN guidelines,[193,194] although some guidelines recommend more lenient thresholds in elderly patients[195] or more stringent thresholds in high-risk patients, such as African Americans.[171] Following the largest HTN trial thus far, the SPRINT,[196] which showed a clear benefit of targeting a BP goal lower than previously recommended, led to a complete overhaul of prior HTN guidelines, with lower treatment targets and a risk-based tailoring of optimal treatment goals.[197] These latest guidelines have been both praised as a long overdue step to more aggressive HTN treatment but they have also been criticized as too aggressive, with the argument that lower treatment targets should translate in a decrease of the disease burden of hypertensive heart disease. However, there has been a long-standing debate about the actual harm of HTN overtreatment, specifically with regard to lowering diastolic BP too much. The first observational data suggesting an increase in MI in patients whose diastolic BP was reduced to less than 90 mm Hg were reported by Stewart[198] and later Cruickshank and colleagues.[199,200] This phenomenon was termed the "J-curve," which describes the decrease in cardiovascular events with lowering of elevated BP down to a threshold point of BP below which mortality increases progressively. Polese and colleagues[201] demonstrated that the lowering of diastolic BP to less than 90 mm Hg with intravenous nitroprusside causes a progressive fall in coronary sinus blood flow in hypertensive patients with LVH, whereas the reduction of diastolic BP to less than 70 mm Hg had no effect on coronary sinus flow in hypertensive patients without LVH. This finding suggests that the (rapid) lowering of BP in patients with hypertensive heart disease may be deleterious, especially in those with LVH (**Fig. 25.10**). Whether, however, the same principle applies to the chronic treatment of HTN is unknown. One explanation for this finding is that an abnormal myocardial microvasculature, which does not keep up with the LV hypertrophic response to pressure overload and neurohumoral stimulation, loses the ability to maintain coronary blood flow with acute drops in BP.

Clinical evidence in favor of the J-curve comes from post hoc analyses of randomized clinical trials. In the INVEST (International Verapamil SR/T Trandolapril) trial of hypertensive patients with established CAD, the incidence of cardiovascular death decreased progressively in patients whose diastolic BP was lowered from 120 to 80 to 89 mm Hg and then increased progressively in those with achieved diastolic BP below 80 mm Hg (see also Fig. 25.10).[202] The J-curve was less pronounced in patients who had undergone coronary revascularization and much more pronounced for diastolic than systolic BP and for MI rather than stroke, consistent with the notion that the coronaries are perfused only in diastole, so that diastolic BP constitutes coronary perfusion pressure. In the PRoFESS (Prevention Regimen for Effectively Voiding Second Strokes) trial of secondary stroke prevention with telmisartan (vs. placebo), the risk of a second stroke (or cardiovascular events) gradually declined when systolic BP was reduced from a baseline of >150 mm Hg to either 130 to 139 mm Hg or 120 to 129 mm Hg but increased again when it was reduced below 120 mm Hg.[203]

Although this observational evidence on the existence of a J-curve phenomenon is concerning and should be considered in the treatment of hypertensive heart disease, several counterarguments have been proposed that weaken the clinical significance of this debate, as recently reviewed by Verdecchia and colleagues:[204] (1) Post hoc observational analysis loses the intended balance of baseline characteristics in the original randomized design such that patients with the lowest achieved BP sometimes were the sickest to begin with, leading to *reverse causality* (i.e., patients with the most advanced illness—whether severe heart failure or cancer and thus the highest mortality rates—had lower BP rather than aggressive antihypertensive therapy

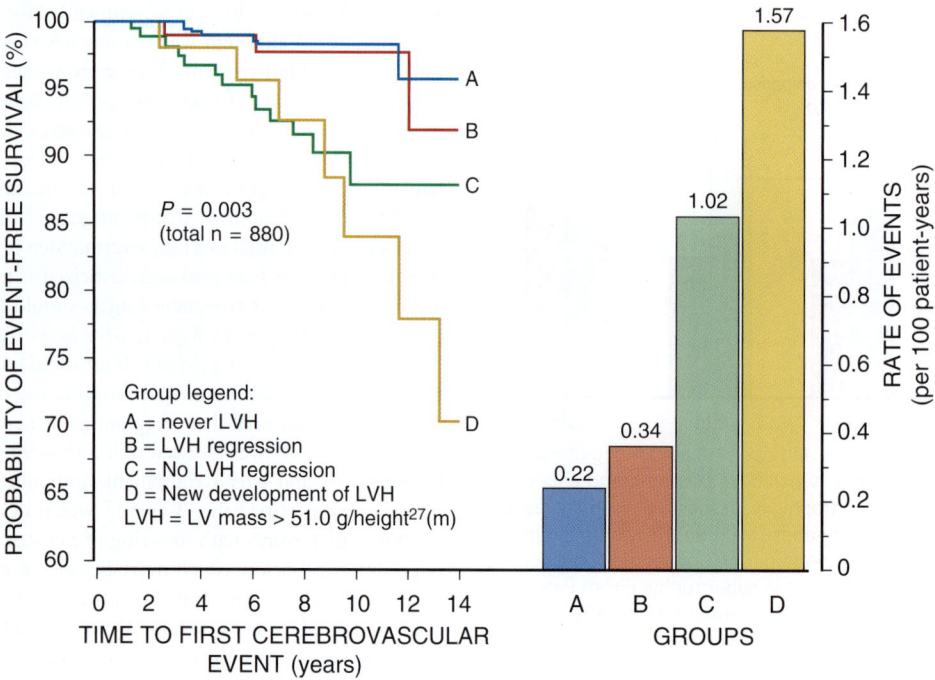

Fig. 25.9 Dynamic Changes of Left Ventricular Mass and Risk of Stroke. Patients who never had left ventricular hypertrophy *(LVH)* and patients who have on-treatment regression of LVH had a similar risk of stroke during up to 14 years of follow-up, whereas those whose LVH did not regress or those who developed LVH while on treatment had the highest risk of stroke. (From Verdecchia P, Angeli F, Gattobigio R, et al. Regression of left ventricular hypertrophy and prevention of stroke in hypertensive subjects. *Am J Hypertens.* 2006;19:493–499.)

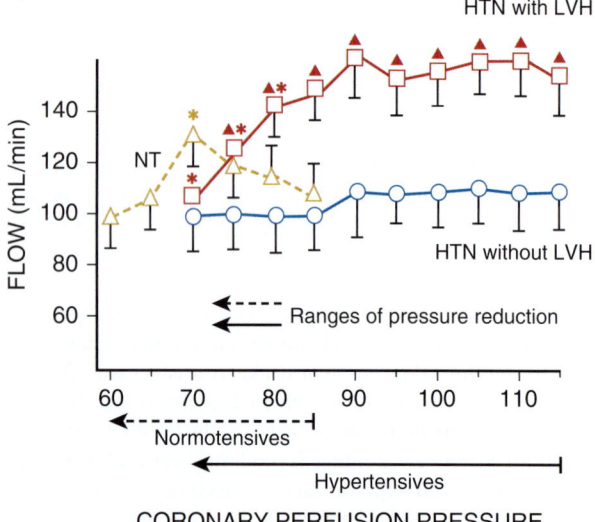

Fig. 25.10 Coronary Blood Flow During Acute Blood Pressure Reduction. In normotensive patients and hypertensive patients without left ventricular hypertrophy *(LVH)*, coronary blood flow is maintained despite acute blood pressure reduction with nitroprusside. In contrast, in hypertensive patients with LVH, coronary blood flow decreases significantly below a coronary perfusion pressure of 90 mm Hg. *HTN,* Patients with hypertension; *NT,* patients with normotension. (Adapted from Polese N, De Cesare N, Montorsi P, et al. Upward shift of the lower range of coronary flow autoregulation in hypertensive patients with hypertrophy of the left ventricle. *Circulation.* 1991;83:845–853.)

causing cardiovascular death from diastolic ischemia). The fact that in some papers the J-shaped association of lower BP was eliminated or at least reduced by multivariate analyses supports this hypothesis.

(2) Most observational data on the J-curve suffer from low sample size in the low BP range and thus have wide confidence margins.[202] In clinical practice, too low a BP is rarely a problem but uncontrolled high BP often is. (3) Diastolic J-curves have been seen in post hoc analyses even in the placebo arms of randomized trials because low diastolic BP is characteristic of elderly patients with isolated systolic HTN, which carries a high risk of cardiovascular events. (4) A post hoc analysis of the diastolic subgroup of INVEST did not show a J-curve in cardiovascular events but did show a systolic J-curve for all-cause mortality, which argues against treatment-induced ischemia.[205] (5) Another post hoc analysis of the diabetic subgroup of Ongoing Telmisartan Alone and in Combination with Ramipril Trial (ONTARGET) showed a progressive reduction in stroke risk down to an achieved systolic BP of 110 mm Hg with no evidence of a J-curve, and there was no J-curve for MI and cardiovascular events from lowering systolic BP below 130 mm Hg but also no benefit.[206] (6) Similarly, in the prospective Valsartan Antihypertensive Long-term Use Evaluation (VALUE) trial, patients were randomized to valsartan or amlodipine regimens and followed for 4.2 years (mean) with no difference in the primary cardiovascular end point. There was no increased risk of MI in patients whose diastolic BP fell below 70 mm Hg. However, this study did observe a stroke but no MI benefit in patients with lower achieved BP.[207] (7) In the Action to Control Cardiovascular Risk in Diabetes (ACCORD) trial,[208] diabetic patients randomized to more intense BP control (achieved systolic BP 119 mm Hg) compared with less intense BP control (achieved systolic BP 133 mm Hg) had no benefit, but also no harm (i.e., absence of a J-curve) regarding cardiovascular events but more hypotensive events and acute renal insufficiency. (8) In the large ONTARGET trial of patients who had very high cardiovascular risk but were not all hypertensive, the lowering of BP reduced (numerically, but not statistically) the incidence of MI with treatment (ramipril, telmisartan, or both) down to a threshold of 116/68.[209] (9) In the aforementioned SPRINT trial,

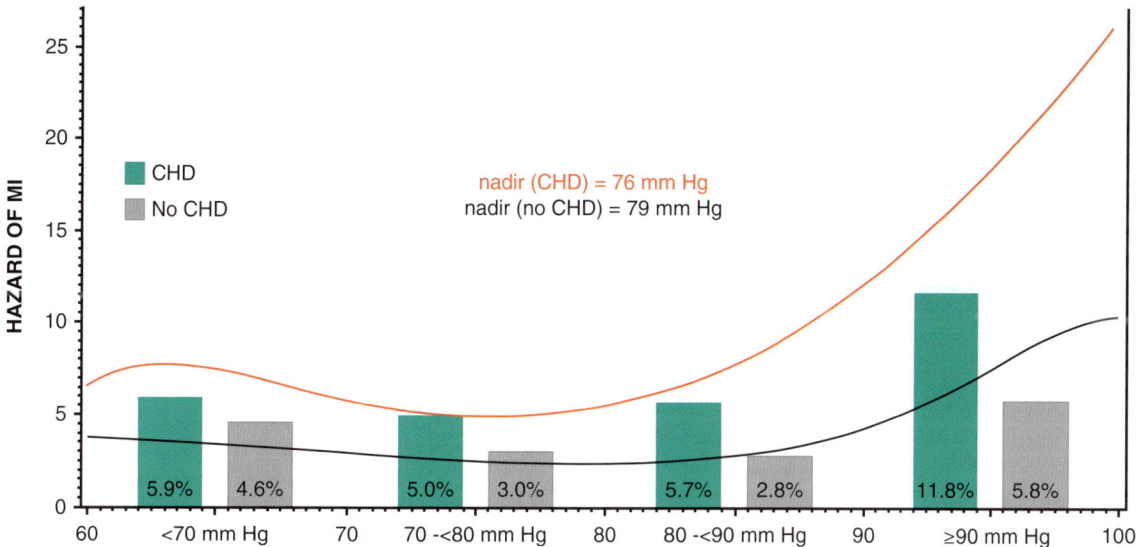

Fig. 25.11 Observational Evidence for Absence of a J-Curve in the Treatment of Hypertension. These data indicate that lowering of diastolic blood pressure decreases the risk for death down to a nadir of 76 mm Hg in patients with coronary heart disease, below which mortality remained nearly constant. *CHD,* Coronary heart disease; *MI,* myocardial infarction. (Adapted from Kjeldsen SE, Berge E, Bangalore S, et al. No evidence for a J-shaped curve in treated hypertensive patients with increased cardiovascular risk: The VALUE trial. *Blood Press.* 2016;25[2]:83–92.)

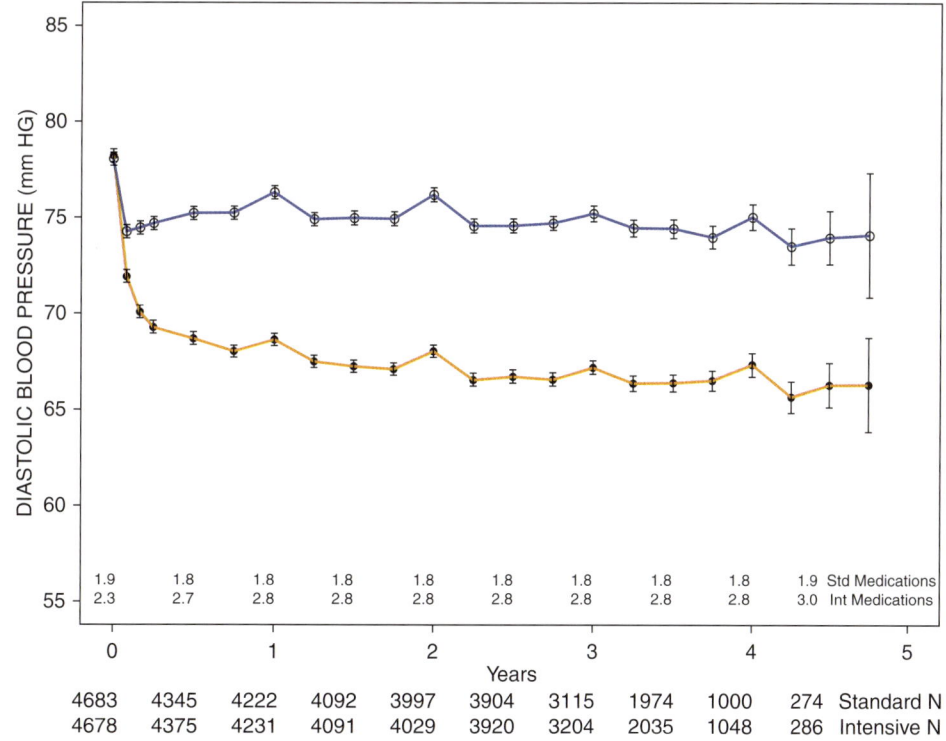

Fig. 25.12 Achieved Diastolic Blood Pressure in the Systolic Blood Pressure Intervention Trial (SPRINT). Mean diastolic blood pressure *(BP)* values (plus standard error bars) in the intensive treatment arm are shown in *yellow,* those in the standard treatment arm in *blue.* (Adapted from SPRINT Research Group. A Randomized Trial of Intensive versus Standard Blood-Pressure Control. *N Engl J Med.* 2015;373:2103–2116.)

the mean diastolic BP was 69 mm Hg in the intensive treatment arm versus 76 mm Hg in the comparison arm. This achieved lower diastolic BP was associated with better overall cardiovascular outcomes, a similar incidence of acute coronary syndromes, and a numerically (but not statistically) significant lower incidence of MI ($P = .19$) (**Figs. 25.11** and **25.12**).[196]

In Memoriam

Dr. Ronald Victor's scientific contributions to the treatment of high blood pressure, which is the subject of this chapter, are legion. He died from metastatic pancreatic cancer at the age of 66, leaving behind a rich legacy defined by a passion for addressing health disparities, particularly high blood pressure in the African-American community. His seminal contribution, which involved recruiting African-American barbers to take part in screening their clients for hypertension, showed that thousands of lives could be saved annually if barbers were enlisted to help fight the epidemic of high blood pressure in the African-American community. He was also responsible for pioneering stem cell research in the treatment of young men and boys with Duchenne muscular dystrophy. He will be remembered by friends and colleagues as a humble, kind, and caring individual. Ron will be sorely missed, and the editors dedicate this chapter in his memory.

KEY REFERENCES

6. Liu L, An Y, Chen M, et al. Trends in the prevalence of hospitalization attributable to hypertensive diseases among United States adults aged 35 and older from 1980 to 2007. *Am J Cardiol.* 2013;112:694–699.
11. Drazner MH. The progression of hypertensive heart disease. *Circulation.* 2011;123:327–334.
16. Levy D, Garrison RJ, Savage DD, Kannel WB, Castelli WP. Prognostic implications of echocardiographically determined left ventricular mass in the Framingham Heart Study. *N Engl J Med.* 1990;322:1561–1566.
20. Pierdomenico SD, Cuccurullo F. Risk reduction after regression of echocardiographic left ventricular hypertrophy in hypertension: a meta-analysis. *Am J Hypertens.* 2010;23:876–881.
38. Ganau A, Devereux RB, Roman MJ, et al. Patterns of left ventricular hypertrophy and geometric remodeling in essential hypertension. *J Am Coll Cardiol.* 1992;19:1550–1558.
40. Heckbert SR, Post W, Pearson GD, et al. Traditional cardiovascular risk factors in relation to left ventricular mass, volume, and systolic function by cardiac magnetic resonance imaging: the Multiethnic Study of Atherosclerosis. *J Am Coll Cardiol.* 2006;48:2285–2292.
50. Peterson GE, de Backer T, Gabriel A, et al. Prevalence and correlates of left ventricular hypertrophy in the African American Study of Kidney Disease Cohort Study. *Hypertension.* 2007;50:1033–1039.
51. Hill JA, Olson EN. Cardiac plasticity. *N Engl J Med.* 2008;358:1370–1380.
87. Gaasch WH, Zile MR. Left ventricular structural remodeling in health and disease: with special emphasis on volume, mass, and geometry. *J Am Coll Cardiol.* 2011;58:1733–1740.
179. Fagard RH, Celis H, Thijs L, Wouters S. Regression of left ventricular mass by antihypertensive treatment: a meta-analysis of randomized comparative studies. *Hypertension.* 2009;54:1084–1091.

The full reference list for this chapter is available on ExpertConsult.

Heart Failure as a Consequence of Valvular Heart Disease

Dominik M. Wiktor, John D. Carroll

OUTLINE

Valvular heart disease (VHD) is not simply a disease of the valve.[1,2] Cardiac valves are the major determinants of the direction of blood flow in the circulation that consists of a system of vessels that distribute and collect blood, and cardiac chambers that create the propelling force for blood movement. VHD causes a disruption of the entire circulatory system. In addition, there is a complex interplay between VHD and comorbid diseases, along with systemic changes seen with aging.

VHD therapy has recently experienced a transformation by changes in its principal etiology in many countries, the medical complexities of many of the patients with VHD, and the introduction of the disruptive technologies of transcatheter treatments. Management of VHD had few major changes for several decades, other than refinements in the techniques for surgical correction of various valve lesions and the replacement of invasive characterization of valve lesions by echocardiography. In the 2006 Guidelines for Management of VHD, there was only one class 1a indication for VHD therapies; mitral balloon commissurotomy for rheumatic mitral stenosis (MS) had positive evidence from multiple randomized trials comparing this first transcatheter VHD treatment to various surgical techniques.[3]

In the past, new knowledge in VHD was primarily driven by single-center studies. Currently a robust multicenter and multinational clinical trial network has been activated in VHD.[4] A learning health care system has also been created with the gathering of comprehensive patient-level data including long-term outcomes and patient-reported health status for all patients in the United States undergoing transcatheter valve therapies

(TVTs) in the Society of Thoracic Surgeons (STS) and American College of Cardiology TVT Registry.[5] The national coverage decision for TVTs by Centers for Medicare and Medicaid Services (CMS) requires entry of patient data into an approved national registry as a condition of coverge.[6]

Finally, the process of evaluation and treatment of VHD patients using the heart team approach has also followed the lead of the multidisciplinary teams used in advanced heart failure for decision-making for transplantation and mechanical support.[7] Shared decision-making and decision-aids have also emerged in VHD.[8,9]

VALVULAR HEART DISEASE AS A TREATABLE CAUSE OF HEART FAILURE

VHD can be definitively treated, in terms of the valve abnormality, with surgery or transcatheter valve repair and replacement, but this often does not occur until patients become symptomatic, as recommended in major guidelines.[10,11] As a result of this interventional timing late in the natural history of VHD, many patients have persistent issues requiring ongoing management, as will be described.

ETIOLOGIES, EPIDEMIOLOGY, AND DEMOGRAPHICS OF VALVULAR HEART DISEASE

Age-associated VHD has replaced rheumatic heart disease (RHD) as the dominant etiology of VHD in countries with medium to high personal income levels. Aortic valve sclerosis is an age-associated valve abnormality in which the valve cusps are thickened or calcified but not hemodynamically impactful.[12] In a study with a mean patient age of 81 years, the prevalence of aortic valve sclerosis had reached 42%.[13] Degenerative changes in the aortic and mitral valve resulting in a moderate to severe hemodynamic impact emerge in 14% of the population by the age of 75.[14] Hemodynamically significant mitral regurgitation has a prevalence of 9.3% in the United States for individuals older than the age of 75 years. Functional mitral regurgitation, typically in the setting of left ventricular dysfunction, is the dominant form.[15,16] VHD in the elderly may be complicated by cardiac amyloidosis, recently reported to occur in 14% of patients with severe aortic stenosis, with a mean age of 86 years.[17]

These facts on VHD associated with aging need to be coupled with the profound demographic change of rapid population aging in the United States and other countries predominantly as a result of increases in life expectancy.[18-20] As a consequence, and on a very practical level, the number of patients potentially needing a valve intervention, such as aortic valve replacement for severe aortic stenosis, is expected to see a major surge in the next decade.[21] Therefore heart failure as a consequence of VHD is demographically programed to increase.

RHD has not disappeared; its global impact remains enormous. RHD was present in 2010 in an estimated 34 million people worldwide and is disproportionately felt in many countries with limited health care budgets and in individuals with low personal income levels.[22] Acute rheumatic fever in the United States has disappeared, and chronic rheumatic VHD, such as MS, in the United States is predominantly found in recent immigrants from countries with a persistent pool of individuals who had rheumatic fever in childhood.[23] Bicuspid aortic valve, the most common congenital heart defect, continues to occur in approximately 0.9% to 1.36% of live births throughout the world and often leads to clinical manifestations from valve malfunction in all age groups.[24-26] Nearly all patients with bicuspid aortic valves will require valve intervention during their lifetimes. A congenital etiology is the leading cause for pulmonic valve abnormalities and has received much attention in the adult congenital heart disease community with the development and widespread use of transcatheter pulmonary valve replacement.[27]

PATHOPHYSIOLOGY OF VALVULAR HEART DISEASE

This section will review broad pathophysiologic concepts and findings applicable to most forms of VHD.

Mechanisms Involved in Producing Stenotic and Regurgitant Heart Valves

In primary VHD the pathologic process from which a valve becomes stenotic or regurgitant is multifactorial and differs with the specific causes, including congenital, rheumatic, infectious, and degenerative. As shown in **Fig. 26.1**, leaflet calcification is pronounced in aortic stenosis and follows a process of inflammation and fibrosis.[2] The pathology also includes lipid deposition and an inflammatory process leading to bulky leaflets not capable of opening fully and increasingly require a higher ventricular pressure to open. The renin-angiotensin-aldosterone system (RAAS) is activated in this process (**see also Chapter 5**) and contributes to pathologic alterations of the leaflet structure and function. Myxomatous degeneration occurs in mitral valve prolapse leading to leaflet redundancy and malcoaptation which produces valve insufficiency. New insights into disease progression, genetics, and molecular alterations have occurred to enhance our understanding of its pathophysiology.[28]

Primary VHD typically is a progressive disease process of the valve, with the hemodynamic burden of pressure or volume overload increasing over time. This process may be gradual, as with aortic stenosis, for which the rate of progression has been studied.[29] It may also

be rapid as in some patients with degenerative mitral regurgitation, in which chordal rupture can cause a sudden increase in the degree of mitral regurgitation.

Genetics Aspects of Valvular Heart Disease

There are four congenital abnormalities of cardiac valves that have a defined genetic basis and are currently being investigated for candidate mutations.[30] Bicuspid aortic valve, myxomatous mitral valve regurgitation, pulmonic valve stenosis, and Ebstein anomaly of the tricuspid valve are the focus of linking these congenital valvulopathies to human genetics. Some evidence has emerged linking adult-onset VHD to genetic influences on the process of valvular calcification and production of aortic stenosis.[31]

Quantification of Valve Lesion Severity

The quantification of valvular stenosis and regurgitation is now routinely performed noninvasively, with echocardiography playing the major role because of availability, accuracy, information about mechanism, assessment of changes in chamber size and function, semiquantitative metrics of pulmonary hypertension, and well-defined metrics of lesions severity (**see also Chapter 32**). Noninvasive evaluation of native valve regurgitation now has guidelines and standards for both echocardiography and cardiovascular magnetic resonance (CMR).[32] Currently there is a trend to use CMR to assess not only the severity of mitral regurgitation but understand pathophysiology in terms of chamber sizes and interstitial fibrosis.[33]

Quantification of the degree valve stenosis is also a first step in characterizing these forms of VHD and understanding subsequent remodeling of anatomy and function of affected structures and is a major component of determining the timing of interventions.[34] Problematic areas in stenosis quantification often involve low flow states that require means of augmenting flow, such as with exercise and intravenous agents that are either positive inotropic or vasodilating agents to determine if Doppler gradients reach thresholds of lesion severity. There has also been renewed interest in better understanding the severity of aortic stenosis by studying individual patient's pressure versus flow curves while undergoing dobutamine infusion.[35] The heterogeneity of the responses indicated that the fixed orifice model initially proposed by Gorlin often breaks down.

Impact on Chamber Size, Function, and Myocardial Hypertrophy

The traditional approach to pathophysiology of VHD focused on the hemodynamic principles of pressure and volume overload produced by stenotic and regurgitant valve lesions. These abnormalities of valve function do lead to changes in chamber size, myocardial hypertrophy, and modifications of systolic and diastolic function. Most recently there has been a renewed interest in understanding changes in left ventricular pressure–volume relationships after the reduction of mitral regurgitation using the most widely used transcatheter reparative technique, MitraClip, that reduces the regurgitant orifice by holding together the edge of the posterior and anterior mitral leaflets where the regurgitation originates.[36] These acute changes in left ventricular preload, unchanged contractility, and reduced regurgitant volume are free of the confounding impact of cardiopulmonary bypass used in surgical mitral interventions.

Myocardial hypertrophy, whether eccentric or concentric, remains as a central feature in the pathophysiology of VHD because it represents a response to the increased work load imposed by stenotic and regurgitant valves. The degree of hypertrophy can be assessed with echocardiography and CMR. The relationship of the degree of hypertrophy to valve lesion severity is variable, and other factors modifying the hypertrophic response include age, gender, obesity, polymorphisms of the

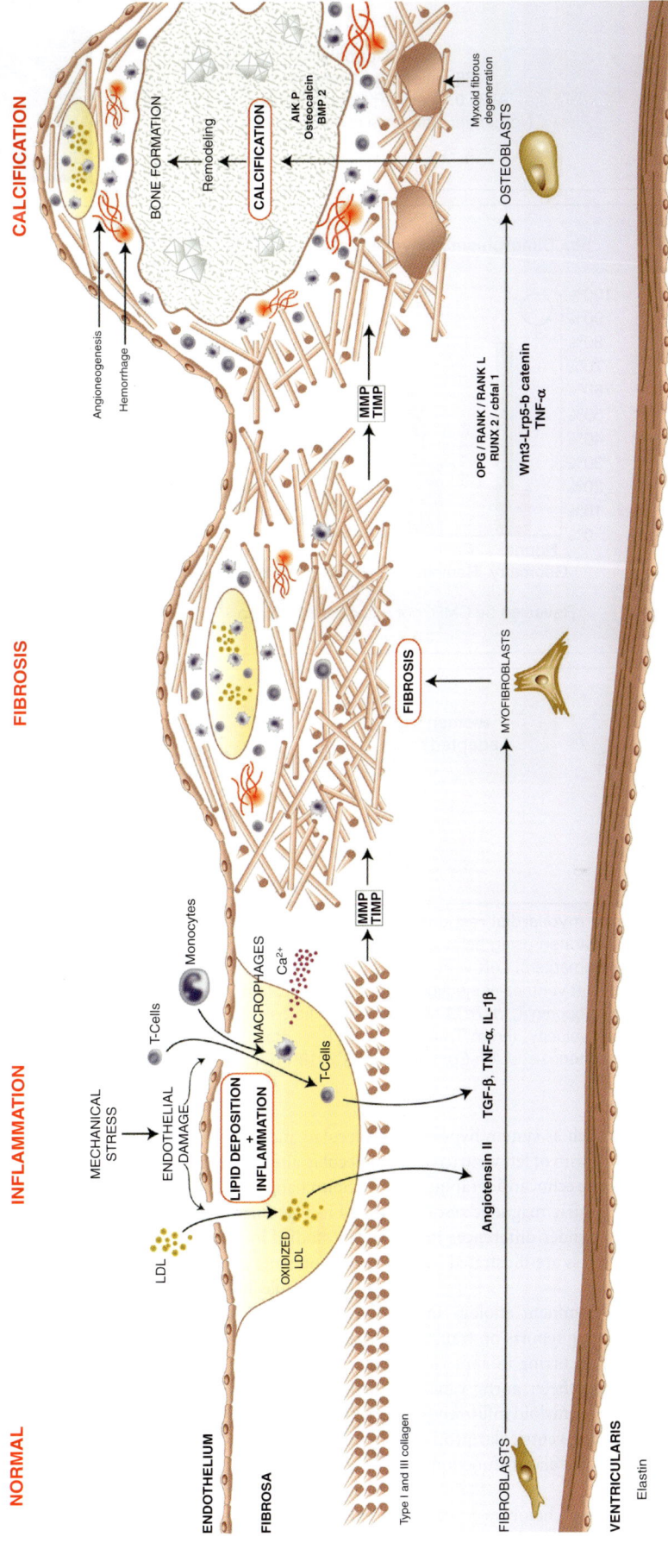

Fig. 26.1 Summary of the pathologic processes occurring within the valve during aortic stenosis. The pathophysiology of degenerative aortic stenosis is outlined in this figure highlighting the cascade of events starting with mechanical stress, endothelial damage, infiltration of lipid, inflammatory cells, followed collagen, microcalcification, and then extensive calcification. The underlying molecular and humoral mechanisms are also detailed. *IL-1β*, interleukin-1β; *LDL*, low-density lipoprotein; *MMP*, matrix metallaoproteinase; *TGF*, transforming growth factor, *TIMP*, tissue inhibitor of metalloproteinase; *TNF*, tumor necrosis factor. (From Dweck MR, Boon NA, Newby DE. Calcific aortic stenosis: a disease of the valve and the myocardium. *J Am Coll Cardiol.* 2012;60(19):1854–1863.)

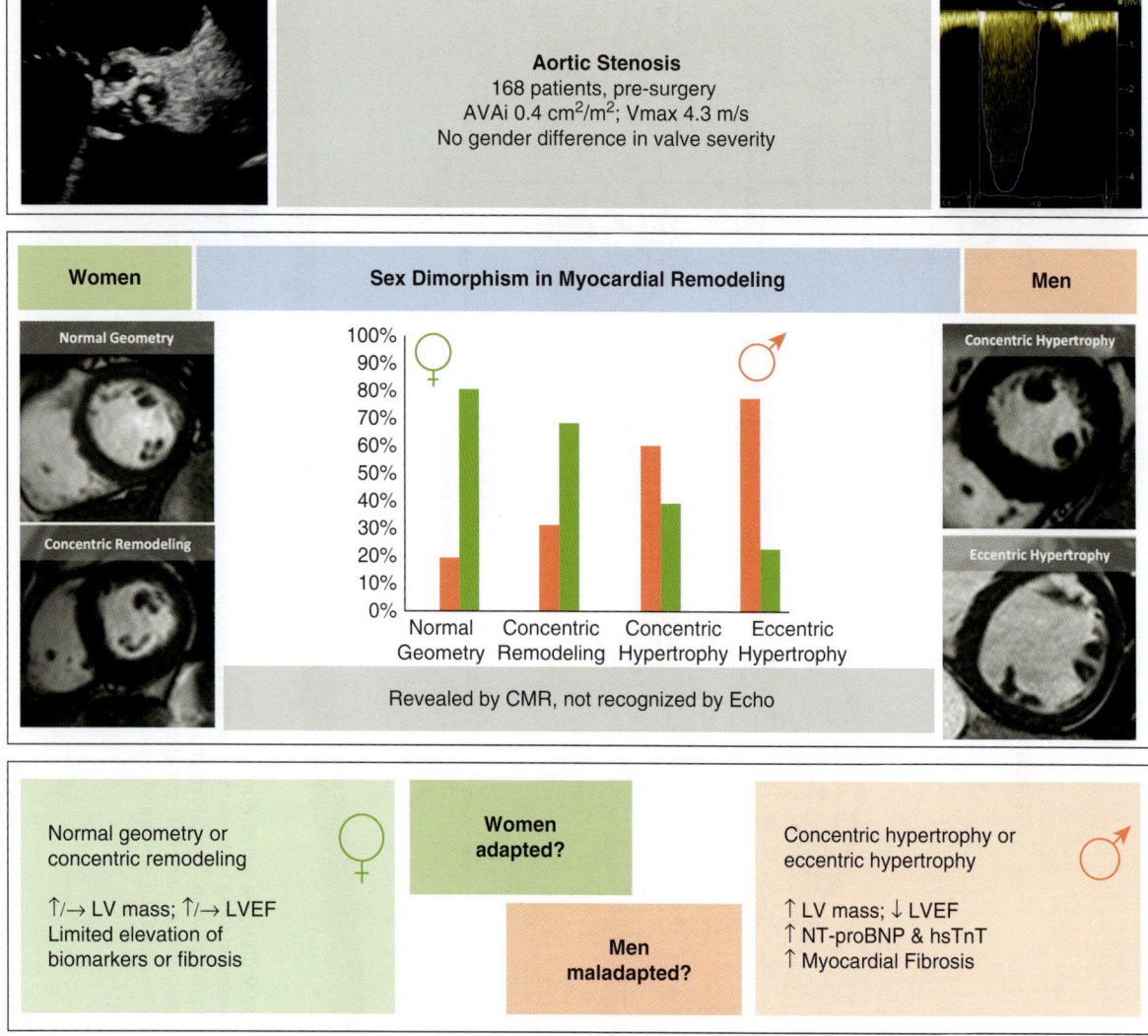

Fig. 26.2 Sex dimorphism in myocardial response to aortic stenosis. Sex differences play a role in disease phenotyping and are illustrated using echocardiography (echo) but more importantly by cardiac magnetic resonance *(CMR)* and biomarkers. Left ventricular *(LV)* remodeling pattern was more adverse in men with more LV dysfunction (by left ventricular ejection fraction *[LVEF]*, N-terminal pro–brain natriuretic peptide *[NT-proBNP]*, high-sensitivity troponin T *[hsTnT]*) and myocardial fibrosis (focal and diffuse). AVAi, Indexed aortic valve area; *Vmax*, peak velocity. (From Treibel T, Kozor R, Fontana M, et al. Sex dimorphism in the myocardial response to aortic stenosis. *J Am Coll Cardiol Img.* 2018;11[7]:962–973).

ACE 1/D gene, and other hemodynamic loads such as system hypertension.[2,37] In aortic stenosis there is a sex dimorphism of left ventricular adaption to aortic stenosis, first described using echocardiographic techniques and recently studied in depth with cardiac magnetic resonance imaging (MRI), shown in **Fig. 26.2**.[37,38] Gender differences in left ventricular fractional shortening and wall stress are illustrated in **Fig. 26.3**.

Since VHD in the elderly has become the dominant etiology in many countries, it is not surprising to see emerging reports on transthyretin cardiac amyloid (**see also Chapter 22**) occurring in approximately one in seven patients undergoing transcatheter aortic valve replacement (TAVR) for severe aortic stenosis.[39,70] Amyloid infiltrative cardiomyopathy will alter diastolic and systolic left ventricular properties but, in contrast to those alterations due to valvular dysfunction, will not regress after relief of stenosis.[17]

Chronic pressure and volume overload of cardiac chambers as seen in VHD also has quantifiable effects on the underlying myocardial molecular and cellular structure and function. These fundamental molecular alterations translate over time to directly observable macroscopic changes in cardiac chamber structure and function. As illustrated in **Fig. 26.4**, these transitions have become most apparent and widely studied in aortic stenosis, where it has been demonstrated that chronic pressure overload of the left ventricle leads to both reversible and irreversible alterations in myocardial structure and function.[40-42] These changes include increases in myocardial cellular hypertrophy, increases in extracellular matrix volume, and both diffuse and focal interstitial fibrosis. Later changes include declines in ventricular myocardial function, including reduction in left ventricular ejection fraction (LVEF) along with ventricular dilation. Myocardial cellular hypertrophy and diffuse fibrosis and increased extracellular matrix volume regress after aortic valve replacement, whereas left atrial enlargement and areas of focal fibrosis appear to be unimpacted.[43,44]

This chapter identifies heart failure as a consequence of VHD, but it is also true that primary myocardial disease and coronary artery

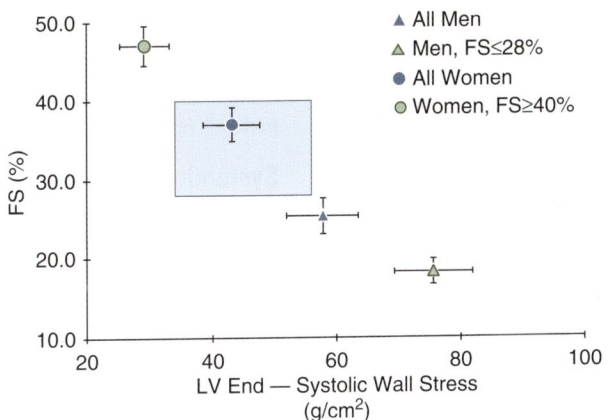

Fig. 26.3 Gender differences in fractional shortening *(FS)* and meridional end-systolic wall stress in aortic stenosis. The gray zone denotes the normal range of this stress-shortening relation. Women with aortic stenosis fall within this normal zone, but men, on average, have reduced FS with elevated stress. Very elevated wall stress was present in the large group of men with subnormal ejection performance. Reduced wall stress was present in those women with supernormal ejection performance. *LV,* Left ventricular. (Reprinted with permission. From Carroll JD, Carroll EP, Feldman T, et al. Sex associated differences in left ventricular function in aortic stenosis of the elderly. *Circulation.* 1992;86[4]:1099–1107. ©1992 American Heart Association, Inc.)

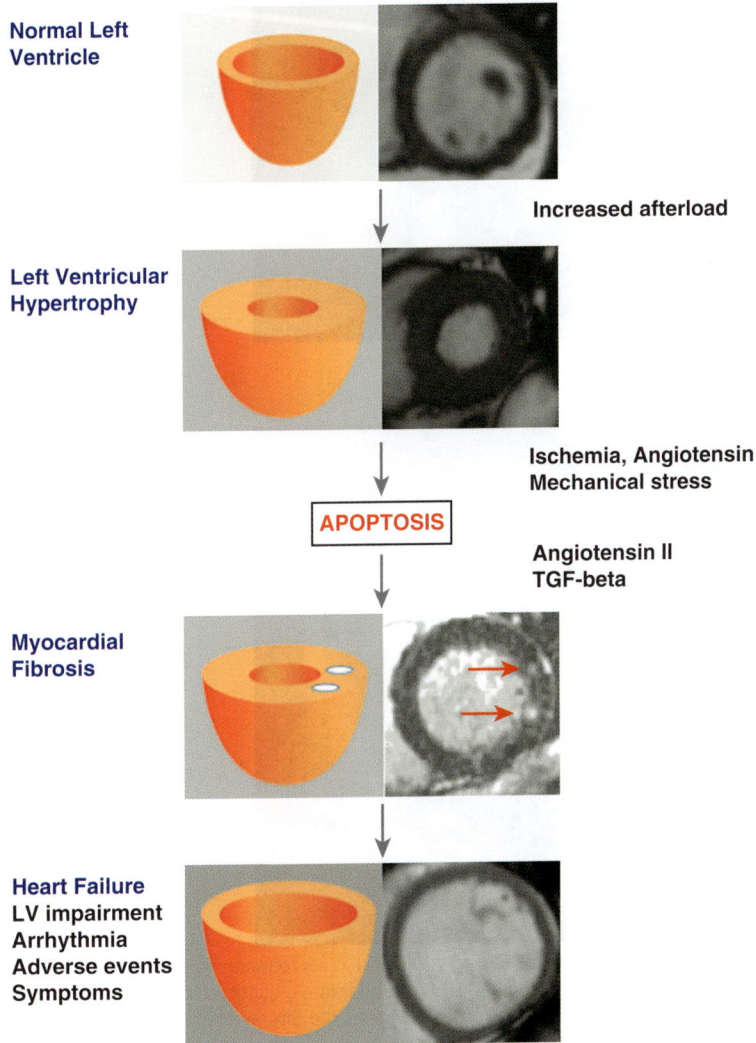

Fig. 26.4 Development and subsequent decompensation of left ventricular *(LV)* hypertrophy in response to aortic stenosis pressure overload leads to left ventricular hypertrophy that often normalizes wall stress and ventricular performance. Subsequent progression leads to functional decompensation associated with myocyte apoptosis that is a response to ischemia and angiotensin. Fibrosis occurs due to profibrotic mediators such as angiotensin and transforming growth factor *(TGF)-β*. The magnetic imaging late gadolinium enhancement technique is useful in detecting and quantifying this progressive process. (*Red arrows* show regions of mid-wall fibrosis on short-axis views of the left ventricle). (From Dweck MR, Boon NA, Newby DE. Calcific aortic stenosis: a disease of the valve and the myocardium. *J Am Coll Cardiol.* 2012;60[19]:1854–1863.)

disease (CAD) with ventricular dysfunction can result in secondary or functional valvular regurgitation. Left ventricular dysfunction leading to alterations in valvular and subvalvular geometry leads to functional mitral regurgitation (**Fig. 26.5**).[15,45] In addition, tricuspid regurgitation is often functional in nature (i.e., with a normal tricuspid valve apparatus) and is caused by disorders producing right ventricular dysfunction whether isolated or in the context of pulmonary vascular disease.

The binary approach to mitral regurgitation as either being primarily a valve function issue versus valvular regurgitation secondary to ventricular dysfunction is convenient in organizing pathophysiology and has therapeutic implications. However, it also can be misleading as it becomes apparent that VHD needs to be understood from a pathophysiologic perspective of the complex interplay between the valve abnormality, the associated vascular properties that determine preload and afterload, and left ventricular structure and function. Changes in both the arterial system (i.e., increased resistance and decreased compliance)

and left ventricle (various forms of hypertrophy, increasing interstitial fibrosis, and myocyte dysfunction) may precede and impact on the patient's response to the development of a severe valve abnormality.[1]

Systemic and Pulmonary Arterial Systems in Valvular Heart Disease

The arterial properties of both the pulmonary and the systemic arterial system are underappreciated aspects of hemodynamic load in VHD. These arterial properties impact on the remodeling associated with VHD. The traditional metric of arterial properties has been the resistance component, but the compliance of larger arteries also produces a hemodynamic load, modifies pressure waveforms, and may mitigate the reverse remodeling after correction of the valve abnormality. The vascular resistance component is most commonly quantified as the pressure gradient across both the pulmonary and systemic vascular bed divided by the flow.

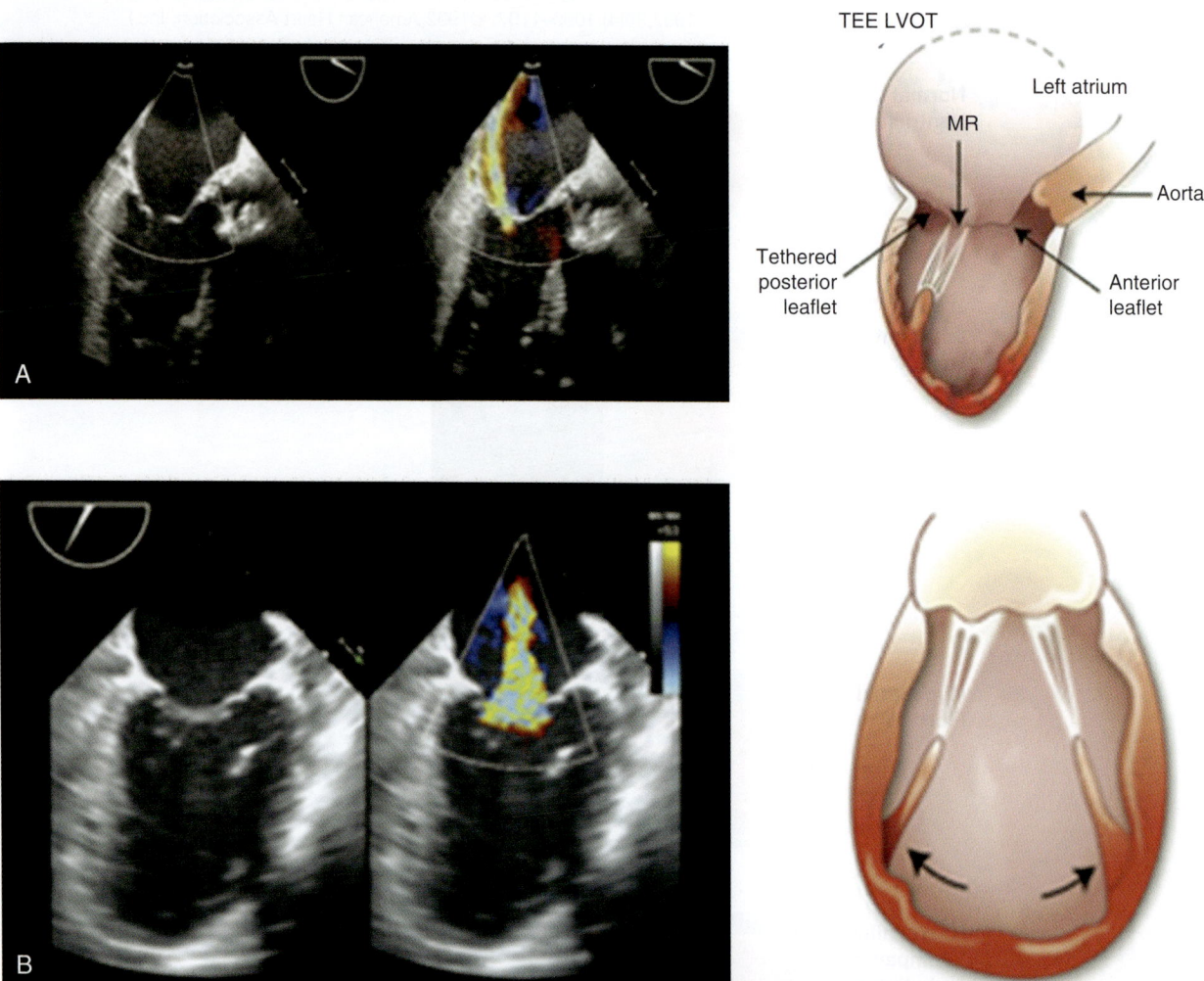

Fig. 26.5 Left Panel: Functional mitral regurgitation. (A) A representative echocardiogram and diagram of ischemic MR, with a posteriorly directed jet. (B) A representative echocardiogram and diagram of MR due to idiopathic dilated cardiomyopathy, with a central jet. Note the lateral displacement of the papillary muscles *(arrows)*. Apical displacement is also typically present, although less well demonstrated in these views. *LVOT,* Left ventricular outflow tract; *MR,* mitral regurgitation; *TEE,* transesophageal echocardiography. Right Panel *(Top):* Freedom from death or heart failure *(HF)* hospitalization in 1256 patients according to the degree of functional mitral regurgitation *(FMR).* *(Bottom)* Freedom from death according to the degree of FMR in patients with ischemic *(lower left)* and nonischemic *(lower right)* cardiomyopathy. (From Asgar AW, Mack MJ, Stone GW. Secondary mitral regurgitation in heart failure: pathophysiology, prognosis, and therapeutic considerations. *J Am Coll Cardiol.* 2015;65[12]:1231–1248.)

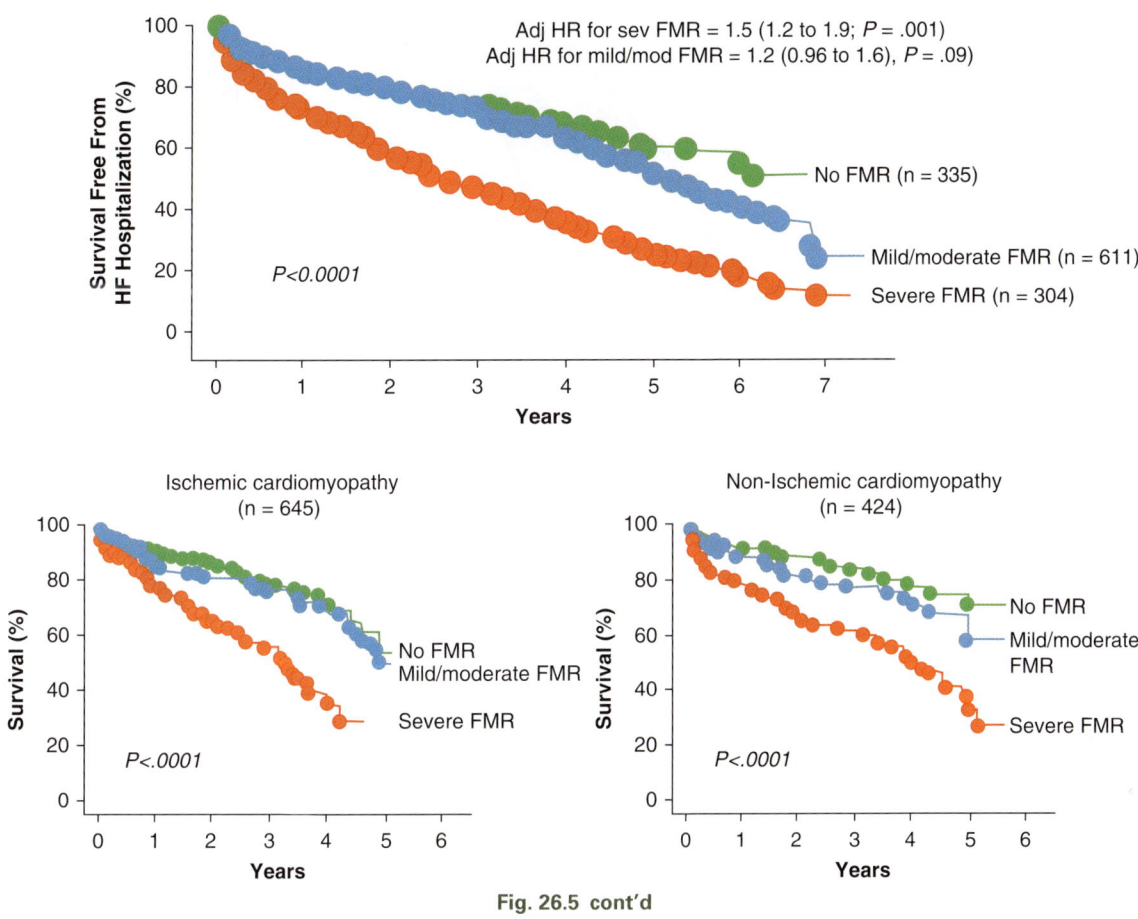

Fig. 26.5 cont'd

Quantification of large arterial hemodynamic properties requires novel methodologies.[46] These include measurement of pulse wave velocity and pulse pressure and various approaches to quantifying large artery compliance including aortic input impedance and arterial elastance.

A dominant influence on large arterial compliance in the systemic circulation is the impact of aging and the additive effects of common disease processes such as systemic hypertension and atherosclerosis. The changes in arterial stiffness due to aging modify the response to vasodilator therapy in heart failure.[47] These aging-related changes in arterial properties add to age-related myocardial changes to modify the manifestations of a variety of cardiovascular diseases, including VHD.[48] Systolic hypertension and widened pulse pressure are associated with aging and relate to increases in aortic stiffness. Large artery stiffness is due to increased collagen and decreased elastin produced by variations in activity of various elastases, including matrix metalloproteinases.[49] The major increase in aortic pulse wave velocity associated with aging can be observed in those with degenerative aortic stenosis. After aortic valve replacement that relieves obstruction at the valvular level, the left ventricle then faces an increase in arterial load as reflected by augmented forward and backward compression waves with frequent unmasking of systemic hypertension and a reduction in stroke volume in the majority of the elderly patients undergoing TAVR (**Fig. 26.6**).[50]

Pulmonary hypertension (**see also Chapter 43**) is a common pathophysiologic consequence of left-sided VHD (**Fig. 26.7**).[51] The increase in venous pressure produces a postcapillary form of pulmonary hypertension. With chronicity hand severity of left-sided VHD there may be both alveolar-capillary stress failure and the development of precapillary pulmonary hypertension. The major pathophysiologic components of pulmonary hypertension in VHD are illustrated in **Fig. 26.8**. Pulmonary hypertension can also lead to right ventricular dilatation, failure, and functional tricuspid regurgitation. These various manifestations for pulmonary hypertension from left-sided VHD can become irreversible and may significantly limit recovery following left-sided valve repair or replacement.

Reverse Remodeling After Correction of Valvular Heart Disease

Postoperative studies after surgical valve replacement and repair have provided an extensive understanding of the reverse remodeling process. More recent studies have shown how TAVR and MitraClip transcatheter therapies have reversed the heart failure syndrome.[52] In aortic stenosis treated with valve replacement, the irreversible and reversible elements of interstitial fibrosis have been identified using cardiac MRI.[44] Further insights into postoperative diastolic dysfunction in patients with VHD have been produced by echocardiographic studies showing typical abnormalities of diastolic dysfunction persisting after valve replacement and requiring medical therapy.[53]

CLINICAL MANIFESATIONS OF VALVULAR HEART DISEASE

The major etiologies, clinical manifestations, prognosis, therapeutic issues, and emerging markers of disease severity of the major isolated valve lesions are presented subsequently.

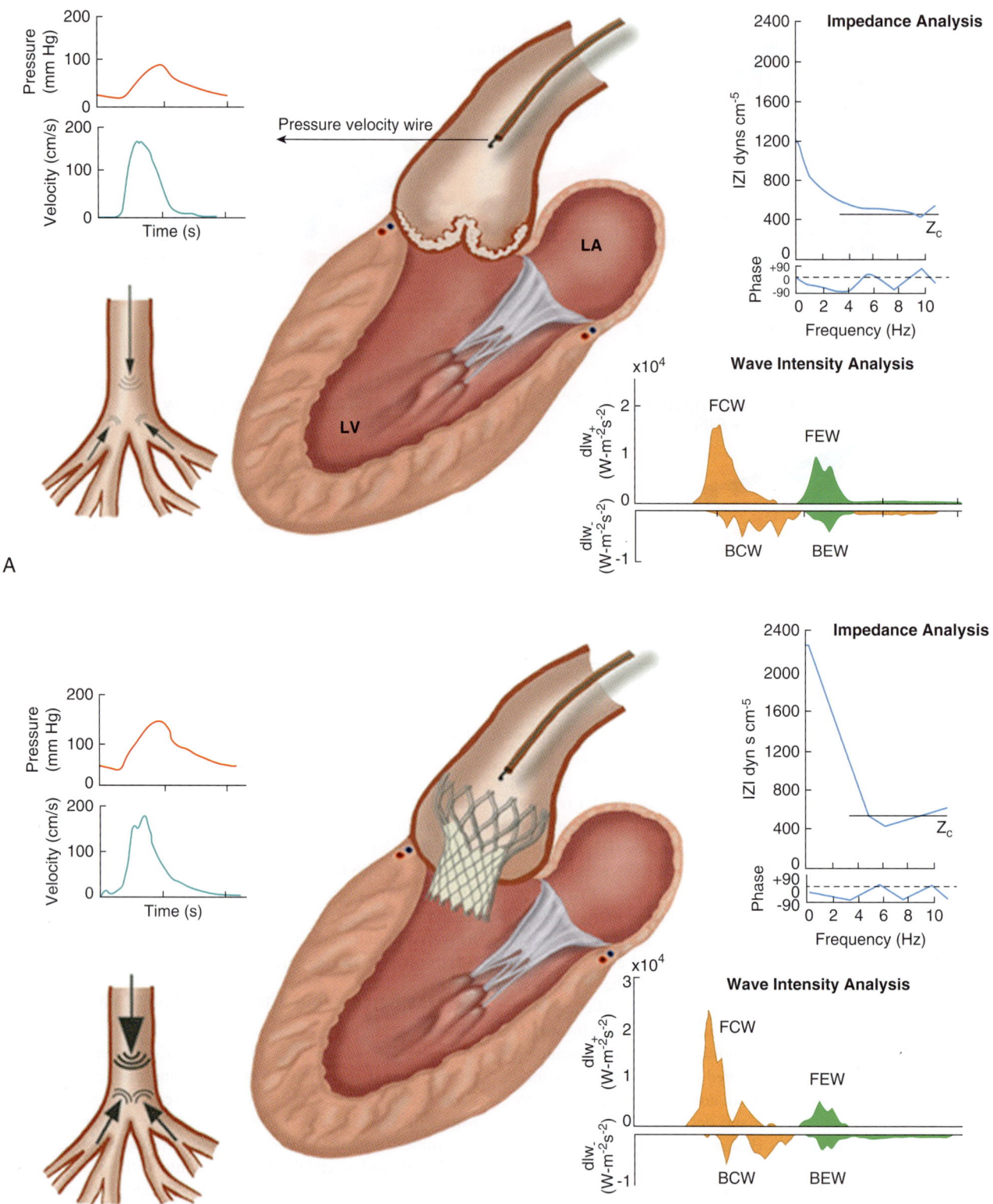

Fig. 26.6 Systemic vascular load in aortic stenosis. Relief of the valvular obstruction exposes the left ventricle to a load from systemic arterial properties. Aortic impedance and wave intensity analysis are shown in a patient before (A) and after (B) transcatheter aortic valve replacement (TAVR). Using both pressure and velocity waveforms, Fourier decomposition reveals the impedance spectrum (Z) that increases after TAVR. Forward (dlw.) and backward (dlw–) traveling pressure waves are illustrated. Compression waves *(salmon)* increase pressure, and expansion waves *(green)* decrease aortic pressure. *BCW,* Backward compression wave; *BEW,* backward expansion wave; *dlw,* wave intensity; *FCW,* forward compression wave; *FEW,* forward expansion wave; *LA,* left atrium; *LV,* left ventricle; *SVR,* systemic vascular resistance. (From Yotti R, Bermejo J, Gutiérrez-Ibañes E, et al. Systemic vascular load in calcific degenerative aortic valve stenosis: insight from percutaneous valve replacement. *J Am Coll Cardiol.* 2015;65[5]:423–433.)

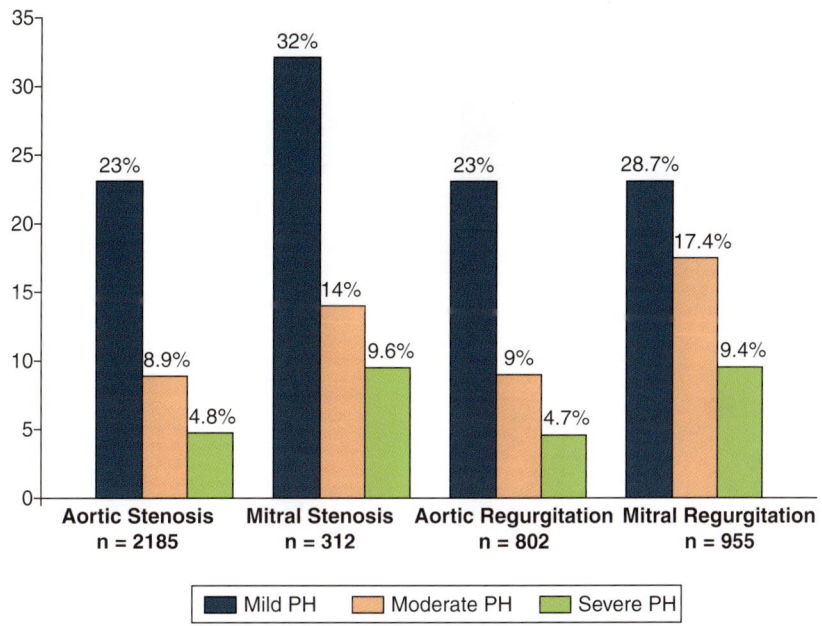

Fig. 26.7 Prevalence of mild, moderate, and severe pulmonary hypertension *(PH)* according to left-sided valvular heart disease (VHD). Pulmonary hypertension is common in VHD. These findings were derived from right heart cardiac catheterization. Mild, moderate, and severe pulmonary hypertension were defined as a mean of greater than 25 mm Hg, 35 mm Hg, and 45 mm Hg, respectively. (From Magne J, Pibarot P, Sengupta PP, et al. Pulmonary hypertension in valvular disease: a comprehensive review on pathophysiology to therapy from the HAVEC group. *J Am Coll Cardiol Img.* 2015;8[1]:83–99.)

Specific Valve Lesions

Aortic Stenosis

Aortic stenosis (**Table 26.1**) is generally a chronic and slowly progressive valvulopathy which leads to pressure overload on the left ventricle. In aortic stenosis, there is progressive narrowing of the outflow of the left ventricle such that higher left ventricular pressure is required to overcome this obstruction to maintain normal systemic aortic pressure leading to a pressure gradient through the narrowed aortic valve. In the early stages of the disease, mild narrowing of the left ventricular outflow carries few apparent consequences and patients are asymptomatic. As the degree of narrowing progresses, compensatory mechanisms become more active to maintain cardiac output and systemic blood pressure. The main compensatory mechanism is that of left ventricular hypertrophy (LVH). As left ventricular myocyte hypertrophy progresses, there is an increase in left ventricular wall thickness and left ventricular mass. These alterations lead to increased left ventricular stiffness and need for higher filling pressures (preload) to achieve adequate filling of the left ventricle, leading to diastolic dysfunction. Diastolic dysfunction alone may lead to symptoms in patients with AS even with normal systolic function. The issue of systolic dysfunction and the mechanisms which lead to it are still incompletely understood. As LVH progresses, along with increases in left ventricular diastolic pressure, coronary perfusion to the subendocardium decreases (coronary perfusion pressure = aortic diastolic pressure − left-ventricular end-diastolic pressure [LVEDP]).[2] One component of progressive left ventricular systolic dysfunction can be attributed to chronic subendocardial ischemia leading to decreases in fractional shortening and global left ventricular systolic function (LVSF).

Aortic Regurgitation

Aortic regurgitation or insufficiency (**Table 26.2**) can broadly be characterized into acute and chronic because the manifestations of this lesion are generally related to the severity, abruptness of onset, and duration of the regurgitation. During diastole, the aortic valve prevents backflow of aortic blood into the left ventricle. In aortic insufficiency, there is leakage of blood through the incompletely closed aortic valve and into the left ventricle. Aortic insufficiency leads to increase ventricular preload (usual filling plus regurgitant volume), which results in volume overload of the ventricle. Chronic aortic insufficiency generally begins with mild leakage through the incompetent aortic valve, such that there is progressive increase in left ventricular preload. Over time, this leads to increases in left ventricular mass due to eccentric hypertrophy and left ventricular dilation. The increase in LV mass leads to increases in wall tension and myocardial oxygen demand, which contributes to symptoms and may ultimately lead to alterations in systolic function.

Mitral Regurgitation

In general, mitral regurgitation (**Table 26.3**) has typically been classified as degenerative (or primary) and functional (or secondary). In degenerative MR, there are characterizable structural alterations of the mitral valve leaflets which lead to abnormalities in how the valve closes and result in backward flow of blood into the left atrium. This backflow of blood leads to a volume load into the left ventricle which eventually causes dilation of the left ventricle, and ventricular systolic dysfunction in late stages of the disease. These structural alterations can lead to worsening regurgitation due to dilation of the mitral annulus and tethering of the subvalvular mitral apparatus worsening regurgitation and clinical decline. In contrast, functional mitral regurgitation is due to abnormalities of the left ventricle, along with the supporting subvalvular mitral apparatus, which leads to malcoaptation of the normal valve leaflet tissue and leakage of blood back into the left atrium during systole (Fig. 26.5). Severe functional MR has negative prognostic implications in patients with severe LV dysfunction.[15] In contrast to degenerative MR in which treatment is aimed at repairing the abnormal mitral valve leaflets, the basis for treatment of functional MR is aimed at reversing the underlying left ventricular dysfunction and optimizing heart failure therapies for heart failure with reduced ejection fraction

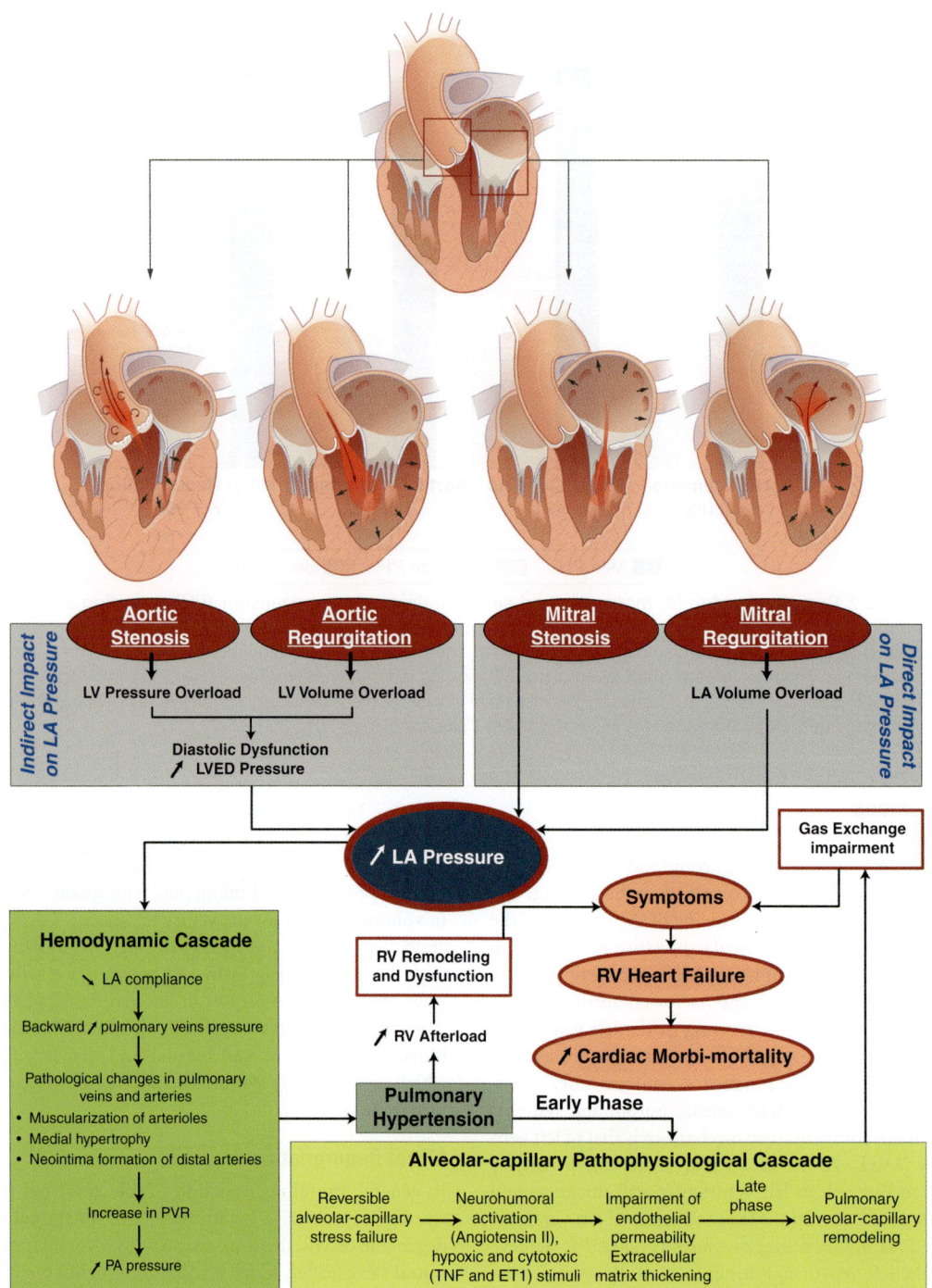

Fig. 26.8 Mechanisms and pathophysiology of pulmonary hypertension in patients with valvular heart disease (VHD). This figure provides an overview of the various factors and subsequent outcomes related to pulmonary hypertension in different forms of VHD. *ET1*, Endothelin-1; *LA,* left atrium; *LV,* left ventricle; *LVED,* left ventricular end-diastolic; *PA,* pulmonary arterial; *PH,* pulmonary hypertension; *PVR,* pulmonary vascular resistance; *RV,* right ventricle; *TNF,* tumor necrosis factor; *VHD,* valvular heart disease. (From Magne J, Pibarot P, Sengupta PP, et al. Pulmonary hypertension in valvular disease: a comprehensive review on pathophysiology to therapy from the HAVEC group. *J Am Coll Cardiol Img.* 2015;8[1]:83–99.)

(HFrEF) because surgical mitral valve repair/replacement has not been shown to dramatically alter the clinical course of patients with severe LV dysfunction and resultant severe mitral regurgitation.[15,54,55]

However, despite these negative surgical results, the recently published results of the COAPT trial have reignited enthusiasm for transcatheter mitral valve repair in FMR. Patients with heart failure and symptomatic, moderate to severe MR were shown to have a significant decrease in heart failure hospitalizations and death following percutaneous edge to edge mitral valve repair compared with those treated with optimal guideline directed medical therapy alone. This trial highlights the importance of aggressive medical therapy for HFrEF and opens the door for targeted therapy in patients with a significant burden of MR complicating and contributing to left ventricular systolic dysfunction and volume overload.[55a]

TABLE 26.1	**Severe Aortic Stenosis**
Major etiologies	• Degenerative • Rheumatic • Congenital
Major symptoms	• Dyspnea on exertion, fatigue, angina, exertion presyncope and syncope, sudden cardiac death
Typical physical examination	• Late peaking systolic murmur, single second heart sound, LV heave, reduced cardiac upstroke (younger patients)
Criteria to meet severe	• Peak velocity >4 m/sec, mean gradient >40 mm Hg, extensive leaflet calcification
Commonly associated cardiovascular findings	• Left ventricular hypertrophy, conduction system abnormalities, pulmonary hypertension in small percent
Prognosis	• 50% mortality at 2 years from symptom onset

Therapeutic issues	• No medical therapy that alters disease progression
	• Diuretic therapy if congestion
	• Indications for valve replacement:
	  • Stage D for high % of patients
	  • Stage C1 for very high gradients, reduced LV systolic function, abnormal exercise test parameters
	• Forms of valve replacement
	  • Surgical AVR with and without root enlargement and ascending aorta replacement
	  • Transcatheter AVR for intermediate or higher risk for SAVR

Important variations	• Recovery of depressed LV systolic function possible after AVR
Novel assessments of disease at stage C (presymptomatic)	• BNP elevation • MRI interstitial fibrosis of LV

AVR/SAVR, Aortic valve replacement/surgical aortic valve replacement; *BNP*, brain natriuretic peptide; *LV*, left ventricle; *MRI*, magnetic resonance imaging.

TABLE 26.2	**Severe Aortic Regurgitation**
Major etiologies	• Congenital (including bicuspid) • Infective endocarditis • Aortoannular disease • Rheumatic
Major symptoms	• Exertional dyspnea • Volume overload (pulmonary edema, lower extremity edema) • Fatigue • Angina
Typical physical examination	• Early systolic decrescendo murmur • S3 gallop • Systolic flow murmur due to increased stroke volume • Peripheral signs of severe AI (water-hammer pulse)
Criteria to meet severe	• Vena contracta ≥0.6 cm • Pressure half-time <200 ms • Effective regurgitant orifice (ERO) >0.3 cm^2 • Regurgitant fraction >50% • Descending aorta holodiastolic flow reversal
Commonly associated cardiovascular findings	• Left ventricular dilation and systolic dysfunction • Left ventricular hypertrophy (eccentric)
Prognosis	• Risk of death is low (0.2%/year) in asymptomatic patients with normal LVSF • Once symptoms or LV systolic dysfunction develops, survival rates dramatically decline

Therapeutic issues	• Afterload reduction can reduce regurgitant fraction and limit negative LV remodeling
	• Surgical AVR is preferred
	• TAVR for pure AI may be technically feasible in high risk patients, with attenuated long-term benefit as compared to TAVR for severe AS
	• Indications for valve replacement:
	  • Most frequently stage D
	  • Stage C if LVEF <50%, or EF ≥50% with LVESD >50 mm/LVEDD >65 mm

Important variations	• Acute AI is poorly tolerated and often requires urgent AVR
Assessments of disease at stage C (presymptomatic)	• Exercise stress testing is reasonable to confirm symptom status • cMRI to clearly define LVEF, systolic and diastolic volumes and measurement of AI severity

AI, Aortic insufficiency; *AVR*, aortic valve replacement; *cMRI*, cardiac magnetic resonance imaging; *EF*, ejection fraction; *LV*, left ventricular; *LVEDD*, left ventricular end-diastolic diameter; *LVEF*, left ventricular ejection fraction; *LVESD*, left ventricular end-systolic diameter; *LVSF*, left ventricular systolic function; *MRI*, magnetic resonance imaging; *TAVR*, transcatheter aortic valve replacement.

Mitral Stenosis

The most frequently encountered etiology leading to severe MS (**Table 26.4**) is RHD. The prevalence of severe rheumatic MS has declined in the developed world such that it is infrequently encountered in many practices; however, worldwide, RHD remains a leading cause of MS, with a relatively high prevalence.[22,23,56] In severe MS, there is obstruction of inflow from the left atrium to the left ventricle which leads to increasing left atrial pressures to maintain flow across the narrowed valve. As left atrial pressure increases, there are concomitant increases in pulmonary artery pressures which leads to symptoms of pulmonary congestion. In addition, there are decreases in cardiac output because forward flow cannot be maintained against the fixed and narrowed mitral valve orifice. Treatment of severe MS requires anatomic correction of the stenotic mitral valve either with percutaneous mitral balloon commissurotomy (in suitable anatomy) or surgical mitral valve replacement. Left ventricular dysfunction in MS may occur.[57] In late stages of the disease, there may be right ventricular failure due to chronic pressure overload related to pulmonary hypertension.

Tricuspid Regurgitation

Tricuspid regurgitation (TR) (**Table 26.5**) is most commonly due to functional alterations of the right ventricle (as in pulmonary hypertension), tricuspid annulus and supporting structure of the tricuspid valve, or pathologic interaction of right ventricular pacing/implantable cardioverter defibrillator (ICD) leads with tricuspid valve leaflets. Less commonly, congenital abnormalities (i.e., Ebstein anomaly) affect the tricuspid leaflets. Incompetence of the tricuspid valve leads to backward flow of blood into the right atrium during ventricular systole, which imparts a chronic volume load on the right ventricle. This leads to right ventricular and tricuspid annular dilation, which in turn causes progressive increases in the degree of TR. Chronic tricuspid regurgitation leads directly to elevations of right atrial and systemic venous pressures. This chronic venous hypertension results in clinical manifestations of severe TR, namely lower extremity edema, ascites, and liver and renal dysfunction. Despite being a common finding on

TABLE 26.3	**Severe Mitral Regurgitation**
Major etiologies	• Degenerative (including rheumatic) • Functional
Major symptoms	• Exertional dyspnea • Volume overload (pulmonary edema, lower extremity edema) • Fatigue
Typical physical examination	• Holosystolic murmur at cardiac apex • Displaced PMI • Loud P2 (related to pulmonary hypertension)
Criteria to meet severe	• Effective regurgitant orifice (ERO) >0.4 cm^2 (>0.2 cm^2 in fMR) • Regurgitant fraction >50% • Vena contracta ≥0.7 cm • Pulmonary vein systolic flow reversal • Prominent flail segment or wall-impinging jet
Commonly associated cardiovascular findings	• Left ventricular dilation and systolic dysfunction • Pulmonary hypertension • Atrial fibrillation

Prognosis	• Indolent course
	• Variable prognosis depending on etiology
	  • Excellent survival in surgically repaired dMR
	  • Functional MR, poor outcomes generally related to LV systolic dysfunction (5-year mortality 50%–60%)

Therapeutic issues	• Limited role for medical therapy in primary MR
	  • Afterload reduction in hypertensive patients or in patients with symptomatic MR in whom surgical repair is not planned
	• Diuretic therapy if congestion
	• Indications for valve replacement:
	  • Most frequently stage D
	  • Stage C if evidence of exercise-induced PH, in patients with LVEF >60% in whom there is high likelihood of successful repair
	• Valve repair favored approach versus mitral valve replacement
	  • Surgical mitral valve repair
	  • Transcatheter mitral valve repair (currently Mitra-Clip) in high-risk patients

Important variations	• Acute worsening in LV systolic function following MV repair/replacement
Assessments of disease at stage C (presymptomatic)	• Exercise echocardiography (assess increase in PA pressures)

dMR, Degenerative mitral regurgitation; *fMR,* functional mitral regurgitation; *LV,* left ventricular; *LVEF,* left ventricular ejection fraction; *MR,* mitral regurgitation; *MV,* mitral valve; *PA,* pulmonary artery; *PH,* pulmonary hypertension; *PMI,* point of maximum impulse.

TABLE 26.4	**Severe Mitral Stenosis**
Major etiologies	• Rheumatic • Calcific • Congenital
Major symptoms	• Exertional dyspnea • Fatigue • Palpitations • Volume overload (pulmonary edema, lower extremity edema) • Hemoptysis
Typical physical examination	• Low-pitched diastolic rumble at cardiac apex • Opening snap • Loud P2 (related to pulmonary hypertension)
Criteria to meet severe	• Mitral valve area <1.5 cm^2 • Mean mitral valve gradient ≥10 mm Hg
Commonly associated cardiovascular findings	• Pulmonary hypertension • Atrial fibrillation
Prognosis	• General prognosis following treatment with percutaneous balloon or surgical commissurotomy is good (80%–90% 5-year complication free survival)

Therapeutic issues	• Rate control and maintenance of NSR
	• Anticoagulation for patients in AF given very high risk of thromboembolic complications
	• Percutaneous mitral balloon commissurotomy (PMBC) is preferred if mitral valve anatomy is favorable
	• Indications for intervention:
	  • Mainly for stage D
	  • In stage C, intervention is indicated in very severe MS (MVA < 1.0 cm^2) or if new onset of AF with severe MS
	  • PMBC may be considered in symptomatic patients with MVA >1.5 if evidence of hemodynamically significant MS during exercise
	• Percutaneous mitral valve replacement emerging as option for patients with unfavorable anatomy for PMBC who are at increased risk for surgical MVR

Important clinical considerations	• Nonrheumatic (calcific) mitral valve/annular stenosis is not amenable to PMBC • LV is uninvolved in pathogenesis of CHF in MS, thus treatment algorithms for CHF in advanced disease may not be applicable
Assessments of disease at stage C (presymptomatic)	• Exercise echocardiography (assess increase in MV gradients and PA pressures)

AF, Atrial fibrillation; *CHF,* congestive heart failure; *MS,* mitral stenosis; *MV,* mitral valve; *MVA,* mitral valve area; *MVR,* mitral valve replacement; *NSR,* normal sinus rhythm; *PA,* pulmonary artery.

transthoracic echo, TR is oftentimes overlooked. However, TR severity greater than mild is associated with poor long-term outcomes and increased mortality.[58] The importance of treatment of underlying causes of TR (i.e., pulmonary hypertension) cannot be overemphasized. To date, surgical tricuspid valve repair/replacement has been the mainstay of anatomic treatment of severe TR. Transcatheter therapies have been used with variable success; however, there has been increasing focus of development of percutaneous technologies, specifically designed for treatment of severe TR, and there is optimism in the field as more devices become available.[59]

Changing Manifestations of Valvular Heart Disease Related to Comorbid Conditions and Aging

VHD manifestations are typically those common to heart failure syndrome but often become mixed with signs and symptoms of diseases of other organ systems and changes associated with aging. In the 2016 annual report of the Society of Thoracic Surgery/American College of Cardiology TVT Registry, patients undergoing TAVR had a median age of 83 years.[60] Patients had a broad spectrum of comorbid conditions, including prior stroke (11.7%), peripheral vascular disease (28.7%), systemic hypertension (90.5%), diabetes mellitus (38.1%), and chronic

TABLE 26.5 Severe Tricuspid Regurgitation

Major etiologies	• Functional/secondary • Congenital • Endocarditis • Carcinoid	
Causes of secondary TR	• Pacemaker/ICD lead • Post RV biopsy	• Severe PH • Annular dilation • Abdominal distension • Anorexia
Major symptoms	• Fatigue • Lower extremity edema	
Typical physical examination	• Holosystolic murmur over left sternal border • Jugular venous distension with prominent V-wave • Pulsatile liver • Right ventricular heave and S3 gallop	
Criteria to meet severe	• Vena contracta >0.7 cm • Central jet >10 cm^2 • Hepatic vein flow reversal	
Commonly associated findings	• Right ventricular dilation • Pulmonary hypertension • Ascites • Liver cirrhosis	
Prognosis	• 40% mortality at 1 year • Severe TR is a predictor of mortality independent of age, pulmonary pressure, or biventricular function	

Therapeutic issues	• No medical therapy that alters disease progression
	• Diuretic therapy for ascites or LE edema
	• RV lead revision may be indicated if TR is secondary to leaflet tethering
	• Aggressive management of left heart failure and pulmonary hypertension
	• Indications for surgical valve repair or replacement
	  • Main indication is concomitant TV annuloplasty or replacement at time of left-sided valve surgery
	  • Even in primary TR with normal right heart size and pulmonary pressures, outcomes following TVR are sobering	

Novel approaches to management	• Transcatheter tricuspid valve repair and replacement approaches are emerging as a possible option	

ICD, Implantable cardioverter defibrillator; *LE,* lower extremity; *PH, pulmonary hypertension; RV,* right ventricular; *TR,* tricuspid regurgitation; *TV,* tricuspid valve; *TVR,* tricuspid valve replacement.

lung disease (41.3%). Aging by itself involves shifts in genetic pathways that influence cardiovascular health and adaptation to VHD.[48,49]

Isolated Valve Lesions Versus Multivalvular Heart Disease

Multiple valves are often involved in many VHD patients of the current era, and heart failure syndrome as a consequence of VHD may have protean clinical manifestations.[61] Mixed valvular involvement is also seen in RHD but with presentation at a young to middle age. In patients undergoing TAVR due to severe aortic stenosis in the United States, 31% also had moderate to severe mitral regurgitation and 22% had moderate to severe tricuspid regurgitation.[62] The etiology of the mitral valve disease in this elderly cohort is often related to mitral annular calcification (MAC) or left ventricular dysfunction producing functional mitral regurgitation. Therefore, to understand heart failure as a consequence of VHD in the current era, we must move away from only considering isolated valve lesions in people with no other serious medical disease and toward understanding the complex interplay of multiple and mixed valvular lesions along with multisystem alterations related to other diseases and the aging process.

CLINICAL EVALUATION OF PATIENTS WITH VALVULAR HEART DISEASE

VHD and HF produce clinical manifestations that broadly overlap (**see also Chapter 31**). Heart failure and VHD both can present with the symptoms and signs of volume overload that to the patient and often to the clinician are the same. The classical sign of VHD is a pathologic

heart murmur, which, in symptomatic VHD, may be subtle or easily missed. It is often only after an echocardiogram that the clinician appreciates that the primary issue may be a valvular lesion.

Many symptoms and signs on physical examination are similar in VHD to those found in the heart failure syndrome from other causes. Left-sided valve lesions are dominated by the symptoms of dyspnea and fatigue (Tables 26.1–26.4). Most dyspnea is exertional and then may progress to orthopnea and overt pulmonary congestion. Right-sided lesions, particularly tricuspid regurgitation, result in symptoms related to peripheral edema and ascites (Table 26.5).

Syncope and presyncope are hallmarks of aortic stenosis when they occur in association with exertion when the physiologic vasodilation cannot be matched by increased cardiac output. When the diagnosis is late or the patient has not sought medical attention for a prolonged period, severe VHD can present as cachexia, with muscle wasting found to occur in 13% of patients undergoing valve surgery.[63]

Certain physical examination findings distinguish heart failure as a consequence of VHD from other causes. These relate to examination of the jugular veins, the carotid impulse, detection of cardiac heaves, murmurs, and changes in valve opening and closing sounds.

Diagnostic Modalities

The evaluation and testing of patients with aortic stenosis and mitral regurgitation have been reviewed in expert consensus documents that summarize the purpose, utility, and subsequent steps in patient management.[45,64]

The purpose of testing revolves around the need to establish a diagnosis, assess the severity of the valve lesions, and understand the associated structural and function changes as a result of the valve lesion. This is supplemented with clarifying associated rhythm and conduction issues. The two essential tests needed in all VHD patients are the transthoracic echocardiogram (TTE) and the 12-lead electrocardiogram. The AP and lateral chest x-ray are often useful, but it sometimes bypassed when a cardiac/chest computed tomography (CT) scan is ordered.

The use of echocardiography in VHD is fundamental and has replaced the need for invasive hemodynamics and angiography in the vast majority of patients.[32,45] The advent of three-dimensional (3D) echocardiography, both TTE and transesophageal echocardiogram (TEE), has enabled the development and efficient performance of the growing number of TVTs.[34,65]

Cardiac CT has become the "gold standard" for the assessment of patients with aortic valve disease. TAVR sizing, detection of other key anatomic characteristics, and assessment of access via the femoral artery, as well as alternative access sites, are standard uses of CT.[66] The ascending aorta when calcified (i.e., the porcelain aorta) is a reason for TAVR rather than SAVR. The finding of aortopathy in the setting of bicuspid aortic stenosis is a reason for SAVR and ascending aorta replacement. Cardiac CT is also essential for assessing the feasibility and planning for many emerging transcatheter mitral valve procedures. These include valve-in-valve procedures for degenerated mitral bioprosthesis, valve-in-ring procedures for treatment of recurrent severe mitral regurgitation after surgical annular ring repair, valve-in-MAC for severe mitral regurgitation and/or MS, and for the upcoming transcatheter mitral valve replacement technologies for predominantly functional mitral regurgitation that must be sized and assessed for whether or not left ventricular outflow obstruction is likely.[67-69]

Cardiac MRI has had less penetration as a standard test in VHD but has provided important insights regarding chamber remodeling, hypertrophy, and interstitial fibrosis.[69] Its role in the assessment of regurgitant lesions has recently been reviewed with an associated guideline.[33]

Most patients undergoing an evaluation for VHD need an evaluation for the presence and severity of CAD. Often in elderly patients with VHD the extent of coronary calcification precludes the accurate assessment of coronary stenoses with cardiac computed tomography angiogram (CTA). Therefore catheter-based coronary angiography is often performed.

Right heart catherization (**see also Chapter 34**) is frequently needed because pulmonary hypertension complicates many forms of VHD, impacts on prognosis, and may require treatment after correction of the valve lesion.

Because atrial fibrillation may be paroxysmal and accompany many valve lesions, prolonged monitoring may be needed to understand symptoms, to assess the potential need for anticoagulation, and to direct the use of rhythm and rate control medications.

Laboratory Testing

The routine blood work that is part of the initial evaluation and subsequent clinic visits in heart failure patients is also justified in VHD patients. Renal and liver abnormalities may accompany more advanced stages of VHD. Anemia is relatively common in an elderly population, and a variety of causes need to be understood because they may impact on treatment decisions. Abnormalities of coagulation are key to characterize before surgical and transcatheter interventions.

Biomarkers are increasingly needed to assess patients with VHD (**see also Chapter 33**).[71] They may be useful in assessing the cause of dyspnea and when it may indicate the patient is entering a decompensated stage of VHD. Natriuretic peptides, specifically brain natriuretic peptide (BNP), provide a unique insight into VHD severity of symptomatic status and may be useful in predicting outcomes.[71] Prospective studies are needed to see if they should be used in the determination of the timing of valve interventions.[72] The role of high-sensitivity troponins has also been studied as to their ability to characterize the

patient's response to VHD and as a potential determinant of timing of VHD intervention.[73,74] The role of biomarkers following surgical or transcatheter correction is quite variable and not well understood. For example, in patients with severe mitral regurgitation who are treated with percutaneous edge-to-edge mitral valve repair with MitraClip, there was no significant decrease in NT-proBNP level after reduction in the degree of MR with MitraClip.[75] In addition, NT-proBNP levels and their change did not correlate with baseline LVEF, LV dimension, NYHA class, or clinical events on follow-up.

Functional Testing (see also Chapter 31)

There are several purposes of performing functional testing in VHD, with exercise and dobutamine infusion being common modalities.[76,77] The 6-minute walk test is used in chronic mitral regurgitation patients to assess functional exercise capacity.[78] Exercise testing in mitral regurgitation helps to clarify symptoms and may indicate prognosis.[79] An exercise evaluation can clarify in MS if a low resting transmitral gradient significantly rises with the increase in heart rate and cardiac output with exercise. Exercise in asymptomatic patients with aortic stenosis may unmask functional limitations and show worrisome signs such as a fall in blood pressure, electrocardiographic signs of ischemia, and ventricular aarythmias.[80] Dobutamine is given to aortic stenosis patients with low resting gradients in the setting of LV systolic dysfunction or low stroke volume index to assess whether gradients reach a severity threshold meeting interventional indications. Exercise testing after surgical valve replacement may also be used to evaluate patient's response to intervention.[81]

Functional assessment of VHD also has been expanded with the use of the Kansas City Cardiomyopathy Questionnaire (KCCQ) to assess patient reported limitations in activities. Both baseline scores and changes after valve replacement were initially used in pivotal device trials but now have become part of routine care.[5,6,82] TAVR has a durable benefit on the KCCQ score even in patients who were considered inoperable.[83]

Gait velocity and grip strength have become routine in the assessment of frailty in older adults with VHD.[5,6,84]

STAGES OF VALVULAR HEART DISEASE AND STAGES OF HEART FAILURE

The stages of VHD and HF have many similarities of definitions and the transitions that signify progression in disease severity. These are outlined in **Table 26.6**. Both approaches reflect progression of the underlying disease, transitions from asymptomatic to symptomatic states, and the occurrence of chamber remodeling.

The stages of HF are also indicative of the potential spectrum of outcomes that may occur after treatment of the primary valve abnormality. Many patients who are post valve intervention are assumed to be in stage A but actually are often stage B as methods are applied showing incomplete reverse remodeling and persistent interstitial fibrosis after valve replacement.[44] Some VHD patients have irreversible changes in chamber and myocardial function that will place them into stage C HF, and even some may transition into stage D.

TREATMENT OF VALVULAR HEART DISEASE

There is no medical therapy that impacts on the progressive nature of the various forms of chronic primary VHD. Multiple randomized trials failed to show a benefit of statins in reducing the rate of progression of aortic stenosis.[85]

Guideline-Directed Medical Therapy (GDMT) should be standard for all risk factors for cardiovascular disease, especially in patients with VHD. Treatment of systemic hypertension is important in patients with asymptomatic aortic or mitral regurgitation but also in aortic stenosis, with care

TABLE 26.6 Stages of Valvular Heart Disease Compared With Stages of Heart Failure Per Professional Society Guidelines

Stage	Definition	Description
Valvular Heart Disease Stages		
A	At risk	Patients with risk factors for development of VHD
B	Progressive	Patients with progressive VHD (mild-to-moderate severity and asymptomatic)
C	Asymptomatic severe	Asymptomatic patients who have the criteria for severe VHD: C1: Asymptomatic patients with severe VHD in whom the left or right ventricle remains compensated C2: Asymptomatic patients with severe VHD with decompensation of the left or right ventricle
D	Symptomatic severe	Patients who have developed symptoms as a result of VHD
Heart Failure Stages		
A	High risk for developing HF	Hypertension, CAD, diabetes mellitus, family history of cardiomyopathy
B	Asymptomatic HF	Previous MI, LV systolic dysfunction, asymptomatic valvular heart disease
C	Symptomatic HF	Known structural heart disease. Shortness of breath and fatigue. Reduced exercise tolerance
D	Refractory End-Stage HF	Marked symptoms at rest despite maximal medical therapy

CAD, Coronary artery disease; *HF,* heart failure; *LV,* left ventricular; *MI,* myocardial infarction; *VHD,* valvular heart disease.
Stages of VHD from Nishimura RA, Otto CM, Bonow RO, et al. 2014 AHA/ACC guideline for the management of patients with valvular heart disease: a report of the American College of Cardiology/American Heart Association Task Force on Practice Guidelines. *J Am Coll Cardiol.* 2014;63(22):e57–e185. Stages of HF from Yancy CW, Jessup M, Bozkurt B, et al. 2013 ACCF/AHA guideline for the management of heart failure: a report of the American College of Cardiology Foundation/American Heart Association Task Force on Practice Guidelines. *Circulation.* 2013;128(16):e240–e327.

to not excessively lower blood pressure.[86] Medical therapies including diuretics and vasodilators are often used with the onset of symptoms and during hospitalization for severe decompensation. Optimal medication therapy, resynchronization, and revascularization are mainstays of managing patients with functional mitral regurgitation.[15]

Early identification of VHD provides a potential opportunity for institution of medical therapy that may delay or arrest the progression of both valve abnormalities and the molecular alterations of the myocardium seen in volume and pressure overload including myocardial fibrosis. Currently no medical therapies achieve these goals, but the search continues. Lipid-lowering therapy, antihypertensive medications, anticalcific therapy, and RAAS inhibition have been studied.[87] Other targets for medical therapy in patients with aortic stenosis include the plasma lipoprotein-associated phospholipase A2, the CACNA1C gene, the apolipoprotein A-I/high-density lipoprotein receptors LOX-1 and SR-B1, the enzyme autotaxin, the endocannabinoid system, and the nonglucocorticoid antioxidant steroid lazaroid U-74389G.[87] The impact of beta-blockers on left ventricular function in degenerative mitral regurgitation represents another investigative avenue.[88] Secondary mitral

regurgitation is an example of VHD that can occasionally be effectively treated by advanced heart failure therapies, and the role of surgery or interventional valve therapies is an area of intensive investigation.[15]

There is often the need to treat VHD-associated issues involving rhythm disturbance, conduction abnormalities, and thromboembolic risks. Recommendations for the management of these issues are well-outlined in the guidelines regarding VHD.[11,86,89]

Timing of Interventions

An ongoing challenge in VHD management is when to correct the valve abnormalities either by traditional surgery or by new transcatheter techniques. One of the pioneers in VHD clinical management, Dr. Eugene Braunwald, articulated in 1990 this issue as follows: "The most important decision in the management of patients with aortic stenosis, or in patients with any valvular lesion, is when to refer them for surgical treatment. This decision must be based on an understanding of the risks and long-term outcome of operative treatment on the one hand, and of the natural history of the condition when treated medically on the other. The former information is ordinarily readily available, but the latter has been more difficult to elicit."[90]

Symptom onset in VHD is often the timepoint in VHD when an intervention to correct the valve abnormality is considered. An updated perspective considers symptom onset as a transitional time in the natural history of VHD when compensatory mechanisms fail and multiple partially to completely irreversible changes may have occurred at different levels (i.e., from cellular to the chamber level).

Two experts in mitral regurgitation management have outlined the rationale for early surgery for asymptomatic patients with severe mitral regurgitation, assuming that the valve is reparable.[91] Early repair is recommended when mitral regurgitation is severe, even in the asymptomatic patient, to reduce the chance of irreversible changes occurring in left ventricular function, left atrial size and proclivity to atrial fibrillation, and pulmonary hypertension. Postoperative mortality after mitral surgery increases if surgery is delayed until symptoms emerge or signs of left ventricular systolic dysfunction emerge. If surgery is earlier and repair, rather than replacement, is performed with an operative mortality less than 1%, then patients are returned to a life expectancy of the general population.[92] This approach has not been subjected to a randomized trial.

A key question is whether this approach can be applied to other valve lesions as new effective and safe treatments become available and the evidence base grows. The data for indications for surgery for both mitral regurgitation and aortic regurgitation were reviewed by Dr. Robert Bonow, who drew a similar conclusion for early intervention in mitral regurgitation as the other authors but showed that the evidence is lacking to justify early intervention in aortic regurgitation.[93]

More recently, data have suggested that underlying biochemical and molecular myocardial alterations far precede development of symptoms in patients with severe aortic stenosis. In addition, functional myocardial changes including subtle declines in ejection fraction (EF), happen quite early in the progression of aortic stenosis, and in fact these changes accelerated before aortic stenosis became severe by standard definitions.[94] There may be new and more sensitive markers of deteriorating function that may replace or complement low EF to justify early intervention in VHD.

The major modifiers of this new paradigm of early correction of severe valve abnormalities are whether or not the treatments are well-enough developed and executed by skilled clinicians with very high likelihood of a safe and effective outcomes and where patient characteristics and personal preferences are suitable for early intervention. Finally, the patient must prefer this strategy over conservative management and watchful waiting after a comprehensive shared decision-making process.

Current State of Transcatheter Therapies for Valvular Heart Disease

TVTs have impacted on a broad spectrum of patients of all ages. Transcatheter treatments have addressed the 30% of patients with moderately severe to severe valvular dysfunction who were not offered surgical intervention, generally on the basis of comorbidities.[95] Older children and young adults with congenital heart disease now are frequently treated with Food and Drug Administration (FDA)-approved transcatheter pulmonic valve replacement for recurrent issues arising after numerous open surgical corrective operations often starting in infancy.[27] Middle-aged adults infrequently are treated with transcatheter mitral and aortic therapies unless they have other medical conditions making cardiac surgery high or prohibitive risk such as prior radiation for thoracic malignancies.[96,97]

Adults older than the age of 75 years have undergone the largest transition in VHD management because the development and commercial release of transcatheter therapies have occurred in older adults with degenerative aortic stenosis and mitral regurgitation. In 2017 in the United States there were 84,095 aortic valve replacements reported to the TVT Registry and the STS database.[98] Of these, 42,605 were via TAVR, 25,580 were SAVR, and an additional 15,910 were SAVR plus coronary bypass grafting. The growth of TAVR over the preceding 4 years was 161%, whereas SAVR declined 14%. Currently in the United States, TAVR is approved for patients who are at intermediate, high, or prohibitive risk for SAVR. Two major randomized clinical trials comparing TAVR and SAVR outcomes in patients at low risk for SAVR have completed enrollment in 2018 and will be reported in 2019 to 2020.

The transcatheter valve revolution is now starting in the mitral and tricuspid valve space.[59,99] Currently in the United States, there are three approved transcatheter treatments for mitral valve disease. The Inoue mitral balloon catheter is FDA approved for the treatment of rheumatic MS, and percutaneous balloon mitral valvuloplasty is extensively used for rheumatic MS around the world.[56] The MitraClip technology is FDA approved for patients with symptomatic, hemodynamically severe degenerative mitral regurgitation if surgery carries a prohibitive risk.[100] The Edwards Sapien 3 transcatheter valve is approved for treatment of degenerated bioprosthetic mitral valves in patients at high risk for redo cardiac surgery.[101]

Current State of Surgical Therapies for Valvular Heart Disease

The decades of experience and documentation of outcomes with surgical approaches to treatment of VHD will continue to provide the majority of patients who are at low risk for surgery with effective and safe treatments. The advantages of surgical approaches to treating VHD include their known durability, the ability to repair valves with a myriad of techniques, to perform other concomitant treatments such as left atrial appendage occlusion, the maze procedure in those with atrial fibrillation, ascending aortic replacement in those with aortopathy, multivalvular repair/replacement, and coronary bypass surgery in those with extensive CAD or anatomic subsets unsuitable for percutaneous coronary intervention.[102]

Treatment of Valvular Heart Disease the Heart Team and Shared Decision Making

An increasing proportion of patients with VHD require a heart team approach in which both surgical and transcatheter approaches need to be considered. Patients who have treatment options are able to make informed choices that incorporate their preferences and goals.

The use of effective decision aids and incorporation of shared decision making into clinical practice have emerged into routine VHD management.[9]

Treatment of Valvular Heart Disease Patients After Interventions

Medical therapy after both surgical and transcatheter treatments is needed in all patients. Often, ongoing treatment of hypertension and other underlying conditions is required. Other medical therapies are being studied that may facilitate the reverse remodeling process, promote hypertrophy regression, and manage persistent diastolic dysfunction such as RAAS inhibition, ACE inhibition, and angiotensin receptor blockade. The prevalence of myocardial transthyretin amyloid in elderly patients with aortic stenosis may approach 25%, and its clinical impact on patients in the post–valve replacement period is being studied.[103]

Prosthetic valve dysfunction can take multiple forms.[104] Anticoagulation of mechanical valves reduces but does not eliminate risk of valve thrombosis, and anticoagulation for bioprosthetic valves may be needed to prevent and treat leaflet thrombosis that appears to be more common in transcatheter aortic valves than surgically implanted valves.[105] Patient-prosthetic mismatch is a problem more with surgical aortic valve replacement and may impact on myocardial hypertrophy regression and suitability for future intervention.[106,107] Transcatheter treatment of degenerated surgically implanted prosthetic valves in the aortic and mitral position has been FDA approved, is increasingly common, and occasionally requires balloon-induced fracture of the sewing ring of a small surgical prosthesis when there is patient-prosthetic mismatch in addition to valve degeneration.[108]

KEY REFERENCES

2. Dweck MR, Boon NA, Newby DE. Calcific aortic stenosis: a disease of the valve and the myocardium. *J Am Coll Cardiol*. 2012;60(19):1854–1863.

6. Carroll JD, Shuren J, Jensen TS, et al. Transcatheter valve therapy registry is a model for medical device innovation and surveillance. *Health Aff (Millwood)*. 2015;34(2):328–334.

15. Asgar AW, Mack MJ, Stone GW. Secondary mitral regurgitation in heart failure: pathophysiology, prognosis, and therapeutic considerations. *J Am Coll Cardiol*. 2015;65(12):1231–1248.

29. Otto CM, Prendergast B. Aortic-valve stenosis—from patients at risk to severe valve obstruction. *N Engl J Med*. 2014;371(8):744–756.

41. Barone-Rochette G, Pierard S, De Meester de Ravenstein C, et al. Prognostic significance of LGE by CMR in aortic stenosis patients undergoing valve replacement. *J Am Coll Cardiol*. 2014;64(2):144–154.

44. Treibel TA, Kozor R, Schofield R, et al. Reverse myocardial remodeling following valve replacement in patients with aortic stenosis. *J Am Coll Cardiol*. 2018;71(8):860–871.

49. Paneni F, Diaz Canestro C, Libby P, Luscher TF, Camici GG. The aging cardiovascular system: understanding it at the cellular and clinical levels. *J Am Coll Cardiol*. 2017;69(15):1952–1967.

55. Lavall D, Hagendorff A, Schirmer SH, Bohm M, Borger MA, Laufs U. Mitral valve interventions in heart failure. *ESC Heart Fail*. 2018;5:552–561.

70. Treibel TA, Fontana M, Gilbertson JA, et al. Occult transthyretin cardiac amyloid in severe calcific aortic stenosis: prevalence and prognosis in patients undergoing surgical aortic valve replacement. *Circ Cardiovasc Imaging*. 2016;9(8):e005066.

94. Ito S, Miranda WR, Nkomo VT, et al. Reduced left ventricular ejection fraction in patients with aortic stenosis. *J Am Coll Cardiol*. 2018;71(12):1313–1321.

The full reference list for this chapter is available on ExpertConsult.

Heart Failure as a Consequence of Congenital Heart Disease

Eric V. Krieger, Anne Marie Valente

Adults with congenital heart disease (CHD) have multiple mechanisms placing them at risk for heart failure, leading one author to refer to CHD as "the original heart failure syndrome."[1] These mechanisms include chronic pressure and/or volume loading, inadequate myocardial preservation during prior surgeries, myocardial fibrosis, surgical injury to a coronary artery, and neurohormonal activation. The number of heart failure–related admissions for adult congenital heart disease (ACHD) patients has increased steadily[2] and heart failure–related complications are the most common cause of death in these patients.[3,4] However, ACHD patients are commonly excluded from heart failure clinical trials and there are few data to guide therapy in this growing population. Due to the increasing recognition of this problem, in 2016, the American Heart Association published two scientific statements focused on chronic heart failure and transplant and mechanical circulatory support in the CHD population.[5,6] This chapter will discuss the growing number of ACHD patients at risk for heart failure, unique aspects of diagnostic testing and therapies in this group, and highlight several types of CHD at the highest risk for the development of heart failure.

EPIDEMIOLOGY

Due to tremendous advances in the diagnosis and management of CHD, there are now more adults than children alive with CHD; the prevalence of CHD is approximately 4/1000 adults.[7] These advances have shifted mortality away from infants and towards adults living with CHD.[5] The number of adults with CHD living in the United States is estimated to be at least 1.4 million, and at least 300,000 of these people have complex forms of CHD.[8]

There is also an increased recognition of heart failure–related complications in ACHD patients, and certain centers have developed specialized ACHD-HF dedicated clinics. However, the reported prevalence of heart failure in ACHD patients is likely an underestimate due

to challenges in making the diagnosis and the gaps in care for ACHD patients.[9] The prevalence of heart failure is highest in patients with complex anatomy, including single ventricle physiology, transposition of the great arteries (TGA), tetralogy of Fallot (TOF), and pulmonary hypertension (**Fig. 27.1**).[10-12] Risk factors for the development of heart failure include high disease complexity, older age, more reoperations, and right ventricular dysfunction.[10]

Heart failure is the leading cause of death in ACHD patients, particularly those with complex anatomy (**Fig. 27.2**).[3, 11-13] In a cohort of 188 ACHD patients with a systemic right ventricle (RV) or single ventricle, 15-year mortality for symptomatic patients was much greater than those without symptoms (47.1% vs. 5%).[14] Zomer reported that ACHD patients admitted for heart failure had a five-fold higher risk of mortality than patients who were not hospitalized (HR = 5.3; 95% CI 4.2–6.9). One- and three-year mortality after the first heart failure admission were 24% and 35%, respectively.[15] In a single-center, retrospective study of almost 7000 adult patients with CHD with a median follow-up of over 9 years, the median age of death was 47 years, and the leading cause of death was heart failure.[4] Additionally, heart failure in ACHD patients is associated with increased morbidities and health care resource utilization. In an analysis of the Nationwide Inpatient Sample (NIS), the number of heart failure–related admissions increased 82% from 1998 to 2005 in adults with CHD.[2] More recently, a review of the 2007 NIS reported that heart failure accounted for 20% of the total ACHD admissions, and that heart failure–related hospitalizations were associated with a three-fold increased risk of death compared to non-heart-failure admissions.[16]

DIAGNOSIS

Heart failure symptoms in ACHD patients may manifest as systolic and/or diastolic dysfunction of a morphological left, right, or single

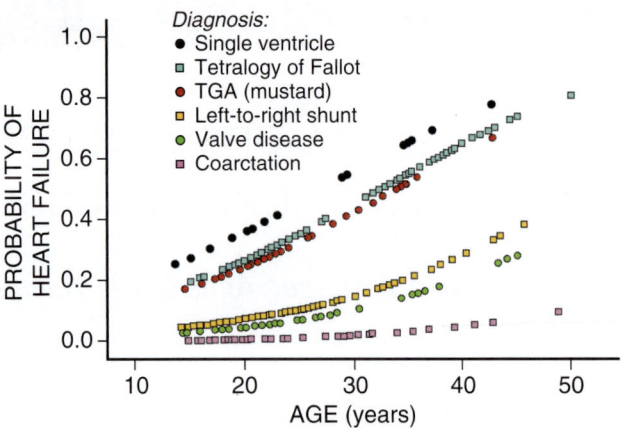

Fig. 27.1 The probability of heart failure based on age and type of congenital heart defect. *TGA*, Transposition of the great arteries. (Adapted from Norozi K, Wessel A, Alpers V, et al. Incidence and risk distribution of heart failure in adolescents and adults with congenital heart disease after cardiac surgery. *Am J Cardiol*. 2006;97:1238–1243.)

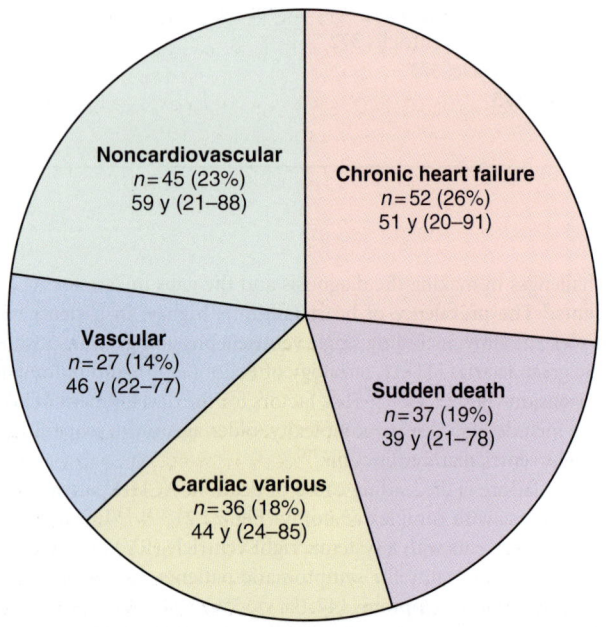

Fig. 27.2 Modes of death in adult congenital heart patients. (Adapted from Verheugt CL, Uiterwaal CS, van der Velde ET, et al. Mortality in adult congenital heart disease. *Eur Heart J*. 2010;31:1220–1229.)

ventricle. Other CHD patients may have normal ventricular function, but signs of end-organ dysfunction, such as the adult single ventricle patient with Fontan physiology, and significant liver disease.

The diagnosis of heart failure in ACHD patients is often challenging. Patients with CHD, having lived their lives with cardiac disease, may not detect subtle changes in their exercise capacity. By the time they notice symptoms, the extent of ventricular dysfunction and valve disease may be severe and irreversible. Compared to patients with acquired heart disease, patients with CHD are more likely to overestimate their functional capacity and underreport heart failure symptoms.[17] Therefore, objective measures of ventricular function through imaging, exercise testing, and serum biomarkers can be helpful in these patients. Exercise testing can be useful to uncover early signs of heart failure, even in patients who report that they are asymptomatic

(**Fig. 27.3**).[18] Patients with CHD and heart failure should be referred to a center with expertise in the care of these patients.[19]

Imaging (see also Chapter 32)

The imaging diagnosis of heart failure in ACHD patients may be challenging, and a multimodality approach is often utilized. The goals of diagnostic imaging in ACHD patients are to evaluate ventricular performance, identify anatomic and functional abnormalities, assess their severity, and provide information that informs clinical decisions. This includes identifying residual hemodynamic issues, such as valve dysfunction and shunts, and evaluating for pulmonary hypertension.

Echocardiography

Echocardiography remains the first-line modality in CHD imaging; however, acoustic windows are often poor in older patients and those with multiple prior cardiac surgeries. It is often challenging to visualize certain parts of the right heart, which limits assessment of RV size and function.

Assessment of ventricular size and function is important in the ACHD patient. Left ventricular (LV) function is most often calculated as the ejection fraction (EF) based on the biplane Simpson or area–length method, both of which assume an ellipsoid shape of the ventricle. These methods are not applicable to the RV or single ventricle patient due to the nonellipsoid shape of the ventricle. There are various echocardiographic techniques that can be used to evaluate RV function. A normal RV fractional area change is >35%. Three-dimensional echocardiography may provide a more accurate and reproducible quantification of RV volumes and function. However, it underestimates RV volumes and may overestimate EF, which is a discrepancy that may increase as the ventricle enlarges.[20]

Cardiac Magnetic Resonance Imaging

The role of CMR is steadily increasing in the ACHD population and CMR has become the gold standard for quantification of RV volumes and function.[21] Phase-velocity imaging is utilized for the assessment of cardiac output and valvular regurgitation. An additional strength of CMR is the ability to characterize myocardial tissue abnormalities. Specifically, late gadolinium enhancement suggestive of myocardial fibrosis has been associated with adverse clinical outcomes in patients with repaired TOF,[22] systemic RV,[23] and Fontan procedures.[24] Quantification of the extracellular volume fraction using the modified look–locker inversion recovery sequence may identify areas of more diffuse fibrosis.[25,26] However, the clinical significance in ACHD patients is unknown.

Cardiopulmonary Exercise Testing

Cardiopulmonary exercise testing is a valuable tool in the assessment of ACHD patients at risk for heart failure. Objective testing is important in this population, as ACHD patients commonly overestimate their actual measured exercise capacity and are unaware of functional limitations.[17] Cardiopulmonary exercise testing is predictive of morbidity and mortality in CHD patients.[27] In a recent single-center experience of cardiopulmonary exercise testing in 1375 ACHD patients (age 33±13 years), decreased peak oxygen consumption (VO_2) and heart rate reserve were predictive of death over a median follow-up of 5.8 years. Additionally, an elevated minute ventilation/volume of carbon dioxide (VE/VCO_2) slope was associated with an increased risk of death in noncyanotic patients.[27] Diller reported the results of objective exercise testing in 335 ACHD patients, and demonstrated that these patients, with a mean age of 33 years, had a similar distribution of heart failure symptoms and exercise capacity to a noncongenital heart failure population at a mean age of 49 years (see Fig. 27.3).[18]

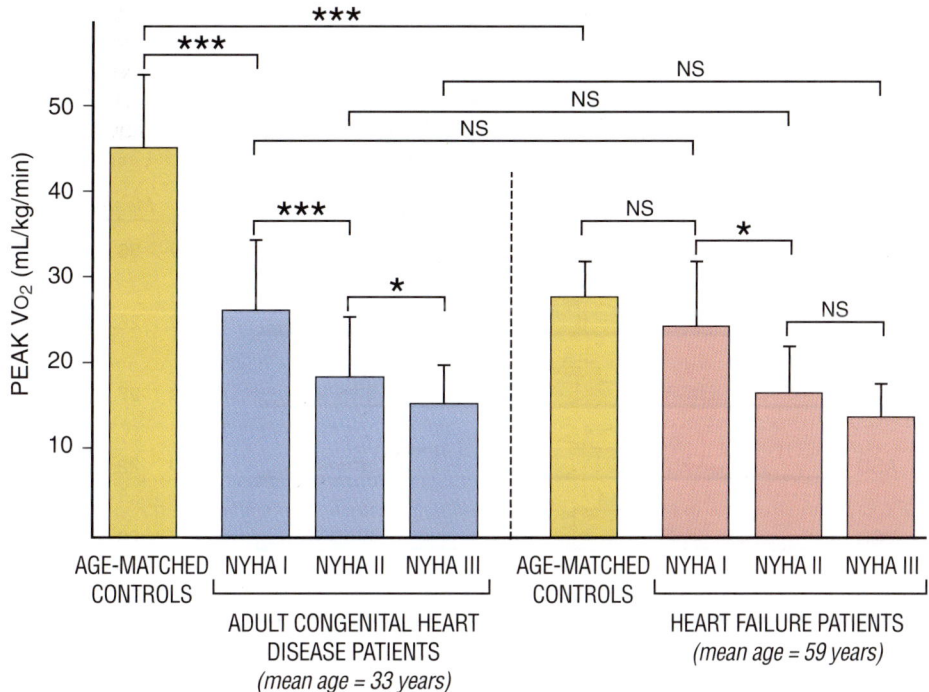

Fig. 27.3 Peak oxygen consumption according to the New York Heart Association (NYHA) class for adult congenital heart patients, chronic heart failure patients, and corresponding reference subjects. *, $P < .05$; ***, $P < .001$; *NS*, not significant. (Adapted from Diller GP, Dimopoulos K, Okonko D, et al. Exercise intolerance in adult congenital heart disease: comparative severity, correlates, and prognostic implication. *Circulation.* 2005;112:828–835.)

ACHD patients may have limited exercise capacity due to both cardiac and non-cardiac etiologies. Ventricular dysfunction (both systolic and diastolic) and electromechanical dyssynchrony are increasingly recognized in ACHD patients. Residual hemodynamic lesions are common in ACHD patients, as almost no one who undergoes CHD surgery is "cured." Chronotropic incompetence is common in ACHD patients, often secondary to injury of the conduction system during surgery, intrinsic conduction abnormalities, or medications, and is associated with increased mortality.[28] Adults with CHD may have noncardiac limitations to exercise capacity. Restrictive lung disease is very common in those who have undergone thoracotomies. Obstructive lung disease, diaphragmatic paralysis (due to phrenic nerve injury), liver dysfunction, skeletal muscle dysfunction, and hematological derangements can also limit exercise capacity.

One of the challenges in interpreting the results and prognostic significance of cardiopulmonary exercise testing in ACHD patients is that the group is very heterogeneous. Kempny has published age- and gender-specific reference values for peak VO_2 for groups of ACHD patients with various congenital heart conditions (**Fig. 27.4**).[29] ACHD patients have elevations in the VE to VCO_2 production slope, and this finding is an independent predictor of mortality.[30] An elevated VE/VCO_2 slope may be in seen in repaired TOF patients, when there is abnormal pulmonary blood flow distribution due to branch pulmonary artery stenosis.[31] However, an elevated VE/VCO_2 slope is not associated with increased mortality in single ventricle patients who have undergone a Fontan procedure, where the elevation in the slope is a consequence of nonpulsatile pulmonary blood flow.[32] Additionally, Fontan patients commonly have a depressed oxygen pulse, even in the absence of ventricular dysfunction, indicating a failure of the Fontan to increase preload to the systemic ventricle during exercise.

Biomarkers (see also Chapter 33)

ACHD patients with heart failure experience neurohormonal activation similar to those patients with heart failure from acquired heart disease. However, because of the diversity of CHD and the various mechanisms of heart failure in ACHD patients, there is no consistent association of individual serum biomarkers to outcomes, which can be generalized across all ACHD patients. Even asymptomatic ACHD patients may have significant neurohormonal activation, which demonstrates the occult nature of ventricular dysfunction in this group of patients.[33] Over the past decade, multiple investigators have reported results of abnormal biomarkers in ACHD patients that have been associated with mortality.[34,35] However, since natriuretic peptides are influenced by age, gender, and hypoxia, it is difficult to define normal levels for a diverse population of ACHD patients. N-terminal pro b-type natriuretic peptide (NT-proBNP) levels vary considerably by the type of underlying CHD, with the highest levels seen in patients with complex CHD such as Fontan physiology and systemic RV.[36] Elevated NT-proBNP levels are predictive of adverse events across a broad range of congenital heart diagnoses.[13] Patients with low levels have excellent clinical outcomes. Patients with high NT-proBNP have worse outcomes and can be further risk stratified by the level of high-sensitivity troponin-T and growth-differentiation factor 15.[37]

The utility of serum biomarkers in patients with Fontan physiology remains uncertain. In these patients, symptoms of heart failure may occur despite normal systolic ventricular function and unremarkable biomarker values. BNP values have not been shown to correlate with ventricular systolic dysfunction in this group of patients.[38,39] In one study of 106 Fontan patients, elevated BNP was found to be an independent predictor of Fontan failure and mortality in adulthood.[40] Biomarkers also have not been effective as screening tools for Fontan-associated liver disease; FibroSure and hyaluronic acid levels are

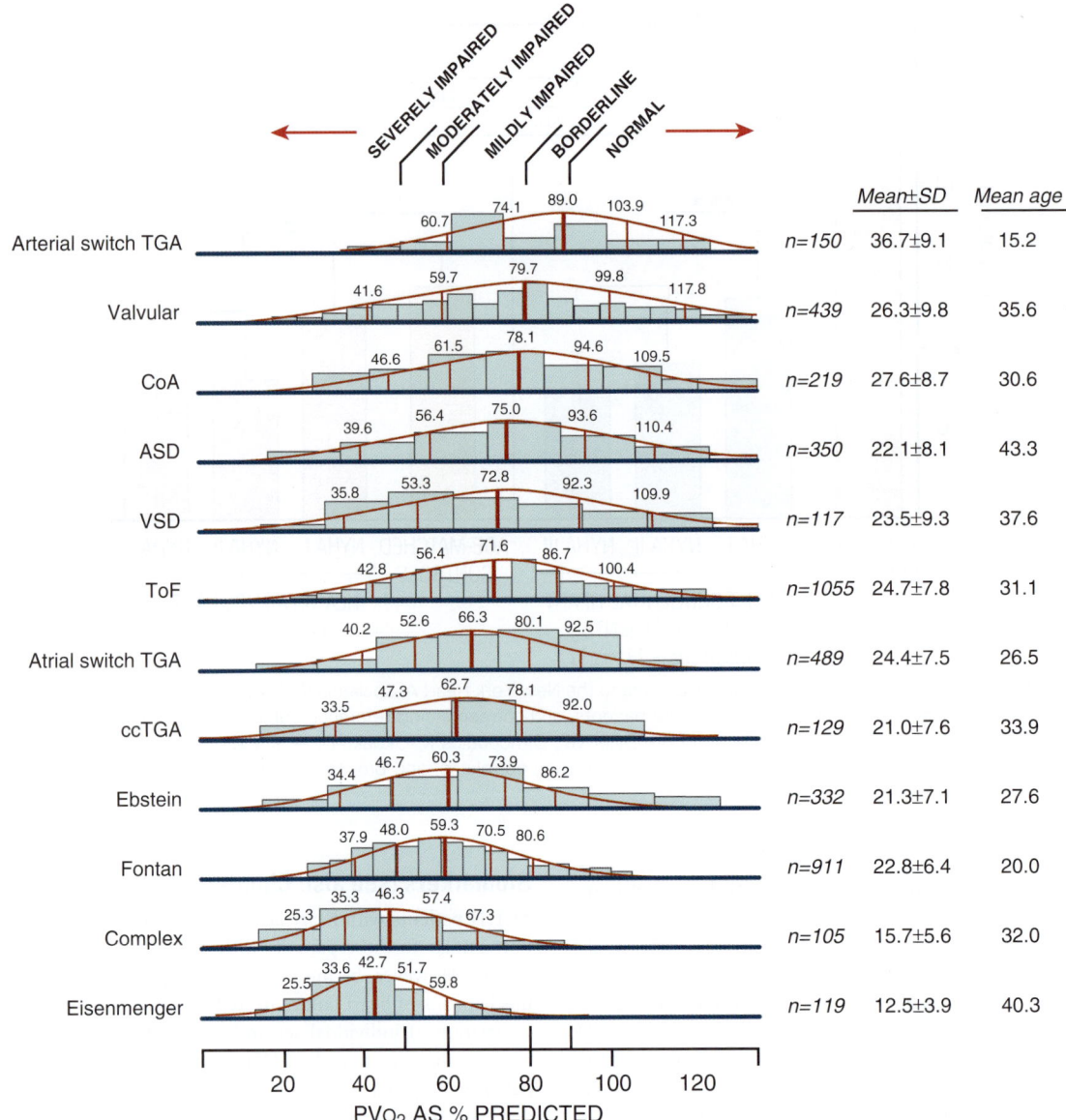

Fig. 27.4 Peak oxygen uptake (peak VO$_2$) for various forms of congenital heart disease, expressed as a percentage of predicted value. The density lines above histograms and the numbers to the right of the graph relate to all patients with a given diagnosis. The numbers above the density lines indicate percentage peak VO$_2$ values for the 10th, 25th, 50th, 75th, and 90th percentile. *ASD*, Atrial septal defect; *ccTGA*, congenitally corrected TGA; *CoA*, coarctation of aorta; *Complex*, complex congenital heart disease (including univentricular hearts); *Ebstein*, Ebstein anomaly; *Eisenmenger*, Eisenmenger syndrome; *Fontan*, patients after Fontan palliation; *TGA*, transposition of the great arterial; *ToF*, tetralogy of Fallot; *Valvular*, mixed collective of patients with congenital valvular heart disease; *VSD*, ventricular septal defect. (Reproduced from Kempny A, Dimopoulos K, Uebing A, et al. Reference values for exercise limitations among adults with congenital heart disease. Relation to activities of daily life—single centre experience and review of published data. *Eur Heart J.* 2012;33:1386–1396.)

elevated in most patients with Fontan circulation, but the levels do not correlate with the degree of hepatic fibrosis.[41]

TREATMENT

ACHD patients are commonly excluded from heart failure clinical trials and there are few data to guide therapy in this growing population. It may be tempting to simply extrapolate from established heart failure guidelines; however, this is dangerous because the mechanism of heart failure

is often very different in ACHD than in the noncongenital population. For example, ACHD patients may have a systemic RV or a single ventricle. Additionally, ACHD patients are more likely to have a correctable anatomic abnormality causing heart failure—such as baffle obstruction, stenotic conduits—so standard medical therapy for heart failure may not be appropriate. Therefore the evaluation of new heart failure symptoms in an ACHD patient must be tailored to the patient's anatomy and surgical repair. It should include evaluation for residual shunts, baffle stenosis, valvular or conduit dysfunction, and collateral vessels; each of these may be

TABLE 27.1   Selected Studies of Medical Therapy Trials in Adult Congenital Heart Patients

Author	Year	Study design	Agent	N	Duration (months)	Endpoints	Results
Tetralogy of Fallot							
Norozi	2007	PDB-RCT	Bisoprolol	33	6	NT-proBNP, RVEF, LVEF	Negative
Babu-Nararyan	2012	PDB-RCT	Ramipril	64	6	RVEF	Negative
Bokma	2017	PDB-RCT	Losartan	95	21	RVEF, RV and LV volume, LVEF, VO₂max, NT-proBNP, QOL	Negative for all predefined primary and secondary endpoints
Systemic RV							
Dore	2005	PDB-COT	Losartan	29	3.5	VO₂max, RVEF, NT-proBNP	Negative
Giardini	2007	Prospective uncontrolled trial	Carvedilol	8	12	RVEF, LVEF, VO₂max, exercise duration	Positive: In this very small uncontrolled trial, carvedilol led to improvements in biventricular size and function
Doughan	2007	Retrospective	Carvedilol or metoprolol	60	Retrospective	NYHA class, RV size	Positive: In this retrospective uncontrolled trial beta blockers led to improvement in NYHA class in patients with systemic right ventricle
Therrien	2008	PDB-RCT	Ramipril	17	12	RVEF, RVEDV	Negative
van der Bom	2013	PDB-RCT	Valsartan	88	36	Primary: RVEF Secondary: RVEDV, VO₂max, QOL	Negative except for small benefit on RVEDV
Fontan							
Kouatli	1997	PDB-COT	Enalapril	18	2.5	VO₂max, exercise duration	Negative
Giardini	2008	PDB-RCT	Sildenafil	27	Single dose	VO₂max, cardiac output, pulmonary blood flow	Positive: Fontan patients who received a dose of sildenafil had an improvement in VO₂max while patients who received a placebo did not
Goldberg	2011	PDB-COT	Sildenafil	28	1.5	Primary: VO₂max Secondary: VE/VCO₂ slope	Negative for primary outcome; Sildenafil improved VE/VCO₂ slope, the secondary outcome
Hebert	2014	PDB-RCT	Bosentan	65	3	VO₂max	Positive: Patients who received Bosentan had improvement in VO₂max, exercise duration, and NYHA class while patients taking placebo did not
Rhodes	2013	PDB-RCT	Iloprost	18	Single dose	VO₂max, O₂ pulse	Positive: Fontan patients who received a single dose of iloprost had improvement in VO₂max and O₂ pulse while patients who took placebo had no improvement

LVEF, Left ventricular ejection fraction; *NT-proBNP,* N-terminal pro b-type natriuretic peptide; *NYHA,* New York Heart Association; *PDB-COT,* prospective double-blind crossover trial; *QOL,* quality of life; *RV,* right ventricle; *RVEDV,* right ventricular end-diastolic volume; *RVEF,* right ventricle ejection fraction; *VCO₂,* volume of carbon dioxide; *VE,* minute ventilation; *VO₂max,* maximal oxygen uptake.

amenable to interventions. The effectiveness of medical therapy for heart failure in specific ACHD populations is discussed in more detail below.

All ACHD patients with new onset heart failure also should be evaluated for pulmonary vascular disease. In a population-based study of greater than 38,000 adults with CHD, subjects with pulmonary hypertension had a more than twofold higher risk of all-cause mortality and three-fold higher risk of heart failure and arrhythmias compared to those without pulmonary hypertension.[42]

The treatment of heart failure in the ACHD patient also must address modifiable risk factors such as hypertension, diabetes, and obesity.[43]

Potential therapies for heart failure in ACHD patients include medical therapies, device therapies, and surgical interventions, such as mechanical assist devices and transplantation. The existing data for medical therapies in ACHD patients are limited, as no adequately powered clinical trials have been performed. Individual studies focused on medical therapies will be discussed in the lesion-specific section below and are listed in **Table 27.1**.[43a-43c,132]

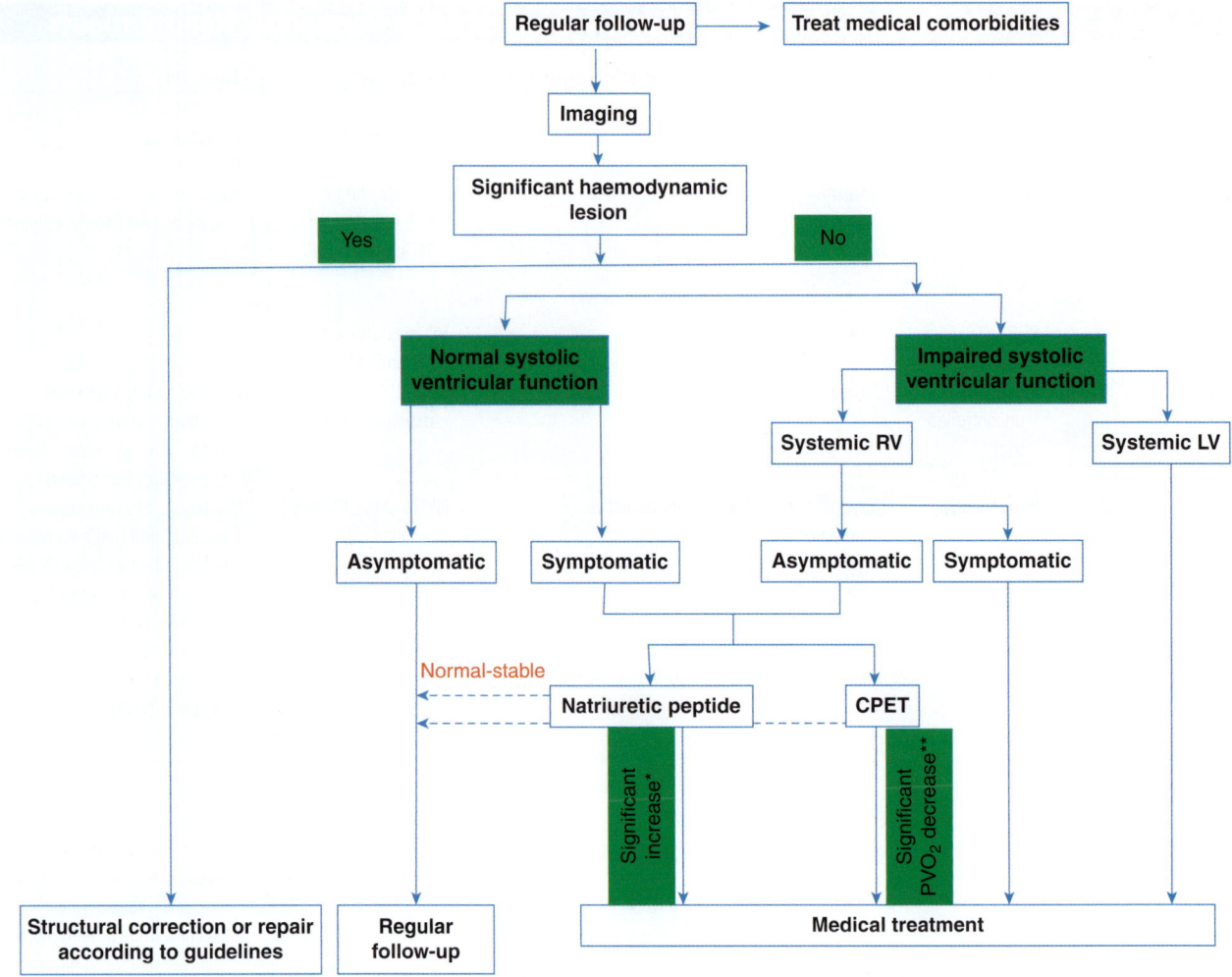

Fig. 27.5 A proposed algorithm for the diagnosis and treatment of heart failure in patients with adult congenital heart disease. *Two-fold increase of baseline natriuretic peptide value within 6 months. **Greater than 25% decrease of peak oxygen consumption. *CPET,* Cardiopulmonary exercise test; *PVO₂,* peak oxygen consumption; *LV,* left ventricle; *RV,* right ventricle. (From Budts W, Roos-Hesselink J, Radle-Hurst T, et al. Treatment of heart failure in adult congenital heart disease: a position paper of the working group of grown-up congenital heart disease and the heart failure association of the European society of cardiology. *Eur Heart J.* 2016;37[18]:1419–1427.)

While the etiology and treatment options for heart failure are diverse in CHD, one proposed algorithm for evaluation and treatment is shown in **Fig. 27.5.**[44]

Cardiac Resynchronization Therapy and Implantable Defibrillators in Adult Congenital Heart Disease (see also Chapter 38)

In patients with chronic systolic heart failure and prolonged QRS duration, cardiac resynchronization therapy (CRT) improves symptoms, and reduces hospitalizations and all-cause mortality.[45] However, there are comparatively few data on CRT in patients with CHD. There are various reasons why it may not be appropriate to apply standard CRT guidelines to ACHD patients. ACHD patients are considerably more heterogeneous than the population studied in the large resynchronization trials, so extrapolation is difficult. Patients with CHD are more likely to have predominantly right-sided heart disease, systemic RV or single ventricle physiology, and the benefits of CRT are not well established in these groups. Additionally, due to shunts or variations in venous anatomy, patients with CHD are more likely to require epicardial pacing or defibrillation that increases the risk of implantation, reduces device longevity, and alters the risk–reward ratio of implanting a CRT device.

Most of the larger series of CRT in CHD are retrospective uncontrolled case series (**Table 27.2**).[46-50] The patients were younger and most studies included children. The procedural complication rate ranged from 9% to 29% and included lead complications, infection, pocket hematomas, blood loss, and, rarely, procedural mortality. Approximately half of the devices were implanted with epicardial leads, although this is less common in older patients. As expected, patients who received CRT had a reduction in QRS width with the greatest reduction in those being converted from single ventricular pacing. The overall rate of clinical response ranged from 32% to 87% of treated patients, and, depending on the study, response was variably defined as an improvement in systemic ventricular EF or improvement in New York Heart Association (NYHA) class.[47-50] Approximately one-third of patients had a robust clinical response.[48]

TABLE 27.2 Selected Studies of Cardiac Resynchronization Therapy Response in Pediatric and Congenital Heart Disease Patients

	Cecchin et al	Dubin et al	Janousek et al	Koyak et al
Year	2009	2005	2009	2018
Number of patients	60	103	109	48
Median age (years)	15	13	17	47
Baseline data				
NYHA class I (%)	27	14	Median NYHA Class 2.5	73% were NYHA III–IV
NYHA class II (%)	42	48		
NYHA class III–IV (%)	32	38		
Systemic ventricular EF (%)	36	26	27	<35
Congenital heart disease (%)	77	71	80	100
Single ventricle (%)	22	7	4	0
Systemic RV (%)	12	17	33	23
QRS (ms)	149	166	160	181
Post-CRT data				
Change NYHA class	NR	NR	Decreased 1.5 grades	NR
Systemic ventricular EF (%)	43	40	Median change +12	NR
QRS (ms)	120	126	130	~172
Improvement in EF or NYHA class (%)	87	76	72	77
Predictors of poor CRT response	Systemic RV	Higher baseline EF	Dilated cardiomyopathy, high baseline NYHA class	NR

CRT, Cardiac resynchronization therapy; *EF*, ejection fraction; *RV*, right ventricle; *NR,* not reported; *NYHA*, New York Heart Association.
Adapted in part from van der Hulst AE, Delgado V, Blom NA, et al. Cardiac resynchronization therapy in paediatric and congenital heart disease patients. *Eur Heart J.* 2011; 32:2236–2246.

A few critically ill patients who were dependent on intravenous inotropic support could be weaned to oral therapy after CRT.[47] Only one large study on CRT in CHD has focused on adult patients. In this study, 48 patients (median age 47 years) underwent CRT. After 2.6 years of follow-up, 77% were CRT responders, improving NHYA functional class, ventricular function, or both.[50]

Cardiac Resynchronization Therapy in Specific Populations

Tetralogy of Fallot

Patients with repaired TOF often have right bundle branch block due to RV dilation and myocardial fibrosis. QRS prolongation has been associated with poor exercise capacity and low cardiac output.[51,52] For this reason some have speculated that CRT may be beneficial. Right bundle branch block pattern is common in repaired TOF; therefore RV pacing with fusion of the spontaneous wave-front is theoretically appealing. Acutely, RV CRT improves myocardial mechanics, improves contractile efficiency, and improves RV contractile performance.[53,54] Generally, the results in CRT trial patients with right bundle branch block have been disappointing compared to those with left bundle branch block.[55] Recent retrospective data showed clinical improvement in 85% of patients with TOF and dyssynchrony who were treated with CRT.[50] In patients with TOF and LV dysfunction, CRT may be reasonable for conventional indications. While CRT cannot be routinely recommended for all patients with right bundle branch block (RBBB), there may be a role for patients in whom a dyssynchronous, failing RV is causing heart failure symptoms.[56]

Systemic Right Ventricle

Many patients with TGA have a morphologic RV that functions as the systemic ventricle. These patients are predisposed to ventricular dysfunction and heart failure, as described elsewhere in this chapter.

Approximately 40% of patients with a systemic RV have a wide QRS or echocardiographic features of dyssynchrony.[54,57,58] Up to 9% of patients with a systemic RV meet conventional indications for CRT (reduced EF, NYHA class ≥ II, sinus rhythm and QRS >120 msec).[57] While it is possible that this population may benefit from CRT, robust data are lacking due to small numbers; in a report of 11 patients with systemic RV who underwent CRT, 55% had clinical improvement.[50] In another report of seven patients with systemic RV who underwent CRT, the results were encouraging; all patients had improved markers of dyssynchrony, improvement in NYHA class, and an improved exercise capacity.[59] Other studies have been less consistent. Approximately 20% of the patients in the studies by Janousek,[49] Cecchin,[48] and Dubin[47] had a systemic RV. Dubin found comparable improvement in those with systemic right and left ventricles. However, Janousek and Cecchin found that patients with systemic RV had less improvement compared with those with systemic LV. The authors speculate that the lack of improvement may be due to these patients' older age, or systemic atrioventricular (tricuspid) valve regurgitation that did not improve after CRT. At this point the literature is conflicting, and there is insufficient evidence to routinely recommend CRT for patients with systemic RV dysfunction; each case must be considered on an individual basis. CRT can be technically challenging in these patients due to variations in the location and drainage of the coronary sinus ostium in patients with TGA.

Single Ventricle

In patients with a functional single ventricle, the systemic ventricle can be either a morphologic left or right depending on the initial cardiac anatomy. Patients with a Fontan operation who require ventricular pacing require an epicardial system to minimize the risk of stroke associated with thrombus formation on a lead in the systemic ventricle. Placement of multisite epicardial leads for CRT is also nonstandardized, and the optimal lead position is unknown, although an effort is made to place the CRT lead 180 degrees from the first pacing lead.[60]

In young children undergoing the Fontan operation, CRT acutely improves postoperative cardiac performance, as measured by echocardiographic markers of dyssynchrony and invasive hemodynamics.[61] Case reports have documented clinical improvement after multisite pacing in the failing Fontan circulation.[62] In the series by Janousek and Cecchin, most Fontan patients had improvement in NYHA class. Cecchin demonstrated, on average, greater than 10% improvement in EF after CRT.[48,49]

Transplantation and Mechanical Support (see also Chapters 44 and 45)

Myocardial dysfunction is common in patients with CHD and is a frequent cause of death in this population.[3,11,12] Therefore, for many patients with CHD, heart transplantation becomes the only potential treatment option. As with other forms of heart disease, transplantation is appropriate for patients with heart failure refractory to conventional medical therapy.

Approximately 3% of adults who undergo heart transplantation have CHD and the proportion is growing over time.[63,64] The most likely congenital diagnoses to result in transplantation include single ventricle anatomy, TGA, and right ventricular outflow tract (RVOT) lesions. Most patients have had at least one prior corrective surgery.[65] Most, but not all,[65] studies have shown that transplanted patients with CHD have higher early mortality than patients without CHD.[66] The most frequent causes of early posttransplant mortality in patients with CHD are hemorrhage and acute graft failure.[67] Longer ischemic times are common in ACHD patients, which is likely due to technically difficult dissections, and are a risk factor for early postoperative death.[66] One-year mortality rates in the CHD population are approximately 20%.[68,69] Older recipient age, older donor age, longer ischemic times, and prior Fontan operation appear to be risk factors for early mortality.[65] The operative risk in CHD patients is somewhat balanced by better long-term survival among those who survive 30 days, so late survival is similar.[70,71]

For patients with CHD who survive greater than 3 months from the time of transplant, long-term survival is similar [64,72] to patients without CHD who receive heart transplantation, suggesting that the increased risk of mortality is related to peritransplant issues.[67] Outcomes for ACHD transplantation and risk factors for adverse outcomes in selected studies are shown in **Table 27.3**.[64-66,68,73-80] A recent systematic review of the literature has shown that although ACHD patients have high early mortality, long-term survival is superior to non-CHD transplant recipients.[70]

Selecting appropriate CHD patients for cardiac transplantation is difficult. Risk models exist to predict the need for transplantation in acquired heart disease,[81] but these models are not validated in patients with ACHD. Therefore it can be difficult to decide when it is appropriate to list a patient with CHD for transplantation. Appropriate timing for listing patients with Eisenmenger syndrome pose an additional challenge as these patients have improved survival compared to other patients with severe pulmonary arterial hypertension, and require combined heart-lung transplantation, which carries a relatively poor prognosis.[82,83] In patients with Eisenmenger syndrome, it is appropriate to consider transplantation for patients with repeated hospitalizations, signs of refractory RV failure, arrhythmias, or worsening cyanosis.

Congenital patients often have complex postsurgical anatomy that can pose technical challenges at the time of transplantation. Systemic or pulmonary veins may need to be surgically redirected in patients with atrial situs inversus. Patients with TGA may require that additional length of great arteries be harvested at the time of donor organ procurement. Many patients with repaired CHD may have pulmonary vascular disease or distorted pulmonary artery anatomy due to prior shunts, branch pulmonary artery stenosis, or stents, which can increase RV afterload and predispose to early graft failure.

An additional barrier to transplantation in adult congenital patients is alloimmunization as a consequence of prior transfusions, homografts, or pregnancies. Patients with elevated preformed reactive antibodies have increased rejection-reduced posttransplant survival. This can make it difficult to find a suitable donor organ. A panel of reactive antibodies should be checked early in the transplant evaluation to determine if the patient is appropriate for transplant listing and if a desensitization protocol is required. Most patients with CHD and end-stage heart failure who are considered for transplantation are never listed for transplantation due to high reactive antibodies, anatomic barriers, perceived surgical risk, or other reasons.[84]

Patients with CHD who are listed for transplant are more likely to be listed at a lower urgency status than patients with acquired heart disease; 64% of patients with CHD are listed as status 2, while only 44% of patients with acquired heart disease are listed as status 2. This discrepancy is, in part, due to the infrequent use of ventricular assist devices (VADs) (which increase urgency status) in patients with CHD and end-stage heart failure. Therefore, listed patients with CHD have a longer time to transplantation and are less likely to receive a transplant once listed. Despite the lower listing priority, patients with CHD were more likely to experience cardiovascular death than patients with acquired heart disease.[85] In addition, ACHD patients listed at the highest priority status are more likely to die or be delisted due to clinical worsening, highlighting the fact that they are listed too late in the disease process.[86] The apparent penalty of transplant listing in patients with CHD could potentially be remedied by more judicious use of implantable defibrillators and VADs in CHD patients,[85] or by changing the urgency status upgrade given to patients with VADs.[87] The United Network for Organ Sharing is transitioning to a new organ allocation system. In the newer seven-tier system, ACHD patients are to be assigned to status 4, grouped with patients with infiltrative cardiomyopathy, ambulatory left VAD patients, and those with intractable angina. It is unknown how the new allocation system will affect patients with CHD.

Fontan patients undergoing transplantation require careful consideration. As discussed above, these patients are likely to have multiple prior palliative surgeries, complex anatomy, collateral vessels, and multiorgan dysfunction manifest by congestive hepatopathy, renal insufficiency, and coagulopathy.[88] They are also more likely to be cachectic and edematous. Fontan patients are therefore at increased risk of perioperative bleeding, postoperative hepatorenal syndrome, or serious infection. Fontan patients may also have in situ pulmonary artery thrombus, which can increase the risk of acute graft failure. Pulmonary vascular resistance is usually low in patients with Fontan physiology, but in the context of a failing Fontan it may be modestly elevated and can be difficult to calculate using standard techniques. Fontan patients appear to have an increased posttransplant risk of death and a higher risk of death from infection.[65,89,90] Careful patient selection is critical to ensure acceptable transplant outcomes in Fontan circulation. Some studies suggest that posttransplant outcomes are best in Fontan patients with reduced EF compared with other causes of failing Fontan circulation.[91,92]

TABLE 27.3 Outcomes of Heart Transplantation in Patients With Congenital Heart Disease

Study	Transplant period	No	Age (years)	1-year survival	5-year survival	10-year survival	Predictors of mortality	Outcomes
Besik, 2016; Single center Czech Republic	1999–2014	25	38	88%	77%	NR	Long donor ischemic time	Mortality: 30 days, 1 year, 5 years, 10 years
Bhama, 2013; Single center United States	2001–2011	19	39	84%	70%	NR	Long donor ischemic time	Mortality: 30 days, 1 year, 5 years
Chen, 2004; Single center United States	1984–2004	106	≥18	78% overall, 83% after 2000	71% overall, recent data NR	58% overall, recent data NR	Early era of operation	Mortality: 1 year, 5 years, 10 years
Davies, 2011; UNOS study United States	1995–2009	129	35	~80%	NR	53%	Transplant performed at low-volume pediatric heart transplant centers. Previous sternotomy.	Mortality: 30 days, 1 year, 5 years, 10 years[d] Morbidity: reoperation, dialysis
Davies, 2011; Single Center Fontan study United States	1984–2007	43	16	62%	59%	48%	Renal dysfunction, operative bleeding	
Irving, 2010; Single center United Kingdom	1988–2009	37	34	~68% overall, 80% after 2002	~58% overall, 69% after 2002	~52% overall	Early era of operation	Mortality: 30 days
Karamlou, 2010; UNOS study United States	1990–2008	575	28	76%	NR	52%	Younger age, Status I, Long ischemic time	Mortality: 1 year, 5 years, 10 years[d] Cause-specific mortality: hemorrhage, malignancy
Paniagua Martin, 2012; Spanish Heart Registry study Spain	1984–2009	55	26	~75%	~68%	~62%	Not reported	Mortality: 30 days, 1 year, 5 years, 10 years Cause-specific mortality: primary graft failure, rejection, infection, CAV + SD, malignancy
Patel, 2009; UNOS study United States	1987–2006	689	>17	80%	69%	57%	Preoperative pulmonary hypertension, elevated panel of reactive antibodies	Mortality: 30 days, 1 year, 5 years, 10 years Cause-specific mortality: primary graft failure, rejection, infection, stroke

CAV, Cardiac allograft vasculopathy; *NR,* not reported; *SD,* standard deviation; *UNOS,* United Network for Organ Sharing.
Adapted in part from Doumouras BS, Alba AC, Foroutan F, Burchill LJ, Dipchand AI, Ross HJ. Outcomes in adult congenital heart disease patients undergoing heart transplantation: a systematic review and meta-analysis. *J Heart Lung Transplant.* 2016;35(11):1337–1347.

A common dilemma is to determine when Fontan patients with concomitant liver disease require combined heart–liver transplantation as nearly all adult Fontan patients have evidence of liver fibrosis on imaging and biopsy; however, there is no consensus on this question. Patients with clinical cirrhosis are usually precluded from single-organ transplantation. However, carefully selected patients with imaging (rather than clinical) findings of cirrhosis may fare well with isolated heart transplant as cirrhotic changes seen on computed tomography were not associated with worse transplant outcomes in a single center study of 32 Fontan patients.[93] At experienced centers, combined heart-liver transplantation can have acceptable outcomes in Fontan patients.[94]

VADs (**see also Chapter 45**) have not gained widespread use in adult patients with CHD.[85] Most reports of VAD use in adult patients with CHD are limited to case reports or small case series of carefully selected patients. A systematic review of VAD therapy in CHD reported on short-term outcomes of 66 CHD patients treated with mechanical circulatory support (MCS). In contrast to MCS in acquired heart disease, CHD patients tend to be critically ill, often INTERMACS 1 or 2.[95] In a recent analysis of the INTERMACS database, 128 ACHD patients were propensity-matched with 512 non-ACHD patients. Although the ACHD group suffered a higher early mortality after mechanical circulatory support, survivors had similar improvements in functional capacity and quality of life, as well as similar adverse event rates compared to the non-ACHD group.[96] There are numerous potential barriers to VAD use in patients with CHD. These include the higher frequency of right-sided heart failure in patients with CHD, a higher prevalence of pulmonary vascular disease, multiple prior chest surgeries, and multiorgan dysfunction with coagulopathy and renal dysfunction.

Exercise Training in CHD

In acquired HF, cardiopulmonary rehabilitation and exercise training improves outcomes; it is safe and supported by guidelines.[97,98]

Compared with acquired HF, there are relatively few data in patients with CHD. Noncompetitive exercise training is safe in patients with CHD[99] and exercise training appears to improve physical capacity, exercise tolerance, and quality of life in patients with CHD. [44,100,101] One trial of exercise training in patients with a systemic RV showed that exercise training improved exercise capacity and heart failure symptoms without any negative impact on RV function.[102] Cardiac rehabilitation and exercise prescriptions are likely underutilized in patients with CHD and should be considered for most patients with CHD and heart failure.

SPECIFIC CONDITIONS

Tetralogy of Fallot

TOF is the most common cyanotic CHD with a prevalence of 0.3 to 0.5 per 1000 live births and accounts for 7% of CHD. It is characterized by deviation of the infundibular septum creating a malalignment ventricular septal defect, aortic override, RVOT obstruction and ventricular hypertrophy. Complete repair involves closure of the ventricular septal defect and relief of RVOT obstruction (**Fig. 27.6**).

Despite excellent early surgical outcomes, multiple residual hemodynamic burdens can predispose to heart failure later in life. Often, pulmonary valve function is not preserved during repair that leads to pulmonary valve regurgitation. Prior to the 1990s, surgery was most commonly performed through a large right ventriculotomy and a sizeable RVOT patch was used to relieve the obstruction. Free pulmonary valve regurgitation was considered to be an inevitable and acceptable tradeoff for complete relief of RVOT obstruction. The large transannular patch contributes to late pulmonary regurgitation and predisposes to lower RV EF later in life.[103]

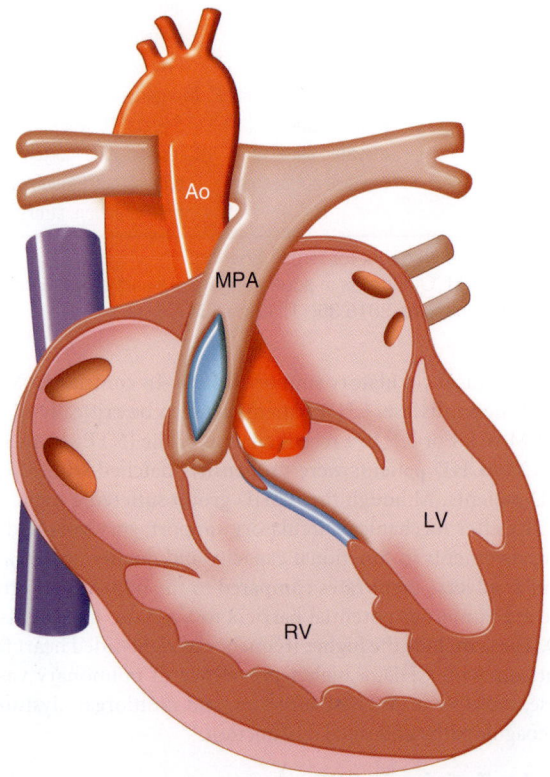

Fig. 27.6 Diagrammatic representation of repaired tetralogy of Fallot. There is a patch across the right ventricular outflow tract and a patch closure of the ventricular septal defect. *Ao,* Aorta; *LV,* left ventricle; *MPA,* main pulmonary artery; *RV,* right ventricle.

As a consequence of ongoing pulmonary regurgitation, many patients developed progressive RV dilation and systolic dysfunction. While free pulmonary regurgitation is initially well tolerated in childhood, changes in RV compliance and pulmonary artery capacitance as well as slower heart rates (allowing for more time in diastole) result in worsening regurgitation in adulthood. This often leads to RV dilation, functional tricuspid valve regurgitation, RV systolic dysfunction as well as atrial and ventricular arrhythmias if left untreated.[104] RV function typically deteriorates and limits exercise tolerance and may cause overt right heart failure, usually in the third and fourth decades of life.

Pulmonary valve replacement (PVR), if done prior to overt RV failure, leads to beneficial RV remodeling characterized by a reduction in end-diastolic volume and stabilization or improvement of RV EF.[105-107] However, not all authors have found an improvement in EF or exercise performance following surgery.[105,107-109] Earlier valve replacement may allow for greater improvement in function and exercise parameters,[110,111] yet patients who undergo PVR prior to meeting consensus guideline criteria may be at increased risk of heart failure, atrial arrhythmia, and nonsustained ventricular tachycardia (VT).[112] The optimal timing for valve replacement remains controversial: the benefits of early pulmonary valve replacement in maximizing ventricular remodeling need to be weighed against the finite lifespan of prosthetic valves. While optimal timing of pulmonary valve replacement in asymptomatic tetralogy patients remains controversial, various authors have demonstrated good short-term outcomes if surgery is done in the context of normal RV function, RV end-diastolic volumes less than 160 to 170 mL/m^2, and end-systolic volume of less than 80 to 90 mL/m^2.[104, 105,109-111,113]

Current data do not suggest that renin-angiotensin-aldosterone system (RAAS) inhibition is effective at improving RV function in repaired TOF. A small trial of ramipril did not show improvement in RV EF in patients with repaired TOF, although those with restrictive RV filling seemed to derive benefit.[114] The larger REDEFINE trial was a double-blind, placebo-controlled study of losartan versus placebo in patients with repaired TOF, and found no benefit of losartan on RV function or clinical status.[115]

LV dysfunction is increasingly recognized in patients with TOF and appears to be an important determinant of outcome. Approximately 20% of adults with repaired TOF have LV systolic dysfunction.[116] Patients with LV dysfunction have more arrhythmias and worse outcomes than TOF patients with preserved LV systolic function.[116-118] The reason for LV dysfunction in patients with TOF is not fully understood but may be caused by interventricular interactions, chronic bundle branch block, aortic regurgitation, neonatal cyanosis, LV volume overload from palliative shunts, or be a consequence of neurohormonal activation from RV failure.[33,116,119]

Systemic Right Ventricle

A systemic RV is one in which the morphologic RV delivers systemic output through the aorta (**Fig. 27.7**). There is no standard definition for systemic RV dysfunction; therefore its prevalence in ACHD patients is unknown, and the response to medical therapies is difficult to interpret. These patients are at high risk for sudden cardiac death and heart failure. Additionally, much of the available literature concerning medical therapies in systemic RV patients includes both TGA (D-loop TGA) and physiologically corrected TGA (c-TGA; also called L-loop TGA, cc-TGA) patients. TGA and c-TGA patients may have very different responses to medical therapies. For example, TGA patients that have undergone an atrial switch procedure often have sinus node dysfunction, whereas c-TGA patients are at high risk for progressive atrioventricular block. Therefore, each group's responses to beta-blockade may be quite different. The current ACHD guidelines recommend imaging every year, or at least every other year, to assess systemic RV function.[19]

TGA (D-loop TGA) results from ventricular–arterial discordance so the aorta connects to the RV pumping deoxygenated blood systemically and the pulmonary artery connects to the LV pumping oxygenated blood back to the lungs, which is a physiology incompatible with life without the presence of a shunt. From the 1960s to 1980s, the most common surgical procedure for this condition was the atrial switch procedure (Mustard or Senning operation), which directed deoxygenated blood via baffles to the LV and out of the pulmonary artery, and directed oxygenated blood to the RV and out of the aorta. These procedures relieved the cyanosis, yet resulted in the RV ejecting to systemic pressure. RV dysfunction is common following atrial switch. The mechanisms for systemic RV dysfunction are incompletely understood but may include suboptimal myofiber arrangement, myocardial ischemia from supply/demand mismatch, and a less robust conduction system. Additionally, these patients have rigid atrial baffles that limit preload augmentation, so these patients may not be able to increase their ventricular stroke volume with exercise, resulting in abnormal atrioventricular coupling.

Patients with c-TGA (L-loop TGA, cc-TGA) have atrioventricular discordance and ventricular arterial discordance, so deoxygenated blood passes thru the LV and out the pulmonary artery while oxygenated blood passes to a systemic RV that pumps out the aorta; therefore these patients are not cyanotic. However, most patients with c-TGA have associated cardiac anomalies including ventricular septal defect, pulmonary stenosis, or dysplastic tricuspid (systemic atrioventricular) valves. The prevalence of systemic RV dysfunction in this condition varies based on associated anomalies. In one large multicenter study of adults with c-TGA, systemic RV dysfunction and heart failure were higher with increasing age, the presence of significant associated cardiac lesions, a history of arrhythmia, pacemaker implantation, and prior cardiac surgery.[120] Tricuspid (systemic atrioventricular) valve

regurgitation contributes to systemic RV failure in c-TGA patients. Surgical replacement of the tricuspid valve should be considered before the RV EF falls below 40% and the pulmonary artery systolic pressure rises above 50 mm Hg.[121]

There have been several small case series examining the effectiveness of beta blockers in patients with a systemic RV, with a limited number of patients and follow-up, and variable results (Table 27.1).[122] The studies are underpowered, which makes it difficult to draw definitive conclusions.

The data for use of agents to inhibit the RAAS in patients with systemic RV are also limited (Table 27.1). Therrien reported the results of a prospective, double blind, randomized, placebo-controlled clinical trial of ramipril for 1 year in 17 adults with TGA who had undergone an atrial switch procedure, and found no significant increase in the systemic RV EF.[123] Small trials of angiotensin receptor blockers have also showed conflicting results. Recently, van der Bom reported the results of a multicenter, double-blind, randomized, controlled trial of valsartan compared with placebo in patients with a systemic RV. There was no significant treatment effect of valsartan on RV EF, exercise capacity, or quality of life during the 3-year follow-up.[124] This study concluded that there is no evidence for the routine use of angiotensin receptor blockers in asymptomatic patients with a systemic RV.

Single Ventricle

Most patients with a single functional ventricle undergo the Fontan operation whereby systemic venous return is diverted to the pulmonary arteries without the aid of a subpulmonic pumping chamber (**Fig. 27.8**). This physiology requires chronic elevations in central venous pressure in order to maintain adequate blood flow through the pulmonary circulation. Heart failure is common after the Fontan operation and is more likely in older patients, those with conduction abnormalities, and those who had their surgery in an older era of Fontan operation.[125] Rather than being a single disease, the failing

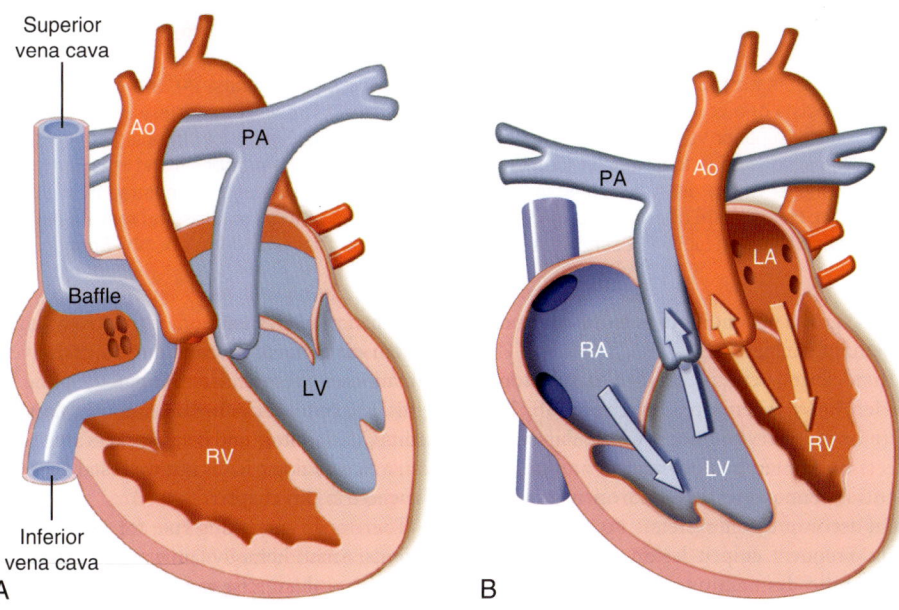

Fig. 27.7 Diagrammatic representation of two types of systemic right ventricles. (A) Complete transposition of the great arteries, status post an atrial switch (Mustard or Senning) procedure. (B) Congenitally corrected transposition of the great arteries, with atrioventricular discordance and ventricular arterial discordance resulting in deoxygenated blood passing from the left ventricle to the pulmonary artery and oxygenated blood reaching the aorta through the systemic right ventricle. *Ao,* Aorta; *LA,* left atrium; *LV,* left ventricle; *PA,* pulmonary artery; *RA,* right atrium; *RV,* right ventricle. (Modified from Libby P. *Essential Atlas of Cardiovascular Disease.* New York, NY: Springer; 2009.)

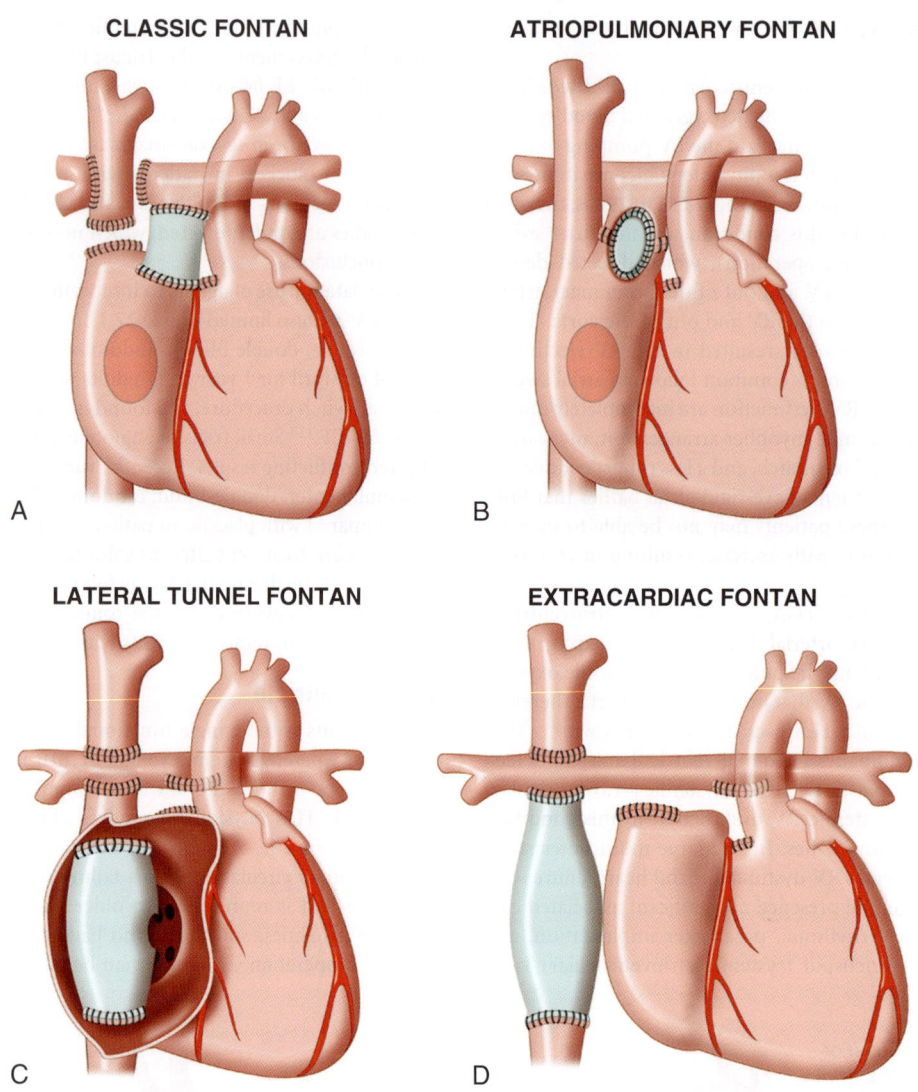

CLASSIC FONTAN

ATRIOPULMONARY FONTAN

A

B

LATERAL TUNNEL FONTAN

EXTRACARDIAC FONTAN

C

D

Fig. 27.8 Diagrammatic representation of the various types of Fontan surgeries. (A) The classic style Fontan, which consists of a conduit from the inferior vena cava to the left pulmonary artery and a classic right Glenn procedure (superior vena cava to the right pulmonary artery). (B) The atriopulmonary connection has been largely abandoned due to dilation of the right atrium predisposing to thrombosis and atrial arrhythmias. (C) Lateral tunnel is widely used, which is, in part, due to the ease of creating a fenestration in this type. (D) Extracardiac conduits are often used as it does not create extensive atrial sutures and may be performed off bypass. (Modified from Libby P. *Essential Atlas of Cardiovascular Disease*. New York, NY: Springer, 2009.)

Fontan circulation is a diverse group of conditions with varying presentation and underlying pathophysiology.[126]

In the Fontan circulation, central venous pressure drives blood through the lungs to the left heart. Therefore, any condition that elevates left atrial pressure or increases pulmonary vascular resistance has deleterious effects on Fontan hemodynamics and necessitates either a rise in central venous pressure, a drop in cardiac output, or the formation of decompressing systemic venous to pulmonary venous collaterals. Frequent culprit lesions that increase Fontan pressure include systolic dysfunction, restrictive ventricular physiology, pulmonary vein stenosis (particularly the left lower pulmonary vein), obstruction within the Fontan circuit (e.g., branch pulmonary artery stenosis), or pressure loss due to hemodynamic inefficiencies in the Fontan circuit. These hemodynamic perturbations are poorly tolerated in Fontan circulation; therefore pathway obstruction and valve dysfunction should be aggressively sought out and treated if found.

Ventricular dysfunction is relatively common in patients with Fontan circulation, perhaps due to excessive afterload and resulting alterations in ventricular-vascular coupling.[127] In patients with systemic LV systolic dysfunction, conventional heart failure treatment with ACE inhibitors and beta blockers are used. Their utility in patients with a morphologic RV is not well established and is discussed in detail elsewhere in this chapter.

There is an increasing role for pulmonary vasodilators in Fontan patients. Small hemodynamic studies have shown improved hemodynamics and exercise performance after a single dose of sildenafil or iloprost.[128,129] The TEMPO trial was a randomized, double-blind, placebo-controlled trial of bosentan in patients with Fontan circulation. After 14 weeks of treatment, subjects on bosentan had a significantly greater improvement in VO$_2$max and exercise time than patients treated with placebo. Of the patients treated with bosentan 25% improved at least one NYHA functional class compared with none of the patients treated with placebo. Importantly, patients in this trial were not required to have pulmonary hypertension or elevated pulmonary vascular resistance prior to enrollment.[130]

Many patients with Fontan circulation have clinical deterioration for reasons other than ventricular dysfunction or pathway obstruction. Atrial tachyarrhythmias, most commonly intraatrial reentrant tachycardia or ectopic atrial tachycardia, are common in patients who had older style Fontan completion prior to the 1990s. Atrial arrhythmias are poorly tolerated in Fontan circulation and should be treated with cardioversion, antiarrhythmic medications, ablation, or surgical conversion to a modern extracardiac Fontan by a center with expertise in the management of arrhythmias in CHD.

Liver disease is common in Fontan patients due to a combination of high central venous pressure, reduced hepatic blood flow, and perioperative liver injury.[88] Liver dysfunction can manifest as radiologic evidence of fibrosis or as overt cirrhosis with ascites and varices. The presence of significant liver dysfunction carries a poor prognosis[131] and should prompt a hemodynamic evaluation. Unfortunately, the presence of significant liver disease can be a barrier to heart transplantation in Fontan patients. Patients with cirrhosis are at risk for perioperative complications such as hepatorenal syndrome, infection, and bleeding. There is no consensus on whether resolution of liver disease is expected after heart transplantation. Multidisciplinary care with an adult CHD doctor, a transplant team, and a hepatologist is needed.

SUMMARY

Heart failure is increasingly recognized in ACHD patients and heart failure–related complications are the most common cause of death in these patients.[3] The prevalence of heart failure is highest in patients with complex anatomy, including single ventricle physiology, TGA, TOF, and those with pulmonary hypertension. The diagnosis of heart failure in ACHD patients may be challenging because patients with CHD, having lived their lives with cardiac disease, may not detect subtle changes in their exercise capacity and may underreport their symptoms. By the time they notice symptoms, the extent of ventricular dysfunction and valve disease may be severe and irreversible. Objective measures of ventricular function through imaging, exercise testing, and serum biomarkers can be very helpful in these patients. The evaluation of heart failure symptoms in an ACHD patient must be tailored to the patient's anatomy and surgical repair, and should include evaluation for residual shunts, baffle stenosis, valvular or conduit dysfunction, and collateral vessels, which may be amenable to interventions. Potential therapies for heart failure in ACHD patients include medical therapies, device therapies, and surgical interventions, such as mechanical assist devices and transplantation. However, guidelines for the management of acquired heart failure are often not applicable to the patient with CHD due to disease heterogeneity, unusual

mechanisms of heart failure, and unique comorbidities in the ACHD patient. Multicenter trials are needed to better define the appropriate therapies for this growing group of patients and a multidisciplinary team with expertise in ACHD and advanced heart failure is required to manage this challenging population.

KEY REFERENCES

4. Diller GP, Kempny A, Alonso-Gonzalez R, Swan L, Uebing A, Li W, et al. Survival prospects and circumstances of death in contemporary adult congenital heart disease patients under follow-up at a large tertiary centre. *Circulation.* 2015;132(22):2118–2125.

6. Stout KK, Broberg CS, Book WM, Cecchin F, Chen JM, Dimopoulos K, et al. Chronic heart failure in congenital heart disease: a scientific statement from the American Heart Association. *Circulation.* 2016;133(8):770–801.

27. Inuzuka R, Diller GP, Borgia F, Benson L, Tay EL, Alonso-Gonzalez R, et al. Comprehensive use of cardiopulmonary exercise testing identifies adults with congenital heart disease at increased mortality risk in the medium term. *Circulation.* 2012;125(2):250–259.

73. Davies RR, Russo MJ, Yang J, Quaegebeur JM, Mosca RS, Chen JM. Listing and transplanting adults with congenital heart disease. *Circulation.* 2011;123(7):759–767.

86. Alshawabkeh LI, Hu N, Carter KD, Opotowsky AR, Light-McGroary K, Cavanaugh JE, et al. Wait-list outcomes for adults with congenital heart disease listed for heart transplantation in the U.S. *J Am Coll Cardiol.* 2016;68(9):908–917.

93. Simpson KE, Esmaeeli A, Khanna G, White F, Turnmelle Y, Eghtesady P, et al. Liver cirrhosis in Fontan patients does not affect 1-year post-heart transplant mortality or markers of liver function. *J Heart Lung Transplant.* 2014;33(2):170–177.

115. Bokma JP, Winter MM, van Dijk AP, Vliegen HW, van Melle JP, Meijboom F, et al. Effect of Losartan on RV dysfunction: results from the Double-Blind, randomized REDEFINE trial in adults with repaired tetralogy of Fallot. *Circulation.* 2017.

121. Mongeon FP, Connolly HM, Dearani JA, Li Z, Warnes CA. Congenitally corrected transposition of the great arteries ventricular function at the time of systemic atrioventricular valve replacement predicts long-term ventricular function. *J Am Coll Cardiol.* 2011;57(20):2008–2017.

124. van der Bom T, Winter MM, Bouma BJ, Groenink M, Vliegen HW, Pieper PG, et al. Effect of valsartan on systemic right ventricular function: a double-blind, randomized, placebo-controlled pilot trial. *Circulation.* 2013;127(3):322–330.

130. Hebert A, Mikkelsen UR, Thilen U, Idorn L, Jensen AS, Nagy E, et al. Bosentan improves exercise capacity in adolescents and adults after Fontan operation: the TEMPO [Treatment With Endothelin Receptor Antagonist in Fontan Patients, a Randomized, Placebo-Controlled, Double-Blind Study Measuring Peak Oxygen Consumption] study. *Circulation.* 2014;130(23):2021–2030.

The full reference list for this chapter is available on ExpertConsult.

Heart Failure as a Consequence of Viral and Nonviral Myocarditis

Dennis M. McNamara

In the attempt to diagnose heart disease more accurately, the term myocarditis is wisely being abandoned in large part; we must remember, nevertheless, that there does exist such a condition as myocarditis. . . .

Paul Dudley White[1]

Dr. White's concerns about the "abandonment" of the term *myocarditis* were unfounded, and over half a century after his initial observations, myocarditis remains an important pathologic term defining of diverse set of cardiac disorders involving primary myocardial inflammation. For his readership in the 1950s, the primary infectious causes of myocardial inflammation were rheumatic fever and diphtheroids, for which effective antibiotic therapies were later developed. In the present day, an ever-changing group of viral etiologies has proven much more difficult to eradicate. Acute myocardial inflammation plays a critical role in viral clearing, but in chronic pathologic states inflammation may play a role in the pathogenesis of nonischemic cardiomyopathy. While immune suppression plays a therapeutic role in specific subsets of myocarditis, for the majority of cases there is no proven benefit.

Although infectious causes remain important, the category of myocarditis includes a diverse set of disorders for which there is no discernible infectious cause, from transient myocardial dysfunction with allergic eosinophilic myocarditis to the progressive myocyte destruction that characterizes giant cell myocarditis (GCM). This chapter will discuss the pathogenesis of heart failure from viral and nonviral forms of myocarditis, the current practice of supportive heart failure treatment, the hope for future targeted therapeutics, and in the case of fulminant myocarditis, the role of mechanical therapy as a bridge to recovery. Despite decades of clinical and basic investigation since Paul Dudley White's initial observations,[1] the diagnosis and treatment of myocarditis remain extremely challenging.

HISTORY

The French pathologist Corvisart described "carditis" in 1806 as an important clinical syndrome, which most commonly was acute and fatal, but could develop into more "chronic organic disease."[2] The term *carditis* was later refined to *myocarditis*, first introduced by Sobernheim in 1837,[3] to describe the myocardial inflammation presumed to be the cause of most nonvalvular cardiac dysfunction. By the latter part of the nineteenth century it was increasingly recognized that primary myocardial inflammation was responsible for only a small subset of nonvalvular cardiac dysfunction, because coronary disease and hypertensive heart disease were far more common causes. In contrast to the previous nondiscriminant use of the term, attempts at more accurate cardiac diagnosis of myocarditis in the twentieth century led to a marked diminishment in its recognition.

The emergence of endomyocardial biopsy (EMB) in the 1960s as a diagnostic tool[4] allowed clinicians to delineate cellular inflammation of the myocardium, and fueled the hope that this heterogeneous group of disorders could now be classified into histopathologic subsets with distinct therapies and outcomes. The Dallas criteria[5] were developed in 1986 by leading cardiac pathologists to standardize the histologic definition of lymphocytic myocarditis (LM), the most commonly observed form of cellular inflammation. They defined *borderline myocarditis* as mononuclear cell infiltrates without myocyte necrosis (**Fig. 28.1**) and *myocarditis* as cellular infiltration with myocyte necrosis (**Fig. 28.2**). Despite the wide acceptance of these histologic criteria for the pathologic assessment of myocarditis, significant variation in interpretation remained in the practical application.[6] A decade later, the World Health Organization task force defined inflammatory cardiomyopathy as "myocarditis in association with myocardial dysfunction. Myocarditis is an inflammatory disease of the myocardium and is diagnosed by established histologic, immunologic, and immunohistochemical criteria."[7] This task force expanded the definition by adding both quantitative and

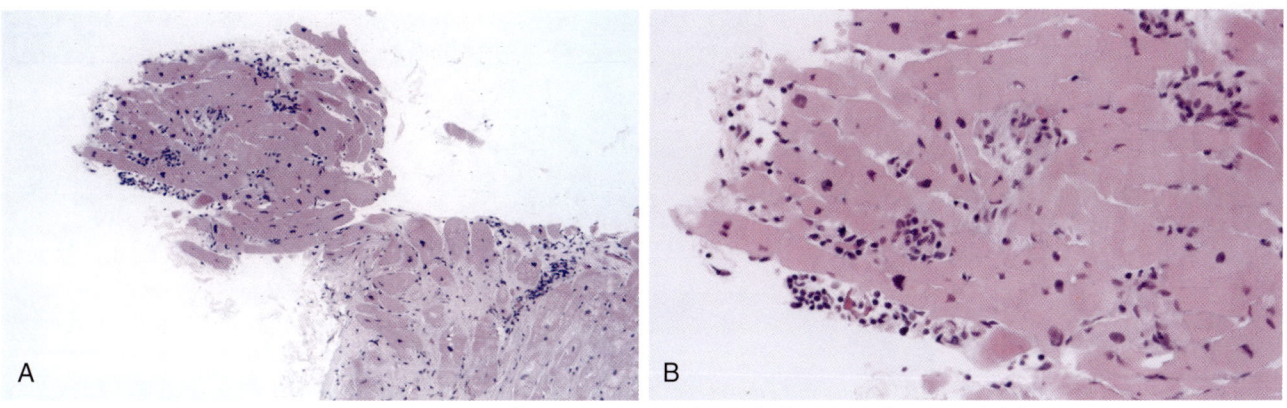

Fig. 28.1 Histopathologic appearance of borderline myocarditis by Dallas criteria (lymphocytic infiltrates without myocyte necrosis) with routine staining with hematoxylin and eosin (H&E) under (A) low power (100×) and (B) high power (350×).

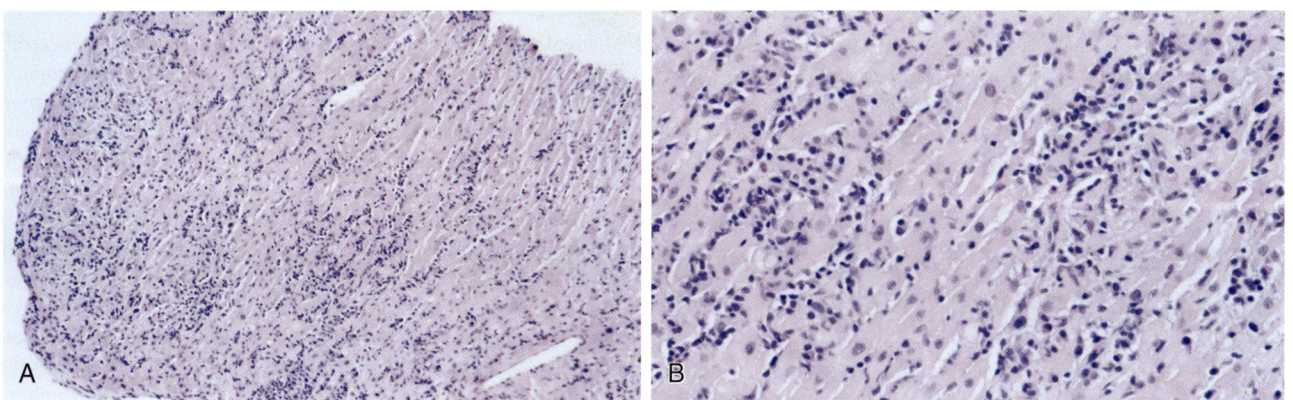

Fig. 28.2 Histopathologic appearance of myocarditis by Dallas criteria (lymphocytic infiltrates with myocyte necrosis) with routine staining with hematoxylin and eosin under (A) low power (100×) and (B) high power (350×).

immunohistochemical criteria for detection of cellular infiltrates and expression of human leukocyte antigen (HLA) class II molecules.

The observed histologic similarity of LM to cardiac allograft rejection led to the hypothesis that a therapeutic strategy of immunosuppression would improve clinical outcomes. When the Myocarditis Treatment Trial (MTT) demonstrated no benefit,[8] the absence of a histologically guided therapy led to a diminished role for EMB, and native cardiac biopsy is not commonly performed in the United States. Efforts continue to improve the diagnostic utility of EMB with the addition of molecular diagnostics to detect viral nucleic acids and routine immunohistochemistry to improve the specificity, but this is only performed at selected centers.[9] The histologic and clinical diversity of myocarditis remains a challenge in terms of the development of targeted therapeutics.

VIRAL ETIOLOGIES

The most common infectious agents initiating myocarditis in North America are viral pathogens (**Table 28.1**), although the dominant viral species continues to evolve over time. Enteroviruses were first described in clinical and serologic studies decades ago[10] and remain a major cause of myocarditis in infants and children.[11] In adults, adenovirus, influenza A and B, and herpesviruses also have been implicated as important viral pathogens,[12-14] whereas hepatitis C has been implicated in Asia,[15] but less commonly reported in case series in the United States. Over the past decade, influenza Heand erythroviruses, such as parvovirus B19,[16] emerged as two important pathogens associated with

TABLE 28.1 Viral Causes of Inflammatory Cardiomyopathy and Myocarditis
Parvovirus (Parvovirus B19)
Adenoviruses
Influenza A and B
Enteroviruses (coxsackie A and B)
Herpesvirus (human herpesvirus-6)
Varicella-zoster
Cytomegalovirus
Epstein-Barr virus
Hepatitis B and C virus
Human immunodeficiency virus
Poliovirus
Variola virus (smallpox)
Rubella virus
Echovirus
Polio

myocarditis. The changing viral milieu represents a considerable challenge for developing therapeutic efforts targeting specific viral pathogens. Effective viral therapies can diminish viral pathogenesis. For example, human immunodeficiency virus (HIV) infection has been associated with myocarditis and dilated cardiomyopathy (DCM)[17]; however, the incidence of HIV-associated cardiomyopathy has been diminished with more aggressive antiviral therapies against HIV.[18]

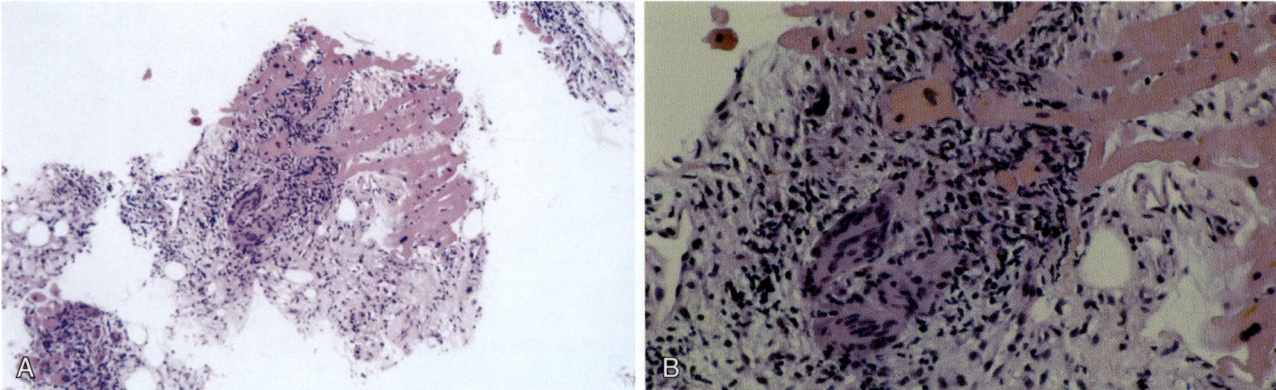

Fig. 28.3 Histopathologic appearance of giant cell myocarditis (multinucleated giant cell) with routine staining with hematoxylin and eosin under (A) low power (100×) and (B) high power (350×).

In the developing world, bacterial pathogens remain important causes as myocarditis as a complication of rheumatic fever and diphtheroids is much more prevalent.[19,20] In Central and South America, the most common infectious agent is the protozoa *Trypanosoma cruzi*, the causative agent for Chagas' disease, which is endemic in certain areas[21] and may affect 15 to 20 million people.[22] This disorder is not seen in North America without a travel history to endemic areas. In immunocompromised hosts, other pathogens, such as toxoplasmosis[23] and aspergillus,[24] can cause myocardial inflammation but generally in the setting of a systemic infection and not as isolated myocarditis.

AUTOIMMUNE (NONVIRAL) ETIOLOGIES

There are several autoimmune forms of myocardial inflammation for which no infectious agent can be identified. For certain diagnoses, histopathology combined with the clinical setting can point toward targeted treatments. Multinucleated giant cells in the myocardium in the setting of fulminant myocarditis suggests the diagnosis of GCM (**Fig. 28.3**), a progressive and destructive form of myocarditis with a high mortality rate on conventional therapy[25] but responsive to immunosuppressive therapy.[26] Finding similar multinucleated granulomas in the myocardium, but with few other inflammatory cells in a more compensated patient, may suggest systemic sarcoidosis, a disorder responsive to treatment with corticosteroids.[27]

Eosinophilic predominance of inflammatory cells in the myocardium with new myocardial dysfunction may suggest an allergic hypersensitivity myocarditis.[28-30] Several pharmacologic agents, including tricyclic antidepressants, antipsychotics, and cephalosporin, have been implicated as triggering eosinophilic myocarditis. This disorder is generally self-limited, and the myocardium will recover with removal of the triggering agent. For persistent myocarditis in the setting of peripheral eosinophilia, a short course of corticosteroids can be considered. Chronic peripheral eosinophilia without a clear initiating agent should merit consideration of a systemic syndrome such as Churg–Strauss vasculitis[31] or hypereosinophilic syndrome (HES),[32] for which immunosuppressive therapy is generally indicated.

Myocarditis may also be a clinical feature of several systemic autoimmune disorders. Systemic lupus erythematosus (SLE),[33] dermatopolymyositis,[34] and rheumatoid arthritis[35] also have been associated with inflammatory myocarditis. In general, immunosuppressive therapy is directed toward the systemic autoimmune disorder and will result in the recovery of myocardial function as well. EMB is rarely performed, except in cases where the systemic disorder is quiescent and the finding of myocardial inflammation may be the only indication for immunosuppressive therapy.

PATHOGENESIS IN MURINE MODELS

Much of what is known of the basic pathogenesis of viral myocarditis is derived from murine models of inoculation with the cardiotropic coxsackie group B virus[36] or encephalomyocarditis virus[37] into susceptible strains. The viral particles are taken up by myocytes via receptor-mediated endocytosis. Translation of viral proteins and replication of viral particles can result in cell lysis within 3 days (**Fig. 28.4**) before the initiation of myocardial inflammation. Macrophage activation results in cytokine expression, including interferon-γ[38,39] and the activation of natural killer (NK) cells,[40] both of which limit viral replication. Infiltrates of antigen-specific T lymphocytes including T-helper (CD4+) cells and cytotoxic T lymphocyte (CD8+) cells are seen within 7 days of infection.[41] Recognition of viral peptides by cytotoxic T cells results in cellular toxicity of virally infected cells.[42] Up to 20% of infiltrating lymphocytes are B cells, and neutralizing antibodies are important in viral clearing although not in cytotoxicity. Viral particles are no longer evident within 15 days of the initial inoculation, although inflammatory infiltrates may persist for 90 days.[43] Viral nucleic acid can be detected after 90 days in only a small percentage of virally infected mice; however, long-term ventricular dilation and remodeling may develop and are associated with myocardial fibrosis. Myocardial inflammation followed by ventricular dilation and fibrosis occurs in transgenic mice overexpressing TNF-α,[44] and in murine models using antimyosin antibodies,[45] demonstrating the role of chronic inflammation in the pathogenesis of nonischemic DCM.

CLINICAL PRESENTATION

Acute myocarditis will typically present with a variety of symptoms, including dyspnea, chest pain, palpitations, syncope, and near syncope, and when associated with left ventricular (LV) dysfunction, most commonly presents with signs of heart failure.[46] A presentation with dyspnea or chest pain associated with electrocardiogram abnormalities[47] or an elevation of cardiac enzymes[48,49] may be the first sign of a possible myocarditis or myopericarditis. The cardiac examination may be unremarkable or may reveal a pericardial rub. Tachycardia, relative hypotension, jugular venous distention, and peripheral edema may suggest more significant hemodynamic compromise. Chest examination may reveal congestion, and decreased breath sounds are suggestive of pleural effusions.

Electrocardiographic findings are generally diffuse and nonspecific. PR depression and global ST elevation may be seen in cases with an associated pericarditis. Low voltage may be evident, particularly in subjects with an associated pericardial effusion. Heart block, ventricular tachycardia, or a new bundle branch block are all suggestive of a more fulminant disorder. Evaluation of biomarkers may reveal an

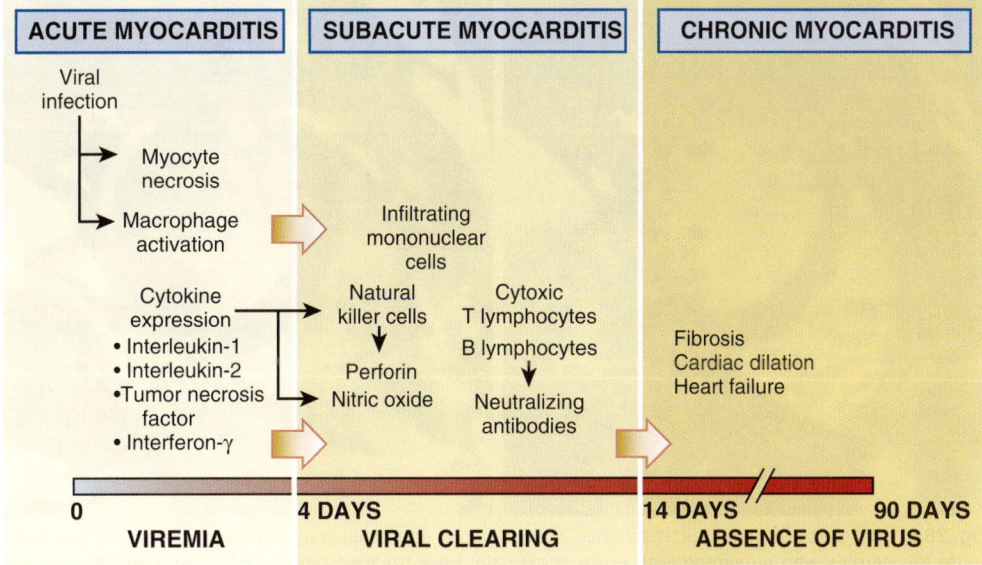

Fig. 28.4 Timeline of progression in murine models from initial viral inoculation to acute myocarditis to subacute myocarditis to chronic myocarditis. (From Feldman AM, McNamara D. Myocarditis. *N Engl J Med.* 2000;343[19]:1388–1398.)

elevation in cardiac troponin and brain natriuretic peptide. More fulminant myocarditis may be associated with elevated liver function tests and a compromise of renal function. Chest x-ray may be unremarkable or show evidence of heart failure and cardiomegaly.

CARDIAC IMAGING (SEE ALSO CHAPTER 32)

Transthoracic echocardiography remains a critically important tool in the evaluation of myocarditis[50,51] and frequently provides the first evidence of ventricular impairment. Systolic dysfunction is generally global; however, it may be segmental and can mimic ischemic disease. Pericardial effusion may be present and provide supportive evidence of an inflammatory process. In severe myocarditis, the ventricular walls may be thickened due to edema; however, routine echocardiography is limited in terms of characterization of the myocardial tissue itself. The dimensions of the LV diameter generally demonstrate minimal LV enlargement and remodeling for an acute presentation, although remodeling may be more evident in more chronic insidious forms.

Cardiac magnetic resonance (CMR) imaging has had an increasing role in the diagnostic evaluation of myocarditis given its ability to characterize cardiac tissue and assess for inflammation (**Fig. 28.5**).[52,53] The use of gadolinium on T1-weighted images allows for assessment of hyperemia and capillary leak with early enhancement, and more significant tissue injury and necrosis with late gadolinium enhancement (LGE). The anatomic distribution of gadolinium enhancement also assists in diagnosis, because an epicardial distribution of gadolinium enhancement is suggestive of myocarditis, whereas an endocardial predominance is more consistent with ischemic injury. The addition of T2-weighted images provides an assessment of myocardial water, and increased content is likely a marker of ongoing edema and inflammation.

The diagnostic criteria for myocarditis by CMR were established by a consensus panel, and the "Lake Louise" criteria were published in 2009.[54] These criteria noted that combining data from all three tissue markers, early and LGE on T1-weighted images and myocardial edema by global and regional T2 relaxation times (**Table 28.2**), increased the utility of CMR and that myocardial inflammation could be predicted with a diagnostic accuracy of 78%. When only gadolinium

TABLE 28.2 Cardiac Magnetic Resonance Imaging Criteria for Myocarditis (Lake Louise Consensus Criteria)

In the clinical setting of suspected myocarditis, the cardiac magnetic resonance (CMR) imaging findings consistent with the diagnosis of myocardial inflammation (at least 2 of 3 criteria) are:

1. Regional or global myocardial increase in signal intensity in T2-weighted images
2. Increased global myocardial early gadolinium enhancement ratio between myocardium and skeletal muscle in gadolinium-enhanced T1-weighted images
3. At least one focal lesion with nonischemic regional distribution in inversion recovery-prepared gadolinium-enhanced T1-weighted images (late gadolinium enhancement [LGE])

CMR is consistent with myocyte injury and/or scar caused by myocardial inflammation, if:

- Criterion 3 is present.

Repeat CMR study between 1 and 2 weeks after the initial CMR study is recommended, if:

- None of the criteria is present, but the onset of symptoms has been very recent, and there is strong clinical evidence for myocardial inflammation.
- One of the criteria is present.
- The presence of left ventricular dysfunction or pericardial effusion provides additional, supportive evidence for myocarditis.

Modified from Friedrich MG, Sechtem U, Schulz-Menger J, et al. for the International Consensus Group on Cardiovascular Magnetic Resonance in Myocarditis. Cardiovascular magnetic resonance in myocarditis: a JACC White Paper. *J Am Coll Cardiol.* 2009;53(17):1475–1487.

enhancement on T1 images was used, CMR assessment would still yield an accuracy of 68%. The time required for data acquisition and the need to transport the patient to the imaging facility limits the ability of CMR to assess the most critically ill subjects. In addition, contrast imaging with gadolinium essential to the evaluation of myocardial inflammation cannot be performed in subjects with renal dysfunction.

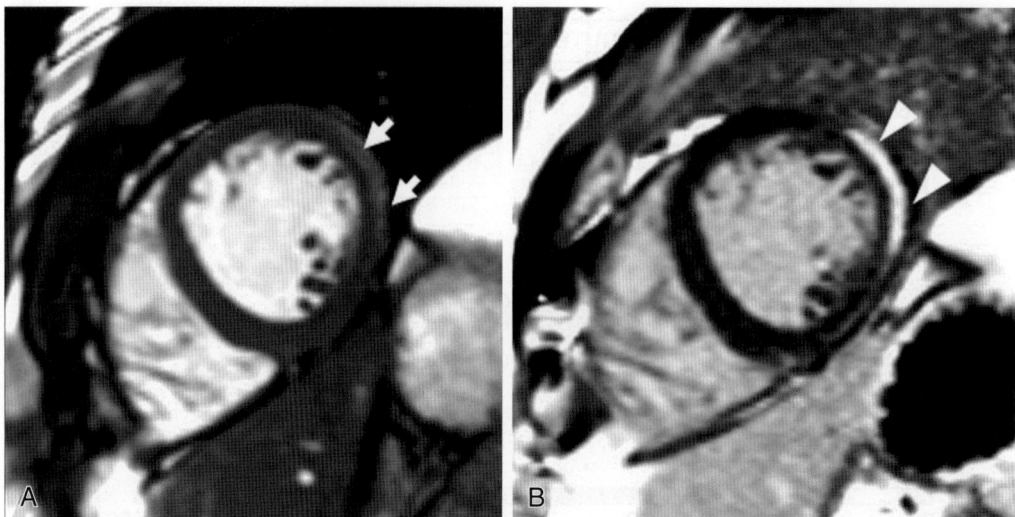

Fig. 28.5 Cardiovascular magnetic resonance midventricular short-axis images from a 21-year-old man with acute myocarditis who presented with acute chest pain, peak troponin I of 15 ng/mL, and angiographically normal-appearing coronary arteries. (A) Myocardial edema *(white arrows)* in the epicardial portion of the inferolateral wall on T2-weighted images. (B) Necrosis on late gadolinium enhancement images in the same region *(white arrowheads)* with uptake of contrast due to loss of cell membrane integrity (20 minutes following 0.2 mmol/kg of gadoteridol). (Courtesy Timothy C. Wong, MD, MS, and Erik B. Schelbert, MD, MS.)

ENDOMYOCARDIAL BIOPSY (SEE ALSO CHAPTER 34)

Although the evaluation of myocardial histology by EMB remains the gold standard for the diagnosis of myocarditis, the diagnostic yield of biopsy remains low. In the large published biopsy series of over 2000 subjects screened for the MTT with EMB, the prevalence of LM was only 10%.[8] Myocardial histology generally does not affect treatment strategies, and although there are notable exceptions, such as GCM, this is far less prevalent than LM and evident in no more than 2% of subjects who had biopsies[55] in published series. The current American Heart Association (AHA) and the European Society of Cardiology guidelines[56] for the indication for EMB are driven by the need to detect histologic diagnoses, such as GCM, which change therapeutic recommendations. These guidelines give the strongest recommendation for EMB in cases of acute fulminant myocarditis (acute myocarditis associated with hemodynamic compromise) and in acute myocarditis associated with ventricular tachycardia or heart block (**Table 28.3**). Although the enhancement of EMB through molecular diagnostics remains an area of research, the role of therapies guided by molecular diagnostics remains uncertain.

EMB does have defined risks, most notably the risk of cardiac perforation and tamponade, which can occur in up to 1% of subjects. These risks are diminished when performed by an experienced operator. The risks of the procedure are increased by the hemodynamic instability of suspected fulminant myocarditis, and EMB in this scenario should be performed by an experienced operator at a tertiary center with the ability to provide mechanical support if required.

MYOCARDITIS MIMICKING ACUTE CORONARY SYNDROME

With the management of myocardial infarction and acute coronary syndromes emphasizing early angiography, the syndrome of myocardial infarction with *nonobstructive* coronary artery disease (MINOCA) is increasingly recognized, and represents 5% to 10% of all subjects presenting with myocardial infarction.[57] While there are multiple potential etiologies for MINOCA including coronary spasm, resolving thrombus, and Takotsubo cardiomyopathy, acute myocarditis

TABLE 28.3 Major Indication for Endomyocardial Biopsy
1. New-onset heart failure of less than 2 weeks' duration associated with a normal size or dilated left ventricle and hemodynamic compromise: recommendation class I, level of evidence B.
2. New-onset heart failure of 2 weeks' to 3 months' duration associated with a dilated left ventricle and new ventricular arrhythmias, second- or third-degree heart block, or failure to respond to usual care within 2 to 3 weeks: recommendation class 1, level of evidence B.
3. Heart failure of greater than 3 months' duration associated with a dilated left ventricle and new ventricular arrhythmias, second- or third-degree heart block, or failure to respond to usual care within 2 to 3 weeks: recommendation class IIa, level of evidence C.
4. Heart failure associated with a DCM of any duration associated with suspected allergic reaction of eosinophilia: recommendation class IIa, level of evidence C.

Class 1 recommendation, condition for which there is evidence of general agreement that a given procedure is beneficial, useful, and effective; *Class IIa,* condition for which there is conflicting evidence but for which the weight of evidence/opinion is in favor of usefulness/efficacy; *level of evidence B,* limited number of randomized trials, nonrandomized studies, and registries; *level of evidence C,* primarily expert opinion. *DCM,* Dilated cardiomyopathy.
Modified from Cooper LT, Baughman KL, Feldman AM, et al. The role of endomyocardial biopsy in the management of cardiovascular disease: a scientific statement from the American Heart Association, the American College of Cardiology, and the European Society of Cardiology. Endorsed by the Heart Failure Society of America and the Heart Failure Association of the European Society of Cardiology. *J Am Coll Cardiol.* 2007;50(19):1914–1931.

is the most common etiology documented, particularly in younger patients.[58] In subjects with MINOCA who undergo CMR, more than one-third typically have imaging results consistent with acute myocarditis.[59] Early myocardial recovery within the index hospitalization is common for cases of MINOCA found to be the result of myocarditis. EMB is used only selectively for more fulminant cases with hemodynamic compromise for which the possible diagnosis of GCM has both prognostic and therapeutic implications.

MEDICAL THERAPY

For myocarditis associated with LV dysfunction, therapy is supportive. Treatment with β-receptor antagonists and with either angiotensin-converting enzyme (ACE) inhibitors or angiotensin receptor antagonists remains the mainstay of therapy.[60] Digoxin should be avoided, as it has been shown to worsen injury in animal models.[61] Diuretics can be used for congestion and fluid overload. For subjects with severe LV dysfunction, anticoagulation should be considered and is definitively indicated for those subjects with evidence of LV thrombus or those presenting with a thromboembolic event.

For subjects with suspected myocarditis and LV dysfunction, the management of potential arrhythmias should be tempered by the possibility of recovery. Treatment with an implantable cardioverter defibrillator (ICD) should be deferred, given the potential for resolution.[62] An ICD is indicated for subjects presenting with "aborted sudden death," in which the placement of an ICD is required for secondary prevention. For subjects presenting with complex ventricular arrhythmias without sudden death, a temporary external defibrillator or life vest can be considered as an alternative to a more permanent device.

Systolic function recovers rapidly within weeks to months in many subjects with recent onset cardiomyopathy,[63] and the role of long-term therapy with ACE inhibitors and β-blockers in subjects who have recovered remains controversial. In subjects who have complete normalization of systolic function after a documented transient episode of myocarditis, medical therapy with ACE inhibitors and β-receptor antagonists can be gradually weaned off and discontinued with careful monitoring for subsequent declines in left ventricular ejection fraction (LVEF). Subjects with persistent abnormalities of either systolic function or remodeling (increased LV diastolic diameter) should be treated long-term with heart failure therapy with either ACE inhibitors,

β-receptor antagonists, or both. In subjects whose systolic function has completely recovered, abnormalities of diastolic function may persist for months[64] and may result in persistent symptoms of exertional dyspnea and fluid retention.

IMMUNOSUPPRESSIVE THERAPY

The role of immunosuppressive therapy remains controversial. While anecdotal reports or small case series may suggest benefit from immunosuppressive therapy, these must be viewed with caution given the high rate of spontaneous recovery for most subjects with suspected myocarditis. In several previous randomized trials, the role of immunosuppressive or immune modulatory therapy was evaluated in acute myocarditis or recent-onset nonischemic cardiomyopathy (with and without myocarditis) and failed to provide evidence of therapeutic benefit (**Table 28.4**).

The first randomized trial of immune suppression for inflammatory heart disease was a National Heart, Lung and Blood Institute-sponsored investigation of several months of oral prednisone for subjects with heart failure caused by DCM. The results demonstrated a modest but significant improvement in LV ejection fraction for subjects treated with steroid therapy with an "inflammatory" biopsy; however, the impact was modest, was not sustained after discontinuing treatment, and did not appear to warrant the side effects of therapy.[65] The MTT evaluated treatment with prednisone and cyclosporine in subjects with biopsy-proven LM. In the MTT, there was no benefit evident for immune suppression, and both the LV function ejection fraction at 6 months and overall survival during follow-up were statistically no different in the treatment group receiving cyclosporine and prednisone from those receiving the placebo.[8]

Immune globulin was reported to be effective for the treatment of pediatric myocarditis in a large single-center series with historical controls.[66] This led to the exploration of its use in adults and reports of efficacy in case series with recent-onset nonischemic cardiomyopathy[67] and peripartum cardiomyopathy (PPCM).[68] The

TABLE 28.4	Randomized Trials of Immune Modulation or Immune Suppression in Myocarditis and Inflammatory Cardiomyopathy					
Reference	**Entry Criteria**	**Agent Studied**	**Randomized**	**Outcome Measures**	**Result**
Parrillo et al.[65]	Subjects with dilated cardiomyopathy divided into reactive versus nonreactive based on biopsy	Prednisone	102	Change in EF at 3 months	Modest benefit overall (4 EF units vs. 2 EF units with placebo); no benefit in nonreactive patients
Mason et al.[8] (Myocarditis treatment trial)	Lymphocytic myocarditis	Prednisone and cyclosporine	111	Change in EF at 6 months	No significant effect (increase of 10 EF units vs. 7 EF units with placebo)
McNamara et al. (IMAC Trial)[69]	History <6 months; subjects with recent onset with and without myocarditis	Immune globulin	62	Change in EF at 6 months	No treatment effect (increase of 14 EF units in both groups)
Wojnicz et al.[72]	History >6 months; increased HLA expression on biopsy	Azathioprine and prednisone	84	LVEF after 3 months	Significant difference in LVEF (0.36 with immune suppression vs. 0.27 with placebo, $P < .001$)
Frustaci et al.[73] (TIMIC study)	History >6 months; lymphocytic myocarditis and viral negative	Azathioprine and prednisone	85	LVEF at 6 months	Significant difference in 6 months (0.46 with immune suppression vs. 0.21 with placebo, $P < .001$)

EF, Ejection fraction; *HLA*, human leukocyte antigen; *IMAC*, Intervention in Myocarditis Virand Acute Cardiomyopathy; *LVEF*, left ventricular ejection fraction; *TIMIC*, Tailored Immunosuppression in Inflammatory Cardiomyopathy (TIMIC) study.

Intervention in Myocarditis and Acute Cardiomyopathy (IMAC) trial evaluated the efficacy of intravenous immune globulin in adults in a multicenter placebo-controlled investigation and failed to demonstrate benefit.[69] The MTT and IMAC investigations targeted very acute subjects, and in both investigations spontaneous recovery in the placebo group limited the study power to determine the efficacy.

ACUTE VERSUS CHRONIC INFLAMMATORY CARDIOMYOPATHY

The inability to improve outcomes with immune suppression in acute myocarditis trials may reflect the fact that acute inflammation plays a beneficial role in viral clearing. Indeed, subjects with the histologically most severe form of LM—so-called fulminant myocarditis—have better long-term outcomes than more subacute indolent forms.[70] In fulminant myocarditis, the clinical inflammation generally resolves rapidly and LV systolic function recovers in parallel. This potential for full recovery with fulminant LM with only supportive care supports the concept that inflammation in the acute setting indeed may be protective. In contrast, in later stages, persistent chronic inflammation may plays a more pathologic role. In a large study from Germany of subjects with chronic DCM undergoing myocardial biopsy, those with evidence of persistent inflammation by cell markers and immunohistochemistry had poorer outcomes overall than those without inflammation.[71]

Two single-center studies from Europe evaluated immunosuppression in more chronic inflammatory heart disease and demonstrated potential benefit for therapeutic intervention in this context (see Table 28.4). The first study from Poland performed EMB on 202 subjects with a nonischemic DCM of at least 6 months' duration, and performed immunohistochemical staining for the expression of HLA antigens. The 84 subjects with strong expression of HLA antigens were defined as "inflammatory" and randomized to 3 months of treatment with either steroids plus azathioprine or a placebo, and were followed for up to 2 years.[72] There was no difference in hospitalization-free survival; however, LVEF improved significantly by 3 months with immune suppression compared with placebo, and this improvement was maintained for the 2-year follow-up. In a second Italian study in chronic myocarditis, the Tailored Immunosuppression in Inflammatory Cardiomyopathy (TIMIC) study,[73] 85 subjects with chronic heart failure (>6 months) and an EMB that demonstrated both active LM and no evidence of viral nucleic acids were randomized to azathioprine plus prednisone for 6 months versus a placebo. LVEF at 6 months improved almost 20 ejection fraction (EF) units in the treatment group and declined in the placebo group. These single-center investigations in cohorts with chronic nonischemic cardiomyopathy support the hypothesis that immune suppression may be more beneficial in the chronic pathologic phase of myocardial inflammation.

VIRAL DIAGNOSTICS AND TARGETED THERAPEUTICS

Molecular diagnostics have been used over the past two decades to evaluate for the presence of viral nucleic acids in EMB specimens. In several European investigations, these data have been used to triage subjects into therapeutic pathways. In the TIMIC trial, only patients with myocarditis who were "virus negative" were randomized to immune suppression. In subjects who were "viral positive" on EMB, small series have attempted to tailor therapy to the specific virus detected.[74,75] In the absence of controlled data, current European guidelines note the potential for antiviral therapy but do not advocate specific treatments.[76] The European Study of Epidemiology and Treatment of Cardiac Inflammatory Diseases

(ESETCID) is a multicenter investigation initiated almost two decades ago to provide controlled data for the efficacy of molecular-targeted therapeutic strategies. This placebo-controlled, multiple-arm therapeutic trial randomized viral-negative subjects into immune suppression with azathioprine and prednisone, enteroviral-positive patients to interferon-α, cytomegalovirus-positive subjects to high-dose immune globulin, and adenoviral or parvo B19-positive subjects to intermediate-dose immune globulin.[77] Reports of the first 3000 subjects screened by EMB for this complicated randomization strategy found eligible subjects with myocarditis and reduced left ventricular ejection fraction in only 6%, and viral nucleic acid in only 11%.[78] A randomized trial of interferon beta-1b in subjects with chronic DCM and EMB confirmation of viral genomes (adenovirus, enterovirus, or parvovirus B19) was recently completed.[79] This investigation suggested treatment with interferon-β facilitated viral clearance and improved heart failure symptoms. A randomized trial evaluating the impact of high dose immune globulin on improvement in LVEF in subjects with chronic cardiomyopathy and parvovirus B19 genomes on EMB is ongoing.[80] The complexity of these molecular diagnostic strategies has limited the ability to validate these targeted strategies, and prevented their adoption outside of specialized centers.

European guidelines emphasize the utility of EMB for the diagnose of myocarditis as well as for "safe (infection negative) immunosuppression and antiviral therapy."[76] US guidelines are more selective,[81] and most cases of myocarditis are diagnosed by clinical criteria and CMR[82] and do not undergo EMB. Enhancements of peripheral diagnostics have improved the ability to determine viral etiologies in cases with acute myocarditis. This has fueled an increase in anecdotal reports of viral-specific therapies in fulminant cases, including influenza B treated with oseltamivir,[83] parvovirus B19 with immune globulin,[84] and CMV with ganciclovir.[85] Despite these reports, the role of targeted antiviral therapy remains uncertain.

MECHANICAL SUPPORT AND RECOVERY

In cases of fulminant myocarditis, mechanical support has been used to provide hemodynamic support and to allow full recovery (**see also Chapter 45**). Subjects with fulminant myocarditis often present with cardiogenic shock and associated multisystem failure. Such patients may require full cardiac support, which can be instituted using either temporary biventricular device support or extracorporeal membrane oxygenation (ECMO). Even in such critically ill patients, mechanical support can allow successful cardiac rescue, with most subjects surviving to leave the hospital with normal cardiac function.[86]

The timetable for recovery from fulminant myocarditis varies from weeks to months, and when support is anticipated for more than several weeks, a chronic long-term left ventricular assist device (LVAD) is required. Factors predicting a greater likelihood of recovery include a short duration of symptoms before LVAD support and the absence of LV remodeling preimplant (i.e., a smaller LV end-diastolic diameter).[87] In a recent multicenter study of ventricular recovery on LVAD, 8 of 11 subjects with recent-onset cardiomyopathy with less than 4 months of symptoms at the time of LVAD implant were successfully recovered and explanted.[88]

PEDIATRIC MYOCARDITIS

There is a greater likelihood of infectious viral causes in pediatric myocarditis, in part because the prevalence of noninfectious causes is much lower in children. Children are more likely to have an inflammatory biopsy and have a greater probability of recovery.[89,90] The specific viral species involved have changed over time and closely mirror those seen in adults. While enteroviruses were once predominant, they were later surpassed first by adenoviruses[91]and more recently by erythroviruses, in particular parvovirus B19.[92] Notably, children have not been included in previous randomized trials of immune suppression or immune modulation. As a result, case series and anecdotal experience dictate practice, and children are more likely to be treated with either steroids or immune globulin. Despite the absence of controlled data on the effectiveness of immune modulatory therapies in children, the use of these therapies remains common practice,[93] with immune globulin used in more than 70% of cases in a recent study of tertiary referral centers, and prednisone used in 25% to 30%.[94]

PERIPARTUM CARDIOMYOPATHY (SEE ALSO CHAPTER 20)

PPCM is a form of nonischemic cardiomyopathy that occurs in women in the peripartum period. An autoimmune pathogenesis has been postulated,[95] triggered by fetal or placental antigens rather than viral. PPCM, which presents at the time maternal cellular immunity is rebounding from the downregulation required for fetal tolerance. The frequency of LM on EMB appears similar to other forms of acute cardiomyopathy.[96] Therapy remains supportive and there is a high probability of ventricular recovery[97] during the first few months postpartum. A recent multicenter investigation of PPCM, Investigation of Pregnancy Associated Cardiomyopathy (IPAC), demonstrated that women presenting with more severe LV dysfunction (an initial LVEF <0.30) had poor outcomes with complete recovery evident in only 37% (**Fig. 28.6**).[98] Analysis of a subset of the IPAC cohort by CMR did not demonstrate evidence of myocardial injury or myocarditis for the majority of women.[99] Examination of circulating cell subsets in women presenting with PPCM demonstrated a decrease in NK cells, but no other changes in cellular immunity.[100] Prolactin plays an important role in the resetting of maternal immunity, and the inhibition of prolactin with the drug bromocriptine has been reported to improve recovery in women with PPCM in case reports[101] and a small, randomized pilot in South Africa.[102] A recent randomized trial in Germany compared treatment with bromocriptine for 1 week to treatment with bromocriptine for 8 weeks, and demonstrated similar recovery in both groups.[103] As this study did not incorporate any standard therapy control group, the actual benefit of bromocriptine therapy beyond standard therapy could not be addressed.

GENOMICS OF MYOCARDITIS AND INFLAMMATORY CARDIOMYOPATHY

Recent analysis of children with acute myocarditis revealed an increased prevalence of homozygous mutations in cardiomyopathy-associated genes, which were present in 12% of the myocarditis cohort compared to less than 1% of controls (**Fig. 28.7**).[104] Prospective studies of subjects with mutations of dystrophin demonstrate a high prevalence of myocarditis by CMR.[105] Whether an increased risk of myocarditis for subjects with cytoskeletal mutations plays a role in the progression to DCM remains unknown. An examination of genomic background in women with PPCM also reveals a high prevalence of cardiomyopathy-associated mutations (15%) with the majority in the structural protein titin.[106] This is consistent with an earlier report of a high prevalence of titin mutations (18%) in subjects with sporadic DCM.[107] These emerging data on the overlap between genetic and inflammatory etiologies demonstrates the complex interplay of genomic predisposition and acquired stressors (e.g., viral infections or pregnancy) in the pathogenesis of myocarditis and DCM.

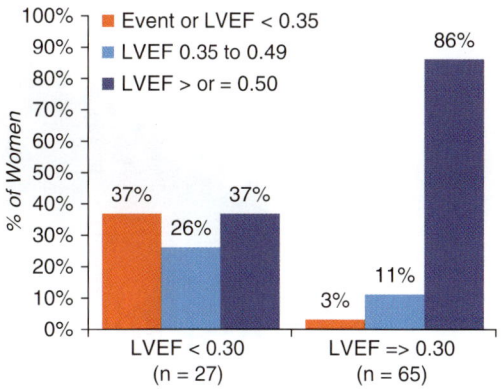

Fig. 28.6 The final outcomes for women presenting with peripartum cardiomyopathy in the Investigation of Pregnancy Associated Cardiomyopathy, based on their initial left ventricular ejection fraction *(LVEF)*. For women with an initial LVEF less than 0.30, only 37% recovered to an LVEF ≥0.50 *(dark blue bars)*, and 37% experienced the poorest outcome *(red bars*, percentage of women with either an event of death or left ventricular assist device implantation, or persistent cardiomyopathy with a final LVEF <0.35). By comparison for women with an LVEF at entry =>0.30, 86% recovered completely and only 3% had the poorest outcomes. From McNamara DM, Elkayam U, Alharethi R, et al. Clinical outcomes in peripartum cardiomyopathy in North America: results of the IPAC study [Investigations of Pregnancy Associated Cardiomyopathy]. *J Am Coll Cardiol*. 2015;66[8]:905–914.

SUMMARY AND FUTURE THERAPEUTIC DIRECTIONS

Myocarditis from both viral and nonviral causes remains an important cause of myocardial dysfunction and heart failure. Current therapy for acute myocarditis with LV dysfunction remains the medical treatment for heart failure, and the role of immune suppression is limited to patients with GCM or those with a systemic autoimmune disorder. Although many subjects with acute myocarditis recover completely with no long-term sequelae, a percentage are left with chronic nonischemic cardiomyopathy and the clinical consequence of progressive heart failure.

The high spontaneous recovery rate of acute myocarditis on contemporary therapy limits the ability to evaluate novel therapies designed to facilitate myocardial recovery. Therefore recent clinical trials have focused on subjects with more chronic myocarditis for whom spontaneous recovery is much less evident. These studies have generally sought evidence on EMB of either chronic inflammation or persistence of viral genomes as targets for intervention. The results of these innovative investigations have been promising, but need to be replicated in larger multicenter trials to determine their therapeutic potential. The ability to delineate subjects with viral persistence or chronic myocardial inflammation was a critical component for these investigations and is an essential requirement for targeted immune suppression in the future.

As genomic investigations continue to advance, it is increasingly recognized that the genetic background plays a crucial role in determining the susceptibility to myocarditis and other forms of inflammatory cardiomyopathy. Mutations in cytoskeletal proteins responsible for familial DCM are increased in frequency in subjects with myocarditis and PPCM. Whether this genomic analysis can assist in predicting clinical outcomes and targeting therapeutics will remain a subject for future investigations.

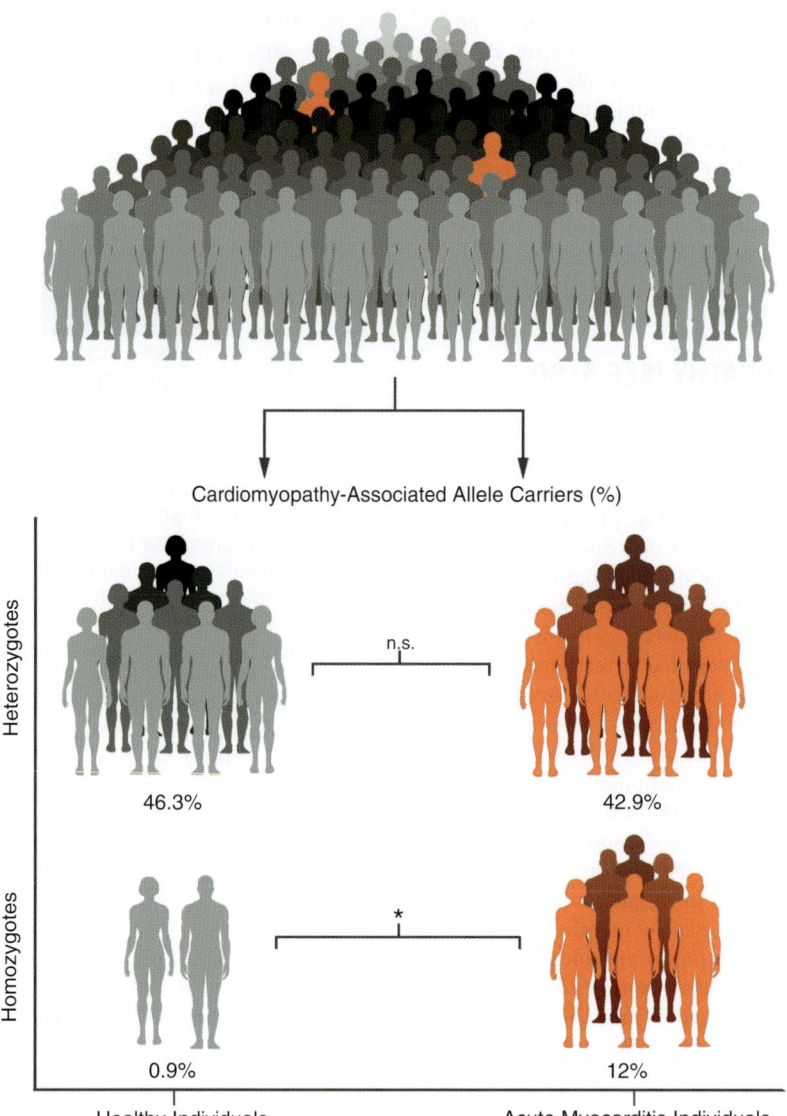

Fig. 28.7 Genomic analysis of a pediatric cohort with acute myocarditis (n = 42) and a control population (n = 1164) comparing the percentage of subjects who are either heterozygous or homozygous for mutations in a panel of 47 cardiomyopathy-associated genes (genes previously linked to arrhythmic right ventricular cardiomyopathy, dilated cardiomyopathy, or left ventricular noncompaction). Homozygous mutations were found in 12% of the children with acute myocarditis, significantly higher than the 0.9% evident in the control population (*P = .002). From Belkaya S, Kontorovich AR, Byun M, et al. Autosomal recessive cardiomyopathy presenting as acute myocarditis. *J Am Coll Cardiol.* 2017;69(13):1653–1665.

KEY REFERENCES

5. Aretz HT, Billingham ME, Edwards WD. Myocarditis, a histopathologic definition and classification. *Am J Cardiovasc Pathol.* 1987;1:3–14.

8. Mason JW, O'Connell JB, Herskowitz A, et al. for the Myocarditis Treatment Trial investigators: a clinical trial of immunosuppressive therapy for myocarditis. *N Engl J Med.* 1995;333:269–313.

25. Cooper LT, Berry GJ, Shabetai R, et al. Idiopathic giant-cell myocarditis—natural history and treatment. *N Engl J Med.* 1997;336:1860–1866.

39. Feldman AM, McNamara D. Myocarditis. *N Engl J Med.* 2000;343:1388–1398.

54. Friedrich MG, Sechtem U, Schulz-Menger J, et al. for the International Consensus Group on Cardiovascular Magnetic Resonance in Myocarditis. Cardiovascular magnetic resonance in myocarditis: a JACC White Paper. *J Am Coll Cardiol.* 2009;53:1475–1487.

56. Cooper LT, Baughman KL, Feldman AM, et al. The role of endomyocardial biopsy in the management of cardiovascular disease: a scientific statement from the American Heart Association, the American College of Cardiology, and the European Society of Cardiology. *J Am Coll Cardiol.* 2007;50:1914–1931.

70. McCarthy RE, Boehmer JP, Hruban RH, et al. Long-term outcome of fulminant myocarditis as compared with acute (nonfulminant) myocarditis. *N Engl J Med.* 2000;342:690–695.

76. Caforio AL, Pankuweit S, Arbustini E, et al. European Society of Cardiology Working Group on Myocardial and Pericardial Diseases. Current state of knowledge on aetiology, diagnosis, management, and therapy of myocarditis: a position statement of the European Society of Cardiology Working Group on Myocardial and Pericardial Diseases. *Eur Heart J.* 2013;34:2636–2648.

80. Heymans S, Eriksson U, Leatonen J, Cooper LT. The quest for new approaches in myocarditis and inflammatory cardiomyopathy. *J Am Coll Cardiol.* 2016;68:2348–2364.

88. Boehmer JP, Starling RC, Cooper LT, et al. for the IMAC Investigators. Left ventricular assist device support and myocardial recovery in recent onset cardiomyopathy. *J Card Fail.* 2012;18:755–761.

The full reference list for this chapter is available on ExpertConsult.

Heart Failure in the Developing World

Karen Sliwa, Simon Stewart

HEART FAILURE: A GLOBAL PERSPECTIVE

At any one time it has been estimated there are approximately 26 million cases of heart failure globally.[1] Although many of these cases reside in the developing world, our understanding of heart failure is largely framed by studies undertaken in high-income countries. The characteristics and consequences of heart failure have also been framed by its clinical diagnosis (with normal values for cardiac indices largely derived from Caucasian populations)[2] and the pivotal clinical trials (e.g., the recent PARADIGM Trial)[3] that have led to the introduction of new treatment modalities. **Table 29.1** summarizes some of the key definitions that have shaped our collective perceptions of heart failure,[4] from a predominantly "systolic dysfunction" phenomenon mainly affecting men, to one that acknowledged neurohormonal activation and wider systemic responses to a "failing heart" and, more latterly, the concept of both impaired and preserved systolic dysfunction affecting both sexes.[5]

The concept of heart failure as more than just a product of coronary artery disease and predominantly affecting men is critical when considering heart failure in the developing world. Accordingly, preliminary data from the developed world suggest there are many different pathways to the syndrome. Based on a number of important factors, including different risk factors (including high levels of communicable disease and exposure to indoor pollutants), high levels of poverty and malnutrition, and suboptimal access to health care systems, it is not surprising that the pattern of heart failure in vulnerable communities in the developing world is different—with potentially more women than men being affected, and with much younger cases typically presenting with more advanced heart disease.

This chapter outlines the pattern of heart failure from a developing world perspective while clearly acknowledging the challenge of comparing data from heterogeneous sources and the variety of methods/definitions used to detect and report on heart failure in low-resource settings.[6] Even if a coherent picture of heart failure is not entirely possible, it is important to note the enormous burden the syndrome imposes on the developing world. This burden is likely to rise as the influence of the traditional killers (malnutrition and infectious diseases) decline and many individuals adopt the lifestyle behaviors (e.g., smoking, high fat diets, and sedentary behaviors) that have fueled an epidemic of heart failure in the developed world.

GLOBAL BURDEN OF HEART FAILURE IN THE DEVELOPING WORLD

Based on different risk factor prevalence among the wide spectrum of ethnic groups influenced by socioeconomic factors, it is inevitable that the epidemiological and clinical profile of heart failure will vary across the globe. Moreover, differential coding of the syndrome, coupled with nuanced differences in defining cases, defies simple regional comparisons, particularly from a developed world perspective. For example, the current International Classification of Diseases system classifies heart failure as an intermediate and not an underlying cause of death.[7] The recently published Global Burden of Disease (GBD) studies, undertaken in 1990 and 2000, reported global death for 235 causes, including cardiovascular and circulatory diseases such as rheumatic heart disease, ischemic heart disease, cardiomyopathy, and others, and list heart failure as a nonfatal health outcome only.[8] Left-sided and right-sided symptomatic heart failure was one of the 289 impairments included in the GBD cause–sequelae list in many locations.[9] Contrasting with more conservative estimates, worldwide an estimate of 37.7 million cases of prevalent heart failure was recorded in 2010, leading to 4.2 years lived with disability (YLDs). Heart failure was distributed across a number of causes (**Table 29.2**). In stark contrast to clinical trial cohorts, more than two-thirds (68.7%) of heart failure globally was attributable to four underlying causes: ischemic heart disease, chronic obstructive pulmonary disease, and hypertensive and rheumatic heart disease. As expected, there were marked regional differences, with hypertensive heart disease, rheumatic heart disease, cardiomyopathy, and myocarditis making a larger contribution in developing countries.

TABLE 29.1   A Historical Perspective on Heart Failure Definitions

Wood, 1968	"A state in which the heart fails to maintain an adequate circulation for the needs of the body despite a satisfactory venous filling pressure."
Braunwald & Grossman, 1992	"A state in which an abnormality of cardiac function is responsible for the failure of the heart to pump blood at a rate commensurate with the requirements of the metabolizing tissues or, to do so only from an elevated filling pressure."
Packer, 1988	"A complex clinical syndrome characterized by abnormalities of left ventricular function and neurohormonal regulation which are accompanied by effort intolerance, fluid retention, and reduced longevity."
Poole-Wilson, 1987	"A clinical syndrome caused by an abnormality of the heart and recognized by a characteristic pattern of hemodynamic, renal, neural, and hormonal responses."
AHA/ACC Heart Failure Guidelines, 2005[100]	"Heart failure is a complex clinical syndrome that can result from any structural or functional cardiac disorder that impairs the ability of the ventricle to fill with or eject blood."
ESC Heart Failure Guidelines, 2005	"A syndrome in which the patients should have the following features: symptoms of heart failure, typically breathlessness or fatigue, either at rest or during exertion, or ankle swelling and objective evidence of cardiac dysfunction at rest."
AHA/ACC Heart Failure Guidelines, 2009 (Update)	Definition essentially unchanged, with reinforcement of these stages of heart failure (see legend below; note that the first two stages are not heart failure) and the central importance of the following statement: "The single most useful diagnostic test in the evaluation of patients with heart failure is the comprehensive two-dimensional echocardiogram coupled with Doppler flow studies to determine whether abnormalities of myocardium, heart valves, or pericardium are present and which chambers are involved. Three fundamental questions must be addressed: (1) Is the LV ejection fraction preserved or reduced? (2) Is the structure of the LV normal or abnormal? (3) Are there other structural abnormalities such as valvular, pericardial, or right ventricular abnormalities that could account for the clinical presentation?"
ESC Heart Failure Guidelines, 2012 (Update)[56]	"A syndrome in which patients have typical symptoms (e.g., breathlessness, ankle swelling, and fatigue) and signs (e.g., elevated jugular venous pressure, pulmonary crackles, and displaced apex beat) resulting from an abnormality of cardiac structure or function."

The AHA/ACC guidelines provide a map of the natural history of heart failure (from a developed world perspective) in respect to four distinct stages: **Stage A:** Those at risk for heart failure, but who have not yet developed structural heart changes (i.e., those with diabetes or coronary disease without prior infarct). **Stage B:** Individuals with structural heart disease (i.e., reduced ejection fraction, left ventricular hypertrophy, chamber enlargement); however, no symptoms of heart failure have ever developed. **Stage C:** Patients who have developed clinical heart failure. **Stage D:** Patients with refractory heart failure requiring advanced intervention (biventricular pacemakers, left ventricular assist device, or transplantation). *AHA/ACC,* American Heart Association/American College of Cardiology.
Data adapted from Krum H, Jelinek MV, Stewart S, et al. 2011 update to National Heart Foundation of Australia and Cardiac Society of Australia and New Zealand Guidelines for the prevention, detection and management of chronic heart failure in Australia, 2006. *Med J Aust.* 2011;194:405–409.

TABLE 29.2   Global Years Lived With Disability for Heart Failure From a Comprehensive List of 289 Causes and Select Sequelae in 1990 and 2010 for All Ages, Both Sexes Combined, and per 100,000

Cause of HF	ALL AGES YLDS (THOUSANDS)			YLDS (PER 100,000)		
	1990	2010	% Δ	1990	2010	% Δ
Cardiovascular and circulatory diseases	14,373 (11,094–18,134)	21,985 (16,947–27,516)	53.0%	271 (209–342)	319 (246–399)	17.7
Rheumatic HD	290 (191–412)	420 (278–592)	45.1%	5 (4–8)	6 (4–9)	11.6
Ischemic HD	894 (609–1236)	1518 (1038–2128)	69.9%	17 (11–23)	22 (15–31)	30.8
Hypertensive HD	292 (202–412)	460 (315–639)	57.4%	6 (4–8)	7 (5–9)	21.1
HF due to cardiomyopathy and myocarditis	272 (183–378)	394 (269–551)	44.8%	5 (3–7)	6 (4–8)	11.4
HF due to endocarditis	42 (28–59)	61 (42–87)	45.8%	1 (1–1)	1 (1–1)	12.2
HF due to other circulatory diseases	183 (123–259)	268 (180–372)	46.3%	3 (2–5)	4 (3–5)	12.6

HD, Heart disease; *HF,* heart failure; *YLDs,* years lived with disability.
Data from Vos T, Flaxman AD, Naghavi M, et al. Years lived with disability (YLDs) for 1160 sequelae of 289 diseases and injuries 1990–2010: a systematic analysis for the Global Burden of Disease Study 2010. *Lancet.* 2012;380:2163–2196.

What Do We Know About the Variation of Risk Factor Prevalence?

A systematic review of worldwide risk factors for heart failure by Khatibzadeh and colleagues[7] found 53 full-text surveys of heart failure patients eligible for inclusion and, after excluding 15 full-text papers, sorted 38 studies by region, using them for a qualitative synthesis. From these surveys it was found that ischemic heart disease was the major risk factor for heart failure in more than 50% of patients in Western high-income regions, as well as Eastern and Central European regions. In contrast, it contributed to 30% to 40% of heart failure cases in East Asia, Asia Pacific high-income regions, Latin America, and the Caribbean. At the lowest end of the scale, in sub-Saharan Africa, ischemic heart disease contributed to less than 10% of cases.

Hypertension proved to be a more consistent contributor to heart failure globally (17% or more crude prevalence among all cases). However, after age and gender adjustment, hypertension was distinctly more common in Eastern and Central Europe (35%, range 32.7%–37.3%) and sub-Saharan Africa (32.6%, range 29.6%–35.7%). Of the other two commonly reported antecedents, rheumatic heart disease was particularly prevalent in East Asia (34%) and sub-Saharan Africa (14%) cases. The heterogeneous group of cardiomyopathy, which can include numerous causes such as familial, peripartum, infectious, infiltrative, autoimmune, postmyocarditis, idiopathic, and many others, were particularly prevalent in sub-Saharan Africa (age- and gender-adjusted prevalence 25.7%, range 22.8%–28.5%). Latin America and the Caribbean, as well as Asia Pacific high-income countries, had a prevalence of 19.8% (16.5%–23.4%) and 16.5% (12.8%–20.6%). Notably, this review relied on data from many studies that exclude younger patients and those with preclinical heart failure, while rarely documenting duration of heart failure symptoms.

What Do We Not Know?

As data from many regions of the world are scarce, there is a particular lack of data estimating urban/rural differences as well as change in contributing factors to heart failure over time. There is an overall underreporting on the specific factors contributing to the spectrum of cardiomyopathy because these investigations are costly and there is a shortage of diagnostic facilities in those areas where, in particular, infectious causes of cardiomyopathy occur. In general, right heart failure per se, or as a contributing factor to left-sided heart failure, is poorly documented and there is a paucity of detailed description of the subtypes of valvular heart disease, such as different types of rheumatic

valve disease or function valve disease. Congenital heart disease, either operated or not operated, usually gets lumped in the category "other causes contributing to heart failure" and warrants further investigation. This is particularly important as the proportion of cases with operated congenital heart disease is increasing and congenital heart disease altogether is more commonly diagnosed.[10] The early stages of heart failure need to be diagnosed in a timely manner as they can be managed in multidisciplinary teams using pharmacologic or nonpharmacologic interventions.

PRIMARY CAUSE AND TYPE OF HEART FAILURE IN THE DEVELOPING WORLD

Heart failure in the developing world is mainly due to non-ischemic causes, such as hypertensive heart disease, valvular heart disease as a result of rheumatic fever and its sequelae, and heart muscle disease caused by infectious or unknown agents. This includes region-specific cardiomyopathies, such as endomyocardial fibrosis (EMF) in Africa, Chagas disease in South America (profiled in **Fig. 29.1**), and peripartum cardiomyopathy (PPCM), which has a particularly high prevalence in the black African population. Cardiac manifestations of HIV include forms of HIV cardiomyopathy.[11] Reporting on the etiology and primary cause of heart failure was, in the past, only clinically based and only in the past 10 to 20 years it has been supported by echocardiography. In addition, the focus is mainly on the causes of heart failure due to systolic dysfunction. Reporting on heart failure with preserved systolic function, as commonly seen due to hypertensive heart disease or in addition to systolic heart failure, is rare from the developing world.[12,13] This needs to be addressed in future studies, because it is likely that the profile of heart failure will also change in those regions as a result of the shifts in population demographics, the prevalence of specific risk factors, and the influence of the evolution of and access to therapeutic options.

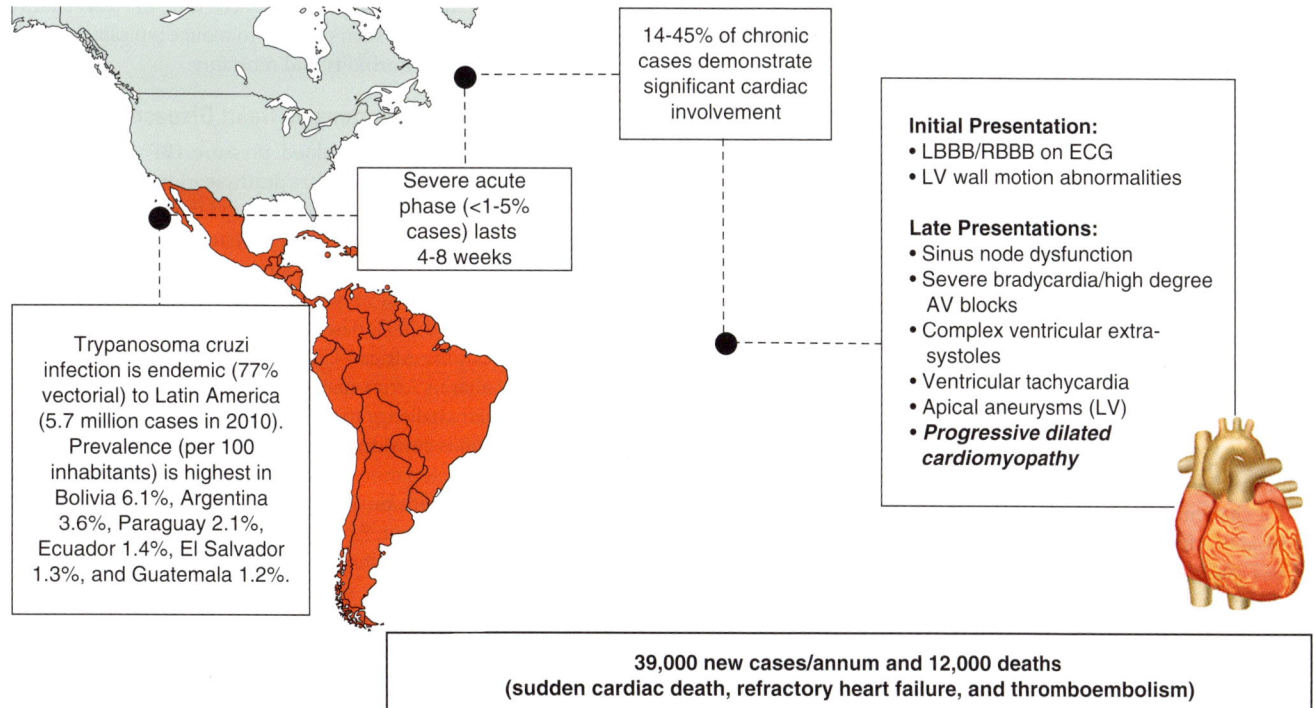

Fig. 29.1 Epidemiology and clinical aspects of Chagas disease. *AV,* Atrioventricular; *ECG,* electrocardiogram; *LBBB,* left bundle branch block; *LV,* left ventricular; *RBBB,* right bundle branch block.

The contribution of communicable disease, including HIV/AIDS (see below) to the overall burden of heart failure in the developing world cannot be underestimated. For example, in the Global Rheumatic Heart Disease Registry Cohort of 3343 predominantly younger individuals (two-thirds female and median age 28 years) patients recruited from 25 centers in 14 low- and middle-income countries in Africa and Asia, heart failure was a major contributor to observed mortality.[14] Overall, 2-year mortality was 17%, and concurrent heart failure conveyed a twofold increased risk of death (adjusted hazard ratio of 2.16, 95% confidence interval [CI] 1.70–2.72). Those cases from the lowest socioeconomic backgrounds had the worse outcomes at a younger age.

SPECIFIC ASPECTS OF HEART FAILURE IN KEY REGIONS IN THE DEVELOPING WORLD

Sub-Saharan Africa

Cardiomyopathy and rheumatic heart disease have historically been considered to be the major causes of heart failure in sub-Saharan Africa, accounting for almost half of all cases presenting to hospitals in the period between 1957 and 2005.[15,16] They pose a great challenge even in the context of the increasing burden of other cardiovascular diseases (CVDs), such as hypertensive heart disease, because they are difficult to diagnose in resource-poor environments as a result of the lack of specialized facilities and access to echocardiography. There is also a limit in effective interventions, such as pharmacotherapy, device-based therapies, valve replacement, and heart transplantation. There has, at least, been important new research on the epidemiology, pathogenesis, and prognosis of heart failure and cardiomyopathy in Africa in the past decade, as well as a few outcome studies.

Heart Failure Overall

Acute decompensated heart failure is the most common primary diagnosis for patients admitted to a hospital with heart disease in Africa.[17,18] Recent data from the Sub-Saharan Africa Survey of Heart Failure (THESUS-HF), the first and largest multicenter registry of acute heart failure in Africa to date, have characterized the causes and short-term outcomes in 1006 Africans with heart failure, from 12 tertiary cardiology centers in nine countries in sub-Saharan Africa.[17] The diagnosis of heart failure in THESUS-HF was based on the presence of dyspnea associated with physical findings of congestive heart failure (CHF), necessitating admission to a hospital in a patient who was 12 years of age or older. Echocardiography was used in all patients included in the study. One of the most striking features is the relative youth of the African patients affected by acute heart failure (mean age 52 years). Acute heart failure therefore strikes the generation of breadwinners and caregivers in African patients, thereby having major economic implications. The younger African patients with acute heart failure have a lower frequency of ischemic heart disease, hypertension, diabetes mellitus, atrial fibrillation, and renal insufficiency compared with elderly heart failure sufferers in developed countries. Compared with a summary of the causes of heart failure in sub-Saharan Africa, based on the case series published between 1957 and 2005,[19] THESUS-HF shows a changing trend in the epidemiology of acute heart failure in sub-Saharan Africa. There was a rise in the contribution of hypertension as a cause of heart failure (from 23% to 45%), a reduction in the role of rheumatic heart disease (from 22% to 14%), and an apparent increase in recognition of ischemic heart disease as a cause of heart failure (from 2% to almost 8%). The high incidence of hypertension and relatively low rate of coronary artery disease have also been observed in other single-center studies, such as the Heart of Soweto Study, where less than 10% of cases of heart failure were attributed to ischemic cardiomyopathy.[20]

A recent publication by Ojji et al.[21] reported on carefully characterized, consecutively captured patients residing in Abuja/Nigeria ($n = 1515$), comparing them to 4626 patients from the Heart of Soweto project, South Africa,[18] showing that hypertension contributed to even 60% of all cases presented with heart failure in Abuja versus 33% in Soweto. In the Soweto cohort, 66% had multiple risk factors versus only 12% in Abuja. On an age- and sex-adjusted basis, compared with the Soweto cohort, the Abuja cohort were more likely to present with a primary diagnosis of hypertension (adjusted odds ratio [OR] 2.10, 95% CI 1.85–2.42) or hypertensive heart disease/failure (OR 2.48, 95% CI 2.18–2.83); $P < .001$ for both. However, they were far less likely to present with coronary artery disease (OR 0.04, 95% CI 0.02–0.11) and right heart failure (2.5% vs. 27%).

Heart failure with systolic dysfunction appears to be the most common form in Africa.[22,23] However, most of the larger hospital- and community-based studies on heart failure were performed before the emphasis on heart failure with preserved ejection fraction. Data on treatment pattern are limited. In a registry in South Africa,[20] medication prescribed for patients presenting with systolic dysfunction ($n = 417$) was appropriately prescribed as loop diuretics (85%), angiotensin-converting enzyme (ACE) inhibitors (70%), β-blocker (64%), aldosterone inhibitors (60%), and digitalis (19%). In the same cohort study, 373 patients had heart failure with preserved ejection fraction and received therapy with diuretics (43%), β-blocker (25%), aldosterone antagonists (22%), and a calcium antagonist (18%). The THESUS Study[17] showed an inappropriately high prescription of aspirin and digitalis. Data on compliance are limited but, if available, were comparable with other regions.[17,24]

A further report from the THESUS Study demonstrated that simple clinical parameters measured at baseline and prior to discharge (including baseline orthopnea, rales, edema, oxygen saturation and changes in physical status from admission to discharge) has the capacity to identify patients at high risk for 6-month mortality.[25] A currently planned, multicenter trial of nurse-led, multidisciplinary heart failure management strategy adapted to the African context (the Pan-African Nurse-led And Community Enhanced cAre in Heart Failure—PANACEA-HF) will target such patients to reduce typically high levels of heart failure–related morbidity and mortality.

Heart Failure Due to Hypertensive Heart Disease

The global impact of elevated blood pressure (BP)/hypertension is profound, being responsible for more deaths worldwide than any other risk factor, including tobacco use, obesity, and lipid disorders (**see also Chapter 25**).[26] Taking Africa as a whole, a systematic review by Ibrahim and Damasceno[26] estimate that the prevalence of hypertension (BP >160/95 mm Hg) in adults 55 years or older increased from 54% to 78% between 1998 and 2003. Based on the change in lifestyle (adopting Western lifestyles), the African Union estimates that 10 to 20 million people in sub-Saharan Africa may currently experience hypertension, providing a similar challenge to HIV/AIDS. Hypertension in the black African population is considered to be a distinct biologic entity.[27] Not only do Africans develop more hypertension, but compared with other ethnic groups, hypertension in Africans is often more severe[28] and more resistant to treatment,[29] often leading to heart failure.

Studies on possible pathophysiologic mechanisms are not yet conclusive, particularly with respect to gender-based heterogeneity. However, observed gender-based differences in the underlying prevalence and characteristics of hypertension are often marked in black Africans. In the Heart of Soweto registry,[18,30,31] detailed information was captured on more than 6000 de novo presentations (5328 with confirmed heart disease) presenting to the cardiology unit of the Baragwanath Hospital, which services a community in profound epidemiologic transition. African women were the single biggest contributors to case presentations (2863 or 54%), with 575 (20%) presenting with a primary diagnosis of hypertension and a further 1196 (42%) with a secondary diagnosis of hypertension. Among the latter, hypertensive heart failure (682/1196 or 57%, mean age 60 ± 14 years) was the most common manifestation of hypertensive heart disease.[30] Interestingly, the level of education and noncommunicable risk factors, such as family history of CVD, smoking, obesity, and type 2 diabetes, correlated with advance disease.

A recent analysis of 320 cases of hypertensive heart failure (43% female and mean age 58–60 years) identified via the Abeokuta Heart Failure Registry in Nigeria provides further insights into this condition from an African perspective. Most cases presented as NYHA III/IV and one-third with preserved systolic function. The median length of hospital stay was 9 days, and the 6-month mortality was 12% (renal dysfunction being an independent modulator of survival). Compared to equivalent patients from neighboring Cameroon,[32] Nigerian cases were older (+5 years). Alternatively, on average they were 2 years younger than South African cases[20] and markedly younger than equivalent cases from North America.[33]

Heart Failure Due to Cardiomyopathies

In adult Africans, cardiomyopathy accounts for 20% to 30% of cardiac cases and is a major cause of heart failure.[17,19] Dilated cardiomyopathy (DCM) refers to a heterogeneous group of heart muscle diseases of diverse causes (see also Chapter 20). Presentation is usually with progressive heart failure. Important causes in Africa include PPCM, EMF, HIV-related cardiomyopathies, genetic causes, and idiopathic cardiomyopathies.[34]

Data from studies in Europe and North America have, for a long time, indicated that as many as 20% to 50% of patients with DCM may have familial disease,[35] but little is known about the frequency and clinical genetics of this disease in Africa (see also Chapter 24). Ntusi and coworkers found that familial DCM affected at least a quarter of African patients with DCM.[36] Patients presented at a young age (29 years old) compared with patients with idiopathic DCM (39 years old). Furthermore, this was associated with PPCM (7%) and followed an autosomal dominant pattern of inheritance in most families. This was the first study to report on the frequency and the probable mode of inheritance of familial DCM in patients who presented at a tertiary center in Cape Town. The recommendation for family screening for familial DCM in all cases of unexplained DCM, including patients with PPCM, to African patients with the disease[37] is supported by these findings.

Studies from South Africa have shown an association with HLA-DR1 and DRw10 antigens, as well as mitochondrial polymorphisms with idiopathic DCM.[38] Isolated left ventricular noncompaction (ILVNC)[39] is probably often unrecognized as a cause of heart failure and stroke.

The first population-based study of the epidemiologic features and early stages of EMF were reported by Mocumbi and coworkers.[40] In a random sample (1063 subjects) of all age groups from rural Mozambique, the prevalence of EMF (19.8% overall) was determined by transthoracic echocardiography. Patients 10 to 19 years old presented with the highest prevalence of EMF (28.1%), and EMF was higher in male compared to female subjects. Biventricular EMF was found to be the most common form (prevalence 55.5%), followed by right-sided EMF (prevalence 29.0%), with most affected patients displaying mild to moderate structural and functional echocardiographic abnormalities, and only 48 being symptomatic with signs of heart failure (22.7%).

HIV/AIDS and its therapy can have effects on the cardiovascular system on several levels leading to heart failure (Fig. 29.2) (see also

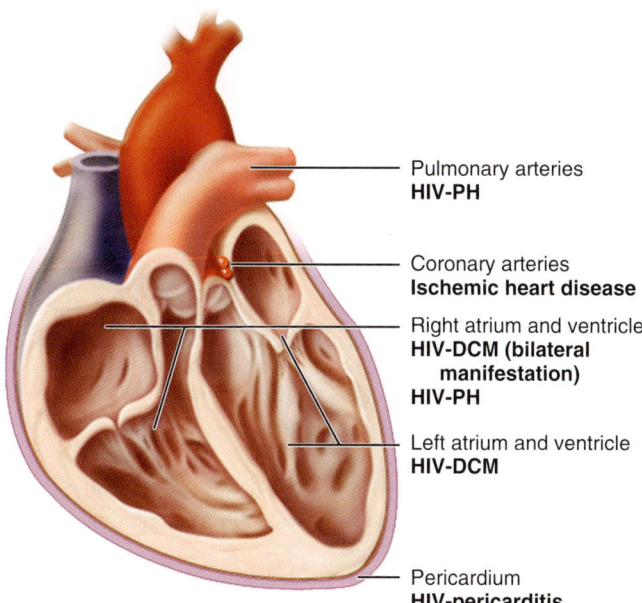

CARDIAC MANIFESTATIONS OF HIV INFECTION

Pulmonary arteries
HIV-PH

Coronary arteries
Ischemic heart disease

Right atrium and ventricle
HIV-DCM (bilateral manifestation)
HIV-PH

Left atrium and ventricle
HIV-DCM

Pericardium
HIV-pericarditis

Fig. 29.2 Effects of HIV on the heart. *DCM*, Dilated cardiomyopathy; *PH*, pulmonary hypertension.

Chapter 30). Cardiomyopathy in HIV-seropositive patients is associated with a longer duration of HIV infection, low total lymphocyte count, low CD4 count, and high HIV-1 viral load.[11,42] A prospective study of 157 patients from Kinshasa showed that almost 50% of the patients developed a cardiac abnormality over a 7-year period.[43] A significant proportion of patients with HIV-associated cardiomyopathy are free of specific cardiac signs and symptoms. In the Heart of Soweto cohort, 24% of patients with HIV-associated cardiomyopathy had asymptomatic left ventricular (LV) dysfunction.[44] Fortunately, the majority of HIV-positive patients in Africa now have access to antiretroviral therapy; although such therapy markedly improves the survival of those with HIV-associated cardiomyopathy it can by itself have negative cardiac effects leading to heart failure.[41]

PPCM is a relatively rare idiopathic disease associated with severe heart failure and occurs toward the end of pregnancy or in the months following delivery (see also Chapter 20).[45,46] Recently published data from the PPCM EORP registry (ESC EURObservational Research Programme [http://eorp.org]) on 411 patients have shown that the condition occurs in women from different ethnic backgrounds globally. However, despite marked differences in socio-economic backgrounds, the mode of presentation was largely similar.[47] Accurate data on the incidence of PPCM are unavailable as few population-based registries exist. Recent studies suggest a wide variation in the estimated incidences of PPCM (Table 29.3).

Novel molecular mechanisms of PPCM have been identified through research performed in the past 10 years. Studies using plasma from African patients with newly diagnosed PPCM have shown that elevated proinflammatory serum markers, such as sFas/Apo1, C-reactive protein, interferon gamma, and interleukin-6, point to proinflammatory processes that are involved in the induction and the progression of PPCM, and possibly influence survival rates.[48,49] Moreover, the findings of Hilfiker-Kleiner and colleagues point to possible involvement of a pathophysiologic circuit involving unbalanced oxidative stress and subsequent enhanced cleavage of the prolactin into an angiostatic and proapoptotic 16-kDa sub fragment, leading to endothelial damage and ventricular dysfunction.[49] The significant role

TABLE 29.3	Incidence of Peripartum Cardiomyopathy in Developing Countries					
Author	Year	Country	Incidence	Cohort	Definition of peripartum cardiomyopathy	Echocardiographic assessment
Fett[101]	2002	Haiti	1 in 400 live births	Afro-Caribbean	1. CHF 1 month before to 5 months after delivery 2. No preexisting heart disease 3. No other cause identified for the CHF	EF <45%
Fett[102]	2005	Haiti	1 in 300 live births	Afro-Caribbean	1. CHF 1 month before to 5 months after delivery 2. No preexisting heart disease 3. No other cause identified for the CHF	EF <45%
Desai[103]	1995	South Africa	1 in 1000 live births	Black Africans	1. CHF 1 month before to 5 months after delivery 2. No preexisting heart disease 3. No other cause identified for the CHF	EF <45%

Only studies using echocardiography have been included.
CHF, Congestive heart failure; *EF*, ejection fraction.

of endothelial damage is further supported by the significantly elevated endothelial microparticles found in acute PPCM, exhibiting apoptosis with impaired microcirculation.[50]

Hilfiker-Kleiner and coworkers went on to dissect the downstream effects of 16-kDa prolactin in PPCM. They discovered that 16-kDa prolactin, which is not signaling through the prolactin receptors, induces the expression of microRNA-146a (miR-146a) in endothelial cells.[51]

The angiogenic imbalance in PPCM as well as preeclampsia may not only depend on 16-kDA prolactin, but may rely on other factors such as soluble fms-like tyrosine kinase (sFlt-1).[52,53]

Bromocriptine, a prolactin-blocker, has recently emerged as a very promising therapeutic approach for the treatment of patients with PPCM,[54,55] based on the concept of enhanced cleavage of the nursing hormone prolactin into a deleterious, antiangiogenic, and proapoptotic form. A proof-of-concept pilot study with 20 African patients with PPCM showed that mortality was reduced and cardiac function improved in patients treated with bromocriptine for 2.5 mg for 2 weeks followed by 2.5 mg daily for 4 weeks, in contrast to patients receiving a placebo. That therapeutic option has been highlighted in the current European Society Guidelines on Cardiac Disease in Pregnancy[56] and received further support from a recently published study on a large multicenter cohort study of PPCM patients.[57]

The findings of this study supported the potential benefit of bromocriptine in addition to standard heart failure therapy. It appears that a short, low-dose bromocriptine therapy aiming to stop lactation is sufficient for most patients with PPCM.[57]

Other forms of heart failure occurring commonly in Africa include heart failure associated with pericardial disease due to late recognition of and poorly managed rheumatic valvular disease and right heart failure. Building on earlier findings from the Heart of Soweto Study,[58] the Pan-African Pulmonary Hypertension Cohort Study of 220 consecutive patients (97% African descent), derived from nine specialist centers in four African countries, highlighted the important contribution of diverse pathways to heart failure on the continent—with significant components of right heart failure arising from pulmonary disease. The three most common causes of pulmonary hypertension (with significant right heart evident in two-thirds of cases) were left heart disease (69%), pulmonary arterial hypertension (16%), and 11% directly attributable to lung disease; indoor and outdoor pollution was a likely factor in many cases. Overall, 21% patients died within 6 months with the combined presence of right atrial/ventricular hypertrophy (46% mortality) conferring an almost threefold risk of death on an adjusted basis.[59]

South America

Heart failure is the main cause of hospitalization based on available data from about 50% of the South American population.[12] With the Latin American countries undergoing marked epidemiologic changes with a marked increase in coronary artery disease due to an increasing prevalence of the traditional risk factors, such as obesity, diabetes, hypertension, and aging population, coronary artery disease is now the main cause of CHF in Latin Americans.[60] However, infectious diseases, such as Chagas disease (see Fig. 29.1) and rheumatic heart disease—common causes of CHF in Latin America—still remain frequent in this region and contribute to the burden of disease.

A number of studies reported data on cause and outcome in patients with acute and chronic heart failure from South America versus other regions of the world. These are the Eplerenone Post-AMI Heart Failure Efficacy and Survival Study[61] and the EVEREST study,[62] comparing in particular North and South America. For example, the recently published data from the EVEREST study reported on the regional differences of the baseline demographics of patients with acute heart failure in regions such as North America (n = 1251), South America (n = 699), Western Europe (n = 564), and Eastern Europe (n = 1619). With a mean age of 62.2 years, the patients in South America were significantly younger compared with the other regions (P < .001), with the same dominance of males (74.5%), but only half of the patients reporting were of white ethnicity (P < .001). There were marked differences in the baseline characteristics with patients from South America having less coronary artery disease (39.9% vs. 77.6%), less chronic obstructive pulmonary disease (5.7% vs. 18.1%), less diabetes (29.9% vs. 51.5%), and less frequent myocardial infarction (29.5% vs. 55.6%) compared with patients in North America (for all P < .001). Therefore there was a significantly lower percentage of patients having had a coronary artery bypass graft (CABG) (13.3% in South America vs. 41.4% in North America, P < .001), and having had less frequently percutaneous coronary intervention (PCI) (12.3% vs. 32.6%). There was also a difference in the use of medical therapy with patients in South America having a particularly high use of ACE inhibitors (93% vs. 75%), higher use of aldosterone blockers (65% vs. 35%), but a lower use of β-blockers (56% vs. 78%). In general, patients in South America were younger, had longer hospitalizations, and had lower PCI and CABG use, and there were some differences in event rates, risk factors, and therapeutic management. Some of the regional differences in drug use, cardiovascular interventions, and severity of the diseases appear to be related to economic factors.

Robust data on prevalence and outcome of heart failure in inpatients are also available from the Brazilian Ministry of Health (DATASUS).[12]

Of the 743,763 hospitalizations due to CVD in 2007, 39.4% were associated with heart failure. The mean period in the hospital was 5.8 days, with a mortality range from 6.5% to 6.9%.[12] Studies from Brazil (REMADHF),[63] Argentina (GESICA),[64] and Mexico[65] on outpatients reported high prevalence of ischemic cause, ranging from 22% to 47%, followed by hypertension and valvular disease.[66] AcqGlobal summarized the specific challenges and opportunities to scale up CVD secondary prevention, including appropriate management of heart failure in Latin America, in an expert consensus document.

As noted earlier, Chagas disease in Latin America remains common. The RAMADHF and GESICA studies reported the prevalence of Chagas disease as a cause of heart failure between 10% and 28%. Disease control programs have significantly reduced the number of infected individuals from approximately 16 to 18 million in the early 1990s to 10 to 12 million in the early 2000s.[67,68] Chagas disease is usually acquired during childhood as a result of *Trypanosoma cruzi* present in the feces of Reduviidae insects penetrating the skin or conjunctiva of people living in rural areas. The disease has an acute phase, presenting as a nonspecific febrile illness lasting several weeks, and is becoming clinically manifest in less than 1% of the infected subjects. Acute myocarditis leading to heart failure only occurs in 1 to 5 of every 10,000 infected people and is commonly (>50%) associated with a significant pericardial effusion.[69]

Chronic Chagas cardiomyopathy evolves over several decades after infection. A recent review by Acquatella reported on the echocardiographic features in Chagas heart disease. More than half of the chronic Chagas cardiomyopathy subjects remain asymptomatic. Early Doppler abnormalities include prolongation of isovolumic contraction and relaxation times. Systolic function frequently is normal, but dysfunction can be provoked by stress testing. More than half of the symptomatic patients have LV apical aneurysm and other contractile abnormalities. Other forms presenting with a generally dilated heart are indistinguishable from other cardiomyopathies. Patients presenting with heart failure in NYHA Class II and III commonly present with arrhythmias, an embolism, and sudden death. The heart is commonly dilated, and LV systolic and diastolic parameters are usually abnormal. Mitral and tricuspid valve regurgitation may be present.[70] The estimated 10-year survival is 75% to 85%. Patients presenting as NYHA FC IV have only a 50% chance of survival.[85] Recent studies reported prognostic variables by echocardiography. Chagas-related electrocardiogram abnormalities, LV systolic and diastolic parameters, and LVEF were predictors of events. Overall, the prognosis of patients with Chagas heart disease is worse in comparison with other causes.[70] Morillo et al[71] conducted a prospective, multicenter randomized study involving 2854 patients with Chagas's cardiomyopathy who received benznidazole or placebo for up to 80 days and were followed for a mean of 5.4 years. The trypanocidal therapy significantly reduced serum parasite detection but did not significantly reduce cardiac clinical deterioration though 5 years of follow-up. Heart transplantation is effective but is associated with reactivation of the *T. cruzi* infection.[72] Altogether key challenges surrounding the effective management of Chagas disease still need to be addressed, and specific trials are necessary to identify cost-effective therapeutics specific to the disease and its cardiac manifestations.

Asia and the Pacific Region

This large and heterogeneous region represents some of the most populous countries in the world, many of which are classified as lower-income with high poverty levels. The region includes the populous giants of China (population 1.3 billion) to India (1.2 billion) and Indonesia (250 million). Despite emerging literature focusing on heart failure around the globe there is still a paucity of regional data

compared to that derived from Europe and North America—particularly from midsize countries, such as Vietnam (population ≈90 million) and Malaysia (28 million).

Regardless of the baseline prevalence of heart failure, any progressive ageing of this populous region will inevitably increase its burden. Accordingly, in South Asia alone (low- to middle-income countries) the projected number of individuals aged 60 years or older will increase more than three-fold from 133 million to close to 500 million within the next 50 years.[73] Based on North American data (heart failure prevalence of 1.9%[74]), it has been estimated that in 2011 there were 30 million cases of heart failure (22 million of which were in India).[73] The potential for new/incident cases of heart failure in the region to steadily add to its underlying burden (particularly in the setting of favorable survival outcomes) is highlighted by a contemporary report from Sri Lanka that showed that 60% of case presentations being de novo.[75] Alternatively, it is unknown whether the most common contributory conditions within this hospital cohort (including anemia [41%], acute ischemic cardiomyopathy [37%], and respiratory disease [10%]) will rise or fall in Sri Lanka. In neighboring Pakistan, ischemic cardiomyopathy is reported to be the predominant cause of heart failure admissions, with >75% presenting with HFrEF.[73]

Overall, ischemic cardiomyopathy appears to be the predominant cause of heart failure in South Asians both living in their country and following migration to other parts of the world.[76] As in sub-Saharan Africa, infectious diseases also contribute to the burden of disease. For example, 4% of patients in a leptospirosis outbreak in Sri Lanka developed heart failure. Additionally, as in the poorer regions of Africa, EMF is endemic to some parts of India.[77,78]

Attempting to use projections from a particular region to the national population is fraught with uncertainty in many countries with diverse socioeconomic conditions and cultures. For example, a study of >1000 medical admissions to a major hospital in Kuala Lumpur (the capital of Malaysia) revealed that heart failure accounted for 7% of these; with coronary artery disease (50% of cases) and hypertension (20%) the main overall risk factors.[79] However, the Malaysian population (including the predominant Malay people plus significant portions of people from Chinese and Indian descent) is ethnically heterogeneous. Accordingly, causative factors varied according to ethnicity (e.g., markedly more diabetes in those of Indian descent).[79] Although one might expect a less complex picture of heart failure in Vietnam (perhaps with northern vs. southern differentials based on cultural and socioeconomic factors), there is a dearth of data to confirm this. Indeed, the most obvious report on heart failure represents the personal experiences of a visiting US student with very little insight into the nature of the problem in that country.[80] There are many such gaps regarding describing heart failure in the largest (i.e., Indonesia) and smallest (the Pacific Islands) populations in the region.

East Asia

In China alone it is estimated that just over 4 million individuals (only 1 million less than the United States but clearly at lower prevalence levels) currently have heart failure.[81] Guo and colleagues recently completed a systematic review of the literature relating to heart failure in East Asia.[82] This and other papers in a series seeking to provide a global picture of heart failure (see South Asia discussion later) provide the most contemporary and up-to-date picture of heart failure in developing countries (albeit mixed with summaries of developed countries in those regions). However, the same caveat regarding lack of standardized data and enormous gaps in the literature (given the size of population) needs to be considered.

Using best available data (reports from China being a predominant feature), they concluded that the prevalence of heart failure in

Malaysia was as high as 6.7% compared with 1.3% in China (with an associated incidence rate of 0.7–0.9 per 1000 per annum).[82] In comparison, the estimated prevalence of heart failure in the highly developed country of Singapore was estimated to be 4.5%.[83] As expected, profound socioeconomic dynamics continue to shape the underlying causes of an evolving burden of heart failure in the region. As such the reported presence of coronary artery disease in heart failure cases across the region ranged from as low as 25% to 47%.[82] In comparison, concurrent hypertension ranged from a low of 19% in Malaysia[84] to a high of 74% in the high-income country of Japan,[85] with markedly different figures in mainland China depending on the region (23%–47%).[86-88] Notably, concurrent cases of valvular disease varied across the region with fewer cases reported in East Asia; in most countries this figure ranged from 15% to 35%, but was only 4% in Malaysia.[82] Reports of heart failure associated with preserved systolic function and heart failure-related survival are few and far between, with almost all reports derived from high-income countries; perhaps not surprisingly given the high prevalence of hypertensive heart failure, Japanese reports dominate the former.

Regional Comparisons

Given the historical paucity of comparable data, the ADHERE (Acute Decompensated Heart Failure National Registry),[89] comprising 10,171 hospitalized cases of heart failure captured via an observational database (2006–2008), was noteworthy for comparing and contrasting the characteristics of heart failure on an international basis. Apart from those higher-income countries (including Australia, Hong Kong, Singapore, and Taiwan), a number of developing countries in the region were included—comprising Thailand (20% of clinical cases), Indonesia (17%), Malaysia (9%), and the Philippines (7%). **Fig. 29.3** compares the median age of heart failure cases for the developing countries with the developed countries included in the registry. Although not providing a perfect correlation, it is evident that in high-income countries in this region with associated high human development index scores, typical heart failure patients present with a median age older than 75 years and with profiles similar to the Western world. Alternatively, as with other regions around the world, such as sub-Saharan Africa, the median age of heart failure cases is markedly lower. More contemporary comparisons derived from the prospective INTER-CHF Study[90] reinforce these observations. Overall, 5813 patients (mean age 59 years, 39% female and 31% rural-dwelling) with heart failure were enrolled from 108 centers across 16 countries in Africa, Asia, the Middle East, and South America. As highlighted by **Table 29.4**, African patients (closely followed by Asian patients) were much younger while still more likely to be clinically advanced (NYHA Class IV). At the other end of the spectrum, South American patients (along with those from Middle Eastern countries) were older and yet less likely to present as NYHA Class IV. Overall, coronary artery disease was the main driver of heart failure within the INTER-CHF cohort with the notable exception of African patients in whom hypertensive heart disease was most common. As expected, given the critical difference in the etiology and characteristics of heart failure, there were regional differences in the clinical management of patients (see Table 29.4). Subsequent follow-up of the INTER-CHF Study cohort demonstrated that baseline differences in the pattern and management of heart failure also translated into substantive differences in outcomes on a regional basis. Overall, 1-year mortality was highest in Africa (34%, mean age at death 56 years) and India (23%, 57 years) compared to just 9% in South America (72 years). Moreover, more than half of all heart failure cases were unexplained in multivariate models.[91] On an adjusted basis, heart failure patients in India were 2.5-fold more at risk of a cardiac death with 1 year compared to those in South America (reference

group) with equivalent hazard ratios being 2.3 and 2.0 for heart failure patients recruited in Africa and Southeast Asia, respectively. For those patients in the Middle East and China there was no difference in outcome compared to their South American counterparts.[91]

Indigenous Peoples

Any commentary on the burden of heart failure in this widely dispersed region is not complete without some consideration of Indigenous populations living in countries otherwise designated as "developed." For example, New Zealand (population ≈4.5 million) has significant numbers of Pacific Islander people who have similar health profiles to those living in the developed world. Data derived from these vulnerable populations share the same characteristics of relatively younger cases and more women affected with more diverse pathways to the syndrome.[92] Carr and colleagues[93] undertook a retrospective, national analysis of mortality and morbidity data attributed to heart failure (data period 1988–1998) in Māori and non-Māori men and women aged 45 years or older. They found that heart failure-related case fatality was almost 9 times and 3.5 times higher, respectively, in Māori men aged 45 to 64 years and older than 65 years, with similar patterns in women. A similar pattern (of markedly increased risk) was found regarding the rate of heart failure admissions. Sopoaga and colleagues[94] demonstrated that previously observed disparities remain high relative to the rest of the population, with Māori people being six times more likely to be admitted to hospital with cardiomyopathy, and four to five times more likely to present with rheumatic heart disease. Across the Tasman Sea in Australia, McGrady[95] and colleagues undertook a population survey of heart failure in the isolated communities of Central Australia (≈15,000 Aboriginal people). Of 436 adults screened (mean 44 years and 64% women), a high proportion (relative to wider population estimates) were diagnosed with heart failure (5.3%) and asymptomatic left ventricular dysfunction (13%). The main drivers of heart failure were obesity (42%), hypertension (41%), and diabetes (40%). Rheumatic heart disease (7% of cases) was a key contributor to the burden of heart failure given its virtual absence in the non-Indigenous population. A follow-up study of heart failure hospitalizations in Central Australia demonstrated that the annual prevalence of any heart failure hospitalization was much higher within the Indigenous population (1.9%; 95% CI 1.7–2.1) compared to the rest of the population (0.5%; 95% CI 0.4–0.6).[96] Importantly, the greatest difference was found in Indigenous women. Moreover, Indigenous cases were significantly younger (mean age 51 years compared to 69 years) and clinically more complex compared to their non-Indigenous counterparts.

KEY CONSIDERATIONS FOR THE PREVENTION AND MANAGEMENT OF HEART FAILURE IN THE DEVELOPING WORLD

An increasing number of initiatives both at the local regional level[97] and the broader global level (e.g., the INTER-CHF Study)[91] are slowly but surely providing more reliable information on the characteristics and burden of heart failure from a developing world perspective. Overall, however, epidemiological studies, particularly those examining the antecedents and natural history of heart failure beyond those who have already developed an advanced form of the syndrome and require hospital treatment, are expensive and logistically difficult to undertake. As such, investment in these types of studies remains extremely scarce, despite the urgency to generate data specific to many diverse communities across the globe.

As expected, emerging reports focusing on heart failure in the developing world confirm and highlight the fact that geographically

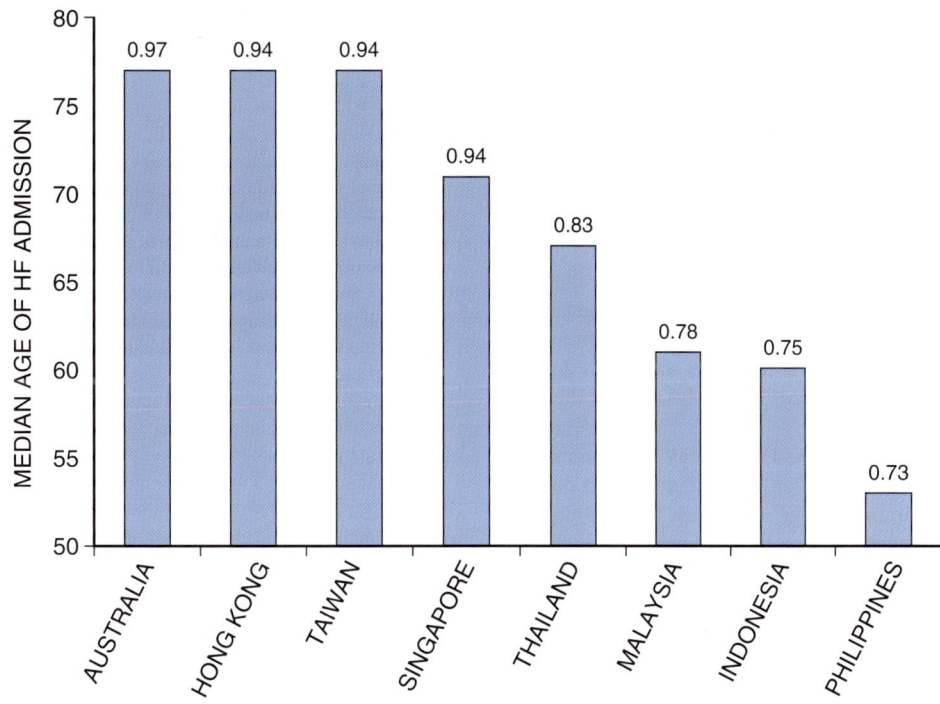

Fig. 29.3 Median age of heart failure (HF) cases in the Acute Decompensated Heart Failure National Registry in countries of the Asia Pacific region, with the number above each bar representing the human development index. (Data from Atherton JJ, Hayward CS, Wan Ahmad WA, et al. Patient characteristics from a regional multicenter database of acute decompensated heart failure in Asia Pacific [ADHERE International-Asia Pacific]. *J Card Fail.* 2012;18:82–88.)

TABLE 29.4	**Regional Comparisons of Heart Failure Within the INTER-CHF Study**			
	Africa (n = 1294)	**Asia (n = 2661)**	**Middle East (n = 1000)**	**South America (n = 885)**
Male, %	52	59	72	61
Mean age, years	53.4	60.0	56.4	67.1
NYHA III/IV, %	57	42	37	31
Preserved LVEF, %	29	41	11	29
HF admission (past 12 months), %	36	28	22	27
Hypertension, %	62	59	68	74
Past myocardial infarction, %	8.2	22	19	18
Diabetes, %	17	26	57	49
Valve disease, %	57	40	48	47
Chronic kidney disease, %	3.8	7.1	12	12
ACEi/ARB therapy, %	77	68	88	75
Beta-blocker therapy, %	48	61	86	73
Diuretic therapy, %	94	62	88	78

ACEi/ARB, Angiotensin-converting enzyme inhibitor/angiotensin receptor blocker; *CHF,* Congestive heart failure; *HF,* heart failure; *LVEF,* left ventricular ejection fraction; *NYHA,* New York Heart Association.
Adapted from Dokainish H, Teo K, Zhu J, et al. Heart failure in Africa, Asia, the Middle East and South America: the INTER-CHF study. *Int J Cardiol.* 2016;204:133–141.

and ethnically diverse populations generate a much more diverse spectrum of heart failure with nonischemic etiology, younger individuals, and proportionately more women than men affected than are typically found in developing countries. It is on this basis that it still remains unclear if current management guidelines developed by the European Society of Cardiology and the American Heart Association, for example, readily apply to developing world patients. Unfortunately, as highlighted by the BA-HEF Study[98] of combination

of hydralazine/nitrate therapy versus placebo in acute heart failure patients recruited from nine sub-Saharan African countries, successfully funding and conducting randomized heart failure trials is just as challenging as that of conducting epidemiological studies. Without providing definitive evidence, this trial suggested that the active combination therapy being tested might have clinical benefits for the types of heart failure and individuals of African origin typically managed on the continent.

What Is Needed for a Global Heart Failure Prevention Strategy?

As highlighted by a report from the INTER-CHF Study,[91] in many regions patients are dying of heart failure from preventable causes.[94] A key challenge highlighted by the INTER-CHF Study is addressing differential mortality outcomes through a better understanding of what actually causes the majority of cases of heart failure in the developing world.[91] In some regions, for example, Brazil, Argentina, and South Africa, a large portion of the health care resources are spent on paying for high-complexity cardiac surgeries, and limited funds are allocated to prevention. Some regions have no specific prevention programs for rheumatic heart disease. As shown by the poor health outcomes associated with the rheumatic heart disease (much of which was directly attributable to heart failure) in the REMEDY Study cohort,[14] this is of concern.

Implementing what is known, tackling obesity, and preventing diabetes, and subsequently hypertension and ischemic heart disease, is probably the most important strategy worldwide. It is on this basis that greater investment in health services to implement what is already available (in terms of primary and secondary prevention strategies) is likely to deliver the most cost-effective outcomes. As articulated by Ojii and colleagues, this must include a key role for primary care services—particularly in rural areas where transportation is impractical and unaffordable. Based on a strong community-orientated approach, with facilities equipped with nonphysician personnel supervised by trained physicians and applying basic screening tools (e.g., point-of-care devices), there is strong potential for primary care to tackle the source of many forms of heart failure. Accordingly, even the most basic of primary care services has the potential to facilitate early diagnosis of the risk factors for heart failure (e.g., hypertension)[99] via simple and affordable diagnostic tools, and could prevent communicable and emerging noncommunicable causes and lead to the use of already affordable pharmacologic therapy, such as, in particular, ACE inhibitors and β-blockers.

KEY REFERENCES

17. Damasceno A, Mayosi BM, Sani M, et al. The causes, treatment, and outcome of acute heart failure in 1006 Africans from 9 countries. *Arch Intern Med.* 2012;172:1386–1394.
18. Sliwa K, Wilkinson D, Hansen C, et al. Spectrum of heart disease and risk factors in a black urban population in South Africa (the Heart of Soweto Study): a cohort study. *Lancet.* 2008;371:915–922.
20. Stewart S, Wilkinson D, Hansen C, et al. Predominance of heart failure in the Heart of Soweto Study cohort: emerging challenges for urban African communities. *Circulation.* 2008;118:2360–2367.
21. Ojji D, Stewart S, Ajayi S, Manmak M, Sliwa K. A predominance of hypertensive heart failure in the Abuja Heart Study cohort of urban Nigerians: a prospective clinical registry of 1515 de novo cases. *Eur. J. Heart Fail.* 2013;15:835–842.
36. Ntusi NB, Badri M, Gumedze F, et al. Clinical characteristics and outcomes of familial and idiopathic dilated cardiomyopathy in Cape Town: a comparative study of 120 cases followed up over 14 years. *S Afr Med J.* 2011;101:399–404.
40. Mocumbi AO, Ferreira MB, Sidi D, Yacoub MH. A population study of endomyocardial fibrosis in a rural area of Mozambique. *N Engl J Med.* 2008;359:43–49.
45. Sliwa K, Hilfiker-Kleiner D, Petrie MC, et al. Current state of knowledge on aetiology, diagnosis, management, and therapy of peripartum cardiomyopathy: a position statement from the Heart Failure Association of the European Society of Cardiology Working Group on peripartum cardiomyopathy. *Eur J Heart Fail.* 2010;12:767–778.
59. Thienemann F, Dzudie A, Mocumbi AO, et al. The causes, treatment, and outcome of pulmonary hypertension in Africa: insights from the Pan African Pulmonary Hypertension Cohort (PAPUCO) Registry. *Int J Cardiol.* 2016;221:205–211.
71. Morillo CA, Marin-Neto JA, Avezum A, et al. Randomized trial of benznidazole for chronic chagas' cardiomyopathy. *N Engl J Med.* 2015;373:1295–1306.
90. Dokainish H, Teo K, Zhu J, et al. Heart failure in Africa, Asia, the Middle East and South America: the INTER-CHF study. *Int J Cardiol.* 2016;204:133–141.

The full reference list for this chapter is available on ExpertConsult.

Heart Failure and Human Immunodeficiency Virus

Gerald S. Bloomfield, Matthew J. Feinstein, Chris T. Longenecker

WHAT IS HUMAN IMMUNODEFICIENCY VIRUS-ASSOCIATED HEART FAILURE?

As antiretroviral therapy (ART) has become widely adopted, acquired immune deficiency syndrome (AIDS)–defining infections and malignancies have become less common, and the burden of chronic noncommunicable diseases has increased. Parallel to this transition, human immunodeficiency virus (HIV)–associated heart failure (HF) has evolved from an end-stage AIDS-related complication to a more heterogeneous disease state representing diverse HIV-related pathophysiologies. HF is more common among people living with HIV (PLWH) than in the HIV-uninfected, even after adjustment for demographic and relevant clinical factors.[1] Worse immune function and more HIV viral replication exacerbate HIV-associated HF risk. Traditional cardiovascular risk factors for HF, ranging from hypertension to smoking, are also more common in PLWH, underscoring the role of both traditional and HIV-specific factors in HF pathogenesis.[2] While there is no uniform definition for HIV-associated HF, most society guidelines and recommendations acknowledge that HIV infection carries with it a risk for a unique HF syndrome differentiated from others by the role of HIV infection, immune dysfunction, or ART on the development of HF.[3,4]

HISTORICAL PERSPECTIVE

Since the first reports of HF due to AIDS-related cardiomyopathy in the mid-1980s,[5] HF has been a known complication of HIV. The initial case reports of cardiac involvement in HIV were notable in that these cases occurred in the absence of Kaposi sarcoma, in which cardiac involvement was common.[5] Throughout the 1980s and 1990s, the presence of HF in PLWH was mainly in the context of myocarditis, opportunistic infections, nutritional deficiencies and/or severe immunosuppression.[6] Most patients had concomitant opportunistic infections. Numerous terms were introduced to describe this syndrome, including AIDS cardiomyopathy, HIV-associated cardiomyopathy, HIV-associated dilated cardiomyopathy, HIV-associated HF, and HIV-associated left ventricular (LV) dysfunction.

In the pre-ART era, HIV-associated HF was classically defined by progressive HIV/AIDS and associated global LV systolic dysfunction. In an observational study of 136 Italian PLWH followed with serial echocardiography from 1988 through 1992, seven (5.1%) developed symptomatic global LV dysfunction over a mean follow-up of 415 days. All patients with incident HF had AIDS, and myocarditis was a prominent feature.[7] In the pre-ART era, very low CD4 count (<100 cells/mm^3) was a common factor associated with LV dysfunction and HF. Overall, the prevalence of HIV-associated cardiomyopathy was 30% to 40% based on clinical-pathological studies in the pre-ART era with an annual incidence of 15.9 per 1000 patients.[8]

Prognostically, the syndrome was initially characterized by severe symptoms and high mortality. Median survival was 101 days for patients with dilated cardiomyopathy, compared to 472 days for patients with normal findings on echocardiogram at a similar level of immunosuppression.[9] Gross autopsy findings demonstrated striking four-chamber dilatation, myofibrillar loss, and focal myocarditis. In the wake of this ostensibly new syndrome, researchers at the time foreshadowed, "Cardiac disease secondary to multiple causes can be expected to complicate the clinical course of these patients."[5]

Although the relative contribution of AIDS cardiomyopathy to HIV-associated HF has declined with wide ART adoption, ART access and adherence are not ubiquitous. Therefore, AIDS cardiomyopathy remains a relevant disease state, particularly in settings with low ART uptake. Sub-Saharan Africa (SSA), for example, accounts for 12% of the global population but is disproportionately affected by HIV with 69% of all adults and 90% of all children living with HIV residing in the region (see also Chapter 29).

CONTEMPORARY SHIFTS IN EPIDEMIOLOGY

Access to effective ART has significantly altered the epidemiology of HF in HIV (Table 30.1). The syndrome has shifted from a severe, dilated cardiomyopathy to one that is often minimally symptomatic and accompanied by mildly decreased LV systolic function. While the prevalence of severe systolic dysfunction has definitely diminished, data from the US Veterans Aging Cohort Study (VACS) show that PLWH on ART remain at higher risk of developing HF compared to the uninfected for HF with preserved, reduced, or borderline ejection fraction (EF).[1] HF risk was greater among PLWH despite having a lower burden of traditional risk factors, including hypertension, diabetes, high low-density lipoprotein (LDL) cholesterol, and obesity. In subgroup analyses adjusted for numerous clinical variables, the most common HF phenotype for white, black, and young (<40 years of age) veterans was HF with reduced EF (HFrEF). PLWH with consistently low CD4+ T-cell counts had significantly elevated risk for HFrEF (hazard ratio [HR] 1.87; 95% confidence interval [CI] 1.36–2.57) and HF with preserved EF (HFpEF) (HR 1.87; 95% CI 1.28–2.73) in comparison to PLWH with higher CD4+ T-cell counts; however, compared with uninfected patients, HF risk among PLWH with CD4+ T-cell count greater than 500 cells/mm³ remained elevated (HR 1.25; 95% CI 1.08–1.43). Consistently detectable viremia was associated with increased risk for HFrEF (HR 1.63; 95% CI 1.28–2.08). In sensitivity analyses, the risk of HF attributed to HIV persisted after restricting the dataset to those without hypertension, alcohol or cocaine abuse, and never smokers, and adjusted for incident myocardial infarction (MI).

Recent analyses suggest that HFpEF is becoming an increasingly common manifestation of HIV-associated HF. In contrast to the global LV dysfunction-predominant manifestation of HF in the pre-ART era, investigators found that HFrEF comprised only 37.1% of incident HF among HIV-infected veterans.[1] Another US Department of Veterans Affairs (VA) study suggests that the HIV-associated risk of HF may be even higher among women (incidence rate ratio 2.5; 95% CI 1.5-4.5, HIV vs. control).[10] Similarly, higher risks were seen for women in an analysis of a large nationally representative electronic health records database (Fig. 30.1).[11]

A substantial portion of PLWH have abnormal diastolic parameters, with or without symptoms. Investigations into asymptomatic cardiac dysfunction among PLWH show a higher prevalence of diastolic dysfunction and higher LV mass index compared with controls. These differences are not solely explained by differences in traditional risk factors and are independently associated with HIV infection.[12]

PATHOPHYSIOLOGY OF HEART FAILURE IN HUMAN IMMUNODEFICIENCY VIRUS

HF reflects a final common pathway of various cardiovascular and systemic disorders. These diverse pathophysiologies are particularly apparent when examining HIV-associated HF. Here, we outline several mechanisms that appear to contribute to HIV-associated HF.

Poor Human Immunodeficiency Viral Control, Opportunistic Infections, and Human Immunodeficiency Virus/Acquired Immune Deficiency Syndrome Cardiomyopathy

Progressive infection and resulting low CD4+ T-cell counts, often less than 100 cells/mm,³ make PLWH particularly vulnerable to opportunistic infection, which may in turn contribute to infectious myocarditis. In a study from the pre-ART era, which included necropsy results from five HIV-infected persons who died from acute systolic HF, three of the patients were found to have acute lymphocytic myocarditis and one was found to have cryptococcal myocarditis.[7] The role of myocarditis in AIDS cardiomyopathy was further reinforced by an autopsy study of 60 Scandinavian patients with AIDS and no known heart disease, which found myocarditis in 25 patients (42%) and diffuse myocardial fibrosis in 40 patients (67%).[13]

Myocardial dysfunction in advanced HIV/AIDS may also relate to nutritional deficiencies common in this condition. AIDS-related deficiencies in micronutrients including L-carnitine and selenium have been proposed as contributors to cardiomyopathy among AIDS patients.[14] There is no clear consensus on whether HIV itself directly infects the myocardium or whether advanced HIV/AIDs merely predisposes to infectious, immune dysregulatory, and inflammatory conditions that lead to myocardial damage.

TABLE 30.1   **Features of Human Immunodeficiency Virus-Associated Heart Failure in the Eras Pre- and Postantiretroviral Therapy**

Characteristics	Pre-ART	With access to ART[a]
Causes	Myocarditis, viral and nonviral opportunistic infections, tuberculous myopericarditis, micronutrient deficiency	Cardiac autoimmunity, chronic inflammation, ART toxicity
Presentation	Predominantly severe systolic dysfunction and advanced heart failure	Mild systolic dysfunction, diastolic dysfunction
Clinical	Symptomatic	Symptomatic or asymptomatic
Echocardiographic Features	Dilated cardiomyopathy, Reduced ejection fraction	Reduced, borderline or preserved ejection fraction, abnormal myocardial strain
Mortality	Median survival ~100 days after diagnosis	Unknown

[a]Features can mimic those in pre-ART era in patients who are not taking ART and with ischemic etiologies that progress to severe systolic dysfunction.
ART, Antiretroviral therapy.

The Role of Atherosclerosis, Thrombosis, and Myocardial Infarction

Persistent inflammation, immune activation, endothelial dysfunction, and dyslipidemia occur commonly in chronic HIV infection, even when well controlled.[15-17] Most studies evaluating associations of HIV-related inflammation and immune dysfunction with cardiovascular events have focused primarily on atherosclerotic and thrombotic endpoints (which may lead to myocardial dysfunction) rather than HF itself. Dyslipidemia is common among persons with treated HIV, particularly those taking protease inhibitors (PIs), and is associated with atherosclerosis in HIV.[18] Chronic inflammation and immune activation are hallmarks of chronic HIV infection and persist even with effective ART.[19] A seminal analysis of the Strategies for Management of Anti-Retroviral Therapy (SMART) study of PLWH and the multi-ethnic study of atherosclerosis (MESA) of uninfected persons demonstrated that high-sensitivity C-reactive protein (hsCRP), interleukin 6 (IL-6), and D-dimer were significantly elevated among PLWH and remained persistently elevated even after effective HIV viral suppression on ART.[20] Elevated levels of inflammatory and coagulation markers have, in turn, been associated with higher risks of MI and overall mortality among PLWH.[17,21] Perhaps not surprisingly, several large cohort studies have found elevated rates of MI among PLWH that persist after accounting for demographics and traditional cardiovascular risk factors.[22,23] Low CD4+ T-cell count, in particular, has been associated with greater rates of MI.[24] Although data regarding ischemic etiologies of HF in HIV are sparse, it is reasonable to infer that these elevated rates of HIV-associated MI may contribute to elevated rates of HF in HIV, as has been described.[25] The contribution of ischemic heart disease to HF in HIV may be particularly important given the potential role of T regulatory cells in myocardial wound healing,[26] and the findings that PLWH may have larger scars following MI than uninfected persons.[27]

Inflammation, Immune Dysfunction, and Diastolic Dysfunction in Human Immunodeficiency Virus

In addition to contributing to atherosclerosis and MI, chronic HIV-related inflammation may contribute directly to myocardial dysfunction. In a cross-sectional study of 196 HIV-infected adults and 52 uninfected controls without known cardiovascular disease, HIV-infected adults had 2.4-fold greater odds of diastolic dysfunction after adjustment for age and traditional cardiovascular risk factors, as well as significantly higher LV mass index.[12] Persons with a history of advanced HIV-associated immune suppression have a higher risk of left ventricular hypertrophy and diastolic dysfunction compared with those with preserved immune function.[12a] Another potential contributor to impaired or restrictive patterns of myocardial relaxation in HIV is subepicardial/pericardial fat, which has been associated with inflammation and atherosclerosis among PLWH.[28] Extensive fibrosis has been demonstrated in persons with well-controlled HIV as well, and may contribute to myocardial dysfunction in HIV. A cross-sectional study evaluating cardiac magnetic resonance imaging (MRI) for 90 PLWH and 39 age-matched controls, all of whom had no known cardiovascular disease, found that myocardial fibrosis was present in 76% of PLWH versus 13% uninfected persons; PLWH also had higher intramyocardial lipid levels.[29] In a separate study of PLWH without known cardiovascular disease, markers of cardiac stress and fibrosis (soluble ST2 and growth differentiation factor 15) were independently associated with diastolic dysfunction and mortality.[30] In light of these findings, it is not surprising that a large study of HIV-infected and uninfected veterans in the United States demonstrated a significantly elevated risk of HFpEF among PLWH.[1] Low CD4+ T-cell count was associated with greater risk for HFpEF and HFrEF among PLWH, further underscoring the potential contribution of immunosuppression to HF in HIV.

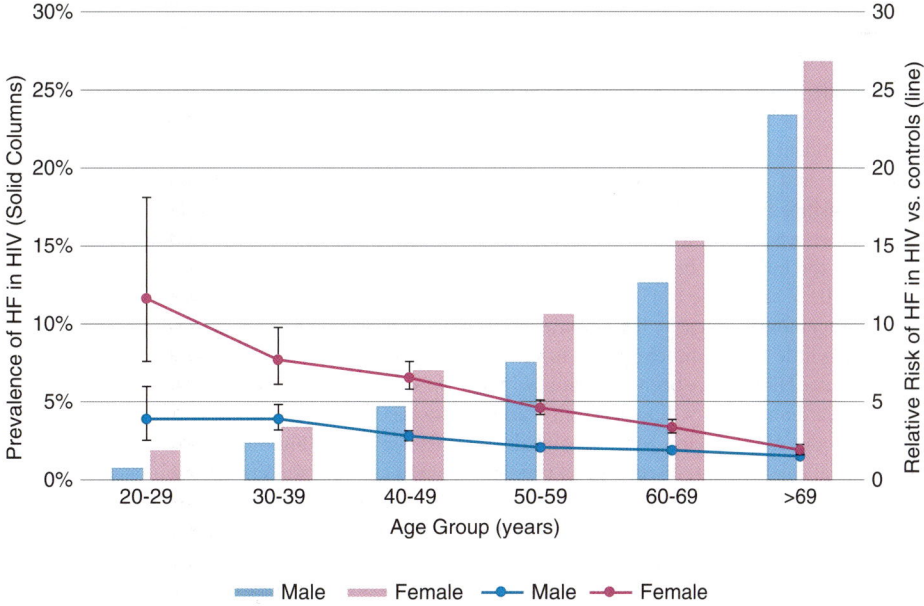

Fig. 30.1 Prevalence of heart failure *(HF)* in human immunodeficiency virus *(HIV)* patients *(solid columns)* and relative risk of HF compared to uninfected controls *(lines)* by age group and gender. (From Al-Kindi SG, El Amm C, Ginwalla M, et al. Heart failure in patients with human immunodeficiency virus infection: epidemiology and management disparities. *Int J Cardiol.* 2016;218:43–46. https://doi.org/10.1016/j.ijcard.2016.05.027.)

Pulmonary Arterial Hypertension

Pulmonary arterial hypertension is significantly more common among PLWH than uninfected persons. Pulmonary arterial hypertension, a recognized complication of HIV in the pre-ART era, has persisted in the modern ART era.[31] Several factors appear to contribute to pulmonary arterial hypertension in HIV, including polymorphisms in the HIV-Nef protein, chronic immune activation, endothelial dysfunction, and coinfection with other viruses.[32,33] Few large studies have evaluated the contribution of pulmonary arterial hypertension to right ventricular dysfunction and failure in HIV. Nevertheless, one may infer that the outsize contribution of pulmonary arterial hypertension in HIV also leads to elevated risks for right ventricular dysfunction and failure.

CARDIAC EFFECTS OF ANTIRETROVIRAL THERAPY

Few interventions in the history of medicine have so dramatically changed the course of human disease as the discovery of effective combination ART for HIV/AIDS. Since the first ART "cocktails" were introduced in the mid-1990s, data from the Centers for Disease Control indicate mortality due to HIV has plummeted from an annual age-adjusted death rate of ~17 per 100,000 in 1995 to ~2 per 100,000 in 2014 (https://www.cdc.gov/hiv/statistics/index.html). The first generations of these drugs were associated with significant metabolic toxicities, including cardiotoxicity; however, more metabolically friendly regimens composed of new drug classes, such as integrase inhibitors, have since been developed (**Table 30.2**).

Randomized trials such as SMART[34] (continuous vs. intermittent ART) and START (Strategic Timing of AntiRetroviral Treatment)[35] (early vs. delayed initiation of ART), have consistently pointed to improved outcomes with ART. The benefit appears to extend to cardiovascular disease specific outcomes, although HF is a rare outcome in these trials of younger patients. Thus, despite some toxicity, dramatic declines in clinical cardiomyopathy cases since the pre-ART era would suggest that on balance ART reduces the risk of HF. Here, we review the toxicities and potential benefits of specific ART drugs and drug-classes.

Nucleoside Reverse Transcriptase Inhibitors

The cardiotoxicity of nucleoside reverse transcriptase inhibitors (NRTIs) is thought to be primarily due to the effect on mitochondrial function. The heart is highly dependent on mitochondria to efficiently generate adenosine triphosphate and to perform other metabolic functions, and is thus highly sensitive to mitochondrial toxic drugs. Commercially licensed NRTIs are associated with varying degrees of mitochondrial dysfunction in the following order of toxicity: zalcitabine (ddC) > didanosine (ddI) > stavudine (d4T) > zidovudine (AZT).[36] Other NRTIs, such as tenofovir, abacavir, lamivudine, and emtricitabine, are associated with little to no mitochondrial toxicity. Accordingly, the mitochondrial toxic NRTIs have been associated with clinically significant myopathy, cardiomyopathy, lipodystrophy, and other complications in animal models and humans. More specifically, AZT and ddC cause mitochondrial enlargement, disruption of crystal architecture, and decreased mitochondrial DNA in cardiomyocytes leading to cardiomyopathy.[37] Currently, the clinical use of these drugs is extremely limited. They may be encountered among patients with highly resistant virus, or among patients who are resistant to changing an ART regimen that has been working for many years.

Other mechanisms besides mitochondrial toxicity are relevant to HF risk profile of certain NRTIs, and this is particularly relevant for two of the most widely prescribed NRTIs: abacavir and tenofovir. Recent use of abacavir and didanosine have been associated with MI risk in the Data Collection on Adverse Events of Anti-HIV Drugs

(D:A:D) study with relative rates of MI of 1.90 (95% CI 1.47–2.45) and 1.49 (95% CI 1.14–1.95), respectively, compared to those without recent use of those drugs.[38] Subsequent observational analyses from this cohort and others appear to confirm the association with abacavir, but a meta-analysis of randomized trial evidence showed no effect of abacavir on MI.[39] Although there is some debate, most experts advise avoidance of abacavir among those with high cardiovascular risk. On the other hand, cumulative tenofovir disoproxil fumarate (TDF) use was recently associated with a 21% lower risk of HF per year of use among US veterans.[40] The finding was consistent across a number of different statistical models, patient subgroups, and sensitivity analyses, and merits future investigation into the mechanism. It is unknown whether the benefit will be seen among users of the newer generation tenofovir alafenamide, which has been associated with lower rates of nephrotoxicity compared to TDF.

Protease Inhibitors

PIs are now widely known for their adverse metabolic effects and drug interactions with commonly prescribed cardiovascular disease therapies such as statins. Older PIs have been associated with risk of MI,[41] but this may not be true for atazanavir, a newer generation PI.[42] PIs may also contribute to HF risk through alterations in glucose metabolism in the heart; although few studies[40] have been powered to test the effect of ART drugs and drug classes on HF outcomes in HIV. There are no long-term data available on the risk of HF due to therapies such as integrase inhibitors.

Cardiac Effects of Antiretroviral Therapy in Children

Cardiac toxicity of ART remains an important consideration for children who are at potentially greater risk of toxicity due to a lifetime of exposure.[43] Fetuses exposed to ART in utero tend have greater chamber and wall size, and more pericardial effusions compared with fetuses not exposed to ART.[44] In addition, there is in utero evidence of worse systolic (by mitral systolic annular peak velocity) and diastolic (by isovolumic relaxation time) function. In one study, zidovudine use was the only factor significantly associated with these structural cardiac changes.[44] Furthermore, many children—especially in high-prevalence regions of SSA—are exposed to ART in utero, even if they are not ultimately infected with HIV (i.e., HIV-exposed uninfected). HIV-exposed uninfected children appear to have subtly reduced LV mass and mildly reduced diastolic function but no significant differences in systolic function.[45] For children who are infected with HIV, treatment with modern combination ART is associated with better LV structure and function by echo over time compared to single-drug regimens or no ART.[46]

COMORBIDITIES AND BEHAVIORAL FACTORS

Multiple medical comorbidities and behaviors potentially confound the association of HIV with HF or may be on the causal pathway to HIV-associated HF (**Fig. 30.2**). Additionally, it is likely that these factors interact in complex ways to contribute to HF risk. However, large cohorts of PLWH often lack granularity on comorbidities and lifestyle factors, and smaller studies that include this granularity lack statistical power.

Hypertension

Untreated HIV infection is typically associated with lower blood pressure. Then, when ART is initiated, blood pressures tend to rise. Thus, treated HIV infection is associated with high rates of clinical hypertension.[47] As expected, systolic hypertension is associated with the risk of MI among PLWH even when blood pressure is only modestly elevated (120–140 mm Hg). However, there is no evidence that the

TABLE 30.2	Major Classes of Antiretroviral Therapy and Known Cardiovascular Side Effects	
Class and Name of ART	Known Effects on Myocardial Dysfunction	Other Cardiovascular Side Effects
Nucleoside reverse transcriptase inhibitors (NRTIs)		
Abacavir (ABC)	No	± Myocardial infarction, dyslipidemia, inflammation
Didanosine (ddl)	Yes	Myocardial infarction
Emtricitabine (FTC)	No	
Lamivudine (3TC)	No	
Stavudine (d4T)	Yes	Dyslipidemia
Tenofovir (TDF)	±	
Zalcitabine (ddC)	Yes	
Zidovudine (AZT)	Yes	Dyslipidemia
Protease inhibitors (PIs)		
Atazanavir (ATV)	No	PR prolongation when given with RTV
Darunavir (DRV)	No	± cardiovascular events
Fosamprenavir (FPV)	No	± cardiovascular events
Indinavir (IDV)	No	Myocardial infarction
Lopinavir/ritonavir (LPV/r)	No	Myocardial infarction, PR and QT prolongation
Nelfinavir	No	± Dyslipidemia
Ritonavir (RTV)	No	All RTV "boosted" PIs carry risk of dyslipidemia
Saquinavir (SQV)	No	± Dyslipidemia, PR prolongation when given with RTV, QT prolongation
Tipranavir	No	
Non-nucleoside reverse transcriptase inhibitors (NNRTIs)		
Efavirenz (EFV)	No	Dyslipidemia, QT prolongation
Nevirapine	No	Dyslipidemia
Rilpivirine (RPV)	No	QT prolongation

ART, Antiretroviral therapy.

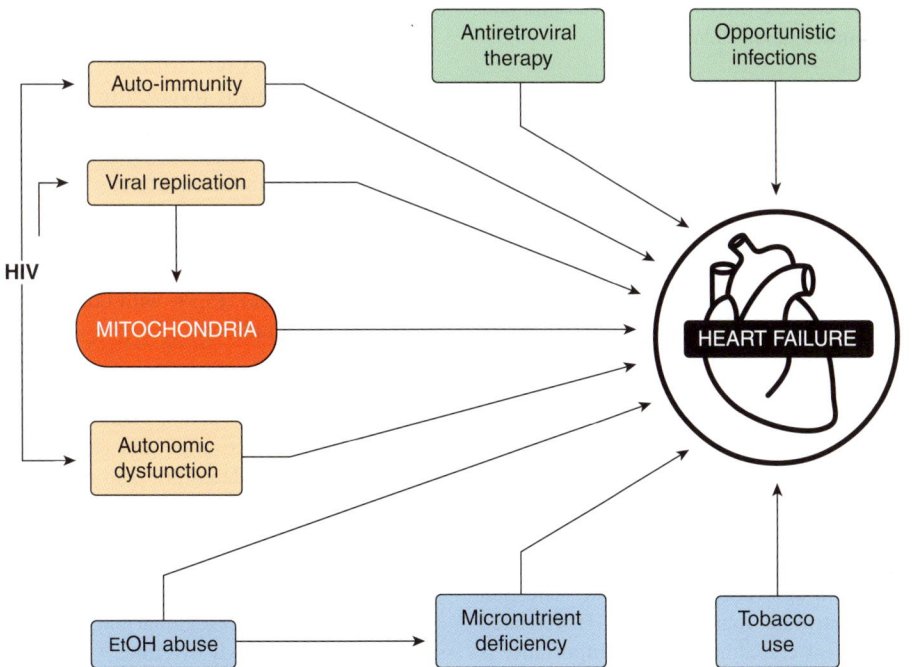

Fig. 30.2 Pathways of human immunodeficiency virus *(HIV)*–associated heart failure. *EtOH,* Ethanol. (From Bloomfield GS, Alenezi F, Barasa FA, et al. Human immunodeficiency virus and heart failure in low- and middle-income countries. *JACC Heart Fail.* 2015;38:579–590. https://doi.org/10.1016/j.jchf.2015.05.003.)

strength of this association is larger than in HIV-uninfected persons.[48] Although HIV is associated with increased LV mass and the risk of HFpEF,[49] the extent to which hypertension mediates these outcomes is not fully understood. A recent meta-analysis of data from around the globe demonstrated that ~35% of all HIV-infected adults on ART have hypertension, compared to approximately ~13% of the HIV-infected ART-naïve adults.[50] Among ART-experienced individuals older than 50 years, more than 50% have hypertension. Hypertension in this group leads to risk of MI[48] and all-cause mortality,[51] suggesting that diastolic dysfunction may be a harbinger of future cardiac risk.

Diabetes

HIV infection and its treatment are also associated with insulin resistance and clinical diabetes, although the magnitude of association may be declining over time with earlier treatment and less metabolically toxic ART. Ischemic and nonischemic HF are well-recognized complications of diabetes. Although diabetes is associated with HF risk independent of HIV (HR 2.0; 95% CI 1.5–2.5)[52] and PLWH may have higher rates of diabetes when HF is clinically adjudicated,[2] to our knowledge, whether diabetes is a more or less important risk factor in PLWH compared with uninfected persons has not been described.

Hepatitis C

Rates of coinfection with hepatitis C virus (HCV) among PLWH are high, though they are decreasing where many are able to access curative HCV treatment. Among US veterans in the VACS, for example, 29% of PLWH had HCV versus 13% among age-, gender-, and race/ethnicity-matched HIV-uninfected control subjects.[1] Hepatitis C can cause myocarditis and cardiomyopathy. Although it is likely that HCV contributes to HF risk in PLWH, few studies have specifically examined structural heart disease or HF risk in HIV monoinfection versus HIV/HCV coinfection. One small pilot MRI study suggested higher LV mass among those with coinfection.[53] Treatment of HCV with interferon-based regimens in PLWH have not been shown to decrease cardiac events, although there is a beneficial effect on cardiovascular risk factors.[54] In the modern HCV curative therapy era, there are no data on long-term cardiovascular outcomes in PLWH.

Kidney Disease

Kidney disease is a well-known risk factor for HF. Over 40% of end-stage renal disease (ESRD) patients have a diagnosis of HF, and HF accounts for 5.4% of all ESRD deaths.[55] Chronic kidney disease (CKD) is common and multifactorial among PLWH. Some ART—specifically tenofovir and PIs—may cause tubulopathy or a decreased glomerular filtration rate. Additionally, comorbidities, such as diabetes and hypertension, are increasingly contributing to CKD among PLWH on treatment. Similar to hypertension or diabetes, the degree to which comorbid kidney disease contributes to HF risk in HIV is incompletely understood. Although TDF is associated with CKD, most studies suggest it is associated with lower HF risk than other antiretrovirals.[40] Finally, the clinical characteristics and prognostic importance of cardiorenal syndrome among PLWH with HF have not been described.

Substance Abuse

Substance abuse is particularly common among PLWH and roughly half endorse present or prior drug or alcohol use disorders.[56] Alcohol, tobacco, and illicit drugs contribute substantially to HIV-related HF risk in the modern treatment era, although their importance is greater in wealthy nations compared to low- and middle-income countries. Heavy alcohol use causes cardiomyopathy and is prevalent in 8% to 42% of PLWH depending on the population surveyed (e.g., in the VACS it is ~25%).[57] Heavy alcohol use is a stronger predictor

of coronary heart disease among PLWHIV than among uninfected controls[57]; however, the risk of HF associated with HIV in the VACS was essentially unchanged when those with alcohol or cocaine abuse/dependence were excluded (HR 1.41 vs. 1.43, included vs. excluded).[1]

Tobacco use is also highly prevalent among PLWH (40%–74% prevalence) and contributes to ischemic heart disease risk.[58] In a Danish cohort, for example, HIV was more strongly associated with MI among smokers compared to nonsmokers, and the population attributable fraction of smoking for MI was 72% among PLWH compared to 24% among uninfected controls.[59] Yet, similar to alcohol use, the risk of HF associated with HIV in the VACS persisted even when smokers were excluded (HR 1.41 vs. 1.33, included vs. excluded).[1]

Stimulants are used more commonly in PLWH than among uninfected persons, most commonly cocaine and methamphetamine (prevalence ~15%–35% depending on the population surveyed).[58] These sympathomimetic drugs can cause cardiomyopathy, MI, and sudden death. Injection drug use—especially heroin—is on the rise in the United States and remains an important driver of HIV transmission in some populations. Importantly, illicit drug use may also be associated with poor disease-management behaviors, such as poor ART adherence, which indirectly affect HF risk.

MANIFESTATIONS OF HEART FAILURE

Low Left Ventricular Ejection Fraction

The pathways between HIV and clinical HF are numerous. Clinical features germane to specific etiologies in the general population (e.g., coronary artery disease, alcohol toxicity, micronutrient deficiency) will present similarly in those with HIV infection. Routine investigations with imaging, invasive or laboratory markers perform as well in the HIV-infected population as in the general population. Asymptomatic HCV/HIV coinfected patients have higher levels of B-type natriuretic peptide (BNP) compared to HIV monoinfected patients.[60] However, it is unclear if this portends greater future HF risk or impacts the interpretation of BNP levels in the HCV/HIV coinfected population.

Symptomatic HF in PLWH was historically associated with ventricular systolic dysfunction, but symptomatic systolic HF has become less common for PLWH, with an 8% prevalence of systolic dysfunction in one systematic review.[61] In an observational cohort study of 98,015 US veterans followed from 2003 through 2012, researchers found elevated risks for HF with HFrEF and HFpEF among HIV-infected versus uninfected veterans.[1] In contrast to the global LV dysfunction-predominant manifestation of HF in the pre-ART era, the investigators found that HFrEF (EF < 40%) comprised only 37.1% of incident HF among HIV-infected veterans, compared to 34.6% with HFpEF (EF > 50%), 15.5% with borderline HFpEF (EF 40%–49%), and 12.8% with unknown EF.

Myocardial Strain and Fibrosis

Among the numerous pathophysiological pathways to LV dysfunction in HIV, immune activation and chronic inflammation are thought to lead to collagen deposition and myocardial fibrosis.[29] Myocardial fibrosis, in turn, leads to diastolic dysfunction and eventual clinical HF. Global longitudinal strain, acquired through speckle-tracking imaging, is lower in PLWH with normal EF compared to matched uninfected controls.[62] Lower CD4+ T-cell count and higher HIV viral load correlate with worse global longitudinal strain,[63] and these abnormalities progress slowly overtime.[64] Cardiac MRI has further demonstrated that HIV infection is associated with subclinical myocardial edema and fibrosis.[65] These results are consistent with other studies demonstrating decreased radial and circumferential strain associated with increased lipid levels and diffuse myocardial fibrosis.[66]

TABLE 30.3 Rates of Cardiac Transplantation or Implantation of Left Ventricular Assist Devices According to Human Immunodeficiency Virus Status from Selected North American Centers

Center Region	Number of Centers	Performed Transplant in HIV+ Patients	HIV Infection as a Contraindication to Transplant	Implanted LVAD in HIV+ Patients	HIV Infection as a Contraindication to LVAD
Northeast	17	3 (18%)	7 (41%)	5 (29%)	1 (6%)
Midwest	17	1 (6%)	10 (59%)	4 (24%)	5 (29%)
West	17	2 (12%)	10 (59%)	3 (18%)	5 (29%)
South	30	1 (3%)	20 (67%)	7 (23%)	6 (20%)
Canada	8	0 (0%)	3 (38%)	0 (0%)	1 (13%)

HIV, Human immunodeficiency virus; *LVAD*, left ventricular assist devices.
Adapted from Uriel N, Nahumi N, Colombo PC, et al. Advanced heart failure in patients infected with human immunodeficiency virus: is there equal access to care? *J Heart Lung Transplant.* 2014;33(9):924–930. https://doi.org/10.1016/j.healun.2014.04.015.

Poor Inotropic Contractile Reserve

Studying PLWH with EF less than 45%, researchers identified that patients with inotropic contractile reserve on dobutamine stress echocardiography had better outcomes than patients without inotropic contractile reserve. The absence of cardiac inotropic contractile reserve had a specificity of 88% and a sensitivity of 74% for cardiac death over a median of 2.4 years.[67] Contractile reserve was also associated with improvement in left ventricular ejection fraction (LVEF). Improved LVEF was more common in patients with inotropic contractile reserve (70%) compared to those without inotropic contractile reserve (22%). Of note, patients with inotropic contractile reserve had healthier immune function and had lower viral loads compared to patients without inotropic contractile reserve. These data suggest that LV dysfunction in PLWH may be reversible, and that inotropic contractile reserve predicts improvement in EF.

Diastolic Dysfunction

Diastolic dysfunction is often present in minimally symptomatic individuals in the ART era. Diastolic dysfunction can be found in 26% to 50% of PLWH, which is nearly 10× greater than the general population in the same age range.[61,68] Diastolic dysfunction is often predated by increased LV mass index, LV hypertrophy, hypertension, and increased filling pressures which, in turn, lead to elevated pulmonary arterial pressures, all of which are common in PLWH.[12,69,70]

CLINICAL MANAGEMENT OF PATIENTS WITH HUMAN IMMUNODEFICIENCY VIRUS AND HEART FAILURE

In light of the evolving nature and unclear mechanisms of HIV-associated HF, few studies have evaluated HF management among PLWH. It is imperative that health care providers are aware of the burden of HF in HIV as well as potential drug-drug interactions when considering diagnostic and therapeutic options. Regarding HF diagnosis, there are insufficient data at present to recommend for or against routine screening for HF among PLWH.

Regarding HF therapies, there are insufficient HIV-specific data to warrant strong recommendations for therapeutic approaches other than those used in the general HF population. Fortunately, several essential HF therapies do not appear to have severe drug-drug interactions with HIV therapies. Diuretics, renally excreted beta blockers, angiotensin-converting enzyme (ACE) inhibitors, and angiotensin II receptor blockers (ARBs), with the exception of losartan and irbesartan, do not appear to have prohibitive drug-drug interactions with most antiretroviral medications.[71] Nevertheless, providers should pay particular attention to HF drugs with cytochrome P450 3A4

(CYP3A4) metabolism when initiating them in PLWH due to the potential for drug-drug interactions with boosted ART regimens that are "boosted" with a CYP3A4 inhibitor such as ritonavir or cobicistat.

HUMAN IMMUNODEFICIENCY VIRUS-SPECIFIC MANAGEMENT

For a patient presenting with advanced AIDS and symptomatic systolic HF, he/she should be started on ART in consultation with an HIV specialist. For those with treated HIV who present with a new diagnosis of LV dysfunction or cardiomyopathy, the ART regimen should be reviewed and any cardiotoxic ART—such as AZT and/or abacavir—should be changed if possible. The patient's primary HIV specialist may have additional considerations that would preclude a switch, such as the ART resistance profile derived from HIV genotyping.

CORONARY ARTERY BYPASS SURGERY

In general, PLWH with well-controlled HIV infection on ART can safely undergo cardiac surgery. In an analysis of over 1600 PLWH and propensity-matched uninfected controls from the Nationwide Inpatient Sample, mortality after cardiac surgery was similar (6.1% vs. 6.2%, HIV vs. control, $P = .915$), and HIV was associated with only a modestly increased rate of any complication (37% vs. 33%, HIV vs. control, $P = .038$; mostly blood transfusions and pneumonia).[72]

DEVICES AND ADVANCED HEART FAILURE THERAPIES

HIV infection is associated with a high rate of sudden cardiac death compared to the general population.[73] Thus, PLWH may derive benefit from implantable cardiac defibrillators (ICDs) if the risk of infection or other complications is not extraordinarily high. There are no published data regarding the safety and efficacy of defibrillators and cardiac resynchronization therapy in this population.

A survey of 89 US and Canadian heart transplant centers, conducted in 2012,[74] revealed that less than 10% had performed heart transplant in a PLWH and 57% considered HIV a contraindication for heart transplant. Only 17% had performed at least one left ventricular assist device (LVAD) implant on a patient with HIV, and 20% considered HIV a contraindication for LVAD. The authors conclude that PLWH have poor access to advanced therapies. Nonetheless, many centers who perform heart transplantation or implant LVADs explicitly consider HIV infection as a contraindication or have never treated PLWH with advanced HF therapy (**Table 30.3**). In a separate analysis of INTERMACS data from 2006 to 2013, HIV infection was associated with modestly worse outcomes among a small sample of 13 PLWH and 7828 uninfected controls.[75]

SUMMARY AND FUTURE DIRECTIONS

HIV-associated HF remains a significant comorbidity for the millions of individuals living with HIV infection worldwide. Since the widespread availability of ART, the clinical presentation, causes, and phenotype of HF have shifted to a disease marked by HFrEF and HFpEF, in contrast to earlier in the history of HIV when severe HFrEF was the most common form. Subclinical, diastolic dysfunction, abnormal myocardial strain, and hemodynamics are being seen more frequently in PLWH with adequate viral control. Numerous questions remain unanswered as to the etiology of myocardial dysfunction and the degree to which HIV viremia, opportunistic infections, atherosclerosis, thrombosis, myocardial infarction, inflammation, immune dysfunction, substance abuse, and ART interrelate and cause HF in this group. Concurrently, guidelines for screening for HF, diagnostic criteria for HIV-associated HF, and treatment recommendations particular to this group have yet to be outlined.

KEY REFERENCES

1. Freiberg MS, Chang C-CH, Skanderson M, et al. Association between HIV infection and the risk of heart failure with reduced ejection fraction and preserved ejection fraction in the antiretroviral therapy era: results from the veterans aging cohort study. *JAMA Cardiol.* 2017;2(5):536–546. https://doi.org/10.1001/jamacardio.2017.0264.
6. Bloomfield GS, Alenezi F, Barasa FA, Lumsden RH, Mayosi BM, Velazquez EJ. Human immunodeficiency virus and heart failure in low- and middle-income countries. *JACC: Heart Fail.* 2015;3(8):579–590. https://doi.org/10.1016/j.jchf.2015.05.003.
11. Al-Kindi SG, ElAmm C, Ginwalla M, et al. Heart failure in patients with human immunodeficiency virus infection: epidemiology and management disparities. *Int J Cardiol.* 2016;218:43–46. https://doi.org/10.1016/j.ijcard.2016.05.027.
12. Hsue PY, Hunt PW, Ho JE, et al. Impact of HIV infection on diastolic function and left ventricular mass. *Circ: Heart Fail.* 2010;3(1):132–139. https://doi.org/10.1161/CIRCHEARTFAILURE.109.854943.
29. Holloway CJ, Ntusi N, Suttie J, et al. Comprehensive cardiac magnetic resonance imaging and spectroscopy reveal a high burden of myocardial disease in HIV patients. *Circulation.* 2013;128(8):814–822. https://doi.org/10.1161/CIRCULATIONAHA.113.001719.
30. Secemsky EA, Scherzer R, Nitta E, et al. Novel biomarkers of cardiac stress, cardiovascular dysfunction, and outcomes in HIV-infected individuals. *JACC: Heart Fail.* 2015;3(8):591–599. https://doi.org/10.1016/j.jchf.2015.03.007.
52. Butt AA, Chang CC, Kuller L, et al. Risk of heart failure with human immunodeficiency virus in the absence of prior diagnosis of coronary heart disease. *Arch Intern Med.* 2011;171(8):737–743. https://doi.org/10.1001/archinternmed.2011.151.
61. Cerrato E, D'Ascenzo F, Biondi-Zoccai G, et al. Cardiac dysfunction in pauci symptomatic human immunodeficiency virus patients: a meta-analysis in the highly active antiretroviral therapy era. *Eur Heart J.* 2013;34(19):1432–1436. https://doi.org/10.1093/eurheartj/ehs471.
68. Sliwa K, Carrington MJ, Becker A, Thienemann F, Ntsekhe M, Stewart S. Contribution of the human immunodeficiency virus/acquired immunodeficiency syndrome epidemic to de novo presentations of heart disease in the heart of soweto study cohort. *Eur Heart J.* 2012;33(7):866–874. https://doi.org/10.1093/eurheartj/ehr398.
69. Mondy KE, Gottdiener J, Overton ET, et al. High prevalence of echocardiographic abnormalities among HIV-infected persons in the era of highly active antiretroviral therapy. *Clin Infect Dis.* 2011;52(3):378–386. https://doi.org/10.1093/cid/ciq066.

The full reference list for this chapter is available on ExpertConsult.

Clinical Evaluation of Heart Failure

Barry Greenberg, Paul J. Kim, Andrew M. Kahn

INTRODUCTION AND GOALS OF CLINICAL EVALUATION

Optimal implementation of heart failure therapy requires expeditious and accurate diagnosis as well as determination of the severity of the disease and, wherever possible, identification of its cause. The earlier in the clinical course that providers recognize the presence and stage of heart failure, the more likely that appropriate treatments will be initiated in a timely manner. In addition, since the clinical course of heart failure and the response to therapy are greatly influenced by a wide variety of risk factors and comorbid conditions, establishing a comprehensive medical, psychological, and social profile of the patient is essential for deciding on the most appropriate management strategies. As outlined in **Table 31.1**, the primary goals of the clinical evaluation are to confirm that the constellation of signs and symptoms that brought the patient to medical attention are indeed due to heart failure, determine the cause and severity of cardiac dysfunction, assess functional limitations and impairment in lifestyle, define the underlying etiology of heart failure, consider the various comorbidities and psychosocial issues that could influence the natural history of the disease, and also determine the success of various therapies and assess prognosis.

There is no single symptom, physical finding, or test that can achieve all these goals. Recognition and staging of heart failure is compounded by the influence of age, gender, etiology, comorbidities, the time course over which cardiac dysfunction develops, and both physiologic and psychologic adaptations to the presence of this disease. The clinical evaluation of heart failure is based on integrating information from a variety of sources, and when done effectively, it enables clinicians to initiate appropriate therapies in an expeditious and cost-effective manner. In the remainder of the chapter, we describe the modalities used for the clinical assessment of heart failure. The recommendations that are offered are based on information in the medical literature, available guidelines, and our own clinical experience in managing heart failure patients over the years.

HISTORY AND PHYSICAL EXAMINATION: THE CORE OF THE EVALUATION

Performance of a thorough history and physical examination received a class I recommendation in both the American College of Cardiology/American Heart Association (ACC/AHA) and the European Society of Cardiology (ESC) heart failure guidelines based predominantly on expert

TABLE 31.1   Key Questions to Be Addressed by the Heart Failure Evaluation

1. Does the patient have heart failure or are the presenting signs and symptoms caused by another condition?
2. What are the abnormalities in cardiac function resulted in heart failure? How severe are they?
3. To what extent does abnormal cardiac function impair the patient's ability to function?
4. What is the etiology of cardiac dysfunction?
5. What are the risk factors or conditions that resulted in the development of heart failure?
6. Are there comorbidities that are influencing the patient's clinical course? Will these comorbid conditions impact proposed heart failure therapies?
7. What is the patient's perception of their disease? Is it realistic and appropriate?
8. What is the patient's social situation? How might this influence their ability to comply with the therapeutic regimen?
9. What is the patient's prognosis? Should advanced therapies be considered? Is palliative or hospice care appropriate at this point in the patient's disease trajectory?

TABLE 31.2   Symptoms of Heart Failure

Fatigue
Shortness of breath at rest or during exercise
Discomfort while breathing (dyspnea)
Rapid breathing (tachypnea)
Difficulty in breathing while bending (bendopnea)
Orthopnea
Paroxysmal nocturnal dyspnea
Cough
Wheeze
Diminished exercise capacity
Nocturia
Weight gain or weight loss
Abdominal pain (particularly confined to the right upper quadrant)
Loss of appetite or early satiety
Increasing abdominal girth or bloating
Edema (of the extremities, scrotum, or elsewhere)
Palpitations
Syncope
History of Cheyne-Stokes respirations during sleep (often reported by the family rather than by the patient)
Somnolence, confusion or diminished mental acuity
Depression

TABLE 31.3   Questions That Are Useful in Coaxing the History from the Patient

1. Is your level of activity less now than in the past?
2. Can you keep up with your peers (e.g., spouse, friends) during activities?
3. Have you changed your activities, modified your participation, or avoided some activities that you enjoy and used to do?

opinion (Level of Evidence, C) in both documents.[1-3] In fact, it is hard to imagine defining management strategies for a heart failure patient without information gleaned from the history and physical examination, and even harder to envision these strategies being successful without knowledge of who the patient is and how they live their life. In addition, the encounter between provider and patient during which the history is taken and physical examination is performed is essential for establishing a level of comfort and trust that will almost certainly be needed by both parties as decisions are made during the course of the patient's disease.

The signs and symptoms of heart failure are typically caused by either congestion or impaired perfusion of vital organs. As abnormalities in cardiac function progress, increases in right and left ventricular filling pressures lead to the development of congestion in the pulmonary and systemic circulations, respectively. Impaired perfusion may become manifest in virtually any organ system in heart failure patients but is most often detected clinically by abnormalities in cerebral, cardiac, renal, hepatic, and skeletal muscle function. Tissue perfusion is determined by the pressure difference between the arterial and venous systems. Pressures within these vascular beds are in turn influenced by both the total intravascular volume and the ambient level of vasomotor tone.

Medical History
Symptoms
Patients seek medical advice because they don't feel well and their activities are impaired. **Table 31.2** contains a list of symptoms associated with heart failure. Since heart failure can affect virtually all organs in the body, the symptoms described by patients are protean. It is important to recognize that these symptoms alone are insufficient to define the presence or severity of heart failure. A specific symptom should always be viewed in the context of other symptoms, physical signs, and the clinical setting in general. How somatic symptoms are appreciated by the patient and how they are related to the provider can vary considerably. The description of symptoms can be influenced by a variety of factors, including the patient's threshold for detecting and relating discomfort, their age and previous level of functioning, individual performance goals, and the time course over which symptoms develop. Psychological issues, socioeconomic factors, and differences in the level of education between the patient and the examiner can also influence how a patient relates their symptoms. Needless to say, all these factors

should be taken into account when evaluating an individual patient. Many patients have difficulty defining the impact of their symptoms on their activities. We find that the questions outlined in **Table 31.3** are helpful in eliciting the full extent of a patient's impairment. Another tried and true method of determining the severity of a patient's symptoms is to seek confirmation whenever a family member or significant other accompanies the patient to the examination. The divergence in opinion of the extent of limitation described by the patient and that offered by a more objective source can be quite substantial.

Although none of the symptoms listed in Table 31.2 are sufficient by themselves for determining that heart failure is the cause of the patient's complaints, some are more specific than others. When present, paroxysmal nocturnal dyspnea (PND) is a very strong indicator that symptoms are due to heart failure, particularly when other conditions that result in nocturnal awakening, including postnasal drip, esophageal reflux, and orthopedic issues, are excluded. PND may also be confused with shortness of breath (SOB) that occurs when patients walk to the bathroom at night after having been awakened by the need to urinate. When PND is suggested, the clinician should confirm that the episodes involve abrupt awakening due to "air hunger"—a sensation that causes the patient to move from a recumbent position to a more upright one, remaining upright for at least several minutes in order to catch their breath. Another helpful clue for defining PND is that PND tends to recur nightly at a relatively constant time after the patient lies down. Another congestive symptom that has recently attained prominence is bendopnea, which is defined as SOB when bending forward, as when a patient puts on their shoes. Bendopnea has been reported in 28% of heart failure patients. When present, it is associated with higher levels of pulmonary artery wedge (PAW) and right atrial (RA) pressures.[4] Symptoms due to impaired cerebral perfusion, including somnolence, confusion, diminished mental acuity, or depression, though common in heart failure patients, are not often related by the patient during the interview. As with functional impairment, it is often the patient's family member or significant other who describes the presence of these symptoms.

The New York Heart Association (NYHA) functional classification (**Table 31.4**) is used to quantify symptomatic limitation in heart failure patients and has proved useful for assessing the adequacy of therapy and determining prognosis. It offers a simple and rapid means of detecting changes in the patient's symptomatic status over time or in response to treatment. As such, it has become the "lingua franca" for communication between providers about the patient's clinical status. Evaluation of the NYHA functional class also provides important prognostic information, as there is a stepwise increase in morbidity and mortality risk with increasing functional class.[5] While other means of assessing symptoms such as cardiopulmonary exercise testing more accurately determine whether the patient's subjective complaints are caused by heart failure and can provide a more precise indication of the patient's limitation, NYHA functional class determination is a standard for assessing and communicating symptomatic status because of its ease and economy.

Patients are also classified according to the stage of heart failure,[2] as depicted in **Fig. 31.1.** In contrast to NYHA functional classification, which is based on symptoms alone, the ACC/AHA Heart Failure Staging system incorporates risk factors and changes in the heart's structure and function into the equation. Whereas patients frequently move to higher or lower NYHA classes as their disease waxes and wanes, a patient's stage of heart failure can only advance. Also, within stages C and D heart failure, symptoms can vary considerably over time. For instance, a stage C patient hospitalized for an episode of decompensation may have symptoms that improve from NYHA class IV on admission to class I or II at the time of discharge. The use of this staging system has helped alert providers to the substantial numbers of patients who are at risk for developing heart failure. In a community-based survey carried out in the United States, 56% of adults ≥45 years of age were found to have stage A or B heart failure.[6] Striking differences in mortality as the stage advances were also noted in this population, emphasizing the need for risk factor modification and early intervention in order to prevent progression of disease and improve outcomes.

Information About Past Medical History and Comorbidities

Heart failure patients tend to be older and often have comorbidities that influence the presentation, clinical course, prognosis, and response to therapy. Comorbid conditions may also interfere with the diagnostic process, aggravate symptoms, and contribute to a reduction in quality

TABLE 31.4 New York Heart Association Functional Classification of Heart Failure

Class	Symptoms
Class I (mild)	No limitation of physical activity
	Ordinary physical activity does not cause undue fatigue, palpitation, or dyspnea (shortness of breath)
Class II (mild)	Slight limitation of physical activity
	Comfortable at rest, but ordinary physical activity results in fatigue, palpitation, or dyspnea
Class III (moderate)	Marked limitation of physical activity
	Comfortable at rest, but less than ordinary activity causes fatigue, palpitation, or dyspnea
Class IV (severe)	Unable to carry out any physical activity without discomfort
	Symptoms of cardiac insufficiency at rest
	If any physical activity is undertaken, discomfort is increased

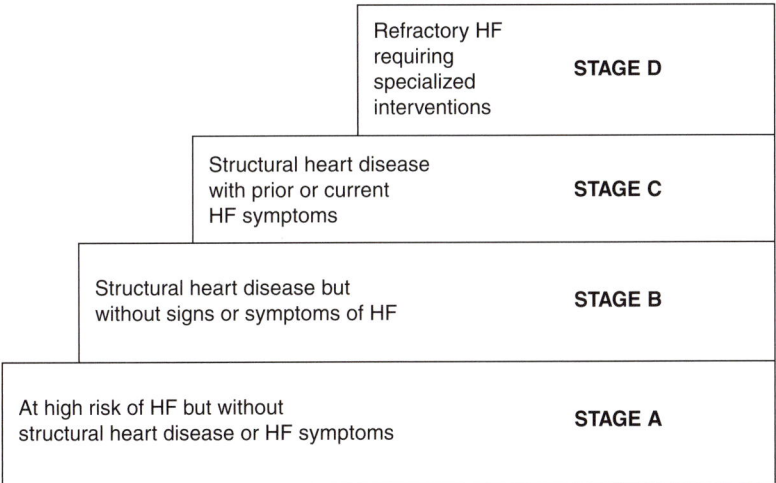

Fig. 31.1 Stages of heart failure. Patients progress through various stages of heart failure beginning with the presence of risk factors to end-stage disease. Whereas symptoms and New York Heart Association Functional Classification may worsen or improve, the stage of heart failure can only remain or progress. (Adapted from Hunt SA, Abraham WT, Chin MH, et al. ACC/AHA 2005 guideline update for the diagnosis and management of chronic heart failure in the adult: a report of the American College of Cardiology/American Heart Association Task Force on Practice Guidelines [Writing Committee to Update the 2001 Guidelines for the Evaluation and Management of Heart Failure]: developed in collaboration with the American College of Chest Physicians and the International Society for Heart and Lung Transplantation: endorsed by the Heart Rhythm Society. *J Am Coll Cardiol.* 2005;46[6]:e1–e82.)

TABLE 31.5 **Comorbid Conditions Commonly Seen in Heart Failure Patients**
Angina
Coronary artery disease
Frailty
Cachexia
Malignancies
Stroke
Peripheral vascular disease
Depression
Diabetes
Gout
Arthritis
Hyperlipidemia
Hypertension
Iron deficiency
Anemia
Chronic kidney disease
Chronic obstructive pulmonary disease
Asthma
Sleep disordered breathing
Obesity
Thyroid disorders (both hypo- and hyperthyroidism)

TABLE 31.6 **Physical Findings Associated with Heart Failure**
Tachycardia
Extra beats or irregular rhythm
Narrow pulse pressure or thready pulse[a]
Pulsus alternans[a]
Tachypnea
Elevated jugular venous pressure
Positive hepatojugular reflux
Dullness and diminished breath sounds at one or both lung bases
Rales, rhonchi, or wheezes
Cardiac apex displaced leftward or inferiorly
Sustained apical impulse
Parasternal lift
S_3 or S_4 (either palpable or audible)
Tricuspid or mitral regurgitant murmur
Hepatomegaly (often accompanied by right upper quadrant discomfort)
Ascites
Presacral edema
Anasarca[a]
Cool or mottled extremities[a]
Pedal edema
Chronic venous stasis changes

[a]These findings are indicative of more severe disease.

of life. Comorbidities of particular importance in the management of heart failure patients are listed in **Table 31.5**. As part of the diagnostic evaluation and, in particular, for designing appropriate management strategies, it is essential for the clinician to have full knowledge of the patient's comorbidities and how they are being treated.

Social and Family History

Understanding the social fabric of the patient's life, including their cultural background, education, work history, current living situation, and social support, will allow the clinician to gain a more thorough assessment of why they may have developed heart failure (e.g., work exposure, travel experience), and how they perceive their current limitations. It will also provide a context for various therapeutic strategies, particularly those that can be offered to patients with advanced heart failure (i.e., mechanical circulatory support and heart transplantation).

Information from family history can provide clues about etiology of heart failure. A history of cardiovascular risk factors or the presence of heart failure in other family members can influence the direction of the diagnostic evaluation. For instance, knowledge that multiple family members have had myocardial infarctions would direct the clinician toward determining whether coronary artery disease is the cause of the patient's heart failure.

Familial Cardiomyopathy and Genetic Testing (see also Chapter 24)

Dilated cardiomyopathy (DCM) is considered to be idiopathic in around half of the cases and approximately a third of these are hereditary.[7,8] Overall, more than 50 genes have been identified as causes of DCM, with the most common ones being genes related to the cytoskeleton (e.g., titin, lamin, and desmin). For patients with DCM, the ACC/AHA Heart Failure Guideline gives a class I recommendation for obtaining a three-generational family history. A history of early onset heart failure or sudden cardiac death in first-degree family members should trigger genetic testing to determine if a familial cardiomyopathy (defined as the presence of DCM in ≥2 relatives) is present.

Physical Examination
Cardiovascular System

Despite the plethora of blood chemistries, biomarker analyses, imaging studies, and other diagnostic tests that all heart failure patients are subjected to in today's medical environment, a carefully performed physical examination provides unique information to the clinician. Oversights in the physical examination are a major contributor to missed or delayed diagnosis, and they lead to exposure to unnecessary tests, initiation of incorrect treatments, and other adverse consequences. In a review of 208 case vignettes, Verghese et al. concluded that physical examination inadequacies are a preventable source of medical error and that adverse events are caused mostly by failure to perform the relevant examination.[9] Clinical signs of congestion have also been shown to be independent predictors of prognosis in heart patients.[10] In a post-hoc analysis of 1376 patients with symptomatic left ventricular systolic dysfunction and a documented recent episode of atrial fibrillation, congestive signs on the physical examination (i.e., peripheral edema, jugular venous distension, a third heart sound, and pulmonary rales) were associated with worse prognosis.[11] Physical findings in heart failure patients have been extensively described by a group of expert clinicians,[12,13] and **Table 31.6** lists the ones that have been found to be most helpful by the authors. A discussion of these signs follows.

1. General. The exam begins when the clinician enters the room, and it uses multiple senses. Visual examination of the patient's body habitus, noting the presence of obesity, cachexia, a neurologic deficit, or orthopedic problem, provides valuable diagnostic information. Vertical head bobbing due to a forceful pulse is seen in patients with chronic aortic insufficiency, while lateral movement from side to side may indicate the presence of severe tricuspid insufficiency. Shortness of breath during normal conversation or when the patient moves to the examining table suggests the presence of pulmonary congestion or underlying lung disease. The clinician should note whether the patient is pale, flushed, perspiring, or in pain, and be alerted to the presence of unusual odors indicating

poor personal hygiene, tobacco, or alcohol use. The astute examiner can detect ketoacidosis by its characteristic fruity odor or advanced liver disease by the "mousy" smell of fetor hepaticus.

2. Vital signs provide extensive information about the patient's current level of well-being, and they may provide clues into the etiology of heart failure. Normal heart rate, blood pressure, respiratory rate, and oxygen saturation are associated with clinical stability, whereas rapid heart rate, low blood pressure (usually below 90 mm Hg), and rapid shallow breathing with reduced oxygen saturation are indicators of decompensation. The patient's pulse rate and characteristics may provide clues regarding etiology of heart failure (e.g., tachycardia induced cardiomyopathy) or the presence of cardiac arrhythmias (e.g., atrial fibrillation). A narrow pulse pressure (less than 25% of systolic blood pressure) is a sign of reduced left ventricular stroke volume, while a wide arterial pulse suggests the presence of a high output state, chronic aortic insufficiency or a stiff, noncompliant vascular bed (as in heart failure with preserved ejection fraction [HFpEF] patients). Peripheral findings indicating a wide pulse pressure (e.g., Quincke or water hammer pulse) are often found in patients with chronic aortic insufficiency, while evidence of poor capillary refill suggests low cardiac output/and or severe vasoconstriction.

3. A low volume carotid pulse is consistent with reduced cardiac output or (when there is delayed rise) aortic stenosis, while a bounding pulse indicates a large stroke volume, stiff noncompliant vascular bed, or (particularly when there is rapid falloff) chronic aortic insufficiency. The contour of the carotid pulse may also contain clues about etiology. A notch or shudder during the upstroke (anacrotic shoulder of aortic stenosis), a double bump in its midportion (bisferiens pulse of chronic aortic insufficiency), or an initially normal carotid upstroke that slows midway through (spike and dome pulse of hypertrophic obstructive cardiomyopathy) are pathognomonic physical findings.

4. The jugular venous pulse is the most useful physical finding for determining a patient's volume status. It has been shown to have better sensitivity and specificity than other signs, such as pulmonary rales or the presence of an S_3. Not only does an elevated JVP detect systemic congestion, but there is good sensitivity (70%) and specificity (79%) between high JVP and elevated left-sided filling pressure.[14] Changes in JVP with therapy usually parallel changes in left-sided filling pressure. Significant interobserver variability regarding the extent of JVP elevation, however, has been noted.[15] Both sensitivity and specificity of the JVP in detecting congestion can be improved by exerting pressure on the right upper quadrant of the abdomen while assessing venous pulsations in the neck (i.e., hepatojugular or abdominojugular reflux).[15] The jugular pulse is best assessed in a warm, well-lighted room with the patient comfortably seated on the exam table with the head elevated at 45 degrees. The venous pulse can be identified by its predominant inward movement that distinguishes it from the sharply outward bounding carotid pulse. When the meniscus of the pulse is identified, the vertical distance to the angle of Louis is measured and 5 cm added to account for the distance to the midpoint of the right atrium. A normal venous pressure is less than 8 cm H_2O. While the position of the meniscus of the venous pulse in the neck will vary according to the patient's degree of elevation, the actual vertical height remains relatively constant so that determination of pulse is theoretically independent of the patient's position. However, at lesser degrees of elevation, the meniscus of the venous pulse may rise to the angle of the jaw, thereby obscuring the true extent of elevated venous pressure. Increasing the elevation of the head of the bed will overcome this limitation. Also, observation

for venous pulsation along the side of the ear above the angle of the jaw can help detect very high levels of venous pressure.

5. Lung examination is used to assess for presence of pulmonary congestion that can be manifest as dullness and diminished breath sounds due to a pleural effusion, fine crackles (rales) due to fluid in the intra-alveolar space, or wheezes due to bronchospasm. When present, rales are specific in confirming that heart failure is present. However, in patients with chronic disease, lymphatic hypertrophy serves to remove fluid buildup in the lungs so that rales are often absent, even when filling pressures are elevated.[15] Rubs indicative of inflammation of the pleural surface can also often be detected by auscultation or even palpation during a deep inspiration.

6. Cardiac examination starts with observation, palpation, and percussion of the chest, which is then followed by auscultation. Chest wall deformities, particularly bowing of the left chest, may occur in patients with congenital abnormalities. The presence of cardiomegaly can often be detected by observing an apical impulse that is displaced laterally in the left precordium. Pulsations in the apical impulse during early and late diastole are the visual analogues of the S_3 and S_4 heart sounds. A visible sternal lift can be appreciated in many patients with pulmonary hypertension, but can also be caused by anterior displacement of the heart by the posteriorly situated left atrium as it fills rapidly during systole, as occurs in patients with severe mitral regurgitation. Percussion of the left cardiac border >8 cm to the left of the midsternal line indicates that the heart is enlarged. Palpation of the precordium builds on the visual evaluation of pulsations at the cardiac apex and over the sternum. It is also used to detect an accentuated second heart sound (as occurs in pulmonary hypertension) and the presence of thrills associated with turbulent flow across a heart valve or due to a structural abnormality such as a ventricular septal defect (VSD). Auscultation for murmurs, gallops, and rubs completes the cardiac examination. While a complete overview of cardiac auscultation is beyond the scope of the chapter, the general focus is to detect the presence of valve abnormalities that could be the cause (e.g., aortic stenosis) or consequence (e.g., mitral or tricuspid insufficiency) of heart failure, get an insight into ventricular filling patterns by listening for the presence of an S_3 and S_4, and determine if other abnormalities (e.g., VSD) or pericardial disease are present. The intensity of heart sounds may also help indicate the presence of cardiac abnormalities. The intensity of S_1 can be diminished by a long PR interval or other conditions (e.g., aortic insufficiency) that lead to left ventricular volume overload while P_2 intensity is increased in patients with pulmonary hypertension.

7. Abnormal physical findings on the abdominal examination due to heart failure are mostly consequences of congestion and include hepatomegaly, splenomegaly, and ascites. The latter is best assessed by testing for shifting dullness, particularly in patients where detection of a fluid wave may be obscured by obesity.

8. Other findings associated with congestion include scrotal edema (grossly underreported, particularly by trainees), presacral edema, and edema of the lower extremities. For the latter, both the depth of indentation caused by pressure of the examiners thumb and how long the pit remains are used determine the grade, which ranges from 1 to 4.

9. While low cardiac output (which may be further accentuated by peripheral arterial constriction) can lead to an abnormally low body temperature, it is more commonly associated with localized reduction in temperature in peripheral tissues. The examiner may detect cool hands, feet, or nose in patients with low cardiac output. Marked reductions in tissue perfusion are characterized by a

dusky mottled appearance of the extremities. Milder degrees of hypoperfusion, however, may be manifest by reduced temperature only in watershed areas such as the knee caps.

10. Low cardiac output and decreased cerebral hypoperfusion can lead to drowsiness, forgetfulness, and other signs of reduced mental acuity. In extreme cases, patients may be judged as having dementia, but the real cause of altered mentation becomes apparent as the patient recovers with treatments that raise cerebral perfusion.

LABORATORY

Essential

A list of routine diagnostic tests used for the evaluation of patients with heart failure is provided in **Table 31.7**. The goal of this testing is to detect reversible or treatable causes of heart failure, determine the patient's suitability for particular therapies, and reveal the presence of comorbidities that might affect treatment strategies. Repeated determination of electrolyte values, renal function, and other variables is also required as the clinical course evolves over time.

Selective

There are a variety of uncommon causes of heart failure, including exposure to toxic substances (e.g., recreational substance abuse, heavy metals), infections (e.g., HIV/AIDS, Chagas disease), infiltrative diseases (e.g., amyloidosis, glycogen storage diseases, lysosomal storage diseases), hormonal abnormalities (e.g., growth hormone, pheochromocytoma), and nutritional deficiencies (e.g., thiamine, L-carnitine, selenium). Testing for these causes for heart failure should be considered when one of them is suspected. The ACC/AHA Guidelines give class IIa recommendations for screening for hemochromatosis or HIV in selected patients who present with heart failure and for obtaining diagnostic tests for rheumatologic diseases, amyloidosis, or pheochromocytoma when there is clinical suspicion of these diseases.[16]

Biomarkers (see also Chapter 33)

Natriuretic peptides, troponins, and numerous additional biomarkers related to inflammation, oxidative stress, vascular dysfunction, and myocardial matrix remodeling have been implicated in heart failure.[17] Natriuretic peptides in particular have assumed an important role in the clinical evaluation of patients. Their measurement in ambulatory patients with dyspnea are given a class I recommendation to support clinical decision making regarding the diagnosis of heart failure.[16] They are most helpful in making the diagnosis in cases where information obtained from the history and physical examination leaves the examiner uncertain about whether or not heart failure is present. As patients with levels below the diagnostic cut-point are highly unlikely to experience heart failure, natriuretic peptide levels are useful in excluding heart failure. In the nonacute setting, values of 35 pg/mL for B-type natriuretic peptide (BNP) and 125 pg/mL for NT-proBNP are considered the upper limit of normal, while in the acute setting these values are increased to 100 pg/mL and 300 pg/mL, respectively. While discordance between natriuretic peptide levels and the rest of the clinical assessment should alert the clinician to the possibility that they may have erred in diagnosing heart failure, it is important to recognize that a number of factors can alter natriuretic peptide levels. These are summarized in **Table 31.8**. Thus natriuretic peptide levels should always be interpreted in the context of the clinical setting. Measurement of natriuretic peptides are also given a class 1 recommendation for use in patients presenting with dyspnea to help support the diagnosis of heart failure and establish disease prognosis or severity in both ambulatory and acutely ill heart failure patients. Measurement of biomarkers of

TABLE 31.7 **Routine Diagnostic Blood Tests Used in the Evaluation of Patients With Heart Failure**

- Hemoglobin and WBC
- Serum electrolytes, including calcium and magnesium
- Urea, creatinine (with estimated GFR)
- Liver function tests (bilirubin, AST, ALT, alkaline phosphatase)
- Glucose, HbA1c
- TSH
- Ferritin, TSAT, TIBC
- Fasting lipid panel
- Natriuretic peptides

ALT, Alanine aminotransferase; *AST*, aspartate aminotransferase; *GFR*, glomerular filtration rate; *HbA1c*, glycosylated hemoglobin; *TIBC*, total iron binding capacity; *TSAT*, transferrin saturation; *TSH*, thyroid-stimulating hormone; *TSAT*, transferrin saturation; *WBC*, white blood cell count.

TABLE 31.8 **Causes of Elevated Concentrations of Natriuretic Peptides**

Cardiac
Heart failure
Acute coronary syndromes
Pulmonary embolism
Myocarditis
Left ventricular hypertrophy
Hypertrophic or restrictive cardiomyopathy
Valvular heart disease
Congenital heart disease
Atrial and ventricular tachyarrhythmias
Heart contusion
Cardioversion, ICD shock
Surgical procedures involving the heart
Pulmonary hypertension
Noncardiac
Advanced age
Ischemic stroke
Subarachnoid hemorrhage
Renal dysfunction
Liver dysfunction (mainly liver cirrhosis with ascites)
Paraneoplastic syndrome
Chronic obstructive pulmonary disease
Severe infections (including pneumonia and sepsis)
Severe burns
Anemia
Severe metabolic and hormone abnormalities (e.g., thyrotoxicosis, diabetic ketosis)

HFpEF, Heart failure with preserved ejection fraction; *HFrEF*, heart failure with reduced ejection fraction; *ICD*, implantable cardioverter defibrillator.

myocardial injury or fibrosis may be considered (class IIb recommendation) for added risk stratification.[16]

The use of natriuretic peptides to screen ACC/AHA stage A patients with risk factors for developing heart failure is given a class IIa recommendation based on the expectation that the presence of elevated levels will be followed by aggressive initiation of guideline directed medical therapy and other life-style strategies designed to prevent further progression of disease.[16] Whether this approach will prove cost-effective and have an impact on quality of life and outcomes, however, requires further study.

THE ELECTROCARDIOGRAM

The electrocardiogram (ECG) is an essential part of the initial evaluation of a patient with new onset or suspected heart failure. In the ACC/AHA guidelines, obtaining an ECG is given a class I recommendation, while the ESC guidelines stress the negative predictive value of a normal ECG in helping exclude the presence of heart failure.[3,16] An ECG should also be obtained whenever there is an episode of acute heart failure or a heart failure patient's condition deteriorates over time. Sinus tachycardia due to sympathetic nervous system activation is seen with advanced heart failure or during episodes of decompensation. The presence of atrial arrhythmias on the ECG may explain why heart failure has worsened, as well as provide a target for therapeutic interventions. Ventricular arrhythmias ranging from isolated PVCs to more complex arrhythmias, including runs of nonsustained ventricular tachycardia, are common in heart failure patients. The presence of ventricular arrhythmias raises concerns about electrolyte abnormalities and also the potential risk of life-threatening rhythm disturbances. A widened QRS complex exceeding 120 milliseconds (msec) in a patient with systolic dysfunction is a useful indicator of ventricular dyssynchrony. The QRS duration is essential in determining whether or not cardiac resynchronization therapy (CRT) should be recommended, with both the QRS pattern and duration used to define the strength of the recommendation for CRT, with the highest level of enthusiasm for patients who have a left bundle branch block (LBBB) pattern with QRS duration ≥150 msec. The P wave morphology helps detect left atrial enlargement (LAE). A biphasic P wave in lead V_1 is a sensitive indicator of LAE, while increased P wave duration in lead II is more specific. An increase in P wave amplitude in lead II suggests that right atrial enlargement may be present. An unusual P wave axis (particularly when coupled with a short PR interval in the setting of atrial arrhythmias) suggests that an ectopic atrial focus or accessory pathway may be present. Increased voltage in lead AVL or in the limb leads should lead to consideration of left ventricular hypertrophy and a search for its causes. A large R wave, prolonged QRS, and ST-T wave changes in the right precordial leads can be a clue that right ventricular hypertrophy is present and should trigger a search for conditions that cause primary or secondary pulmonary hypertension. The presence of Q waves suggests that heart failure may have been caused by a myocardial infarction (or possibly amyloidosis); new or reversible repolarization changes raise concerns that clinical deterioration may be due to worsening myocardial ischemia, even when chest pain is absent. Low QRS voltage suggests the presence of an infiltrative disease, particularly amyloidosis, or pericardial effusion.

CHEST X-RAY

Like the ECG, the chest X-ray plays an integral role in the evaluation of a patient with heart failure, and it also receives a class I recommendation in the ACC/AHA guideline.[16] The chest x-ray helps determine heart size and the presence of pulmonary congestion. It is also useful in detecting alternative cardiac or pulmonary diseases that may be causing or contributing to the patient's symptoms.

Cardiac size is best determined from the posteroanterior projection (PA), with the beam source 6 feet from the patient's back. Radiographs obtained in the anteroposterior projection or with the beam source closer to the patient than usual (both of which are common with portable chest radiography) will magnify the cardiac silhouette, making the determination of cardiac size problematic. The lateral film is quite useful in detecting ventricular enlargement that may not be apparent on the PA projection and to define which ventricle is enlarged. Since the right ventricle is an anterior structure, enlargement is detected by filling in of the retrosternal airspace. Enlargement of the left ventricle extends the lower portion of the cardiac silhouette toward the spine. Pulmonary congestion can be recognized by the presence of a "butterfly" pattern of alveolar opacities that fan out bilaterally from engorged hilar pulmonary arteries to the periphery of the lungs (**Fig. 31.2**). Subtle findings of pulmonary congestion include the presence of Kerley B lines (thin horizontal linear opacities extending to the pleural surface caused by the accumulation of fluid in the interstitial space), peribronchial cuffing detected as a thickened and fuzzy appearance of the walls of small bronchi that are cut *en face* in the PA projection, and evidence of prominent upper lobe vasculature (indicating pulmonary venous hypertension). Pleural effusions or fluid in the right minor fissure may also be seen. Although these findings are quite helpful in making the diagnosis of heart failure when they are present, they are often absent, even when patients present with acute decompensation. The low sensitivity of the chest x-ray to detect worsening in patients with established disease is related to the fact that long-standing elevations in pulmonary capillary pressures lead to the development of lymphatic hypertrophy that prevents fluid from building up in the lung parenchyma.

The chest radiograph can provide clues about the cause of heart failure. For instance, the absence of cardiomegaly suggests that ejection fraction is preserved or that the onset of systolic dysfunction has been recent. Disproportionate enlargement of the left atrium raises the possibility of mitral valve disease or (when there is biatrial enlargement) an infiltrative process. Prominence of the right ventricle without enlargement of other chambers should raise the suspicion of pulmonary hypertension as a cause of right-sided heart failure. The chest radiograph may also provide an indication that heart failure is due to coronary, valvular, or pericardial disease when calcification is noted in the appropriate position.

ECHOCARDIOGRAPHY (SEE ALSO CHAPTER 32)

In the vast majority of cases, transthoracic echocardiography is the initial cardiac imaging test used to evaluate patients with newly diagnosed or suspected heart failure, and its use is given a class I recommendation in both the ACC/AHA and ESC heart failure guidelines.[2,3] This test is essentially harmless, involves no radiation, and can be done at the bedside if necessary. Echocardiography is particularly well-suited for evaluating myocardial structure and function, valvular function, and hemodynamics. Limitations of echocardiography are that available imaging planes and image quality are dependent on acoustic windows.

Cardiac Structure and Systolic Function

A vital early step in the initial evaluation of heart failure patients is the noninvasive assessment of left and right ventricular size and systolic function. Echocardiography provides an assessment of chamber sizes and morphology, as well as left and right ventricular function.

Left Ventricular Volumes and Systolic Function

These are usually quantified using the biplane method and the modified Simpson rule.[18] For patients with suspected heart failure, the finding of severely depressed left ventricular systolic function confirms the diagnosis, and is usually followed by further evaluation to determine the etiology. In patients with suboptimal endocardial definition, intravenous contrast agents can improve measurement accuracy and reproducibility.[19] Three-dimensional echocardiography can be used to quantify regional function and has been shown to provide more accurate and reproducible evaluation of left ventricular systolic

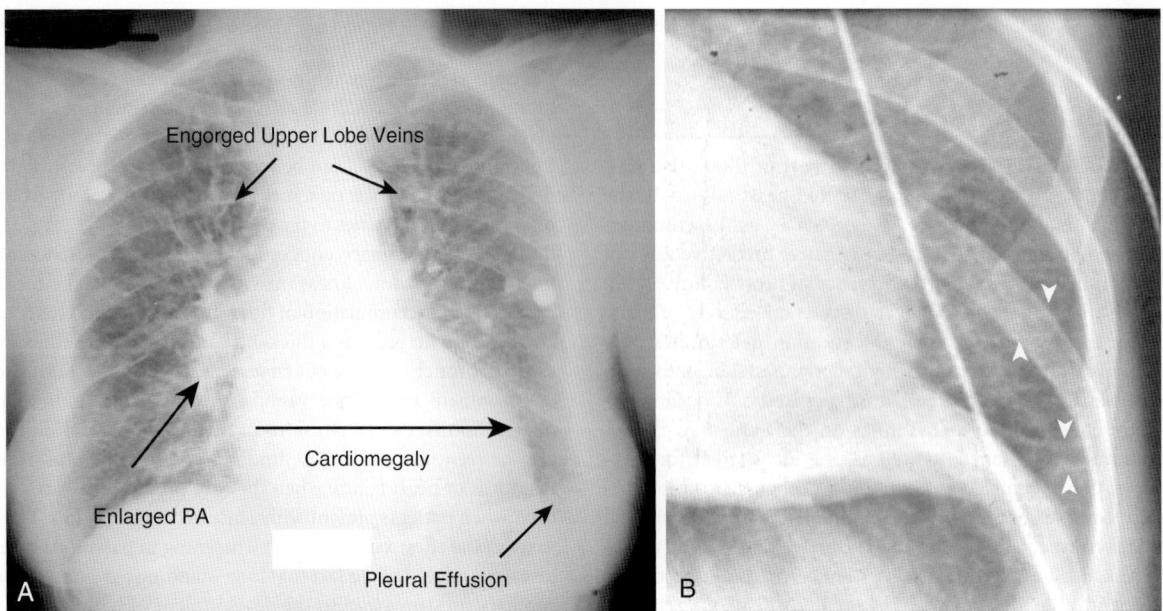

Fig. 31.2 Chest X-ray in a heart failure patient. (A) Cardiac and vascular features of heart failure are depicted. (B) Kerley B lines *(arrows)* are apparent as horizontal linear densities that extend to the pleural surface of the lung. *PA,* Pulmonary artery.

function.[20] In addition, myocardial strain imaging using speckle tracking permits quantitative measurements of local myocardial function independent of translational movement due to tethering.[21] Global longitudinal strain has been shown to be a more sensitive and reproducible measure of myocardial function than ejection fraction, and therefore may be particularly useful in the early detection of cardiomyopathies.[22]

Right Ventricular Systolic Function

Determination of right ventricular systolic function is more difficult to assess by ultrasound due to the shape of the chamber as well as its anterior location, which places it in close proximity to the chest wall. Nevertheless, right ventricular systolic function is increasingly recognized as being prognostically important in patients with heart failure. Right ventricular systolic function can be qualitatively assessed from two-dimensional echocardiographic images and quantitatively measured using the right ventricular fractional area change in the apical four chamber view. Two important commonly used quantitative measures of right ventricular systolic function are tricuspid annular plane systolic excursion (TAPSE), assessed using M-mode imaging, and the tricuspid annular peak velocity (S′), assessed by pulsed tissue Doppler imaging.[23] Three-dimensional echocardiography and strain rate imaging have been shown to provide additional useful quantitative assessments of right ventricular function.[23]

Cardiac Volumes

In addition to the measurement of left and right ventricular systolic function, echocardiographic evaluation includes assessment of cardiac volumes and wall thicknesses. Left ventricular and atrial volumes are both of prognostic significance in patients with heart failure.[24,25] Right-sided volumes are usually characterized qualitatively but can also be quantified from the apical four-chamber view and using three-dimensional echocardiography. The relative sizes of the cardiac chambers and wall thicknesses may suggest specific diagnoses (depicted in **Fig. 31.3A to D**). For example, isolated right ventricular enlargement suggests the presence of an intracardiac shunt or pulmonary hypertension, while detection of concentric left ventricular

hypertrophy with severe biatrial enlargement in the absence of hypertension may be secondary to an infiltrative cardiomyopathy such as amyloidosis.

Diastolic Function and Hemodynamics

The assessment of diastolic function and left-sided filling pressures are especially important in heart failure patients. An increasing number of patients have heart failure due to abnormal filling dynamics with preserved left ventricular systolic function. In addition, the degree of diastolic dysfunction is an independent predictor of morbidity and mortality in heart failure patients with and without systolic dysfunction.[26] The assessment of diastolic filling using Doppler measurements includes analyses of the mitral valve inflow pattern, tissue velocity at the mitral valve annulus, pulmonary vein flow, and the left atrial volume indexed to body surface area. The most recent guideline from the American Society of Echocardiography also includes the peak tricuspid regurgitant velocity.[34] Chronic diastolic dysfunction is associated with structural changes, which may assist in diagnosing and risk-stratifying patients. Indexed left atrial volume is particularly useful because it is less susceptible to changes in loading conditions, and increased left atrial volume is associated with elevated filling pressures, more severe diastolic function, and increased morbidity.[28] The presence of left ventricular hypertrophy should also increase the suspicion for concomitant diastolic dysfunction.

Determination of Pressures

Left ventricular filling pressures can be estimated using the ratio of the peak mitral inflow E wave velocity to that of the mitral annular tissue Doppler e′ wave velocities, with elevated ratios associated with increased likelihood of elevated filling pressures. These ratios should be interpreted in conjunction with the other parameters used to evaluate diastolic filling, and it should be noted that their utility is diminished in specific populations (e.g., patients with acute decompensated systolic heart failure, hypertrophic cardiomyopathy, pericardial disease, severe mitral calcification). Echocardiographic measurements are also used to noninvasively estimate right-sided filling pressures in heart failure patients, specifically right atrial pressures and pulmonary artery systolic and diastolic pressures (see **Chapter 23** for details). Elevated pulmonary artery pressure is seen commonly in patients with heart failure with preserved ejection fraction and can be clue to the presence of diastolic dysfunction.[29] The presence and degree of pulmonary hypertension is an additional negative prognostic factor in patients with heart failure.[30]

Valvular Disease

Examination of the four heart valves is important to rule out primary valvular disease as an etiology for heart failure, and to evaluate the degree of coexisting or secondary abnormalities in valve function. Echocardiography with Doppler imaging is well-suited to evaluate valvular disease and is usually the modality of choice for the initial evaluation of both stenotic and regurgitant valvular heart disease. Chamber dilation and remodeling are often associated with significant chronic regurgitation of the atrial-ventricular valves, and it is important to distinguish this functional regurgitation from regurgitation due to primary valvular disease.

Structural Abnormalities

The evaluation of heart failure patients also includes an assessment for acquired or congenital structural abnormalities, which is typically initially done with echocardiography. In patients with ischemic cardiomyopathy, adverse remodeling after myocardial infarction may result in the formation of ventricular aneurysms, which are most commonly apical.

Pericardial Disease

Pericardial constriction may cause heart failure and often remains undiagnosed until well after patients initially present with symptoms. Thickening of the pericardium is often difficult to directly visualize by ultrasound and is better detected by other imaging modalities. However, a number of clues suggesting pericardial constriction may be seen by echocardiography, including abnormal septal motion on two-dimensional and M-Mode images, characteristic right and left ventricular and hepatic vein filling patterns with respiratory variation reflecting interventricular dependence, and relatively high E wave velocity on tissue-Doppler recordings from the medial mitral valve annulus.[31]

Dyssynchrony Assessment

Multiple techniques and algorithms to assess inter- and intraventricular dyssynchrony have been developed using echocardiography, as well as other imaging modalities. Currently, outcome data are limited, and the optimal protocol is not yet known (see also **Chapter 38**).

Detection of Cardiac Thrombi

Patients with heart failure and left ventricular systolic dysfunction are more prone to having spontaneous cardiac thrombi formation. Two-dimensional echocardiography may detect thrombi, and using an ultrasonic contrast agent increases diagnostic accuracy (see **Fig. 31.3E**).

Performing Repeat Echocardiograms

Although echocardiograms are often repeated at regular intervals in stable heart failure patients, there is little justification for this practice. Repeat echocardiograms should be performed when there is a significant change in clinical status, such as when a patient appears to have recovered cardiac function spontaneously (e.g., viral myocarditis, Takasubo), or following initiation of guideline directed medical therapy. The latter is of particular importance in making recommendations for devices such as ICDs or CRT. A repeat study should also be performed if the patient's condition deteriorates, particularly when advanced therapies are being considered.

Other Imaging Modalities (see also Chapter 32)

Other cardiovascular imaging modalities that can provide important ancillary information to help guide the management of heart failure patients include invasive coronary angiography, computed tomography (CT), magnetic resonance imaging (MRI), and nuclear imaging (**Table 31.9**). The selection of additional imaging modalities should be matched to the diagnoses being considered, specific information hoped to be gained, and local expertise and availability.

Ischemic Evaluation: Coronary Anatomy and Myocardial Viability (see also Chapter 19)

Coronary artery disease is common in heart failure patients, and along with hypertension has the highest population attributable risk.[32] The initial diagnosis of heart failure is often followed by an evaluation for an ischemic cause, particularly in patients with heart failure with reduced ejection fraction (HFrEF), as revascularization can potentially improve left ventricular (LV) systolic function and increase survival.[33] Previously, invasive coronary angiography was used to establish or exclude coronary artery disease in heart failure patients. However, noninvasive imaging modalities, including coronary CT angiography, nuclear imaging, and cardiac MRI, are now increasingly being used for this purpose. Coronary CT angiography has shown to be highly accurate for excluding an ischemic etiology, with a sensitivity of 98%.[34] Assessment of coronary artery calcium alone by cardiac CT, without the need for intravenous contrast, can essentially exclude ischemic cardiomyopathy in patients with an Agatston score of 0.[35] Cardiac CT angiography can also accurately quantify LV ejection fraction and determine regional wall motion abnormalities with minimal increase in radiation exposure. Due to a substantially lower risk of complications compared with invasive coronary angiography, cardiac CT has gained increasing favor as the initial imaging modality for detection of coronary disease in patients with new onset heart failure. This said, invasive coronary angiography remains the gold standard for evaluation of coronary artery disease, and our approach is to perform angiography when there is high likelihood of coronary artery disease based on a typical clinical presentation, ECG or echocardiographic findings suggestive of a prior myocardial infarction, or presence of traditional risk factors, including family history of premature coronary artery disease. Single photon emission computed tomography (SPECT) and positron emission tomography (PET) are also widely used to evaluate for coronary artery disease in heart failure patients.

In patients with known ischemic cardiomyopathy, assessment of viable myocardium is often an important factor in clinical decision making, as territories with viable myocardium have shown reversibility of myocardial dysfunction after revascularization.[36] Myocardial viability can be assessed by Thallium-201 SPECT, fluorine-18 labeled deoxyglucose (FDG) PET, or MRI. FDG-PET is considered one of the most sensitive means of detecting viable myocardium and is preferred over Thallium-201 SPECT. Cardiac MRI using both stress perfusion imaging and late gadolinium enhancement during the same exam has also been used to distinguish ischemic from nonischemic cardiomyopathies. The degree of late gadolinium enhancement from T1-weighted images is evaluated, and <50% transmural extent of late gadolinium enhancement is considered to be indicative of the presence of viable myocardium.[37] Although determination of viability received a class IIa recommendation in ACC/AHA guidelines,[2] it should be noted that whether the results of viability testing can help improve outcomes in heart failure patients remains controversial.[33,38]

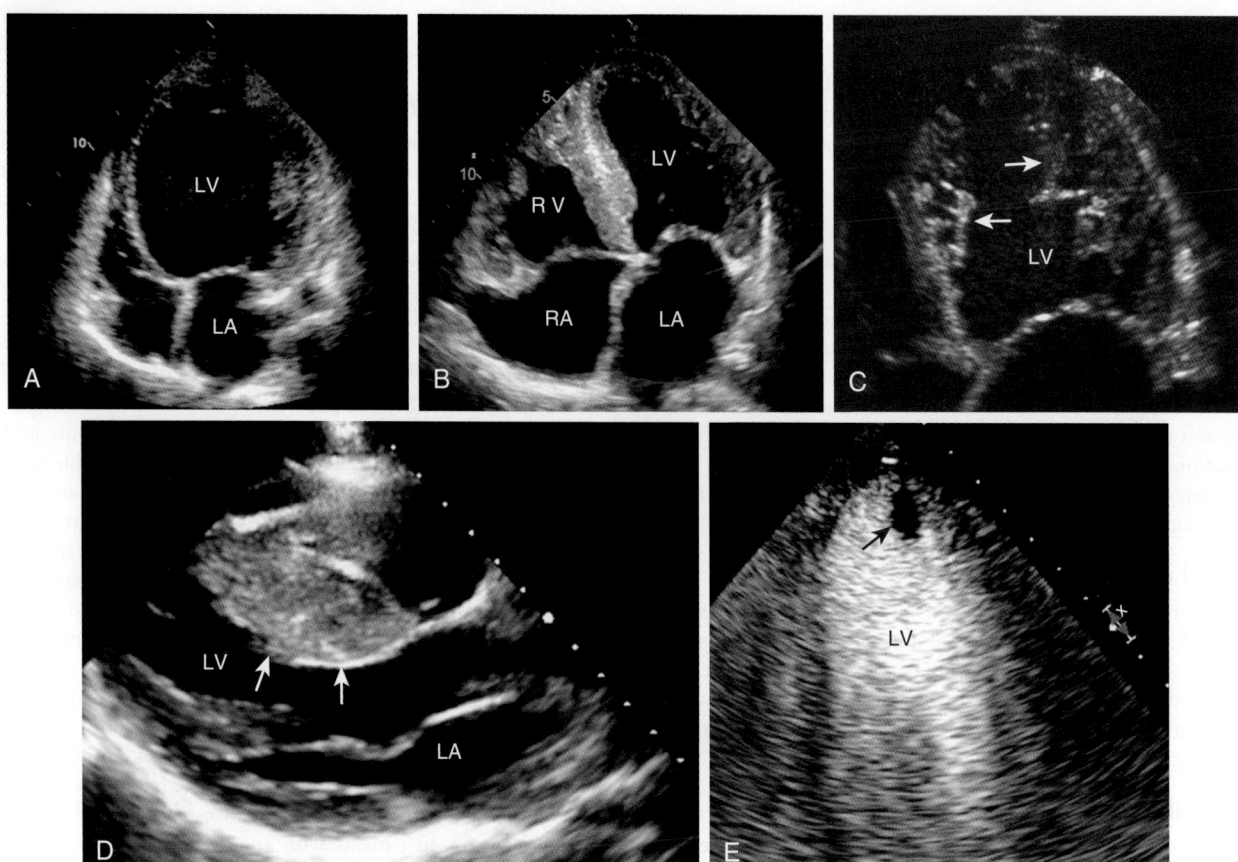

Fig. 31.3 Example echocardiographic images: (A) an apical 4-chamber view from a patient with nonischemic cardiomyopathy, showing left ventricular dilation and concentric remodeling; (B) an apical four-chamber view from a patient with cardiac amyloidosis, showing biventricular hypertrophy, biatrial enlargement, and thickened A-V valves; (C) an apical four-chamber view showing the left ventricle from a patient with noncompaction cardiomyopathy showing extensive trabeculations *(arrows)*; (D) parasternal long view from a patient with hypertrophic cardiomyopathy, showing marked septal hypertrophy *(arrows)*; (E) an apical four-chamber view with contrast from a patient with ischemic cardiomyopathy, showing a filling defect due to an apical thrombus *(arrow)*. *LA,* Left atrium; *LV,* left ventricle; *RA,* right atrium; *RV,* right ventricle.

Morphologic and Functional Evaluation

With the availability of alternative noninvasive imaging options, the use of contrast left ventriculography has largely fallen out of favor for determining LV ejection fraction in patients with new onset heart failure. Cardiac MRI is considered the gold standard for accurate evaluation of right and left ventricular size and function. It is most useful when the morphologic and functional information obtained from echocardiography is equivocal or insufficient due to poor acoustic windows. Cardiac CT also provides accurate biventricular size and function. Both cardiac MRI and CT provide excellent evaluation of the cardiac anatomy, which is particularly important in patients with suspected congenital abnormalities (e.g., partial anomalous pulmonary venous return and atrial or ventricular septal defects), pericardial, and valvular diseases. A multigated acquisition scan (MUGA) has also been shown to provide accurate and reproducible measures of LV ejection fraction. Nuclear assessment of RV ejection fraction can be performed using first-pass planar scintigraphy.[39]

Imaging for Nonischemic Causes of Cardiac Dysfunction

Nuclear cardiac imaging has emerged as an important modality in the initial evaluation of patients with suspected infiltrative cardiomyopathies (see also **Chapters 21 and 22**). In particular, FDG-PET and technetium 99m pyrophosphate SPECT have shown to be extremely helpful in establishing the diagnosis of cardiac sarcoidosis and amyloidogenic transthyretin (ATTR) cardiac amyloidosis, respectively. Diagnosis of cardiac sarcoidosis, a condition associated with considerable morbidity and mortality,[40] previously depended on histopathology of tissue obtained by endomyocardial biopsy. However, given the patchy involvement of cardiac sarcoidosis, the diagnosis could be missed due to inadequate sampling. FDG-PET has markedly improved the ability to make the clinical diagnosis of cardiac sarcoidosis without the need for endomyocardial biopsy in patients who present with cardiac manifestations consistent with cardiac sarcoidosis (**Fig. 31.4**).[41] In addition, FDG uptake can be longitudinally monitored to demonstrate treatment response with immunosuppressive therapy.[42]

SPECT imaging has proved to be quite useful in the diagnosis of cardiac amyloid. Through the use of bone seeking tracers such as technetium 99m pyrophosphate, SPECT has shown high sensitivity (91%) and specificity (92%) for the diagnosis of ATTR cardiac amyloid.[43] Thus a positive technetium 99m pyrophosphate SPECT scan in the absence of an abnormal monoclonal protein allows reliable diagnosis of ATTR cardiac amyloidosis and avoids the need for endomyocardial biopsy.[44] There is also growing interest in the use of ^{18}F-florbetapir or ^{18}F-florbetaben in cardiac PET for the diagnosis of AL cardiac amyloidosis, in addition to ATTR cardiac amyloidosis.[45,46]

TABLE 31.9 Cardiac Imaging Modalities Used to Evaluate Heart Failure Patients

Imaging Modality	Most Useful in Defining	Conditions Where Most Helpful	Advantages	Disadvantages
Coronary angiography	Coronary disease (gold standard)	Suspected coronary artery disease	Intervention can be performed at time of CAD diagnosis	Invasive, exposure to radiation, risk for contrast induced nephropathy
Echocardiography	Biventricular function and chamber assessment, wall motion, valvular lesions and other structural abnormalities, pericardial effusion, estimating atrial and pulmonary pressures	Suspected coronary artery disease, valvular disease, pericardial tamponade, pulmonary hypertension	Versatile, can be done at bedside, no radiation. Provides both functional and hemodynamic information. Most commonly used in initial evaluation of HF	Limited assessment in patients with poor acoustic windows, interreader variability
Computed tomography	Coronary disease, right and left ventricular function and volumes, defining congenital heart disease anatomy	Suspected coronary artery disease and adult congenital heart disease	High negative predictive value for CAD	Exposure to radiation, risk for contrast induced nephropathy, difficult imaging with rapid heart rate
Magnetic resonance	Ischemic versus nonischemic cardiomyopathy, myocardial viability, right and left function and volumes (gold standard), quantifying valvular regurgitation, characterizing different nonischemic cardiomyopathies, defining congenital heart disease anatomy	Identification of ischemic cardiomyopathy, viable myocardium, specific nonischemic cardiomyopathies (e.g., myocarditis, sarcoidosis, amyloidosis, iron overload, arrhythmogenic RV cardiomyopathy, LV non-compaction, and constrictive pericarditis), and adult congenital heart disease	No radiation, evaluates myocardial tissue best among noninvasive modalities, quantification of valvular regurgitation	Limited to magnet compatible metals, is more technically challenging in patients with arrhythmias
Nuclear Imaging				
MUGA	LV function and volumes	Accurate quantification of LV ejection fraction with poor acoustic windows	Highly reproducible measure of LV EF	Exposure to radiation
First-pass radionuclide angiography	RV function and volumes	Reasonable accurate quantification of RV ejection fraction in advanced heart failure	Allows quantification of RV EF where MRI is not possible	Exposure to radiation, relatively more complicated to perform compared to MUGA
SPECT	Myocardial perfusion, LV function and volumes, amyloidosis	Suspected coronary artery disease and amyloidosis	Allows for nonbiopsy diagnosis of amyloidosis	Exposure to radiation, may miss three-vessel CAD
PET	Myocardial perfusion and viability, LV function and volumes, sarcoidosis	Suspected coronary artery disease, "hibernating" myocardium, sarcoidosis	Allows for nonbiopsy diagnosis for sarcoidosis	Exposure to radiation, may miss three-vessel CAD

CAD, Coronary artery disease; *EF*, ejection fraction; *LV*, left ventricle; *MRI*, magnetic resonance imaging; *MUGA*, multigated acquisition scan; *PET*, positron emission tomography; *RV*, right ventricle; *SPECT*, single photon emission computed tomography.

Cardiac MRI has the ability to characterize myocardial and pericardial tissue noninvasively to a degree that cannot be achieved with other noninvasive imaging modalities, and it does so while avoiding radiation exposure. Using late gadolinium contrast enhancement, cardiac MRI can accurately identify infarcted myocardium and distinguish ischemic from nonischemic cardiomyopathy. Cardiac MRI is also used to diagnose nonischemic cardiomyopathies such as hypertrophic cardiomyopathy, left ventricular noncompaction, arrhythmogenic right ventricular cardiomyopathy, iron overload cardiomyopathy, and myocarditis (**Fig. 31.5**). The diagnosis of myocarditis can also be made using the Lake Louise criteria (see also **Chapter 28**).[47] Although MRI imaging can detect the characteristic myocardial findings of cardiac sarcoidosis and cardiac amyloidosis,[48,49] as opposed to FDG-PET, the value of this imaging modality has not been established in following the course of sarcoidosis after treatment. In addition, the high prevalence of pacemakers and defibrillators implanted in patients with cardiac sarcoidosis limits serial cardiac MRI imaging. This limitation,

however, should be obviated in the future with the advent of MRI compatible implantable devices. Additional applications of cardiac MRI include myocardial tagging to evaluate constrictive pericarditis and blood flow velocity assessment by phase contrast to assess regurgitant fraction in valvular heart disease, further improved upon by three-directional velocity-encoded MRI.[50]

Imaging to Determine Prognosis

^{123}I-MIBG (metaiodobenzylguanidine) SPECT can be used to evaluate increased sympathetic function in heart failure patients. Increased myocardial sympathetic activity attributed to decreased norepinephrine reuptake among other mechanisms[51] is well described in heart failure patients and has been correlated with mortality.[123] I-MIBG SPECT can quantify the decreased norepinephrine reuptake by the heart. A decreased late heart/mediastinum ratio of ≤1.68 identified heart failure patients at significantly increased mortality risk, regardless of the LV ejection fraction.[52] In addition to providing prognostic

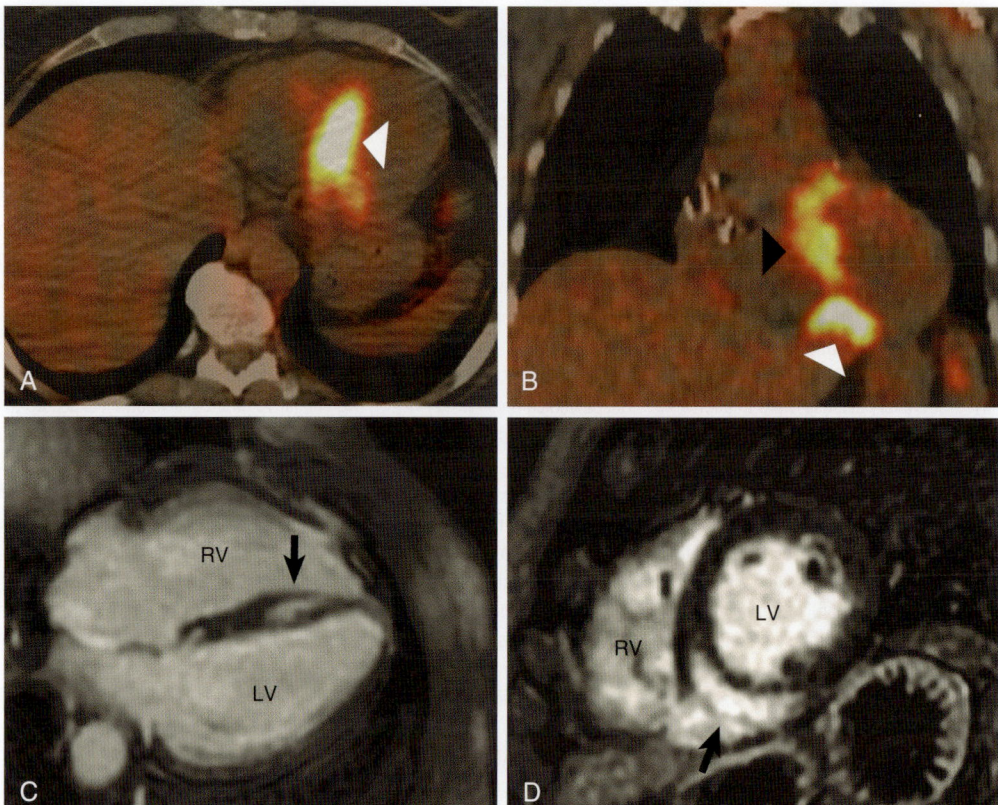

Fig. 31.4 Fluorine-18 labeled deoxyglucose-positron emission tomography (FDG-PET) and cardiac magnetic resonance imaging (MRI) images from a patient with cardiac sarcoidosis presenting with dyspnea on exertion, fatigue, and trifascicular block. Axial (A) and coronal (B) views of FDG-PET demonstrating active inflammation in the inferoseptal *(white arrowhead)* and anteroseptal walls *(black arrowhead)* consistent with cardiac sarcoidosis. Patient preparation performed with high-fat/low-carbohydrate diet and overnight fast to suppress normal myocardial uptake. Cardiac MRI demonstrates corresponding late gadolinium enhancement *(black arrow)* of the inferoseptal wall in four-chamber (C) and short-axis (D) views. *LV*, Left ventricle; *RV*, right ventricle.

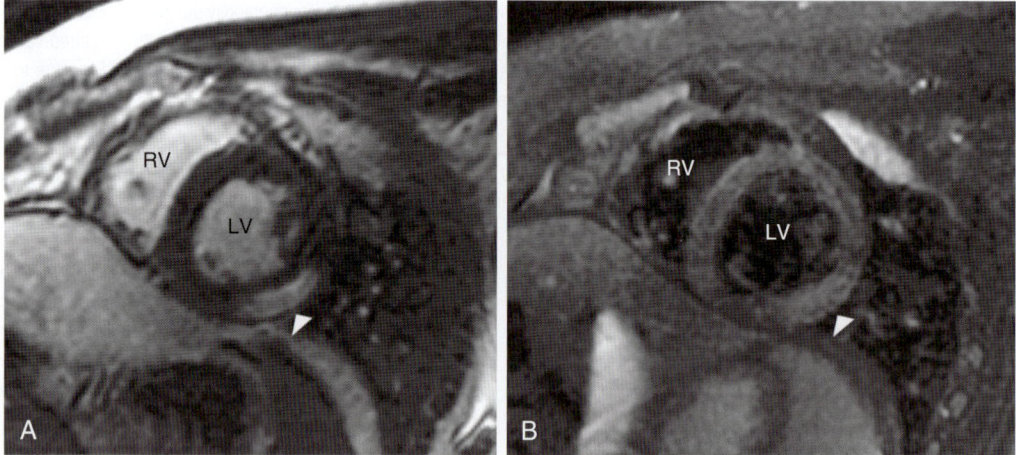

Fig. 31.5 Cardiac magnetic resonance imaging showing short axis views of late gadolinium enhancement (A) of the mid inferolateral wall and adjacent pericardium *(white arrowhead)* in addition to increased myocardial edema (B) consistent with perimyocarditis in a patient with acute onset of chest pain and dyspnea with a viral upper respiratory infection a week prior to presentation. *LV*, Left ventricle; *RV*, right ventricle.

information,[123] I-MIBG SPECT can also predict ventricular arrhythmias and thus help further identify patients who are suitable candidates for implantable cardioverter defibrillator therapy.[53] This imaging modality has also been used to monitor treatment effect, for instance after initiating β-blocker therapy.[54]

The burden of fibrosis, as detected by late gadolinium enhancement on MRI, provides prognostic value in various cardiomyopathies, including ischemic cardiomyopathy,[55] dilated cardiomyopathy,[56] cardiac amyloidosis,[48] and hypertrophic cardiomyopathy.[57]

RIGHT-HEART CATHETERIZATION (SEE ALSO CHAPTER 34)

Measurement of intracardiac pressures and cardiac output (CO) by right-heart catheterization is less commonly performed now than in the past. The diagnosis of heart failure can often be made clinically, and echocardiography provides additional information, including estimation of right and left atrial pressures and right ventricular systolic pressure by noninvasive means. Use of hemodynamic monitoring to guide therapy was evaluated in patients with severe symptomatic heart failure in the Evaluation Study of Congestive Heart Failure and Pulmonary Artery Catheterization Effectiveness (ESCAPE) trial.[58] The results showed that the routine use of right-heart catheterization to help "tailor therapy" failed to reduce mortality and days out of the hospital but was associated with an increased incidence of catheter-related adverse events. A caveat to these results is that the study did not include patients who potentially required inotropic agents. While no longer recommended for routine use, there are specific guideline recommendations for invasive evaluation in heart failure patients (**Table 31.10**).[2] Right-heart catheterization is also often helpful for diagnosing constrictive pericarditis, restrictive cardiomyopathy, and HFpEF, and for confirming the presence and extent of pulmonary hypertension. Patients being evaluated for advanced heart failure therapies require right-heart catheterization to assess pulmonary hypertension and right ventricular failure, as the results are used to determine candidacy as well as plan pre- and postoperative management.

When right-heart catheterization is performed, pressure (both mean and phasic) and flow measurements are obtained. Elevated pulmonary capillary wedge pressure helps in determining pulmonary congestion due to heart failure, and an end-expiratory mean pulmonary capillary wedge pressure (PCWP) ≥15 mm Hg is considered abnormal.[59] The waveforms in the pressure tracing help interpret the findings. A large V wave in the right atrial or pulmonary artery wedge pressure tracing is seen in patients with tricuspid or mitral regurgitation but also can be seen in other settings, including advanced heart failure with a noncompliant atrium. A rapid y-descent of the V wave is characteristic of constrictive pericarditis but also can be seen in restrictive cardiomyopathy, right ventricular failure, and severe tricuspid or mitral regurgitation. In pericardial tamponade, equalization of right and left ventricular filling pressures and a prominent x-descent after the A wave with absence of y-descent after the V wave is characteristically seen.

Cardiac output and index (CI) are also important parameters obtained during a right-heart catheterization. CO can be determined by measuring the mixed venous oxygen (MvO_2) saturation and utilizing the Fick equation or by thermodilution technique. Neither method is perfect, and there are pitfalls for each that need to be recognized. The Fick equation often is limited by assumption of VO_2, as direct measurement is not usually obtained in the catheterization laboratory. Cardiac output can be overestimated if the catheter migrates into the pulmonary wedge position and oxygenated blood is sampled, or when severe mitral regurgitation forces oxygenated blood from the capillaries into the distal pulmonary arteries. Thermodilution is prone to underestimation with tricuspid regurgitation or when CO is very low and the tracer is warmed by surrounding tissue. Thermodilution CI has, however, been shown to better predict mortality (<2.2 L/min/m²) and is thus favored by some over the Fick CI.[60]

Exercise during right-heart catheterization is often helpful in determining the cause of dyspnea in patients who have normal pressures at rest.[61] HFpEF can be an elusive diagnosis, particularly earlier in its course, and right-heart catheterization incorporating exercise hemodynamics increases the sensitivity for identifying HFpEF. A PCWP ≥25 mm Hg is

TABLE 31.10 Recommendations for Right Heart Catheterization in Heart Failure Patients

Class I

Monitoring with a pulmonary artery catheter should be performed in patients with respiratory distress or impaired systemic perfusion when clinical assessment is inadequate

Class IIa

Invasive hemodynamic monitoring can be useful for carefully selected patients with acute heart failure with persistent symptoms despite empiric adjustment of standard therapies and

a. whose fluid status, perfusion, or systemic or pulmonary vascular resistance is uncertain;

b. whose systolic pressure remains low, or is associated with symptoms, despite initial therapy;

c. whose renal function is worsening with therapy;

d. who require parenteral vasoactive agents;

e. who may need consideration for mechanical circulatory support or transplantation

Class III

Routine use of invasive hemodynamic monitoring is not recommended in normotensive patients with acute heart failure.

Modified from Yancy CW, Jessup M, Bozkurt B, et al. 2013 ACCF/AHA guideline for the management of heart failure: a report of the American College of Cardiology Foundation/American Heart Association Task Force on Practice Guidelines. *J Am Coll Cardiol.* 2013;62(16):e147–239.

commonly observed in HFpEF patients during exercise.[59] Abnormalities in patients with mitral stenosis can also be dynamic, and measurement of hemodynamics during exercise can be useful in determining the severity of this condition.[62] Similarly, the magnitude of pulmonary hypertension may not be apparent unless the patient is exercised. Right-heart catheterization can also help distinguish between pulmonary hypertension caused by changes in the pulmonary vasculature, as opposed to that which occurs as a consequence of elevated pressures on the left side of the heart. The response to pulmonary arterial vasodilating agents, such as nitroprusside or milrinone, helps determine whether a patient with pulmonary hypertension will be acceptable for heart transplantation.

ENDOMYOCARDIAL BIOPSY

The AHA, ACC, and the ESC have defined clinical circumstances in which endomyocardial biopsy provides meaningful information regarding prognosis or for guiding therapies.[63] The eight scenarios with class IIa or greater recommendation for endomyocardial biopsy are summarized in **Table 31.11**. Endomyocardial biopsy is usually performed in patients with specific presentations of acute heart failure. It is not commonly indicated in the evaluation of chronic heart disease, other than in cases where an infiltrative etiology is being considered and imaging fails to provide a definitive diagnosis. Broader application of endomyocardial biopsy is not recommended, due to the limited diagnostic information that is gained. For instance, in patients with initially unexplained cardiomyopathy, a specific histologic diagnosis was provided in only 15% of the patients.[64] The limited use of endomyocardial biopsy in the community is based on these limited benefits, which are weighed against the 3% to 8% adverse event risk of this invasive procedure. Fortunately, biopsy-related deaths are very rare.[65] Strong consideration of endomyocardial biopsy, however, should be given when there is a clinical picture consistent with fulminant

---

TABLE 31.11 Clinical Scenarios for Indications for Endomyocardial Biopsy (Class of Recommendation IIa or Greater)

Class I

- New-onset heart failure of <2 weeks' duration associated with a normal-sized or dilated left ventricle and hemodynamic compromise
- New-onset heart failure of 2 weeks' to 3 months' duration associated with a dilated left ventricle and new ventricular arrhythmias, second- or third-degree heart block or failure to respond to usual care within 1–2 weeks

Class IIa

- Heart failure of ≥3 months' duration associated with a dilated left ventricle and new ventricular arrhythmias, second- or third-degree heart block, or failure to respond to usual care within 1–2 weeks
- Heart failure associated with a dilated cardiomyopathy of any duration associated with suspected allergic reaction and/or eosinophilia
- Heart failure associated with suspected anthracycline cardiomyopathy
- Heart failure associated with unexplained restrictive cardiomyopathy
- Suspected cardiac tumors
- Unexplained cardiomyopathy in children

---

myocarditis (see also **Chapter 28**). This entity is defined by a distinct onset of severe heart failure symptoms within 2 weeks of presentation with hypotension or cardiogenic shock necessitating inotropes, vasopressors, or mechanical circulatory support.[66] Since the prognosis of giant cell myocarditis or acute necrotizing eosinophilic myocarditis is especially poor, diagnosis must be quickly established to guide immunosuppressive therapy that can be life-saving.[67-69] Concurrent evaluation for urgent heart transplantation is also undertaken in patients who do not respond to immunosuppression because of the high mortality in patients with giant cell myocarditis with a fulminant presentation.[70] Since giant cell myocarditis is clinically indistinguishable from lymphocytic fulminant myocarditis, a condition with a better prognosis,[71] histologic diagnosis provides meaningful prognostic information as well as guidance in clinical management. A practical note is that empiric treatment with steroids while awaiting biopsy results in patients with fulminant presentation and does not appear to affect accurate diagnosis as long as endomyocardial biopsy is pursued within a reasonably short timeframe (e.g., ≤24 hours after steroid initiation).[72]

In patients with a nonfulminant presentation, the Dallas criteria are commonly used to confirm diagnosis of lymphocytic myocarditis. These criteria, however, have low to moderate sensitivity, and establish a diagnosis in only 20% to 30%[73] of suspected myocarditis patients. Sampling limitations due to patchy inflammation, as in lymphocytic myocarditis, contribute to the low sensitivity.[74] Immunohistochemical staining with a large panel of monoclonal and polyclonal antibodies, including anti-CD3 (T lymphocytes), anti-CD68 (macrophages), and anti HLA-DR, is recommended to increase the diagnostic sensitivity.[75] Molecular analysis with DNA-RNA extraction and reverse transcriptase–polymerase chain reaction (RT-PCR) amplification of viral genomes, including enteroviruses, adenoviruses, influenza A virus, cytomegalovirus, Epstein-Barr virus, parvovirus B19, and human herpes virus-6, further improves diagnostic sensitivity for myocarditis. However, the lack of convincing evidence for changing treatment outcomes other than in giant cell or eosinophilic myocarditis continues to temper the enthusiasm for more widespread use of endomyocardial biopsy, particularly in less experienced centers.[74]

Although the role of endomyocardial biopsy for diagnosing infiltrative disease has diminished with advancements in cardiovascular imaging, it is still used in patients with suspected glycogen and lysosomal storage diseases.

ASSESSING EXERCISE CAPACITY

Objective assessment of exercise capacity is extremely helpful when caring for patients with dyspnea and/or fatigue as classification based on subjective complaints may not reliably determine the extent of exercise incapacity nor the contribution of heart failure to the patient's limitation. Formal exercise testing can confirm the extent of limitations experienced by patients in the course of their daily activities and assess the effectiveness of treatments such as cardiac resynchronization therapy. It can also assess prognosis and confirm that the patient has progressed to refractory ACC/AHA stage D heart failure. Advancement of a patient to stage D heart failure (which is associated with truncated survival) should trigger discussion with the patient regarding their goals of care and in selected patients raise the question of potential candidacy for advanced therapies such as heart transplant or durable mechanical circulatory support.

The 6-minute walk test is a simple but valuable tool for assessing submaximal exercise capacity that can easily be administered in the clinic or office setting. The distance walked in 6 minutes has been shown to be inversely correlated to mortality and hospitalizations.[76] The ability to walk <300 meters is most commonly used as a cutpoint to indicate the risk of increased mortality and hospitalizations.[77] However, the 6-minute walk test does not discriminate between the causes (e.g., cardiac or pulmonary) of impaired exercise capacity or determine if low levels of exercise are influenced by patient (or examiner) motivation, neurologic, orthopedic, or other medical problems; nor does it account for the effects of conditioning or age. Despite these limitations, the ease of administration and reproducibility of results make the 6-minute walk test a valuable tool for assessing the functional capacity of heart failure patients.

In comparison to the 6-minute walk test, cardiopulmonary exercise (CPX) testing is a much more robust and precise tool. It is considered the gold standard for assessing exercise capacity. In the United States, functional capacity is typically measured using a motorized treadmill. A stationary cycle ergometer can also be used in patients with gait or balance instability, orthopedic limitations, severe obesity, or when simultaneous cardiac imaging is planned. Patients breathe through a mask or a mouthpiece, and using rapidly responding O_2 and CO_2 sensors, the CPX system directly measures oxygen uptake (VO_2) and carbon dioxide output (VCO_2) at rest, during exercise, and during recovery. Important parameters obtained by CPX include peak VO_2 obtained at maximal effort, peak respiratory exchange ratio (RER), ventilatory efficiency by VE/VCO_2 slope, anaerobic or ventilatory threshold, and exercise breathing reserve. In addition, standard parameters of exercise testing such as heart rate, blood pressure, pulse oximetry, and electrocardiographic changes are obtained.

Evidence of an adequate exercise effort is based on measurement of the peak RER in addition to the maximal heart rate response (age predicted maximal heart rate = 220 minus age). RER is defined as the ratio between VCO_2 and VO_2. With progression to higher exercise intensities, lactic acid buffering contributes to increased VCO_2. A peak RER of ≥1.05 is used as the cutoff to demonstrate adequate patient effort was achieved.[78] Thus RER provides a more accurate and reliable index of maximal patient effort than target heart rate and is not confounded by medications such as β-blockers.[79] Peak VO_2 indicates oxygen consumption at maximal effort and has been consistently shown to be a reliable prognostic indicator.[79] It is typically indexed to body weight to facilitate intersubject comparisons. A peak VO_2 less than 14 mL/kg/min (or 12 mL/kg/min for patients on β-blockers) is associated with a poor prognosis and is considered an indication for referral for advanced therapies.[78] However, as these thresholds were previously determined in older men, using ≤50% peak VO_2 in young patients (<50 years) and

TABLE 31.12 Weber-Janicki Classification of Functional Impairment during Incremental Treadmill Testing in Heart Failure

Class	Severity	Peak VO$_2$ (mL/kg/min)	Anaerobic Threshold	Maximal Cardiac Index (L/min/m^2)
A	None to mild	>20	>14	>8
B	Mild to moderate	16–20	11–14	6–8
C	Moderate to severe	10–16	8–11	4–6
D	Severe	6–10	5–8	2–4
E	Very severe	<6	<4	<2

Adapted from Weber KT, Kinasewitz GT, Janicki JS, Fishman AP. Oxygen utilization and ventilation during exercise in patients with chronic cardiac failure. *Circulation.* 1982;65(6):1213–1223.

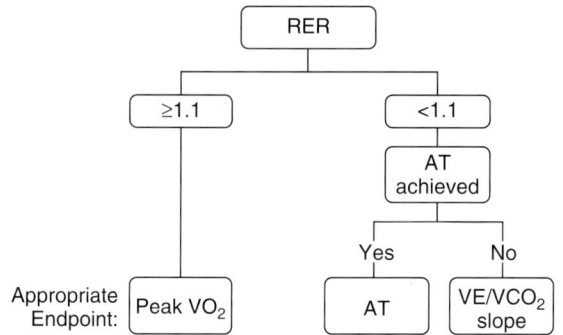

Fig. 31.6 Flow chart for determining appropriate metabolic endpoint to interpret cardiopulmonary exercise. Refer to Table 31.12 for determination of functional impairment. *RER*, Respiratory exchange ratio. (Modified from Milani RV, Lavie CJ, Mehra MR. Cardiopulmonary exercise testing: how do we differentiate the cause of dyspnea? Cir*culation.* 2004;110[4]:e27–31.)

women as the threshold to guide transplant listing has been advocated.[80] In addition, VO$_2$ at the anaerobic threshold has also been shown to have valuable prognostic value, and the corresponding heart rate and workload can be used to prescribe individualized patient exercise training intensity (**Table 31.12**).[81] VE/VCO$_2$ slope is steeper in advanced heart failure patients and may be of even greater prognostic value than peak VO$_2$. A VE/VCO$_2$ slope >35 is associated with poor prognosis.[82] Both VE/VCO$_2$ and anaerobic threshold VO$_2$ are reproducible parameters independent of the patient achieving maximal effort and thus are important measures that should be analyzed in conjunction with peak VO$_2$ (**Fig. 31.6**). Finally, exercise breathing reserve provides an assessment of respiratory limitation where the peak minute ventilation is calculated as a percentage of maximum voluntary ventilation. When greater than 80% of maximum voluntary ventilation is achieved at peak exertion, pulmonary limitation should be considered, particularly with other ancillary findings, including decrease in oxygen saturation by pulse oximetry and ≥15% decrease in FEV$_1$ post exercise.[81]

KEY REFERENCES

13. Leier CV, Chatterjee K. The physical examination in heart failure--Part II. *Congest Heart Fail.* 2007;13(2):99–104.
16. Yancy CW, Jessup M, Bozkurt B, et al. 2017 ACC/AHA/HFSA Focused Update of the 2013 ACCF/AHA guideline for the management of heart failure: a report of the American College of Cardiology/American Heart Association Task Force on Clinical Practice Guidelines and the Heart Failure Society of America. *J Am Coll Cardiol.* 2017;70(6):776–803.
22. Tops LF, Delgado V, Marsan NA, Bax JJ. Myocardial strain to detect subtle left ventricular systolic dysfunction. *Eur J Heart Fail.* 2017;19(3):307–313.
38. Ling LF, Marwick TH, Flores DR, et al. Identification of therapeutic benefit from revascularization in patients with left ventricular systolic dysfunction:inducible ischemia versus hibernating myocardium. *Circ Cardiovasc Imaging.* 2013;6(3):363–372.
53. Zhou W, Chen J. I -123 metaiodobenzylguanidine imaging for predicting ventricular arrhythmia in heart failure patients. *J Biomed Res.* 2013;27(6):460–466.
56. Halliday BP, Gulati A, Ali A, et al. Association between midwall late gadolinium enhancement and sudden cardiac death in patients with dilated cardiomyopathy and mild and moderate left ventricular systolic dysfunction. *Circulation.* 2017;135(22):2106–2115.
59. Borlaug BA, Nishimura RA, Sorajja P, et al. Exercise hemodynamics enhance diagnosis of early heart failure with preserved ejection fraction. *Circ Heart Fail.* 2010;3(5):588–595.
62. Nishimura RA, Carabello BA. Hemodynamics in the cardiac catheterization laboratory of the 21st century. *Circulation.* 2012;125(17):2138–2150.
71. Magnani JW, Danik HJ, Dec GW, DiSalvo TG. Survival in biopsy-proven myocarditis:a long-term retrospective analysis of the histopathologic, clinical, and hemodynamic predictors. *Am Heart J.* 2006;151(2):463–470.
74. Heymans S, Eriksson U, Lehtonen J, Cooper LT. The quest for new approaches in myocarditis and inflammatory cardiomyopathy. *J Am Coll Cardiol.* 2016;68(21):2348–2364.

The full reference list for this chapter is available on ExpertConsult.

Cardiac Imaging in Heart Failure

Martin St. John Sutton, Alan R. Morrison, Albert J. Sinusas, Victor A. Ferrari

DEFINITION OF HEART FAILURE

Heart failure can be defined as a clinical syndrome caused by an abnormality of cardiac structure or function that results in failure to deliver oxygen at a rate commensurate with the needs of the body tissues (systolic failure), or failure to receive blood at normal filling pressures (diastolic failure).[1] The diagnosis of heart failure may be difficult to establish clinically, especially during its early stages because the symptoms and physical signs are nonspecific, consisting of dyspnea, effort intolerance, fatigue, elevated jugular venous pressure, and lower extremity edema (**see also Chapter 31**). As a result, cardiac imaging has assumed a pivotal role in supporting early diagnosis and in guiding optimal management of patients with heart failure from acquired and congenital heart disease.[2,3]

EPIDEMIOLOGY OF HEART FAILURE (SEE ALSO CHAPTER 18)

Heart failure currently affects approximately 30 million people worldwide, nearly six million of whom reside in the United States.[3] One in nine deaths in 2009 were attributable to heart failure, and about half of the patients with heart failure die within 5 years[3]. There are an additional 650,000 new cases of heart failure diagnosed each year in the United States, which is, in part, due to improved noninvasive cardiac imaging methods such as transthoracic two-dimensional (2D) echocardiography (TTE).[4] The incidence of heart failure increases with advancing age, so that approximately 10% of all males and females over 70 years of age have heart failure.[5] In addition, heart failure is the most frequent hospital discharge diagnosis in patients >65 years old. Heart failure costs the nation an estimated $30.7 billion each year, including costs related to health care services, diagnostic imaging, medications, and missed days of work.[6] Furthermore, the increase in life expectancy over the last three decades predicts that by the year 2035 there will be approximately 70 million subjects in the United States over 75 years of age, of whom 7 million (10%) will have heart failure. For this reason, heart failure has been targeted as a major health care initiative.

OBJECTIVES OF CARDIAC IMAGING IN HEART FAILURE

There are three major objectives of cardiac imaging in the setting of heart failure. The primary objective of noninvasive and invasive cardiac imaging is to establish the definitive cardiac diagnosis *de novo*, or to confirm the clinically suspected diagnosis. The secondary objective is to acquire reproducible high-quality, high-resolution images that enable accurate quantitative assessment of cardiac chamber size, architecture, global, and regional left ventricular (LV) function. The tertiary objective is to relate metrics of cardiac chamber size and function to risk stratification and long-term clinical outcome.

The aims of this chapter are to discuss the optimal and appropriate use of the panoply of multi-modal cardiovascular imaging techniques that are currently used routinely in patients with heart failure. We do not wish to compare and contrast the individual strengths and weaknesses of each of the various imaging modalities in each clinical situation, but rather to describe the most efficacious contemporary use of imaging modalities for a range of specific etiologies of heart failure. Special attention is given to a number of different pathoetiologies of heart failure that include (1) systolic and diastolic heart failure, (2) valvular heart disease, (3) myocardial viability and ventricular remodeling postinfarction, (4) detection of myocardial fibrosis, (5) selection of patients for device deployment, (6) dilated cardiomyopathy (DCM), and (7) right heart failure.

Choosing the cardiovascular imaging modality best suited to resolve the clinical differential diagnoses and to safely guide therapy can be challenging. This is because many of the cardiovascular symptoms in heart failure are nonspecific and correlate poorly with the degree of ventricular dysfunction.

COST OF IMAGING TESTS

Cardiac imaging is a frequent costly component of cardiovascular health care. Thus, when choosing a cardiovascular imaging modality it is important to be cognizant of the cost effectiveness of each modality relative to the clinical question.[2] For example, echocardiography is the method of choice in patients with suspected HF for reasons of accuracy, availability (including portability), safety, and cost.[4,7] However, echocardiography is frequently complemented by other modalities based on the specific clinical questions. Adherence to the American College of Cardiology Foundation/American Heart Association (AHA) guidelines for the diagnosis and treatment of heart failure should dovetail with the appropriate use of multimodal imaging. The ultimate aims of cardiovascular imaging are to maximize diagnostic accuracy and to improve patient care and clinical outcomes cost effectively, using evidence-based medicine to guide the appropriate use of our limited health care system resources.[8,9]

HEART FAILURE WITH REDUCED EJECTION FRACTION VERSUS HEART FAILURE WITH PRESERVED EJECTION FRACTION

Recent studies place the prevalence of heart failure with preserved ejection fraction (HFpEF) at around 54% with a range from 40% to 71%[10]

(see also Chapter 39). Clinical presentation of patients presenting with the new onset of heart failure and reduced LV ejection fraction (HFrEF/systolic heart failure) cannot always be reliably distinguished clinically from HFpEF patients. Exam findings, such as lateral displacement of the LV apical impulse, as a clinical clue to LV dilatation often cannot be appreciated in HFrEF due to body habitus, chronic lung disease, or a diffuse and weak apical impulse. LV dilatation can be easily confirmed by chest x-ray (CXR) or TTE. LV dilatation and decreased ejection fraction (EF) are crucial for the diagnosis of HFrEF. There is a preponderance of elderly women with systemic hypertension in HFpEF as compared with HFrEF.[11,12] More than two thirds of patients with HFrEF have an ischemic etiology for their LV dysfunction.[1] The diagnosis of HFpEF can strictly only be made by the combination of clinical demographics and computational image analysis, which provides an estimation of EF and an assessment of the severity of LV diastolic dysfunction with TTE. HFpEF has only recently been acknowledged as a discrete pathophysiologic entity because formerly it was considered to be a benign condition for which there is still no specific treatment. However, studies have demonstrated that HFpEF is a discrete entity with a significant annual morbidity and mortality, and a readmission rate for acute exacerbations of heart failure.[13] Doppler echocardiographic imaging can distinguish HFpEF from HFrEF because in HFrEF there is obligatory LV dilatation to maintain a normal stroke volume as LVEF declines.[14] In contrast, LV cavity size in HFpEF is normal or small and there is usually mild to moderate concentric hypertrophic remodeling (**Fig. 32.1**A and B) induced by concomitant hypertension (HTN), with preserved left ventricular ejection fraction (LVEF) (≥50%).

EVALUATION OF LEFT VENTRICULAR DIASTOLIC DYSFUNCTION

Diastolic dysfunction is the underlying pathophysiologic abnormality that typifies HFpEF.[15] Diastolic LV dysfunction as assessed by echocardiography includes an abnormal transmitral peak E wave, a peak A wave that ranges from delayed relaxation to irreversible restrictive physiology, and severely elevated filling pressures (**Fig. 32.2**). (E/e′), reduced e′ myocardial velocities by tissue Doppler imaging in the septum and lateral wall, are consistent with delayed relaxation and an enlarged left atrium.[16,17] In addition, there is consistently abnormal pulmonary venous flow (see Fig. 32.2). Diastolic ventricular function also can be assessed with nuclear techniques from ventricular volume curves in terms of LV peak filling rate (PFR), time to PFR, and filling fractions. However, there is no single echo, Doppler, or nuclear parameter that is sufficiently robust to diagnose the presence of LV diastolic dysfunction.

The reason for distinguishing HFpEF from HFrEF patients is because they have different LV morphology, epidemiology, and mechanisms of heart failure systolic and diastolic LV function—all of which are evident by 2D and 3D transthoracic echocardiographic imaging. Furthermore, patients with HFpEF do not derive a clear benefit from traditional heart failure therapy, which includes β-adrenergic receptor blockers, angiotensin converting enzyme inhibitors, angiotensin receptor blockers, and mineralocorticoids inhibitors.[18-20] Heart size in HFpEF remains stable although LV hypertrophy may increase, and diastolic dysfunction may worsen over time. In contrast, heart size in HFrEF is increased at the time of diagnosis and increases progressively thereafter (**Fig. 32.3**). The prognosis of HFpEF is better than in HFrEF, although the rate of hospital readmission for recurrent heart failure is similar. Echocardiographic changes in LV size, geometry, hypertrophy, and function have been reported prospectively in multiple studies of systolic heart failure/HFrEF for more than three decades. By comparison there is a paucity of Doppler echocardiographic information on HFpEF available for assessment of diastolic LV function over time, except for studies from the Framingham database.[12,21]

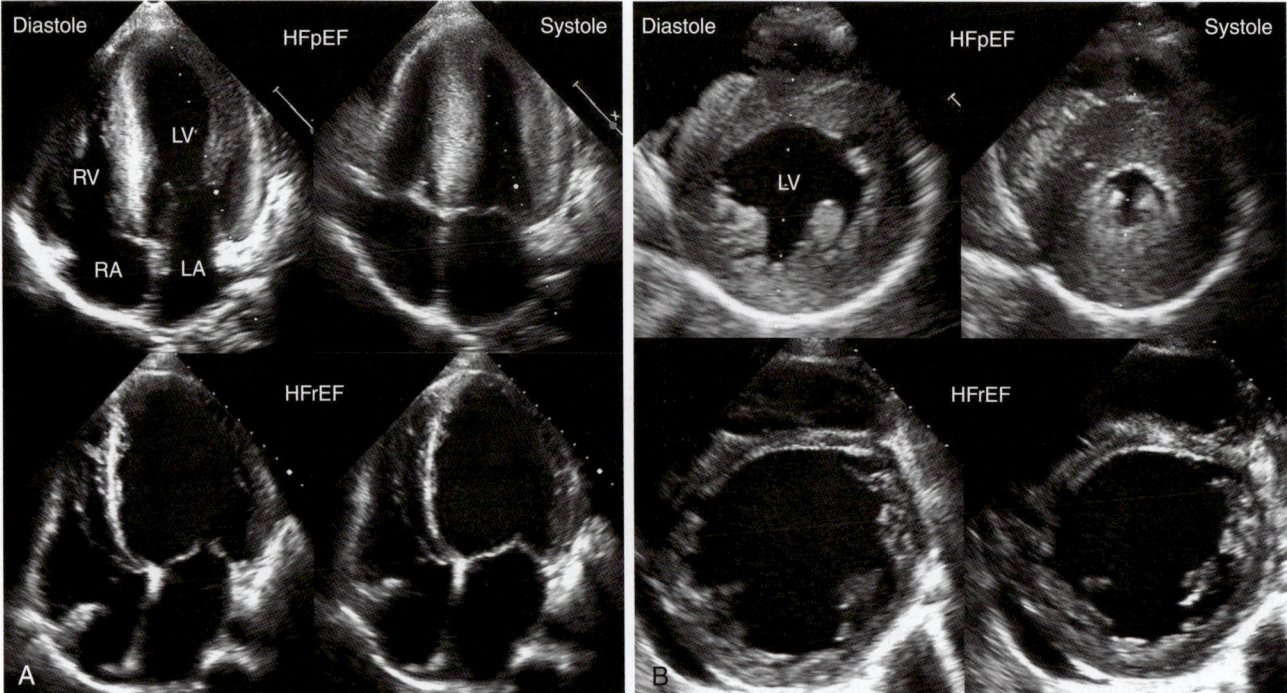

Fig. 32.1 (A) Transthoracic echocardiogram *(TTE)* of the apical 4-chamber view at end-diastole *(top left panel)* and end-systole *(top right panel)* from a patient with HFpEF showing normal left ventricular *(LV)* cavity size and with an ejection fraction of 53%, moderate concentric LV hypertrophy, and an enlarged left atrium. The apical 4-chamber view from a patient with HFrEF is seen at end-diastole *(bottom left panel)* and at end-systole *(bottom right panel)*. In contrast to the patient in the top panels, the patient with HFrEF has a markedly enlarged LV with severely decreased function (EF of 20%), a distal septal scar from a remote myocardial infarction indicating an ischemic etiology for the LV dysfunction, and an enlarged left atrium. (B) TTE of the same two patients above showing images of the LV short-axis views at the level of the tips of the mitral valve leaflets at end-diastole *(top left panel)* and at end-systole *(top right panel)* with HFpEF *(top panels)* with marked concentric hypertrophy. The HFrEF patient shown at end-diastole *(bottom left panel)* and at end-systole *(bottom right panel)* has a much larger LV with poor function (EF 20%) and thinning of the septum. *EF,* Ejection fraction; *HFpEF,* heart failure with preserved ejection fraction; *HFrPF,* heart failure with reduced ejection fraction; *RV,* right ventricular.

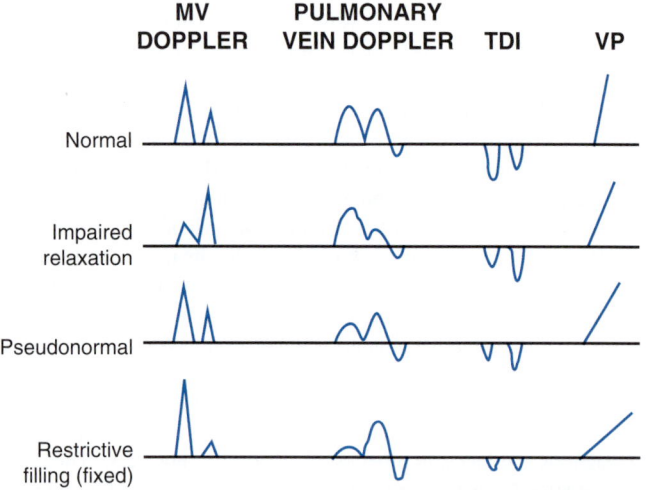

Fig. 32.2 Doppler Assessment of Diastolic Function. HFpEF is primarily a disorder of left ventricular diastolic function ranging from impaired myocardial relaxation to fixed restrictive filling manifest by abnormal transmitral blood flow velocities, pulmonary vein flow, tissue Doppler imaging *(TDI)*, and a progressive decrease in propagation velocity. *HFpEF,* Heart failure with preserved ejection fraction; *MV,* mitral valve; *VP,* velocity of propagation.

MULTIPLE MODALITY CARDIAC IMAGING

Cardiac diagnostic imaging techniques are used routinely in heart failure and range from simple assessment of overall heart size, cardiac silhouette, and the presence of pulmonary congestion by CXR to real-time 3D-Doppler echocardiographic reconstruction of the heart and the great vessels, or CMR perfusion showing delayed gadolinium enhancement due to myocardial fibrosis. Although computed tomography (CT) provides spectacular high-resolution cardiac imaging, the doses of ionizing radiation and of iodinated contrast agents precludes serial studies that are required in patients with heart failure undergoing LV remodeling.

CXR is obtained in all heart failure patients for the detection of cardiomegaly, individual chamber and great vessel enlargement, pulmonary venous congestion, and pericardial and pleural effusions that are frequent accompaniments of decompensated heart failure. Even minor hemodynamically irrelevant pericardial effusions in heart failure are associated with increased risk of cardiac mortality.[22]

Echocardiography is the imaging modality of choice in all causes of heart failure because it is portable, safe, and provides accurate quantitative information at the bedside, which includes LV volumes, chamber architecture, regional and global systolic and diastolic function, valve function, and pulmonary artery systolic pressure, all of which

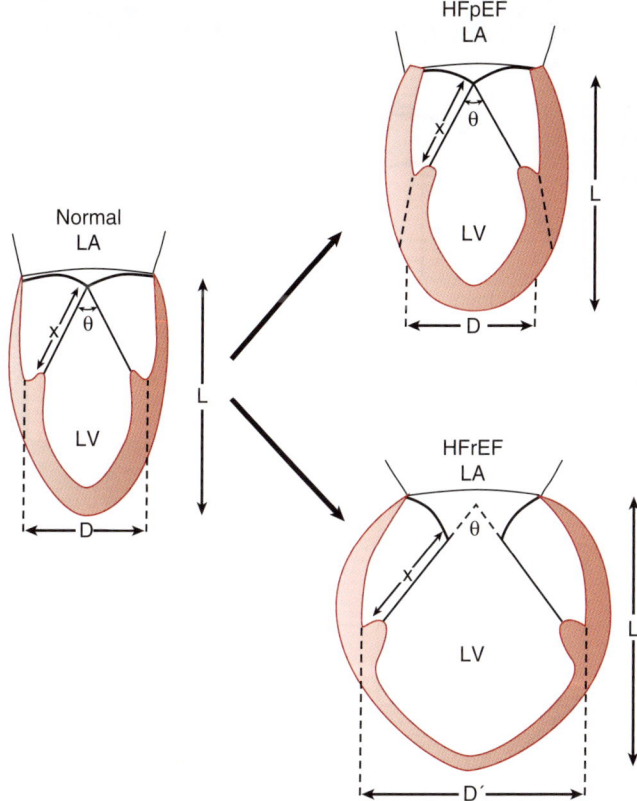

Fig. 32.3 Remodeling-Associated Left Ventricular *(LV)* Geometry Changes. Schema showing the cavity geometry in the normal heart *(left panel)*, a heart of a patient with HFpEF *(top right panel)* showing normal LV cavity dimensions and moderate LV hypertrophy consistent with concentric remodeling. The heart in the bottom right panel represents a heart with HFrEF that is typified by severe cavity dilatation, distorted LV geometry, separation of the papillary muscles with an increase in the angle "θ" causing mal-coaptation of the mitral valve leaflets and mitral regurgitation. *HFpEF,* Heart failure with preserved ejection fraction; *HFrPF,* heart failure with reduced ejection fraction; *LA,* left atrium.

correlate with clinical outcomes. In addition, Doppler measures of intracardiac blood flow velocities and myocardial velocities permit the calculation of myocardial strain and torsion/rotation that enable the complete assessment of global and regional myocardial mechanics. A great advantage of 2D and 3D echocardiography is that all of this information regarding myocardial mechanics is immediately available at the bedside and, furthermore, can be repeated safely as needed. However, misgivings have been expressed recently regarding the use of 2D echocardiography to assess LV volumes, EF, and LV mass in serial studies because of the poor test and retest reproducibility and the magnitude of the standard deviations derived from a meta-analysis, which involved a large number of studies.[23] However, these findings are discordant with a number of recent studies in which serial echoes were performed and consistently demonstrated important reproducible changes in LV size, mass, and function following intervention.[24-26]

Assessment of Left Ventricular Function by Echocardiography

M-Mode echocardiography has been used for measurements of LV size, mass, and loading conditions (end-systolic meridional and circumferential wall stress), and myocardial function (fractional and mid-wall shortening and velocity of circumferential fiber shortening peak). However, M-Mode echo assessments of LV function are limited

because it is assumed that there is uniform wall thickness and normal concentric wall motion, whereas the majority of patients with HFrEF have coronary artery disease (CAD) and ischemic cardiomyopathy[1] in which the hallmarks of CAD are LV wall motion abnormalities and variations in LV wall thickness. Thus M-Mode echo measurements of LV size and function are not admissible in over two-thirds of the HFrEF population. LV linear dimensions are still used in randomized clinical trials in hypertension that require serial measurements with or without an intervention as the primary outcome measure.

TTE is the most frequently used, and clinically the most important, diagnostic imaging modality in HFrEF and in HFpEF.[28] LV end-systolic, end-diastolic volumes and stroke volume can be calculated from biplane orthogonal images of the LV in the apical 4-chamber and the apical 2-chamber planes using Simpson's method of discs.[29] LV mass (LVM) also can be estimated from measurements of end-diastolic wall thickness, LV cavity diameter/2 and LV length (5/6 short-axis area × length). The important fundamental relation between LV volume and mass can be examined. Estimates of LV volumes, LVM, and EF by 2D echo provide insight into the structural, geometric, and functional changes in the left ventricle as the heart remodels and the severity of heart failure progresses. 2D Doppler echocardiography has played a major role in elucidating our current understanding of the different natural histories and etiological mechanisms involved in HFpEF and HFrEF.

In addition to TTE determination of LV volumes, mass (LVH as increased relative wall thickness), LV shape, and EF have proved to be powerful predictors of clinical outcome in patients with heart failure.[30,31] LV stroke volume can be calculated from LV volumes (EDV − ESV = SV) by 2D and 3D TTE, and by Doppler measurement of intracardiac blood flow velocities in the LV outflow tract (LVOT). Blood volume flow in unit time can be assessed as the product of the time velocity integral (TVI) and the cross-sectional area (CSA) of the flow stream (TVI × CSA). When recorded from the LVOT, stroke volume correlates closely with stroke volume estimated from LV volumes. Recently, the LVOT has been shown to be elliptical rather than circular by transesophageal echocardiography (TEE), CMR, and CT, especially in the presence of LVH that protrudes into the LVOT in patients with hemodynamically important aortic stenosis (AS) and severe systemic hypertension. The influence of an abnormal LV outflow tract cross-sectional shape can be minimized by planimetry analysis of the cross-section directly.[32]

Myocardial Strain and Strain Rate

Measurement of myocardial strain is a relatively new concept that describes global and regional ventricular systolic function using speckle-tracking echocardiography or magnetic resonance with myocardial tagging. Speckle tracking echocardiography depends upon the temporal and spatial tracking of naturally occurring intramyocardial reflectors of ultrasound (speckles) within the 2D echocardiographic images of the LV walls. Displacement of these speckles is due to myocardial deformation[33] from which myocardial strain is calculated. Strain is defined as the change in myocardial segment length (ΔL) divided by resting segment length (L_0): $S = \Delta L / L_0$. The insonating beam is directed parallel to the LV long axis. Myocardial strain is assessed in three planes: longitudinal, circumferential, and radial.

Longitudinal strain is calculated from the LV long axis, and the radial and circumferential strains from the LV short-axis images obtained at the LV mid-cavity level (**Fig. 32.4**). Estimates of myocardial strains by speckle tracking echocardiography have been validated in man by CMR with myocardial tagging and in animals by sonomicrometry.[33] Global systolic strains can be assessed in addition to simultaneous assessment of myocardial strains in each segment using the

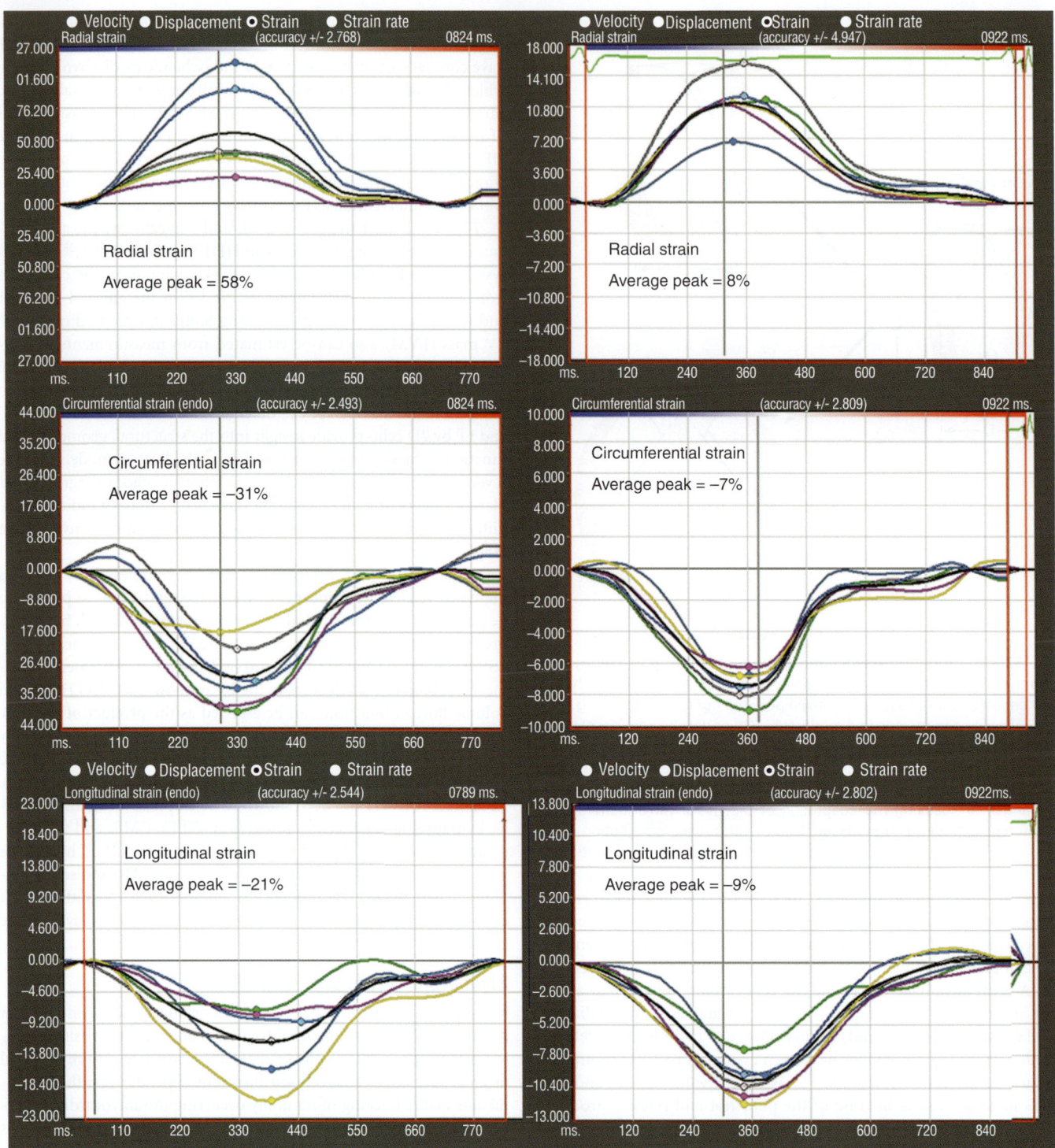

Fig. 32.4 Left Ventricular *(LV)* Strain—Normal Versus Cardiomyopathy. This six-panel figure shows radial strain in a normal subject with an average peak value of +58% *(top left panel)* and severely reduced average peak radial strain of +8% in a heart failure patient *(top right panel*, note difference in scale). Of note, there was no evidence for LV dyssynchrony in either subject/patient. In the middle and lower panels, the average peak circumferential strain and average peak longitudinal strain are shown with the normal in the left panels and the heart failure patient in the right panels. Note the major reduction in the average peak radial, circumferential, and longitudinal strains in heart failure without evidence for dyssynchrony.

16- or 17-segment model of the LV. Myocardial strains can be recorded simultaneously from the interventricular septum and from the lateral LV wall in each of three myocardial segments (apical, mid, and proximal) from the apical 4-chamber, 2-chamber, and apical long-axis views (see Fig. 32.4). Strain analysis can be quantified after acquisition

of the echo images. Measurement of the time period from onset of QRS to peak strain for each myocardial segment provides insight as to the coordination of contraction and the degree of dyssynchrony. Strain can detect mild perturbations in LV function before any change is detectable in LV volumes or EF. The strain rate is the rate of change of strain, which has not always proved as robust or reproducible as the measurement of deformation due to a number of confounding factors.

3D echocardiography: Numerous studies have demonstrated the correlations between LV volumes, mass, and EF estimated by 2D and CMR. Still closer correlations have been demonstrated between real time 3D echocardiography and CMR with less variability about the mean.[34]

Real time 3D echocardiographic assessment of LV volumes, mass, and LVEF (**Fig. 32.5**) correlates more closely to CMR than 2D Echo, with less variability than with 2D.[35] However, the greater precision of measurement of LV mass and EF by CMR is the reason that CMR has become the standard of reference for quantification of LV mass and LV volumes.

A proportion of echocardiograms in heart failure patients are technically limited because endocardial definition is incomplete, resulting in poor image quality, necessitating interpolation of extensive regions of the LV endocardium. This occurs especially in patients with emphysema or morbid obesity that may even preclude quantitative analysis. However, endocardial definition is improved with harmonic imaging and can be further enhanced with intravenous echo contrast so that a proportion of poor-quality studies can be recovered for quantitative analysis.

TEE: When image quality is poor, switching to TEE or to an alternative imaging modality, such as CMR, for better image quality may be a better strategy. However, there is a trade-off for the exquisite image quality attained by TEE, and that is that quantitation of LV volumes from biplane TEE images consistently underestimates volumes calculated by TTE. This occurs because of unavoidable foreshortening of the LV long axis in the apical imaging planes with TEE. This foreshortening artifact results in the underestimation of LV volumes, EF, and longitudinal strain.

TEE is not indicated in the routine assessment of patients with heart failure except in special circumstances, which include poor image quality, suspected vegetative endocarditis, assessment of magnetic resonance due to papillary muscle infarction, and occasionally to measure left atrial size.

An additional important role performed by 2D echocardiography is the detection of LV cavity thrombus (**Fig. 32.6**) adherent to severely hypokinetic or akinetic myocardial segments. Thrombus formation also occurs in the left atrial cavity and/or appendage, especially in patients with left atrial enlargement and atrial fibrillation. In patients with unexplained worsening symptoms, 2D echocardiograms should be performed to rule out significant pericardial effusion, pleural effusion, or the onset of atrial fibrillation, which is a common dysrhythmia in heart failure.

Nuclear Cardiology: Radionuclide SPECT and PET

Single photon emission computed tomography (SPECT) and positron emission tomography (PET) imaging have become standard approaches for quantitative physiologic imaging in patients with HF. Radiotracer techniques have been widely used to evaluate regional and global ventricular function, and to detect myocardial ischemia, hibernation, infarction, and ventricular remodeling. Nuclear imaging techniques also are well suited for in vivo molecular imaging because of their high sensitivity, spatial resolution, and availability of new hybrid instrumentation and molecular targeted probes.[36] Molecular imaging offers a novel approach for detecting molecular or cellular changes in vivo before the development of any physiological or anatomic changes. Recently dedicated hybrid imaging systems combining nuclear detector systems with high resolution structural imaging modalities such as x-ray CT or magnetic resonance imaging have been introduced into routine clinical practice. In addition to aiding the interpretation of the

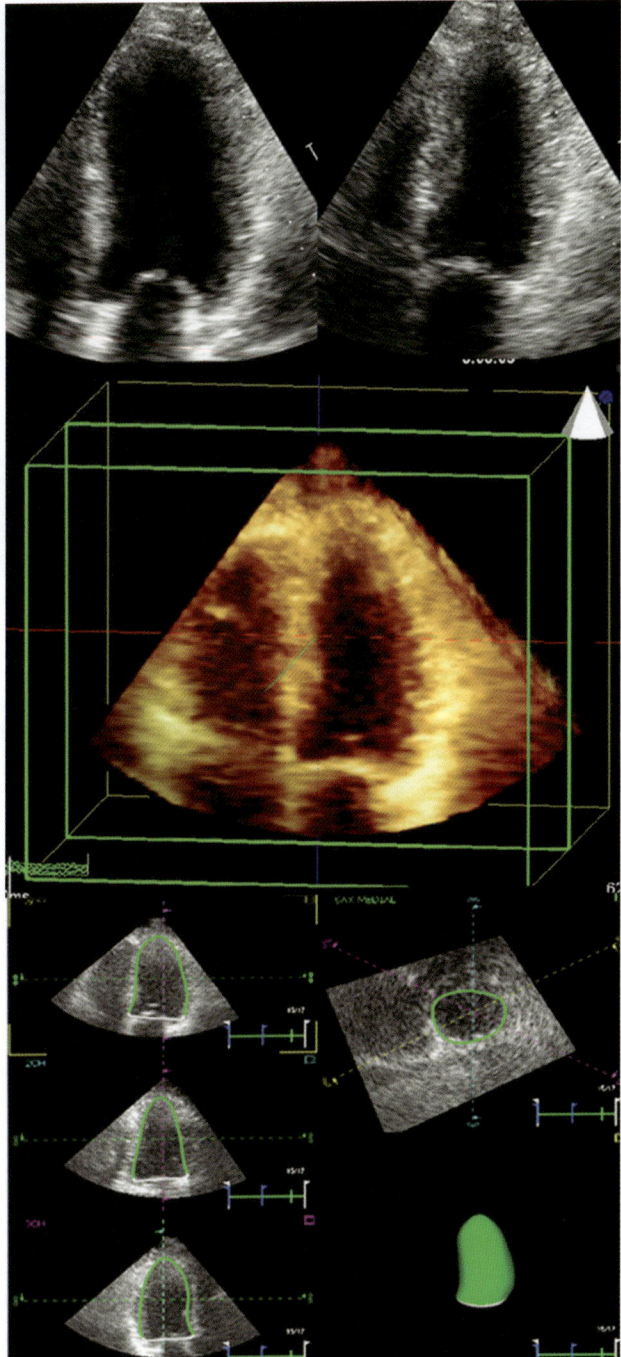

Fig. 32.5 Three-Dimensional *(3D)* Echocardiography. 3D echocardiogram showing acquisition and processing of apical images of the LV from a normal subject. These 3D echocardiograms allow for quantification of LV volumes and LV mass that compare favorably with those calculated from cardiac magnetic resonance *(CMR)* images. CMR has become the reference standard for quantitative analysis of LV geometry and function. *LV,* Left ventricular.

SPECT/PET findings, anatomical information in hybrid imaging facilitates correction for attenuation, scatter, and partial volume effects, resulting in enhanced image quality, dose reduction, and radiotracer quantification. Beyond this, hybrid systems have the potential to provide independent and real-time synergistic data that improve disease characterization and patient care, as recently described for PET/magnetic resonance hybrid scanners.[37]

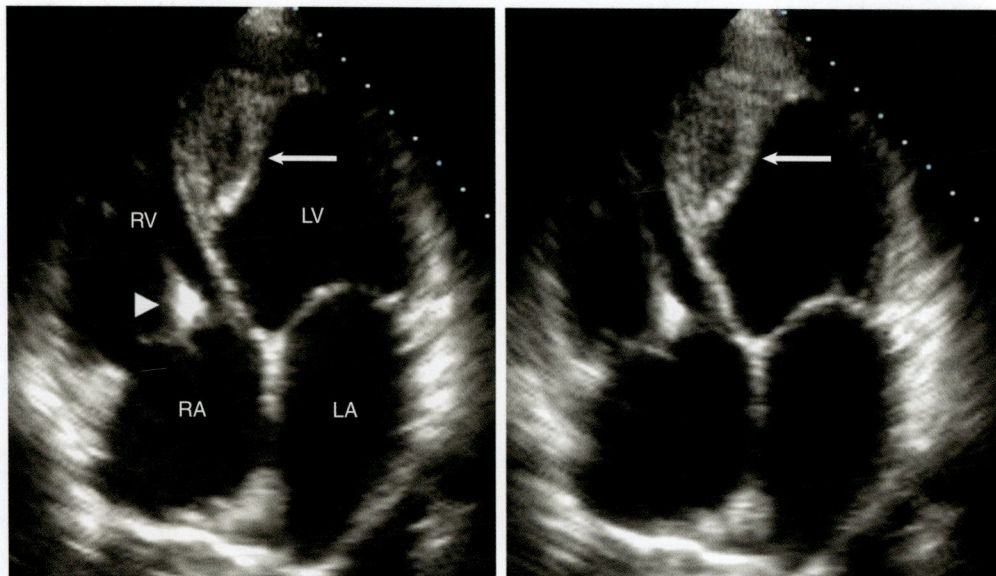

Fig. 32.6 Left Ventricular *(LV)* Dysfunction With an Apical Thrombus. 2D TTE showing an apical 4-chamber view at end-diastole *(left panel)* and at end-systole *(right panel)* in a 60-year-old female who became acutely short of breath 2 weeks ago with easy fatigue, who previously walked to work 5 days per week. She did not seek medical help until she sustained a near syncopal episode. The LV is enlarged and there is severe hypokinesis of the mid-septum to the apex of the LV with a large adherent thrombus attached to the distal septum with liquefaction necrosis at the center *(arrows)*. *2D,* Two-dimensional; *RV,* right ventricular; *TTE,* transthoracic echocardiogram.

Assessment of Physiologic Ischemia

In the evaluation of patients with heart failure it is important to rule out ischemic heart disease as the etiology of the LV dysfunction because of the potential to impact ventricular dysfunction by revascularization (**see also Chapter 19**). This can be accomplished by an assessment of stress-induced changes in regional perfusion or function. Rest and stress myocardial perfusion imaging can be accomplished with either SPECT or PET perfusion imaging. Importantly, radionuclide myocardial perfusion imaging effectively visualizes regional changes in myocardial blood flow, which is a principal target of many therapies in patients with CAD. Rest and stress radiotracer studies continue to play a major role in the diagnosis of CAD, which is the major cause of HF. Thus, stress/rest SPECT perfusion imaging can effectively separate ischemic from nonischemic cardiomyopathy.

The care of patients with acute myocardial infarction (MI) is directed at establishing early coronary reperfusion, since aborting ischemia may result in myocardial salvage. Myocardial salvage results in preservation of LV function, which is the most important predictor of long-term survival postinfarction. Radiotracer imaging has proved effective in estimation of infarct size and salvage of cardiomyocytes after MI. The radiotracer technique also provides a reliable estimation of residual LV function. There is a well-established relationship between survival and global RV and LV function in patients undergoing reperfusion with thrombolytic therapy or percutaneous coronary intervention (PCI).[38]

Assessment of Right and Left Ventricular Volumes and Function

The traditional radiotracer approaches to assess ventricular function included first-pass radionuclide angiocardiography, and equilibrium radionuclide angiocardiography (ERNA), which use imaging of Tc99m-labeled red blood cells (RBCs). The first-pass technique permits assessment of global right and left ventricular size and function, but is inadequate for the evaluation of regional LV function, because only a single projection of the ventricle is obtained. To assess RV and LV functional reserve by the first-pass technique, separate injections of the radiotracer are made at rest and during peak exercise. The first-pass technique has been replaced by ERNA, which, in turn, has been superseded by gated SPECT blood pool angiography[39] and gated SPECT perfusion imaging.[40] Analysis of temporal changes in count density from 4D SPECT images provides an index of regional LV wall thickening.[41] New 3D radiotracer-based imaging approaches offer a more comprehensive evaluation of regional and global LV function.[42] Serial equilibrium blood pool imaging can be performed at rest and during various levels of exercise or after pharmacologic perturbations to evaluate ventricular functional reserve. Gated SPECT perfusion imaging is primarily restricted to the evaluation of resting function.

LV end-diastolic (LVED) and end-systolic volumes can be evaluated serially using nuclear approaches in patients with HF and can be used to track LV remodeling and to monitor therapy. Volumes from gated blood pool images are calculated based on radiotracer count density and are therefore relatively independent of alterations in regional geometry. Simple count-based techniques allow volume measurements to be made without the confounding technical issues of accurate measurement of attenuation.[43,44] These estimates of volumes can be improved by applying 3D imaging techniques.

Assessment of diastolic function is also important in the evaluation of patients with HFpEF and with HFrEF in the elderly with hypertension and/or CAD. ERNA results have high reproducibility because there are no geometric assumptions and there is much less operator dependence in image acquisition. Diastolic parameters, such as filling rate, time to peak filling, and filling fractions, can be readily assessed from the ventricular volume curve.[45] Studies have demonstrated good correlation between echocardiography and ERNA for reliable determination of diastolic parameters. In patients with diastolic dysfunction, there will be a prolongation of isovolumic relaxation time, a delay in the onset of rapid filling, a decrease in slope of rapid filling phase, and an exaggerated atrial kick. The lower limit of normal PFR is 2.50

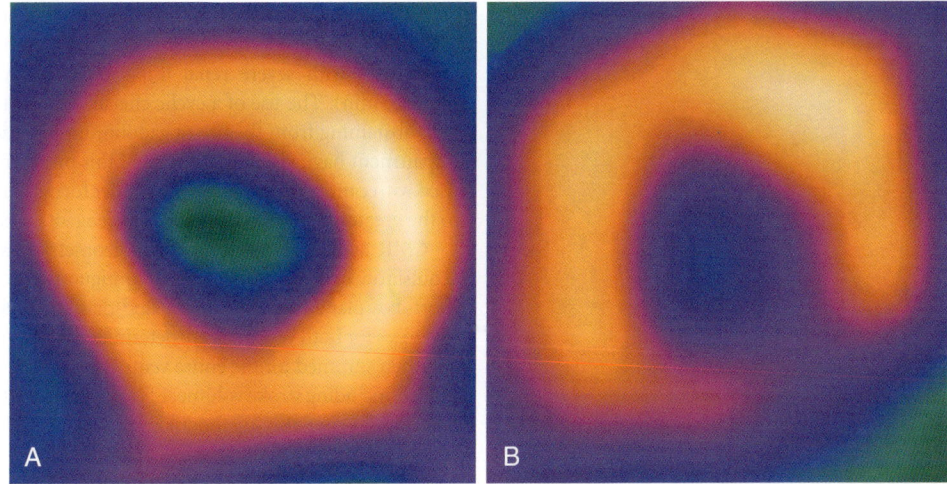

Fig 32.7 Resting Myocardial Perfusion and Late 123I MIBG Myocardial Imaging in a Patient With Reduced Left Ventricular Ejection Fraction. The patient demonstrates normal resting myocardial perfusion (A), but abnormal regional 123-I meta-iodobenzylguanidine (123I-MIBG) imaging (B). A correlation has been demonstrated between the size of the 123I-MIBG defect and the risk of ventricular arrhythmias. This relatively large area of abnormal sympathetic function accurately predicted this patient's appropriate implantable cardioverter defibrillator therapy (antitachycardia pacing) after 18 months of follow-up. (Modified from Boogers MJ, Borleffs CJ, Henneman MM, et al. Cardiac sympathetic denervation assessed with 123-iodine metaiodobenzylguanidine imaging predicts ventricular arrhythmias in implantable cardioverter-defibrillator patients. *J Am Coll Cardiol.* 2010;55:2769–2777.)

end-diastolic volumes per second (EDV/s). In addition, time to PFR can be expressed in milliseconds and is expected to be less than 180 milliseconds in normal subjects. The PFR and the atrial filling rate have been shown to correspond to the E and A waves of Doppler echocardiographic mitral velocity wave forms. When ERNA is used, such measurements should be routine in the assessment of heart failure in the presence or absence of CAD.

Imaging Autonomic Dysfunction

Cardiac autonomic dysfunction is associated with an increased risk of ventricular arrhythmia and sudden cardiac death in heart failure (**see also Chapter 42**). Alterations in pre- and postsynaptic cardiac sympathetic function can be assessed noninvasively using both SPECT and PET radiotracers.[46-48] The most widely used SPECT radiotracers for imaging of presynaptic function is ^{123}I-meta-iodobenzylguanidine (^{123}I-MIBG), which shares many cellular uptake and storage properties with norepinephrine. Many studies have demonstrated the clinical value of ^{123}I-MIBG imaging for both diagnostic and prognostic purposes in patients with heart failure. In these patients, ^{123}I-MIBG scans typically show a reduced heart-to-mediastinal uptake ratio (HMR), heterogeneous distribution within the myocardium, and increased ^{123}I-MIBG wash-out from the heart. HMR is a marker of specific sympathetic nerve terminal tracer retention and has prognostic value in heart failure.[49] The wash-out ratio of ^{123}I-MIBG predicts sudden cardiac death, independent of LVEF.[50] A large prospective study of ^{123}I-MIBG imaging demonstrated a significant relationship between the heart failure related events and the HMR, which was independent of LVEF and BNP.[51] This clinical study also showed an association between myocardial sympathetic neuronal dysfunction and the risk for subsequent cardiac death. Moreover, the size of the MIBG defect on delayed SPECT imaging also predicts ventricular arrhythmias (**Fig. 32.7**).

Presympathetic function also can be assessed by PET imaging with ^{11}C-meta-hydroxyephedrine (^{11}C-HED).[52] In nontransmural MIs, the HED imaging defect can exceed the perfusion defect, but it is not clear whether this is associated with higher ventricular arrhythmia risk. In patients with nonischemic cardiomyopathy, there is decreased HED

uptake, and in a recent retrospective study, global HED uptake was an independent predictor of adverse outcomes in patients with New York Heart Association (NYHA) class II and III heart failure (**Fig. 32.8**).[53] This PET sympathetic imaging approach is under evaluation in patients with CAD and depressed LVEF. A recently completed single site prospective clinical study (PAREPET) showed that quantitative ^{11}C-HED PET imaging was one of the best predictors of sudden cardiac death, independent of LVEF and infarction size.[54,55]

Computed Tomography

CT and CMR imaging both produce exquisite image quality with and without contrast enhancement and allow comprehensive quantitative assessment of LV and RV architecture and function as well as delineation of the coronary artery anatomy. The disadvantage of CT is the exposure to both ionizing radiation and iodinated contrast agents. Recently, attempts have been made to minimize radiation exposure during CT and have had a modicum of success.

Cardiac Magnetic Resonance Imaging

The acquisition of such high-fidelity image quality is the reason that CMR has become the standard of reference for quantification of LV volumes, LVEF, and LV mass (**Fig. 32.9A**). The accuracy and reproducibility of CMR makes it the ideal tool for serial assessment of ventricular size and function, and at the same time it reduces the sample sizes necessary in clinical trials.[56,57] However, a substantial proportion of heart failure patients have ICDs, permanent pacemakers, and there is an increasing number of CRT device implants in whom CMR imaging is currently contraindicated. The numerical data generated in healthy normal subjects and in acute and chronic heart failure by CMR are commonly used to risk stratify patients with heart failure. Serial imaging of the heart in patients with heart failure is frequently used to assess the rate of disease progression, and the response to pharmacologic agents, devices, and surgical and cellular therapies. Serial evaluation of large patient cohorts has also been used to assess the efficacy of novel pharmacologic agents and device therapies for heart failure in large, randomized, clinical trials. Gadolinium-containing CMR contrast agents have been used safely in many millions

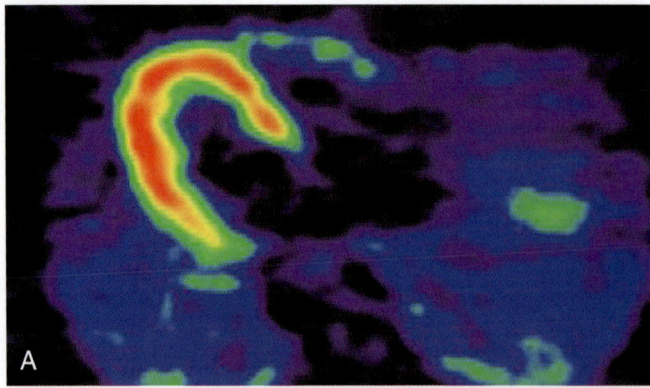

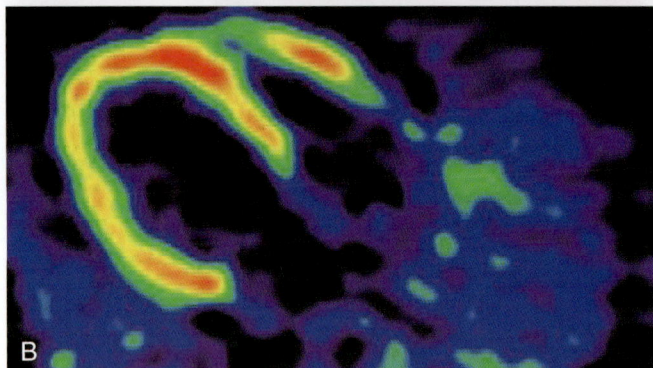

Fig 32.8 Myocardial 11C HED Uptake in a Healthy Subject and a Heart Failure Patient. The healthy subject (A) shows normal 11C HED uptake, while the patient with dilated cardiomyopathy (B) demonstrates reduced 11C HED uptake on quantitative evaluation. (Modified from Pietila M, Malminiemi K, Ukkonen H, et al. Reduced myocardial carbon-11 hydroxyephedrine retention is associated with poor prognosis in chronic heart failure. *Eur J Nucl Med.* 2001;28:373–376.)

of patients. A rare disorder known as nephrogenic sclerosing fibrosis was reported as a potential side effect following high-dose contrast use in patients with severe renal impairment (glomerular filtration rate <30 mL/min). The use of a cyclic chelate-based gadolinium agent along with abstaining from the use of gadolinium in patients with severe renal impairment have virtually eliminated this problem. These agents can be used with caution in patients with milder forms of renal impairment, due to the greater risks of iodinated contrast agents used in cardiac CT.

CMR avoids errors imposed by geometric assumptions during the acquisition of 3D stacked sets of contiguous cine slices, usually in the short-axis plane (see Fig. 32.9B). End-diastolic and end-systolic volumes and mass for both ventricles are determined by the planimetry of each slice and then summed for the entire ventricle. Measures of ventricular performance, including stroke volume, EF, and cardiac output, may be accurately quantified using this methodology. Similarly, calculation of abnormal hemodynamic states resulting from coronary artery, valvular, and congenital heart disease causing left- or right-sided heart failure may be performed routinely. The high quality of the data allows indexation to important variables such as body surface area, gender, and age. These data demonstrate that indexation is important for the confident diagnosis of conditions in their early stages; for example, dilated or hypertrophic cardiomyopathy.[58] LV diastolic function also can be assessed by CMR. However, echocardiography is used routinely, is readily available, and has been the preferred imaging modality of choice in large, randomized clinical trials.

VALVULAR HEART DISEASE AND HEART FAILURE (SEE ALSO CHAPTER 26)

Mitral Valve Regurgitation

Mitral regurgitation (MR) is more frequently associated with chronic HFrEF than with HFpEF, occurring in approximately 50% of patients, ranging in severity from mild to severe. MR is readily detected by Doppler because color flow velocity mapping is exquisitely sensitive

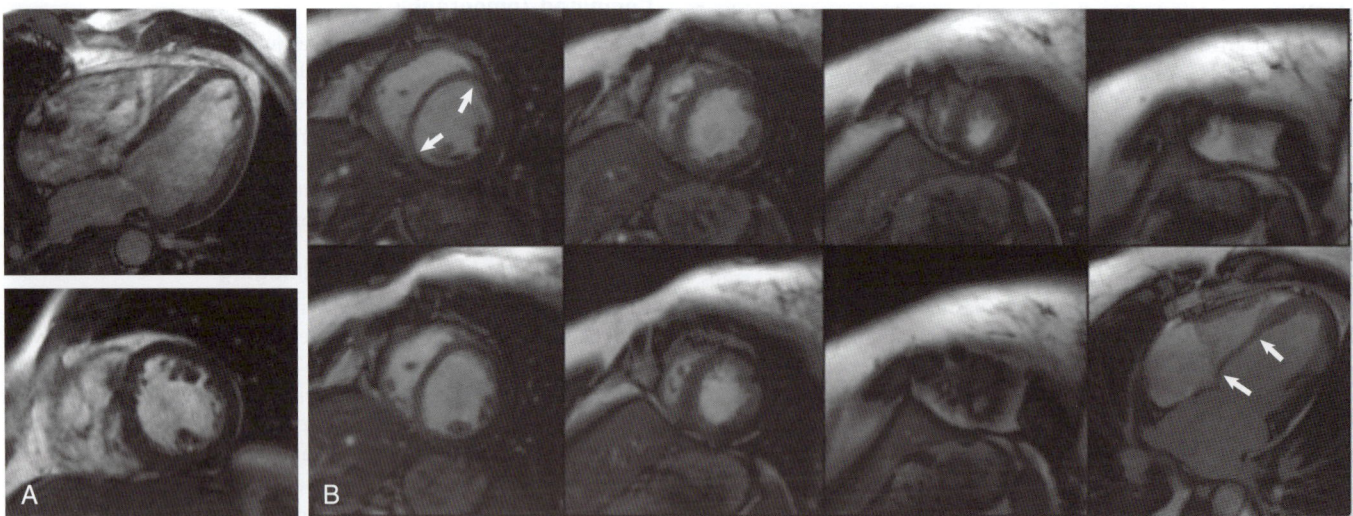

Fig. 32.9 Short-Axis and Long-Axis CMR Images—Normal Versus Heart Failure. Representative single slice short-axis and 4-chamber CMR images are shown in Panel A. Note the excellent soft tissue contrast and depiction of intracardiac vs. extracardiac structures. Panel B shows a series of end-diastolic short-axis images from base to apex in a chronic heart failure patient following remote Giant cell myocarditis, as well as a 4-chamber view *(lower right)*. The more basal short-axis slices show thinning of the septum from the base to the mid-ventricle, which is confirmed by the 4-chamber image *(arrows)*. Note detailed depiction of the right ventricular as well as left ventricular anatomy. *CMR,* Cardiovascular magnetic resonance.

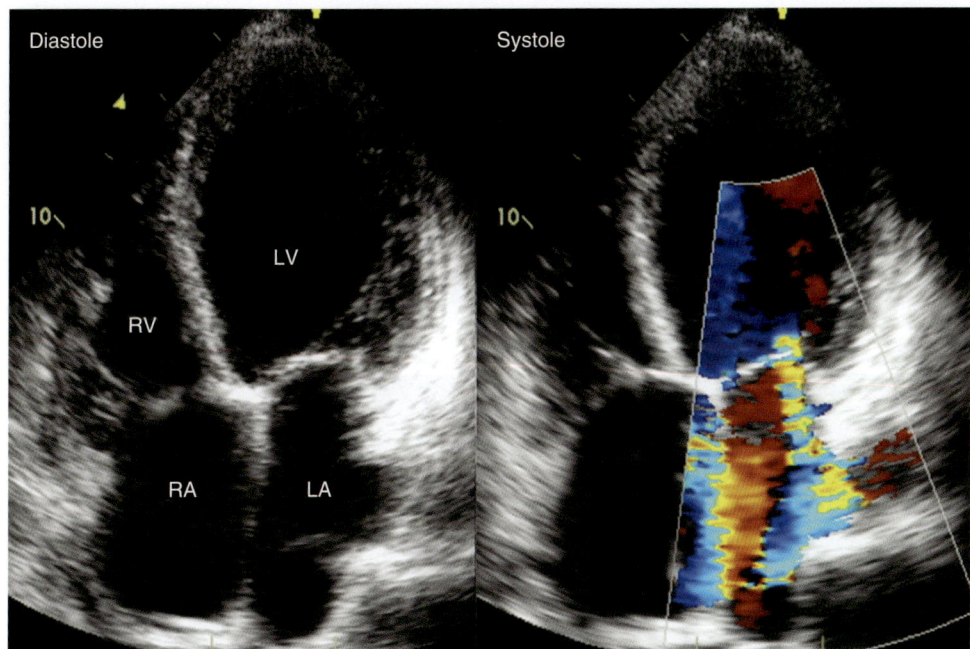

Fig. 32.10 Cardiomyopathy With Mitral Regurgitation Depicted by Echocardiography. A 2D transthoracic echocardiogram in the apical 4-chamber view from a patient with HFrEF at end-diastolic *(left panel)* and in systole with color flow Doppler *(right panel)* shows moderately severe left ventricular enlargement and poor function *(left panel)*. In the right panel color flow Doppler demonstrates two mitral regurgitant jets and moderately severe MR jet with proximal iso-velocity surface area. *2D,* Two-dimensional; *AO,* aorta; *HFrPF,* heart failure with reduced ejection fraction; *LA,* left atrium; *MR,* mitral regurgitation.

even to trivial MR. The underlying mechanism of MR in HFrEF can be appreciated by 2D and 3D TTE imaging, which demonstrates distortion of the geometry of the mitral subvalve apparatus, stretching of the mitral annulus preventing adequate coaptation of the mitral valve leaflets caused by progressive LV cavity enlargement, which results in MR (**Fig. 32.10**; see Fig. 32.3). Compared to HFrEF that undergoes eccentric remodeling, LV cavity size in HFpEF is not prone to dilatation but instead undergoes concentric hypertrophic remodeling that only rarely results in severe MR.

Evaluation of the presence and severity of MR in heart failure is hemodynamically important because the excessive volume handling from MR increases LV loading conditions, causing further deterioration in LV function as predicted by the inverse relationship between load and ejection phase indices. This shows that the greater the increase in LV load, the greater the reduction in LVEF. The corollary of this relationship provides the rationale for the chronic use of vasodilator therapy to reduce load and improve refractory heart failure. Another cause of MR, which is also more frequent in HFrEF than HFpEF, is due to recurrent episodes of myocardial ischemia triggered by the worsening of regional myocardial blood flow that may cause severe sudden onset MR and flash pulmonary edema/acute heart failure. This can be documented by stress echo, radionuclide stress, or CMR perfusion studies.

The clinical question that often needs resolution occurs when HFrEF and MR coexist, is whether MR is the primary cause of the heart failure or whether the heart failure is the cause of the secondary MR. Since the majority of HFrEF have an ischemic etiology, the development of MR is the result of postinfarction remodeling. When the MR is moderate to severe following remote MI and the mitral valve leaflets and mitral annulus are intrinsically normal, it is more likely that the MR is secondary due to alteration of LV architecture by cavity dilatation and remodeling, which causes the failure of normal coaptation of the mitral leaflets in heart failure. In contrast, when the mitral valve

leaflets are rheumatically thickened with commissural fusion or when the leaflets are myxomatous and degenerative, it is more than likely that the MR is primary and the heart failure is secondary to hemodynamically significant MR. The mitral valve can be imaged in exquisite detail by TTE and TEE, such that there is little doubt as to its normality or abnormality. In a small minority of patients, it is not possible to determine which is the primary event. However, care should be taken to inspect the mitral valve leaflets, commissures, and subvalve tensor apparatus for undisclosed ruptured chordae tendineae from excessive traction. The hemodynamic severity of MR should be quantified noninvasively using the proximal iso-velocity surface area (PISA) and not by visual estimation alone.

When MR is severe, it may spuriously increase LVEF causing delay in urgently needed surgical mitral valve repair or replacement. The presence of even trivial MR can be demonstrated by Doppler color flow velocity mapping. However, color flow mapping describes velocity distribution and not regurgitant volume flow. The severity of MR should be quantified by PISA, which relies upon the principle that blood flow velocity increases as it approaches a restrictive orifice forming a series of hemispheric iso-velocity shells. The finite orifice is the mitral regurgitant orifice with the velocity shells forming on the ventricular side of the regurgitant orifice. The conservation of mass dictates that the flow rates at each of the hemispherical iso-velocity shells are equal to the flow rates at the mitral regurgitant orifice. The flow rate can be calculated as the surface area of a hemisphere $2\pi r^2 \times$ aliasing velocity, where r = the radius of the hemisphere which is the only Doppler parameter that needs to be measured. The severity of MR can be evaluated comprehensively by a number of echo parameters derived from PISA, including: effective regurgitant orifice area which equals flow rate/peak mitral regurgitant jet velocity; regurgitant volume which is the product of effective mitral regurgitant orifice area and the TVI of the mitral regurgitant jet; and regurgitant fraction, which is the ratio of regurgitant volume to stroke volume.

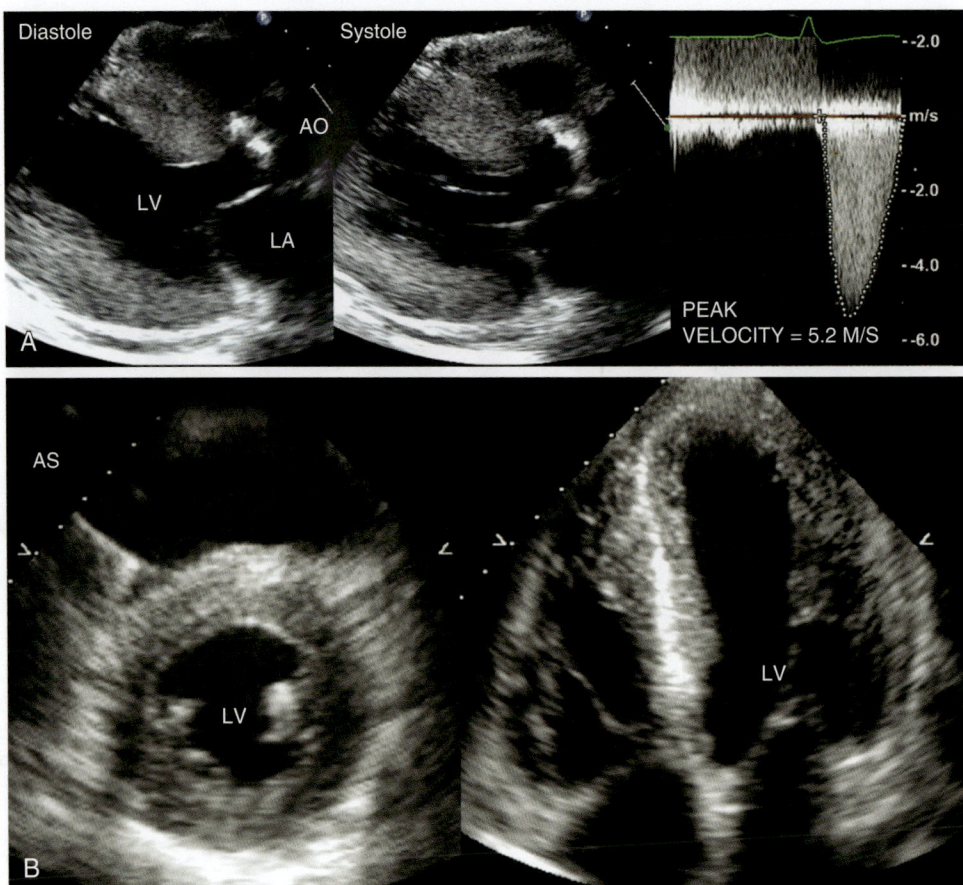

Fig. 32.11 (A) Aortic Stenosis *(AS)*: 2D and Doppler Evaluation: A left parasternal TTE in an octogenarian with heart failure symptoms due to previously undiagnosed critical AS showing top normal LV size with severe LV hypertrophy, *(left and middle panels)* and a heavily calcified immobile aortic valve with a transaortic peak systolic valve gradient of >100 mm Hg *(right panel)* by continuous wave Doppler. The aortic valve area was 0.7 cm². (B) LV Remodeling in AS: A TTE from a patient in the seventh decade with normal LV dimensions but with at least moderate concentric LV hypertrophy shown in the LV short-axis view *(left panel)* and the apical 4-chamber view *(right panel)* with typical concentric remodeling. *2D*, Two-dimensional; *LV,* left ventricular; *TTE*, transthoracic echocardiogram.

Aortic Valve Disease as a Cause of Heart Failure

Aortic Stenosis

Subjects with congenital AS present in their late teens to early 20s with chest pain, syncope, or symptoms of heart failure for valvuloplasty or open-chest valve replacement. Adult onset/acquired severe "senile" calcific AS occurs from the sixth to ninth decade. Bicuspid valves require surgical intervention for valve replacement on average a decade earlier than stenotic trileaflet aortic valves. TTE is the diagnostic imaging modality of choice for aortic valve stenosis and enables the precise assessment of the severity of AS in terms of the aortic valve effective orifice area, and the peak and mean trans-aortic valve gradients and LVEF (**Fig. 32.11**). A proportion of adults with severe or critical AS develop heart failure, which is associated with a poor prognosis. If critical AS is not recognized and the LV is allowed to dilate, the trans-aortic gradient falls as LV function deteriorates so the aortic valve orifice area must be calculated by 2D or 3D echo. There is an increasingly recognized subgroup of symptomatic patients with severe AS who have low transvalvular gradients due to LV systolic dysfunction, known as low-flow AS.[59] It is important to identify these elderly patients because they do well clinically with trans-cutaneous intervention. Hemodynamically, chronic decompensated calcific AS associated with LV dilatation and decreased LVEF must be differentiated from idiopathic dilated cardiomyopathy with concomitant age-related calcification of the aortic valve. This can

be achieved with 2D Doppler echo of the apical long axis and the apical 5-chamber view (see Fig. 32.11). 2D, 3D, or TEE are the imaging modalities of choice for the diagnosis and quantification of severity of AS. Bicuspid aortic valves (BAVs) are associated with ascending aortic aneurysm formation that is independent of the hydraulics across the aortic valve.[60,61] The extent and severity of the aortopathy should ideally be assessed by either CT angiography (CTA) or CMR with contrast, and if the maximal dimension distal to the sinuses of Valsalva at the sinotubular junction is >4.5 cm, surgical repair or endovascular stenting should be considered, irrespective of symptoms.[62] The anatomy of the commissures can be determined best by 2D, TEE, or 3D echo. Once the diagnosis of hemodynamically significant AS is established, management should follow the American College of Cardiology (ACC)/AHA Guidelines.[63] Ascending aortic aneurysms need to be carefully monitored by serial measurements of maximal diameter and growth rate that determine the timing of surgery or endovascular stenting. Dilatation of the aortic root with effacement of the sinuses of Valsalva may disrupt the architecture of the aortic valve leaflets resulting in secondary rather than primary aortic regurgitation (AR).

Chronic AR has become a less common cause of congestive heart failure in the Western hemisphere because of the decline in incidence of rheumatic heart disease. The diagnosis of AR is easily made by documenting the regurgitant diastolic blood flow reversal in the LVOT flow

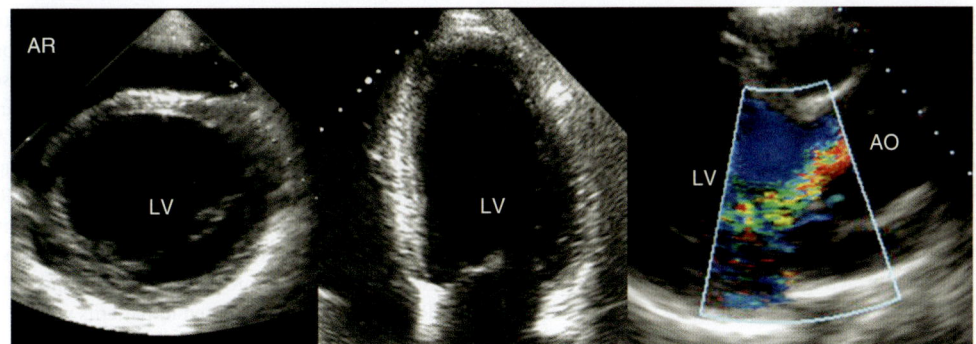

Fig. 32.12 Echocardiographic Findings in Aortic Regurgitation *(AR).* Chronic aortic regurgitation in a young female (aged 39) who presented with fatigue and heart failure symptoms for almost 1 year. LV short axis *(left panel)* shows marked LV dilatation but only mildly reduced contractile function *(middle panel)* consistent with eccentric LV remodeling and preserved systolic function and showing the appearance of an early diastolic color flow Doppler velocity signal of moderate aortic regurgitation *(right panel).*

by Doppler color flow velocity mapping, which is extremely sensitive even to trivial AR. The etiology of AR is due either to abnormalities of the aortic valve leaflets or to abnormalities of the aortic root geometry. The aortic valve is bicuspid in 1% of all live births and undergoes calcification, becoming stenotic and/or regurgitant. BAV may be associated with ascending aortopathy, which is independent of the hemodynamic severity of the aortic valve pathology.[60,61] The valve leaflet morphology may vary from rheumatic-like thickening with calcified commissural fusion to floppy myxomatous leaflets that fail to coapt. Moreover, the geometry of the aortic root may be altered by aneurysmal dilation or effacement of the sinuses of Valsalva, as seen in Marfan syndrome, resulting in secondary AR.

In heart failure due to chronic severe AR, the LV is markedly dilated with moderate to severe eccentric hypertrophy, and though there may be preserved function early in the course, systolic function gradually deteriorates (**Fig. 32.12**). One-third of patients with moderate to severe AR do not develop cardiovascular symptoms, and become symptomatic late in the natural history of their disease when irreversible LV dysfunction develops. This emphasizes an important role for imaging with Doppler echocardiography in AR. The severity of the AR can be accurately quantified by Doppler echo assessment of the deceleration rate of the regurgitant aortic jet, by the diameter of the *vena contracta*, regurgitant volume, regurgitant fraction, and the effective regurgitant orifice area. Clinical decision-making to recommend aortic valve replacement (AVR) is based largely on echo measurements of LV cavity size (end-systolic and end-diastolic dimensions) and function (see Fig. 32.12) in conjunction with symptoms as recommended in the ACC/AHA 2014 Guidelines for the management of patients with valvular heart disease.[63] Thus, TTE imaging provides the requisite information regarding LV size, geometry, and hemodynamic assessment necessary to confidently advocate AVR to remove the regurgitant volume, which is important in the appropriate management of patients with chronic AR and congestive heart failure.

Cardiovascular Magnetic Resonance Assessment of Valvular Heart Disease

CMR may be a useful alternative to echocardiography in patients with valvular disease with limited image quality, or those with conflicting or inconclusive results. Tissue characterization may help physicians to determine the etiology and potential therapy of valvular heart disease (e.g., ischemic vs. nonischemic MR). While regurgitant and stenotic jets are evident in cine images, a more complete valvular disease assessment requires a quantitative evaluation of flow and flow velocity data that have been previously validated.[64,65]

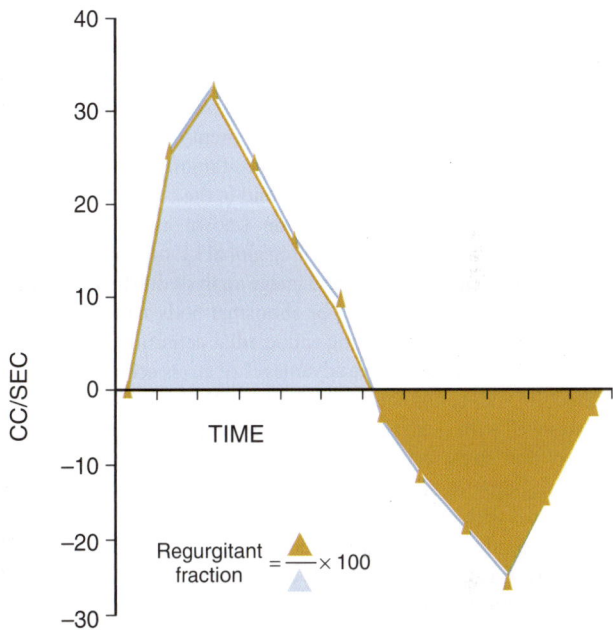

Fig 32.13 Cardiac Magnetic Resonance Assessment of Chronic Aortic Regurgitation. Forward *(gray curve)* and reverse *(yellow curve)* flow across the aortic valve is depicted in this graph. The forward stroke volume is calculated as the total blood flow across the valve in systole [Velocity-time integral via phase contrast images × blood vessel cross-sectional area = Blood flow in cc/sec], while the regurgitant fraction is the integral of the reverse flow over time divided by the forward flow multiplied by 100. (Courtesy Mark Fogel, MD.)

The regurgitant volume and regurgitant fraction in MR may be measured by comparing the LV stroke volume with the systolic aortic flow. More recent applications have used quantitative assessment of MR jets in adjudicating the severity of MR, which has informed therapeutic decision making and impacted outcomes. CMR was able to better predict patients with severe MR than TTE or TEE, especially in those patients with highly eccentric jets.[66]

In AR, the regurgitant fraction is measured by integrating the diastolic flow across the aortic valve, and comparing it to the systolic forward flow (**Fig. 32.13**). CMR can accurately quantify the effective cardiac output and provide an important objective parameter of heart failure related to low output states.

In stenotic valvular disease, flow quantification can be used to identify increased transvalvular flow velocity and to calculate pressure gradients.[67] By visualizing the stenotic orifice, CMR offers reliable aortic valve area quantification and avoids limitations related to oblique or turbulent jets and unreliable pressure gradients, particularly in low output states.[2,68-70]

MYOCARDIAL VIABILITY

HFrEF patients who have an ischemic etiology may present with angina, shortness of breath, reduced exercise capacity, and a low LVEF due to the presence of noncontracting but viable myocardium (**see also Chapter 19**). There are three noninvasive imaging methods commonly used for assessing myocardial viability: stress echocardiography, nuclear imaging, and CMR perfusion studies.

Stress Echocardiography

Viable noncontracting myocardium in heart failure can be detected by exercise and/or pharmacologic (e.g., low-dose dobutamine) stress echocardiography. The purpose of identifying viable myocardium in selected heart failure patients is because restoration of myocardial perfusion targeted to the ischemic regions can potentially translate into increased regional and global (LVEF) function. There are three nonoverlapping phasic responses to dobutamine stress echocardiography. First, at low levels of stress there is recruitment of myocardial shortening that is lost as the level of stress (dobutamine dosage) increases, described as a "biphasic response." Second is the continued improvement in regional and global function known as the "contractile reserve." Third is a plateau or worsening global LV function. Technical limitations in image acquisition and image analysis due to lung disease, enhanced respiratory excursion, or abnormal body habitus (obesity) can be minimized by augmenting endocardial definition with intravenous echo contrast agents. The advantages of stress echocardiography for detecting viable, noncontracting myocardium are that stress echo correlates well with nuclear imaging, yet it does not involve radiation exposure, and stress echo is relatively inexpensive. Patients with a biphasic response to stress benefit from revascularization more than those patients with contractile reserve. In contrast, those with a flat or negative response to stress usually do not benefit from revascularization and are at high risk for adverse clinical cardiovascular outcomes. In chronic ischemic heart disease there may be a history of remote transmural MI that can be identified as a hyper-echoic (highly echo reflective) region of the free LV wall or septum that is thinner than normal wall thickness (<6 mm) and does not contract or change in thickness with increasing work load during stress echo testing.

A prerequisite for the diagnosis of viability and ischemic myocardium with noninvasive imaging tools is the acquisition of high-quality images at rest but especially during stress testing. CMR studies provide complete and continuous endocardial surfaces. By contrast, the 2D and 3D TTE images often need to be interpolated, although the need for major interpolation has diminished since the introduction of harmonic imaging and the use of intravenous echo contrast for the express purpose of enhancing endocardial definition. Myocardial viability also can be detected by radionuclide angiography and CMR perfusion studies.

Radiotracer-Based Assessment of Myocardial Viability and Remodeling

Serial SPECT perfusion imaging can be used for the assessment of myocardial viability and salvage following reperfusion,[71-74] and later following PCI.[75,76] These indices of myocardial salvage derived from nuclear imaging are predictive of the long-term outcome.

Nuclear imaging techniques also have been used specifically to predict LV remodeling. [201]Tl and ^{99m}Tc-labeled perfusion images also have been used to assess infarct size, and this radiotracer-based estimation of myocardial viability has correlated with subsequent LV remodeling. ^{99m}Tc-sestamibi imaging has been used to assess infarct size early post-MI in patients and these perfusion-based estimates of infarct size have correlated with LV volumes at 1 year.[77,78] Another study suggested that infarct severity on ^{99m}Tc-sestamibi imaging maybe a better predictor of remodeling than infarct size alone.[78] Radionuclide assessment of viability was also shown to predict LV remodeling in a study of patients with ischemic cardiomyopathy.[80] In this study, viability was assessed with serial nitrate enhanced ^{201}Tl and ^{99m}Tc-sestamibi imaging. Remodeling was prevented in patients with at least five viable segments who underwent revascularization at the 21-month follow-up.[80] The direct relationship between the extent of ^{201}Tl defects and collagen content in severe ischemic cardiomyopathy was assessed in a study of hearts excised after cardiac transplantation. There was greater collagen content in segments with irreversible ^{201}Tl defects compared to segments with reversible defects or normal ^{201}Tl perfusion. Furthermore, noninfarcted segments in the hearts with cardiomyopathy also had elevated collagen content compared to control hearts.[81]

Cardiovascular Magnetic Resonance Stress

CMR can also be used to predict post-revascularization recovery of LV function, using late gadolinium enhancement (LGE) and low-dose dobutamine stress testing. The degree of transmural LGE predicts regional functional recovery, and improvement in LVEF frequently occurs when there is hibernation of >20% of the global LV myocardium. On a regional basis, LGE has an 80% positive predictive value for recovery in segments demonstrating no infarction, and a 90% negative predictive valve for no improvement in segments with >50% transmural scar.[82] Other work suggests that low-dose dobutamine stress CMR (DSMR) may be more sensitive for viability assessment, and additional clinical experience is accumulating. LGE demonstrates myocardium with nontransmural scar that is destined not to recover function despite revascularization (**Fig. 32.14**). Failure of functional improvement also may be due to incomplete revascularization, persistent hibernation early post-revascularization, or abnormal wall mechanics, which may be recruitable with dobutamine or exercise stress. CMR also predicts the response to beta-blockers in heart failure patients, and demonstrates lower response rates in patients with larger MIs.[83]

Detection of Myocardial Ischemia with Cardiovascular Magnetic Resonance

CMR may be used for ischemia assessment using either a first-pass stress myocardial perfusion strategy or dobutamine stress wall motion imaging, as alternatives to myocardial perfusion SPECT and stress echocardiography, respectively. DSMR is a technique that has been performed in a number of centers that have demonstrated its diagnostic accuracy and prognostic capability. DSMR studies may be used at low dose for viability, or at high dose (with or without atropine) for demonstrating supply/demand mismatch ischemia. Stress perfusion CMR has been proven accurate in multicenter studies, and has several advantages over conventional nuclear perfusion methods.[84] CMR does not suffer from the "roll-off" or plateau effect at high myocardial perfusion rates seen with SPECT, and the higher resolution CMR methods permit depiction of nontransmural ischemia, which is easily detectable by visual inspection. Recent clinical trials, including the multicenter, multiple vendor Magnetic Resonance Imaging for Myocardial Perfusion Assessment in Coronary Artery Disease Trial (MR-IMPACT) involving over 240 patients, have shown that perfusion CMR performs comparably or better than perfusion SPECT for the detection of CAD.[85] Greater clinical utility will come from direct comparison between modalities,

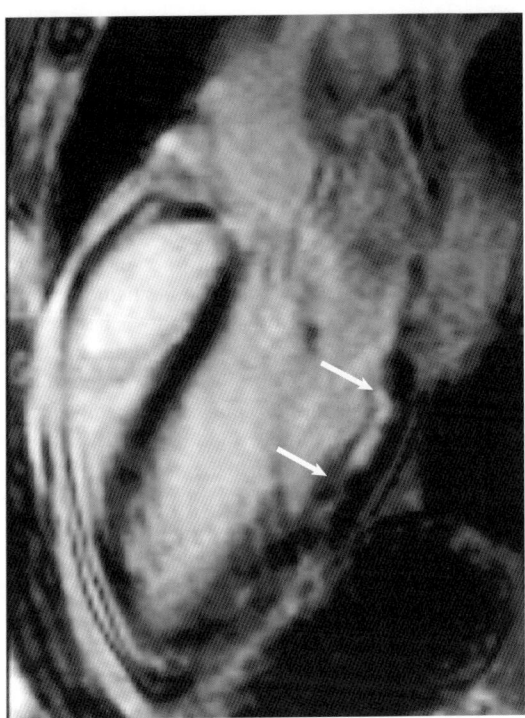

Fig. 32.14 CMR Nontransmural Scar. Note the nontransmural area of increased signal intensity (late gadolinium enhancement) at the basal inferolateral wall, which represents nonviable myocardial tissue at the subendocardial level *(arrows)*.

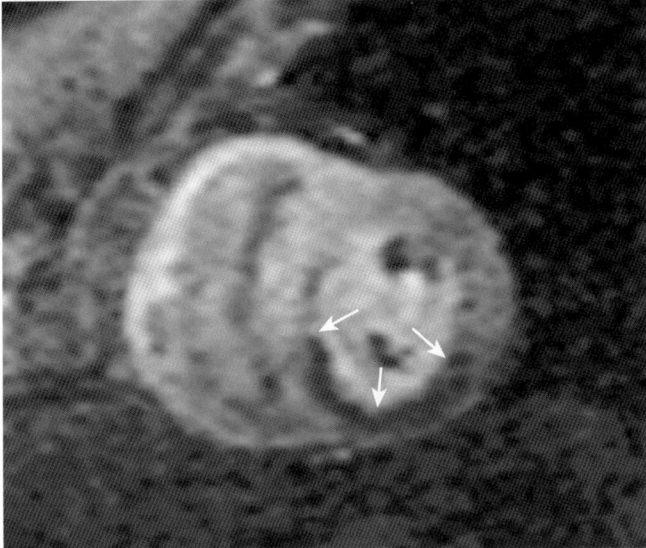

Fig. 32.15 Nontransmural Ischemia. The darker area in this image represents hypoperfused (less contrast agent delivery) subendocardial tissue resulting from poststress perfusion imaging of a patient with an epicardial vessel stenosis of >70% *(arrows)*.

such as the recent Clinical Evaluation of Magnetic Resonance imaging in Coronary heart disease (CE-MARC) trial, which performed a head-to-head comparison of adenosine stress perfusion CMR and adenosine stress ^{99}Tc tetrofosmin in 752 patients with angina and suspected coronary artery disease. The sensitivity and negative predictive value for CMR were greater than SPECT, while the specificity and positive predictive value were similar.[86]

The negative predictive value for cardiac events is excellent with a normal stress CMR, and cardiac risk increases corresponding to greater degrees of ischemia.[87] By adding myocardial tagging to stress CMR to measure myocardial strain, interobserver variability is reduced, accuracy may be improved, and new physiological information may be obtained.[88-90] The addition of perfusion imaging to tagging provides a more complete characterization of the state of the myocardium, particularly at greater field strengths, that is, 3T.[91] Clinical experience is increasing with CMR stress techniques, and protocols are being harmonized, such that variability between interpreters and centers may be minimized. Detection of nontransmural ischemia with stress DSMR perfusion techniques by abnormal wall motion will likely endorse these methods as valuable clinical tools (**Fig. 32.15**).

Detection of Infarction with Cardiovascular Magnetic Resonance I

LGE techniques have matured to the point where high-quality, reproducible detection of both nontransmural and transmural MIs are achievable 10 minutes after intravenous injection of a gadolinium-containing contrast agent. The greater volume of distribution of the diseased tissue produces higher regional gadolinium concentration, which appears bright and readily identifiable on T1-weighted CMR pulse sequences. The LGE techniques depict both acute and chronic infarction, and focal as well as diffuse fibrosis, and are highly accurate and reproducible as demonstrated by a recent large multi-center clinical trial.[92] LGE has advanced the assessment of MIs because

the technique shows greater sensitivity than SPECT perfusion and wall motion abnormality imaging techniques, due to the vagaries of spatial resolution and endocardial detection, as well as other potential artifacts.[93] Studies focused on the prognostic impact of unrecognized infarctions have demonstrated additional incremental value over conventional risk measures in patients with clinically suspected CAD but no known previous infarction.[94] LGE has an important role in the assessment of heart failure patients in particular. In a series of 150 consecutive heart failure patients with an LVEF <50% and contemporaneous echo evaluation, CMR had a significant clinical impact in 65%—including a new diagnosis in 30%—predominantly related to the detection of LGE.[95] LGE techniques also play an important role in heart failure related to infiltrative disorders. Diseases such as amyloidosis and sarcoidosis may be detected by their unique patterns on LGE imaging. Beyond LGE, CMR can detect and permit serial noninvasive evaluation of another important systemic disorder causing heart failure—hemochromatosis. Local myocardial iron concentration changes the signal properties such that greater tissue iron concentrations result in greater signal alterations. CMR thus becomes a tool to follow chelation or other therapies in order to optimally treat affected patients.

TRANSITION FROM MYOCARDIAL INFARCTION TO HEART FAILURE WITH REDUCED EJECTION FRACTION

More than two-thirds of HFrEF patients have occlusive CAD or previous MI in whom ischemia may be ongoing, resulting in maladaptive changes not only in the surviving cardiomyocytes but also in the extracellular matrix. MI results in almost immediate cessation of myocardial contraction in the territory subtended by the occluded nutrient coronary artery. Echocardiographic imaging in acute MI shows a region of the LV wall that is akinetic or severely hypokinetic with altered acoustic impedance that is spatially congruent with the infarct location and coronary artery perfusion defect at cardiac catheterization. The non-contracting infarct zone thins due to stretching by actively contracting myocardium contiguous and remote to the infarction zone, resulting in LV dilatation and increased wall stress. Failure to normalize the increased wall stress is a trigger for progressive LV dilatation and an adverse outcome (**see also Chapter 12**). Disproportionate LV dilatation causes an increase in load that results in further deterioration in LV function. A number of factors are involved in the transition from the initial infarction to chronic HFrEF that includes the initial infarct size, infarct location and transmurality, patency of the culprit infarct artery, activation of the neurohumoral RAAS and sympathetic nervous system, changes in the extracellular matrix (ECM), and local tropic factors. In this dynamic process of ventricular remodeling, a balance is sought between increased wall stress causing LV dilatation and opposing restraining forces from the viscoelastic collagen scaffold formed by the ECM. When equilibrium between these opposing forces is not attained, progressive remodeling leads to further LV dilatation, poor LV function, and the insidious onset of heart failure—a course that portends a poor prognosis. When equilibrium is achieved, myocardial repair begins with formation of a collagenous scar with a high enough tensile strength to prevent further infarct expansion and LV cavity dilatation. Old MIs are detectable by the highly echo reflective, thin (wall thickness <0.6 cm) noncontracting region of myocardium. The progressive structural and functional remodeling in HFrEF has been well characterized by 2D TTE in a number of randomized clinical trials of chronic heart failure.[30,31,96-98] The changes in LV structure and function postinfarction described by serial TTE can be followed by serial CMR in HFrEF. Much less is known about the natural history of HFpEF except that the LV usually does not dilate, LV hypertrophy may increase (consistent with hypertrophic concentric remodeling), and diastolic dysfunction may worsen with time. Randomized control trials have shown that echocardiography-determined LV volumes, mass, shape, and EF are powerful predictors of clinical outcome.[30] Although LVEF is used for clinical decision making more than any other metric in the management of heart failure, it is not a measure of contractility and varies widely with changes in loading conditions. LV stroke volume is more robust and can be estimated from LV volumes and from Doppler velocity signals and diameters recorded from the LVOT. However, stroke volume in HFrEF has been shown by quantitative 2D TTE to remain unchanged until LVEF falls to 20% or below, at which point the LV can no longer modulate stroke volume by structural remodeling.[14,99] Increases in cardiac output are achieved either by increasing resting heart rate or by ejecting a smaller fraction of a larger end-diastolic volume. These two mechanisms work in concert to maintain cardiac output as EF falls.

The introduction of angiotensin converting enzyme inhibitors (ACEi) and the angiotensin receptor blockers was followed by several large randomized controlled trials in which serial TTE imaging was used to assess their efficacy in reducing adverse events.[31,96] Quantitative TTE demonstrated that ACEi, beta adrenergic receptor blockers, and aldosterone antagonists resulted in symptomatic benefit and improved clinical outcomes associated with structural and functional reverse remodeling mediated by attenuating neurohumoral activation.[97]

A variety of imaging modalities including echo, nuclear, and CMR have since been used in multiple prospective, randomized, clinical trials in HFrEF testing the efficacy of novel pharmacologic agents, surgical interventions, and device placement over long-term follow-up. The control arms of these trials are useful data repositories that demonstrate changes in LV architecture and function and extent of LV remodeling over 5-year follow-up with serial quantitative analysis of echocardiographic images at 6-month intervals.[100] Studies involving large numbers of HFrEF patients of all NYHA symptom classes have shown the strong predictive value of the echocardiographic metrics for clinical outcomes.

As our understanding of the causative mechanisms of heart failure has improved, the number of treatment options for heart failure patients has diversified such that there are now specific therapies for selected patient populations. Cardiac imaging modalities have proved useful in identifying patients for consideration of orthotopic heart transplantation, ventricular assist device placement, cardiac resynchronization therapy (CRT), internal cardiac defibrillator placement, and detection of hemodynamically severe MR requiring surgical repair or replacement.

Cardiac Magnetic Resonance Infarction II

CMR provides much greater detail of infarcted myocardium and tissue that has experienced ischemia/reperfusion injury. In acute infarction, CMR can depict areas of microvascular obstruction—generally a subendocardial dark area on LGE—which identifies tissue with extremely long gadolinium inflow times. This abnormality is best detected 1 to 2 minutes after gadolinium contrast injection, and is known as early gadolinium enhancement (EGE) imaging. Microvascular obstruction portends a poorer prognosis, more unfavorable remodeling, and is a negative prognostic indicator above and beyond LVEF.[101] Of note, microvascular obstruction is not seen in the chronic state due to infarct involution and collagen remodeling, and is present only in the first few weeks after infarction. EGE imaging is also more accurate than echocardiography for the detection of LV thrombi, which are of low signal intensity in contrast to the brighter adjacent infarcted myocardium.

Other unique aspects of CMR include its ability to noninvasively depict areas of reversible ischemia, area at risk, and myocardial hemorrhage. A T2-weighted CMR pulse sequence is used to detect cellular edema, which distinguishes areas of recent ischemia/reperfusion injury from irreversibly injured tissue.[102] This method also allows for calculation of the area at risk following reperfusion of an acute infarction (the edematous area), while the salvaged myocardium corresponds to the difference between the infarcted territory (depicted by LGE), and the edematous area.[103] These changes can be seen for days or weeks after infarction or reperfusion, but SPECT methods have a narrow time window of only a few hours. T2* CMR may also detect intramyocardial hemorrhage related to acute infarction and the functional outcome of this process.[104]

CARDIAC RESYNCHRONIZATION THERAPY (SEE ALSO CHAPTER 38)

Enrollment criteria for randomized clinical CRT trials of patients with chronic refractory heart failure have been consistent and included a prolonged QRS duration >120 ms, LV dilatation (LVED >5.5 cm), and dysfunction (LVEF <35%) determined echocardiographically. Between 30% and 50% of HFrEF patients have a high degree of atrioventricular infra-Hisian conduction delay most commonly with left bundle branch block (LBBB) morphology. There is a close relation between mortality and duration of the QRS, so that the longer the QRS duration the higher the mortality.

LBBB occurs in approximately 70% of patients with idiopathic dilated cardiomyopathy and is associated with LV dyssynchrony, which involves reversed septal motion and loss of coordinated systolic inward wall motion. There is also a delay in the temporal acquisition of peak myocardial velocities in the 17-segment model of the LV by Doppler echocardiography. LV dyssynchrony was initially regarded as being synonymous with prolonged QRS duration. A number of attempts were made using Doppler parameters to identify patients who responded and benefited before device deployment.[105] CRT was associated with symptomatic improvement due to LV reverse remodeling in approximately 65% to 70% of patients in all NYHA Classes from I through IV heart failure.[98,106,107] The beneficial impact on mortality when CRT was combined with an implantable cardioverter-defibrillator was greater than with CRT alone. HFrEF patients with nonischemic LV dysfunction experienced threefold greater reverse remodeling than patients with ischemic heart failure. This salutary impact of CRT on reverse remodeling is sustained for at least 5 years of follow-up.[24,108]

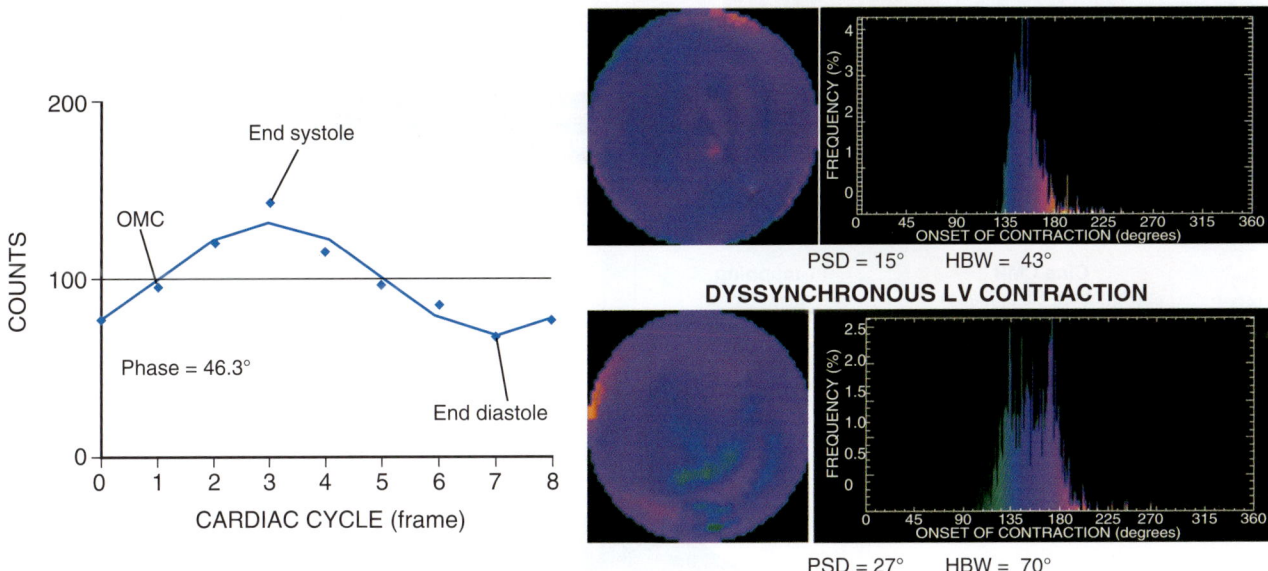

Fig. 32.16 Single Photon Emission Computed Tomography *(SPECT)* Approach to Left Ventricular *(LV)* Dyssynchrony. The left panel shows the time–activity curve from a single myocardial segment. Based on the partial volume effect, this is essentially a thickening curve. The low fidelity curve based on 8-bin gating is converted to a continuous curve by Fourier transformation. For the purposes of comparing thickening among all myocardial segments, the point of inflection of the thickening curve on a horizontal line representing the average segmental counts during one cardiac cycle (the onset of mechanical contraction) *(OMC)*, is chosen as the reference point. The right panel shows the creation of a histogram and phase polar map of OMC from the approximately 600 myocardial segments acquired during a standard SPECT study. *Top panel* shows a narrow histogram and uniform phase polar map indicative of synchronous LV contraction. *Bottom panel* shows a wide histogram and nonuniform phase polar map indicative of dyssynchronous LV contraction. The automated measures of synchrony, which have been validated, are the phase standard deviation *(PSD)* (the standard deviation of the phase distribution) and the histogram bandwidth *(HBW)* (the range of phases which encompasses 95% of the OMCs).

Nuclear Imaging for Cardiac Resynchronization Therapy

CRT reduces both the morbidity and the mortality of HF patients who present with a wide QRS and who become refractory to medications. ERNA provides high temporal resolution, greater reproducibility, and biventricular volumetric analysis, and allows the depiction of both intraventricular and interventricular synchrony. Alternatively, gated SPECT blood pool and perfusion imaging have recently been shown to be beneficial in the evaluation of resynchronization therapy (CRT) in patients with end-stage heart failure.[109,110] The degree of intra- and interventricular dyssynchrony demonstrated by these nuclear modalities is assessed by phase analysis. For gated SPECT blood pool imaging the combination of a baseline LVEF greater than 15% with significant interventricular dyssynchrony were the best predictors for improvement in LV systolic function after 6 months of CRT.[111] Gated SPECT perfusion imaging is unique in allowing the simultaneous assessment of the degree of LV dyssynchrony and the site of the latest activation along with the assessment of scar burden from perfusion imaging. Thus, a single image acquisition provides a means for predicting CRT response in heart failure patients (**Fig. 32.16**).

Cardiovascular Magnetic Resonance for Resynchronization Therapy

The disappointing response rate to CRT for patients with DCM (~30% with LBBB/wide QRS) motivated a search for novel imaging indicators to identify potential responders. Studies have shown reduced response rates and poorer outcomes in patients with LV inferolateral scar.[112] Technical aspects of the procedure such as avoiding areas of lateral wall scar during LV lead placement have increased response rate in small groups of patients.[113] However, the presence of midwall fibrosis appears to be an even stronger marker of potential responders to CRT. A recent study demonstrated a marked increase in both cardiovascular mortality and major adverse cardiac events, and a low rate of LV reverse remodeling (nonresponse rate) in those patients demonstrating midwall LGE.[114]

IDIOPATHIC DILATED CARDIOMYOPATHY

Idiopathic dilated cardiomyopathy (IDCM) accounts for approximately one-quarter to one-third of all patients presenting with HFrEF and one-third of the prevalence of ischemic cardiomyopathy (**see also Chapter 20**). Seventy percent of these DCM patients develop conduction delay that is typically of LBBB morphology with major prolongation of the QRS duration often become refractory to pharmacologic therapy. It is important to identify these patients because they are typically young with very low LVEF who respond especially well to resynchronization therapy. These patients are easy to diagnose by 2D TTE that reveals massive LV cavity dilatation, inadequate LV hypertrophy, usually with severe dyssynchrony. The majority of these patients with IDCM and especially those with LBBB respond favorably to CRT therapy. Moreover, there is a threefold greater reduction in LV volumes and more than a threefold greater increase in EF in idiopathic DCM than in patients with ischemic cardiomyopathy indicating that more extensive reverse LV remodeling can be achieved in patients with nonischemic DCM.[98]

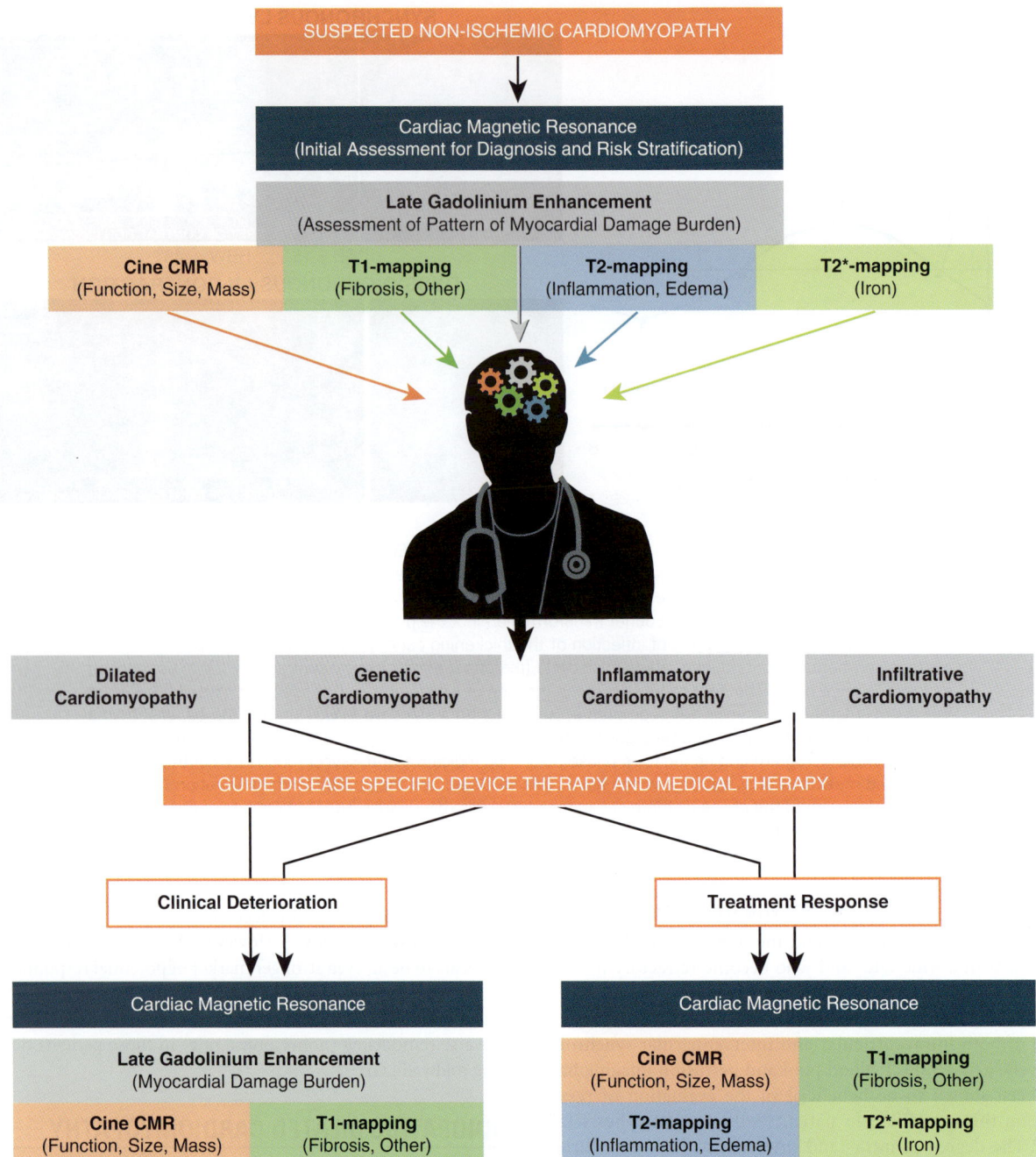

Fig 32.17 Proposed Pathway for Evaluation of Suspected Nonischemic Cardiomyopathy With Cardiovascular Magnetic Resonance *(CMR)*. The use of multiple CMR pulse sequences not only allows for depiction of chamber sizes, mass, and function, but also detection of focal and diffuse fibrosis, inflammation and edema, and infiltrative diseases. The diagnosis, management, and reassessment of these parameters may be performed throughout the follow up period as well. (From Patel A, Kramer CM. Role of cardiac magnetic resonance in the diagnosis and prognosis of nonischemic cardiomyopathy. *JACC Cardiovasc Imaging.* 2017;10:1180–1193.)

However, only two-thirds of all heart failure patients respond to CRT and attempts to preselect patients who respond to CRT using a number of Doppler echo parameters or clinical demographics by any imaging modality in the PROSPECT trial has not been successful.[105]

MISCELLANEOUS CAUSES OF HEART FAILURE (SEE ALSO CHAPTER 21 AND 22)

A staged approach to patients who present with a suspected nonischemic cardiomyopathy with CMR has been suggested by Patel using CMR techniques (**Fig. 32.17**).[115]

By using a combination of LGE, cine MR (for size, function, and mass), T1 mapping for fibrosis, T2 mapping for inflammation/edema, and T2* mapping for iron (when appropriate), the data are synthesized along with clinical data by the interpreting physician into one of the major categories for cardiomyopathy: dilated CM, familial CM, inflammatory CM, or infiltrative CM. Management may then be guided toward an initial disease-specific device and/or medical therapy, as well as chronic management to assess response to therapy or evaluate patients who clinically deteriorate. Additional testing may be performed as indicated to confirm diagnoses that may have an atypical presentation. In **Fig. 32.18**, the CMR image shows diffuse, patchy

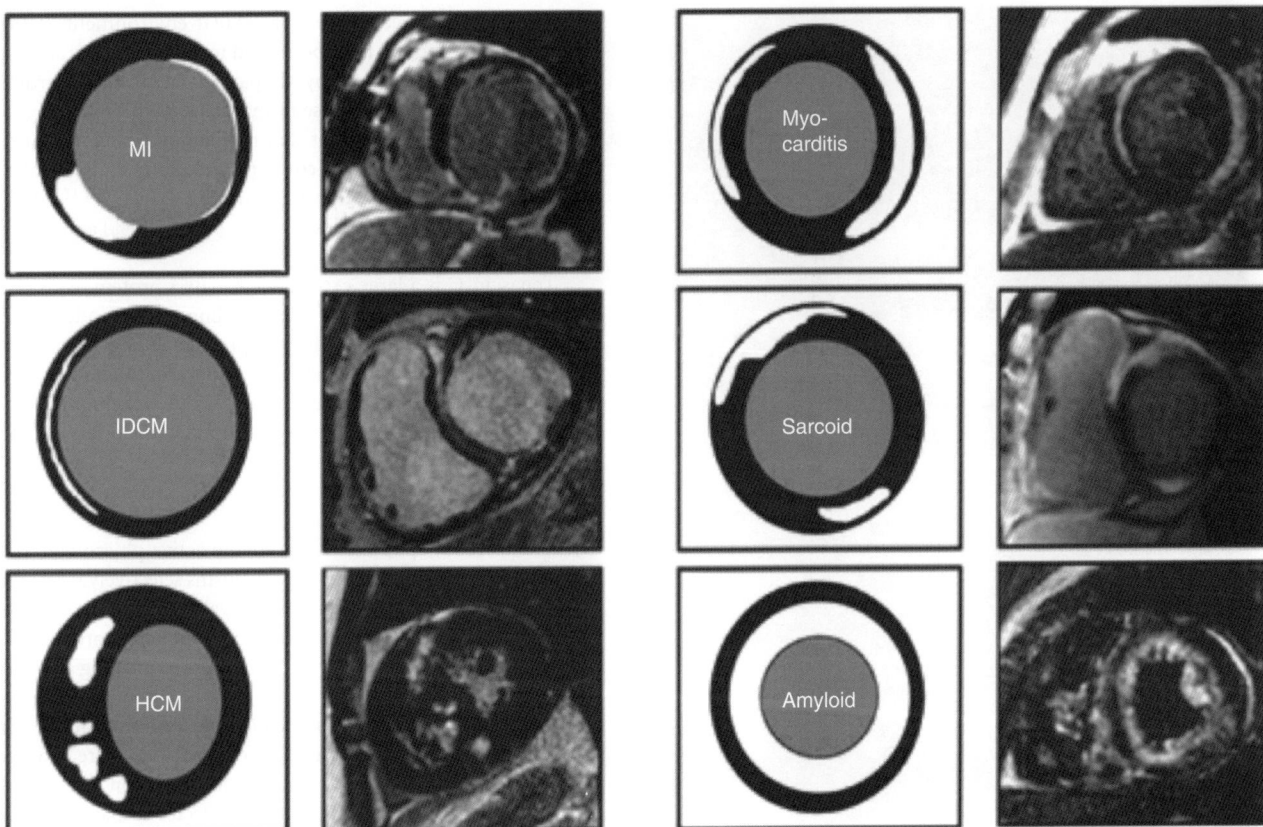

Fig. 32.18 Schematic Diagram of the Typical Patterns of Late Gadolinium Enhancement *(LGE)* for Various Types of Cardiomyopathies.

fibrosis in a patient with longstanding poorly controlled hypertension and an LVH with strain pattern on electrocardiogram. A more typical pattern of diffuse LV and RV LGE is seen in amyloidosis (**Fig. 32.19**), often with difficulty nulling the myocardium on LGE exams. In this case, a Tc-99m pyrophosphate scan was performed, demonstrating vigorous tracer uptake by the myocardium, consistent with ATTR cardiac amyloidosis (**see also Chapter 22**). CMR has also demonstrated prognostic value in detection and management of cardiac sarcoidosis.[116]

There are two additional causes of heart failure that both have a poor prognosis and yet should not be overlooked. These are (1) vegetative endocarditis, and (2) partial rupture of an LV papillary muscle from ischemia. Both of these should be diagnosed unequivocally by 2D TTE, 3D TTE, or ideally by TEE imaging.

(1) Vegetative endocarditis may destroy the mitral or aortic valve leaflets resulting in severe MR or AR, causing myocardial abscess and congestive heart failure especially when the definitive diagnosis and appropriate antibiotic therapy are delayed. The diagnosis may be obscured because no organism is identified due to earlier administration of an inappropriately short course of antibiotics before the diagnosis of endocarditis was entertained. Severe MR or AR may also result when the causative microorganism is especially virulent, or resistant to the antibiotic therapy or when the vegetations are large and excessively mobile. Excessively mobile valve vegetations put increased traction on the leaflets and mitral tensor apparatus causing leaflet tears or avulsion of the valve and recurrent systemic embolization of septic vegetative material.

Diagnostic uncertainty regarding rupture of the chordae tendineae resulting in severe MR with flail or partially flail leaflets should be clarified by 3D TTE or TEE (**Fig. 32.20**) prior to surgical intervention. TEE provides essential information regarding the morphology of large

vegetations prone to embolization and whether there is evidence of intramyocardial or valve ring abscess. These echocardiographic findings impact directly on the timing of surgical intervention, the choice of the size and type of prosthesis.

(2) Another valvular cause of acute hemodynamic instability is partial or complete rupture of a papillary muscle (inferior > anterior) causing severe MR. The increased mobility of the ruptured heads of a papillary muscle are often not well visualized by TTE or by contrast LV angiography. When the diagnosis of ruptured papillary muscle is entertained, urgent TEE should be performed as the imaging modality of choice. TEE lays out the anatomy and pathophysiology that facilitates complete diagnosis. Ischemic injury or rupture of a papillary muscle is more commonly associated with LV inferobasal rather than lateral wall hypokinesis.

ASSESSMENT OF RIGHT VENTRICULAR FUNCTION

The complex shape of the normal RV does not easily conform to simple mathematical models like the LV, and this poses difficulties in quantifying ventricular volumes and RV cavity function. Two-dimensional echo is limited to the measurement of percentage change of RV cavity areas at end-diastole and end-systole as indicators of RV size, while RV function is limited to percentage change in LV area. The RV is important in heart failure because it is a strong and independent predictor of clinical outcome in HFrEF patients.[117] Quantification of RV volumes and EF with CTA or CMR imaging can be achieved with much greater precision than by Doppler echo.[118] In addition, CMR can quantify the regurgitant fraction across both the pulmonary and tricuspid valves, which is of great value in congenital heart disease as well as in adults.

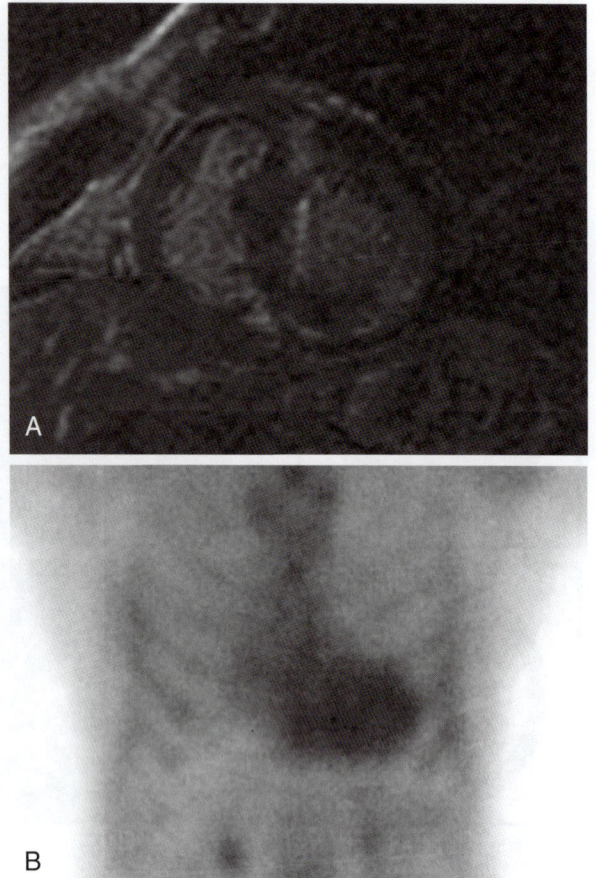

Fig. 32.19 (A) Cardiovascular magnetic resonance *(CMR)* image showing patchy, diffuse uptake, but not in a classic cardiac amyloid pattern. (B) A Tc-99m pyrophosphate image demonstrates avid uptake (darker image = greater concentration of tracer), consistent with ATTR cardiac amyloidosis.

COMPLICATIONS OF HEART FAILURE

Detection of complications of heart failure is important and includes hemodynamic compromise caused by large pericardial and pleural effusions, the onset of atrial fibrillation with rapid ventricular response, the development of acute severe MR, and the increased stroke risk associated with intracardiac thrombus within the left heart chambers.[22] In idiopathic dilated and ischemic cardiomyopathies the combination of dilated chambers and decreased amplitude of left atrial and LV wall motion results in low velocity intracardiac blood flow which predisposes to thrombus formation with the attendant risk of thrombus propagation to the systemic circulation, especially with the onset of atrial fibrillation, which is common in heart failure. The presence of left heart thrombus necessitates anticoagulation that has additional significant morbidity and mortality.

FUTURE DIRECTIONS IN CARDIAC IMAGING

Nuclear Imaging

Injury and Inflammation

Myocardial injury and inflammation lead to the disruption of cellular membranes and the release of myosin heavy chain. Necrosis is a nonregulated process that results in cell membrane disruption and the loss and release of intracellular content into the extracellular environment. As such, necrosis-targeted tracers cliave been developed to target intracellular components (e.g., myosin, histones, phosphatidylserine [PS])

not normally exposed to the extracellular environment. ^{111}In-labeled antimyosin antibodies have been used to visualize myocardial damage in patients with HF caused by idiopathic and alcoholic cardiomyopathies. They have also been used to visualize myocyte damage in acute MI.[119,120] It became apparent that noninvasive imaging of this extracellular exposure of myosin could provide early diagnostic as well as longer-term prognostic information (**Fig. 32.21**).[121,122] Antimyosin antibody imaging has a high sensitivity (91%–100%) and high negative predictive value (93%–100%).[123]

Tenascin-C is a large extracellular matrix protein expressed in the heart during inflammation, wound healing, and remodeling.[124] Serum tenascin-C levels provide additional prognostic information to BNP in heart failure.[125] ^{111}In-antitenascin-C monoclonal antibody fragments have also been used in a dual isotope SPECT imaging technique with ^{99m}Tc-MIBI to assess early inflammation in vivo during postinfarction remodeling.

Apoptosis and Cell Death

Unlike necrosis, apoptosis is the highly active physiologic process of programmed cell death whereby organisms selectively target cells to be eliminated. Potential targets for the evaluation of myocellular apoptosis include Annexin V and the critical apoptotic protease family of caspases. Pyrophosphate- and glucarate-based imaging allows for evaluation of necrotic cell death.

Cardiovascular disorders including cardiomyopathy, heart failure, myocarditis, and MI are all associated with increased apoptosis. Apoptotic signaling pathways trigger the activation of caspases, cysteine proteases, and in particular the key effector caspase-3.[126] Caspase-3 disrupts the processes that regulate various subregions of the cell membrane, leading to increased PS on the outer cell membrane.[127] Exposure of PS to the cell surface makes it an excellent target for imaging via the PS-binding protein annexin V.

[99m]Tc-labeled annexin V was utilized to detect in vivo cell death in patients presenting with MI and who underwent PCI.[128] Revascularized patients had early ^{99m}Tc-labeled annexin V SPECT imaging and subsequent ^{99m}Tc-sestamibi-based perfusion imaging. Early regional retention of ^{99m}Tc-labeled annexin V correlated well with the perfusion defect. [99m]Tc labeled annexin V also appears to have predictive value in terms of deterioration of LV function in patients with known cardiomyopathy (**Fig. 32.22**).[129] In addition to nuclear imaging approaches, Annexin-V has been linked to small paramagnetic iron oxide (SPIO) nanoparticles and gadolinium-based contrast agents for higher spatial resolution and detection of apoptosis with CMR. AnxCLIO-Cy5.5, an Annexin V cross-linked SPIO that is also tagged with the fluorescein probe, Cy5.5, has been demonstrated to have high affinity for apoptotic cardiomyocytes in vivo in rodent models of ischemia-reperfusion (I/R) injury and chronic HF (**Fig. 32.23**).[130-132] In addition, annexin-V has been linked to magnetic resonance imaging (MRI) contrast agent (gadolinium diethylenetriamine pentaacetate)-coated liposomes, and permits the detection of early apoptotic myocytes in vivo following I/R injury in rodents with CMR.[133,134]

Heart transplant rejection is characterized by perivascular and interstitial mononuclear inflammatory infiltrates associated with myocyte apoptosis and necrosis (**see also Chapter 44**). In a study of 18 patients undergoing apoptotic imaging within 1 year of cardiac transplantation, Annexin-V retention correlated with the severity of rejection.[135] All patients with a negative scan had a concomitant negative biopsy. The authors suggested that serial annexin V imaging for apoptotic cells could be used as a surrogate for the detection of allograft rejection in place of serial biopsies in patients post-heart transplant. As an alternative to visualizing apoptosis, several studies have demonstrated that certain agents allow the visualization of ongoing myocardial necrosis

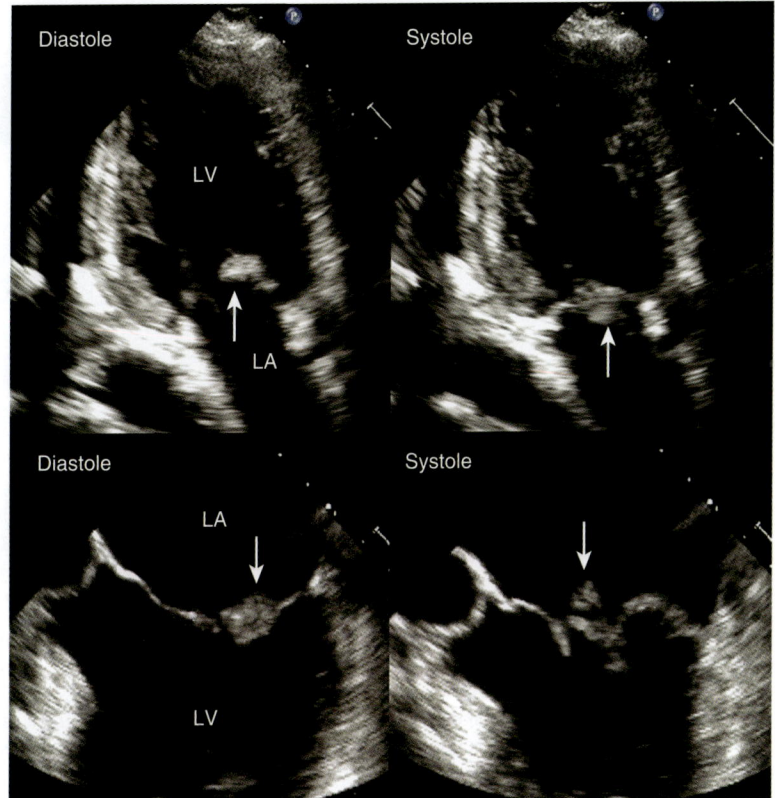

Fig. 32.20 Mitral Valve Vegetation by Transesophageal Echocardiography (TEE). TEE of the apical long-axis view showing mitral valve thickening that was mobile but was initially thought to be nonspecific in a 70-year-old male who developed spiking fevers, symptoms of heart failure and increasingly severe mitral regurgitation with positive blood cultures. A TEE was performed that revealed a discrete vegetation on the mitral valve with ruptured chordae allowing mild prolapse of the posterior valve leaflet and acute severe mitral regurgitation that worsened with stress. *LV*, Left ventricular; *TTE*, transthoracic echocardiogram.

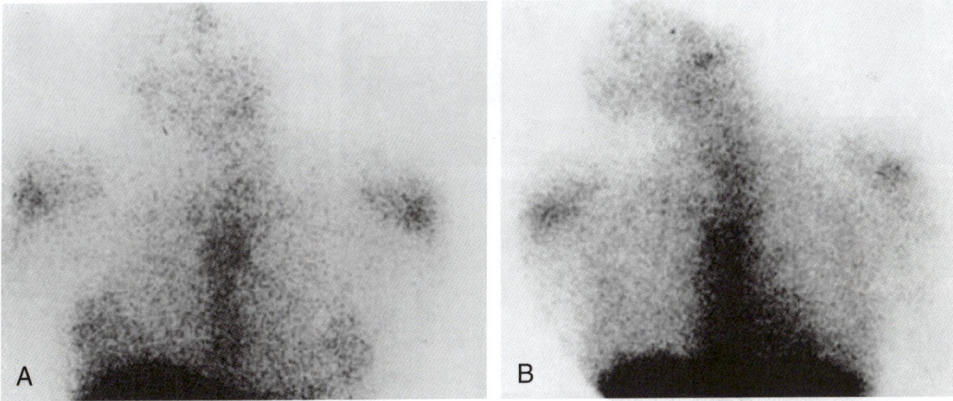

Fig. 32.21 ^{111}In-Antimyosin Antibody Uptake in Myocarditis. (A) No myocardial antimyosin uptake is seen in the left panel (heart to lung ratio [HLR] = 1.4) in a scan with normal findings. (B) Moderate myocardial antimyosin uptake (HLR 1.8) in a patient with active myocarditis. (Modified from Martin ME, Moya-Mur JL, Casanova M, et al. Role of noninvasive antimyosin imaging in infants and children with clinically suspected myocarditis. *J Nucl Med.* 2004;45:429–437.)

as a mechanism of identifying acute infarction potentially even in the presence of prior MI. ^{99m}Tc-glucarate enters necrotic cells by passive diffusion following breakdown of the sarcolemma and binds to exposed histones in cardiomyocyte nuclei, making it a useful an alternative to ^{99m}Tc-pyrophosphate.[136] Canine models for ischemia and infarction reveal a high affinity of ^{99m}Tc-glucarate for necrotic tissue versus ischemic but viable myocardium. Initial data in patients revealed that ^{99m}Tc-glucarate is able to diagnose MI noninvasively in patients presenting with chest pain with a sensitivity, which is dependent on time of presentation, specifically within the first 9 hours of symptom onset.[137]

Imaging Inflammation

[111]In-Oxine allows for the radiolabeling of cells and has been widely used to label leukocytes. Interestingly, the biphasic recruitment of specific monocytes to the myocardium post-MI was elucidated with

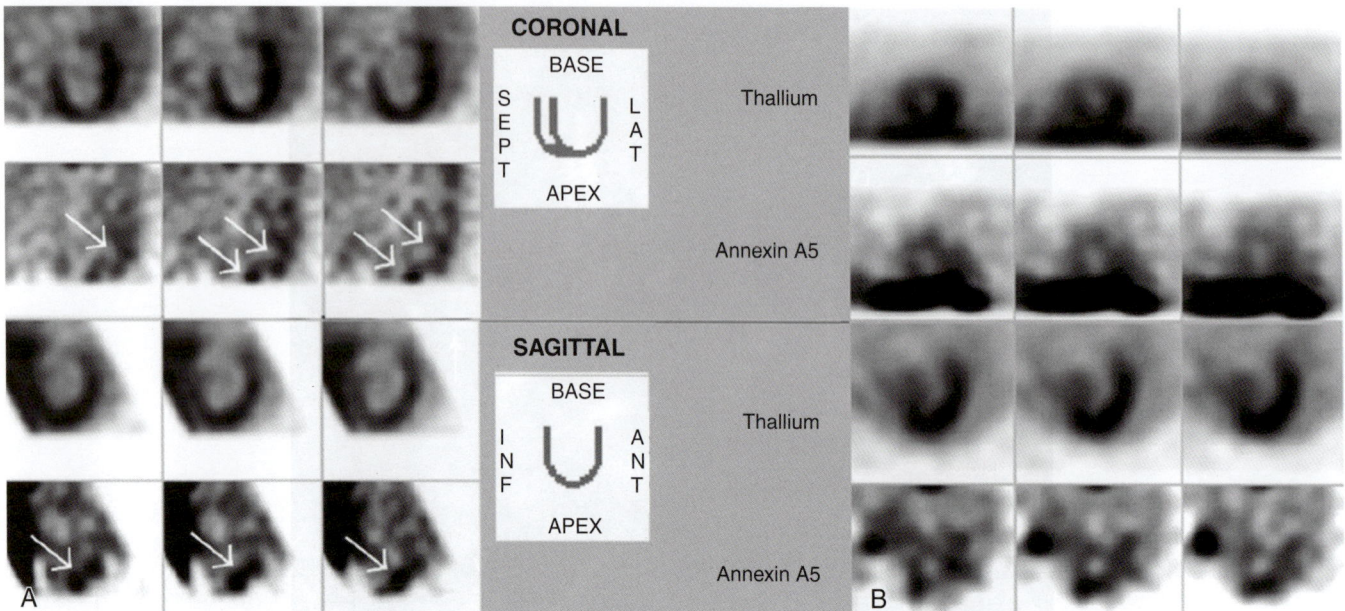

Fig. 32.22 Dual Isotope Imaging With ^{201}Tl for Left Ventricular *(LV)* Myocardial Border Detection and [99]mTc-Labeled Annexin V in Dilated Cardiomyopathy *(DCM).* (A) DCM patient with rapid deterioration of LV function. There is apical and lateral wall focal uptake, and mild septal uptake *(arrows).* (B) DCM patient with acute heart failure. There is global uptake of the tracer. *ANT,* Anterior; *INF,* inferior; *LAT,* lateral; *SEPT,* septal. (Modified from Kietselaer BL, Reutelingsperger CP, Boersma HH, et al. Noninvasive detection of programmed cell loss with 99mTc-labeled annexin A5 in heart failure. *J Nucl Med.* 2007;48:562–567.)

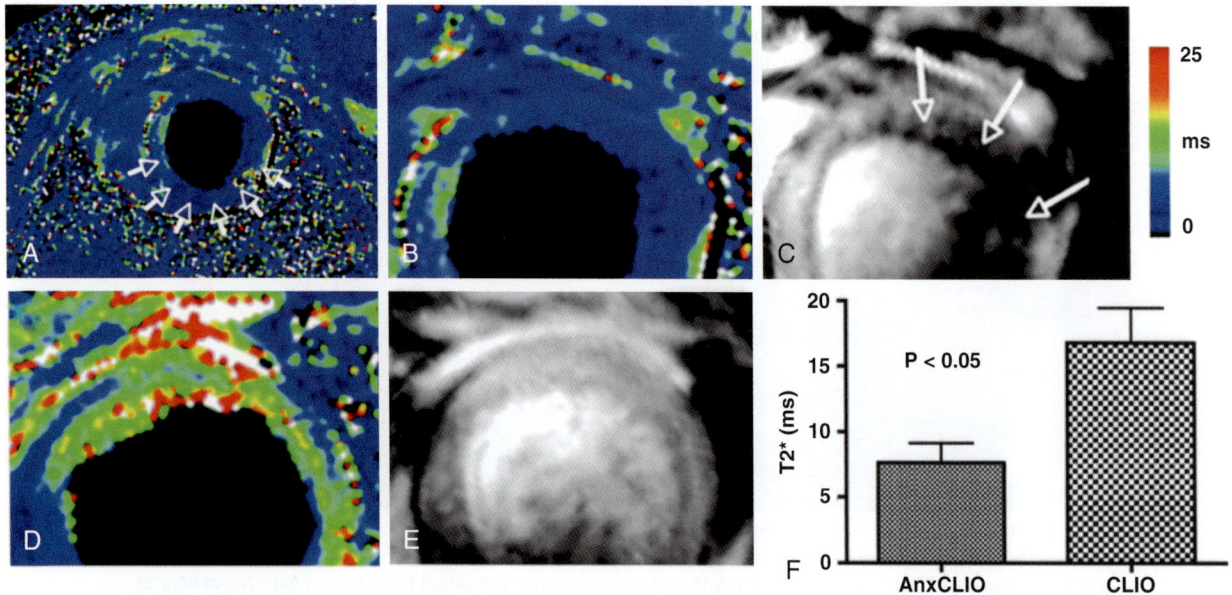

Fig. 32.23 Molecular Magnetic Resonance Imaging of Cardiomyocyte Apoptosis In Vivo. (A) In vivo T2* map in a mouse with Gaq overexpression (model of heart failure) injected with 10 mg Fe/kg of AnxCLIO-Cy5.5. Susceptibility artifacts from the lungs and the iron oxide–laden liver precluded interpretation of the T2* maps over the inferior portion of the left ventricle *(arrows).* These areas were thus excluded from the analysis. (B) Magnified view of the T2* map shown in A. (C) T2*-weighted image in the mouse (injected with AnxCLIO-Cy5.5) at an echo time *(TE)* of 8 ms. (D) T2* map, and (E) T2*-weighted image (TE, 8 ms) in a mouse injected with CLIO-Cy5.5. Numerous discrete foci of signal hypointensity *(arrows,* C), consistent with probe uptake, were seen in the mice injected with AnxCLIO-Cy5.5 (C) but not in the mice injected with CLIO-Cy5.5 (E). (F) T2* was significantly lower in the mice injected with AnxCLIO-Cy5.5 (n5) than in those injected with CLIO-Cy5.5 (n=5). The uptake of AnxCLIO-Cy5.5 *(arrows,* C) was frequently most prominent in the subendocardium. (From Sosnovik DE, Nahrendorf M, Panizzi P et al. Molecular MRI detects low levels of cardiomyocyte apoptosis in a transgenic model of chronic heart failure. *Circ Cardiovasc Imaging.* 2009;2:468–475.)

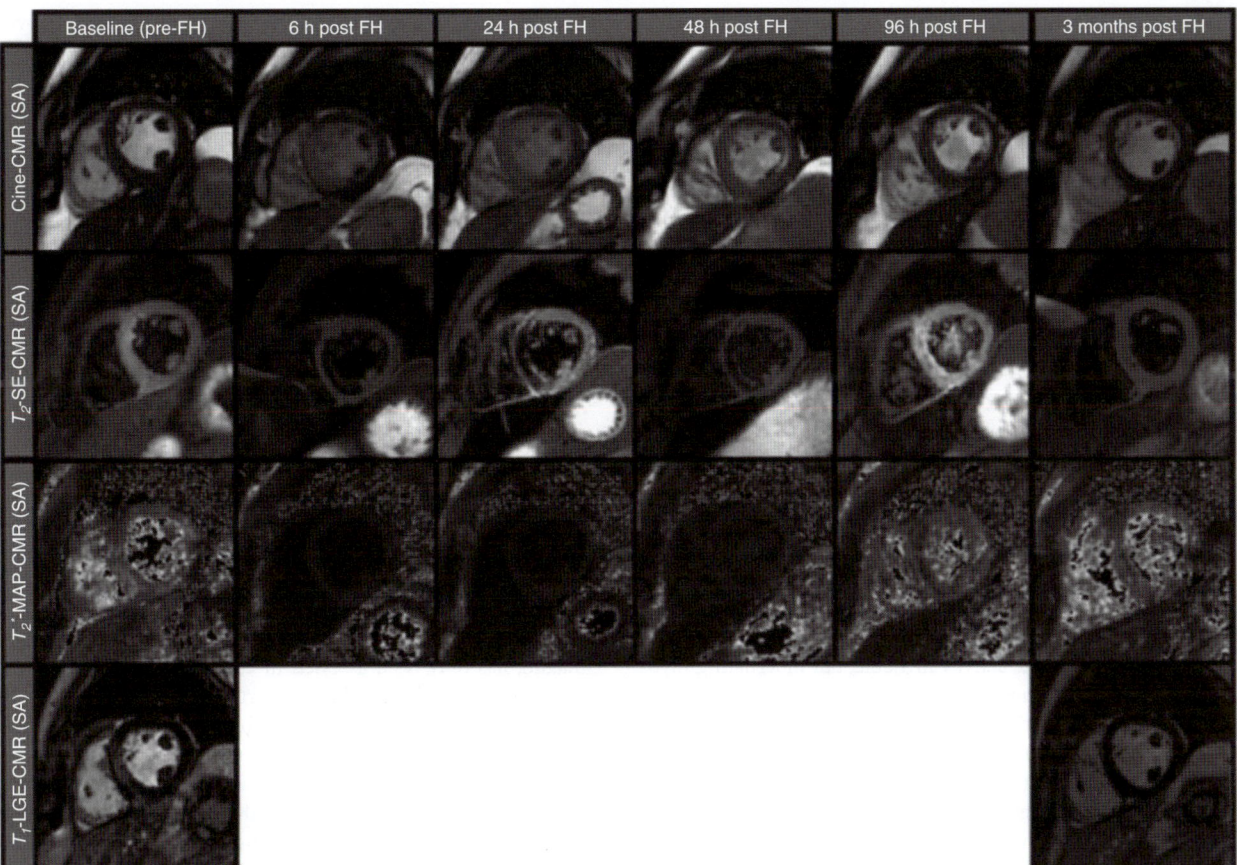

Fig. 32.24 Exemplary cardiovascular magnetic resonance *(CMR)* images in the short-axis view of a study patient with a septal myocardial infarction who received a single dose of ferumoxytol (Feraheme *[FH]*) injection within 1 week following acute ST elevation myocardial infarction. This patient underwent pre-FH (baseline) and post-FH (after 6, 24, 48, 96, and 3 months) CMR imaging studies. The first row shows cine-CMR images over time with visible hyperenhancement in the septal wall at 6–48 hr post-FH. The second row shows T2-weighted short-tau inversion recovery-spin echo images over time with evidence of hypoenhancement in the septal wall at 6–48 hr post-FH. The third row shows T2*-mapping images at different time points with evidence of "signal void" in the septal wall at 6–48 hr post-FH. The fourth row shows LGE images at baseline and 3 months. (From Yilmaz A, Dengler MA, van der Kuip H, et al. Imaging of myocardial infarction using ultrasmall superparamagnetic iron oxide nanoparticles: a human study using a multi-parametric cardiovascular magnetic resonance imaging approach. *Eur Heart J.* 2013;34:462–475.)

[111]In-Oxine radio-labeling of isolated Ly-6C[High] and Ly-6C[Low] monocyte subtypes in rodent myocardium. On day 2 after acute myocardial infarction (AMI), the accumulation of ^{111}In-Oxine labeled-Ly-6C[High] cells were visualized in vivo with microSPECT/CT, and ex vivo autoradiography, co-registered with 2,3,5-triphenyltetrazolium chloride staining, confirmed accumulation of Ly-6C[High] in the infarct and border zone of the myocardium.[138]

Iron oxide-based nanoparticles (especially ultra-SPIOs, or USPIOs) are readily taken up by macrophages; therefore, imaging these nanoparticles with MRI provides a unique opportunity to track in vivo monocyte/macrophage recruitment to the myocardium. Preclinical studies provided the first evidence that USPIO accumulation and consequent image hypoenhancement was directly proportional to the number of infiltrated macrophages in the infarcted myocardium.[139,140] The translation of these findings to AMI patients was facilitated by recent US Food and Drug Administration approval of the novel USPIO probe, ferumoxytol, to treat anemia in chronic kidney disease. Initial small studies in acute STEMI patients observed signal hypo-enhancement on T2-weighted images and a signal void on T2*-maps in the infarct area early post-MI (within 7 days) following ferumoxytol administration (**Fig. 32.24**). In addition, a substantial drop in T2* values, albeit to a lesser extent, was detected in the periinfarct zone and in the remote myocardium in these patients, indicating a global influx of inflammatory macrophages to the myocardium that extend beyond the area at risk (see Fig. 32.24).[141,142] Recently, the safety profile and therapeutic potential of ferumoxytol use in post-MI patients was established.[143] Taken together, these studies demonstrate the feasibility of detecting the in vivo infiltration of macrophages to myocardium post-MI with MRI.

Imaging Inflammatory Cell Activity

[18]F-fluorodeoxyglucose (FDG), a glucose analog, also has been applied in the setting of targeted inflammatory cell imaging in atherosclerosis and following an AMI, since proinflammatory cells, such as M1 macrophages metabolize glucose.[144] However, the specificity of this tracer for inflammatory cells postinfarct is complicated by the switch in myocardial substrate usage from fatty acids to glucose during ischemia and in both phenotypes of chronic HF.[145] Nonetheless, early preclinical studies showed an increase in ^{18}F-FDG uptake in vivo on PET imaging 7 days following I/R injury in mice, which corresponded to an abundance of macrophages in the infarct region on ex vivo immunohistochemical evaluation.[146] However, considerable background myocardial

^{18}F-FDG uptake was apparent on these studies. Other preclinical studies, which use myocardial glucose suppression, have demonstrated increased ^{18}F-FDG uptake in vivo on PET in the infarct and border zone early post-MI (5–7 days) and confirmed that the imaging signal was associated with elevated monocyte and macrophage populations in these same regions with postmortem biochemical analyses.[147,148] Importantly, the value of ^{18}F-FDG imaging of postinfarct inflammation and in predicting LV remodeling has been recently described in a small number of patients (*n* = 29) following an AMI (**Fig. 32.25**).[149] Higher ^{18}F-FDG uptake in the infarct region (expressed as SUV_{mean}) 5 days following reperfusion after an AMI was independently predictive of adverse LV remodeling (Δ EF, Δ end-diastolic volume, Δ end-systolic volume) after 6 months when accounting for MR derived infarct size (LGE extent, % left ventricle) and circulating leukocyte levels. Interestingly, peak circulating leukocytes, $CCR2^+$ monocytes (inflammatory) and $CD14^{High}$ $CD16^+$ (intermediate inflammatory monocytes) were associated with LV ^{18}F-FDG uptake extent (^{18}F-FDG uptake ≥50% of maximum), while $CD14^{High}$ $CD16^+$ (inflammatory) and $CD14^{Low}$ $CD16^+$ (noninflammatory) monocyte subtypes were not associated with this ^{18}F-FDG uptake. Indeed, larger studies are needed to corroborate and substantiate these results.

As mentioned above, ^{18}F-FDG is a nonspecific radiotracer that may also represent metabolic activity in viable, but hibernating myocardium. Therefore, there has been an effort to apply more specific inflammatory tracers in the postinfarct setting. ^{11}C-methionine is a positron emitting amino acid tracer, which is routinely used to assess protein synthesis for oncological applications. Early studies in MI patients within 2 weeks of reperfusion demonstrated elevated ^{11}C-methionine uptake in the infarct area relative to the remote myocardium, with the magnitude of ^{11}C-methionine uptake being greater in patients imaged closer to reperfusion.[150] A series of elegant in vitro and in vivo preclinical studies further elucidated these early findings and demonstrated selective uptake of ^{11}C-methionine for polarized M1 macrophages, neutrophils, monocytes, T cells, and natural killer cells, but not for M2 macrophages, nor B cells. In addition, in vivo microPET imaging of ^{11}C-methionine in mice following left anterior descending occlusion showed significantly elevated ^{11}C-methionine uptake in the infarct region relative to the remote myocardium and control mouse myocardium at 3 and 5 days post-MI.[151] Similarly, the chemokine receptor, CXCR4, which is believed to be involved in leukocyte recruitment to injured myocardium, has been imaged with PET and ^{68}Ga-pentixafor in the early postinfarct setting in mice and humans. In mice, ^{68}Ga-pentixafor uptake followed a similar temporal uptake pattern in the infarct region as ^{11}C-methionine post-MI, that is ^{68}Ga-pentixafor uptake peaked in the infarct region relative to the remote myocardium at 3 days post-MI and thereafter fell to levels observed in the remote region on day 7. Ex vivo studies associated myocardial ^{68}Ga-pentixafor uptake to inflammatory cell infiltration. In a small pilot study, ^{68}Ga-pentixafor showed a wide range of uptake magnitude in the infarct region of AMI patients early (within 5 days) postreperfusion (**Fig. 32.26**).[152] The value of ^{11}C-methionine and ^{68}Ga-pentixafor in predicting LV remodeling in patients post-MI is presently under investigation.

Ventricular Remodeling

Ventricular remodeling is a complex biological process that involves angiogenesis, wound repair, and scarring. Several cell types modulate this adaptive remodeling process in ischemic and nonischemic cardiomyopathies. Vascular endothelial growth factor (VEGF) receptors, integrins, and matrix metalloproteinases are all potential new targets to modulate remodeling because of their association with neovascularization, and turnover of the ECM.

VEGF receptors are potential targets for visualization of ventricular remodeling-associated angiogenesis. A PET tracer, [64]Cu-6DOTA-$VEGF_{121}$, was developed for this express purpose in patients with MI.[153] The tracer is detectable by immunofluorescence microscopy in the infarct region and peaks with the changing levels of VEGFR expression in the tissue. ^{18}F-FHBG is a cardiac-specific reporter probe for use with micro-PET imaging in small animals. The reporter system was linked to VEGF to detect the impact of angiogenic therapy with an imaging-based approach.[154] Increased capillary density and small blood vessels were seen in the VEGF-treated myocardium prior to detectable increases in regional organ perfusion. These results provide evidence that a molecular reporter system can be developed in tandem with vasculogenic therapy.

During angiogenesis, there is up-regulation of adhesion molecules such as $\alpha_v\beta_3$ integrin. An ^{111}In-labeled quinolone (^{111}In-RP748) with high affinity and selectivity for $\alpha_v\beta_3$ integrin showed increased relative ^{111}In-RP748 uptake in acute myocardial infarcts, which persisted for at least 3 weeks postreperfusion (**Fig. 32.27**).[155] The imaging of $\alpha_v\beta_3$ integrin by the PET imaging tracer, ^{18}F-Galakto-RGD, in a 35-year-old patient 2 weeks after a transmural MI, demonstrates the feasibility of utilizing integrin-based imaging in human myocardial tissue (**Fig. 32.28**).[156] Despite widespread preclinical use, ^{18}F-galactco-RGD imaging has only been assessed in case reports and small studies in early post-MI patients. These reports have shown ^{18}F-galacto-RGD uptake in some, but not all, patients following an AMI.[157] ^{68}Ga-PRGD2 is another $\alpha_v\beta_3$ targeted PET tracer that has shown clinical feasibility. ^{68}Ga-PRGD2 showed peak focal uptake in the infarct and border regions early (~1 week) after an AMI that was elevated, to a lesser extent, in some patients for up to 2.5 months after an AMI.[158] At this time, it is unknown whether ^{18}F-galactco-RGD and ^{68}Ga-PRGD2 uptake early post-MI correlates with clinical outcome and ventricular remodeling. On the other hand, ^{18}F-fluciclatide, an $\alpha_v\beta_3$ and $\alpha_v\beta_5$ selective radiotracer, has been shown to be taken up into the infarct region early (~2 weeks) post-acute STEMI and the magnitude of ^{18}F-fluciclatide uptake was related to functional recovery of myocardial segments with wall hypokinesis at 9 months follow-up (**Fig. 32.29**).[159] In line with animal studies, ^{18}F-fluciclatide uptake was higher in patients with subendocardial infarction, with no uptake in a subset of patients with prior infarction.

Since collagen deposition and fibrosis in the failing heart are mediated by myofibroblasts, markers that indicate increased myofibroblast recruitment and activity are of interest. Myofibroblasts demonstrate an up-regulation of integrins, leading to use of the ^{99m}Tc-labeled cy5.5-RGD peptide analogue, CRIP, to image upregulated $\alpha_v\beta_3$ integrins in a murine model of MI.[160] A subgroup of animals was treated with either captopril or a combination of captopril and losartan to positively affect ventricular remodeling and to visualize the effect on the CRIP- $\alpha_v\beta_3$ integrin signal. Ex vivo SPECT imaging of CRIP revealed lower signal intensity images in the treated hearts and correlated with smaller infarct size and increased LVEF, demonstrating the potential of integrin-targeted imaging in tracking response to therapy.

Collagen type I, and to a lesser extent type III, are the main components of cardiac fibrosis. Since collagen is entirely extracellular, and can increase to 10-fold or more during fibrosis development, nontargeted imaging using tracers that are trapped in ECM space but are not taken up in cells has been used as a surrogate to visualize scar/fibrosis. Gadolinium (Ga)-DOTA is an MR agent that is most widely used ECM targeted agent for assessing infarct size and viability after an MI.[161,162] Similar PET tracers, such as ^{64}Cu-DOTA, have been developed and confirmed the microdistribution of DOTA localization in the infarct region, which included collagen, myocytes, and expanded ECM compared to the remote myocardium following an MI.[163] Indeed,

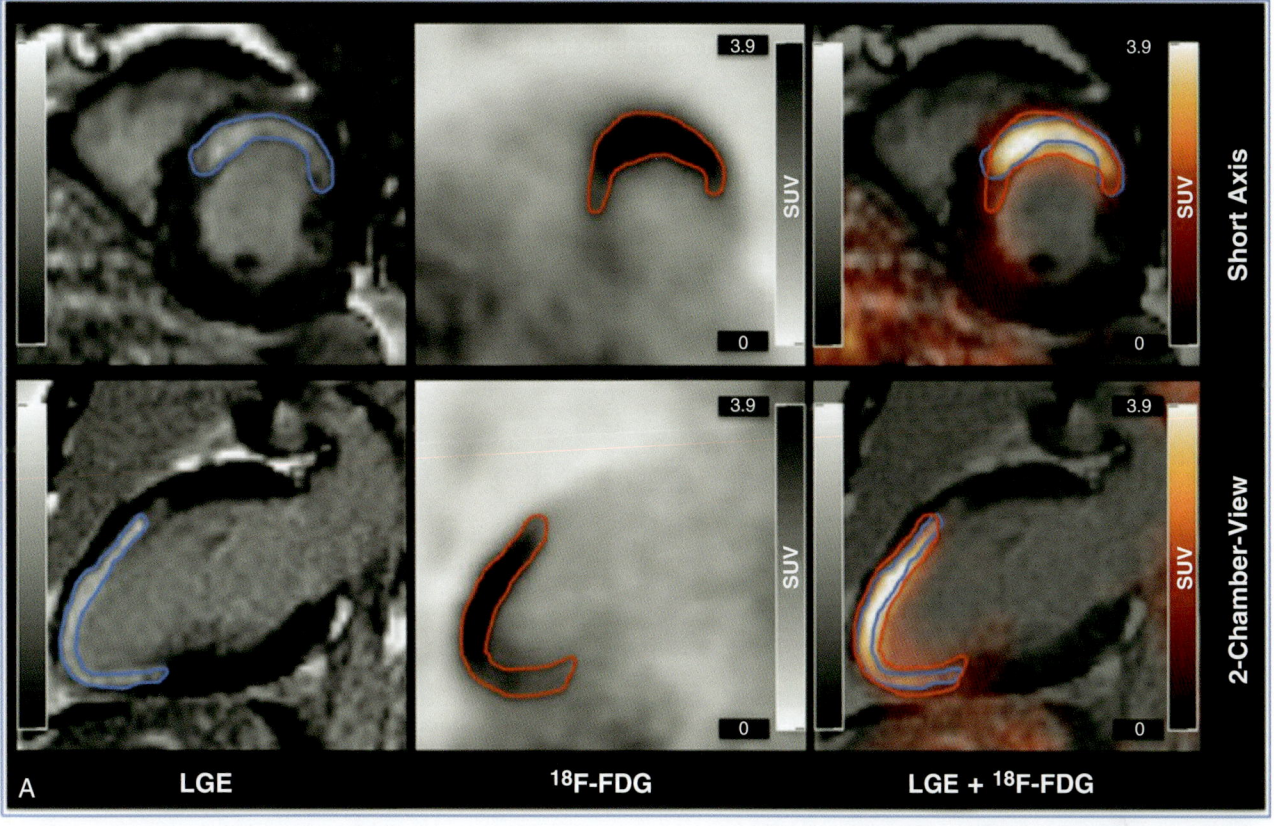

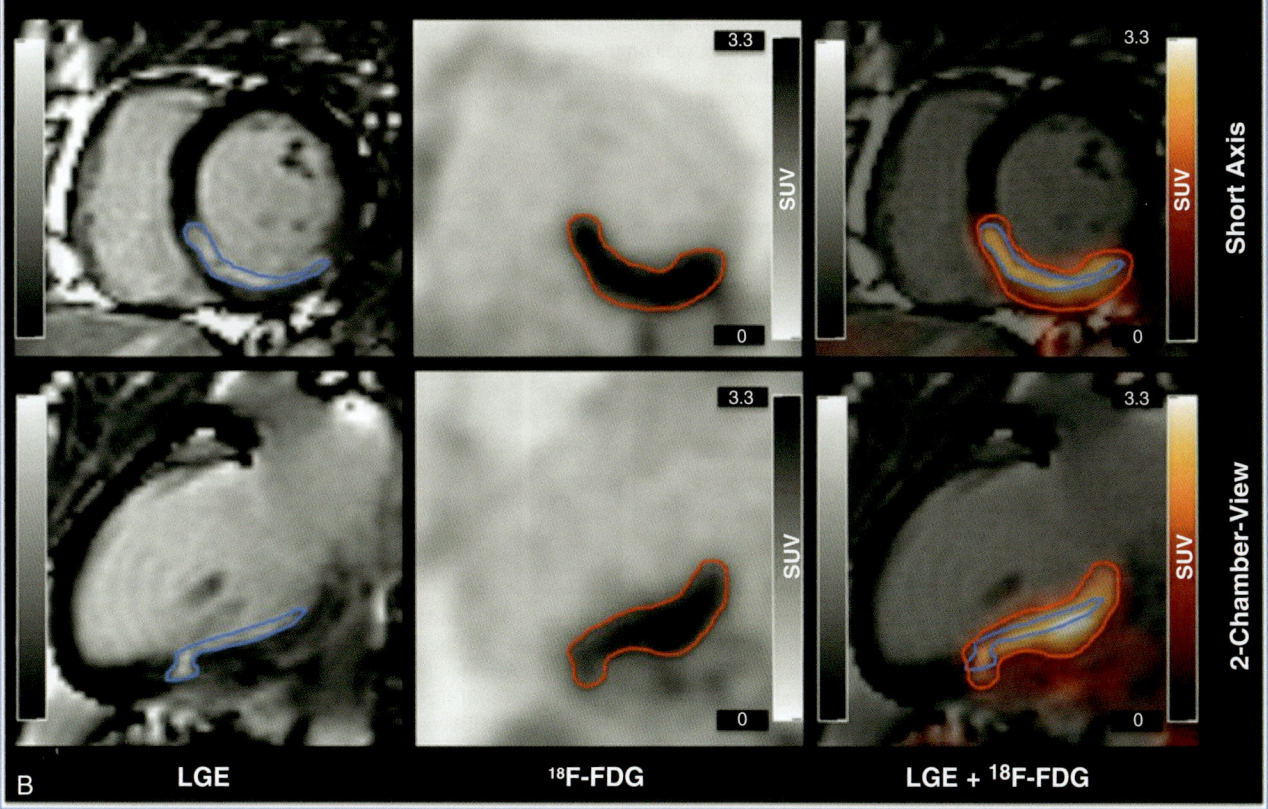

Fig. 32.25 ^{18}F-Fluorodeoxyglucose *(18F-FDG)* positron emission tomography *(PET)*/magnetic resonance images *(MRI)* of two patients shortly after acute myocardial infarction. Short- and long-axis views of late gadolinium enhancement *(LGE)* MRI *(left)*, ^{18}F-FDG–PET images *(middle)*, and overlay *(right)* of patients with anterior (A) or inferior (B) myocardial infarction. (From Rischpler C, Dirschinger RJ, Nekolla SG et al. Prospective evaluation of 18 F-fluorodeoxyglucose uptake in postischemic myocardium by simultaneous positron emission tomography/magnetic resonance imaging as a prognostic marker of functional outcome. *Circ Cardiovasc Imaging.* 2016;9(4):e004316.)

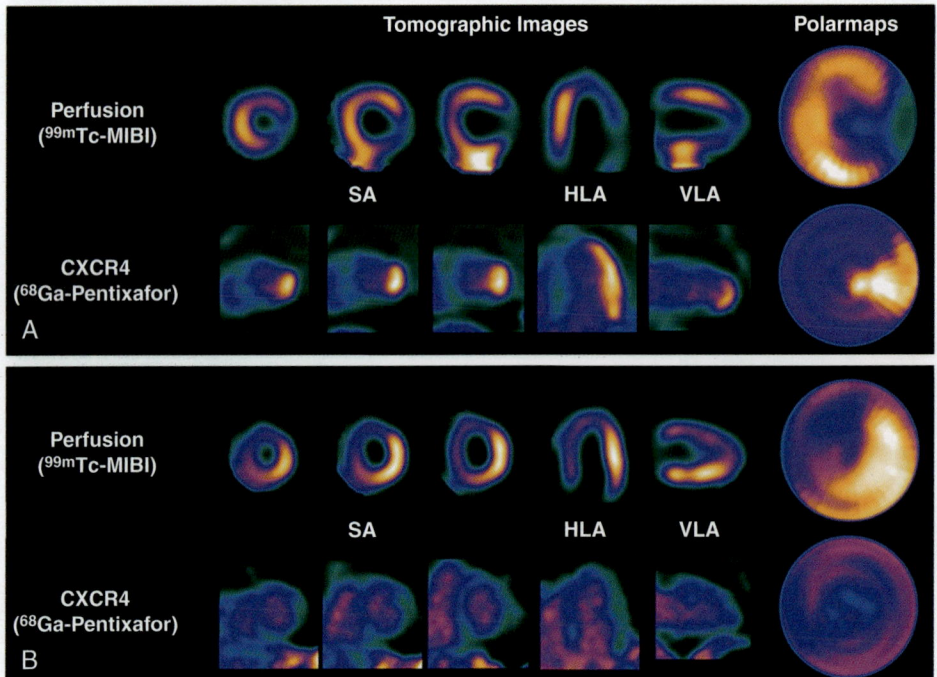

Fig 32.26 Targeted Imaging Identifies Various Levels of CXCR4 Expression in Patients After an Acute Myocardial Infarction. Tomographic images of perfusion and uptake of the CXCR4-ligand ^{68}Ga-pentixafor in two representative cases with intermediate size infarcts. (A) Lateral wall perfusion defect (summed rest score 17) with high corresponding pentixafor uptake in the defect region in a patient studied at 4 days after reperfusion. (B) Anteroseptal wall perfusion defect (summed rest score 16) with very low, almost absent pentixafor uptake in the defect region in a patient studied at 7 days after reperfusion. Polar maps display entire left ventricle myocardial activity with the base in the periphery, the apex in the center, the anterior wall on top, the inferior wall on bottom, the lateral wall on the right, and the septum on the left. *HLA,* Horizontal long axis; *SA,* short axis; *VLA,* vertical long axis. (From Thackeray JT, Derlin T, Haghikia A et al. Molecular imaging of the chemokine receptor CXCR4 after acute myocardial infarction. *JACC Cardiovasc Imaging.* 2015;8:1417–1426.)

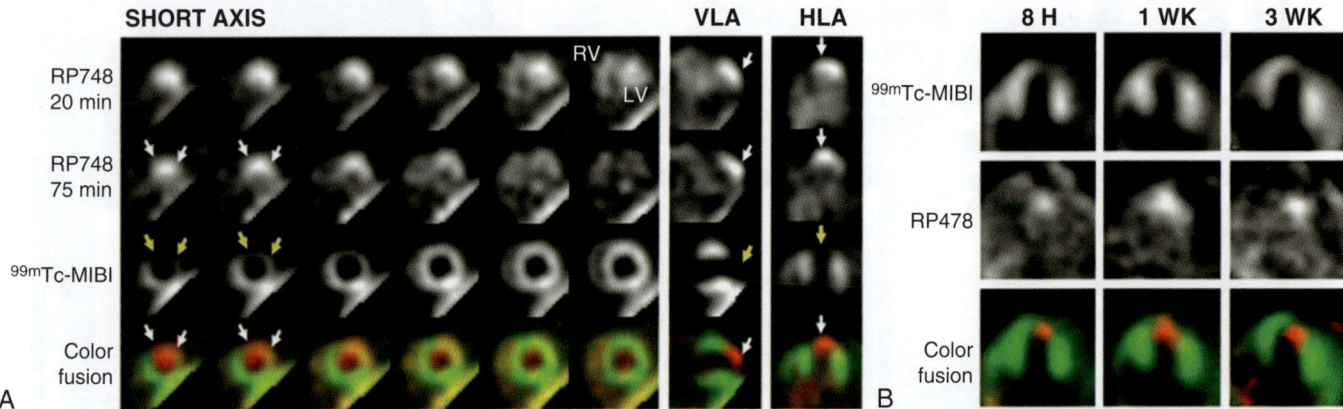

Fig. 32.27 Angiogenesis Demonstrated by In Vivo ^{111}In-RP748 and ^{99m}Tc-Sestamibi *(^{99m}Tc-MIBI)* Images From Dogs With Chronic Infarction. (A) Serial in vivo canine ^{111}In-RP748 SPECT short-axis, vertical long-axis (VLA), and horizontal long-axis *(HLA)* images 3 wk post LAD infarction at 20 min, and 75 min postinjection. ^{111}In-RP748 SPECT images are shown registered with ^{99m}Tc-MIBI perfusion images *(third row).* The 75 min ^{111}In-RP748 SPECT images were colored red and fused with MIBI images *(green)* to show localization of ^{111}In-RP748 activity within the heart *(color fusion, bottom row).* Right ventricular *(RV)* and left ventricular *(LV)* blood pool activities are seen at 20 min *(top row).* White arrows indicate region of increased ^{111}In-RP748 uptake in anterior wall. This corresponds to the anteroapical ^{99m}Tc-MIBI perfusion defect *(yellow arrows).* (B) Sequential ^{99m}Tc-MIBI *(top row)* and ^{111}In-RP748 in vivo SPECT HLA images at 90 min postinjection *(middle row)* from a dog at 8 hr, and 1 and 3 wk post-LAD infarction. Increased myocardial ^{111}In-RP748 uptake is seen in the anteroapical wall at all three time points (though appears greatest 1 wk postinfarction). Color fusion ^{99m}Tc-MIBI *(green)* and ^{111}In-RP748 *(red)* images *(bottom row)* demonstrate ^{111}In-RP748 uptake within ^{99m}Tc-MIBI perfusion defect. (From Meoli DF, Sadeghi MM, Krassilnikova S, et al. Noninvasive imaging of myocardial angiogenesis following experimental myocardial infarction. *J Clin Invest.* 2004;113:1684–1691.)

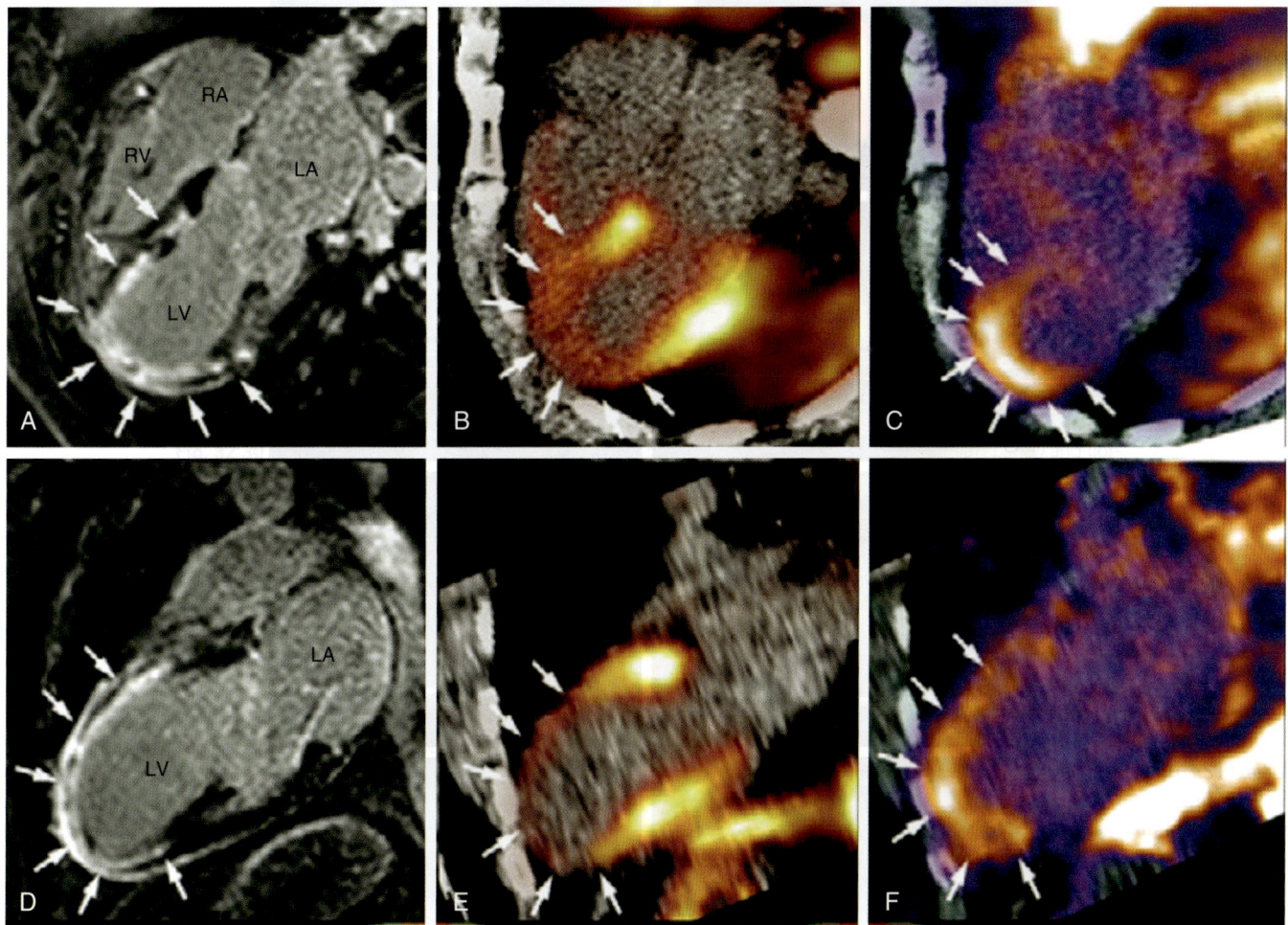

Fig. 32.28 **18F-Galakto-RGD Positron Emission Tomography Imaging.** Cardiac magnetic resonance *(CMR)* image with extensive late gadolinium enhancement *(arrows)* from the anterior wall to the apical region in the 4- (A) and 2-chamber (D) views. Panels B and E show severely reduced myocardial blood flow using 13N-ammonia in similarly-oriented images, corresponding to the regions of CMR delayed enhancement *(arrows)*. Panels C and F show focal 18F-RGD signal co-localized to the infarcted area. This signal likely reflects angiogenesis in the healing area *(arrows)*. (From Makowski MR, Ebersberger U, Nekolla S, Schwaiger M. In vivo molecular imaging of angiogenesis, targeting alphavbeta3 integrin expression, in a patient after acute myocardial infarction. *Eur Heart J.* 2008;29[18]:2201.)

the nonspecificity and kinetics of these tracers are not suitable for the assessment of diffuse fibrosis that is commensurate with reactive fibrosis in pressure/volume overload and certain cardiomyopathies.

In addition to nuclear probes, gadolinium has been conjugated to EP-3533, a type I collagen specific peptide that is freely diffusible to the extracellular space and binds to type I collagen with high affinity. In a mouse model of chronic MI, dynamic weighted MRI showed that EP-3533 had significantly longer retention rate in scarred myocardium when compared to a commercial gadolinium-based contrast agent (**Fig. 32.30**).[164] In addition, the collagen binding protein, CNA-35, has been attached to paramagnetic/fluorescent micellar nanoparticles for the MRI detection of collagen in abdominal aortic aneurysms, but has yet been applied in the post-MI setting.

By radiolabeling molecules that target matrix metalloproteinases (MMPs), like pharmacological inhibitors that specifically bind to the catalytic domain, MMP activation postinfarct can be visualized in vivo (**Fig. 32.31**).[165,166] Preclinical imaging studies were carried out utilizing 99mTc-labeled compound (99mTc-RP805) targeting MMP activation and hybrid SPECT/CT imaging with a dual isotope imaging protocol that combined 99mTc-RP805 imaging with adjunctive 201Tl perfusion imaging. These dual isotope imaging studies revealed significant MMP

activation within the perfusion defect region, as well as lesser degrees of MMP activation in periinfarct and remote areas of the heart. This suggests that MMP activation is taking place throughout the heart and supports the concept that molecules that target MMP activation might be utilized to evaluate ventricular remodeling.

Further imaging studies have been performed using 99mTc-labeled analog of RP782 (99mTc-RP805) and hybrid SPECT/CT imaging with a dual isotope protocol involving 99mTc-RP805 imaging and adjunctive 201Tl-perfusion imaging. The dual isotope imaging studies showed MMP activation within the perfusion defect region, suggesting that MMP activation is taking place primarily within areas of injury, and supports the concept that targeting MMP activation with imaging approaches might be utilized to evaluate ventricular remodeling. Other broad-spectrum MMP inhibitors (CGS 27023A) have been labeled with both 11C and 18F for PET imaging, but the value of these tracers in postinfarct remodeling is still under investigation.

Metabolism and Ischemic Memory

Under normal physiological conditions, myocardial energy demand is primarily met by fatty acid oxidation. However, pronounced changes in oxygen supply (ischemia) or demand (pressure/volume overload) during

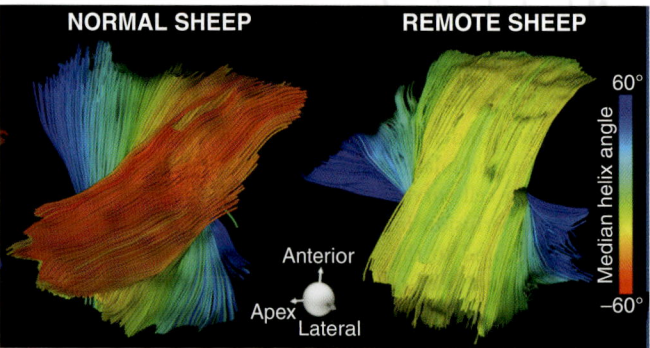

Fig. 32.35 Noninvasive Assessment of Myocardial Fiber Orientation with Cardiac Magnetic Resonance. These images identify the normal transmural fiber orientation pattern *(left)* and the altered fiber orientation pattern postinfarction on the right. The color pattern identifies both the layer (endo- or epicardial) and the direction of the fibers in that layer. Note the greater dispersion of fiber angles in the infarcted heart.

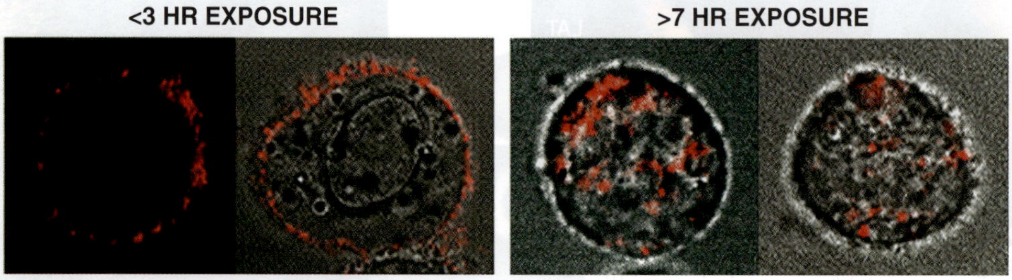

Fig. 32.36 Cardiac Magnetic Resonance Molecular Imaging to Assess Myocyte Apoptosis. Time lapse confocal microscopy show the Annexin cross-linked iron oxide nanoparticle bound predominantly to the apoptotic cell surface at <3 hr postincubation, but becomes internalized into the cells with more than 7 hr of exposure. Since the iron oxide is the component producing the signal in the Annexin-bound nanoparticle complex, either location (surface or intracellular) will produce a contrast effect.

KEY REFERENCES

4. Kirkpatrick JN, Vannan MA, Narula J, Lang RM. Echocardiography in heart failure: applications, utility, and new horizons. *J Am Coll Cardiol.* 2007;50:381–396.

17. Nagueh SF, Smiseth OA, Appleton CP, et al. Recommendations for the evaluation of left ventricular diastolic function by echocardiography: an update from the american society of echocardiography and the european association of cardiovascular imaging. *J Am Soc Echocardiogr.* 2016;29:277–314.

33. Amundsen BH, Helle-Valle T, Edvardsen T, et al. Noninvasive myocardial strain measurement by speckle tracking echocardiography: validation against sonomicrometry and tagged magnetic resonance imaging. *J Am Coll Cardiol.* 2006;47:789–793.

66. Uretsky S, Argulian E, Narula J, et al. Use of cardiac magnetic resonance imaging in assessing mitral regurgitation: current evidence. *J Am Coll Cardiol.* 2018;71:547–563.

115. Patel A, Kramer CM. Role of cardiac magnetic resonance in the diagnosis and prognosis of nonischemic cardiomyopathy. *JACC Cardiovasc Imaging.* 2017;10:1180–1193.

116. Coleman GC, Shaw PW, Balfour Jr PC, et al. Prognostic value of myocardial scarring on CMR in patients with cardiac sarcoidosis. *JACC Cardiovasc Imaging.* 2017;10:411–420.

148. Lee WW, et al. PET/MRI of inflammation in myocardial infarction. *J Am Coll Cardiol.* 2012;59(2):153–163.

149. Rischpler C, et al. Prospective evaluation of 18 F-fluorodeoxyglucose uptake in postischemic myocardium by simultaneous positron emission tomography/magnetic resonance imaging as a prognostic marker of functional outcome. *Circ Cardiovasc Imaging.* 2016;9:e004316.

161. Perea RJ, et al. T1 mapping: characterisation of myocardial interstitial space. *Insights into Imaging.* 2015;6:189–202.

168. Saraste A, Knuuti J. PET imaging in heart failure: the role of new tracers. *Heart Failure Rev.* 2017;22:501–511.

The full reference list for this chapter is available on ExpertConsult.

Biomarkers and Precision Medicine in Heart Failure

Nasrien E. Ibrahim, Hanna K. Gaggin, James L. Januzzi Jr.

The underlying mechanisms in the development and progression of heart failure (HF) are complex and involve an intricate interplay of cardiac strain and injury, tissue inflammation, neurohumoral activation, oxidative stress, and ventricular remodeling, all compounded by the impact of comorbidities such as cardiorenal interactions and other medical conditions. Traditionally, diagnostic evaluation of patients suspected of having HF has involved history, physical examination, and chest x-ray (**see also Chapter 31**). However, the complex diagnosis of HF by clinical presentation alone may be challenging because patients often present with signs and symptoms that are vague and nonspecific. In fact, isolated findings from history or physical examination correlate poorly with objective methods of cardiac function, and clinical criteria that combine relevant findings perform poorly in accurately diagnosing HF (sensitivity 50%–73% and specificity 54%–78%). This challenge is associated with delays in definitive diagnosis and treatment, increased health care expenditures, and ultimately with poor prognosis. Although noninvasive and invasive diagnostic studies complement the initial history and physical examination in the evaluation of the HF patient, such methods, including echocardiography and right heart catheterization, have limitations and the routine use of these methods are associated with significant cost and potential risk.

Given the complexity of HF biology—which includes processes that are not easily detectable with physical examination or imaging techniques—increased interest has been given to the use of biomarkers to supplement clinical judgment; many biomarkers are conveniently measured and easily interpretable and may support clinical evaluation, while at the same time reflecting important pathophysiology involved in HF presence, severity, and prognosis.

In addition, beyond the traditional clinical roles played by biomarkers in HF patients (e.g., diagnosis, prognosis estimation, and therapy monitoring), biomarkers are playing an increasing role in the development of therapies for diagnosis. It is likely that testing of biomarker signatures may inform more precise application of therapies.

BIOMARKERS: DEFINITION AND GUIDELINES FOR EVALUATION

Although biomarkers may be measured from multiple sources, most frequently they are obtained from blood or urine samples; this chapter will focus on biomarkers derived from such sources. In general, a biomarker is typically a protein compound, quantifiable, easily available (at a reasonable cost and turnaround time), and indicative of the biologic process underlying the disease, providing a special insight into the microcosms surrounding the disease.

As articulated by Ibrahim and Januzzi,[1] measurement of an HF biomarker should be easily achieved through the use of assays with acceptable analytical precision and provide accurate results with well-defined biologic variation. The biomarker candidate should primarily reflect important processes involved in HF pathophysiology and should not recapitulate clinical information already available at the bedside. The study of HF biomarkers should be appropriate to the clinical use being evaluated, and design should be rigorous; new assays should be evaluated across a wide range of HF patients, and the statistical methods used to evaluate the biomarker (relative to clinical variables and other biomarkers) should be contemporary and robust.

MAJOR SOCIETY GUIDELINES

Several major societies have set forth clinical practice guidelines for the diagnosis, prognosis, and treatment of HF, including the recent update by the American Heart Association (AHA)/American College of Cardiology (ACC)/Heart Failure Society of America (HFSA) writing group on HF.[2] The use of B-type natriuretic peptide (BNP) and N-terminal B-type natriuretic peptide (NT-proBNP) is now recommended in the routine evaluation of HF for the purposes of diagnosis and in determining prognosis, but other novel applications are now supported.

TABLE 33.1   2017 American College of Cardiology/American Heart Association Heart Failure Guideline Recommendations for the Use of Biomarkers in Heart Failure[2]

Biomarkers		Class of Recommendation	Level of Evidence
BNP or NT-proBNP	Diagnosis	I	A
	Hospital admission prognosis	I	A
	Prevention	IIa	B
	Hospital discharge prognosis	IIa	B
	Guided-therapy (chronic HF)	IIb	B
Troponin T or I (myocardial injury)	Hospital admission prognosis	I	A
Soluble ST2, Galectin-3 (myocardial fibrosis)	Prognosis (chronic HF)	IIb	B

BNP, B-type natriuretic peptide; *HF*, heart failure; *NT-proBNP*, N-terminal pro–brain natriuretic peptide.

The most established applications for BNP and NT-proBNP, as noted, are for establishment of diagnosis and estimation of prognosis in HF. The most recent ACC/AHA/HFSA guideline update (**Table 33.1**) has given natriuretic peptide testing a class I (level of evidence A) for both applications. In patients with acute HF syndromes, the guidelines also put a new emphasis on use of natriuretic peptide testing to estimate risk for adverse events after discharge (class IIa, level of evidence B). As well, the guidelines also added use of BNP or NT-proBNP to identify community-based patients as at risk for new-onset HF (class IIa, level of evidence B–R). As will be discussed later, clinical practice guideline updates have also considered the role of more novel biomarkers; troponin testing for risk assessment was given a class I (level of evidence A), whereas both soluble (s)ST2 and galectin-3 (biomarkers of myocardial fibrosis) were given a class II recommendation.[2]

HEART FAILURE BIOMARKERS

A vast number of biomarkers in HF have been examined to date (examples are shown in **Table 33.2**). No single, standardized categorization of HF biomarkers exists, although several have been proposed. Braunwald suggested that markers may be considered in the following categories: (1) myocardial stretch, (2) myocyte injury, (3) extracellular matrix remodeling, (4) inflammation, (5) renal dysfunction, (6) neurohumoral activation, and (7) oxidative stress (**Fig. 33.1**).[3] Clearly, significant overlaps among these various processes exist, which may allow further simplification of biomarker categories to (1) myocardial insult, (2) neurohormonal activation, (3) myocardial remodeling, and (4) markers of comorbidity.

Myocardial Insult

Various myocardial insults are among the initiating event in the cascade of changes that occur in HF. Within the context of myocardial insult are subcategories of biomarkers that reflect myocardial stretch, myocyte necrosis, and oxidative stress.

TABLE 33.2   Biomarkers of Heart Failure

Myocardial Insult
- Myocyte stretch
  - BNP, NT-proBNP, MR-proANP
- Myocardial necrosis
  - Troponin T, troponin I, myosin light-chain kinase I, heart-type fatty-acid protein, CKMB
- Oxidative stress
  - Myeloperoxidase, uric acid, oxidized low-density lipoproteins, urinary biopyrins, urinary and plasma isoprostanes, plasma malondialdehyde

Neurohormonal Activation
- Sympathetic nervous system
  - Norepinephrine, Chromogranin A, MR-proADM
- Renin angiotensin system
  - Renin, angiotensin II, aldosterone
- Arginine vasopressin system
  - Arginine vasopressin, copeptin
- Endothelins

Remodeling
- Inflammation
  - C-reactive protein, TNF-α, Fas, soluble TNF receptors, interleukins (1, 6, and 18) osteoprotegerin
- Hypertrophy/fibrosis
  - Soluble ST2, galectin-3
- Extracellular matrix remodeling
- Collagen propeptides (PINP, PIIINP), matrix metalloproteinases (MMP-2, MMP-4, MMP-8), tissue inhibitors of MMP
- Apoptosis
  - GDF-15
- Miscellaneous
  - MicroRNA, quiescin Q6, soluble fms-like tyrosinekinase-1 (also known as VEGFR-1)

Markers of Comorbidity
- Renal biomarkers
  - Renal function
- Creatinine, BUN, eGFR, cystatin C, β trace protein
  - Renal injury markers
- NGAL, KIM-1, NAG, liver-type fatty acid binding protein, IL-18
  - Hematologic biomarkers
- Hemoglobin, RDW
- Liver function tests
- Albumin
- Adiponectin

BNP, B-type natriuretic peptide; *BUN*, blood urea nitrogen; *CKMB*, creatinine kinase, myocardial bound; *eGFR*, estimated glomerular filtration rate; *GDF*, growth differentiation factor; *KIM*, kidney injury molecule; *MMP*, matrix metalloproteinases; *MR-proANP*, midregional propeptide assay for atrial natriuretic peptide; *MR-proADM*, midregional proadrenomedullin; *NAG*, N-acetyl β-(D)-glucosaminidase; *NGAL*, neutrophil-gelatinase associated lipocalin; *NT-proBNP*, N-terminal pro–brain natriuretic peptide; *PINP*, procollagen type I amino-terminal; *PIIINP*, procollagen type III amino-terminal; *RDW*, red blood cell distribution width; *TNF*, tumor necrosis factor; *VEGFR*, vascular endothelial growth factor receptor.

Myocardial Stretch

Dense granules were noted in tissue derived from the atria of the heart by electron microscopy in the 1950s. Furthermore, stretching of the canine left atrium was shown to increase urine output, and injection

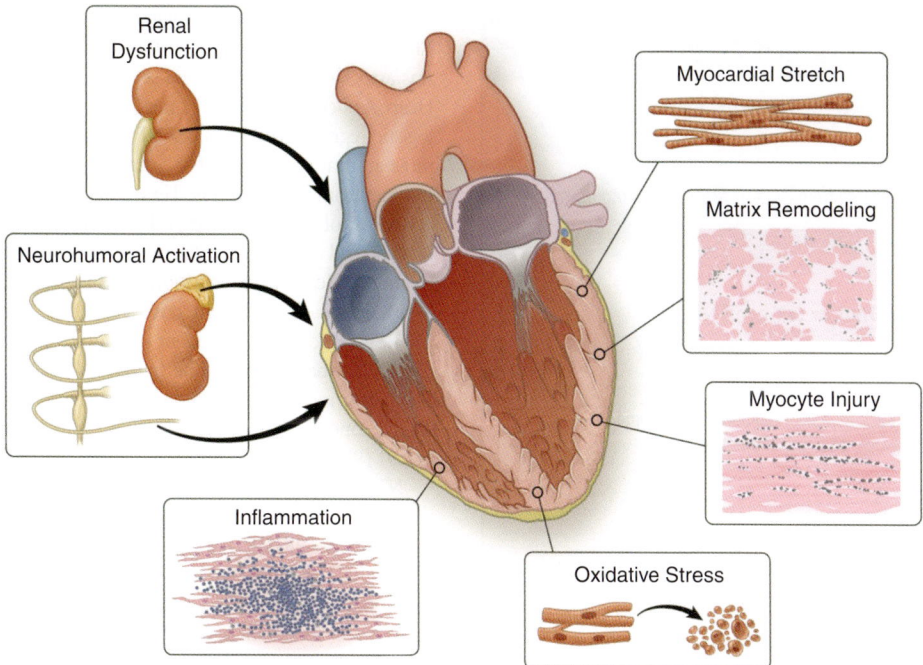

Fig. 33.1 Schema for HF Biomarker Classification.[1,3] (From Ibrahim NE, Januzzi JL. Beyond natriuretic peptides for diagnosis and management of heart failure. *Clin Chemistry*. 2017;63:211–222.)

of atrial homogenates into rats caused diuresis and natriuresis. Atrial natriuretic peptide (ANP) was subsequently purified, sequenced, and reproduced. In the 1980s, a homologous peptide with similar biologic activity was discovered in porcine brain and named BNP. Soon other natriuretic peptides, sharing similar structural features, were discovered: urodilatin (a renally active isoform of ANP), C-type natriuretic peptide, and Dendroaspis natriuretic peptide, the latter found in snake venom. Although each of the natriuretic peptide family of markers is of potential use in the evaluation and management of the patient with HF, BNP and NT-proBNP are most studied, and ANP has been increasingly examined.

BNP and NT-proBNP. Left ventricular (LV) wall stretch from increased pressure or volume is the most potent inducer of BNP gene transcription. One of the early products of the BNP gene is a 108–amino acid peptide, $proBNP_{1-108}$, which is subsequently cleaved into the biologically active 32–amino acid peptide, BNP, and a biologically inert 76 amino acid peptide, NT-proBNP. Both BNP and NT-proBNP are released into the blood stream within minutes of their synthesis. In addition, varying amounts of uncleaved $proBNP_{1-108}$ are released. Although the cause of this observation is not understood, it is now known that such concentrations of $proBNP_{1-108}$ are produced in increasing degrees in more advanced HF. Furthermore, the conventional assays for BNP or NT-proBNP measurement cross-react with circulating $proBNP_{1-108}$, which means that the overall measured natriuretic peptide value in patients evaluated clinically contains a mixture of cleaved and uncleaved peptide.

BNP binds to membrane-bound natriuretic peptide receptors (NPRs) type A and B, activating intracellular cyclic guanosine monophosphate (cGMP), beginning a cascade of events leading to natriuresis, diuresis, vasodilation, inhibition of renin and aldosterone, and inhibition of fibrosis. Besides being removed by receptor-mediated mechanisms (including by the NPR C), BNP is also degraded by various enzymatic processes, including neprilysin, meprin-A, and dipeptidyl peptidase-IV. In addition, BNP is cleared passively by numerous organs, such as the kidneys, with high blood flow. Due to the multitude of means by which BNP is removed from circulation, the half-life

of BNP is approximately 20 minutes. In contrast, NT-proBNP is only passively cleared by multiple organs, including the kidneys.

A major misconception about clearance of BNP and NT-proBNP regards to the degree of dependence on renal function for their removal from the circulation. Mechanistic studies actually suggest the degree of renal clearance to be identical for both BNP and NT-proBNP, with approximately 25% of both being cleared by renal mechanisms, down to an estimated glomerular filtration rate (eGFR) of less than 15 mL/min/1.73 m².

Extensive studies have established BNP and NT-proBNP as the "gold standard" biomarkers for the diagnosis and prognostication of HF, and emerging data suggest value for their use in the management of patients with HF.

Diagnosis. In healthy adults, circulating concentrations of BNP are quite low and women tend to have slightly higher values than men (14 vs. 8 pg/mL), with similar findings observed with NT-proBNP (<300 pg/mL). Other conditions that affect concentrations of natriuretic peptides beyond cardiac structure and function include factors that may lead to higher values (advancing age, renal dysfunction), as well as those that may lead to lower than expected values (obesity). These factors are discussed later (**Table 33.3** and **33.4**). In the context of pressure or volume overload states such as acutely decompensated HF (ADHF), BNP or NT-proBNP concentrations typically dramatically increase and sex-dependent differences becomes less relevant.

When considering the interpretation of BNP or NT-proBNP, numerous data exist currently to suggest that their concentrations reflect multiple aspects of physiology. Thus, although wall stress is a prime factor responsible for their release, a broad range of cardiac structural and functional abnormalities may trigger elevation in BNP or NT-proBNP (see Table 33.4). Appropriate interpretation of these natriuretic values in the context of each patient is crucial. **Table 33.5** details the recommended cutoff points for natriuretic peptide testing in HF.

BNP and NT-proBNP: ADHF diagnosis. In 1586 patients presenting to the emergency department with acute dyspnea, the Breathing Not Properly Study Multinational Study[4] showed that patients diagnosed with ADHF had

TABLE 33.3 Factors Influencing the Clinical Interpretation of BNP or NT-proBNP Values

Factors That Decrease BNP or NT-proBNP

- Obesity
- Flash pulmonary edema
- Heart failure etiology upstream from LV (e.g., acute mitral regurgitation, mitral stenosis)
- Cardiac tamponade
- Pericardial constriction

Factors That Increase BNP or NT-proBNP

Left ventricular dysfunction
  Hypertrophic heart muscle diseases
  Infiltrative myocardiopathies, such as amyloidosis
  Acute cardiomyopathies, such as apical ballooning syndrome
  Inflammatory, including myocarditis and chemotherapy
  Valvular heart disease
Previous heart failure
Arrhythmia
  Atrial fibrillation and flutter
Acute coronary syndromes
Cardiotoxic drugs
  Anthracyclines and related compounds
Significant pulmonary disease
  Acute respiratory distress syndrome, lung disease with right-sided heart failure, obstructive sleep apnea, pulmonary hypertension
  Pulmonary embolism
Advanced age
Renal dysfunction
Anemia
Critical illness
  Burns
  Stroke
High output states
  Sepsis
  Cirrhosis
  Hyperthyroidism

BNP, B-type natriuretic peptide; *LV*, left ventricular; *NT-proBNP*, N-terminal pro–brain natriuretic peptide.

TABLE 33.4 Cardiac Abnormalities Associated With Increased Natriuretic Peptide Concentrations

Myocardial dysfunction	• Systolic dysfunction
	• Diastolic dysfunction
	• Fibrosis/scar
	• Hypertrophy
	• Infiltrative diseases
Valvular abnormalities	• Mitral stenosis, regurgitation
	• Aortic stenosis, regurgitation
	• Tricuspid regurgitation
	• Pulmonic stenosis
Cardiac chamber size	• Ventricular enlargement
	• Atrial enlargement
Filling pressures	• Atrial, ventricular
	• Pulmonary
Ischemic heart disease	• Coronary artery ischemia
Heart rhythm abnormalities	• Atrial fibrillation, flutter
Pericardial diseases	• Constriction, tamponade
Congenital abnormalities	• Shunts, stenotic lesions

higher BNP levels compared with those without HF (mean, 675 ± 450 vs. 110 ± 225 pg/mL; $P < .001$). Furthermore, increasing concentration of BNP was associated with increasing severity of HF as evidenced by New York Heart Association (NYHA) functional class ($P < .001$). In a multivariable logistic regression analysis, a BNP greater than 100 pg/mL was the single most accurate predictor of the diagnosis of ADHF than any other single findings from history, physical examination, chest x-ray, or laboratory tests. A BNP cutoff value of 100 pg/mL had overall sensitivity of 90%, specificity of 76%, and accuracy of 85%, performing better than either the NHANES (National Health and Nutrition Examination Survey) criteria (accuracy, 67%) or the Framingham criteria for the diagnosis of HF (accuracy, 73%). BNP added independent and additive information in the diagnosis of ADHF when added to the traditional evaluation of patients with HF. The performance of BNP in the diagnosis of HF can be summarized by its receiver operating characteristic (ROC) curve area under the curve (AUC) of 0.91 (95% confidence interval [CI] 0.90–0.93; $P < .001$).

NT-proBNP has also been shown to be useful to aid in the diagnosis of ADHF. In the ProBNP Investigation of Dyspnea in the Emergency Department (PRIDE) study,[5] patients with ADHF had much higher NT-proBNP values compared with patients without HF (median, 4054 [interquartile range 1675–10028] vs. 131 [interquartile range 46–433] pg/mL; $P < .001$), increasing NT-proBNP correlated well with increasing severity of HF ($P = .001$) and was the strongest predictor of ADHF diagnosis, compared with any other single traditional findings. Despite the excellent diagnostic performance of NT-proBNP (AUC, 0.94) compared with clinical judgment alone (AUC, 0.90), the best approach in the evaluation of patients suspected of HF is a combination of both the NT-proBNP and clinical judgment (AUC, 0.96), as shown in **Fig. 33.2**. Although an NT-proBNP cutoff value of 900 pg/mL provided identical performance to that reported for a BNP of 100 pg/mL in the Breathing Not Properly Multinational Study, the International Collaborative on NT-proBNP (ICON) investigators reported that age stratification of NT-proBNP reference limits (≥450, ≥900, and ≥1800 pg/mL for ages <50, 50–75, and >75 years) improved performance even further.[6] Importantly, an NT-proBNP threshold value of less than 300 pg/mL was found to exclude ADHF with high negative predictive value. The ICON Re-evaluation of Acute Diagnostic Cut-Offs in the Emergency Department (ICON-RELOADED) Study has affirmed the value of NT-proBNP for diagnostic evaluation of ADHF in a contemporary population.[7]

Important insights from these studies include the fact that BNP and NT-proBNP were superior to radiographic standards for HF diagnosis, and both may also identify unsuspected HF in patients with underlying lung disease. Although renal function may impair the diagnostic performance of both BNP and NT-proBNP (as discussed later), with careful adjustment of reference limits, careful analyses suggest both retain utility for evaluation of patients with acute dyspnea.

As 50% of modern HF is composed of patients with preserved left ventricular ejection fraction (LVEF), it is helpful to understand the performance of BNP and NT-proBNP in those with heart failure and preserved ejection fraction (HFpEF) versus those with heart failure and reduced ejection fraction (HFrEF). Given the generally smaller LV chamber size in HFpEF, there tends to be less wall stress in such patients; accordingly, natriuretic peptide concentrations are typically lower in those with HFpEF; however, lower BNP or NT-proBNP concentrations are not pathognomonic for HFpEF by any means. The same cutoff values for BNP and NT-proBNP are recommended for the diagnosis of HF in patients with HFpEF as well as HFrEF, with the recognition that the sensitivity may be reduced in those with preserved LV function.[8,9] In this setting, values of BNP or NT-proBNP are rarely normal, but if "low," they are more likely in a range between the "rule-out" and "rule-in" thresholds (the so-called gray zone; see later). It is important to know the normal or baseline values of BNP or NT-proBNP in comparison for a given patient.

TABLE 33.5 Suggested Natriuretic Peptide Cut-Points in Heart Failure

	Cutoff Value	Sensitivity	Specificity	Positive Predictive Value	Negative Predictive Value
To Exclude Acutely Decompensated HF:					
BNP	<30–50 pg/mL	97%	–	–	96%
NT-proBNP	<300 pg/mL	99%	–	–	99%
MR-proANP	<57 pmol/L	98%	–	–	97%
To Identify Acutely Decompensated HF:					
Single cutoff point strategy					
BNP	<100 pg/mL	90%	76%	79%	89%
NT-proBNP	<900 pg/mL	90%	85%	76%	94%
MR-proANP	<127 pmol/L	87%	79%	67%	93%
Multiple cut-point strategy					
BNP, "gray zone" approach	<100 pg/mL to exclude	90%	73%	75%	90%
	100–400 pg/mL, "gray zone"	–	–	–	–
	>400 pg/mL, to rule in	63%	91%	86%	74%
NT-proBNP, "age-stratified" approach	<450 pg/mL for age <50 years	90%	84%	88%	66%
	<900 pg/mL for age 50–75 years				
	<1800 pg/mL for age >75 years				
MR-proANP, "age-stratified" approach	<104 pmol/L for age <65 years	82%	86%	75%	91%
	214 pmol/L for age ≥65 years				
Outpatient Application					
BNP	20 pg/mL (asymptomatic)	–	–	–	96%
	or 40 pg/mL (symptomatic)				
NT-proBNP, "age stratified" approaches	<125 pg/mL for age <75 years	–	–	–	98%
	<450 pg/mL for age ≥75 years	–	–	–	91%
	or				
	<50 pg/mL for age <50 years	–	–	–	98%
	<75 pg/mL for age 50–75 years	–	–	–	98%
	<250 pg/mL for age >75 years	–	–	–	93%
MR-proANP	Unknown	Unknown	Unknown	Unknown	Unknown

BNP, B-type natriuretic peptide; *HF*, heart failure; *MR-proANP*, midregional propeptide assay for atrial natriuretic peptide; *NT-proBNP*, N-terminal pro–brain natriuretic peptide.

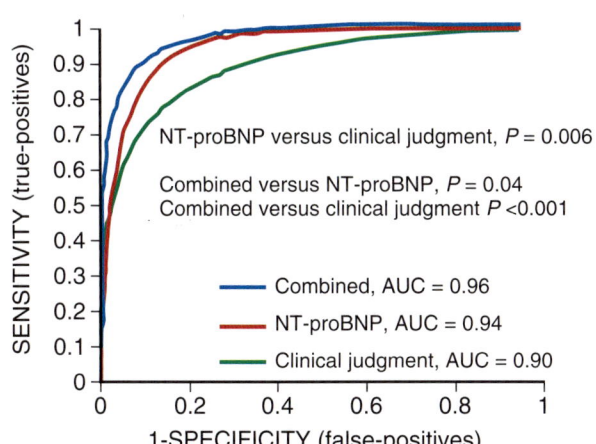

Fig. 33.2 Comparison of NT-proBNP Versus Clinical Judgment for the Diagnosis of Acutely Decompensated Heart Failure. (From Januzzi JL, Jr, Camargo CA, Anwaruddin S, et al. The N-terminal Pro-BNP investigation of dyspnea in the emergency department [PRIDE] study. *Am J Cardiol.* 2005;95:948–954.)

Relative to the added value of natriuretic peptide testing when put together with standard clinical evaluation, the B-type natriuretic peptide for Acute Shortness of breath EvaLuation (BASEL),[10] the Improved Management of Patients With Congestive Heart Failure (IMPROVE-CHF),[11] and the NT-proBNP for EValuation of dyspneic patients in the Emergency Room and hospital (BNP4EVER)[12] studies all indicated an advantage to use of either BNP or NT-proBNP when added to clinical judgment. For example, in both BASEL and IMPROVE-CHF, the use of BNP and NT-proBNP, respectively, led to considerable cost savings, findings echoed by Siebert and colleagues in a report from the PRIDE study.[13] In BASEL, the use of BNP was associated with less use of intensive care unit admission, without excess hazard with such care. In the IMPROVE-CHF study, not only was NT-proBNP–supplemented evaluation superior diagnostically, but patients in the NT-proBNP arm also had better short-term outcomes.

When considering the appropriate application of BNP or NT-proBNP for diagnostic evaluation of ADHF, it is worth reviewing the circumstances where testing is most valuable. As shown by Green and colleagues,[14] indecision when evaluating patients with acute dyspnea occurs in approximately 30% of cases seen in the emergency department and is associated with considerably higher short-term risk. Results by Steinhart and colleagues from the IMPROVE-CHF study lend important clarity regarding the importance of natriuretic peptide testing in this setting;

although NT-proBNP correctly (and significantly) reclassified diagnoses in patients judged with confidence in this study, the value of the biomarker was considerably greater in those with uncertain diagnosis. These findings inform the current class I guideline recommendations for use of BNP or NT-proBNP for ADHF diagnosis.[2]

BNP and NT-proBNP: chronic HF diagnosis.

Not surprisingly, both BNP and NT-proBNP have been shown to be useful in the diagnosis of HF in the outpatient setting. However, in contrast to the diagnostic application of BNP or NT-proBNP in the acute environment, both peptides have been mainly examined relative to their negative predictive value to exclude the diagnosis, rather than to confirm it. In this regard, the optimal reference limits for use in this setting are considerably lower than in patients with acute dyspnea (see Table 33.5). For NT-proBNP, the ICON-Primary Care group[15] showed that age stratification again improves diagnostic accuracy in this setting. If a patient is found to be greater than the BNP or NT-proBNP cutoffs, further diagnostic testing such as echocardiography is likely needed. Causes of falsely low BNP or NT-proBNP in the outpatient setting are comparable to those with acute dyspnea.

Another potential use of BNP or NT-proBNP in the nonacute setting is for screening at-risk patients for the presence of underlying structural heart disease. Although influenced by numerous cardiac correlates (see Table 33.4), a single measurement of BNP or NT-proBNP may be able to identify reduced LV function in asymptomatic individuals; in addition, in recognition of their dependence on diastolic indices, as well for their concentrations, both peptides may be useful also in screening for diastolic ventricular dysfunction.

Natriuretic peptides: caveats.

Despite the promising information conveyed by BNP or NT-proBNP in the evaluation of HF patients, there are several important limitations that need to be considered in the interpretation of their results; several factors have been shown to alternately lead to higher than expected BNP or NT-proBNP values, as well as lower than expected values (see Table 33.3). Beyond age, as discussed previously, a number of diagnoses have been associated with increased natriuretic peptide levels, as detailed in Table 33.3.[16] Clinical judgment when interpreting natriuretic peptide concentrations is crucial: as with any diagnostic test, a differential diagnosis should be kept in mind when interpreting an elevated BNP or NT-proBNP value.

Although discussed previously, the importance of renal function in the interpretation of BNP or NT-proBNP deserves more detail. Patients with chronic kidney disease typically have higher BNP and NT-proBNP values. Mechanistically, this is due both to peptide accumulation, as well as increased release of BNP or NT-proBNP due to shared comorbidities such as hypertension, LV hypertrophy, and chronic volume overload. In patients with renal insufficiency (GFR <60 mL/min/1.73 m^2), a BNP cutoff of 200 pg/mL or NT-proBNP of 1200 pg/mL provides good diagnostic performance; alternatively, the age-stratified NT-proBNP cutoffs may be used with good accuracy and without adjustment.[17] Furthermore, both BNP and NT-proBNP are considerably prognostic in patients with chronic kidney disease, even in the absence of overt cardiovascular disease; NT-proBNP may even predict progression of renal dysfunction in population studies.

Notably, BNP and NT-proBNP levels are lower in overweight and obese patients. This phenomenon is hypothesized to be due to suppression of synthesis or release of natriuretic peptides in obese subjects. However, regardless of body mass index (BMI), BNP, or NT-proBNP concentrations are typically higher in patients with HF compared with patients without, and age-adjusted cutoff points retain usefulness for the diagnosis of acute HF. In the PRIDE study of acute dyspnea patients,[18] ROC analyses of NT-proBNP for diagnosis of acute HF had AUC of 0.94 for lean, 0.95 for overweight, and 0.94 for obese patients. An NT-proBNP value less than 300 pg/mL still had excellent diagnostic performance in ruling out acute HF across all BMI categories.

When a patient has a BNP or NT-proBNP between the optimized cutoff to exclude HF and the optimized cutoff to diagnose it, this is referred to as a "gray zone" result. van Kimmenade and colleagues reported that patients with a gray zone NT-proBNP in ICON were more likely to have ADHF when physical findings, such as elevated jugular venous pressure or pulmonary rales, were present.[19] In addition, although complicating biomarker-based evaluation of the patient with suspected HF, gray zone values have prognostic meaning, above that of patients with lower concentrations of BNP or NT-proBNP. This informs another strength of BNP and NT-proBNP: the estimation of prognosis across the spectrum of HF.

An important development has been approval of a novel class of HF therapy, the angiotensin receptor/neprilysin inhibitor (ARNI; e.g., sacubitril/valsartan); this drug was recently embedded as a class I, level of evidence (LOE) B-R therapy into HF treatment guidelines (**see also Chapter 37**).[2] The mechanism of action of this class of drug includes blockade of the angiotensin II receptor together with neprilysin. The latter is a ubiquitous zinc-dependent metalloproteinase involved in degradation of numerous vasoactive peptides involved in cardiovascular regulation, including biologically active natriuretic peptides. Thus concentrations of ANP, BNP, and C-type natriuretic peptide (CNP) are all thought to be affected by inhibition of neprilysin; in the context of therapy with sacubitril/valsartan, concentrations of BNP tend to rise. In contrast, NT-proBNP is not a substrate for neprilysin, so its concentrations tend to fall in the setting of neprilysin inhibition.

In the phase 2 Prospective Comparison of ARNI with ARB on Management of HFpEF (PARAMOUNT) trial, 301 patients with chronic HFpEF, NYHA class II–III symptoms, and elevated natriuretic peptide concentrations were treated with sacubitril/valsartan versus valsartan alone. At 12 weeks, ARNI therapy reduced NT-proBNP and increased BNP concentrations compared with valsartan alone.[20] More recently, in the Angiotensin-Neprilysin Inhibition versus Enalapril in Heart Failure (PARADIGM-HF) trial,[21] measurement of BNP and NT-proBNP concentrations in patients with HFrEF were made at baseline, 4 weeks, and 8 months. A significant increase in measured BNP concentrations was seen at 4 weeks after treatment with sacubitril/valsartan, and at 8 months patients treated with neprilysin inhibition still had higher concentrations of BNP when compared with those treated with enalapril. Conversely, those treated with sacubitril/valsartan had early and sustained reduction in NT-proBNP across the duration of the study.

A post hoc analysis of 2080 patients in the PARADIGM-HF demonstrated that higher posttreatment NT-proBNP concentrations predicted outcomes such as cardiovascular death or HF hospitalization. Those HFrEF patients with significant posttreatment NT-proBNP reductions had lower subsequent rates of such adverse outcomes, independent of whether the patients were treated with angiotensin-converting enzyme inhibition (i.e., enalapril) or with neprilysin inhibition (i.e., sacubitril/valsartan).[22]

Uncertainties abound with respect to how neprilysin inhibits BNP, including vagaries about how much "rise" is expected from treatment alone, whether the peptide remains prognostic in those taking sacubitril/valsartan, and how durable the effect of the "rise" in BNP may be over time. In addition, to the extent the numerous available BNP immunoassays are based on different antibody pairs, it is not even certain all assays are affected similarly by neprilysin inhibition; given that neprilysin degrades the BNP in multiple sites (**Fig. 33.3**), it is reasonable to suspect differences will be modest, but this is presently unknown.

Given these uncertainties, although data are limited, it is fair to suggest NT-proBNP as the preferred biomarker when measuring natriuretic peptides in patients taking sacubitril/valsartan.

BNP and NT-proBNP: prognosis.

Concentrations of BNP or NT-proBNP are strong predictors of future clinical outcomes in a variety of populations spanning all stages of HF articulated by the ACC/AHA guidelines: from patients without any cardiac dysfunction

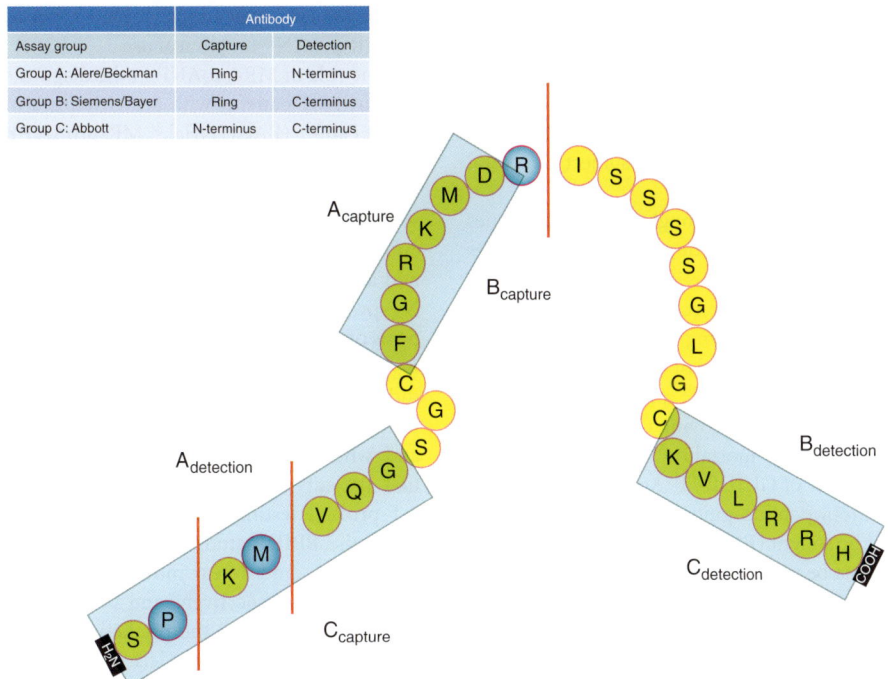

	Antibody	
Assay group	Capture	Detection
Group A: Alere/Beckman	Ring	N-terminus
Group B: Siemens/Bayer	Ring	C-terminus
Group C: Abbott	N-terminus	C-terminus

Fig. 33.3 The structure of BNP, the zones bound by typical immunoassays used clinically for BNP and NT-proBNP measurement, and the areas where neprilysin cleaves the BNP ring. Boxes indicate sites of binding of either the capture or detection antibodies for the tests used for BNP measurement, while the cleavage sites identified by the blue amino acid target for neprilysin along with where the peptide is divided.

but at high risk of developing HF in the future (stage A), through patients with asymptomatic LV dysfunction (stage B), to symptomatic HF (stage C) and advanced HF (stage D).

The largest body of data supporting the use of BNP and NT-proBNP is in patients with ADHF. The Acute Decompensated Heart Failure National Registry (ADHERE)[23] showed that higher admission BNP values were associated with increased in-hospital mortality among 48,629 patients admitted to the hospital with ADHF. Moreover, there was a linear relationship between increasing quartile of BNP and in-hospital mortality, even after adjusting for potential confounders such as age, gender, systolic blood pressure, pulse, renal function, sodium, and dyspnea in both HFpEF and HFrEF patients. In a similar manner, admission NT-proBNP concentrations were found to be strongly predictive of both short- and long-term clinical outcomes.[6,24] NT-proBNP values greater than 986 pg/mL predicted death at 1-year ($P < .001$, 79% sensitivity and 68% specificity), even after adjusting for relevant traditional factors. Some studies have examined the role of follow-up BNP or NT-proBNP measurement compared with admission. Indeed, discharge natriuretic peptides obtained after inpatient treatment for ADHF appeared to be even more predictive of future mortality and/or rehospitalization when compared with admission values. This application for hospital discharge risk assessment is discussed further, later.

In chronic HF, serial assessment with BNP and NT-proBNP for prognosis has been shown to be of value. In a large population of ambulatory patients with chronic stable HF enrolled in the Valsartan Heart Failure Trial (Val-HeFT) study, NT-proBNP was measured at baseline and at 4 months; although baseline values were prognostically important, changes in NT-proBNP concentrations over 4 months and relationship to all-cause mortality were more important in providing prognostic information.[25] Thus, in analogy to those patients with acute symptoms, serial assessment of BNP or NT-proBNP appears to provide incremental data regarding likelihood for adverse outcome. Mechanistically, elevated values of NT-proBNP in chronic HF not only predict adverse outcome but also identify patients at highest risk for deleterious LV remodeling.

An emerging application for BNP or NT-proBNP is to predict cardiovascular risk in apparently unaffected patients in the population. In 3346 asymptomatic subjects without HF from the Framingham Offspring Study,[26] baseline elevated concentrations of BNP or NT-proBNP strongly predicted future clinical outcomes, including all-cause mortality, first major cardiovascular event, HF, atrial fibrillation, and stroke or transient ischemia attack; most notably, BNP levels greater than 80th percentile (20.0 for men and 23.3 pg/mL for women) were associated with a 62% increase in the risk of death, 76% increase in first cardiovascular event, and 307% increase in the risk of HF (all $P < .05$). Similar results were found with NT-proBNP, where values greater than 80th percentile (497 for men and 541 pg/mL for women) were associated with a 76% increase in the risk of death, 52% increase in first cardiovascular event, and 502% increase in the risk of HF (all $P < .05$). Much as in acute and chronic coronary syndromes, serial measurement of natriuretic peptides in the community may inform risk for future HF better than a single assessment. For example, among ambulatory elderly patients without prevalent HF at baseline, DeFilippi and colleagues demonstrated that a baseline NT-proBNP greater than 190 pg/mL predicted incident HF during follow-up; however, a second measurement added considerable prognostic information; those with rising concentrations of NT-proBNP had substantial risk for incident HF (adjusted hazard ratio [HR] 2.13; 95% CI 1.68–2.71) and cardiovascular death (HR 1.91; 95% CI 1.43–2.53) compared with those with sustained low concentrations.[27]

BNP and NT-proBNP: management of HF. Coupled with their dynamic and prognostically meaningful behavior in the context of HF treatment is the interesting observation that natriuretic peptide concentrations appear to fall in the context of treatment with therapies shown to improve long-term mortality in HF, including beta-blockers, angiotensin-converting enzyme inhibitors, angiotensin II receptor blockers, and mineralocorticoid receptor antagonists, as well as cardiac resynchronization therapy.[28] Significant reduction in BNP or NT-proBNP concentrations typically occur within 2 to 4 weeks of successful therapy titration, allowing for a defined window for resampling and assessment for benefit of therapy. The obvious exception to this rule is if patients are treated with an ARNI, wherein a rise in BNP is expected, with reduction in NT-proBNP.

The concept of using BNP or NT-proBNP as a "guide" to HF care, with a goal of achieving excellent guideline-derived medical therapy plus natriuretic peptide suppression, has been the subject of several clinical trials.

Following the seminal pilot study by Troughton and colleagues from the Christchurch Cardioendocrine Group,[29] numerous studies have explored the topic of BNP- or NT-proBNP–guided HF care, with mixed outcomes.[30] The largest and most recent of these studies was the Guiding Evidence Based Therapy Using Biomarker Intensified Treatment in Heart Failure (GUIDE-IT) trial of 894 high-risk patients with chronic HFrEF. This study did not find NT-proBNP–guided therapy more effective than usual care in improving outcomes including HF hospitalization and cardiovascular mortality.[31]

Caveats exist about the result of GUIDE-IT. Aggregate experience would dictate that for natriuretic peptide–guided HF care to be successful, a low target value must be sought (BNP <100 pg/mL; NT-proBNP <1000 pg/mL), therapies must be titrated to lower the natriuretic peptide concentrations, and significant lowering of the biomarkers must occur. In those trials that had these three characteristics, substantial improvement in outcomes was observed.[29,32,33] In GUIDE-IT, no differences were seen with respect to guideline-directed medical therapy (GDMT) and no differences in achieved NT-proBNP concentration: 46% of participants in the biomarker-guided arm and 40% of the usual care group achieved an NT-proBNP less than 1000 pg/L at 12 months (P = .21). To achieve this substantial NT-proBNP lowering in the "usual care" arm, patients were seen nearly monthly, on average. In addition, most of the GUIDE-IT study investigators practiced at academic tertiary care referral centers. Thus it remains uncertain if the "usual care" in GUIDE-IT was a fair representation of usual HFrEF care in nonacademic centers.

Meta-analyses combining findings from existing studies have shown a 20% to 30% mortality reduction associated with biomarker-guided HF management over standard HF care, nonetheless suggesting merit of this approach.[34] The GUIDE-IT study suggests aggressively managed, frequently seen patients may not profit from this approach; future studies focusing the intervention on patients treated in a more typical fashion are needed.

Biomarkers have also been used to identify at-risk patients who may benefit from aggressive titration of guideline-directed medical therapies. Huelsmann and colleagues examined 300 patients with type 2 diabetes and an elevated NT-proBNP (<125 pg/mL) but free of cardiac disease and determined that those randomized to the intensified group who had uptitration of renin-angiotensin system antagonists and beta-blockers in a cardiologist's office had significant reduction in the primary endpoint of hospitalization/death due to cardiac disease at 2 years compared with the control group (HR 0.351; 95% CI 0.127–0.975; P = .044). The same was true for other end points: all-cause hospitalization and unplanned cardiovascular hospitalizations/death (P < .05 for all).[35]

Emerging natriuretic peptide tests: MR-proANP. In parallel to the B-type peptides, circulating levels of ANP rapidly increase with cardiac stretch; unlike BNP, whose production is induced after myocyte stretch, ANP is premade and stored in the myocardium, predominantly in the atrium. However, reliable detection of circulating ANP is challenging because its half-life is only 2 to 5 minutes due to effects of neprilysin. However, its immediate precursor protein, proANP, is stable and has a longer half-life, which makes serum measurement possible. The development of a midregional propeptide assay for atrial natriuretic peptide (MR-proANP) assay has led to the examination of

its use for HF applications. Table 33.5 details suggested cutoff points for MR-proANP for clinical use.

The role of MR-proANP in the diagnosis of ADHF was first examined in 1641 patients with acute dyspnea in the Biomarkers in Acute Heart Failure (BACH) trial.[36] MR-proANP performed well in diagnosing ADHF and was noninferior to BNP or NT-proBNP; a MR-proANP cutoff point of greater than or equal to 120 pmol/L had a sensitivity of 97% and specificity of 60% with accuracy of 74%, whereas BNP with a cutoff point of 100 pg/mL had a sensitivity of 96%, specificity of 62%, and accuracy of 73%. In the PRIDE study analysis of MR-proANP,[37] NT-proBNP performed slightly better than MR-proANP in the diagnosis of ADHF (AUC of 0.94 for NT-proBNP vs. 0.90 for MR-proBNP; P = .001 for difference); however, MR-proANP was found to be an independent predictor of HF diagnosis even with NT-proBNP in a multivariable model (odds ratio, 4.34; 95% CI 2.11–8.92; P < .001) and when added to NT-proBNP measurement, correctly reclassified patients who had false-negative and false-positive results by NT-proBNP testing alone.

In the PRIDE study,[37] MR-proANP strongly and independently predicted 1- and 4-year mortality (adjusted HR 2.99, P < .001, and 3.12, P < .001, respectively) and addition of NT-proBNP to these models did not attenuate the predictive power of MR-proANP. Adding MR-proANP to base models containing NT-proBNP significantly improved the C-statistic at 1 and 4 years and reclassified mortality risk as a part of a multimarker strategy in determining prognosis.

In chronic HF, the Gruppo Italiano per lo Studio della Sopravvivenza nell'Insufficienza Cardiaca–Heart Failure (GISSI-HF) study[38] examined the predictive power of MR-proANP in stable chronic HF patients. Investigators found that an MR-proANP greater than or equal to 278 pmol/L had the best prognostic accuracy for 4-year mortality among several novel and established biomarkers including NT-proBNP, midregional proadrenomedullin (MR-proADM), C-terminal provasopressin (copeptin), and C-terminal pro-endothelin-1 (AUC of 0.74, 95% CI 0.70–0.76). In addition, MR-proANP added independent prognostic information beyond NT-proBNP and relevant clinical characteristics in a reclassification analysis. Using the same biomarkers, only the change in MR-proANP over 3 months was found to be significant in predicting mortality.

Although initial data from the BACH study suggested that MR-proANP was less likely to be affected by covariates that reduce diagnostic accuracy of BNP or NT-proBNP (such as age, renal function, or obesity), subsequent data from other sources suggest that factors influencing BNP or NT-proBNP are quite likely to exert a similar effect on MR-proANP.[37] As an example, Richards and colleagues recently reported that atrial fibrillation reduced the diagnostic accuracy of MR-proANP for ADHF diagnosis just as much as it did BNP or NT-proBNP.[39]

Cardiac Necrosis

Cardiac troponins. In the context of cardiomyocyte necrosis, disruption of normal cardiomyocyte membrane results in the inner contents of the damaged cells to be released into the extracellular space; a variety of cellular and structural proteins such as troponin, creatine kinase, myoglobin, and cardiac fatty acid binding protein is released into circulation and become detectable in peripheral blood. Of these, cardiac troponins have rapidly become the standard of care biomarker in diagnosing myocardial infarction (MI). Cardiac troponins levels have also been found to be elevated in nonacute MI settings; one such setting is in HF.

The exact mechanism behind the release of troponins in HF is unclear but may be related to either increased myocyte membrane permeability or necrosis. A variety of HF mechanisms are involved in the release of troponin: inflammation, neurohormonal activation, ventricular stretch, increased wall tension, supply-demand mismatch, cytotoxicity, cellular necrosis, apoptosis, or autophagy. Regardless, increased circulating levels of cardiac troponins in HF patients have been shown to be closely linked to future clinical outcomes. With the development and application of highly sensitive cardiac troponin (hsTn) assays that can accurately detect even minute concentrations, most patients with HF are found to have detectable levels of cardiac troponins with a substantial percentage demonstrating concentrations of the biomarker above the upper reference limit for a normal patient population, even in the absence of ischemic heart disease.

In the ADHERE,[40] 4240 patients (6.2%) out of 69,259 patients with ADHF had an elevated troponin, and in this context, higher in-hospital mortality (8.0% vs. 2.7%, $P < .001$) was observed, with an adjusted odds ratio for death of 2.55 (95% CI 2.24–2.89, $P < .001$) compared with patients with negative troponin measurement. Using an hsTnT assay,[41] 30.6% of patients with ADHF were found to have elevated troponin values. In a multivariable model that included NT-proBNP and the interleukin (IL) receptor family member, sST2, hsTnT remained a significant and independent predictor of all-cause mortality with an HR of 1.16 (95% CI 1.09–1.24, $P < .001$). In a multimarker strategy, patients with all three biomarkers less than their optimal cutoff point had the best survival (0% death) at a median follow-up of 739 days, whereas 53% of those with elevation of all three biomarkers died. In integrated discrimination analyses, the use of all three markers in a multimarker approach was the best model for mortality prediction. As might be expected, the use of a highly sensitive assay was particularly helpful in determining the prognosis in patients with undetectable conventional TnT concentrations.

Although the prognostic ramification of an elevated troponin in patients with ADHF is clear, the therapeutic steps to follow with such an elevated value remain less well defined. Nonetheless, given the great importance of acute MI in the precipitation of ADHF, current position statements recommend the universal measurement of troponin in patients with acute symptoms, to primarily diagnose or exclude an ischemic cause for the presentation.[42]

In chronic HF, cardiac troponin levels are also frequently increased, and in analogy to ADHF, such elevations are prognostic. When using a conventional assay, only approximately 10% of patients had detectable TnT out of the 4035 stable chronic HF patients in the Val-HeFT study.[43] Not surprisingly, detectable troponin concentration was associated with an increased risk of death (HR 2.08, 95% CI 1.72–2.52) and first hospitalization for HF (HR 1.55, 95% CI 1.25–1.93) at 2 years in a model that adjusted for traditional risk factors. When hsTnT was measured in this same cohort, troponin was detectable in 92% of the cohort and predicted future adverse outcomes (HR 1.05, 95% CI 1.04–1.07, $P < .001$) as well as LV remodeling. Adding hsTnT to a baseline model including BNP and relevant clinical predictors significantly improved prognostic discrimination. Combining patients from both the Val-HeFT study and the GISSI-HF study, investigators looked at the role of serial hsTnT measurement in 5284 patients with chronic HF.[44] Increases in hsTnT over 3 to 4 months of follow-up strongly predicted all-cause mortality (adjusted HR 1.59, 95% CI 1.39–1.82 and 1.88, 95% CI 1.50–2.35 after adjustment for traditional risk factors, baseline hsTnT, and baseline NT-proBNP), but improvement in test performance was only modest over a single baseline measurement of hsTnT.

Concentrations of troponin—particularly when measured with a highly sensitive method—may be of use to predict the onset of HF in apparently healthy individuals. For example, hsTnT measurement was found to be useful in predicting future development of HF in 4221 older, community-dwelling adults; hsTnT >12.94 pg/mL was associated with

HF incidence rate of 6.4 per 100 person-years (95% CI 5.8–7.2) and an adjusted HR of 2.48 (95% CI 2.04–3.00).[45] An elevated hsTnT was also predictive of future cardiovascular death (incidence rate of 4.8, 95% CI 4.3–5.4 and adjusted HR 2.91, 95% CI 0.9–1.2 compared with those with undetectable hsTnT). A repeat hsTnT measurement in 2 to 3 years showed that among patients with detectable hsTnT at baseline, greater than 50% change in hsTnT was associated with an even higher risk for HF (adjusted HR 1.61, 95% CI 1.32–1.97) and cardiovascular death (adjusted HR 1.65, 95% CI 1.35–2.03), whereas a decrease in hsTnT was associated with a lower risk for developing HF and having cardiovascular death. In a lower risk cohort from the Framingham Heart Study, Wang and colleagues similarly demonstrated the prognostic importance of hsTnI for predicting death and HF onset, even when extensively adjusted for relevant covariates, including other biomarkers.[46]

Oxidative Stress

Reactive oxygen species (ROS) are the by-product of normal aerobic metabolism and are involved in a variety of intracellular proteins and signaling pathways, including vital proteins involved in myocardial excitation-contraction coupling and myocyte growth. Under normal circumstances, ROS are scavenged and neutralized by antioxidants. However, in pathologic conditions such as HF, free radicals are present in relative excess to the antioxidants, creating a state of oxidative stress, which can exert direct toxic effect on myocardial structure and function. An important biomarker of oxidative stress is myeloperoxidase (MPO), a 150-kDa protein. MPO is found in blood neutrophils, and through its activity produces hypochlorous acid, a potently oxidative cytotoxic compound. MPO appears to be prognostic in both acute and chronic HF; in acute settings, MPO may be additively prognostic to BNP for forecasting death by 1 year. In chronic HF, Tang and colleagues reported that MPO values were prognostic, even when adjusted for relevant covariates.[47] Reichlin et al. showed that MPO concentrations greater than 99 pmol/L were associated with significantly increased 1-year mortality (HR 1.58, $P = .02$). The combination of MPO and BNP improved the prediction of 1-year mortality (HR 2.80, $P < .001$).[48]

Uric acid. Xanthine oxidase is an important source of ROS, including superoxide anion and hydrogen peroxide. Serum uric acid has been shown to reflect the degree of xanthine oxidase activation in HF; in addition, uric acid may be a marker of cell death when other purines are degraded. When elevated, uric acid appears to predict HF onset; in 4912 unaffected participants from the Framingham Offspring Study, incident HF was approximately six times higher in patients with the highest quartile of serum uric acid level (≥6.3 mg/dL) compared with those at the lowest quartile (<3.4 mg/dL), with an adjusted HR of 2.1 (95% CI 1.04–4.22).[49]

Beyond its link to incident HF, there is a strong association of serum uric acid with severity of the diagnosis with a particularly important role for prognostication. For example, among 112 patients with chronic HF, in a multivariable Cox model containing relevant clinical, biochemical, and mechanical characteristics, uric acid remained independently predictive of clinical outcomes ($P < .0001$), although to less extent after adjustment. This association is less likely due to uric acid itself, but rather indicative of uric acid's role in xanthine oxidase activation; decreasing uric acid levels with a uricosuric agent, probenecid, did not improve endothelial function in HF, but inhibition of xanthine oxidase with allopurinol did.[50] Disappointingly, strategies to reduce ROS have not shown clinical benefit in HF outcomes in randomized controlled trials. In the Oxypurinol Therapy in Congestive Heart Failure (OPT-CHF) study,[51] oxipurinol, a xanthine oxidase inhibitor, reduced uric acid levels but failed to show improvement in the composite primary end point that included hospitalization and cardiovascular death.

Neurohormonal Activation

Cardiac insults such as reduced LV function trigger production of biologically active neurohormones to compensate for reduced myocardial function; the net effect of these peptides is to increase retention of salt and water, peripheral arterial vasoconstriction, and contractility. These effects are responsible for raising blood pressure, improving perfusion of vital organs, and activation of inflammatory mediators responsible for cardiac repair and remodeling. However, overexpression and prolonged activation of the same proteins ultimately lead to deleterious long-term effects on the heart and the circulation and end up contributing to progression of HF.

Sympathetic Nervous System

One of the first responses to cardiac and circulatory dysfunction is the activation of the sympathetic nervous system and inhibition of the parasympathetic tone, resulting in relative excess function of the adrenergic nervous system.

Norepinephrine. Activation of the sympathetic nervous system in HF results in an increased circulating concentration of the potent adrenergic neurotransmitter, norepinephrine. Elevated norepinephrine results in increased heart rate and myocardial contraction, as well as peripheral vasoconstriction, but at the expense of increased energy requirement. Interestingly, in advanced HF patients, there is a paradoxical decline in myocardial concentration of norepinephrine as HF progresses. The mechanism behind this phenomenon of norepinephrine depletion is unclear but may be related to decreased stimulation with prolonged adrenergic activation, deregulation of the synthesis of norepinephrine, or decreased reuptake of norepinephrine.

Chromogranin A. Chromogranin A (CgA) is a major component of chromaffin granules that are stored and released together in the adrenal glands with catecholamines such as norepinephrine. CgA has also been found in the heart and colocalized to the atrial and ventricular myocardium with ANP and BNP. It has been shown that CgA is the precursor of several biologically active proteins, including vasostatin-1 and catestatin, and is intimately involved in the regulation of the adrenergic system activation. However, the exact mechanism and effect on the heart remain to be resolved. CgA levels are elevated in both acute and chronic HF syndromes and are directly related to severity of HF, although its ability to diagnose ADHF is poor.

Adrenomedullin. Adrenomedullin is a potent vasodilator with cyclic adenosine monophosphate (AMP)–independent inotropic properties that was originally found to be produced by pheochromocytoma cells, arising from the adrenal medulla. Adrenomedullin concentrations are elevated in patients with chronic HF, in those with diastolic LV dysfunction, and restrictive filling, and adrenomedullin concentrations increase with HF severity. However, adrenomedullin itself is a target for neprilysin and is thus biologically unstable rendering it difficult to reliably measure; to address this, a novel assay measuring the midregion of a more stable prohormone, proadrenomedullin, was recently developed (MR-proADM). Much like its parent compound, MR-proADM is elevated in patients with HF and has been found to be a remarkably strong predictor of early mortality, adding value beyond BNP or NT-proBNP.[36,37]

In a study of chronic HF, MR-proADM was a strong and independent predictor of 18-month all-cause mortality (risk ratio 3.92, 95% CI 1.76–8.7) and HF hospitalization (risk ratio 2.4, 95% CI 1.3–4.5) even after a full adjustment for other biomarkers and clinical factors.[52] Notably, in this analysis from the Australia–New Zealand HF study, an interaction was found between carvedilol treatment and MR-proADM concentrations; in patients with greater than the median values of MR-proADM, treatment with carvedilol significantly reduced the risk of death or HF hospitalizations. Shah et al. showed that among patients

with acute dyspnea MR-proADM had high AUC for mortality during the first year from enrollment (0.792); other biomarkers were more powerfully predictive for later death, although MR-proADM remained independently prognostic of mortality to 4 years of follow-up.[53] More information is needed regarding MR-proADM before routine clinical use can be recommended.

Renin-Angiotensin-Aldosterone System

Most components of the renin-angiotensin-aldosterone system can be measured in patients with HF; however, circulating concentrations of these hormones do not necessarily reflect the local tissue activities of these entities, and their measurement is complicated and costly. Plasma renin activity and aldosterone concentration are often normal in patient with chronic stable HF, despite evidence of increased local activity of angiotensin II and angiotensin-converting enzyme in the heart. In the setting of ADHF, circulating levels of renin, angiotensin II, and aldosterone appear to increase but, again, may not fully reflect the tissue activities of these entities.

Arginine vasopressin. Sympathetic stimulation can also lead to increased release of arginine vasopressin (AVP), also known as vasopressin or antidiuretic hormone, from the posterior pituitary. AVP plays a central role in the regulation of free water clearance and plasma osmolality by increasing absorption of water from the collecting ducts of the kidneys. It also increases peripheral vasoconstriction and endothelin production, which further increases arterial blood pressure.

Circulating levels of AVP are elevated in patients with severe HF, but reliable measurement is quite challenging, similar to challenges posed by measurement of ANP or adrenomedullin. However, the C-terminal segment of the precursor of provasopressin, copeptin, is a reliable surrogate marker for AVP and has been reported to be a suitable surrogate, predictive of adverse outcomes in patients with ADHF, and predicts cardiovascular outcomes in patients with chronic HF independent of NT-proBNP and troponin. Although it is tempting to speculate that elevated concentrations of copeptin might identify those HF patients most likely to benefit from therapy with vasopressin receptor antagonists, this concept has yet to be comprehensively explored.

Endothelin. Endothelins are vasoconstrictive peptides that may play a role in the development and exacerbation of HF, as well as pulmonary hypertension. Big endothelin-1 is a 39–amino acid propeptide that is cleaved into the biologically active endothelin-1; both have been shown to be elevated in patients with HF and predict the presence of elevated pulmonary pressures, as well as mortality. In the VAL-HeFT trial, concentrations of both big endothelin-1 and endothelin-1 were prognostic, even when adjusted for other relevant biomarkers and clinical factors. Although it is possible that measurement of endothelin-1 might be useful to predict benefit from drugs that oppose its biological activity, such data are not yet available. Data from the Catheter Sampled Blood Archive in Cardiovascular Diseases (CASABLANCA) trial[54] shows that endothelin-1 may be predictive of incident HF in patients undergoing coronary angiography for various indications.

Myocardial Remodeling

Activation of the neurohormonal system does not fully explain the continued progression of HF in patients whose neurohormonal system appears to have stabilized. Ventricular remodeling is a deleterious process by which cellular and structural changes occur in the LV myocardium, resulting in dilation and reduced function; eventually, if unchecked, remodeling may result in worsening LVEF and progressively worse prognosis. Conversely, beneficial therapies for HF such as angiotensin-converting enzyme (ACE) inhibitors or angiotensin II receptor blockers, beta-blockers, mineralocorticoid inhibitors, or cardiac resynchronization therapy may result in favorable "reverse" remodeling.

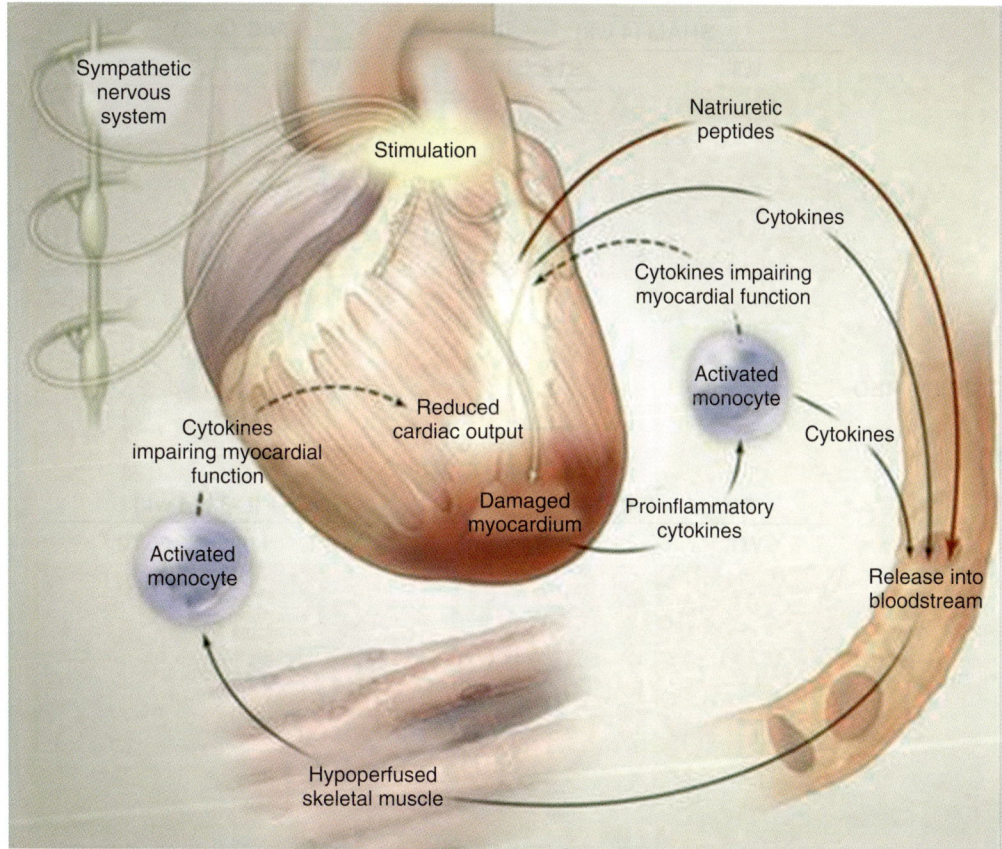

Fig. 33.4 Role of Inflammation in Heart Failure. (From Braunwald E. Biomarkers in heart failure. *N Engl J Med*. 2008;358:2148–2159.)

Several classes of biomarkers have been linked to myocardial remodeling; a theorized advantage of biomarker testing to predict remodeling is that such measurement might identify those patients with ongoing biologic changes likely to lead to deleterious remodeling before the structural changes of the LV have occurred. In this, directed therapy intervention might be more effective.

Inflammation

Several of the proteins involved in the inflammatory pathways are strongly recruited after myocardial insult and are thought to initiate the repair process. However, when these proinflammatory cytokines such as tumor necrosis factor (TNF) and IL are activated for prolonged period of time, they also appear to contribute to the progression of adverse cardiac remodeling (**Fig. 33.4**).[55] Cardiac remodeling involves not just the cardiomyocytes but also nonmyocytes and myocardial extracellular matrix. There is also a close connection between proinflammatory proteins and neurohormonal activation, and both processes often lead to further myocardial insult.

Multiple studies have consistently linked inflammation, as assessed with various biomarkers, with outcomes in HF. Indeed, beyond C-reactive protein (CRP), elevated values for multiple members of the IL family (such as IL-1, IL-6, and IL-18), as well as TNF-α (and related compounds, such as Fas, a proapoptotic hormone linked to remodeling), are elevated in a prognostic fashion in patients with HF; whether these inflammatory biomarkers are by-product markers or mediators of disease remains unclear. In the largest study to date, circulating levels of TNF, soluble TNF receptors, and IL-6 levels were obtained in patients with chronic HF and found to be associated with increased risk of mortality, even after adjusting for all traditional risk factors and

characteristics (all $P < .05$). Even in older patients without any cardiovascular disease, IL-6 and TNF-α, but not CRP, were significantly and independently associated with incident HF in a model that included traditional risk factors.[56]

In exploring a process as widespread and nonspecific as inflammation, it becomes very important to adjust for potential covariates that may influence the level of proinflammatory proteins. A further compounding problem with the measurement of inflammatory biomarkers is poor understanding of the triggers for their release, very little understanding of their biologic variability, and lack of relevant clinical tools for treating an elevated inflammatory biomarker concentration. It has been suggested that gut translocation of bacterial products may, in part, explain associations between inflammation and HF, particularly when the right heart is congested.[57]

Microbiome. There is evidence that translocation of gut flora and their toxins to the blood stream is a possible trigger of inflammation associated with HF. To better understand this association, Pasini and colleagues studied 60 patients with HF and showed that compared with normal controls, HF patients had intestinal overgrowth of pathogenic bacteria and *Candida* species. Intestinal permeability was higher in those with moderate to severe HF compared with those with mild HF; and intestinal permeability and right atrial pressure were mutually interrelated.[57]

It has been shown that higher plasma concentrations of dietary-induced, gut microbia–derived metabolites such as choline, betaine, and trimethylamine-*N*-oxide (TMAO) were found in patients experiencing major adverse cardiac events compared with those without. Circulating TMAO levels are influenced by dietary intake of foods that are high in substrates of TMAO production, such as

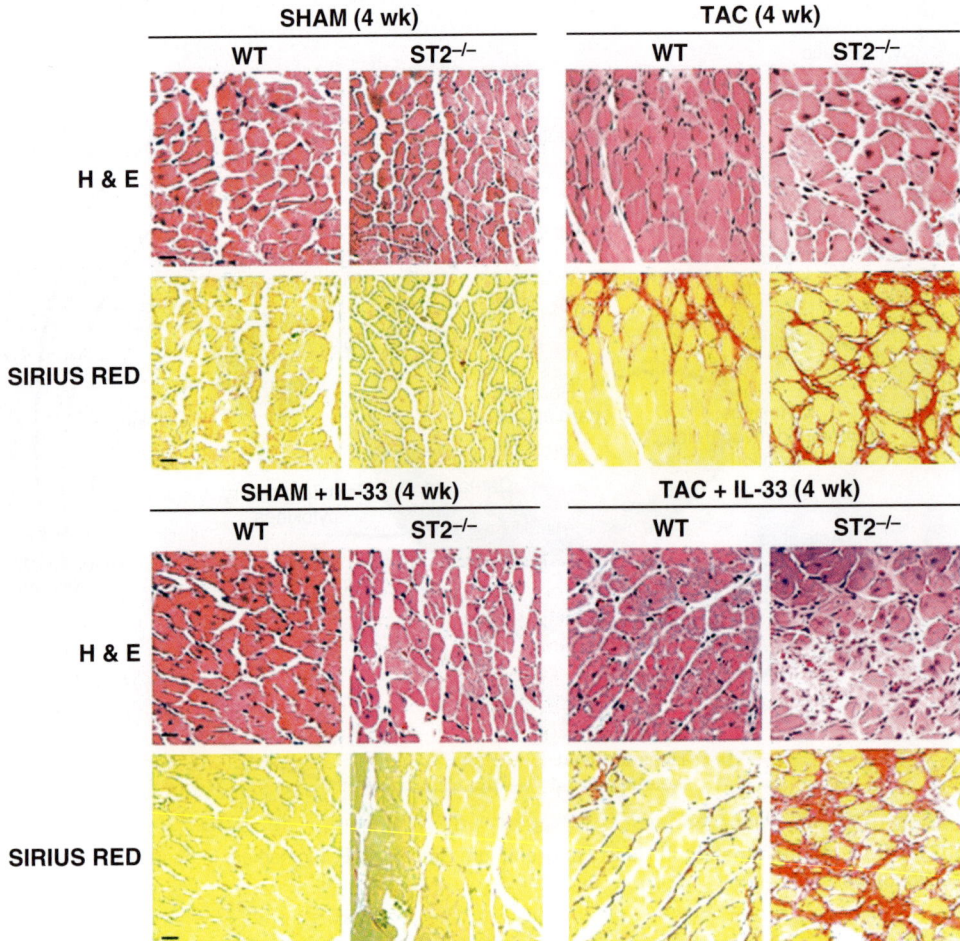

Fig. 33.5 Importance of sST2 and IL-33 Signaling in Animal Models of Pressure Overload. Substantial myocyte hypertrophy and fibrosis occurs in the setting of thoracic aortic constriction, a finding that is rescued by IL-33 infusion in wild-type but not ST2 knock-out animals. *H&E*, Hematoxylin and eosin stain; *IL*, interleukin; *TAC*, thoracic aortic constriction; *WT*, wild type. (From Sanada S, Hakuno D, Higgins LJ, et al. IL-33 and ST2 comprise a critical biomechanically induced and cardioprotective signaling system. *J Clin Invest.* 2007;117:1538–1549.)

phosphatidylcholine or L-carnitine. In a study by Tang and colleagues, higher TMAO concentrations were observed in patients with HF and higher TMAO concentrations predicted 5-year mortality risk after adjustment of traditional risk factors and BNP concentrations (HR 2.2, 95% CI 1.42–3.43, $P < .001$).[58] Higher TMAO concentrations were also shown to portend increased risk of HF hospitalization; and choline, betaine, and TMAO correlated with BNP concentrations. TMAO was also found to be a predictor of CKD. As such, TMAO may play a role in the pathogenesis of HF.

Hypertrophy/Fibrosis

Soluble ST2. The IL-1 receptor family member ST2 was originally described in the context of inflammation, cell proliferation, and autoimmune diseases involving T helper type 2 lymphocyte responses. Since then, ST2 is now known as a unique biomarker with pluripotent effects in vivo, including a powerful role in cardiovascular disease. In the setting of mechanical cardiomyocyte and cardiac fibroblasts stretch, the ST2 gene is strongly induced and the resulting ST2 proteins are closely linked with cardiac remodeling and fibrosis in HF. In its interaction with IL-33, a protein with antifibrosis and antiremodeling effects, ST2 actively participates in inducible pathways in mitigating biomechanical stress.

The ST2 system includes a membrane-bound ligand receptor (ST2L) and the freely circulating sST2; both can bind with IL-33. When IL-33 binds to ST2L, it transduces favorable effects that mitigate ventricular remodeling in volume overloaded states. On the other hand, excessive sST2 acts as a decoy receptor and IL-33 is no longer able to bind to ST2L, blocking the favorable effects from this ST2L. In experimental models, interruption of ST2L expression or infusion of high concentrations of sST2 leads to unchecked ventricular hypertrophy, fibrosis, remodeling, and higher risk for death (**Fig. 33.5**).[59] These findings are recapitulated clinically, where elevated concentrations of sST2 have been closely associated with the phenotype of cardiac decompensation and remodeling and very strongly linked to adverse clinical outcomes in HF. An advantage of ST2 is that its concentration is not affected by age, renal function, or BMI, unlike natriuretic peptides. sST2 testing for risk prediction in both acute and chronic HF has received a class II recommendation in the recent ACC/AHA HF guidelines.[2]

Studies show that sST2 is a consistently strong determinant of HF prognosis, adding independent information to the information already provided by natriuretic peptides and other biomarkers. Increased circulating concentrations of sST2 are associated with HF severity as assessed by LVEF and NYHA functional class, and elevated sST2 concentrations predict mortality in ADHF patients in adjusted multivariable analysis, providing prognostic information superior to (and additive with) NT-proBNP (HR 9.3, *P* = .003; AUC for 1-year mortality 0.80, *P* < .001).[60] The prognostic information provided by sST2 was equivalent in those with HFrEF and HFpEF, and when measured serially in ADHF, sST2 provides incremental information beyond the baseline value; percent change in sST2 during treatment for ADHF is strongly predictive of 90-day mortality (AUC, 0.783; *P* < .001), again superior to natriuretic peptides.[61] In a recent large-scale analysis of multiple biomarkers in a large, international analysis, sST2 values were among the strongest predictors of death by 30 days and 1 year, substantially reclassifying risk beyond clinical variables and other biochemical markers.[62] A recent meta-analysis pooling multiple studies of sST2 in ADHF reaffirmed the independent value of the biomarker for prognosis.[63]

In a chronic HF, similarly consistent data support measurement of sST2. For example, in a study of 1100 chronic HF patients,[64] those with elevated sST2 had a 3.2-fold risk increase in adverse outcomes (95% CI 2.2–4.7, *P* < .0001). In comparison with NT-proBNP, sST2 had similar prognostic ability, but again the best strategy was to combine the information from both biomarkers. Adding sST2 and NT-proBNP to the Seattle Heart Failure Model improved reclassification. Much as in ADHF, a meta-analysis of chronic HF studies emphasized importance of sST2 to add unique prognostic information in chronic HF.[65]

It is noteworthy that serial measurement of sST2 adds incremental prognostic information compared with a single baseline measure. For example, in ADHF, Manzano-Fernandez showed those patients with sST2 less than or equal to 76 ng/mL at presentation and less than or equal to 46 ng/mL on day 4 had the lowest mortality rates (3%), whereas those with both sST2 values greater than these cutoff points had the highest mortality (50%).[66] In a similar fashion, Gaggin et al. showed importance of serial sST2 measurement in chronic HF; notably, in this head-to-head serial measurement comparison of NT-proBNP, growth differentiation factor (GDF)-15, hsTnT, and sST2, only sST2 serial measurement independently added to the risk model (odds ratio: 3.64; 95% CI 1.37–9.67; *P* = .009) and predicted reverse myocardial remodeling (odds ratio: 1.22; 95% CI 1.04–1.43; *P* = 01).[67] In 447 patients with ADHF, ST2 concentrations were lower in patients with HFpEF (0.55 vs. 0.38 ng/mL, *P* < .001) but remained an independent predictor of mortality regardless of the LVEF. In the adjusted analyses that included NT-proBNP, elevated ST2 concentrations were associated with a greater mortality risk in both populations (HFpEF, per ng/mL, HR 1.41, 95% CI 1.14–1.76, *P* = .002; and HFrE per ng/mL, HR 1.20, 95% CI 1.10–1.32, *P* < .001).[68]

Other applications of sST2 testing include prediction of incident HF and risk for death in those with acute MI; for example, in the Thrombolysis in Myocardial Infarction 36 trial, an elevated sST2 value at presentation identified patients at highest risk for incident HF by 30 days; similar data for death were also noted.[69] Concordant with these results, following acute MI, Weir and colleagues demonstrated concentrations of sST2 predict ventricular remodeling. In this same analysis, the benefits of mineralocorticoid receptor antagonism with eplerenone were explored. Only those patients with elevated sST2 concentrations showed protection from remodeling from eplerenone therapy, whereas those with low sST2 values did not.[70]

The potential role of sST2 to prognosticate HF onset in apparently well patients is also present. In a healthy cohort from the Framingham Heart study,[46] sST2 concentrations were measurable in 100% of subjects and, when elevated predicted onset of hypertension[71] and incident HF, even after exhaustively adjusting for other novel and established biomarkers, as well as clinical variables.

Galectin-3. Galectin-3 is a member of the lectin family found in a wide variety of cells and tissues, including the heart. In the heart, it is closely involved in the initiation of the inflammatory cascade following cardiac insult and contributes to ventricular remodeling by the way of tissue repair, myofibroblast proliferation, and fibrogenesis. Soon after the galectin-3 gene was found to be induced in rat HF models, investigators demonstrated that instillation of galectin-3 in the pericardium resulted in considerable collagen deposition. Galectin-3 genetic knockout mouse models are resistant to LV pressure and volume overload, with a slower progression to LV dysfunction or HF.

In a cohort of patients with acute dyspnea,[72] circulating levels of galectin-3 were higher in patients with ADHF compared with those without (*P* < .001) and were prognostic for short-term hazard; since then, galectin-3 measurement has been shown to be predictive of clinical outcomes in patients with both acute and chronic HF syndromes. Serial measurement of galectin-3 in chronic HF adds significantly to baseline values[73]; however, there are no known therapeutic interventions yet identified to respond to elevated galectin-3 values. Despite suggestion of a pathophysiologic link between galectin-3 and aldosterone-mediated fibrosis, retrospective analyses of mineralocorticoid receptor antagonist therapy did not reveal a significant benefit in patients with increased galectin-3 levels[74]; conversely recent data suggest that any benefit of aldosterone antagonist use would be seen primarily in patients with low galectin-3 concentrations.[75] In patients with HFpEF, galectin-3 concentrations greater than the median of 13.8 ng/mL were shown to be an independent predictor of the primary end point of all-cause mortality and/or readmission at 1-year follow-up after adjustment for several clinical factors and natriuretic peptides (HR 1.43, 95% CI 1.07–1.91 *P* = .015).[76] Similar to sST2, galectin-3 testing received a class II recommendation in the ACC/AHA HF guidelines for risk prediction in HF.[2]

Extracellular Matrix Remodeling

An important component of the nonmyocardial tissue in the heart includes connective tissue and extracellular matrix. Cardiac fibroblasts comprise greater than 90% of the nonmyocyte cells in the heart and are responsible for the secretion of most extracellular matrix such as collagens, laminin, and fibronectin. As such, fibroblasts are involved in fibrosis and scar formation in response to cardiac insult, neurohormonal activation, or remodeling itself; indeed, histologically, one of the hallmarks of advanced HF is increased fibrosis as marked by increased collagen content. The N-terminal procollagens such as type I amino-terminal (PINP) and procollagen type III amino-terminal (PIIINP) serve as markers of collagen turnover and elevated circulating concentrations of both have been detected in HF patients. This finding is accompanied by loss of normal structural integrity of collagens and the resulting progressive LV enlargement, increased myocardial stiffness, and increased substrate for arrhythmias. The discovery of the matrix metalloproteinases (MMPs), a set of enzymes capable of breaking down collagens, and tissue inhibitors of matrix metalloproteinases (TIMPs) that regulate the activities of MMPs has informed further knowledge of matrix biology; increased MMP (coupled with TIMP) activities have been reported in LV myocardium of dilated cardiomyopathies and linked to adverse clinical outcomes. In another study, a profile of extracellular matrix biomarkers that included MMP-2, MMP-4, PIIINP, and MMP-8 has been shown to be characteristic of HFpEF.[77]

Evaluation of therapeutic agents with close links to collagen synthesis and fibrosis such as aldosterone antagonists showed a reduction of PINP and PIIINP concentrations and improved outcomes in HF and may demonstrate how biomarkers can be leveraged to help guide therapy.

MicroRNA. MicroRNAs (miRNAs) are small noncoding RNA molecules that are closely involved in the transcriptional and posttranscriptional regulation of gene expression. miRNAs were first described in both animal and human HF models by van Rooij and colleagues.[78] Since then, promising data suggest that they play an important role in the pathogenesis of structural alternations of the failing heart through their ability to regulate the expression of genes that are closely involved in cardiac remodeling.

Because miRNAs are remarkably stable and disease specific, several miRNAs have been demonstrated to be fairly accurate in the diagnosis of HF in small pilot studies; miR-423-5p was most strongly diagnostic of HF, with AUC of 0.91 from healthy controls and 0.83 from acutely dyspneic patients, and closely linked with HF severity including LVEF and NYHA.[79] One of the characteristics of an ideal biomarker is a change in the biomarker level with a change in clinical status, especially in response to therapy; levels of two of the identified miRNAs, miR-499-5p and miR-423-5p, changed in response to therapy that improved measures of cardiac remodeling and survival.[80] The small number of subjects in studies of miRNA limits the wider implication of these results; more research is needed to confirm these findings.

Apoptosis

Progressive loss of myocytes in HF contributes further to LV dysfunction and remodeling in a vicious cycle. The loss of myocyte can take several forms and apoptosis appears to play a prominent role in HF progression.

Growth differentiation factor-15. GDF-15 is a protein that belongs to the transforming growth factor-β family, with a role in regulating response to injury in a broad array of tissues. In the heart, GDF-15 appears to participate in the modulation of myocardial strain, remodeling, and apoptosis. The gene for GDF-15 is robustly induced in cardiomyocytes after metabolic stress such as cardiac ischemia (nitric oxide dependent) or increased cardiac tension such as HF; induction of GDF-15 expression in this setting occurs in an angiotensin II–dependent manner.

Elevation of circulating GDF-15 levels is common in patients with chronic HF. Marked elevation in GDF-15 level is associated with worsening HF severity, but similar to many other HF biomarkers, the proposed utility of GDF-15 measurement in HF appears to be in its ability to independently forecast prognosis beyond the established natriuretic peptides. Increasing levels of GDF-15 in chronic HF was associated with increasing risk of adverse outcomes (risk of mortality of 10.0%, 9.4%, 33.4%, and 56.2% in increasing quartiles of GDF-15, $P < .001$). After adjusting for NT-proBNP and other traditional risk factors, GDF-15 was still predictive of mortality with an adjusted HR for 1 unit increase in the natural log scale of 2.26 (95% CI 1.52–3.37, $P < .001$).

In a study of 1734 patients from the Val-HeFT study,[81] a trial that randomized study participants to valsartan or placebo in chronic HF patients, GDF-15 measurement was performed at baseline and after 12 months of study follow-up. In a comprehensive multivariable Cox regression model that included an exhaustive list of baseline characteristics, GDF-15 remained an independent predictor of all-cause mortality; however, its predictive power was minimal (HR 1.007, 95% CI 1.001–1.014, $P = .02$). Such results suggest that most of the prognosis can be explained by already available baseline characteristics. GDF-15 levels rose over time (145 ng/L in the placebo group vs. 173 ng/L in the valsartan group, $P = .94$), and such an increase was associated with increased risk of death and first morbid event even after adjustment for other baseline characteristics. Contrary to the theoretical link between GDF-15 and angiotensin II receptor, there was no significant interaction between clinical outcomes and valsartan treatment.

Concentrations of GDF-15 may be prognostic in HFpEF. Recently, Chan et al. demonstrated that GDF-15 was a significant independent predictor for composite outcome even after adjusting for important

clinical predictors, including high sensitivity troponin and NT-proBNP (adjusted HR 1.76 per 1 Ln U, 95% CI 1.39–2.21, $P < .001$) in both HFrEF and HFpEF (P interaction =.275).[82] In patients with atrial fibrillation, GDF-15 was significantly associated with major bleeding and all-cause mortality (HR 1.72, 95% CI 1.30–2.29, $P < .005$), and it improved the C-index of both the HAS-BLED (hypertension, [uncontrolled systolic blood pressure >160 mm Hg], abnormal renal and/or liver function, previous stroke, bleeding history or predisposition, labile international normalized ratios, elderly, and concomitant drugs and/or alcohol excess) (0.62–0.69) and ORBIT-AF (Outcomes Registry for Better Informed Treatment of Atrial Fibrillation) (0.68–0.71) bleeding risk scores.[83] In patients with acute coronary syndromes, baseline GDF-15 concentrations predicted major noncoronary artery bypass grafting–related major bleeding, spontaneous MI, and stroke, as well as cardiovascular and noncardiovascular death. Similarly, elevated GDF-15 concentrations at 1 month after an acute coronary syndrome was shown to be associated with an increased risk of noncoronary artery bypass grafting–related major bleeding (3.9% vs. 1.2%; HR 3.38; 95% CI 1.89–6.06), independent of baseline GDF-15.[84]

Insulin-like growth factor binding protein-7. The importance of tissue aging has been recently recognized in numerous cardiovascular and noncardiovascular illnesses. The senescence-associated secretome is a group of autocrine, paracrine, and endocrine substances whose release is induced by transformation of injured tissue to the senescence-associated secretory phenotype; the aggregate effect of this group of peptides is cell-cycle arrest, with the teleologic goal of preventing division of cells with damaged genetic material.

Among the substances in the senescence secretome is insulin-like growth factor binding protein-7 (IGFBP7); this peptide hormone potently induces G_1 cell cycle arrest and is linked to numerous disease states, including risk for acute kidney injury (AKI), as well as diabetes, obesity, and HF. It is noteworthy that HFpEF is a disorder of older, obese patients with diabetes, and indeed concentrations of IGFBP7 are significantly associated with myocardial diastolic abnormalities. Gandhi and colleagues first reported, in patients with HFrEF, concentrations of IGFBP7 were correlated with left atrial volume index ($\varrho = 0.237$, $P = .008$), transmitral E/A ratio ($\varrho = 0.304$, $P = .001$), E/E′ ratio ($\varrho = 0.257$, $P = .005$), and right ventricular systolic pressure ($\varrho = 0.316$, $P = .001$).[85] IGFBP7 has now been repeatedly associated with diastolic dysfunction in those with HFpEF as well.[86] For example, among 160 patients with HFpEF, higher baseline IGFBP7 was modestly correlated with worse diastolic function: higher E velocity (Spearman correlation [ϱ] = 0.40), E/E′ ($\varrho = 0.40$), left atrial volume index ($\varrho = 0.39$), and estimated right ventricular systolic pressure ($\varrho = 0.41$; all $P < .001$) and weakly correlated with transmitral E/A ($\varrho = 0.26$; $P = .006$). Change in IGFBP7 was also significantly correlated with change in E, E/A, E/E′, and right ventricular systolic pressure. Elevated baseline IGFBP7 was associated with lower baseline Vo2max (13.2 vs. 11.1 mL/min/kg; $P < .001$), and change in IGFBP7 was inversely correlated with change in Vo2max ($\varrho = -0.19$; $P = .01$). Concentrations of IGFBP7 are also prognostic in patients with HF. These data support the role of IGFBP7 as a candidate biomarker of senescence in HF.

Markers of Comorbidity
Renal Biomarkers

Renal function markers. Abnormal renal function is one of the most prognostic comorbidities in patients with both acute and chronic HF syndromes (**see also Chapter 15**). HF and abnormalities are so tightly intertwined that the term "cardiorenal syndrome" has been coined to describe this deleterious intersection.

It is well-established that standard measures of renal function such as serum creatinine, eGFR, or blood urea nitrogen (BUN) are important predictors of outcome in patients with HF. For example, among those with ADHF in the ADHERE, both creatinine and BUN were independent predictors of hospital death; a classification and regression tree model containing both measures plus the presence of low blood pressure were useful to partition patients into various risk groups, with rates of death ranging from 2.1% to 21.9%.[87] Thus the value of renal function estimates to predict prognosis is additive (and frequently superior) to many risk factors in HF. Relative to other biomarkers, eGFR has been shown to be additive to natriuretic peptides for forecasting adverse outcome[88]; it has been postulated the definition of "cardiorenal syndrome" should be based on conjoined measurement of a cardiac biomarker such as NT-proBNP, plus a renal function marker such as eGFR.[89]

Beyond standard measures such as creatinine, newer methods to estimate renal function have been examined. Of these, cystatin C appears most promising. Cystatin C is a 13-kDa protein produced at a constant rate by all nucleated cells that is filtered and then catabolized by tubular cells. The CKD-EPI (Chronic Kidney Disease Epidemiology Collaboration) creatinine-cystatin equation has been shown to be superior to other methods for eGFR rate in those with ADHF and is superior for predicting mortality and/or HF hospitalization. In addition, the combination of NT-proBNP and eGFR calculated with the CKD-EPI equation predicted outcomes better in patients with ADHF than either biomarker alone. In studies of HF prognosis, cystatin C has been consistently shown to be superior to creatinine.[90] In patients with chronic stable HF, cystatin C remained an independent predictor of major adverse cardiovascular events after adjustment for traditional risk factors and BNP ($P < .001$). Similarly, in ADHF, cystatin C predicted mortality and morbidity better than traditional measures of renal function. Cystatin C concentrations in patients with HFpEF were found to be a strong and independent predictor for all-cause mortality and/or readmission in patients with acute HF, regardless of renal function. Patients in the highest quartile of cystatin C concentration were at the highest risk (HR 3.40; 95% CI 1.86–6.21; $P < .0001$).[91]

Renal injury markers. Rather than focusing on renal function, biomarkers that predict the presence of AKI may be of particular value. This is because standard markers of renal function do not become abnormal until days after renal injury. Several early markers of renal injury have been discovered that appear to reflect the close interaction between the heart and the kidneys in cardiorenal dysfunction, whether from advanced HF and poor renal perfusion or due to excessive diuretic use and subsequent renal dysfunction.

Several biomarkers linked to AKI have been examined in patients with HF. Among these are neutrophil gelatinase–associated lipocalin (NGAL), kidney injury molecule (KIM)-1, N-acetyl β-(D)-glucosaminidase (NAG), liver-type fatty acid binding protein, IL-18, and the ratio of urinary TIMP2 and IGFBP7.

NGAL is a siderophore protein involved in response to injury of epithelial cells, such as those in the kidneys. Concentrations of urine or serum NGAL have been suggested to be reflective of renal injury; notably, concentrations of NGAL are elevated in those with ADHF and prognosticate the onset of renal dysfunction in this setting. However, the accuracy of NGAL to forecast imminent AKI was modest, with 68% sensitivity and 70% specificity (AUC 0.71, 95% CI 0.58–0.84), and after adjustment for baseline renal function, the odds ratio (OR) for AKI was 3.73 (95% CI 1.26–11.01). Reflective of the poor prognosis in cardiorenal syndrome, patients with elevated NGAL had poor prognosis; NGAL greater than 167.5 ng/mL was associated with 2.7-fold increase in the risk of death and a 2.9-fold risk of death or hospitalization.[92] Similar findings were seen with urinary NGAL. The role of NGAL remains uncertain because conflicting evidence relative to its value exists.

Fewer data exist for KIM-1 or NAG in HF. KIM-1 is a glycoprotein expressed in the proximal tubule. Urinary levels of KIM-1 have been shown to be an early indication of tubular injury in AKI. In patients with chronic HFrEF, urinary KIM-1 concentrations were reported to be higher than in those without HF (1460 vs. 56 pg/mL) and KIM-1 values correlated with LVEF and NYHA functional class.[93] NAG was originally described as a biomarker of AKI several years ago; it is a glycosidase found in renal tubular epithelia whose urinary concentrations are reasonably linked to acute tubular necrosis. Similar to KIM-1, concentrations of NAG correlate with LV function and HF severity in patients with chronic HF.[93] In 2130 patients from the GISSI-HF trial, NGAL, KIM-1, and NAG were independently associated with the combined end point of all-cause mortality and HF hospitalizations (NGAL, HR 1.10, 95% CI 1.00–1.20, $P = .04$; KIM-1, HR 1.13, 95% CI 1.02–1.24, $P = .02$; NAG, HR 1.22, 95% CI 1.10–1.36, $P < .001$); this association remained true even in patients with normal eGFR.

The NephroCheck Test uses the urine TIMP2/IGFBP7 ratio to predict AKI. In two multicenter observational studies of critically ill patients, TIMP2 and IGFBP7 together demonstrated an AUC of 0.80 (0.76 and 0.79 alone, respectively). Urine TIMP2/IGFBP7 was significantly superior to all previously described markers of AKI ($P < .002$), none of which achieved an AUC greater than 0.72. In addition, TIMP2/IGFBP7 significantly improved risk stratification when added to a nine-variable clinical model and remained significant and superior to all other markers regardless of changes in reference creatinine method.[94] More recently, Heung and colleagues demonstrated that the performance of TIMP2/IGFBP7 was not affected by the presence of a variety of common comorbid conditions.[95]

Hematologic Biomarkers

Abnormalities of hematologic indices are exceedingly common in patients with HF and are of considerable prognostic importance. Anemia is caused by a multitude of abnormalities, including renal dysfunction, inflammation, and iron deficiency; it is typically defined as a serum hemoglobin less than 13 g/dL in men and less than 12 g/dL in women, is associated with worse HF symptomatology and adverse outcomes in patients with both HFrEF and HFpEF, and is additive to NT-proBNP for prognostication. Studies focused on use of intravenous iron to treat HF are ongoing.

Beyond hemoglobin, a curious association between red blood cell distribution width (RDW) and outcome in HF has been found. Felker and colleagues originally noted that for each increase in RDW in the Candesartan in HF: Assessment of Reduction in Mortality and Morbidity study, a 17% increase in risk for morbidity and mortality was observed.[96] In ADHF, RDW remained in adjusted models that included renal function and NT-proBNP, predicting death to 1 year from presentation. Data from the Study of Anemia in a HF Population registry suggest the link between RDW, and outcomes may be explained by inflammation and impaired iron mobilization.[97]

Liver Function Tests and Serum Albumin

Abnormalities of hepatic function such as elevated aminotransferases are common in patients with severe HF. This usually indicates significant congestion of the hepatic venous system consequent to right heart congestion; however, low blood pressure may contribute. In a similar fashion, low serum albumin (e.g., <3.4 g/dL) is common in patients with HF, independent of BMI, possibly reflecting protein loss from enteral congestion due to right-sided HF. Both abnormal liver function tests and hypoalbuminemia in the context of HF are independently prognostic, even when considered in the context of natriuretic peptide measurement.

Adipokines

Adiponectin is a 244–amino acid peptide involved in fatty acid metabolism, as well as glucose regulation. Concentrations of adiponectin are inversely related to BMI and may play a role in suppression of the metabolic disarray associated with obesity and metabolic syndrome. Elevated values of adiponectin have been reported in patients with cardiac cachexia and may be prognostic in HF.

Neprilysin

As noted, neprilysin plays an important role in the metabolism of vasoactive compounds active in HF.[1] Recent attention has focused on soluble neprilysin as a biomarker in HF; in a study of 350 patients with acute HF, admission neprilysin concentrations were associated with short- and long-term outcomes, including HF hospitalization and cardiovascular death.[98] In a larger cohort of 1069 patients, Bayes-Genis and colleagues were able to show soluble neprilysin significantly associated with both the cardiovascular death or hospitalization (HR 1.18; 95% CI 1.07–1.31; $P = .001$) and cardiovascular death (HR 1.18; 95% CI 1.05–1.32; $P = .006$).

FUTURE DIRECTIONS: PROTEOMICS, METABOLOMICS, AND MULTIMARKER TESTING

With the rapid advancement in proteomic and genomic technologies and a growing fund of knowledge relative to the existing biomarkers currently available, the potential role of biomarkers in HF is likely to grow exponentially. Rather than focusing on the information provided by a single biomarker, it is likely that phenotyping patients using a mixture of biomarkers that provide "orthogonal" information will be of benefit. Technological advances have allowed for the isolation of proteins that allows for more in-depth analysis of the cardiac proteome. Proteins associated with cardiovascular disease represent pathways in inflammation, wound healing and coagulation, proteolysis and extracellular matrix organization, and handling of cholesterol. Two novel examples have recently been developed. The SOMAscan is a multiplexed, highly sensitive proteomic platform that may measure up to 1300 proteins in a single sample of blood, using aptamer technology. In patients with coronary heart disease, results from the SOMAscan were found to better predict cardiovascular events than the refit Framingham secondary event risk score.[99] Similarly, Olink is a proteomic platform that offers different panels, one of which is a 92 cardiovascular disease–related protein biomarker panel targeted at improvement in the diagnosis and prognostication of cardiovascular disease. Much like the SOMAscan, the technology used by Olink provides high sensitivity and a broad range of possible analytes. Due to their technology, both SOMAscan and Olink methods do not provide absolute biomarker concentrations; only relative concentrations are generated.

Metabolomic profiling identifies novel biomarkers and mechanisms involved in cardiovascular disease. Metabolomics is focused on analysis of small molecules that reflect the state of an organism in a certain point of time. Metabolomic profiling aims to comprehensively measure biomarkers in a fast, cost-effective, and clinically informative manner, and advanced statistical methods allow for identification of signature profiles in particular cohorts. As such, metabolomics has the potential to identify new pathophysiologic pathways and, consequently, therapeutic targets, to assist in improved risk-stratification and personalized cardiac management. Such metabolomic profiles may represent the metabolic fingerprint of individual patients and may serve as diagnostic and/or prognostic tools that have the potential to significantly alter the management of cardiovascular disease. For instance, Vaarhorst and colleagues defined a weighted metabolite score consisting of 13 proton nuclear magnetic resonance signals that was associated with prevalent coronary heart disease independent of traditional risk factors (OR = 1.59, 95% CI 1.19–2.13); in addition, it was moderately predictive of incident coronary heart disease (C-index 0.75, 95% CI 0.70–0.80).[100]

Multimarker strategies have the potential to better personalize the care of patients with HF. As a proof of concept, Ky and colleagues examined a panel of biomarkers among 1513 patients with chronic HF including BNP, CRP, MPO, soluble fms-like tyrosine kinase receptor-1, hsTnI, sST2, creatinine, and uric acid.[101] The score derived from this panel was independent (adjusted HR 6.80, 95% CI 8.75–21.5), additive to the established clinical risk score from the Seattle Heart Failure Model, with an improvement in the AUC of 0.803 from 0.756 ($P = .003$) and improved reclassification (net reclassification improvement of 25.2%, 95% CI 14.2%–36.2%, $P < .001$) (**Fig. 33.6**). In a similar fashion, Gaggin and colleagues studied 115 patients with chronic HF and found that a model containing traditional risk factors and several biomarkers including ET-1, NT-proBNP, hsTnI, and ST2 best predicted cardiovascular events, and ET-1 improved classification. Percent time spent with ET-1 of less than or equal to 5.90 pg/mL was predictive of fewer cardiovascular events (OR=0.75; 95% CI 0.62–0.91), and ET-1 reduction over time was associated with a lower rate of cardiovascular events compared with increasing or stable ET-1 (24.4% vs. 50.0%).[102] As such, ET-1 complemented other biomarkers, and serial measurements had additive prognostic value.

FUTURE DIRECTIONS: PRECISION MEDICINE IN HEART FAILURE

Despite great promise in oncology, the use of precision approaches in HF remain unrealized. In theory, using biologic signatures to identify the "right therapy for the right patient at the right time" remains a goal that is sought but not achieved. This is greatly influenced by the current dogmatic approach to HF therapy, which argues for applying the same therapies at the same doses in every affected patient. Until the medical community is ready to move beyond this approach, individualizing care in patients with the diagnosis will remain challenging.

There are different roles biomarkers may play for "precision" medicine in HF. On the one hand, biomarkers might be useful to better characterize patients into phenotypic subgroups with varying responses to standard HF therapies. On the other hand, biomarkers might identify specific pathways in HF that might be targeted for superior outcome. An important distinction must be made between biomarkers that are prognostic of outcome versus those that are predictive of therapy response. The former category informs risk for deleterious outcome in a diagnosis but may not identify a specific therapy option; a prime example of this would be GDF-15 or galectin-3. In contrast, predictive biomarkers may or may not be prognostic, but their results either identify response to therapy a specific therapy that would be of benefit in treating HF. Predictive markers may be directly associated with disease mechanism

To date, most conceptual and clinical application of biomarkers for "precision" care has focused on their use to provide a more detailed "phenotype" among groups of affected patients. This has generally focused on use of biomarkers that inform presence and significance of abnormal pathways involved in HF presence, severity, and outcome. For example, using machine learning that incorporated clinical characteristics with other aspects such as biomarker results, Ahmad and colleagues identified "clusters" of HF phenotypes with differential outcome.[103] In a similar fashion, one may use biomarkers for more refined characterization of HF. This may be of specific value in HF syndromes with more heterogeneous causes such as HFpEF.

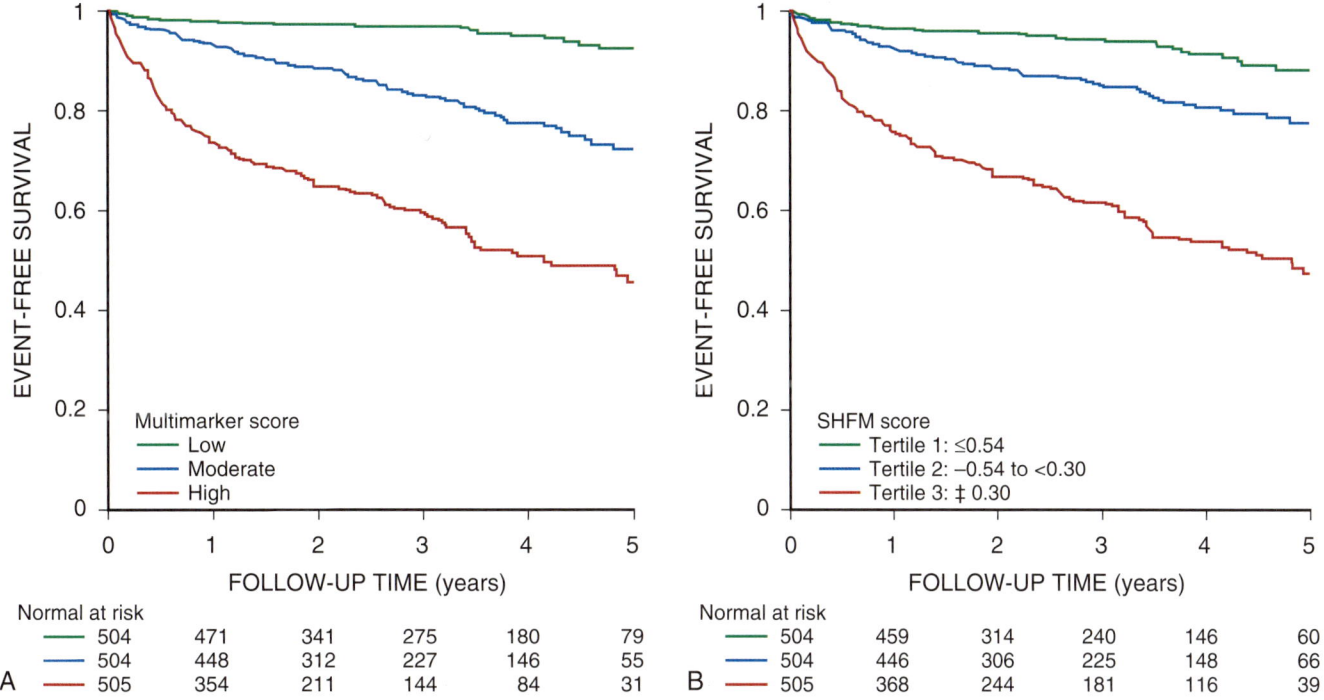

Fig. 33.6 Event-free survival by multimarker score category (A) and tertiles of the Seattle Heart Failure Model (SHFM) score (B). (From Ky B, French B, Levy WC, et al. Multiple biomarkers for risk prediction in chronic heart failure. *Circ Heart Fail.* 2012;5:183–190.)

TABLE 33.6 **Summary of Signaling Molecule Polymorphism Effects by Drug or Device Class, Irrespective of Race**

Drug or Class	Polymorphism (Effects on Response in HF)
Standard beta-blockers	*GRK5* Gln41Leu (↓ by Leu carriers) [1]; *ADRB2* Gln27Glu (carvedilol ↑ in Glu genotypes) [2,3] *ACE* Del/intron16/Ins (↑ in Del homozygotes) [4]
Bucindolol (beta-blocker/sympatholytic)	*ADRB1* Arg389Gly (↑in Arg homozygotes,[5] ↓ in {389Gly + *ADRA2C* 322-325Del} genotypes;[6] *EDN1* Lys198Asn (gene dose-related ↓ in Asn genotypes)[7]; *ECE1* Thr341Ile (↓ in Ile genotypes)
Angiotensin-converting enzyme inhibitors	*ACE* Del/intron16/Ins (↑ in Del homozygotes)[8]
Angiotensin AT-1 receptor blockers	↑ biomarker (NT-proBNP) response in *AGTR1* 1166C genotypes[9]
Mineralocorticoid receptor blockers	No effects reported
Hydralazine/isosorbide dinitrate	*NOS3* Glu298Asp (↑ in Glu homozygotes)[10]; *CYP11B2* T-344C (↑ in −344T homozygotes)[11]; *GNB3* 825T(↑ in TT homozygotes)[12]
Cardiac resynchronization therapy	*ADRB2* Gln27Glu (↑ in Glu homozygotes)[13]; *NR3C2* Ile180Val(↑ in Ile homozygotes)[14]
ICD appropriate discharge for VT/VF	*SCN5A* Ser1103Tyr (↑ events in Tyr carriers)[15]

References are given in the online supplement.
HF, Heart failure; *ICD,* implantable cardioverter defibrillator; *NT-proBNP,* N-terminal pro–brain natriuretic peptide; *VF,* ventricular fibrillation; *VT,* ventricular tachycardia.
Adapted from Taylor MR, Sun AY, Davis G, et al. Race, common genetic variation, and therapeutic response disparities in heart failure. *JACC Heart Fail.* 2014;2:561–572.

In contrast to simply using biomarkers to phenotype patients is the idea of using biomarkers to specifically identify abnormal pathways in HF that might be specifically targeted. The topic of precision pharmacotherapy for HF has been recently reviewed. Although presently specifically focused on understanding variability in response to therapies based on genetic variation (**Table 33.6**),[104] it is reasonable to expect the future to hold ability to measure circulating predictive biomarkers identifying specific therapy choices and monitor patients so treated.

Acknowledgments

Dr. Ibrahim is supported in part by the Dennis and Marilyn Barry Fellowship in Cardiology Research. Dr. Gaggin is supported in part by the Ruth and James Clark Fund for Cardiac Research Innovation. Dr. Januzzi is supported in part by the Hutter Family Professorship.

KEY REFERENCES

1. Ibrahim NE, Januzzi JL. Beyond natriuretic peptides for diagnosis and management of heart failure. *Clin Chem.* 2017;63:211–222.
5. Januzzi Jr JL, Camargo CA, Anwaruddin S, et al. The N-terminal Pro-BNP investigation of dyspnea in the emergency department (PRIDE) study. *Am J Cardiol.* 2005;95:948–954.
6. Januzzi JL, van Kimmenade R, J Lainchbury, et al. NT-proBNP testing for diagnosis and short-term prognosis in acute destabilized heart failure: an international pooled analysis of 1256 patients: the International Collaborative of NT-proBNP Study. *Eur Heart J.* 2006;27:330–337.

7. Gaggin HK, Chen-Tournoux AA, Christenson RH, et al. Rationale and design of the ICON-RELOADED study: international collaborative of N-terminal pro-B-type natriuretic peptide re-evaluation of acute diagnostic cut-offs in the emergency department. *Am Heart J.* 2017;192:26–37.

9. O'Donoghue M, Chen A, Baggish AL, et al. The effects of ejection fraction on N-terminal ProBNP and BNP levels in patients with acute CHF: analysis from the ProBNP Investigation of Dyspnea in the Emergency Department (PRIDE) study. *J Card Fail.* 2005;11:S9–S14.

13. Siebert U, Januzzi Jr JL, Beinfeld MT, Cameron R, Gazelle GS. Cost-effectiveness of using N-terminal pro-brain natriuretic peptide to guide the diagnostic assessment and management of dyspneic patients in the emergency department. *Am J Cardiol.* 2006;98:800–805.

37. Shah RV, Truong QA, Gaggin HK, et al. Mid-regional pro-atrial natriuretic peptide and pro-adrenomedullin testing for the diagnostic and prognostic evaluation of patients with acute dyspnoea. *Eur Heart J.* 2012;33:2197–2205.

85. Gandhi PU, Gaggin HK, Sheftel AD, et al. Prognostic usefulness of insulin-like growth factor-binding protein 7 in heart failure with reduced ejection fraction: a novel biomarker of myocardial diastolic function? *Am J Cardiol.* 2014;114:1543–1549.

89. van Kimmenade RRJ, Pinto Y, Januzzi JL. When renal and cardiac insufficiencies intersect: is there a role for natriuretic peptide testing in the 'cardio-renal syndrome'? *Eur Heart J.* 2007;28:2960–2961.

102. Gaggin HK, Truong QA, Gandhi PU, et al. Systematic evaluation of endothelin 1 measurement relative to traditional and modern biomarkers for clinical assessment and prognosis in patients with chronic systolic heart failure: serial measurement and multimarker Testing. *Am J Clin Pathol.* 2017;147:461–472.

The full reference list for this chapter is available on ExpertConsult.

Hemodynamics in Heart Failure

Jose Nativi-Nicolau, John J. Ryan, James C. Fang

The first right heart catheterization (RHC) in humans was performed in 1929 by Dr. Werner Forssmann (on himself), who ultimately shared in the 1956 Nobel Prize in Medicine with Andre Cournand and Dickinson Richards for their work in cardiac catheterization. RHC was further refined by the work of Drs. Bradley and Fife, and in 1969 Drs. Scheinman, Abbot, and Rapaport reported their use of a flow-directed right heart catheter. Following their report of a bedside balloon flotation catheter by Drs. Swan and Ganz in the *New England Journal of Medicine* in 1970, RHC became widespread both in the catheterization laboratory and in intensive care units for critically ill and unstable patients.[1] Despite advances in noninvasive hemodynamic assessment with echocardiography and cardiac magnetic resonance imaging (MRI), RHC and left heart catheterization (LHC) remains the gold standard for hemodynamic assessment in heart disease.[2] Today, the three predominant reasons to obtain invasive hemodynamics in heart failure include:

1. To resolve diagnostic uncertainty in patients with cryptic symptoms.
2. To assess the suitability for advanced therapies in chronic heart failure.
3. To investigate pulmonary hypertension (PH).

The Society for Cardiovascular Angiography and Interventions and the Heart Failure Society of America Clinical Expert Consensus Document on the Use of Invasive Hemodynamics for the Diagnosis and Management of Cardiovascular Disease summarize the recommendations for invasive hemodynamics for specific clinical scenarios in **Table 34.1**.[3]

TECHNICAL ISSUES

It is important to recognize that invasive hemodynamics are traditionally measured at rest, in the sedated state, and in a supine position. These limitations should be appreciated when invasive hemodynamics are used to reconcile cryptic symptoms, assess prognosis, or prepare patients for advanced therapies. However, most of our contemporary understanding of heart failure hemodynamics is derived from these resting, supine, and sedated studies. Traditional and novel hemodynamic formulas are illustrated in **Fig. 34.1**. Exercise and upright hemodynamics can be obtained in a properly prepared laboratory and are often necessary in certain clinical situations, but are not commonly performed on a routine basis in most clinical catheterization laboratories. The hemodynamic response to various physiologic and/or pharmacologic challenges should also be considered at the time of RHC to maximize the information obtained during this invasive procedure. Finally, it should be appreciated that traditionally obtained hemodynamic measurements lack concomitant measurements of cardiac and/or intravascular volume, so pressure is used as a surrogate for volume.

Pressure measurements in cardiac catheterization are recorded using fluid-filled catheters connected to strain-gauge pressure transducers using the principle of the Wheatstone bridge. Because of the need for pressure transmission to record a signal, a time delay is inherent and should be accounted for when assessing instantaneous pressure differences (e.g., gradients). Moreover, fluid-filled systems are influenced by various factors, including transducer height, patient position, catheter length, air bubbles, fluid frequency response/damping (e.g., catheter whip artifacts), and open connections.

These issues can be avoided by using micromanometer catheters that use high fidelity pressure sensors at the point of measurement (Millar Instruments, Houston, TX). Such systems can also be combined with special conductance catheters to provide simultaneous volume measurements, but their use is confined to research laboratories. These systems provide more sophisticated measures of ventricular performance such as contractility, diastolic function, and ventricular pressure-volume (PV) relationships.[4]

The impact of respiration on intracardiac pressures should be considered. The dynamic changes in intrathoracic pressures associated with respiration are usually modest (e.g., −1 to 5 mm Hg) but can be quite dramatic (e.g., severe obesity, obstructive pulmonary disease) and will have a significant influence on intracardiac pressures. However, it is common in both clinical practice and investigation that mean pressure measurements rather than respirophasic ranges are reported, which can lead to important misinterpretations. For example, the pulmonary capillary wedge pressure (PCWP) averaged over the duration of the respiratory cycle may underestimate the true end-expiratory left ventricular end-diastolic pressure (LVEDP) and lead to an erroneous diagnosis of World Health

TABLE 34.1   Key Clinical Recommendations for Invasive Hemodynamic Evaluation

Hypertrophic Cardiomyopathy

1. For symptomatic patients being considered for septal reduction therapy, invasive hemodynamic assessment with characterization of the dynamic LVOT obstruction should be performed for those in which the noninvasive imaging studies are inconclusive.
2. In the cardiac catheterization laboratory, transseptal assessment is preferred for characterization of dynamic LVOT obstruction.
3. Dynamic LVOT obstruction at rest and with provocation should be examined.

Valvular heart disease

1. An invasive hemodynamic evaluation is recommended to resolve discrepancies between clinical findings and noninvasive imaging data in patients with valvular disease when surgical or catheter-based therapy is being considered.
2. Invasive hemodynamic studies of patients with valvular disease should be performed with simultaneous measurement of multiple central cardiac chambers.
3. Invasive hemodynamic evaluations are beneficial for patients with valvular regurgitation in certain scenarios, such as eccentric jets with difficult quantitation, prosthetic valves with possible acoustic shadowing, and acute lesions in which color flow Doppler might be limited.

Ventricular Function

1. Although diastolic function is most comprehensively assessed by measuring ventricular stiffness and relaxation, the commonly available methods of catheterization with direct measurement of left- and right-sided ventricular filling pressures provide incremental diagnostic data on diastolic function.
2. In patients presenting exercise intolerance, in which noninvasive and resting invasive measurements are inconclusive, provocative testing in the cardiac catheterization laboratory should be considered to determine the presence of a cardiac etiology. Cycle ergometry exercise is the most physiologically relevant and sensitive stressor and is preferred over other maneuvers such as saline loading or arm exercise.

Pericardial Disease

1. An invasive hemodynamic evaluation should be strongly considered for all patients with suspected constrictive pericarditis due to the frequently complex pathophysiology and the need for high diagnostic specificity when considering surgery.
2. Invasive studies for constrictive pericarditis should entail examination of the dynamic respiratory criteria.
3. An invasive hemodynamic study is typically not required for the diagnosis of cardiac tamponade.

Pulmonary Hypertension and the Right Ventricle

1. Invasive assessment of pulmonary hemodynamics is required for patients with pulmonary hypertension who are being considered for vasodilator therapy and cardiac transplantation.
2. Invasive assessment of pulmonary hemodynamics should be considered when there is diagnostic uncertainty regarding pulmonary hypertension based on noninvasive data. This assessment should establish the diagnosis according to WHO classification.
3. Invasive assessment of pulmonary hemodynamics should be performed to monitor and assess the effectiveness of pulmonary hypertension therapies.
4. Invasive assessment of pulmonary hemodynamics can be used to assess the risk of right ventricular failure with advanced heart failure therapies.
5. In the appropriate setting, a properly performed and interpreted exercise hemodynamic assessment can be a highly useful tool to elucidate a cause of dyspnea or mechanism of PH.

Congenital Heart Disease

1. Cardiac catheterization should be performed for patients with shunts when there is evidence of elevated pressures, chamber enlargement, or symptoms that are out of proportion to the size of the congenital lesion, and prior to closure of shunts.
2. Cardiac catheterization should be performed to assess the hemodynamics of congenital heart disease patients with known or suspected right ventricular failure, especially in palliated single ventricle physiology.
3. Cardiac catheterization should be performed to determine the severity of obstructions in series.

Cardiogenic shock and circulatory support devices

1. Invasive hemodynamic assessment, with measurement of ventricular filling pressures, cardiac output, and systemic vascular resistance, is recommended for the diagnosis of cardiogenic shock.
2. Continuous hemodynamic monitoring with a pulmonary artery catheter is recommended for acute management of patients receiving therapy with mechanical circulatory support.
3. Pulmonary artery catheterization is useful to guide withdrawal of mechanical circulatory and pharmacologic support in patients with myocardial recovery from cardiogenic shock.
4. In patients without recovery of myocardial and end-organ function, hemodynamic monitoring is useful to assess candidacy for and transition to advanced heart failure therapies, including durable mechanical circulatory support and heart transplantation.

LVOT, Left ventricular outflow tract; *PH,* pulmonary hypertension; *WHO,* World Health Organization.
Adapted from Sorajja P, Borlaug BA, Dimas VV, et al. SCAI/HFSA clinical expert consensus document on the use of invasive hemodynamics for the diagnosis and management of cardiovascular disease. *Catheter Cardiovasc Interv.* 2017;89:E233–E247.

Organization (WHO) group 1 rather than group 2 or mixed PH.[5] It is optimal to manually measure end-expiratory pressures since the effects of negative intrathoracic pressures required for ventilation on intracardiac pressures are minimal at end expiration. A breath hold can be useful if done at end expiration as long as a Valsalva maneuver does not ensue.

RHC is generally safe, but its routine use in heart failure management should be tempered by complications associated with any invasive procedure. Serious complications, such as pneumothorax, pulmonary embolism, and pulmonary arterial rupture are rare. In the ESCAPE (Evaluation Study of Congestive Heart Failure and Pulmonary Artery

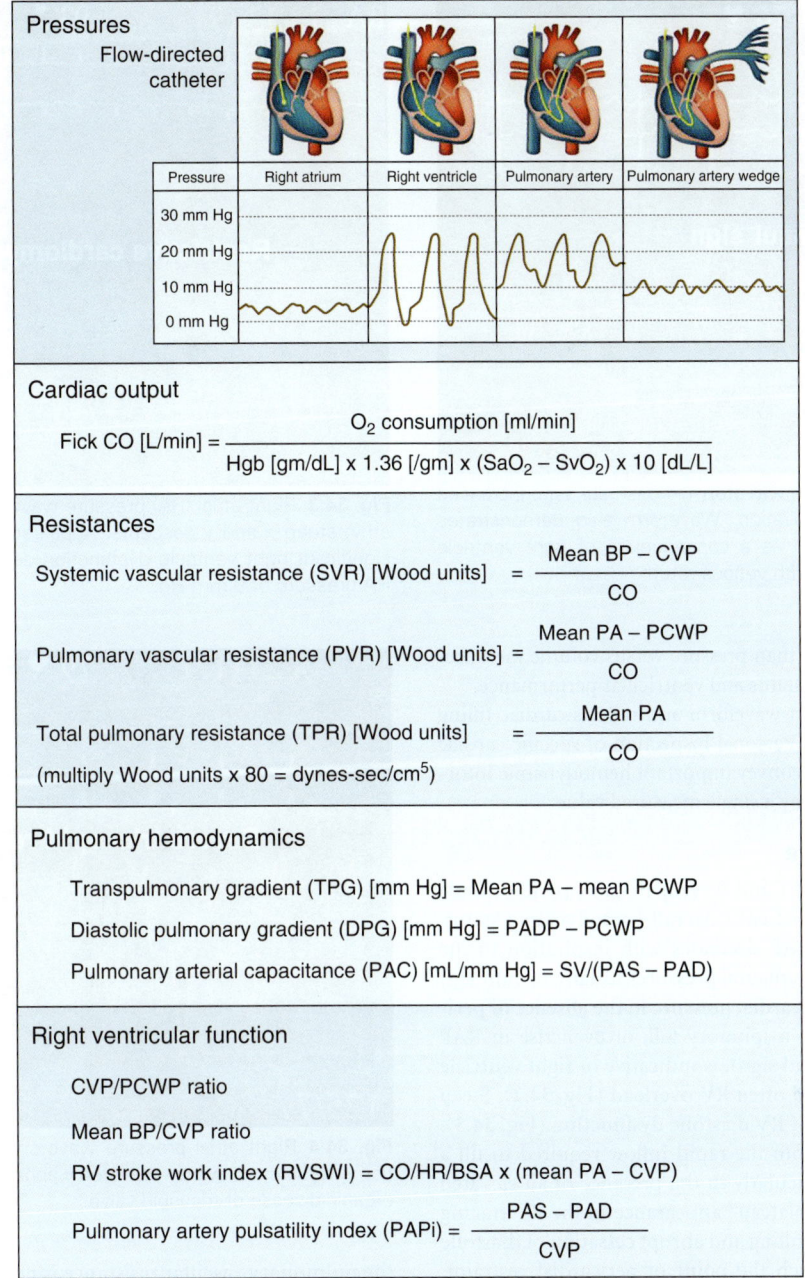

Pressures

Flow-directed catheter

Pressure	Right atrium	Right ventricle	Pulmonary artery	Pulmonary artery wedge
30 mm Hg				
20 mm Hg				
10 mm Hg				
0 mm Hg				

Cardiac output

$$\text{Fick CO [L/min]} = \frac{O_2 \text{ consumption [ml/min]}}{\text{Hgb [gm/dL]} \times 1.36 \text{ [/gm]} \times (SaO_2 - SvO_2) \times 10 \text{ [dL/L]}}$$

Resistances

$$\text{Systemic vascular resistance (SVR) [Wood units]} = \frac{\text{Mean BP} - \text{CVP}}{\text{CO}}$$

$$\text{Pulmonary vascular resistance (PVR) [Wood units]} = \frac{\text{Mean PA} - \text{PCWP}}{\text{CO}}$$

$$\text{Total pulmonary resistance (TPR) [Wood units]} = \frac{\text{Mean PA}}{\text{CO}}$$

(multiply Wood units $\times$ 80 = dynes-sec/cm^5)

Pulmonary hemodynamics

Transpulmonary gradient (TPG) [mm Hg] = Mean PA − mean PCWP

Diastolic pulmonary gradient (DPG) [mm Hg] = PADP − PCWP

Pulmonary arterial capacitance (PAC) [mL/mm Hg] = SV/(PAS − PAD)

Right ventricular function

CVP/PCWP ratio

Mean BP/CVP ratio

RV stroke work index (RVSWI) = CO/HR/BSA × (mean PA − CVP)

$$\text{Pulmonary artery pulsatility index (PAPi)} = \frac{\text{PAS} - \text{PAD}}{\text{CVP}}$$

CO = cardiac output, BP = blood pressure, CVP = central venous pressure,
PA = pulmonary artery, LA = left atrial, PCWP = pulmonary capillary wedge pressure,
Hb = hemoglobin, Sa = arterial saturation, Sv = mixed venous saturation,
PAS = pulmonary artery systolic, PAD = pulmonary artery diastolic,
HR = heart rate, BSA = body surface area

Fig. 34.1 Hemodynamic formulas and calculations. *BP,* Blood pressure; *BSA,* body surface area; *CO,* cardiac output; *CVP,* central venous pressure; *Hgb,* hemoglobin; *HR,* heart rate; *LA,* left atrial; *PA,* pulmonary artery; *PAD,* pulmonary artery diastolic; *PAS,* pulmonary artery systolic; *PCWP,* pulmonary capillary wedge pressure; *RV,* right ventricle; *Sa,* arterial saturation; *Sv,* mixed venous saturation.

Catheterization Effectiveness) trial, in-hospital adverse events were more common among patients in the RHC group compared with the clinical assessment group (22% vs. 11.5%; *P* = .04).[6] Adverse events due to the pulmonary artery catheter (PAC) occurred in 4% (n = 9) of the RHC group. The most common complication was access site bleeding. There were no hospital deaths attributed to the PAC. Adverse events included PAC-related infection, catheter knotting, pulmonary infarction and hemorrhage, and ICD shocks. Pulmonary arterial rupture and RBBB (with subsequent complete heart block in the setting of

a baseline LBBB) did not occur. Pulmonary artery (PA) rupture is rare in clinical practice, but risk factors include severe PH, anticoagulation, mitral valve disease, and advanced age.[7,8]

HEMODYNAMIC WAVEFORMS

In clinical practice, it is difficult to measure LV volume throughout the cardiac cycle rendering the use of PV loops for clinical care impractical. The difficulty in obtaining PV loops has resulted in a dependence

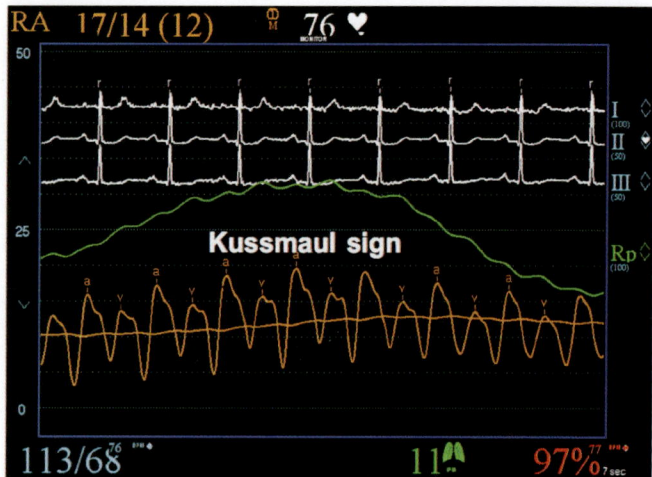

Fig. 34.2 Right atrial pressure waveform. Kussmaul sign: increased right atrial pressure with inspiration. Waveform also demonstrates dynamic tricuspid regurgitation as a consequence of right ventricle enlargement and dysfunction with venous return.

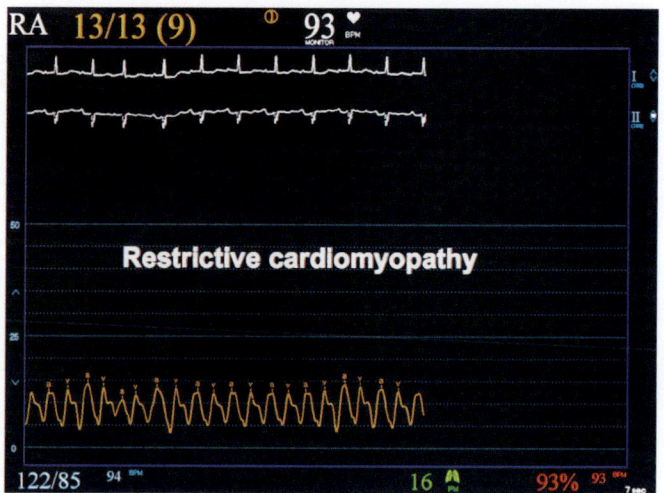

Fig. 34.3 Right atrial (RA) pressure waveform. Restrictive cardiomyopathy: steep *x* and *y* descents. Appearance of the waveform conveys significant right ventricle dysfunction despite the minimal increase in RA pressure of 9 mm Hg.

on pressure versus time rather than pressure versus volume measurements to assess hemodynamic status and ventricular performance.

Each chamber has a distinct waveform and reflects cardiac filling as well as ventricular ejection. Personal inspection of specific cardiac chamber waveforms can often convey important hemodynamic information that is not appreciated by a single measured value.

Right Atrium and Ventricle

The right atrial pressure (RAP) and waveform can provide simple yet important insight into a patient's overall hemodynamic status. During normal respiration, RAP decreases with inspiration to the same degree as the drop in intrapleural pressure (usually <5 mm Hg) and generally reflects intrapericardial pressure in the absence of pericardial constraint. Lack of an inspiratory fall, or even rise in RAP with inspiration (e.g., Kussmaul sign), is indicative of right ventricle (RV) diastolic dysfunction and often RV overload (**Fig. 34.2**). Steep *y* descents are also indicative of RV diastolic dysfunction (**Fig. 34.3**). The steep *y* descent results from the rapid inflow required to fill a stiff RV in early diastole, particularly in the presence of an elevated RAP. Similarly, the "dip and plateau" appearance in the RV tracing indicates rapid, early diastolic filling and abrupt cessation of diastolic inflow as the LV and RV reach the point of pericardial restraint. Such findings are commonly found in conditions associated with RV dysfunction, including advanced heart failure with reduced ejection fraction (HFrEF), restrictive cardiomyopathies, heart transplantation, and RV infarction. A prominent *v* wave is noted in severe tricuspid regurgitation, regardless of chronicity (**Fig. 34.4**). The central venous pressure may also be approximated by the venous pressure in a peripheral vein with appropriate establishment of the phlebostatic zero reference.[9]

The RV is a low-pressure chamber in normal individuals. A small systolic gradient between the RV systolic pressure (RVSP) and PA systolic pressure (PASP) facilitates forward flow in this low-pressure system. The RV waveform can be distinguished from the PA waveform by the rise in pressure during diastole in contrast to the fall in pressure in the PA tracing. The rise in the RVSP over time, dP/dt, can be used to estimate the PA diastolic pressure (ePAD) since pulmonic valve opening will occur at the end of isovolumic contraction or maximum dP/dt (**Fig. 34.5**). The ePAD will approximate the PCWP (e.g., within 2–3 mm Hg) as long as

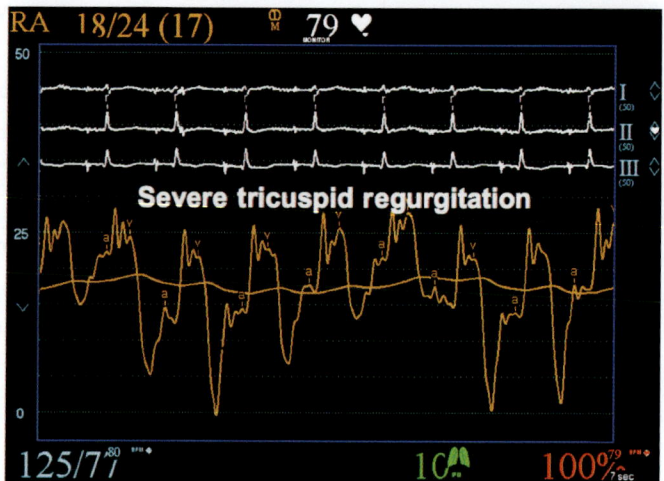

Fig. 34.4 Right atrial pressure waveform. Severe tricuspid regurgitation: prominent *v* wave. Waveform appears ventricularized due to the organic disease of tricuspid valve.

the pulmonary vascular resistance is normal. This strategy was used for the CHRONICLE device to provide a continuous estimate of the PCWP.[10]

Pulmonary Capillary Wedge

A common concern in RHC is whether a true PCWP has been obtained (**Fig. 34.6**). Fluoroscopy and a visible change in the waveform is typically used to confirm the PCWP position. Loss of the pulmonary arterial waveform and a change to a "flattened" appearance with attenuated deflections usually signifies the PCWP. A prominent *v* wave can also be seen with a true PCWP but can be easily confused with the PASP. The *v* wave of PCWP occurs well after the T wave of the ECG, whereas the peak systolic wave of PASP occurs before or within the T wave. Difficulty in distinguishing between PCWP and PASP is particularly problematic in patients with prominent *v* waves (e.g., acute severe mitral regurgitation, ventricular septal defects, and severe diastolic dysfunction).

Hybrid tracings between PCWP and actual pulmonary artery pressure (PAP) result in an overestimation of PCWP and should be

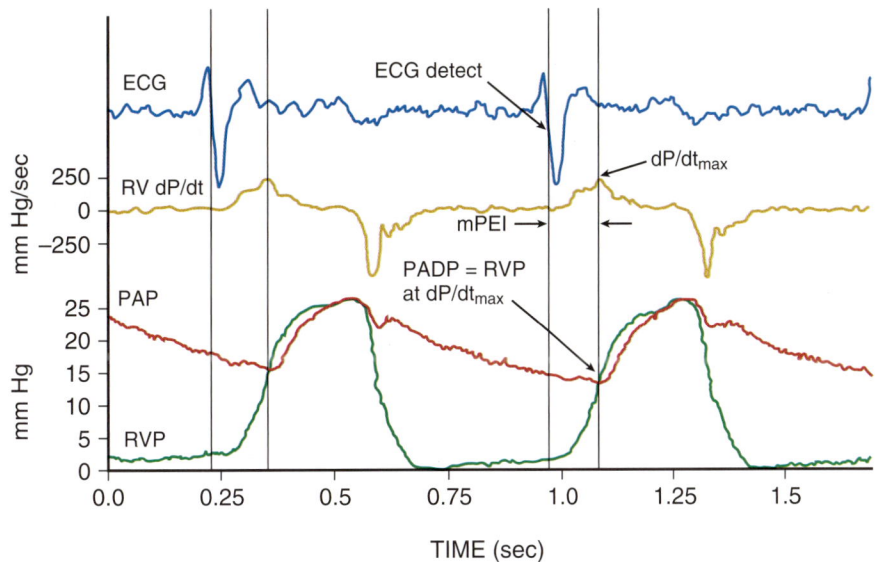

Fig. 34.5 Schematic illustration of computer detection of the QRS complex *(ECG Detect)*, maximal first derivative of right ventricular pressure *(dP/dtmax)* and modified preejection interval *(mPEI)*. Pulmonary artery diastolic pressure *(ePAD)* equals right ventricular pressure at maximal first derivative of pressure measured over time *(dP/dt)*. PAP, pulmonary artery pressure; RV, right ventricle; RVP, right ventricular pressure. (From Reynolds DW, Bartelt N, Taepke R, Bennett TD. Measurement of pulmonary artery diastolic pressure from the right ventricle. *J Am Coll Cardiol.* 1995;25:1176–1182.)

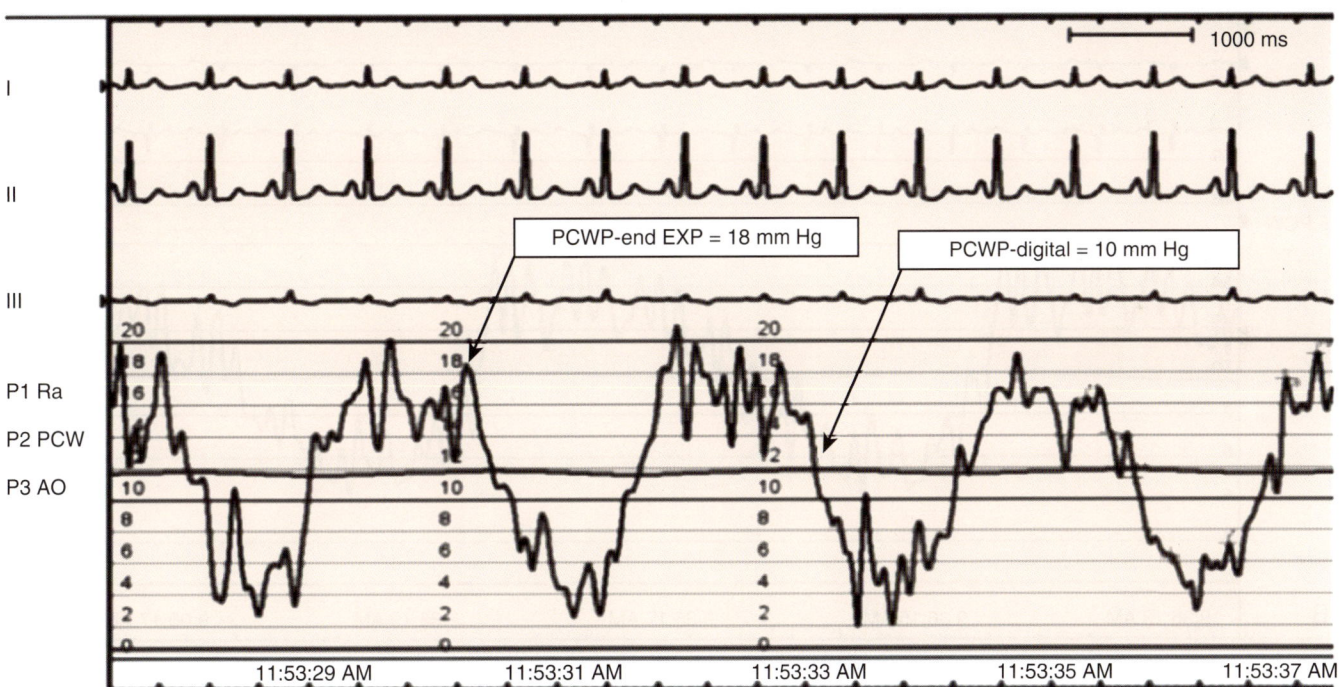

Fig. 34.6 **Errors in pulmonary capillary wedge pressure.** Tracing illustrates the respirophasic waveforms with the digitized means. The difference between pulmonary capillary wedge pressure *(PCWP)*–end expiration versus PCWP-digital suggests misclassification of the type of pulmonary hypertension. (From Ryan JJ, Rich JD, Thiruvoipati T, Swamy R, Kim GH, Rich S. Current practice for determining pulmonary capillary wedge pressure predisposes to serious errors in the classification of patients with pulmonary hypertension. *Am Heart J.* 2012;163:589–594.)

suspected when the PCWP exceeds the PA diastolic pressure (**Fig. 34.7**). Damping of the hemodynamic waveform should also be considered. Underdamping, which is often referred to as ringing or "whip" artifact, can lead to inaccurate pressure recordings and can be rectified by drawing a small amount of blood or contrast into the catheter to

increase the viscosity of the fluid. In patients with severe right ventricular enlargement and dysfunction, caution must be used when it comes to interpreting an elevated PCWP or LVEDP. Right ventricular pressure overload from pulmonary artery hypertension (PAH) can result in elevated LVEDP due to impaired relaxation of the LV secondary to

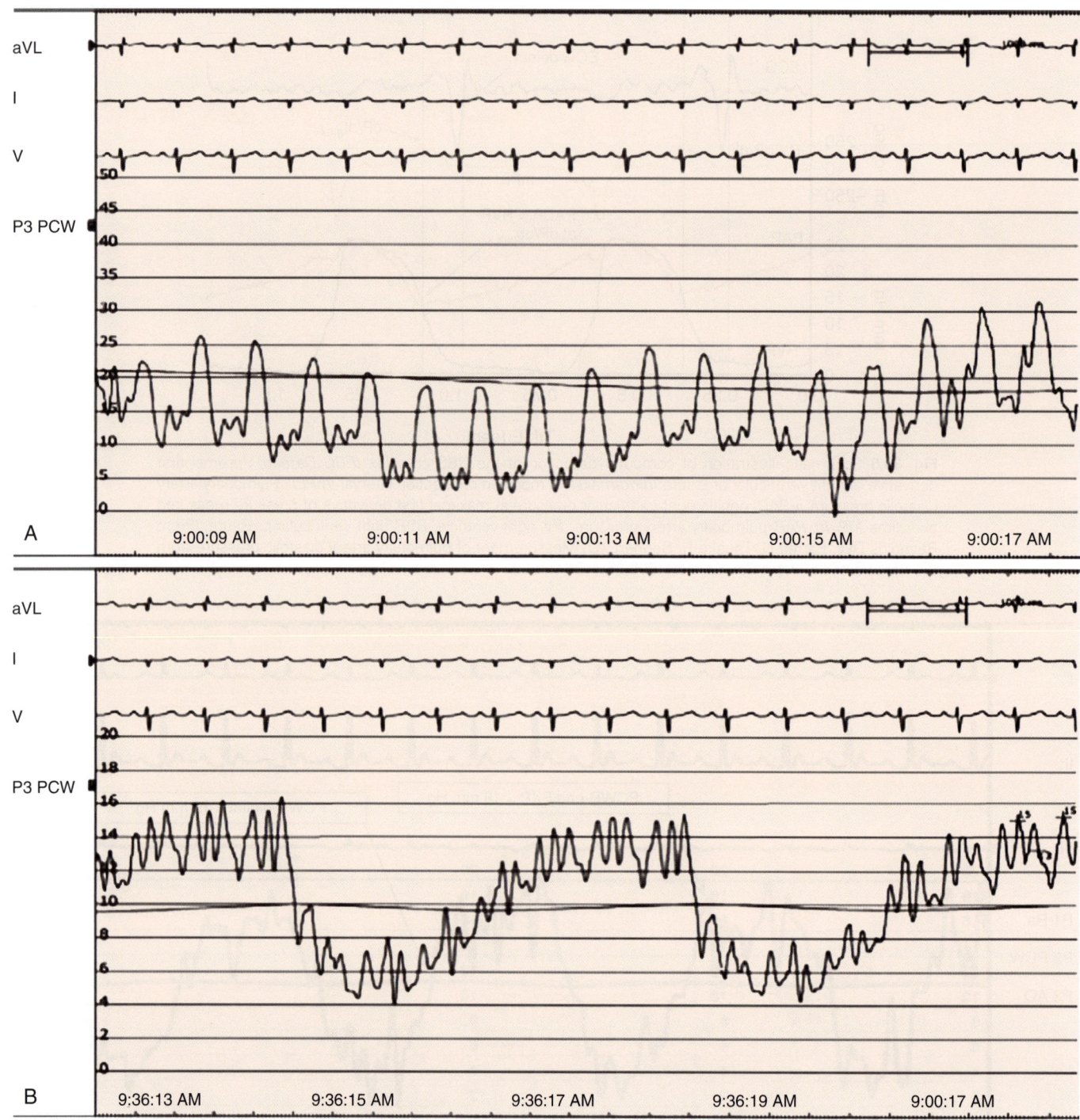

Fig. 34.7 Errors in pulmonary capillary wedge pressure. (A) Hybrid tracing of pulmonary artery pressure and wedge tracing overestimating wedge pressure. (B) Actual pulmonary capillary wedge pressure tracing once the balloon is deflated and allowed to wedge in a smaller, more distal branch of the pulmonary artery. *PCW*, Pulmonary capillary wedge. (From Guillinta P, Peterson KL, Ben-Yehuda O. Cardiac catheterization techniques in pulmonary hypertension. *Cardiol Clin.* 2004;22:401–415.)

RV enlargement as well as pericardial restraint (see also later discussion). In this setting, LV diastolic dysfunction is a consequence and not independent of the primary abnormality (PAH).

If there is still uncertainty about the accuracy of the measured PCWP, it is best confirmed by other means. A common strategy is to use the O_2 saturation from a blood sample obtained from the PCWP position.[5] In the true PCWP position, the O_2 saturation from the PCWP blood sample should have an O_2 saturation comparable to systemic arterial saturation (in the absence of intracardiac shunts). Wedge position can also be confirmed by cautious injection of contrast to document true wedging of the balloon. LVEDP should be directly measured if uncertainty exists as to the accuracy of the PCWP as a surrogate for left ventricular filling. In circumstances where accurate assessment of left atrial pressure (LAP) is critical, consideration should be given to directly measuring LAP across the atrial septum.

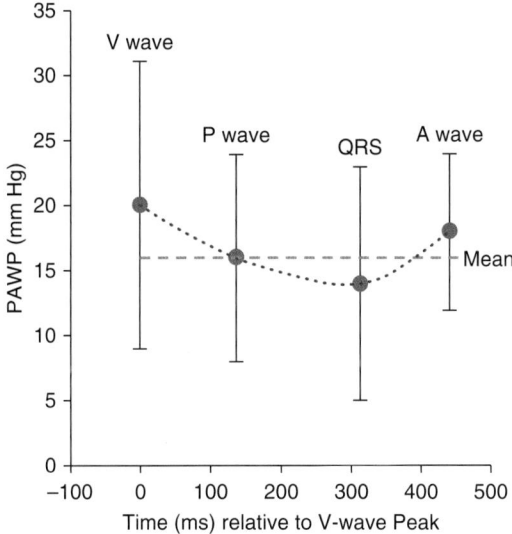

Fig. 34.8 Pulmonary artery wedge pressure *(PAWP)* and time coordinates during diastole. In a subset of 42 patients in sinus rhythm, pressures relevant to the diastolic conduit phase of the left atrium were manually measured beat-by-beat in the PAWP tracing, along with corresponding time intervals within the cardiac cycle. These measurements included the peak V-wave PAWP (i.e., end-systolic PAWP), the pressure at the onset of the ECG P wave (i.e., mid-diastolic PAWP), the pressure at the onset of the ECG QRS-complex (i.e., late-diastolic PAWP), and the peak A-wave PAWP (i.e., peak contraction pressure). For each measurement, the time of the event within that cardiac cycle was recorded to establish pressure-time coordinates. Measurements were repeated over 8–10 cardiac cycles, and averaged. (From Wright SP, Moayedi Y, Foroutan F, et al. Diastolic pressure difference to classify pulmonary hypertension in the assessment of heart transplant candidates. *Circ Heart Fail.* 2017;10:e004077.)

The PCWP waveform is similar to that seen in the left atrium with well characterized *a* and *v* waves, in addition to *x* and *y* descent (*c* waves are less apparent in PCWP tracings). PCWP waveforms are also slightly damped and delayed compared to that seen in the LA because of transmission of the pressures through the lung parenchyma. As noted earlier, in the absence of increased pulmonary vascular resistance, PA diastolic pressure is similar to mean PCWP (e.g., within 2–3 mm Hg). If there is PH, the PA end-diastolic pressure will be markedly higher than PCWP.[11] Furthermore, when pulmonary vascular resistance is increased by pulmonary venous hypertension or mitral stenosis, PCWP may overestimate LVEDP.[12] PCWP may also underestimate LVEDP since PCWP is an intrathoracic pressure that is an indirect assessment of LVEDP and is not a direct measurement of LV filling pressure. In one study, PCWP was more than 5 mm Hg lower than LVEDP in about a third of cardiac patients.[13] Therefore when it is critical to have a definitive measure of LV filling pressure, direct measurement of LVEDP is necessary.

The height of the *v* wave should be reported separately from the mean PCWP, particularly when it exceeds the height of the *a* wave by greater than 50%. The height of the *v* wave is determined by left atrial chamber compliance and distending blood volume. Although most commonly associated with acute severe mitral regurgitation (due to the sudden retrograde volume overwhelming the compliance of the left atrium), it is also characteristic of a large volume ventricular septal defect and can be seen in severe left ventricular diastolic dysfunction.

Large *v* waves augment the mean PCWP and can lead to overestimation in LAPs, as in **Fig. 34.8**.[14-16] In this setting, the mean *a* wave pressure should be reported, in addition to the mean PCWP and height

of the *v* wave, to reflect the end-diastolic PCWP. Another approach is to use the onset of the QRS, complex to define the end-diastolic PCWP.[16]

Measuring Cardiac Output

The two most commonly used methods for measuring cardiac output (CO) are the thermodilution and Fick methods. Both methods are limited by technical issues and physiologic assumptions. The indication-dilution technique is rarely used in contemporary clinical practice but forms the basis for the thermodilution method.

In the thermodilution method, a known volume of cold saline or dextrose is injected at a known temperature into the proximal port of the PAC. The subsequent change in temperature of this solution is measured by a thermistor at the distal end of the catheter. The change in temperature of the injectate allows measurement of the CO. If the temperature does not change markedly and remains close to the temperature at which it was injected, this reflects a high CO because there is insufficient time for the surrounding structures to transfer heat energy to the fluid. In contrast, if the CO is low, there will be ample time to transfer heat energy from the blood to the injectate before it passes the thermistor at the distal end of the catheter. In this setting, the temperature of the injectate will change markedly and will be reflective of a decreased CO. The CO is calculated using an equation that incorporates a calibration factor plus the volume, the specific gravity, and the temperature of the injectate along with the temperature and specific gravity of the blood. The CO is inversely related to the area under the thermodilution curve (e.g., change in temperature over time) with a larger area reflective of a lower CO. Accuracy of the CO measurement is improved by a greater difference between the temperature of the injectate and the temperature of the blood. The thermodilution technique overestimates flow in patients with low output states. Concern is frequently raised regarding the accuracy of thermodilution in patients with severe tricuspid regurgitation, but it remains remarkably useful even in this setting. A large retrospective analysis of more than 1200 patients who underwent RHC demonstrated modest agreement between thermodilution and Fick CO (using an assumed oxygen consumption) (r = 0.65), with 38% of patients having a difference of more than 20%. However, the thermodilution CO was associated with a greater mortality risk (thermodilution hazard ratio [HR] 1.71 [95% confidence interval (CI) 1.47–1.99], Fick HR 1.42 [95% CI, 1.22–1.64]) (**Fig. 34.9**).[17]

The Fick method is based upon the principle that oxygen (O_2) consumption equals the product of O_2 delivery rate (e.g., CO) and O_2 extraction (e.g., the difference in O_2 content between the arterial and venous circulation). Thus CO equals the ratio of O_2 consumption to O_2 extraction and is therefore directly proportional to O_2 consumption. Measurement of O_2 consumption requires specialized equipment (e.g., a metabolic cart) to measure the content of O_2 in expired air. Since most clinical laboratories lack the capacity to make this measurement, most clinical laboratories assume a uniform normalized O_2 consumption (e.g., 125 cc/min/m²) for all patients. Corrections for metabolic state, age, and gender are generally not made, and errors in O_2 consumption can be as high as 50% since O_2 consumption varies widely between patients and clinical status. Such issues are compounded during exercise hemodynamics.[18] Errors in the Fick method can also occur if the mixed venous O_2 content is inaccurately measured due to contamination of the pulmonary arterial sample with blood from the PCWP. Blood from the PA is recommended for accurate assessment of the mixed venous oximetry as it mixes the O_2 content from the superior vena cava, inferior vena cava, and cardiac veins. Blood samples from the superior vena cava and right atrium are often used as surrogates for the mixed venous O_2,[19] but may not be adequate estimations in patients with sepsis, shunts, fistulas, and normal cardiac index. Peripheral venous oximetry can also be used to follow trends in CO, assuming oxygen consumption

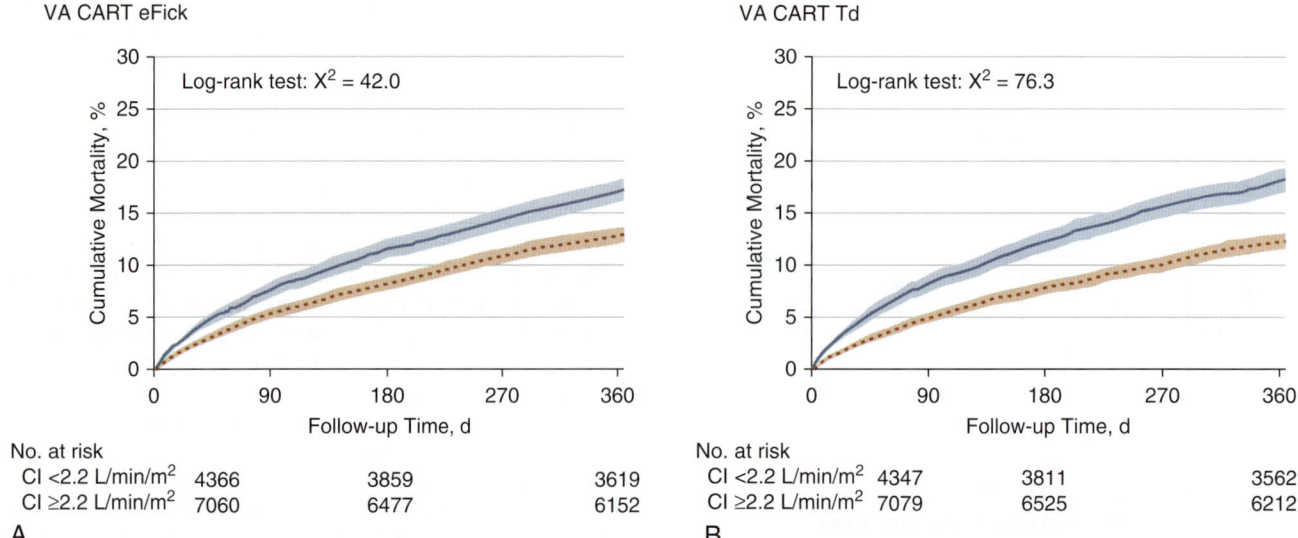

Fig. 34.9 Cumulative mortality through 90 days and 1-year follow-up, classified by normal and low thermodilution *(Td)* and estimated oxygen uptake Fick *(eFick)* cardiac index categories. (Adapted from Opotowsky AR, Hess E, Maron BA, et al. Thermodilution vs. estimated fick cardiac output measurement in clinical practice: an analysis of mortality from the Veterans Affairs clinical assessment, reporting, and tracking [VA CART] program and Vanderbilt University. *JAMA Cardiol.* 2017;2:1090–1099.)

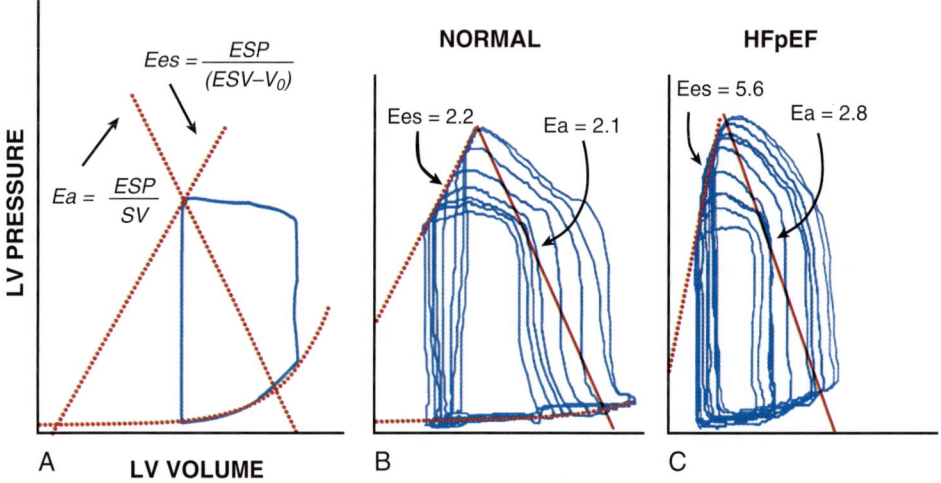

Fig. 34.10 (A) Left ventricular end-systolic elastance *(Ees)* is described by the slope and intercept of the end-systolic pressure–volume relationship; arterial elastance *(Ea)* is defined by the negative slope between the end-systolic pressure–volume point and end-diastolic volume. (B) A normal adult has relatively low Ees and Ea, with a coupling ratio around unity, whereas older aged, hypertensive subjects with heart failure with preserved ejection fraction (HFpEF) subjects (C) display marked increases in ventricular and arterial elastance. *ESP*, End-systolic pressure; *ESV*, end-systolic volume; *LV*, left ventricle; *SV*, stroke volume (From Borlaug BA, Kass DA. Ventricular-vascular interaction in heart failure. *Cardiology Clin.* 2011;29:447–459.)

is relatively constant over time.[9] Inaccurate assessment of hemoglobin content will also lead to measurement errors, and simultaneous measurement of hemoglobin concentration should be obtained if possible. If O_2 consumption is accurately measured, the Fick method is more accurate than the thermodilution method in patients with low CO.

HEMODYNAMICS OF HEART FAILURE WITH REDUCED EJECTION FRACTION

The hemodynamic interaction between the left ventricle and the vascular system (e.g., ventricular-vascular coupling) for any degree of intrinsic myocardial contractility is best described with PV loops.[4] In a PV loop,

load-independent contractility is characterized by the slope of the end-systolic pressure-volume relationship (ESPVR) curve, or end-systolic elastance (Ees), which is also influenced by chamber size. Vascular afterload is characterized by arterial stiffness or elastance (Ea) and determined from the negative slope of the line through the end-systolic and end-diastolic volumes (**Fig. 34.10**); this measurement integrates the resistive and pulsatile components of afterload and is heart-rate dependent.[20] Ejection fraction, systolic blood pressure, stroke volume, and stroke work can all be derived from end diastolic volume (EDV) and these elastances.

The ratio of these two measurements represents ventricular-arterial coupling (Ea/Ees) and describes the "matching" of vascular load to myocardial function.[20-22] Experimental studies suggest an

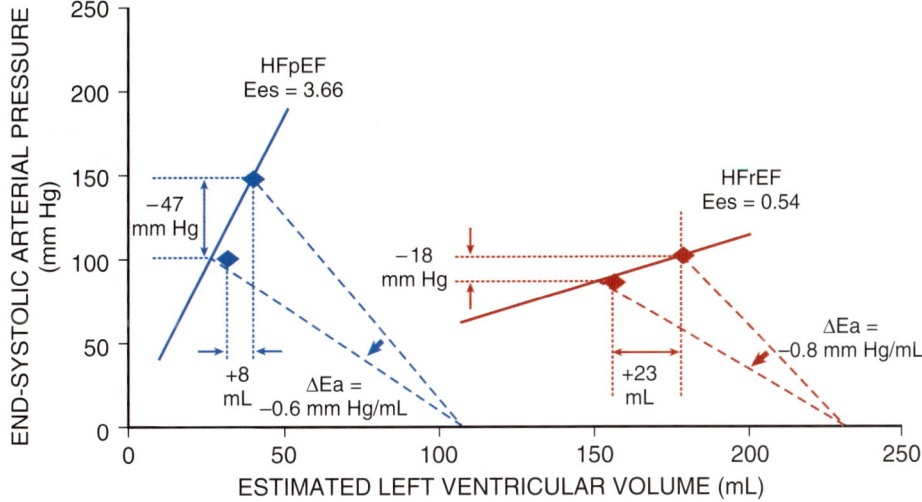

Fig. 34.11 Differential effect of afterload reduction in heart failure with preserved ejection fraction *(HFpEF)* vs. heart failure with reduced ejection fraction *(HFrEF)*. In HFpEF *(blue)*, a reduction in afterload (Ea = −0.6 mm Hg/cc) with a vasodilator produces a large decrease in BP (−47 mm Hg) but only modest increase in stroke volume (+8 cc) since Ees is steep (3.66). In contrast, comparable vasodilation (Ea = −0.8 mm Hg/cc) produces only a modest decrease in blood pressure (−18 mm Hg) but a large increase in stroke volume (+23 cc) due to the shallow Ees (0.54) in HFrEF *(red)*. E_a, Elastance; *Ees*, end-systolic elastance. (From Schwartzenberg S, Redfield MM, From AM, et al. Effects of vasodilation in heart failure with preserved or reduced ejection fraction implications of distinct pathophysiologies on response to therapy. *J Am Coll Cardiol* 2012;59:442–451.)

optimal Ea/Ees ratio is 0.6 to 1.2, which maximizes the efficient transfer of blood from the heart into the systemic circulation. In patients with HFrEF, this ratio is increased since ventricular elastance (Ees) is depressed from the underlying cardiomyopathy and arterial elastance (Ea) is increased from neurohormonal activation and vasoconstriction.[21] This afterload "mismatch" has prognostic implications independent of EF and can be a target for therapy (see later discussion). In a recent noninvasive multicenter study of HFrEF patients, an Ea/Ees ratio greater than 2.34 was found an independent risk factor of all-cause mortality, cardiac transplantation, or VAD implantation (HR 2.1, 95% CI 1.3–3.3).[23]

It is important to note that systemic blood pressure and systemic vascular resistance (SVR) do not adequately describe afterload in a pulsatile system. In clinical practice, the resistive load is described by the SVR ([MAP—CVP]/CO); the pulsatile load is usually not described. The pulsatile load can be quantified by the total systemic arterial compliance (C_a) (Stroke Volume Index/aortic pulse pressure). Because the aorta provides the majority of this pulsatile load, central pulsatile load (or characteristic impedance, Zc = change in pressure/change in flow in early systole) better characterizes the work that must be overcome by the LV during ejection and is elevated in HFrEF.[24] Although not practical for routine clinical use, the effective arterial elastance (Ea = ESP/SV, where ESP, end systolic pressure; SV = stroke volume) combines the resistive and pulsatile components of LV afterload and best describes the impact of ventricular-vascular coupling to LV performance.

In HFrEF, vasodilation can dramatically improve stroke volume since the reduced contractile state is particularly afterload sensitive and characterized by an increased Ea/Ees ratio (e.g., afterload "mismatch"). Vasodilator therapy takes advantage of the inverse relationship between CO and impedance. In HFrEF, the afterload sensitive nature of the failing LV is reflected by the relatively flat ESPVR, for example, shallow Ees. This flat ESPVR accounts for the marked improvement in stroke volume that occurs with vasodilator therapy without a significant drop in blood pressure (**Fig. 34.11**).

HEMODYNAMICS FOR ASSESSMENT AND MANAGEMENT

A hemodynamically directed clinical assessment is prognostic. The 1-year risk of mortality or urgent transplantation increases with worsening hemodynamic status. With bedside evaluation of filling pressures and perfusion, the patient can be classified as Profile A (Warm and Dry), B (Warm and Wet), C (Cold and Wet), and L (Cold and Dry).[25] Congested patients (profile B) are at greater risk for death or transplant than those compensated (profile A) (HR 1.84; P = .02); the highest risk is associated with congestion and poor perfusion (profile C) (HR 2.48; P = .03).[26] Drazner and coworkers confirmed that a bedside clinical assessment (e.g., orthopnea, jugular venous distension, impression of inadequate perfusion) did parallel invasively obtained hemodynamics in a group of patients with advanced heart failure. Moreover, invasively obtained hemodynamics in this population did identify those at increased risk of morbidity and mortality.[27] The CVP is particularly useful since it is easy to obtain at the bedside or invasively. An elevated CVP is the hemodynamic abnormality most commonly associated with the cardiorenal syndrome.[28] An increased CVP/PCWP ratio is also associated with more RV dysfunction and poorer outcomes in patients with advanced heart failure treated with left ventricular assist device therapy (**see Chapter 45**).[29]

The hemodynamic profile can be used to guide therapy. Most patients with decompensated heart failure present congested but well perfused (**see also Chapter 36**). Vasodilators and decongestion with diuretics or mechanical fluid removal are recommended for symptom relief but this hemodynamic profile rarely requires invasively obtained hemodynamics to guide therapy. In contrast, selected patients with clinical evidence of inadequate perfusion (e.g., hypotension, end-organ dysfunction, lack of improvement with empiric therapy) may benefit from invasive hemodynamics to guide therapy. This approach can be particularly useful when there is hypotension since the cause may be vasoplegic (e.g., low SVR) rather than due to poor perfusion (e.g., low cardiac index, high SVR). In this setting, if an inadequate CO is confirmed (and hypovolemia is not present), subsequent therapy can be "tailored" to the total hemodynamic

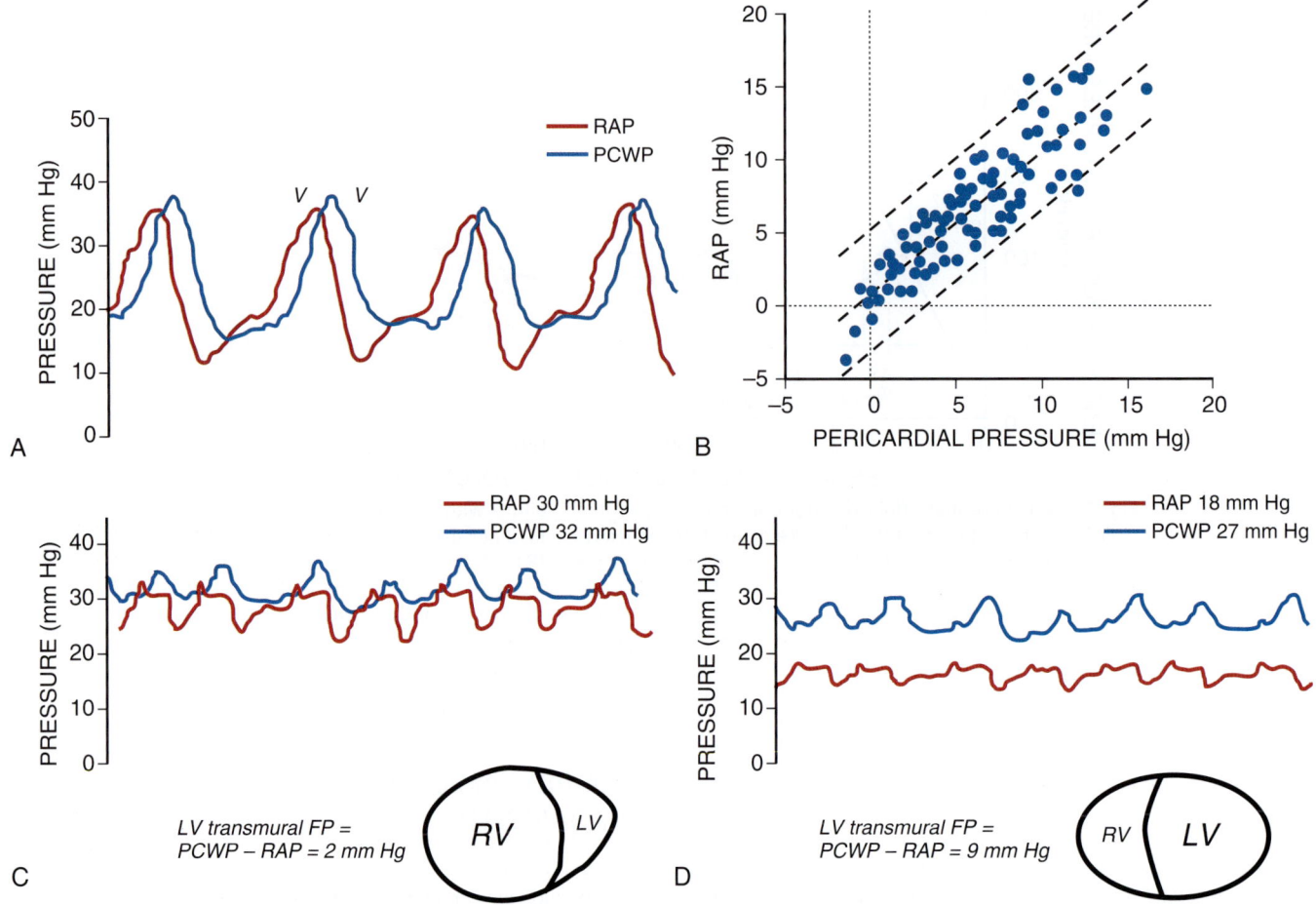

Fig. 34.12 Ventricular interdependence in right heart failure from group 2 pulmonary hypertension. (A) Typical equalization in right atrial pressure (RAP) and pulmonary capillary wedge pressure (PCWP) from enhanced interdependence in a patient with biventricular heart failure and severe functional tricuspid insufficiency. Note the prominent V wave in the PCWP that tracks closely with the right atrium (RA) V wave, even in the absence of significant mitral insufficiency. This is caused by pressure changes in the RA being transmitted to the left atrium across the interatrial septum. (B) External pericardial pressure, which restrains left heart filling, can be estimated by RAP. Thus when RA pressure is elevated near PCWP, true left ventricle (LV) preload volume may be reduced despite marked elevation in left PCWP, because transmural pressure is reduced. (C) and (D) Unloading of right heart congestion in this circumstance may enhance left-sided preload, even if PCWP drops, because transmural pressure increases. FP, Filling pressure; RV, right ventricle. (From Guazzi M, Borlaug BA. Pulmonary hypertension due to left heart disease. *Circulation.* 2012;126:975–990.)

picture.[30,31] In the ESCAPE trial, the RA decreased from 14 ± 10 to 10 ± 7 mm Hg, PCW fell from 25 ± 9 to 17 ± 7 mm Hg, the CI rose from 1.9 ± 0.6 to 2.4 ± 0.7 L/min/m², and the SVR fell from 1500 ± 800 to 1100 ± 500 dynes-sec-cm⁻⁵ with tailored therapy.[6] Reasonable hemodynamic goals include an RA less than 10 mm Hg, PCWP less than 15 mm Hg, and an SVR less than 1200 dynes-sec-cm⁻⁵ to maximize the forward CO while maintaining a mean BP greater than 65 to 70 mm Hg or a systemic systolic blood pressure of at least 80 to 90 mm Hg. These goals are physiologically based; there is no randomized evidence to support these targets to improve symptoms or impact clinically important outcomes.

These hemodynamic goals are generally achieved with diuretic management and vasodilators. This approach is preferred over inotropic management when the cardiac index is low and SVR is elevated due to the increase in mortality associated with inotropic agents.[2] Often intravenous rather than oral vasodilators are elected to achieve rapid hemodynamic goals, which minimizes the duration of PA line placement. Sodium nitroprusside (SNP) is ideal in this regard because its effects are rapid in onset and it is rapidly cleared and is recommended in numerous guidelines.[2,30-32] Its balanced vasodilator effect is particular useful when filling pressures are high, SVR is increased (e.g., >2000 dynes-sec-cm⁻⁵)

and the cardiac index is low. In an observational experience from the Cleveland Clinic, use of tailored therapy with SNP was associated with improved survival in patients presenting with a low cardiac index (1.6 ± 0.2 L/min/m²) and elevated SVR (1846 ± 567 dynes-sec-cm⁻⁵), without worsening renal function or need for inotropic support.[31] Randomized experiences with SNP in chronic heart failure however are lacking. Nitroglycerin and nesiritide can also be used for "tailored" therapy.

An effective reduction in mitral regurgitation and an increase in forward stroke volume also occurs with vasodilators due to a reduction in left ventricular volume and mitral annular orifice size.[33] In addition, relieving right heart congestion leads to improved LV filling through reduction in the pericardial constraint imposed by an over-distended RV "crowding out" the LV.[34] In fact, almost half of the measured intraventricular diastolic pressure is a consequence of external forces from the pericardium and RV.[35,36] Diastolic ventricular interaction is most evident when RA pressure (an estimate of pericardial pressure) equals PCWP, effectively decreasing LV transmural pressure as in LV preload.[37] "Release" of the pericardial constraint by decompressing the RV paradoxically increases LV transmural pressure, thereby optimizing LV preload (**Fig. 34.12A–D**).

TABLE 34.2 Recommendations for Invasive Evaluation

Recommendations	COR	LOE
Monitoring with a pulmonary artery catheter should be performed in patients with respiratory distress or impaired systemic perfusion when clinical assessment is inadequate	1	C
Invasive hemodynamic monitoring can be useful for carefully selected patients with acute HF with persistent symptoms and/or when hemodynamics are uncertain	IIa	C
When ischemia may be contributing to HF, coronary arteriography is reasonable	IIa	C
Endomyocardial biopsy can be useful in patients with HF when a specific diagnosis is suspected that would influence therapy	IIa	C
Routine use of invasive hemodynamic monitoring is not recommended in normotensive patients with acute HF	III: No Benefit	B[6]
Endomyocardial biopsy should not be performed in the routine evaluation of HF	III: Harm	C

COR, Class of Recommendation; HF, heart failure; LOE, level of evidence.
Adapted from Yancy CW, Jessup M, Bozkurt B, et al. 2013 ACCF/AHA guideline for the management of heart failure: a report of the American College of Cardiology Foundation/American Heart Association Task Force on Practice Guidelines. *J Am Coll Cardiol.* 2013;62:e147–e239.

Hemodynamic profiles have changed over time. Due to the routine use of aggressive oral vasodilators in chronic systolic heart failure, it is relatively less common to see patients with a low cardiac index and extremely elevated SVR. In advanced heart failure, a low cardiac index may be associated with an "abnormally" normal SVR (e.g., <1200 dynes-sec-cm^{-5}) or vasoplegic state. In this situation, inotropic support, with or without vasopressors, may be necessary in the acute setting. Unless there is another reason to explain the inappropriate vasoplegia (e.g., infection, adrenal insufficiency), this hemodynamic profile is difficult to treat, associated with poor outcomes, and should initiate a consideration of advanced therapies.

Despite the potential use of hemodynamics for "tailored" therapy, the *routine* utilization of invasive hemodynamics for the treatment of heart failure is not recommended. The 2013 ACCF/AHA guidelines for the management of heart failure observe that RHC and PA catheter is best reserved for situations where a particular therapeutic or clinical question is being addressed, such as inadequate clinical assessment and uncertain hemodynamics in patients with inadequate systemic perfusion and/or respiratory distress (**Table 34.2**).[2] The ESCAPE trial was a multicenter randomized controlled trial of PA catheter-guided management in acute decompensated heart failure patients with a left ventricular ejection fraction (LVEF) less than 30%.[6] Compared to patients treated without a PA catheter, the use of invasive hemodynamics to guide therapy achieved no significant difference in mortality (10% vs. 9%; P = .35) or days hospitalized (8.7 vs. 8.3 days; P = .67). PA catheter guided therapy was associated with more in-hospital adverse events as described above. Use of PA catheter to guided therapy remains a reasonable approach in patients not responding to initial therapy or with deteriorating clinical status. An analysis of the National Inpatient Sample demonstrated significant temporal and hospital variations in the utilization of PA across the United States.[38] From 2001 to 2006 there was a significant decline in the use of PA catheters; however from 2007 to 2012 there was disproportionate increase in utilization of PA catheters, mainly in hospitals with large capacity, teaching programs, and advanced heart failure services (**Fig. 34.13**). There was also a significant decline in the mortality among patients treated with PA catheters, with at-risk–adjusted odds ratio of 1.66 (95% CI 1.60–1.74) from 2001 to 2003 that fell to 1.04 (95% CI 0.97–1.12) from 2010 to 2012 (**Fig. 34.14**).

HEMODYNAMICS AND ADVANCED HEART FAILURE

Hemodynamic assessment in advanced heart failure is necessary to evaluate PH, RV function, and candidacy for advanced therapies. The primary hemodynamic considerations when faced with PH and heart failure are to confirm its presence and severity, delineate etiology, and assess reversibility (**Fig. 34.15**) (**see also Chapter 43**). Excluding WHO Group 1, PH is crucial; it is defined by a mean PAP ≥25 mm Hg and a resting PCWP less than 15 mm Hg. Therefore accurate measurement of PCWP is critical. If there is uncertainty regarding this measurement, LVEDP should be obtained directly. A fluid challenge or a selective pulmonary vasodilator (e.g., inhaled nitric oxide) can be used to selectively assess the LV filling pressure response to an increase in volume.[39]

The PH of heart failure is defined by a mean PAP ≥25 mm Hg with resting PCWP ≥15 mm Hg, for example, as in WHO Group 2 PH. In heart failure, the chronically elevated pressures of the left heart are passively transmitted back into the pulmonary circulation leading to elevated pulmonary arterial pressures, variably referred to as passive, postcapillary, or secondary PH.

Although PH in heart failure has been defined by mean PAP, a PASP ≥35 mm Hg is a valid surrogate for a mean PAP ≥25 mm Hg.[40] In heart failure, PH is commonly increased out of proportion to the predicted PH relative to the increase in left heart filling pressure, as in "mixed," reactive, or combined precapillary and postcapillary PH. It is defined by a mean PAP ≥25 mm Hg, PCWP ≥15 mm Hg, transpulmonary gradient (TPG) ≥12 to 15 mm Hg, and PVR ≥2.5 to 3.0 Wood units.[41] Recent observations suggest pathophysiologic overlap with WHO Group 1 PH.[42] In HFrEF, mixed PH is not easily predicted from clinical profiles but is associated with greater disease severity and increased mortality.[40,43] Due to its independent association with disease severity and mortality, PH and specifically mixed PH may be a novel target for therapy.

The pulmonary arterial diastolic pressure gradient (DPG) (PAD—PCWP) may also be used to clarify which patients with mixed PH are at greater risk for mortality.[44] The DPG is free of the influence of flow and PCWP for its calculation (in contrast to the measurement of pulmonary vascular resistance [PVR]) and may therefore be a better reflection of the pulmonary vascular system. In the setting of an elevated TPG greater than 10–12 mm Hg, a DPG greater than 7 mm Hg has been associated with increased mortality.

These clinical observations may be explained by the unique pathophysiology of PH in heart failure. Left-side diastolic dysfunction increases the RV afterload to a greater extent than the simple passive transmission of back pressure into the pulmonary circulation. In the pulmonary vasculature, arterial compliance is high and is evenly distributed across the lungs. The main PA contributes relatively little to overall compliance and is minimally affected by age, which contrasts with the aorta which accounts for more than 75% of the compliance of the systemic circulation.[45] There are also 10 times more vessels in the pulmonary bed than in the systemic circulation and vascular resistance is 10-fold lower in the lung than in the systemic circulation. Therefore the distal pulmonary vessels contribute to both vascular resistance and compliance. These circumstances lead to premature pulmonary arterial

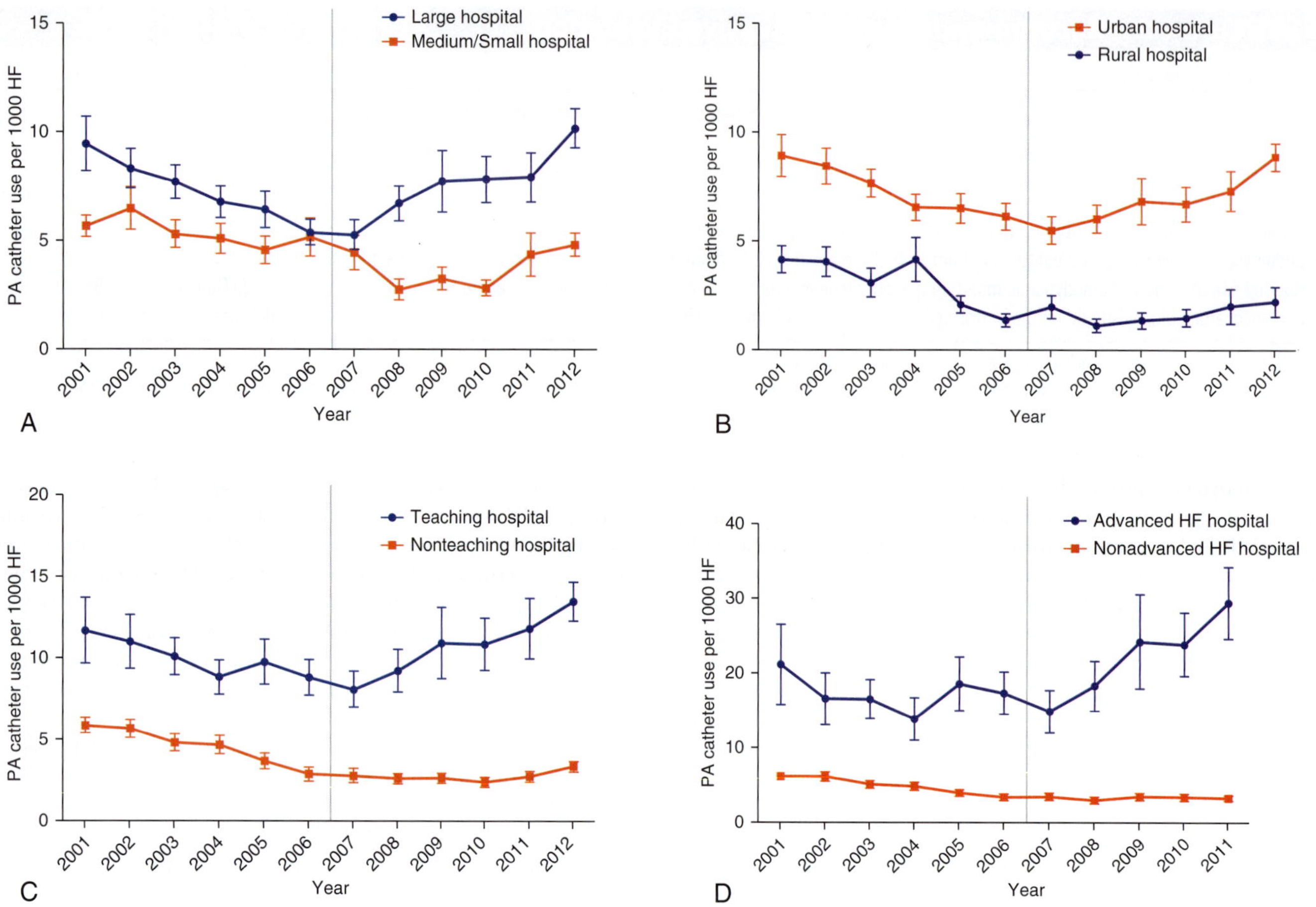

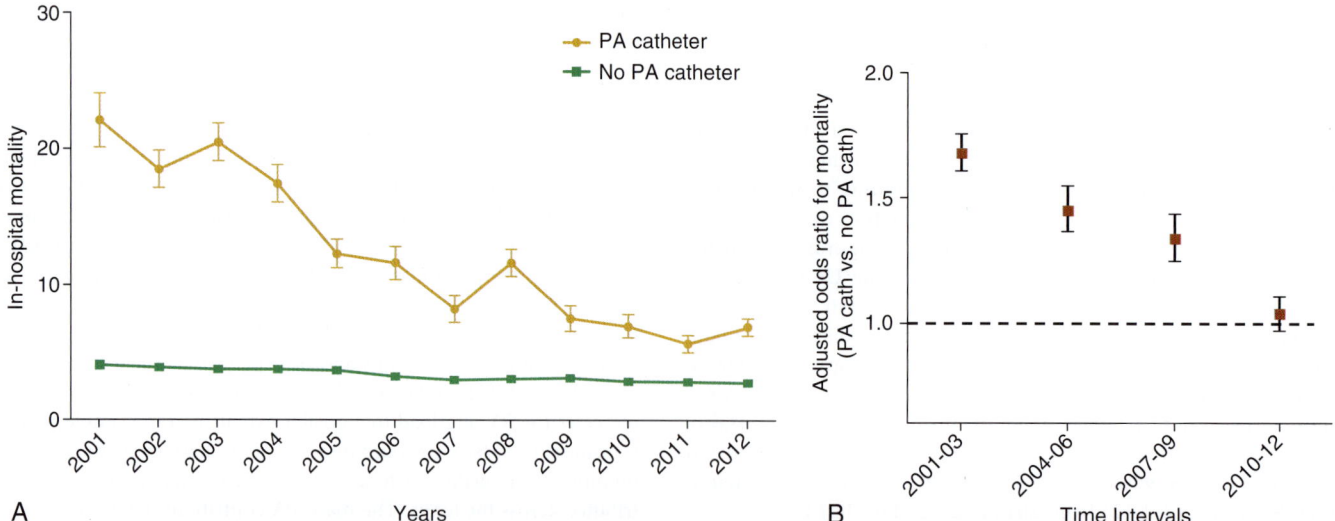

Fig. 34.13 Trends in pulmonary artery *(PA)* catheter utilization in heart failure *(HF)* by hospital characteristics. (A) Hospital capacity, (B) urban versus rural location, (C) teaching status, and (D) advanced HF facilities. (From Khera R, Pandey A, Kumar N, et al. Variation in hospital use and outcomes associated with pulmonary artery catheterization in heart failure in the United States. *Circ Heart Fail.* 2016;9:e003226.)

Fig. 34.14 Trends in mortality in patients with pulmonary artery *(PA)* catheterization in heart failure. (A) Overall and (B) risk-adjusted odds ratios for mortality in propensity-matched analysis in different temporal cohorts. (From Khera R, Pandey A, Kumar N, et al. Variation in hospital use and outcomes associated with pulmonary artery catheterization in heart failure in the United States. *Circ Heart Fail.* 2016;9:e003226.)

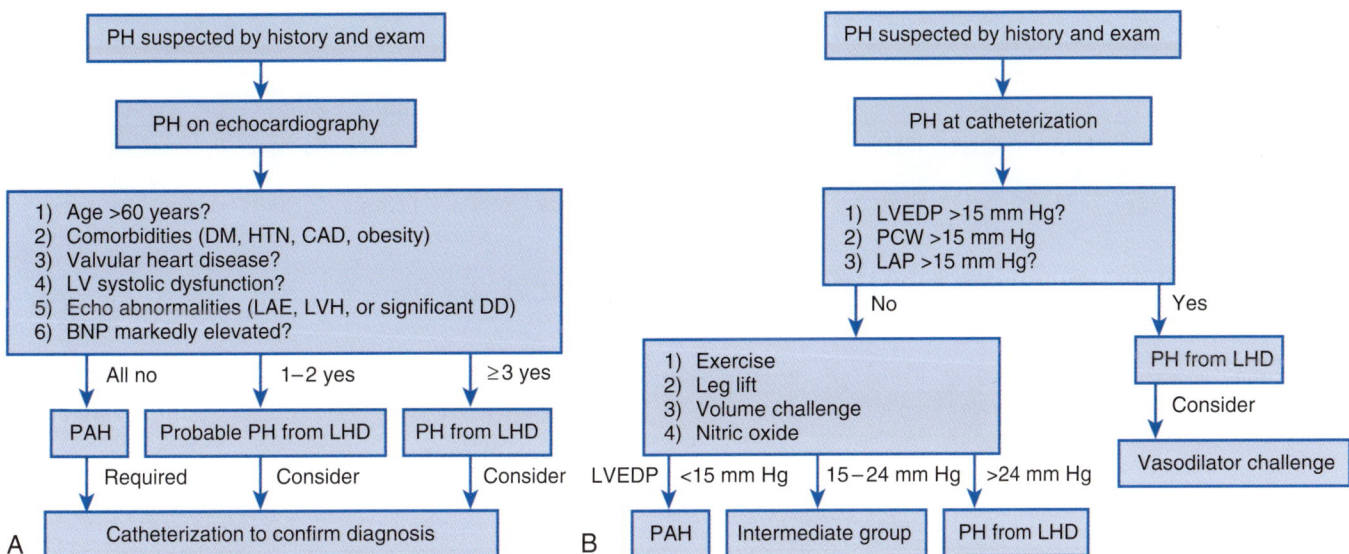

Fig. 34.15 Echocardiographic (A) and hemodynamic (B) approach to pulmonary hypertension *(PH). CAD,* Coronary artery disease; *DD,* diastolic dysfunction; *DM,* diabetes mellitus; *HTN,* hypertension; *LAE,* left atrial enlargement; *LAP,* lipid accumulation product; *LHD,* left heart disease; *LV,* Left ventricle; *LVDP,* left ventricular developed pressure; *LVH,* left ventricular hypertrophy; *PAH,* pulmonary artery hypertension; *PCW,* pulmonary capillary wedge.

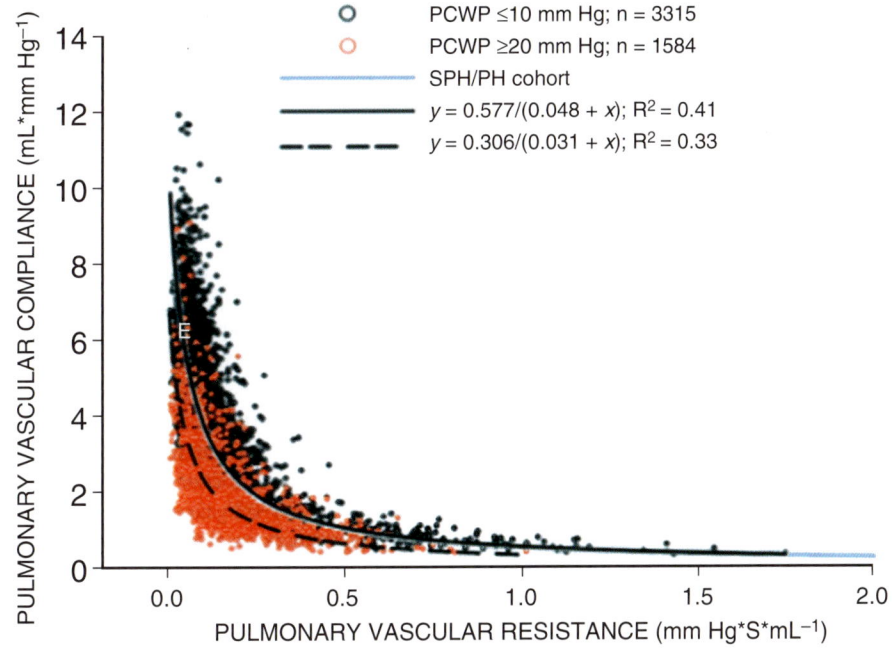

Fig. 34.16 **Inverse relationship between compliance and resistance in pulmonary circulation.** Increased pulmonary capillary wedge pressure *(PCWP) (red)* moves this relationship to the left *(dotted line). PH,* Pulmonary hypertension; *SPH,* severe portal hypertension. (From Tedford RJ, Hassoun PM, Mathai SC, et al. Pulmonary capillary wedge pressure augments right ventricular pulsatile loading. *Circulation.* 2012;125:289–297.)

wave reflections, augmentation of the systolic PAP, and increases in the mean PAP. This combination of resistance and compliance in the same bed explains why elevations in PCWP result in both direct and indirect increases in mean PAP.

For a given LAP, the product of resistance and compliance has been shown to be constant and not significantly altered by PH.[45] Increases in LAP shift the resistance/compliance relationship to the left, such that compliance is lower at any given PVR (**Fig. 34.16**). This increases the pulsatile component of RV afterload (e.g., impedance) relative to the resistive load, to which the normal RV is extremely sensitive. Therefore RV hydraulic efficiency is compromised to a greater extent in patients with PH due to left heart disease as a consequence of this abnormal ventricular-vascular coupling and afterload mismatch. This impact on RV efficiency suggests increased pulmonary arterial compliance in heart failure could affect outcomes. Some have suggested that a PA compliance greater than 2.0 cc/mm Hg is associated with increased mortality, but there are few studies that have systematically addressed this parameter with partition values.

TABLE 34.3	Selective Intravenous Pulmonary Vasodilators											
Agent	Route	$T_{1/2}$	Dose	Increase	mPAP	PVR	TPG	PCWP	SBP	SVR	CI	Side effects
Nitric Oxide	Inhaled	15–30 s	10–40 ppm	10 ppm	Decrease	Decrease	Decrease	Increase	No effect	No change	Decrease	Increased LV pressure
Adenosine	Intravenous	5–10 s	50–150 mcg/kg/min	50 mcg/kg/min	Decrease	Decrease	Decrease	Possible increase	Decrease	No change	Increase	Chest pain, AV block
Epoprostenol	Intravenous	3 min	2–12 ng/kg/min	2 ng/kg/min	Decrease	Decrease	Decrease	Decrease	Decrease	Decrease	Increase	Headache, nausea
Nitroprusside	Intravenous	2 min	0.25–3 µg/kg/min	0.25 µg/kg/min	Decrease	Decrease	Decrease	Decrease	Decrease	Decrease	Increase	Flushing, hypotension
Milrinone	Intravenous	2.5 hr	50 µg/kg IV bolus	Maintenance: 0.375–0.75 µg/kg/minute	Decrease	Decrease	Decrease	Decrease	Decrease	Decrease	Increase	Atrial and ventricular arrhythmia

AV, Atrioventricular; *CI,* cardiac index; *IV,* intravenous; *LV,* left ventricular; *mPAP,* mean pulmonary artery pressure; *PCWP,* pulmonary capillary wedge pressure; *PVR,* peripheral vascular resistance; *SBP,* systolic blood pressure; *SVR,* systemic vascular resistance; *T½,* half life; *TPG,* transpulmonary gradient.
Adapted from Fang JC, DeMarco T, Givertz MM, et al. World Health Organization Pulmonary Hypertension group 2: pulmonary hypertension due to left heart disease in the adult—a summary statement from the Pulmonary Hypertension Council of the International Society for Heart and Lung Transplantation. *J Heart Lung Transplant.* 2012;31:913–933.

Heart Transplantation

An elevated PVR is an independent risk factor for RV failure and early mortality after heart transplantation (**see also Chapter 44**). Cardiac surgery alone may also exacerbate an elevated PVR through cardiopulmonary bypass, transfusions, and hypoxia. However, if PH is predominantly driven by an increase in PCWP and the PVR is reversible, successful transplantation is possible. The magnitude of PVR elevation does not appear to impact heart transplant outcomes as long as the PH is reversible.[46]

The ISHLT Cardiac Transplant Guidelines recommend assessment of pulmonary pressures and resistance in all transplant candidates.[47] A vasodilator challenge is advised when the PASP ≥50 mm Hg, the TPG ≥15 mm Hg, or PVR ≥3 Wood units (or 240 dynes-sec-cm⁻⁵). In the 1992 classic study at Stanford University, "reversible" PH was defined by a decrease in PVR to ≤2.5 Wood units without excessive hypotension (e.g., asymptomatic systolic BP ≥85 mm Hg) and was associated with a posttransplant mortality of 3.8%.[48] In that series, the inability to acutely achieve this goal (using SNP) suggested "fixed" PH and an unacceptable posttransplant mortality (e.g., 20%–40%). More contemporary experiences have confirmed those early observations. In 217 heart transplant patients from Germany, survival in the 22.6% patients with reversible PH with prostacyclin (PVR <2.5 Wood units; TPG <12 mm Hg) was comparable to patients without PH, despite more early right heart failure.[49] An upper limit to PVR for transplantation has not been established although most centers will not consider patients with fixed PVR greater than 5 Wood units, PASP greater than 60 mm Hg, or TPG greater than 15 to 20 mm Hg without some chronic attempt to lower the PVR (e.g., chronic inotropes, IABP, VAD).[50] An analysis from the United Network for Organ Sharing registry of patients listed for heart transplantation with high PVR (>5 wood units [WU]) demonstrated that VADs and inotropes can provide a similar reduction in PVR (−1.71 vs. −1.85 WU, respectively; *P* = .52). However, PVR normalization (PVR <2.5) occurred in only 30% to 35% of patients. Despite an average pretransplant PVR of 4.0 WU in the inotrope group and 3.5 WU in the VAD group, the wait-list mortality was similar, although posttransplant survival was not assessed.[51] Regular surveillance RHC is also recommended since PH often gets worse with time, although this practice has little evidence base.

Several agents are available to assess pulmonary vasoreactivity (**see** previous discussion of SNP, **Table 34.3**). Bolus milrinone is useful since titration is not necessary and hypotension is uncommon; 50 mcg/kg over 1 minute is well tolerated and produces its peak effect within minutes. The effects of inotropy and vasodilation produce a fall in PVR of 30%, although there is usually minimal change in TPG. Selective pulmonary vasodilators (e.g., inhaled nitric oxide) can be used, but can precipitate acute pulmonary edema if the diastolic compliance of the LV is overwhelmed with the sudden increase in transpulmonary flow. If the resting PCWP is greater than 20 to 25 mm Hg, milrinone, nitroprusside, or nitroglycerin are preferable for this reason. In contrast, sildenafil is well tolerated in chronic systolic heart failure when given acutely.[52]

Chronic lowering of LV filling pressures, whether by mechanical circulatory support (MCS) or transplant, may ultimately reverse the PH and allow transplantation (**see Chapter 44**).[41] Retrospective studies have shown reduction in pulmonary pressures with prolonged MCS in patients with HF and "fixed" PH.[53] Sildenafil has been used as an adjuvant in this setting to help lower the pulmonary pressures.[54]

Most posttransplant resting hemodynamics normalize within months following transplantation.[55] In 24 heart transplant recipients, the mean PAP fell from 38 ± 9 mm Hg to 19 ± 5 mm Hg and the PVR fell from 2.5 ± 1.1 Wood units to 1.2 ± 0.4 Wood units 1 year after heart transplantation. However, there may be significant acute diastolic dysfunction of the LA and LV, manifest by large *v* waves in the PCW tracing (in the absence of significant mitral regurgitation) in the immediate days to weeks after transplant. LV compliance improves but does not normalize; there is generally a rapid rise in LVEDP with exercise.[56] In some instances, an increase in filling pressures and low index may be associated with severe cellular rejection but rejection is generally hemodynamically silent.[57]

Left Ventricular Assist Devices

All patients who are evaluated for MCS should have invasive hemodynamics obtained to confirm the severity of heart failure, to measure pulmonary pressures and vascular resistance, and to assess RV function. Severe preimplant irreversible RV failure is a contraindication for

LVAD implantation (**see also Chapter 45**). Physiologically, the LVAD depends on adequate left ventricular loading from the RV and therefore adequate RV function is required. In the case of bridging to transplant, consideration should be given to biventricular VADs or a total artificial heart if RV function is not adequate.

RV function may also suffer post implant due to the effects of cardiopulmonary bypass, transfusions, and ischemic injury to the RV and pulmonary vasculature during surgery. Post implant, RV failure can be defined by (1) the need for at least 14 days of continuous inotropic support or (2) the need for a right ventricular assist device (RVAD). The thresholds for these interventions are extremely variable among centers and clinicians and contribute to the wide range of post-implant RV failure rates from 4% to 40%.[58,59] Post-implant RV dysfunction is likely when there is a low mean PA pressure (with an elevated CVP), increased CVP or CVP/PCWP ratio, and a low right ventricular stroke work index (RVSWI). A low mean PAP with an elevated CVP suggests lack of RV preload recruitable stroke work and a RV that is not capable of generating enough PA pressure to overcome an elevated PVR. An elevated CVP, particularly in relation to the PCWP (e.g., CVP/PCWP ratio), suggests significant RV dysfunction; a CVP/PCWP ratio greater than 0.63 is an independent risk factor for RV failure.[58] The MAP/CVP ratio integrates an assessment of the systemic circulation relative to the pulmonary circulation; a value of less than 7.5 has been associated with early RV failure and mortality after LVAD implantation.[60]

A more load independent measure of RV function is reflected in the RVSWI, which describes RV contractile performance for a given afterload/preload and is based upon the use of a PV loop. The right ventricular stroke work is calculated by multiplying stroke volume (indexed by body surface area [BSA]) and the pressure generated by the RV while ejecting that stroke volume (e.g., mean PAP—CVP).

In a single center LVAD study, post-implant RV failure was rare if the RVSWI was greater than 900 mm Hg-mL-m^{-2} (3%) but common when less than 600 mm Hg-mL-m^{-2} (29%–38%).[61] Risk scores have been proposed to determine the risk of RV failure after LVAD implantation and are dependent on specific hemodynamics as well as other measures of RV function such as tricuspid annular plane systolic excursion (TAPSE), RVEF, tricuspid regurgitation, and RV size.[62] However, all such risk scores have been limited by only modest predictive ability[63] and post-LVAD RV failure has continued to be an important clinical problem.

The pulmonary artery pulsatility index (PAPi) defined as [(systolic PA pressure − diastolic PA pressure)/central venous pressure], has been used as a hemodynamic index of right ventricular function and may predict RV failure after inferior MI[64] and after LVAD implantation. In a single center study, lower PAPi values of less than 2.0 were identified in 74% of patients who required RVAD support and no patients with PAPi values above 3.1 required a RVAD. A PAPi cutoff of 2.0 demonstrated an area under the curve of 0.77 to predict RVAD support with a sensitivity of 74% and specificity of 67%.[65]

Echocardiography, using a ramp protocol,[66] is commonly used to optimize LVAD speed with evaluations of septal position, AV opening, and the degree of mitral regurgitation. However, invasive hemodynamics have shown that only approximately 40% of patients have normal hemodynamics at baseline, using echocardiographic-derived speeds.[67] The combination of simultaneous invasive hemodynamics and echocardiography, to tailor the CVP and PCWP to near normal values, may be used to improve LVAD speed optimization.[67] During such a protocol, the relationship between the PAD and PCW (DPG) may provide incremental hemodynamic information. In a single-center report, close to half of patients evaluated in this manner had inappropriate "decoupling" of the diastolic pulmonary pressure gradient (DPG) defined as greater than 5 mm Hg between the diastolic PA

pressure and PCWP.[68] This decoupling suggests the presence of pre-capillary PH, and has been associated with worse outcomes in patients with LVADs. Invasive ramp studies targeting normalization of the decoupling was associated with higher 1-year heart failure readmission–free survival rate compared with the non-normalized group (n = 19, 100% vs. 53%; *P* = .035).[68]

With longer support times, the continuous flow design of contemporary LVADs has led to other hemodynamic derangements, in particular the development of aortic insufficiency (AI). After 2 years of support, approximately 30% of patients develop at least moderate AI (using conventional echocardiographic techniques),[69] often requiring modifications in diuretics, speed settings, and in severe cases, valve replacement or heart transplantation. Traditional echocardiographic measures for AI do not account for the continuous nature of the regurgitant flow and are known to underestimate the severity of AI.[70] A hybrid (e.g., simultaneous echo + catheterization) approach has recently been described that quantifies regurgitant fraction by subtracting right-sided CO measured by catheterization from left-sided total systemic CO (flow across the LVAD added to flow across the aortic valve) measured by echocardiography.[71]

THE HEMODYNAMICS OF HEART FAILURE WITH PRESERVED EJECTION FRACTION (SEE ALSO CHAPTER 39)

Initial studies in HFpEF were focused on the presence of diastolic dysfunction as the primary hemodynamic determinant of symptoms and pathophysiology. More recently, there is growing evidence for other pathophysiologic mechanisms to explain the dyspnea and exertional intolerance of these patients with multiple comorbidities.[72]

The hemodynamic characteristics of HFpEF can be characterized using a PV loop. Elegant studies by Kass and others have demonstrated that a steep ESPVR and noncompliant EDPVR combine to limit stroke volume.[73] Moreover, increased end-systolic stiffness (Ees) is associated with an increased effective arterial elastance (Ea). The hemodynamic consequences of a stiff ventricular-arterial system is a larger increase in blood pressure in response to increases in end-diastolic volume; similarly larger falls in blood pressure occur with modest decreases in end-diastolic volume.[74] However, the ventricular-arterial coupling (Ea/Ees) is comparable to age-matched asymptomatic and hypertensive subjects, although the absolute values for Ea and Ees are increased.[20] Stiffening of the aorta also leads to early wave reflection and an increased vascular load late into systole, prolonging relaxation and increased LVEDP.[75]

Some hemodynamic correlate of diastolic dysfunction is common but not necessary in HFpEF. European heart failure guidelines recommend the documentation of diastolic dysfunction, either invasively or noninvasively.[76] However, the hemodynamic nature of the diastolic dysfunction may not be uniform and may be associated with any of the four phases of diastole (isovolumic relaxation, early ventricular filling, diastasis, or atrial contraction). Moreover, diastolic dysfunction is not always associated with symptomatic heart failure.[77]

In clinical practice, the hemodynamic abnormality most commonly associated with HFpEF is an abnormally elevated filling pressure in the setting of a relatively normal LV volume, implying a steep end-diastolic pressure volume relationship (EDPVR). In study of predominantly middle-aged men with HFpEF, the end-diastolic pressure was higher (25 ± 6 vs. 8 ± 2 mm Hg; *P* < .001) and the end-diastolic volume was lower (103 ± 22 mL vs. 115 ± 9 mL; *P* = .01), displacing the entire EDPVR upward and left.[77] Patients with HFpEF also have higher stiffness constant compared to controls. Ventricular relaxation can also be quantified using the mono-exponential rate of isovolumic pressure decay (Tau) and is prolonged in HFpEF. Contractile reserve is blunted in HFpEF. Vasodilation during exercise (reduction in arterial elastance [Ea] and systemic vascular resistance index [SVRI]) is also impaired in HFpEF. These factors contribute to abnormal ventricular-arterial coupling responses (**Fig. 34.17**).[78] However, these sophisticated measures of diastole are not obtained in clinical practice due to the complexity of making such measurements. Volume loading in the catheterization laboratory has been proposed to unmask diastolic dysfunction when resting PCWP less than 15–20 mm Hg and can be accomplished with bolus saline infusion or leg raising (see later discussion).

PH is also frequently noted HFpEF. In fact, the most common etiology of PH in the setting of a preserved ejection fraction is HFpEF. In a community-based echocardiographic study, 83% of the HFpEF population had a PASP greater than 35 mm Hg and was also more severe than predicted from an estimate of the PCWP.[79]

HEMODYNAMIC CHALLENGES: EXERCISE AND VOLUME LOADING

In patients with cryptic exertional dyspnea or exertional intolerance and normal resting hemodynamics, invasive hemodynamics with exercise or volume challenge may uncover HFpEF or PH.[80]

Technical Considerations

Exercise hemodynamics are usually obtained in the supine position in most clinical catheterization laboratories; some academic laboratories have the technical expertise to perform upright studies and concomitant measurement of oxygen consumption (e.g., metabolic cart). Supine or upright bicycle ergometry is favored due to the ability to

incrementally increase workload with a conventional activity. Upper extremity exercise with weights or straight leg raising for several minutes or until symptoms appear has been used by some investigators. However, published guidelines do not address how hemodynamic assessment during exercise should be performed nor what the goal of exercise should be. However, it is reasonable to (1) start at a low level of exercise; (2) titrate upwards at fixed intervals until symptoms; and (3) measure hemodynamics at rest, peak exercise, and, if possible, after each stage. During exercise, there can be dramatic fluctuations in intracardiac pressures secondary to wide swings in intrathoracic pressures and measurements should be made at end-expiration. Heart rate response should also be noted since chronotropic incompetence may be more relevant than the hemodynamic response as an explanation for exertional intolerance.

The normal response to exercise consists of an increase in mean systemic and pulmonary arterial pressures, as well as heart rate and myocardial contractility.[80] SVR decreases with exercise (despite the increase in mean arterial pressure); there is also a slight decrease in pulmonary vascular resistance with exercise. Oxygen consumption increases with exercise and is facilitated by an increase in CO as well as an increase in tissue oxygen extraction. An increase in PCWP is expected (e.g., preload recruitable stroke work) as venous return increases, but the magnitude should be modest (e.g., <20–25 mm Hg) and the rise in pressure gradual. Eighty percent of the increase in PCWP during supine exercise occurs early and at low levels of exertion. There is some debate as to what constitutes a normal response of intracardiac and pulmonary pressures to exercise. Previous definitions have relied on younger populations to define a normal response to exercise; a conservative definition is an exertional PCWP (at end-expiration) elevation of less than 25 mm Hg.[81] However, healthy cohorts show that

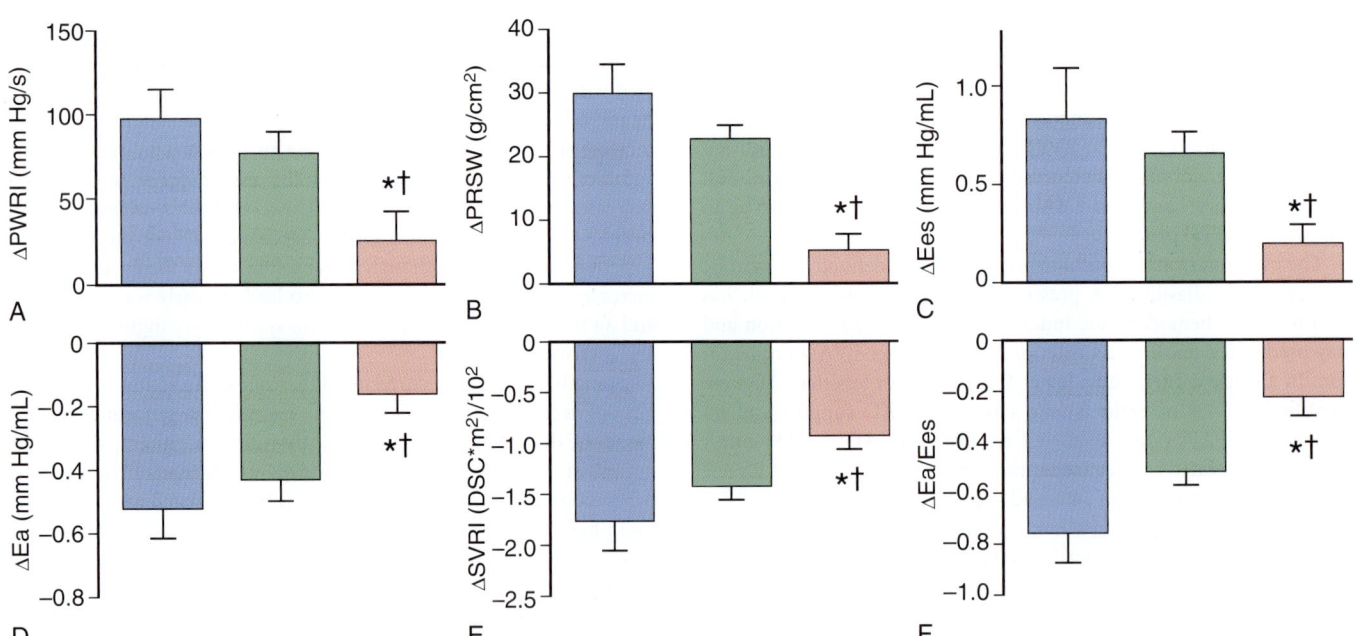

Fig. 34.17 Contractile, vascular, and coupling reserve with low-level exercise (20 W). (A–C) Compared with both control subjects *(blue bars)* and hypertensive subjects *(green bars)*, contractile reserve was blunted in heart failure with preserved ejection fraction (HFpEF) *(red bars)* at 20 W, evidenced by blunted increases in end-systolic elastance *(Ees)*, preload recruitable stroke work *(PRSW)*, and peak power index *(PWRI)*. (D and E) Vasodilation (reduction in arterial elastance *[Ea]* and systemic vascular resistance index *[SVRI]*) was also impaired in HFpEF. (F) These deficits led to abnormal ventricular-arterial coupling responses in HFpEF subjects compared with controls and hypertensive subjects. [a]*P* < .05 versus hypertension; [b]*P* < .05 versus control. (From Borlaug BA, Olson TP, Lam CS, et al. Global cardiovascular reserve dysfunction in heart failure with preserved ejection fraction. *J Am Coll Cardiol.* 2010;56:845–854.)

the elevation in PCWP during exercise increases with age (**Fig. 34.18**), and 30% of healthy adults with age ≥60 years demonstrated values above 25 mm Hg in PCWP.[82]

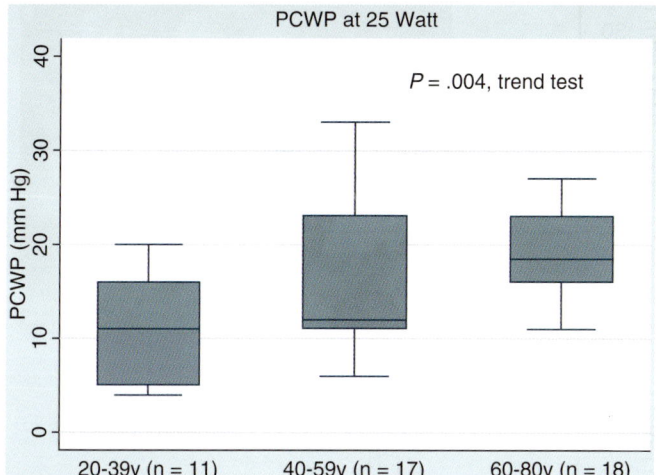

Fig. 34.18 Box plot of pulmonary capillary wedge pressure *(PCWP)* in those who achieved a workload of 25 W across all age categories. (From Wolsk E, Bakkestrøm R, Thomsen JH, et al. The influence of age on hemodynamic parameters during rest and exercise in healthy individuals. *JACC Heart Fail.* 2017;5:337–346.

LV diastolic compliance can also be assessed with a volume challenge and may unmask occult pulmonary venous hypertension when PH is present.[83] Volume loading can be accomplished by leg raising or the rapid infusion of saline. Leg raising provides 250 to 500 cc of blood volume into the chest within seconds. Infusion of warm isotonic saline can also be used but should be rapid (100–200 cc/min up to 1–2 L), and use of a pressurized bag is recommended. In healthy subjects, the PCWP increases from 10 ± 2 to 16 ± 3 mm Hg after 1 L and to 20 ± 3 mm Hg after 2 L. Older healthy women have a greater increase in PCWP relative to infused volume (e.g., 16 ± 4 mm Hg/L/m²; $P < .019$) than men and younger women; there is also a greater increase in mean PAP relative to CO in women compared to men, regardless of age.

Selective volume loading of the LV can also be accomplished by administering selective pulmonary vasodilators (e.g., inhaled nitric oxide) if there is increased pulmonary vascular resistance and normal PCWP or LVEDP.

Specific Clinical Scenarios

In HFrEF, intracardiac pressures also rise but more rapidly and with a blunted CO response. There is also a concomitant rapid rise in pulmonary pressures and TPG (**Fig. 34.19**). In some HFrEF patients, the rise in PA pressures plateau with exercise (**Fig. 34.20**). The steep increase in PA pressures and the plateau pattern are associated with reduced peak VO₂, inability to augment RV stroke work, and increased mortality.[84]

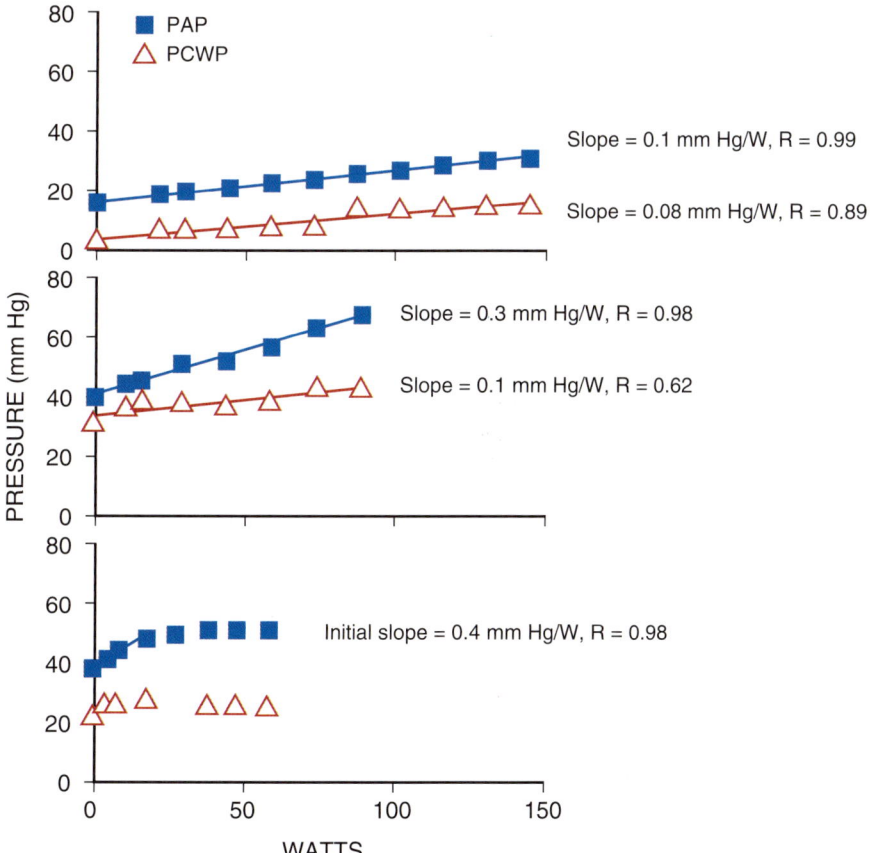

Fig. 34.19 Representative patterns of pulmonary arterial pressure *(PAP)* and pulmonary capillary wedge pressure *(PCWP)* responses to exercise in controls *(top)*, patients with left ventricular systolic dysfunction *(LVSD)* with a linear PAP increment with exercise *(middle)*, and patients with LVSD with a PAP plateau pattern during exercise *(bottom)*. (From Lewis GD, Murphy RM, Shah RV, et al. Pulmonary vascular response patterns during exercise in left ventricular systolic dysfunction predict exercise capacity and outcomes. *Circ Heart Fail* 2011;4:276–285.)

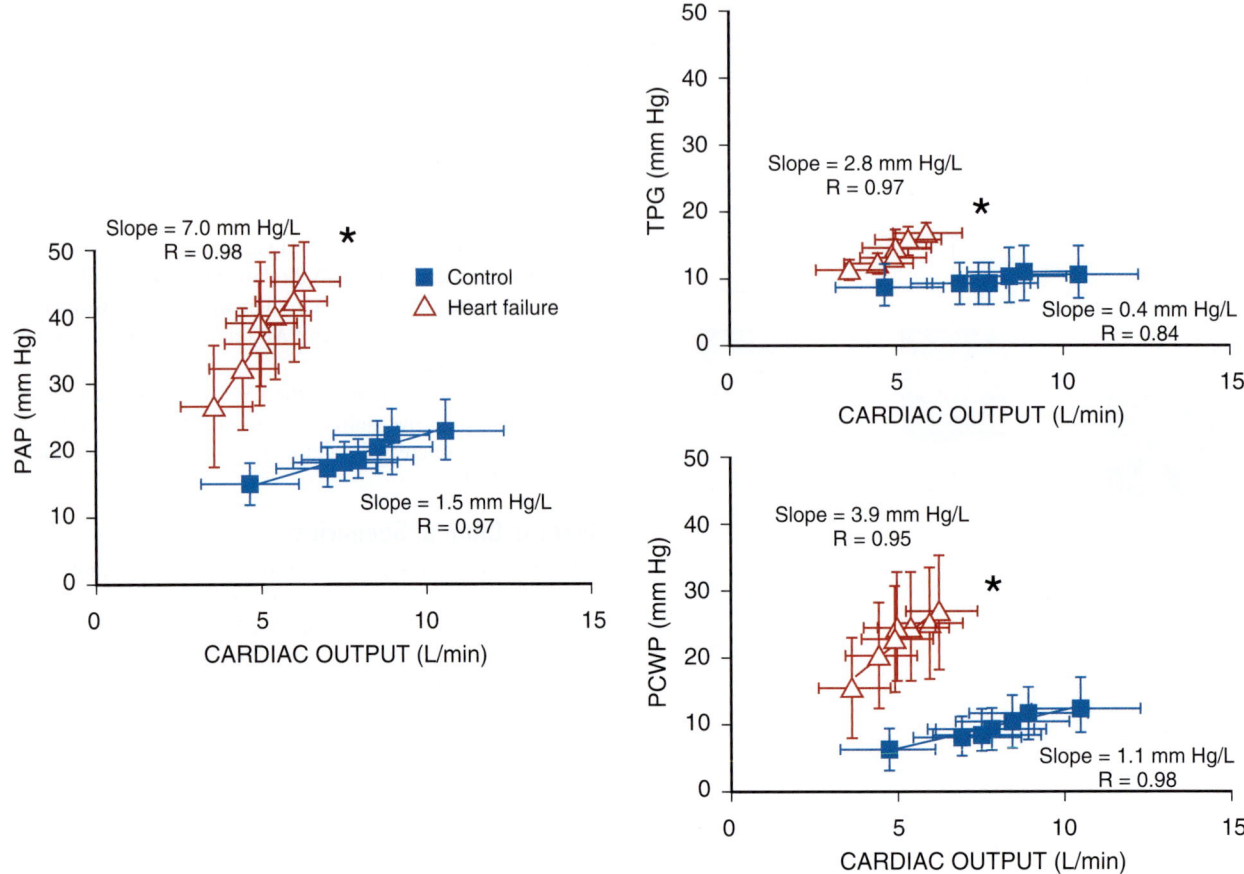

Fig. 34.20 Mean pulmonary arterial pressures *(PAP)* relative to cardiac outputs (CO) during incremental exercise in patients with left ventricular systolic dysfunction *(LVSD)*. Transpulmonary gradient *(TPG)* and pulmonary capillary wedge pressure *(PCWP)* responses to exercise relative to cardiac output in patients with LVSD. [a]*P* < .005 for the comparison of pressure changes in patients with LVSD with pressure changes in controls. (From Lewis GD, Murphy RM, Shah RV, et al. Pulmonary vascular response patterns during exercise in left ventricular systolic dysfunction predict exercise capacity and outcomes. *Circ Heart Fail.* 2011;4:276–285.)

In patients with LVEF greater than 50%, exercise-induced HFpEF is defined as an increase in PCWP to greater than 20–25 mm Hg with exercise and consistent with an inability to accommodate the venous return without an increase in left ventricular end-diastolic volume, limiting preload recruitable stroke work.[80] This response can also be elicited with leg raising or volume loading.[81] In HFpEF patients, rapid infusion of saline (100–200 cc/min up to 1–2 L) results in a steeper increase in PCWP (25 ± 12 mm Hg/L/m^2) than healthy younger (12 ± 3 mm Hg/L/m^2) and older subjects (14 ± 5 mm Hg/L/m^2). An increase in PCWP greater than 18 mm Hg suggests diastolic dysfunction,[85] although some investigators prefer more conservative values such as greater than 25 mm Hg. In HFpEF, exercise testing also demonstrates a decrease in peak oxygen consumption due to reduced peak CO secondary to blunted inotropic, chronotropic, and vasodilator reserve. Other mechanisms of inadequate oxygen transport may also be present. Poor oxygen delivery across the lungs, inadequate CO, decreased skeletal muscle oxygen diffusion, or combinations of these defects have been described.[86]

When the mean PAP exceeds 30 mm Hg in the setting of a PCWP less than 20 mm Hg during exercise, a diagnosis of exercise-induced PAH should be considered (**Fig. 34.21**). In a study by Tolle et al., 406

patients with dyspnea on exertion underwent upright cardiopulmonary exercise testing with hemodynamic monitoring. Exercise-related PAH was associated with a significant impairment in oxygen consumption (66.5% ± 16.3% of controls) and comparable to PAH.[87] However, the clinical relevance of exercise-induced PH in asymptomatic subjects is not clear. For example, elite athletes demonstrate a higher increase in mean PA pressure compared to healthy controls because of the marked increase in stroke volume with exercise.[88] It appears that coupling an increase in mean PAP to greater than 30 mm Hg with an increase in total pulmonary resistance (mean PA/CO) to greater than 3 WU during exercise helps to distinguish the exercise PH of left heart disease and early pulmonary vascular disease from a normal physiologic response.[89]

The exercise hemodynamics of severe tricuspid regurgitation were described by Andersen et al.[90] Compared to healthy controls, patients with severe tricuspid regurgitation generated lower exercise CO (6.4 vs. 10.3 L/min; P = .001), despite a threefold increase in RAP (27 vs. 8 mm Hg; P < .0001) and 1.7-fold increase in PCWP (27 vs. 16 mm Hg; P = .0003). During exercise, 80% of the patients demonstrated a Kussmaul sign and absent (x) descent (ventricularization) of the RAP tracing (**Fig. 34.22**), suggesting the limits of RV diastolic capacity was being exceeded.

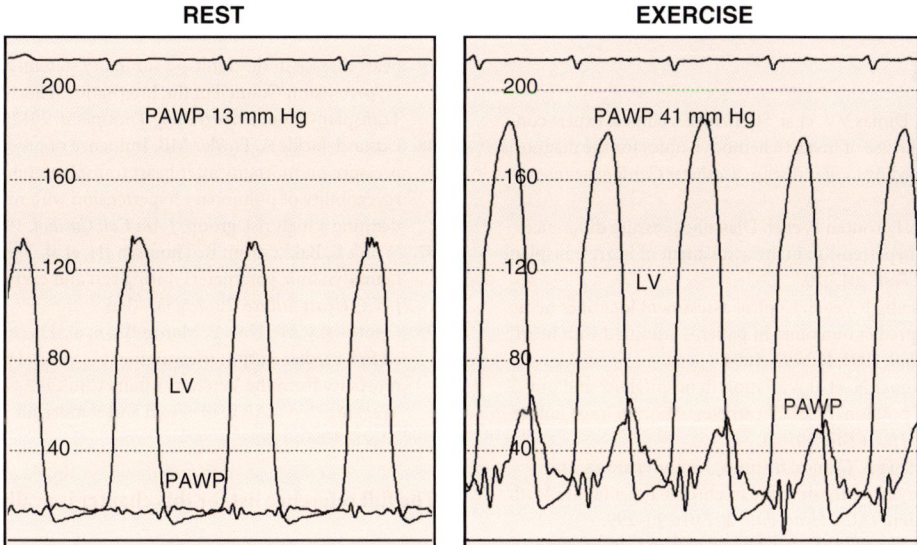

Fig. 34.21 Effect of exercise in a patient with normal resting hemodynamics but significant exertional dyspnea and normal left ventricular ejection fraction. At a low level of supine bicycle exercise, there was a marked increase in pulmonary artery wedge pressure *(PAWP)* to 41 mm Hg with a large *v* wave. There was not significant mitral regurgitation by simultaneous echocardiography, indicating that these symptoms were due to noncompliance of the left atrium and left ventricle. (From Nishimura RA, Carabello BA. Hemodynamics in the cardiac catheterization laboratory of the 21st century. *Circulation.* 2012;125:2138–2150.)

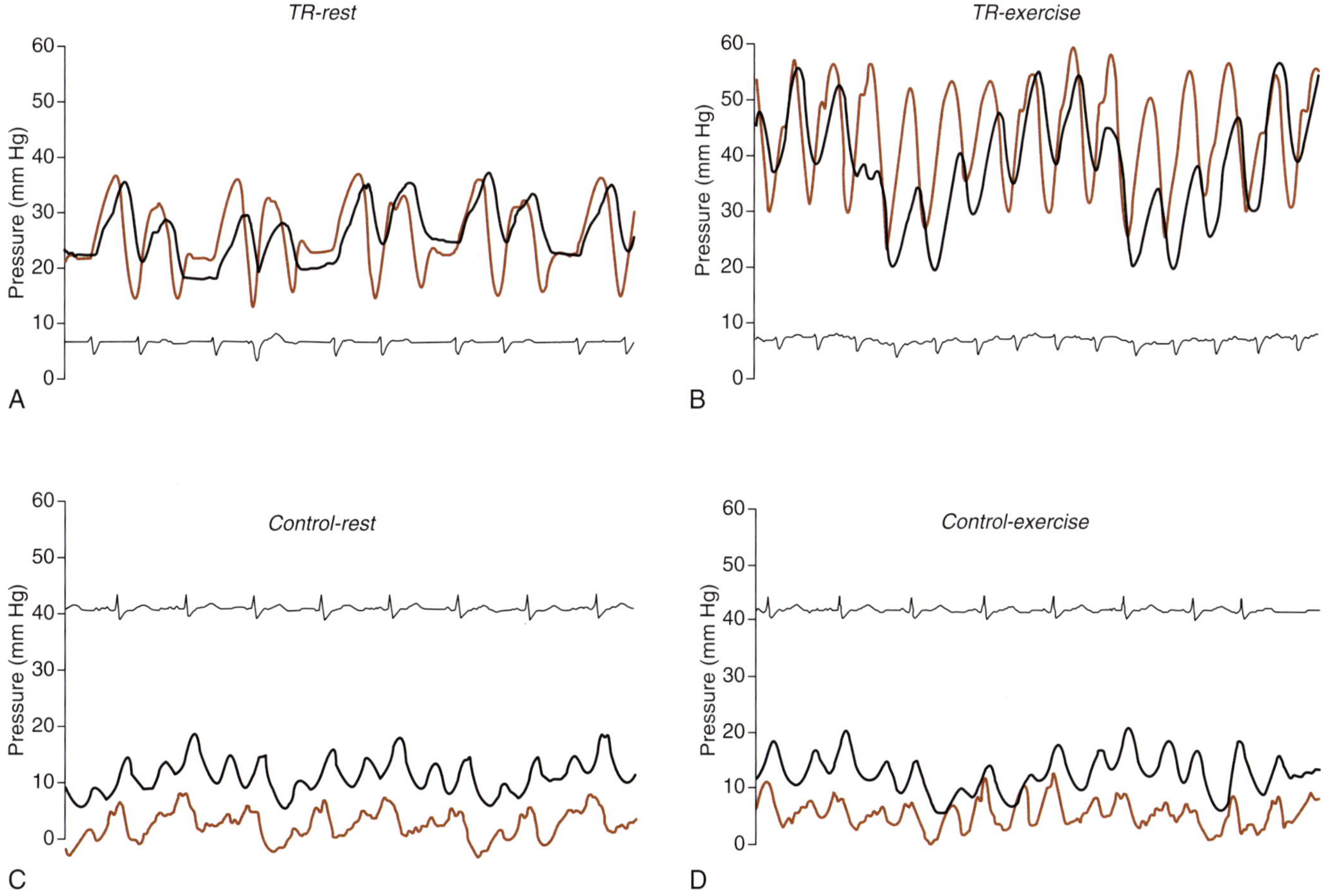

Fig. 34.22 Typical right atrial (RA; *red*) and pulmonary capillary wedge pressure (PCWP; *black*) tracings in a patient with severe tricuspid regurgitation at rest (A) and with exercise (B) and in a control patient at respective states (C and D). Note the prominent C–V waves with absent-descent (ventricularized waveforms) and near-equalization of right and left heart pressures in the tricuspid regurgitation (TR) patient. During inspiration, there is no drop in RA pressure (RAP; Kussmaul sign) despite reduction in PCWP associated with the drop in intrathoracic pressure, such that the transmural pressure gradient becomes transiently negative. In the control patient, PCWP and RAP are normal at rest and with exercise, and PCWP consistently exceeds RAP. (From Andersen MJ, Nishimura RA, Borlaug BA. The hemodynamic basis of exercise intolerance in tricuspid regurgitation. *Circ Heart Fail.* 2014;7:911–917.)

KEY REFERENCES

3. Sorajja P, Borlaug BA, Dimas VV, et al. SCAI/HFSA clinical expert consensus document on the use of invasive hemodynamics for the diagnosis and management of cardiovascular disease. *Catheter Cardiovasc Interv*. 2017;89:E233–E247.

16. Wright SP, Moayedi Y, Foroutan F, et al. Diastolic pressure difference to classify pulmonary hypertension in the assessment of heart transplant candidates. *Circ Heart Fail*. 2017;10.

26. Nohria A, Tsang SW, Fang JC, et al. Clinical assessment identifies hemodynamic profiles that predict outcomes in patients admitted with heart failure. *J Am Coll Cardiol*. 2003;41:1797–1804.

38. Khera R, Pandey A, Kumar N, et al. Variation in hospital use and outcomes associated with pulmonary artery catheterization in heart failure in the United States. *Circ Heart Fail*. 2016;9.

40. Miller W, Grill D, Borlaug B. Clinical features, hemodynamics, and outcomes of pulmonary hypertension due to chronic heart failure With reduced ejection graction. *JACC Heart Fail*. 2013;1:290–299.

41. Fang JC, DeMarco T, Givertz MM, et al. World Health Organization pulmonary hypertension group 2: pulmonary hypertension due to left heart disease in the adult—a summary statement from the Pulmonary Hypertension Council of the International Society for Heart and Lung Transplantation. *J Heart Lung Transplant*. 2012;31:913–933.

48. Costard-Jackle A, Fowler MB. Influence of preoperative pulmonary artery pressure on mortality after heart transplantation: testing of potential reversibility of pulmonary hypertension with nitroprusside is useful in defining a high risk group. *J Am Coll Cardiol*. 1992;19:48–54.

82. Wolsk E, Bakkestrom R, Thomsen JH, et al. The influence of age on hemodynamic parameters during rest and exercise in healthy individuals. *JACC Heart failure*. 2017;5:337–346.

93. Opotowsky AR, Hess E, Maron BA, et al. Thermodilution vs estimated fick cardiac output measurement in clinical practice: an analysis of mortality from the Veterans Affairs Clinical Assessment, Reporting, and Tracking (VA CART) program and Vanderbilt University. *JAMA Cardiol*. 2017;2:1090–1099.

The full reference list for this chapter is available on ExpertConsult.

Disease Prevention in Heart Failure

Viorel G. Florea, Jay N. Cohn

Prevention of heart failure is an urgent public health need with national and global implications. Despite recent advances in the therapy of cardiovascular disorders, heart failure remains a challenging disease with a high prevalence (**Fig. 35.1**) and a dismal long-term prognosis.[1] On the basis of data from the National Health and Nutrition Examination Survey (NHANES) 2011 to 2014, an estimated 6.5 million Americans 20 years of age or older had heart failure.[1] This represents an increase from an estimated 5.7 million United States adults with heart failure based on the NHANES 2009 to 2012.[1] The "aging of the population" and improved survival and "salvage" of patients with acute myocardial infarction are believed to be some factors contributing to this growing burden of heart failure. Projections show that the prevalence of heart failure will increase 46% from 2012 to 2030, resulting in greater than 8 million people 18 years of age or older with heart failure (**see also Chapter 18**).[2]

It becomes evident that the heart failure burden will not be eliminated by an improvement in the survival of patients who are already affected with the disease; instead, a drastic reduction in the incidence of heart failure is required to prevent an increase in the heart failure burden. It is therefore important that we develop a population-level strategy to prevent the lifetime risk of heart failure that applies to the large number of "at-risk" individuals. Such a strategy would complement our current approaches that are aimed at intensive management of patients with manifest heart failure (**Fig. 35.2**). The burden of heart failure risk factors and the effect of their prevention and treatment on incident heart failure are examined in this chapter. Because the primary mechanisms of the development of heart failure may be cardiac (structural remodeling, impaired contractility, decreased compliance) or peripheral (arterial stiffening, impaired arterial vasodilator reserve,

fluid retention), this discussion is an attempt to characterize the specific mechanisms of the effect of the predisposing conditions and their treatment on the development of heart failure.

Given the sizeable public health burden posed by heart failure and limited health care resources, it is critical to identify the primary "drivers" of this problem. In 2001 a new approach to the classification of heart failure was adopted by the American College of Cardiology/American Heart Association which emphasized both the evolution and progression of the disease and which included **stage A** patients who are at high risk for developing heart failure but have no structural disorder of the heart and **stage B** patients with structural disorders of the heart but who have never developed symptoms of heart failure.[3] This new classification scheme adds a useful dimension to our understanding of heart failure, recognizing that there are established risk factors and structural prerequisites for the development of heart failure and that therapeutic interventions performed even before the appearance of left ventricular dysfunction or symptoms can prevent the development of heart failure. The progression of the structural changes that lead to heart failure mandates that an all-out effort be made to slow or halt this progression. The best time to intervene would probably be in stage B, when the early structural changes can be identified but they have not yet progressed to the symptomatic phase of the disease.

PRIMORDIAL PREVENTION OF CARDIOVASCULAR DISEASE AND HEART FAILURE

Functional and structural changes of the cardiovascular system progress with aging in all individuals. The rate of this progression is under the influence of genetic and environmental contributors. These

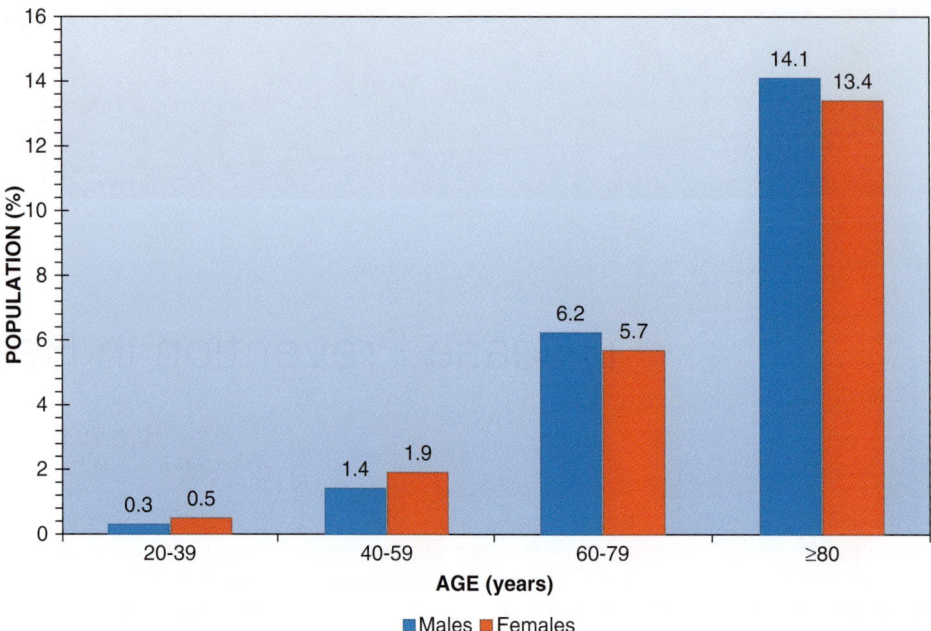

Fig. 35.1 Prevalence of heart failure for adults 20 years or older by sex and age (Reprinted with permission. National Health and Nutrition Examination Survey: 2011–2014). (National Center for Health Statistics and National Heart, Lung, and Blood Institute. From Benjamin EJ, Blaha MJ, Chiuve SE, et al. Heart disease and stroke statistics-2017 update: a report from the American Heart Association. *Circulation.* 2017;135[10]:e146–e603.)

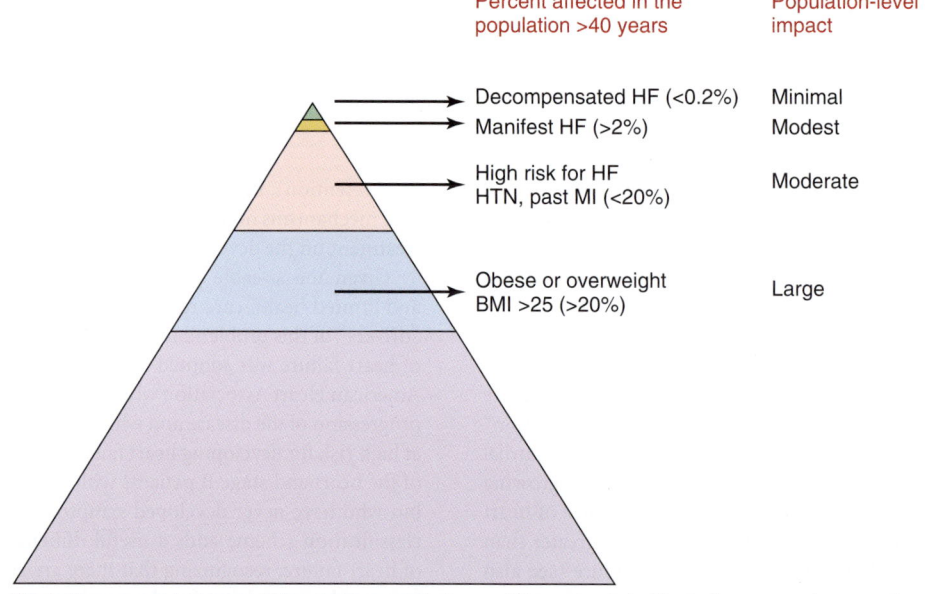

Fig. 35.2 The pyramid of heart failure in the population and the potential effect of a range of preventive and treatment strategies in lowering age-specific mortality rates. *BMI,* Body mass index; *HF,* heart failure; *HTN,* hypertension; *MI,* myocardial infarction. (From Young J, Narula J. Preface: prevention should take center stage. *Cardiol Clin.* 2007;25:xi–xiii; data from Yusuf S, Pitt B. A lifetime of prevention: the case of heart failure. *Circulation.* 2002;106:2997–2998.)

functional and structural changes will eventuate in a morbid event if other factors do not end life before the cardiovascular changes have reached their symptomatic stage. Most morbid events are complications of progressive changes in the artery walls, whereas heart failure represents a complication of functional and structural changes in the myocardium.

Certain risk factors have been statistically associated with the early development of cardiovascular diseases, thus implying that these risk factors may accelerate the age-related changes in the health of

the arteries or heart. The role of heredity versus environment on the development of these risk factors remains uncertain. Blood pressure, cholesterol, obesity, and even smoking may be related to genetic and environmental factors. Pharmacologic management of blood pressure and cholesterol have been shown in prospective trials to slow progression of disease and delay morbid events, but the efficacy of dietary and exercise interventions have not been documented. Preventing or treating these risk factors has nonetheless been a mission of American health agencies, as reflected in the goals of the American Heart Association to

TABLE 35.1　Seven Health Metrics of Ideal Cardiovascular Health

	Health Metric
1	Nonsmoking
2	Body mass index <25 kg/m^2
3	Physical activity at goal levels
4	Dietary pattern that promotes cardiovascular health
5	Untreated total cholesterol <200 mg/dL
6	Untreated blood pressure <120/<80 mm Hg
7	Fasting blood glucose <100 mg/dL

Data from Lloyd-Jones DM, Hong Y, Labarthe D, et al., American Heart Association Strategic Planning Task F and Statistics C. Defining and setting national goals for cardiovascular health promotion and disease reduction: the American Heart Association's strategic impact goal through 2020 and beyond. *Circulation.* 2010;121(4):586–613.

reduce the burden of disease (**Table 35.1**). Public health efforts to promote a healthy environment and healthy lifestyle might therefore delay progression of disease in at least some individuals, but for the health care professional the goal is to identify individuals in need of pharmacologic intervention to slow disease progression.

Therefore, in regard to heart failure, the public health efforts to prevent risk factors may be viewed as a prudent effort to forestall the symptomatic phase of the disease, but intervention pharmacologically to slow the progressive structural changes in the left ventricle (stage B heart failure) is the responsibility of the medical profession.

Although prevention of heart failure in individuals with stage A heart failure who already have known risk factors is important, once predisposing conditions are present, substantial elevations in long-term and lifetime risks for cardiovascular disease and heart failure are largely unavoidable. It is therefore important to focus on prevention before the development of risk factors. Prevention of cardiovascular disease and heart failure should start with healthy lifestyle education. In 2010 the American Heart Association created a new set of national goals for cardiovascular health promotion and disease reduction.[4] Specifically the American Heart Association committed itself to achieving the following central organizational goals: *"By 2020, to improve the cardiovascular health of all Americans by 20%, while reducing deaths from cardiovascular diseases and stroke by 20%."*[4] These goals require new strategic directions for the American Heart Association in its research, clinical, public health, and advocacy programs for cardiovascular health promotion and disease prevention in the current decade and beyond. The goals introduce the concept of *ideal cardiovascular health,* which is defined by the absence of clinically manifest cardiovascular disease together with the simultaneous presence of optimal levels of seven health metrics (see Table 35.1), including four health behaviors (nonsmoking, body mass index less than 25 kg/m^2, physical activity at goal levels, and pursuit of a diet consistent with current guideline recommendations) and three ideal health factors (untreated total cholesterol <200 mg/dL, untreated blood pressure <120/<80 mm Hg, and fasting blood glucose <100 mg/dL).[4] Greater adherence to the American Heart Association's Life's Simple 7 guidelines was shown to be associated with a lower lifetime risk of heart failure and better cardiac structure and functional parameters by echocardiography.[5] Among 20,900 male physicians in the Physicians Health Study, healthy lifestyle habits (normal body weight, not smoking, regular exercise, moderate alcohol intake, consumption of breakfast cereals, and consumption of fruits and vegetables) were individually and jointly associated with a lower lifetime risk of heart failure, with the highest risk in men adhering to none of the six lifestyle factors and the lowest risk in men adhering to four or more desirable factors.[6] These data confirm an association between lifestyle and disease, but they do not document cause and effect. Such documentation would require an expensive and robust intervention trial, which has not yet been successfully conducted. Because prevention of cardiovascular disease should ideally start in childhood, the American Heart Association developed the Life's Simple 7 for kids to help children understand how small lifestyle choices might affect their cardiovascular health.

The potential importance of nonsmoking, healthy dietary pattern, and physical activity for the ideal cardiovascular health have been reviewed extensively elsewhere.[4] Here, the existing evidence is provided as it relates to the prevention of cardiovascular disease and heart failure.

Smoking

Tobacco use is a major risk factor for cardiovascular disease and appears to have a multiplicative effect with the other major risk factors for coronary artery disease, such as high serum levels of lipids, untreated hypertension, and diabetes mellitus.[1] Since the first report on the health dangers of smoking was issued by the United States Surgeon General in 1964, age-adjusted rates of smoking among adults have declined, from 51% of males smoking in 1965 to 16.7% in 2015 and from 34% of females in 1965 to 13.7% in 2015.[1] The decline in smoking, along with other factors (including improved treatment and reductions in the prevalence of risk factors such as uncontrolled hypertension and high cholesterol), is a contributing factor in the sharp decline in the heart disease death rate during this period.[1]

Although the majority of ex-smokers report that they quit without any formal assistance,[7] cessation medications (including sustained-release bupropion, varenicline, and nicotine gum, lozenge, nasal spray, and patch) are effective for helping smokers quit.[8] In addition to medications, smoke-free policies, increases in tobacco prices, cessation advice from health care professionals, and quit-lines and other counseling have contributed to smoking cessation.[9]

Physical Activity

Being physically active is associated with good health, and being inactive is associated with poorer health. Physical activity may improve risk factors for cardiovascular disease (such as blood pressure and cholesterol level) and reduce the likelihood of coronary artery disease, type 2 diabetes mellitus, myocardial infarction, stroke, and premature mortality.[1]

The American Heart Association guidelines on physical activity recommend that children get at least 60 minutes of physical activity daily and that adults get at least 150 minutes of moderate intensity or 75 minutes of vigorous-intensity aerobic activity per week and perform muscle strengthening activities at least 2 days/week.[1] In the Health Professionals Follow-Up Study, for every 3-hour-per-week increase in vigorous-intensity activity reported, there was a 22% lower risk of myocardial infarction, and this could be explained in part by beneficial effects of physical activity on high-density lipoprotein cholesterol, vitamin D, apolipoprotein B, and hemoglobin A$_{1c}$.[10] A meta-analysis of nine cohort studies, representing 122,417 patients, found that as little as 15 minutes of daily moderate to vigorous physical activity was associated with reduced all-cause mortality in adults 60 years of age or older. This potential protective effect of physical activity appeared to be "dose dependent," because the greatest reduction in mortality per minute of greater physical activity was for those at the lowest levels of physical activity. These findings suggest that older adults may benefit from physical activity time far below the amount recommended by the federal guidelines.[11]

Moderate physical activity is associated with a lower long-term incidence of heart failure, preventing cardiac injury and neurohormonal activation.[12] In patients with heart failure, intense activity (an aerobic interval-training program three times per week for 12 weeks) was associated with a an improvement in left ventricular ejection fraction and decreases in pro-B-type natriuretic peptide (proBNP), left ventricular end-systolic and end-diastolic volumes compared with control and endurance-training groups.[13] Exercise training in patients with heart failure with preserved ejection fraction was associated with improved exercise capacity and favorable changes in diastolic function.[14]

Healthy Dietary Pattern

Dietary habits affect multiple cardiovascular risk factors, including both established risk factors (systolic blood pressure, diastolic blood pressure, low-density lipoprotein cholesterol levels, high-density lipoprotein cholesterol levels, glucose levels, and obesity/weight gain) and novel risk factors (e.g., inflammation, cardiac arrhythmias, endothelial cell function, triglyceride levels, lipoprotein[a] levels, and heart rate).[1] Sodium linearly raises blood pressure in a dose-dependent fashion, with stronger effects among older people, hypertensive people, and African Americans,[15] and induces additional blood pressure–independent damage to renal and vascular tissues.[16] Estimated sodium intake of more than 3.7 g/day was associated with adverse cardiac remodeling and worse systolic strain and diastolic e' velocity, which may predispose to heart failure.[17]

Among 17 leading risk factors in the United States in 2010, suboptimal dietary habits were most prominently associated with mortality.[18] In 2010 a total of 678,000 deaths of all causes were associated with suboptimal diet.[1] A previous investigation reported the estimated mortality effects of several specific dietary risk factors in 2005 in the United States. High dietary salt consumption was estimated to be potentially responsible for 102,000 annual deaths, low dietary omega-3 fatty acids for 84,000 annual deaths, high dietary trans fatty acids for 82,000 annual deaths, and low consumption of fruits and vegetables for 55,000 annual deaths.[19]

The 2015 US Dietary Guidelines Advisory Committee summarized the evidence for benefits of healthful diet patterns on a range of cardiometabolic and other disease outcomes.[20] They concluded that a healthy dietary pattern is higher in vegetables, fruits, whole grains, low-fat or nonfat dairy, seafood, legumes, and nuts; moderate in alcohol (among adults); lower in red and processed meat; and low in sugar-sweetened foods and drinks and refined grains. Greater versus lower adherence to a Mediterranean dietary pattern, characterized by higher intakes of vegetables, legumes, nuts, fruits, whole grains, fish, and unsaturated fat and lower intakes of red and processed meat, was associated with a lower risk of incident coronary heart disease and stroke.[21] Although higher conformity with the Mediterranean dietary pattern has been associated with lower risk of cardiovascular mortality in a primary prevention cohort,[22] adherence to the Mediterranean diet in patients already afflicted with heart failure did not influence long-term mortality after an episode of acute heart failure, but it was associated with decreased rates of rehospitalization during the next year.[23]

During recent decades, consumption of red meat has been increasing globally, especially in developing countries. At the same time, there has been growing evidence that high consumption of red meat, especially of processed meat, may be associated with an increased risk of major chronic diseases, including type 2 diabetes mellitus, cardiovascular disease, and cancer, and increased mortality risk.[24]

Recent years have brought interesting insights into the human gut microbiota and have highlighted its potential impact on cardiovascular diseases, including heart failure. Changes in composition of gut microbiota, called dysbiosis, can trigger systemic inflammation, which is known to be involved in the pathophysiology of heart failure. Studies

have suggested a role for the intestinal microbiota in the pathogenesis of atherosclerosis in patients with a diet rich in phosphatidylcholine (with major sources including eggs, liver, beef, and pork) through the formation of the metabolite trimethylamine and conversion to trimethylamine-N-oxide (TMAO).[25] The production of TMAO from dietary phosphatidylcholine is dependent on metabolism by the intestinal microbiota (**Fig. 35.3**). Increased TMAO levels are associated with an increased risk of incident major adverse cardiovascular events such as heart failure, chronic kidney disease, myocardial infarction, stroke, or death.[26,27]

Recent evidence suggests that adherence to a healthy plant-based diet is associated with lower risk of coronary heart disease[28] and heart failure.[29] Eating at least five servings of fruit and vegetables every day while avoiding processed foods (which have high salt content) and fried foods, and eating lean meats like fish and poultry provide a well-balanced, heart-healthy diet.[29] Although an increasing number of studies showed an inverse association of certain dietary components such as nut consumption[30] or moderate alcohol consumption[31] with cardiovascular disease and heart failure, the evidence that these and other lifestyle choices affect cardiovascular disease progression in an individual patient is not persuasive.

DISEASE PREVENTION IN STAGE A HEART FAILURE

Stage A heart failure is defined as people without heart failure symptoms or structural heart disease but with predisposing conditions for heart failure. This classification is used to identify high-risk patients to prevent progression to structural heart disease or symptomatic heart failure. It is estimated that one-third of the US adult population is living with predisposing conditions for heart failure (i.e., are in stage A heart failure), many of whom are not adequately recognized or being appropriately or adequately treated for their risk factors.[32]

A number of risk factors have been identified that may lead to heart failure. These exert their adverse effects through functional and structural influence on the left ventricle, characterized as ventricular remodeling and defined as progressive ventricular hypertrophy, enlargement, and cavity distortion over time.[33,34] The clinical syndrome of heart failure usually results from both impaired left ventricular performance and congestion secondary to sodium and fluid retention.

The risk factors for heart failure include hypertension, diabetes mellitus, atherosclerotic disease, metabolic syndrome, obesity, chronic kidney disease, and the use of many therapeutic and recreational agents that can exert cardiotoxic effects. Coronary heart disease, hypertension, smoking, diabetes mellitus, and obesity appear to be responsible for 52% of incident heart failure cases in the population, with their population attributable risks shown in **Table 35.2**.[35] Valvular heart disease is responsible for an additional 2% of incident heart failure cases in the population.[36] The pathogenetic role of predisposing conditions/comorbidities in the development of heart failure with preserved ejection fraction is illustrated in **Fig. 35.4**. As shown, comorbidities induce systemic inflammation. Chronic inflammation, in turn, affects the lungs, myocardium, skeletal muscle, and kidneys, leading to diverse heart failure with preserved ejection fraction phenotypes.[37] These predisposing conditions/comorbidities are, by and large, preventable with currently known and available strategies. A recent study on 34,736 participants in the Women's Health Study showed that women with new-onset atrial fibrillation who achieved or maintained optimal risk factor control (obesity, smoking, elevated blood pressure, and diabetes mellitus) exhibited a lower heart failure risk.[38]

Hypertension and Heart Failure (see also Chapter 25)

Considerable evidence from experimental and clinical studies and epidemiologic investigations indicates the critical role of hypertension in

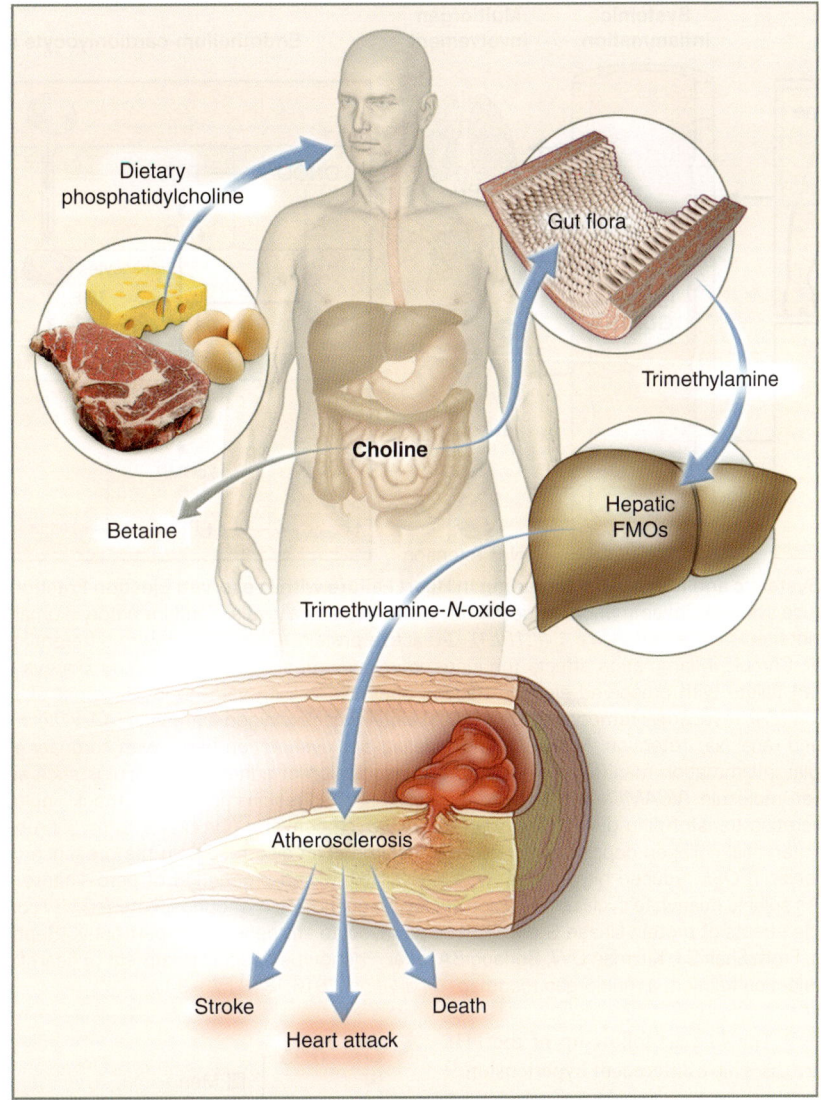

Fig. 35.3 Pathways Linking Dietary Phosphatidylcholine, Intestinal Microbiota, and Incident Adverse Cardiovascular Events. Ingested phosphatidylcholine (lecithin), the major dietary source of total choline, is acted on by intestinal lipases to form a variety of metabolic products, including the choline-containing nutrients glycerophosphocholine, phosphocholine, and choline. Choline-containing nutrients that reach the cecum and large bowel may serve as fuel for intestinal microbiota (gut flora), producing trimethylamine (TMA). TMA is rapidly further oxidized to trimethylamine-N-oxide (TMAO) by hepatic flavin-containing monooxygenases *(FMOs)*. TMAO enhances the accumulation of cholesterol in macrophages, the accumulation of foam cells in artery walls, and atherosclerosis, all factors that are associated with an increased risk of heart attack, stroke, and death. Choline can also be oxidized to betaine in both the liver and kidneys. Dietary betaine can serve as a substrate for bacteria to form TMA and presumably TMAO. (From Tang WH, Wang Z, Levison BS, et al. Intestinal microbial metabolism of phosphatidylcholine and cardiovascular risk. *N Engl J Med.* 2013;25;368[17]:1575–1584.)

TABLE 35.2 **Heart Failure Risk Factors**	
Risk Factor	**Population Attributable Risk (%)**
Coronary heart disease	20
Hypertension	20
Cigarette smoking	14
Diabetes mellitus	12
Obesity	12
Valvular heart disease	2

Data from Dunlay SM, Weston SA, Jacobsen SJ, Roger VL. Risk factors for heart failure: a population-based case-control study. *Am J Med.* 2009;122(11):1023–1028.

the pathogenesis of heart failure. In an observational study including more than 1 million adult patients 30 years of age or older, higher systolic blood pressure and diastolic blood pressure were associated with increased risk of cardiovascular disease incidence and angina, myocardial infarction, heart failure, stroke, peripheral artery disease, and abdominal aortic aneurysm, each evaluated separately.[39] Higher blood pressure in midlife is a harbinger of increased risk of heart failure in later life,[40] thus suggesting that early risk factor modification may decrease heart failure burden. Data from the Framingham Heart Study (FHS) indicate that recent (within the past 10 years) and remote antecedent blood pressure levels could be an important determinant of cardiovascular disease and heart failure risk over and above the

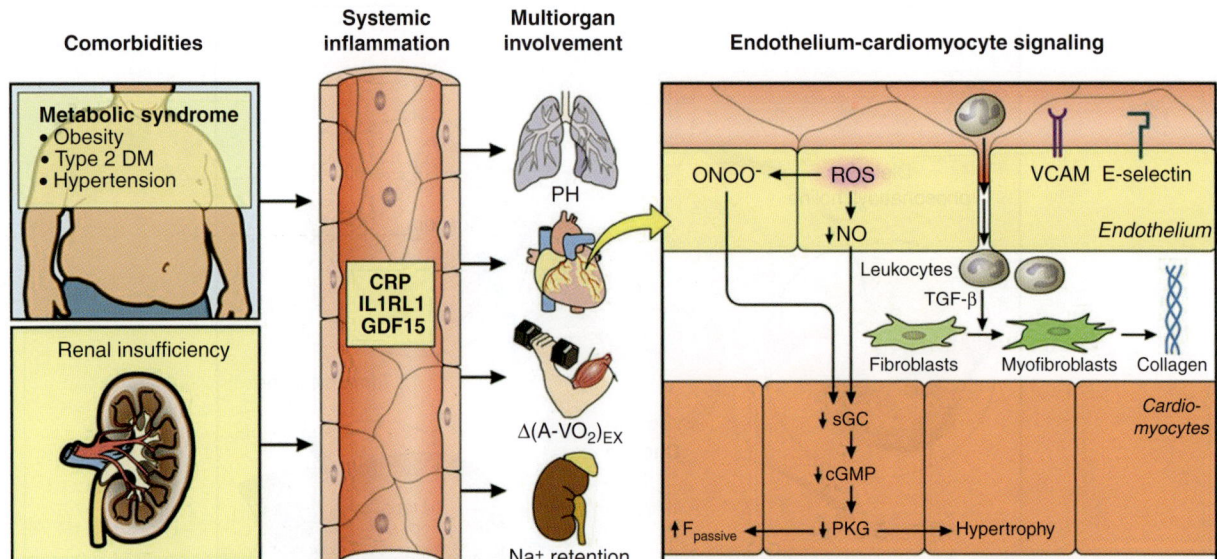

Fig. 35.4 Systemic and Myocardial Signaling in Heart Failure with Preserved Ejection Fraction. Comorbidities induce systemic inflammation, evident from elevated plasma levels of inflammatory biomarkers such as soluble interleukin 1 receptor–like 1 *(IL1RL1)*, C-reactive protein *(CRP)*, and growth differentiation factor 15 *(GDF15)*. Chronic inflammation affects the lungs, myocardium, skeletal muscle, and kidneys leading to diverse heart failure with preserved ejection fraction phenotypes with variable involvement of pulmonary hypertension *(PH)*, myocardial remodeling, deficient skeletal muscle oxygen extraction *(ΔA-VO2)* during exercise *(Ex)*, and renal Na+ retention. Myocardial remodeling and dysfunction begin with coronary endothelial microvascular inflammation manifest from endothelial expression of adhesion molecules such as vascular cell adhesion molecule *(VCAM)* and E-selectin. Expression of adhesion molecules attracts infiltrating leukocytes secreting transforming growth factor-β *(TGF-β)*, which converts fibroblasts to myofibroblasts with enhanced interstitial collagen deposition. Endothelial inflammation also results in the presence of reactive oxygen species *(ROS)*, reduced nitric oxide *(NO)* bioavailability, and production of peroxynitrite *(ONOO⁻)*. This reduces soluble guanylate cyclase *(sGC)* activity, cyclic guanosine monophosphate *(cGMP)* content, and the favorable effects of protein kinase G *(PKG)* on cardiomyocyte stiffness and hypertrophy. (Reprinted with permission. From Shah SJ, Kitzman DW, Borlaug BA, et al. Phenotype-specific treatment of heart failure with preserved ejection fraction: a multiorgan roadmap. *Circulation.* 2016;134[1]:73–90.)

current blood pressure level.[40,41] The 44-year follow-up of the FHS showed that 75% of heart failure cases have antecedent hypertension.[42] In addition, hypertension is frequently accompanied by metabolic risk factors and obesity, which themselves increase the risk of heart failure.[40] Hypertension is the most powerful pathogenetic factor in the development of heart failure with preserved ejection fraction.[43] This strong relationship has led some authors to propose that heart failure with preserved ejection fraction may be a later stage of hypertensive heart disease.[44]

Although many genes or gene combinations influence blood pressure,[45] poor diet, physical inactivity, and excess intake of alcohol, alone or in combination, may be an important contributor to hypertension.[46] Some of the diet-related factors associated with high blood pressure include overweight and obesity, excess intake of sodium, and insufficient intake of potassium, calcium, magnesium, protein (especially from vegetables), fiber, and fish fats.[47,48]

Progression from chronic hypertension to structural ventricular changes, and then to asymptomatic diastolic and systolic ventricular dysfunction, is well established by natural history investigations from longitudinal epidemiologic cohort studies, such as the FHS.[49] Elevated blood pressure places greater hemodynamic burden on the myocardium and leads to left ventricular hypertrophy (**Fig. 35.5**).[50] Left ventricular hypertrophy is associated with increased myocardial stiffness and decreased compliance, initially during exercise and subsequently at rest.[51] The initial concentric hypertrophy (thick wall, normal chamber volume, and high mass-to-volume ratio), per the Laplace's law, helps to keep wall tension normal despite high intraventricular pressure

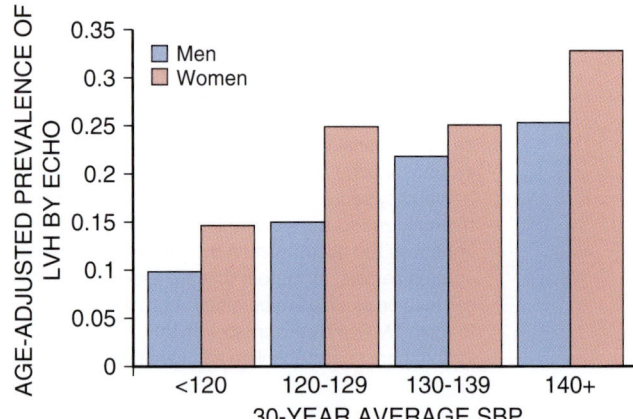

Fig. 35.5 Prevalence of left ventricular hypertrophy *(LVH)*, demonstrated by echocardiography *(ECHO)*, as a function of 30-year average systolic blood pressure *(SBP)*. (From Lauer MS, Anderson KM, Levy D. Influence of contemporary versus 30-year blood pressure levels on left ventricular mass and geometry: the Framingham Heart Study. *J Am Coll Cardiol.* 1991;18[5]:1287–1294.)

(**Fig. 35.6**). Because systolic stress (afterload) is a major determinant of ejection performance, normalization of systolic stress helps to maintain a normal stroke volume despite the need to generate high levels of systolic pressure.[52] Constriction and stiffening of small arteries at branch points and in the microcirculation augment reflected waves

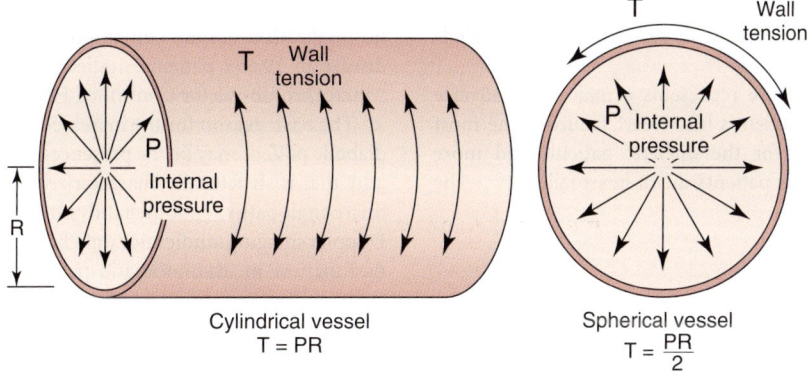

Fig. 35.6 Laplace's Law. The larger the vessel radius *(R)* is, the higher the wall tension *(T)* must be to withstand a given internal fluid pressure *(P)*. For a given vessel radius and internal pressure, a spherical vessel has half the wall tension of a cylindrical vessel.

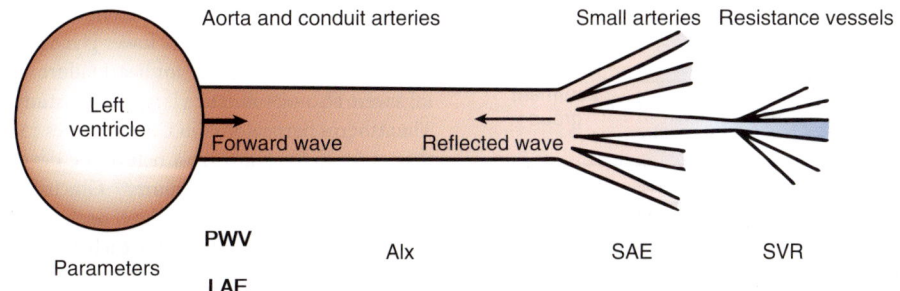

Fig. 35.7 The different parameters of arterial stiffness/elasticity and the information they provide along the arterial system. *AIx,* Augmentation index; *LAE,* large artery elasticity; *PWV,* pulse wave velocity; *SAE,* small artery elasticity; *SVR,* systemic vascular resistance. (From Duprez DA. Arterial stiffness/elasticity in the contribution to progression of heart failure. *Heart Fail Clin.* 2012;8[1]:135–141.)

that may impose a late systolic aortic pressure load on left ventricular emptying that is not detectable in the arm (**Fig. 35.7**).[53] Therapy that relaxes these small arteries may therefore exert a greater benefit than is apparent from standard blood pressure measurement.

A new guideline for the prevention, detection, evaluation, and management of high blood pressure in adults was recently proposed.[46] It changed the definition of hypertension, which is now considered to be a systolic blood pressure of 130 mm Hg or higher or a diastolic blood pressure of 80 mm Hg or higher. According to these new criteria, 46% of adults in the United States have high blood pressure. Strategies to control blood pressure are an integral part of any effort to prevent heart failure.[46]

Prevention of hypertension and treatment of established hypertension are complementary approaches to reducing cardiovascular disease risk in the population, but prevention of hypertension provides the optimal means of reducing risk and avoiding the harmful consequences of hypertension.[54] The updated guideline presents new treatment recommendations for patients with hypertension, which include lifestyle changes and blood pressure–lowering medications. Correcting the dietary aberrations, physical inactivity, and excessive consumption of alcohol that cause high blood pressure is a potentially important approach to prevention and management of high blood pressure, either on their own or in combination with pharmacologic therapy. However, hereditary factors may predominate, and drug management may be necessary to supplement nonpharmacologic interventions such as behavioral strategies aimed at lifestyle change, prescription of dietary supplements, or implementation of kitchen-based interventions that directly modify elements of the diet. At a societal level, policy changes can enhance the availability of healthy foods and facilitate physical activity.[46]

Aggressive blood pressure control may be the most effective approach to reduce the incidence of heart failure in a hypertensive population. A number of clinical trials demonstrate the benefit of treating hypertension in the prevention of heart failure.[55] For instance, Hypertension in the Very Elderly trial showed a 64% relative risk reduction in heart failure with the diuretic indapamide with or without the angiotensin-converting enzyme (ACE) inhibitor perindopril (**Fig. 35.8**).[56]

Diabetes Mellitus and Heart Failure (see also Chapter 48)

On the basis of data from NHANES 2011 to 2014, an estimated 23.4 million adults have diagnosed diabetes mellitus, 7.6 million adults have undiagnosed diabetes mellitus, and 81.6 million adults (33.9%) have prediabetes (e.g., fasting blood glucose of 100 to <126 mg/dL).[1] The number of patients with diabetes mellitus continues to rise, owing mainly to changes in lifestyle (excessive calorie and fat intake and decreased physical activity). The total prevalence of diabetes in the United States is expected to more than double from 2005 to 2050 (from 5.6% to 12.0%) in all age, sex, and race/ethnicity groups.[57] On the basis of NHANES 2011 to 2014 data for adults with diabetes mellitus, 20.8% had their diabetes mellitus treated and controlled, 46.4% had their diabetes mellitus treated but uncontrolled, 9.9% were aware they had diabetes mellitus but were not treated, and 22.9% were undiagnosed and not treated (**Fig. 35.9**).

Diabetes mellitus is a major risk factor for cardiovascular disease, such as coronary heart disease, stroke, peripheral artery disease, heart failure, and atrial fibrillation.[58] In the Multi-Ethnic Study of Atherosclerosis (MESA), diabetes mellitus was associated with a twofold increased adjusted risk of incident heart failure among 6814 individuals free of cardiovascular disease at baseline over a mean follow-up of 4 years.[59]

The occurrence of heart failure represents a major and adverse prognostic turn in a diabetic patient's life. Heart failure is the most common admission diagnosis for the diabetic patient, and more than one-third of type 2 diabetic patients die of heart failure.[60,61] The

presence of diabetes mellitus conferred a greater risk for heart failure hospitalization despite contemporary management of cardiovascular disease in 19,699 patients studied in the international REduction of Atherothrombosis for Continued Health (REACH) registry.[62]

The basic reason for the increased prevalence of heart failure in the diabetic patient may be the presence of a distinct diabetic cardiomyopathy that is structurally characterized by cardiomyocyte hypertrophy, microangiopathy, endothelial dysfunction, and myocardial fibrosis.[63] Doppler imaging studies not only have confirmed evidence of diastolic dysfunction in asymptomatic patients with diabetes but also have shown a direct relationship between the extent of diastolic dysfunction and glycemic control (**Fig. 35.10**).[64]

Although neither the Diabetes Control and Complications Trial (DCCT) in type 1 diabetes nor the UK Prospective Diabetes Study (UKPDS) in type 2 diabetes showed a reduction in cardiovascular events with intensive glycemic control,[65,66] a prospective, observational component of UKPDS revealed a continuous relationship between glycemic exposure and the development of heart failure with no threshold of risk, such that for each 1% lower glycosylated hemoglobin (HbA_{1c}), there was a 16% lower risk for heart failure (**Fig. 35.11**).[67] Similar findings were also reported in a large cohort study from the United States.[68] The Atherosclerosis Risk in Communities (ARIC) study demonstrated that chronic hyperglycemia before the development of diabetes contributed to risk of heart failure.[69] Glucose levels predict hospitalizations for congestive heart failure, with a 10% increase in the risk of heart failure hospitalization for each 18-mg/dL (1-mmol) increase in fasting glucose level.[70]

Although controlling other metabolic risks in patients with diabetes is of plausible potential importance, the Look AHEAD (Action for Health in Diabetes) trial found that intensive lifestyle intervention focusing on weight loss did not reduce the risk of cardiovascular morbidity or mortality compared with a control program of diabetes support and education in overweight or obese adults with type 2 diabetes.[71] Attaining optimal glycemic control should be a goal in both the prevention and treatment of heart failure in patients with diabetes.

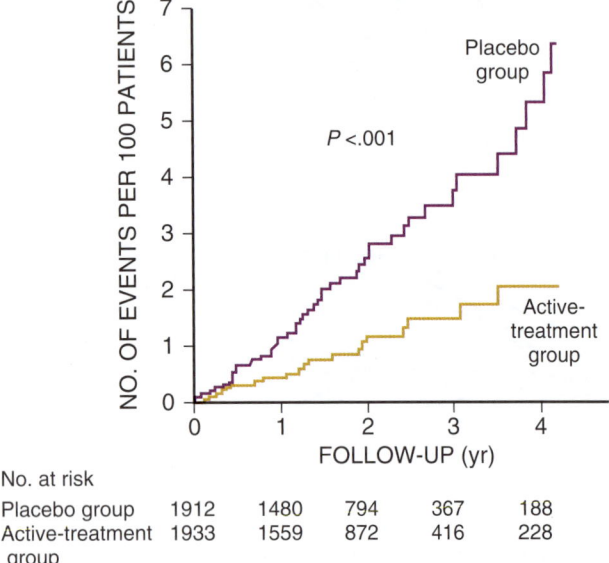

No. at risk					
Placebo group	1912	1480	794	367	188
Active-treatment group	1933	1559	872	416	228

Fig. 35.8 Kaplan-Meier estimates of the rate of heart failure according to study group in the hypertension in the very elderly trial. For subjects receiving active treatment, in comparison with those receiving a placebo, the unadjusted hazard ratio was 0.36 (95% confidence interval, 0.22–0.58). (From Beckett NS, Peters R, Fletcher AE, et al. Treatment of hypertension in patients 80 years of age or older. *N Engl J Med.* 2008;358[18]:1887–1898.)

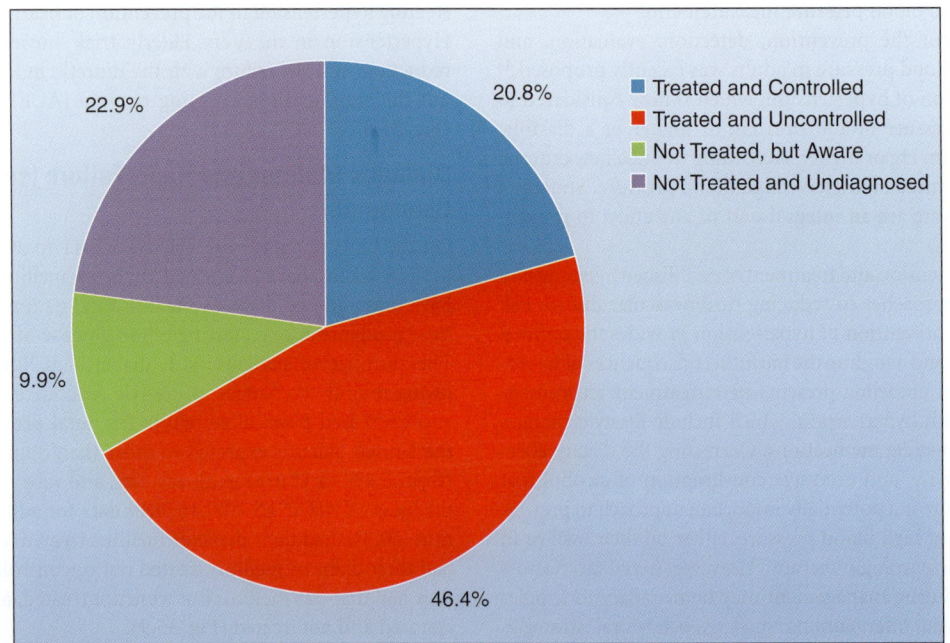

Fig. 35.9 Diabetes mellitus awareness, treatment, and control in adults 20 years of age or older (National Health and Nutrition Examination Survey 2011–2014). (Reprinted with permission. From Benjamin EJ, Blaha MJ, Chiuve SE, et al. Heart disease and stroke statistics-2017 update: a report from the American Heart Association. *Circulation.* 2017;135[10]:e146–e603.)

Standard therapies for diabetes mellitus, such as use of ACE inhibitors or angiotensin receptor blockers, can prevent the development of other risk factors for heart failure, such as renal dysfunction,[72,73] and may themselves directly lower the likelihood of heart failure.[74-76] Recent evidence showed that treatment of patients with type 2 diabetes mellitus with sodium-glucose cotransporter-2 inhibitor (SGLT-2i) versus other glucose-lowering drugs was associated with a lower risk of hospitalization for heart failure and death.[77]

Atherosclerotic Disease and Heart Failure (see also Chapter 19)

Patients with known atherosclerotic disease (e.g., of the coronary, cerebral, or peripheral arteries) are at increased risk of developing heart

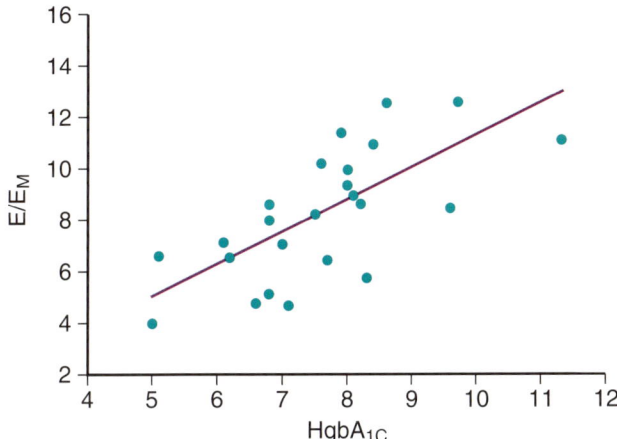

Fig. 35.10 Relationship between glycosylated hemoglobin (*HgbA₁c*) and left ventricular diastolic function in patients with type 1 diabetes and without overt heart failure (r = 0.68, P <.0002). E/Em = relation of peak early diastolic transmitral flow *(E)* to myocardial relaxation velocity during early diastole *(Em)*. (From Shishehbor MH, Hoogwerf BJ, Schoenhagen P, et al. Relation of hemoglobin A₁c to left ventricular relaxation in patients with type 1 diabetes mellitus and without overt heart disease. *Am J Cardiol.* 2003;91[12]:1514–1517.)

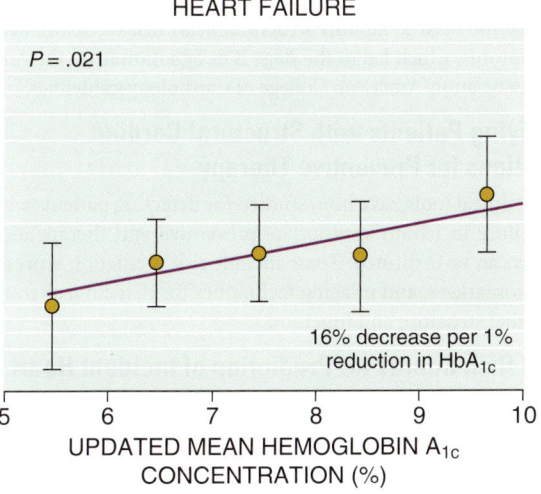

Fig. 35.11 Relative risk of heart failure in relation to glycosylated hemoglobin (HgbA₁c) in the UK prospective diabetes study. (From Stratton IM, Adler AI, Neil HA, et al. Association of glycaemia with macrovascular and microvascular complications of type 2 diabetes [UKPDS 35]: prospective observational study. *BMJ.* 2000;321[7258]:405–412.)

failure. The role of coronary artery disease and myocardial infarction as major antecedents of heart failure has been well established.[1]

Myocardial infarction stimulates cardiac remodeling[78] and contributes to the development of heart failure. The percentage of people with a first myocardial infarction who will have heart failure in 5 years at 45 years of age or older is 16% of men and 22% of women.[1] Even in heart failure patients classified clinically as "nonischemic cardiomyopathy," up to a fourth may have evidence of coronary artery disease at autopsy.[79] Indeed, patients with "nonischemic cardiomyopathy" may develop clinical ischemic events, an observation that suggests that coronary disease may not be just an "innocent bystander" in these patients.[80] In addition to epicardial disease, microvascular coronary disease is also both widespread and often underrecognized.[81]

The risk of coronary artery disease and myocardial infarction can be reduced by modification of risk factors. Hydroxymethylglutaryl–coenzyme A reductase inhibitors (statins) reduce cardiovascular events in patients with myocardial infarction and the occurrence of heart failure in patients with coronary heart disease.[82] ACE inhibitors reduce incidence of heart failure by 23% among patients who have coronary artery disease and normal systolic function and by 37% among patients who have reduced left ventricular systolic function.[83] In one large-scale trial, long-term treatment with an ACE inhibitor decreased the risk of the primary end point of cardiovascular death, myocardial infarction, and stroke in patients with high-risk established vascular disease who were without evidence of heart failure or reduced left ventricular ejection fraction.[76] Among patients with stable coronary artery disease and no heart failure, ACE inhibitor therapy significantly reduced the incidence of death, myocardial infarction, or cardiac arrest.[84]

Metabolic Syndrome and Heart Failure

Metabolic syndrome is a multicomponent risk factor for cardiovascular disease and type 2 diabetes mellitus. Although several different clinical definitions for metabolic syndrome have been proposed, the International Diabetes Federation and others recently proposed a harmonized definition for metabolic syndrome.[85] By this definition, metabolic syndrome is diagnosed when three or more of the following five risk factors are present (**Table 35.3**): (1) fasting plasma glucose of 100 mg/dL or more or undergoing drug treatment for elevated glucose, (2) high-density lipoprotein cholesterol less than 40 mg/dL in men or less than 50 mg/dL in women or undergoing drug treatment for reduced high-density lipoprotein cholesterol, (3) triglycerides of 150 mg/dL or more or undergoing drug treatment for elevated triglycerides, (4) waist circumference 102 cm or more in men or 88 cm or more in women, and (5) blood pressure 130 mm Hg or more systolic or 85 mm Hg or more diastolic or undergoing drug treatment for hypertension.

TABLE 35.3 Metabolic Syndrome

	Risk Factor
1	Fasting plasma glucose ≥100 mg/dL or undergoing drug treatment for elevated glucose
2	High-density lipoprotein cholesterol <40 mg/dL in males or <50 mg/dL in females or undergoing drug treatment for reduced high-density lipoprotein cholesterol
3	Triglycerides ≥150 mg/dL or undergoing drug treatment for elevated triglycerides
4	Waist circumference >102 cm in males or >88 cm in females
5	Blood pressure ≥130 mm Hg systolic or ≥85 mm Hg diastolic or undergoing drug treatment for hypertension

Metabolic syndrome is diagnosed when any 3 of the 5 risk factors are present.

On the basis of data from NHANES 1999 to 2010, the age-adjusted prevalence of metabolic syndrome in the United States peaked in the 2001 to 2002 cycle and declined in the 2009 to 2010 NHANES cycle.[86] In the 1999 to 2000 cycle, the age-adjusted prevalence of metabolic syndrome was 25.5%. In 2001 to 2002 the age-adjusted prevalence peaked at 27.4%. In 2009 to 2010, the age-adjusted prevalence was 22.9%.

The prevalence of metabolic syndrome increases with greater cumulative life-course exposure to sedentary behavior and physical inactivity,[87] frequent television viewing,[88] fast food intake,[89] short sleep duration,[90] and intake of sugar-sweetened beverages.[91] Each of these risk factors is reversible with lifestyle change.

A recent meta-analysis of prospective studies concluded that metabolic syndrome increased the risk of developing cardiovascular disease.[92] It is estimated that 13.3% to 44% of the excess cardiovascular disease mortality in the Unites States can be explained by metabolic syndrome or metabolic syndrome–related existing cardiovascular disease.[93] Metabolic syndrome has been associated with incident atrial fibrillation[94] and heart failure.[95]

Mechanisms underlying elevated cardiovascular risk associated with metabolic syndrome appear to involve subclinical target organ damage.[96] Metabolic syndrome has been shown to be closely related to high-risk coronary plaque features including increased necrotic core,[97] impaired coronary flow reserve,[98] abnormal indices of left ventricular strain,[99] left ventricular diastolic dysfunction,[100] left ventricular dyssynchrony,[101] and subclinical right ventricular dysfunction.[102]

Identification of metabolic syndrome represents a call to action for the health care provider and patient to address the need for pharmacotherapy and the underlying lifestyle-related risk factors, including abdominal obesity, physical inactivity, and atherogenic diet, as well as clinical management to address the characteristic atherogenic dyslipidemia, elevated blood pressure, elevated glucose, and the prothrombotic state that are common to people with metabolic syndrome. A multidisciplinary team of health care professionals is desirable to adequately address these multiple issues in patients with the metabolic syndrome.

Obesity and Heart Failure

Obesity continues to be a leading public health concern in the United States. According to NHANES 2013 to 2014, 37.7% of United States adults were obese (35.0% of males and 40.4% of females).[103] Overweight and obesity are major risk factors for cardiovascular disease, including type 2 diabetes mellitus, hypertension, and dyslipidemia,[104] subclinical atherosclerosis,[105] stroke,[106] atrial fibrillation,[107] and venous thromboembolism.[108] Overweight and obesity are also associated with increased risk of heart failure (**Fig. 35.12**)[109,110] and mortality.[111] Whether the culprit is the obesity itself or if genetic factors that may underlie obesity are contributory remains uncertain in the absence of prospective controlled intervention trials. The MESA[112] and the more recent Dallas Heart Study[113] both used cardiac magnetic resonance imaging (MRI) in large multiethnic cohorts of adults and demonstrated an association between adiposity and concentric left ventricular remodeling (characterized by increased mass-to-volume ratio due to a greater increase in left ventricular mass relative to end-diastolic volume) without change in ejection fraction. Importantly, the Dallas Heart Study showed a dynamic relationship between changes in multiple indices of adiposity and left ventricular remodeling over 7 years.[113] These findings further support the importance of preventing obesity as primary prevention for concentric remodeling and eventual heart failure.

Despite the known association between overweight/obesity and the development of cardiovascular diseases, numerous studies, including in heart failure, have demonstrated an "obesity paradox," in that obese patients with established cardiovascular diseases appear to have a more favorable clinical prognosis in heart failure, hypertension, coronary heart disease, and atrial fibrillation than do their leaner counterparts with the same cardiovascular diseases.[114,115] In the Atrial Fibrillation Follow-up Investigation of Rhythm Management (AFFIRM) study, a multicenter trial of atrial fibrillation, obese patients had lower all-cause mortality than normal-weight patients after multivariable adjustment over a 3-year follow-up period.[116] In another study in patients with new-onset diabetes mellitus, adults who were normal weight at the time of incident diabetes had higher mortality than adults who were overweight or obese.[117]

The reasons for the obesity paradox remain unclear. The simplest explanation is that obesity precipitates symptomatic heart failure at an earlier stage of the ventricular remodeling process. However, because heart failure is a catabolic state, obese patients may have more metabolic reserve, and there is no doubt that cachexia is associated with adverse prognosis in heart failure.[118] Various cytokines and neuroendocrine profiles of obese patients may be protective.[118] Adipose tissue is known to produce soluble tumor necrosis factor-α receptors, which could have a protective effect in obese patients with heart failure by neutralizing the adverse biologic effects of tumor necrosis factor-α.[119] In addition, higher circulating lipoproteins in obese patients may bind and detoxify lipopolysaccharides that play a role in stimulating the release of inflammatory cytokines, all of which may serve to protect obese heart failure patients.[115,120]

Although weight reduction clearly has beneficial cardiovascular effects and efforts to promote optimal body weight are likely to have an impact on a number of risk factors for heart failure and other cardiovascular diseases, only limited data are available to base current recommendations for intentional weight loss in patients with established heart failure.[114] Although the "weight" of evidence supports intentional weight reduction in heart failure, especially for those with more significant obesity,[114] better clinical studies are needed to define optimal body composition in patients with heart failure.

DISEASE PREVENTION IN STAGE B HEART FAILURE

The pivotal studies of Survival and Ventricular Enlargement (SAVE) of patients after myocardial infarction[121] and Studies of Left Ventricular Dysfunction (SOLVD)[122] of asymptomatic patients with left ventricular dysfunction showed that neurohormonal inhibition of the renin-angiotensin system reduces the progression to manifest heart failure. This generated the need to identify structural heart disease before heart failure symptoms, which led to the stage B designation from the American Heart Association/American College of Cardiology guidelines.[3]

Identifying Patients with Structural Cardiac Alterations for Preventive Therapy

Several clinical tools have been studied for detecting patients with early heart failure in whom appropriate preventive and therapeutic interventions can be instituted. These include risk prediction scores, circulating biomarkers, and imaging techniques for detecting alterations in myocardial structure and function.

Use of Risk Scores for Prediction of Incident Heart Failure

Two epidemiology studies have developed heart failure risk prediction scores that generally have only a moderate discriminative value for identifying whether or not an individual will develop overt heart failure. The original FHS heart failure prediction score was developed in the late 1990s in individuals with hypertension, coronary heart disease, or valve disease and used simple clinical data available from the medical record. This risk score identified patients with incremental risk of

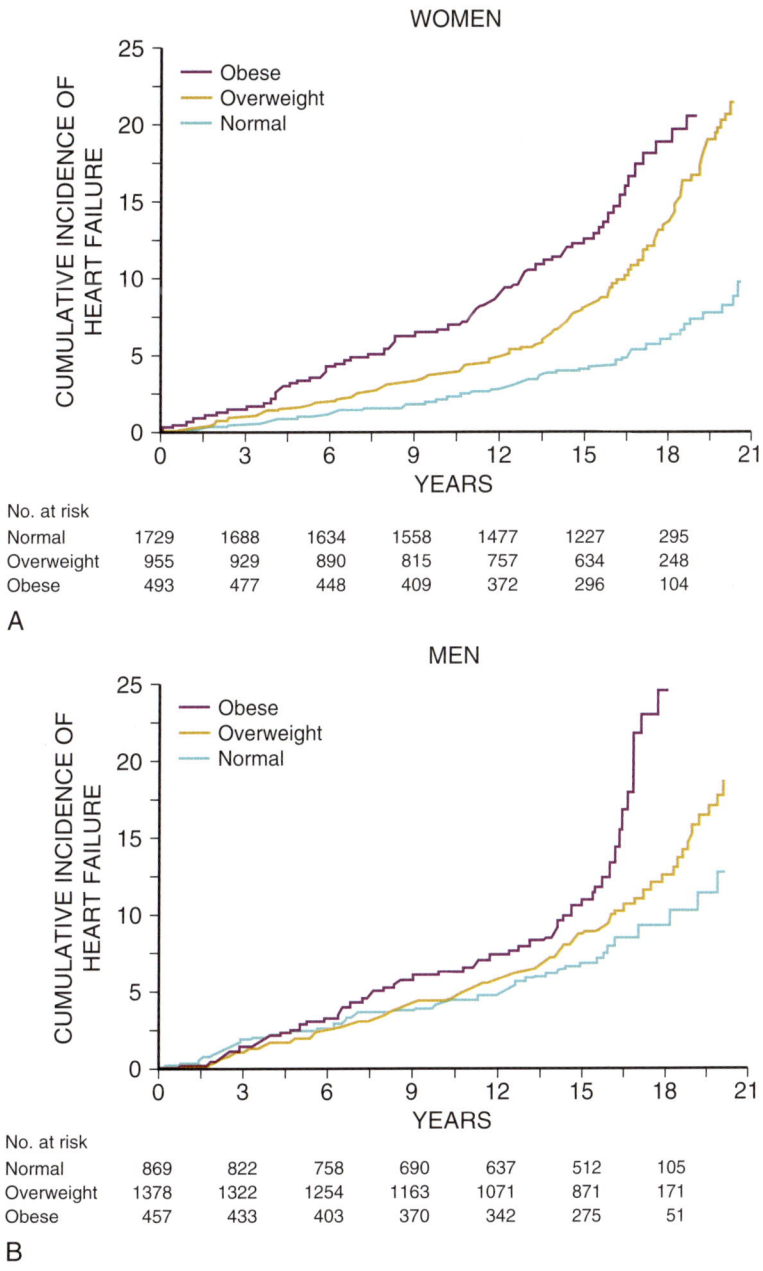

WOMEN

CUMULATIVE INCIDENCE OF HEART FAILURE

Obese
Overweight
Normal

YEARS

No. at risk
Normal	1729	1688	1634	1558	1477	1227	295
Overweight	955	929	890	815	757	634	248
Obese	493	477	448	409	372	296	104

A

MEN

CUMULATIVE INCIDENCE OF HEART FAILURE

Obese
Overweight
Normal

YEARS

No. at risk
Normal	869	822	758	690	637	512	105
Overweight	1378	1322	1254	1163	1071	871	171
Obese	457	433	403	370	342	275	51

B

Fig. 35.12 Cumulative incidence of heart failure in women (A) and men (B) according to category of body mass index at the baseline examination. The body mass index was 18.5 to 24.9 in normal subjects, 25.0 to 29.9 in overweight subjects, and 30.0 or more in obese subjects. (From Kenchaiah S, Evans JC, Levy D, et al. Obesity and the risk of heart failure. *N Engl J Med.* 2002;347[5]:305–313.)

future heart failure.[123] The Health Aging and Body Composition (ABC) study derived another risk score predictive of incident heart failure at 5 years.[124] The ABC risk score was superior to the FHS score but still provided only moderate discrimination for incident heart failure. The ABC heart failure model was externally validated in the Cardiovascular Health Study (CHS).[125] The ABC study and CHS define the numbers of older individuals without prevalent heart failure who have low (<5%), average (5%–10%), high (10%–20%), and very high (>20%) risk of overt heart failure over 5 years and thus provide insight into the number of persons who would be suitable for an intervention to prevent incident heart failure. Findings in the ABC study and CHS indicate that approximately 40% of older individuals have a risk of more than 5% of heart failure over 5 years and that approximately 75% of heart failure events occur in these individuals. Thus intervening with a

heart failure prevention strategy in those at a risk of more than 5% of developing heart failure would limit the application of the intervention to 40% of the older population and offer the potential to affect 75% of future heart failure events. Intervening in those at more than 10% risk of developing heart failure would limit the application of the intervention to 20% of the older population and offer the potential to affect 50% of future heart failure events.

Use of Biomarkers for Screening and Prevention of Heart Failure (see also Chapter 33)

Biomarkers encompass an expanding array of biochemical variables, the levels of which may reflect various aspects of the pathophysiology of heart failure. Putative biomarkers can be broadly classified into (a) biomarkers of neurohormonal activation, (b) myocyte injury,

(c) extracellular matrix remodeling, (d) inflammation, (e) oxidative stress, and (f) newer biomarkers whose pathophysiologic associations are less well defined.[126]

Most of the early studies of natriuretic peptides have focused on the role of BNP or *N*-terminal proBNP (NT-proBNP) testing among patients presenting with signs and symptoms of heart failure ("stage C and D heart failure"). The diagnostic and prognostic utility of plasma natriuretic peptide levels in the overt heart failure setting has prompted interest in evaluation of these biomarkers as screening tools for patients with risk factors for heart failure and asymptomatic left ventricular dysfunction ("stage A and B heart failure").

Data from Olmsted County, Minnesota, showed that in stage A and B heart failure, plasma NT-proBNP values greater than age-/sex-specific 80th percentiles were associated with increased risk of death, heart failure, cerebrovascular accident, and myocardial infarction even after adjustment for clinical risk factors and structural cardiac abnormalities.[127] Higher NT-proBNP levels have also been associated with the greater likelihood of detecting incident heart failure in a population with stable coronary artery disease.[128] Investigations from the FHS reported that plasma natriuretic peptide levels predicted the risk of death and first cardiovascular event including heart failure, atrial fibrillation, and stroke or transient ischemic attack (**Fig. 35.13**).[129]

Both the FHS and the ABC study have explored the ability of several biomarkers to enhance clinical scores for heart failure risk assessment. In the FHS, BNP and the urinary albumin to creatinine ratio (but not C-reactive protein, plasminogen activator inhibitor 1, homocysteine, or aldosterone to renin ratio) increased the discrimination of a clinical heart failure prediction score modestly.[130] In the ABC study, the additive value of inflammatory markers (interleukin-6, tumor necrosis factor-α, and C-reactive protein) to the ABC clinical risk score was assessed. Interleukin-6 provided modest but statistically significant additive discrimination and improved the risk stratification.[131] These studies suggest that heart failure risk stratification can be improved by biomarkers that might be useful if a prevention strategy was targeting those with increased heart failure risk.

The Dallas Heart Study included a cardiac magnetic resonance (CMR) examination in 2339 participants aged 30 to 65 years and found that 12.5% of participants met the definition of stage B heart failure defined as the presence of left ventricular hypertrophy, reduced ejection fraction, or prior myocardial infarction.[132] They then examined the ability of the ABC heart failure risk score, BNP, NT-proBNP, and the combination of BNP or NT-proBNP and clinical risk score to detect stage B heart failure. The combination of a high clinical risk score and an elevated BNP or NT-proBNP had the best predictive characteristics for identifying stage B heart failure, but positive predictive values were quite low and indicate that 70% of imaging studies obtained in response to screening would not identify left ventricular hypertrophy or systolic dysfunction.[132]

The Olmsted County Heart Study examined the potential utility of plasma BNP as a stand-alone screening intervention to detect asymptomatic left ventricular systolic dysfunction in the general population.[133] The predictive characteristics of BNP for detection of ejection fraction of 40% or less were better than for detection of ejection fraction of 50% or less, but even focusing on detection of EF of 40% or less, the burden of imaging and yield on imaging would preclude a biomarker-only strategy from becoming widely accepted because most follow-up study results would be negative. A similar analysis with NT-proBNP in the same cohort was largely identical.[134] Similar findings were found in the FHS.[135] Although other investigators postulate that natriuretic peptides could be cost effective,[136] the low prevalence of systolic dysfunction provides a very high bar for using natriuretic peptides as screening biomarkers.

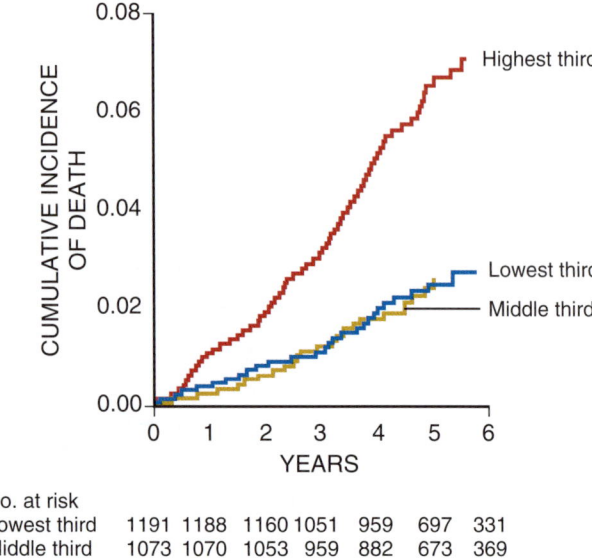

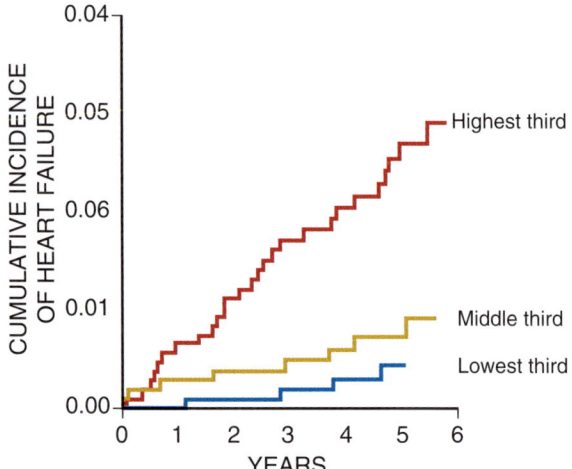

Fig. 35.13 Cumulative incidence of death (A) and heart failure (B), according to the plasma B-type natriuretic peptide level at baseline. (From Wang T, Larson M, Levy D, et al. Plasma natriuretic peptide levels and the risk of cardiovascular events and death. *N Engl J Med.* 2004;350[7]:655–663.)

New data suggest that natriuretic peptide biomarker screening and early intervention may prevent heart failure. In a large-scale unblinded single-center study (STOP-HF [The St Vincent's Screening to Prevent Heart Failure]),[137] patients at risk of heart failure (identified by the presence of hypertension, diabetes mellitus, or known vascular disease [e.g., stage A heart failure]) but without established left ventricular systolic dysfunction or symptomatic heart failure at baseline were randomly assigned to receive screening with BNP testing or usual primary care. Intervention-group participants with BNP levels of ≥50 pg/mL underwent echocardiography and were referred to a cardiovascular specialist who decided on further investigation and management. All patients received further coaching by a specialist nurse who emphasized individual risk and the importance of adherence to medication and healthy lifestyle behaviors. BNP-based screening reduced the composite end point of asymptomatic left ventricular dysfunction

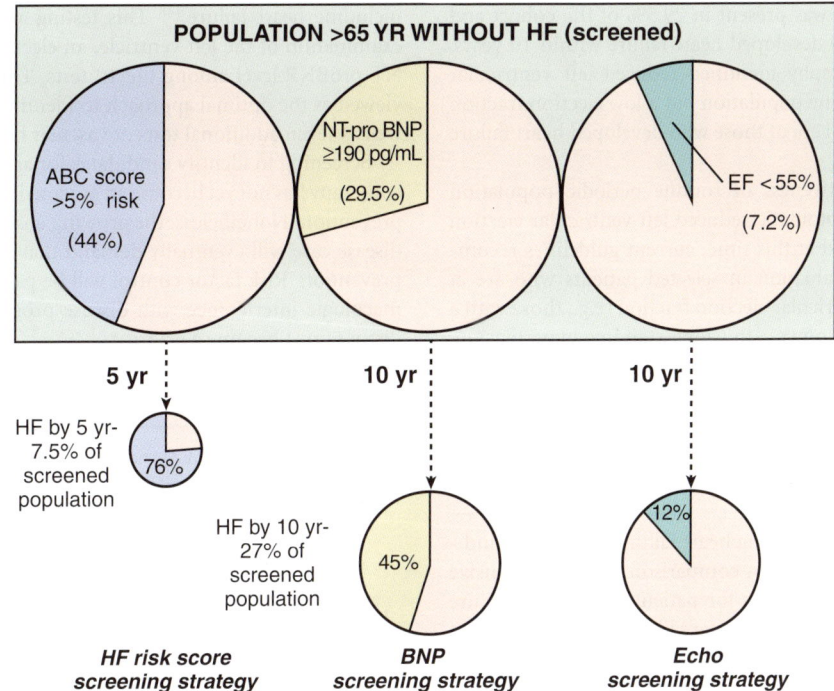

Fig. 35.14 The Health Aging and Body Composition *(ABC)* Heart Failure risk score, N-terminal pro-B-type natriuretic peptide *(NT-proBNP)* levels, and echocardiography-based screening in the Cardiovascular Health Study cohort. The percentage of the cohort with a positive screening result, the percentage of the cohort who went on to develop incident heart failure, and the percentage of the patients who developed heart failure who would have been identified by the screening intervention are shown (see text for details). *EF,* Ejection fraction; *HF,* heart failure. (From Redfield MM. Strategies to screen for stage B as a heart failure prevention intervention. *Heart Fail Clin.* 2012;8[2]:285–296.)

(systolic or diastolic) with or without newly diagnosed heart failure.[137] Similarly, in another small, single-center randomized clinical trial, accelerated uptitration of renin-angiotensin-aldosterone system antagonists and beta-blockers reduced cardiac events in patients with diabetes mellitus and elevated NT-proBNP levels but without cardiac disease at baseline.[138] As a result, the recent 2017 update of the guideline for the management of heart failure supports natriuretic peptide biomarker-based screening for patients at risk of developing heart failure, followed by guideline-directed management and therapy, as a useful approach (class IIa Recommendation) to prevent the development of left ventricular dysfunction (systolic or diastolic) or new-onset heart failure.[139]

Use of Imaging for Evaluation of Newly Suspected or Potential Heart Failure

In patients with signs and symptoms that raise suspicion of heart failure, assessment of left ventricular systolic and diastolic function is important and can be performed with a variety of imaging techniques. The same holds true for patients who are at risk for heart failure, such as patients after acute myocardial infarction, those with hypertension and left ventricular hypertrophy, those who are exposed to potentially cardiotoxic chemotherapeutic agents,[140] and first-degree relatives of those with an inherited cardiomyopathy. The main objectives of imaging for heart failure evaluation revolve primarily around understanding both cardiac structure and function, and secondarily in determining the underlying cause, so that proven therapies may be targeted to appropriate patients.

Although the prevalence of asymptomatic left ventricular systolic dysfunction in the general adult population (3%–6%) may be too low to advocate use of traditional imaging techniques as a primary screening modality, population studies have identified subsets with sufficient prevalence of systolic dysfunction (elderly men with prevalent cardiovascular disease in whom the prevalence of asymptomatic left ventricular ejection fraction of 50% or less was 17%) that may warrant a primary imaging strategy.[141]

There are many diagnostic procedures used to evaluate patients with newly suspected or potential heart failure. Resting electrocardiogram or chest x-rays are part of the routine data collected with general history and physical examinations when appropriate. More advanced procedures include both rest and stress tests for echocardiography, radionuclide imaging (including radionuclide ventriculography [RNV], single-photon emission computed tomography [SPECT], positron emission tomography [PET], and cardiovascular magnetic resonance [CMR]). Recently, coronary artery calcium (CAC) has emerged as a predictor of future major adverse atherosclerotic cardiovascular events in asymptomatic individuals.[142] In addition, imaging of cardiac structures and coronary anatomy with coronary computed tomography angiography may be considered to facilitate initiation of cardioprotective medications.[143] The use of these procedures should prudently take into account their possible technical capabilities, safety, and cost effectiveness.[144]

Fig. 35.14 shows the utility of the ABC Heart Failure risk score, NT-proBNP levels, and echocardiography in detecting incident heart failure in the CHS population.[141] The percentage of the cohort with a positive screening result, the percentage of the cohort who went on to develop incident heart failure, and the percentage of the patients who developed heart failure who would have been identified by the screening intervention are shown. The ABC Heart Failure risk score indicated higher (>5%) risk of heart failure at 5 years in 44% of the cohort and identified 76% of those who developed heart failure by 5 years. An abnormal NT-proBNP level was present in 29.5% of the cohort and identified 45% of those who developed heart failure within 10 years. The screening echocardiography identified reduced left ventricular ejection fraction in 7.2% of the population but a low ejection fraction on screening identified only 12% of those who developed heart failure within 10 years.

Although the cost effectiveness of routine periodic population imaging screening for asymptomatic reduced left ventricular ejection fraction is not recommended at this time, current guidelines recommend echocardiographic evaluation in selected patients who are at high risk of reduced left ventricular ejection fraction (e.g., those with a strong family history of cardiomyopathy, long-standing hypertension, previous myocardial infarction, or those receiving cardiotoxic therapies) and in those with suspected valvular abnormalities or congenital heart lesions.[145]

FUTURE DIRECTIONS

Thus far, research aimed at preventing heart failure in high-risk individuals has been relatively modest in comparison with the extensive efforts at discovering new treatments for patients after heart failure has developed. Because preventive efforts are likely to be applicable to much larger numbers of individuals, such efforts could lead to greater population-level benefits. It is therefore important that we develop a strategy of prevention of heart failure that applies to the large number of "at-risk" individuals. Such a strategy would complement our current approaches that are aimed at intensive management of patients with manifest heart failure. Implementation of our current knowledge of both prevention and treatment of hypertension, obesity, and atherosclerotic vascular disease has the potential to have a large impact on the incidence and mortality from heart failure.

The ability to identify noninvasively early abnormalities of cardiovascular function and structure has led to the concept that it would be preferable to screen for and treat abnormalities that lead to all cardiovascular morbid events, not only heart failure. Because heart failure is a manifestation of chronic progression of these functional and structural defects, and some of these same abnormalities may lead to myocardial infarction, stroke, renal failure, peripheral vascular disease, and other morbid cardiovascular events, efforts to reduce the prevalence of all these events would appear to be more cost effective than focusing specifically on heart failure.[146] One approach to this effort is the disease score for detection of early cardiovascular disease developed by Cohn and colleagues.[147] This method of performing 10 noninvasive tests of vascular and cardiac health has led to a scoring system that has been remarkably sensitive and specific in predicting future morbid events,

including heart failure.[148] This testing array includes an ultrasound examination of the left ventricle, an electrocardiogram, and a plasma NT-proBNP level among the 10 tests. Thus it includes what may be viewed as the optimal approach to identifying early cardiac disease, as well as seven additional tests of vascular health.

Screening to identify candidates for aggressive preventive pharmacotherapy has not yet become an accepted standard approach to disease prevention. Nonetheless, the growing cost of advanced cardiovascular disease care will eventually demand that more effort be expended on prevention. Risk factor control will be part of that strategy, but pharmacologic interference with disease progression for those with early disease must become a priority.

KEY REFERENCES

6. Djousse L, Driver JA, Gaziano JM. Relation between modifiable lifestyle factors and lifetime risk of heart failure. *JAMA.* 2009;302:394–400.
11. Hupin D, Roche F, Gremeaux V, Chatard JC, Oriol M, Gaspoz JM, et al. Even a low-dose of moderate-to-vigorous physical activity reduces mortality by 22% in adults aged >/=60 years: a systematic review and meta-analysis. *Br J Sports Med.* 2015;49:1262–1267.
14. Edelmann F, Gelbrich G, Dungen HD, et al. Exercise training improves exercise capacity and diastolic function in patients with heart failure with preserved ejection fraction: results of the Ex-DHF [Exercise training in diastolic heart failure] pilot study. *J Am Coll Cardiol.* 2011;58:1780–1791.
21. Fung TT, Rexrode KM, Mantzoros CS, et al. Mediterranean diet and incidence of and mortality from coronary heart disease and stroke in women. *Circulation.* 2009;119:1093–1100.
23. Miro O, Estruch R, Martin-Sanchez FJ, Group I-SR, et al. Adherence to Mediterranean diet and all-cause mortality after an episode of acute heart failure. Results of the MEDIT-AHF Study. *J Am Coll Cardiol HF.* 2017:1–11.
25. Wang Z, Klipfell E, Bennett BJ, et al. Gut flora metabolism of phosphatidylcholine promotes cardiovascular disease. *Nature.* 2011;472:57–63.
37. Shah SJ, Kitzman DW, Borlaug BA, van Heerebeek L, Zile MR, Kass DA, et al. Phenotype-specific treatment of heart failure with preserved ejection fraction: a multiorgan roadmap. *Circulation.* 2016;134:73–90.
44. Messerli FH, Rimoldi SF, Wilhelm M. Heart failure with preserved ejection fraction: a late stage of hypertensive heart disease. *J Am Coll Cardiol.* 2017;70:2458.
71. Look ARG, Wing RR, Bolin P, et al. Cardiovascular effects of intensive lifestyle intervention in type 2 diabetes. *N Engl J Med.* 2013;369:145–154.
144. Anand IS, Florea VG, Solomon SD, Konstam MA, Udelson JE. Noninvasive assessment of left ventricular remodeling: concepts, techniques, and implications for clinical trials. *J Card Fail.* 2002;8:S452–S464.

The full reference list for this chapter is available on ExpertConsult.

Acute Heart Failure

Peter S. Pang, Marco Metra

OUTLINE

Nearly one third of acute heart failure (AHF) patients die or are rehospitalized within 90 days after discharge in the United States, with similar numbers in Europe.[1-3] Despite a decade of intensive research efforts, substantially improving outcomes remains an elusive goal.[3] Reducing morbidity and mortality remains the greatest current challenge of AHF management.

BACKGROUND AND EPIDEMIOLOGY

More than 6.5 million Americans have heart failure (HF), with more than 1 million new diagnoses each year.[4] By 2030, the prevalence of HF is projected to increase 46%, with HF related costs exceeding 70 billion US dollars (**see also Chapter 18**).[5] Despite the increasing prevalence, AHF admissions have stayed relatively flat or even decreased, at least by primary discharge diagnosis. Approximately 1 million hospitalizations with a primary discharge diagnosis of AHF occur every year.[4] Although the trajectory of primary discharge diagnoses has stayed flat, when all diagnoses are considered, AHF hospitalizations are rising (**Fig. 36.1**). Already, AHF is the most common and costliest cause of hospitalization and rehospitalization for older Americans.[6]

While rehospitalization rates have marginally improved, both rehospitalization and mortality rates remain high. In 2008, for Medicare beneficiaries, 30-day readmissions were 23.5% with a 7.9%

postdischarge mortality.[3] By 2014, 30-day readmissions had decreased to 22.7%, with an 8.6% postdischarge mortality.[3] Within 5 years, 75% of patients hospitalized with HF will be dead, irrespective of a reduced or preserved ejection fraction (EF) (**Fig. 36.2**).[7]

Amid such poor outcomes and high health care costs are health inequities; disparities evident by race, gender, and socioeconomic status. For first episodes of AHF, black males and females have the highest incidence (**Fig. 36.3**). For socioeconomically disadvantaged patients, initial admissions and readmissions are markedly higher.[8,9]

In 2003, Dr. Braunwald described HF as the "last great battleground in cardiology."[10] Ironically, as more and more patients live longer with cardiovascular disease—a testament to the tremendous advances in reducing the burden of ischemic heart disease and sudden cardiac death—such patients are at risk for developing HF (**Fig. 36.4**). As the population ages, unless outcomes improve, the burden of AHF will increase. Disparities may also worsen.

DEFINITION: WHAT IS ACUTE HEART FAILURE? WHY DOES THE DEFINITION MATTER?

AHF is a clinical diagnosis. No single test or physical exam feature definitively "rules in" or "rules out" AHF. Thus there is no diagnostic "gold standard." Perhaps unsurprisingly, there is neither a universal,

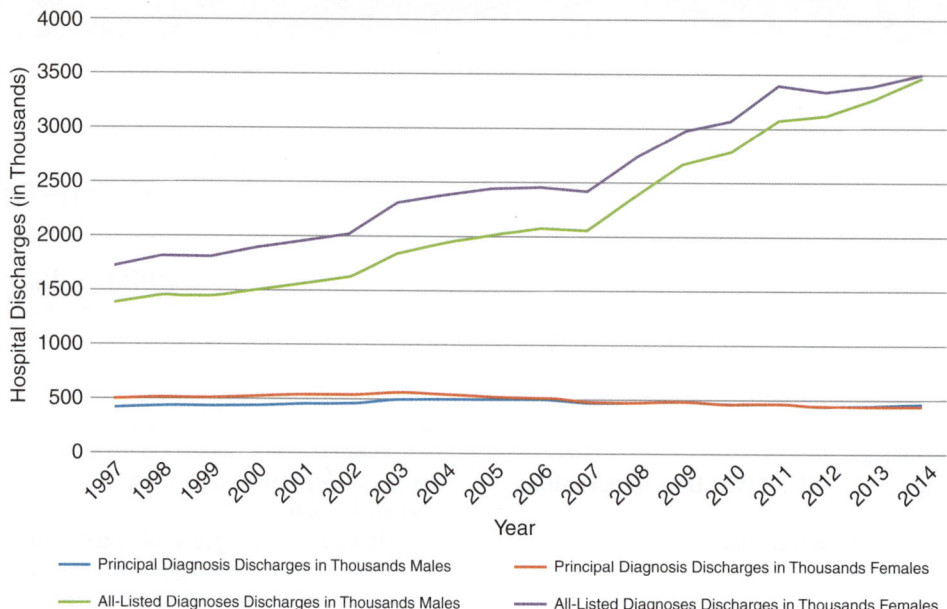

Fig. 36.1 Hospital Discharges for Heart Failure by Sex. (Reprinted with permission. From Benjamin EJ, Virani SS, Callaway CW, et al. Heart disease and stroke statistics—2018 update: a report from the American Heart Association. *Circulation.* 2018;137[12]:e67–e492. ©2018 American Heart Association, Inc.)

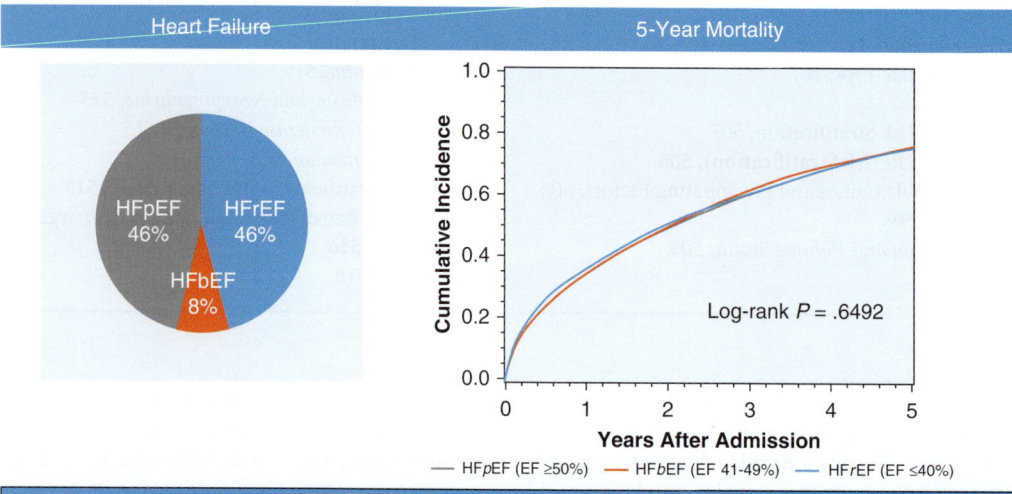

Outcomes - 5-Year Event Rates (%)					
	Mortality	Readmission	CV Readmission	HF Readmission	Mortality/Readmission
HFrEF	75.3	82.2	63.9	48.5	96.4
HFbEF	75.7	85.7	63.3	45.2	97.2
HFpEF	75.7	84.0	58.9	40.5	97.3

Fig. 36.2 Five-year outcomes in patients hospitalized for acute heart failure by ejection fraction. *CV,* Cardiovascular; *HF,* heart failure; *HFbEF,* HF with borderline EF; *HFpEF,* heart failure with preserved ejection fracture; *HFrEF,* Heart failure with reduced ejection fraction. (From Shah KS, Xu H, Matsouaka RA, et al. Heart failure with preserved, borderline, and reduced ejection fraction: 5-year outcomes. *J Am Coll Cardiol.* 2017;70[20]:2476–2486.)

well-accepted definition of AHF, nor a nomenclature to describe the various AHF syndromes.[11] Various names have been used, including acute decompensated heart failure (ADHF), hospitalization for heart failure (HHF), and acute heart failure syndromes (AHFS). Currently, AHF is the most widely used and is the current terminology in several consensus guidelines.[12,13]

Agreement upon a definition is not an academic exercise; it has significant clinical implications. Describing AHF in an 85-year-old female with no past history of HF and a systolic blood pressure at presentation of 210/120 mm Hg does not appropriately describe the 65-year-old male with known ischemic heart disease, EF of 10%, on maximal guideline recommended HF therapies awaiting transplantation. Such

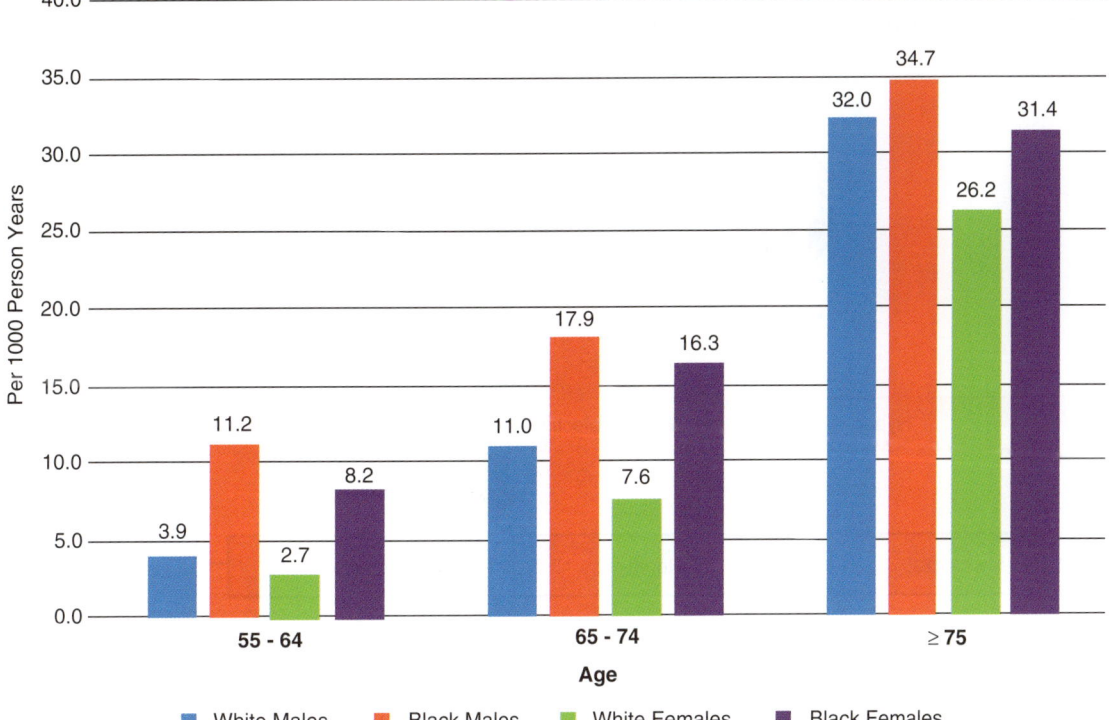

Fig. 36.3 First acute decompensated heart failure annual event rates per 1000 from ARIC (atherosclerosis risk in communities studied) community surveillance. (Reprinted with permission. From Benjamin EJ, Virani SS, Callaway CW, et al. Heart disease and stroke statistics—2018 update: a report from the American Heart Association. *Circulation.* 2018;137[12]:e67–e492. ©2018 American Heart Association, Inc.)

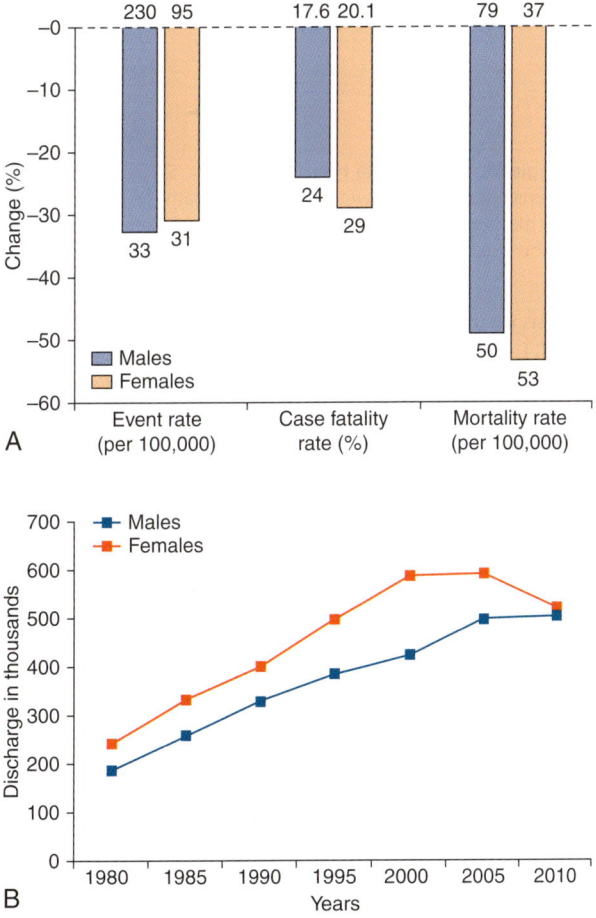

Fig. 36.4 Reduction in Myocardial Infarction and Increase in Heart Failure. (A) Percentage changes in event rate, case fatality rate, and mortality rate for acute myocardial infarction in England from 2002 to 2010. The numbers at the top of the bars are the values for 2002. Note the striking reductions in all three indicators during a relatively short period. (B) Hospital discharges for heart failure by sex in the United States from 1980 to 2010. Note the steady rise from 1980 to 2000 and then a plateau. (A, Adapted from study data by Smolina K, Wright FL, Rayner M, and Goldacre MJ. B, Source from National Hospital Discharge Survey/National Center for Health Statistics and National Heart, Lung and Blood Institute. From Braunwald E. The war against heart failure: the Lancet lecture. *Lancet.* 2015;385[9970]:812–824.)

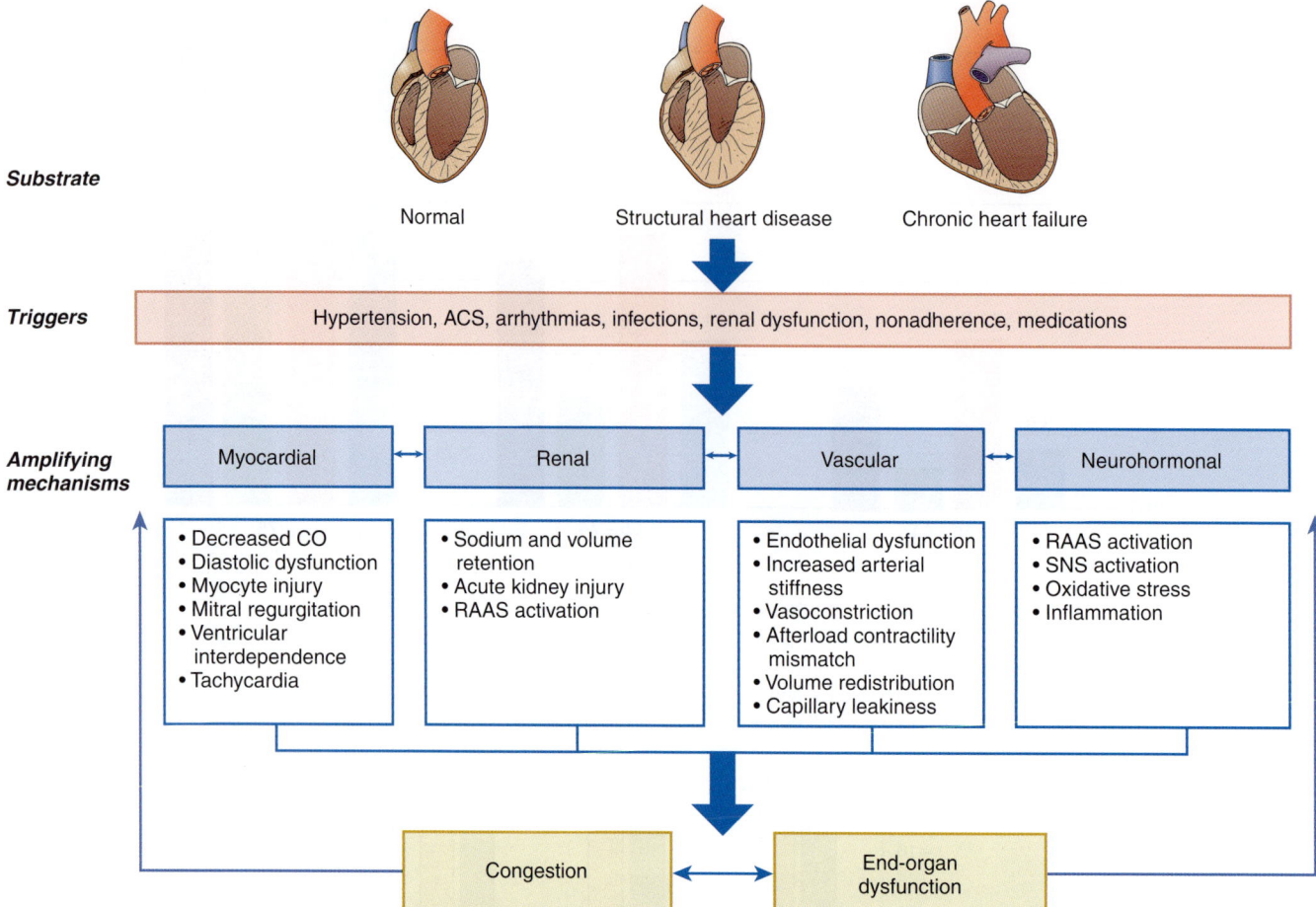

Fig. 36.5 A Pathophysiologic Model of Acute Heart Failure. *ACS,* Acute coronary syndrome; *CO,* cardiac output; *RAAS,* renin-angiotensin-aldosterone system; *SNS,* sympathetic nervous system. (From Felker GM, Teerlink JR. Diagnosis and management of acute heart failure. In Zipes DP, et al. eds. *Braunwald's Heart Disease,* 11th ed. Philadelphia, PA: Elsevier; 2019.)

heterogeneity of the AHF presentation broadens when comorbid conditions and precipitants of AHF are considered. Lack of consensus on a definition hinders both policy and research; the slow rate of progress to reduce morbidity and mortality may be directly related to the inability to define exactly what problem we are addressing.

Unfortunately, no universal definition is proposed. For the purposes of this chapter, AHF is defined as "signs of symptoms of heart failure requiring urgent or emergent therapy."[11]

PATHOPHYSIOLOGY OF ACUTE HEART FAILURE

Unlike chronic HF with reduced ejection fraction (HFrEF), the pathophysiology of AHF is less well understood. In chronic HF, neurohormonal activation (renin-angiotensin-aldosterone—sympathetic nervous system), adverse hemodynamic conditions, energetics, and inflammation, are all well-established, overlapping pathophysiologic constructs. While these mechanisms are undoubtedly also present in AHF, their relative contribution to the AHF presentation is less well known.

A conceptual model for understanding the complexity of the pathophysiology of AHF is shown in **Fig. 36.5**. An AHF episode most likely occurs on top of a structural/functional cardiac abnormality (Stage B HF). A precipitant triggers or incites the initial AHF event. This precipitant, combined with the underlying structural/functional abnormality—complicated by other comorbid conditions—ultimately

leads to AHF. Once AHF has begun, a cascade of other abnormalities occurs, affecting the heart itself, vasculature, neurohormonal system, kidneys, and liver, as well as inciting inflammatory pathways. These mechanisms act as potential amplifiers, exacerbating the current AHF episode.

Related to this pathophysiological construct is the concept of organ injury. It is common to see myocardial injury in the form of troponin release or acute kidney injury in the setting of AHF. Whether such organ injury contributes to the AHF episode, results from it, or both has not been definitively established.[14] What is clear is the association of organ injury with worse outcomes.[15,16] **Fig. 36.6** graphically demonstrates this concept, as well as the idea that prevention of such injury may alter the patient's outcome. This concept gained momentum in the RELAX-AHF-1 (Serelaxin, recombinant human relaxin-2, for treatment of acute heart failure) trial, where marked and congruent differences in biomarkers were observed, suggesting such prevention of injury may have resulted in improved 180-day mortality.[17,18] Unfortunately, the mortality benefits were not replicated in a confirmatory trial.[19]

Ultimately, to what extent and severity each of these overlapping pathways contributes to AHF, remains to be defined. We do not yet know what exactly to target in each patient that will result in improved outcomes. We do know that certain pathologic conditions—such as elevated left ventricular end diastolic filling pressures—are a hallmark of AHF and associated with worse outcomes. However, acutely improving hemodynamics has yet to result in less

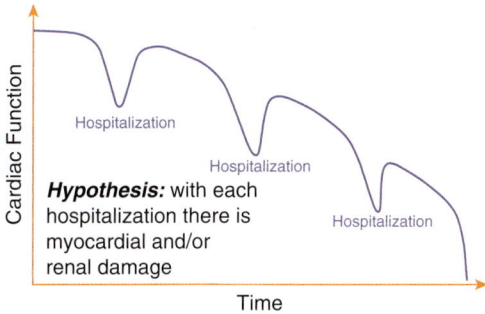

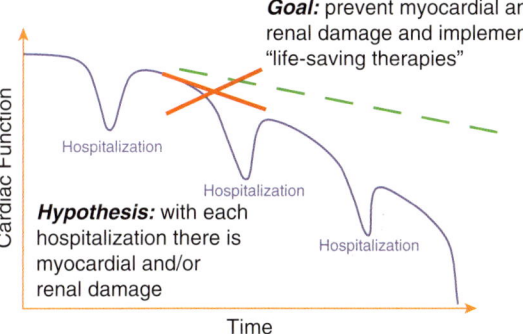

Fig. 36.6 (A) Contribution of each hospitalization to the progression of heart failure. (B) Potential impact of halting organ injury during an acute heart failure hospitalization. (Modified from Gheorghiade M, De Luca L, Fonarow GC, et al. Pathophysiologic targets in the early phase of acute heart failure syndromes. *Am J Cardiol.* 2005;96[6A]:11G–17G.)

morbidity or mortality.[20] At present, identifying markers associated with worse outcomes has yet to translate into targets for therapy.

Comorbid Conditions

The presence of comorbid conditions adds another layer of complexity to the AHF presentation. The "pure" AHF phenotype, however defined, is rare. Rather, the patient with other underlying medical comorbid conditions (i.e., hypertension, chronic obstructive pulmonary disease, diabetes, ischemic heart disease; **see also Chapter 48**) and social determinants of health (i.e., insurance status, caregiver support, adequate nutrition, lack of housing) is by far the norm. Whether these conditions contribute to AHF or are worsened by AHF is not always clear. During both initial and inpatient management, each potential comorbid condition must be accounted for, as described later.

It is doubtful a single, universal construct exists to encompass the entire pathophysiology of AHF. Although patients present with similar signs and symptoms, their underlying biology is unique. Perhaps this desire to lump all of AHF phenotypes together, rather than divide, has contributed to our limited ability to improve outcomes.

INITIAL MANAGEMENT

Despite the heterogeneity of the AHF patient, general principles of initial management may be applied and are outlined as follows. Prompt diagnosis, initial decongestive management, as well as management of comorbid conditions, and robust transitional care—followed by guideline adherent disease management—form the foundation of AHF care.

Previously proposed classifications of AHF patients to facilitate initial management categorize patients once; we recommend reassessment and reclassification during the entire course of a patients' hospital stay. Such reassessments recognize the dynamic nature of AHF.

TABLE 36.1 Approach to the Acute Heart Failure Patient in the Emergency Department
1. Is emergent action necessary?
2. Am I certain of the diagnosis? Diagnosis and treatment commonly occur in parallel, unlike the classic teaching of a history, followed by physical examination, followed by orders for ancillary testing, initial differential, revised differential based on test results, then treatment.
3. What is the underlying cause of the current episode of AHF?
4. What is the patient's volume status? Is it primarily volume overload or volume re-distribution? (Based on initial assessment, begin treatment)
5. Has the patient responded to initial treatment?
6. Have I addressed the precipitant or the reason why the patient went into AHF?
7. After reassessment of the patient, do they need hospitalization?

AHF, Acute heart failure.

Emergency Department Management

The majority of hospitalized AHF patients initially present to the emergency department (ED). The traditional axiom of airway, breathing, circulation (ABCs) applies; however, most patients do not present in extremis. The two polar archetypes are the flash pulmonary edema patient, typically due to hypertension, and the cardiogenic shock patient. After ensuring the ABCs, elucidating and managing the precipitant is paramount—for example, AHF secondary to a massive myocardial infarction (MI) or valve rupture. Although such presentations are not common, this principle of management applies to even less urgent cases. **Table 36.1** approaches the AHF patient in the ED as a series of clinical questions. **Fig. 36.7** shows an algorithmic approach toward the AHF patient in the ED or clinic setting.

Diagnosis

Delays in diagnosis and subsequent treatment are associated with worse outcomes.[21-23] Patients rarely present with a diagnosis, however; rather, they present with a "chief complaint." Thus determining whether the patient's reported "shortness of breath" is due to AHF or an alternative diagnosis relies on history and physical examination, combined with ancillary studies (**see also Chapter 31**). Unfortunately, the history and physical exam lack sensitivity. Paroxysmal nocturnal dyspnea and orthopnea should be assessed, but they lack specificity.[24] An S3 gallop (remarkably challenging to hear in a busy ED) and jugular venous distention are the most specific, but insensitive and clinician dependent.[24] Despite congestion being the *sine qua non* of AHF, measuring congestion reliably, with robust intra- and interobserver agreement, is challenging.[25,26] Nevertheless, a thorough history (especially a past history of HF) and physical exam, combined with traditional ancillary studies of chest x-ray, EKG, basic metabolic profile, and complete blood count, are recommended.

Chest X-Ray and Lung Ultrasound

One of the greatest clinical benefits of the chest x-ray (CXR) is identifying alternative diagnoses; the sensitivity and specificity are less than 80% for the diagnosis of AHF.[27] The imaging modality recommended at the bedside is lung ultrasound (**Fig. 36.8**). More than any other test, including natriuretic peptides (NPs), lung ultrasound (LUS) has the most robust likelihood ratio (LR) + 7.4 (95% CI 4.2–12.8) and LR − 0.16 [95% CI 0.05–0.51]), to aid in diagnosis. Sonographic detection of pulmonary edema is represented by B-lines, discrete artifacts resulting from the reverberation of sound waves off of fluid-filled pulmonary interstitium. In the

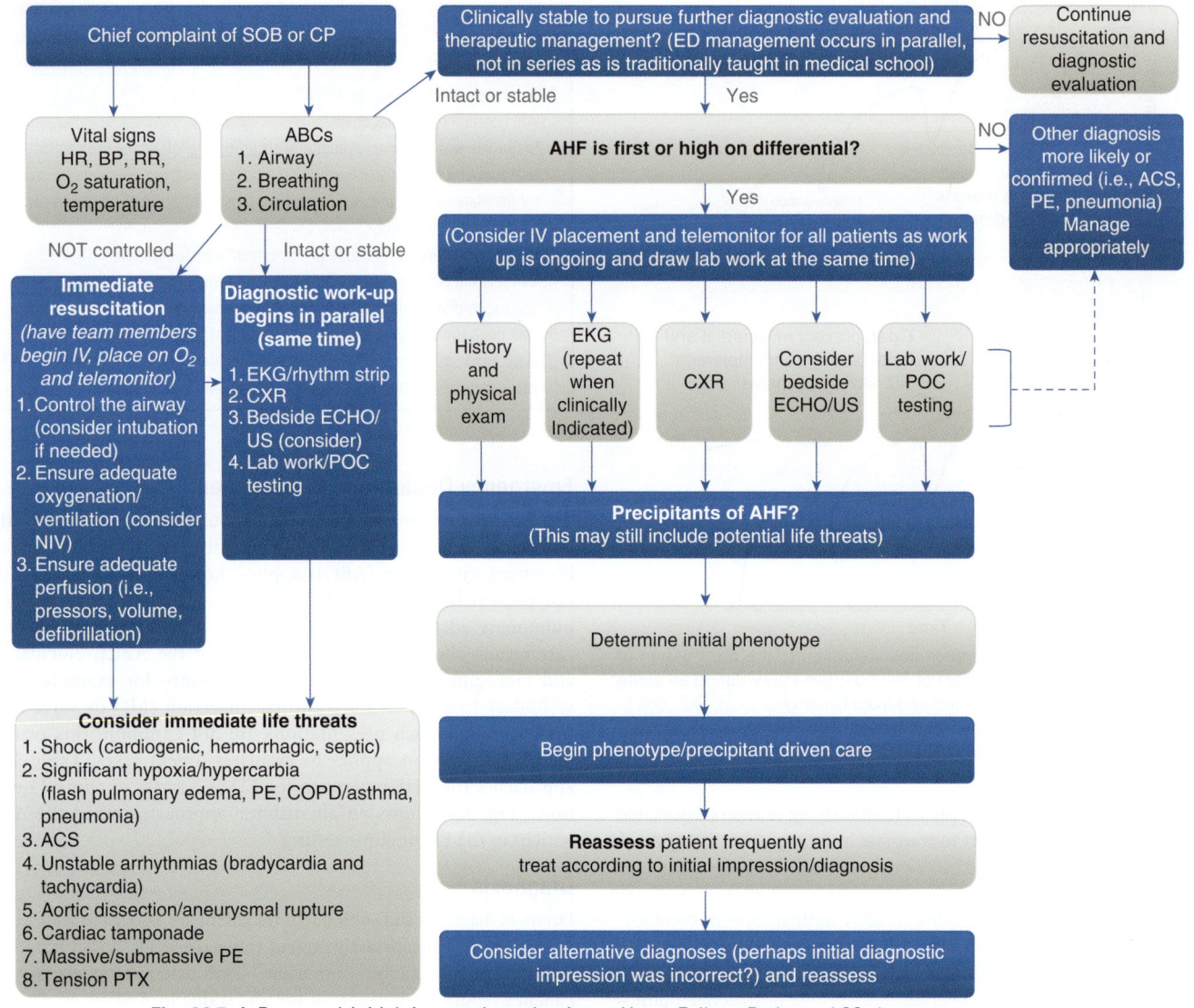

Fig. 36.7 A Proposed Initial Approach to the Acute Heart Failure Patient. *ACS,* Acute coronary syndrome; *AHF,* acute heart failure; *BP,* blood pressure; *COPD,* chronic obstructive pulmonary disease; *CP,* cor pulmonale; *CXR,* chest X-ray; *ECHO,* echocardiogram; *ED,* emergency department; *EKG,* electrocardiogram; *HR,* heart rate; *IV,* intravenous; *NIV,* noninvasive ventilation; *PE,* pulmonary embolism; *POC,* point-of-care; *PTX,* pneumothorax; *RR,* respiratory rate; *SOB,* shortness of breath; *US,* ultrasound. (From Pang PS, Collins SP, Miró Ò, et al. Editor's choice-the role of the emergency department in the management of acute heart failure: an international perspective on education and research. *Eur Heart J Acute Cardiovasc Care.* 2017;6[5]:421–429.)

proper clinical setting, B-lines represent pulmonary edema. The most recent European Society of Cardiology (ESC) guidelines now include LUS as an adjunct to diagnosis.[28]

Focused Ultrasound

Formal echocardiography is rarely done in the United States in the ED setting. This does not obviate its value. For patients with worsening HF, reassessment of myocardial structure and function is recommended,[12] especially if a clear etiology or precipitant is not identified. While point-of-care ultrasound does not replace formal echocardiography, point-of-care ultrasound or FoCUS (focused ultrasound) is often performed by noncardiologists at the bedside. This rapid approach is recommended by cardiology and noncardiology societies.[29,30] For

example, qualitative assessments of right and left ventricular function, identification of tamponade, and hypovolemia may be critical to aid in the management of the shock patient.[29,30] The European Association of Cardiovascular Imaging outlines three broad frameworks for emergency FoCUS echocardiography: (1) diagnostic, (2) symptom or sign based, and (3) resuscitative.[30] However, FoCUS does not replace formal echocardiography.

Natriuretic Peptides and Troponin (see also Chapter 33)

NPs facilitate diagnosis.[13] In addition, NPs are excellent discriminators of risk (i.e., prognosis). Despite their value and guideline recommendation, recent meta-analysis suggests their greatest value is in excluding AHF. While very high values help rule in AHF, intermediate values

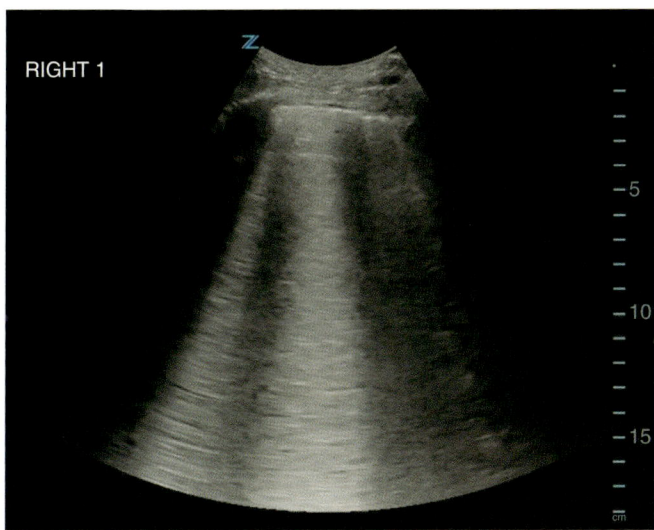

Fig. 36.8 Representation of B-lines by Lung Ultrasound.

have less diagnostic discrimination. Using thresholds of 100 pg/mL for BNP and 300 pg/mL NTproBNP, a low value significantly reduces the posttest probability of AHF (LR = 0.1).[24]

Guidelines also recommend troponin testing in AHF.[31,32] Not only does this aid in identification of occult MI, troponin discriminates higher risk patients.[14-16] With the advent of higher sensitivity assays, the proportion of AHF patients with evidence of myocardial injury outside of ACS exceeds 90%.[16]

Initial Classification

Once the diagnosis of AHF has been made, the algorithm (**Fig. 36.9**) outlined by the European Society of Cardiology outlines a pragmatic approach to initial classification and management of the AHF patient. The vast majority of patients present as "Wet and Warm," based on the hemodynamic profiles established by Nohria and Stevenson (**Fig. 36.10**).[33,34] Thus most AHF management algorithms predominantly focus on this category. While the "Wet and Cold" patient is only a small fraction of AHF presentations, these are the most challenging to manage. In the classification scheme presented as follows, specific doses and types of medications are not discussed, as they will be reviewed in greater detail later in this chapter.

Warm and Wet—Vascular Type

As highlighted in Fig. 36.9, elevated systolic blood pressure is common. Contemporary registries, such as Get With The Guidelines HF and EurObservational, note mean systolic blood pressure (SBP) of 140 and 133 mm Hg, respectively.[31,32] These patients benefit from both vasodilators and IV loop diuretic therapy. The flash pulmonary edema patient represents the prototypical AHF patient with elevated blood pressure. Such patients present in extremis, sitting bolt upright (tripod position), gasping, with systolic blood pressures commonly above 180 mm Hg. Jugular venous distention, diffuse crackles, and minimal to no lower extremity edema are common findings. Rapid noninvasive ventilation (assuming an appropriate mental status), sublingual nitrates followed by IV vasodilators, and a small dose of IV loop diuretics often results in dramatic improvement.

Warm and Wet—Cardiac Type

This presentation is best represented by the patient with a history of HFrEF who slowly worsens over time. Gradual weight gain, progressive peripheral edema, and worsening dyspnea on exertion are common

historical features. Such patients demonstrate more total volume overload instead of the volume redistribution seen in the vascular type presentation. For such patients, aggressive decongestion, starting with IV loop diuretics, are recommended. Such patients might also benefit from vasodilatation.

Cold and Wet

Advanced HF patients—defined as those with persistent signs and symptoms of HF despite maximal guideline directed therapy—may have a low (<90 mm Hg) systolic blood pressure at baseline with narrow pulse pressures (<25% of the systolic blood pressure). For clinicians who do not routinely care for advanced HF patients, this presentation can be quite alarming. Furthermore, assessing volume status is challenging given the chronic state of congestion; this challenge is compounded when the physician has never seen the patient before and who presents for a perceived or true emergency. Finally, treatment is not benign! Inotropes or inodilators are associated with worse longer-term outcomes.[12,13,35] Thus "treating a number" (i.e., low SBP that is baseline and sufficient for organ perfusion) is not recommended. In this setting, we propose the following clinical question to guide next steps: Is immediate and emergent action needed or is there some time to ascertain what is baseline? In the former case, all emergent actions should be undertaken (**see also Chapter 45**). If emergent action is not necessary, urgent evaluation is critical. This should focus on volume status and potential precipitants of decompensation, including worsening HF.

Emergency Department Risk Stratification

After initial stabilization and management, the conclusion of the ED phase of management is disposition (what happens to the patient next?). In the United States, more than 80% of AHF patients who present to the ED are hospitalized.[36] However, retrospective data suggest up to 50% of patients might be discharged or observed for a brief period of time.[37] Given the high financial costs of hospitalizations, the impact of hospitalization itself on patients (i.e., safety, deconditioning), identifying patients safe for discharge would be of tremendous value to both patients and the health care system.[38,39]

Most risk scores are designed to identify higher risk patients, allowing clinicians and health care systems to focus limited resources to those in greatest need. However, for the ED, high-risk is not the primary concern; those patients are hospitalized. Rather, it is identifying patients safe to go home, despite the high postdischarge morbidity and mortality. Several ED-based risk instruments show promise, yet none are quite ready for universal use.[40-42] One example is the use of high-sensitive troponin assays; absence of myocardial injury may identify a lower risk cohort.[16] A biomarker approach to risk-stratification, a risk-score, or a combined approach will eventually be realized; for the time being, we recommend the absence of high-risk features as an initial approach. However, the complexity of HF patients (i.e., polypharmacy, social determinants of health, multiple comorbidities) often overwhelms the compressed time frame of ED management (on average 4–6 hours, usually less). Use of observation status or an observation unit as a "bridge" may be more realistic then direct discharge.[38,39] Given the high proportion of patients currently hospitalized, expecting patients to be sent home may be impractical; using observation to first demonstrate that hospitalization is not necessary for lower risk patients may ultimately lead to more directly discharges.[39] **Fig. 36.11** is one proposed algorithm to aid in disposition decision-making.

using measurements of volume status such as body weight and fluid balance. Hence, diuretic resistance has been defined as the weight loss per unit of 40 mg furosemide or equivalent, or as the net fluid loss per milligram of loop diuretic or as the ratio of urinary sodium to urinary furosemide.[68] Measurements such as body weight and urinary output allow, however, only a rough estimate of the change in the volume status. A spot urine sample collected 1 to 2 hours after loop diuretic administration has been recently used to predict the natriuretic response at 6 hours and diuretic resistance. In the following days, however, urine may tend to become more hypotonic during hospitalization.

Independent of how diuretic response is measured, diuretic resistance is a major challenge of AHF management. It is caused by multiple mechanisms whose contribution may vary from patient to patient (**Table 36.5**). Hemodynamic factors, associated with congestion, have a pivotal role. Thus diuretic resistance begets itself through persistent congestion and may ultimately lead to refractory kidney failure and death, if not counteracted on time.

Increased sodium reabsorption at the tubular level, rather than reduced glomerular filtration rate, may be the main determinant of diuretic resistance.[70] When diuretic response is inadequate and the patient has persistent symptoms and signs of congestion, the initial intravenous dose of loop diuretic may be doubled. If the diuretic response remains inadequate, concomitant administration of other diuretics acting at different sites of action, such as thiazides or metolazone, is indicated.[68,69,71] A proposed pharmacologic approach to the problem of diuretic resistance is shown in **Table 36.6**.

Nonloop Diuretics and Aquaretics

Thiazide and thiazide-like diuretics block the sodium chloride cotransporter in the distal convoluted tubule. Thus they may, at least partially, counteract the increased sodium reabsorption associated with chronic loop diuretic use.[67,69] The thiazide-like diuretics, metolazone and chlorthalidone, have a slower gastrointestinal absorption and a longer half-life, compared with thiazides. They all induce a significant potassium excretion; their administration is associated with an increased risk of hypokalemia, hyponatremia, and renal dysfunction.

TABLE 36.4 Echocardiographic Estimates of Ventricular Filling Pressures

Hemodynamic Parameter	Echocardiographic Measurement
Left atrial pressure	
Normal or low	• E/A ratio <0.8
	• E/e′ <8
• Increased	• E/A ratio ≥2
	• Deceleration half-time <160 msec
	• E/e′ >14
	• Increased systolic pulmonary artery pressure estimated by continuous wave Doppler tricuspid regurgitation systolic jet velocity
Right atrial pressure	
Normal or low	• Inferior vena cava (IVC) diameter <2.1 cm that collapses >50% with a sudden inspiratory maneuver (i.e., sniff)
	• IVC ≤12 mm (in patients with positive pressure ventilation in whom degree of IVC collapse cannot be used)
	• Systolic predominance of hepatic vein flow pattern
Increased	• IVC diameter >2.1 cm that collapses <50% with a sniff
	• Lost systolic predominance of hepatic vein flow

Modified from Harjola VP, Parissis J, Brunner-La Rocca HP, et al. Comprehensive in-hospital monitoring in acute heart failure: applications for clinical practice and future directions for research. A statement from the Acute Heart Failure Committee of the Heart Failure Association [HFA] of the European Society of Cardiology [ESC]. *Eur J Heart Fail.* 2018;20[7]:1081–1099.

TABLE 36.5 Causes of Diuretic Resistance in Acute Heart Failure

Pharmacokinetic factors[59]
- Slow diuretic absorption caused by gut edema
- Impaired excretion of the diuretic into the tubular lumen
  - Chronic kidney disease
  - Drugs (e.g., nonsteroidal antiinflammatory drugs)

Hemodynamic factors
- Increased renal venous pressure[63]
- Increased intra-abdominal pressure[114]
- Kidney hypoperfusion

Neurohormonal activation
- Reduced glomerular perfusion pressure
- Proximal and distal tubule hyperfunction
  - Renin-angiotensin system
  - Sympathetic nervous system
  - Vasopressin

Nephron remodeling[115]
- Distal tubule hypertrophy

See references 59, 67–69.

TABLE 36.6 Stepped Care Pharmacologic Approach

Level	Previous Oral Furosemide Dose[a]	Bolus + Infusion Rate	Metolazone[b]
1	≤80 mg	40 mg + 5mg/hr	No
2	81–160 mg	80 mg + 10 mg/hr	5 mg daily
3	161–240 mg	80 mg + 20 mg/hr	5 mg BID
4	>240 mg	80 mg + 30 mg/hr	5 mg BID

[a]A dose of 40 mg of furosemide is considered equivalent to 1 mg bumetanide or 20 mg torsemide.
[b]Chlorthalidone or hydrochlorothiazide may be administered alternatively.
Goal of treatment is a urine output of 3–5 L daily until the achievement of euvolemia. Moving to a further level is indicated when daily urine output is less than 3 L/day. At 48 hours, the addition of intravenous inotropes or vasodilators or mechanical support may be indicated. Alternatively, the administration of 2.5 times the previous oral daily dose of furosemide may be divided into two equal doses per day.[60]
Modified from Ellison DH, Felker GM. Diuretic treatment in heart failure. *N Engl J Med.* 2017;377[20]:1964–1975; and Bart BA, Goldsmith SR, Lee KL, et al. Ultrafiltration in decompensated heart failure with cardiorenal syndrome. *N Engl J Med.* 2012;367[24]:2296–2304.

Metolazone is generally preferred, as it remains effective in patients with a low glomerular filtration rate. However, recent data suggest other nonloop diuretics may also be effective in patients with renal dysfunction.[72]

When used at high doses, mineralocorticoid receptor antagonists (MRA) have natriuretic effects. They may also counteract the contribution of increased aldosterone secretion as a cause of diuretic resistance and hypokalemia. The Aldosterone Targeted Neurohormonal Combined with Natriuresis Therapy in Heart Failure (ATHENA-HF) trial compared the efficacy and safety of high dose spironolactone, 100 mg daily, versus placebo or spironolactone 25 mg daily, in 360 patients with AHF. Though well tolerated, the high-dose MRA regimen had no favorable effects on either the primary efficacy endpoint (NT-proBNP plasma levels) or any secondary endpoints, including symptoms' relief, signs of congestion, weight changes, worsening HF, and 30-day mortality.[73] Despite these results, combined administration of spironolactone may still be considered in patients who are resistant to loop diuretics and/or to counteract hypokalemia.[28,69]

The carbonic anhydrase inhibitor acetazolamide inhibits sodium reabsorption in the proximal tubules. The proximal tubule reabsorbs 65% to 70% of tubular sodium. The increased chloride delivery to the macula densa, following acetazolamide administration, may inhibit renin secretion. Small preliminary studies suggested beneficial effects by the coadministration of acetazolamide to patients with AHF. The Acetazolamide in Patients with Decompensated Heart Failure and Volume Overload (ADVOR) trial is a multicenter, randomized, double-blind trial that will evaluate the efficacy of combined acetazolamide administration to patients with AHF (ClinicalTrials.gov Identifier: NCT03505788).

Vasopressin secretion is activated in AHF leading to free water retention and hyponatremia. The efficacy of tolvaptan, a selective V2-receptor antagonist, was tested in the Efficacy of Vasopressin Antagonism in HF Outcome Study with Tolvaptan (EVEREST). Tolvaptan was associated with an improvement in some signs and symptoms of congestion in the absence of a change in global clinical status and long-term outcomes.[74,75] In another recent trial, the early addition of tolvaptan to a standardized furosemide regimen in patients with AHF and fluid overload did not improve symptoms or need of rescue therapy, compared with placebo, despite greater body weight and fluid loss.[76] Similar results were obtained in another trial enrolling patients with AHF with concomitant renal dysfunction or hyponatremia or diuretic resistance.[77] Vasopressin antagonist may, however, still be indicated in patients with fluid overload and severe hyponatremia.[13]

Ultrafiltration

Ultrafiltration removes plasma water from whole blood across a semipermeable membrane in response to a pressure gradient. Different from loop diuretics, which produce hypotonic urine, the fluid removed by ultrafiltration is isotonic with plasma. Thus a relatively larger amount of sodium is removed with ultrafiltration, compared with loop diuretics.[78] Despite initial favorable results, the largest trial to date, the Cardio-Renal Rescue Study in Acute Decompensated Heart Failure (CARRESS-HF), failed to show efficacy over an intense pharmacological regimen.[71] In this trial, 188 patients with AHF and worsening renal function were randomized to ultrafiltration, at a fixed rate of 200 mL/hr, versus a stepped care regimen of pharmacologic therapy. The reduction in body weight was similar with ultrafiltration, compared with pharmacological treatment, though with higher serum creatinine values at 96 hours and with more side effects.[71] The interpretation of the results is, however, complicated by the relatively high crossover rate. In a subsequent per protocol analysis, ultrafiltration was associated with greater fluid loss compared with pharmacologic

therapy.[79] Another trial comparing ultrafiltration with standard therapy was prematurely stopped for slow enrollment.[80] Another trial, the Peripheral Ultrafiltration for the Relief from Congestion in Heart Failure (PURE-HF), is ongoing (ClinicalTrials.gov Identifier: NCT03161158). In the current guidelines, ultrafiltration is indicated when diuretic strategies are unsuccessful.[13,28]

Vasodilators

A summary of commonly used vasoactive medications in the setting of AHF is shown in **Table 36.7**. Intravenous vasodilators are the second most frequently used drugs for the treatment of AHF.[81] They are indicated for symptomatic treatment when systolic blood pressure is greater than 110 mm Hg. Although high doses have been used in hypertensive patients,[82] they should generally be started at low doses and titrated to effect. Caution should be taken to avoid hypotension, and extreme caution must be adopted in patients with valve stenosis.

The rationale for the administration of vasodilators is twofold: one, to reduce excessive left ventricular afterload and mitral regurgitation, when present (arterial vasodilation); and two, to decrease excessive preload caused by the increase in venous return. This second mechanism may be particularly important in patients where the main cause of acute decompensation is not fluid retention but redistribution from the splanchnic venous bed capacitance to the IVC and the central circulation.[83-85] Physiologically, splanchnic capacitance veins act as a blood reservoir to maintain a stable cardiac preload. Up to 27% of total blood volume can be mobilized from the splanchnic venous bed by sympathetic stimulation.[86] Because of the peculiar distribution of the adrenergic receptors in the splanchnic bed, sympathetic stimulation causes α-receptors–mediated vasoconstriction of splanchnic capacitance veins with concomitant β_2-adrenergic receptors–mediated vasodilation of the hepatic veins, and may therefore squeeze blood into the central circulation with an effect that has been compared with that of an autotransfusion from the splanchnic capacitance veins.[85]

Nitrates

Sodium nitroprusside, nitroglycerin, and the other nitrates act as an exogenous source of nitric oxide (NO) that binds to soluble guanylate cyclase (sGC), producing cyclic GMP (cGMP) and vascular smooth muscle relaxation. At low doses, nitrates act predominantly on the venous circulation, resulting in increased venous capacitance and reduced systemic preload. At higher doses they dilate arteries, including the coronary arteries, and decrease left ventricular afterload. Sodium nitroprusside has more balanced effects on the arterial and venous systems and is therefore effective in patients with concomitant arterial hypertension and mitral regurgitation. Careful hemodynamic monitoring is warranted.[58]

Nitrates are currently recommended in the ESC and American College of Cardiology and American Hospital Association (ACC/AHA) guidelines.[13,28] A much more restrictive approach, however, is advanced by the UK National Institute for Health and Care Excellence, based on the minimal evidence of their efficacy.[87] Small trials showed a benefit of a strategy based on nitrates and small doses of furosemide versus the use of high doses of furosemide.[82] A Cochrane meta-analysis issued in 2013 found only four controlled studies eligible for inclusion; the authors concluded that "there is a lack of data to draw any firm conclusions concerning the use of nitrates in AHF because current evidence is based on few low-quality studies."[88] Another systematic literature review, including 35 of 2001 published studies, concluded intravenous nitrovasodilators improve short-term symptoms and are safe, though no data suggest an effect on mortality.[89] A more recent analysis, conducted using propensity matching in a prospective, multicenter cohort, failed to show any improvements in patients receiving

TABLE 36.7   Intravenous Vasoactive Agents for Treatment of Acute Heart Failure

Intravenous Medication	Initial Dose	Effective Dose Range	Comments (including potential adverse effects)
Vasodilators			
Nitroglycerin; glyceryl trinitrate	20 µg/min	40–400 µg/min	Hypotension, headache Tolerance with continuous use after 24 hr
Isosorbide dinitrate	1 mg/hr	2–10 mg/hr	Hypotension, headache Tolerance with continuous use within 24 hr
Nitroprusside	0.3 µg/kg/min	0.3–5 µg/kg/min (usually <4 µg/kg/min)	Caution in patients with active myocardial ischemia Hypotension; cyanide side effects (nausea, dysphoria); thiocyanate toxicity; light sensitive
Nesiritide[a]	2 µg/kg bolus with 0.010–0.030 µg/kg/min infusion[b]	0.010–0.030 µg/kg/min[c]	Uptitration: 1 µg/kg bolus, then increase infusion rate by 0.005 µg/kg/min no more frequently than every 3 hr, up to maximum of 0.03 µg/kg/min Hypotension, headache (less than with organic nitrates)
Inotropes			
Dobutamine	1–2 µg/kg/min	2–20 µg/kg/min	For inotropy and vasodilation; hypotension, tachycardia, arrhythmias are potential AE, potential increased risk of death; ?mortality
Dopamine	1–2 µg/kg/min	2–4 µg/kg/min	For inotropy and vasodilation; hypotension, tachycardia, arrhythmias; ?mortality
	4–5 µg/kg/min	5–20 µg/kg/min	For inotropy and vasoconstriction; tachycardia, arrhythmias; ?mortality
Milrinone	25–75 µg/kg bolus over 10–20 min[b] followed by infusion	0.10–0.75 µg/kg/min	For vasodilation and inotropy; hypotension, tachycardia, arrhythmias; renal excretion; ?mortality
Enoximone[a]	0.25–0.75 mg/kg	1.25–7.5 µg/kg/min	For vasodilation and inotropy; hypotension, tachycardia, arrhythmias; ?mortality
Levosimendan[a]	12–24 µg/kg bolus over 10 min followed by infusion	0.1–0.2 µg/kg/min	For vasodilation and inotropy; active metabolite present for ~84 hr; hypotension, tachycardia, arrhythmias; ?mortality
Epinephrine		0.05–0.5 µg/kg/min	For vasoconstriction and inotropy; tachycardia, arrhythmias, end-organ hypoperfusion; ?mortality
Norepinephrine		0.2–1.0 µg/kg/min	For vasoconstriction and inotropy; tachycardia, arrhythmias, end-organ hypoperfusion; ?mortality

[a]Not approved for use in all countries.
[b]Some clinicians do not administer a bolus dose, to decrease the risk of hypotension. Bolus not recommended in patients with hypotension.
[c]Lower doses have also been effective in some small studies.
AE, Adverse effect; *?mortality,* these agents have been associated with an increased risk of death.
From Felker GM, Teerlink JR. Diagnosis and management of acute heart failure. In Zipes DP, et al., eds. *Braunwald's Heart Disease.* 11th ed. Philadelphia, PA: Elsevier; 2019.

nitrates in regards to multiple endpoints, including mortality.[90] The Goal-Directed Afterload Reduction in Acute Congestive Cardiac Decompensation Study (GALACTIC; NCT00512759) is a 770-patient trial testing the hypothesis that early treatment with nitrates and hydralazine to a target systolic blood pressure of 90 to 110 mm Hg can improve outcomes and be safe in patients with AHF.

Nesiritide

In addition to nitrates and sodium nitroprusside, nesiritide is another vasodilator to be considered in patients with AHF.[13] It is available in the United States but only a minority of European countries. It is a recombinant form of human BNP, acting as a balanced arterial and venous vasodilator when infused intravenously. In the VMAC (Vasodilation in the Management of Acute Congestive Heart Failure) trial, nesiritide caused a larger and more persistent reduction of the pulmonary artery wedge pressure than nitrates and slightly improved dyspnea relief versus placebo.[91] It was then tested versus placebo in the large multicenter trial ASCEND-HF (Acute Study of Clinical Effectiveness of Nesiritide in Decompensated Heart Failure), aimed at the assessment of its safety and efficacy on short- and long-term outcomes.[92] The trial showed nesiritide safety and slight efficacy on dyspnea relief at 6 and 24 hours, although this improvement did not meet the prespecified statistical significance. There was no difference between nesiritide and placebo in the coprimary endpoint of 30-day mortality or HF hospitalization.[92] Lastly, low-dose nesiritide failed to improve diuresis, renal function,

and outcomes, compared with placebo, in the Renal Optimization Strategies Evaluation (ROSE) trial.[93]

Recent Agents Tested in Acute Heart Failure Clinical Trials

Given the limited evidence base of traditional therapies, combined with high postdischarge event rates, multiple novel agents have been tested in AHF. We highlight three of the most recent AHF trials.

Serelaxin is recombinant human relaxin-2, present in both sexes, contributing to many of cardiovascular and renal function changes observed during pregnancy. It has vasodilatory and antifibrotic, antiinflammatory, antiapoptotic, and organ protective effects, potentially useful for the treatment of AHF. Compared with placebo, it had favorable effects on signs of congestion, in-hospital worsening HF, and mortality in two trials, enrolling 234 and 1161 patients, respectively.[17,18,94] Based on these data, the larger serelaxin in AHF-2 (RELAX-AHF-2) trial, powered to detect a significant effect on mortality with the inclusion of 6800 patients, was designed.[19] The trial failed to show any effect of serelaxin on cardiovascular mortality as well as in-hospital worsening HF, the second coprimary endpoint, which was reduced numerically by 11% ($P = .19$).

Ularitide is the synthetic form of urodilatin, a peptide formed via alternative splicing of atrial natriuretic peptide (ANP) with four additional amino acids at its N-terminal extension. It is synthesized in the distal renal tubular cells. It stimulates guanylate cyclase activity and increases cGMP levels similarly to nitrates and nesiritide. Compared with nesiritide, it has been associated with a greater activity on the renal tubular cells with natriuretic and diuretic effects.[81,95] After small, promising studies, ularitide was tested in the large randomized, double-blind Phase III Trial of Ularitide's Efficacy and Safety in Patients with Acute Heart Failure (TRUE-AHF) enrolling 2157 patients with AHF. Pharmacologic activity was shown by the decrease in blood pressure and plasma NT-proBNP levels with ularitide versus placebo. However, ularitide had no significant effects on the two coprimary endpoints: (1) cardiovascular death, during a median follow-up of 15 months, and (2) a hierarchical composite endpoint that evaluated the initial 48-hour clinical course. A post hoc analysis excluding patients identified before the database lock as ineligible for the trial showed a benefit of ularitide with respect of the hierarchical clinical composite outcome ($P = .03$).[96]

A β-arrestin-biased angiotensin II type 1 receptor blocker, TRV120027, has failed to show efficacy versus placebo in a phase IIb clinical trial.[97] CXL-1427 is a second-generation nitroxyl (HNO) donor. In addition to vasodilatory effects mediated by increased cGMP and other mechanisms, it also has direct myocardial inotropic and lusitropic effects. It has been tested in a small hemodynamic study, and a phase IIB trial is ongoing (ClinicalTrials.gov Identifier: NCT03357731).[98]

Inotropic Agents

Administration of intravenous inotropic agents is indicated only for the treatment of patients with left ventricular systolic dysfunction and low cardiac output not caused by hypovolemia, along with peripheral and end-organ hypoperfusion. These patients commonly have low blood pressure, probably the best sign of low cardiac output in AHF, and may have congestion secondary to cardiac dysfunction ("cold and wet" patients). Inotropes are not indicated for general use; they may cause tachycardia, especially in patients with concomitant atrial fibrillation, tachyarrhythmias, myocardial ischemia, and increased mortality.[13,28]

Dobutamine

Dobutamine is the prototype of the traditional inotropic agents. It has high affinity for the β1-adrenergic receptors with mild β2-receptor and α1-adrenergic receptor agonist properties. β1-adrenergic receptors stimulation causes an increase in intracellular cyclic AMP concentration with secondary protein kinase activation, sarcolemma calcium channels opening, and sarcoplasmic reticulum calcium release. Calcium binding to troponin C removes the inhibitory effect of troponin I and allows actin myosin interaction and sarcomere contraction.

Dobutamine administration has beneficial short-term hemodynamic effects with an increase in cardiac output and decrease in pulmonary artery wedge pressure in patients with AHF. However, it also increases heart rate and atrioventricular node conduction velocity, with further tachycardia in patients with atrial fibrillation. Dependency on β1-adrenergic receptors density and activity is a major limitation of dobutamine. Its hemodynamic response can be blunted by concomitant β-blocker therapy and by β-adrenergic receptors downregulation. This may cause large interindividual variability in response to dobutamine. Tolerance development secondary to β1-receptors downregulation after prolonged exposure has been described after days of continuous dobutamine infusion.[99-102]

Dobutamine administration is associated with an increased risk of death. In the Flolan International Randomized Survival Trial (FIRST), a randomized, controlled trial of continuous intravenous epoprostenol plus conventional therapy versus conventional therapy alone, in patients with advanced HF, the trial was prematurely halted for a strong trend towards decreased survival in epoprostenol treated patients. Further analysis showed dobutamine infusion (mean dose 9 μg/kg/min, range 5–12 μg/kg/min, median duration 14 days) treated patients had higher rates of adverse events (worsening HF, need for vasoactive medications, resuscitated cardiac arrest, myocardial infarction, and total mortality, 85.3 vs. 64.5%; $P = .0006$) and a higher mortality (70.5

vs. 37.1%; $P = .0001$).[103] Further studies and a meta-analysis suggested an increased risk of death associated with dobutamine infusion.[104] It is, however, likely that this occurs mostly with prolonged infusions and/or the administration of relatively high doses (i.e., >5 μg/kg/min). Although this may be related to the lack of valid alternatives, dobutamine remains useful for the short-term treatment of patients with low cardiac output and peripheral hypoperfusion,[13,28] despite its limitations.

Dopamine

When administered at low doses (0.5–3 μg/kg/min), dopamine stimulates dopamine 1 and dopamine 2 receptors, resulting in splanchnic and renal vasodilation and an increase in renal blood flow. At higher doses (3–5 μg/kg/min), dopamine binds to β1-adrenergic receptors, increasing norepinephrine release from sympathetic nerve terminals with an increase in cardiac contractility and heart rate. At even higher doses (5–20 μg/kg/min), α1-adrenergic receptor mediated vasoconstriction dominates with an increase in peripheral vascular resistance.[102]

Low-doses of dopamine, so-called "renal doses," are often used to improve diuresis and renal blood flow in patients with AHF and renal dysfunction or at risk of it. In the ROSE trial, randomization to low-dose dopamine had no significant effect on 72-hour diuresis or on the change in renal function, measured by cystatin C levels, as well as other secondary endpoints related to decongestion, renal function, or clinical outcomes.[93]

Epinephrine and Norepinephrine

Epinephrine and norepinephrine are full agonists of the β- and α-adrenergic receptors. They increase cardiac contractility, heart rate, and peripheral vascular resistance. They also are associated with cardiac arrhythmias and ischemia. Significant additional inotropic and blood pressure support can be provided by these agents as a short-term life-saving intervention (see Table 36.7 for initial dosing). These agents may lead to renal or hepatic failure and gangrene through excessive vasoconstriction. Compared with norepinephrine, epinephrine has more affinity for type 2 β-adrenergic receptors, and thus is slightly less likely to cause adverse effects due to intense vasoconstriction. A threefold increase in mortality was, however, found with epinephrine administration, compared with other treatments, in a large meta-analysis.[105] A recent Cochrane database analysis of randomized controlled clinical trials comparing different strategies with inotropic agents or vasodilators for the treatment of low cardiac output syndrome or cardiogenic shock identified 13 studies with 2001 participants.[106] The authors concluded that, "at present, there are no robust and convincing data to support a distinct inotropic or vasodilator drug-based therapy as a superior solution to reduce mortality in haemodynamically unstable people with cardiogenic shock or low cardiac output syndrome" so that "there remains a great need for large, well-designed randomised trials on this topic."[106] In a recent prospective, double-blind, multicenter trial, 57 patients with postinfarction cardiogenic shock were randomized to epinephrine or norepinephrine. Changes in blood pressure and cardiac index were similar between the two groups. However, the incidence of refractory shock was higher with epinephrine versus norepinephrine (37% vs. 7%; $P = .008$), and other endpoints including heart rate and metabolic indexes were not favorably affected by epinephrine.[107]

Phosphodiesterase Inhibitors

Phosphodiesterase 3 inhibitors (PDE3-Is) increase cAMP level by inhibiting its breakdown within the cell. Thus their mechanisms of action and effects on cardiac function are similar to those of β1-AR agonists. PDE3-Is act, however, downstream from the β1-AR, and thus their actions are independent from β1-ARs density, but not from cAMP concentrations.[102] PDE-Is also have greater vasodilating activity, compared with dobutamine, mediated by direct effects of cAMP in the vascular smooth muscle cells. This vasodilatory activity may cause hypotension and worsen end-organ perfusion in patients who are already hypotensive at baseline and with low ventricular filling pressures.

In the Outcomes of a Prospective Trial of Intravenous Milrinone for Exacerbations of Chronic HF (OPTIME-CHF), the effects of a PDE-I, milrinone, were assessed with a prospective, double-blind, parallel group, randomized, placebo-controlled design in 951 patients with AHF.[35] No difference was found between the milrinone and placebo groups with respect to the total number of days hospitalized for cardiovascular causes, in-hospital mortality, 60-day mortality, or the composite incidence of death or readmission. However, patients on milrinone, compared with those on placebo, had more treatment failures caused by adverse events, as well as episodes of sustained hypotension requiring intervention (10.7% vs. 3.2%; $P < .001$) and new atrial arrhythmias (4.6% vs. 1.5%; $P = .004$).[35] A further analysis showed that milrinone may increase mortality in patients with concomitant coronary artery disease.[108]

A major limitation of OPTIME-HF, necessitated by the placebo-controlled trial design, patients required to receive inotropic therapy, such as those with shock, lactic acidosis or hypotension, were excluded from the study. Accordingly, patients randomized had a relatively high blood pressure (120/71 mm Hg), and few patients were on concomitant dobutamine therapy (9.3% on placebo vs. 11.5% on dobutamine).[35]

Levosimendan

Levosimendan has two main mechanisms of action: calcium sensitization of the contractile proteins, through enhanced Ca^{2+} binding by troponin C, and opening of ATP-dependent K^+ channels in the smooth muscle vascular cells causing arteriolar and venous dilation. No favorable effects on outcomes were shown with levosimendan compared with placebo or dobutamine, respectively, in large randomized trials. In the placebo-controlled trials, levosimendan was associated with an improvement in the composite clinical primary endpoint, with less episodes of worsening HF and a larger BNP decrease.[109] However, levosimendan was associated with more frequent hypotension (50% vs. 36%; ventricular tachycardia, 25% vs. 17%; and atrial fibrillation, 9% vs. 2%).[109] In the trial comparing levosimendan with dobutamine in 1327 patients with AHF, 180-days mortality was similar between the two study groups (26% with levosimendan vs. 28% with dobutamine, $P = .40$). BNP decrease was larger in the patients assigned to levosimendan and the rate of worsening HF was greater in the dobutamine group, whereas the rate of new onset atrial fibrillation was greater in the levosimendan group.[110]

Despite these disappointing results, it is possible the design and conduct of the trial may have influenced the results. Peripheral vasodilation and hypotension is a potential major limitation of levosimendan. An interaction was found between baseline blood pressure and the effects on mortality of levosimendan versus placebo, with an increased risk of death in patients with a baseline systolic blood pressure less than 100 to 105 mm Hg and vice versa.[109] Further, only patients with an insufficient response to diuretics and/or vasodilators were eligible and thus were on maximal doses of diuretics and/or vasodilators. This combined with a relatively high dose of levosimendan, 12 μg/kg IV, administered as a bolus before the continuous infusion at 0.1 μg/kg/min, could have favored the neutral results. A bolus dose of levosimendan is currently not commonly used in clinical practice. Intermittent administration of intravenous levosimendan has been tested in small randomized clinical trials with favorable results in NT-proBNP levels (primary endpoint), quality of life, and HF hospitalizations.[111]

Other Treatments in the Acute Phase

Thrombosis/thromboembolism prophylaxis, for example with low-molecular-weight heparin, is recommended for patients hospitalized with AHF who are not anticoagulated and with no contraindication to anticoagulation in order to reduce the risk of deep vein thrombosis and pulmonary embolism. It is the only recommendation for which there is a class I recommendation, as based on randomized clinical trials.[13,28] Cardioversion may be required when tachyarrhythmias are the cause of AHF. Control of a rapid ventricular rate may be required in patients with atrial fibrillation. Noninvasive positive pressure ventilation is recommended for patients in respiratory distress (for example, respiratory rate >25 breaths/min, SpO_2 <90%) who have an appropriate mental status. Given that it is noninvasive, it should be started as soon as possible to decrease respiratory distress.[28,88]

Evidence-Based Treatment and Predischarge Assessment

Treatment of the initial phase of AHF is based on therapies with little robust evidence. However, during the hospitalization for AHF, proven *chronic* HF evidence-based treatment should be maintained and implemented before discharge whenever possible. Inhibitors of the renin-angiotensin aldosterone system may be less tolerated during AHF due to hypotension and risk for worsening renal function and electrolyte disturbances. β-blockers may be less tolerated for hypotension as well, along with their acute negative inotropic effects. However, maintenance of these therapies during the AHF hospitalization may be associated with better outcomes, though these findings may be confounded by a less severe presenting condition.

Predischarge optimization of evidence-based therapies both with respect to their initiation and uptitration to target doses is associated with better postdischarge outcomes.[112,113] If not maintained during hospitalization, neurohormonal antagonists and, namely, β-blockers should be initiated at low doses, to be gradually titrated in the next days following discharge.[13]

Close postdischarge follow-up must be scheduled and multidisciplinary HF disease-management programs should be adopted, especially for patients at high risk for hospital readmission. Volume status should be closely monitored, ideally by both the physician and the care team.

CONCLUSION

The public health burden of AHF continues to grow, with an increasing prevalence worldwide and dismal postdischarge outcomes. Neither traditional therapies nor attempts at novel therapies definitively improve outcomes. At present, prompt diagnosis, decongestion, recognition and treatment of precipitants and comorbid conditions, along with frequent in-hospital assessment, followed by optimization of guideline directed chronic heart failure therapies predischarge are the mainstays of AHF management. Much more work is needed to improve outcomes for AHF patients.

KEY REFERENCES

2. Gheorghiade M, et al. Systolic blood pressure at admission, clinical characteristics, and outcomes in patients hospitalized with acute heart failure. *JAMA.* 2006;296(18):2217–2226.
20. Binanay C, et al. Evaluation study of congestive heart failure and pulmonary artery catheterization effectiveness: the ESCAPE trial. *JAMA.* 2005;294(13):1625–1633.

26. Gheorghiade M, et al. Assessing and grading congestion in acute heart failure: a scientific statement from the acute heart failure committee of the heart failure association of the European Society of Cardiology and endorsed by the European Society of Intensive Care Medicine. *Eur J Heart Fail*. 2010;12(5):423–433.

33. Nohria A, et al. Clinical assessment identifies hemodynamic profiles that predict outcomes in patients admitted with heart failure. *J Am Coll Cardiol*. 2003;41(10):1797–1804.

35. Cuffe MS, et al. Short-term intravenous milrinone for acute exacerbation of chronic heart failure: a randomized controlled trial. *JAMA*. 2002;287(12):1541–1547.

53. Testani JM, et al. Potential effects of aggressive decongestion during the treatment of decompensated heart failure on renal function and survival. *Circulation*. 2010;122(3):265–272.

60. Felker GM, et al. Diuretic strategies in patients with acute decompensated heart failure. *N Engl J Med*. 2011;364(9):797–805.

62. Metra M, et al. Is worsening renal function an ominous prognostic sign in patients with acute heart failure? The role of congestion and its interaction with renal function. *Circ Heart Fail*. 2012;5(1):54–62.

74. Gheorghiade M, et al. Short-term clinical effects of tolvaptan, an oral vasopressin antagonist, in patients hospitalized for heart failure: the EVEREST Clinical Status Trials. *JAMA*. 2007;297(12):1332–1343.

92. O'Connor CM, et al. Effect of nesiritide in patients with acute decompensated heart failure. *N Engl J Med*. 2011;365(1):32–43.

The full reference list for this chapter is available on ExpertConsult.

Guidelines
The Hospitalized Patient[a]

The most significant addition to the 2009 American College of Cardiology and American Hospital Association (ACC/AHA) updated guidelines was the inclusion of specific new recommendations regarding the hospitalized patient (**Table 36G.1**). Although there were a number of new class I indications involving the diagnosis of heart failure, the use of B-type natriuretic peptide and N-terminal pro-B natriuretic peptide (NT-proBNP), recognition of acute coronary syndromes, recognition of potential precipitating factors, use of supplemental oxygen, use of intravenous inotropic or pressure agents in patients with clinical evidence of hypotension with hypoperfusion, use of pulmonary artery catheters, and transition of intravenous to oral diuretics, the level of evidence supporting each of these recommendations was based on consensus opinion or standard use of care (i.e., level of evidence, C). Stronger class I recommendations (level of evidence, B) were provided for the use of intravenous diuretics to decongest patients, initiation of ACE inhibitors/ARBs, and β-blockers before hospital discharge, as well as the importance of postdischarge systems of care.

The updated guidelines offer qualified support (class IIa) for the use of urgent catheterization and revascularization, the use of vasodilators (intravenous nitroglycerin, nitroprusside, nesiritide), invasive hemodynamic monitoring, and ultrafiltration. More muted support (class IIb) was given for the use of inotropic agents (dopamine, dobutamine, or milrinone) in patients with severe left ventricular dysfunction, low blood pressure, and evidence of low cardiac output. In contrast, the use of inotropic agents in patients without evidence of decreased organ perfusion, as well as the routine use of invasive hemodynamic monitoring, was not recommended (class III indication).

---

[a] Felker GM, Teerlink JR. Guidelines: The Hospitalized Patient. In Zipes DP, et al, editors: *Braunwald's Heart Disease: A Textbook of Cardiovascular Medicine,* ed 11. Philadelphia, Elsevier, 2019.

TABLE 36G.1	ACC/AHA Recommendations for the Hospitalized Patient with Heart Failure	
Class	**Indication**	**Level of Evidence**[a]
I	Thorough history and physical examination to evaluate for adequacy of systemic perfusion, volume status, contribution of precipitating factors and/or comorbidities, and whether HF is associated with preserved ejection fraction	C
	Concentrations of B-type natriuretic peptide (BNP) or N-terminal pro-B-type natriuretic peptide (NT-proBNP) to evaluate dyspnea if the contribution of heart failure is not known	A
	Acute coronary syndrome should be promptly identified by electrocardiogram and cardiac troponin testing and treated as appropriate for the overall condition and prognosis of patient.	C
	Oxygen therapy should be administered to relieve symptoms related to hypoxemia.	C
	Improve systemic perfusion in patients who present with rapid decompensation and hypoperfusion associated with decreasing urine output and other manifestations of shock.	C
	Treatment of significant fluid overload with intravenous loop diuretics. The diuretic dose should be titrated to relieve symptoms and to reduce extracellular fluid volume excess.	B, C
	Monitor the effects of therapy with careful measurement of fluid intake and output, vital signs, body weight, and symptoms of systemic perfusion and congestion.	C
	Intensify the diuretic regiment when the diuresis is inadequate to relieve congestion.	C
	Intravenous inotropic or vasopressor drugs should be administered to maintain systemic perfusion and preserve end-organ performance in patients with clinical evidence of hypotension associated with hypoperfusion and elevated cardiac filling pressures.	C
	Invasive hemodynamic monitoring to guide therapy in patients who are in respiratory distress or with clinical evidence of impaired perfusion if filling pressures cannot be determined from clinical assessment	C
	Medications should be reconciled and adjusted as appropriate on admission to and discharge from the hospital.	C
	Maintenance treatment with oral therapies known to improve outcomes (ACE inhibitors or ARBs and β-blocker therapy) in the absence of hemodynamic instability or contraindications	C
	Initiation of treatment with oral therapies known to improve outcomes (ACE inhibitors or ARBs and β-blocker therapy) in stable patients prior to hospital discharge	B
	During transition from intravenous to oral diuretic therapy, patient should be monitored carefully for supine and upright hypotension, worsening renal function, and HF signs/symptoms.	C
	Comprehensive written discharge instructions for patients and their caregivers is strongly recommended.	C
	Postdischarge systems of care, if available, should be used to facilitate the transition to effective outpatient care.	B
IIa	Urgent cardiac catheterization and revascularization in patients with acute HF with known or suspected acute myocardial ischemia due to occlusive coronary disease when there are signs and symptoms of inadequate systemic perfusion and revascularization are likely to prolong meaningful survival.	C
	Intravenous nitroglycerin, nitroprusside, or nesiritide for patients with evidence of severely symptomatic fluid overload in the absence of systemic hypotension	C
	Ultrafiltration for patients with refractory congestion not responding to medical therapy	B
IIb	Intravenous inotropic drugs (dopamine, dobutamine, or milrinone) for patients presenting with documented severe systolic dysfunction, low blood pressure, and evidence of low cardiac output, with or without congestion, to maintain systemic perfusion and preserve end-organ performance	C
III	Use of parenteral inotropes in normotensive patients with acute decompensated HF without evidence of decreased organ perfusion.	B
	Routine use of invasive hemodynamic monitoring in normotensive patients with acute decompensated HF and congestion with symptomatic response to diuretics and vasodilators.	B

[a]See guidelines text for definition of level of evidence categories.

ACC, American College of Cardiology; *ACE*, angiotensin-converting enzyme; *AHA*, American Heart Association, *ARBs*, angiotensin receptor blockers; *HF*, heart failure.

Contemporary Medical Therapy for Heart Failure Patients with Reduced Ejection Fraction

Robert J. Mentz, G. Michael Felker

Heart failure (HF) is a complex clinical syndrome that represents a final common pathway for many types of cardiovascular disease. Multiple overlapping frameworks for classifying HF exist (**see also Chapters 18 and 31**). HF can be viewed as a continuum that is comprised of four interrelated stages as defined by the American College of Cardiology and the American Heart Association (ACC/AHA) Guidelines (**Fig. 37.1**).[1] Stage A patients represent the largest group, defined as patients who are at high risk for developing HF, but who do not yet have evidence of structural heart disease or symptoms of HF (e.g., patients with diabetes or hypertension; **see also Chapter 35**). Stage B includes patients who have structural heart disease, but without symptoms of HF (e.g., patients with a previous myocardial infarction [MI], left ventricular [LV] hypertrophy, or asymptomatic LV dysfunction). Stage C includes patients who have structural heart disease and have developed symptoms of HF. Stage D includes patients with refractory HF requiring special interventions (e.g., patients who may be candidates for advanced surgical therapies (LV assist devices or cardiac transplantation; **see also Chapters 44 and 45**) or palliative care and hospice (**see also Chapter 50**).

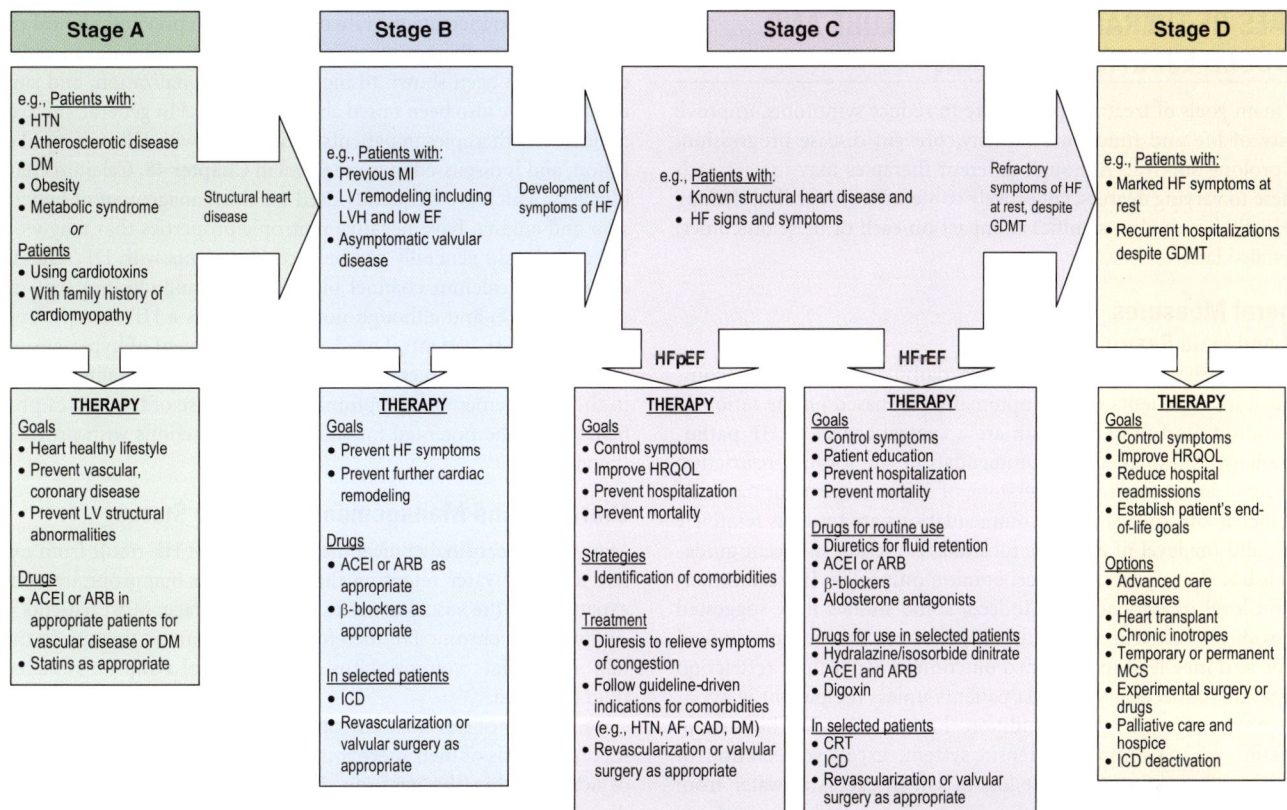

Fig. 37.1 American College of Cardiology and the American Heart Association stages of heart failure. *ACEI,* Angiotensin-converting enzyme inhibitor; *AF,* atrial fibrillation; *ARB,* angiotensin receptor blocker; *CAD,* coronary artery disease; *CRT,* cardiac resynchronization therapy; *DM,* diabetes mellitus; *EF,* ejection fraction; *GDMT,* guideline-directed medical therapy; *HF,* heart failure; *HRQOL,* health-related quality of life; *HTN,* hypertension; *ICD,* implantable cardioverter-defibrillator; *LV(H),* left ventricular hypertrophy; *MCS,* mechanical circulatory support; *MI,* myocardial infarction. (Modified from Hunt SA, Abraham WT, Chin MH, et al. 2009 focused update incorporated into the ACC/AHA 2005 guidelines for the diagnosis and management of heart failure in adults: a report of the American College of Cardiology Foundation/American Heart Association task force on practice guidelines: developed in collaboration with the International Society for Heart and Lung Transplantation. *J Am Coll Cardiol.* 2009;53:e1–e90; and Yancy CW, Jessup M, Bozkurt B, et al. 2013 ACCF/AHA guideline for the management of heart failure: a report of the American College of Cardiology Foundation/American Heart Association task force on practice guidelines. *J Am Coll Cardiol.* 2013;62:e147–e239.)

Epidemiologically, a large (and growing) proportion of patients with symptomatic HF have normal or near normal ejection fraction (EF), so-called heart failure with preserved ejection fraction, or HFpEF. This clinical entity, for which effective therapies have yet to be developed with the possible exception of mineralocorticoid receptor antagonists (MRAs) in appropriately selected patients, is covered in detail in **Chapter 39.** Similarly, acute decompensated HF leading to hospitalization is a major public health problem and is covered in detail in **Chapter 36.** In the current chapter, we will focus on contemporary medical therapy for patients with symptomatic heart failure and reduced ejection fraction (HFrEF), with a focus on both the biologic rationale and the clinical evidence supporting contemporary treatment. Notably, few areas in medicine have seen as much progress in the development of effective new therapies over recent decades as has the treatment of HFrEF, with multiple classes of agents and devices (which are covered separately in **Chapter 38**) having demonstrated major improvements in morbidity and mortality over this period. Cumulatively, contemporary guideline-directed medical therapy has reduced mortality in HFrEF by more than 60% over the last 30 years (**Fig. 37.2**).

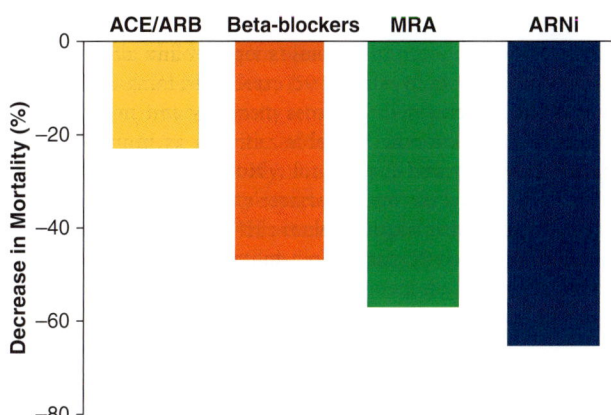

Fig. 37.2 Mortality improvements for contemporary heart failure and reduced ejection fraction medications. *ACE* Angiotensin-converting enzyme inhibitor; *ARB,* angiotensin receptor blocker; *ARNi,* angiotensin receptor-neprilysin inhibitor; *BB,* β-blocker; *MRA,* mineralocorticoid receptor antagonist.

GOALS OF THERAPY IN HEART FAILURE AND REDUCED EJECTION FRACTION

The main goals of treatment in HF are to reduce symptoms, improve quality of life and functional capacity, prevent disease progression, and prolong survival. Although different therapies may impact each of these to varying degrees, collectively contemporary medical therapy for HFrEF has made a significant impact on each of these outcomes, as detailed later.

General Measures
Diet and Fluid Restriction

Dietary restriction of sodium (2–3 g daily) is commonly recommended in all patients with symptomatic HF, based on the rationale that sodium and fluid retention are a central aspect of HF pathophysiology. Although the recommendation for sodium restriction has been a long-standing cornerstone of HF management, the body of evidence on which these recommendations are based is relatively scant, and the level of evidence for fluid restriction in recent guidelines is based primarily on expert opinion only (class IIa recommendation, level of evidence C).[1] Indeed, some studies have suggested that sodium restriction may actually worsen the neurohormonal profile and may lead to worsened outcomes.[2] Strict fluid restriction is generally unnecessary in most patients unless the patient is hyponatremic (<130 mEq/L), a condition that may develop because of activation of the renin-angiotensin system, excessive secretion of arginine vasopressin (AVP), or loss of salt in excess of water from prior diuretic use. Fluid restriction (<2 L day) should be considered in hyponatremic patients or for those patients whose fluid retention is difficult to control despite high doses of diuretics and sodium restriction.

Activity

Regular physical activity or exercise training is recommended for HF patients (class I, level of evidence A) by the current ACC-AHA guidelines.[1] This recommendation is based on studies and meta-analyses suggesting that exercise training improves functional capacity, quality of life, and clinical outcomes in patients with HF. Unlike many lifestyle interventions, exercise training has been rigorously studied in a large randomized outcomes trial of patients with HFrEF. HF-ACTION (A Controlled Trial Investigating Outcomes of Exercise Training) was a large multicenter randomized controlled study of exercise training that enrolled patients with an EF of 35% or less and New York Heart Association (NYHA) class II to IV symptoms with a primary endpoint of all-cause mortality and all-cause hospitalization.[3] In this study, structured exercise training demonstrated a modest improvement in all-cause mortality and hospitalizations after adjustment for other variables, as well as improvements in functional capacity and quality of life. Notably, in the HF-ACTION study there was no evidence that exercise training in HF was unsafe, even in patients with relatively severe HF symptoms. Based on the results of HF-ACTION, cardiac rehabilitation for patients with HF is covered by the Centers for Medicare and Medicaid Services in the United States.

Therapies to Avoid

Several common classes of medications may exacerbate symptoms of HF, potentially lead to disease progression, and thus should be avoided in patients with heart failure. Nonsteroidal antiinflammatory drugs (NSAIDs) inhibit the synthesis of prostaglandins, lead to sodium and fluid retention, and may lead to worsening HF. Thiazolidinediones are a class of antidiabetic agents that may lead to fluid retention and have

been shown to increase the rate of HF events in previous clinical trials. The antidiabetic therapy saxagliptin in the DPP-4 inhibitor medication class has also been shown to increase HF hospitalization, and similar concerns have also been raised about alogliptin.[4] In general, the area of antidiabetes therapies in patients at risk for or with HF is in rapid evolution, and is discussed in more detail in **Chapter 48**. Calcium channel blockers, which are frequently used for the management of hypertension and angina, have negative inotropic properties that may worsen HF and should generally not be used in patients with HF. The dihydropyridine calcium channel blockers (e.g., amlodipine) have been studied in HF, and although not efficacious as a HF therapy, appear to be safe in HF patients if needed for management of hypertension or angina.[5] The use of dietary supplements should generally be avoided in the management of symptomatic HF because of the lack of proven benefit and the potential for significant interactions with proven HF therapeutics.

Diuretics and Management of Volume Status

Many of the cardinal clinical manifestations of HF result from excessive salt and water retention that leads to an inappropriate volume expansion of the vascular and extravascular space. Most patients with symptomatic chronic HF therefore require diuretic therapy to maintain appropriate volume status and to control symptoms related to fluid retention.

A number of classification schemes have been proposed for diuretics on the basis of their mechanism of action and their anatomic locus of action within the nephron. The most common classification for diuretics employs an admixture of chemical (e.g., "thiazide" diuretic), site of action (e.g., "loop" diuretics), or clinical outcomes (e.g., "potassium-sparing" diuretics).

Loop Diuretics

The loop diuretics are the primary form of diuretic used in patients with HF.[6] These agents increase sodium excretion by up to 20% to 25% of the filtered load of sodium, enhance free water clearance, and maintain their efficacy unless renal function is severely impaired. The agents in this class, which include furosemide, bumetanide, and torsemide, act by reversibly inhibiting the Na^+-K^+-$2Cl^-$ symporter (cotransporter) on the apical membrane of epithelial cells in the thick ascending loop of Henle (**Fig. 37.3**), resulting in decreased urine sodium and chloride reabsorption with natriuresis and diuresis. The increase in delivery of Na^+ and water to the distal nephron segments also markedly enhances K^+ excretion, particularly in the presence of elevated aldosterone levels. Loop diuretics have a sigmoidal-shaped dose response relationship (**Fig. 37.4**).[6] Importantly, in both HF and renal insufficiency, the dose response for the loop diuretics curve shifts downward and to the right, thereby necessitating a higher dose to achieve the same effect and diminishing the likely maximal diuretic effect. The plasma concentration of loop diuretics also varies in peak value and duration of effect whether given intravenously or orally.

Because furosemide, bumetanide, and torsemide are bound extensively to plasma proteins, delivery of these drugs to the tubule by filtration is limited. However, these drugs are secreted efficiently by the organic acid transport system in the proximal tubule and thereby gain access to their binding sites on the Na^+-K^+-$2Cl^-$ symporter in the luminal membrane of the ascending limb. Thus the efficacy of loop diuretics is dependent upon sufficient renal plasma blood flow and proximal tubular secretion to deliver these agents to their site of action. Although these drugs have similar mechanisms of action, they differ in terms of bioavailability and pharmacokinetics in ways that may have important clinical implications (**Table 37.1**).[7]

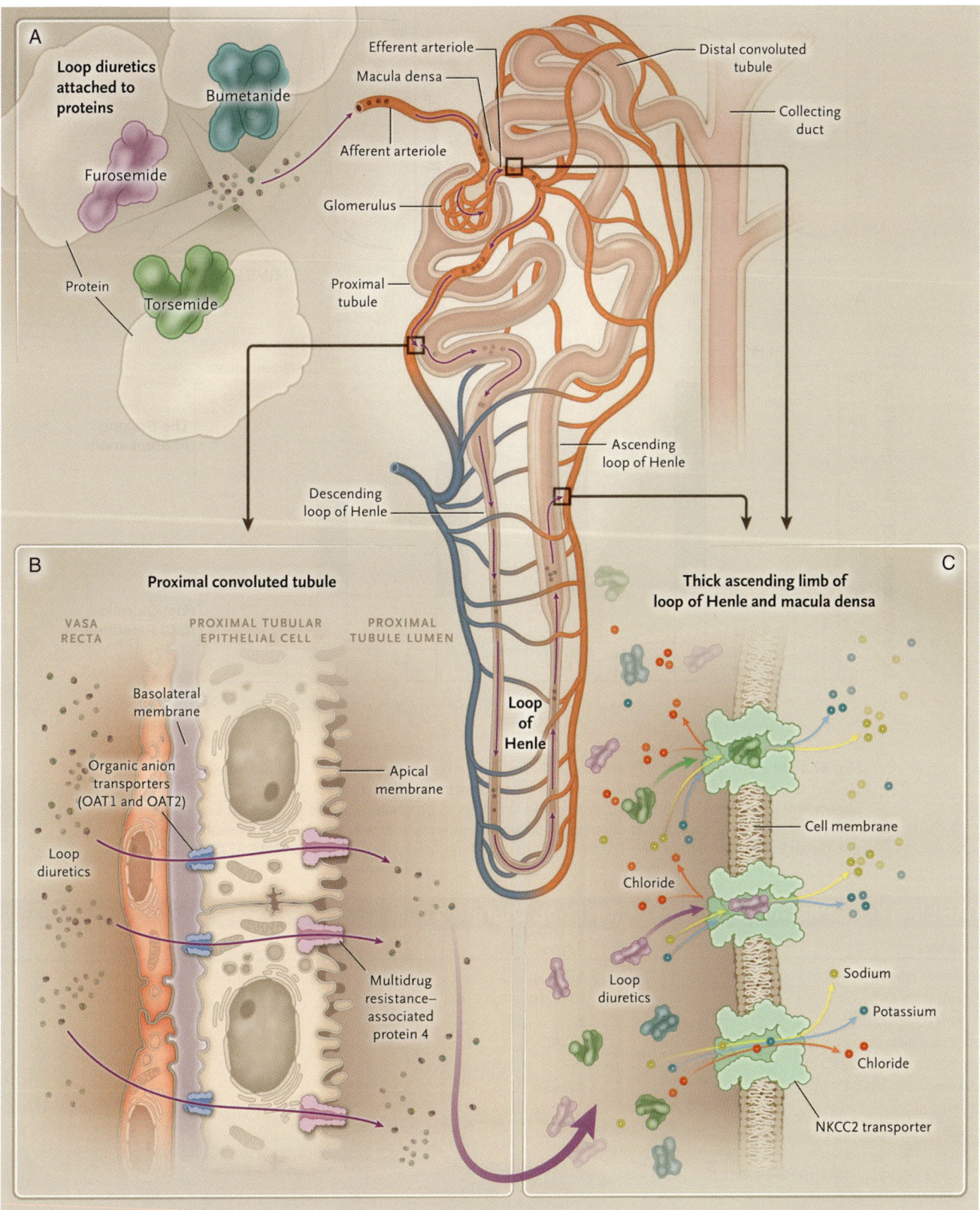

Fig. 37.3 Mechanisms of Loop Diuretic Action and Resistance. As shown in panel A, loop diuretics circulate bound to protein. As shown in panel B, they are secreted into the tubule lumen by organic anion transporters (OAT1 and OAT2) at the basolateral membrane and by multidrug resistance–associated protein 4 (and others) at the apical membrane. As shown in panel C, diuretics compete with chloride for binding to sodium–potassium–chloride cotransporter 2 (NKCC2), which is also present at the macula densa. Abnormalities at each step can mediate diuretic resistance. (From Ellison DH, Felker GM. Diuretic treatment in heart failure. *N Engl J Med.* 2017;377:1964–1975.)

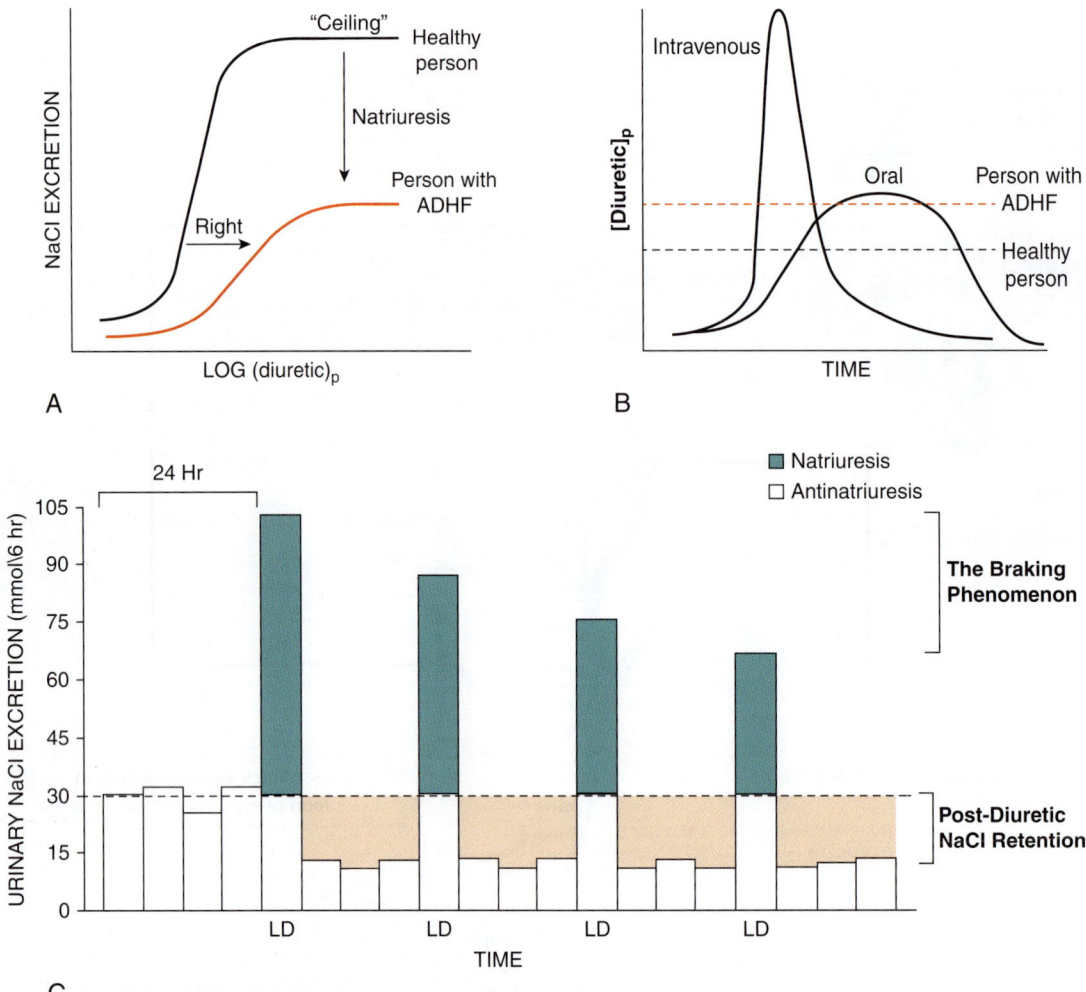

Fig. 37.4 (A) Dose response curves of loop diuretics in normal versus patients with heart failure. (B) Comparison of pharmacokinetics of oral versus intravenous loop diuretics (LD). (C) An example of the braking phenomenon, whereby each additional dose of LD results in progressively less natriuresis. Each period of natriuresis is followed by a period of postdiuretic sodium retention. ADHF, Acute decompensated heart failure. (From Ellison DH, Felker GM. Diuretic treatment in heart failure. *N Engl J Med.* 2017;377:1964–1975.)

TABLE 37.1 Pharmacokinetics of the Loop Diuretics

Property	Furosemide	Bumetanide	Torsemide
Relative IV potency	40 mg	1 mg	20 mg
Bioavailability (%)	10–100 (average = 50)	80–100	80–100
PO to IV conversion	2:1	1:1	1:1
Initial outpatient PO dose (mg)	20–40	0.5–1	5–10
Maintenance outpatient PO dose (mg)	40–240	1–5	10–20
Maximum daily IV dose (mg)	400–600	10	200
Onset (min)			
Oral	30–60	30–60	30–60
Intravenous	5	2–3	10
Peak serum concentration after PO administration (hr)	1	1–2	1
Affected by food	Yes	Yes	No
Metabolism	50% renal conjugation	50% hepatic	80% hepatic
Half-life (hr)			
Normal	1.5–2	1	3–4
Renal dysfunction	2.8	1.6	4–5
Hepatic dysfunction	2.5	2.3	8
Heart failure	2.7	1.3	6
Average duration of effect (hr)	6–8	4–6	6–8

From Felker GM, Mentz RJ. Diuretics and ultrafiltration in acute decompensated heart failure. *J Am Coll Cardiol.* 2012;59:2145–2153.

Thiazides and Thiazide-Like Diuretics

Thiazide-type diuretics inhibit the Na/Cl cotransporter in the distal tubule, thus blocking sodium resorption.[8] Commonly used drugs in this class include hydrochlorothiazide, chlorthalidone, chlorothiazide, and metolazone (which is not technically a thiazide but has similar properties). Thiazides have been shown to be a potentially powerful adjunct to loop diuretics (so-called sequential nephron blockade), especially in patients demonstrating a substantial degree of diuretic resistance and/or with significant renal dysfunction. The potential benefits imparted by the addition of a thiazide-type diuretic must be balanced against the potential risks, specifically the risk of resulting electrolyte and metabolic abnormalities. Hypokalemia in particular is a frequent consequence of the sequential nephron blockade that results from combining a thiazide-type diuretic with a loop diuretic. Other electrolyte abnormalities, such as hyponatremia and hypomagnesemia, are also common and may be severe. Use of these agents as an adjunct to loop diuretics in the outpatient setting should generally be done with caution and only with careful monitoring.

Mineralocorticoid Receptor Antagonists and Potassium-Sparing Diuretics

MRAs, such as spironolactone and eplerenone, are relatively weak diuretics at commonly used doses, but are generally used in HF patients as neurohormonal antagonists rather than for their diuretic properties (as described in detail later). High doses of MRAs (e.g., doses of spironolactone of 100 mg/day or more) may induce substantial diuresis, and can be considered for use as a therapy for refractory diuretic resistance, although careful monitoring of potassium and renal function is required.[9] A recent study of high-dose spironolactone for 96 hours in the acute HF setting was safe but did not improve natriuretic peptide levels, congestion, or clinical outcomes.[10] Potassium-sparing diuretics such as triamterene are mild diuretics, but are typically not effective in HF patients and are seldom used clinically in this population.

Vasopressin Antagonists

Increased circulating levels of the pituitary hormone AVP contribute to increased systemic vascular resistance and positive water balance in HF patients. The cellular effects of AVP are mediated by interactions with three types of receptors: V_{1a}, V_{1b}, and V_2. Selective V_{1a} antagonists block the vasoconstricting effects of AVP in peripheral vascular smooth muscle cells, whereas V_2 selective receptor antagonists inhibit recruitment of aquaporin water channels into the apical membranes of collecting duct epithelial cells, thereby reducing the ability of the collecting duct to resorb water. The AVP antagonists or *vaptans* were developed to selectively block the V_2 receptor (tolvaptan) or nonselectively block both the V_{1a}/V_2 receptors (conivaptan). These agents are not diuretics per se, but have been termed *aquaretics* because they lead to excretion of free water rather than natriuresis. Long-term therapy with the V_2 selective vasopressin antagonist tolvaptan did not improve mortality but appears to be safe when given chronically after a HF hospitalization.[11] Several recent studies explored a potential role for improved short-term symptoms of dyspnea and measures of congestion with tolvaptan in the setting of acute HF, but these were neutral.[12,13] The two vasopressin antagonists (conivaptan and tolvaptan) that are currently approved by the US Food and Drug Administration (FDA) are not specifically approved for HF, but are approved for the treatment of hyponatremia in patients with HF.

Practical Issues in the Use of Diuretics in Heart Failure

Patients with evidence of volume overload or a history of fluid retention should be treated with a diuretic to relieve their symptoms. In patients who have moderate to severe HF symptoms and/or renal insufficiency, a loop diuretic is generally required. Diuretics should generally be titrated as needed to relieve signs and symptoms of fluid overload. One commonly used method for finding the appropriate dose is to double the dose until the desired effect is achieved or the maximal dose of diuretic is reached. Patients with chronic HF can be instructed on parameters for self-adjustment of diuretics based on daily weights and symptoms (**see also Chapter 47**). Although furosemide is the most commonly used loop diuretic, bumetanide or torsemide may be preferable in selected patients because of their increased bioavailability (see Table 37.1) and the potential antifibrotic effect of torsemide. Changing to torsemide in particular may induce diuresis in patients seemingly refractory to oral furosemide. With the exception of torsemide, the commonly used loop diuretics are short acting (<3 hours). For this reason, loop diuretics are usually more effective when given at least twice daily to minimize periods where the concentration in the tubular fluid declines below a therapeutic level, which may produce postdiuretic sodium retention or "rebound."[6] Infrequent dosing may therefore lead to sodium retention that exceeds natriuresis, especially if dietary sodium intake is not restricted. An ongoing large outcomes trial is investigating the strategy of torsemide versus furosemide in a broad population of patients with HF (ClinicalTrials.gov Identifier: NCT03296813).

Risks of Diuretic Use

Observational studies have shown associations between loop diuretics, especially at higher doses, and adverse clinical outcomes in patients with HF.[14] These observations are confounded by the fact that patients receiving higher doses of diuretics tend to have greater disease severity or comorbidity, making it difficult to determine whether higher doses of diuretics are simply a marker for greater HF severity or are actually causing harm in HF patients. Postulated mechanisms for worse outcomes with loop diuretics include stimulation of the renin-angiotensin-aldosterone system (RAAS) and sympathetic nervous system, electrolyte disturbances, and deterioration of renal function. Although randomized data on the use of diuretics in HF are limited, the largest randomized study to date of diuretics in patients with acute decompensated HF (the DOSE study) did not suggest that higher doses of diuretics were associated with significant harm (**see also Chapter 36**).[15]

Patients with HF who are receiving diuretics should be monitored for complications of diuretics on a regular basis. The major complications of diuretic use include electrolyte and metabolic disturbances, volume depletion, and worsening azotemia. The interval for reassessment should be individualized based on severity of illness and underlying renal function; the use of concomitant medications such as angiotensin-converting enzyme (ACE) inhibitors, angiotensin receptor blockers (ARBs), and MRAs; the past history of electrolyte imbalances; and/or need for more aggressive diuresis.

Diuretic use can lead to potassium depletion, which can predispose the patient to significant cardiac arrhythmias and sudden death. Renal potassium losses from diuretic use can also be exacerbated by the increase in circulating levels of aldosterone observed in patients with advanced HF, and by the marked increases in distal nephron Na^+ delivery that follow use of loop or distal nephron diuretics. Serum potassium levels should generally be maintained between 4.0 and 5.0 mEq/L. Hypokalemia can be prevented by increasing the dietary intake of KCL, although most patients on significant doses of loop diuretics will require oral potassium supplementation. Diuretics may be associated with multiple other metabolic and electrolyte disturbances, including hyponatremia, hypomagnesemia, metabolic alkalosis, hyperglycemia, hyperlipidemia, and hyperuricemia.

Diuretic Resistance and Management

One inherent limitation of diuretics is that they achieve water loss via excretion of solute at the expense of glomerular filtration, which in turn activates a set of homeostatic mechanisms that ultimately limit their effectiveness. The term *diuretic resistance* typically defines a clinical scenario with progressively diminished responsiveness to diuretics despite persistent signs and/or symptoms of volume excess. One common cause of diuretic resistance is the so-called braking phenomenon to the effect of loop diuretics—this results from hemodynamic changes at the glomerulus mediated by the RAAS and sympathetic nervous system and adaptive changes in the distal nephron.[6] Additionally, as mentioned previously, most loop diuretics, with the exception of torsemide, are short-acting drugs. Accordingly, after a period of natriuresis, the diuretic concentration in plasma and tubular fluid declines below the diuretic threshold. In this situation, renal Na$^+$ reabsorption is no longer inhibited and a period of antinatriuresis or postdiuretic NaCl retention ensues. If dietary NaCl intake is moderate to excessive, postdiuretic NaCl retention may overcome the initial natriuresis in patients with excessive activation of the adrenergic nervous system and renin-angiotensin system. Other potential contributors to apparent diuretic resistance include changes in cardiac or renal function or patient noncompliance with their diuretic regimen or diet. Concurrent use of drugs that adversely affect renal function, such as NSAIDs and cyclooxygenase-2 (COX-2) inhibitors, may contribute to diuretic resistance.

Management of patients with progressive resistance to diuretics requires careful consideration of potential causes. Increasing doses of diuretics to ensure that therapeutic concentrations are achieved in the tubule is the typical initial step. Another common method for treating the diuretic-resistant patient is to administer two classes of diuretic concurrently ("sequential nephron blockade"). Most commonly, this involves adding a thiazide-like diuretic to a loop diuretic. Many clinicians choose metolazone because its half-life is longer than that of some other distal collecting tubule diuretics, and because it has been reported to remain effective even when the glomerular filtration rate is low. As noted previously, careful monitoring of fluid status, renal function, and electrolytes is critical with this approach, because sequential nephron blockade can be associated with dramatic fluid shifts and electrolyte disturbances.

Neurohormonal Antagonists in the Management of Heart Failure

Maladaptive chronic activation of the renin-angiotensin-aldosterone axis and sympathetic nervous system is central to modern understanding of the pathophysiology of HF (**see Chapters 5** and **6**). The clinical development of drugs that antagonize these axes has been the most fundamental and important development in the management of chronic HF, establishing for the first time the ability of medical therapy to change the natural history of the disease process. In this regard, inhibitors of the RAAS (ACE inhibitors, ARBs [with and without neprilysin inhibition], and MRAs) and β-blockers have emerged as cornerstones of modern HF therapy for patients with HFrEF (see Fig. 37.1). The ability of therapies to effectively intervene on ventricular remodeling has been consistently shown to be the most reliable surrogate for predicting subsequent efficacy in improving clinical outcomes (**Fig. 37.5**). These classes of agents, often collectively referred to as *neurohormonal antagonists,* have been shown to arrest, prevent, and even (particularly for β-blockers) potentially reverse the process of progressive ventricular remodeling that is associated with disease progression in HF (**Fig. 37.6**). As described in detail later, these agents have a large evidence base definitively establishing their efficacy in improving morbidity and mortality in patients with chronic HF and reduced EF, which is summarized in the current ACC/AHA guidelines as "guideline-directed evaluation and management," or GDEM (see Fig. 37.1).

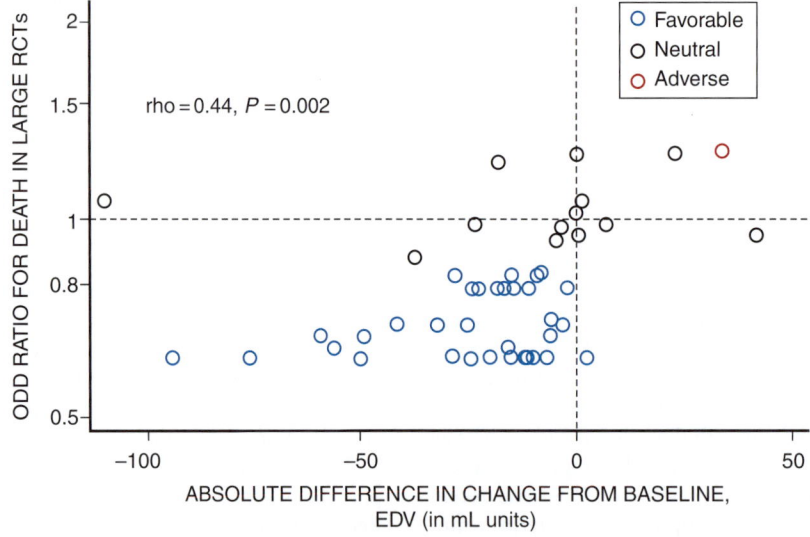

Fig. 37.5 Relationship between drug effect on ventricular remodeling and mortality in randomized trials. Quantitative relationship between drug effects on end-diastolic volume and mortality: each data point represents a placebo-corrected change in end-diastolic volume *(EDV)* from an individual remodeling trial plotted against the mortality odds ratio (OR) for the specific therapy. Interventions were classified as favorable *(blue circles)* if the upper limit of the 95% confidence interval (CI) of the OR for death from the mortality trials was less than 1, neutral *(black circles)* if the 95% CI crossed 1, and adverse *(red circles)* if the lower limit of the 95% CI was greater than 1. There were significant correlations between short-term therapeutic effects on EDV and longer-term therapeutic effect on mortality. *RCTs,* Randomized clinical trials. (From Kramer DG, Trikalinos TA, Kent DM, et al. Quantitative evaluation of drug or device effects on ventricular remodeling as predictors of therapeutic effects on mortality in patients with heart failure and reduced ejection fraction: a meta-analytic approach. *J Am Coll Cardiol.* 2010;56:392–406.)

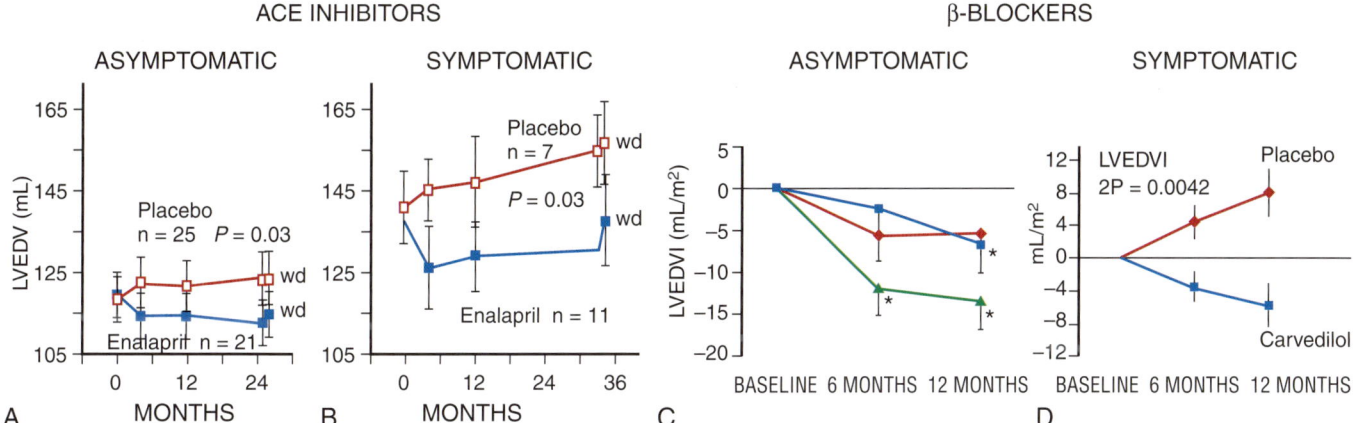

Fig. 37.6 The effect of angiotensin-converting enzyme *(ACE)* inhibitors and β-blockers on ventricular remodeling. (A) and (B) Left ventricular end-diastolic volumes *(LVEDV)* (mean ± SE) in enalapril and placebo patients within the prevention trial and the previously reported treatment trial who had measurements made at all five time points. Measurements are at baseline, 4 months, 1 year, and at study end (mean of 25 months and 33 months for prevention trial and treatment trial patients, respectively). The final data point on each graph is after withdrawal *(wd)* of study drug for a minimum of 5 days. *P* values shown are for comparison of placebo and enalapril groups by repeated-measures analysis applied to all time points. Baseline volumes were significantly higher in treatment trial patients (*P* < .005). In the prevention trial and the treatment trial, placebo-treated patients manifested progressive increases in ventricular volumes, whereas enalapril-treated patients showed an early and sustained reduction in LV volumes. Treatment difference between the placebo and enalapril groups was significantly greater within the treatment trial than within the prevention trial (*P* < .02 at 1 year). (C) Effect of metoprolol succinate on LV volumes. Shown are the least square mean changes *(SE)* in LVEDVI (B) compared with the baseline for patients receiving metoprolol succinate 200 mg *(triangles)*, 50 mg *(squares)*, or placebo *(diamonds)*. **P* < .05 versus baseline. (D) Changes in LVEDVI from baseline *(BL)* to 6 months (6M) and 12 months (12M). Data are presented as mean value ± SE. *P* values comparing carvedilol and placebo are for repeated measures multivariate analysis of variance *(MANOVA)* over 12 months of treatment. (A and B, From Konstam MA, Kronenberg MW, Rousseau MF, et al. Effects of the angiotensin converting enzyme inhibitor enalapril on the long-term progression of left ventricular dilatation in patients with asymptomatic systolic dysfunction. SOLVD [Studies of Left Ventricular Dysfunction] Investigators. *Circulation.* 1993;88:2277–2283. C, From Colucci WS, Kolias TJ, Adams KF, et al. Metoprolol reverses left ventricular remodeling in patients with asymptomatic systolic dysfunction: the REversal of VEntricular Remodeling with Toprol-XL (REVERT) trial. *Circulation.* 2007;116:49–56. D, From Doughty RN, Whalley GA, Gamble G, et al. Left ventricular remodeling with carvedilol in patients with congestive heart failure due to ischemic heart disease. Australia-New Zealand Heart Failure Research Collaborative Group. *J Am Coll Cardiol.* 1997;29:1060–1066.)

Angiotensin-Converting Enzyme Inhibitors and Angiotensin Receptor Blockers
Rationale/Pathophysiologic Basis for Use

Activation of the RAAS plays a key role in the pathophysiology of the development and progression of HF. The fundamental biology of this neurohormonal axis as it relates to HF is covered in **Chapter 5**. The RAAS may be inhibited at many levels: renin inhibition, inhibition of the conversion of angiotensin I to angiotensin II, antagonism of one or more angiotensin II receptors, and blockade of the primary target of aldosterone, the mineralocorticoid receptor.

Angiotensin-converting enzyme inhibitors. ACE inhibitors were the first agents clinically available for inhibiting the RAAS and continue to be the most widely used in clinical practice. ACE inhibitors interfere with the renin-angiotensin system by inhibiting the enzyme that is responsible for the conversion of angiotensin I to angiotensin II. These agents act by inhibiting one of several proteases responsible for cleaving angiotensin I to form angiotensin II. However, alternative enzymatic pathways have become recognized as playing a major role in angiotensin II production in humans. For example, in the failing human heart, angiotensin II formation is only partially inhibited by an ACE inhibitor but almost completely blocked by an inhibitor of chymase, another protease that catalyzes the formation of angiotensin II from angiotensin I.[16]

Accordingly, ACE inhibitor therapy achieves only partial inhibition of angiotensin II production.

To the extent that ACE inhibitors reduce production of angiotensin II, effects attributable to angiotensin II are diminished regardless of which receptor mediates the particular effect (i.e., both AT_1 and AT_2 receptors). ACE not only cleaves angiotensin I to form angiotensin II, but is also the principal protease that degrades bradykinin; thus ACE inhibition leads to increased levels of bradykinin within the circulation and at the tissue level. The hemodynamic effects of ACE inhibitors may be mediated in part through increases in regional bradykinin levels. Bradykinin stimulates endothelial release of nitric oxide (NO) and vasodilator prostaglandins, contributing to the vasodilator effects of ACE inhibitors. In some animal models of myocardial injury or pressure overload, the beneficial effects of ACE inhibitors mitigating cardiomyocyte hypertrophy and fibroblast hyperplasia within the myocardium are blocked by a bradykinin antagonist.[17] Thus, reduction of bradykinin metabolism, resulting in potentiation of local bradykinin levels, potentially contributes to the therapeutic benefit of ACE inhibitors.

Angiotensin Receptor Blockers. Although ACE inhibitors and ARBs both inhibit RAAS, they do so by different mechanisms. ARBs block the effects of angiotensin II on the angiotensin type 1 receptor, the receptor subtype that is responsible for virtually all the adverse biologic effects relevant to angiotensin II on cardiac remodeling. In contrast to ACE inhibitors, effects of angiotensin II receptor antagonists limit the responses specifically mediated by that receptor. Because most of the clinically relevant effects of angiotensin II appear to be mediated through the AT_1 receptor, AT_1 receptor antagonists mirror the actions anticipated through the blockade of angiotensin II production. However, loss of feedback inhibition results in increased angiotensin II levels after administration of an AT_1 receptor antagonist, which leads to overstimulation of alternative angiotensin II receptors. The unopposed activation of non-AT_1 receptors may mediate some of the clinically relevant effects attributable to AT_1 receptor blockade. For example, stimulation of the AT_2 receptor may be responsible for the antiproliferative and antifibrotic effects of AT_1 antagonists within the cardiovascular system, although unopposed activation of the AT_2 receptor may also promote apoptosis.[18]

Effects on Hemodynamics

The primary acute hemodynamic effect of both ACE inhibitors and ARBs is vasodilation. Early investigations of ACE inhibitors demonstrated that these agents produced dose-dependent decreases in right atrial pressure, pulmonary capillary wedge pressure, and systemic vascular resistance, with a resultant increase in cardiac index.[19] In addition, inhibition of neurohormonal activation over time is evident from decreases in heart rates and plasma catecholamine levels at rest and with exercise.[20] Similarly, ARBs produce dose-dependent decreases in right atrial pressure, pulmonary capillary wedge pressure, and systemic vascular resistance in association with increased cardiac index, which are sustained over time in the absence of tachyphylaxis.[21] These hemodynamic effects of ARBs occur without increases in heart rate or neurohormonal activation. Beneficial hemodynamic and clinical effects of irbesartan were reported by Havranek and colleagues in patients already taking ACE inhibitors.[22]

Effects on Ventricular Structure

In addition to a wealth of experimental evidence supporting the important role of the RAAS in the pathophysiologic processes of ventricular remodeling (**see Chapter 5**), clinical evidence also supports this premise. Sharpe and associates demonstrated that captopril initiated within 48 hours after Q wave MI reduced the increase in LV end-diastolic volume after only 3 months of therapy.[23] Similarly, in the multicenter Survival and Ventricular Enlargement (SAVE) trial, captopril improved survival among patients after MI with reduced left ventricular ejection fraction (LVEF) (<40%) and mitigated the degree of LV chamber dilation after the first year of therapy.[24] ACE inhibitors prevent progressive LV remodeling in patients with LV systolic dysfunction with or without symptoms of HF (see Fig. 37.6).[25] In a substudy of the Studies of Left Ventricular Dysfunction (SOLVD) trial, the placebo recipients exhibited LV dilation over the span of this study (1 year), whereas the enalapril recipients exhibited the opposite, which was consistent with a decrease in LV chamber size for a given LV pressure. This study demonstrated clinically that ACE inhibition prevents, and perhaps reverses, the extent of ventricular remodeling in patients with LV systolic dysfunction.

The precise effect of AT_1 receptor antagonists on ventricular remodeling is not as well studied. In the Evaluation of Losartan in the Elderly (ELITE) radionuclide substudy, researchers compared the effect of losartan, an AT_1 antagonist, with that of the ACE inhibitor captopril on LV remodeling in elderly patients with HF and systolic dysfunction (EF < 40%).[26] After 48 weeks of therapy, captopril and losartan demonstrated statistically equivalent effects in reducing LV

end-diastolic and end-systolic volumes, although there was a trend toward a greater beneficial effect of captopril in this study. Perhaps the largest study of whether combination therapy with an ACE inhibitor and ARB produces greater reduction in LV remodeling has been the Valsartan in Acute Myocardial Infarction Trial (VALIANT), in which investigators examined the effect of valsartan alone, captopril alone, and their combination in patients after an acute MI complicated by HF, LV dysfunction, or both.[27] Although the patient population in this trial differed from that in HF trials (after MI, mean LVEF among the groups was 39%), the degree of LV remodeling (increase in LV end-diastolic volume and change in LVEF) was similar among all three groups of patients.[28] The results of the VALIANT substudy do not support the view that combination therapy in patients with HF or LV dysfunction after MI exerts a greater effect in limiting LV remodeling than either class of agent alone.

Effects on Functional Capacity and Symptoms

Angiotensin-Converting Enzyme Inhibitors. Reduced functional capacity in patients with HF caused by systolic dysfunction results from a variety of cardiac and noncardiac factors. ACE inhibitors have variably been shown to improve exercise capacity in patients with HF and systolic dysfunction, presumably through their sustained hemodynamic benefits, as described previously. However, the improvement in exercise capacity noted with ACE inhibitors is often modest in clinical trials. The lack of more dramatic improvements in exercise capacity in clinical trials may result in part from improved survival among patients with advanced HF being treated with ACE inhibitors. For example, in the Vasodilators in Heart Failure Treatment (V-HeFT) II trial, in which ACE inhibition was compared with the combination of hydralazine and isosorbide dinitrate, subjects receiving the latter regimen had a more pronounced improvement in exercise capacity as judged by peak exercise oxygen consumption.[29] However, the survival rate among patients treated with the ACE inhibitor was better than that among subjects taking hydralazine and isosorbide, which raised the question of whether more differentially better survival among patients treated with enalapril may have diluted any improvements in exercise capacity.

A number of studies have demonstrated that ACE inhibitors improve exercise time and ameliorate symptoms of HF.[30,31] Taken together, these clinical data demonstrate that ACE inhibitors favorably influence symptoms of HF and exercise capacity in patients with LV systolic dysfunction.

Angiotensin Receptor Blockers. ARBs also improve exercise capacity and symptoms in patients with HF. Losartan has been shown to improve symptoms of HF after 12 weeks of therapy in patients with reduced LVEF (<45%).[32] In a comparative trial with the ACE inhibitor enalapril, losartan-treated patients demonstrated similar exercise capacity and symptoms of HF after 12 weeks of treatment.[33]

Riegger and colleagues studied the effects of various doses of the ARB candesartan (4, 8, and 16 mg) in patients with HF and LV systolic dysfunction.[34] In this study, ACE inhibitors were withdrawn 2 weeks before the placebo run-in period. With all three doses of candesartan, patients demonstrated an improved HF symptoms score and improved exercise capacity in comparison with placebo-treated patients. Researchers in the Randomized Evaluation of Strategies for Left Ventricular Dysfunction (RESOLVD) pilot study compared candesartan alone, enalapril alone, and their combination over a 43-week period.[35] Each agent resulted in similar improvements in exercise capacity and quality of life. Thus, available studies suggest that ARBs produce improvements in exercise capacity and HF symptoms that are similar to those produced by ACE inhibitors, either historically or in a direct, individual manner.

TABLE 37.2   Key Randomized Trials of Angiotensin-Converting Enzyme Inhibitors and Angiotensin Receptor Blockers in Heart Failure

Trial Name	Agent	NYHA Class	No. of Subjects Enrolled	12-Month Placebo Mortality (%)	12-Month Effect Size (%)	P Value 12 Months (Full F/U)
ACEIs						
HF						
CONSENSUS-1	Enalapril	IV	253	52	↓31	.01 (.0003)
SOLVD-Rx	Enalapril	I–III	2569	15	↓21	.02 (.004)
SOLVD-Asx	Enalapril	I, II	4228	5	0	.82 (.30)
Post-MI						
SAVE	Captopril	—	2231	12	↓18	.11 (.02)
AIRE	Ramipril	—	1986	20	↓22	.01 (.002)
TRACE	Trandolapril	—	1749	26	↓16	.046 (.001)
ARBs						
HF						
VAL-HeFT	Valsartan	II–IV	5010	9	0	NS (.80)
CHARM-Alternative	Candesartan	II–IV	2028	NS	NS	NS (.02)
CHARM-Added	Candesartan	II–IV	2547	NS	NS	NS (.11)
HEAAL	Losartan	II–IV	3846	NS	NS	NS (.24)

ACEI, Angiotensin-converting enzyme inhibitor; *ARB*, angiotensin receptor blocker; *CHARM*, Candesartan Heart Failure: Assessment of Reduction in Mortality and Morbidity; *CONSENSUS*, Cooperative North Scandinavian Enalapril Survival Study; *HEAAL*, Heart Failure Endpoint Evaluation of Angiotensin II Antagonist Losartan; *HF*, heart failure; *MI*, myocardial infarction; *NYHA*, New York Heart Association; *SOLVD*, Studies of Left Ventricular Dysfunction; *TRACE*, Trandolapril Cardiac Evaluation; *VAL-HeFT*, Valsartan Heart Failure Trial.

Effects on Morbidity and Mortality

Although the hemodynamic and clinical effects of ACE inhibitors are notably similar to those of ARBs, these two classes of agents should not be considered interchangeable, inasmuch as they possess both overlapping and distinct effects. Clinical evidence for the benefit of ACE inhibitors exceeds that for ARBs, a finding that is strongly influenced by the earlier development of ACE inhibitors. Results of clinical trials, both early and more recent, have helped determine whether, and under what circumstances, these agents can be used interchangeably or in combination.

Angiotensin-Converting Enzyme Inhibitors. ACE inhibitors were the first class of agents shown to significantly alter the natural history of HF, as demonstrated by a reduction in the frequency of death and of other morbid events. Most of these data have been accumulated from patients with reduced LVEF, and clinicians have therefore recognized the necessity for measuring ventricular systolic function and prescribing ACE inhibitors to patients with reduced EF (e.g., ≤35%) as standards of care for patients with HF. **Table 37.2** lists the key trials demonstrating the benefit of ACE inhibitors in this population. These trials recruited a broad variety of patients, including women and the elderly, and patients with a wide range of causes and severity of LV dysfunction.

The consistency of data from the SOLVD Prevention Study,[36] SAVE,[37] and Trandolapril Cardiac Evaluation (TRACE)[38] has shown that asymptomatic patients with LV dysfunction (stage B) have less remodeling and a reduced risk of progressing to symptomatic HF when treated with ACE inhibitors. ACE inhibitors have also consistently shown benefit for patients with symptomatic LV dysfunction (stage C). All significant placebo-controlled ACE inhibitors in HFrEF patients have demonstrated a reduction in mortality. Further, the absolute benefit is greatest in patients with the most severe HF. Indeed, the patients with NYHA class IV HF in the Cooperative

North Scandinavian Enalapril Survival Study (CONSENSUS I)[39] had a much larger effect size than the SOLVD Treatment Trial,[40] which in turn had a larger effect size than the SOLVD Prevention Trial.[36] Although only three placebo-controlled mortality trials have been conducted in patients with chronic HF, the aggregate data suggest that ACE inhibitors reduce mortality in direct relation to the degree of severity of chronic HF. A pooled analysis of placebo-controlled trials of ACE inhibitors suggested a 23% reduction in mortality and a 35% reduction in the combined endpoint of death or HF hospitalization compared with a placebo.[41] The V-HeFT-II trial provided evidence that ACE inhibitors improve the natural history of HF through mechanisms other than vasodilation, inasmuch as subjects treated with enalapril had significantly lower mortality than subjects treated with the vasodilatory combination of hydralazine plus isosorbide dinitrate (which does not directly inhibit neurohormonal systems).[29] Although enalapril is the only ACE inhibitor that has been used in placebo-controlled mortality trials in chronic HF, multiple ACE inhibitors have proven to be roughly equally effective when administered in oral form within the first week of the ischemic event in MI trials, supporting the general notion that the ACE inhibitor effect is a class effect in HF. In a direct randomized comparison study of high dose (≈35 mg of lisinopril) compared with low dose (≈5 mg of lisinopril), the Assessment of Treatment with Lisinopril and Survival (ATLAS) study suggested that mortality was similar, although higher doses were associated with lower rates of HF hospitalization.[42]

Importantly, it should be emphasized that patients with low blood pressure (<90 mm Hg systolic) or impaired renal function (serum creatinine greater than 2.5 mg/mL) were not recruited or represent a small proportion of patients who participated in these trials. Thus the efficacy of these agents for these patient populations is less well established.[43]

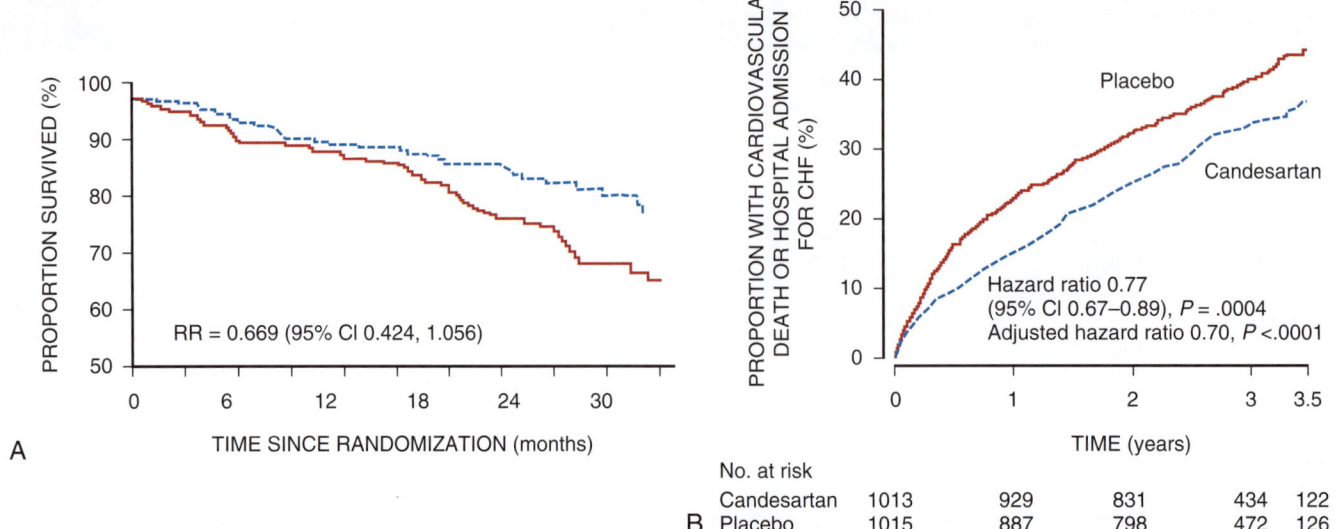

Fig. 37.7 Outcomes with ARBs compared with the placebo in heart failure. (A) Kaplan-Meier curves for mortality in the valsartan *(dotted line)* and placebo *(solid line)* groups (*n* = 185 and 181, respectively) without angiotensin-converting enzyme *(ACE)* inhibitor background therapy (*P* = .017 by log-rank test) in the Valsartan Heart Failure Trial (Val-HeFT). (B) Kaplan-Meier cumulative event curves for the primary outcome (all-cause mortality, cardiovascular death, or hospitalization) in the Candesartan Heart Failure: Assessment of Reduction in Mortality and Morbidity trial (CHARM-Alternative) in ACE-intolerant patients. (A, From Maggioni AP, Anand I, Gottlieb SO, et al. Effects of valsartan on morbidity and mortality in patients with heart failure not receiving angiotensin-converting enzyme inhibitors. J Am Coll Cardiol. 2002;40:1414–1421; B, From Granger CB, McMurray JJ, Yusuf S, et al. Effects of candesartan in patients with chronic heart failure and reduced left-ventricular systolic function intolerant to angiotensin-converting-enzyme inhibitors: the CHARM-Alternative trial. Lancet. 2003;362:772–776.)

Mechanisms Underlying These Effects

The original hypothesis behind investigation of ACE inhibitors in patients with HF was that these agents would reduce the progression of clinical HF through vasodilation. As noted previously, direct comparison between ACE inhibitors and other vasodilatory regimens (e.g., nitrates and hydralazine in the V-HeFT studies) support the concept that ACE inhibitors alter the natural history of HF via mechanisms distinct from their hemodynamic effects, including direct effects on the cellular mechanisms responsible for progressive changes in the myocyte and the interstitium. Beyond an effect on clinical events linked to progressive HF, both the SOLVD and SAVE studies demonstrated significant reductions in the incidence of MI, which potentially contributed to the overall influence of ACE inhibitors on mortality. Furthermore, within the SOLVD population, enalapril caused a significant reduction in the number of patients hospitalized for unstable angina. These findings provided, for the first time, evidence of an influence of ACE inhibitors on the pathogenesis of acute coronary syndromes, an influence potentially mediated by effects on the arterial wall, on the balance between thrombosis and thrombolysis, or on both.

Angiotensin Receptor Blockers. In symptomatic HF patients who were intolerant of ACE inhibitors, the aggregate clinical data suggest that ARBs are roughly as effective as ACE inhibitors in reducing HF morbidity and mortality. Candesartan significantly reduced all-cause mortality, cardiovascular death, or hospitalization in ACE-intolerant patients in the Candesartan Heart Failure: Assessment of Reduction in Mortality and Morbidity (CHARM-Alternative) trial.[44] Similar findings were shown with valsartan in the small subgroup of patients not receiving an ACE inhibitor in the Valsartan Heart Failure Trial (Val-HeFT) (**Fig. 37.7**).[45,46] A direct comparison of ACE inhibitors and ARBs was assessed in the Losartan

Heart Failure Survival Study (ELITE-II), which showed that losartan was not associated with improved survival in elderly HF patients when compared with captopril, but was significantly better tolerated.[47] Two trials have evaluated ARBs compared to ACE inhibition in post-MI patients who developed LV dysfunction or signs of HF. The direct comparison of losartan with captopril indicated that losartan was not as effective as captopril on all-cause mortality, whereas valsartan was shown to be noninferior to captopril on all-cause mortality in the VALIANT study.[27] The combination of captopril and valsartan produced no further reduction in mortality in VALIANT, although the number of adverse events increased. When given in addition to ACE inhibitors in general cohorts of patients with symptomatic HF, the effects of ARBs were shown to have a modest beneficial effect in the CHARM-Added trial.[48] However, the addition of valsartan to ACE inhibitors had no beneficial effect on mortality in Val-HeFT, although the combined endpoint mortality and morbidity was significantly (13.2%) lower with valsartan than with the placebo because of a reduction in the number of patients hospitalized for HF.[45] The question of high-dose versus low-dose angiotensin receptor antagonism on clinical outcomes was evaluated in the Heart Failure Endpoint Evaluation of Angiotensin II Antagonist Losartan (HEAAL) trial.[49] This study showed that the use of a high-dose losartan was not associated with a significant reduction in the primary endpoint of all-cause death or admission for HF (hazard ratio [HR] 0.94, 95% confidence interval [CI] 0.84–1.04, *P* = .24) when compared with low-dose losartan, but was associated with a significant reduction in HF admissions (HR 0.94, 95% CI 0.84–1.04, *P* = .24), suggesting that uptitration of ARBs may confer clinical benefit.

Although one meta-analysis suggests that ARBs and ACE inhibitors have similar effects on all-cause mortality and HF hospitalizations,[50] and although ARBs may be considered as initial therapy rather than ACE inhibitors following MI, the general consensus is that ACE inhibitors remain the first-line therapy for the treatment of HF, whereas ARBs are recommended for ACE inhibitor-intolerant patients. Importantly, a recent ACC/AHA/Heart Failure Society of America (HFSA) guideline update highlights that ACE inhibitors, ARBs, and now also angiotensin receptor-neprilysin inhibitors (ARNIs) have a class I recommendation for use in patients with chronic HFrEF in conjunction with other GDEMs (see further discussion later).[51] Combination therapy with ACE inhibitors and ARB can be considered in persistently symptomatic patients, although the risk of side effects is higher (see later discussion), particularly in patients also treated with MRAs (the triple combination of ACE inhibitors, ARBs, and MRAs is specifically discouraged; class III recommendation for harm) in current guidelines.[1]

Side Effects, Complications, and Drug Interactions

Angiotensin-Converting Enzyme Inhibitors. Most of the adverse effects of ACE inhibitors are related to suppression of the renin-angiotensin system. The decreases in blood pressure and mild azotemia that are often seen during the initiation of therapy are, in general, well tolerated and do not require a decrease in the dose of the ACE inhibitor. However, if hypotension is accompanied by dizziness or if the renal dysfunction becomes severe, it may be necessary to decrease the dose of the diuretic if significant fluid retention is not present, or alternatively, decrease the dose of the ACE inhibitor if significant fluid retention is present. Hyperkalemia may also become problematic if the patient is receiving potassium supplements or a potassium-sparing diuretic. Potassium retention that is not responsive to these measures may require a reduction in the dose of ACE inhibitor or (rarely) discontinuation. The side effects of ACE inhibitors that are related to kinin potentiation include a nonproductive cough (10%–15% of patients) and angioedema (1% of patients). In patients who cannot tolerate ACE inhibitors because of cough or angioedema, ARBs are the next recommended line of therapy. Patients intolerant to ACE inhibitors because of hyperkalemia or renal insufficiency are likely to experience the same side effects with ARBs. The combination of hydralazine and an oral nitrate should be considered for these latter patients (see later discussion).

Early clinical evidence suggested that aspirin use may prevent or limit the hemodynamic and survival benefits of ACE inhibitors. Importantly, contemporary studies derived from registry data and population-based cohorts have refuted these earlier concerns related to a potential aspirin and ACE inhibitor interaction. In multiple recent systematic reviews of ACE inhibitor trials, improvement in clinical outcomes continued to be evident in patients receiving aspirin at baseline, although the magnitude of the benefit tended to be lower.[52]

Angiotensin Receptor Blockers. ARBs are well tolerated and highly efficacious in patients who are intolerant of ACE inhibitors because of cough, skin rash, and angioedema and should therefore be used in symptomatic and asymptomatic patients with an EF less than 40% who are ACE inhibitor-intolerant for reasons other than hyperkalemia or renal insufficiency. Both ACE inhibitors and ARBs have similar effects on blood pressure, renal function, and potassium. Therefore, the problems of symptomatic hypotension, azotemia, and hyperkalemia will be similar for both of these agents. Although less frequent than with ACE inhibitors, angioedema has also been reported in some patients who receive ARBs. In patients who are intolerant to ACE inhibitors and ARBs, the combined use of hydralazine and isosorbide dinitrate may be considered as a therapeutic option in such patients.

Practical Tips

Angiotensin-Converting Enzyme Inhibitors. Starting and target doses for commonly used ACE inhibitors and ARBs are shown in **Table 37.3**. Because fluid retention can attenuate the effects of ACE inhibitors, it is preferable to optimize the dose of diuretic first before starting the ACE inhibitor. However, it may be necessary to reduce the dose of diuretic during the initiation of an ACE inhibitor to prevent symptomatic hypotension. ACE inhibitors should be initiated in low doses, followed by increments in dose if lower doses have been well tolerated. Titration is generally achieved by doubling doses every 3 to 5 days. The dose of ACE inhibitors should be increased until the doses used are similar to those that have been shown to be effective in clinical trials or to the maximally tolerated dose. Higher doses are more effective than lower doses in preventing hospitalization based on the ATLAS trial.[42] For stable patients, it is acceptable to add therapy with β-blocking agents before full target doses of ACE inhibitors are reached. Blood pressure (including postural changes), renal function, and potassium should be evaluated within 1 to 2 weeks after initiation of ACE inhibitors, especially in patients with preexisting azotemia, hypotension, hyponatremia, diabetes mellitus, or in those taking potassium supplements. Abrupt withdrawal of treatment with an ACE inhibitor may lead to clinical deterioration and should therefore be avoided in the absence of life-threatening complications (e.g., angioedema, hyperkalemia).

Angiotensin Receptor Blockers. Multiple ARBs that are approved for the treatment of hypertension are now available to clinicians. Three of these, losartan, valsartan, and candesartan, have been extensively evaluated in the setting of HF. ARBs should be initiated with the starting doses shown in **Table 37.3**, which can be uptitrated every 3 to 5 days by doubling the dose of ARB. As with ACE inhibitors, blood pressure, renal function, and potassium should be reassessed within 1 to 2 weeks after initiation and followed closely after changes in dose.

Angiotensin–Neprilysin Inhibition

Neprilysin is a neutral endopeptidase (NEP) that degrades several peptides in the neurohormonal axis, including natriuretic peptides, bradykinin, and adrenomedullin. NEP inhibition increases levels of these vasoactive peptides and counters adverse vasoconstriction, sodium retention, and ventricular remodeling. Neprilysin inhibition was initially combined with ACE inhibition in the medication omapatrilat. Data in HF animal models demonstrated that combined ACE and NEP inhibition with omapatrilat was more effective than ACE inhibition alone in preventing adverse changes in LV geometry.[53] In the Omapatrilat Versus Enalapril Randomized Trial of Utility in Reducing Events (OVERTURE) conducted in 5770 chronic HF patients, omapatrilat reduced cardiovascular death or hospitalization (HR 0.91, 95% CI 0.84–0.99, $P = .024$), but there was no difference between the therapies for the primary endpoint of death or HF hospitalization ($P = .187$).[54] However, studies with omapatrilat in patients with hypertension demonstrated an increased risk for serious angioedema and the compound was not developed further.

Sacubitril/valsartan, which consists of the ARB valsartan and the NEP inhibitor sacubitril, was developed to minimize the risk of angioedema. This medication class is referred to as an angiotensin receptor–neprilysin inhibitor or ARNI. In the phase 2 study, Prospective comparison of ARNI with ARB on Management Of heart failUre with preserved ejectioN fracTion (PARAMOUNT) ($N = 301$), sacubitril/valsartan led to greater reductions in N-terminal pro-B-type natriuretic peptide (NT-proBNP) than valsartan at 12 weeks and was well tolerated.[55] The effect of sacubitril/valsartan on morbidity and mortality in HFrEF was evaluated in the Prospective

TABLE 37.3 Starting and Target Doses for Guideline-Recommended Drugs for Heart Failure and Reduced Ejection Fraction

Drug	Initial Daily Dose(S)	Maximum Dose(S)	Mean Doses Achieved IN Clinical Trials
ACE Inhibitors			
Captopril	6.25 mg 3 times	50 mg 3 times	122.7 mg/day
Enalapril	2.5 mg twice	10–20 mg twice	16.6 mg/day
Fosinopril	5–10 mg once	40 mg once	N/A
Lisinopril	2.5–5 mg once	20–40 mg once	32.5–35.0 mg/day
Perindopril	2 mg once	8–16 mg once	N/A
Quinapril	5 mg twice	20 mg twice	N/A
Ramipril	1.25–2.5 mg once	10 mg once	N/A
Trandolapril	1 mg once	4 mg once	N/A
ARBs			
Candesartan	4–8 mg once	32 mg once	24 mg/day
Losartan	25–50 mg once	50–150 mg once	129 mg/day
Valsartan	20–40 mg twice	160 mg twice	254 mg/day
Aldosterone Antagonists			
Spironolactone	12.5–25.0 mg once	25 mg once or twice	26 mg/day
Eplerenone	25 mg once	50 mg once	42.6 mg/day
β-Blockers			
Bisoprolol	1.25 mg once	10 mg once	8.6 mg/day
Carvedilol	3.125 mg twice	50 mg twice	37 mg/day
Carvedilol CR	10 mg once	80 mg once	N/A
Metoprolol succinate extended release (metoprolol CR/XL)	12.5–25 mg once	200 mg once	159 mg/day
Hydralazine and Isosorbide Dinitrate			
Fixed-dose combination	37.5 mg hydralazine/20 mg isosorbide dinitrate 3 times daily	75 mg hydralazine/40 mg isosorbide dinitrate 3 times daily	≈175 mg hydralazine/90 mg isosorbide dinitrate daily
Hydralazine and isosorbide dinitrate	Hydralazine: 25–50 mg, 3 or 4 times daily and isosorbide dinitrate: 20–30 mg 3 or 4 times daily	Hydralazine: 300 mg daily in divided doses and isosorbide dinitrate: 120 mg daily in divided doses	N/A

ACE, Angiotensin-converting enzyme; *ARB*, angiotensin receptor blocker; *HFrEF*, heart failure with reduced ejection fraction; *N/A*, not applicable. From Yancy CW, Jessup M, Bozkurt B, et al. 2013 ACCF/AHA guideline for the management of heart failure: a report of the American College of Cardiology Foundation/American Heart Association task force on practice guidelines. *J Am Coll Cardiol*. 2013;62:e147–e239.

Comparison of ARNI with ACE inhibitors, to Determine Impact on Global Mortality and Morbidity in Heart Failure (PARADIGM-HF) trial.[56] PARADIGM-HF was a double-blind randomized controlled trial of enalapril versus sacubitril/valsartan in 8442 patients with NYHA class II-IV symptoms and an LVEF ≤40% with a primary endpoint of cardiovascular death or HF hospitalization. For inclusion in the trial, participants had to be taking a stable dose of ACE or ARB equivalent to at least 10 mg of enalapril daily for at least 4 weeks. In addition, prior to randomization, patients had to tolerate a single-blind run-in period of enalapril 10 mg twice daily followed by sacubitril/valsartan uptitrated to 97/103 twice daily. The trial was stopped early by the Data Safety Monitoring Board with a median follow-up of 27 months given the overwhelming evidence for a clinically important benefit of sacubitril/valsartan on cardiovascular mortality. There was a 20% relative reduction in the primary endpoint with sacubitril/valsartan compared with enalapril (**Fig. 37.8**). The benefits with sacubitril/valsartan were consistent across study endpoints, including all-cause mortality (HR 0.84, 95% CI 0.76–0.93, $P < .001$), cardiovascular mortality (HR 0.80, 95% CI 0.71–0.89, $P < .001$), and HF hospitalization (HR 0.79, 95% CI 0.71–0.89,

$P < .001$). Patients receiving sacubitril/valsartan had more symptomatic hypotension and nonserious angioedema, but less renal impairment, hyperkalemia, and cough than the enalapril group. The findings of this large clinical trial provide strong support for using sacubitril/valsartan instead of ACE inhibitors in the treatment of chronic HF. The recent ACC/AHA guideline update now includes a class I recommendation for replacing ACE inhibitors or ARB therapy in patients with chronic symptomatic HFrEF (NYHA class II or III) to further reduce morbidity and mortality.[51]

The use of sacubitril/valsartan was also shown in the PARADIGM-HF trial to result in modest benefits in health-related quality of life compared with enalapril.[57] Specifically, the change in Kansas City Cardiomyopathy Questionnaire (KCCQ) score from baseline to 8 months demonstrated less worsening in the sacubitril/valsartan group. The between-group difference was 1.64 points (95% CI of 0.63–2.65; $P = .001$). This benefit was observed across different age groups in the study population (**Fig. 37.9**).[58] Additional post hoc analyses of the PARADIGM-HF trial have demonstrated that sacubitril/valsartan, as compared with enalapril, results in substantial reductions in time to first hospitalization for HF during the first 30 days of use and that mortality benefits are in large part

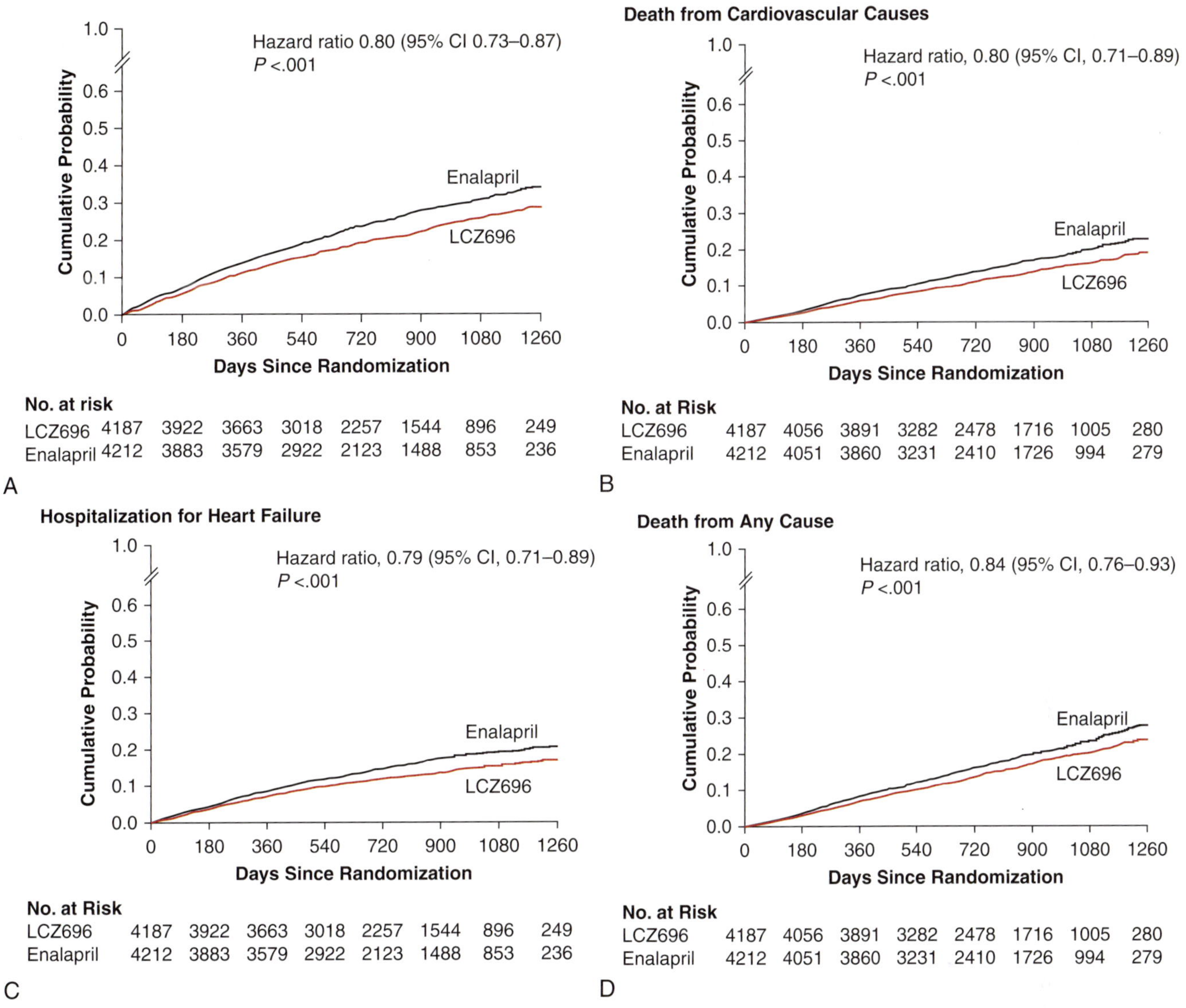

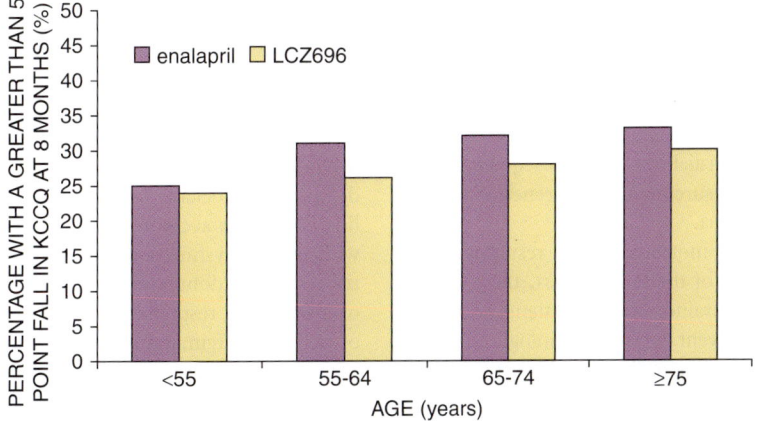

Fig. 37.8 Kaplan-Meier curve for *Panel A*, the primary composite endpoint (death from cardiovascular causes or first hospitalization for heart failure), *Panel B*, cardiovascular death, *Panel C*, Hospitalization for heart failure, *Panel D*, all-cause mortality, according to treatment with either sacubitril-valsartan *(red line)* or enalapril *(blue line)*. (From McMurray JJ, Packer M, Desai AS, et al.; For the PARADIGM-HF Investigators and Committees. Angiotensin-neprilysin inhibition versus enalapril in heart failure. *N Engl J Med.* 2014;371:993–1004.)

Fig. 37.9 Change in quality of life between treatment with sacubitril-valsartan *(hatched lines)* versus enalapril *(solid boxes)* in the PARADIGM-HF study, stratified by age. (From Jhund PS, Fu M, Bayram E, et al. Efficacy and safety of LCZ696 (sacubitril-valsartan) according to age: insights from PARADIGM-HF. *Eur Heart J.* 2015;36:2576–2584.)

due to reductions in sudden death and worsening HF death.[59] Recently, the PIONEER-HF (Comparison of Sacubitril–Valsartan versus Enalapril on Effect on NT-proBNP in Patients Stabilized from an Acute Heart Failure Episode) trial demonstrated that sacubitril/valsartan initiation during a hospitalization for acute decompensated HF as compared with enalapril initiation resulted in greater reduction in NT-proBNP through weeks 4 and 8 and was safe in terms of worsening renal function, hyperkalemia, and symptomatic hypotension.[59a] A number of ongoing clinical trials are addressing gaps in knowledge around the use of sacubitril/valsartan including use in those with advanced symptoms (LIFE [Entresto (LCZ696) In Advanced Heart Failure]) and in patients with HFpEF (PARAGON [Efficacy and Safety of LCZ696 Compared to Valsartan, on Morbidity and Mortality in Heart Failure Patients With Preserved Ejection Fraction]).

Practical Tips

Angiotensin Receptor-Neprilysin Inhibitor. The recommended starting dose for sacubitril/valsartan is 49/51 mg twice daily with doubling of the dose after 2 to 4 weeks to a target of 97/103 mg twice daily. Per the medication label, the dose should be reduced to 24/26 mg twice daily for ACE inhibitor–or ARB-naïve patients, for those taking lower doses, and for those with severe renal impairment (estimated glomerular filtration rate [eGFR]<30 mL/min/1.73 m^2) or moderate hepatic impairment. Sacubitril/valsartan lowers blood pressure and may cause symptomatic hypotension. Volume status and salt depletion should be corrected prior to starting the medication, and diuretic reduction may also be needed if patients are relatively euvolemic at the time of initiation. If hypotension occurs after addressing these other considerations, then the dose should be reduced or temporarily discontinued. Blood pressure (including postural changes), renal function, and potassium should be evaluated within 1 to 2 weeks after initiation of sacubitril/valsartan, especially in patients with preexisting azotemia, hypotension, hyponatremia, diabetes mellitus, or in those taking potassium supplements. Sacubitril/valsartan should not be administered concomitantly with ACE inhibitors or within 36 hours of the last dose of an ACE inhibitor (class III recommendation).

β-Blockers

Rationale/Pathophysiologic Basis for Use

A detailed description of the role of the adrenergic system in HF is included in **Chapter 6**. Early studies demonstrating that the failing heart was subjected to too much adrenergic stimulation provided the rationale for β-blocker therapy. To address the question of whether adrenergic activity and β-adrenergic signaling were increased or decreased in the failing human heart, end-stage failing hearts from cardiac transplant recipients were compared with nonfailing unused organ donor hearts; in failing hearts, β-receptor density and signaling were found to be markedly reduced, which was interpreted as evidence of exposure to increased adrenergic activity and of a mechanism responsible for compromised myocardial reserve.[60] Subsequent observations clearly showed, by direct measurement, that adrenergic activity is increased in the failing human heart.[61]

Because of their acute negative inotropic effects resulting from interruption of adrenergic support of the failing heart, these agents were initially considered to be contraindicated in patients with HF. However, β-blocking agents also prevent the adverse biologic effects of chronically elevated adrenergic signaling in the failing heart, which is the basis for their salutary therapeutic effects. β-blockers competitively antagonize one or more adrenergic receptors (α_1, β_1, and β_2). Although there are a number of potential benefits to blocking all three receptors, most of the deleterious effects of sympathetic activation are mediated by the β_1-adrenergic receptor. Indeed, demonstration of the beneficial effects of β-blocking agents on cardiac function and outcomes is the final proof of the hypothesis that chronic adrenergic activation is a major determinant of the progressive clinical course of HF. In addition, detailed functional, structural, and gene expression analyses have demonstrated that with β-blocker treatment, the dysfunctional, remodeled left or right ventricle can improve in HF patients.

When given in concert with ACE inhibitors, β-blockers reverse the process of LV remodeling, improve patient symptoms, prevent hospitalization, and prolong life (see Figs. 37.2 and 37.6). Indeed, the effects of β-blockade on remodeling and clinical events are probably the most dramatic of any single intervention in HF. Therefore, β-blockers are routinely indicated for all patients with symptomatic or asymptomatic HF and LVEF less than 40%.

Effects on Ventricular Structure

Multiple studies have consistently shown the beneficial effects of chronic β-blocker therapy on LV function and structure (see Fig. 37.6).[62,63] Long-term benefits include an increase in LVEF, a decrease in LV volumes and in mitral regurgitation (when present), and a reversion of the left ventricle to a more elliptical shape. Improvement in load-independent indices of myocardial contractility has also been shown, which demonstrates that the improvement is related to changes in the intrinsic properties of the myocardium. LV diastolic function and right ventricular function are also improved by long-term β-blocker therapy. Although RAAS inhibitors have also been shown to impact LV remodeling, the effects of β-blocker therapy are generally more dramatic and include "normalization" or near normalization of ventricular structure and LV function in a minority of patients.

The functional effects of β-blocker therapy on the failing heart are biphasic.[64] Administration of β-blockers may be associated with an early, short-term deterioration in cardiac function, which is consistent with the negative inotropic effects of adrenergic drive withdrawal and is enhanced in the failing heart because of its dependence on adrenergic support. Carefully performed studies with serial echocardiography have shown a decrease from baseline in LVEF in the first few days of treatment, followed by return to baseline values after 1 month.[64] An increase in LVEF from baseline values starts to become apparent after 3 to 4 months of treatment and tends to improve further for at least another year. At 3 to 4 months, a decrease in LV volumes and favorable changes in shape also become apparent. From a clinical standpoint, this initial deterioration in LV function is generally not apparent if β-blocker therapy is initiated gradually and slowly uptitrated in patients who are relatively euvolemic.

Predictors of changes in parameters of LV function have been identified and are rather consistent across multiple studies. Predictors of an improvement in LVEF include a nonischemic cause of HF, higher blood pressure at baseline, the administration of a higher β-blocker dose, and higher baseline heart rates.[65] Patients with a nonischemic cause generally show a greater contractile reserve. Higher heart rate at baseline and the administration of a higher, rather than lower, β-blocker dosage are related to the level of adrenergic drive and the degree of β-blockade, respectively. A higher blood pressure at baseline is a rather accurate index of contractile reserve in left ventricles with systolic dysfunction. Accordingly, the demonstration of contractile reserve by dobutamine echocardiography is an excellent predictor of a favorable response to β-blocker therapy.[66] In patients with HF of ischemic origin, a direct relation exists between the number of LV segments showing myocardial hibernation and change in LVEF after β-blocking treatment.[67] The basis of all these observations is the fact that the magnitude of the improvement in LV function after chronic β-blockade is directly related to the amount of viable myocardium present at baseline. Changes in LV function are related to subsequent prognosis.[68] Patients with the greatest increase in LVEF and reduction in volumes have an excellent long-term prognosis.

Effects on Functional Capacity/Symptoms

The impairment of exercise capacity in patients with HF is related to myocardial dysfunction and to the abnormalities in β-adrenergic receptor signal transduction that result in reduced cardiac sensitivity to sympathetic stimulation.[69] β-Blocker therapy improves myocardial function and, on that basis, would be expected to improve exercise performance. However, if β-adrenergic receptors are blocked by higher doses of β-blocking agents or are not upregulated by therapy, then exercise tolerance may not improve. This is because the failing heart is dependent on increasing heart rate for improving exercise capacity, more so than is the nonfailing heart. Thus, despite the improvement in cardiac function and stroke volume, both at rest and during exercise, the β-blocker–related reduced chronotropic response to exercise may prevent cardiac output from rising sufficiently during exercise to allow an improvement in exercise capacity.

In general, β_1-selective β-blocking agents, such as metoprolol, which at lower doses do not block myocardial β_2-adrenergic receptors and upregulate myocardial β_1-receptors, slightly improve maximal exercise capacity. In contrast, agents such as carvedilol and bucindolol—which may not alter myocardial β_1-adrenergic receptor density, have slower offset kinetics from β_1-adrenergic receptors, and also block β_2-adrenergic receptors—may not allow an increase in peak exercise cardiac output and heart rate sufficient to improve exercise capacity and peak VO$_2$. Multicenter trials have also generally failed to show any change in submaximal exercise capacity.[70]

In contrast to direct measurements of exercise capacity, most controlled studies have shown a significant improvement in symptoms and functional class in patients with HF treated with β-blockers.[71] Data suggest that patients treated with a β-blocker were 32% more likely to experience an improvement and 30% less likely to experience a worsening in NYHA class.[72] Direct assessment of HF symptoms, and global clinical assessment (a quality-of-life measurement) by either the patient or the physician, have been similarly sensitive, showing an improvement in clinical status.[71] The interpretation of the functional capacity and symptom outcomes of these studies is that β-blockade does not worsen exercise capacity, and the improvement in cardiac function is associated, albeit indirectly, with an improvement in symptoms and quality-of-life measures.

Effects on Morbidity and Mortality

Three β-blockers have been shown to be effective in reducing the risk of death in patients with chronic HF: bisoprolol and sustained-release metoprolol succinate competitively block the β_1 receptor, and carvedilol competitively blocks the α_1, β_1, and β_2 receptors. A summary of the major outcome trials of β-blockers is provided in **Table 37.4**.

The first placebo-controlled multicenter trial with a β-blocking agent was the Metoprolol in Dilated Cardiomyopathy (MDC) trial, which used the shorter-acting tartrate preparation at a target dose of 50 mg three times a day in symptomatic HF patients with idiopathic dilated cardiomyopathy.[73] Metoprolol tartrate at an average dose of 108 mg/day reduced the prevalence of the primary endpoint of death or need for cardiac transplantation by 34%, which did not quite reach statistical significance ($P = .058$). The benefit was due entirely to a reduction by metoprolol in the morbidity component of the primary endpoint, with no favorable trends in the mortality component of the primary endpoint.

A more efficacious formulation of metoprolol was subsequently developed, metoprolol (succinate) CR/XL, which has a better pharmacologic profile than metoprolol tartrate because of its controlled-release profile and longer half-life. In the Metoprolol CR/XL Randomized Intervention Trial in Congestive Heart Failure (MERIT-HF), metoprolol CR/XL provided a significant relative risk reduction in mortality of 34% in subjects with mild to moderate HF and moderate to severe systolic dysfunction when compared with the placebo group.[74] Importantly, metoprolol CR/XL reduced mortality from both sudden death and progressive pump failure. Further, mortality was reduced across most demographic groups, including older versus younger subjects, nonischemic versus ischemic causes, and lower versus higher EFs.

Bisoprolol is a second-generation β_1 receptor-selective blocking agent with approximately 120-fold higher affinity for human β_1 versus β_2 receptors. The first trial performed with bisoprolol was the Cardiac Insufficiency Bisoprolol Study I (CIBIS-I) trial, which examined the effects of bisoprolol on mortality in subjects with symptomatic ischemic or nonischemic cardiomyopathy.[75] CIBIS-I showed a nonsignificant 20% risk reduction for mortality at 2 years' follow-up ($P = .22$). Because the sample size for CIBIS-I was based on an unrealistically high expected event rate in the control group, a follow-up trial with more conservative effect size estimates and sample size calculations was conducted. In CIBIS-II, bisoprolol reduced all-cause mortality by 32% (11.8% vs. 17.3%, $P = .002$), sudden cardiac death by 45% (3.6% vs. 6.4%, $P = .001$), HF hospitalizations by 30% (11.9% bisoprolol vs. 17.6% placebo, $P < .001$), and all-cause hospitalizations by 15% (33.6% vs. 39.6%, $P = .002$).[76] The CIBIS-III trial addressed the important question of whether an initial treatment strategy using the β-blocker bisoprolol was noninferior to a treatment strategy of using an ACE inhibitor (enalapril) first, among patients with newly diagnosed mild to moderate HF.[77] The two strategies were compared in a blinded manner with regard to the combined primary endpoint of all-cause mortality or hospitalization,

TABLE 37.4 Key Randomized Placebo-Controlled Trials of β-Blockers in Heart Failure

Trial Name	Agent	NYHA Class	No. of Subjects Enrolled	12-Month Control Mortality (%)	12-Month Effect Size (%)	P Value 12 Months (Full F/U)
Heart Failure						
CIBIS-I	Bisoprolol	III, IV	641	21	↓20	NS (.22)
US Carvedilol	Carvedilol	II, III	1094	8	↓66	NS (<.001)
ANZ Carvedilol	Carvedilol	I–III	415	NS	NS	NS (>.1)
CIBIS-II	Bisoprolol	III, IV	2647	12	↓34	NS (.001)
MERIT-HF	Metoprolol CR	II–IV	3991	10	↓35	NS (.006)
BEST	Bucindolol	III, IV	2708	23	↓10	NS (.16)
COPERNICUS	Carvedilol	Severe	2289	28	↓38	NS (.0001)
Post-MI						
CAPRICORN	Carvedilol	I	1959		↓23	NS (.03)
BEAT	Bucindolol	I	343	NS	↓12	NS (.06)

MI, Myocardial infarction; *NS,* not specified; *NYHA,* New York Heart Association.

and with regard to each of the components of the primary endpoint individually. Although the per-protocol primary endpoint analysis of death or rehospitalization did not meet the prespecified criteria for noninferiority, the intent-to-treat analysis showed that bisoprolol was noninferior to enalapril (HR 0.94, 95% CI 0.77–1.16, P = .019 for noninferiority). Although CIBIS-III did not provide clear-cut evidence to justify starting with a β-blocker first, the overall safety profile of the two strategies was similar. Current guidelines continue to recommend starting with an ACE inhibitor first, followed by the subsequent addition of a β-blocker.

Of the three β-blockers that are approved for the treatment of HF, carvedilol has been studied most extensively. The phase III US Trials Program, composed of four individual trials managed by a single Steering and Data and Safety Monitoring Committee, was stopped prematurely because of a highly significant 65% reduction in mortality by carvedilol that was observed across all four trials (P < .0001).[68] This was followed by a second study, the Australia-New Zealand Heart Failure Research Collaborative Group Carvedilol Trial (ANZ-Carvedilol), which showed there was a significant improvement in LVEF (P < .0001) and a significant (P = .0015) reduction in LV end-diastolic volume index in the carvedilol treated group at 12 months, and a significant relative risk reduction of 26% in the clinical composite of death or hospitalization for the carvedilol group at 19 months.[78] Rates of hospitalization were also significantly lower for patients treated with carvedilol (48%) compared with the placebo (58%). The Carvedilol Prospective Randomized Cumulative Survival (COPERNICUS) study extended these benefits to patients with more advanced HF.[79] In COPERNICUS, patients with advanced HF symptoms had to be clinically euvolemic and have an LVEF less than 25%. When compared with placebo, carvedilol reduced the mortality risk at 12 months by 38% and the relative risk of death or HF hospitalization by 31%. Carvedilol has also been evaluated in a post-MI trial in which patients had to exhibit LV dysfunction. The Carvedilol Post-Infarct Survival Controlled Evaluation (CAPRICORN) trial was a randomized, placebo-controlled trial designed to test the long-term efficacy of carvedilol on morbidity and mortality in patients with LV dysfunction after MI who were already treated with ACE inhibitors.[80] Although carvedilol did not reduce the prespecified primary endpoint of mortality plus cardiovascular hospitalization, it did significantly reduce total mortality by 23% (P = .03), cardiovascular mortality by 25% (P < .05), and nonfatal MI by 41% (P = .014). Finally, in the Carvedilol or Metoprolol European Trial (COMET) carvedilol (target dose, 25 mg twice daily) was compared with immediate-release metoprolol tartrate (target dose, 50 mg twice daily) with respect to the primary endpoint of all-cause mortality.[81] In COMET, carvedilol was associated with a significant 33% reduction in all-cause mortality when compared with metoprolol tartrate (33.9% vs. 39.5%, HR 0.83, 95% CI 0.74–0.93, P = .0017) (**Fig. 37.10**). Based on the results of the COMET trial, short-acting metoprolol tartrate is not recommended for use in the treatment of HF. The results of the COMET trial emphasize the importance of using doses and formulations of β-blockers that have been shown to be effective in clinical trials. There have been no head-to-head trials to ascertain whether the survival benefits of carvedilol are greater than those of metoprolol (succinate) CR/XL when both drugs are used at the appropriate target doses.

Not all studies with β-blockers have been universally successful, suggesting that the effects of β-blockers should not necessarily be viewed broadly as a class effect. Indeed, early studies with the first generation of nonspecific $β_1$ and $β_2$ receptors without ancillary vasodilating properties (e.g., propranolol) resulted in significant worsening of HF and death. The Beta-blocker Evaluation of Survival Trial (BEST) evaluated the third-generation β-blocking agent bucindolol, which is a completely nonselective $β_1$ and $β_2$ blocker with some $α_1$-receptor blockade properties.[82] Although the BEST trial showed that there was a nonsignificant (P = .10) 10% reduction in total mortality in the bucindolol-treated

group, there was a statistically significant 19% reduction in mortality in white patients (P = .01). The differential response of bucindolol in white patients has been suggested to be secondary to a polymorphism (Arginine 389) in the $β_1$-adrenergic receptor that is more prevalent in white patients.[83] There is ongoing investigation into whether genetically guided therapy with bucindolol may be appropriate in some patients for treatment of HF and/or prevention of atrial fibrillation (GENETIC-AF; clinicaltrials.gov identifier: NCT01970501). Nebivolol is a selective $β_1$ receptor antagonist with ancillary vasodilatory properties that are mediated, at least in part, by NO. In the Study of Effects of Nebivolol Intervention on Outcomes and Rehospitalization in Seniors with Heart Failure (SENIORS), nebivolol significantly reduced the composite outcome of death or cardiovascular hospitalizations (HR 0.86, 95% CI 0.74–0.99, P < .04), which was the primary endpoint of the trial, but did not reduce mortality.[84] Although approximately 35% of the patients in SENIORS had an LVEF greater than 35%, more than half of these patients had an EF ranging from 35% to 50% and thus would not be considered as HFpEF patients. Nebivolol is not currently FDA approved for the treatment of HF.

Side Effects

The adverse effects of β-blockers are generally related to the predictable complications that arise from interfering with the adrenergic nervous system. These reactions generally occur within several days of initiating therapy, and are generally responsive to adjusting concomitant medications as described earlier. Treatment with a β-blocker can be accompanied by feelings of general fatigue or weakness. In most cases, the increased fatigue spontaneously resolves within several weeks or months; however, in some patients, it may be severe enough to limit the dose of β-blocker or require the withdrawal or reduction of treatment. Therapy with β-blockers can lead to bradycardia and/or exacerbate heart block. Moreover, β-blockers (particularly those that block the $α_1$ receptor) can lead to vasodilatory side effects. Accordingly, the dose of β-blockers should be decreased if the heart rate decreases to less than 50 beats/min and/or second- or third-degree heart block develops, or symptomatic hypotension develops. Continuation of β-blocker

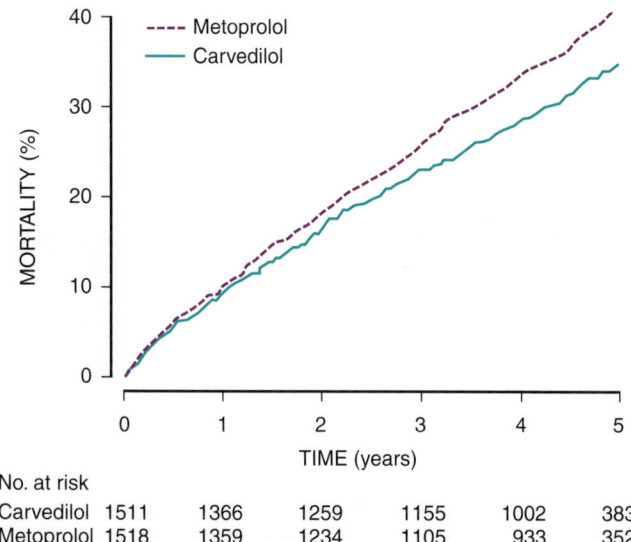

Fig. 37.10 All-cause mortality in the Carvedilol or Metoprolol European Trial *(COMET)* with carvedilol compared with immediate-release metoprolol tartrate. (From Poole-Wilson PA, Swedberg K, Cleland JG, et al. Comparison of carvedilol and metoprolol on clinical outcomes in patients with chronic heart failure in the Carvedilol Or Metoprolol European Trial (COMET): randomised controlled trial. *Lancet.* 2003;362:7–13.)

treatment during an episode of acute HF decompensation has been shown to be safe in randomized trials.[85] β-blockers are not recommended for patients with asthma and active bronchospasm, although they can be tolerated by most patients with chronic lung disease.

Practical Tips

Analogous to the use of ACE inhibitors, β-blockers should be initiated in low doses (see Table 37.3), followed by gradual increments in the dose if lower doses have been well tolerated. The dose of β-blocker should be increased until the doses used are similar to those that have been reported to be effective in clinical trials (see Table 37.3). Furthermore, in patients taking a low dose of an ACE inhibitor, the addition of a β-blocker appears to produce a greater improvement in symptoms and reduction in the risk of death than an increase in the dose of the ACE inhibitor, although this question has never been specifically subjected to randomized trials. However, unlike ACE inhibitors, which may be uptitrated relatively rapidly, the dose titration of β-blockers should proceed no sooner than 2-week intervals, because the initiation and/or increased dosing of these agents may lead to worsening fluid retention because of the abrupt withdrawal of adrenergic support to the heart and the circulation. Therefore, it is important to optimize the dose of diuretic before starting therapy with β-blockers. If worsening fluid retention does occur, it is likely to occur within 3 to 5 days of initiating therapy and will be manifest as an increase in body weight and/or symptoms of worsening HF. The increased fluid retention can usually be managed by increasing the dose of diuretics. Patients need not be taking high doses of ACE inhibitors before being considered for treatment with a β-blocker, because most patients enrolled in the β-blocker trials were not taking high doses of ACE inhibitors.

Randomized trial data from the IMPACT HF study show that β-blockers can be safely started before discharge even in patients hospitalized for HF, provided that the patients are stable and do not require intravenous HF therapy.[86] Contrary to initial concerns, the aggregate results of clinical trials suggest that β-blocker therapy is well tolerated by the great majority of HF patients (>85%), including patients with comorbid conditions, such as diabetes mellitus, chronic obstructive lung disease, and peripheral vascular disease. Nonetheless, there are a subset of patients (10%–15%) who remain intolerant to β-blockers because of worsening fluid retention or symptomatic hypotension and a minority who are intolerant because of reactive airway disease.

Mineralocorticoid Receptor Antagonists
Rationale/Pathophysiologic Basis for Use

Effects of RAAS activation are also mediated through aldosterone, the secretion of which is partially under the control of angiotensin II stimulation of the AT_1 receptor. Even in the presence of angiotensin II inhibition, increases in aldosterone persist in the circulation (endocrine effects) and at tissue levels (autocrine and paracrine effects).[87] Clinical studies have shown a "breakthrough" of aldosterone levels after prolonged treatment with an ARB or an ACE inhibitor in chronic HF.[35] Aside from its effect on renal sodium-potassium exchange, the mineralocorticoid receptor mediates a wide array of effects across the cardiovascular system. There is substantial experimental evidence that mineralocorticoid receptor activation contributes to several adverse myocardial effects, such as increased myocardial fibrosis, inflammation, myocyte hypertrophy, and apoptosis.[88-90] Jaffe and associates reported that mineralocorticoid receptors are expressed in blood vessels and regulate gene transcription in vascular smooth muscle cells.[91] They also reported the intriguing finding that angiotensin II promoted mineralocorticoid receptor–specific effects in the absence of aldosterone; thus, indirect mineralocorticoid receptor activation probably contributes importantly to RAAS-induced pathologic effects throughout the cardiovascular and renal systems.

The fact that the mineralocorticoid receptor may be activated by aldosterone and alternative stimuli, and the multifaceted means through which such activation may accelerate the advance of cardiovascular disease, represents a rationale for exploring the benefits of MRAs, on top of ACE inhibitors or ARBs.

Effects on Ventricular Structure/Hemodynamics

Findings related to the effects of mineralocorticoid receptor inhibition on cardiac remodeling in HF have been mixed. Some studies have suggested a benefit. For example, Hayashi and colleagues demonstrated that administration of the MRA spironolactone prevents postinfarct LV remodeling associated with suppression of a marker of myocardial collagen synthesis.[92] In contrast, Udelson and colleagues found no remodeling effect with the selective MRA eplerenone when added to an ACE inhibitor and β-blocker during 9 months of randomized, controlled treatment in patients with NYHA class II to class III HF and reduced LVEF.[93] It is possible that the reduction in mortality observed with mineralocorticoid receptor blockers in selected populations with HF is at least partly mediated by vascular effects or other pleiotropic effects, as opposed to myocardial effects. Although the mechanism for the beneficial effect of spironolactone has not been fully elucidated, prevention of extracellular matrix remodeling and prevention of hypokalemia are plausible mechanisms.

Effects on Morbidity and Mortality

Three landmark studies demonstrated reduced mortality when patients with HF and reduced LVEF were treated with an MRA (**Fig. 37.11**). The first evidence that MRAs could produce a major clinical benefit in HF was demonstrated by the Randomized Aldactone Evaluation Study (RALES) trial, which evaluated spironolactone (25 mg per day initially, titrated to 50 mg/day for signs of worsening HF) versus a placebo in NYHA class III or IV HF patients with an LVEF less than 35%, who were being treated with an ACE inhibitor, a loop diuretic, and in most cases digoxin.[94] Spironolactone led to a 30% reduction in total mortality when compared with the placebo ($P = .001$). The frequency of hospitalization for worsening HF was also 35% lower in the spironolactone group than in the placebo group.

The Eplerenone in Mild Patients Hospitalization and Survival Study in Heart Failure (EMPHASIS-HF) trial, which was performed in patients with NYHA class II HF with an EF less than 30% (or 35% if the QRS width was >130 msec), demonstrated that eplerenone (titrated to 50 mg/day) led to a significant 27% decrease in cardiovascular death or HF hospitalization (HR 0.63, 95% CI 0.54–0.74, $P < .001$).[95] There were also significant decreases in all-cause death (24%), cardiovascular death (24%), all-cause hospitalization (23%), and HF hospitalizations (43%). Importantly, the effect of eplerenone was consistent across all prespecified subgroups. In contrast to the RALES trial, which was conducted before the widespread adoption of β-blockers, the background therapy for EMPHASIS-HF included ACE inhibitors or ARBs and β-blockers.

The findings in RALES and EMPHASIS-HF are consistent with findings in randomized clinical trials (RCTs) in patients with acute MI and LV dysfunction. The Eplerenone Post-Acute Myocardial Infarction Heart Failure Efficacy and Survival Study (EPHESUS) evaluated the effect of eplerenone (titrated to a maximum of 50 mg/day) on morbidity and mortality among patients with acute MI complicated by LV dysfunction and HF.[96] Treatment with eplerenone led to 15% decrease in all-cause death in the EPHESUS trial (RR 0.85, 95 CI 0.75–0.96, $P = .008$). Based on the results of the RALES and EMPHASIS-HF trials, MRAs are currently recommended for all patients with persistent NYHA class II–IV symptoms and an EF less than 35%, despite treatment with an ACE inhibitor (or an ARB if an ACE inhibitor is not tolerated) and a β-blocker.

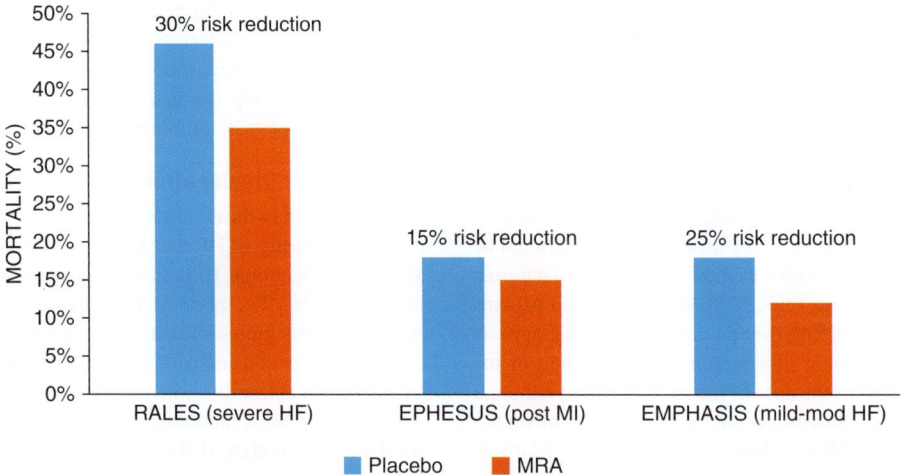

Fig. 37.11 Comparison of treatment effects and risk reduction in mortality for mineralocorticoid receptor antagonists *(MRA)* versus placebo in severe heart failure (RALES), post myocardial infarction heart failure (EPHESUS), or mild to moderate heart failure (EMPHASIS). (Data from Pitt B, Zannad F, Remme WJ, et al. The effect of spironolactone on morbidity and mortality in patients with severe heart failure. Randomized Aldactone Evaluation Study Investigators. N Engl J Med. 1999;341:709–717; Pitt B, Remme W, Zannad F, et al. Eplerenone, a selective aldosterone blocker, in patients with left ventricular dysfunction after myocardial infarction. N Engl J Med. 2003;348:1309–1321; and Zannad F, McMurray JJ, Krum H, et al. Eplerenone in patients with systolic heart failure and mild symptoms. N Engl J Med. 2011;364:11–21.)

Side Effects

The major problem with the use of MRAs is the development of life-threatening hyperkalemia, which is more prone to occur in patients who are receiving potassium supplements or who have underlying renal insufficiency. Aldosterone antagonists are not recommended when the serum creatinine is greater than 2.5 mg/dL (or creatinine clearance is <30 mL/min) or the serum potassium is greater than 5.5 mmol/L. The development of worsening renal function should lead to consideration regarding stopping aldosterone antagonists because of the potential risk of hyperkalemia. Although the rate of significant hyperkalemia is relatively modest in clinical trials (≈2%–3%), outcomes data suggest that it is potentially much higher in clinical practice with less intensive monitoring of potassium.[97] Painful gynecomastia may develop in 10% to 15% of patients who use spironolactone, in which case eplerenone may be substituted.

Practical Tips

The administration of an MRA is recommended for patients with NYHA class II to IV HF who have EF less than 35% and who are receiving standard therapy, including diuretics, ACE inhibitors, and β-blockers. Spironolactone should be initiated at a dose of 12.5 to 25 mg daily, and uptitrated to 25 to 50 mg daily, whereas eplerenone should be initiated at doses of 25 mg/day and increased to 50 mg daily. As noted previously, potassium supplementation is generally stopped after the initiation of aldosterone antagonists, and patients should be counseled to avoid food that have a high potassium content. Potassium levels and renal function should be rechecked within 3 days and again at 1 week after initiation of an aldosterone antagonist. Subsequent monitoring should be dictated by the general clinical stability of renal function and fluid status but should occur at least monthly for the first 6 months.

Hydralazine and Nitrates

Therapy with the combination of hydralazine and isosorbide dinitrate (H-ISDN) has been shown to reduce all-cause mortality and morbidity in African Americans. There are two placebo-controlled (V-HeFT-I and A-HeFT) randomized trials and one active-controlled (V-HeFT-II) randomized trial with H-ISDN.

The biology of nitrate therapy in HF is complex and is complicated by issues such as nitrate tolerance and variations in nitrate dosing.[98] Studies have demonstrated several mechanisms for nitrate tolerance, which occur within several days of initiating therapy.[99] In brief, chronic nitrate therapy increases vascular oxidative stress via production of superoxide from mitochondrial sources, vascular smooth muscle, and endothelium. The resulting reactive oxygen species (ROS) inhibit the bioactivation of administered nitrate into NO. This "quenching of NO" by ROS reduces dilator metabolites.

To combat these mechanisms, radical scavengers and substances, which reduce oxidative stress indirectly, are able to relieve tolerance and endothelial dysfunction. For example, hydralazine is an efficient ROS scavenger, which prevents the development of nitrate tolerance when given concomitantly with nitrates. Additional agents postulated to limit or reverse nitrate tolerance include ACE inhibitors, ARBs, β-blockers, statins, folic acid, and vitamin C.

The Veterans Administration Cooperative Study on Vasodilator Therapy of Heart Failure (V-HeFT-I) investigated 642 male patients with chronic HF treated with digoxin and diuretics. Patients were randomized to H-ISDN, prazosin, or a placebo.[100] Published in 1986, no study patients were treated with β-blockers or ACE inhibitors. H-ISDN increased exercise capacity and LVEF compared with placebo. Treatment with H-ISDN produced a 28% reduction in mortality compared with the placebo. The benefit of H-ISDN was particularly prominent in younger patients with a lower EF. H-ISDN did not reduce hospitalizations.

In V-HeFT-II, 804 men, mainly with NYHA class II or III symptoms, were randomized to enalapril or H-ISDN (300 /160 mg), added to a diuretic and digoxin.[29] No patients were treated with a β-blocker. Enalapril produced more favorable effects on survival. There was a trend in the H-ISDN group toward an increase in all-cause mortality during the overall period of follow-up (mean 2.5 years): relative increase in risk was 28%. However, H-ISDN increased peak oxygen consumption and resulted in a greater increase in LVEF compared with enalapril.

A post hoc retrospective analysis of these vasodilator trials demonstrated particular efficacy of H-ISDN in the African American cohort.[101] Thus a subsequent trial of H-ISDN was conducted that was limited to patients self-described as African American, the African-American Heart Failure Trial (A-HeFT).[102] In A-HeFT, 1050 African American men and women with NYHA class III or IV HF symptoms were randomized to a placebo or a fixed-dose combination H-ISDN. The initial dose of treatment was 37.5 mg hydralazine/20 mg ISDN three times daily, increasing to a target of 75 /40 mg three times daily. Published in 2004, study patients received medical management similar to contemporary guideline recommendations: ACE inhibitor (70%), ARB (17%), β-blocker (74%), and spironolactone (39%). The trial was discontinued prematurely after a median follow-up of 10 months because of a significant reduction in mortality with H-ISDN. The primary endpoint was a weighted composite score of all-cause mortality, first hospitalization for HF, and change in the quality of life. H-ISDN also reduced the risk of HF hospitalization and improved quality of life. Despite these impressive results, uptake of this therapy in African American patients has been modest, with data suggesting that fewer than 10% of eligible patients are treated with this therapy.[103] Many potential factors may contribute to the underutilization of this therapy. The inclusion criteria of only self-identified African American patients has led to some uncertainty, given that this is as much a social construct as a specific genetic population. Additionally, the relatively small RCT (for a phase 3 study), which was terminated early, the complexity of the regimen (and the uncertainty about the suitability of substitution of inexpensive forms of the generic drugs), and access-to-care issues are all potential contributors to low prescription rates for this form of treatment.

Side Effects

The most common adverse effects with H-ISDN in the landmark trials were headache, dizziness/hypotension, and nausea. Arthralgia leading to discontinuation or reduction in dose of H-ISDN occurred in 5% to 10% of patients in V-HeFT I and II. A lupus-like syndrome has also been rarely reported, but a sustained increase in antinuclear antibody occurs in 2% to 3% of patients.

Practical Tips

H-ISDN should not be used in patients who have no prior use of ACE inhibitors/ARBs or β-blockers and should not be substituted for ACE inhibitors/ARBs in patients who are tolerating therapy without difficulty. Adherence to this combination has generally been poor because of the number of daily doses and tablets required, and the side-effect profile including headache and dizziness. However, the benefit of these drugs can be substantial in specific patient populations who have been studied in randomized trials. Therefore, slower titration of the drugs should be performed to enhance tolerance of the therapy. If the fixed-dose combination is available, the initial dose should be one tablet containing 37.5 mg of hydralazine hydrochloride and 20 mg of isosorbide dinitrate three times daily. The dose can be increased to two tablets three times daily for a total daily dose of 225 mg of hydralazine hydrochloride and 120 mg of isosorbide dinitrate. When the two drugs are used separately, both pills should be administered at least three times daily. Initial low doses of the drugs given separately may be progressively increased to a goal similar to that achieved in the fixed-dose combination trial.

Ivabradine

Ivabradine is a heart rate–lowering agent that acts by selectively blocking the cardiac pacemaker If ("funny") current that controls the spontaneous diastolic depolarization of the sinoatrial node. Ivabradine blocks I$_f$ channels in a concentration-dependent manner by entering the channel pore from the intracellular side, and thus can only block the channel when it is open. The magnitude of I$_f$ inhibition is directly related to the frequency of channel opening and would therefore be expected to be most effective at higher heart rates. Initially developed and approved as an antianginal agent in Europe, ivabradine was also shown to improve outcomes in the Systolic Heart failure treatment with the If inhibitor Ivabradine Trial (SHIFT), which enrolled symptomatic patients with an LVEF of 35% or less who were in sinus rhythm with a heart rate of 70 beats/min or more and on standard medical therapy for HF (including β-blockers).[104] SHIFT showed that ivabradine (uptitrated to a maximal dosage of 7.5 mg twice daily) reduced the primary composite outcome of cardiovascular death or HF hospitalization by 18% (HR 0.82, 95% CI 0.75–0.90, $P < .0001$ (**Fig. 37.12**). The composite endpoint was driven primarily by reducing hospital admissions for worsening HF (HR 0.74, CI 0.66–0.83, $P < .0001$), insofar as there was no decrease in cardiovascular deaths (HR 0.91, 95% CI 0.80–1.03, $P = .13$) or all-cause deaths. Given that ivabradine lowered heart rate by approximately 10 beats/min and that only 26% of the patients in the trial were on optimal doses of β-blockers, it is possible that titrating β-blockers to recommended doses may have reduced the HF hospitalizations to a similar degree. Additional safety evidence for ivabradine comes from the morbidity-mortality evaluation of the I$_f$ inhibitor ivabradine in patients with coronary disease and LV dysfunction (BEAUTIFUL) trial, in which more than 10,000 patients with coronary heart disease and an EF less than 40% were randomized to treatment with ivabradine 7.5 mg twice daily.[105] Although this trial did not meet its primary endpoint of reducing cardiovascular death, MI, or HF hospitalization, it was well tolerated in this patient population.

In terms of patient-assessed symptoms and quality of life, there were modest benefits with ivabradine. Patient-reported global assessment improved in 72% of the ivabradine group versus 68% of the placebo group (P-value = .0005). For health-related quality of life via the KCCQ, the clinical and overall summary score values were better in the ivabradine group compared with placebo at 12 months (i.e., more patients experienced improvements and fewer experienced worsening). Ivabradine improved the clinical summary score (CSS) by 1.8 and the overall summary score (OSS) by 2.4 (placebo-corrected, $P = .02$ and $P < .01$, respectively).

Ivabradine use has been incorporated into the current ACC/AHA guideline recommendations.[51] Ivabradine has a class IIa recommendation to reduce HF hospitalization in symptomatic chronic HFrEF patients in normal sinus rhythm with a heart rate greater than 70 bpm who are receiving GDEM including a β-blocker at the maximally tolerated dose.

Unanswered questions regarding the use of ivabradine include the safety and efficacy of initiation in the acute HF setting, whether the benefits can be achieved on a background of more aggressive use of β-blockers, and its applicability in African American populations and in populations with higher use of implantable devices.

Digoxin

Digoxin is the oldest drug (by far) in the HF armamentarium, first described by William Withering in 1775. A derivative of the foxglove plant, digoxin works by inhibiting the Na+/K+ adenosine triphosphatase (ATPase) pump in the sarcomere, leading to increases in intracellular calcium. This results in both positive inotropic properties and negative chronotropic properties, and digoxin has long been used for both HF and rate control in atrial fibrillation. Despite the long clinical experience with digoxin, both its precise mechanism of action and its overall risk-benefit ratio in HF patients remain the subjects of debate. Early studies of digoxin in HF were focused on digoxin withdrawal; because digoxin was then the standard of care (and there were few other therapies other than diuretics), it was thought to be problematic to randomize HF patients to placebo. Early studies such as PROVED (Prospective Randomized Study of Ventricular Failure and the Efficacy of Digoxin) and RADIANCE (Randomized Assessment of [the effect of] Digoxin on Inhibitors of the Angiotensin-Converting Enzyme)

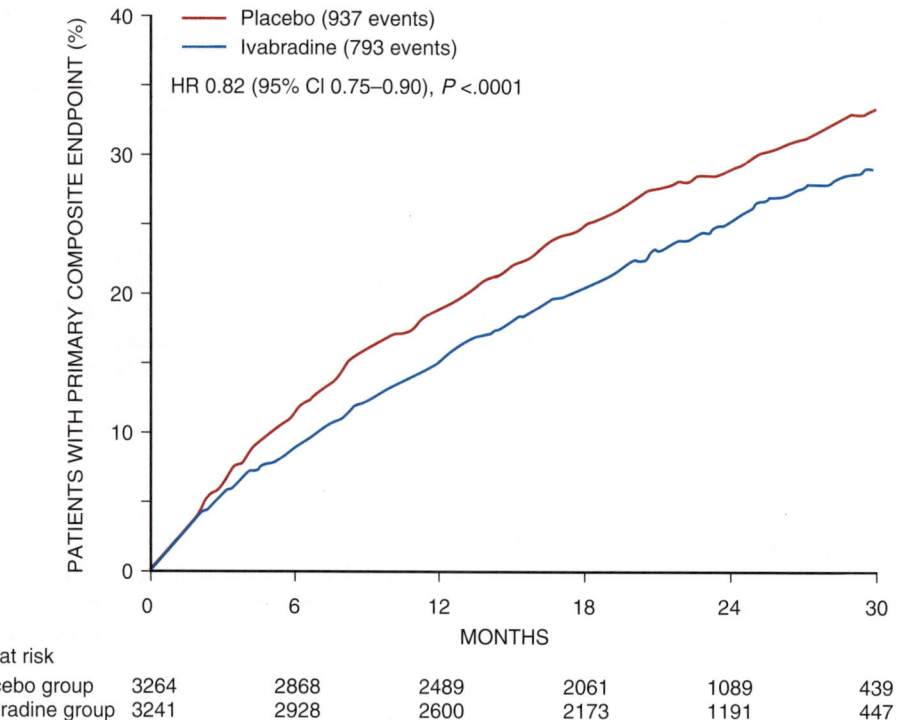

Fig. 37.12 Kaplan-Meier cumulative event curves for the primary composite endpoint of cardiovascular death or hospital admission for worsening heart failure in the Systolic Heart failure treatment with the I*f* inhibitor Ivabradine Trial. (From Swedberg K, Komajda M, Böhm M, et al. Ivabradine and outcomes in chronic heart failure (SHIFT): a randomised placebo-controlled study. Lancet. 2010;376:875–885.)

suggested that patients who had been taking digoxin chronically had clinical deterioration when digoxin was withdrawn.[106,107] The largest and most robust study of digoxin was the DIG (Digitalis Investigation Group) study, which randomized 6800 patients with symptomatic HF (NYHA class II–III) and EF ≤45% to digoxin or placebo.[108] The DIG study did not show a benefit with regard to the primary endpoints (all-cause mortality, HR = 0.99), but did show that digoxin had a favorable impact on recurrent hospitalizations for HF (HR = 0.72, P < .001). A large number of secondary analyses of the DIG trial have focused on the role of serum digoxin concentration (SDC) on the efficacy and safety of digoxin, and have generally concluded that lower SDCs (<1 ng/mL) are associated with a potentially more favorable risk-benefit profile, particularly in women.[109] A variety of nomograms have been developed that aid in calculating both the initial loading dose and maintenance dose of digoxin.[110] A number of observational studies have evaluated the efficacy of digoxin in the setting of more contemporary HF therapy and generally found no evidence of benefit. Despite the limitations of such analyses, given the uncertainty about the benefits and the narrow therapeutic window, digoxin use has generally declined in contemporary HF management. In current guidelines, digoxin is given a class IIa (LOE B) recommendation, and the guidelines note the necessity of careful patient selection and monitoring to avoid toxicity and maximize potential benefit.[1]

FUTURE DIRECTIONS

The progressive development of neurohormonal antagonists for chronic HF with systolic dysfunction has been one of the major success stories of modern cardiology. However, some have questioned whether the field has reached the ceiling benefits that can be provided by progressive neurohormonal blockade. Notably, attempts to intervene on another major pathophysiologic mechanism associated with

HF progression, such as inflammation and oxidative stress, have not yet been successful (**see also Chapters 7** and **8**). Moving forward, therapeutic development for chronic HF is increasingly focused on novel approaches covered elsewhere in this textbook, including modulation of myocardial metabolism (**see Chapter 17**), device therapies (**see Chapter 38**), neuromodulation (**see Chapter 42**), cellular and gene-based therapies (**see Chapter 41**), and mechanical circulatory support (**see Chapter 45**). In addition to ongoing development of new treatments, broad-based implementation of currently proven therapies remains a major unmet public health issue (**Chapter 49**).

KEY REFERENCES

6. Ellison DH, Felker GM. Diuretic treatment in heart failure. *N Engl J Med.* 2017;377:1964–1975.

25. Konstam MA, Rousseau MF, Kronenberg MW, et al. Effects of the angiotensin converting enzyme inhibitor enalapril on the long-term progression of left ventricular dysfunction in patients with heart failure. SOLVD Investigators. *Circulation.* 1992;86:431–438.

36. Investigators S. Effect of enalapril on mortality and the development of heart failure in asymptomatic patients with reduced left ventricular ejection fractions. The SOLVD Investigattors. *N Engl J Med.* 1992;327:685–691.

37. Pfeffer MA, Braunwald E, Moye LA, et al. Effect of captopril on mortality and morbidity in patients with left ventricular dysfunction after myocardial infarction. Results of the survival and ventricular enlargement trial. The SAVE Investigators. *N Engl J Med.* 1992;327:669–677.

52. Latini R, Tognoni G, Maggioni AP, et al. Clinical effects of early angiotensin-converting enzyme inhibitor treatment for acute myocardial infarction are similar in the presence and absence of aspirin: systematic overview of individual data from 96,712 randomized patients. Angiotensin-converting Enzyme Inhibitor Myocardial Infarction Collaborative Group. *J Am Coll Cardiol.* 2000;35:1801–1807.

56. McMurray JJ, Packer M, Desai AS, et al. Angiotensin-neprilysin inhibition versus enalapril in heart failure. *N Engl J Med.* 2014;371:993–1004.

60. Bristow MR, Ginsburg R, Minobe W, et al. Decreased catecholamine sensitivity and β-adrenergic-receptor density in failing human hearts. *New England Journal of Medicine.* 1982;307:205–211.

74. Group M-HS. Effect of metoprolol CR/XL in chronic heart failure: metoprolol CR/XL randomised intervention trial in congestive heart failure (MERIT-HF). *Lancet.* 1999;353:2001–2007.

79. Packer M, Coats AJ, Fowler MB, et al. Effect of carvedilol on survival in severe chronic heart failure. *N Engl J Med.* 2001;344:1651–1658.

94. Pitt B, Zannad F, Remme WJ, et al. The effect of spironolactone on morbidity and mortality in patients with severe heart failure. Randomized Aldactone Evaluation Study Investigators. *N Engl J Med.* 1999;341:709–717.

The full reference list for this chapter is available on ExpertConsult.

Guidelines

Management of Heart Failure with a Reduced Ejection Fraction[a]

This chapter will review guidelines for the management of patients with a reduced ejection fraction (HFrEF). A joint task force of the American College of Cardiology and the American Heart Association (ACC/AHA) published updated comprehensive guidelines for the evaluation and management of heart failure (HF) in 2013.[1] These were updated in two sequential focused guidelines in 2016[2,3] that focused on changes in medical therapies, but did not provide new guidelines for devices for diagnosing and/or treating heart failure. The Heart Failure Society of America has partnered with the ACC and the AHA to provide coordinated recommendations about the 2016 and 2017 guidelines.[5] The European Society (ESC) guidelines for the diagnosis and treatment of chronic heart failure were published 2016,[3] which superseded guidelines in 2012.[4]

The ACC/AHA guidelines classify patients according to four stages: stage A—patients at high risk for developing heart failure but without structural disorders of the heart; stage B—patients with a structural disorder of the heart but no symptoms of heart failure; stage C—patients with past or current symptoms of heart failure associated with underlying structural heart disease; and stage D—patients with end-stage disease who require specialized treatment strategies such as mechanical circulatory support, continuous inotropic infusions, cardiac transplantation, or hospice care. The following guidelines are organized into recommendations for each stage. As with other ACC/AHA guidelines, these recommendations classify interventions into one of three classes of recommendation (COR), including two levels of the intermediate group and two of the no benefit group. Included is the term *guideline-directed medical therapy (GDMT)*, which represents optimal medical therapy as defined by the ACC/AHA guideline recommended therapies.

TREATMENT OF PATIENTS AT HIGH RISK OF DEVELOPING HEART FAILURE (STAGE A)

The 2013 ACC/AHA guidelines for stage A patients (see **Table 37G.1**) are simplified from previous guidelines and continue to provide strong recommendations (class I) for treating hypertension and lipid disorders in accordance with contemporary guidelines in order to lower the risk of HF. The guidelines also suggest that other conditions that may lead to or contribute to HF, such as obesity, diabetes mellitus, tobacco use, and known cardiotoxic agents, should be controlled or avoided.

TREATMENT OF PATIENTS WITH LEFT VENTRICULAR DYSFUNCTION WHO HAVE NOT DEVELOPED SYMPTOMS (STAGE B)

The goal of therapy in stage B HF is to reduce the risk of further damage to the heart and to minimize the rate of progression of LV dysfunction (Table 37G.2). In the absence of contraindications, beta-blockers and ACE (angiotensin-converting enzyme) inhibitors (or ARBs [angiotensin receptor antagonists] in those intolerant of ACE inhibitors) are recommended for all patients with histories of myocardial infarction, regardless of ejection fraction and for all patients with diminished ejection fraction, regardless of history of myocardial infarction (class I, level of evidence A–C). In contrast, the guidelines discourage use of calcium-channel blockers with negative inotropic action in this population. The guidelines also support the use of an ICD (class IIb, level of evidence B) in patients with asymptomatic ischemic cardiomyopathy who have had a recent (>40 days) myocardial infarction with an EF of ≤30%, who are on appropriate medical therapy and have a reasonable expectation of life >1 year.

TREATMENT OF PATIENTS WITH LEFT VENTRICULAR DYSFUNCTION AND CURRENT OR PRIOR SYMPTOMS (STAGE C)

Fig. 37G.1 and **Table 37G.3** summarize the 2017 ACC/AHA/HFSA recommended approach to the treatment of stage C and D HFrEF.[5] Application of the same measures recommended for preventing or minimizing progression of left ventricular dysfunction for stage A and B patients is supported for stage C patients, who have current or prior symptoms attributable to left ventricular dysfunction (Table 37G.3).

The 2017 ACC/AHA/HFSA updated guidelines support the use of beta-blockers (bisoprolol, carvedilol, and sustained release metoprolol succinate) and ACE inhibitors (ARBs for patients who cannot tolerate ACE inhibitors) for all stage C patients, in the absence of contraindications, and use of diuretics for patients with fluid overload. New for the 2017 guidelines is the class I recommendation (level B-R) to replace an ACE inhibitor/ARB by an ARNI to further reduce morbidity and mortality in patients with NYHA class II-III heart failure. When stopping an ACE inhibitor and starting an ARNI it is important to wait at least 36 hours, to avoid the risk of angioedema (class III: Harm, LOE – EO). Of note the 2016 ESC guidelines do not recommend the routine replacement of ACE inhibitor/ARB by an ARNI unless the patient remains symptomatic after an ACE inhibitor (equivalent to 10 bid of enalapril) or ARB, a beta-blocker, and a mineralocorticoid receptor antagonist and had elevated levels of plasma natriuretic peptides (BNP ≥ 150 pg/mL or plasma NT-proBNP ≥ 600 pg/mL) or if there was an HF hospitalization within the past 12 months with an elevated plasma elevated level of plasma natriuretic peptides (BNP ≥ 100 pg/mL or plasma NT-proBNP ≥ 400 pg/mL).[3] The class IIa recommendation for the use

[a]Adapted from Mann DL. Management of heart failure with a reduced ejection fraction. In Zipes DP, et al, editors: *Braunwald's Heart Disease: A Textbook of Cardiovascular Medicine.* 11th ed. Philadelphia: Elsevier; 2019.

TABLE 37G.1   ACC/AHA Guidelines for Treating Patients at High Risk of Developing Heart Failure (Stage A)

Class	Indication	Level of Evidence
I	Hypertension and lipid disorders should be controlled in accordance with contemporary guidelines to lower the risk of HF.	A
I	In patients at increased risk, stage A, the optimal blood pressure in those with hypertension should be < 130/80.	B-R
I	Other conditions that may lead to or contribute to HF, such as obesity, diabetes mellitus, tobacco use, and known cardiotoxic agents, should be controlled or avoided.	C
II	For patients at risk of developing HF, natriuretic peptide biomarker–based screening followed by team-based care, including a cardio-vascular specialist optimizing GDMT, can be useful to prevent the development of left ventricular dysfunction (systolic or diastolic) or new-onset HF	B-R

ACC, American College of Cardiology; *AHA,* American Heart Association.

TABLE 37G.2   ACC/AHA Guidelines for Treatment of Asymptomatic Left Ventricular Systolic Dysfunction (Stage B)

Class	Indication	Level of Evidence
I	In all patients with a recent or remote history of MI or ACS and reduced EF, ACE inhibitors should be used to prevent symptomatic HF and reduce mortality. In patients intolerant of ACE inhibitors, ARBs are appropriate unless contraindicated	A
	In all patients with a recent or remote history of MI or ACS and reduced EF, evidence-based beta-blockers should be used to reduce mortality beta-blockade and ACE inhibition in all patients with a recent or remote history of MI regardless of ejection fraction or presence of heart failure	B
	In all patients with a recent or remote history of MI or ACS, statins should be used to prevent symptomatic HF and cardiovascular events	A
	Blood pressure should be controlled in accordance with clinical practice guidelines for hypertension to prevent symptomatic HF.	A
	ACE inhibitors should be used in all patients with a reduced EF to prevent symptomatic HF	A
	Beta-blockers should be used in all patients with a reduced EF to prevent symptomatic HF	C
IIa	To prevent sudden death, placement of an ICD is reasonable in patients with asymptomatic ischemic cardiomyopathy who are at least 40 days post-MI, have an LVEF of 30% or less, are on appropriate medical therapy, and have reasonable expectation of survival with a good functional status for more than 1 year	B
III: Harm	Nondihydropyridine calcium channel blockers with negative inotropic effects may be harmful in asymptomatic patients with low LVEF and no symptoms of HF after MI.	B

ACC, American College of Cardiology; *ACE,* angiotensin-converting inhibitor; *ACS,* acute coronary syndrome; *AHA,* American Heart Association; *ARB,* angiotensin receptor antagonist; *MI,* myocardial infarction.

of ivabradine in symptomatic patients in sinus rhythm and a heart rate > bpm (at rest) is also new for the 2017 AHA/ACC/HFSA guidelines.

Based on the results of the Eplerenone in Mild Patients Hospitalization and Survival Study in Heart Failure (EMPHASIS-HF), mineralocorticoid receptor antagonists are now recommended for all NYHA class II-IV heart failure patients with an EF < 35% to reduce morbidity and mortality, unless contraindicated (class I, level of evidence A). As with the 2009 guidelines, the use of hydralazine and isosorbide remains a class I indication for self-identified African Americans who remain symptomatic in NYHA class III-IV HF despite optimal therapy. The combination of hydralazine and isosorbide is recommended in patients who are intolerant of an ACE inhibitor or an ARB. Digitalis remains a reasonable approach to decrease hospitalizations in symptomatic patients. Based on the results of the WARCEF (Warfarin Versus Aspirin in Reduced Cardiac Ejection Fraction) trial, anticoagulation is not recommended in patients with chronic HF without atrial fibrillation, a prior embolic event or a cardioembolic source (class III: No Benefit). However, anticoagulation continues to be recommended for patients with chronic HF and permanent/persistent/paroxysmal atrial fibrillation who have an additional risk factor for cardioembolic stroke (class I, level of evidence B). The guidelines explicitly discourage the routine use of a combination of an ACE inhibitor with an ARB and mineralocorticoid receptor

antagonist because of the risk of hyperkalemia; use of an ACE inhibitor with an ARNI because of the risk of angioedema; and calcium-channel blockers, long-term infusion of positive inotropic drugs (except as palliation in patients with end-stage disease, see **Table 37G.3**), use of nutritional supplements, statins as adjunctive therapy for HF, and hormonal therapies other than those needed to replete deficiencies.

TREATMENT OF PATIENTS WITH REFRACTORY END-STAGE HEART FAILURE (STAGE D)

The 2009 ACCF/AHA HF guidelines define stage D as "patients with truly refractory HF who might be eligible for specialized, advanced treatment strategies, such as mechanical circulatory support (MCS [**see Chapter 45**]), procedures to facilitate fluid removal, continuous inotropic infusions, or cardiac transplantation (**see Chapter 44**) or other innovative or experimental surgical procedures, or for end-of-life care, such as hospice" (**see Chapter 50**). The guidelines provide clear indications for the use of inotropic agents and mechanical circulatory support in stage D patients (**Table 37G.4**). The guidelines endorse the use of continuous intravenous inotropic support until definitive therapy can be performed (e.g., MCS, heart transplantation) and/or to maintain systemic perfusion and preserve end-organ performance until the

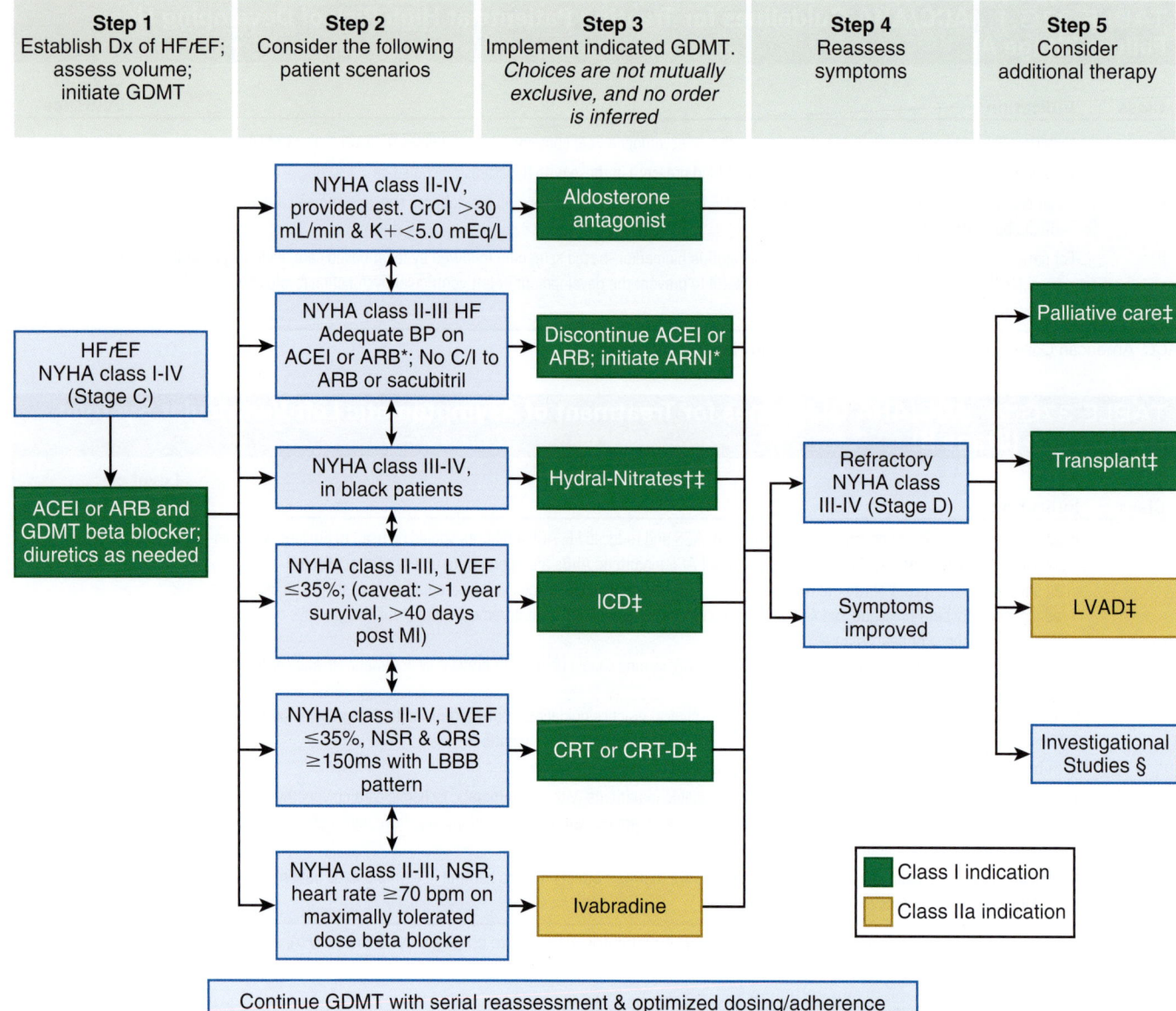

| **Step 1** Establish Dx of HF*r*EF; assess volume; initiate GDMT | **Step 2** Consider the following patient scenarios | **Step 3** Implement indicated GDMT. *Choices are not mutually exclusive, and no order is inferred* | **Step 4** Reassess symptoms | **Step 5** Consider additional therapy |

Fig. 37G.1 Treatment algorithm stage C and D heart failure with a reduced ejection fraction. For all medical therapies, dosing should be optimized and serial assessment exercised. See text in **Chapter 37** for details. Key: *See text for important treatment directions. †Hydral-Nitrates green box: The combination of ISDN/HYD with ARNI has not been robustly tested. BP response should be carefully monitored. ‡See 2013 ACC/AH heart failure guidelines[1] §Participation in investigational studies is also appropriate for stage C and NYHA class II and III HF. *ACEI,* Angiotensin-converting enzyme inhibitor; *ARB,* angiotensin receptor-blocker; *ARNI,* angiotensin receptor-neprilysin inhibitor; *BP,* blood pressure; bpm, beats per minute; *C/I,* contraindication; *CrCl,* creatinine clearance; *CRT-D,* cardiac resynchronization therapy–device; *Dx,* diagnosis; *GDMT,* guideline-directed management and therapy; *HF,* heart failure; *HFrEF,* heart failure with reduced ejection fraction; *ICD,* implantable cardioverter-defibrillator; *ISDN/ HYD,* isosorbide dinitrate hydral-nitrates; *K+,* potassium; *LBBB,* left bundle-branch block; *LVAD,* left ventricular assist device; *LVEF,* left ventricular ejection fraction; *MI,* myocardial infarction; *NSR,* normal sinus rhythm; *NYHA,* New York Heart Association. (Modified from Yancy CW, Jessup M, Bozkurt B, et al. 2017 ACC/AHA/HFSA Focused Update of the 2013 ACCF/AHA Guideline for the Management of Heart Failure: A Report of the American College of Cardiology/American Heart Association Task Force on Clinical Practice Guidelines and the Heart Failure Society of America. *Circulation.* 2017;136:e137–e161.)

acute precipitating problem is resolved (class I, level of evidence C). The guidelines also support inotropic support as "bridge therapy" to GDMT and/or device therapy (class IIa, level of evidence B), as well as short-term continuous intravenous inotropic in hospitalized patients with documented severe systolic dysfunction who present with low blood pressure and significantly depressed cardiac output, in order to maintain systemic perfusion and preserve end-organ performance, or as palliative therapy for symptom control (class IIb, level of evidence B). The guidelines regard long-term use of either continuous or intermittent, intravenous parenteral positive inotropic agents, in the

absence of specific indications or for reasons other than palliative care, as potentially harmful (Class III: Harm, level of evidence B).

The 2013 ACC/AHA guidelines provide qualified support for MCS in carefully selected patients with stage D heart failure with a reduced ejection fraction (HFrEF), in whom definitive management (e.g., cardiac transplantation) or cardiac recovery is anticipated or planned, and also indicate that percutaneous and extracorporeal ventricular assist devices (VADs) are reasonable as a "bridge to recovery" or "bridge to decision" for carefully selected patients with HFrEF with acute profound hemodynamic compromise (class IIb, level of evidence B). The

TABLE 37G.3 ACC/AHA Guidelines for Treatment of Patients with Prior or Current Symptoms of Chronic HFrEF (Stage C)

Class	Indication	Level of Evidence
Nonpharmacologic Interventions		
I	Patients with HF should receive specific education to facilitate HF self-care	B
	Exercise training (or regular physical activity) is recommended as safe and effective for patients with HF who are able to participate to improve functional status	A
IIa	Cardiac rehabilitation can be useful in clinically stable patients with HF to improve functional capacity, exercise duration, HRQOL, and mortality	B
	Sodium restriction is reasonable for patients with symptomatic HF to reduce congestive symptoms	C
	Continuous positive airway pressure (CPAP) can be beneficial to increase LVEF and improve functional status in patients with HF and sleep apnea	B
Pharmacological Interventions		
I	Measures listed as class I recommendations for patients in stages A and B are recommended where appropriate.	A,B,C
	GDMT as depicted in should be the mainstay of pharmacological therapy for HFrEF	A
Diuretics		
I	Diuretics are recommended in patients with HFrEF who have evidence of fluid retention, unless contraindicated, to improve symptoms.	C
ACE/ARBs/ARNIs		
I	The use of ACE inhibitors is beneficial for patients with prior or current symptoms of chronic HFrEF to reduce morbidity and mortality	A
	The use of ARBs to reduce morbidity and mortality is recommended in patients with prior or current symptoms of chronic HFrEF who are intolerant to ACE inhibitors because of cough or angioedema	A
I	ARNIs are recommended in patients with HFrEF unless contraindicated, to reduce morbidity and mortality	B-R
I	ARNIs are recommended in patients with HFrEF NYHA class II or III who are tolerant to an ACE inhibitor or ARB; replacement by an ARNI is recommended to further reduce morbidity and mortality	B-R
IIa	ARBs are reasonable to reduce morbidity and mortality as alternatives to ACE inhibitors as first line therapy for patients with HFrEF, especially for patients already taking ARBs for other indications, unless contraindicated	A
IIb	Addition of an ARB may be considered in persistently symptomatic patients with HFrEF who are already being treated with an ACE inhibitor and a beta-blocker in whom an aldosterone antagonist is not indicated or tolerated	A
IIa	Ivabradine can be beneficial to reduce HF hospitalizations in patients with NYHA class II-III HFrEF (LVEF < 35%) who are receiving GDMT, including a beta-blocker, and who are in sinus rhythm with a heart rate > 70 bpm	B-R
III: Harm	Routinely combining an ACE inhibitor, an ARB, and an aldosterone antagonist	C
III: Harm	ARNI should not be administered concomitantly with ACE inhibitors or within the last dose of an ACE inhibitor	B-R
III: Harm	ARNI should not be administered to patients with a history of angioedema	C-EO
Beta-Blockers		
I	Use of 1 of the 3 beta-blockers proven to reduce mortality (i.e., bisoprolol, carvedilol, and sustained-release metoprolol succinate) is recommended for all patients with current or prior symptoms of HFrEF, unless contraindicated, to reduce morbidity and mortality	A
Aldosterone Receptor Antagonists		
I	Aldosterone receptor antagonists (or mineralocorticoid receptor antagonists) are recommended in patients with NYHA class II-IV and who have LVEF < 35%, unless contraindicated, to reduce morbidity and mortality.	A
I	Aldosterone receptor antagonists are recommended to reduce morbidity and mortality following an acute MI in patients who have LVEF < 40% or less who develop symptoms of HF or who have a history of diabetes mellitus, unless contraindicated.	B
III: Harm	Inappropriate use of aldosterone receptor antagonists is potentially harmful because of life-threatening hyperkalemia or renal insufficiency when serum creatinine is more than 2.5 mg/dL in men or more than 2.0 mg/dL in women (or estimated glomerular filtration rate <30 mL/min/1.73 m^2), and/or potassium more than 5.0 mEq/L	B
Hydralazine and Isosorbide Dinitrate		
I	The combination of hydralazine and isosorbide dinitrate is recommended to reduce morbidity and mortality for patients self-described as African Americans with NYHA class III-IV HFrEF receiving optimal therapy with ACE inhibitors and beta-blockers, unless contraindicated	A

Continued

TABLE 37G.3   ACC/AHA Guidelines for Treatment of Patients with Prior or Current Symptoms of Chronic HFrEF (Stage C)—cont'd

Class	Indication	Level of Evidence
IIa	A combination of hydralazine and isosorbide dinitrate can be useful to reduce morbidity or mortality in patients with current or prior symptomatic HFrEF who cannot be given an ACE inhibitor or ARB because of drug intolerance, hypotension, or renal insufficiency, unless contraindicated	B
Digoxin		
IIa	Digoxin can be beneficial in patients with HFrEF, unless contraindicated, to decrease hospitalizations for HF	B
Anticoagulation		
I	Patients with chronic HF with permanent/persistent/paroxysmal AF and an additional risk factor for cardioembolic stroke (history of hypertension, diabetes mellitus, previous stroke or transient ischemic attack, or ≥75 years of age) should receive chronic anticoagulant therapy	A
I	The selection of an anticoagulant agent (warfarin, dabigatran, apixaban, or rivaroxaban) for permanent/persistent/paroxysmal AF should be individualized on the basis of risk factors, cost, tolerability, patient preference, potential for drug interactions, and other clinical characteristics, including time in the international normalized ratio therapeutic range if the patient has been taking warfarin	C
IIa	Chronic anticoagulation is reasonable for patients with chronic HF who have permanent/persistent/paroxysmal AF but are without an additional risk factor for cardioembolic stroke	B
III: No Benefit	Anticoagulation is not recommended in patients with chronic HFrEF without AF, a prior thromboembolic event, or a cardioembolic source	B
Statins		
III: No Benefit	Statins are not beneficial as adjunctive therapy when prescribed solely for HF	A
Omega-3 fatty acids		
IIa	Omega-3 polyunsaturated fatty acid (PUFA) supplementation is reasonable to use as adjunctive therapy in patients with NYHA class II-IV symptoms and HFrEF or HFpEF, unless contraindicated, to reduce mortality and cardiovascular hospitalizations	B
Drugs of Unproven Value or That May Cause Harm		
III: No Benefit	Nutritional supplements as treatment for HF are not recommended in patients with current or prior symptoms of HFrEF	B
	Hormonal therapies other than to correct deficiencies are not recommended for patients with current or prior symptoms of HFrEF	C
III: Harm	Drugs known to adversely affect the clinical status of patients with current or prior symptoms of HFrEF are potentially harmful and should be avoided or withdrawn whenever possible (e.g., most antiarrhythmic drugs, most calcium channel blocking drugs (except amlodipine), NSAIDs, or thiazolidinediones)	B
	Long-term use of infused positive inotropic drugs is potentially harmful for patients with HFrEF, except as palliation for patients with end-stage disease who cannot be stabilized with standard medical treatment (see recommendations for stage D).	C
Calcium Channel Blockers		
III: No Benefit	Calcium channel blocking drugs are not recommended as routine therapy for patients with HFrEF	A

ACC, American College of Cardiology; *ACE,* angiotensin-converting inhibitor; *AHA,* American Heart Association; *ARB,* angiotensin receptor blocker; *HFpEF,* heart failure with a preserved ejection fraction; *HFrEF,* heart failure with a reduced ejection fraction.

guidelines also provide qualified support for the use of durable VADS to prolong survival in carefully selected patients with stage D HFrEF. As in previous guidelines, cardiac transplantation remains a class I indication (level of evidence C) for carefully selected patients with stage D HFrEF despite GDMT and device and surgical management.

COMORBIDITIES IN HEART FAILURE PATIENTS

The 2013 ACC/AHA practice guidelines recognize the importance of comorbidities in heart failure, including hypertension, anemia, diabetes, arthritis, chronic kidney disease, and depression, but did not provide specific recommendations (**see Chapter 48**). However, the 2017 ACC/AHA/HFSA focused guideline update did provide specific recommendations for the treatment of hypertension, anemia, and sleep disordered breath (**Table 37G.5**)

COORDINATING CARE FOR PATIENTS WITH CHRONIC HEART FAILURE

The guidelines recognize that systems of care designed to support patients with HF and other cardiac diseases can produce significant improvement in outcomes, but indicate that the quality of evidence

TABLE 37G.4   ACC/AHA Guidelines for Treatment of Patients with End-Stage Heart Failure (Stage D)

Class	Indication	Level of Evidence
Nonpharmacological Interventions		
IIa	Fluid restriction (1.5 to 2 L/d) is reasonable in stage D, especially in patients with hyponatremia.	B
Inotropic Support		
I	Until definitive therapy (e.g., coronary revascularization, MCS, heart transplantation) or resolution of the acute precipitating problem, patients with cardiogenic shock should receive temporary intravenous inotropic support to maintain systemic perfusion and preserve end-organ performance.	C
IIa	Continuous intravenous inotropic support is reasonable as "bridge therapy" in patients with stage D refractory to GDMT and device therapy who are eligible for and awaiting MCS or cardiac transplantation.	B
IIb	Short-term, continuous intravenous inotropic support may be reasonable in those hospitalized patients presenting with documented severe systolic dysfunction who present with low blood pressure and significantly depressed cardiac output to maintain systemic perfusion and preserve end-organ performance	B
	Long-term, continuous intravenous inotropic support may be considered as palliative therapy for symptom control in select patients with stage D despite optimal GDMT and device therapy who are not eligible for either MCS or cardiac transplantation	B
III: Harm	Long-term use of either continuous or intermittent, intravenous parenteral positive inotropic agents, in the absence of specific indications or for reasons other than palliative care, is potentially harmful in the patient with HF	B
	Use of parenteral inotropic agents in hospitalized patients without documented severe systolic dysfunction, low blood pressure, or impaired perfusion, and evidence of significantly depressed cardiac output, with or without congestion, is potentially harmful	B
Mechanical Circulatory Support (MCS)		
IIa	MCS is beneficial in carefully selected patients with stage D HFrEF in whom definitive management (e.g., cardiac transplantation) or cardiac recovery is anticipated or planned	B
	Nondurable MCS, including the use of percutaneous and extracorporeal ventricular assist devices (VADs), is reasonable as a "bridge to recovery" or "bridge to decision" for carefully selected patients with HFrEF with acute, profound hemodynamic compromise	
	Durable MCS is reasonable to prolong survival for carefully selected patients with stage D HFrEF	B
Cardiac Transplantation		
I	Evaluation for cardiac transplantation is indicated for carefully selected patients with stage D HF despite GDMT, device, and surgical management	C

ACC, American College of Cardiology; *AHA,* American Heart Association; *GDMT,* guideline-directed medial therapy; *HFrEF,* heart failure with a reduced ejection fraction; *MCS,* mechanical circulatory support.

TABLE 37G.5   ACC/AHA/HFSA Guidelines for Treatment of Comorbidities in Heart Failure

	Hypertension	
I	Patients with HFrEF and hypertension should be prescribed GDMT titrated to attain systolic blood pressure less than 130 mm Hg	C-EO
Anemia		
IIb	In patients with NYHA class II and III HF and iron deficiency (ferritin <100 ng/mL or 100 to 300 ng/mL if transferrin saturation is <20%), intravenous iron replacement might be reasonable to improve functional status and QoL	B-R
III: No Benefit	In patients with HF and anemia, erythropoietin stimulating agents should not be used to improve morbidity and mortality	B-R
Sleep Disordered Breathing		
IIa	In patients with NYHA class II–IV HF and suspicion of sleep disordered breathing or excessive daytime sleepiness, a formal sleep assessment is reasonable	C-LD
IIb	In patients with cardiovascular disease and obstructive sleep apnea, CPAP may be reasonable to improve sleep quality and daytime sleepiness	B-R
III:Harm	In patients with NYHA class II–IV HFrEF and central sleep apnea, adaptive servo-ventilation causes harm	B-R

ACC, American College of Cardiology; *AHA,* American Heart Association; *CABG,* coronary artery bypass grafting; *CAD,* coronary artery disease; *GDMT,* guideline-directed medical therapy; *HFpEF,* heart failure with a preserved ejection fraction; *HFrEF,* heart failure with a reduced ejection fraction.

TABLE 37G.6   Coordinating Care for Patients With Chronic Heart Failure

Class	Indication	Level of Evidence
I	Effective systems of care coordination with special attention to care transitions should be deployed for every patient with chronic HF that facilitate and ensure effective care that is designed to achieve GDMT and prevent hospitalization	B
	Every patient with HF should have a clear, detailed, and evidence-based plan of care that ensures the achievement of GDMT goals, effective management of comorbid conditions, timely follow-up with the healthcare team, appropriate dietary and physical activities, and compliance with Secondary Prevention Guidelines for cardiovascular disease. This plan of care should be updated regularly and made readily available to all members of each patient's healthcare team	C
	Palliative and supportive care is effective for patients with symptomatic advanced HF to improve quality of life	B

ACC, American College of Cardiology; *AHA,* American Heart Association; *GDMT,* guideline-directed medical therapy; *IV,* intravenous; *NYHA,* New York Heart Association.

is mixed for specific components of HF clinical management interventions, such as home-based care, disease management, and remote telemonitoring programs. Hence, the guidelines recommend that interventions should focus on improving adherence to GDMT (**Table 37G.6**). The updated guidelines advocate patient education, and involvement of patients with HF and their families, especially during transitions of care, to ensure effective care that is designed to achieve GDMT and prevent hospitalizations (class I, level of evidence B). The guidelines also recommend that every patient with HF should have a clear, detailed, and evidence-based plan of care that ensures the achievement of GDMT goals, effective management of comorbid conditions, timely follow-up with the healthcare team, appropriate dietary and physical activities, and compliance with Secondary Prevention Guidelines for cardiovascular disease (class I, level of evidence C). The guidelines recommend that the HF and palliative care teams are best suited to help patients and families decide when end-of-life care (including hospice) is appropriate (class I, level of evidence C). The core elements of comprehensive palliative care for HF include expert symptom assessment and management, including symptom control, psychosocial distress, health-related quality of life, preferences about end-of-life care, caregiver support, and assurance of access to evidence-based disease modifying interventions.

REFERENCES

1. Yancy CW, Jessup M, Bozkurt B, et al. 2013 ACCF/AHA guideline for the Management of Heart Failure: A report of the American College of Cardiology Foundation/American Heart Association Task Force on practice guidelines. *Circulation.* 2013;128:e240–e327.

2. Yancy CW, Jessup M, Bozkurt B, et al. 2016 ACC/AHA/HFSA focused update on New Pharmacological Therapy for Heart Failure: An update of the 2013 ACCF/AHA guideline for the Management of Heart Failure: A report of the American College of Cardiology/American Heart Association Task Force on Clinical Practice Guidelines and the Heart Failure Society of America. *J Am Coll Cardiol.* 2016;68:1476–1488.

3. Ponikowski P, Voors AA, Anker SD, et al. 2016 ESC guidelines for the diagnosis and treatment of acute and chronic heart failure: The task force for the diagnosis and treatment of acute and chronic heart failure of the European Society of Cardiology (ESC) developed with the special contribution of the Heart Failure Association (HFA) of the ESC. *Eur Heart J.* 2016;18:891–975.

4. McMurray JJ, Adamopoulos S, Anker SD, et al. ESC guidelines for the diagnosis and treatment of acute and chronic heart failure 2012: The task force for the diagnosis and treatment of acute and chronic heart failure 2012 of the European Society of Cardiology. Developed in collaboration with the Heart Failure Association (HFA) of the ESC. *Eur Heart J.* 2012;33:1787–1847.

5. Yancy CW, Jessup M, Bozkurt B, et al. 2017 ACC/AHA/HFSA focused update of the 2013 ACCF/AHA guideline for the Management of Heart Failure: A report of the American College of Cardiology/American Heart Association Task Force on Clinical Practice Guidelines and the Heart Failure Society of America. *Circulation.* 2017;136:e137–e161.

Management of Arrhythmias and Device Therapy in Heart Failure

John D. Ferguson

Arrhythmias are common in heart failure patients. This chapter will discuss the diagnosis and therapy of arrhythmias in patients with heart failure.

ATRIAL FIBRILLATION

Atrial fibrillation (AF) is the most common sustained cardiac arrhythmia. Its prevalence increases with age and with both systolic and diastolic heart failure.[1-4] It has been reported that up to 25% of patients with chronic heart failure will have permanent AF.[5,7-9] AF is one of the strongest predictors for the development of heart failure. In the Framingham Heart Study, the development of AF was responsible for worsening heart failure symptoms and was seen as the second greatest reason for hospitalization, second to acute heart failure exacerbation.[5] AF is also associated with significant morbidity and mortality, due primarily to the increased risk of thromboembolic events and adverse hemodynamic effects that may result in new onset or worsening heart failure, decreased exercise tolerance, as well as impaired quality of life.[6]

Epidemiology

In the Framingham Heart Study, 2326 men and 2866 women were followed for 2 years, and the risk of developing permanent AF was 8.5% for men and 13.7% for women. Paroxysmal AF was seen in 8.2% of men and 20.4% of women. In those without prior or concurrent congestive heart failure or myocardial infarction, the lifetime risks for AF were approximately 16%.[10] In diastolic heart failure, approximately 25% to 30% of patients have evidence of AF.[11] The prevalence increases with the severity of diastolic heart failure, reaching up to 40% in advanced stages.[12] Sustained high ventricular rates during atrial arrhythmias may result in a tachycardia-induced cardiomyopathy that in the absence of any other myopathic process may be completely reversible. However, in patients who develop AF in the setting of established heart failure, atrial fibrosis with deleterious electrical remodeling is the primary cause for the arrhythmia.

Pathophysiology

The clinical manifestations of AF relate to the loss of atrial systolic function and an irregular, ventricular response whose rate is typically determined by the conduction and refractory properties of the atrioventricular (AV) node. Left atrial systole contributes up to 25% of the cardiac output, and this fraction may increase to 50% in left ventricular failure.[13,14] The loss of atrial systolic function results in impaired hemodynamic function of the heart. AF causes a fall in cardiac stroke volume of about 10% in normal subjects, with a greater decrease seen at fast ventricular rates. This loss becomes more important clinically with increasing age and progressive impairment of left ventricular systolic or diastolic function, because atrial systole makes a greater contribution toward the overall stroke volume in these conditions. In addition to the loss of AV synchrony, the irregular and often inappropriate ventricular rates seen in AF result in suboptimal ventricular filling. These may further compromise cardiac output, an effect particularly seen in patients with mitral stenosis or diastolic dysfunction. Cardioversion of AF with poorly controlled ventricular rates usually improves left ventricular ejection fraction (LVEF) and exercise capacity, but the improvement occurs gradually after the procedure.[13]

Loss of atrial systolic function results in stasis within the left atrium, leading to intra-atrial thrombus formation and an increased risk of stroke and thromboembolism. During episodes of AF, echocardiography can detect spontaneous echo contrast (SEC) as a result of the formation of erythrocyte aggregations and thrombus in the atria. Stasis within the left atrium has been related to hemostatic abnormalities that are suggestive of a hypercoagulable state and that involve coagulation factors and abnormal endothelial and platelet function. These abnormalities of hemostasis have been related to changes in inflammatory indices and growth factors.[14,15] The hypercoagulable state is often exaggerated in low flow states such as left ventricular dysfunction.[15] Hypercoagulability is altered by antithrombotic therapy and gradually by cardioversion of AF to sinus rhythm. Prothrombotic indices in AF have been shown to be prognostically relevant, being predictive of stroke and vascular events, and can be used to refine clinical stroke risk stratification.[16,17] Atrial natriuretic peptide levels are also increased in patients who have AF, which contributes to hemoconcentration and an increased risk for thrombus formation.

Prolonged AF with rapid ventricular rates produces functional, ultrastructural, and microscopic changes within the myocardium that may result in progressive left ventricular dilation and reduction of left ventricular systolic function; this is referred to as *tachycardia-induced cardiomyopathy*. In a patient who has chronic heart failure and is in sinus rhythm, increased intracardiac pressures may lead to atrial stretch and dilation, predisposing to both the development and the recurrence of AF. Several potential electrophysiologic mechanisms may be responsible for AF.[4,18] One postulated mechanism is multiple wavelet reentry, in which wavefronts continuously sweep through the atria in a random fashion. The multiple wavelet hypothesis requires that a minimum number of wavefronts and enough atrial tissue to permit their simultaneous propagation exist. An alternate hypothesis is that there are only one or two primary reentrant circuits or rotors that are constantly forming and disappearing, but the cycle lengths in these circuits are too short to allow the rest of the atria to follow in an organized fashion, resulting in fibrillatory conduction.[18] It has been shown clinically that AF may be produced by rapid tachycardias from either focal sources, commonly found in musculature of the pulmonary veins, or stable reentrant circuits that drive the remaining atrial tissue until degeneration to AF occurs.[18,19] The pulmonary veins, which include muscular sleeves that may be electrically active, and the posterior left atrial wall are considered to be the critical structures involved in the pathogenesis of AF.[19]

Clinical Presentation

The classification of AF focuses on temporal pattern after onset. Paroxysmal AF is a recurrence of AF that terminates spontaneously in 7 days or less. Persistent AF is recurrent AF that lasts longer than 7 days. Patients who undergo cardioversion within 48 hours of onset are described as paroxysmal and persistent if done after 48 hours. Longstanding persistent AF is continuous AF that has lasted longer than 1 year. Permanent AF is when the patient remains in longstanding persistent AF and there is no plan for rhythm control.[20]

Among patients who have recurrent forms of AF, this temporally based clinical classification can assist management strategies, particular in relation to considering rhythm control or rate control. In paroxysmal AF, the episodes are generally self-terminating, and thus the goals of therapy are the prevention of paroxysms and the long-term maintenance of sinus rhythm. In sustained AF, the therapeutic goal is either cardioversion to sinus rhythm or heart rate control. Antithrombotic therapy for moderate or high-risk patients is an important component of both strategies.

The differentiation between these clinical categories is dependent on the history given by the patient, electrocardiogram (ECG) documentation of the episode, and the duration of the most recent previous episode of AF. Although this classification is helpful, there is considerable variability, both between patients and in the same patient, in the temporal pattern of AF episodes, and approaches to therapy must be individualized, especially in relation to symptoms. Furthermore, paroxysmal AF may become permanent (8% at 1 year, 18% at 4 years), especially with increasing age.[21] The EURO Heart Survey showed that hypertension, age older than 75 years, previous transient ischemic attack or stroke, chronic obstructive pulmonary disease, and heart failure were independent predictors of AF progression.[21] These investigators used these factors to develop the HATCH score, which predicts the probability of progression of AF. With an increasing HATCH score, the percentage of patients in whom AF progressed to persistent forms was significantly higher. Fifty percent of the patients with a HATCH score more than five progressed to persistent AF, compared with only 6% of the patients with a HATCH score of 0.[21,22]

Diagnosis

The investigation of a patient with AF requires a careful clinical history (including a past medical history) with emphasis on certain clinical features. The history should cover whether the symptoms are sustained or intermittent and whether any complications (such as heart failure, stroke, or thromboembolism) are present. Other useful data include the date of the first episode, information about acute precipitating factors or chronic conditions linked to AF, how symptoms are relieved, the typical duration of episodes and the typical interval between them, the duration of the current or most recent episode, and current and past drug treatment for both rate and rhythm control.

At the initial consultation, basic blood tests, including full blood count, biochemistry (renal function, electrolytes), and thyroid function tests, are taken. A full blood count is useful to exclude anemia because anticoagulation may be considered. Serum urea and electrolytes are relevant for consideration of drug therapy (e.g., the dose of digoxin would be reduced in renal impairment). The risk of AF is increased by clinical and subclinical hyperthyroidism, and thus the serum thyroid stimulating hormone level should be measured in all patients who have AF, even if there are no symptoms suggestive of thyrotoxicosis.

The arrhythmia should be documented, ideally with a standard 12-lead ECG. The characteristic ECG findings in AF include rapid baseline oscillations or fibrillatory waves that vary in size, shape, and timing; the absence of discrete P waves; and an irregularly irregular ventricular rate.

The ECG may also provide a clue to the electrophysiologic features that may have caused AF (e.g., a previous myocardial infarction, left ventricular hypertrophy, or preexcitation). Often, patients present with previous symptoms suggestive of AF but are in sinus rhythm at the time of their evaluation. If symptoms occur on a daily basis, a 24-hour ambulatory ECG should provide the diagnosis. If symptoms occur less frequently, a patient-activated event recorder or an implanted loop recorder would be more likely to provide a diagnosis. Smartphone apps, smartwatch heart rate monitoring, and home blood pressure monitors are increasingly helping with arrhythmia diagnosis.

An echocardiogram provides important information for the initial evaluation of most patients with AF.[4,23] Either transthoracic echocardiography or transesophageal echocardiography (TEE), or a combination of the two, may be appropriate. The initial goal of the echocardiographic evaluation should be to establish the presence or absence of structural heart disease, including valvular abnormalities, congenital anomalies, chamber dimensions, pericardial thickening or effusions, and ventricular function.

Left atrial size is an important predictor of outcome in patients with AF because the presence of significant left atrial enlargement has been shown to reduce the chances of successful cardioversion and long-term maintenance of sinus rhythm in most series. Left atrial enlargement may also increase the risk of stroke, owing to a greater potential for stasis in the dilated chamber.[4]

Although transthoracic echocardiography is acceptable for assessing chamber size, detection of thrombi or the assessment of left atrial appendage anatomy and function requires the TEE approach. Using TEE, up to 27% of patients with AF of more than 3 days' duration may have detectable thrombi. A prethrombotic finding, SEC (also called "smoke"), is due to erythrocyte aggregation in the low-flow state and is even more commonly seen. Other TEE indices of high stroke risk include the presence of left atrial thrombus, low left atrial appendage velocities, dense SEC, and complex aortic plaque in the descending aorta.[23]

Invasive electrophysiologic studies have only a limited role in the routine evaluation of patients with AF unless catheter ablation is planned. Electrophysiologic studies of AF should be reserved for the following situations: when another arrhythmia (e.g., atrial flutter or atrial or supraventricular tachycardia) is thought to be the cause of the AF, when other electrophysiologic abnormalities or symptoms (e.g., preexcitation, sinus node dysfunction, syncope) require clarification or therapy, or when catheter ablation is planned.

Management of Acute Episodes of Atrial Fibrillation

Successful management of acute episodes of AF requires attention to several issues, including rate control, pharmacologic or electrical conversion, and protection against thromboembolic events. When patients present with new onset or recurrent episodes of AF, the initial step should be to assess their symptoms and hemodynamic status. Rarely, the patient will be so severely compromised that urgent electrical cardioversion will be required despite a high risk for early recurrence. In most patients, however, the first step for stabilization should be to lower the ventricular rate. In an intensive care unit or other monitored setting, intravenous β-blockers are usually the first choice in patients with heart failure and systolic dysfunction. Intravenous digoxin may be a useful adjunct, but its onset of action is delayed and its inability to lower rate is lessened during periods of high sympathetic tone. The non-dihydropyridine calcium channel blockers, diltiazem and verapamil, are effective alternatives in patients with preserved systolic function but must be used with caution, if at all, in patients with known systolic dysfunction. Intravenous amiodarone can play a dual role, since it will both slow ventricular rates and may eventually cardiovert the rhythm. The heart rate target during attempts at rate control will depend on the patient's condition. In a resting, minimally symptomatic patient, one tries to approximate what the average rate would be in sinus rhythm (i.e., 60–100 beats/min). During periods of stress, however, this degree of rate control may not be achievable, and rates up to 110 to 120 beats/min are usually adequate to control symptoms.

Once the patient's rate had been controlled, a decision about possible cardioversion should be made. Anticoagulation issues that will affect this decision will be discussed later. Most patients with new onset AF will be candidates for at least one attempt at cardioversion. Elective direct-current cardioversion without addition of an antiarrhythmic drug is an appropriate strategy for patients with recent onset AF in whom the risk of recurrence is thought to be only moderate or low. After cardioversion, the patient can be followed off antiarrhythmic drugs until a recurrence has been documented. AV nodal blocking agents are often continued at least during the early period after cardioversion. Although intravenous ibutilide and vernakalant (not currently available in the United States) are effective for conversion

of recent onset AF, neither of these agents is advisable in patients with systolic heart failure or left ventricular hypertrophy. Intravenous or oral loading with amiodarone or oral loading with dofetilide is the best approach for pharmacologic cardioversion if long-term therapy is planned in the heart failure patient.[24]

Chemical or electrical cardioversion of AF of more than 2 days' duration is associated with a significant risk (2%–8%) of stroke or systemic thromboembolism in all patients with nonvalvular AF not on anticoagulants.[25] A prudent approach is to start anticoagulation in patients without contraindications scheduled for cardioversion if the cardioversion is to be delayed or if the duration of the episode is uncertain. For episodes of greater than 48 hours' duration, two anticoagulation strategies are acceptable. If early cardioversion is planned, the patient should undergo a transesophageal echocardiogram to exclude the presence of left atrial appendage thrombus. If no thrombus is visualized, anticoagulation is continued and cardioversion may be performed. The alternate strategy is to delay cardioversion until the patient has been adequately anticoagulated for at least 3 weeks. Although warfarin with an international normalized ratio (INR) between 2.0 and 3.0 has long been the anticoagulation standard, preliminary data suggest that a similar duration of anticoagulation with dabigatran, rivaroxaban, and apixaban would be similarly effective. The TEE-guided and delayed treatment approaches were compared in the ACUTE trial. Both approaches were associated with a low rate of thromboembolic events after cardioversion and similar probabilities for sinus rhythm maintenance and bleeding.[26,27]

Chronic Management of Atrial Fibrillation

Patients with recurrent forms of AF will require a treatment program that provides rate control, an assessment of the benefits and feasibility of restoring and maintaining sinus rhythm, and mitigation of the risks for stroke and systemic embolism.

Rate Control Versus Rhythm Control

The first question that must be addressed in patients with recurrent AF is whether a rate control or a rhythm control strategy is most appropriate. Factors that should be considered include the temporal pattern (paroxysmal vs. persistent) of the arrhythmia, the frequency of episodes, the severity of symptoms, patient factors, and the probabilities for maintaining sinus rhythm or effectively controlling ventricular rates.

Although a rhythm control strategy would seem intuitively to be superior to a rate control strategy, a series of randomized trials has been unable to demonstrate this with pharmacologically based therapies. The two most relevant trials for heart failure patients were the AFFIRM trial and the AF-CHF trial.[28,29] AFFIRM randomized 4060 patients, 23% of whom had heart failure, between rate control and rhythm control strategies. No difference in total mortality or stroke was seen between the two strategies, with a slight trend favoring rate control. Patients in whom sinus rhythm was maintained during the study had improved outcomes, but this likely represents a "healthy responder" phenomenon. A second trial, AF-CHF, compared rate control and rhythm control strategies in patients required to have heart failure and depressed left ventricular systolic function. There was no significant difference between the two strategies in the three primary endpoints, mortality, stroke, and heart failure hospitalizations. In addition, even when patients were grouped into those with high and low prevalence of sinus rhythm during the course of the study, no benefit on these outcomes could be demonstrated. However, it must be remembered that entry into all of the rate control versus rhythm control strategy trials required that the patient be a candidate for both approaches. Highly symptomatic patients therefore were unlikely to be

TABLE 38.1	**Rate Control Agents for Primary Rate Control Strategy**			
Drug Class	**Specific Drug**	**Loading Dose**	**Maintenance Dose**	**Adverse Effects**
β-Blockers	Bisoprolol	2.5–20 mg PO daily	Same	Bronchospasm, sinus brady-cardia, AV block, exercise intolerance, hypotension, fatigue, depression
	Carvedilol	3.125–25 mg PO bid or sustained release 10–80 mg PO daily	Same	
	Metoprolol	2.5–5 mg IV or 25–100 mg PO bid or ER 25–200 mg PO daily	Same as PO dose	
	Nebivolol	5–40 mg PO daily	Same	
Calcium channel blockers	Diltiazem[a]	0.25 mg/kg IV bolus followed by 5–15 mg/hr infusion	120–480 mg ER PO daily	Sinus bradycardia, heart failure, AV block, hypotension, digoxin interaction (ver-apamil), peripheral edema
	Verapamil[a]	0.075–0.15 mg/kg IV bolus or 120–480 mg ER PO daily		
Other	Digoxin[b]	0.25 mg IV q4–6 hours (max 1 mg)	0.125–0.25 mg PO daily	Bradycardia, AV block, ventric-ular ectopy

[a]Use only in heart failure with preserved ejection fraction.
[b]Best used in conjunction with β-blocker for rate control.
AV, Atrioventricular; *ER,* extended release; *IV,* intravenous.
From Fuster V, Ryden LE, Cannom DS, et al. ACC/AHA/ESC 2006 guidelines for the management of patients with atrial fibrillation: a report of the American College of Cardiology/American Heart Association task force on practice guidelines and the European Society of Cardiology committee for practice guidelines (writing committee to revise the 2001 guidelines for the management of patients with atrial fibrillation). *J Am Coll Cardiol.* 2006;48:e149–e246.

randomized. Therefore, most clinicians recommend that heart failure patients with persistent symptoms related to their AF should have at least an initial attempt to restore and maintain sinus rhythm with rate control a fallback approach if rhythm control is unsuccessful or poorly tolerated.

Rate Control

The optimal range for ventricular rates during AF is still controversial. In AF-CHF the heart rate goals were 80 beats/min or less at rest and 110 beats/min or less during a 6-minute walk test. Similar heart rate targets were used in AFFIRM. In RACE II, a trial specifically designed to assess strict and lenient rate control, however, no adverse effects were seen with a more lenient heart rate target. RACE II, however, included very few patients with a history of heart failure.[30]

Options for rate control are shown in **Table 38.1**. β-blockers should be first-line therapy for rate control in patients with AF and heart failure. In addition to controlling rates in AF, several β-blockers have been shown to reduce mortality in heart failure patients in general. Non-dihydropyridine calcium channel blockers, verapamil, and dilti-azem may be used in patients with heart failure and preserved systolic function, but their negative inotropic actions make them contraindicated in patients with a depressed ejection fraction. Digoxin remains a potentially useful adjunct to β-blockers for rate control but must be used with caution due to its narrow therapeutic range.

For patients with permanent AF in whom rate cannot be controlled and for those with drug refractory highly symptomatic recurrent episodes, AV junctional ablation can be an effective strategy. The potentially deleterious effects of RV apical pacing must be considered. In some patients, poor rate control alone may be responsible for the low ejection fraction, and these patients may be managed with just RV pacing. If LV function is depressed even when the patient is in sinus rhythm, biventricular pacing for cardiac resynchronization will be the method of choice.

Pharmacologic Rhythm Control

As shown in **Fig. 38.1**, pharmacologic treatment options for maintaining sinus rhythm in patients with heart failure are limited. With the possible exception of disopyramide in patients with hypertrophic cardiomyopathy, class IA agents are not useful due to the high prevalence of side effects. Flecainide and propafenone are contraindicated in patients with heart failure. Dronedarone is similarly contraindicated in heart failure patients based on the data from the ANDROMEDA and PALLAS trials, both of which showed increased mortality with drone-darone therapy in patients with heart failure. Drug selection in patients with left ventricular hypertrophy is also limited by the risk for QT pro-longation and *torsades de pointes* with class III agents like sotalol. These observations frequently leave only dofetilide (not currently marketed in the European Union) and amiodarone as treatment options for heart failure patients. Dofetilide is a relatively pure I_{Kr} blocker that is effective for both converting AF episodes and for maintaining sinus rhythm. In the Diamond-HF trial, dofetilide did not increase overall mortality and improved outcomes in the subgroup with AF, but care-ful attention to dose and effects on the QTc during therapy is required. Heart failure patients with unstable renal function would not be good candidates for dofetilide. Amiodarone, therefore, frequently remains the only reasonable choice for sinus rhythm maintenance in patients with heart failure. Amiodarone was the drug most frequently used in both AFFIRM and AF-CHF. The estimated probability of maintaining sinus rhythm with selective use of electrical cardioversion in patients on amiodarone is 60% to 80% at 2 to 3 years but decreases over time. Amiodarone has many side effects, however, and should be used at the lowest effective chronic dose, usually 200 mg daily.

A number of agents and interventions that do not have classic anti-arrhythmic effects are also likely to be important to the overall management of AF in heart failure. Angiotensin-converting enzyme (ACE) inhibitors, angiotensin receptor blockers (ARBs), β-adrenergic block-ers, and aldosterone antagonists may be useful in this regard because they may both delay the onset of AF initially and act synergistically with more traditional antiarrhythmic drugs long-term. Sleep apnea is another risk factor for AF that should also be treated when present.[32]

Atrial Fibrillation Ablation in Heart Failure

AF ablation may be technically challenging in patients with congestive heart failure. The basic technique of pulmonary vein antral isolation

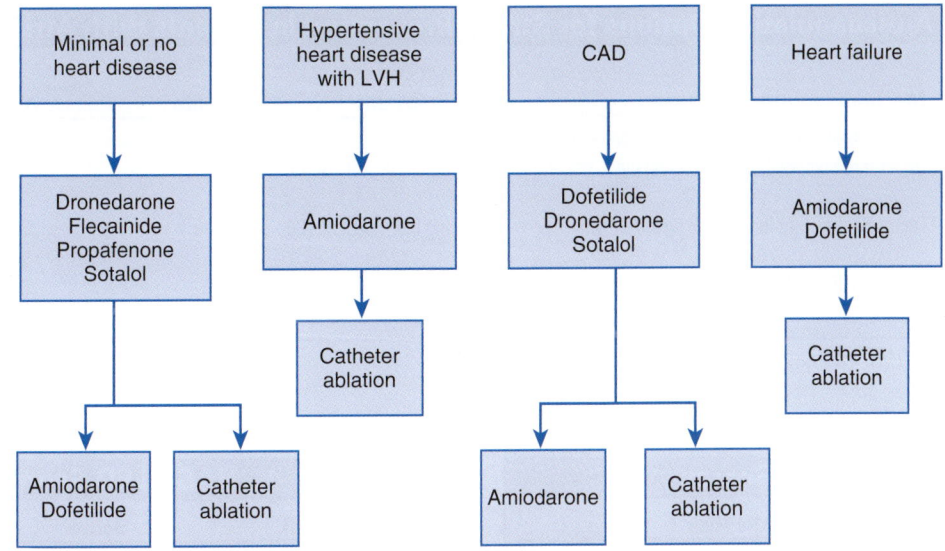

Fig. 38.1 Rhythm control strategies. Choice of antiarrhythmic drug therapy based on comorbidities. *CAD,* Coronary artery disease; *LVH,* left ventricular hypertrophy. (From Camm AJ, Lip GYH, De Caterina R, et al. 2012 focused update of the ESC guidelines for the management of atrial fibrillation. *Eur Heart J.* 2012;33:2719–2747.)

alone is rarely successful due to left atrial enlargement, chronic left atrial hypertension, and diffuse atrial scarring (**Fig. 38.2**). Additional linear lesions, both left and right atrial, and lesions targeting atrial electrograms that are fractionated are often placed with a modest increase in efficacy. Nevertheless, even though only intermediate success rate should be anticipated, catheter or surgical ablation may be a useful option in selected patients.[24] Catheter ablation should probably be attempted before AV junctional ablation in younger patients without AV block because the latter procedure is irreversible and creates a situation of life-long pacemaker dependency.

The Catheter Ablation versus Antiarrhythmic Drug Therapy in Atrial Fibrillation (CABANA) Trial randomized 2204 patients with new onset AF either greater than 65 years or less than 65 years with ≥1 risk factor for stroke to initial therapy with catheter ablation or antiarrhythmic drugs. Congestive heart failure was reported in 15% of this population. The intention to treat analysis showed no difference in the composite endpoint of all-cause mortality, disabling stroke, bleeding, or cardiac arrest. Crossover between groups was substantial with 10% of the ablation group not receiving ablation and 28% of the drug group crossing over to ablation. A secondary analysis of treatment received showed significant reduction in the primary composite endpoint for patients undergoing ablation (7.0%) versus drug treatment (10.9%, HR 0.67). Patients with a history of heart failure did better than those with no prior heart failure.[33]

The Catheter Ablation for Atrial Fibrillation with Heart Failure (CASTLE-AF) Trial randomized patients with systolic heart failure, an LVEF ≤35%, and New York Heart Association (NYHA) class II, III, IV symptoms to catheter ablation or medical therapy (rate or rhythm control). After a mean follow-up of 37.8 months, the composite endpoint of all-cause mortality or hospitalization for worsening heart failure was significantly lower in the ablation group (28.5% vs. 44.6%). There was also a 45% reduction in heart failure hospitalizations in the ablation group.[34]

Anticoagulation in Atrial Fibrillation and Atrial Flutter

Nonrheumatic AF has been associated with a fivefold increase in the risk of ischemic stroke. It has been estimated that 15% of all ischemic strokes occur in patients with AF. Patients with stroke and AF are

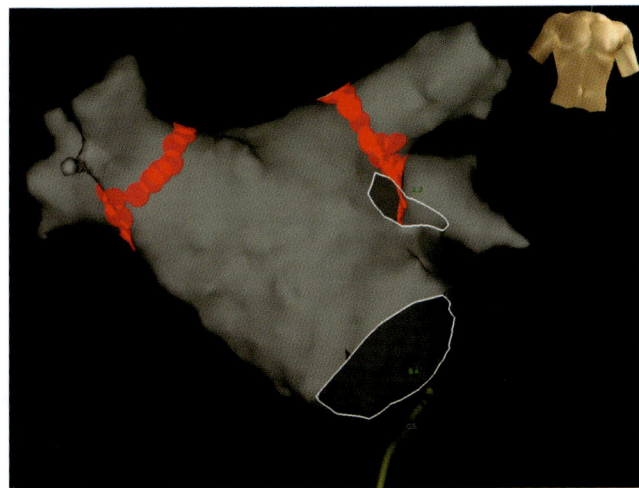

Fig. 38.2 Atrial fibrillation ablation. An anteroposterior view of the left atrium demonstrating radiofrequency ablation lesions around the pulmonary veins.

at higher risk for recurrent stroke and more severe stroke leading to greater disability and loss of independence. Stroke in patients with AF are 1.5 to 3.0 times more likely to be fatal than those in patients in sinus rhythm. Balanced against the increased risk for stroke and systemic embolism in patients with AF is the risk of bleeding associated with long-term anticoagulant therapy. For each patient, these risks must be carefully weighed to achieve optimal outcomes. Several new anticoagulation options are now available in addition to warfarin (see later discussion and **Table 38.2**).

Several scoring systems for stroke risk in patients with AF have been proposed. Although all the proposals have limitations, they remain clinically useful. In North America and Europe, the $CHADS_2$ and CHA_2DS_2-VASc schemes are used most commonly. Heart failure is a risk factor in both these scoring systems, so virtually all patients with heart failure and AF are candidates for chronic anticoagulation. In the absence of contraindications, oral anticoagulation is recommended for patients with CHADS2 or CHADSVASc (**Table 38.3**) scores of 2 or

TABLE 38.2	Anticoagulation Options for Stroke Prevention in Patients with Atrial Fibrillation				
Drug	Mechanism of Action	Dose	Renal Dose Adjustment	Half-life	Elimination
Warfarin	Vitamin K antagonist	Variable INR 2–3	N/A	35–45 hr	Hepatic CYP450
Dabigatran	Direct thrombin inhibitor	150 mg bid	75 mg bid if CrCl 15–30	12–17 hr	80% renal 20% hepatic
Apixaban	Factor Xa direct inhibitor	5 mg bid	2.5 mg bid if CrCl 15–30	8–15 hr	75% hepatic 25% renal
Rivaroxaban	Factor Xa direct inhibitor	20 mg daily	15 mg daily if CrCl 15–50	5–9 hr	66% hepatic 33% renal

CrCl, Creatinine clearance; *INR,* International normalized ratio.
See references 31 and 32.

TABLE 38.3	Stroke Risk Scores		
CHADS$_2$ Risk	Score	CHA$_2$DS$_2$-VASc Risk	Score
CHF	1	CHF (or LVEF ≤ 40%)	1
Hypertension	1	Hypertension	1
Age >75	1	Age ≥75	2
Diabetes	1	Diabetes	1
Stroke or TIA	2	Stroke or TIA	2
		Vascular disease	1
		Age 65–74	1
		Female	1
Maximum	6	Maximum	10

Stroke risk scores estimate the stroke risk based on comorbid conditions to help determine appropriate anticoagulation for patients with atrial fibrillation.
CHF, Congestive heart failure; *LVEF,* left ventricular ejection fraction; *TIA,* transient ischemic attack.
From Camm, AJ, Lip GYH, De Caterina R, et al. 2012 focused update of the ESC guidelines for the management of atrial fibrillation. *Eur Heart J.* 2012;33:2719–2747.

TABLE 38.4	HAS-BLED Scores	
HAS-BLED Risk		Score
Hypertension		1
Abnormal renal and/or liver function (1 point each)		1 or 2
Stroke or TIA		1
Bleeding		1
Labile INR		1
Elderly (Age >65)		1
Drugs and/or alcohol use (1 point each)		1 or 2
Maximum		9

HAS-BLED scores estimate bleeding risk in patients to be placed on systemic anticoagulation.
INR, International normalized ratio; *TIA,* transient ischemic attack.
From Camm, AJ, Lip GYH, De Caterina R, et al. 2012 focused update of the ESC guidelines for the management of atrial fibrillation. *Eur Heart J.* 2012;33:2719–2747.

greater and should be considered for scores of 1. Bleeding risk is also a critical factor in decisions about long-term anticoagulation, and scoring systems to predict risk have also been described. An example, the HAS-BLED score, is shown in **Table 38.4**.[32,35]

Warfarin has long been the primary oral anticoagulant for patients with AF. In a series of randomized trials in patients with nonvalvular AF, warfarin was shown to decrease stroke rate by approximately two-thirds. Similar effects were seen in patients with both paroxysmal and permanent AF. The target INR should be 2.0 to 3.0, with increased rates of stroke clearly seen below an INR of 1.7 and increased bleeding when INR values were more than 4.0. Recently, new oral anticoagulants have been introduced. Dabigatran, a direct thrombin inhibitor, and three factor Xa inhibitors, rivaroxaban, apixaban, and edoxaban, were shown to be noninferior to warfarin in large randomized clinical trials in nonvalvular AF.[32,35,36] Meta-analysis of the 42,411 participants in all four of these pivotal phase 3 clinical trials showed a 19% reduction in stroke or systemic embolic events compared with warfarin, a 10% reduction in all-cause mortality, and a 12% reduction in intracranial hemorrhage but an increase in gastrointestinal bleeding.[36]

Prognosis

AF may adversely influence prognosis both by increasing the risk of thromboembolic events and by aggravating or directly causing heart failure or ischemia. Proarrhythmic responses to drug therapy or bleeding from anticoagulants may also contribute to an increase in mortality

in patients who have AF. In the Framingham study, AF was associated with an odds ratio (OR) for death of 1.5 (95% CI, 1.2–1.8) among men and 1.9 (95% CI, 1.5–2.2) among women after adjustment for multiple clinical parameters.[5] The greatest absolute impact of AF on prognosis is seen when it occurs in patients who have advanced heart disease or other comorbid diseases.[6] In patients who do not have significant heart disease, AF has lesser effects on survival. As strategies for appropriate anticoagulation, effective rate control and heart failure management continue to evolve; it may be that the magnitude of the independent effect of AF will be lessened in the future. AF is the most common sustained arrhythmia in adult populations.[5] Although AF itself is usually not life threatening, it leads to significant patient morbidity and economic costs, and contributes to stroke and heart failure. Clinical decisions in patients who have AF are often difficult, and no uniformly effective therapies are available. In some patients, ventricular rate control and anticoagulation may be preferable to aggressive attempts to maintain sinus rhythm with repeat cardioversions and antiarrhythmic drug therapy. Newer strategies, such as less toxic antiarrhythmic agents, catheter ablation, improved surgical approaches, and new oral anticoagulants, offer promise for the future, but their efficacy and optimal uses still need to be demonstrated.

ATRIAL FLUTTER

Atrial flutter is defined as a rapid, regular atrial rhythm, with an atrial rate of 240 to 350 beats/min. Atrial flutter has an electrophysiologic

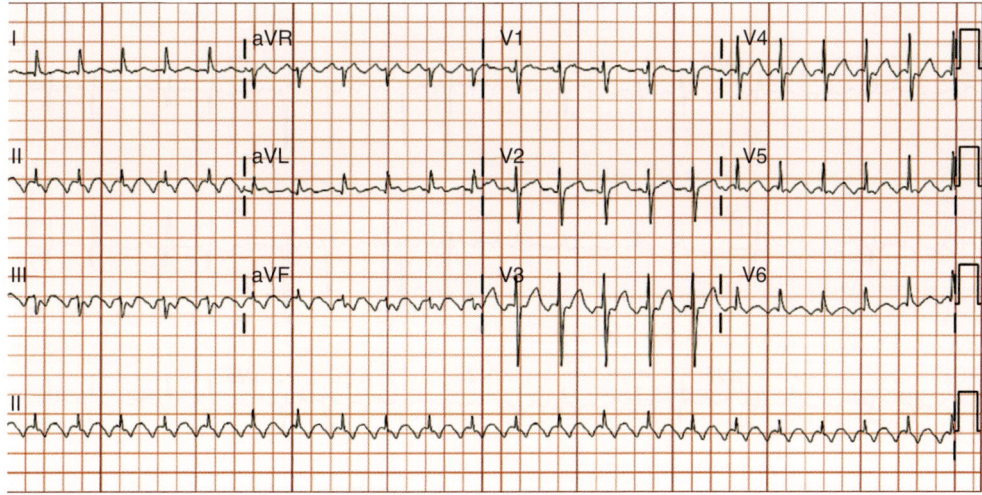

Fig. 38.3 Typical atrial flutter.

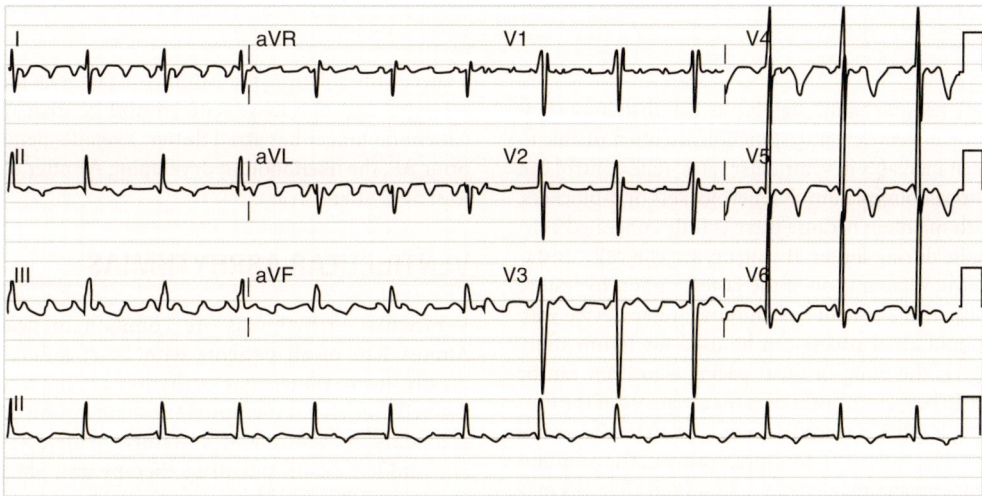

Fig. 38.4 Atypical atrial flutter.

mechanism different from AF but is often caused by the same factors and has a similar overall management strategy. When atrial flutter and AF are documented in the same patient, both will require treatment.

Epidemiology

Using the Marshfield Epidemiological Study Area, Granada and colleagues demonstrated an overall incidence of 88/100,000 person-years. Atrial flutter was found to be 2.5 times more common in men and 3.5 times more common in heart failure patients.[37] The highest rates of atrial flutter are seen post open heart surgery, with a 10% incidence in the first week.[38] This type of atrial flutter may resolve within weeks of the operation and not recur.

Pathophysiology and Diagnosis

The most common electrophysiologic mechanism for atrial flutter is a single macro-reentrant circuit located in the atrium. The rhythm is regular and ranges from 240 to 350 beats/min.[38] The ventricular rate that presents with atrial flutter depends on the AV nodal conduction and refractoriness. AV conduction is often 2:1 or 4:1, but may be variable. In 2:1 atrial flutter, the ventricular rate is often close to 150

beats/min. Atrial flutter is often classified as either typical or atypical. In typical flutter, the atrial impulse travels in a counterclockwise fashion up the right atrial septum, across and down the right atrial free wall, and then along the tricuspid isthmus. The activation sequence results in the classic findings of "sawtooth" flutter waves in the inferior ECG leads and an upright flutter wave in lead V1 (**Fig. 38.3**). Reverse typical flutter is when the atrial impulse travels in the opposite direction, also known as "clockwise" flutter (**Fig. 38.4**). Other macro-reentrant atrial tachycardias are also possible and are frequently seen after cardiac surgery that involves atrial incisions or after ablation procedures for AF (scar-related atrial tachycardias) (**Fig. 38.5**).[38]

The ECG is helpful in the diagnosis of atrial flutter. In typical atrial flutter, the flutter waves are seen in the inferior leads II, III, and aVF, as well as in lead V1 (see Fig. 38.3). Flutter waves should have the same axis and cycle length often resembling a sawtooth pattern. Typical flutter can be identified with negative flutter waves in the inferior leads and positive flutter waves in V1. If atrial flutter is suspected but is difficult to identify, vagal maneuvers or other measures to block the AV node can be used to reveal flutter waves.[38]

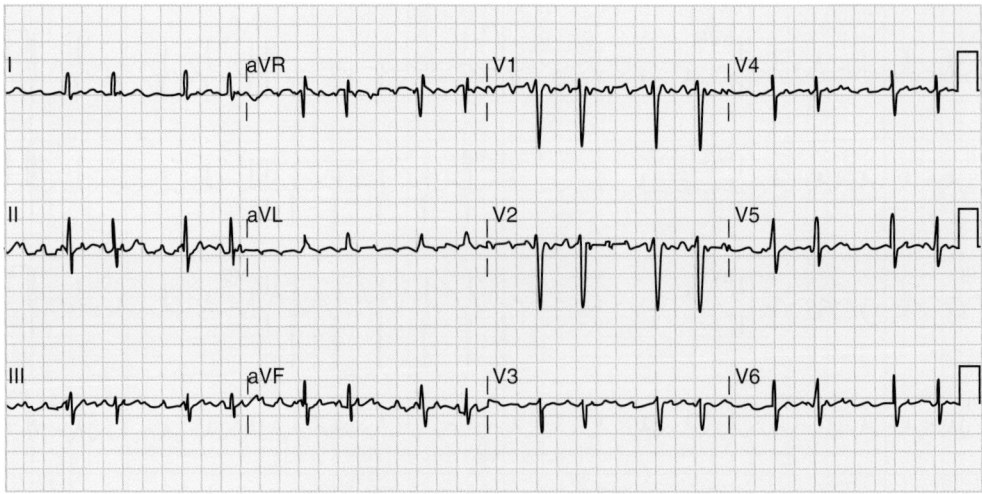

Fig. 38.5 Scar-related atrial tachycardia.

Management

In acute atrial flutter, hemodynamic stability is the first important concern. Patients with left ventricular dysfunction are often unable to compensate for sudden increases in ventricular rates. Rate control can be attempted with intravenous calcium channel blockers or β-blockers, but is often difficult to maintain because there is little concealed conduction in the AV node during flutter. If patients are clinically unstable, direct current cardioversion is often the fastest option to restore hemodynamic stability. If the patient has an intracardiac device with pacing capabilities, rapid atrial pacing can be used for termination. Bipolar atrial pacing via the ramp or burst pacing algorithm can be performed starting at 10 beats/min faster than the atrial rate of the flutter cycle length. Pacing is often performed for at least 10 to 30 seconds until the flutter wave axis in lead II becomes positive. The stimulus strength often needed is greater than 10 mA, and several attempts may be required to terminate.[38]

Before termination of atrial flutter, one must assess the stroke risk associated with return of normal sinus rhythm. Anticoagulation guidelines for cardioversion of atrial flutter are similar to those for cardioversion of AF. If the patient has been anticoagulated for the duration of the arrhythmia, the stroke risk is low. If the patient has been in sustained atrial flutter for less than 48 hours, the risk for thromboembolism is also considered low.

Similar to AF, amiodarone and dofetilide are the only drug options for patients with left ventricular dysfunction. Both have limited success in conversion of patients from atrial flutter to normal sinus rhythm. They may play a role in maintenance of sinus rhythm after electrical cardioversion, especially in patients with recurrence or patients with concomitant AF.

Radiofrequency catheter ablation of atrial flutter has become a safe and effective treatment option for most patients. If the reentrant circuit incorporates the cavotricuspid isthmus, then creating a linear lesion on the isthmus from the tricuspid annulus to the inferior vena cava will terminate the rhythm. Left atrial flutter or scar lesion–related flutter often require detailed mapping before radiofrequency ablation. Due to the high acute success rates of catheter ablation and the side effects of antiarrhythmic medications, radiofrequency ablation is first-line therapy for appropriate patients. Patients with previously documented AF will usually continue to have AF after

a successful ablation for isthmus-dependent flutter and should be managed appropriately. Rate control is often more effective if the patient no longer has atrial flutter. Even if a patient has no history of prior AF, the likelihood of developing AF after a flutter ablation is at least 50% after 3 years.[39]

VENTRICULAR ARRHYTHMIAS

Ventricular arrhythmias are common in heart failure patients. Almost half of all patients with heart failure will die suddenly, mostly from ventricular arrhythmias. Implantable cardioverter-defibrillator (ICD) therapy is the main option for both primary and secondary prevention of sustained ventricular tachycardia (VT) and sudden death, but drug therapy and ablation are frequently important adjuncts.[40]

There is no one mechanism that causes ventricular arrhythmias in patients with heart failure. Instead, multiple elements contribute to the arrhythmogenesis, including increased sympathetic tone, ischemia, myocardial scar, conduction delay, increased diastolic calcium levels, early and delayed afterdepolarizations, electrolyte abnormalities, and drugs. Common drugs that potentiate VT are antiarrhythmics, phosphodiesterase inhibitors, sympathomimetic drugs, and digoxin.[41]

Acute Episodes of Sustained Monomorphic Ventricular Tachycardia

The goal of acute therapy for sustained VT is to restore rapidly a stable rhythm with a physiologically appropriate rate and thereby prevent organ damage or further hemodynamic deterioration. Patients with severe hypotension, chest pain, or evidence for hypoperfusion of critical organs should be considered hemodynamically unstable, and direct current cardioversion is usually the most expeditious method for terminating the arrhythmia. In many patients, however, the tachycardia is not immediately life threatening and the patient is conscious and not in severe distress. In such patients, pharmacologic cardioversion is the procedure of choice.[40,42]

Pharmacologic conversion of sustained monomorphic VT episodes has not been studied in large controlled randomized trials. Observational and limited controlled trial data, however, indicate that

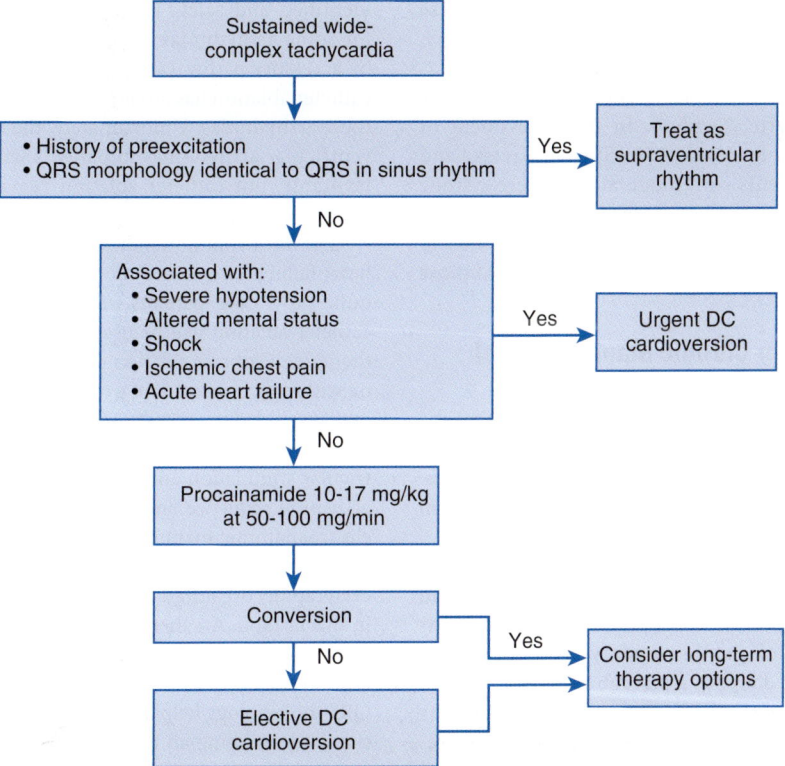

Fig. 38.6 Wide-complex tachycardia management. *DC,* Direct-current.

intravenous procainamide is the most effective agent.[43-45] Because procainamide-induced conversion is related to peak plasma drug concentrations, conversion is more likely with faster infusion rates (50–100 mg/min up to 15–17 mg/kg). These infusion rates, however, may cause hypotension and QT prolongation, so blood pressure and the ECG must be frequently monitored throughout the infusion. Typically the VT cycle length will lengthen, and the slower rate will partially mitigate the vasodilating and negative inotropic effects of the drug. If the cycle length fails to lengthen, the ECG morphology changes, or the patient develops symptomatic hypotension, then the infusion should be immediately stopped and electrical cardioversion considered.

Intravenous lidocaine and β-adrenergic blocking agents have very limited efficacy for terminating episodes of sustained VT in patients with heart failure. Verapamil and diltiazem are contraindicated in wide-complex tachycardias of unknown mechanism in patients with structural heart disease.[40,42] Rarely, if there is a strong possibility that the wide-complex tachycardia is supraventricular in origin, adenosine may be used. In most supraventricular arrhythmias, adenosine will either terminate the tachycardia or provide diagnostic information if AV block occurs. Intravenous amiodarone may be useful to treat recurrent episodes or if incessant monomorphic VT is seen (**Fig. 38.6**).

Nonsustained Ventricular Tachycardia

Nonsustained VT is commonly detected during ECG monitoring in heart failure patients with both ischemic and nonischemic cardiomyopathies.[46] The frequency and complexity of ventricular ectopy are likely to increase during periods of worsening heart failure. A number of trials have tested the hypothesis that antiarrhythmic drug therapy either empirically administered or when guided by arrhythmia suppression during serial ambulatory ECG monitoring would

improve survival and prevent sudden death. The drug most carefully evaluated has been amiodarone. In 1997, the Amiodarone Trials Meta-analysis Investigators reviewed 13 randomized controlled trials comparing amiodarone to placebo in patients with either recent myocardial infractions or congestive heart failure.[47] They estimated that prophylactic amiodarone would reduce arrhythmic/sudden death by 29% and total mortality by 13%. The studies included in this meta-analysis were completed before modern therapy for heart failure, including aggressive revascularization, renin-angiotensin system, β-adrenergic blockade, and aldosterone antagonism, was widely practiced. In the Sudden Cardiac Death-Heart Failure Trial (SCD-HeFT), which was completed in 2004, empiric amiodarone had no advantage over a placebo in patients with NYHA class II symptoms and actually increased mortality in patients with class III symptoms. A more recent meta-analysis of 15 randomized trials showed that prophylactic amiodarone had no overall benefit regarding mortality.[48] In most situations, asymptomatic ventricular ectopy should be considered a risk factor for future events and not as a target for therapy. However, in patients with very high frequency monomorphic premature ventricular contractions (PVCs) and VT, mapping and ablation of the site of origin may improve function and eliminate symptoms.

Sudden Cardiac Death in Patients with Heart Failure

The risk of sudden cardiac death (SCD) in heart failure patients is a major contributor to morbidity and mortality in this population. The annual incidence varies according to observational data, but ranges from 200,000 to 460,000. In the Metoprolol CR/XL Randomized Intervention Trial in Congestive Heart Failure (MERIT-HF), 64% of patients in NYHA class II who died had SCD, compared with 59% of patients in class III and 33% of patients in class IV. The reasons for the elevated risk of SCD in heart failure patients are unknown, but multiple theories have arisen. These include subendocardial ischemia, left ventricular hypertrophy, myocardial stretch, increased sympathetic tone, and aberrant baroreceptor response increasing ventricular arrhythmias, electrolyte abnormality, and coronary artery emboli. In the Assessment of Treatment with Lisinopril and Survival (ATLAS) trial, Uretsky and associates looked at 3164 patients with moderate to severe systolic heart failure. There were a total of 1382 deaths (43.7%) during the follow-up period of 36 to 60 months. Autopsy was performed in 188 patients, and acute coronary causes were found in 54% of those with SCD.

Pharmacologic Therapy for Chronic Management of Ventricular Tachycardia

Although ICD therapy has evolved into the primary therapeutic modality to prevent death from ventricular arrhythmias, frequent ICD shocks are painful and may cause significant psychological distress. Therefore, concomitant antiarrhythmic drugs are often prescribed in an effort to reduce shock frequency.

Amiodarone and sotalol are the drugs most commonly used as adjuncts to ICD therapy in patients with structural heart disease and heart failure.[49-51] Pacifico and associates randomized 302 patients with prior sustained arrhythmias and secondary prevention ICDs to either sotalol (160–320 mg daily) or a placebo.[49] Sotalol resulted in a 48% reduction of the primary endpoint of death from any cause or delivery of first shock for any cause. Overall shock frequency was significantly reduced to 1.43 ± 3.53 shocks per year in the sotalol group from 3.89 ± 10.65 shocks per year in the placebo group. In the Optimal Pharmacological Therapy in Cardioverter Defibrillator Patients Trial (OPTIC), β-adrenergic blockade only, sotalol, and amiodarone plus β-blockade were compared.[50] Sotalol and, to a greater degree, amiodarone plus β-blockade significantly decreased the frequency of shocks, both appropriate and inappropriate. There are, however, more recent data suggesting that antiarrhythmic drug therapy to prevent ICD shocks may not always be beneficial. Kowey and colleagues reported a phase II dose-ranging study of celivarone, a noniodinated analog of amiodarone, in patients with ICDs.[52] Celivarone had no significant effect on ICD shock frequency or mortality in this trial. The study included a small calibrator group treated with amiodarone. Although the amiodarone group had fewer ICD shocks, they also had a higher mortality. Patients with class III heart failure on amiodarone also had a higher mortality than placebo patients in SCD-HeFT. Until more definitive data on the value of adjunct antiarrhythmic therapy become available, it seems reasonable to restrict such therapy to only ICD patients with frequent, symptomatic episodes of atrial or ventricular arrhythmias.

In addition to the known extracardiac side effects of antiarrhythmic drugs, the potential for drug-ICD interactions must be considered. Antiarrhythmic drugs with sodium channel blocking properties may increase the defibrillation threshold. Pure class III agents are unlikely to do so and may actually decrease defibrillation energy requirements. Pacing thresholds may rarely be affected. Antiarrhythmic drugs frequently prolong VT cycle lengths and may require changes in programmed detection zones. Antiarrhythmic drugs may result in sinus bradycardia or worsen AV conduction, increasing the need for atrial and/or ventricular pacing.[53,54]

Catheter Ablation of Ventricular Tachycardia

Catheter ablation works best when a single structure or site not required for normal function but critical for the arrhythmia can be identified and safely ablated. Success rates with catheter ablation for some arrhythmias (e.g., supraventricular tachycardias mediated by accessory pathways or dual AV nodal pathways) are so high that catheter ablation has largely supplanted drug therapy in patients with these arrhythmias. Unfortunately, the results of catheter ablation for ventricular arrhythmias in patients with heart failure are much less favorable, but catheter ablation remains an important option for many patients.

The most common indication for catheter ablation in patients with heart failure is sustained monomorphic VT. Unless the tachycardia is quite slow, most patients will have an ICD for primary therapy and catheter ablation will be used to decrease the need for frequent ICD therapies. Catheter ablation may be used in these patients either alone or with concomitant antiarrhythmic drug therapy. Catheter ablation may be guided in several ways. If the VT is well tolerated, the arrhythmia is induced at electrophysiologic study with programmed ventricular stimulation and critical portions of the VT circuit defined by activation sequence and entrainment mapping. A three-dimensional electroanatomic mapping system is typically used to help guide catheter positioning. If circulatory support is used during the procedure, even rapidly organized tachycardias can usually be mapped and ablated in this fashion. An alternate technique uses voltage mapping to define areas of myocardial scarring and then places linear ablation lesions around the border zone of the scar. Pace mapping to match a known QRS morphology helps guide the region to be isolated. Most VT ablation is done using an endocardial approach, but recent observations suggest that epicardial ablation may be required, particularly for patients with nonischemic forms of cardiomyopathy. Unfortunately, many patients either will have multiple VT circuits at the time of their initial ablation attempt or will manifest new VTs during long-term follow-up, and the overall success rate for complete elimination of VT may be only 40% to 60%.[55] Despite this, decreasing the frequency of required ICD therapies may be an important part of patient management (**Figs. 38.7** and **38.8**).

The second most common indication for VT ablation in patients with heart failure is when frequent PVCs by themselves compromise ventricular function and result in a tachycardia-induced cardiomyopathy. This is usually seen with extremely high-density PVCs in patients without other forms of heart disease, with a threshold for onset at about 10,000 PVCs per day. If the PVC morphology is stable, the site of origin can usually be mapped and identified by activation mapping, confirmed with pace mapping, and ablated with local radiofrequency (RF) energy delivery. For patients without disease that causes myocardial scarring, this type of PVC ablation may be curative and their LVEF may return to normal.[56]

Finally, several groups have reported success in eliminating recurrent episodes of ventricular fibrillation (VF) by targeting a PVC focus whose firing triggers recurrent episodes. For this to be effective, the patient should have multiple VF episodes triggered by a PVC with a single morphology.

Risks of catheter ablation for VT are considerably higher than those for most other arrhythmias. In patients with peripheral vascular disease, vascular complications at access sites or inability to access the left ventricle may be problems. Valve or coronary artery damage, embolic events, cardiac perforations, bleeding, and hemodynamic compromise from the mapping procedure are also potential complications.[55]

Device Therapy
Implantable Cardioverter-Defibrillator

The first clinical use of a totally implanted defibrillator was reported in 1980.[57] In the ensuing years, the ICD has developed into the most important therapy for preventing sudden death and treating sustained

TABLE 38.6 Selected Cardiac Resynchronization Therapy Trials

Trial	Randomization	Year	Patients	Entry Criteria	CRT Outcomes
MIRACLE[92]	CRT versus OMT, 6 months	2002	453	NYHA class III–IV and LVEF ≤35% with QRS ≥130	Improved NYHA class, LVEF, QoL, and 6MWD; reduced LVEDD and MR
MIRACLE-ICD[97]	CRT-D versus ICD, 6 months	2003	369	NYHA class III–IV and LVEF ≤ 35% with QRS ≥130	Improved, NYHA class, QoL, and peak Vo_2
CONTAK-CD[98]	CRT-D versus ICD, 6 mo	2003	490	NYHA class II–IV with LVEF ≤ 35% and QRS ≥ 120	Improved 6MWD, NYHA class, QoL, and LVEF with reduced LV volume
COMPANION[99]	OMT versus CRT-P or versus CRT-D, 15 months	2004	1520	NYHA class III–IV with LVEF ≤ 35% and QRS ≥120	Reduced all-cause mortality and hospitalization
CARE-HF[75]	OMT versus CRT-P, 29.4 mo	2005	813	NYHA class III–IV with LVEF ≤ 35% and QRS ≥ 120	Reduced all-cause mortality and hospitalization; improved NYHA class and QoL
REVERSE[100]	CRT-ON versus CRT-OFF, 12 months	2008	610	NYHA class I–II with LVEF ≤ 40% and QRS ≥ 120	CRT did not reduce all-cause mortality but reduced LVESV index and hospitalization [a]
MADIT-CRT[86]	CRT-D versus ICD, 12 mo	2009	1820	NYHA class I–II with LVEF ≤ 30% and QRS ≥ 130	34% reduction in the risk of death or heart failure events[a]
RAFT[101]	CRT-D versus ICD, 40 months	2010	1798	NYHA class II–III with LVEF ≤ 30% and QRS ≥ 120	Reduced all-cause mortality and hospitalization

[a]Benefits largely in NYHA class II.
6MWD, Six-minute walk distance; *CRT-D,* cardiac resynchronization therapy defibrillator; *CRT-P,* cardiac resynchronization therapy pacemaker; *ICD,* implantable cardioverter-defibrillator; *LVEDD,* left ventricular end-diastolic dimension; *LVEF,* left ventricular ejection fraction; *LVESV,* left ventricular end-systolic volume; *MADIT-CRT,* Multicenter Automatic Defibrillator Implantation Trial cardiac resynchronization therapy; *MIRACLE,* Multicenter InSync Randomized Clinical Evaluation trial; *MR,* mitral regurgitation; *NYHA,* New York Heart Association; *OMT,* optimal medical therapy; *QoL,* quality of life.

distance walked in 6 minutes or improvement in NYHA functional class 3 to 6 months after CRT implantation. Studies have defined response to CRT as a combination of several clinical measures or as a combination of both clinical and echocardiographic measures.

In the Multicenter InSync Randomized Clinical Evaluation (MIRACLE) trial, there was a 67% improvement in the group randomized to CRT using a clinical composite score to determine which patients were improved, unchanged, or worsened.[92] Intriguingly, a more recent Frequent Optimization Study Using the QuickOpt Method (FREEDOM) trial, designed to assess strategies for AV and interventricular (VV) interval optimization, reported a 67.5% improvement after CRT using the same clinical composite score.[93] Despite advances in knowledge and experience with CRT, the proportion of patients considered clinical nonresponders has remained at roughly 30%.

In nonresponders, first the ECG can be checked with and without pacing to confirm left ventricular pacing. If the underlying QRS is narrower than the paced QRS, pacing may not benefit. Next the device should be interrogated to ensure optimal pacing with close to 100% biventricular pacing. If the percentage of biventricular pacing is less than 98.5%, the reason should be determined and corrected. Most frequently, this is due to atrial or ventricular arrhythmia. Next the lead position should be confirmed on posteroanterior and lateral chest x-ray. It is generally recommended to implant the LV lead in a basal to midlateral or posterolateral branch of the coronary sinus, if there is an eligible vein. Lead reposition can be changed if there are options for a more suitable vein position. The onset of the QRS to the LV electrogram, the QLV, can be measured at implant or during subsequent device interrogation and has become a useful measure to predict response to CRT. A QLV greater than 95 milliseconds had the best improvement in EF, ESV, EDV, and QOL measures at 6 months.[94] LV fusion pacing has been introduced to allow fusion of the LV stimulation with intrinsic ventricular activation. This form of CRT, effective in patients who do not have AV block, has been shown to be noninferior to standard CRT, and a superiority trial is now underway. Echocardiographic assessment immediately after the device implantation or during the follow-up procedures provides further information on the reasons for response and nonresponse to CRT. The transmitral filling profile improves acutely in most patients with the initiation of CRT. If it remains below 40% to 45% of the corresponding cycle length, changing the AV-delay of the device programming can optimize it. The SMART AV trial showed that patients with normal AV-delay did not derive benefit from echo-guided or device-guided AV-optimization compared with the empiric settings; however, patients with prolonged AV-conduction were not included in this prospective, randomized study.[95] The presence or even worsening of intraventricular dyssynchrony is a common problem in CRT nonresponders. VV-optimization is a useful tool to correct intraventricular dyssynchrony by device programming. Optimal VV-delay settings are highly variable in CRT patients, and therefore echocardiography-guided VV-optimization is recommended. Echocardiography can also be used to optimize LV lead placement. Speckle-tracking echocardiography to identify the latest site of peak contraction free of scar for optimal LV lead placement resulted in improved reverse ventricular remodeling compared with nontargeted patients in the TARGET trial of 220 patients.[96]

Arrhythmias Associated with Left Ventricular Assist Device Therapy (see Chapter 45)

A general schematic approach to arrhythmia management in patients with advanced heart failure is shown in **Fig. 38.10**. Left ventricular assist devices (LVADs) have become more common in the treatment of advanced heart failure patients. With the advancement of these mechanical circulatory support systems, they can be used not only for a bridge to heart transplant but also for destination therapy.[102,103]

Atrial arrhythmias are common in patients with LVADs. AF is the most common atrial arrhythmia in patients with LVADs. Treatment for this is the same as in any patient with heart failure. β-blockers are the preferred treatment, namely metoprolol tartrate, because carvedilol may cause a significant drop in blood pressure. Calcium channel blockers should be avoided, because they are contraindicated in most

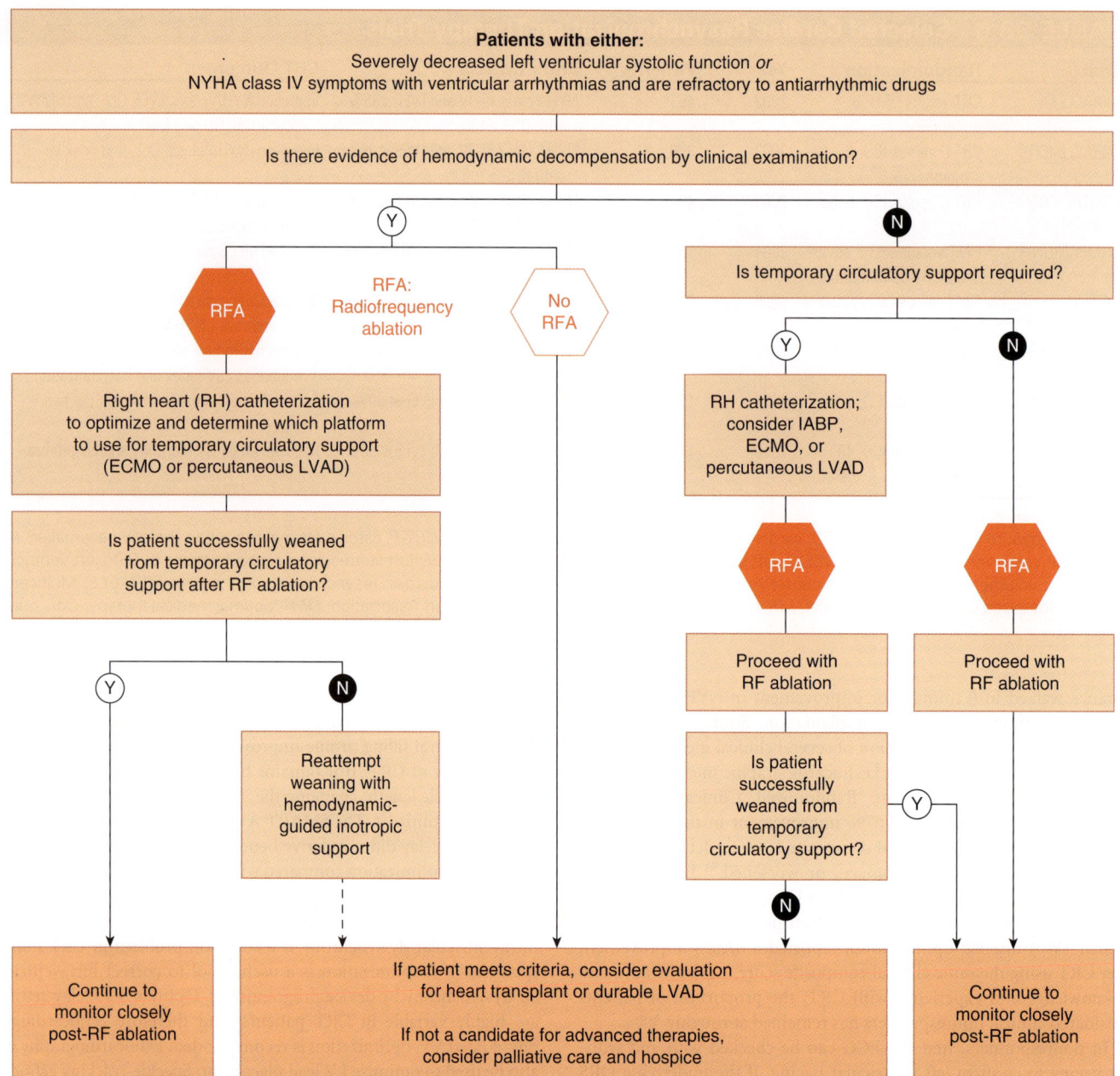

Fig. 38.10 General approach to arrhythmias management in patients with advanced heart failure. *ECMO,* Extracorporeal membrane oxygenation; *IABP,* intra-aortic balloon pump; *LVAD,* left ventricular assist device; *RF,* radiofrequency; *RFA,* radiofrequency ablation; *RH,* right heart. (From Santangeli P, Rame JE, Birati EY, Marchlinski FE. Management of ventricular arrhythmias in patients with advanced heart failure. *J Am Coll Cardiol.* 2017;69(14):1842–1860.)

heart failure patients due to the negative inotropic response. Catheter ablation in this population may be difficult and has not been studied in a prospective trial. All patients with LVADs are typically anticoagulated; thus the risk of thromboembolism because of AF is low.[104]

Ventricular arrhythmias are common in patients with end-stage heart failure. The substrate causing these arrhythmias does not change with the placement of an LVAD; thus the risk of developing ventricular arrhythmias is unchanged. There is a theoretical reduction of VT as the left ventricular end-diastolic pressure is lowered, thereby decreasing the risk of ventricular arrhythmias. However, with the addition of an inflow cannula inserted into the left ventricle, the risk of developing ventricular arrhythmias greatly increases. This occurs when the left ventricle is underfilled, especially when the inflow cannula touches any of

the endocardial structures, most commonly the septal wall. This occurs any time the patient loses intracardiac volume, as with diuresis, significant blood loss, or increased LVAD speed, resulting in overpumping and collapse of the ventricle. Treatment involves resolving the underlying issue by turning the LVAD speed down, replacing blood loss, or reducing diuretics. Drug therapy includes β-blockers, amiodarone, or dofetilide. Mexiletine can be added if breakthrough occurs.[105] Limited data suggest that ranolazine may reduce ventricular arrhythmia burden in antiarrhythmic drug refractory cases.[106] Catheter ablation has been performed on patients with drug refractory ventricular arrhythmias. Ablation should be a secondary treatment because it is more difficult due to the presence of an inflow cannula as well as increased blood flow (**Fig. 38.11**).[107]

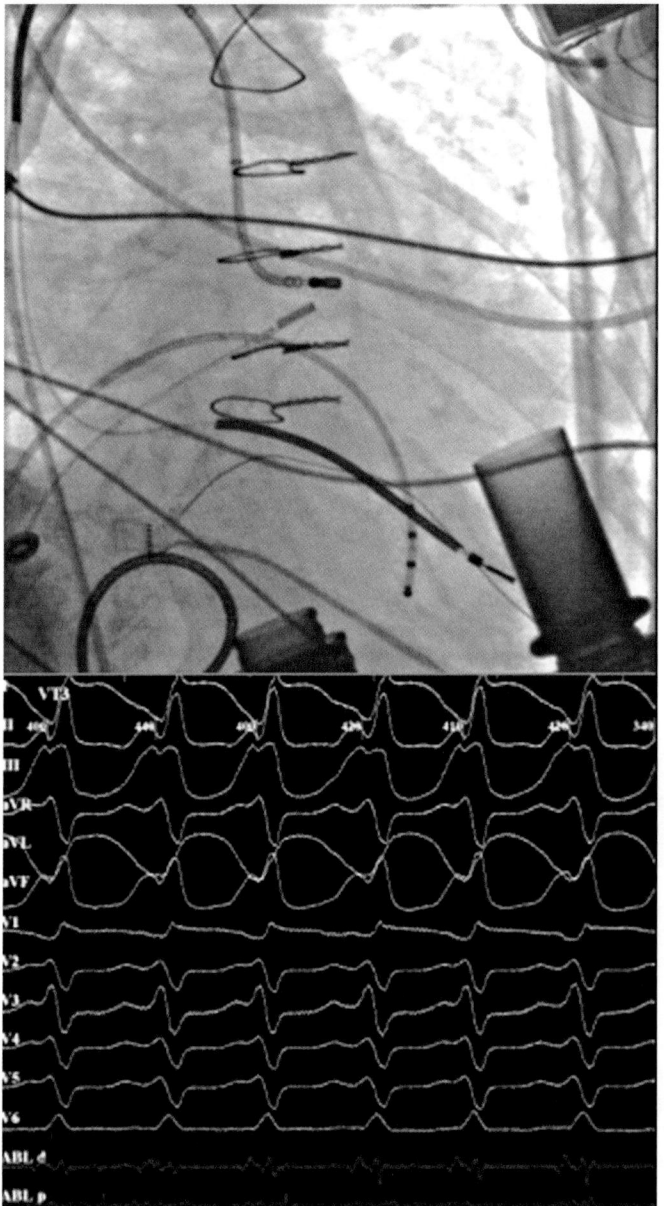

Fig. 38.11 Ventricular tachycardia ablation in a patient with a left ventricular assist device. Notice the early ventricular signals on the intracardiac electrograms from the ablation catheter.

Arrhythmia Management After Heart Transplantation

Improved outcomes after heart transplantation have led to a median survival time exceeding 10 years. The fact that patients live longer has led to increased occurrence of arrhythmias.

Sinus node ischemia, graft ischemia, drug effects, and sympathetic denervation all predispose patients to postsurgical bradycardia. Temporary pacing is often established via epicardial wires to keep ventricular rates greater than 90 beats/min. Permanent pacemaker implantation is reserved for symptomatic bradycardia or sinus node dysfunction.[108]

Atrial arrhythmias range in incidence from 0.3% to 24% for AF and 2.8% to 30% for atrial flutter after heart transplantation. AF is the most common, especially early after surgery. Atrial flutter and other atrial tachycardias are more common later in the course after transplant. Interestingly, AF within 2 weeks has been associated with rejection, and atrial flutter after 3 weeks is the most common arrhythmia associated with rejection. Management of these arrhythmias is similar to other patients; however, prolonged antiarrhythmic drug therapy is not usually indicated.[108]

Nonsustained VT is somewhat common in the early postoperative period. This will typically become less frequent after transplant. If VT occurs late after heart transplant, severe cardiac allograft vasculopathy should be suspected. These patients may need antiarrhythmic therapy and should be considered for ICD placement. Up to 25% of patients with ventricular arrhythmias may have SCD, and this is the most common cause of death after heart transplantation.[108]

KEY REFERENCES

10. Lloyd-Jones DM, Wang TJ, Leip EP, et al. Lifetime risk for development of atrial fibrillation: the Framingham Heart Study. *Circulation.* 2004;110:1042–1046.
20. Calkins H, Kuck KH, Cappato R, et al. 2012 HRS/EHRA/ECAS expert consensus statement on catheter and surgical ablation of atrial fibrillation. *Heart Rhythm.* 2012;9(4):632–696.
28. Wyse DG, Waldo AL, DiMarco JP, et al. A comparison of rate control and rhythm control in patients with atrial fibrillation. *N Engl J Med.* 2002;347:1825–1833.
34. Marrouche NF, Brachmann J, Andresen D, et al. Catheter ablation for atrial fibrillation with heart failure. *N Engl J Med.* 2018;378(5):417–427.
55. Stevenson WG, Soejima K. Catheter ablation for ventricular tachycardia. *Circulation.* 2007;115:2750–2760.
61. Bardy GH, Lee KL, Mark DB, et al. for the Sudden Cardiac Death in Heart Failure Trial (SCD-HeFT) Investigators. Amiodarone or an implantable cardioverter-defibrillator for congestive heart failure. *N Engl J Med.* 2005;352:225–237.
75. Cleland JG, Daubert JC, Erdmann E, et al. for the CARE-HF Study Investigators. The effect of cardiac resynchronization on morbidity and mortality in heart failure. *N Engl J Med.* 2005;352:1539–1549.
86. Moss AJ, Hall WJ, Cannom DS, et al. Cardiac-resynchronization therapy for the prevention of heart failure events. *N Engl J Med.* 2009;361:1329–1338.
92. Abraham WT, Fisher WG, Smith AL, et al. Cardiac resynchronization in chronic heart failure. *N Engl J Med.* 2002;246:1845–1853.
101. Tang AS, Wells GA, Talajic M, et al. Cardiac-resynchronization therapy for mild-to-moderate heart failure. *N Engl J Med.* 2010;363:2385–2395.

The full reference list for this chapter is available on ExpertConsult.

Guidelines
Cardiac Resynchronization Therapy and Implantable Cardioverter-Defibrillators for Heart Failure with a Reduced Ejection Fraction[a]

In 2012 the ACC/AHA/HRS updated the 2008 guidelines for device-based therapy of cardiac rhythm abnormalities.[1] These revised guidelines were incorporated into the 2013 American College of Cardiology Foundation and American Heart Association (ACCF/AHA) heart failure guidelines.[2] The revised guidelines (**Table 38G.1**) include a comprehensive revision of CRT indications based on all available studies through 2013. The guidelines expand the indications for CRT to some NYHA class II and very select class I patients, limit CRT indications by QRS morphology and QRS duration, and attempt to harmonize indications across NYHA classes when possible. The most certain indications are for those patients who have LVEF ≤35%, sinus rhythm, LBBB with a QRS duration ≥150 milliseconds, and NYHA class II, III, or ambulatory IV symptoms on optimal medical treatment.

Patients with reduced LVEF are at increased risk for ventricular tachyarrhythmias leading to sudden cardiac death. Patients who have had sustained ventricular tachycardia, ventricular fibrillation, unexplained syncope, or cardiac arrest are at the highest risk for recurrence. Indications for ICD therapy as secondary prevention of sudden cardiac death are also discussed in the 2013 ACCF/AHA guidelines for heart failure (**Table 38G.2**),[2] as well as the ACCF/AHA/HRS device-based therapy guidelines.[3]

TABLE 38G.1 American College of Cardiology Foundation and American Heart Association Guidelines for Cardiac Resynchronization

Class	Indication	Level of Evidence
I	CRT is indicated for patients who have LVEF of 35% or less, sinus rhythm, LBBB with a QRS duration of 150 msec or greater, and NYHA class II, III, or ambulatory IV symptoms on GDMT.	Level of Evidence A for NYHA class III/I, Level of Evidence: B for NYHA class II
IIa	CRT can be useful for patients who have LVEF of 35% or less, sinus rhythm, a non-LBBB pattern with a QRS duration of 150 msec or greater, and NYHA class III/ambulatory class IV symptoms on GDMT.	A
	CRT can be useful for patients who have LVEF of 35% or less, sinus rhythm, LBBB with a QRS duration of 120–149 msec, and NYHA class II, III, or ambulatory IV symptoms on GDMT.	B
	CRT can be useful in patients with AF and LVEF of 35% or less on GDMT if (a) the patient requires ventricular pacing or otherwise meets CRT criteria and (b) atrioventricular nodal ablation or pharmacologic rate control will allow near 100% ventricular pacing with CRT.	B
	CRT can be useful for patients on GDMT who have LVEF of 35% or less, and are undergoing placement of a new or replacement device with anticipated requirement for significant (>40%) ventricular pacing.	C
IIb	CRT may be considered for patients who have LVEF of 35% or less, sinus rhythm, a non-LBBB pattern with QRS duration of 120–149 msec, and NYHA class III/ambulatory class IV on GDMT.	B
	CRT may be considered for patients who have LVEF of 35% or less, sinus rhythm, a non-LBBB pattern with a QRS duration of 150 msec or greater, and NYHA class II symptoms on GDMT.	B
	CRT may be considered for patients who have LVEF of 30% or less, ischemic etiology of HF, sinus rhythm, LBBB with a QRS duration of 150 msec or greater, and NYHA class I symptoms on GDMT.	C
III: No Benefit	CRT is not recommended for patients with NYHA class I or II symptoms and non-LBBB pattern with QRS duration less than 150 msec.	
	CRT is not indicated for patients whose comorbidities and/or frailty limit survival with good functional capacity to less than 1 year.	

AF, Atrial fibrillation; *CRT*, cardiac resynchronization therapy; *GDMT*, guideline-directed medical therapy; *LBBB*, left bundle branch block; *LVEF*, left ventricular ejection fraction; *NYHA*, New York Heart Association.

---

[a]From Abraham WT. Guidelines: cardiac resynchronization therapy and implantable cardioverter-defibrillators for heart failure with a reduced ejection fraction. In Zipes DP, et al, editors: *Braunwald's Heart Disease: A Textbook of Cardiovascular Medicine.* 11th ed. Philadelphia: Elsevier; 2019.

TABLE 38G.2 American College of Cardiology Foundation and American Heart Association Guidelines for Indications for Implantable Cardioverter-Defibrillators

Class	Indication	Level of Evidence
I	ICD therapy is recommended for primary prevention of SCD in selected patients with HFrEF at least 40 days post MI with LVEF <35% and NYHA class II or III symptoms on chronic GDMT, who are expected to live >1 year.	A
I	ICD therapy is recommended for primary prevention of SCD in selected patients with HFrEF at least 40 days post MI with LVEF <30% and NYHA class I symptoms while receiving GDMT, who are expected to live >1 year.	B
IIa	To prevent sudden death, placement of an ICD is reasonable in patients with asymptomatic ischemic cardiomyopathy who are at least 40 days post MI, have an LVEF of 30% or less, are on appropriate medical therapy, and have reasonable expectation of survival with a good functional status for more than 1 year.	B
IIb	ICD therapy to prevent SCD in patients with nonischemic cardiomyopathy who are at least 40 days post MI, have an LVEF <35%, with NYHA functional class II or III symptoms while undergoing chronic optimal medical therapy, and who have reasonable expectation of survival for more than 1 year with good functional status.	B
	The usefulness of implantation of an ICD is of uncertain benefit to prolong meaningful survival in patients with a high risk of nonsudden death as predicted by frequent hospitalizations, advanced frailty, or comorbidities such as systemic malignancy or severe renal dysfunction.	B

GDMT, Guideline-directed medical therapy; *HFrEF,* heart failure with a reduced ejection fraction; *ICD,* implantable cardioverter-defibrillator; *LVEF,* left ventricular ejection fraction; *MI,* myocardial infarction; *NYHA,* New York Heart Association; *SCD,* sudden cardiac death.

REFERENCES

1. Tracy CM, Epstein AE, Darbar D, et al. 2012 ACCF/AHA/HRS focused update of the 2008 guidelines for device-based therapy of cardiac rhythm abnormalities: a report of the American College of Cardiology Foundation/American Heart Association task force on practice guidelines and the Heart Rhythm Society [corrected]. *Circulation.* 2012;126:1784–1800.
2. Yancy CW, Jessup M, Bozkurt B, et al. 2013 ACCF/AHA guideline for the management of heart failure: a report of the American College of Cardiology Foundation/American Heart Association task force on practice guidelines. *Circulation.* 2013;128:e240–e327.
3. Epstein AE, DiMarco JP, Ellenbogen KA, et al. ACC/AHA/HRS 2008 guidelines for device-based therapy of cardiac rhythm abnormalities: a report of the American College of Cardiology/American Heart Association task force on practice guidelines (writing committee to revise the ACC/AHA/ NASPE 2002 guideline update for implantation of cardiac pacemakers and antiarrhythmia devices) developed in collaboration with the American Association for Thoracic Surgery and Society of Thoracic Surgeons. *J Am Coll Cardiol.* 2008;51:e1–e62.

39

Treatment of Heart Failure with Preserved Ejection Fraction

Savitri Fedson, Arunima Misra, Anita Deswal

Over the past two decades, it has become increasingly apparent that approximately 50% of patients with heart failure (HF) have a normal or almost normal ejection fraction (**see also Chapter 11**), referred to variably as *diastolic HF* or *HF with preserved ejection fraction* (HFpEF).[1-3] The prevalence of this condition is likely to keep increasing as the prevalence of the elderly with comorbid conditions increases.[4,5] Although the rates of mortality and morbidity associated with HFpEF and compared with HF with reduced ejection fraction (HFrEF) or systolic HF have varied, there is consensus that HFpEF is associated with substantial morbidity and mortality and the frequency of clinical events increases markedly once a patient is hospitalized for HF.[1,3] In addition, patients with left ventricular ejection fraction (LVEF) between 40% and 49% are now referred to as HF with "borderline" or "midrange" ejection fraction (HFbEF and HFmrEF, respectively). These patients share characteristics and outcomes between HFpEF and HFrEF and, in some studies, appear to have similar demographics as those with HFpEF but with a higher incidence of coronary artery disease.[6-8] Several clinical trials have included at least a part of this patient group as having HFpEF. Until recently, most randomized clinical trials for HF underrepresented these populations. A study examining secular trends in HF within Olmstead County found that survival improved significantly over time among patients with HFrEF (likely related to use of evidence-driven therapies), but no such trend toward improvement was noted for patients with HFpEF.[3] Therefore there exists an urgent need to identify effective treatment strategies for the management of patients with this condition.

DEVELOPMENT OF TREATMENT STRATEGIES BASED ON THE PATHOPHYSIOLOGY OF HEART FAILURE WITH PRESERVED EJECTION FRACTION

The development of treatment strategies for HFpEF is based on our evolving understanding of the pathophysiology of this condition (reviewed in detail in **Chapter 11**). HFpEF commonly afflicts elderly patients with comorbidities of hypertension, left ventricular (LV) hypertrophy, diabetes mellitus, myocardial ischemia, and obesity. Of these risk factors, hypertension and subsequent concentric LV hypertrophy are the most prevalent and highly associated with HFpEF. Less commonly, HFpEF may occur as a result of restrictive and infiltrative cardiomyopathies and transplant rejection.[9] In the presence of the aforementioned conditions, clinical symptoms and signs of HF are commonly precipitated by concomitant anemia, pulmonary disease, renal insufficiency, atrial fibrillation, infection, and uncontrolled hypertension. In patients with HFpEF, in the absence of significant valvular or pericardial disease, diastolic dysfunction consisting of abnormalities of LV relaxation and increased LV stiffness have long been thought to be the central pathophysiologic abnormality contributing to the development of HF.[10,11] This led to the term *diastolic HF* to describe this condition. Even though mechanistic studies demonstrate that abnormalities of diastolic function are invariably present in HFpEF, there is some disagreement concerning the relative contribution of diastolic dysfunction to clinical HF in an elderly comorbid population in whom there is a high prevalence of diastolic dysfunction even in the absence of clinical HF. It is likely that these elderly patients frequently experience clinical decompensation when the precipitants listed previously occur in the presence of the underlying substrate of diastolic dysfunction. Decompensated HF would be unlikely when the same precipitants occur in patients without underlying diastolic dysfunction.

Furthermore, factors other than diastolic dysfunction have also been suggested as contributors to the development of HFpEF and include both central (cardiac) and peripheral (skeletal muscle and vasculature) abnormalities. These include increased vascular and LV systolic stiffness, early systolic dysfunction, endothelial dysfunction, volume overload secondary to renal disease with abnormal renal sodium handling, atrial dysfunction, neurohumoral (specifically renin-angiotensin-aldosterone system [RAAS]) activation, reduced vasodilator reserve, chronotropic incompetence during exercise, and impaired right ventricular-pulmonary artery coupling and have all been related to the HFpEF syndrome.[12-18] Cardiometabolic diseases, including obesity, hypertension, and diabetes are thought to induce a systemic proinflammatory state, which in turn may trigger systemic and coronary microvascular inflammation. This results in reduction of nitric oxide (NO) bioavailability downstream, which promotes myocyte and myocardial hypertrophy, cardiomyocyte stiffness, and interstitial fibrosis.[19] Aging is associated with a reduction in the elastic properties of the heart and vasculature associated with an increase in systolic blood pressure. Aging and the higher prevalence of comorbidities likely contribute to the much higher prevalence of HFpEF in the elderly.

The following sections in this chapter will provide an overview of therapeutic modalities that could be effective in patients with HFpEF, based either on symptomatic benefit or on targeting pathophysiologic mechanisms. The clinical approach to management of these patients with HFpEF will then be summarized based on current evidence and consensus opinion.

TREATMENT OF VOLUME OVERLOAD AND CONGESTION

In HFpEF, diuretics reduce ventricular filling pressures and are therefore useful in providing symptomatic benefit in patients presenting with pulmonary vascular congestion and peripheral edema. It should be noted that some patients who fit the classic profile of "diastolic heart failure" with significant concentric left hypertrophy and small LV volumes may exhibit a fall in cardiac output with rapid diuresis, resulting in hypotension and prerenal azotemia. This results from the fact that these patients have a very steep LV diastolic pressure-volume curve such that a small change in diastolic volume causes a large change in pressure and cardiac output.[20] In addition, right ventricular characteristics may affect this relationship. In one small study of HFpEF patients, worsening renal function during acute HF hospitalization was associated with reduced right ventricular function and increased right ventricular free wall thickness compared with matched patients with no worsening renal function.[21] It is known that the right ventricle forms the external pressure for approximately one-third of the surface area of the left ventricle.[9,22] Therefore elevation of right-heart diastolic pressures can constrain the filling of the left ventricle. In some patients, reduction of right-sided diastolic pressures by diuretics may unload the interventricular septum, improving LV distensibility,[23] and may therefore be associated with a reduction in pulmonary venous pressures while maintaining LV filling and cardiac output. More recently, Maurer and colleagues have demonstrated that in a subgroup of patients with hypertensive HFpEF, the LV end-diastolic pressure-volume relationship may be shifted rightward with somewhat increased end-diastolic volumes (in contrast to the classic paradigm of diastolic HF with a leftward- and upward-shifted end-diastolic pressure volume relationship and smaller LV volume).[14] This may be a result of a volume overload state contributed to by extracardiac factors such as renal dysfunction with abnormal renal sodium handling, obesity, and anemia. This could also represent a group of patients who would also respond more favorably to diuretic therapy. In addition, low-dose diuretics, especially thiazide diuretics, are useful in the treatment of hypertension, a key pathophysiologic factor in HFpEF.[24] Some patients with HFpEF and severe volume overload may also be candidates for ultrafiltration (**discussed in Chapter 36**).

Furthermore, renal dysfunction is a key pathogenic process leading to HFpEF.[25] Abnormal renal function is also likely required to produce salt-sensitive hypertension,[26] seen very frequently in HFpEF in older patients. Inappropriate salt and water retention with sodium and volume overload contribute to renal and cardiovascular (CV) dysfunction in a vicious cycle. In animal models, a high-salt diet results in hypertension, severe ventricular hypertrophy, and cardiac fibrosis, as well as proteinuria, glomerulosclerosis, and renal inflammation. Importantly, these effects were attenuated with the use of a thiazide diuretic. Fluid overload may be even more important than the hypertension, in that in patients with chronic kidney disease, CV events are more likely in those with modest degrees of fluid overload, with or without concomitant hypertension.[27] Therefore adequate treatment of patients with volume-optimizing strategies may offer more than just symptomatic benefit.

NITRATES AND NITRITES

Therapy with nitrates may provide symptomatic benefit in patients with HFpEF with pulmonary vascular congestion. Nitrates are primarily venodilators, with some arterial vasodilating action. They may benefit patients with HFpEF by reducing preload, thus leading to a reduction in ventricular filling pressures and pulmonary congestion. In acute decompensated HF, they can be used intravenously and may improve symptoms by reducing filling pressures, as well as by controlling systemic hypertension. Again, as with diuretics, caution is required when nitrates are used in patients without hypertension or with severe diastolic dysfunction with monitoring for a significant reduction in cardiac output and blood pressure as a result of preload reduction. Theoretically, by releasing NO, nitrates may also improve the diastolic distensibility of the ventricle.[28]

The *Nitrate's Effect on Activity Tolerance in Heart Failure with Preserved Ejection Fraction* (NEAT-HFpEF) trial evaluated the effects of nitrates on daily activity in 110 ambulatory patients with HFpEF (**Table 39.1**). This trial was a 6-week dose-escalation regimen of isosorbide mononitrate (from 30 mg to 60 mg to 120 mg once daily) or placebo, with subsequent crossover to the other group for 6 weeks. The primary end point was the daily activity level, quantified as the average daily accelerometer units. In the group receiving the 120-mg dose of isosorbide mononitrate, as compared with the placebo group, there was a nonsignificant trend toward lower daily activity and a significant decrease in hours of activity per day. During all dose regimens, activity in the nitrate group was lower than that in the placebo group. There were no significant between-group differences in the secondary end points of 6-minute walk distance, quality-of-life scores, or N-terminal pro-B type natriuretic peptide (NT-proBNP) levels.[29] Although this trial did not demonstrate benefit of nitrates across patients with chronic HFpEF, selective use of nitrates during acute hospitalization for HFpEF, especially in the setting of uncontrolled hypertension, or the use of nitrates chronically as antianginal therapy in HFpEF with concomitant coronary artery disease may still be beneficial.

Although nitrates improve hemodynamics with vasodilation and thus reduce systemic vascular resistance, they are subject to tolerance over a period of time. In contrast, nitrites can continue to produce sustained vasodilation with long-term exposure.[30] Omar et al. explored the pharmacologic properties of nitrites in the human circulation, reporting that nitrite vasodilates not only the arteriolar and venous circulation but also the conduit blood vessels, an effect similar to that observed with nitroglycerin. This effect was associated with a reduction in central systolic blood pressure, augmentation index, and pulsed wave velocity, which represent hemodynamic effects that might show therapeutic promise in the setting of HFpEF.[31]

Importantly, because nitrite is a stable metabolic product of NO and is readily reduced back to NO in hypoxic and acidic environments,

TABLE 39.1   Study Characteristics of Selected Multicenter Clinical Trials in Heart Failure with Preserved Ejection Fraction with Nonmortality–Morbidity End Points

	RELAX[83]	Aldo-DHF[56]	PARAMOUNT[64]	NEAT-HFpEF[29]	INDIE-HFpEF[35]	Kitzman et al.[126]
HF trial population	N = 190 NYHA class II-IV LVEF ≥50% BNP >200 pg/mL or NT-BNP >400 pg/mL Abnormal peak VO$_2$ Median age: 69 years Male 52%	N = 422 NYHA class II-III LVEF ≥50% Diastolic dysfunction Mean age: 67 years Male 48%	N = 301 NYHA class II-III LVEF >45% NT-proBNP >400 pg/mL Mean age: 71 years Male 47%	N = 110 NYHA class II-IV LVEF ≥50% Prior HF hospitalization or cath: elevated LV filling pressures or elevated NT-proBNP >400 pg/mL or BNP >200 pg/mL or diastolic dysfunction on echo Mean age: 69 years Male 53%	N = 105 NYHA class II-IV LVEF ≥50% Prior HF hospitalization or cath: elevated LV filling pressures or elevated NT-proBNP >400 pg/mL or BNP >200 pg/mL or diastolic dysfunction on echo + loop diuretic Mean age: 68 years Male 44%	N = 100 NYHA class II, III LVEF ≥50% BMI ≥30 kg/m^2 Mean age ~66.5 years
Selected exclusion criteria	GFR <20 mL/min/1.73 m^2 On nitrates or alpha antagonists Morbid obesity	Significant CAD, Potassium ≥5.1 mmol/L eGFR <30 mL/min/1.73 m^2 Concomitant therapy with potassium-sparing diuretics	Potassium >5.2 meq/L eGFR <30 mL/min/1.73 m^2	eGFR <20 mL/min/1.73 m^2 Systolic blood pressure <110 mm Hg or >180 mm Hg Resting HR >110	eGFR <20 mL/min/1.73 m^2 Systolic blood pressure <115 mm Hg seated or <90 mm Hg standing just prior to test dose Resting HR >110	
Protocol: [a]Double-blind randomized	[a]Sildenafil versus placebo Target dose 60 mg thrice daily Duration: 24 weeks	[a]Spironolactone (25 mg daily) versus placebo Duration: 12 months	[a]LCZ696 (target 200 mg twice daily) versus valsartan (target 160 mg twice daily) Duration: 12 weeks main; 24 weeks extension	[a]Isosorbide mononitrate (from 30 mg to 60 mg to 120 mg once daily) or placebo Duration: 6 weeks then crossover	[a]Inhaled, nebulized inorganic sodium nitrite versus inhaled, nebulized placebo at a dose of 80 mg (or maximally tolerated dose) administered three times daily Duration: 4 weeks then crossover	Randomized to exercise, hypocaloric diet, diet + exercise, or control Duration: 20 weeks
Primary end point	Exercise tolerance: peak oxygen consumption	Coprimary: peak oxygen consumption and diastolic function (E/E′)	Change in NT-proBNP from baseline to 12 weeks	Daily activity level, quantified as the average daily accelerometer units assessed by patient-worn accelerometers	Exercise tolerance: peak oxygen consumption	Coprimary: exercise tolerance by peak oxygen consumption and quality of life

[a]Randomized control trial.

BMI, Body mass index; *CAD,* coronary artery disease; *cath,* catheter; *DHF,* diastolic heart failure; *eGFR,* estimated glomerular filtration rate; *GFR,* glomerular filtration rate; *HF,* heart failure; *HFpEF,* heart failure with preserved ejection fraction; *HR,* heart rate; *INDIE-HFpEF,* Inorganic Nitrite Delivery to Improve Exercise Capacity in Heart Failure with Preserved Ejection Fraction; *LV,* left ventricular; *LVEF,* left ventricular ejection fraction; *NEAT-HFpEF,* Nitrate's Effect on Activity Tolerance in Heart Failure with Preserved Ejection Fraction; *NT-proBNP,* N-terminal pro B-type natriuretic peptide; *NYHA,* New York Heart Association; *PARAMOUNT,* Prospective Comparison of ARNI with ARB on Management Of heart failUre with preserved ejectioN fraction; *PEP-CHF,* Perindopril in Elderly People with Chronic Heart Failure.

its use in HFpEF to improve exercise capacity is a potentially promising. Experiments in mice show that nitrite therapy increased NO levels, and it prevented cardiac dysfunction and improved LV dimensions in HF models.[32] A study done in humans using inhaled sodium nitrite via a nebulizer showed that acute administration of inhaled sodium nitrite reduced biventricular filling pressures and pulmonary artery pressures at rest and during exercise in HFpEF.[33]

The *Inorganic Nitrite Delivery to Improve Exercise Capacity in Heart Failure with Preserved Ejection Fraction* (INDIE-HFpEF) trial was designed to study the effectiveness of inhaled inorganic nitrite on exercise capacity in patients with HFpEF (**see Table 39.1**). Inorganic nitrite functions as an important in vivo reservoir for NO generation, particularly under hypoxic and acidotic conditions. As such, inorganic nitrite becomes most active at times of greater need for NO signaling, as during exercise when LV filling pressures and pulmonary artery pressures increase.[34] The trial enrolled 105 HFpEF patients with a median age of 68 years, LVEF ≥50% with New York Heart Association (NYHA) class II to IV with objective evidence of HF. Patients were randomly assigned to receive a placebo or the inorganic nitrite administered with a nebulizer three times a day for 4 weeks and then crossed over. Preliminary results showed that inhaled nitrite was not effective in improving exercise capacity measured by peak oxygen consumption (VO_2) or other indices of clinical status of HFpEF including levels of NT-proBNP, nor did it improve quality-of-life scores. Thus currently the data do not support the use of inhaled nitrite for symptomatic relief in HFpEF.[35] Further studies looking at different dosing, methods of delivery, or length of therapy using nitrites will be needed to fully evaluate if nitrites will be useful in the treatment of HFpEF.

TREATMENT OF HYPERTENSION (SEE ALSO CHAPTER 25)

Of the various risk factors for the development of HFpEF, hypertension, and subsequent LV hypertrophy are the most prevalent and highly associated with the condition. The significant contribution of hypertensive heart disease to the development of diastolic dysfunction and HFpEF (reviewed in Hoit and Walsh)[36] implies that treating hypertension should be beneficial not only for the treatment but also for the prevention of HFpEF. In addition, the increased afterload imposed by significant arterial hypertension reduces LV relaxation and filling rates.[37] Stiffening of the aorta and the left ventricle, as occurs in elderly patients with HFpEF, increases the tightness of the coupling of arterial systolic and left atrial pressures, with an increase in systolic arterial pressure resulting in elevation of left atrial pressures.[13,38] Controlling systolic hypertension could allow the left ventricle to eject to a smaller end-systolic volume, thus allowing the ventricle to operate with a smaller diastolic volume and reduced left atrial pressure. Lowering the systolic pressure allows the left ventricle to relax more rapidly, enhancing early filling.[39] In addition, concentrically hypertrophied hearts demonstrate increased passive stiffness and impaired relaxation independent of hemodynamic loads and have limited coronary vascular reserve that can contribute to myocardial ischemia even in the absence of epicardial coronary artery disease. Adequate control of hypertension should benefit patients with HFpEF by favorably altering loading conditions in the short term and, in the long term, by leading to regression of LV hypertrophy. Although there may be some additional benefits of using one class of drugs versus others,[40] the most important goal is achieving an adequate reduction in blood pressure. Several trials evaluating reduction of blood pressure using angiotensin-converting enzyme (ACE) inhibitors or angiotensin receptor blockers (ARBs), compared with other agents have suggested that ultimately blood pressure control rather than the specific class of antihypertensive agents used may be the major determinant of regression of hypertrophy and improvement in diastolic function.[24,41,42] Moreover, trials have definitively demonstrated approximately 50% reduction in the incidence of HF in patients treated for hypertension, especially in the elderly population.[43,44] Based on the totality of the data available, the most recent update of the American College of Cardiology and American Heart Association (ACC/AHA) HF guidelines recommend that in patients at increased risk (stage A HF) the optimal blood pressure in those with hypertension should be less than 130/80 mm Hg. In addition, patients with established HFpEF and persistent hypertension after management of volume overload should be prescribed guideline directed therapy titrated to attain a systolic blood pressure less than 130 mm Hg.[8]

Drugs such as beta-blockers and calcium channel blockers that reduce blood pressure and heart rate and thus indirectly improve diastolic function, as well as increase diastolic filling time, may be beneficial in patients with HFpEF. In contrast, the direct myocardial effects of slowing the relaxation rate of the ventricle and the negative inotropic actions of these drugs may be detrimental with respect to diastolic function.[9] In addition, a recent study demonstrated that during exercise, patients with HFpEF achieved

less of an increase in heart rate (inadequate chronotropic response) and thus a blunted cardiac output despite a similar rise in end-diastolic volume, stroke volume, and contractility compared with matched subjects with hypertensive cardiac hypertrophy.[12] These data suggest possible deleterious effects of heart rate–reducing drugs, such as beta-blockers and certain calcium channel blockers, in patients who may already have reduced exercise capacity resulting from reduced chronotropic reserve.

Over the years, a number of small studies evaluating calcium channel blockers, beta-blockers, ACE inhibitors, and ARBs variably suggested modest benefit in exercise capacity, NYHA class, quality of life, and diastolic function in patients with HFpEF. Since then, large, randomized multicenter trials evaluating the benefit on longer-term outcomes have been performed.

Given that several patients with HFpEF have uncontrolled, drug-resistant hypertension and that hypertension is a major driver of incidence and exacerbation of HFpEF, strategies other than medications that could aid in better blood pressure control are attractive in the prevention and treatment of HFpEF. Although the role of the baroreflex system in long-term blood pressure control has been debated, studies suggest that the system is important in chronic hypertension and that renal sympathoinhibition with a resultant increase in natriuresis may be one of the mechanisms by which the baroreflex participates in long-term blood pressure control. Animal and human studies have demonstrated a safe and effective lowering of blood pressure with chronic electrical stimulation of the carotid sinus. The postulated mechanism is that activation of the baroreceptors is interpreted by the brain as elevation in blood pressure, with resultant activation of the cardiac parasympathetic tone and diminished sympathetic outflow to the heart, kidneys, and peripheral vasculature.[45,46] A systematic review/meta-analysis examined the efficacy of baroreflex activation therapy (BAT) (through implantable baroreceptor stimulating devices) in patients with resistant hypertension. Twelve studies, including 1 randomized clinical trial and 11 prospective studies, were evaluated, of which 5 prospective studies were selected for meta-analysis. The data analysis showed that office systolic blood pressure and diastolic blood pressure decreased by BAT treatment and that the effect on systolic blood pressure was significant in both the Barostim neo device and the Rheos System. However, the available evidence was limited by risk of bias, small sample size, and few randomized trials, with the conclusion that there is presently insufficient evidence to fully evaluate the efficacy and safety of BAT for patients with resistant hypertension.[47] If BAT is proven to be successful in treating resistant hypertension, the resultant treatment option contributing to a sustained improvement of blood pressure in patients with HFpEF and resistant hypertension could translate into improvement in HFpEF outcomes.

RENIN-ANGIOTENSIN-ALDOSTERONE BLOCKADE

Angiotensin-Converting Enzyme Inhibitors and Angiotensin Receptor Blockers

As in HFrEF, preclinical and clinical evidence suggests that the activation of the RAAS is a contributing factor in the development of HFpEF, principally through the trophic effects of angiotensin II on the vasculature and myocardium, but perhaps also through myocardial fibrosis mediated by aldosterone (see also Chapter 5).[48,49] In addition, angiotensin II slows LV relaxation resulting in elevation of LV diastolic pressure.[50] Therefore agents such as ACE inhibitors and ARBs, with their antihypertensive and angiotensin II–attenuating effects, were attractive options in the treatment of HFpEF. Furthermore, clinical trials have shown ACE inhibitors and ARBs to be effective in improving CV outcomes in populations with diabetes, coronary artery disease, vascular disease, and hypertension,[50,51] comorbidities that are frequently present in and contribute to the development of HFpEF.

TABLE 39.2   Study Characteristics of Large Multicenter Clinical Trials Evaluating Morbidity and Mortality in Heart Failure with Preserved Ejection Fraction

	CHARM-Preserved[53]	PEP-CHF[52]	I-PRESERVE[54]	TOP-CAT[58]	PARAGON-HF[65]
HF trial population	N = 3023 LVEF >40% NYHA class II–IV NYHA III/IV: 39% Mean age: 67 years >75 years: 23% Male: 60%	N = 850 LVEF >40% NYHA class I–IV NYHA III/IV: 24% Mean age: 75 years ≥70 years: 100% Male: 45% Diastolic dysfunction and/ or LVH or LA dilation	N = 4128 LVEF ≥45% NYHA class II–IV NYHA III/IV: 79% Mean age: 72 years ≥60 years: 100% Male 40% HF hospitalization or substrate for HF (LVH or LA dilation)	N = 3445 LVEF ≥45% NYHA class II–IV NYHA III/IV: 34% Mean age: 69 years Male: 48% HF hospitalization or BNP >100 pg/mL or NT-proBNP ≥360 pg/mL	Estimated N = 4600 LVEF ≥45% NYHA class II–IV Age ≥50 years Structural heart disease: LVH or LA dilation NT-proBNP ≥200 pg/mL with HF hospitaliza- tion within 9 months otherwise NT-proBNP >360 pg/mL
Major exclusion criteria	Significant hypotension Creatinine >3 mg/dL Serum K >5.5 meq/L	Systolic bp <100 mmHg Creatinine >2.3 mg/dL Serum K >5.4 meq/L	Systolic bp <100 or >160 mmHg Creatinine >2.5 mg/dL	GFR <30 mL/min/1.73 m² or creatinine ≥2.5 mg/dL Serum K ≥5.0 meq/L Uncontrolled hypertension	GFR <30 mL/min/1.73 m² Serum K ≥5.2 meq/L Uncontrolled hypertension History of angioedema
Use of ACE inhibitors/ ARBs at baseline	ACE inhibitor use allowed	No concomitant ACE inhibitor/ARB	ACE inhibitors allowed in ⅓ patients when indicated for diabetes or vascular disease	ACE inhibitor/ARB allowed	No concomitant ACE inhibitor/ARB
Protocol: ªDouble-blind random- ized	ªCandesartan versus placebo, uptitrated to target 32 mg/day Median follow-up: 36.6 months	ªPerindopril versus placebo, uptitrated to target 4 mg/day Median follow-up: 25.2 months	ªIrbesartan versus placebo, uptitrated to target 300 mg/day Mean follow-up: 49.5 months	ªSpironolactone versus placebo uptitrated to target 45 mg/day Mean follow-up:	ªValsartan target 160 mg twice daily or sacubitril/ valsartan target 97/103 mg twice daily. All patients with sequen- tial single-blind run-in periods to ensure toler- ability of both drugs at half target doses (i.e., valsartan titrated to 80 mg twice daily followed by sacubitril/valsartan 49/51 mg twice daily) Results not yet reported
Primary end point	Composite of CV mortality or HF hospitalization	Composite of all-cause mortality or HF hospi- talization	Composite of all-cause mortality or CV hospi- talization	Composite of CV mor- tality, aborted cardiac arrest or HF hospital- ization	Composite of CV death, or total (first and recurrent) HF hospitalizations

ªRandomized control trial.

ACE, Angiotensin-converting enzyme; *ARB,* angiotensin receptor blockers; *bp,* blood pressure; *CV,* cardiovascular; *HF,* heart failure; *LA,* left atrial; *LVEF,* left ventricular ejection fraction; *LVH,* left ventricular hypertrophy; *NYHA,* New York Heart Association.

On the basis of a strong theoretical rationale for RAAS block-ade in patients with HFpEF, three large randomized clinical trials were designed specifically to evaluate ACE inhibitors and ARBs in patients with HFpEF. These include the Candesartan in Heart fail-ure Assessment of Reduction in Mortality and morbidity-Preserved (CHARM-Preserved) trial, the Perindopril in Elderly People with Chronic Heart Failure (PEP-CHF) trial,[52,53] and the Irbesartan in Heart Failure with PRESERVED Ejection Fraction (I-PRESERVE) trial.[54] The characteristics of the patient populations evaluated in these trials are summarized in **Table 39.2**.

Of the 3023 patients enrolled in the CHARM-Preserved trial, almost 20% were on ACE inhibitors and 56% on beta-blockers at the time of randomization to candesartan or placebo.[53] After a median follow-up of approximately 37 months, the primary end point (CV or HF hospitalization) occurred in 22% of the candesartan and 24% of the placebo group (hazard ratio [HR] 0.89, 95% confidence

interval [CI] 0.77–1.03, *P* = .118; covariate-adjusted HR 0.86, 95% CI 0.74–1.00, *P* = .051) (**Fig. 39.1**). The difference, which was of bor-derline statistical significance only for the adjusted hazard ratios, was driven mostly by a difference in HF hospitalizations between the can-desartan- and placebo-treated groups (HR 0.85, 95% CI 0.72, 1.01, *P* = .072), with almost identical CV mortality rates between the two groups (**Fig. 39.2**). In addition, the total number of HF hospitaliza-tions was noted to be significantly lower in the candesartan group. Of note, at 6 months into the trial, the blood pressure was significantly more reduced in the candesartan group (6.9 mm Hg systolic and 2.9 mm Hg diastolic) compared with the placebo group (*P* < .0001). It is therefore difficult to tease out whether the modest 15% relative reduction in HF hospitalizations with candesartan compared with a placebo in patients with HFpEF was mostly a result of blood pressure reduction versus any other more specific angiotensin-blocking effects of candesartan and whether any other drugs causing similar blood pressure reduction would have led to similar effects. The lack of a greater benefit from the use of the ARB in CHARM-Preserved may also have been contributed to by the fact that ACE inhibitors were allowed for patients in the trial, with 20% of patients being on ACE inhibitors even at the beginning of the trial, and the relatively lower than expected annual event rates of the primary composite outcome of 9.1% in the placebo group.

The PEP-CHF trial of perindopril in HFpEF was conducted in a more elderly patient population compared with the CHARM-Preserved trial (see Table 39.2). However, the results of the study were neutral with respect to the primary outcome (composite of all-cause mortality and unplanned HF-related hospitalization) and demonstrated only a trend toward modest benefit in other end points.[52] As compared with the CHARM-Preserved trial, the

PEP-CHF study enrolled only 850 patients with HFpEF, who, in addition to having relatively preserved LVEF, also had objective evidence of diastolic dysfunction at enrollment. The mean follow-up of 26 months was shorter than the CHARM-Preserved trial. The event rate was much lower than expected, and, despite much longer follow-up than originally intended, only 46% of the expected events occurred, giving the study only 25% power to show a difference in the primary end point. Furthermore, a large number of patients stopped their assigned treatment after 1 year, and most of them started taking open-label ACE inhibitors (discontinuation rate of 38% at 18 months, approximately 36% of patients on open-label ACE inhibitor treatment by the end of the study). Over the total duration of follow-up, perindopril was not associated with an improvement in the primary composite end point of death or HF hospitalization (HR 0.92, 95% CI 0.70–1.21, P = .55; **Fig. 39.3A**). However, if analysis was confined to 1 year of follow-up, at which point most patients were still taking the assigned medication, perindopril was associated with a statistically borderline significant 31% relative reduction in the primary end point (HR 0.69, 95% CI 0.47–1.01, P = .055). Similarly, although perindopril was not associated with a benefit in HF hospitalization over the entire duration of the trial (see **Fig. 39.3B**), at 1 year of follow-up, the perindopril group had a lower rate of HF hospitalizations (HR 0.63, 95% CI 0.41–0.97, P = .03). Thus, although perindopril did not have a beneficial effect on the overall primary outcome, there was a suggestion of reduction in HF hospitalizations at 1 year when patients were on assigned treatment.[52] In addition, significant improvements were observed compared with the placebo group in some other secondary end points, including the proportion of patients in NYHA functional class I and change in 6-minute-walk distance at 1 year. Similar to the observation in the CHARM-preserved trial, the active arm of perindopril had a significantly greater reduction in systolic blood pressure (mean difference = 3 mm Hg, P = .03) compared with the placebo arm. Furthermore, it was noted that patients with a higher baseline blood pressure appeared to have a greater benefit with perindopril. Therefore, similar to the CHARM-preserved trial, it is not possible to rule out a significant contribution of the blood pressure–lowering effect of the ACE inhibitor as opposed to

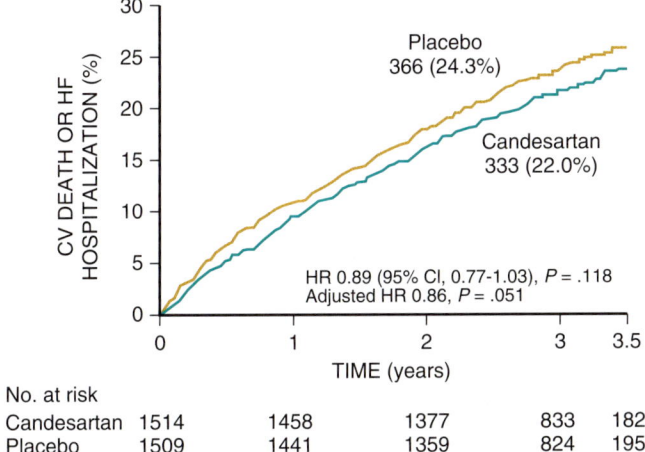

Fig. 39.1 Kaplan-Meier curves for time to first occurrence of the primary end point in patients with heart failure with preserved ejection fraction in the CHARM-Preserved Trial. *CI,* Confidence interval; *CV,* cardiovascular; *HF,* heart failure; *HR,* hazard ratio. (From Yusuf S, Pfeffer MA, Swedberg K, et al. Effects of candesartan in patients with chronic heart failure and preserved left-ventricular ejection fraction: the CHARM-Preserved Trial. *Lancet.* 2003;362[9386]:777–781.)

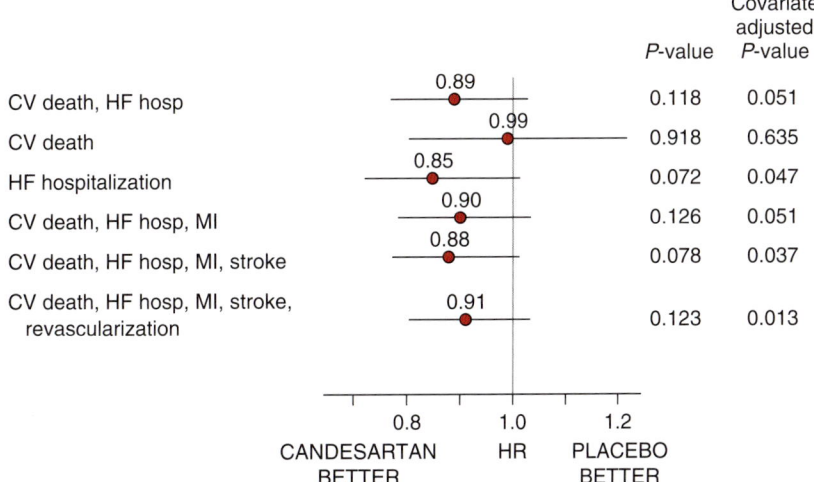

Fig. 39.2 Hazard ratios and 95% confidence intervals for candesartan versus placebo for selected secondary end points in the CHARM-Preserved Trial. *CV,* Cardiovascular; *HF,* heart failure; *HR,* heart rate; *MI,* myocardial infarction. (From Yusuf S, Pfeffer MA, Swedberg K, et al. Effects of candesartan in patients with chronic heart failure and preserved left-ventricular ejection fraction: the CHARM-Preserved Trial. *Lancet.* 2003;362[9386]:777–781.)

other RAAS-blocking actions of perindopril toward the observed short-term beneficial effect on HF hospitalizations. In addition, both trials illustrate the encountered difficulty of lower event rates of patients enrolled in clinical trials compared with those seen in the general population. The switch over to open-label ACE inhibitors illustrates the many existing indications for the use of ACE inhibitors or ARBs in patients with vascular disease, diabetes, and hypertension, the same group of comorbidities that are frequently encountered in patients with HFpEF, thus potentially limiting the opportunities to add ACE inhibitors or ARBs specifically for HFpEF.

The largest trial, I-PRESERVE, enrolled 4128 patients with HFpEF (**see Table 39.2**).[54] The patients were randomly assigned to ARB, irbesartan, or placebo. During a mean follow-up of 49.5 months, there was no significant difference in the occurrence of the primary outcome (death from any cause or hospitalization for a CV cause [i.e.,

HF, myocardial infarction, unstable angina, arrhythmia, or stroke]) between irbesartan and the placebo (HR 0.95; 95% CI 0.86–1.05; P = .35; **Fig. 39.4**). Overall rates of death were also similar (HR 1.00; 95% CI 0.88–1.14; P = .98), as were rates of CV hospitalization, HF hospitalization, and other secondary outcomes. Although, compared with the CHARM-preserved trial, the I-PRESERVE trial studied a greater number of patients, with slightly better preserved EF (≥45% vs. >40% in CHARM-Preserved), greater specificity of the substrate for HfpEF, and a greater proportion of older patients and women (i.e., a study cohort more representative of the "real world" HFpEF population), this trial did not provide any evidence for overall benefit of ARBs on CV outcomes in HfpEF patients.

Thus apart from the modest signal of 15% relative reduction in HF hospitalizations with candesartan compared with a placebo in HfpEF patients observed in the CHARM-Preserved trial and a possible benefit on HF hospitalizations and functional class at an intermediate time-point in PEP-CHF (in the absence of benefit over the entire duration of follow-up), neither ACE inhibitors nor ARBs has been proven to have a convincing beneficial effect on clinical outcomes in HfpEF.

In addition, of note, RAAS inhibitors can induce renal dysfunction in both HfrEF and HfpEF. However, in contrast to patients with HfrEF, where mortality increase with worsening renal function is small, HfpEF patients with RAAS inhibitor-induced worsening renal function may have an increased mortality risk, without experiencing improved outcome with RAAS inhibition.[55]

Aldosterone Receptor Antagonists

Mineralocorticoid receptor activation by aldosterone contributes to the pathophysiology of HF through several mechanisms, including sodium retention, potassium loss, endothelial dysfunction, vascular inflammation, fibrosis, and hypertrophy. Smaller trials of aldosterone receptor antagonists suggested benefit on diastolic function without improvement in functional capacity. The Aldosterone Receptor Blockade in Diastolic Heart Failure (ALDO-DHF) trial was a prospective, randomized, double-blind, placebo-controlled trial evaluating the effect of spironolactone on diastolic function and exercise capacity in 422 patients with HfpEF (**see Table 39.1**).[56] At the end of 12 months of treatment, compared with a placebo, spironolactone use resulted in improvement in echocardiographic parameters of diastolic dysfunction (mitral annular E/e′ adjusted mean difference between the placebo and spironolactone −1.5;

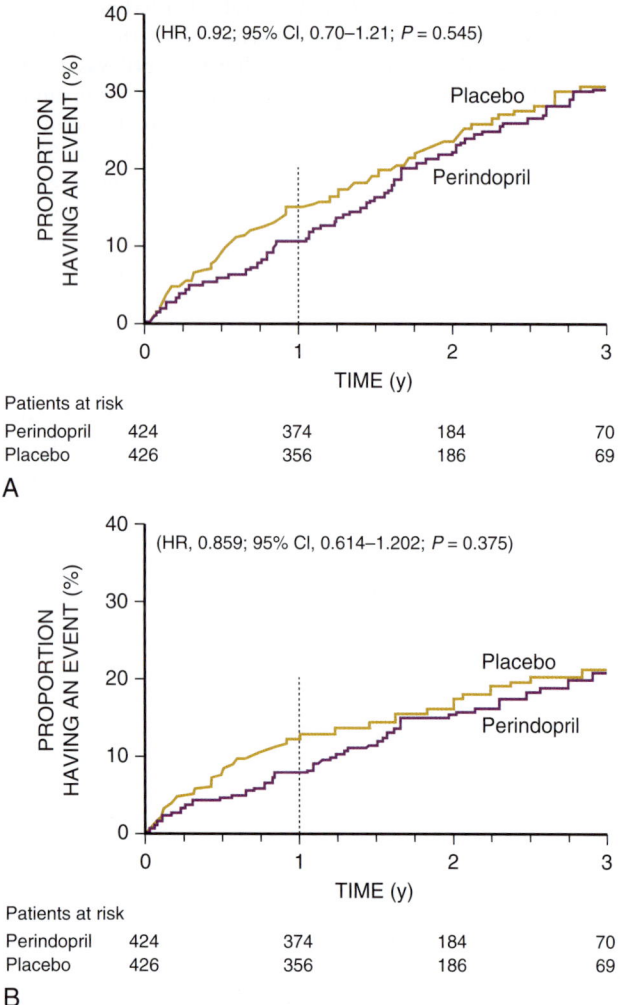

Fig. 39.3 The Perindopril in Elderly People with Chronic Heart Failure (PEP-CHF) Trial. (A) Kaplan-Meier curves of time to first occurrence of the primary end point, all-cause mortality, or unplanned HF hospitalization in the PEP-CHF trial. The *red line* points out the occurrence of the end point at 1 year of follow-up. (B) Kaplan-Meier curves of time to first occurrence of the secondary end point of unplanned HF hospitalization in the PEP-CHF trial. The *red line* points out the occurrence of the end point at 1 year of follow-up. *CI*, Confidence interval; *HF*, heart failure; *HR*, hazard ratio. (From Cleland JG, Tendera M, Adamus J, et al. The perindopril in elderly people with chronic heart failure [PEP-CHF] study. *Eur Heart J.* 2006;27[19]:2338–2345.)

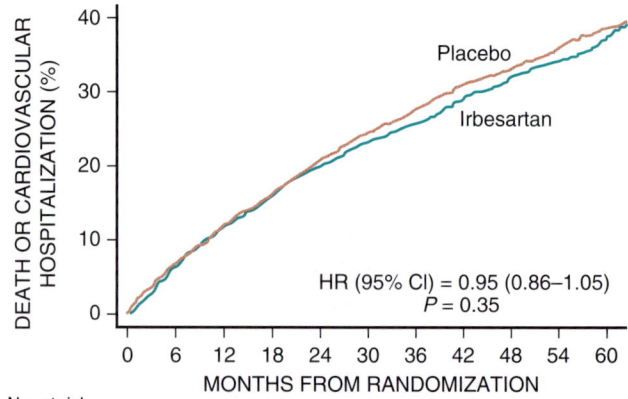

Fig. 39.4 Kaplan-Meier curves of time to first occurrence of the primary end point in the I-PRESERVE trial. *CI*, Confidence interval; *HR*, hazard ratio. (From Massie BM, Carson PE, McMurray JJ, et al. Irbesartan in patients with heart failure and preserved ejection fraction. *N Engl J Med.* 2008;359[23]:2456–2467.)

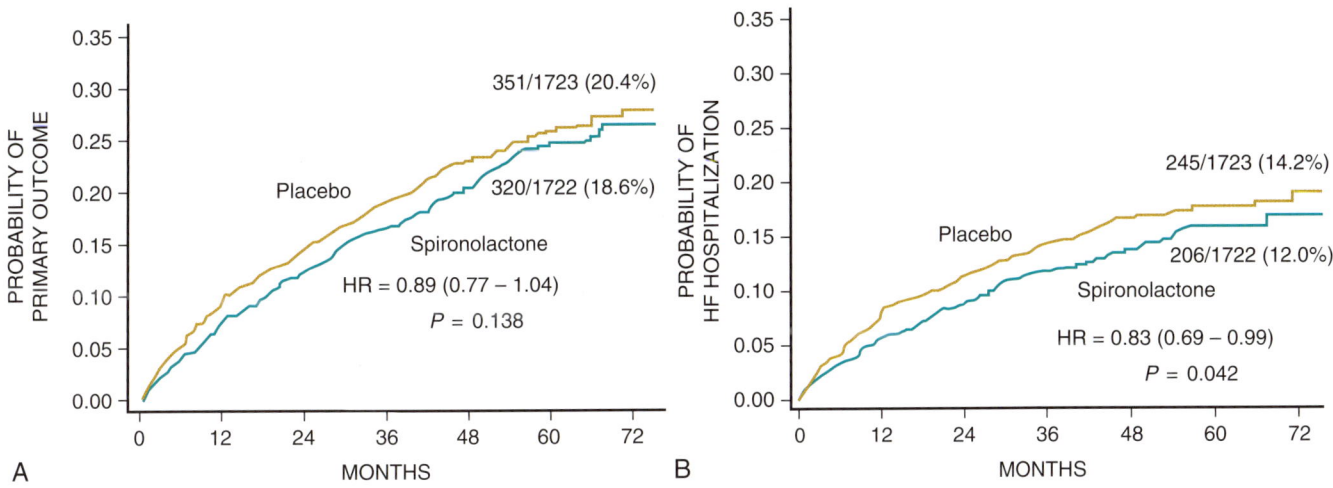

Fig. 39.5 Kaplan-Meier curves of time to first occurrence of the primary end point of cardiovascular death, heart failure hospitalization, or resuscitated cardiac arrest (A) and of HF hospitalization (B) in the TOPCAT trial. *HF,* Heart failure; *HR,* hazard ratio; *TOPCAT,* Treatment of Preserved Cardiac Function Heart Failure with an Aldosterone Antagonist. (From Pitt B, Pfeffer MA, Assmann SF, et al, TOPCAT Investigators. Spironolactone for heart failure with preserved ejection fraction. *N Engl J Med.* 2014;370[15]:1383–1392.)

95% CI −2.0 to −0.9, *P* < .001), neuroendocrine activation (NT-proBNP geometric ratio 0.86, 95% CI 0.75–0.99, *P* = .03), and induced reverse remodeling (decline in LV mass index; difference −6 g/m², 95% CI −10 to −1 g/m²; *P* = .009) but did not improve HF symptoms or quality of life and slightly reduced the 6-minute walking distance, with no effect on hospitalizations. The lack of clinical improvement despite improvement in echocardiographic and laboratory parameters may have been caused by the relatively younger and healthier patient cohort (86% NYHA class II, ≈50% on diuretics and baseline median NT-proBNP 158 ng/mL), a low event rate, and shorter follow-up. Similarly, another smaller study, the Randomized Aldosterone Antagonism in Heart Failure with Preserved Ejection Fraction (RAAM-PEF) trial, evaluated the effects of the more selective aldosterone receptor blocker, eplerenone, compared with a placebo on 6-minute walk distance, diastolic function, and markers of collagen turnover after 6 months of treatment. The use of eplerenone was associated with improvement in diastolic dysfunction (E/e′, *P* ≤ .01) and reduced collagen turnover but no change in 6-minute walk distance (*P* = .91) as compared with a placebo.[57]

The large multicenter double-blind, placebo-controlled trial, Treatment of Preserved Cardiac function heart failure with an Aldosterone Antagonist (TOPCAT), evaluated the effects of spironolactone on morbidity and mortality in 3445 patients with HFpEF (LVEF ≥45%; see Table 39.2).[58] Overall, the primary end point of CV death, HF hospitalization, or resuscitated cardiac arrest was similar between the spironolactone and the placebo arms (18.6% vs. 20.4%, HR 0.89, 95% CI 0.77–1.04, *P* = .14; Fig. 39.5A), as were the individual components of CV mortality and aborted cardiac arrest. However, HF hospitalizations were lower (12.0% vs. 14.2%, *P* = .042; see Fig. 39.5B); all-cause hospitalizations were similar (*P* = .25). Hyperkalemia (18.7% vs. 9.1%, *P* < .001) and renal failure, defined as serum creatinine ≥ times the baseline value and above the upper limit of the normal range, were both significantly higher in the spironolactone arm. Therefore, in the TOPCAT trial, spironolactone was not overall superior to placebo in improving CV outcomes in patients with HFpEF, with a significantly higher rate of hyperkalemia and renal failure in patients treated with spironolactone. Most of these patients were already on an ACE inhibitor/ARB. The reduction in HF hospitalizations with spironolactone was encouraging, but this finding should be approached with caution because all-cause hospitalizations were similar between the placebo and spironolactone arms.

An interesting post hoc analysis revealed a disparity in outcomes between the centers in North and South America and those in Eastern Europe. In the United States, Canada, Brazil, and Argentina, where the rate of the primary composite outcome was 31.8% in the placebo group, spironolactone had a significant benefit on the primary end point (HR 0.82, 95% CI 0.69–0.98). However, in Russia and the Republic of Georgia, where the primary outcome occurred in only 8.4% of patients taking the placebo, spironolactone did not have any effect (HR 1.10, 95% CI 0.79–1.51; Fig. 39.6).[59] Given that there are no current therapies that have been demonstrated to significantly improve clinical outcomes in HFpEF populations, it has been suggested that higher-risk HFpEF populations similar to those enrolled in the TOPCAT trial in the Americas, aldosterone receptor antagonists might be considered to reduce the risk of hospitalizations (see Table 39G.1).[8]

Angiotensin Receptor/Neprilysin Inhibitors

Natriuretic peptides have been associated with potent natriuresis, vasodilation, and inhibition of the RAAS and may have antifibrotic and antisympathetic effects (see also Chapter 9).[60,61] Neprilysin (neutral endopeptidase 24–11) inhibition leads to increased circulating levels of natriuretic peptides by preventing their breakdown with consequent cardiac, vascular, and renal protective effects. In addition, the augmentation of active natriuretic peptides increases generation of myocardial cyclic guanosine monophosphate (cGMP), which improves myocardial relaxation and decreases hypertrophy. However, neprilysin inhibition also prevents breakdown of vasoconstrictors like angiotensin II, thus diminishing the beneficial effects of neprilysin inhibition. Concomitant inhibition of the RAAS, along with neprilysin inhibition, helps to overcome this limitation and is the basis of dual-acting vasopeptidase inhibitors (Fig. 39.7). Previous studies showed promising effects of a combination drug with neutral endopeptidase and an ACE inhibitor (omapatrilat) for treatment of patients with hypertension and HF.[62] However, further development of this agent was stopped due to increased occurrence of angioedema, likely from increased bradykinin levels from neprilysin and ACE inhibition. ARBs are associated with a lower incidence of angioedema as compared with ACE inhibitors and were substituted for ACE inhibitors in the development of a new dual vasopeptidase inhibitor, LCZ696 (combination of an ARB, valsartan, and a neprilysin inhibitor, sacubitril), with higher antihypertensive potency as compared with

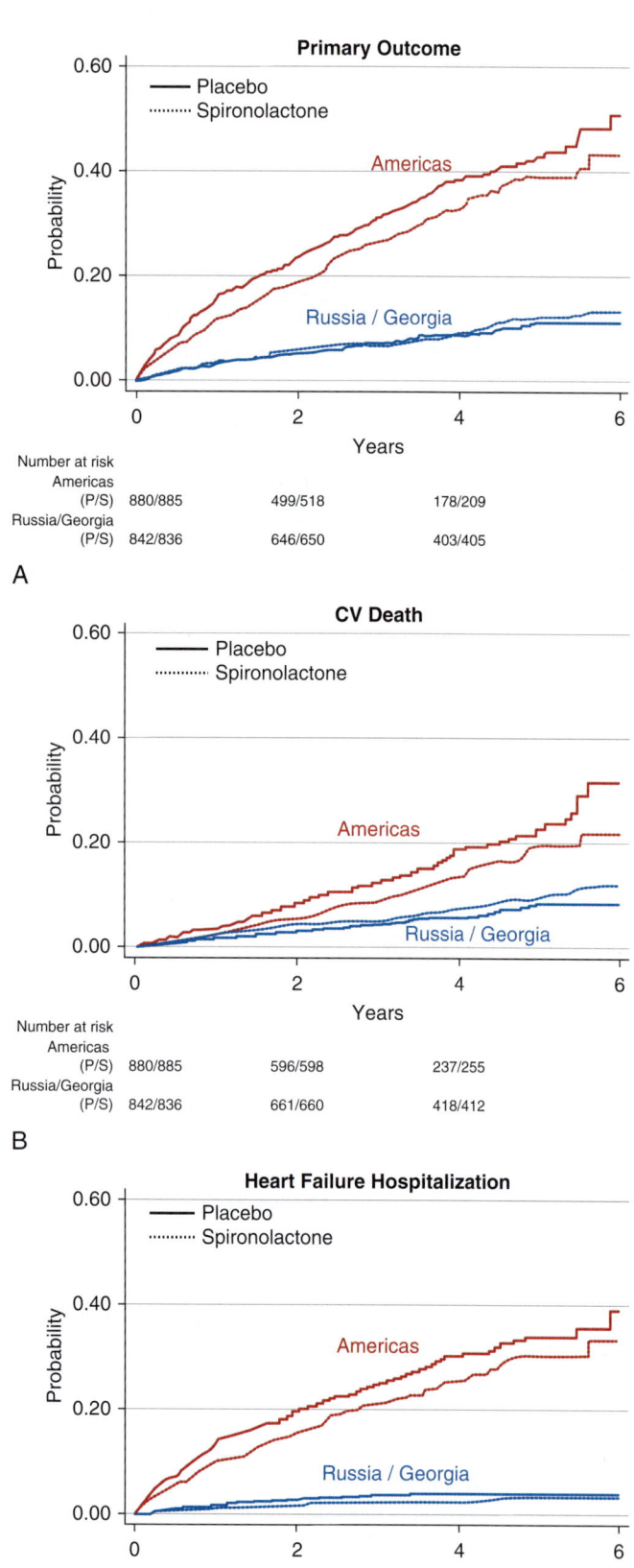

A

Number at risk
Americas
(P/S)   880/885   499/518   178/209
Russia/Georgia
(P/S)   842/836   646/650   403/405

B

Number at risk
Americas
(P/S)   880/885   596/598   237/255
Russia/Georgia
(P/S)   842/836   661/660   418/412

C

Number at risk
Americas
(P/S)   880/885   502/518   180/209
Russia/Georgia
(P/S)   842/836   646/649   403/404

valsartan and similar tolerability. The use of this ARB-neprilysn inhibitor or angiotensin receptor/neprilysin inhibitor (ARNI) was associated with a significant morbidity and mortality benefit in patients with HFrEF.[63]

This combination of sacubitril-valsartan was also evaluated in a phase II double-blind, randomized, parallel group trial, the Prospective Comparison of ARNI with ARB on Management Of heart failUre with preserved ejectioN fracTion (PARAMOUNT) trial.[64] The trial evaluated 301 patients with NYHA class II to III HFpEF (LVEF ≥ 45%) and NT-proBNP ≥400 pg/mL and randomized patients to LCZ696 titrated to 200 mg twice daily or valsartan titrated to 160 mg twice daily and treated for 36 weeks (**see Table 39.1**). The primary end point, a decrease in NT-proBNP from baseline to 12 weeks, was significantly greater in the LCZ696 group compared with the valsartan group (ratio of change LCZ696/valsartan at 0.77, 95% CI 0.64–0.92, $P = .005$; **Fig. 39.8**). Although, NT-proBNP remained significantly reduced at 36 weeks compared with baseline, the difference between the two treatment groups was no longer statistically significant ($P = .2$). However, left atrial volume ($P = .003$) and left atrial dimension ($P = .034$) were significantly reduced and NYHA class improved at 36 weeks in patients in the LCZ696 group. No other echocardiographic parameters (including measures of diastolic function) differed between the treatment groups. The effect of LCZ696 on NT-proBNP appeared greater in subgroups of patients with systolic blood pressure higher than 140 mm Hg (possibly related to a greater blood pressure–lowering effect of this agent compared with ARBs and ACE inhibitors) and in diabetic patients.

The ongoing phase III trial will determine the effects of LCZ696 on clinical outcomes. The Prospective Comparison of ARNI with ARB on Management of Heart Failure with Preserved Ejection Fraction (PARAGON-HF) has completed enrollment of nearly 5000 patients with chronic HFpEF who are being followed for the cumulative number of primary composite events of CV death and total (first and recurrent) HF hospitalizations (**see Table 39.2**; **Fig. 39.7**). The trial has enrolled subjects with symptoms of HF on diuretics with LVEF ≥45%, evidence of structural heart disease (left atrial enlargement or LV hypertrophy), and elevated natriuretic peptides (NT-proBNP).[65]

Neprilysin is also one of several proteases that plays a role in the degradation of amyloid-β proteins, and concern has therefore been raised about the theoretical possibility that long-term neprilysin inhibition could influence the development of Alzheimer disease. However, the specific role of neprilysin in the pathogenesis of Alzheimer disease remains unclear. In addition to the likely redundancy in the enzymes that break down amyloid-β, individuals with truncating mutations in the gene encoding for neprilysin, who have total neprilysin deficiency, appear to lack any phenotypic consequence.[66] A multicenter randomized double-blind study to evaluate the effects of LCZ696 compared with Valsartan on cognitive function in patients with chronic HFpEF, Prospective Evaluation of Cognitive Function in Heart Failure: A Randomized Double-blind Study in Patients with Preserved Ejection Fraction Cardiac Failure Treated with Valsartan or Entresto (PERSPECTIVE) trial, which started enrollment of approximately 500 participants in 2016, will provide data on possible effects of LCZ696 on

Fig. 39.6 Kaplan-Meier plots of time to the first primary outcome event and two major components in the TOPCAT trial according to geographic area. (A) Time to primary outcome. (B) Time to cardiovascular (CV) death. (C) Time to first confirmed hospitalization for heart failure (HF). *CI,* Confidence interval; *R,* hazard ratio; *TOPCAT,* Treatment of Preserved Cardiac Function Heart Failure with an Aldosterone Antagonist. (From Pfeffer MA, Claggett B, Assmann SF, et al. Regional variation in patients and outcomes in the treatment of preserved cardiac function heart failure with an aldosterone antagonist [TOPCAT] trial. *Circulation.* 2015;131[1]:34–42.)

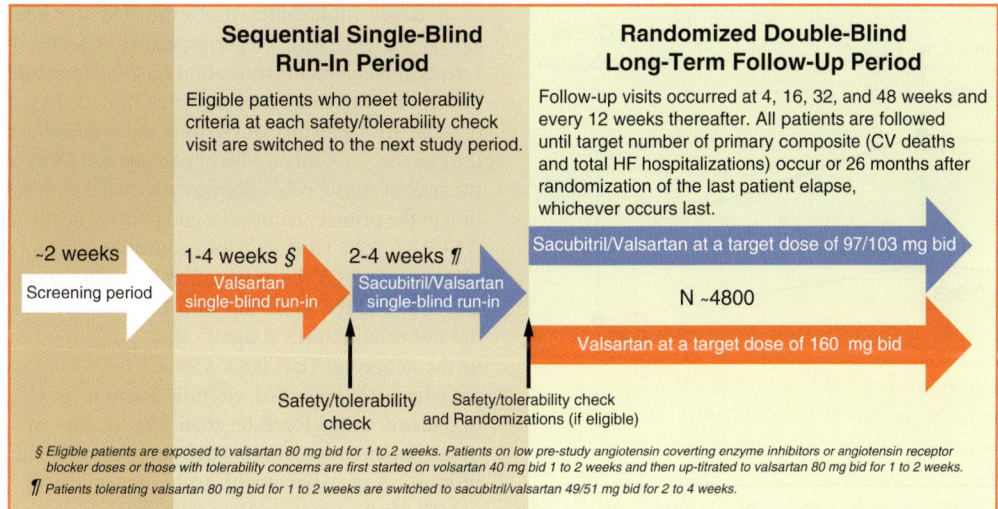

MECHANISM OF ACTION

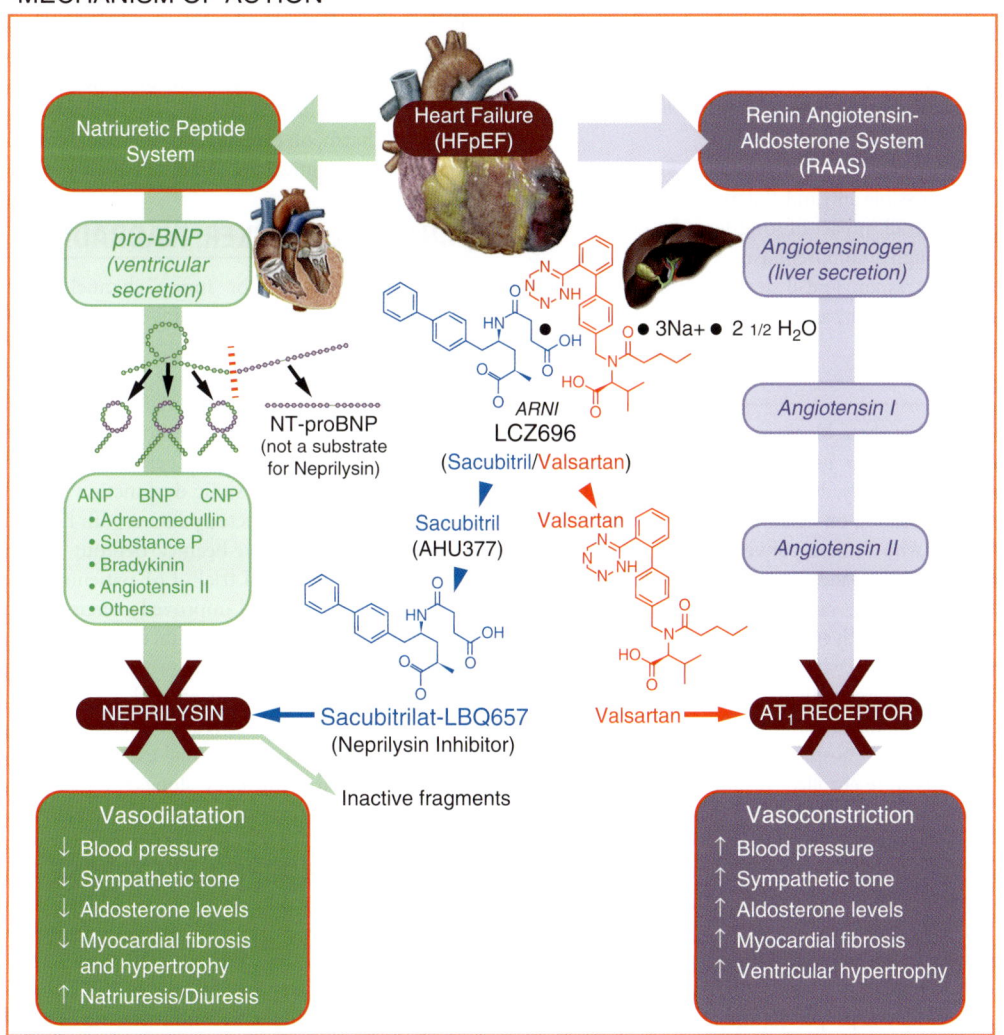

Fig. 39.7 Study design of PARAGON-HF and mechanism of action of sacubitril/valsartan. *ANP,* Atrial natriuretic peptide; *ARNI,* Angiotensin receptor/neprilysin inhibitor; *CNP,* C-type natriuretic peptide; *CV,* cardiovascular; *HF,* heart failure; *HFpEF,* heart failure with preserved ejection fraction; *NT-proBNP,* N-terminal pro B-type natriuretic peptide. (From Solomon SD, Rizkala AR, Gong J, et al. Angiotensin receptor neprilysin inhibition in heart failure with preserved ejection fraction: rationale and design of the PARAGON-HF trial. *JACC Heart Fail.* 2017;5[7]:471–482.)

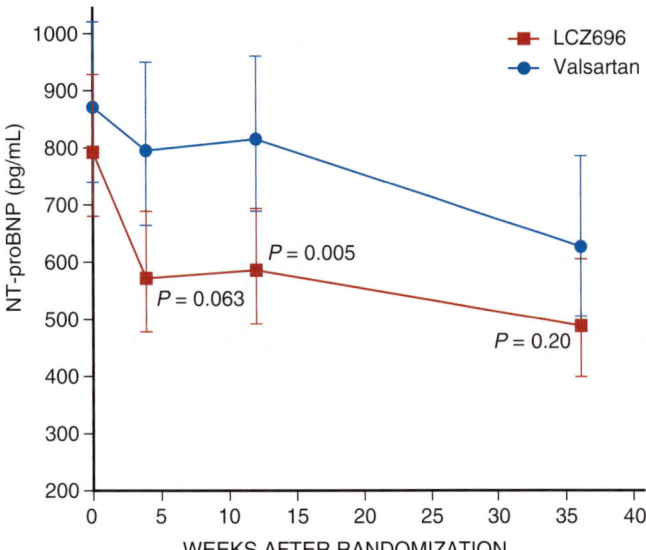

Fig. 39.8 PARAMOUNT trial: NT-proBNP at 4, 12, and 36 weeks in the LCZ696 and valsartan groups. (From Solomon SD, Zile M, Pieske B, et al. The angiotensin receptor/neprilysin inhibitor LCZ696 in heart failure with preserved ejection fraction: a phase 2 double-blind randomized controlled trial. *Lancet.* 2012;380[9851]:1387–1395.)

cognitive function due to possible amyloid-β deposition in the brain.[67] This trial will assess the overall impact of long-term LCZ696 therapy on cognitive function through a comprehensive battery of neuropsychological tests and will assess amyloid-β deposition in the brain by using positron emission tomography amyloid imaging.[68]

BETA-BLOCKADE

No large definitive trials of beta-blockers in HFpEF have been performed. A smaller trial of 95 patients, the Swedish Doppler-echocardiographic study (SWEDIC), demonstrated no significant benefit of the beta-blocker, carvedilol, on diastolic function patients with mild HFpEF (LVEF >45%) who also met conventional Doppler criteria for diastolic dysfunction.[69] The Japanese Diastolic Heart Failure Study (J-DHF) trial was a multicenter, randomized, placebo-controlled, open, blinded–end point trial, which evaluated the effects of carvedilol in 245 patients with HFpEF (LVEF >40%) during a median follow-up of 3.2 years. There was no difference in the primary composite outcome of CV death or HF hospitalization or in the secondary composite outcome of CV death or any CV hospitalization. However, only 245 of the planned 800 patients were enrolled, resulting in the trial being underpowered.[70] Another smaller trial, the Effects of the Long-term Administration of Nebivolol on the clinical symptoms, exercise capacity, and LV function of patients with Diastolic Dysfunction: (ELANDD) study evaluated 116 patients with NYHA class II to III symptoms, LVEF greater than 45%, and echocardiographic signs of LV diastolic dysfunction. The patients were randomized to 6 months of treatment with nebivolol or a placebo. Nebivolol is a beta$_1$ selective blocker that also has vasodilating and antioxidative properties and improves endothelial dysfunction via its effects on the endothelial NO synthase. However, in the trial, no differences were demonstrated in the 6-minute walk distance or peak oxygen consumption between the nebivolol or placebo groups. The resting and peak blood pressure decreased in patients on nebivolol; there was a significant interaction between change in peak exercise heart rate and peak oxygen consumption (r = 0.391, P = .003), and it was postulated that the negative chronotropic effect of the beta-blocker may have contributed to the neutral results of the study.[71]

A larger multicenter trial evaluated the effects of nebivolol in elderly patients with HF, irrespective of LVEF. In the Study of the Effects of Nebivolol Intervention on Outcomes and Rehospitalizations in Seniors with heart failure (SENIORS), 2128 patients aged 70 years or older with a history of HF were randomized to receive nebivolol or the placebo.[72] Of these, 35% of patients had LVEF greater than 35%. In the overall study, nebivolol was associated with a modest 14% reduction in the primary composite end point of death or CV hospitalization (HR 0.84, 95% CI 0.74–0.99), contributed to by a reduction in both mortality and CV hospitalization. A similar magnitude of reduction was noted in the subgroup with LVEF greater than 35%; however, it did not reach statistical significance, possibly a result of fewer patients in the subgroup (HR 0.82, 95% CI 0.63–1.05). Although labeled as patients with preserved ejection fraction or HFpEF, this subgroup of patients with EF greater than 35% clearly consisted of a heterogeneous patient population with both preserved and reduced LVEF. The proportion of patients with truly preserved LVEF (≥50%) was small (<15% of all patients in the trial). Therefore, although the overall trial suggests a modest CV benefit of the beta-blocker, nebivolol, in elderly patients with HF, the results did not convincingly demonstrate a benefit in elderly patients with HFpEF.

In summary, these trials of the beta-blockers carvedilol and nebivolol, although limited by sample size, have not demonstrated definitive benefits, or harm, on exercise and functional capacity, on diastolic dysfunction, or on clinical outcomes in patients with HFpEF.

I$_F$ CHANNEL BLOCKER: IVABRADINE

Ivabradine inhibits the I$_f$ or "funny" channel, which is highly expressed in the sinoatrial (SA) node, and involves a mixed Na$^+$–K$^+$ inward current, which is one of the most important ionic currents for regulating pacemaker activity in the SA node. Ivabradine selectively inhibits the I$_f$ current in a dose-dependent manner. Blocking this channel selectively decreases the sinus rate without any effects on cardiac contractility.[73] Trials of the I$_f$ channel blocker ivabradine have predominantly enrolled patients with systolic dysfunction or ischemic heart disease with a proven role in selected patients with HFrEF. Two small trials in patients with HFpEF have been carried out, with a combined total of 83 patients. In the initial trial of 61 patients, patients randomized to ivabradine for 7 days had improved exercise capacity, increased peak VO$_2$, and improved diastolic function with exercise (reduced exercise-induced rises in E/e').[74] However, in the later but smaller trial, ivabradine significantly reduced peak heart rate in the HFpEF group but also significantly worsened the change in VO$_2$ peak in HFpEF and significantly reduced submaximal exercise capacity, as determined by the oxygen uptake efficiency slope.[75] Whether use of ivabradine in HFpEF has a long-term role in patients remains unclear.

SELECTIVE PHOSPHODIESTERASE TYPE 5 INHIBITION

Selective inhibitors of phosphodiesterase-5 (PDE5) are known to enhance NO-mediated vasodilation by inhibiting degradation of cyclic GMP, a key intracellular second messenger (**see also Chapters 1 and 2**).[76] Although inhibitors of the cyclic adenosine monophosphate (cAMP)–specific phosphodiesterase-3 or PDE3 (including inotropic agents, such as milrinone and enoximone) augment intracellular levels of cyclic AMP and increase mortality in patients with HF (**see Chapter 36**),[77] selective inhibitors of PDE5 such as sildenafil are highly selective for human PDE5, do not increase cyclic AMP, and lack inotropic effects. Therefore they are thought to not share the toxicity associated with PDE3 inhibition.

Several experimental observations suggest that sildenafil may be beneficial in the treatment of patients with HFpEF. In mice exposed to sustained pressure overload, chronic PDE5A inhibition led to attenuation of cardiac and myocyte hypertrophy and interstitial fibrosis and improved cardiac functioning.[78] Sildenafil treatment applied to well-established hypertrophic cardiac disease in mice also prevented further cardiac and myocyte dysfunction, as well as progressive remodeling.[79] The investigators demonstrated that PDE5 is upregulated in the heart in response to pressure overload and that the effects of PDE5 inhibition are not mediated by an effect on blood pressure. In addition, PDE5 inhibition has been associated with an improvement in large artery stiffness in hypertensive men.[80] Beneficial effects on pulmonary vasculature with reduction in pulmonary pressures, as well as reduction in right ventricular hypertrophy, have been demonstrated with patients with pulmonary hypertension.[81] Furthermore, PDE5 inhibition may restore renal responsiveness to natriuretic peptides in several states of abnormal sodium handling including HF.[82] These beneficial effects, along with the fact that PDE5 is upregulated in CV disease states such as HF, with resultant greater susceptibility to PDE5 inhibition in these diseases, make selective PDE5 inhibition an attractive therapeutic target in the treatment of patients with HFpEF.

This hypothesis was tested in the PhosphodiesteRasE-5 Inhibition to improve cLinical status And eXercise Capacity in Diastolic Heart Failure (RELAX) trial. This study was a multicenter, double-blind, placebo-controlled, randomized clinical trial of 216 stable outpatients with HFpEF (LVEF ≥ 50%), elevated NT-proBNP or elevated invasively measured filling pressures, and reduced exercise capacity (**see Table 39.1**). Patients were randomized to a placebo or sildenafil 20 mg thrice daily for 12 weeks followed by 60 mg thrice daily for the next 12 weeks. The primary outcome—a change in peak oxygen consumption after 24 weeks of therapy and secondary end points, including change in 6-minute walk distance and a composite clinical status score—was not significantly different between the two groups at 24 weeks. In addition, no differences were noted in Doppler assessed LV diastolic function parameters or in the pulmonary arterial systolic pressures between the two treatment groups. Serious adverse events occurred in 22% of sildenafil patients and 16% of placebo patients. Unexpectedly, there was modest but statistically significant worsening of renal function observed in patients treated with sildenafil, which was associated with concordant increases in NT-proBNP, uric acid, and endothelin-1, suggesting that the decline in renal function was physiologically significant. There were more (not statistically significant) patients who withdrew consent, died, or were too ill to perform the cardiopulmonary exercise test in the sildenafil treatment group, potentially accentuating the lack of benefit observed, particularly if those who withdrew did so due to adverse effects or poor clinical status.[83] The lack of clinical benefit in the RELAX study was in contrast to a smaller prior study of sildenafil in HFpEF (n = 44), which had demonstrated significant reductions in pulmonary artery and right heart pressures, right ventricular function, and some benefits for left heart diastolic pressures and diastolic function.[84] No exercise testing was performed in that study. Importantly, compared with the RELAX trial, HFpEF patients in that study had fewer comorbidities and significantly higher blood pressure, LV mass, pulmonary arterial hypertension, profound right ventricular systolic dysfunction, and right ventricular failure. Thus it can be hypothesized that the primary therapeutic effects of PDE5 inhibitors in HF involve the drugs' ability to dilate the pulmonary vascular bed, enhance right ventricular contractility, and reduce ventricular interdependence and that pulmonary arterial hypertension and right ventricular failure must be significant to observe clinical benefit in HFpEF.

OTHER TARGETS FOR MEDICAL THERAPY

Endothelin Antagonists

Experimental studies suggested that selective antagonists of endothelin type A (ETA) could exert beneficial effects in diastolic HF through attenuation of the progression of LV hypertrophy and fibrosis with resultant improvement in diastolic function.[85] In addition, in patients with moderate to severe HF, acute ETA receptor blockade with sitaxsentan caused selective pulmonary vasodilation. Therefore sitaxsentan was thought to be of potential value in the treatment of patients with pulmonary hypertension secondary to chronic HF. Based on these considerations, a smaller trial with a selective ETA antagonist, sitaxsentan, randomized 192 HFpEF patients (EF ≥ 50%) 2:1 to sitaxsentan 100 mg/day (n = 128) versus placebo (n = 64) for 24 weeks. Treatment with sitaxsentan increased exercise tolerance (treadmill time) but did not improve any of the secondary end points such as LV mass, diastolic function, or functional status.[86] Subsequently, in a murine model of HFpEF, dual ETA/ETB receptor inhibition with macitentan improved HFpEF by abrogating adverse cardiac remodeling via antihypertrophic mechanisms and by reducing stiffness.[87] However, in a small group of patients with HFpEF and pulmonary hypertension, the dual ETA/ETB receptor antagonist, bosentan, did not result in any improvement with even a signal for worsening in exercise capacity or pulmonary hypertension.[88]

Advanced Glycation End Products Cross-Link Breakers

Increased LV and arterial stiffness, which may be involved in the pathophysiology of HFpEF (**see Chapter 11**), especially in elderly subjects and in patients with diabetes,[13,89] is at least partially contributed to by nonenzymatic cross-links that develop between advanced glycation end products (AGEs) on long-lived proteins, such as collagen and elastin. Alagebrium chloride (ALT-711) nonenzymatically breaks AGE cross-links and has been shown to improve LV distensibility and arterial compliance in elderly subjects with systolic hypertension.[90] A small open-label study that evaluated the use of alagebrium in elderly patients with stable HFpEF found that alagebrium was associated with a reduction of LV mass, improved tissue Doppler indices of diastolic function (e′), and improved quality of life. However, there was no change in blood pressure, pulse pressure, peak oxygen consumption, or aortic distensibility.[91] Although a number of trials with this agent in HF including HFpEF were initiated, the studies were terminated without completion.

Novel Hypoglycemic Agents

Diabetes mellitus is a major risk factor for CV disease in general and for HFpEF. A selective inhibitor of the sodium-glucose cotransporter-2 (SGLT-2), empagliflozin, was associated with improved glycemic control, weight loss, and improved blood pressure in diabetic patients. The Empagliflozin Cardiovascular Outcome Event Trial in Type 2 Diabetes Mellitus Patients (EMPA-REG Outcome) trial in patients with diabetes was designed to look at its CV effects with a primary end point of CV death, nonfatal myocardial infarctions, and stroke. Besides a significant benefit on the primary outcome, empagliflozin reduced HF hospitalizations by nearly a third and reduced HF-related deaths.[92] Approximately 10% of the 7020 patients enrolled in the trial had baseline HF (without specification of LVEF), and the reduction in CV death and HF hospitalization were similar in patients with and without HF. In addition, there was a decreased rate of loop diuretic use in patients treated with empagliflozin compared with placebo.[93] Similarly, another SGLT2 inhibitor, canagliflozin, was evaluated in a large trial program of patients at high CV risk and diabetes, the Canagliflozin Cardiovascular Assessment Study (CANVAS program) of canagliflozin or placebo. Again, CV death or hospitalized HF was significantly reduced in those treated with canagliflozin compared with placebo, as was fatal or hospitalized HF (HR, 0.70; 95% CI, 0.55–0.89) and hospitalized HF alone (HR, 0.67; 95% CI, 0.52–0.87). At baseline, 14.4% of patients had HF, and the benefit on CV death or hospitalized HF may be greater in patients with a prior history of HF (HR, 0.61; 95% CI, 0.46–0.80) compared with those without HF at baseline (HR, 0.87; 95% CI, 0.72–1.06; p interaction = 0.021).[94] Although the data for LVEF are absent in both trials, certainly SGLT-2 inhibitors could be considered as an additional agent in treating patients with diabetes with HF and at risk for HF.

There may be a beneficial effect of the SGLT-2 inhibitors in HF, which is separate from its effect on glycemic control. The benefits for HF outcomes appeared early during follow-up in the clinical trials, suggesting a mechanism driven primarily by volume and hemodynamic effects. However, other mechanisms have also been hypothesized. Reductions in preload and afterload resulting from natriuresis, systemic blood pressure lowering, modification of the intrarenal renin angiotensin axis, reduction in arterial stiffness, and preservation of renal function may all contribute to the benefits observed. Others have hypothesized that the main driver of benefit might be the unique effects of SGLT-2 inhibitors on renal sodium and glucose handling, which leads to improvements in diabetes-related maladaptive afferent renal arteriolar vasoconstriction. Furthermore, direct positive effects of SGLT-2 inhibition on cardiac metabolism that are attributable to a shift from fatty acids to ketone bodies as the substrate for myocardial energy generation with resultant improvement in myocardial efficiency and function may contribute.[94,95] Large randomized clinical trials are ongoing to evaluate the benefit of SGLT-2 inhibitors on clinical outcomes in patients with HFpEF with or without baseline diabetes.

Metabolic Modulators

Several alterations in cardiac energy metabolism have been identified in HF and contribute to the severity of HF. Some alterations may be specific to the type of HF, such as HFpEF, and are also dependent on the coexistence of comorbidities, such as obesity and diabetes, as noted in the preceding section. Other metabolic abnormalities identified in HFpEF include reduced mitochondrial oxidative capacity, increased fatty acid oxidation, decreased glucose oxidation, and an uncoupling between glucose uptake and oxidation, resulting in an increased rate of glycolysis.[96] Therefore there is interest in metabolic modulators energy substrate such as perhexiline in HFpEF; however, at this time no definitive data of clinical benefit of such agents in HFpEF are available, and this remains an area of potential research.

Antiinflammatory Agents

Enhanced inflammation is associated with worsening outcomes in HF patients and may play a direct role in disease progression (**see Chapter 7**). Interleukin-1β (IL-1β) is a proinflammatory cytokine that is chronically elevated in HF and has been associated with adverse ventricular-vascular remodeling, pressure overload–induced cardiac hypertrophy, and negative inotropy, as well as reduced β-adrenergic receptor responsiveness.[97] A paradigm for HFpEF development that has been proposed identifies a systemic proinflammatory state induced by comorbidities as the cause of myocardial structural and functional alterations.[19] Therefore the agent Anakinra, an IL-1 receptor antagonist, was studied in a small crossover pilot study of 12 patients with HFpEF and systemic inflammation high sensitivity C-reactive protein [hs CRP] > 2 mg/L) in the Diastolic Heart failure Anakinra Response Trial (D-HART). Anakinra given for 14 days led to a statistically significant improvement in peak oxygen consumption (+1.2 mL/kg/min, P = .009) and a significant reduction in plasma CRP levels (−74%,

P = .006). The reduction in CRP levels correlated with the improvement in peak oxygen consumption (R = −0.60, P = .002).[98] Based on this pilot study, the D-HART2 trial will test the hypothesis that IL-1 blockade with anakinra improves cardiorespiratory fitness, diastolic dysfunction, and elevated inflammation in patients with HFpEF.[99]

Lusitropic Agents

Ranolazine is an antiischemic drug that inhibits the late sodium current in cardiac myocytes. In patients with HF, the late sodium current is increased,[100] leading to increased sodium accumulation, which reverses the direction of the Na^+/Ca^{2+}-exchanger, contributing to a Ca^{2+} overload in the cell. By inhibiting the late Na^+ current (INa), ranolazine is expected to prevent (or reduce) sodium accumulation in the myocyte, thus improving calcium extrusion through the Na^+/Ca^{2+}-exchanger and thereby improve relaxation of the myocardium.[101] Data from in vitro, ex vivo, and animal studies indicate that ranolazine improved diastolic function of the myocardium.[102] A proof of concept, small single-center clinical trial, the RAnoLazIne for the Treatment of Diastolic Heart Failure (RALI-DHF) was conducted in HFpEF. Patients with LVEF greater than 45%, echo E/e′ greater than 15, NT-proBNP greater than 220 pg/mL, left ventricular end diastolic pressure (LVEDP) greater than 18 mm Hg, and time constant of relaxation tau greater than 50 milliseconds were randomized to receive an infusion of ranolazine for 24 hours followed by 1000 mg twice daily for 14 days (n = 12) or placebo (n = 8). There was a significant decline in LVEDP (P = .04), as well as pulmonary capillary wedge pressure (PCWP) (P = .04) 30 minutes after infusion of ranolazine but not with placebo.[103] Mean pulmonary artery pressure showed a trend toward a decrease in the ranolazine group that was significant under pacing conditions at 120 beats/min (P = .02) but not for the placebo group. These changes occurred without changes in LV end-systolic pressure or systemic or pulmonary resistance but in the presence of a small but significant decrease in cardiac output (P = .04). Relaxation parameters were unaltered. Echocardiographically, the E/e′ ratio did not significantly change after 22 hours. After 14 days of treatment, no significant changes were observed in echocardiographic or cardiopulmonary exercise test parameters without significant changes in NT-proBNP levels. The clinical significance of the results of this small short-term study with ranolazine improving some hemodynamic measures but without any improvement in relaxation parameters remains uncertain at this time.

DEVICE-BASED THERAPIES

Treatment of Obstructive Sleep Apnea

Unlike HFrEF, where a number of studies have shown an increased prevalence of central sleep apnea, HFpEF may be more often associated with obstructive sleep apnea (OSA). In one study, sleep-disordered breathing was reported in greater than 50% of patients with HFpEF, with most patients having OSA.[104] Patients with HFpEF and sleep-disordered breathing had worse diastolic dysfunction compared with patients without sleep-disordered breathing. Several theoretical mechanisms are postulated for the contribution of OSA toward the development of diastolic dysfunction and HF.[105] The most direct mechanism may be through long-standing OSA causing hypertension, a major risk factor for the development and progression of HFpEF. LV hypertrophy may be more closely linked to hypertension during sleep than during wakefulness. In patients with HF, the coexistence of OSA may also be associated with higher sympathetic nerve activity and higher systolic blood pressure during wakefulness, despite more intense antihypertensive therapy. Responses to cytokines, catecholamines, endothelin, and other growth factors produced in OSA may also contribute to ventricular hypertrophy independently of hypertension. In addition, nocturnal oxygen desaturation is an independent

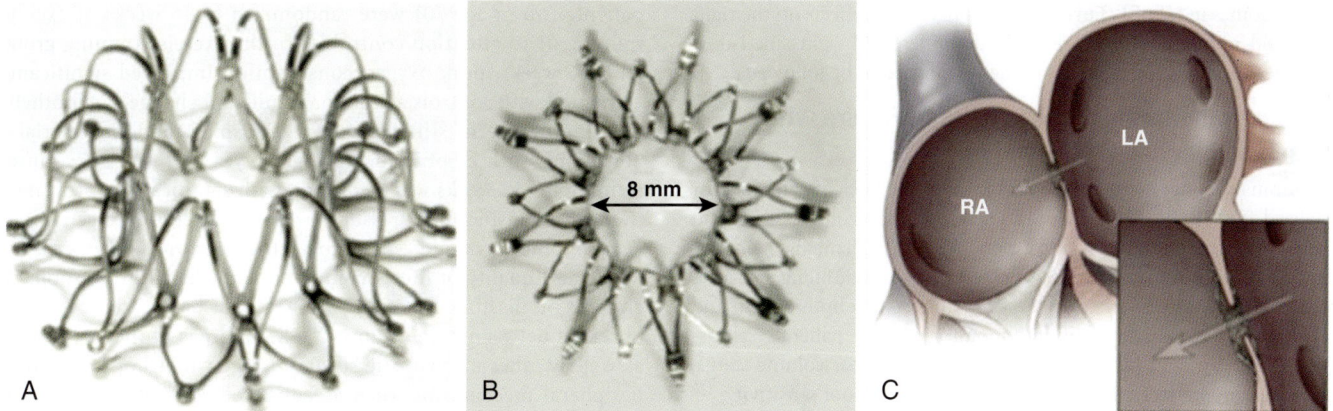

Fig. 39.9 Interatrial shunt device. (A) Corvia Interatrial Shunt Device (IASD) System II. (B) Enface view of the IASD System II (internal diameter, 8 mm). (C) The IASD creates an interatrial shunt that unloads the left atrium *(LA)* by shunting blood from the higher pressure LA to the lower pressure right atrium *(RA)*. (From Feldman T, Mauri L, Kahwash R, et al. Transcatheter interatrial shunt device for the treatment of heart failure with preserved ejection fraction [REDUCE LAP-HF I (reduce elevated left atrial pressure in patients with heart failure)]: a Phase 2, randomized, sham-controlled trial. *Circulation.* 2018;137[4]:364–375.)

predictor of impaired ventricular relaxation. Long-term exposure to markedly subatmospheric pressure during OSA could also promote hypertrophy and diastolic dysfunction. Furthermore, a leftward shift of the interventricular septum due to overdistention of the right ventricle during OSAs may limit LV filling and thus decrease cardiac output. Some of these CV changes may be reversible with effective continuous positive airway pressure (CPAP) treatment.

Although theoretically appealing, along with small studies suggesting benefit of CPAP on diastolic function, apneic-hypopneic episodes, and blood pressure,[106,107] little direct clinical evidence is available regarding the benefit of CPAP on HF outcomes in patients with HF, specifically HFpEF. Based on current evidence, as stated in the most recent AHA/ACC guideline update for HF, in patients with CV disease and OSA, CPAP may be reasonable to improve sleep quality and daytime sleepiness (**see Table 39G.1**).[8,108] Larger clinical outcome trials are needed to examine the clinical benefit of treatment of sleep apnea on clinical outcomes in patients with HFpEF.

Pacemakers

Patients with HFpEF also have chronotropic incompetence in response to exercise that may contribute to significant limitation of their physical activity. Borlaug and colleagues showed that at matched low-level workload, as well as at peak workload, patients with HFpEF had less of an increase in heart rate and cardiac output and less systemic vasodilation than control subjects, despite a similar rise in end-diastolic volume, stroke volume, and contractility.[12] Although these findings first question the conventional wisdom of using beta-blockers, which are negative chronotropic agents, in HFpEF patients, especially the elderly, they also provide a potential target for treatment of HFpEF. Although trials have been designed to evaluate the effects of atrial rate-responsive pacing on exercise capacity and quality of life in patients with HFpEF, no results are currently available for this strategy based on difficulties with patient enrollment.

Mechanical Targeting of Left Atrial Pressure Reduction

Elevation in left atrial pressure either at rest or especially with exertion is a common finding in patients with HFpEF and is causal in symptoms of dyspnea and exercise intolerance and correlate with outcomes. In the setting of mitral stenosis, the presence of an atrial septal defect (Lutembacher syndrome) is associated with fewer symptoms; this was

the theoretical rationale for a trial of an interatrial shunt device (IASD; Corvia Medical, Tewksbury, MA; **Fig. 39.9**). The REDUCe Elevated Left Atrial Pressure in Patients with Heart Failure (REDUCE LAP-HF) is a trial of an iatrogenic interatrial shunt to decrease left atrial pressures during exercise. The 8-mm shunt (IASD, Corvia Medical) was evaluated in an open-label phase I trial of 68 patients; the shunt remained patent at 1 year as demonstrated by echo or oximetry. It was associated with a reduction in exercise pulmonary capillary wedge pressure and demonstrated improvement in NYHA class, quality of life, and 6-minute walk distances at 6 months.[109] One year after interatrial septal shunt device implantation, there were sustained improvements in NYHA class, quality-of-life scores, and 6-minute walk distance. Echocardiography showed a small, stable reduction in LV end-diastolic volume index, with a concomitant small stable increase in the right ventricular end-diastolic volume index. Invasive hemodynamic studies performed in a subset of patients demonstrated a sustained reduction in the workload corrected exercise pulmonary capillary wedge pressure.[110] Simulation studies have shown that an 8-mm internal diameter for the shunt device is optimal in maximally reducing left atrial pressure without overloading the right heart (i.e., keeping pulmonary-to-systemic flow relatively low at a 1.2–1.3 range).[111] Subsequently, a phase II study randomized 44 patients (1:1) with NYHA class III or ambulatory class IV HFpEF, LVEF ≥40%, exercise PCWP ≥25 mmHg, and PCWP-right atrial pressure gradient ≥5 mm Hg to either the procedural arm with IASD or to the sham arm. The mean age of the study subjects was 70 years, and 50% were women. At 1 month, the IASD resulted in a greater reduction in pulmonary capillary wedge pressure compared with sham control (*P* = .028 accounting for all stages of exercise). The peak PCWP decreased by 3.5 ± 6.4 mm Hg in the treatment group versus 0.5 ± 5.0 mm Hg in the control group (*P* = .14). There were no periprocedural or 1-month major adverse cardiac, cerebrovascular, and renal events in the IASD group.[112] In addition, there was a greater reduction in mean pulmonary artery pressure and pulmonary vascular resistance in the IASD treatment arm compared with the control arm, although these differences did not achieve statistical significance. Other device systems such as the V-Wave implantable shunt (V-Wave Ltd, Or Akiva, Israel) are also being tested for similar effects.[113] It remains to be seen in larger randomized sham-controlled trials whether the short-term reduction in pressures with IASDs will be sustained and whether they will translate into sustained improvements in symptoms and outcomes in HFpEF. Furthermore, longer-term effects on the right heart and right-sided pressures related to increased right-sided flow with the iatrogenic shunt, albeit modest, will need to be followed.

Pressure Monitoring Devices in Heart Failure with Preserved Ejection Fraction

Symptoms of congestion are present in more than 90% of patients hospitalized for HF including HFpEF. Therefore body volume shifts and changes are a major concern, and experience with implantable hemodynamic monitors has suggested that an increase in cardiac filling pressures precedes HF events by ≥1 to 2 weeks in patients with both HFrEF and HFpEF.[114,115] Although traditional monitoring with patient's self-assessment and weight monitoring are useful to monitor volume status, these measurements are limited by inaccuracies and poor sensitivity.[116]

An example of potential utility of therapy guided by implantable hemodynamic monitors in HFpEF was provided by a small prespecified subgroup analysis from the CardioMEMS Heart Sensor Allows Monitoring of Pressure to Improve Outcomes in NYHA Class III Heart Failure Patients (CHAMPION) trial.[117] After permanent implantation of a microelectromechanical system–based pressure sensor in the pulmonary artery, patients with HFpEF defined by LVEF ≥40% were randomly assigned to a treatment group (n = 62) in which standard HF management was combined with pressure-based adjustment of medical therapy of diuretics and vasodilators. The control group (n = 57) was managed using standard clinical approaches (without access to daily uploaded pulmonary artery pressures). After an average follow-up of 17 months, patients in the treatment group had 50% fewer HF hospitalizations compared with the control group (HR 0.50; 95% CI, 0.35–0.70; $P < .0001$). A further smaller subgroup analysis of patients with LVEF ≥50% also had significantly lower hospitalization rates (HR 0.30, 95% CI 0.18–0.48; $P < .0001$). Most adjustments in response to changes in pulmonary artery pressures were with diuretic dose adjustment, with only a small proportion using changes in vasodilator (nitrate) therapy. Although holding promise, more data are needed before recommending more widespread use of this strategy to reduce HF hospitalizations in large numbers of HFpEF patients that are cared for in diverse outpatient practices. The findings do underscore the effectiveness of diuretics when carefully used to prevent acute exacerbations in this patient group.

EXERCISE TRAINING IN HEART FAILURE WITH PRESERVED EJECTION FRACTION

Exercise intolerance is often one of the debilitating symptoms in patients with HFpEF (**see also Chapters 11 and 16**). A meta-analysis of five studies evaluated the benefit of exercise training in patients with HFpEF. Three randomized controlled trials, one non-randomized controlled trial, and one prepost study were included (total n = 228).[118-123] The combined duration of exercise programs and follow-up ranged from 12 to 24 weeks. Exercise was found to be safe with no deaths, hospital admissions, or serious adverse events observed during or immediately following exercise training. In four trials that used peak oxygen uptake as an end point, compared with control, the change in exercise capacity was higher with exercise training (between-group mean difference: 3.0 mL/kg/min, 95% CI 2.4–2.6). In the four studies using the Minnesota Living with HF questionnaire, there was evidence of a larger gain in health-related quality of life with exercise training (7.3 units, 95% CI 3.3–11.4). The largest study showed some evidence of improvement in the echocardiographic E/e′ ratio with exercise training, but this was not confirmed in the other studies. In the Prospective Aerobic Reconditioning Intervention Study (PARIS), a total of 63 HFpEF

patients (mean age 70) were randomized to 16 weeks of exercise training or to attention control.[123] In the exercise training group, after 16 weeks, peak oxygen consumption improved significantly compared with controls, without a significant change in endothelial function or arterial stiffness. In another small randomized trial of 26 patients with HFpEF (median age 73 years), inspiratory muscle training for 12 weeks was associated with significant improvement in maximal inspiratory pressure, peak Vo_2, exercise oxygen uptake at anaerobic threshold, ventilatory efficiency, 6-minute walk distance, and quality of life as compared with the control group. No changes on diastolic function parameters or biomarker levels were observed between both groups.[124] The findings of these two trials, as well as other mechanistic studies, suggest that improvement in peripheral mechanisms, such as enhanced skeletal muscle perfusion and/or oxygen use, rather than central CV mechanisms, may be responsible for the exercise-mediated increase in peak Vo_2 in older HFpEF patients.[125] The training programs used in these trials are described in **Table 39.3**. Kitzman and colleagues subsequently examined whether 20 weeks of caloric restriction (diet) or aerobic

TABLE 39.3 **Exercise Regimens Used in Clinical Trials in Heart Failure with Preserved Ejection Fraction**

Study	Exercise Regimen Used
Edelman et al.[119]	Supervised center-based, 24-week aerobic (cycling) exercise: Weeks 1–4: 2 sessions/week, 20–40 min/session, 50%–60% peak VO₂. Weeks 5–12: 3 sessions/week, 20–40 min/session, 70% peak VO₂ plus resistance training
Gary et al.[129]	Self-monitored community based, 12-week aerobic (walking) exercise: 3 sessions/week 30–40 min/session, 40%–70% THR
Kitzman et al.[120]	Supervised center-based, 16-week aerobic (cycling) exercise: 3 sessions/week, 1 hr/session, 40%–70% HRR
Kitzman et al.[123]	Supervised: 3 sessions/week, 1 hr/session for 16 weeks Aerobic (track and cycle ergometry) and isolated arm ergometry. 40%–70% HRR
Korzeniowska-Kubacka et al.[121]	Supervised center-based, 18-week aerobic (cycling and gymnastics) exercise: 3 sessions/week, 40 min/session, 80% maximum HR
Smart et al.[122]	Supervised center-based, 16-week aerobic (cycling) exercise: 3 sessions/week, 1 hr/session, 60%–70% peak VO₂ plus resistance training weeks 8–16
Kitzman et al.[126]	1-hour supervised exercise sessions 3 times per week consisting primarily of walking exercise using an individualized exercise prescription based on the exercise test results, and intensity level was progressed as tolerated, based primarily on heart rate reserve

HR, Heart rate; *HRR*, heart rate reserve; *THR*, target heart rate; *VO₂*, oxygen consumption.

exercise training (exercise) improve exercise capacity and quality of life in obese older patients with HFPEF (**see Table 39.1**).[126] Of the 100 enrolled participants, 26 participants were randomized to exercise, 24 to diet, 25 to exercise and diet, and 25 to control. Of these, 92 participants completed the trial. Exercise attendance was 84%, and diet adherence was 99%. Exercise capacity as measured by peak VO_2 was increased significantly by both interventions: exercise (1.2 mL/kg/min; 95% CI, 0.7 to 1.7, $P < .001$) and diet (1.3 mL/kg/min, 95% CI, 0.8 to 1.8, $P < .001$). The combination of exercise and diet was additive for peak VO_2 (joint effect, 2.5 mL/kg/min). There was no significant improvement in quality of life with exercise or diet. The change in peak VO_2 was positively correlated with the change in percent lean body mass and the change in thigh muscle to intermuscular fat ratio. Body weight decreased by 7% in the diet group, 3% in the exercise group, 10% in the exercise and diet group, and 1% in the control group. Another approach with home-based cardiac rehabilitation was demonstrated to be promising in an initial feasibility study for 12 weeks in the Rehabilitation EnAblement in CHronic Heart Failure (REACH-HF) trial in 50 patients with HFpEF.[127] Study retention (90%) and intervention uptake (92%) were excellent. At 6 months, data from 45 patients showed a potential direction of effect in favor of the intervention group, including quality-of-life scores. Improvements were also seen in a number of intervention caregivers' mental health and burden compared with control.

Based on benefit noted in these relatively smaller trials, larger multicenter randomized trials evaluating the benefits of exercise training with or without diet on functional and clinical outcomes in HFpEF are awaited.

CURRENT RECOMMENDATIONS FOR THE MANAGEMENT OF PATIENTS WITH HEART FAILURE WITH PRESERVED EJECTION FRACTION (GUIDELINE RECOMMENDATIONS)

The clinical diagnosis of HFpEF depends on the presence of clinical symptoms and signs of HF with preserved LVEF (≥45% or 50%) measured by any cardiac imaging technique. The presence of diastolic abnormalities, evidence of elevated LV filling pressures and left atrial enlargement, as well as substrate for diastolic dysfunction (i.e., LV hypertrophy) on echocardiography, may provide supportive evidence. Although considered rudimentary, the clinical confirmation of the diagnosis of HF is key, especially in ruling out other causes of symptoms such as lung disease and obesity. Several conditions need to be considered in the differential diagnosis before treating for the prototypic "diastolic heart failure" or HFpEF. The algorithm suggested in a prior version of the Heart Failure Society of America Heart Failure Practice Guidelines still provides a useful guiding framework for the initial work-up of these patients (**Fig. 39.10**).[128] Conditions that require specific intervention need to be identified, such as valvular heart disease, coronary artery disease, pericardial disease, isolated right HF due to primary pulmonary conditions, or contributing systemic conditions such as anemia and thyrotoxicosis. Once these conditions are ruled out or treated, patients with HFpEF should be managed based on the general recommendations provided by the American College of Cardiology Foundation (ACCF)/AHA Guideline for the Management of Heart Failure (**see Table 39G.1**).[8] Treatment considerations can be broadly grouped under the following categories: treatment of volume overload; aggressive control of hypertension;

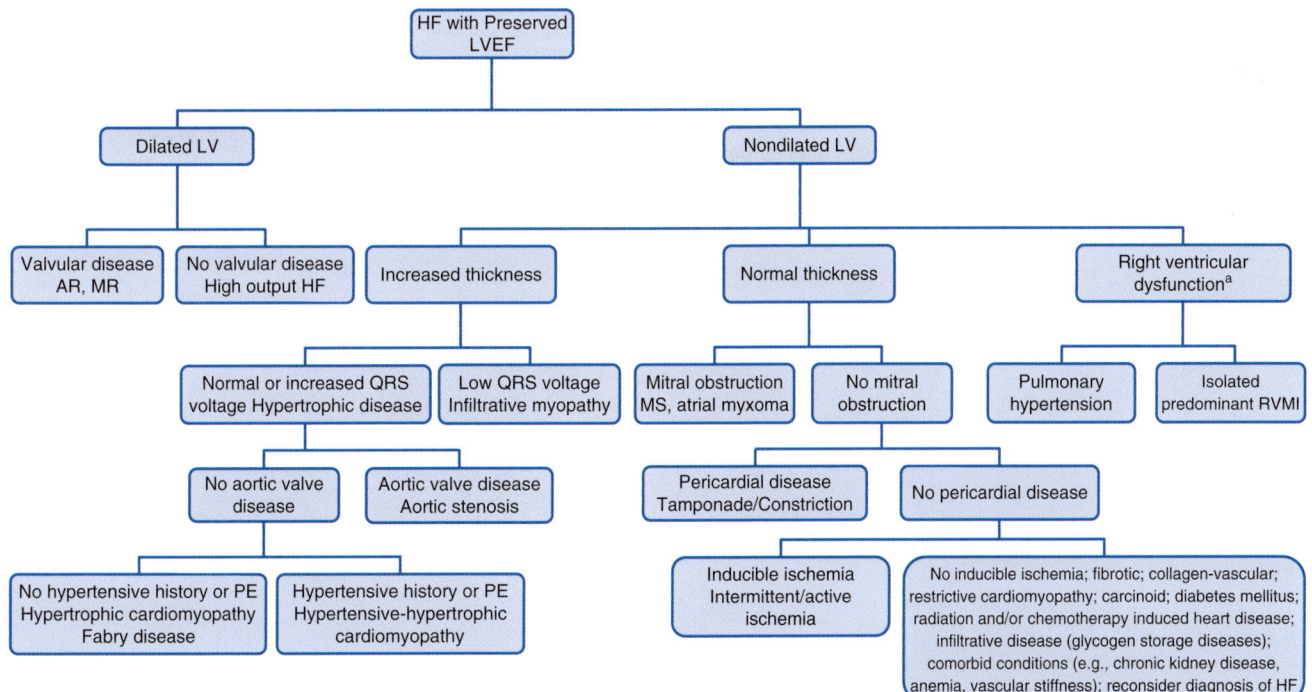

Fig. 39.10 Diagnostic algorithm for patients with heart failure with preserved ejection fraction. [a]Some patients with RV dysfunction have LV dysfunction due to ventricular interaction. *AR*, Aortic regurgitation; *HF*, heart failure; *LV*, left ventricular; *LVEF*, left ventricular ejection fraction; *MR*, mitral regurgitation; *MS*, mitral stenosis; *PE*, pulmonary embolism; *QRS*, electrocardiographic ventricular depolarization; *RVMI*, right ventricular myocardial infarction. (From Lindenfeld J, Albert NM, Boehmer JP, et al. HFSA 2010 comprehensive heart failure practice guideline. *J Card Fail*. 2010;16[6]:e1–e194.)

treatment of factors contributing to decompensation, most commonly atrial fibrillation; uncontrolled hypertension, ischemia, anemia, and infections; and therapies based on associated CV diagnoses or risk factors including obesity. Of note in the practice guidelines, none of the recommendations are based on strong level of evidence A, and most recommendations are based on consensus opinion of experts. In addition, the general principles of treatment of HF can be applied to patients with HFpEF in regard to fluid and salt restriction and avoidance of potentially harmful drugs, such as nonsteroidal antiinflammatory agents and thiazolidinediones. In contrast to patients with HFrEF, nondihydropyridine calcium channel blockers with potential negative inotropic effects such as diltiazem and verapamil could be considered to treat hypertension and angina and to control the rate in atrial fibrillation in patients with HFpEF.

SUMMARY AND FUTURE DIRECTIONS

The recognition of the high prevalence of HFpEF, with its associated substantial morbidity and mortality, has initiated a quest for effective therapy for the condition. Unlike in HFrEF, where RAAS blockers have been proven to have definite beneficial effects on mortality and morbidity, none of the clinical trials to date with ACE inhibitors or ARBs has demonstrated definitive benefit in clinical outcomes in patients with HFpEF. A number of novel therapies that are being currently tested for HFpEF are targeting alternate pathophysiologic mechanisms. At present, recommended therapy is aimed at relief of symptoms, control of hypertension, and management of other contributory comorbidities. Although RAAS blockers and beta-blockers are not routinely recommended at present specifically for the treatment of HFpEF, their use will remain important for proven indications for other comorbid conditions that frequently coexist. We may need to reconsider traditional end points such as mortality for the efficacy evaluation of therapies in patients with HFpEF, a highly comorbid population with many competing risks for mortality; we may need to consider whether hospitalization and exercise capacity are more meaningful end points in this patient population. In addition, because of the heterogeneity of patients with HFpEF, it may be difficult to prove a "one-size-fits-all" therapeutic agent, and there is a need to study relevant interventions in more homogeneous subgroups of patients.

KEY REFERENCES

8. Yancy CW, Jessup M, Bozkurt B, et al. 2017 ACC/AHA/HFSA Focused Update of the 2013 ACCF/AHA Guideline for the Management of Heart Failure: a Report of the American College of Cardiology/American Heart Association Task Force on Clinical Practice Guidelines and the Heart Failure Society of America. *J Card Fail*. 2017;23(8):628–651.

34. Reddy YNV, Lewis GD, Shah SJ, et al. INDIE-HFpEF (Inorganic Nitrite Delivery to Improve Exercise Capacity in Heart Failure With Preserved Ejection Fraction): rationale and design. *Circ Heart Fail*. 2017;10(5). pii: e003862.

54. Massie BM, Carson PE, McMurray JJ, et al. Irbesartan in patients with heart failure and preserved ejection fraction. *N Engl J Med*. 2008;359(23):2456–2467.

58. Pitt B, Pfeffer MA, Assmann SF, et al. Spironolactone for heart failure with preserved ejection fraction. *N Engl J Med*. 2014;370(15):1383–1392.

59. Pfeffer MA, Claggett B, Assmann SF, et al. Regional variation in patients and outcomes in the Treatment of Preserved Cardiac Function Heart Failure With an Aldosterone Antagonist (TOPCAT) trial. *Circulation*. 2015;131(1):34–42.

83. Redfield MM, Chen HH, Borlaug BA, et al. Effect of phosphodiesterase-5 inhibition on exercise capacity and clinical status in heart failure with preserved ejection fraction: a randomized clinical trial. *JAMA*. 2013;309(12):1268–1277.

93. Fitchett D, Zinman B, Wanner C, et al. Heart failure outcomes with empagliflozin in patients with type 2 diabetes at high cardiovascular risk: results of the EMPA-REG OUTCOME(R) trial. *Eur Heart J*. 2016;37(19):1526–1534.

112. Feldman T, Mauri L, Kahwash R, et al. Transcatheter interatrial shunt device for the treatment of heart failure with Preserved Ejection Fraction (REDUCE LAP-HF I [Reduce Elevated Left Atrial Pressure in Patients With Heart Failure]): a Phase 2, Randomized, Sham-Controlled Trial. *Circulation*. 2018;137(4):364–375.

117. Adamson PB, Abraham WT, Bourge RC, et al. Wireless pulmonary artery pressure monitoring guides management to reduce decompensation in heart failure with preserved ejection fraction. *Circ Heart Fail*. 2014;7(6):935–944.

126. Kitzman DW, Brubaker P, Morgan T, et al. Effect of caloric restriction or aerobic exercise training on peak oxygen consumption and quality of life in obese older patients with heart failure with preserved ejection fraction: a randomized clinical trial. *JAMA*. 2016;315(1):36–46.

The full reference list for this chapter is available on ExpertConsult.

TABLE 39G.1 Guideline Recommendations for the Treatment of Patients with Heart Failure with a Preserved Ejection Fraction

Class of Recommendation	Level of Evidence	Recommendations
I	B	Systolic and diastolic blood pressure should be controlled in patients with HFpEF in accordance with published clinical practice guidelines to prevent morbidity.
I	C	Diuretics should be used for relief of symptoms due to volume overload in patients with HFpEF.
IIa	C	Coronary revascularization is reasonable in patients with CAD in whom symptoms (angina) or demonstrable myocardial ischemia is judged to be having an adverse effect on symptomatic HFpEF despite GDMT.
IIa	C	Management of AF according to published clinical practice guidelines in patients with HFpEF is reasonable to improve symptomatic HF.
IIa	C	The use of beta-blocking agents, ACE inhibitors, and ARBs in patients with hypertension is reasonable to control blood pressure in patients with HFpEF.
[a]IIb	B-R	In appropriately selected patients with HFpEF (with EF ≥45%, elevated BNP levels or HF admission within 1 year, estimated glomerular filtration rate >30 mL/min, creatinine <2.5 mg/dL, potassium <5.0 mEq/L), aldosterone receptor antagonists might be considered to decrease hospitalizations.
IIb	B	The use of ARBs might be considered to decrease hospitalizations for patients with HFpEF.
[a]III—No benefit	B-R	Routine use of nitrates or phosphodiesterase-5 inhibitors to increase activity or QoL in patients with HFpEF is ineffective.
III—No benefit	C	Routine use of nutritional supplements is not recommended for patients with HFpEF.
[a]I	B-R	In patients at increased risk, stage A HF, the optimal blood pressure in those with hypertension should be less than 130/80 mmHg
[a]I	C-LD	Patients with HFpEF and persistent hypertension after management of volume overload should be prescribed GDMT titrated to attain systolic blood pressure less than 130 mm Hg.
[a]IIa	C-LD	In patients with NYHA class II–IV HF and suspicion of sleep-disordered breathing or excessive daytime sleepiness, a formal sleep assessment is reasonable.
[a]IIb	B-R	In patients with cardiovascular disease and obstructive sleep apnea, CPAP may be reasonable to improve sleep quality and daytime sleepiness.

[a]New recommendations in the 2017 update of the 2013 ACC/AHA Guideline.[8]
Strength of recommendations: Class I: recommendation that treatment is useful or effective; Class IIa: recommendation in favor of treatment being useful or effective; Class IIb: greater conflicting evidence from multiple randomized trials or meta-analyses.
Level of evidence: A, data derived from multiple randomized clinical trials or meta-analyses; B, data derived from a single randomized clinical trial or nonrandomized studies; C, only consensus opinion of experts, case studies, or standard of care.
ACE, Angiotensin-converting enzyme; *AF*, atrial fibrillation; *ARB*, angiotensin receptor blockers; *BNP*, brain natriuretic peptide; *CAD*, coronary artery disease; *CPAP*, continuous positive airway pressure; *GDMT*, guideline-directed medical therapy; *HF*, heart failure; *HFpEF*, heart failure with a preserved ejection fraction; *NYHA*, New York Heart Association; *QoL*, quality of life.

REFERENCE

Yancy CW, Jessup M, Bozkurt B, et al. 2017 ACC/AHA/HFSA focused update of the 2013 ACCF/AHA guideline for the management of heart failure: a report of the American College of Cardiology/American Heart Association Task Force on Clinical Practice Guidelines and the Heart Failure Society of America. *J Cardiac Fail.* 2017;23(8):628–651.

40

Management of Heart Failure in Special Populations: Older Patients, Women, and Racial/Ethnic Minority Groups

Susan M. Joseph, Angela L. Brown, Michael W. Rich

While heart failure (HF) affects all segments of the population, older patients, women, and racial and ethnic minority groups have been markedly underrepresented in most major HF trials. This chapter provides a brief summary of the epidemiology, clinical features, and management of HF in these large and important subgroups of the HF population.

HEART FAILURE IN OLDER ADULTS

Epidemiology (see also Chapter 18)

HF is predominantly a disorder of older adults with prevalence and incidence rates that increase progressively with age. Of the nearly 6.5 million adults with HF in the United States, 50% are at least 75 years of age, and prevalence among those over the age of 80 years exceeds 13% in both men and women.[1] The disparity between sexes seen in younger adults is abolished at advanced age with a slightly higher prevalence in women than men.[1] The prevalence and incidence of HF are similar in older whites and African Americans.

In addition to age, risk factors for the development of HF in the older population include ischemic heart disease, systolic hypertension, widened pulse pressure, diabetes,[2] chronic lung disease, renal dysfunction, atrial fibrillation, left ventricular hypertrophy,[2] and obesity. Of these risk factors, systolic hypertension has the greatest population attributable risk, especially among women, for the development of HF. HF has a profound impact on the quality of life in older adults, and is an independent risk factor for cessation of driving[3] and loss of functional capacity as evidenced by a decline in activities of daily living (ADLs) and independent ADLs (IADLs).[4]

Incident HF in older adults is predominantly characterized by the phenotype of HF with normal or preserved ejection function (HFpEF) (**see also Chapter 39**). More than 50% of older patients with HF have HFpEF, and the proportion increases with age.[5,6] There is also a female preponderance in HFpEF. Women with HFpEF are more likely than men to be older and obese, and to have chronic kidney disease and hypertension, but less likely to have an ischemic cause, atrial

TABLE 40.1 **Heart Failure in Older Adults**

Characteristic	Older Adults	Middle Aged
Prevalence	~10%	<1%
Incidence (per 1000)	>10	2–3
Sex	Predominately Women	Predominately Men
Primary etiology	Hypertension	Coronary Artery Disease
Clinical features	Atypical	Typical
LV systolic function	Normal or Preserved	Impaired
Comorbidities	Multiple	Few

LV, Left ventricular.

TABLE 40.2 **Challenges to the Diagnosis of Heart Failure in Older Adults**

Atypical symptoms	Malaise, confusion, irritability, anorexia, sleep disturbance, decreased activity, abdominal complaints
Alternative explanations for symptoms and signs	Fluid retention: drugs (NSAIDs), chronic kidney disease Dyspnea: chronic lung disease, anemia, pneumonia, deconditioning Fatigue: anemia, hypothyroidism, obesity, deconditioning, depression, poor sleep quality Lower extremity edema: calcium channel blockers, venous insufficiency
Minimize symptoms or attribute to "normal" aging	"I just can't get around; I'm 87."
Fewer exertional symptoms	Sedentary lifestyle, osteoarthritis, sarcopenia, poor balance, poor vision

NSAIDs, Nonsteroidal antiinflammatory drugs.

fibrillation, or chronic obstructive pulmonary disease.[7] Thus, the profile of the typical older person with HF contrasts with that of middle-aged patients enrolled in HF trials (**Table 40.1**).

Prognosis

Older age is an independent predictor of reduced survival in patients with HF, as it is with any chronic illness. In addition, common age-associated comorbidities, such as anemia, chronic kidney disease, and cognitive impairment, contribute to increased mortality after adjusting for age, sex, and race.[8]

Despite major advances in HF therapy over the past two to three decades, overall mortality rates among patients with HFpEF have not declined (**see also Chapter 39**).[9] In the Framingham Heart Study, the annual mortality rate for HFpEF was 8.9%, which is approximately two-fold higher than age-matched controls, but only half that reported for HF with reduced ejection fraction (HFrEF) (19.6%). However, among patients hospitalized for HF, mortality is similar in HFpEF and HFrEF. Additionally, hospitalization for HFpEF is increasing relative to HFrEF.[10] Among Medicare beneficiaries, HF is associated with the highest 30-day readmission rate, with approximately one in five individuals being rehospitalized at 30 days.[11] Among older patients discharged with HF, a majority of 30-day readmissions are for conditions other than HF, suggesting that interventional strategies will need to be patient-centered rather than HF-specific.[12,13]

Data from community-dwelling older subjects with HF suggest that the cause of death differs between patients with HFpEF versus HFrEF. Among patients with HFpEF, noncardiovascular conditions are the leading cause of death (49%), whereas coronary heart disease accounts for the greatest proportion (43%) in patients with HFrEF.

Pathophysiology

The pathophysiology of HF differs in older compared with younger adults due to age-related alterations in left ventricular filling dynamics and declines in cardiovascular reserve. As a result, mild to moderate stressors that would be relatively well tolerated in younger patients can precipitate acute HF in older adults. Age-related changes in other organ systems can also impair the ability of older adults to compensate for HF and can alter the response to pharmacologic therapy. The superimposition of normal aging means that at equivalent levels of impairment in cardiac function the clinical severity of HF is more advanced in older patients (i.e., higher New York Heart Association [NYHA] functional class). In addition, multimorbidity and geriatric syndromes are the rule rather than the exception in older adults with HF, and recent evidence suggests that these coexisting conditions likely contribute to the pathophysiology of HFpEF.[14]

Diagnosis and Clinical Features

Older adults with HF have chronic exercise intolerance, reduced quality of life, frequent hospitalizations, and high health care costs.

Importantly, morbidity in older adults with HFrEF or HFpEF is similar, with comparable exercise intolerance and impairments in quality of life.[14]

The diagnosis of HF is challenging in older adults who are more likely to have other conditions that mimic the symptoms and signs of HF. A reliable history may be more difficult to obtain due to cognitive dysfunction or sensory impairment, making corroborating history from a family member or caregiver particularly helpful. Atypical presentations are more common in older adults, in whom HF may manifest as somnolence, confusion, disorientation, weakness, fatigue, gastrointestinal disturbances, or failure to thrive. Older adults may fail to perceive a gradual but progressive decline in exercise tolerance, and physicians often attribute this to advancing age or other conditions, thereby limiting early identification of HF. Care must be taken to exclude other potential causes for the signs and symptoms of HF (**Table 40.2**). Serial assessments of functional capacity using standard tests (e.g., 6-minute walk distance or gait speed)[15] and evaluation of ADLs and IADLs can be helpful adjuncts in quantifying and monitoring functional capacity. Both chest radiography and echocardiography have lower specificity for diagnosing HF in older patients, thus contributing to diagnostic uncertainty. Natriuretic peptide assays aid in diagnosing HF, assessing disease severity, and evaluating response to treatment. However, natriuretic peptide levels increase mildly with aging, are higher in women than in men, and are affected by renal function, anemia, and obesity; thus, the predictive accuracy of the assays is reduced in older patients.[16] These difficulties notwithstanding, the diagnosis of HFpEF should be based on symptoms and/or signs of HF in combination with a left ventricular ejection fraction (LVEF) ≥50%, exclusion of other primary causes of the symptom complex, and with or without evidence for diastolic dysfunction or elevated natriuretic peptides.[17]

Frailty and Cognitive Dysfunction

Frailty is a systemic syndrome characterized by impaired physiologic reserve, slowness, weakness, and wasting. It is associated with, but distinct from, aging, disability, and comorbid illness. Frailty and cognitive dysfunction are highly prevalent in older patients with HF, ranging from 25% to 80%, which is nearly double the prevalence in age-matched cohorts without HF.[18,19] Both entities independently predict mortality in patients with HF, and the magnitude of effect is similar to traditional measures such as ejection fraction or systolic blood pressure.[20] The relationship between HF and both frailty and cognitive dysfunction is bidirectional so that patients with HF are at significantly increased risk for frailty and dementia.[21] Due to the variable manifestations of these syndromes in patients with HF, particularly in the early stages, periodic screening for frailty and cognitive dysfunction is recommended.

Since HF is a chronic condition, and successful management is contingent on effective self-care[22] (i.e., adherence to a complex and ever-changing medical regimen, the need to follow dietary restrictions, monitoring of symptoms, engaging in exercise or physical therapy, and keeping follow-up appointments with multiple providers), impaired cognitive function can contribute to unfavorable outcomes, including recurrent hospitalizations and mortality.[23] Yet, despite the negative impact of cognitive dysfunction on outcomes, these deficits often go unrecognized.[24,25] Accordingly, implementing strategies to improve recognition of cognitive impairment (e.g., through routine screening) and tailoring treatment to individuals with cognitive dysfunction may enhance patient care and outcomes.[26]

Identification of cognitive impairment in older adults with HF should prompt interventions to maximize adherence to self-management programs and to minimize the hazards of complex medical regimens. As the risk for adverse drug effects increases exponentially with the number of drugs prescribed, all unnecessary (and perhaps even some indicated) medications should be discontinued.[27] Basic principles of transitional care dictate that early clinical follow-up is essential in this vulnerable group of patients. Clear written instructions and communication of medication changes to individuals assisting cognitively impaired older adults with HF is mandatory. If mobility limits an older adult's ability to attend an office visit, then an early postdischarge home health visit by trained allied health professionals should be scheduled to reduce unplanned readmissions or death.

Treatment

Goals of therapy in older HF patients include relief of symptoms, improvement in functional capacity and quality of life, reduction in hospital admissions, and improved survival. In older patients, preservation of independence and maintenance of a satisfactory quality of life may be more important than survival.[28] Optimal management requires a systematic approach comprising: (1) accurate diagnosis, (2) search for reversible or treatable etiologies, (3) judicious use of medications, (4) management of risk factors, (5) patient and caregiver education, (6) enhancement of self-management skills, (7) coordination of care across disciplines, and (8) close follow-up.

A recent meta-analysis demonstrated the efficacy of a multidisciplinary approach to HF care in reducing hospitalizations, improving quality of life, reducing total costs, and increasing survival (**see also Chapter 47**).[29] Many such studies included older patients who are ideal candidates for multidisciplinary care. One randomized trial involving patients aged 70 and older with either HFpEF or HFrEF demonstrated a 56% reduction in 90-day HF rehospitalizations.[30] Other important strategies in HF disease management include: (1) smoking cessation, (2) moderation in alcohol use, (3) administration of pneumococcal and influenza vaccinations, (4) control of polypharmacy and over-the-counter medications, (5) consideration of cardiac rehabilitation, and (6) palliative care and end-of-life planning. **Table 40.3** outlines potential members of a multidisciplinary team and their roles in promoting optimal patient care.

Biomarker Guided Therapy (see also Chapter 33)

Given the high prevalence of chronic HF in older adults coupled with the fact that HF is associated with the highest rate of 30-day readmissions of all chronic conditions,[12] there has been considerable interest in

TABLE 40.3	**Multidisciplinary Team for Older Adults With Heart Failure**
Potential Consultants	**Roles**
Geriatrician	Provides comprehensive evaluation and management strategy for all medical, social and psychological issues
Palliative care consultation	Provides evaluation and management strategy to address palliative care needs, including but not limited to pain, dyspnea, depression, and end-of-life issues
Nurse practitioner	Provides ongoing patient and family education, disease management
Medical subspecialists	Assist in managing comorbid conditions including renal insufficiency, arthritis, chronic lung disease, etc.
Psychiatrist	Evaluate for and treat comorbid psychiatric conditions including depression, delirium, and dementia
Pharmacist	Systematically evaluate for medication appropriateness, proper dosing, and drug-drug interactions
Physical therapist	Evaluate rehabilitation potential, and develop individualized physical therapy program, assess home safety
Occupational therapist	Evaluate home and determine safety of environment, provide alternative approaches to perform activities and enhance function
Nutritionist	Evaluate current dietary intake, modify diet to limit salt intake, manage calorie content, and develop appropriate diets for patients with comorbid conditions, including obesity, diabetes, and chronic renal disease
Social worker	Evaluate psychosocial situation, assist in family counseling, ensure optimal use of health care services, and engage in long-term care planning

the use of biomarkers to guide therapy. The TIME-CHF investigators demonstrated that HF therapy guided by N-terminal B-type natriuretic peptide (BNP) did not improve overall clinical outcomes or quality of life compared with symptom-guided treatment in a cohort of older adults.[31] A meta-analysis of 12 randomized studies demonstrated that the use of cardiac peptides to guide pharmacologic therapy significantly reduced mortality and HF hospitalizations in patients with chronic HF.[32] However, there was a strong interaction with age, such that outcomes were significantly improved by natriuretic peptide-guided therapy in younger patients ($\leq$75 years; OR 0.45, 95% CI 0.21–0.97, $P = .043$), but not in older patients (>75 years; OR 0.80, 95% CI 0.42–1.51, $P = .493$).[32] More recently, the GUIDE-IT trial failed to demonstrate a beneficial effect of N-terminal pro B-type natriuretic peptide (NT-proBNP)–guided therapy on cardiovascular mortality or time to first HF hospitalization relative to usual care, with similar findings in patients younger or older than age 75.[33]

Pharmacologic Interventions for HFrEF (see also Chapter 37)

While clinical trials have demonstrated the beneficial effects of ACE inhibitors in patients with HFrEF, older patients have been underrepresented and there have been no trials specifically evaluating outcomes in this age group. However, a meta-analysis of published trials with stratification by age (<55 years, 55–64 years, 65–74 years, ≥75 years) demonstrated no heterogeneity in treatment effects by age for the combined outcomes of death, or myocardial infarction (MI) and death, or readmission for HF, suggesting a consistent benefit across age groups, although the magnitude of benefit appeared to be less among those over the age of 75 years.[34] The use of ACE inhibitors in older patients may be complicated by preexisting renal dysfunction, renal artery stenosis, orthostatic hypotension, and increased susceptibility to side effects due to concomitant therapy; for example, drug interactions with nonsteroidal antiinflammatory drugs (NSAIDs) or other medications.

Angiotensin-receptor blockers (ARBs) are a reasonable alternative to ACE inhibitors in chronic HF but combination therapy with an ACE inhibitor and ARB is not recommended due to the increased risk for adverse events without clear benefit.

Several large randomized trials have shown that long-term beta-blockade is beneficial in patients with HFrEF. Patients up to age 80 have been included in these trials, and subgroup analyses indicate that beta-blockers are as effective in older as in younger adults. Older patients often have relative contraindications to beta-blockers, such as bradycardia, heart block, bronchospastic lung disease, or severe peripheral arterial disease. Nonetheless, indications for beta-blockers are similar in older and younger patients with HFrEF, although initiation and dose titration should be more cautious.

In the Randomized Aldactone Evaluation Study (RALES), subgroup analysis showed similar mortality benefits in patients ≥67 years of age (relative risk 0.68) compared to those less than 67 years of age (relative risk 0.74). Since significant hyperkalemia is more common in older adults prescribed spironolactone in usual care settings, close monitoring for side effects, including renal impairment and hyperkalemia, is warranted.

The Digitalis Investigation Group (DIG) study demonstrated similar effects of digoxin in younger and older patients, but toxicity was more common in older adults. The volume of distribution and renal clearance of digoxin decline with age, so that lower doses, e.g., 0.125 mg daily or less, are needed to achieve a therapeutic effect in older adults.

In the PARADIGM-HF trial, valsartan-sacubitril was associated with 20% reduction in the primary outcome of death from cardiovascular causes or hospitalization for HF (HR 0.80, 95% CI 0.73–0.87, $P < .001$) compared to enalapril among patients with NYHA class II-IV HF and an LVEF ≤40%.[35] All-cause mortality was also reduced by 16% (HR 0.84, 95% CI 0.76–0.93, $P < .001$). Among patients ≥75 years of age (N = 1563, 18.5% of trial population), results were similar to those in younger patients (**Fig. 40.1**).[35]

In the SHIFT study, patients with symptomatic HF, an LVEF ≤35%, and a resting heart rate ≥70/minute despite maximally tolerated beta-blockers were randomized to ivabradine or placebo and followed for a median of 22.9 months.[36] Ivabradine reduced the primary composite outcome of cardiovascular death or hospitalization for worsening HF by 18% (HR 0.82, 95% CI 0.75–0.90, $P < .0001$), with similar findings in patients older versus younger than age 65, although there was a slight trend to lower efficacy in older patients (P for interaction by age .099) (**Fig. 40.2**).[36]

Device Therapy for HFrEF

Although implantable cardioverter-defibrillators (ICDs) reduce mortality from sudden cardiac death in patients with HF and an LVEF ≤35% (**see Chapter 38**), few older patients were enrolled in the ICD trials, and a meta-analysis concluded that the benefit of ICDs in reducing mortality is lower in older compared to younger patients.[37] This age-associated decline in benefit is most likely attributable to the higher risks of death from both nonarrhythmic causes and "nonshockable"

rhythms (i.e., asystole and pulseless electrical activity) in older patients. In addition, major complications related to ICD implantation are twice as common in patients ≥80 years than in younger patients.[38] Although current guidelines do not advocate age-based criteria for ICD implantation, it is acknowledged that data are limited in older patients and a shared decision-making process is recommended when considering ICD therapy, especially in patients with competing comorbidities or frailty.[39] Patients should be advised about the potential benefits and risks of ICD implantation, including the possibility of an adverse effect on quality of life. Although many older patients elect to forego ICD implantation after an informed discussion, those who desire an ICD should not be denied a device solely on the basis of age. In these patients, it is appropriate to discuss circumstances under which the patient would want to have the device deactivated, especially at the end of life due to progressive HF or other terminal illness.[40]

Cardiac resynchronization therapy (CRT) improves symptoms, exercise tolerance, quality of life, and survival in selected patients with advanced HFrEF, persistent limiting symptoms despite conventional medical therapy, and dyssynchronous left ventricular contraction. Although few older patients have been enrolled in the CRT trials, observational studies indicate that the benefits of CRT are age-independent. Since a primary objective of CRT is to improve symptoms and quality of life, it is appropriate to offer CRT, with or without an ICD, to older patients who meet criteria for device implantation.

Implantable left ventricular assist devices (LVADs) reduce symptoms, increase exercise tolerance, and improve quality of life and survival in selected patients with advanced HFrEF, including adults in their 70s and 80s (**see also Chapter 45**). Originally developed as a "bridge" to heart transplantation, LVADs are now often implanted as "destination therapy" in patients who are not transplant candidates. As a result, an increasing number of older adults are receiving LVADs, and this trend is likely to accelerate as the safety and efficacy of these devices continue to improve. Older patients are at increased risk for LVAD-related complications, particularly gastrointestinal bleeding and stroke, and patients with advanced comorbidities or frailty may not be suitable candidates. Notably, however, a recent study demonstrated that frailty decreased in approximately half of older adults (mean age 70 years) after 6 months of LVAD therapy.[41] In addition, small studies of LVADs in highly selected septuagenarians and octogenarians have reported favorable effects on quality of life and survival,[42] so age alone should not be considered an absolute contraindication to LVAD implantation.

Pharmacologic Interventions for HFpEF

Pharmacological therapies for HFpEF have been reviewed in detail in **Chapter 39**. Although there have now been multiple trials testing diverse pharmacologic agents in predominantly older patients with HFpEF, none have been shown to reduce mortality, and the effects of these agents on other clinical outcomes, including hospitalizations, exercise tolerance, and quality of life, have been modest. Several additional trials are ongoing, including PARAGON-HF, which compares sacubitril-valsartan to valsartan alone in patients with HFpEF (NCT 01920711), and a series of studies evaluating sodium-glucose co-transporter-2 (SGLT-2) inhibitors in patients with HF, but at the present time there are no proven pharmacologic therapies for the treatment of HFpEF.

Nonpharmacologic Interventions for HFpEF

While pharmacologic interventions for HFpEF in older adults have been disappointing, nonpharmacologic approaches, including diet and exercise, are emerging as promising therapeutic targets. In one study, exercise training improved peak oxygen consumption in

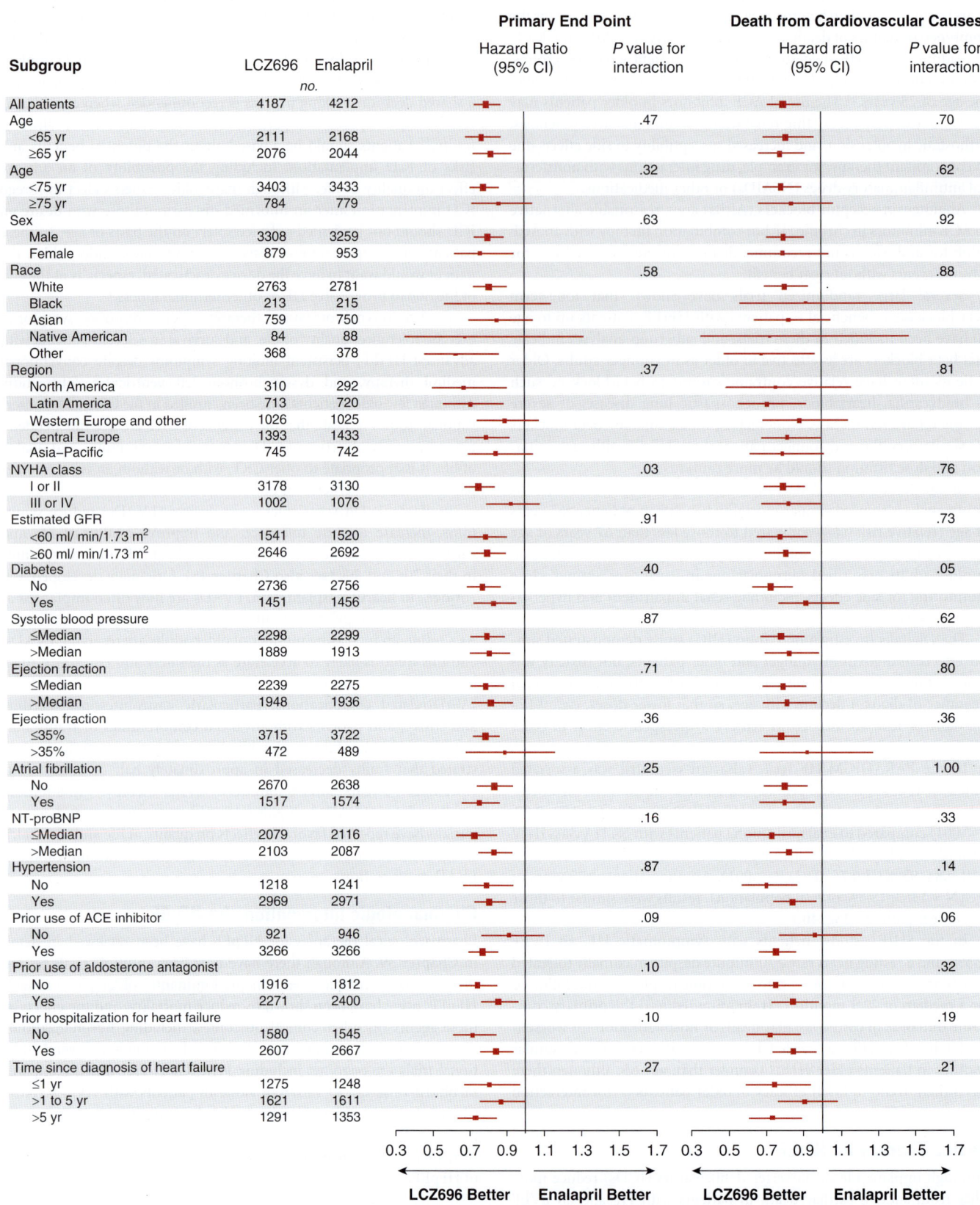

Fig. 40.1 Effect of sacubitril-valsartan on the primary composite endpoint and on death from cardiovascular causes in prespecified subgroups. *GFR*, Glomerular filtration rate; *NT-proBNP*, N-terminal pro B-type natriuretic peptide; *NYHA*, New York Heart Association. (From McMurray JJV, Packer M, Desai AS, et al. Angiotensin-neprilysin inhibition versus enalapril in heart failure. *N Engl J Med.* 2014;371[11]:993–1004.)

patients with HFpEF, an effect mediated primarily by an increase in peak arterial–venous oxygen difference.[43] This suggests that peripheral mechanisms (i.e., improved microvascular and/or skeletal muscle function) contribute to improved exercise capacity after exercise training in HFpEF. Dietary interventions have been understudied in older adults, especially those with HFpEF. In animal models, salt sensitivity is associated with a low renin state accompanied by renal dysfunction, hypertension, and obesity. In a small study in patients with HFpEF, the DASH/sodium restriction diet reduced systolic blood pressure, arterial stiffness, and oxidative stress, and improved diastolic function, ventricular-arterial coupling, and submaximal exercise tolerance.[44,45] More recently, a 20-week intervention combining calorie restriction and exercise training was found to be more effective than either intervention alone in improving peak oxygen consumption in obese older adults with HFpEF, although there was no significant effect on patient-reported quality of life.[46]

HEART FAILURE IN WOMEN

Epidemiology (see also Chapter 18)

More than 40% of patients with HF are women, and among older adults the prevalence of HF is greater in women than in men.[1] Women with HF are twice as likely to have HFpEF compared to men, and women with HFrEF tend to have a higher LVEF than men. In the Atherosclerosis Risk in Communities Study, white women had the lowest age-adjusted rate of developing HF at 3.4 per 1000 person-years, as compared with white men (6.0), black women (8.1), and black men (9.1).[47] In Olmstead County, Minnesota, the incidence of HF increased 8% in women and 3% in men from 1979 to 2000,[48] while the Framingham investigators reported an increase in HF incidence for both women and men from 1980 to 1999.[49] During both time periods, age-adjusted 5-year mortality rates declined for both sexes. Although age-adjusted HF incidence is higher in men than in women, men also have shorter survival. However, the female survival advantage is limited to patients with nonischemic HF.

Clinical Features

In the Studies of Left Ventricular Dysfunction (SOLVD) database, women with chronic HF and impaired LV systolic function were more likely than men to have dependent edema, jugular venous distension, and an S_3 gallop. However, women (n = 54,674) in the ADHERE registry for acute decompensated HF (impaired and preserved systolic function) did not differ from men (n = 50,713) with respect to the frequency of HF symptoms and signs.[50]

Comorbidities differ between men and women. Compared to men, women with HF are more likely to have hypertension, whereas men are more likely to have coronary artery disease (CAD) and a history of smoking. In the A-HeFT trial, African-American women had lower hemoglobin and more diabetes but less renal insufficiency than men.[51] Thyroid disease is more frequent in women with acute decompensated HF, while chronic obstructive lung disease, peripheral arterial disease, and renal insufficiency are more common in men.[50] Pregnancy-related cardiomyopathy, a condition unique to women, is discussed in **Chapter 20**.

BNP and NT-proBNP tend to be modestly higher in women than men, but data regarding sex differences in other HF biomarkers are scarce. One study demonstrated that levels of biomarkers related to inflammation, including C-reactive protein and interleukin-6, were

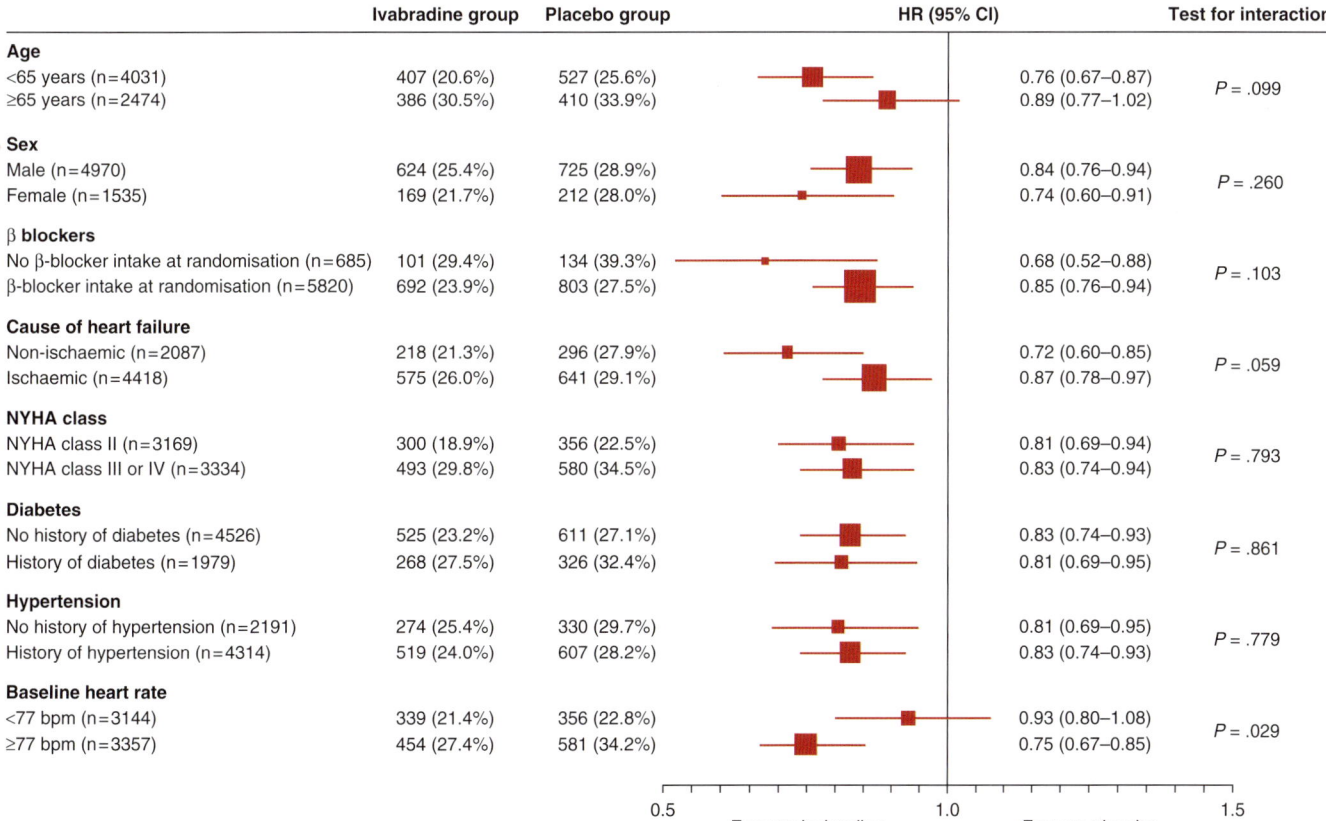

	Ivabradine group	Placebo group	HR (95% CI)	Test for interaction
Age				
<65 years (n=4031)	407 (20.6%)	527 (25.6%)	0.76 (0.67–0.87)	P = .099
≥65 years (n=2474)	386 (30.5%)	410 (33.9%)	0.89 (0.77–1.02)	
Sex				
Male (n=4970)	624 (25.4%)	725 (28.9%)	0.84 (0.76–0.94)	P = .260
Female (n=1535)	169 (21.7%)	212 (28.0%)	0.74 (0.60–0.91)	
β blockers				
No β-blocker intake at randomisation (n=685)	101 (29.4%)	134 (39.3%)	0.68 (0.52–0.88)	P = .103
β-blocker intake at randomisation (n=5820)	692 (23.9%)	803 (27.5%)	0.85 (0.76–0.94)	
Cause of heart failure				
Non-ischaemic (n=2087)	218 (21.3%)	296 (27.9%)	0.72 (0.60–0.85)	P = .059
Ischaemic (n=4418)	575 (26.0%)	641 (29.1%)	0.87 (0.78–0.97)	
NYHA class				
NYHA class II (n=3169)	300 (18.9%)	356 (22.5%)	0.81 (0.69–0.94)	P = .793
NYHA class III or IV (n=3334)	493 (29.8%)	580 (34.5%)	0.83 (0.74–0.94)	
Diabetes				
No history of diabetes (n=4526)	525 (23.2%)	611 (27.1%)	0.83 (0.74–0.93)	P = .861
History of diabetes (n=1979)	268 (27.5%)	326 (32.4%)	0.81 (0.69–0.95)	
Hypertension				
No history of hypertension (n=2191)	274 (25.4%)	330 (29.7%)	0.81 (0.69–0.95)	P = .779
History of hypertension (n=4314)	519 (24.0%)	607 (28.2%)	0.83 (0.74–0.93)	
Baseline heart rate				
<77 bpm (n=3144)	339 (21.4%)	356 (22.8%)	0.93 (0.80–1.08)	P = .029
≥77 bpm (n=3357)	454 (27.4%)	581 (34.2%)	0.75 (0.67–0.85)	

0.5   1.0   1.5
Favours ivabradine   Favours placebo

Fig. 40.2 Effect of ivabradine on cardiovascular death or worsening heart failure in prespecified subgroups. *NYHA*, New York Heart Association. (From Swedberg K, Kamajda M, Bohm M, et al. Ivabradine and outcomes in chronic heart failure (SHIFT): a randomised placebo-controlled study. *Lancet.* 2010;376[9744]:875–885.)[36]

significantly lower in women than in men.[52] In this study, mortality was also lower in women compared to men, independent of differences in clinical characteristics.

Women with HF tend to have lower quality of life than men with greater impairment in functional capacity,[53] more HF hospitalizations,[50,53] and more depression.[54] While women are more likely than men to have HFpEF, long-term mortality rates are similar for patients with HFpEF or HFrEF.

Ischemic Heart Failure in Women

Women develop ischemic heart disease at an older age than men. Although CAD is a less common cause of HF in women than in men, the presence of CAD is a more potent risk factor for HF than hypertension in both sexes. Diabetes mellitus is common in both men and women with HF,[50] and it is a strong risk factor for the development of HF in women with CAD.

Therapy in Women

Although women have been included in clinical trials in greater numbers than minorities, they have still been significantly underrepresented. Nonetheless, evidence-based treatment guidelines for HF therapy provide similar recommendations for men and women.[39] Accordingly, most studies have shown that women hospitalized with HF receive HF medications at similar rates as men,[55,56] but women may be less likely to reach target doses of medications. Notably, the Get with the Guidelines HF Registry demonstrated that women and men were treated equally with respect to most guideline-recommended HF therapies, and that the use of ACE inhibitors and beta-blockers approached 90% in both sexes.[57]

Angiotensin Converting Enzyme Inhibitors

A meta-analysis of 30 ACE-inhibitor studies that included a total of 1587 women with HF demonstrated trends toward improved survival (13.4% vs. 20.1%) and in the combined endpoint of survival and hospitalization (20.2% vs. 29.5%) among women randomized to ACE-inhibitors (**Table 40.4** and **Fig. 40.3**).[58,59]

Angiotensin Receptor Blockers

Sex-specific data for ARBs are limited. Pooled data from the CHARM-Alternative and the CHARM-Added trials that included 1188 women with NYHA functional class II-IV HF and LVEF ≤40% showed that candesartan reduced the combined endpoint of cardiovascular death or HF hospitalization in women. In the CHARM-Overall population, reduction in the combined endpoint was similar for men and women (**Fig. 40.4**).[60]

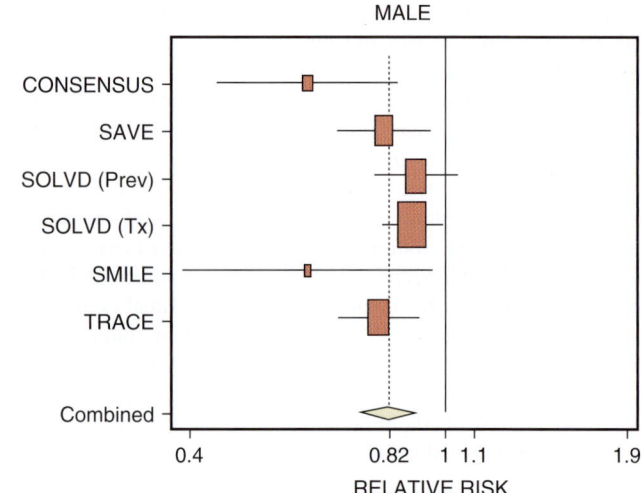
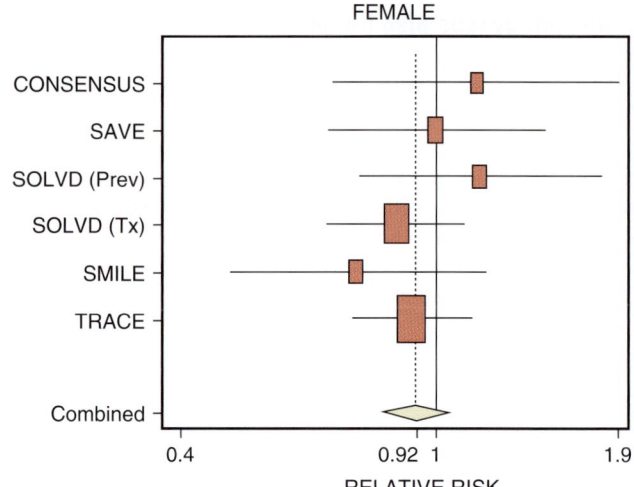

Fig. 40.3 Effect of angiotensin-converting enzyme inhibitors in the management of left ventricular systolic dysfunction according to race, gender, and diabetic status. *SOLVD*, Studies of Left Ventricular Dysfunction. (Reproduced with permission from Shekelle PG, Rich MW, Morton SC, et al. Efficacy of angiotensin-converting enzyme inhibitors and beta-blockers in the management of left ventricular systolic dysfunction according to race, gender, and diabetic status: a meta-analysis of major clinical trials. *J Am Coll Cardiol.* 2003;41[9]:1529–1538.)

TABLE 40.4	Effect of Angiotensin-Converting Enzyme Inhibitors on Mortality by Sex			
Study Name	**Male N**	**Female N**	**RR Male (95% CI)**	**RR Female (95% CI)**
CONSENSUS	179	74	0.61 (0.44–0.85)	1.14 (0.68–1.90)
SAVE	1841	390	0.80 (0.68–0.95)	0.99 (0.67–1.47)
SMILE	1128	428	0.61 (0.39–0.96)	0.74 (0.47–1.18)
SOLVD-Prevention	3752	476	0.90 (0.77–1.05)	1.15 (0.74–1.78)
SOLVD-Treatment	2065	504	0.89 (0.80–0.99)	0.86 (0.67–1.09)
TRACE	1248	501	0.79 (0.68–0.91)	0.90 (0.74–1.11)
Random effects pooled estimate	*10,213*	*2373*	*0.82 (0.74–0.90)*	*0.92 (0.81–1.04)*

CI, Confidence interval; *RR,* relative risk.
From Shekelle PG, Rich MW, Morton SC, et al. Efficacy of angiotensin-converting enzyme inhibitors and beta-blockers in the management of left ventricular systolic dysfunction according to race, gender, and diabetic status. *J Am Coll Cardiol.* 2003;41(9):1529–1538.

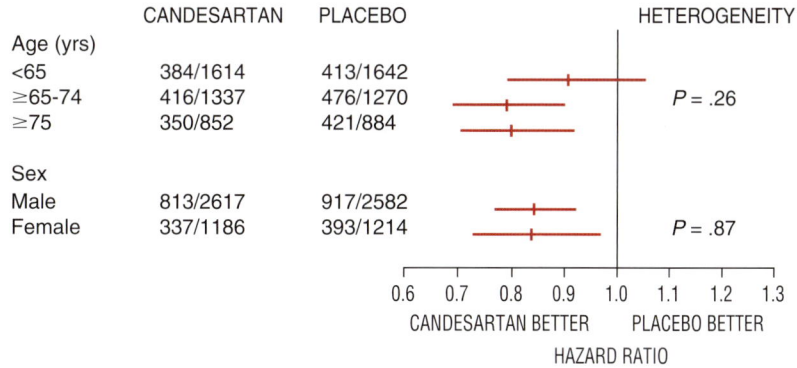

Fig. 40.4 Effects of candesartan on cardiovascular death or heart failure hospitalizations in the CHARM study. (Reproduced with permission from Pfeffer MA, Swedberg K, Granger CB, et al. Effects of candesartan on mortality and morbidity in patients with chronic heart failure: the CHARM-Overall programme. *Lancet.* 2003;362[9386:759–766.)[60]

Beta-Blockers

As with ACE-Is and ARBs, meta-analyses of beta-blocker trials suggest that these agents are equally beneficial in women and men with HFrEF (**Table 40.5**).[59]

Aldosterone Antagonists

Subgroup analysis of the RALES trial with spironolactone and the EPHESUS trial with eplerenone revealed similar mortality benefits for men and women with systolic HF.

Hydralazine/Isosorbide Dinitrate

The early Veterans Administration HF trials using the combination of hydralazine/isosorbide dinitrate were limited to men. In the A-HeFT study, combination hydralazine/isosorbide dinitrate was added to ACE inhibitor/ARB and beta-blocker therapy in 1050 self-identified African Americans with NYHA functional class III-IV HF (420 women). Survival benefits were noted for both women (HR 0.33, 95% CI 0.16–0.71, P = .003) and men (HR 0.79, 95% CI 0.46–1.35, P = .385) with no significant treatment interaction by sex.[51]

Digoxin

In a post-hoc subgroup analysis of the DIG trial, women with HF and impaired systolic function (LVEF <45%) were reported to have increased mortality when treated with digoxin compared to placebo (adjusted HR 1.23, 95% CI 1.02–1.47), whereas in men digoxin had no effect on mortality (adjusted HR 0.93, 95% CI 0.85–1.02). However, subsequent analysis of the DIG trial data showed that digoxin at serum concentrations of 0.5 to 0.9 ng/mL was safe and effective for both women and men.[61]

Valsartan–Sacubitril and Ivabradine

Subgroup analyses of the PARADIGM-HF and SHIFT trials of val-sartan–sacubitril and ivabradine, respectively, found no treatment interaction by sex (**see Fig. 40.1** and **Fig. 40.2**).[35,36] Notably, however, women comprised only 21.8% of the PARADIGM-HF trial population and 23.6% of the SHIFT population.

Cardiac Resynchronization Therapy

Although few studies have reported sex-specific data, there is some evidence that women may derive greater benefit from CRT compared to men. In the MADIT-CRT trial, which randomized 1367 men and 453 women with an LVEF ≤30% and NYHA class II HF to CRT plus ICD versus ICD alone, CRT was associated with better outcomes and greater degree of reverse remodeling in women compared to men.[62]

TABLE 40.5 Effect of Beta-Blockers on Mortality by Sex

Study Name	Male N	Female N	RR Male (95% CI)	RR Female (95% CI)
CIBIS-II	2132	515	0.71 (0.58–0.87)	0.52 (0.30–0.89)
COOPERNICUS	1822	465	0.68 (0.54–0.86)	0.63 (0.39–1.04)
MERIT-HF	3093	898	0.63 (0.50–0.78)	0.93 (0.58–1.49)
US Carvedilol HF	838	256	0.44 (0.24–0.82)	0.32 (0.11–0.93)
Random effects pooled estimate	*7885*	*2134*	*0.66 (0.59–0.75)*	*0.63 (0.44–0.91)*

CI, Confidence interval; *RR*, relative risk.
From Shekelle PG, Rich MW, Morton SC, et al. Efficacy of angiotensin-converting enzyme inhibitors and beta-blockers in the management of left ventricular systolic dysfunction according to race, gender, and diabetic status. *J Am Coll Cardiol.* 2003;41(9):1529–1538.

In the Comparison of Medical Therapy, Pacing, and Defibrillation in Heart Failure (COMPANION) study, which included 299 women, women receiving CRT had a significant reduction in the combined endpoint of all-cause mortality or hospitalization for any cause compared to women randomized to medical therapy, and there was no interaction by sex.[63]

Implantable Cardioverter Defibrillator

Guideline recommendations for ICD implantation to prevent sudden death are based on many multicenter studies, but women have been underrepresented and few studies have provided adequate sex-specific data. The limited analyses available for women do not clearly demonstrate a mortality benefit. In the Sudden Cardiac Death in HF Trial (SCD-HeFT) trial, which included 382 women with NYHA class II–III HF and LVEF ≤35% (ischemic and nonischemic cardiomyopathy), ICD therapy did not reduce mortality in women (HR 0.96, 95% CI 0.58–1.61); however, the trial was not powered to detect sex differences. In the MADIT-II study, which included 119 women with ischemic cardiomyopathy and LVEF ≤30%, there was a nonsignificant trend toward lower mortality in women receiving an ICD (adjusted

STUDY NAME	HAZARD RATIO	(95% CI)	NO. OF WOMEN	*P* VALUE
MUSTT	1.64	(0.92–2.92)	68	.09
MADIT II	0.57	(0.28–1.18)	192	.12
DINAMIT	1.00	(0.49–2.04)	160	>.99
DEFINITE	1.14	(0.50–2.64)	132	.76
SCD-HeFT	0.90	(0.56–1.43)	382	.66
Combined	**1.01**	**(0.76–1.33)**	**934**	**.95**

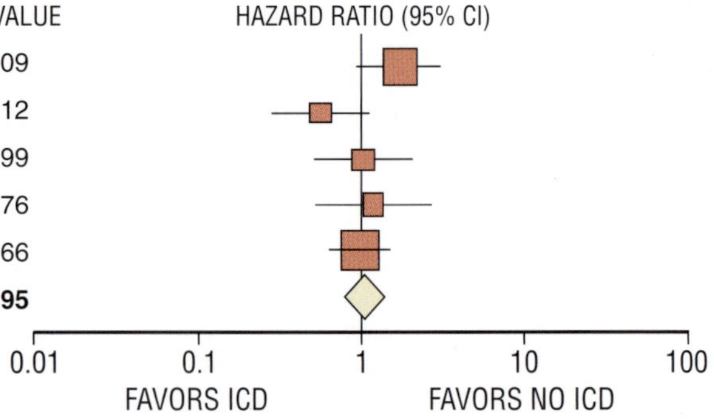

HAZARD RATIO (95% CI)

0.01   0.1   1   10   100
FAVORS ICD   FAVORS NO ICD

Fig. 40.5 Mortality among women with systolic dysfunction randomized to implantable cardioverter-defibrillator *(ICD)* implantation versus medical therapy for the primary prevention of sudden cardiac death. Error bars indicate 95% confidence intervals *(CIs)*. Diamonds designate overall effect and squares, the effect for each individual study; both represent the width of the confidence interval. *DEFINITE*, Defibrillators in Non-Ischemic Cardiomyopathy Treatment Evaluation; *DINAMIT*, Defibrillator In Acute Myocardial Infarction Trial; *MADIT*, Multicenter Automatic Defibrillator Implantation Trial; *MUSTT*, Multicenter Unsustained Tachycardia Trial; *SCD-HeFT*, Sudden Cardiac Death in Heart Failure Trial. (From Ghanbari H, Dalloul G, Hasan R, et al. Effectiveness of implantable cardioverter-defibrillators for the primary prevention of sudden cardiac death in women with advanced heart failure: a meta-analysis of randomized controlled trials. *Arch Intern Med.* 2009;169[16]:1500–1506.)

HR 0.57, *P* = .132), suggesting that women with ischemic cardiomyopathy may benefit. A meta-analysis of ICD therapy in women found no overall benefit (**Fig. 40.5**).[64] Due to the low inclusion of women in clinical trials and the lower utilization of ICDs in women, current data are insufficient to support differential use of ICDs by sex.

Left Ventricular Assist Devices (see also Chapter 45)

Implantable LVADs are being used more frequently for the treatment of end-stage refractory HF. Although there are no sex differences in the surgical techniques for implanting LVADs, small individuals with body surface area (BSA) less than 1.5 m² have historically had limited LVAD options because the devices require a minimum body size in order to fit properly. However, current devices fit in most individuals with BSA >1.3 m². FDA-approved continuous-flow devices, including the HeartMate II, the HeartWare HVAD, and the more recent HeartMate 3 (for short-term use) are smaller, making implantation feasible in most adults, and in many children and adolescents. Nonetheless, women continue to be underenrolled in LVAD clinical trials. Women have similar survival rates compared to men with LVAD therapy.[65,66] However, women tend to have a higher incidence of both bleeding and stroke than men after LVAD placement.[65,67,68]

Heart Transplantation (see also Chapter 44)

Based on data from the International Society of Heart and Lung Transplantation registry, women received 23.7% of the 17,868 heart transplants performed from 2006 to June 2011, representing significant increases from 22.3% and 19.3% in the prior 5- and 10-year periods.[69] Overall survival rates are now similar in both women and men, although female recipients of a male donor heart may be at higher risk of 1-year mortality than male recipients from a male donor.[69] Reasons for lower rates of transplantation in women are not clear, but may be partially explained by higher levels of reactive antibodies in parous women, making it more challenging to find a suitable donor. Women also tend to be older, possibly decreasing their candidacy for transplantation.

HEART FAILURE IN RACIAL/ETHNIC MINORITY GROUPS

Despite advances in therapy, racial and ethnic disparities persist in HF prevalence and outcomes. The complex interaction of genetics, social factors, environment, and lifestyle may affect pathophysiologic and therapeutic observations seen in these racial and ethnic populations, which exhibit considerable heterogeneity.[70] Because these groups are underrepresented in clinical trials, specific recommendations are derived from extrapolated data or post hoc analyses that lack statistical power and methodological rigor.[71]

Prevalence

As discussed in **Chapter 18**, the prevalence of HF varies by sex and race/ethnicity.[1] African Americans have a disproportionately high prevalence of HF compared with the general population and other racial groups. The prevalence for Hispanics is less than that of non-Hispanic whites and blacks, but greater than non-Hispanic Asian men and women.[1] The prevalence of HF in minority populations is projected to increase substantially by the year 2030, reflecting demographic shifts in the US population (**Fig. 40.6**).[72]

In the Multi-Ethnic Study of Atherosclerosis, which included 6814 participants (38.5% white, 27.8% African American, 21.9% Hispanic, and 11.2% Chinese American), the 5-year risk for HF by race/ethnicity was highest in African Americans, followed by Hispanics, non-Hispanic whites, and Chinese Americans (**Fig. 40.7**).[73]

Clinical Features

HF in African Americans occurs at an earlier age and is more frequently associated with hypertension and diabetes than with ischemic heart disease.[74] Hispanics with HF are younger than other racial groups and have higher rates of diabetes and renal disease.[75] Rates of ischemic cardiomyopathy are intermediate between non-Hispanic white and African-American populations.

HF data for Asian populations are limited. A review of Asian populations residing in Canada found that South Asian patients with HF tend to be younger and are more likely to have diabetes and lower body mass index.[76] In the Strong Heart Study, an observational study of American Indians with high prevalence of diabetes, obesity, and metabolic syndrome, the incidence of HF was 6.4 per 1000 person-years during 11 years of follow-up. Higher levels of C-reactive protein and fibrinogen were associated with increased risk.[77]

Observed racial differences in morbidity from HF may be related to differences in comorbid conditions (e.g., hypertension, diabetes, renal disease), effectiveness of treatment, socioeconomic factors

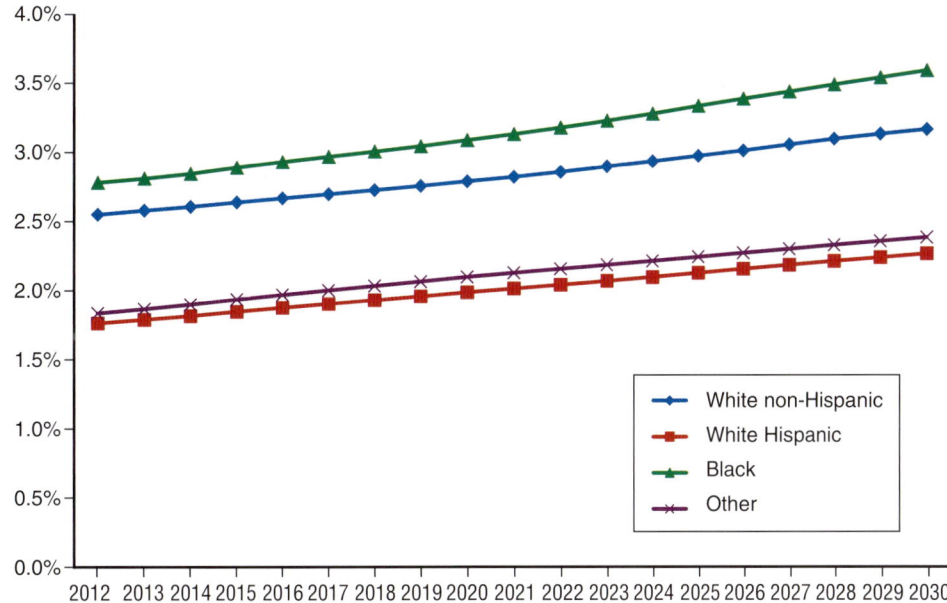

Fig. 40.6 Projected US prevalence of heart failure from 2012 to 2030 for different races. (From Heidenreich PA, Albert NM, Allen LA, et al. Forecasting the impact of heart failure in the United States: a policy statement from the American Heart Association. *Circ Heart Fail*. 2013;6[3]:606–619.)

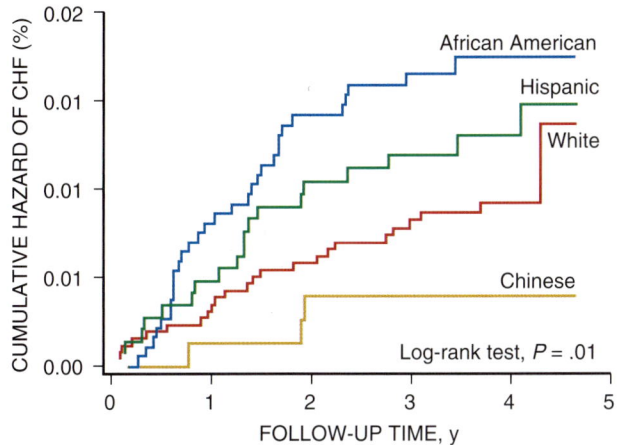

Fig. 40.7 Cumulative hazards ratio for the development of heart failure by racial/ethnic group in the MESA (Multi-Ethnic Study of Atherosclerosis) study. *CHF*, Congestive heart failure. (Reproduced with permission Bahrami H, Kronmal R, Bluemke DA, et al. Difference in the incidence of congestive heart failure by ethnicity: the multi-ethnic study of atherosclerosis. *Arch Intern Med*. 2008;168[19]:2138–2145.)

(access to insurance and specialty care), lifestyle, and health-care–seeking behaviors (time between symptom onset and presentation for care). Data from Medicare enrollees showed that compared with white Americans, HF hospitalization was 50% more likely for African Americans and 20% more likely for Hispanics, but 50% less likely for Asian patients.[78] African Americans and Hispanics with HF have higher hospitalization and readmission rates compared with whites (**Fig. 40.8**).[78] Length of stay is highest among non-Hispanic whites, intermediate among Hispanics, and shortest in African Americans.[78]

Mortality data for African Americans with HF are conflicting,[79] due in part to differences in study period, methodology (registries, observational databases, administrative databases, or randomized clinical trials), pathophysiology (HFpEF vs. HFrEF), and patient age.

However, death certificate data for any-mention HF show higher rates in African-American men and women.[1]

Data from a meta-analysis of studies reporting mortality by race after hospitalization for HF showed that mortality in African Americans was 32% lower during short-term follow-up and 16% lower during long-term follow-up compared with white patients.[80] Hispanics have also been reported to have lower in-hospital and short-term mortality compared with whites.[75] Mechanisms for differences in outcomes by race/ethnicity are poorly understood and more data are needed.

Pathophysiology

Evolving data suggest that African Americans may have altered nitric oxide–dependent vascular function and less responsiveness to renin-angiotensin system inhibition.[81] African Americans have lower norepinephrine levels, a trend toward lower plasma renin activity, and reduced nitric oxide availability compared with other racial groups.[82,83] This imbalance may contribute to adverse ventricular remodeling (**see Chapters 5 and 6**). There is also evidence that NT-proBNP levels are significantly lower in African Americans than in whites, which may affect the reliability of specific NT-proBNP thresholds for diagnosing HF in African Americans.[84] However, the relationship between natriuretic peptide levels and mortality is similar in African Americans and whites.[84]

Certain genetic markers have been shown to exist in linkage disequilibrium in African American populations (**see also Chapter 24**). African Americans who are homozygous for polymorphisms in gene encoding for both β_1-adrenergic receptors and α_2-adrenergic receptors are at 10-fold greater risk for HF.[85] Overexpression of transforming growth factor β_1 may imply worse prognosis,[86,87] and overexpression of other polymorphisms (e.g., endothelial nitric oxide synthase [eNOS], aldosterone synthase, and the G protein 825-T allele) may influence HF risk. Although the study of gene variants represents an expanding area for research, caution must be employed when considering race as a surrogate for disease expression or response to therapy.

Although HFpEF is more prevalent in African Americans, data on prognosis are limited. In a middle-aged African-American cohort of

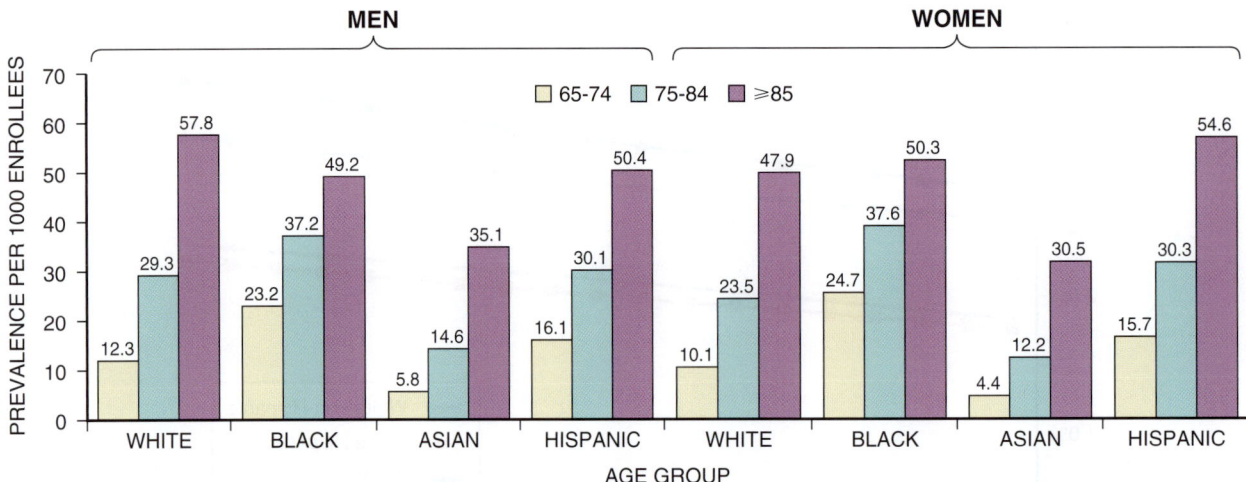

Fig. 40.8 Age-specific prevalence of hospitalization with a first-listed diagnosis of heart failure among Medicare enrollees aged ≥ 65 years by sex and race/ethnicity. (Modified from Brown DW, Haldeman GA, Croft JB, Giles WH, Mensah GA. Racial or ethnic differences in hospitalization for heart failure among elderly adults: Medicare, 1990 to 2000. *Am Heart J.* 2005;150[3]:448–454.)

the Atherosclerosis Risk in Communities study, HFpEF was the most common form of HF and was associated with better prognosis compared with HFrEF.[88]

Racial Differences in Response to Drug Treatment

Few clinical trials in HF prespecified subgroup analysis by race/ethnicity or included sufficient numbers of subjects for meaningful statistical analysis. Retrospective analyses suggest differences between African-American and white populations in response to HF pharmacotherapy, but few data exist for Hispanics and Asians. Despite this, evidence-based guidelines do not differ in recommendations based on race/ethnicity except for use of the hydralazine/isosorbide dinitrate combination in African Americans.[39]

ACE Inhibitors

Pooled data from the SOLVD prevention and treatment trials found that enalapril therapy was associated with similar reductions in mortality in African-American and white patients, although overall mortality and mortality due to pump failure, stroke, and pulmonary embolism were all higher in African Americans.[89,90] Enalapril was also associated with a significant reduction in the risk of hospitalization for HF among white patients but not among African-American patients. African Americans assigned to receive enalapril experienced a 44% greater risk of HF hospitalization (7.9 more admissions per 100 person-years of follow-up) compared with white patients assigned to enalapril.[90] In whites treated with enalapril, significant reductions in both systolic (5 ± 17.1 mm Hg) and diastolic blood pressure (3.6 ± 10.6 mm Hg) were observed, whereas no reduction in blood pressure was seen in African Americans. In a post hoc analysis of the SOLVD prevention study, enalapril delayed the progression from asymptomatic LV dysfunction to symptomatic HF in both African-American and white subjects.[91] However, despite the comparable relative reduction in risk for the development of symptomatic HF, differences in baseline risk were such that African Americans randomized to enalapril were at higher risk than whites randomized to placebo for progression to clinical HF. Furthermore, this difference persisted after adjusting for potential confounders, including LVEF, NYHA class, serum sodium, and cause of LV dysfunction (**Fig. 40.9**).[91]

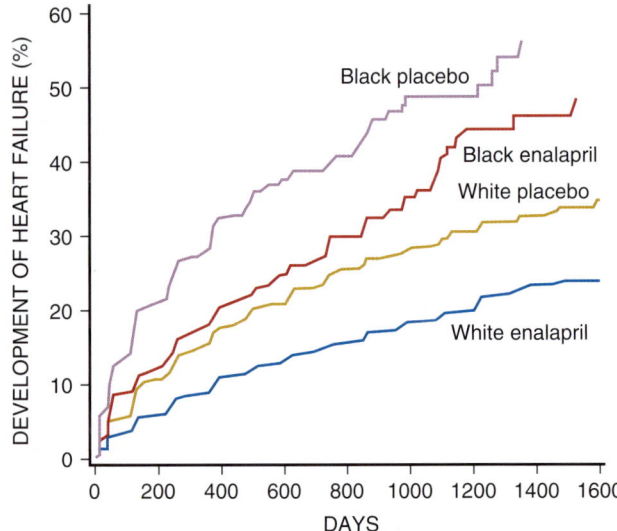

Fig. 40.9 Effect of angiotensin-converting enzyme inhibition on the prevention of development of symptomatic heart failure in black and white patients with asymptomatic left ventricular dysfunction. (Adapted from Dries D, Strong M, Cooper R, Drazner MH. Efficacy of angiotensin-converting enzyme inhibition in reducing progression from asymptomatic left ventricular dysfunction to symptomatic heart failure in black and white patients. *J Am Coll Cardiol.* 2002;40[2]:311–317.)

β-Blockers

Although β-blockers are of proven benefit in HFrEF, enrollment of African Americans in clinical trials has been limited. Post hoc analyses show trends toward beneficial effects in African Americans for carvedilol and metoprolol, but hazard ratios failed to reach statistical significance due to low sample size.[92]

In the Beta-blocker Evaluation of Survival Trial (BEST), the only trial prospectively stratified by African-American or white race, bucindolol significantly reduced the risk of death or hospitalization among white patients, but was associated with a nonsignificant increase in the risk of serious clinical events in African Americans (**Fig. 40.10**).[93]

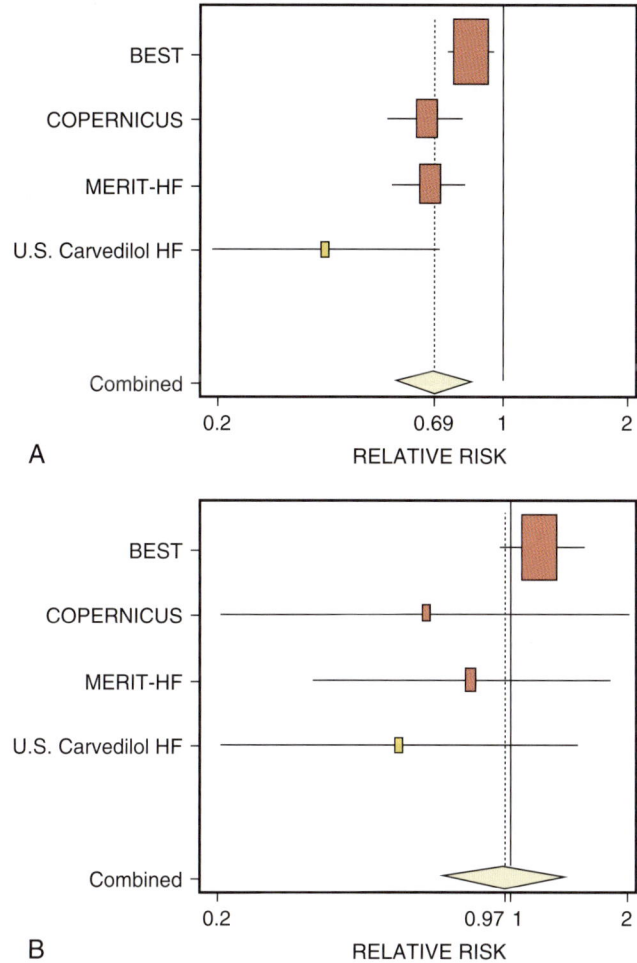

Fig. 40.10 Effect of β-Blocking Agents in Black and White Patients. (A) Effects of β-blocking agents in white patients. (B) Effects of β-blocking agents in black patients. (Adapted from Shekelle PG, Rich MW, Morton SC, et al. Efficacy of angiotensin-converting enzyme inhibitors and beta-blockers in the management of left ventricular systolic dysfunction according to race, gender, and diabetic status: a meta-analysis of major clinical trials. *J Am Coll Cardiol.* 2003;41[9]:1529–1538.)

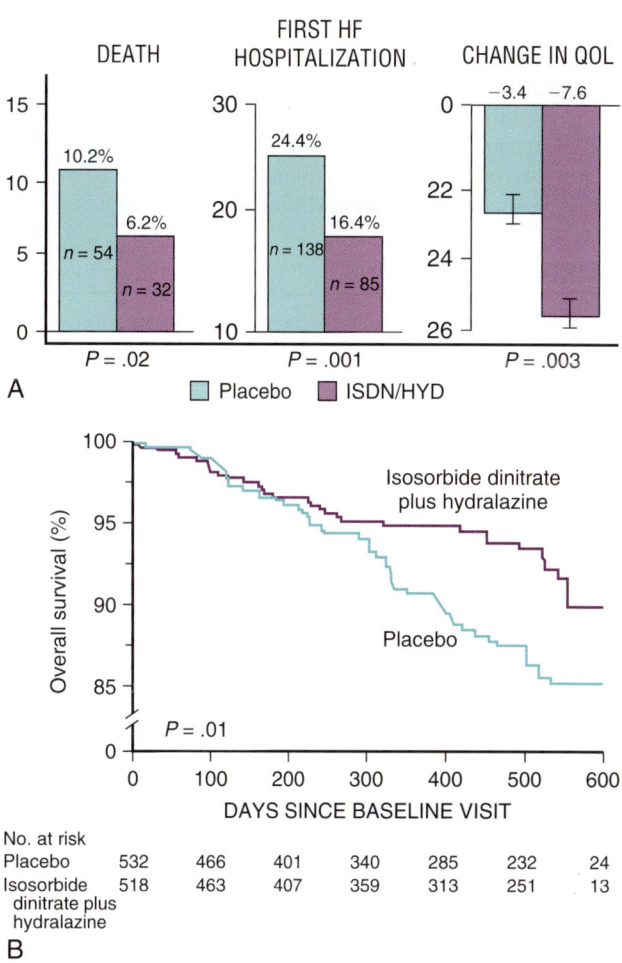

Fig. 40.11 Clinical Outcomes in the African-American HF Trial (A-HeFT). (A) Components of composite score in A-HeFT. (B) Effect of fixed dose hydralazine isosorbide on mortality in A-HeFT. *HF,* Heart failure; *HYD,* hydralazine; *ISDN,* isosorbide dinitrate; *QOL,* quality of life. (Modified from Taylor AL, Ziesche S, Yancy C, et al. Combination of isosorbide dinitrate and hydralazine in blacks with heart failure. *N Engl J Med.* 2004;351[20]:2049–2057.)

Hydralazine/Isosorbide Dinitrate

Retrospective analyses of the Vasodilator HF Trials (V-HeFT I and II), which included 28% to 30% African Americans, suggested racial differences in response to treatment.[82] In V-HeFT I, which compared the combination of hydralazine/isosorbide dinitrate to prazosin or placebo, a mortality benefit was observed in African American but not in white patients treated with hydralazine and isosorbide dinitrate. In the V-HeFT II trial, which compared enalapril with hydralazine/isosorbide dinitrate, a survival advantage of enalapril was observed only in white patients; in African Americans, mortality was similar in those randomized to enalapril or hydralazine/isosorbide dinitrate. The African-American HF Trial (A-HeFT) tested the hypothesis that the addition of hydralazine/isosorbide dinitrate to background neurohormonal blockade would improve HF outcomes in African-American patients with low ejection fractions and advanced symptoms.[94] Compared with placebo, hydralazine/isosorbide dinitrate significantly reduced mortality by 43% and the rate of first hospitalization by 33% in self-identified African-American men and women (**Fig. 40.11**).[94] Hydralazine/isosorbide dinitrate is recommended for African Americans with HFrEF in combination with renin-angiotensin system inhibitors and β-blockers.[39] The impact of this strategy in other populations requires further study.

Angiotensin Receptor Blockers, Aldosterone Antagonists, Digoxin

Clinical trials of these pharmacotherapeutic agents included small numbers of racial/ethnic minorities and do not permit conclusions regarding treatment by race.

Valsartan–Sacubitril and Ivabradine

Due to limited trial data, no conclusions can be drawn regarding the use of valsartan-sacubitril or ivabradine by race/ethnicity, although data from the PARADIGM-HF trial suggest similar effects of sacubitril-valsartan across racial/ethnic groups (**see Fig. 40.1**).[35,36]

Implantable Cardioverter Defibrillators and Cardiac Resynchronization Therapy

Minorities have been under-represented in trials testing the utility of ICDs and CRT, as well as in registries tracking the use of these devices.[95-97] The SCD-HeFT enrolled 23% minorities and showed similar benefits in African Americans and whites.[98] Subsequent observational data have shown improved mortality and no interaction by racial/ethnic group.[99,100]

Heart Transplantation

Retrospective analysis of data from the Organ Procurement and Transplantation database revealed that although 6-month survival has improved with time in all racial/ethnic groups, the risk of death or retransplant remains higher in African Americans.[101] Furthermore, longer-term survival (i.e., beyond 6 months) has not improved over time for African-American or Hispanic/Latino transplant recipients.[101,102]

SUMMARY

HF in older patients, women, and racial/ethnic minority groups is often associated with distinct differences in prevalence, pathophysiology, clinical features, and response to treatment relative to HF in younger white men (i.e., the demographic group with highest enrollment in most clinical trials). Additional studies are needed to define optimal strategies for prevention and treatment of HF in these populations.

KEY REFERENCES

14. Upadhya B, Pisani B, Kitzman DW. Evolution of a geriatric syndrome: pathophysiology and treatment of heart failure with preserved ejection fraction. *J Am Geriatr Soc.* 2017;65:2431–2440.

22. Riegel B, Moser DK, Buck HG, et al. Self-care for the prevention and managmeent of cardiovascular disease and stroke. A scientific statement for healthcare professionals from the American Heart Association. *J Am Heart Assoc.* 2017;6:e006997. https://doi.org/10.1161/JAHA.117.006997.

37. Santangeli P, Di Biase L, Dello Russo A, et al. Meta-analysis: age and effectiveness of prophylactic implantable cardioverter-defibrillators. *Ann Intern Med.* 2010;153. 592–529.

40. Lampert R, Hayes DL, Annas GJ, et al. HRS expert consensus statement on the management of cardiovascular implantable electronic devices (CIEDs) in patients nearing end of life or requesting withdrawal of therapy. *Heart Rhythm.* 2010;7:1008–1026.

46. Kitzman DW, Brubaker P, Morgan T, et al. Effect of caloric restriction or aerobic exercise training on peak oxygen consumption and quality of life in obese older patients with heart failure with preserved ejection fraction: a randomized clinical trial. *JAMA.* 2016;315:36–46.

62. Arshad A, Moss AJ, Foster E, et al. Cardiac resynchronization therapy is more effective in women than in men: the MADIT-CRT (Multicenter Automatic Defibrillator Implantation Trial with Cardiac Resynchronization Therapy) trial. *J Am Coll Cardiol.* 2011;57(7):813–820.

64. Ghanbari H, Dalloul G, Hasan R, Daccarett M, Saba S, David S, et al. Effectiveness of implantable cardioverter-defibrillators for the primary prevention of sudden cardiac death in women with advanced heart failure: a meta-analysis of randomized controlled trials. *Arch Intern Med.* September. 2009;169(16):1500–1506.

84. Bajaj NS, Gutierrez OM, Arora G, et al. Racial differences in plasma levels of N-terminal pro-B-type natriuretic peptide and outcomes. *JAMA Cardiol.* 2018;3:11–17.

88. Gupta DK, Shah AM, Castagno D, et al. Heart failure with preserved ejection fraction in African Americans. *J Am Coll Cardiol Heart Fail.* 2013;1:156–163.

99. Ziaeian B, Zhang Y, Albert NM, et al. Clinical effectiveness of CRT and ICD therapy in heart failure patients by racial/ethnic classification: insights from the IMPROVE HF registry. *J Am Coll Cardiol.* 2014;64(8): 797–807.

The full reference list for this chapter is available on ExpertConsult.

Stem Cell-Based and Gene Therapies in Heart Failure

Kenta Nakamura, W. Robb MacLellan

CARDIAC CELL THERAPY

Myocardial infarction (MI), despite significant advances in acute reperfusion and chronic pharmacotherapy, remains a major cause of heart failure in the United States.[1] The lost myocardium is replaced by fibrotic scar leading to progressive left ventricular (LV) remodeling and further dysfunction. Although limited myocyte turnover in the adult mammalian heart[2,3] has been reported to occur at baseline,[4] this intrinsic regenerative capacity is limited and inadequate to restore function following injury.[5,6] Thus healing following loss of myocardium is achieved through myocyte hypertrophy and scar formation.[7] In contrast, lower vertebrates and even mammals in the early postnatal period have robust regenerative capacity, suggesting regenerative therapies are a viable approach to restore function, enhance quality of life, and improve mortality.

Although pharmacologic approaches have been responsible for significant reductions in mortality and slow the progression of ventricular remodeling, they do not address the underlying etiology of heart failure, namely, the loss of contractile myocardium. Despite the compelling need for regenerative therapies in heart failure and two decades of concerted effort, such treatments have yet to transform contemporary cardiovascular practice. A multitude of cell-based (adult and progenitor cells, pluripotent and multipotent cell-derived cardiomyocytes, stromal cells, engineered tissues), gene-based (noncoding RNA, episomes), and cell-free (secretomes, growth factors, biomaterials) therapies have been proposed (**Fig. 41.1**). The most promising of the cell- and gene-based investigational therapies will be reviewed in this chapter.

Mechanisms of Action for Cardiac Cell Therapy

Cell therapy broadly aims to achieve two distinct but complementary goals: (1) direct cell replacement through implantation of cells or grafting of tissues into the injured myocardium and (2) stimulation of endogenous repair processes such as angiogenesis, inflammation, apoptosis, and fibrosis (**see Fig. 48.1**). Direct cell or tissue replacement offers the most intuitive strategy to replace cardiac myocytes ("remuscularization") and restore function following acute MI; however, it has also been the most elusive. Remuscularization may be the only effective strategy for irreversible fibrosis or remodeling associated with chronic injury, a larger albeit more complex indication than acute injury. However, replacement therapies remain exploratory at this stage in development. Whether adult stem cells are even capable of forming new cardiac muscle is an area of great debate (**see also Chapter 3**).[8-12] In contrast, replacement strategies based on pluripotent stem cells can clearly remuscularize infarcted myocardium in preclinical models,[13-17] but have their own set of challenges that will need to be overcome before they are a viable clinical strategy.

The first cell type investigated for cardiac cell replacement therapy was adult skeletal myoblasts over two decades ago.[18,19] Although initially thought to transdifferentiate into cardiomyocytes, this has been conclusively shown not to occur,[20] and the cells themselves do not couple electrically with the host myocardium. Clinical trials of autologous skeletal myoblast transplantation in patients with heart failure did not improve regional or global LV function and caused ventricular arrhythmias, prompting abandonment of this cell type for therapy.[21] More recently, efforts have shifted to other adult sources of cells purporting regenerative benefit through cell-cell and paracrine mechanisms, activating and stimulating endogenous regeneration and modulating repair mechanisms. Numerous autologous and allogeneic adult cell types have been investigated clinically, including adult stem cells of cardiac origin such as cardiac stem/progenitor cells (CSCs/CPCs) and noncardiac origin such as cardiosphere-derived cells (CDCs), as well as various bone marrow (BM)-derived cells (e.g., BM-derived mononuclear stem cells [BM-MNCs], and BM-derived mesenchymal stem cells [BM-MSCs]) (**Table 41.1**). These so-called first-generation cell types have been further refined as "second-generation" cells composed of highly purified subpopulations or modified to potentiate their regenerative capacity. Development of these adult cell types has been accelerated to numerous phase II/III clinical trials within the past

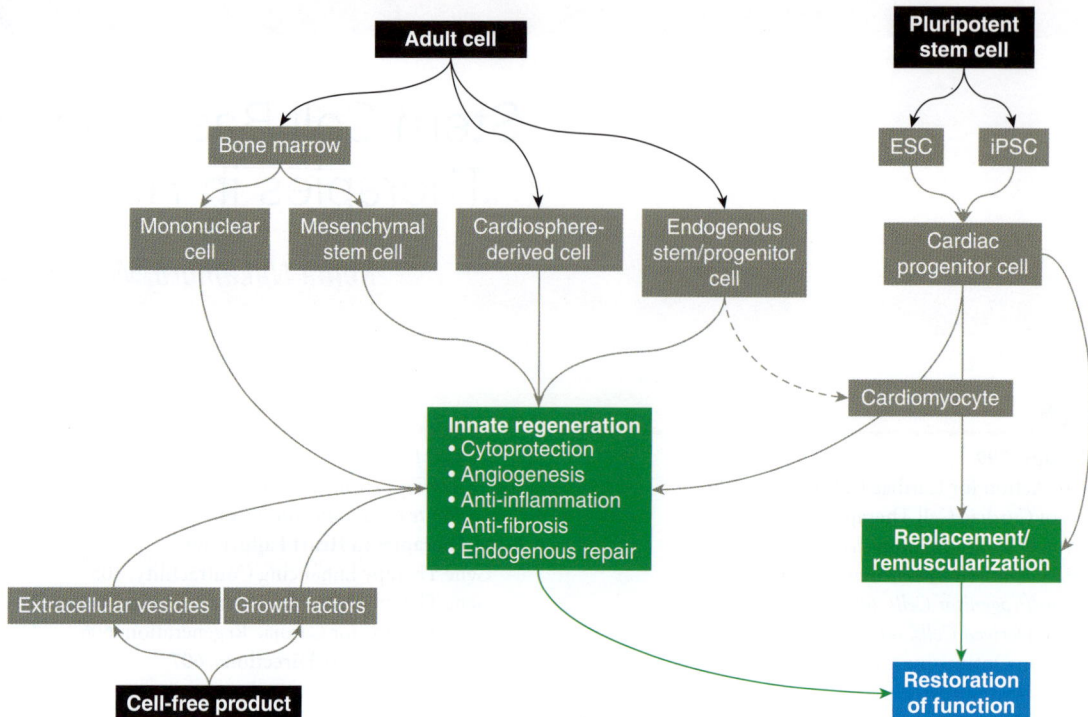

Fig. 41.1 Proposed cell types for therapeutic cardiac regeneration. (*ESC,* Embryonic stem cell; *iPSC,* induced pluripotent stem cell.)

decade.[22,23] With the realization that cell therapy has multiple effects in addition to regeneration, including cell-cell interaction and paracrine secretion of cardioactive cytokines and growth factors, investigators have expanded the indications for cell therapy from acute MI to ischemic and nonischemic cardiomyopathy to refractory angina,[24] peripheral artery disease,[25] and stroke.[26] Recently, it has been recognize that cell-free preparations are capable of replicating the beneficial effects of cell therapy; these secretomes consist of extracellular vesicles/exosomes[27-29] and growth factor-enriched myocardial matrixes.[30,31] Whether they account for all of the benefits of cellular therapy and whether they are equally efficacious will need to await further clinical development.

Given their proven potential to remuscularize infarcted tissue, there is great interest in pluripotent stem cells such as human embryonic stem cells (ESCs) as a renewable source of differentiated cardiomyocytes. First isolated in 1998,[32] human ESCs are isolated from the inner cell mass of the blastocyst in the early stages of embryogenesis. These cells retain the potential to differentiate into any somatic cell type given the appropriate stimulation. Initially, there was hope that the heart milieu itself could provide either critical cell-cell cues or growth factors to guide ESCs to a cardiac phenotype and integrate into host myocardium. This notion was quickly dispelled as injected ESCs into mouse myocardium formed teratomas rather than mature cardiomyocytes,[33] in addition to eliciting immunogenicity and graft rejection.[34] However, cardiomyocytes derived from ESCs can be transplanted and survive in normal rodent hearts[35] and electrically couple with existing cardiomyocytes in porcine models.[36] When transplanted into recipient rodent models after MI, there was a reproducible and durable improvement in LV function and electrical coupling with the host myocardium.[37-39] Efficient methods for high-purity, clinical-grade cardiomyocyte production from ESCs now allow extension of replacement cell strategies into preclinical large animal studies. Upward of one billion human ESC-derived human cardiomyocytes (hESC-CMs), approximating the cell loss during anterior MI, have been successfully implanted in

postinfarction, nonhuman primates.[15] In this seminal study by Chong et al. and Murry et al., hESC-CMs were engrafted into infarcted primate hearts via epicardial injection, resulting in significant remuscularization. The human graft became vascularized and electromechanically coupled with the host myocardium within 2 weeks posttransplant and remained durable up to 2 months, albeit with significant immunosuppression to prevent xenograft rejection. A more recent example demonstrated the effectiveness of allogenic transplantation of 400 million primate induced pluripotent stem cell (iPSC)-derived cardiomyocytes into major histocompatibility complex (MHC) haplotype homozygous matched primates.[14] As expected with significant engraftment of ectopic ventricular tissue, ventricular arrhythmias were observed in both studies, albeit transient and hemodynamically tolerated. Arrhythmogenicity of such grafts appears be proportional to graft size and the size of the host heart (no ventricular arrhythmias were noted in preceding small-model studies) and can be expected to pose a challenge in large animal studies. Although these preclinical proof-of-concept studies show promise and are grounded in more than three decades of basic science scholarship transitioning from in vitro and small animal models to more relevant large animal studies,[40] significant challenges to clinical translation remain. Efficient and reproducible cell production and processing, avoidance or suppression of ventricular arrhythmias, graft survival without prohibitive immunosuppression, and currently surgical epicardial delivery must be addressed prior to broad clinical acceptance. To circumvent many of these issues, an alternative strategy using a surgically placed epicardial patch seeded with ESC-derived CPCs is already enrolling a first-in-human trial,[41] despite recent evidence suggesting that cardiac progenitors do not durably engraft and any benefit is mediated through transient paracrine mechanisms.[12]

The discovery of an alternative pluripotent stem cell, iPSCs, by Takahashi and Yamanaka et al. has markedly accelerated pluripotent stem cell research and translation into potential therapies. Overexpression of four genes (c-Myc, Oct3/4, SOX2, and Klf4) known to maintain pluripotency in stem cells reprogramed somatic cells back

TABLE 41.1 Summary of Select Randomized Control Trials for Cardiac Regenerative Therapy

Study	Design	Number of Subjects T	Number of Subjects C	Cell Type	Route	Cell Number (×10⁶)	Timing (Post-AMI)	Follow-up (Months)	Primary Outcome	Result
Acute Myocardial Infarction										
Wollert et al. (BOOST)[58]	SC, OL	30	30	Allo BM-MNC	IC	2460	5–7 days	6	Global LVEF	Positive
Schachinger et al. (REPAIR–AMI)[101]	MC, DB	95	92	Auto BM-MNC	IC	236 ± 174	3–6 days	4	Global LVEF	Positive
Janssens et al. (Leuven–AMI)[102]	SC, DB	33	34	Auto BM-MNC	IC	172 ± 72	24 hours	4	Global LVEF	Negative
Huikuri et al. (FINCELL)[103]	MC, DB	39	38	Auto BM-MNC	IC	402 ± 196	3 days	6	Global LVEF	Positive
Tendera et al. (REGENT)[104]	SC, OL	97	20	Auto BM-MNC or CD34+CXCR4+ BM-MNC	IC	178 (BMMNC) 1.90 (CD34+CXCR4+ BMCs)	3–12 days	6	Global LVEF	Negative
Roncalli et al. (BONAMI)[105]	MC, OL	52	49	Auto BM-MNC	IC	98.3 ± 8.7	9 days	3	Myocardial viability	Negative
Hirsch et al. (HEBE)[106]	MC, OL	69	65	BM-MNC/PB-MNC	IC	296 ± 164 (BM) 287 ± 137 (PB)	5–7 days	4	Global or regional LVEF	Negative
Traverse et al. (LateTIME Trial)[107]	MC, DB	58	29	Auto BM-MNC	IC	150	2–3 weeks	6	Global LVEF	Negative
Traverse et al. (TIME)[108]	MC, DB	79	41	Auto BM-MNC	IC	147 ± 17	3 or 7 days	6	Global or regional LVEF	Negative
Choudry et al. (REGENERATE-AMI)[109]	MC, DB	55	45	Auto BM-MNC	IC	60	<24 hours	12	Global LVEF	Negative
Sürder et al. (SWISS-AMI)[110]	MC, DB	95	55	Auto BM-MNC	IC	152	5–7 days or 3–4 weeks	12	Global LVEF	Negative
Quyyumi et al. (PreSERVE-AMI)[63]	MC, DB	78	83	Auto BM-MSC	IC	10 ± 2	9 days	6	Resting myocardial perfusion	Negative
Wollert et al. (BOOST-2)[59]	SC, OL	151	37	Allo BM-MNC	IC	700–2080	8.1 ± 2.6 days	6	Global LVEF	Negative
Mathur et al. (BAMI, NCT01569178)[111]	MC, DB	~175	~175	Auto BM-MNC	IC		2–8 days	24	All-cause mortality	Recruiting, estimated completion 2019
Ischemic Cardiomyopathy										
Menasche et al. (MAGIC)[21]	MC, DB	67	30	Skeletal myoblasts	TEP	400 or 800	>1 month		Global or regional LVEF	Negative
Perin et al. (FOCUS-HF)[112]	SC, OL	20	10	Auto BM-MNC	TEN	178	>3 months	12	QOL, MLHFQ LVESV, VO₂ max, SPECT reversibility	Positive
Perin et al. (FOCUS-CCTRN)[113]	MC, DB	61	31	Auto BM-MNC	TEN	100	>1 month	6	Global or regional LVEF	Negative
Assmus et al. (CELLWAVE)[114]	SC, DB	82	40	Auto BM-MNC	IC	205 ± 110	>3 months	4	Global LVEF	Positive
Patel et al. (ixCell-DCM)[64]	MC, DB, sham control	58	51	Proprietary auto BM-MSC and M2 macrophages	TEN		>3 months	12	Composite (all-cause death, cardiovascular hospitalizations, and worsening HF)	Positive

Continued

TABLE 41.1   Summary of Select Randomized Control Trials for Cardiac Regenerative Therapy—cont'd

Study	Design	Number of Subjects T	Number of Subjects C	Cell Type	Route	Cell Number (×10⁶)	Timing (Post-AMI)	Follow-up (Months)	Primary Outcome	Result
Bartunek et al. (CHART-1)[74]	MC, DB, sham control	120	151	Auto BM-CpSC	TEN	24	>3 months	40	Composite (all-cause death, worsening HF, MLHFQ, 6MWT, LVESV, and LVEF)	Negative
Choudhury et al. (REGENERATE-IHD)[115]	SC, DB	70	35	G-CSF/auto BM-MNC	IC or TEN	115.1	>3 months	12	Global LVEF	Positive for TEN
CONCERT-HF (NCT02501811)	MC, DB	~72	~72	Auto BM-MSC/c-kit⁺ CSC	TEN			12	Global LVEF, VO₂ max, 6MWT, etc.	Recruiting, estimated completion 2018
DREAM HF-1 (NCT02032004)	MC, DB	~300	~300	Auto BM-MPCs	TEN			12	Time to HF exacerbation	Recruiting, estimated completion 2018
CHART-2 (NCT02317458)	MC, DB, sham control	~200	~200	Auto BM-CpSC	TEN			52	Composite (CV death, worsening HF, MLHFQ)	Recruiting, estimated completion 2020
Assmus et al. (REPEAT, NCT01693042)[61]	MC, OL	~334	~334	Auto BM-MNC	Repeated IC			24	All-cause mortality	Recruiting, estimated completion 2022

6MWT, 6-minute walk test; AMI, acute myocardial infarction; allo, allogeneic; auto, autologous; BM, bone marrow; BMC, bone marrow cell; CpSCs, cardiopoietic stem cells; CSC, cardiac stem cells; CV, cardiovascular; DB, double-blind; G-CSF, granulocyte-colony stimulating factor; HF, heart failure; IC, intracoronary; LVEF, left ventricular ejection fraction; LVESV, left ventricular end-systolic volume; MLHFQ, Minnesota Living with Heart Failure questionnaire; MNC, mononuclear cell; MSC, mesenchymal stem cell; MPC, mesenchymal precursor cell; MC, multicenter; PB, peripheral blood; OL, open-label; QOL, quality of life; SC, single-center; SPECT, single-photon emission computed tomography; TEN, transendocardial; TEP, transepicardial; VO₂ max, maximal oxygen consumption.

to a state of pluripotency.[42,43] The process has been validated using a full spectrum of somatic cells, including cells isolated from a single hair follicle or a sample of blood. iPSCs offer benefits over ESCs such as autologous source, allowing patient-specific human leukocyte antigen (HLA) compatibility, potentially obviating the need for immunosuppression, and avoiding the societal issues surrounding blastocyst and embryo research. However, the reprograming process has been reported to result in genomic abnormalities and incomplete reprograming, leaving residual epigenetic marks that are of uncertain clinical significance.[44] However, cardiomyocytes generated from iPSCs appear functionally indistinguishable from cardiomyocytes derived from ESCs and native cardiomyocytes, although they are phenotypically immature.[45,46] Engineered sheets of iPSC-derived cardiomyocytes have been ectopically transplanted onto failing postinfarction hearts in pig with benefit,[47,48] although the clinical relevance of such an approach is unclear given that such grafts failed to couple electromechanically or vascularize with the host myocardium.

Clinical Trials of Cardiac Cell Therapy

The first cardiac cell therapy trials were performed more than 20 years ago,[49] with intracoronary delivery of BM-MNCs. There have now been more than 100 clinical trials of cell therapy for MI, more than 90 for chronic ischemic cardiomyopathy, and 25 for nonischemic cardiomyopathy.[50] Trials to date have generally used heterogeneous populations of adult cell types and have consistently shown safety regardless of the specific investigational cell product, delivery approach, dosing protocol, or patient characteristics. Individual trials initially suggested efficacy, but these early trials were small without randomization, standardized enrollment criteria, or end points. More recent trials with larger cohorts and superior study design have generally failed to convincingly show benefit over guideline-directed medical therapy (see Table 41.1).[22,50-52] A recent Cochrane meta-analysis of 38 randomized control trials capturing 1907 post-MI patients concluded the current body of evidence for cell therapy to be low quality and lacking evidence for benefit by composite end point of mortality, nonfatal MI, and/or heart failure readmission.[53] Long-term mortality greater than 12 months and incidence of nonfatal MI were individually reduced with cell therapy but confounded by relatively low event rates, small study cohorts, and nonstandardized trial designs and adjudication. Numerous challenges remain for the clinical translation of cardiac cell therapy (Fig. 41.2).[22] Several representative trials of cell therapy are presented here to highlight these challenges facing cardiac cell therapies.

Bone Marrow–Derived Mononuclear Cells

BM-derived stem cells encompass a diverse cell population, of which BM-MNCs and MSCs have been studied the most clinically. In one of the original and most controversial papers in the field, Orlic et al.[10] reported myocardial regeneration with new myocyte formation following acute MI with BM-MNC therapy in mice, which was rapidly extended into large animal and human studies.[40] To date, this study has not been reproduced, and there is no direct evidence that any BM cell derivative can differentiate into a mature cardiomyocytes. [54] Nevertheless, given the proposed alternative beneficial effect through cell-cell or paracrine mechanisms of action, clinical trials of BM-MNCs particularly in post-MI patients have continued to increase. The trials have generally yielded inconclusive or conflicting results likely due to the small size of phase I/II studies, heterogeneity of cell isolation, preparation, dosing, timing of therapy, baseline patient characteristics, end point adjudication, and study design. Routinely, modest and inconsistent but promising results in pilot and single-center phase I trials have not been reproduced in larger, multicenter phase II trials.[55-57] For example, the original BOne marrOw transfer to enhance ST elevation infarct regeneration (BOOST, NCT00224536) trial of autologous intracoronary BM-MNCs randomized 60 ST-segment elevation myocardial infarction (STEMI) patients to therapy or placebo and showed improvement in LV systolic function[58] but was not supported in the follow-up BOOST-2 trial (ISRCTN17457407)[59,60] of 153 STEMI patients randomized to cell therapy or placebo. To definitively answer the role of BM-MNCs as cardiac cell therapy, the Bone marrow–derived mononuclear cells on all-cause mortality in Acute MI (BAMI, NCT01569178) trial represents the culmination of more than a decade of investigation in BM-MNCs for acute MI and LV dysfunction. BAMI is the first phase III trial designed to show benefit in all-cause mortality; however, enrollment has been significantly reduced from the initial 3000 to 350 patients due to challenges with recruiting patients. Given the significant reduction in enrollment, it is unclear whether the trial will have sufficient statistical power to demonstrate the beneficial effects of adjunctive intracoronary infusion of autologous BM-MNCs in addition to revascularization and guideline-directed medical therapy in patients with acute MI and impaired left ventricular ejection fraction (LVEF) (≤45%). Recruitment for the multinational, open-label, randomized controlled trial commenced in 2016 and is anticipated to conclude in 2019 after 2-year minimum follow-up. For postinfarction ischemic cardiomyopathy, REpetitive Progenitor cEll therapy in Advanced chronic hearT failure (REPEAT, NCT01693042), is a multicenter, open-label, randomized controlled trial of single versus repeat

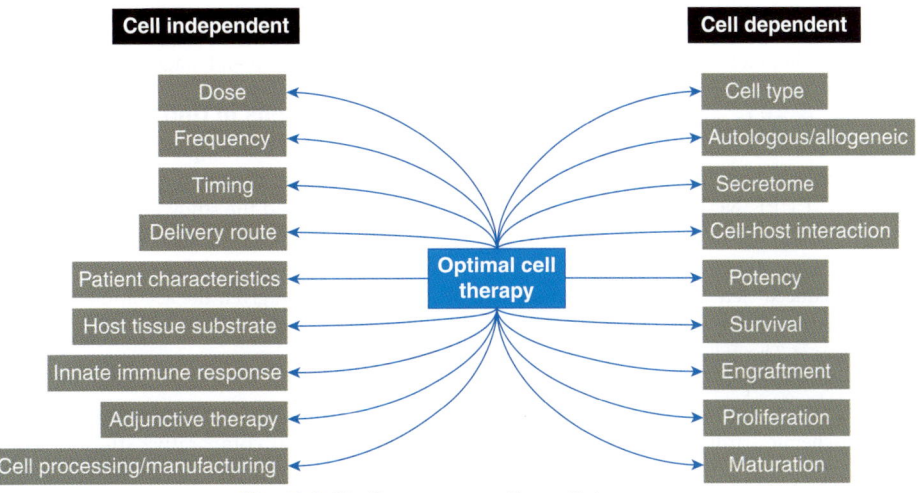

Fig. 41.2 Challenges to cardiac cell therapy.

intracoronary infusion of BM-MNCs powered for all-cause mortality at 2 years currently enrolling for an anticipated completion in 2022.[61] If the BAMI and REPEAT trials are successfully completed, their outcomes will help to more definitively answer the efficacy of BM-MNCs in acute MI and ischemic cardiomyopathy, respectively.

Bone Marrow–Derived Mesenchymal Stem Cells

The Prospective Randomized Study of Mesenchymal Stem Cell Therapy in Patients Undergoing Cardiac Surgery (PROMETHEUS, NCT00587990) trial[62] randomized nine patients undergoing cardiac surgical revascularization to intravenous BM-MSC therapy or placebo and provided early safety data and signal towards long-term benefit at 18 months. More recent studies have continued to demonstrate safety but generally negative primary outcomes, including the PreSERVE-AMI trial of intracoronary infusion of autologous CD34+ BM-MSCs following acute STEMI with impaired LV function.[63] Notably, the multicenter, double-blind, sham-controlled trial ixCELL-DCM studying a proprietary therapeutic cell product consisting of autologous BM-MSCs and M2 macrophages in 126 patients with dilated ischemic cardiomyopathy demonstrated a positive impact on the primary composite end point of all-cause death, cardiovascular hospitalizations, and heart failure decompensation at 1 year, although driven primarily by increased heart failure events in the sham control cohort.[64]

Cardiac Stem/Progenitor Cells

Several groups have reported that multipotent CSCs/CPCs exist in the heart and proposed they can effect true regeneration,[65] either directly or through stimulation of endogenous regenerative capacity and CSC niches,[66] although this has been disputed.[67,68] The potency of these cells declines with age due to accumulation of DNA damage and telomere attrition[69,70] and is, unfortunately, inversely related to the incidence and severity of cardiac disease. The Stem Cell Infusion in Patients with Ischemic cardiomyopathy (SCIPIO, NCT00474461)[71] trial was the first randomized study of intracoronary autologous CSCs/CPCs in ischemic cardiomyopathy. The small study of 20 treatment and 13 control patients with LVEF less than 40% randomized to cell therapy or placebo at 4 months post MI at the time of surgical revascularization demonstrated improved LVEF from 30% at baseline to 38% and 42% at 1 and 2 years, respectively, while the placebo control experienced a 3.7% absolute improvement in LVEF at 2 years. Additional end points such as infarct size and New York Heart Association (NYHA) functional classification were improved at 1 year and sustained at 2 years post therapy. Initial enthusiasm at the positive results have been tempered by controversy and a statement of concern issued by the host journal.[72] Nevertheless, the study has spurred further research into a subpopulation of CSCs/CPCs with high expression of Nkx2.5, Tbx5, Mesp-1, and Mef2C, so-called cardiopoietic stem cells (CpSCs) which are thought to be particularly reparative. Lineage-specification of BM-MSCs using growth factors to guide cardiopoiesis and to enrich the CpSC subpopulation led to the first clinical trial of these so-called second-generation adult stem cell products in the Cardiopoietic Stem Cell Therapy in Heart Failure (C-CURE, NCT00810238) trial.

The C-CURE trial used BM-CpSCs in ischemic cardiomyopathy, demonstrating safety and suggestion of efficacy including significantly improved LVEF, reduced left ventricular end-systolic volume (LVESV), and improved 6-minute walk test (6MWT) compared with the standard of care.[73] The follow-up study, European-based Congestive Heart Failure Cardiopoietic Regenerative Therapy (CHART-1, NCT01768702) trial, is a double-blind, sham-controlled study of 315 patients with ischemic cardiomyopathy treated with an endomyocardial injection of CpSCs.[74] Although safety was again demonstrated, the trial failed to achieve the prespecified primary composite end point (all-cause death, worsening heart failure, LVEF, LV end-diastolic volume, 6MWT), compared with sham control. The negative result of CHART-1, the largest trial of its kind to date, has raised several questions including the choice of cell type (autologous source with comprised regenerative capacity), untested dosing and delivery, and insufficient statistical power. The North American counterpart, CHART-2, (NCT02317458) is now evaluating whether transendocardial injection of CpSCs is effective in a subgroup of patients with more advanced heart failure and an end-diastolic volume of 200 to 370 mL.

Additional studies of second-generation cell products are currently ongoing. Combination therapy of intramyocardial injection of BM-MSCs and CSCs/CPCs is being studied in the multicenter phase II trial Combination of Mesenchymal and C-Kit+ Cardiac Stem Cells as Regenerative Therapy for Heart Failure (CONCERT-HF, NCT02501811) of 144 patients with ischemic cardiomyopathy randomized to BM-MSCs alone, CSCs/CPCs alone, combination MSCs and CSCs/CPCs, or placebo. The multicenter phase II trial Efficacy and Safety of Allogeneic Mesenchymal Precursor Cells (Rexlemestrocel-L) for the Treatment of Heart Failure (DREAM HF-1, NCT01569178) will randomize 600 patients with ischemic cardiomyopathy to mesenchymal precursor cells or placebo (study completion date of 2019). Finally, the phase I/II Transendocardial Autologous Cells in Heart Failure Trial (TAC-HFT, NCT02503280) will investigate combined MSCs and CSCs/CPCs or placebo in idiopathic dilated cardiomyopathy and is intended to start enrollment in 2020.

Cardiosphere-Derived Cells

A unique, heterogeneous population of endogenous cells derived from heart explants called CDCs have undergone extensive preclinical and clinical testing. Cardiospheres are heterogeneous spheroid-forming colonies of nonmyocyte cells that are formed from adult heart tissue in culture, which include MSCs, smooth muscle cells, endothelial cells, cardiac fibroblasts, and presumably CPCs. In preclinical studies, CDCs improved LV function when transplanted into infarcted myocardium.[75] The single-center Cardiosphere-Derived Autologous Stem Cells to Reverse Ventricular Dysfunction (CADUCEUS, NCT00893360)[76] trial randomized patients post MI with impaired LVEF less than 40% to cell therapy or placebo. At 12 months, therapy failed to improve functional end points of LVEF or NYHA functional classification, although scar size was reduced 12.3% at 12 months compared with placebo. The follow-up multicenter phase II trial Allogeneic Heart Stem Cells to Achieve Myocardial Generation (ALLSTAR, NCT01458405)[77] was recently terminated early for futility to achieve the primary end point of scar size by magnetic resonance imaging (MRI) after interim analysis at 6 months. CDC therapy is currently being investigated for dilated cardiomyopathy in end-stage Duchenne muscular dystrophy.

Open Questions in Optimizing Cardiac Cell Therapy

The modest and/or frequent negative results of cardiac cell therapy trials have been attributed to a number reasons, both specific to the therapy itself and the study design used.[22,78] However, although each of these interacting variables could have significant influence on the efficacy of cell therapy, it is not clear if, or how, these vexing issues will ever be resolved given the accumulating negative trials in the field of adult cell therapy.[79]

Cell Source

Multiple competing cell types have been proposed for cardiac cell therapy without comparative study to assess superiority or clearly defining the mechanisms of action for benefits (regenerative versus paracrine). Combination therapy could also provide additive benefits given the diverse mechanism of action of the various cell types but has not been studied systematically. Although combination therapy is being pursued in the ongoing CONCERT and TAC-HFT trials, it is questionable whether sufficient preclinical data exist to identify the most effective combinations. Another important variable is autologous versus allogeneic source. Although autologous source avoids the immunocompatibility issues of allogeneically sourced cells, patient comorbidities such as advanced age, diabetes, smoking, and obesity may limit the biologic potency of harvested cell components. Allogeneic cells also allow for "off-the-shelf" product development under strict quality-controlled conditions and ease of scalability.

Cell Dose

For replacement therapies such as proposed with pluripotent stem cell-derived cardiomyocytes, dose escalation until lost myocardium is fully remuscularized seems logical. Accordingly, preclinical studies have described administration of upwards of one billion ESC-derived cardiac myocytes, although full dosing studies in appropriate human-sized models have not occurred.[15] For adult stem cell products with primarily paracrine effects, the appropriate dosing is unclear. A reverse dose response has been reported in the POSEIDON trial[80] likely due to vascular obstruction and maladaptive neoangiogenesis with intracoronary administration, whereas higher doses appeared beneficial for transendocardial delivery, as observed in the TRIDENT trial.[81] Variable cell potency further complicates the issue of cell dosing, particularly for autologously sourced cells. In the absence of well-powered and appropriately controlled dose response trials, optimal dosing remains unknown.

Timing of Therapy

Although often reported interchangeably, administration of cells in the acute, subacute, or chronic phases following MI would be expected to work by significantly different mechanisms and require different properties. Acute administration aims to modulate inflammation and apoptosis, whereas subacute or chronic therapy aims to augment myocardial repair and regeneration. Although not studied systematically, a meta-analysis of adult cell therapy suggests that 2 to 8 days post MI is the most favorable window to modulate injury response and potentiate repair mechanisms.[56] Interestingly, preclinical studies have generally focused on the subacute phase, occurring at 2 weeks after the resolution of acute phase inflammation and reperfusion injury that may be hostile to engraftment. Indeed, ESC-derived cardiac myocyte transplantation is beneficial only in this subacute phase, insofar as limited studies in chronic cardiomyopathy have been negative.[82,83]

Route of Administration

Several routes of cell administration have been studied preclinically, including intravenous, percutaneous endomyocardial, intracoronary, transcoronary endocardial, retrograde intracoronary sinus with antegrade coronary obstruction, and open surgical epicardial. By far the most common route of adult cell delivery post MI is intracoronary infusion, given the central role for catheter-based revascularization in contemporary practice. However, intracoronary cell delivery is associated with rapid washout and little retention of cells, which may be sufficient for paracrine effects but not for remuscularization. Intramyocardial injection, whether epicardially or endocardially delivered, is superior for cell engraftment[84] but poses a higher risk of arrhythmia and perforation of the infarcted myocardium after MI and thus may be more appropriate for subacute and chronic therapy where remuscularization is the goal. More granular issues of optimal target

tissue, such as periinfarct versus intrainfarct myocardium or transmural infarcted versus stunned/hibernating myocardium, are largely unexplored.

Patient Characteristics. The myriad of patient characteristics affecting myocardial substrate have not been studied yet undoubtedly impact response to cell therapy, particularly for autologous cell products where poor patient parameters impair both cell potency and host receptivity have not been investigated. Patient comorbidities such as advanced age, diabetes, and injury-related features such as ischemia time, reperfusion, revascularization strategy, and reperfusion burden are highly variable between patients and influence the natural history of infarction and subsequent heart failure. Given the small size of existing studies and heterogeneity with respect to inclusion criteria, it is unlikely this will be resolved soon.

GENE THERAPIES IN HEART FAILURE

As the molecular basis of developmental and disease processes are elucidated with greater clarity (**see Chapters 1** and **2**), advancements in genetic and epigenetic modulation now allow for regulation of gene expression and function to repair the failing heart experimentally[85] and clinically (**Table 41.2**).[86] Current approaches in heart failure seek to enhance calcium handling, stem cell chemotaxis, angiogenesis, and cytoprotection to prevent or repair cardiomyopathies with defined genetic lesions.[87] However, multiple obstacles remain before clinical approaches will be feasible, including the technical challenge of engineering viral and nonviral constructs with tissue-specificity and safety, transfection efficiency, product production and cost, and patient selection. The most developed cardiac gene therapy for heart failure targets the sarcoplasmic/endoplasmic reticulum Ca^{2+}-ATPase (SERCA2a) to enhance cardiac contractility and overexpression of stromal cell-derived factor 1 (SDF-1) to enhance stem cell homing.[88]

Gene Therapy Enhancing Contractility

The SERCA2a Ca^{2+} cycling protein regulates cardiomyocyte contractility and relaxation by transporting Ca^{2+} from the cytosol into the sarcoplasmic reticulum during diastole in preparation for systolic contraction.[89] Downregulation of SERCA2a occurs with heart failure progression, and correction of SERCA2a deficiency improves function in vitro.[90] In the first-in-human phase I/II trial Calcium Upregulation by Percutaneous Administration of Gene Therapy in Cardiac Disease (CUPID, NCT00454818), 39 patients with LVEF less than 40% were randomized to intracoronary infusion of recombinant adeno-associated virus (AAV) delivery of SERCA2a or placebo and showed a trend for improved long-term functional end points.[91] However the subsequent randomized, multicenter, double-blind, placebo-controlled phase II trial (CUPID 2, NCT01643330) of 250 patients with advanced heart failure LVEF ≤ 35%, intracoronary infusion of AAV/SERCA2a failed to improve achieve the primary end point of time to recurrent HF-related events. CUPID 2 is the largest clinical trial of gene therapy in heart failure to date, with several ongoing studies mostly involving calcium homeostasis and stem cell homing (see Table 41.2). In an alternative approach to improve cardiac contractility, adenovirus-mediated gene transfer of human adenylyl cyclase type 6 (AC6) was studied 56 patients randomized to gene therapy or placebo. Although there was a transient increase in LVEF at 4 months, the benefit was not sustained at 12 months, and the primary end point of improved exercise duration was not different from the placebo control. A pivotal multicenter double-blind, randomized, phase III Heart *F*ailure with *R*educed *L*eft *V*entricular *E*jection *F*raction: One-time *G*ene *T*ransfer *U*sing *R*T-100– *I*ntracoronary Administration of Adenovirus 5 encoding *H*uman AC6 (FLOURISH, NCT03360448) trial is anticipated to start in 2018.

TABLE 41.2   Summary of Randomized Clinical Trials for Cardiac Gene Therapy for Heart Failure

Trial	NUMBER OF PATIENTS		Gene Target	Vector	Route	Study Design	Patient	Primary Endpoint	Follow-up (Months)	Outcome
	T	C								
Jessup et al. (CUPID)[116]	25	14	SERCA2a	AAV-1	IC	MC, DB	NYHA class III/IV, LVEF ≤35%	Composite of NYHA, 6MWT, VO₂ max NT-proBNP, QOL	6	Positive
Greenberg et al. (CUPID 2)[117]	123	127	SERCA2a	AAV-1	IC	MC, DB	NYHA class III/IV, LVEF ≤35%	Time to recurrent CV event	12	Negative
SERCA-LVAD (NCT00534703)	12	12	SERCA2a	AAV-1	IC	MC, DB	Chronic HF with LVAD	Safety and feasibility		Ongoing
AGENT-HF (NCT01966887)	22	22	SERCA2a	AAV-1	IC	SC, DB	NYHA class III/IV, LVEF ≤35%	LVESV	6	Ongoing
Penn et al. (STOP-HF)[88]	17		Plasmid	SDF-1	TEN	SC, OL	NYHA class III, LVEF ≤40%	MACE	1	Positive
Chung et al. (STOP-HF 2)[86]	62	31	Plasmid	SDF-1	TEN	MC, DB	Ischemic cardiomyopathy, LVEF ≤40%	6MWT	4	Negative
RETRO-HF (NCT01961726)	Phase 1: 12 Phase 2: 20	Phase 2: 20	Plasmid	SDF-1	RCS	Phase 1: SC, OL Phase 2: MC, DB	Ischemic cardiomyopathy, LVEF ≤40%	6MWT	4	Ongoing
Hammond et al. (AC6 Gene Transfer for CHF)[118]	42	14	hAC6	Adenovirus 5	IC	MC, DB	Chronic HF, LVEF ≤40%	Composite exercise time and dobutamine stress echo	3	Negative
FLOURISH (NCT03360448)	~268	~268	hAC6	Adenovirus 5	IC	MC, DB	Chronic HF, LVEF ≥10 to ≤ 35%	Heart failure hospitalizations	12	Planned, estimated completion 2019

6MWT, 6-minute walk test; *AAV,* adeno-associated virus; *CV,* cardiovascular; *DB,* double-blind; *hAC6,* human adenylyl cyclase type 6; *HF,* heart failure; *IC,* intracoronary; *LVAD,* left ventricular assist device; *LVEF,* left ventricular ejection fraction; *LVESV,* left ventricular end-systolic volume; *MACE,* major adverse cardiovascular events; *MC,* multicenter; *NT-proBNP,* N-terminal pro-brain natriuretic peptide; *NYHA,* New York Heart Association; *OL,* open-label; *QOL,* quality of life; *RCS,* retrograde coronary sinus; *SC,* single-center; *SDF-1,* stem cell-derived factor 1; *SERCA2a,* sarcoplasmic reticulum Ca²⁺ ATPase; *TEN,* transendocardial; *VO₂ max,* maximal oxygen consumption.

Gene Therapy Enhancing Stem Cell Homing

The SFD-1/CXC chemokine receptor 4 (CXCR4) mediates trafficking of reparative stem cells to the site of myocardial injury.[92] Overexpression of SDF-1 in the border zone of infarcted myocardium improved cardiac function and promoted angiogenesis.[93] Following a phase I trial of SDF-1 gene therapy using 15 endomyocardial injections of SDF-1–containing plasmids, the double-blind and placebo-controlled phase II trial STOP-HF (NCT01643590)[86] randomized 93 patients with advanced heart failure and failed to achieve the composite primary end point of 6-minute walk test (6MWT) and Minnesota Living with Heart Failure Questionnaire (MLWHFQ) at 4 months. It has been speculated that the neutral results of CUPID2 and STOP-HF may be explained by poor uptake of the respective gene therapy into myocytes in the larger trials. In CUPID 2, the viral uptake ranged from less than 20 to 561 copies of vector per microgram of DNA, corresponding to less than 1% of the myocardium infected, compared with preclinical animal studies with uptake of 20,000 to 350,000 copies of

vector per microgram of DNA. In an attempt to address this limitation, the ongoing RETRO-HF trial uses infusion of a plasmid expressing SDF-1 infused retrograde through the coronary sinus through with simultaneous antegrade coronary obstruction to improve construct uptake.[87] More fundamental changes to improve transduction efficiency, patient selection, and consideration of alternative gene targets may be required for future studies.

Gene Therapy for Cardiac Regeneration

Attempts to reactivate endogenous cardiomyocyte proliferation after injury have proven remarkably difficult. Early studies using overexpression of viral oncogenes induced cardiac myocyte death.[94,95] The observation that the postnatal mammalian cardiomyocyte, in disease states, can replicate DNA but fails to undergo karyokinesis (separation into two cells) is perplexing and provocative. The inability to undergo cell division appears to involve a specific G2/M cell cycle block similar to cellular senescence. The genes responsible for cell division in cardiac myocytes condense and wrap into transcriptionally inactive heterochromatin.[96] When heterochromatin formation is interrupted, cardiomyocytes regained the ability to reenter the cell cycle and divide. However, the process of cellular division requires disassembly and reassembly of the sarcomere with transient loss of contractile function until division is complete. Some experimental models with induced proliferation have resulted in LV dilation and contractile dysfunction, suggesting that even if strategies can be designed to overcome the proliferation block in adult cardiac myocytes,[96] an effective therapy to regenerate the adult heart using endogenous machinery will also require a strategy to mitigate the deleterious effects of sarcomeric disassembly/reassembly on global organ function.

In an alternative approach to cardiac regeneration, investigators have explored whether it is feasible to directly reprogram fibroblasts in scar tissue into cardiac myocytes. Shortly after the discovery of cellular reprogramming to induce somatic cells into pluripotent stem cells, a similar approach was used to reprogram cells into specific cell types such as exocrine pancreatic cells into endocrine cells or neurons.[97] In 2010 a trio of transcription factors (Gata4, Mefc2, and Tbx5) were reported to transdifferentiate mouse fibroblasts into cardiomyocytes,[98] although subsequent reports suggested HAND2 was also required.[99] Infection of the postinfarct murine heart with these transcription factors[99,100] resulted in 4% to 35% of cardiomyocytes in the infarct border zone originating from infected fibroblasts, resulting in nearly a 50% reduction in scar area and improved LV function. Whether these results are translatable to larger animal models will await additional studies, but the approach holds much promise.

These studies represent the best-developed cardiac gene therapy approaches and highlight the barriers to clinical translation, including retroviral infection and integration, low event efficiency, and tissue specificity. Unlike cell-based therapies in general, the mechanisms of cardiac gene therapy to date are well elucidated with convincing preclinical data, although identification of novel molecular targets amendable to genetic manipulation remains a priority. Translation of these insights clinically hinge on the development of next-generation vectors and delivery systems, likely based upon a safe nonviral or plasmid platform with high potency and specificity.

SUMMARY AND FUTURE DIRECTIONS

In this chapter we have reviewed to the clinical application of cell-based therapies for cardiac regeneration, as well as advances in gene therapy for treating heart failure patients. The modest improvement in LV function in cell therapy clinical trials with small numbers of patients, as well as the negative outcomes of larger stem-cell therapy trials, have given rise to a number of important questions regarding the feasibility of the therapy itself, as well as questions about the optimal cell source, cell dose, timing of administration of cell therapy, patient characteristics, and the optimal route of administration of stem cells. For the field of stem cell therapy to move forward, these important issues will need to be carefully addressed. Although gene transfer strategies appear promising in experimental models of HF, a considerable amount of work remains to be done with respect to improvements in vector technology, methods for cardiac gene delivery, and perhaps most importantly, understanding what gene targets are safe to focus on in clinical trials in heart failure patients. Biologic therapeutics hold great promise as novel approaches to treating patients affected by heart failure, but numerous hurdles remain before any of these therapies will become part of our standard approach to care.

KEY REFERENCES

2. Bergmann O, Zdunek S, Felker A, et al. Dynamics of cell generation and turnover in the human heart. *Cell.* 2015;161(7):1566–1575.
6. Senyo SE, Steinhauser ML, Pizzimenti CL, et al. Mammalian heart renewal by pre-existing cardiomyocytes. *Nature.* 2013;493(7432):433–436.
15. Chong JJ, Yang X, Don CW, et al. Human embryonic-stem-cell-derived cardiomyocytes regenerate non-human primate hearts. *Nature.* 2014;510(7504):273–277.
51. Fisher SA, Doree C, Mathur A, et al. Meta-analysis of cell therapy trials for patients with heart failure. *Circ Res.* 2015;116(8):1361–1377.
52. Gyongyosi M, Wojakowski W, Navarese EP, et al. Meta-analyses of human cell-based cardiac regeneration therapies: controversies in meta-analyses results on cardiac cell-based regenerative studies. *Circ Res.* 2016;118(8):1254–1263.
53. Fisher SA, Brunskill SJ, Doree C, et al. Stem cell therapy for chronic ischaemic heart disease and congestive heart failure. *Cochrane Database Syst Rev.* 2016;12:CD007888.
99. Song K, Nam YJ, Luo X, et al. Heart repair by reprogramming non-myocytes with cardiac transcription factors. *Nature.* 2012;485(7400):599–604.
109. Choudry F, Hamshere S, Saunders N, et al. A randomized double-blind control study of early intra-coronary autologous bone marrow cell infusion in acute myocardial infarction: the REGENERATE-AMI clinical trial. *Eur Heart J.* 2016;37(3):256–263.
117. Greenberg B, Butler J, Felker GM, et al. Calcium upregulation by percutaneous administration of gene therapy in patients with cardiac disease (CUPID 2): a randomised, multinational, double-blind, placebo-controlled, phase 2b trial. *Lancet.* 2016;387(10024):1178–1186.
118. Hammond HK, Penny WF, Traverse JH. Intracoronary gene transfer of adenylyl cyclase 6 in patients with heart failure: a randomized clinical trial. *JAMA Cardiol.* 2016;1(2):163–171.

The full reference list for this chapter is available on ExpertConsult.

Neuromodulation in Heart Failure

John Keaney, Jagmeet P. Singh

The autonomic nervous system (ANS) plays a vital role in the management of cardiac function. The subdivisions of the ANS are the parasympathetic nervous system (PNS) and the sympathetic nervous system (SNS; see also Chapter 13). The SNS is the stimulatory pathway. Increased sympathetic tone enhances AV conduction and myocardial contractility. The PNS activation of the heart occurs via the tenth cranial nerve, the vagus. Vagal activation leads to negative inotropic and chronotropic effects, and a reduction in blood pressure. Importantly, it is the beat-to-beat balance between these two opposing limbs of the ANS, which regulates the heart rate, blood pressure, cardiac contractility, and electrical stability of the myocardium.

ANATOMY OF THE AUTONOMIC NERVOUS SYSTEM

The principle regions of ANS control are located within the medulla oblongata, which in turn is subject to control by the hypothalamus and the cerebral cortex. The medulla receives afferent fibers from the glossopharyngeal nerve and the vagus nerve (**Fig. 42.1**), which terminates in the nucleus tractus solitarius (NTS). From here, neurons project to the rostral ventrolateral medulla (RVLM) and the nucleus ambiguous in the brainstem. Sympathetic preganglionic neurons of the intermediolateral cell column of the spinal cord arise in the RVLM and may have either inhibitory or excitatory effects on the sympathetic preganglionic neurons. The balance of stimulation in the fibers descending from the medulla and local spinal inputs determines the nature of the effect of the activity of the sympathetic preganglionic neurons. Sympathetic preganglionic neurons travel via the ventral roots of the spinal cord to the sympathetic chain, where most synapse with the cell bodies of the sympathetic postganglionic fibers. Some extend further and may terminate directly in target organs, such as the adrenal medulla. Axons from postganglionic cell bodies are nonmyelinated and travel in mixed peripheral nerves where they terminate in the outer parts of the tunica media. Arteries and larger arterioles have a rich supply of sympathetic vasoconstrictor fibers, with less dense innervation of veins and smaller arterioles. Noradrenaline released by sympathetic postganglionic neurons act on alpha-adrenoreceptors, leading to vasoconstriction (**see also Chapters 6 and 13**). Cardiac sympathetic fibers travel subepicardially along the main coronary arteries.

Parasympathetic preganglionic fibers leave the CNS via the cranial and sacral spinal outflows. In comparison with the SNS, they terminate on the postganglionic neurons situated in the end-organs themselves, such as the heart. Below the atrioventricular groove, the parasympathetic fibers penetrate the myocardium and are subendocardial in their distribution. There is a greater density of parasympathetic innervation in the atria compared with the ventricles.

CARDIAC REFLEXES

Sympathetic outflow to the heart and peripheral tissues is regulated by cardiovascular reflexes. Increasingly these reflexes have served as the primary targets for ANS modulation as a therapy for the treatment of heart failure. Autonomic fibers carry afferent arms of these reflexes, whereas efferent limbs are formed by either somatic or autonomic nerves.

Baroreceptors are high pressure mechanoreceptors located in high pressure areas, such as the wall of the aortic arch and the carotid body (see Fig. 42.1). Afferent fibers of these receptors relay information regarding arterial pressure to the brainstem, where they terminate in the NTS. Afferents from the aortic arch travel within the vagus, whereas those from the carotid sinus are carried initially by the carotid sinus nerves, which then merge with the glossopharyngeal. The baroreceptors are dynamic receptors that respond to changes in pressure. At normal levels of blood pressure (MAP 90–100 mm Hg), there is only a modest degree of activity in the afferent nerves, which is in phase with the arterial pulse wave. A steep incline in activity occurs as pressure increases between 60 and 180 mm Hg. This afferent information leads to an increase in vagal activity and a decrease in cardiac sympathetic activity. The vagal activity causes a resultant bradycardia, while the reduction in sympathetic vasoconstriction leads to vasodilatation.

The venous mechanoreceptors that are located in the junction of the atria and the pulmonary arteries send their signals via

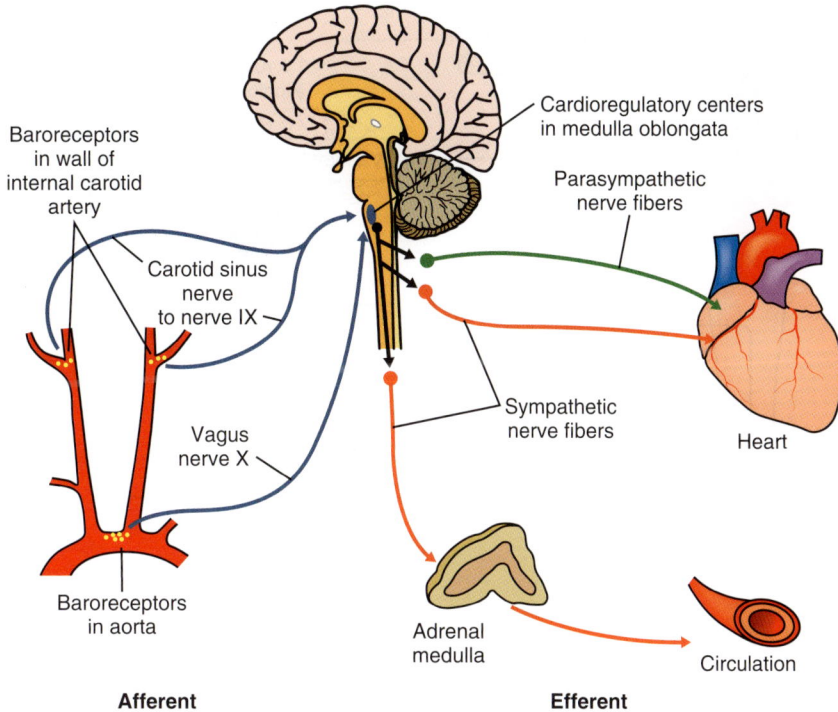

Fig. 42.1 Schematic overview of autonomic regulation of the cardiovascular system. The autonomic outflow to the heart and the peripheral circulation is regulated by cardiovascular reflexes. In humans, the primary mechanism for autonomic modulation is via the baroreflexes. The baroreflex afferents, which are highly specialized stretch-sensitive nerve endings mainly located in the wall of the carotid sinus and in the wall of the aortic arch, change their firing rate with changes in arterial pressure, and project through the glossopharyngeal and vagal nerves to the central nervous systems, where signals are integrated. The baroreflex control of circulatory homeostasis occurs on a negative feedback basis. In general, an increased firing rate of the baroreceptors secondary to a rise in systemic arterial pressure results in increased efferent cardiac vagal activity and decreased sympathetic, which in turn slows down heart rate, decreases cardiac contractility, and decreases peripheral vascular resistance. Opposite hemodynamic changes occur when a decrease in systemic arterial pressure lowers the baroreceptor firing rate, which results in an increase in efferent sympathetic nerve activity, which increases heart rate, increases cardiac contractility, and increases peripheral vascular resistance. (From La Rovere MT, Christensen JH. The autonomic nervous system and cardiovascular disease: role of n-3 PUFAs. *Vascul Pharmacol.* 2015;71:1–10.)

unmyelinated fibers of the vagus nerve as a part of the Bainbridge reflex. The Bainbridge reflex responds to increases of blood volume in venous circulation by increasing heart rate and ventricular contractility via inhibition of efferent vagal fibers. These cardiovascular reflex arcs are intimately related to each other with the Bainbridge reflex serving to counterbalance the baroreceptor reflex; the Bainbridge reflex is dominant when blood volume is increased, and the baroreceptor reflex is dominant when blood volume is decreased.

In the setting of a failing heart, a range of compensatory functions attempt to preserve cardiac function (**Fig. 42.2**). The ANS and renin-angiotensin-aldosterone system (RAAS) are the chief curators of cardiovascular homeostasis.[1] Reduced cardiac output increases afferent stimuli from baroreceptors to the CNS cardioregulatory regions, with subsequent activation of the SNS. Though acutely advantageous, the compensatory mechanisms to maintain cardiac output, which are brought about by the SNS activation, in conjunction with vasoconstriction and sodium and water retention brought about by the RAAS system, are detrimental in chronic cardiac dysfunction.[2] It is now established that alterations of the sympathovagal balance with diminished vagal activity and accelerated sympathetic activity is a predictor of increased mortality in heart failure (**see also Chapter 13**).[3] In addition to being a proarrhythmic state, a shift in the ANS balance toward

heightened SNS activity is associated with nitric oxide (NO) dysregulation, excess cytokine release, and adverse cardiac remodeling.[4-6]

MEASUREMENT OF AUTONOMIC NERVOUS SYSTEM ACTIVITY

Measurement of autonomic activity has been demonstrated to correlate with prognosis in HF. The activity of the SNS can be measured in different ways. Examples are measurement of heart rate, plasma or urinary norepinephrine (NE) level, assessment of local tissue NE spillover, muscle sympathetic nerve activity (MSNA), iodine ^{123}I-metaiodobenzylguanidine (^{123}I-mIBG), or heart rate variability (HRV; **Fig. 42.3**). The simplest assessment of overall ANS function is resting heart rate, which is a marker of SNS activation and PNS withdrawal. The SHIFT trial assessed the efficacy of ivabradine in patients with HF and found that the lowest risk of mortality was in patients with a heart rate of less than 60 beats/min. Guideline documents for the treatment of HF patients recommend treatment the use of β-blockers and ivabradine to reduce heart rate to this target (**see also Chapter 37**).[7,8]

Reduced HRV is a marker of increased mortality in HF patients. The ANS and PNS effect the beat-to-beat variability in different

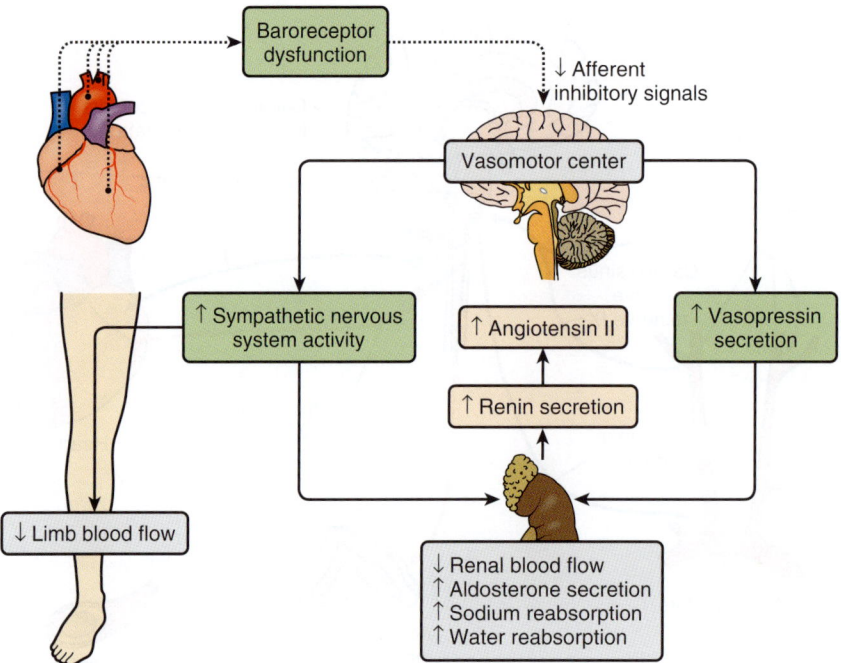

Fig. 42.2 **Activation of neurohormonal systems in heart failure.** Decreased cardiac output in patients with heart failure with reduced ejection fraction results in the unloading of high-pressure baroceptors *(black dots)* in the left ventricle, carotid sinus, and aortic arch. This unloading leads to generation of afferent signals to the central nervous system (CNS) that, in turn, leads to activation of efferent sympathetic nervous system pathways that innervate the heart, kidney, peripheral vasculature, and skeletal muscles. This unloading also leads to afferent signals to the CNS that stimulate cardioregulatory centers in the brain that stimulate the release of arginine vasopressin from the posterior pituitary. (From Hartupee J, Mann DL. Neurohormonal activation in heart failure with reduced ejection fraction. *Nat Rev Cardiol.* 2017;14[1]:30–38; and adapted from Nohria A. Cusco JA, Creager MA. Neurohumoral, renal, and vascular adjustments in heart failure. In: Colucci WS, ed. *Atlas of Heart Failure.* 4th ed. New York: Springer; 2004:101–126.)

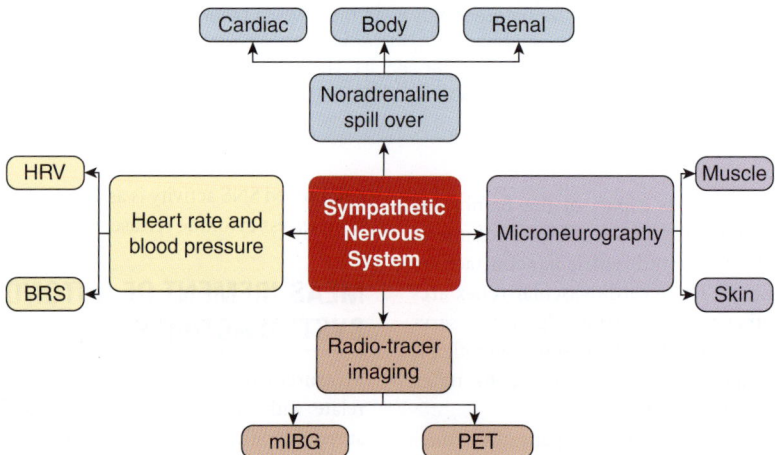

Fig. 42.3 **Different techniques to quantify the sympathetic nervous system in heart failure patients.** There are four different methods for assessing sympathetic nervous system activity in heart failure patients: norepinephrine spillover, heart rate and blood pressure response, radio-tracer imaging, and microneurography. *BRS,* Baroreceptor sensitivity; *HRV,* heart rate variability; *mIBG,* metaiodobenzylguanidine; *PET,* positron emission tomography. (Modified from Patel HC, Rosen SD, Lindsay A, Hayward C, Lyon AR, di Mario C. Targeting the autonomic nervous system: measuring autonomic function and novel devices for heart failure management. *Int J Cardiol.* 2013;170[2]:107–117.)

frequency bands.[9,10] The SNS regulates the low-frequency component of HRV, in contrast to the vagal effects, which modulates the high frequency variance. ANS balance may be assessed by computation of the low frequency/high frequency ratio.[11] Therefore, it may be possible to assess the different contributions of each limb of the ANS. HRV can easily be assessed, requiring just simple measurement of consecutive RR intervals. However, it has a number of limitations. First, the most appropriate technique for HRV measurement remains ill-defined. It can be collected in short (10 minutes) intervals with short-segment electrocardiography or over 24 hours with cardiac monitoring.

Secondly, HRV does not correlate specifically with SNS function. It measures both PNS and SNS activity, including both postsynaptic and presynaptic pathways.[12] Finally, the development of atrial fibrillation, increased ectopy, and the use of biventricular pacing as heart failure advances restricts the measurement of HRV.[13]

Quantification of NE spillover was one of the earliest attempts at assessing ANS activity. Radiotracer techniques that involve measuring radioisotopes dilution with plasma concentration of NE can be used to calculate regional NE spillover.[14] However, there is considerable variability in the way that circulating NE is metabolized by different tissues,[15] contributing to limitations in the use of NE spillover. In addition, NE increases may be related to decreased regional clearance rather than increased secretion. Microneurography facilitates measurement of nerve firing within the skin and local vasculature,[16,17] but its clinical use has been precluded by low reliability.[18]

The radiotracers iodine-labeled metaiodobenzylguanidine (^{123}I-mIBG), which is used for planar and single-photon emission computed topography (SPECT) imaging, and ^{11}C-hydroxyephedrine, which is used for positron emission topography (PET) imaging, can be used to image local SNS activity. Increased LV function has been seen in HF patients with increased sympathetic innervation as assessed by mIBG scan.[19-21] The heart-to-mediastinal (H/M) ratio is the most accepted measure used to image cardiac ANS activity. Reduced H/M ratio correlates with increased risk of arrhythmia and mortality.[22-24] The AdreView Myocardial Imaging for Risk Evaluation in Heart Failure (ADMIRE-HF) study enrolled 961 HF patients. ADMIRE-HF demonstrated that an abnormal mIBG H/M ratio was associated with major adverse cardiovascular events and ventricular arrhythmia.[25] However, other investigators have not been able to demonstrate a clear relationship between mIBG studies and arrhythmia inducibility at during electrophysiology studies.[26]

PHARMACOLOGICAL TARGETING OF AUTONOMIC NERVOUS SYSTEM DYSFUNCTION IN HEART FAILURE

The use of β-blockers to attenuate the effect of NE on Beta-1 and Beta-2 adrenoreceptors is now well established and has been recommended in international HF guidelines for more than 10 years (**see also Chapter 37**).[7,8] Targeting the PNS pharmacologically remains more challenging. Acetylcholine (ACh) is released from the presynaptic membrane and binds to parasympathetic muscarinic receptors. ACh is rapidly hydrolyzed by acetylcholinesterase. One proposed method of increasing PNS stimulation is the use of acetylcholinesterase inhibitors (ChEIs). Donepezil is a centrally acting ChEI that crosses the blood-brain barrier and is used in the treatment of Alzheimer's disease. In a retrospective 2010 study of patients with Alzheimer's disease, 76 patients who were treated with donepezil were compared with 915 who were not. Those treated with donepezil had a significantly lower rate of cardiovascular mortality compared with the control arm.[27] Donepezil has also been shown to attenuate plasma BNP levels in patients with Alzheimer's disease,[28] as well as improve LV function and decrease neurohumoral activation in animal models of HF.[29] The most compelling data on the protective effect of donepezil comes from the Swedish National Dementia Registry. In this registry of more than 7000 patients, the use of donepezil was associated with a 34% reduction in the primary endpoint of myocardial infarction or cardiovascular mortality.[30] Pyridostigmine is another ChEI, but it only acts peripherally. It increased HRV and reduced ventricular arrhythmias in a small study of 23 patients with HF. However, in addition to stimulating PNS activity, ChEI may also increase sympathetic cervical, splanchnic, and lumbar ganglionic neurotransmitters. The short-acting ChEI

edrophonium increases MSNA after administration.[31] Therefore, in addition to the SNS to restore the ANS imbalance in chronic HF, there is potential therapeutic benefit from pharmacologically targeting the PNS. However, the studies conducted on donepezil and pyridostigmine are small, and further, larger trials are required.

DEVICE-BASED MODULATION OF AUTONOMIC NERVOUS SYSTEM DYSFUNCTION IN HEART FAILURE

Interest in research into implantable devices to manipulate the ANS has ignited in recent years (**Table 42.1**). However, though early studies in animal model have demonstrated promise, this potential has not yet been successfully translated into successful clinical trials in patients with HF. In the following section, we will focus on the preclinical and clinical studies that have employed vagus nerve stimulation (VNS), baroreceptor activation therapy (BAT), spinal cord stimulation (SCS), and renal nerve denervation, with the goal of deconstructing these studies in order to better understand why it has been so difficult to translate the encouraging preclinical studies into successful phase II/III clinical trials. The important therapeutic areas of left cardiac sympathetic denervation have been the subject of several recent reviews and will not be discussed herein.

Vagus Nerve Stimulation

VNS is an approved therapy for the treatment of a wide range of medical conditions such as depression[32] and epilepsy.[33] Studies of canines with pacing-induced HF have shown that vagal stimulation leads to a significant reduction in left end-diastolic diameter and an improvement in LV ejection fraction at 4 and 8 weeks. This study, by Zhang et al., noted a marked decrease in CRP, angiotensin II, and NE in the animals treated with VNS versus controls.[33a] Further research in rats with HF from ischemia also demonstrated a reduction in LV end diastolic diameter, and an improved survival at 140 days (86% compared with 50%) in the animals in the treatment arm.[33b] In addition to improved LV function, VNS decreases ventricular arrhythmias in animal models.[34,35]

The postulated mechanisms behind the beneficial effects vary. These include an anti-inflammatory effect supported by the decrease in CRP seen in the study above by Zhang et al. Locally produced cytokines may initiate a reflex afferent response via sensory fibers traveling to the NTS. Vagal stimulates inhibit tumor necrosis factor (TNF) and macrophage activation, reducing this inflammatory response. Efferent vagal fibers cause the release of ACh in the reticuloendothelial system,[36] which inhibits the release of several inflammatory cytokines.[37] NO release is increased following vagal stimulation, and is another mechanism through which VNS can mediate its beneficial effects. NO has a number of diverse and often opposing cardiac effects, but can inhibit ischemia/reperfusion injury and prevent LV remodeling. Finally, vagal blockade increases plasma renin activity,[38] while VNS inhibits renin release.[39]

There are three devices currently available for VNS (**Fig. 42.4**). The CardioFit device (Biocontrol Medical, New Hope, MN) utilizes an RV sensing lead (referred to as a closed-loop system), whereas the other two devices, the Precision (Boston Scientific, Marlborough, MA) and Demipulse (Cyberonics, Houston, TX) do not (referred to as an open-loop system). Following a surgical exposure of the vagus within the carotid sheath, the vagal nerve stimulation cuff is usually positioned 3 cm below the carotid bifurcation (**Fig. 42.5**). In this position, the vagus carries both cardiac and noncardiac fibers. The first human study of VNS was an eight-patient phase II trial undertaken with the CardioFit device. Eight patients were followed for 6 months.[40] VNS was noted to

TABLE 42.1 Trials of Device-Based Modulation of the Autonomic Nervous System in Heart Failure

Trial Name	Device	Trial Design	Patients	Outcomes	Follow-up	Results	References
Vagus Nerve Stimulation							
CardioFit	CardioFit, BioControl Medical.	Multicenter, open-label, noncontrolled	32 Patients; EF ≤35%, NYHA II–III; AF and plan for CRT excluded	1. Procedure related adverse events 2. NYHA, QoL, 6MWT, LV volumes	6 months	3 deaths unrelated to procedure 12 patients had device related pain, cough and dysphonia Improved NYHA, QoL, 6MWT, EF	41
NECTAR-HF	Precision, Boston Scientific	Multicenter, 2:1 randomization, sham-controlled	96 Patients; EF ≤35%, NYHA II–III, LVEDD ≥5.5 cm; AF and planned CRT, or CRT in situ <1 year excluded	1. LVESD 2. LVESV, EF, peak VO2, NT-proBNP, QQL, 6MWT	6 months	No Change in LVESD. Improved QoL and NYHA Device related coughing and facial paresthesia	42
ANTHEM-HF	IPG 103, Cyberonics	Multicenter, open-label, controlled	60 Patients; EF ≤40%, NYHA II–III, LVEDD 5–8 cm, QRS <150 msec	1. Procedure related complications 2. LVESV and EF 3. NYHA, QoL, 6MWT	6 months	1 procedure related death Improved LVESD, EF, NYHA, QoL, 6MWT	43
INOVATE-HF	CardioFit, BioControl Medical	Multicenter, 3:2 randomized, open-labeled	707 Patients; EF ≤40%, NYHA II–III, LVEDD 5–8; AF excluded	1. All-cause mortality or HFH 2. Freedom from procedure related complications 3. NYHA, 6MWT, LVESV, QoL	16 months	- No benefit in reducing mortality/HFH - No safety issues - Improved NYHA, 6MWT, QoL	44
Spinal Cord Stimulation							
SCS Heart Study	Eon Mini, Abbott	Multicenter, 4 patients who did not fulfill study criteria as controls	22 patients; EF 20%–35%, LVEDD 55–80 mm, ICD, NYHA III; Excluded for AF, prior spinal cord stimulator	1. Death due to VT, MI, or SCD 2. HFH 3. Composite score of QoL, VO2, NT-proBNP and others	6 months	Significant improvements in EF, QoL, EF, VO2, and LVESVi - No deaths	56
DEFEAT-HF	PrimeAdvanced Neurostimulator, Medtronic	Multicenter, randomized controlled trial. Patients randomized 3:2 to SCS "on" or "off" initially. All "on" at 6 months.	66 patients; EF ≤35%, QRS <120 ms, NYHA III; CRT patients excluded	1. Changes in LVESVi 2. VO2 max, NT-proBNP	12 months	- No changes in LVESVi. - No significant difference in secondary endpoints	57
Carotid Baroreceptor Stimulation							
Gronda et al.	Barostim neo, CVRx Inc	Single center, open-label, uncontrolled	11 Patients; EF ≤40%, NYHA III; Excluded if no indication for CRT or eGFR <30 mL/min	1. Reduction SNS activity. 2. Safety, BRS, EF, hemodynamics	6 months	Improvements in MSNA and BRS Improved QoL, 6MWT, EF	53
Barostim neo HF, Barostim HOPE4HF	Barostim neo, CVRx Inc	Multicenter, randomized, open-label, controlled	146 Patients; EF ≤35%, NYHA III; Carotid artery stenosis >50%, eGFR <30 mL/min, and recent CRT excluded	1. Safety (MANCE) 2. NYHA, QoL, 6MWT	6 months	Procedure was safe. MANCE free rate 9.2% Improvements in NYHA, QoL, 6MWT	54

TABLE 42.1 Trials of Device-Based Modulation of the Autonomic Nervous System in Heart Failure—cont'd

Trial Name	Device	Trial Design	Patients	Outcomes	Follow-up	Results	References
Renal Nerve Denervation							
REACH-pilot	Simplicity, Medtronic	Single center, open-label, uncontrolled	7 Patients; Systolic HF, NYHA III–IV; eGFR <35 mL/min excluded	Safety	6 months	No safety concerns. 6 MWT improved	65
RDT-PEF	Simplicity, Medtronic	Single center, randomized, open-label	25 Patients; EF >40%, NYHA II–III, BNP >35 ng/L or increased LAV/LVH; Excluded patients with eGFR <45 mL/min or if CMR contraindicated	1. QoL, peak VO$_2$, BNP, E/e´, LAV, LVM. 2. Safety	12 months	A signal for improvement in co-primary endpoints at 3 months, which did not persist at 12 months Renal angioplasty required during procedure in 2 patients	66

6MWT, 6-minute walk test; *AF,* atrial fibrillation; *BRS,* baroreceptor sensitivity; *CMR,* cardiac magnetic resonance imaging; *CRT,* cardiac resynchronization therapy; *EF,* ejection fraction; *eGFR,* estimated glomerular filtration rate; *HFH,* heart failure hospitalization; *LAV,* left atrial volume; *LVEDD,* left ventricular end diastolic diameter; *LVESD,* left ventricular end-systolic diameter; *LVESV,* left ventricular end-systolic volume; *LVH,* left ventricular hypertrophy; *MANCE,* major adverse neurological and cardiovascular events; *MI,* myocardial infarction; *MSNA,* muscle sympathetic nerve activity; *NYHA,* New York Heart Classification; *QoL,* quality-of-life questionnaires; *SNS,* sympathetic nervous system; *VO$_2$,* oxygen uptake; *VT,* ventricular tachycardia.

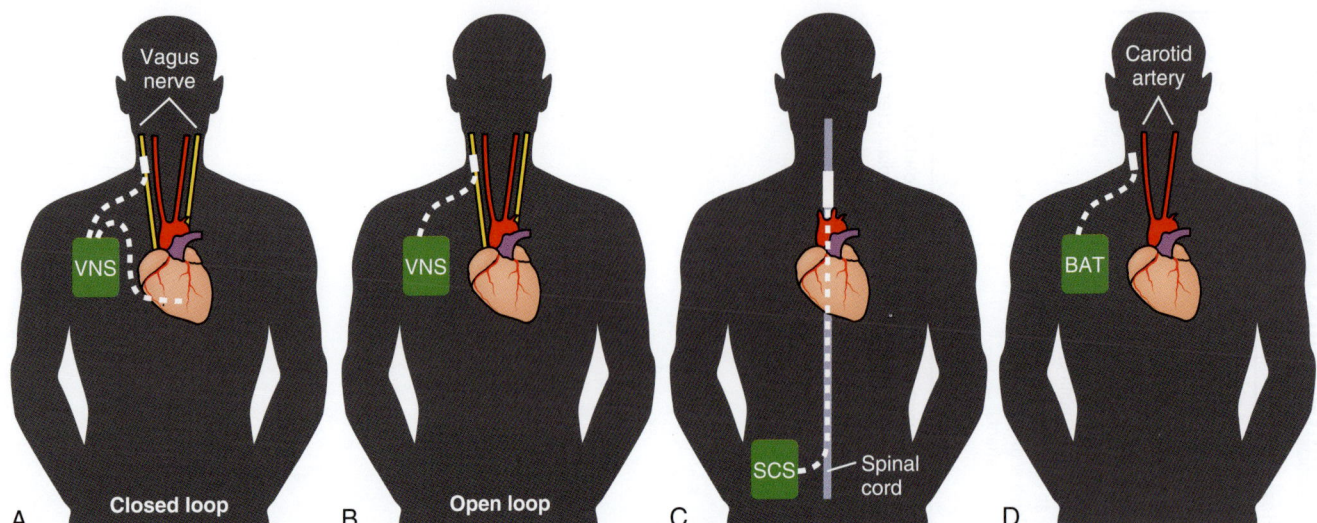

Fig. 42.4 Schematic demonstrating the location and stimulation sites for device-based neuromodulatory activity. (A) Vagus nerve stimulator placed in right subpectoral region with standard transvenous pacing/sensing lead placed in right ventricular *(closed loop)* and vagus nerve stimulating lead *(dotted white lines)* tunneled to cervical vagus region. (B) Vagus nerve stimulator placed in right subpectoral region with vagus nerve stimulating lead *(dotted white line)* tunneled to cervical vagus region *(open loop)*. (C) The spinal cord stimulation generator is implanted in abdomen or paraspinous region with stimulation lead *(blue line)* placed in dorsal epidural space at thoracic level 4. (D) Baroreflex stimulation generator placed in right subpectoral region with bilateral stimulation leads tunneled to the carotid baroreceptor region. *BAT,* Baroreceptor activation therapy; *SCS,* spinal cord stimulation; *VNS,* vagus nerve stimulation. (From Byku M, Mann DL. Neuromodulation of the failing heart: lost in translation? *JACC Basic Transl Sci.* 2016;1[3]:95–106; and modified and adapted from Lopshire JC, Zipes DP. Device therapy to modulate the autonomic nervous system to treat heart failure. *Curr Cardiol Rep.* 2012;14[5]:593–600.)

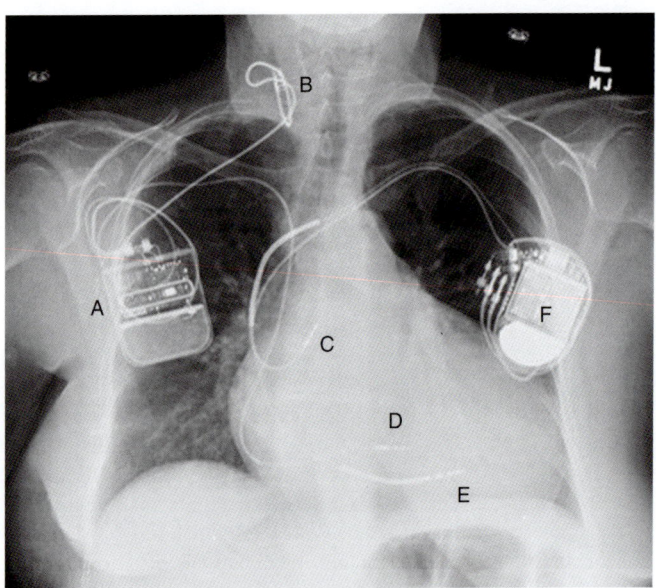

Fig. 42.5 Chest X-ray of a patient following VNS implant. (A) Implanted VNS generator; (B) **cuff** placed around vagus nerve in carotid sheath; (C) ICD right atrial lead; (D) VNS RV lead; (E) ICD RV lead; (F) dual chamber ICD generator. *RV,* Right ventricle; *VNS,* vagus nerve stimulation.

be well tolerated, and was associated with improved NYHA class, LV end-systolic volume, and quality of life. A further multicenter study of 32 patients supported these findings.[41] Neural Cardiac Therapy for Heart Failure (NECTAR-HF) was the first randomized sham-controlled trial designed for VNS. This study assessed VNS using the Boston Scientific

Precision Pulse generator. A total of 96 patients were randomized in a 2:1 fashion to therapy on or off. The NECTAR-HF trial did not meet the primary end point of the trial, which was change in LV end-systolic diameter (LVESD) from baseline after a 6-month period.[42]

The Autonomic Neural Regulation Therapy to Enhance Myocardial Function in Heart Failure (ANTHEM-HF) used different vagus stimulation parameters compared with NECTAR. In ANTHEM, higher amplitudes and frequencies were employed to achieve VNS. ANTHEM randomized 60 patients to left versus right VNS with the Demipulse model 103 (Cyberonics). Over the 6-month follow-up period, 77% of patients improved at least one NYHA class. There were also statistically significant improvements in LVEF, LVESD, and high-sensitivity CRP. The device was well tolerated.[43]

VNS with the CardioFit Monitor (Biocontrol Medical, Israel) was under evaluation in the INNOVATE-HF (Increase of Vagal Tone in Heart Failure) international study of the CardioFit device.[44] It enrolled 707 patients with NYHA III, who were randomized in a 3:2 fashion to VNS or ongoing medical therapy. The primary end point was time to all-cause mortality or first HF hospitalization. The trial was stopped early because of futility at a mean follow-up period of 16 months. The primary end point occurred in 30.3% of the active arm and 25.8% of those with medical therapy, with no difference in survival (**Fig. 42.6**).

Therefore, despite very promising preclinical data supporting the use of VNS in HF, these preclinical studies have not translated to patients. The optimal VNS protocol remains undefined. Further rigorous preclinical work is necessary to clarify other variable parameters of VNS, including stimulation frequency, synchronization to the cardiac cycle, whether the left or right vagus is used, and whether afferent, efferent, or both nerves should be preferentially stimulated. The use of VNS in HF has a strong rationale, and appears feasible and safe; however, the most extensive studies to date have been negative.

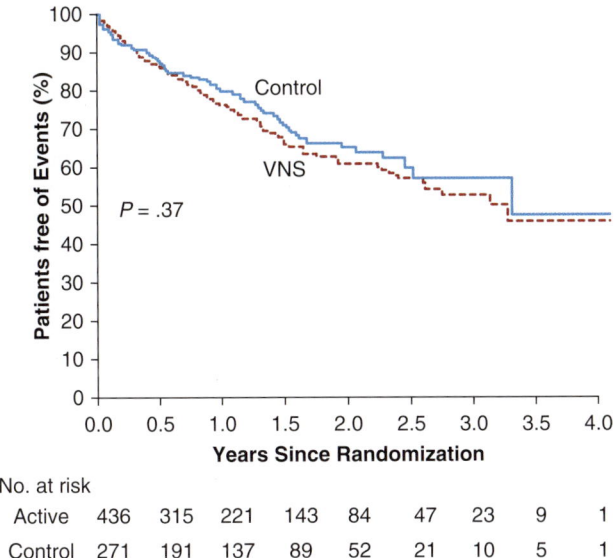

No. at risk								
Active	436	315	221	143	84	47	23	9	1
Control	271	191	137	89	52	21	10	5	1

Fig. 42.6 Primary efficacy end point of the INOVATE-HF trial. There was no significant difference in the primary composite outcome of death from any cause or a worsening heart failure event in the vagus nerve stimulation *(VNS)* treatment arm when compared with the control group (hazard ratio, 1.14; 95% confidence interval, 0.86–1.53; *P* = .37). (From Gold MR, Van Veldhuisen DJ, Hauptman PJ, et al. Vagus nerve stimulation for the treatment of heart failure: the INOVATE-HF trial. *J Am Coll Cardiol.* 2016;68:149–158.)

Carotid Baroreceptor Stimulation

The carotid body is an ovoid organ sitting at the bifurcation of each carotid (see Fig. 42.1). It is innervated by the carotid sinus nerve (a branch of the glossopharyngeal), nerve fibers from the vagus, and sympathetic innervation from nearby ganglia. Chemoreceptors in the carotid body respond to acute hypoxemia, as well as hypoglycemia, acidotic pH, and variations in the arterial carbon dioxide tension. Stimulation of the chemoreceptors increases sympathetic tone. Baroreceptors are also present in the carotid body. Activation of these stretch-sensitive mechanoreceptors reduces sympathetic outflow and increases vagal tone.[45,46] Carotid sinus stimulation was first studied as a treatment for angina and hypertension 60 years ago; however, this work did not progress because of technologic limitations of the time. Baroreceptor dysfunction is a feature of early HF, and may escalate as the disease progresses. Improving baroreflex function may ameliorate the neurohormonal excitation that accompanies HF progression.[3,47] Preclinical work demonstrated that baroreceptor stimulation leads to enhanced survival in dogs with pacing-induced HF.[48] This was associated with a reduction in plasma NE levels. In conjunction with this reduction in NE, other investigators have described a reduction in angiotensin II levels.[45,47,49,50]

Baroreflex stimulator leads are implanted following ultrasound guided exposure of the carotid bifurcation. The electrode is positioned in the carotid sinus, with the optimal location identified by eliciting the hemodynamic response in a number of locations. Leads may be unilateral or bilateral. The leads are then tunneled to the generator, which sits in the infraclavicular area, in a similar position to a pacemaker. The Rheos system (CVRx, Minneapolis, MN) is the most investigated carotid body stimulation (CBS) device to date. It consists of a pulse generator and two electrodes leads, which are connected to the perivascular tissue of the carotid sinuses bilaterally.

The Device Based Therapy of Hypertension Trial (DEBuT-HT) was a phase II, nonrandomized study of CBS in 45 patients with drug-resistant hypertension. After a 2-year follow-up, a significant reduction in BP (33/22 mm Hg) was observed.[51] A prospective substudy of this investigation reported that in patients with early stage HF, the treatment resulted in a significant reduction in left atrial dimensions and a reduction in left ventricular mass.[52]

In a pilot feasibility study of 11 patients with HF, CBS caused a marked and sustained reduction in sympathetic activation.[53] There was a reduction in HF hospitalizations, and an improvement in exercise tolerance and NYHA class. The Barostim HOPE4HF trial randomized 146 patients with NYHA III and EF of less than 35% to treatment with BAT (baroreflex activation therapy) or control. BAT was shown to improve VO$_2$ max, 6-minute walk test, and EF. There was also a reduction in days hospitalized for HF, though this was not significant. There was no change in EF between the two study arms.[54] Overall, BAT appears to be safe, though the evidence to date is limited to two small trials. The Barostim therapy for Heart Failure Study (BeAT-HF, ClinicalTrials.gov ID: NCT 02627196) is currently recruiting. Hopefully this study will further our understanding of the potential role of BAT in HF. This study of BAT in 600 patients with systolic HF, commenced recruitment in 2016 and has an estimated completion year of 2021. In addition to the studies noted, novel strategies of carotid sinus nerve stimulation are being evaluated. This includes the Acute Carotid sinus Endovascular Stimulation study (ACES-II, ClinicalTrials.gov ID: NCT01458483), which is uses a catheter in the internal jugular vein to stimulate the carotid sinus.

Spinal Cord Stimulation

SCS, which involves placement of one or two electrodes within the epidural space (see Fig. 42.4), is an FDA-approved treatment for chronic pain and refractory angina. The beneficial effects of SCS on HF and the risk of arrhythmias have been well described in animal models. SCS administered to a canine model of HF reduced infarct size and ventricular arrhythmias.[55,56] Canine postinfarct models with ICD implanted were randomized to SCS, medical therapy, or a combination of SCS and medical therapy. The SCS groups showed the largest improvement in LVEF and a marked reduction in ventricular arrhythmias, as well as a decline in BNP and plasma NE levels.

The first in-human study was the SCS Heart Study, which involved use of Eon Mini neurostimulation system (Abbott Medical, Lake Bluff IL). Two octrode electrodes were implanted under fluoroscopic guidance in 17 patients with NYHA III to IV HF. The leads were placed from T1 to T3. Four patients who did not consent to the device implantation served as controls. A total 13 of the 17 patients in the treatment arm improved NYHA class. Statistically significant improvements in LVEF (26 ± 6% vs. 37 ± 8%) and LVESV (174 ± 57 mls vs. 137 ± 37 mls) were also seen.[57] Complications noted in the study included back and neck paresthesia in one patient, lead dislodgement requiring repositioning, and inappropriate motor stimulation.

The DEFEAT-HF (determining the feasibility of spinal cord neuromodulation for the treatment of chronic HF) was a phase II randomized trial of 81 patients, again with NYHA class III to IV and EF less than 35%. All patients had SCS implanted and were randomized in a 2:1 fashion to either no treatment for the first 6 months, or active therapy. Unfortunately, over the 6 months of this study, there was no statistically significant reduction in left-ventricular end-systolic volume index (LVESVi); indeed patients randomized to SCS-off tended to have a higher likelihood of reduction in LVESVi (38% vs. 70%) compared with SCS-on.[58]

Renal Sympathetic Denervation

Stimulation of efferent sympathetic nerves increases renin secretion from the juxtaglomerular cells, as well as causing vasoconstriction, which results in reduced glomerular filtration. Activation of afferent nerves stimulates CNS centers, which are involved in ANS regulation. The renal sympathetic nerves course alongside the renal arteries, moving closer to the arterial lumen as they move more distally from the aorta.[59] This proximity of artery and nerves facilitates destruction of the nerves by transcatheter techniques as a target for HF and hypertension.

The early excitement in renal sympathetic denervation (RDN) was stirred by RCTs using a single-electrode Simplicity catheter (Medtronic, Minneapolis, MN) in patients with treatment-resistant hypertension. The initial first-in man studies reported profoundly beneficial effects of RDN on hypertension.[60] However, this enthusiasm was tempered significantly following the SIMPLICITY HTN-3 trial. This blinded, sham-controlled RCT failed to show any benefit.[61]

Surgical denervation in animal models of heart failure surgical renal denervation has resulted in improved renal perfusion and increased ejection fractions.[62] Following infarction in rats, it has been shown to be superior to traditional HF therapies with β-blockers and ACE inhibitors in preventing adverse remodeling.[63] Studies of transcatheter RDN in canines have shown improved EFs, less myocardial fibrosis, as well as reductions in plasma aldosterone, NE, natriuretic peptides, and angiotensin II.[64] In addition, RDN in animals has positive antiarrhythmic effects.[65]

The REACH-pilot was a study of seven patients with HF and an average EF of 43%. The predominant aim of this study was to assess the overall safety of RDN in humans with HF. After a 6-month follow-up, the authors concluded that it was a safe therapy, with no significant hypotension or renal dysfunction. In addition each patient had improved 6-minute walk distances.[66] A total of 25 patients were randomized to RDN or usual care in the Renal Denervation in heart failure with preserved ejection fraction trial (RDT-PEF). At 3 months, improvements in peak oxygen uptake and E/e′ were seen, but these findings did not persist to 12 months and the overall primary composite endpoint was neutral.[67]

SUMMARY AND FUTURE DIRECTIONS

ANS imbalances play a crucial role in the progression of HF. The greater this imbalance, the greater the risk of mortality in patients.[13] Enormous strides have been made in treating HF over recent decades, which has translated into significant improvements in quality of life and prognosis for patients. Pharmacological beta-blockade reduces sympathetic activation is one of the first-line interventions initiated in patients with reduced LV systolic function. Their role in HF demonstrates the positive impact of ANS modulation in HF.

Despite these treatments, the mortality in HF remains unacceptably high. Innovative nonpharmacological strategies have evolved and are under ongoing investigation to facilitate further manipulation of the ANS as therapeutic intervention in HF. The next generation of HF therapies is likely to involve device-based modulation of the ANS. There is a wealth of preclinical studies confirming the great potential of these treatments. However, human studies thus far have faltered in proving to have a significant clinical impact. The poor performance of devices used in human trials of neuromodulation suggests that technologies have progressed at a greater pace than our understanding of ANS physiology. For many therapies, important variables in stimulation, such as timing, frequencies, and current amplitude, remain undefined. Great potential exists, but we are yet to learn how to harness it. Undoubtedly, once these hurdles are overcome, device-based manipulation of the ANS will become a pivotal treatment for patients with HF.

KEY REFERENCES

13. van Bilsen M, Patel HC, Bauersachs J, et al. The autonomic nervous system as a therapeutic target in heart failure: a scientific position statement from the Translational Research Committee of the Heart Failure Association of the European Society of Cardiology. *Eur J Heart Fail.* 2017;19:1361–1378.

30. Nordstrom P, Religa D, Wimo A, et al. The use of cholinesterase inhibitors and the risk of myocardial infarction and death: a nationwide cohort study in subjects with Alzheimer's disease. *Eur Heart J.* 2013;34:2585–2591.

41. De Ferrari GM, Crijns HJ, Borggrefe M, et al. Chronic vagus nerve stimulation: a new and promising therapeutic approach for chronic heart failure. *Eur Heart J.* 2011;32:847–855.

42. Zannad F, De Ferrari GM, Tuinenburg AE, et al. Chronic vagal stimulation for the treatment of low ejection fraction heart failure: results of the neural cardiac therapy for heart failure (NECTAR-HF) randomized controlled trial. *Eur Heart J.* 2015;36:425–433.

44. Gold MR, Van Veldhuisen DJ, Hauptman PJ, et al. Vagus nerve stimulation for the treatment of heart failure: the INOVATE-HF trial. *J Am Coll Cardiol.* 2016;68:149–158.

51. Scheffers IJ, Kroon AA, Schmidli J, et al. Novel baroreflex activation therapy in resistant hypertension: results of a European multi-center feasibility study. *J Am Coll Cardiol.* 2010;56:1254–1258.

54. Abraham WT, Zile MR, Weaver FA, et al. Baroreflex activation therapy for the treatment of heart failure with a reduced ejection fraction. *JACC Heart Fail.* 2015;3:487–496.

57. Tse HF, Turner S, Sanders P, et al. Thoracic Spinal Cord Stimulation for Heart Failure as a Restorative Treatment (SCS HEART Study): first-in-man experience. *Heart Rhythm.* 2015;12:588–595.

58. Zipes DP, Neuzil P, Theres H, et al. Determining the feasibility of spinal cord neuromodulation for the treatment of chronic systolic heart failure: the DEFEAT-HF study. *JACC Heart Fail.* 2016;4:129–136.

66. Davies JE, Manisty CH, Petraco R, et al. First-in-man safety evaluation of renal denervation for chronic systolic heart failure: primary outcome from REACH-Pilot study. *Int J Cardiol.* 2013;162:189–192.

The full reference list for this chapter is available on ExpertConsult.

Pulmonary Hypertension

Hilary M. DuBrock, Shannon M. Dunlay, Margaret M. Redfield

PULMONARY HYPERTENSION: DEFINITION AND CLASSIFICATION

Pulmonary hypertension (PH) is a hemodynamic finding and is considered to be present when the mean pulmonary artery pressure (mPAP) is greater than 20 mm Hg as recently defined by the Sixth World Symposium on Pulmonary Hypertension. Historically, PH has been defined as a mPAP ≥25 mm Hg, but the definition was recently re-evaluated and changed to a mPAP of >20 mm Hg to reflect a value that is two standard deviations above the mean normal value for mPAP. It should be noted, however, that studies referenced in this chapter have used a mPAP ≥25 mm Hg to define PH and that the role of pulmonary hypertension targeted therapy for treatment of PH with a mPAP of 21–24 mm Hg is not known[1] (**Table 43.1**). PH is *suspected* based on clinical features or when echocardiography reveals an elevation in Doppler-derived estimates of PAPs and/or unexplained right ventricular enlargement or dysfunction. When the clinical situation and/or echocardiographic findings raise the suspicion of PH, a

right heart catheterization must be performed to confirm the presence of PH and to determine the specific hemodynamic perturbation causing the elevation of mPAP: precapillary PH (PAH), isolated postcapillary PH, increased cardiac output, or some combination of these patterns (see Table 43.1). Finally, the underlying disease process or processes leading to PH must be defined.

A wide range of diseases can cause PH. The outdated separation of PH into primary and secondary causes has been replaced by a classification where PH is apportioned to five broad groups according to the underlying disease process and specific hemodynamic characteristics (**Table 43.2**). In general, the clinical classification of PH, as defined by the Sixth World Symposium on Pulmonary Hypertension, identifies groups with common pathophysiology and treatment implications, and thus provides a context in which to structure the diagnostic evaluation.[1]

The prevalence of PH and the contribution of each PH group to the global burden of PH have not been well defined, and will vary according to practice setting and adequacy of diagnostic evaluation. An observational cohort study of an echocardiographic laboratory serving a region of Australia reported an estimated minimum prevalence of 326 cases of PH per 100,000 individuals, with the predominance of cases due to left heart disease (**Fig. 43.1**).[2]

CLINICAL FEATURES RAISING THE SUSPICION OF PULMONARY HYPERTENSION

The symptoms of PH are nonspecific and influenced by the hemodynamic type and underlying disease, but PH should be suspected in patients complaining of dyspnea, fatigue, exercise intolerance, chest pain, syncope, or edema. The physical examination

may reveal evidence of PH as well as clues to the etiology of PH (**Table 43.3**).

Enlargement of the central pulmonary arteries with peripheral pruning of the pulmonary vasculature may be present on chest radiograph (CXR) in patients with PAH. In the case of concomitant right ventricular failure, right ventricular enlargement (decrease in retrosternal space) and right atrial enlargement (enlarged right heart border) also may be seen (**Fig. 43.2**). Findings on electrocardiography (ECG) include signs of right ventricular hypertrophy such as right axis deviation, tall R wave in V1, and inverted T waves and ST depression in lead V1 to V3, and tall p waves in lead II due to right atrial enlargement.

TABLE 43.1 Hemodynamic Parameters Defining Types of Pulmonary Hypertension

	True Normal	PAH	Isolated Postcapillary PH	Combined Precapillary and Postcapillary PH	High Output State
Established Parameters					
Mean PAP (mPAP, mm Hg)	<15	>20	>20	>20	>20
Systolic PAP (PASP, mm Hg)	<25	>35–40	>35–40	>35–40	>35–40
Mean PCWP (mm Hg)	<12	≤15	>15	>15	variable
PVR ([mPAP-PCWP]/CO, wood units)	<2	≥3	< 3	≥ 3	<3
Cardiac index (L/min/m^2)	>2.5	variable	variable	variable	>5
Emerging Parameters					
Mean TPG (mPAP-PCWP, mm Hg)	<7	>12	≤12	>12	<12
Diastolic PG (PADP-PCWP, mm Hg)	<5	≥7	<7	≥7	<7
Reactivity testing in Group I PAH	Appropriate Agents			Positive Response	
	Inhaled NO, IV Adenosine, IV Prostacyclin			↓mPAP ≥10 mm Hg *and* to <40 mm Hg without ↓ in CO	

CO, Cardiac output; *IV,* intravenous; *mPAP,* mean pulmonary artery pressure; *NO,* nitric oxide; *PADP,* pulmonary artery diastolic pressure; *PAP,* pulmonary artery pressure; *PAH,* pulmonary arterial hypertension; *PASP,* systolic pulmonary artery pressure; *PCWP,* pulmonary capillary wedge pressure; *PG,* pressure gradient; *PVH,* pulmonary venous hypertension; *PVR,* pulmonary vascular resistance; *TPG,* transpulmonary gradient.

TABLE 43.2 Classification of Pulmonary Hypertension

Group 1 PH: Pulmonary Arterial Hypertension
1.1 Idiopathic (IPAH)
1.2 Heritable or Familial (FPAH)
1.3 Drug and toxin induced
1.4 Associated with (APAH)
    1.4.1 Connective tissue disease
    1.4.2 Human immunodeficiency virus infection
    1.4.3 Portal hypertension
    1.4.4 Congenital heart disease
    1.4.5 Schistosomiasis
1.5 PAH long-term responders to calcium channel blockers
1.6 PAH with overt features of venous/capillaries (PVOD/PCH) involvement
1.7 Persistent PH of the newborn

Group 2 PH: PH Due to Left Heart Disease
2.1 PH due to heart failure with preserved left ventricular ejection fraction
2.2 PH due to heart failure with reduced left ventricular ejection fraction
2.3 Valvular disease
2.4 Congenital or acquired cardiovascular conditions leading to postcapillary PH

Group 3 PH: PH Associated With Lung Disease and/or Hypoxia
3.1 Obstructive lung disease
3.2 Restrictive lung disease
3.3 Other pulmonary diseases with mixed obstructive and restrictive pattern
3.4 Hypoxia without lung disease
3.5 Developmental lung disorders

Group 4 PH: PH due to pulmonary artery obstructions
4.1 Chronic thromboembolic PH
4.2 Other pulmonary artery obstructions

Group 5 PH: Pulmonary Hypertension With Unclear Multifactorial Mechanisms
5.1 Hematological disorders
5.2 Systemic and metabolic disorders
5.3 Others
5.4 Complex congenital heart disease

APAH, Associated pulmonary arterial hypertension; *IPAH,* idiopathic pulmonary arterial hypertension; *PH,* pulmonary hypertension.
Reproduced with permission of the © ERS 2019: European Respiratory Journal 1801913; DOI: 10.1183/13993003.01913-2018 Published 13 December 2018.

DIAGNOSTIC EVALUATION OF PULMONARY HYPERTENSION

In general, evidence of PH is discovered when echocardiography is obtained during the evaluation of known or suspected left heart or lung disease. If the severity of PH at Doppler echocardiography is

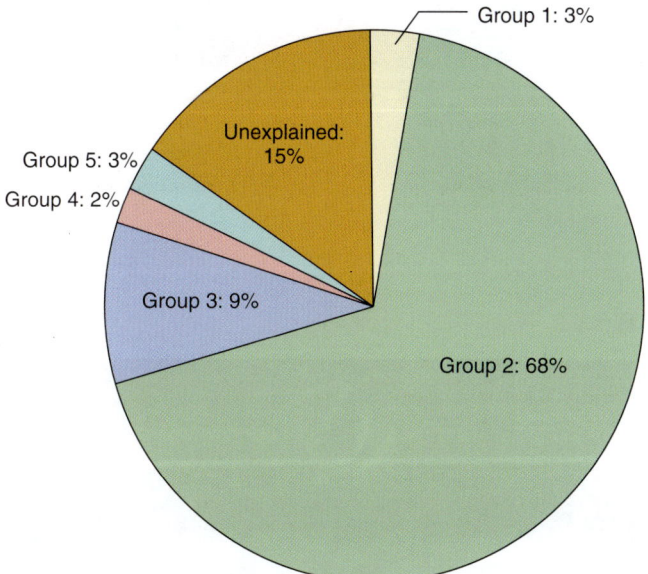

Fig. 43.1 Distribution of the underlying etiology of pulmonary hypertension. The proportions of patients with pulmonary hypertension (PH) classified as group 1 (pulmonary arterial hypertension), group 2 (PH due to left-sided disease), group 3 (PH due to lung disease), group 4 (PH due to chronic thromboembolic disease), group 5 (PH due to rare miscellaneous causes), or unexplained among an Australian cohort are shown. (From Strange G, Playford D, Stewart S, et al. Pulmonary hypertension: prevalence and mortality in the Armadale echocardiography cohort. *Heart*. 2012;98[24]:1805–1811.)

consistent with the severity of known left heart or lung disease, PH is usually attributed to the underlying process without further evaluation. However, if the severity of PH appears out of proportion to the severity of left heart or lung disease or if PH is found in the absence of known cardiopulmonary disease, a rigorous evaluation should be performed to characterize the severity of PH and ascertain the etiology. Guidelines recommend a comprehensive evaluation when the Doppler estimated right ventricular systolic pressure (RVSP) exceeds 40 to 50 mm Hg in the absence of a clear etiology,[3] particularly in the setting of right heart structural and functional abnormalities, and in patient cohorts at an elevated risk of PAH; for example, scleroderma, chronic liver disease, or human immunodeficiency virus (HIV) infection.

Even in the setting of an obvious cause, the potential for an additional process contributing to PH should be entertained to address concomitant and potentially treatable causes of PH. For example, a diagnosis of chronic thromboembolic pulmonary hypertension (CTEPH) (Group 4 PH) should not be missed since this form of PH is potentially curable with surgery. Left heart or pulmonary disease are risk factors for sleep-disordered breathing (Group 3), and patients with pulmonary disease may have unrecognized left heart disease (and vice versa). Understanding the degree of PH expected in patients with left heart or pulmonary disease is required to appreciate when PH is "out of proportion" and suggestive of additional processes.

The accepted diagnostic evaluation of PH is shown in **Table 43.4** and focuses on pivotal tests warranted in the evaluation of patients with PH in whom the etiology is not obvious from the history, physical examination, CXR, and ECG. When pivotal tests are positive, contingent tests are obtained. The order and extent of the evaluation will be influenced by clinical suspicion but echocardiography should be performed in all patients.

Echocardiographic Evaluation of Known or Suspected Pulmonary Hypertension

Echocardiography is a central test in the clinical evaluation of known or suspected PH. The echocardiogram should address three key features. The first is an assessment of pulmonary hemodynamics. With

TABLE 43.3 Physical Examination in Pulmonary Hypertension

Finding	Implications	Finding	Etiologic Insights
Inspection		Clubbing	Congenital HD, PVOD
↑ JVP	RV failure	Central Cyanosis	Hypoxia; R→L shunt
↑ A wave	Early RV failure	Sclerodactyly	Collagen vascular disease
V wave	Tricuspid regurgitation	Telangiectasia	
Ascites	RV failure	Rash	
Edema	RV failure	Raynaud's	
Palpation		Varicose veins	Thromboembolic disease
Right parasternal lift	RV enlargement	Stasis pigment/ulcer	
Hepatomegaly	RV failure	Splenomegaly	Portopulmonary PH
Pulsatile liver	Tricuspid regurgitation	Spider angioma	
Auscultation		Palmar erythema	
↑ S₂P	Elevated PAP	Icterus	
Early systolic click	Elevated PAP	Caput medusa	
Holosystolic murmur RSB	Tricuspid regurgitation	Velcro rales	Interstitial lung disease
Inspiratory accentuation	Tricuspid regurgitation	Left sided murmur	Left heart disease
Diastolic murmur <u>LUSB</u>	Pulmonic regurgitation	Apical S₃ or S₄	
S₃ or S₄ RSB	RV failure	Laterally displaced apex	

JVP, Jugular venous pressure; *LUSB*, left upper sternal border; *PH*, pulmonary hypertension; *PVOD* pulmonary veno-occlusive disease; *RSB*, right sternal border; *RV*, right ventricular; *S₂P*, pulmonic component of the second heart sound.

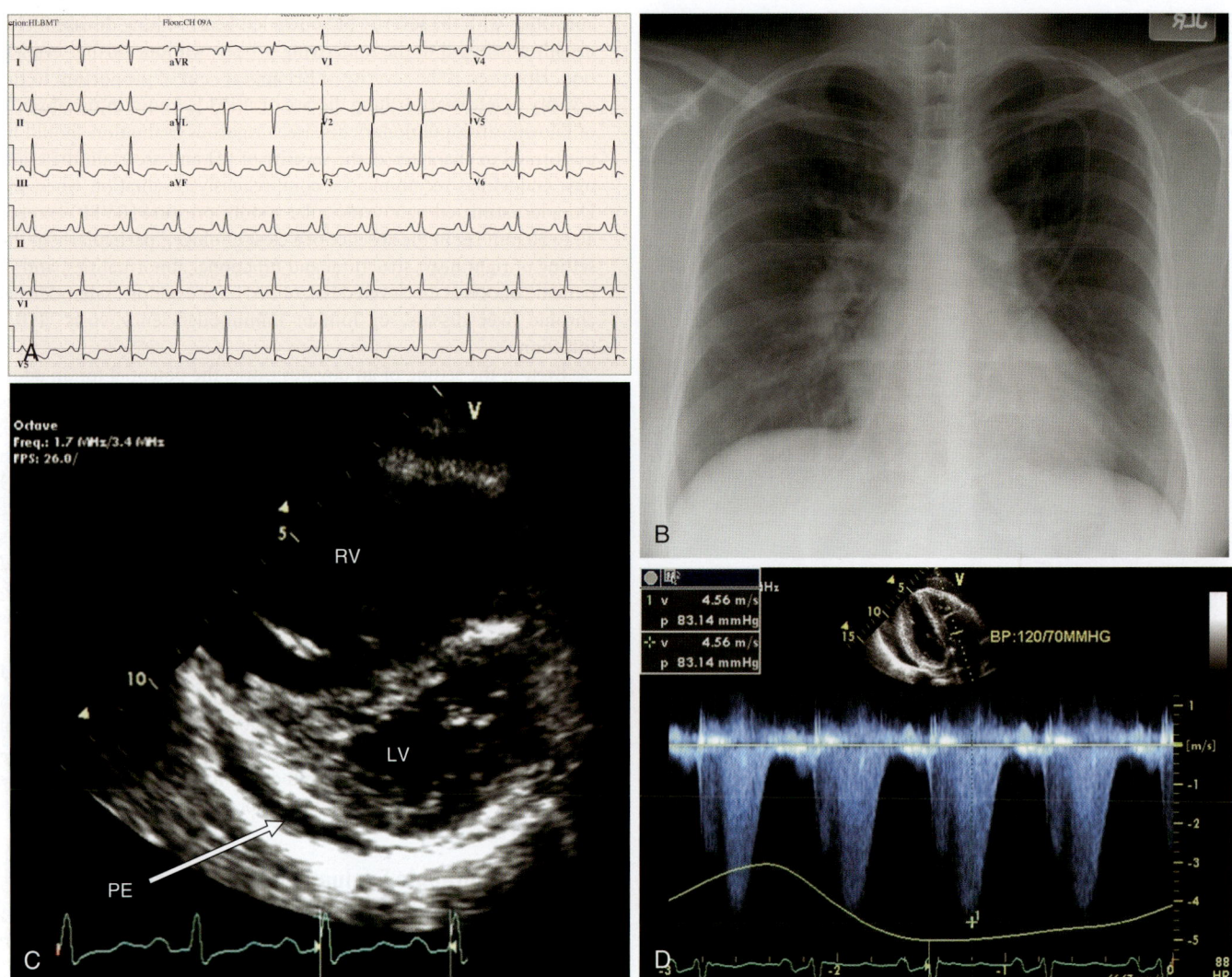

Fig. 43.2 Electrocardiography, chest radiograph, and echocardiographic findings in patients with pulmonary arterial hypertension. Typical electrocardiography findings include right axis deviation, right atrial enlargement, and right ventricular hypertrophy *(Panel A)*. Enlargement of the central pulmonary arteries with peripheral pruning of the vascular and evidence of right sided chamber enlargement may be seen on chest x-ray *(Panel B)*. Right ventricular *(RV)* enlargement, flattening of the intraventricular septum resulting in a D-shaped left ventricle *(LV)* may be seen on echocardiography *(Panel C)*. A pericardial effusion *(PE)* may be present. The peak tricuspid regurgitation velocity can be used to estimate the right ventricular systolic pressure *(Panel D*, elevated at >4 m/sec here). *BP*, Blood pressure.

close attention to technical detail, the echocardiogram may provide reasonable accurate estimates of systolic, mean, and diastolic PAPs based on the Doppler velocity profiles of the peak tricuspid regurgitation (TR) and pulmonary valve regurgitation signals (see **Fig. 43.2**). This information is integrated with a two-dimensional and Doppler estimation of right atrial pressure based on imaging of the inferior vena cava and hepatic veins. Although a suspicion of PH can be based on echocardiographic estimates, the diagnosis *cannot be established* without right heart catheterization.

The second key feature in an echo evaluation of a PH patient is the evaluation for a host of variables that help define the severity of disease. These relate to quantitative assessment of right-sided enlargement and dysfunction.[4] With regard to right ventricular contractility, a key feature to note is that in contrast to the left ventricle the predominant direction of contractility is in the longitudinal plane with the base of the right ventricle moving down

toward the apex. Hence measures of longitudinal contractility, such as the tricuspid annular plane systolic excursion (TAPSE), the peak systolic velocity of the tricuspid annulus by tissue Doppler, and longitudinal systolic strain best reflect right ventricular performance and prognosis.[5,6] Other findings that indicate more severe disease include the presence of a "D-shaped" left ventricle, a delayed relaxation mitral inflow pattern, a high estimated right atrial pressure, more tricuspid valve regurgitation, and right-sided chamber enlargement. The presence of a pericardial effusion, common in PAH, reflects chronic central venous hypertension and/or the presence of connective tissue disease, which are both features that indicate an increased mortality risk in PAH.[7,8]

The third important focus of an echocardiographic study in a patient with PH is the separation of precapillary from postcapillary PH. Indeed, many features of advanced left heart disease, such as significant left-sided valvular stenosis, or regurgitation, or myocardial

TABLE 43.4 Diagnostic Evaluation of Pulmonary Hypertension

Pivotal Tests	Contingent Testing	To Assess....
History, physical exam, CXR and electrocardiogram		Suspect PH
Transthoracic echo	Transesophageal echo (select cases)	Doppler estimated PASP
		RV size and function
		Presence of left heart disease
		Congenital abnormalities
Ventilation/perfusion scan	Pulmonary angiography, CT angiography, coagulopathy evaluation	Chronic thromboembolic disease
		Low probability: no further testing
		Intermediate or high probability: CT or invasive pulmonary angiography
Overnight oximetry	Polysomnography	Sleep-disordered breathing related PH
Pulmonary function testing	Arterial blood gas, chest CT	Lung disease related PH
HIV	Infectious disease evaluation	HIV related PH
Antinuclear antibody	Other CTD serologies, rheumatology evaluation	Connective tissue disease related PH
Liver function tests	Liver ultrasound	Portopulmonary hypertension
6 Minute walk test; BNP or NT-proBNP, CPXT		Prognosis and baseline to assess therapeutic response
Right heart catheterization		Presence, severity, and type of PH (see **Table 43.1**)
		Exclude intracardiac shunt
		PAH—Assess vasodilator response to guide therapy

BNP, Brain natriuretic peptide; *CPXT*, cardiopulmonary exercise test; *CT*, computed tomography; *CTD*, connective tissue disease; *CXR*, chest x-ray; *HIV*, human immunodeficiency virus; *NT-pro BNP*, amino terminal BNP; *PAH*, pulmonary arterial hypertension; *PASP*, systolic pulmonary artery pressure; *PH*, pulmonary hypertension; *RV*, right ventricular.

disease, are easily characterized by echocardiography. While echocardiographic features, including left atrial size, may be helpful, the separation of a patient with heart failure with preserved ejection fraction (HFpEF) and advanced right heart dysfunction from a patient with a restricted pulmonary vascular mechanism of PH can be challenging solely on the basis of echo.

Laboratory Testing

All patients should have a routine chemistry panel, complete blood cell count, liver function tests, and thyroid function tests. Antinuclear antibody titer is used to screen for connective tissue disease. Although 40% of patients with idiopathic pulmonary arterial hypertension (IPAH) have positive but low antinuclear antibody (ANA) titers (≥1:80 dilutions), patients with a substantially elevated ANA or suspicious clinical findings require further serologic assessment and rheumatology consultation. HIV serology should be considered.

Pulmonary Function Testing

Pulmonary function testing (PFT) is used to diagnose and quantify the underlying airway or parenchymal lung disease and should be performed in all patients with PH. The diffusing capacity for carbon monoxide (DLCO) is reduced in patients with PAH. A patient with PAH would be expected to have normal spirometry and lung volumes. In all forms of PAH, desaturation during exercise is typically related to diffusion limitation during exercise and the inability of the right ventricle to augment cardiac output, resulting in further depression of mixed venous oxygen saturation. Overnight oximetry can screen for clinically significant sleep apnea or hypopnea during sleep. In the evaluation of all patients with PH, an assessment of sleep-disordered breathing is recommended.

Right Heart Catheterization

Right heart catheterization is *mandatory* to confirm the diagnosis of PH and should be completed on all patients prior to initiating therapy. Cardiac output, cardiac index, pulmonary vascular resistance (PVR), PA pressure, pulmonary artery wedge pressure (PAWP), and right atrial pressure should all be determined. Intracardiac shunting

should also be excluded and vasodilator testing should be performed in patients with idiopathic PAH.

GROUP 1: PULMONARY ARTERIAL HYPERTENSION

PAH describes a group of various pulmonary hypertensive diseases that have similar histopathology, clinical presentations, and approaches to therapy. These include idiopathic and heritable causes and PH related to a number of associated conditions including: connective tissue diseases, chronic liver disease, HIV infection, schistosomiasis, and exposure to certain drugs or dietary products. In addition, pulmonary veno-occlusive disease (PVOD) and pulmonary capillary hemangiomatosis (PCH) are included as a subgroup in this category of PAH (Group 1.6) because they also are characterized by precapillary PH, pulmonary arteriopathy, similar risk factors, and a genetic predisposition. Persistent PH of the newborn is categorized as a separate subgroup, classified as Group 1.7.[1]

Epidemiology and Clinical Features

PAH, based on the previous definition of an elevated mPAP >25 mm Hg, is considered a rare disease with an estimated prevalence of 15 to 50 cases per million individuals.[9]

Idiopathic Pulmonary Arterial Hypertension

Idiopathic PAH is defined as the presence of precapillary PH in the absence of an underlying risk factor. Idiopathic PAH, previously referred to as "primary pulmonary hypertension" is a rare disease with an annual incidence of 1 to 2 cases per million and occurs more commonly in women than men. In the Western world, idiopathic PAH is the most common subtype of PAH and accounts for almost half of patients with Group 1 PAH.[10] Although previously regarded as a disease of the young, the epidemiology of PAH has changed over recent years with an increase in the average age at diagnosis. Historical registries reported an average age at diagnosis in the fourth decade, whereas more contemporary registries report an average age at diagnosis in the fifth to sixth decades of life.[9] It is not known whether this finding is due to a change in disease phenotype, improved recognition and diagnosis of PAH in older individuals, or misclassification of PH due to left heart disease.

Heritable Pulmonary Arterial Hypertension

Heritable or familial causes of PAH include those patients with either a family history of PAH or those patients with a de novo mutation that imparts a heritable risk. These include alterations in genes from the transforming growth factor beta family, including bone morphogenetic protein receptor type 2 (BMPR2), activin-like kinase 1 (ALK1), Endoglin (ENG), and mothers against decapentaplegic 9 (SMAD9), as well as genes such as Caveolin-1 (CAV1), and potassium channel superfamily K member-3 (KCNK3).[1,11,12] BMPR2 mutations are present in 20% of PAH cases, but have a lifetime penetrance of only 10% to 20%.[12] Testing for BMPR2 mutations is available and should be considered in patients with idiopathic PAH, particularly in those with a family history of PAH, and to relatives of patients with heritable PAH, but should be preceded by genetic counseling.

Pulmonary Arterial Hypertension Associated Conditions
Connective Tissue Disease

PAH associated with connective tissue disease is the most common subtype of associated PAH.[10] PAH can occur in conjunction with all forms of connective tissue diseases but occurs most commonly in systemic sclerosis (typically limited scleroderma and commonly associated with the anticentromere antibody), occurring in approximately 12% of cases.[13] As such, routine screening for PAH with symptom assessment, PFT (evaluating for abnormalities in diffusion capacity), and echocardiography every 1 to 2 years should be considered in patients with systemic sclerosis. Patients with PAH associated with connective tissue diseases often have a less robust response to PAH-specific medications and a poorer prognosis than those with idiopathic PAH.[14] All patients with unexplained PAH should have clinical and autoantibody testing for connective tissue disease.

Congenital Heart Disease (see also Chapter 27)

PAH is a known complication of congenital heart disease, and is frequently associated with systemic to pulmonary shunts. Initially systemic-pulmonary shunts led to a period of high pulmonary flow, but low pulmonary resistance. However, over time the high vascular shear stress related to elevated blood flow induces endothelial damage and progressive irreversible pulmonary vascular remodeling. The term "Eisenmenger syndrome" refers to the irreversible state of PAH mediated through arterial shunts causing pulmonary vasculopathy and ultimately resulting in a right-to-left or bidirectional shunt. The likelihood of PAH developing usually depends on the site and severity of the defect with ventricular septal defects causing PAH more commonly than atrial septal defects or a patent ductus arteriosus. Rarely, PAH may develop even after the defect is corrected.

The early diagnosis of lesions and the appropriate timing of corrective surgery are critical to the prevention of PAH with congenital heart disease. While multifactorial, persistent exposure to increased blood flow can result in progressive endothelial dysfunction, vasoconstriction, and vascular remodeling in the pulmonary circulation, which is not always reversible. Some patients will have residual elevation in PVR and PAH even following repair if irreversible changes have occurred in the pulmonary circulation.[15] Compared with a patient who has idiopathic PAH, a patient with PH associated with congenital heart disease and a comparable degree of PH has a greater probability of longer survival.[16]

Drugs and Toxins

Drugs and toxins have been implicated in the pathogenesis of some cases of PAH, including the use of central nervous system stimulants and appetite suppressants. In the 1960s, the anorexigen aminorex was first reported to be associated with PAH, and was withdrawn from the market in 1972. In the 1980s and 1990s, fenfluramine and dexfenfluramine, were reported to be associated with a marked increase in the risk of PAH if used for greater than 3 months. The fenfluramines act by stimulating serotonin release; serotonin is a potent pulmonary vasoconstrictor and a smooth muscle mitogen.[17] Central nervous system stimulants, such as amphetamine and methamphetamine, may also cause PAH.[18] Severe PH has also been reported in patients treated with dasatinib, a tyrosine kinase inhibitor used in the treatment of chronic myeloid leukemia. In some cases of dasatinib-associated PH, PH may be at least partially reversible with discontinuation of the drug.[19]

Chronic Liver Disease

Patients with both cirrhotic and noncirrhotic portal hypertension have a greatly increased risk of PH. PH in the setting of liver disease may be due to a hyperdynamic circulation, volume overload, or pulmonary vascular remodeling with increased PVR. Right heart catheterization is necessary to distinguish these hemodynamic profiles. Precapillary PH in the setting of portal hypertension affects approximately 5% to 6% of patients with liver disease, and is referred to as portopulmonary hypertension. Portopulmonary hypertension is pathologically indistinct from idiopathic PAH. Untreated moderate to severe PH is associated with high perioperative mortality at the time of liver transplant, so screening transthoracic echocardiogram is recommended in all patients undergoing evaluation for liver transplantation.[20,21]

Pulmonary Venoocclusive Disease and Pulmonary Capillary Hemangiomatosis

These are rare causes of PAH, but are commonly misdiagnosed as idiopathic PAH. Risk factors include connective tissue disease, occupational exposures to organic solvents, and receipt of some chemotherapeutic agents.[22] Pathologically, PVOD is characterized by extensive occlusion of the pulmonary veins by fibrous tissue. In PCH there is proliferation of benign thin-walled capillary vessels in the lung parenchyma. These diseases should be suspected when patients present with precapillary PH, a severely reduced diffusion capacity and abnormalities on chest imaging, such as centrilobular ground glass nodules, mediastinal lymphadenopathy, interlobular septal thickening, and pleural effusions. Patients with PVOD and PCH may also develop pulmonary edema with the initiation of PAH targeted therapies. Typically the PAWP is normal or low. Lung biopsy is required to confirm the diagnosis; however, the procedural risk is often prohibitive. Genetic mutations in eukaryotic initiation factor 2 alpha kinase 4 (EIF2AK4) occur in approximately 20% of patients with sporadic PVOD and PCH and can be helpful in establishing the diagnosis.[23] Prognosis is poor, and there is a variable response to therapy. Lung transplantation is the only successful management strategy.

Pathophysiology of Group I Pulmonary Arterial Hypertension

In PAH, there is a disruption in the balance of vasodilators and vasoconstrictors, smooth muscle mitogens and growth inhibitors, and prothrombotic and anticoagulant compounds (**Fig. 43.3**). As such, it is characterized by vasoconstriction, smooth muscle cell proliferation, and thrombosis.

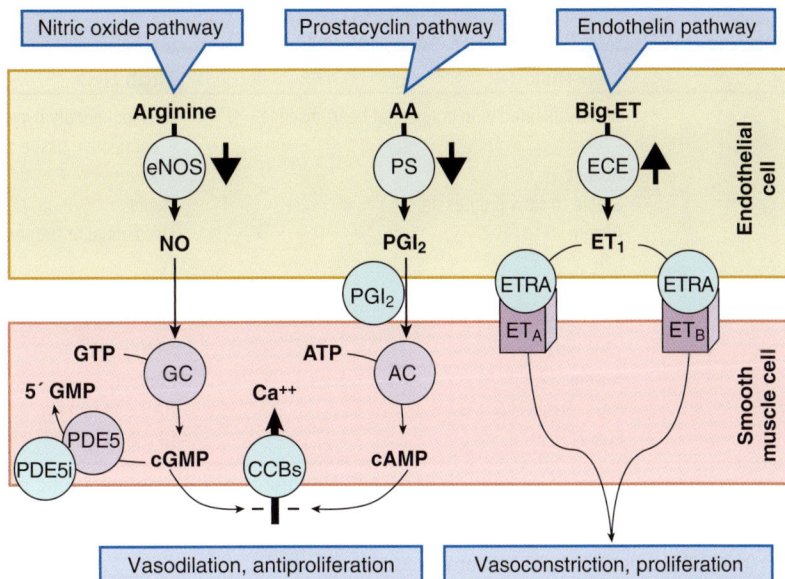

Fig. 43.3 Disturbed mechanistic pathways in patients with pulmonary arterial hypertension. The three mechanistic pathways known to be disturbed in patients with pulmonary arterial hypertension (PAH) are shown. The short, *thick black arrows* depict aberrations observed in these pathways in patients with PAH. The point at which drug treatment affects these mechanistic pathways are shown in *gray circles*. *AA*, Arachidonic acid; *CCB*, calcium channel blocker; *ETRA*, endothelin receptor antagonist; *PDE5i*, phosphodiesterase 5 inhibitor. *Left*, The nitric oxide *(NO)* pathway. NO is created in endothelial cells by type III (i.e., endothelial) NO synthase *(eNOS)*, which in pulmonary arterial smooth muscle cells (PASMCs) induces guanylate cyclase *(GC)* to convert guanylate triphosphate *(GTP)* to cyclic guanylate monophosphate *(cGMP)*. Cyclic GMP is a second messenger that constitutively maintains PASMC relaxation and inhibition of PASMC proliferation by ultimately reducing inward flux of calcium ions *(Ca++)*. Cyclic GMP is removed by the PDE5 enzyme to yield the inactive product 5′GMP. Patients with PAH have reduced expression and activity of eNOS. *Middle*, The prostacyclin pathway. The production of prostaglandin I2 *(PGI2* [i.e., prostacyclin]) is catalyzed by prostacyclin synthase *(PS)* in endothelial cells. In PASMCs, PGI2 stimulates adenylate cyclase *(AC)*, thus increasing production of cyclic adenosine monophosphate *(cAMP)* from adenosine triphosphate *(ATP)*. Cyclic AMP is a second messenger that constitutively maintains PASMC relaxation and inhibition of PASMC proliferation. Patients with PAH have reduced expression and activity of PS. *Right*, The endothelin *(ET)* pathway. Big- (i.e., pro-) ET is converted in endothelial cells to ET1 (a 21–amino acid peptide) by endothelin-converting enzyme *(ECE)*. ET$_1$ binds to PASMC ET$_A$ and ET$_B$ receptors, ultimately leading to PASMC contraction, proliferation, and hypertrophy. Patients with PAH have increased expression and activity of ECE. *GMP*, guanylate monophosphate. (From McGoon MD, Kane GC. Pulmonary hypertension: diagnosis and management. *Mayo Clin Proc.* 2009;84[2:191–207].)

Prostacyclin and thromboxane A2 are arachidonic acid metabolites. Prostacyclin is a potent vasodilator that inhibits platelet activation, and has been shown to be deficient in PAH. Conversely, thromboxane A2 is prothrombotic, and is found in elevated levels in PAH.[24] Nitric oxide is a known vasodilator and inhibitor of smooth muscle proliferation and platelet activation. It is produced by the family of nitric oxide synthase enzymes, which are reduced in the endothelium in PAH.[25] Endothelin-1 is a potent vasoconstrictor and inhibits pulmonary artery smooth muscle cell proliferation. Plasma levels of endothelin-1 are high in PAH,[26] and its clearance is reduced. Additional vascular substances, including serotonin, vasoactive intestinal peptide, and vascular endothelial growth factor, have altered homeostasis in PAH.[27] Autoimmunity and inflammation are also emerging as important processes involved in PAH pathogenesis and disease progression.[28] Autoantibodies are frequently detected in PAH; circulating cytokines are commonly elevated in PAH and are associated with a poor prognosis. Development of novel therapies that target immune dysregulation is an active area of investigation.

Prognosis in Group I Pulmonary Arterial Hypertension

In patients with untreated PAH, the median survival is 2.8 years, with 1-, 3-, and 5-year survival of 68%, 48%, and 34%, respectively.[29] Fortunately, PAH registries across the world have reported overall improved survival in the modern PAH treatment era. According to the US REVEAL registry, which enrolled over 2500 patients with Group 1 PAH between 2006 and 2009, 1-, 3-, and 5-year survival rates from the time of diagnosis were 85%, 68%, and 57%, respectively[10]. Patients with connective tissue disease and portopulmonary hypertension tend to have a worse prognosis, whereas patients with congenital heart disease have more favorable survival. Although female sex is considered a risk factor for PAH, male sex is associated with worse survival, potentially due to differences in right ventricular adaptation.[9] Additional markers of adverse prognosis are shown in **Table 43.5**. Prognosis is best determined in patients with PAH by integration of etiology and functional class with clinical, echocardiographic, and hemodynamic factors.[30,31] A number of integrative prognostic scores are now available to aid the PH physician in this assessment.[32,33]

TABLE 43.5 Risk Assessment in Pulmonary Arterial Hypertension

Determinant of Prognosis	Low Risk	High Risk
PAH subgroup	PAH associated with congenital heart disease	Portopulmonary hypertension, PAH associated with connective tissue disease, familial PAH
Clinical signs of right heart failure	Absent	Present
Progression of symptoms	Stable to slow progression	Rapid
Syncope	Absent	Occasional or frequent
Functional class	I, II	IV
6-minute walk distance	>440 m	<165 m
Percent predicted DLCO	≥80	≤32
NT-proBNP	<300 ng/L	>1400 ng/L
Pericardial effusion	Absent	Present
Hemodynamics	RAP < 8 mm Hg	RAP > 14 mm Hg
	CI ≥ 2.5	CI < 2.0 L/min/m²

CI, Cardiac index; *DLCO*, diffusing capacity for carbon monoxide; *NT-proBNP*, N-terminal pro B-type natriuretic peptide; *PAH*, pulmonary arterial hypertension; *RAP*, right atrial pressure.

Reproduced with permission of the © 2019 European Society of Cardiology & European Respiratory Society. European Respiratory Journal 46 (4) 903–975; DOI: 10.1183/13993003.01032-2015 Published 30 September 2015.

Clinical Assessment

Clinical evidence of right ventricular failure and rapidly progressive symptoms are associated with adverse prognosis in PAH. In particular, syncope, as a sign of poor cardiac output, is an independent predictor of mortality in PAH. The World Health Organization (WHO) functional class categorizes a patient based on their symptoms and functionality (class I, no limitation in physical activity; class II, slight limitation in physical activity; class III, no symptoms at rest but marked limitation in physical activity; class IV, symptoms with any physical activity and possibly at rest). While somewhat controversial,[34] most studies demonstrate that the 6-minute walk test is a good indicator of prognosis and response to therapy; distances greater than 500 m are associated with good prognosis and less than 300 m should trigger consideration of a change in therapy.

Biomarkers (see also Chapter 33)

While several biomarkers have been assessed for their use in determining prognosis in PAH, the most widely tested is brain natriuretic peptide (BNP) and its amino-terminal fragment (NT-pro BNP). Elevated BNP and NT-pro BNP levels reflect right ventricular dysfunction, and are associated with increased mortality risk.[35,36]

Hemodynamics (see also Chapter 34)

Hemodynamic variables that reflect the degree of right ventricular decompensation or integrative parameters of function and load provide critically important prognostic information. These include measures of right atrial pressure, cardiac output, PVR, and compliance. Vasoreactivity testing in Group 1 PAH is routinely performed (see **Table 43.1**). A positive response to acute administration of a pulmonary vasodilator occurs in less than 10% of patients with idiopathic PAH but identifies a cohort that may respond to calcium channel antagonists and has a better prognosis. As described above, echocardiography provides important noninvasive hemodynamic information but also measures of right-sided enlargement and right ventricular dysfunction that reflect disease severity. Computed tomography and magnetic resonance imaging of the right ventricle also provide useful measures of right ventricular enlargement and cardiac output.

Management of Group I Pulmonary Hypertension

Management of PAH includes general lifestyle modifications applicable to patients with all forms of PH as well as PAH targeted therapies, adjuvant therapies, and advanced therapies. Treatment of associated conditions (connective tissue disease, HIV, etc.) is also important but is not discussed here.

Choice of initial therapies for PAH is contingent upon the results of vasoreactivity testing and the assessment of symptoms and prognosis. Patients with functional class IV symptoms should be treated with intravenous (IV) epoprostenol.[22] Combining drugs with upfront or sequential combination therapy has now become the standard of care, and recent guidelines recommend consideration of upfront combination therapy.[22] A recommended flow diagram for treatment is shown in **Fig. 43.4**.

General Treatment Recommendations for Patients with Pulmonary Hypertension

Heart Failure Management. Salt restriction (<2.4 g/day) and diuretic therapy may be needed to avoid volume overload in patients with PAH and right ventricular dysfunction.

Exercise. Low level aerobic exercise, as tolerated, is recommended.[3] Heavy exertion and isometric exercise should be avoided in advanced cases of PH, as they may trigger syncope. Cardiopulmonary rehabilitation programs should be considered in the overall PH management program and are invariably very beneficial.

Oxygen Therapy. Hypoxemia is a potent pulmonary vasoconstrictor and can contribute to the development or progression of PH. It is generally recommended that supplemental oxygen be used to maintain normoxia with oxygen saturations 90% or above, but there is little long-term evidence to support this recommendation. In patients with obstructive sleep apnea (OSA) and PH, treatment of OSA with positive airway pressure therapy should be provided, with the expectation that pulmonary pressures will decrease, although they may not normalize, particularly when PH is more severe.

Pregnancy Avoidance. Pregnancy carries a high associated mortality (30%) in patients with PAH.[37] Several physiologic changes contribute to the potential deterioration during pregnancy, including an increase in hypercoagulability, blood volume, and oxygen consumption, which can contribute to right ventricular dysfunction. As such, pregnancy is not advised in patients with PAH, and nonestrogen-based contraceptive programs are recommended.

Calcium Channel Blockers. Calcium channel blockers have no role in the management of PAH except in the setting of a subset of patients (<10%) with idiopathic PAH and a significant acute response to vasodilatory testing at the time of right heart catheterization. Nifedipine, diltiazem, or amlodipine can be used, but verapamil

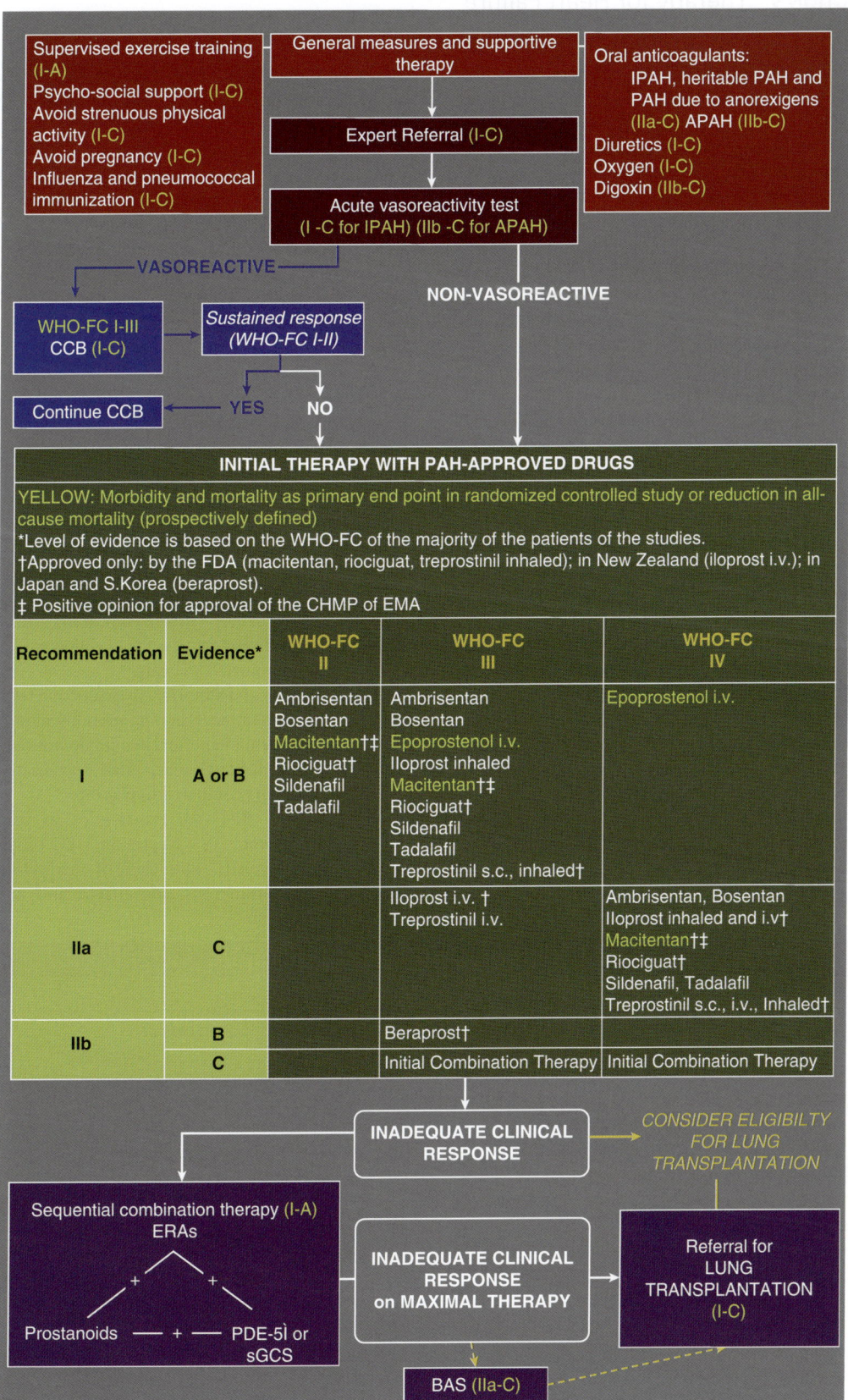

Fig. 43.4 Evidence-based treatment algorithm for the management of pulmonary arterial hypertension. This algorithm summarizes an evidence-based approach to treatment of pulmonary arterial hypertension *(PAH)*. *APAH,* Associated pulmonary arterial hypertension; *BAS,* balloon atrial septostomy; *CCB,* calcium channel blockers; *CHMP,* Committee for Medicinal Products for Human Use; *EMA,* European Medicines Agency; *ERA,* endothelin receptor antagonist; *FDA,* Food and Drug Administration; *IPAH,* idiopathic pulmonary arterial hypertension; *i.v.,* intravenous; *PDE-5i,* phosphodiesterase type-5 inhibitor; *s.c.,* subcutaneous; *sGCS,* soluble guanylate cyclase stimulators; *WHO-FC,* World Health Organization functional class. (From Galiè N, Corris PA, Frost A, et al. Updated treatment algorithm of pulmonary arterial hypertension. *J Am Coll Cardiol.* 2013;62[25 Suppl]:D60–D72.)

should be avoided due to its negative inotropic effects. If the patients fail to reach functional class I or II with calcium channel blocker therapy, then alternative or additional PH-specific medications should be prescribed. While improved systemic blood pressure (BP) control by calcium channel blockers is often indicated in patients with Group 2 PH, there is no proven role for calcium channel blockers to lower pulmonary pressures in other PH settings, and it may be of harm.

Drug Therapy for Group I PAH-PAH Targeted Therapy

Therapy for PAH has rapidly evolved in the last 15 years from the use of unselected vasodilating drugs to the use of therapies that more effectively target pulmonary dilatation and vascular remodeling with an impact on morbidity and mortality. The PAH-targeted therapies are outlined in **Table 43.6** and summarized here.

Phosphodiesterase-5 Inhibitors. The phosphodiesterase-5 (PDE-5) inhibitors, sildenafil and tadalafil, have been shown to be efficacious therapies for patients with PAH. They are selective inhibitors of PDE-5 that degrade cyclic guanosine monophosphate (cGMP) and are found in high concentrations in the pulmonary arteries and corpora cavernosum.[38] Normally, endothelium-derived nitric oxide stimulates intracellular guanylate cyclase resulting in increased levels of cGMP, which then act to mediate smooth muscle relaxation. PDE-5 inhibitors prevent the breakdown of cGMP, thus prolonging its effects.

Sildenafil and tadalafil have been shown to improve exercise capacity and pulmonary hemodynamics in PAH.[39-41] These oral therapies are generally well tolerated, with the most notable adverse effects of headache, nasal congestion, epistaxis, and gastroesophageal reflux. Rare adverse effects of acute visual or auditory loss have been reported. The effects of PDE-5 inhibitors on mortality in PAH are unclear.

Soluble Guanylate Cyclase Stimulators. Riociguat is a soluble guanylate cyclase stimulator that also acts via the nitric oxide pathway to stimulate guanylate cyclase and increase cGMP production. In Group 1 PAH, riociguat improves exercise capacity, PVR, and time to clinical worsening. Riociguat is also approved for treatment of inoperable or residual CTEPH (Group 4 PH).[42,43] Riociguat should not be used in combination with PDE-5 inhibitors or nitrates. Side effects include hypotension, gastroesophageal reflux, and headache.

Endothelin Receptor Antagonists. Endothelin-1 is a potent vasoconstrictor and smooth muscle mitogen, and is overexpressed in several forms of pulmonary vascular disease. Endothelin receptor antagonists (ERA) emerged in the 1990s as important therapies in PAH. Bosentan is a nonselective endothelin-receptor antagonist, while ambrisentan selectively inhibits the type A endothelin-1 receptor. Macitentan, the latest ERA to be approved for PAH, targets both endothelin type A and B receptors and was chemically modified from bosentan to improve tissue targeting.

Bosentan is US Food and Drug Administration–approved for use in WHO functional class II through IV PAH patients, based on its proven efficacy in several randomized, controlled trials.[44-46] In the BREATHE trial, bosentan improved 6-minute walk distance, Borg dyspnea index, and time to clinical worsening compared with placebo in patients with WHO class III or IV PAH.[44] Bosentan also improved 6-minute walk distance and mean PVR in patients with WHO functional class II PAH.[46] Bosentan has been demonstrated to improve survival compared with model-predicted estimates.[47] Ambrisentan improves exercise capacity in PAH. Macitentan was one of the first PAH drugs approved on the basis of a long-term event-driven clinical trial. Macitentan delays PAH disease progression and reduces the likelihood of a composite outcome of morbidity and mortality events.[48]

Hepatotoxicity and abnormal liver function tests is an adverse effect with use of bosentan, necessitating monthly monitoring of liver function tests; ambrisentan and macitentan do not require regular laboratory monitoring, although macitentan is associated with an increased incidence of anemia compared to placebo.

Prostacyclin Analogs. Prostanoids available to treat PAH include epoprostenol (IV), treprostinil (IV, subcutaneous, inhaled), and iloprost (inhaled). This class of medications is expensive, is associated with numerous side effects, and is often reserved for

TABLE 43.6	Pulmonary Arterial Hypertension Targeted Therapies				
Class	**Medication**	**Route**	**Dosage**	**Side Effects**	**Monitoring**
Calcium Channel Blockers				Hypotension, peripheral edema	
	Amlodipine	PO	2.5–10 mg/day		
	Diltiazem	PO	120–900 mg/day		
	Nifedipine	PO	120–240 mg/day		
PDE-5 inhibitors				Headache, hypotension, visual disturbances, gastroesophageal reflux	
	Sildenafil	PO	20–40 mg TID		
	Tadalafil	PO	40 mg/day		
Soluble guanylate cyclase stimulators				Hypotension, headache, gastroesophageal reflux	
	Riociguat PO		0.5–2.5 mg TID		
Endothelin receptor antagonists				Hepatotoxicity, peripheral edema	Monthly AST/ALT monitoring with bosentan
	Bosentan	PO	62.5–125 mg BID		
	Ambrisentan	PO	5–10 mg/day		
	Macitentan	PO	10 mg/day	Anemia	
Prostanoids/IP receptor agonists				Jaw pain, diarrhea, arthralgias, headache	
	Epoprostenol	IV	1–40 ng/kg/min		
	Treprostinil	IV, SC	1.25–40 ng/kg/min	Pain, erythema at SC site with treprostinil	
		INH	18–54 mcg 4 times/day		
		PO	0.25–12 mg BID		
	Iloprost	INH	2.5–5 mcg 6 times/day	Cough	
	Selexipag	PO	200–1600 mcg BID		

ALT, Alanine aminotransferase; *AST, aspartate aminotransferase; BID,* twice a day; *INH,* inhalation; *IV,* intravenous; *PDE-5,* phosphodiesterase-5; *PO,* by mouth; *SC,* subcutaneous; *TID,* three times a day.

patients with more advanced stages of disease. Epoprostenol has been best studied, and is first-line therapy for patients with severe PAH as it is the only therapy that has been shown to improve survival in these patients. It improves functional class, hemodynamics, and survival. In a randomized, multicenter trial of 81 patients, epoprostenol was associated with improved quality of life, a reduction in mPAP, and an improvement in the 6-minute walk distance compared with placebo.[49] Survival at 1, 2, 3, and 5 years is improved with epoprostenol compared with historical PAH controls and equation-predicted survival.[50,51] Therapy is complicated, requiring a central venous catheter for a continuous IV infusion through a portable pump. The half-life is very short (<5 minutes) and hence interruption of therapy may result in life-threatening rebound PH. Treprostinil has a longer half-life and can be administered subcutaneously, as a continuous IV infusion, orally, or in lower doses via inhalation. Iloprost can be delivered by adapted aerosol device. Common dose-dependent adverse effects include headache, jaw pain, diarrhea, nausea, an erythematous rash, and musculoskeletal pains, predominantly involving the legs and feet.

Prostacyclin IP Receptor Agonist. Selexipag is an oral nonprostanoid prostacyclin IP receptor agonist approved to treat Group 1 PAH. In a large clinical trial of 1156 patients with Group 1 PAH and functional class II or III symptoms, selexipag was associated with a significant benefit that was largely driven by a reduction in hospitalizations and disease progression.[52] Adverse effects were similar to the known side effects of prostacyclin therapy.

Choice and Order of Therapy. The choice of therapy is best determined by an experienced PH care team and the patient, based on a host of factors including disease severity, economic, individual capabilities, and family support. In principle, patients with advanced disease at presentation should be considered for parenteral prostanoid therapy with other therapies considered in milder forms of disease or as second-line agents. Studies continue to emerge demonstrating the safety and efficacy of combination therapy in PAH.[53-55] Indeed, as there are multiple biological pathways involved in the pathogenesis of PAH, there is a strong rationale to use upfront or sequential combination medical therapy in its treatment, and this has now become the standard of care.[56] PAH is a very expensive disease, in terms of not only the high patient morbidity and mortality, but also the diagnostic and serial evaluation and the cost of pulmonary vascular-targeted therapies.

Drug Therapy for Group I Pulmonary Arterial Hypertension-Adjuvant Therapy

Anticoagulation. PAH is a prothrombotic state due to an imbalance of the homeostasis of prothrombotic and antithrombotic factors. PAH patients are also at risk for intrapulmonary thrombosis due to sluggish blood flow in the pulmonary circulation and endothelial dysfunction. Given this predisposition, it is generally recommended that patients with idiopathic PAH have systemic anticoagulation with warfarin with a goal international normalized ratio of 1.5 to 2.5.[3] The evidence for this practice is controversial, so decisions regarding anticoagulation should be made on an individual basis after weighing the risks and benefits. Anticoagulation is associated with increased mortality in patients with scleroderma-associated PAH, and is typically not recommended in patients with associated PAH.[57]

Management of Right Heart Failure. Although pulmonary vascular remodeling is the primary pathological process in PAH, right heart failure is the main cause of death and can be challenging to manage. Diuretics are used to manage volume overload in patients with right heart failure; if hospitalized, IV diuretics may be indicated. Digoxin is prescribed in some circumstances as it increases cardiac

output in patients with right heart failure and PAH.[58] However, there are no long-term clinical data to support its use. Inotropes, such as dobutamine or milrinone, can be used in the acute setting to augment right ventricular contractility. Concomitant use of vasopressors, such as norepinephrine or vasopressin, may be necessary to maintain systemic blood pressure. Treatment with β blockers is not recommended due to their potential negative inotropic and pulmonary vasoconstrictive effects. Angiotensin receptor blockers and angiotensin converting enzyme inhibitors may contribute to systemic hypotension and have no current role in the treatment of PAH patients.

Atrial Septostomy. Atrial septostomy is considered in highly specialized centers in selected patients with severe PAH and right ventricular dysfunction. The creation of a right-to-left shunt allows improved left-sided filling and cardiac output at the expense of systemic oxygen desaturation. Careful selection is required as in the presence of very advanced disease (e.g., with severe elevations of right atrial pressure or poor baseline systemic oxygen saturations) periprocedural mortality can be high.[59] There is a carefully selected role as a bridge to transplant or as a palliative procedure when surgical options are not feasible.

Lung Transplantation. Transplantation remains an option in patients with PAH but is generally reserved for those with progressive disease despite advanced medical therapies, or in patients with subtypes of PAH associated with a poor prognosis and response to treatment, such as PVOD.[60] The optimal type of transplant is challenging. Heart–lung transplant is hampered by a shortage of available organs, although it has the advantages of requiring only one airway anastomosis yielding a very low rate of vascular complications, and generally the best hemodynamic outcomes. Patients should be considered for heart–lung transplant if their degree of right ventricular dysfunction is felt to be irreversible with resolution of the PH with lung transplant alone. Single lung transplant is easier than bilateral lung transplant to perform and requires less operative, ischemic, and cardiopulmonary bypass time, but there is the potential for ventilation-perfusion (V/Q) mismatch and reperfusion injury. Bilateral lung transplant may produce better hemodynamics, less V/Q mismatch, fewer early complications, better immediate overall lung function, and possibly improved long-term survival, but the operation is longer and more difficult to perform.[61]

GROUP 2: PULMONARY HYPERTENSION WITH LEFT HEART DISEASE

Patients with left-sided heart disease have PH due to a combination of PVH, pulmonary artery vasoconstriction and pulmonary vascular remodeling. When the transpulmonary gradient and PVR are normal, the PH is passive and a result of elevation in PAWP. This is referred to as isolated postcapillary PH. This is most common in the early stages of heart failure, and may respond to measures to reduce the PAWP such as diuretics and afterload reduction. When the PAWP, PVR, and transpulmonary gradient are elevated, this indicates the presence of combined precapillary and postcapillary PH, and suggests that PVH, pulmonary vasoconstriction, and pulmonary vascular remodeling are contributing to the PH.[62] In addition to transpulmonary gradient and PVR, the diastolic pressure gradient (DPG) may be helpful in differentiating precapillary from postcapillary PH (see **Table 43.1**). The potential reversibility of reactive PH can be tested during a hemodynamic catheterization by administering a nitroprusside challenge and assessing the change in PVR. In the case of reversible reactive PH, lowering of the PAWP with heart failure therapies will result in return of the PVR to normal. If the PVR cannot be reduced to normal with correction of the PAWP, then the reactive PH is fixed but may respond to dramatic sustained unloading with inotropic therapy or left ventricular assist device (LVAD).[63] The reversibility of reactive PH in patients with left-sided heart failure is an important consideration in evaluating patients for heart transplantation.

PH may arise as a result of disease of the left-sided heart valves, left ventricular systolic dysfunction, left ventricular diastolic dysfunction or the left atrium.

Pulmonary Hypertension Due to Left-Sided Valvular Heart Disease

Mitral valve disease results in elevated left atrial pressure, and, as a result, elevation in pulmonary pressures, both due to passive backward transmission of the elevated left atrial pressure and reactive pulmonary artery changes. Mitral stenosis results in an obstruction in blood flow from the left atrium to the left ventricle, and, accordingly, left atrial pressures must rise so that blood flow may continue. The development of PH plays an important role in the recommended timing of intervention in mitral stenosis, as surgical mortality is higher once PH has developed.[64] Mitral regurgitation can lead to PH through volume overload to the left atrium causing passive PVH, which, if longstanding, can trigger vasoconstriction and remodeling in the pulmonary arterial circulation. In mitral regurgitation due to degenerative disease, the development of PH (pulmonary artery systolic pressure ≥50 mm Hg) is common (present in 23% of cases) and increases the risk of all-cause and perioperative death.[65] In asymptomatic moderate or severe mitral regurgitation, exercise-induced PH (pulmonary artery systolic pressure ≥60 mm Hg) is present in 46% of patients, is associated with reduced 2-year symptom-free survival,[66] and represents an important indication for surgery. Aortic stenosis can contribute to PH by promoting left ventricular hypertrophy and diastolic dysfunction, which triggers elevation in left atrial pressures and PVH. Aortic regurgitation can rarely contribute to PH through elevation in left ventricular end diastolic pressure (LVEDP).

Pulmonary Hypertension in Heart Failure With Preserved or Reduced Ejection Fraction (see also Chapter 39)

Both systolic and diastolic dysfunction of the left ventricle can result in elevation in LVEDP, left atrial pressure, and pulmonary venous pressure, and can thus result in PH. The degree of PH in heart failure is thought to be proportional to the duration and intensity of exposure to PVH, which occurs independent of left ventricular ejection fraction (EF),[67] but may also be related to other factors. In heart failure with reduced EF (HFrEF, EF <50%), the prevalence of PH varies depending on the study population and definition used. In one study performed in 377 consecutive patients with heart failure and EF less than 35%, the prevalence of a mPAP greater than 20 mm Hg was 62% and was highly correlated with PAWP.[68] Diastolic dysfunction can also result in PH. Ventricular systolic and diastolic stiffness increases with age, particularly in females.[69] Both diastolic dysfunction prevalence[70] and PAPs[71] increase with age. In HFpEF (EF ≥50%), PH is also quite common. In an Olmsted County community study of patients with HFpEF, the median estimated RVSP by echocardiography was 48 mm Hg and 83% of patients had an RVSP ≥35 mm Hg.[72] Elevation in PAPs is associated with adverse prognosis in both HFpEF and HFrEF.[68,72,73]

The recognition that heart failure can occur in patients with preserved EF and that PH is as common in HFpEF as in HFrEF has complicated the assessment of PH as elderly patients with dyspnea frequently undergo echocardiography and may be found to have normal EF and elevated estimated RVSP. An approach to such patients has been suggested (**Fig. 43.5**).[74]

Pulmonary Hypertension Due to Left Atrial Disease

Reduced left atrial compliance is common in both HFpEF and HFrEF and is manifest by large V waves in the PCWP tracing in the absence of mitral regurgitation. However, isolated or predominant left atrial pathology ("stiff left atrial syndrome" or "left atrial hypertension") can occur following left atrial radiofrequency ablation or surgical MAZE procedure performed for atrial arrhythmias. These patients may present with dyspnea on exertion, elevated PAPs, and large V waves on pulmonary capillary wedge pressure tracings that accentuate with volume load.[75] While little is known about this entity, as it is associated with extensive left atrial scar formation it is difficult to treat.

Treatment

In PH due to left heart disease, treatment of the underlying left heart disease is the mainstay of therapy. In valvular heart disease, surgical repair of the valvular abnormality, if indicated, may resolve the PH. The use of PDE-5 inhibitors to treat residual PH after surgical correction of valvular disease should generally be avoided given a recent study that showed worse clinical outcomes in those treated with sildenafil.[76] In HFrEF, the use of evidence-based medications, such as angiotensin converting enzyme inhibitors, angiotensin receptor blockers, β blockers, aldosterone antagonists, and diuretics, may result in improvement in afterload reduction, reverse remodeling, and improvement in ventricular mechanics and function that will lower LVEDP and PAWP, and thus may reduce PAPs. Control of systemic hypertension and volume optimization are also advocated in HFpEF, though no therapies have been demonstrated to improve outcomes. Aldosterone blockade with spironolactone may be beneficial. In the TOPCAT trial of spironolactone versus placebo, spironolactone did not significantly reduce the primary outcome of death from cardiovascular causes, aborted cardiac arrest, or hospitalization for heart failure, but benefit was observed in some subgroups.[77] If PAPs remain elevated despite hemodynamic optimization and normalization of the PAWP, there are no guidelines for the use of PH-specific therapies in either HFpEF or HFrEF. Despite promising results in animal models and small single-center studies using the endothelin receptor antagonist bosentan, trials have not consistently shown efficacy.[78] There has been recent interest in using PDE-5 inhibitors to treat patients with left ventricular dysfunction, particularly HFpEF. A small single-center study demonstrated improvement in hemodynamics and left ventricular diastolic function with sildenafil.[79] However, the RELAX (PDE-5 Inhibition to Improve Clinical Status and Exercise Capacity in HFpEF) multicenter, randomized, controlled trial found no change in exercise capacity or clinical status after 24 weeks of sildenafil compared with placebo.[80] Subsequently, other trials in HFpEF confirmed no benefit of sildenafil in PH associated with left heart disease, and the COMPERA registry reported decreased tolerance and efficacy of PAH targeted therapy in HFpEF patients relative to idiopathic PAH patients.[62,81] However, this was not a randomized trial.

GROUP 3: PULMONARY HYPERTENSION ASSOCIATED WITH LUNG DISEASES AND/OR HYPOXIA

The respiratory diseases most commonly associated with PH are chronic obstructive pulmonary disease (COPD), interstitial lung disease, mixed obstructive and restrictive abnormalities, and sleep-disordered breathing. PH associated with advanced respiratory diseases is common but usually mild. A mPAP between 25 and 35 mm Hg is often seen in advanced disease and is associated with a worse prognosis. An

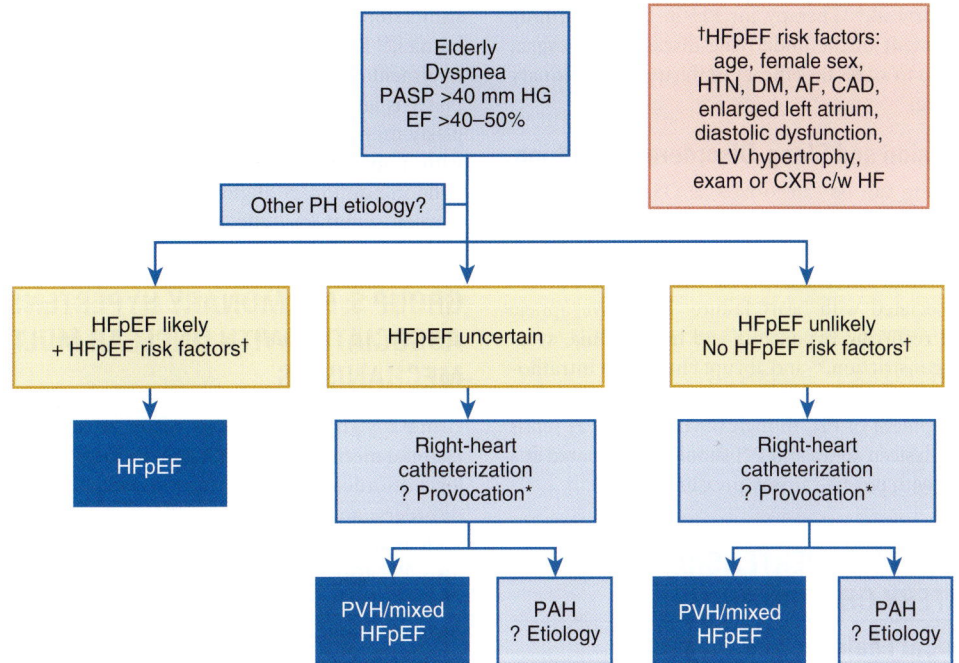

Fig. 43.5 Algorithm to evaluate elderly patients with dyspnea, normal ejection fraction and unexplained pulmonary hypertension at echocardiography. Decision to proceed to right heart catheterization is driven by the severity of pulmonary hypertension *(PH)* and the clinical evidence suggesting the presence of heart failure with preserved ejection fraction *(HFpEF)*. In many cases, the diagnosis of HFpEF can be made on the basis of clinical features and risk factors for HFpEF. In patients in whom the diagnosis of HFpEF is not evident, right heart catheterization should be considered. If resting hemodynamics do not clarify diagnosis, provocative measures* should be considered and may include: normal pulmonary capillary wedge pressure (PCWP) but HFpEF strongly suspected—exercise or volume expansion elevated PCWP and pulmonary vascular resistance (mixed PH)—systemic vasodilator (nipride) particularly if systemic blood pressure is elevated pulmonary arterial hypertension *(PAH)*—pulmonary vasodilator to assess responsiveness and potential for treatment with calcium channel blocker. *AF,* Atrial fibrillation; *CAD,* coronary artery disease; *CXR,* chest x-ray; *DM,* diabetes mellitus; *EF,* ejection fraction; *HF,* heart failure; *HTN,* hypertension; *LV,* left ventricle; *PASP,* systolic pulmonary artery pressure; *PVH,* pulmonary venous hypertension. (Modified from Hoeper MM, Barberà JA, Channick RN, et al. Diagnosis, assessment, and treatment of non-pulmonary arterial hypertension pulmonary hypertension. *J Am Coll Cardiol.* 2009;54[1 Suppl]:S85–S96.)

mPAP greater than 35 mm Hg in the setting of advanced lung disease denotes a very high risk, and such patients should be evaluated in a specialized center with consideration given towards transplantation. In milder forms of disease (e.g., forced expiratory volume in one second >60% predicted, and a forced vital capacity >70%) PH is uncommon and alternate mechanisms should be considered. In the setting of combined pulmonary fibrosis and emphysema, spirometry may be normal and diffusion capacity is often severely reduced. These patients may develop PH associated with lung disease and hypoxia in the absence of significant abnormalities on spirometry. Regardless of the mechanism, attention should be given to aggressively treating hypoxia.

Pulmonary Hypertension Associated With Chronic Obstructive Pulmonary Disease

COPD is a common lung disorder characterized by chronic obstruction of air inflow that is usually progressive and inhibits normal breathing. Chronic hypoxic vasoconstriction of the pulmonary arteries can lead to changes in the pulmonary vasculature, including intimal hyperplasia and smooth muscle hypertrophy. The exact prevalence of PH in COPD is unclear. Among a cohort of COPD patients followed with serial right heart catheterizations, none had PH at baseline, though 25% developed mild to moderate PH over time, which appeared to be associated with

worsening hypoxemia.[82] In patients with severe COPD, approximately two-thirds had elevated RVSP estimated by echocardiography.[83] While most COPD patients have mild PH, there appears to be a group of patients who have severe PH out of proportion to their pulmonary mechanics, suggesting this group may have a genetic predisposition to pulmonary vascular disease, and COPD provides the "second hit." In addition to standard therapies, such as bronchodilators for COPD, oxygen may be beneficial, particularly for those with right ventricular dysfunction.[84] While there has been interest in using PH-specific medications in this population, randomized, controlled trial evidence is lacking. Pulmonary vasodilatation runs the risk of perfusing poorly ventilated areas of the lung, increasing V/Q mismatch and worsening hypoxia.

Pulmonary Hypertension Associated With Interstitial Lung Disease

Interstitial lung disease (also known as diffuse parenchymal lung disease) is a group of clinical disorders affecting the interstitium. While the prevalence of PH has varied widely depending on the patient population and method of measurement, studies which have used right heart catheterization and defined PH as a mPAP of ≥25 mm Hg have demonstrated a prevalence from 8.1% in a cohort with interstitial lung disease.[85] PH in the setting of interstitial lung disease (ILD) is associated with worse survival.[86] Therapy for PH in interstitial lung disease consists of treatment of the underlying disease and oxygen. There are insufficient data to assess the efficacy of the use of pulmonary vasodilators in this setting.

Pulmonary Hypertension and Sleep-Disordered Breathing

Sleep-disordered breathing can be categorized as OSA, where there is cessation of airflow due to mechanical obstruction, or central sleep apnea (CSA), where there is an absence of respiratory effort and airflow. OSA is highly prevalent and is associated with obesity, whereas CSA is most often associated with heart failure. Repetitive apneic events lead to frequent recurring hypoxemia and hypercapnia, sympathetic-mediated vasoconstriction,[87] and abrupt changes in intrathoracic pressure, venous return, and cardiac output.[88] Sleep apnea can contribute to the development of PH, though the degree of PH tends to be mild.[89] Patients with sleep apnea and PH should be evaluated at a sleep center and treated with positive airway pressure therapy.

GROUP 4: PULMONARY HYPERTENSION DUE TO PULMONARY ARTERY OBSTRUCTIONS

Epidemiology, Clinical Features, and Diagnostic Evaluation

CTEPH is defined by PH caused by emboli in the pulmonary arterial system. It is characterized by intraarterial thrombus organization that fibroses and leads to intraluminal obliteration. The inciting event is thought to be a single or multiple recurrent pulmonary emboli (PE), followed by progressive vascular remodeling and fibrous scar formation. The cumulative incidence of CTEPH following a clinical PE approaches 4% at 2 years.[90] Risk factors for CTEPH include a variety of local and host factors, such as younger age, prior PE, idiopathic etiology for PE, a prior history of splenectomy or ventriculoatrial shunt, and elevated levels of antiphospholipid antibodies.[90] However, up to 63% of patients diagnosed with CTEPH never have a history of clinically diagnosed PE.[91]

The pathophysiology of CTEPH is not entirely explained by pulmonary arterial obliteration but rather secondary downstream vascular remodeling due to molecular mechanisms similar to PAH, including inflammation[92] and activation of the endothelin system.[93]

As patients presenting with CTEPH may have no prior diagnosis of PE, it is important to screen for chronic thromboembolic disease as part of the diagnostic evaluation of PH. Ventilation-perfusion lung scanning is recommended for screening as it has a high sensitivity (90%–100%) for the detection of CTEPH, which means that a negative or very low-probability result essentially rules out CTEPH. A segmental unmatched perfusion defect visualized on ventilation-perfusion scanning should be evaluated for definitive assessment with pulmonary angiography. PE-protocol computed tomography scans have a significantly lower sensitivity for CTEPH and should not be used for screening.

Treatment

With the identification of CTEPH the patient should be referred to a specialized center for consideration of surgical pulmonary thromboendarterectomy as the outcome can be dramatically improved by the resection of the fibrotic intraluminal material.[94] All patients should receive lifelong anticoagulation with warfarin to achieve an international normalized ratio goal of of at least 2.0 to 3.0. The goal of anticoagulation is to reduce the risk of further thromboembolic events. Selective use of pulmonary vascular targeted therapies may play a role in patients whose disease is too distal for a surgical approach or in patients who have persistent PH postoperatively. In patients with CTEPH and inoperable disease or residual PH, riociguat, a soluble guanylate cyclase

stimulator led to an improvement in exercise capacity and hemodynamics.[43] Riociguat is currently the only approved medical therapy for treatment of CTEPH. Lastly, percutaneous balloon pulmonary angioplasty is an emerging treatment option.[95] Balloon pulmonary angioplasty may be beneficial as an adjuvant to medical therapy in patients with inoperable disease or in patients with residual PH after surgery. Balloon pulmonary angioplasty is associated with improved hemodynamics, symptoms, and functional capacity, but the optimal timing and long-term outcomes remain to be determined.

GROUP 5: PULMONARY HYPERTENSION ASSOCIATED WITH UNCLEAR MULTIFACTORIAL MECHANISMS

Group 5 is a heterogeneous group of PH associated with unclear multifactorial mechanisms. This group includes PH associated with hematologic disorders, such as chronic hemolytic anemia, myeloproliferative disorders, and splenectomy; PH associated with systemic disorders, such as sarcoidosis, pulmonary histiocytosis, lymphangioleiomyomatosis; PH associated with metabolic disorders, such as glycogen storage disease and thyroid disease; and PH associated with other conditions, such as chronic renal failure. PAH targeted therapy may be beneficial in some patients with Group 5 PH, but there is little evidence to support the use of PAH targeted therapy in this group of PH.[1]

KEY REFERENCES

1. Simonneau G, Montani D, Celermajer DS, et al. Haemodynamic definition and updated clinical classification of pulmonary hypertension. *Eur Resp J.* Published online Dec 13, 2018.

3. McLaughlin VV, Archer SL, Badesch DB, et al. ACCF/AHA 2009 expert consensus document on pulmonary hypertension a report of the American College of Cardiology Foundation Task Force on Expert Consensus Documents and the American Heart Association developed in collaboration with the American College of Chest Physicians; American Thoracic Society, Inc.; and the Pulmonary Hypertension Association. *J Am Coll Cardiol.* 2009;53:1573–1619.

10. Badesch DB, Raskob GE, Elliott CG, et al. Pulmonary arterial hypertension: baseline characteristics from the REVEAL Registry. *Chest.* 2010;137:376–387.

22. Galie N, Humbert M, Vachiery JL, et al. 2015 ESC/ERS guidelines for the diagnosis and treatment of pulmonary hypertension: the Joint Task Force for the Diagnosis and Treatment of Pulmonary Hypertension of the European Society of Cardiology (ESC) and the European Respiratory Society (ERS): Endorsed by: Association for European Paediatric and Congenital Cardiology (AEPC), International Society for Heart and Lung Transplantation (ISHLT). *Europ Resp J.* 2015;46:903–975.

33. Benza RL, Gomberg-Maitland M, Miller DP, et al. The REVEAL Registry risk score calculator in patients newly diagnosed with pulmonary arterial hypertension. *Chest.* 2012;141:354–362.

43. Ghofrani HA, D'Armini AM, Grimminger F, et al. Riociguat for the treatment of chronic thromboembolic pulmonary hypertension. *N Engl J Med.* 2013;369:319–329.

48. Pulido T, Adzerikho I, Channick RN, et al. Macitentan and morbidity and mortality in pulmonary arterial hypertension. *N Engl J Med.* 2013;369:809–818.

52. Sitbon O, Channick R, Chin KM, et al. Selexipag for the treatment of pulmonary arterial hypertension. *N Engl J Med.* 2015;373:2522–2533.

56. Galie N, Barbera JA, Frost AE, et al. Initial use of ambrisentan plus tadalafil in pulmonary arterial hypertension. *N Engl J Med.* 2015;373:834–844.

72. Lam CS, Roger VL, Rodeheffer RJ, Borlaug BA, Enders FT, Redfield MM. Pulmonary hypertension in heart failure with preserved ejection fraction: a community-based study. *J Am Coll Cardiol.* 2009;53:1119–1126.

The full reference list for this chapter is available on ExpertConsult.

Heart Transplantation

Evan P. Kransdorf, Jon A. Kobashigawa

The first human heart transplant (HT) was performed more than 50 years ago, in 1967, by Christiaan Barnard at Groote Schuur Hospital in Cape Town, South Africa.[1] Since that time over 100,000 lives have been saved by this procedure. Despite steady progress in the field of mechanical circulatory support (MCS), HT remains the therapy that provides the best quality of life and long-term survival for patients with end-stage heart failure. The availability of better immunosuppressive agents and other improvements in the care of HT recipients have led to dramatic increases in median survival time after HT, from several days in the beginning to 11 years in the current era.[2] Furthermore, the percentage of HT recipients surviving to 1 year posttransplant has progressively increased over the last 25 years, from 84% for HT performed in 1990 to 90% for HT performed in 2015 (**Fig. 44.1**). Long-term survival has also improved, with the percentage of HT recipients surviving to 10 years posttransplant increasing from 45% for HT performed in 1990 to 56% for HT performed in 2005.

EVALUATION AND MANAGEMENT OF HEART TRANSPLANT CANDIDATES

Indications for Transplant

Given the scarcity of donor hearts available as well as the risks inherent to the procedure, patients with cardiomyopathy should be referred for consideration of HT only once they have developed advanced heart failure symptoms (NYHA class III or greater) refractory to all medical and device therapies. Within this patient population substantial heterogeneity exists with regard to prognosis. Cardiopulmonary exercise testing can serve as an important test to improve risk stratification for adverse outcomes. A peak oxygen consumption (VO_2) of 14 mL/kg per minute or less has traditionally served as one of several thresholds for listing for HT.[3]

Once end-stage cardiomyopathy is present, early referral for consideration of HT is important, given that a prolonged waiting time may be necessary before an organ becomes available. Clinical criteria for referral for HT have been developed and may assist the general cardiologist in the identification of patients who would benefit from HT.[4] Specific indicators include hypotension (systolic blood pressure ≤90 mm Hg, creatinine ≥1.8 mg/dL, hemoglobin ≤12 g/dL, and inability to tolerate a beta-blocker or renin-angiotensin receptor antagonist.)

The demographics of heart failure have changed within the US population over the last 30 years, and indications for HT have paralleled these changes. Most significantly, better treatments for coronary artery disease (CAD) have led to an increased incidence of heart failure due to ischemic heart disease, but fewer of these patients required HT. Comparing 1990 with 2017, the percentage of HT performed for ischemic cardiomyopathy in the United States decreased substantially from 56% to 35% (**Fig. 44.2**).[5] With this, there was an increase in the percentage of HT performed for all other indications, including dilated cardiomyopathy (increased from 40% to 54%), restrictive/hypertrophic cardiomyopathy (increased from 1% to 6%), redo HT (increased from 2% to 3%), and congenital heart disease (increased from 1% to 3%).

Evaluation of the Heart Transplant Candidate

Owing to the scarcity of donor hearts, candidates for HT must undergo a rigorous evaluation process to ensure that they will have good outcomes after HT. Evaluation should be performed with three main goals in mind. The first goal of evaluation is to confirm that the candidate has end-stage heart failure and that there are no alternative therapies other than HT that may be suitable. The next goal is to ensure that the function of noncardiac organs (despite optimal medical therapy) will not affect posttransplant outcomes. This includes a rigorous evaluation of

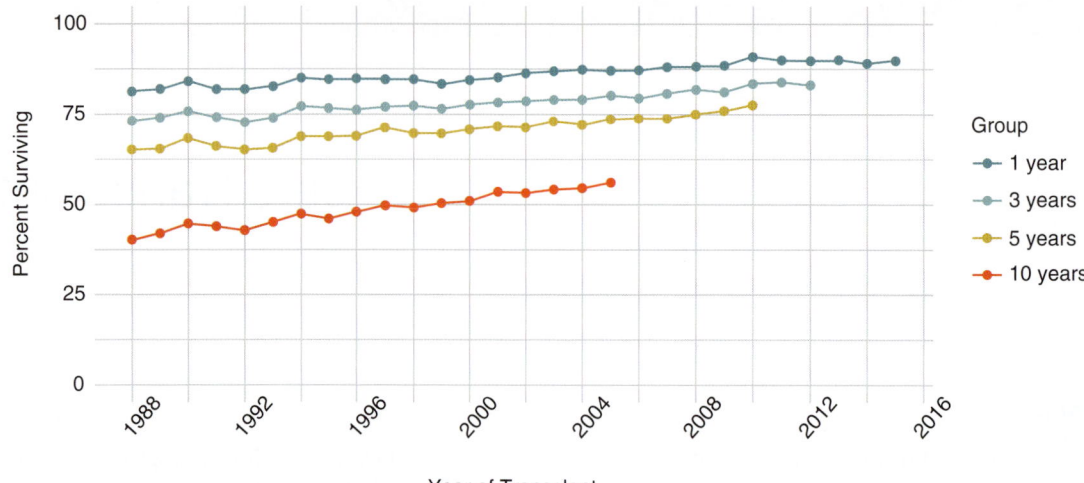

Fig. 44.1 Survival after heart transplantation has improved over successive years between 1988 and 2016. For each year of transplant on the x-axis, the percentage of recipients who survived to 1 year *(dark blue)*, 3 years *(light blue)*, 5 years *(yellow)*, and 10 years *(red)* posttransplant is plotted on the y-axis. (Unpublished data from United Network for Organ Sharing.)

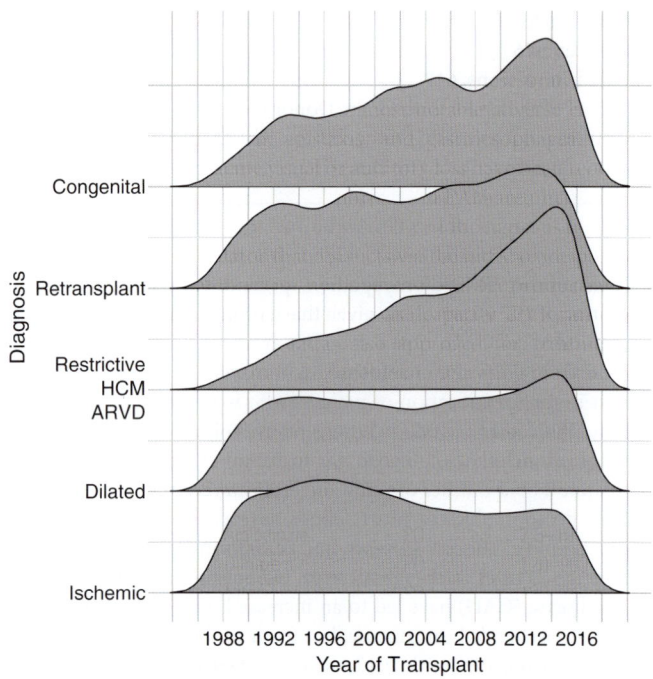

Fig. 44.2 Indications for heart transplantation in the United States between 1988 and 2016. During this 28-year period, 55,844 heart transplants were performed for adult recipients. For cases where the cause of the recipient's cardiomyopathy was known, 45% were performed for ischemic disease, 46% for dilated cardiomyopathy, 4% for restrictive/hypertrophic or right ventricular cardiomyopathy, 3% were retransplants, and 2% were for congenital heart disease. Over this time the percentage of transplants performed for ischemic disease has decreased, while the percentage performed for all other indications has increased. *ARVD,* Arrhythmogenic right ventricular dysplasia; *HCM,* hypertrophic cardiomyopathy. (Unpublished data from United Network for Organ Sharing.)

endocrine, kidney, liver, and lung function to identify potential collateral organ dysfunction that could limit outcomes after HT.[3] The exact testing required varies by transplant program but generally includes specialist consultations as well as laboratory and imaging studies

(**Table 44.1**). Lastly, a history of compliance with medications and medical recommendations must be present as well as adequate social support to help the patient through the HT process.

The unique physiology of the donor heart coupled with the technical aspects of the surgical procedure lead to several issues that require special consideration for HT candidates. First, the presence of pulmonary hypertension in the HT candidate requires careful assessment and management (**see also Chapters 34 and 43**). The donor heart is very sensitive to right ventricular afterload owing to the lack of conditioning to elevated pulmonary pressures as well as the effects of brain death on the right ventricle. Thus pulmonary hypertension is an important risk factor for right ventricular dysfunction of the cardiac allograft early posttransplant.[6]

The criteria for pulmonary hypertension as a contraindication for HT as recommended by the International Society for Heart and Lung Transplantation (ISHLT) include a pulmonary artery systolic pressure ≥50 mm Hg and either a pulmonary vascular resistance of ≥3 Woods units or a transpulmonary gradient ≥15 mm Hg.[3] If elevated pulmonary pressures are identified, a vasodilator challenge should be undertaken using intravenous vasodilator agents such as nitroglycerin, nitroprusside, or milrinone. If the pulmonary hypertension is reversible, then the patient is an acceptable candidate for HT, as the presence of "reversible" pulmonary hypertension does not affect posttransplant outcomes.[3]

Obese HT recipients experience an increased risk of mortality.[7] The ISHLT Listing Criteria for HT recommend that candidates with a body mass index greater than 35 kg/m² undergo weight loss before being listed for HT.[3] As obesity has become increasingly prevalent in the United States, the acceptable limits of body size for HT candidates have become a salient issue. As discussed in more detail further on, size matching is an important factor affecting donor heart selection, and donor weight is typically limited to no less than 30% of recipient weight. As a result, obese HT candidates have longer waiting times and consequently higher mortality on the wait list.

HT candidates who possess circulating anti–human leukocyte antigen (HLA) antibodies, a problem known as allosensitization, have diminished access to transplantation. This is because of the need to exclude from the potential donor pool donors with HLA antigens to which the HT candidate has antibodies in order to prevent the possibility of hyperacute rejection.[8] The degree of a candidate's

TABLE 44.1 Evaluation for Heart Transplantation

Area of Assessment	Specific Testing
Cardiology	*Goal: Confirm that end-stage heart failure is present and there are no further treatment options beyond transplant*
	Echocardiogram
	Right heart catheterization
	Coronary angiogram
	Cardiac magnetic resonance imaging
	Cardiopulmonary exercise test
Cardiac surgery	*Goal: Determine anatomic suitability for transplant and surgical risk assessment*
	ABO type
	Computed tomography of the chest
Dental	*Goal: Confirm the absence of any dental contraindications to transplant*
Endocrine	*Goal: Confirm that there is no active endocrine disease; if present, confirm that diabetes is well controlled*
	Glycated hemoglobin, thyroid-stimulating hormone
Infectious disease	*Goal: Confirm that there are no active infectious diseases present; infectious disease risk assessment*
	Infectious disease serologies including hepatitis viruses
Nutrition	*Goal: Confirm that the patient is not malnourished*
Oncology	*Goal: Confirm there is no active neoplastic disease present*
	Mammogram (women over 40)
	Papanicolaou test/human papillomavirus screening
	Prostate-specific antigen (men)
Psychiatric	*Goal: Confirm that there is no active psychiatric diseases present*
Pulmonary	*Goal: Confirm that there is no active pulmonary disease present*
	Pulmonary function test
Renal	*Goal: Confirm that there is no active renal disease present*
	Glomerular filtration rate
	Assessment of urinary protein
Social work	*Goal: Confirm that the patient has demonstrated compliance with medications and that there is adequate social support for transplantation*
Vascular	*Goal: Confirm that there is no active vascular disease present*
	Carotid ultrasound
	Lower extremity ankle-brachial index and ultrasound
Gastroenterology	*Goal: Confirm that there is no active gastrointestinal/liver disease present*
	Colonoscopy
	Liver ultrasound (if liver function tests abnormal)

allosensitization was originally assessed using the panel-reactive antibody (PRA) assay. The development of solid-phase methods of antibody identification has led to the use of the calculated panel-reactive antibody (CPRA), which uses the gene frequencies of the excluded HLA antigens in historic donors.[9] CPRA summarizes the percentage of the potential donor population with the candidate's unacceptable HLA antigens for both the class I and II specificities as a single numeric value. As the CPRA value increases, HT candidates experience longer waiting times and an increased risk for adverse outcomes such as death and removal from the wait list for worsening condition (**Fig. 44.3**).[10]

There are several strategies to improve access to transplantation for allosensitized candidates. First, careful consideration should be given to the process of identifying which HLA antigens to exclude. Multiple techniques including the traditional cell-based cross-match and solid-phase methods should be used for this purpose.[11] Next, immune-modulating therapies can be utilized to reduce the level of circulating HLA antibodies, a process known as desensitization.[12] The optimal approach for managing allosensitized patients, both prior to and after HT, has not been established.

After optimizing cardiac function, renal dysfunction is common in patients with advanced heart failure and is another important consideration in HT candidates. On the basis of the estimated glomerular filtration rate (eGFR) cutoffs used to define chronic kidney disease,

Habib et al. showed that 46% of HT recipients had a baseline eGFR of less than 60 mL/min per 1.73 m^2.[13] After adjustment for covariates, eGFR consistent with moderate (30–44 mL/min per 1.73 m^2) or severe (<30 mL/min per 1.73 m^2) renal dysfunction was strongly associated with posttransplant mortality. Thus HT candidates with an eGFR of less than 30 to 40 mL/min per 1.73 m^2 should be considered for a combined heart-kidney transplant.

THE HEART TRANSPLANT PROCEDURE

Donor Heart Evaluation and Management

The number of donor hearts that become available is limited; therefore there is a continual excess of candidates waiting for a HT as compared with the number of donor hearts that become available.[14] Thus the careful evaluation and medical optimization of each potential heart donor is of upmost importance. There are several steps in the donor evaluation and management process (**Fig. 44.4**).[15]

Deceased donors are persons that have suffered brain death, most commonly due to traumatic injury or stroke.[16] After brain death has been declared by two separate neurologists, the family is approached regarding the possibility of organ donation by representatives of the clinical team or by representatives of the local organ procurement organization (OPO). OPOs are a group of nonprofit organizations that evaluate and manage donors throughout the United States. If consent for organ donation is granted by the deceased patient's family, representatives of the OPO will begin the donor evaluation and management process.

The general evaluation of deceased donors includes screening for infectious diseases (e.g., human immunodeficiency virus, hepatitis A/B/C, syphilis) and occult malignancy. If the donor is acceptable from this standpoint, cardiac tests such as echocardiography and pulmonary artery catheterization are performed. Coronary angiography is frequently performed for older donors or those with risk factors for CAD. Abnormalities of cardiac function by echocardiography and angiography are strong predictors for rejection of the donor heart.[17] Overall only about 30% of deceased donors become heart donors.[18] The physiologic effects of brain death can lead to cardiac dysfunction, so throughout the donor evaluation process the donor is managed by the OPO to maintain optimal cardiac function.[15]

Donor Heart Allocation

Through the allocation process, donor hearts that become available are assigned to a HT candidate on the wait list. The process begins with the OPO, which generates a list of potential recipients for a donor heart. This list is termed a "match list" and enumerates all potential

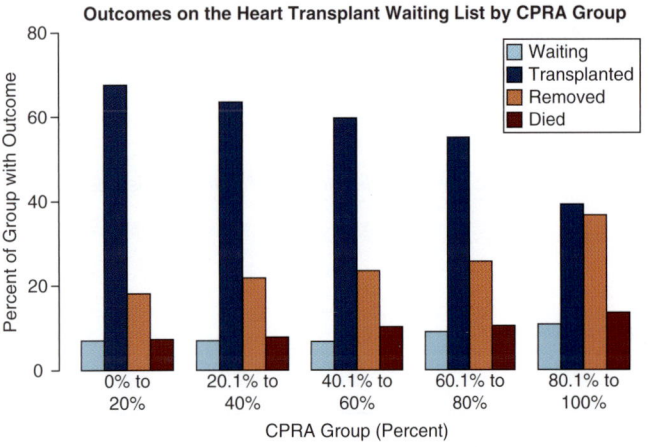

Outcomes on the Heart Transplant Waiting List by CPRA Group

Fig. 44.3 Plot of frequency of waiting list outcomes for sensitized heart transplant candidates grouped by calculated panel reactive antibody (CPRA) value. Candidates were sorted into five groups by their initial CPRA value. As the CPRA increased, the percentage of candidates who received a transplant decreased and the percentage of candidates who were still waiting for a transplant, were removed from the waiting list, or died increased. (From Kransdorf EP, Kittleson MM, Patel JK, Pando MJ, Steidley DE, Kobashigawa JA. Calculated panel-reactive antibody predicts outcomes on the heart transplant waiting list. *J Heart Lung Transplant.* 2017;36[7]:787–796.)

recipients that are compatible with the donor and who could receive the organ. The order of potential recipients on the match list is specified by an allocation algorithm developed by the Organ Procurement and Transplantation Network/United Network for Organ Sharing (OPTN/UNOS), which places potential recipients into priority bins first by geographic location, then medical urgency, and then blood type compatibility.[19]

Medical urgency is assessed using a tiered system composed of six statuses of increasing urgency. Patients in the most urgent tier, status 1, are primarily patients requiring extracorporeal membrane oxygenation (ECMO) (**Fig. 44.5**).[20] Patients in status 2 are mostly those requiring an intra-aortic balloon pump or temporary left ventricular assist device (for 14 days or less). Patients requiring high-dose inotropic agents, who in the previous medical urgency system composed the bulk of the status 1A group, now make up the status 3 group. Status 4, akin to status 1B in the previous medical urgency system, is composed of patients on inotropes without hemodynamic monitoring, those with a dischargeable left ventricular assist device (after using their discretionary 30 days of status 3 time), and those with certain cardiomyopathy diagnoses such as congenital heart disease and restrictive cardiomyopathy. Status 6 is composed of all other candidates, frequently those with ambulatory heart failure.

Within each priority bin, donor hearts are allocated by the accumulated active waiting time (i.e., candidates with longer waiting time will have a lower sequence number on the match list and are more likely to receive the organ) (**Fig. 44.6**). The transplant program for each potential recipient is notified of the potential for allocation to one of the candidates on the wait list and performs an assessment of the quality of the donor heart for that recipient. Numerous parameters are considered during this assessment, but critical elements include the donor-recipient match for size, sex, and age as well as donor factors such as left ventricular function, left ventricular hypertrophy, and ischemic time.[21] To be an acceptable donor, donor weight is recommended to be no more than 30% below that of the recipient[22] except when a female donor is being used for a male recipient, in which case donor weight is recommended to be no more than 20% below that of the recipient. Donor age is frequently kept to age 55 or less.[21,22] As discussed earlier, abnormal left ventricular function that fails to improve during donor management as well as significant left ventricular hypertrophy are common reasons that organs are declined.[15]

If the transplant program finds the organ is appropriate for the recipient, the offer is accepted. Ultimately the donor heart will be placed with the potential recipient with the lowest sequence number whose transplant program accepted the organ offer. The transplant program for the recipient to whom the donor heart was placed will work with the OPO to coordinate the heart procurement.

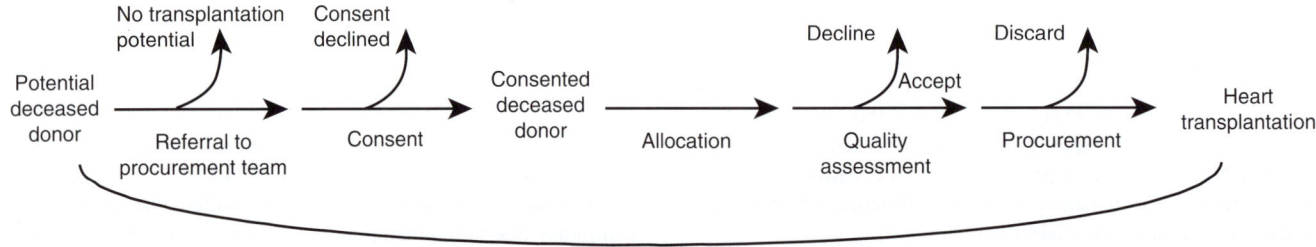

Fig. 44.4 Steps in the donor evaluation process. The process starts with identification of potential organ donors and concludes with transplant of the donor heart into the recipient. (From Kransdorf EP, Stehlik J. Donor evaluation in heart transplantation: the end of the beginning. *J Heart Lung Transplant.* 2014;33[11]:1105–1113.)

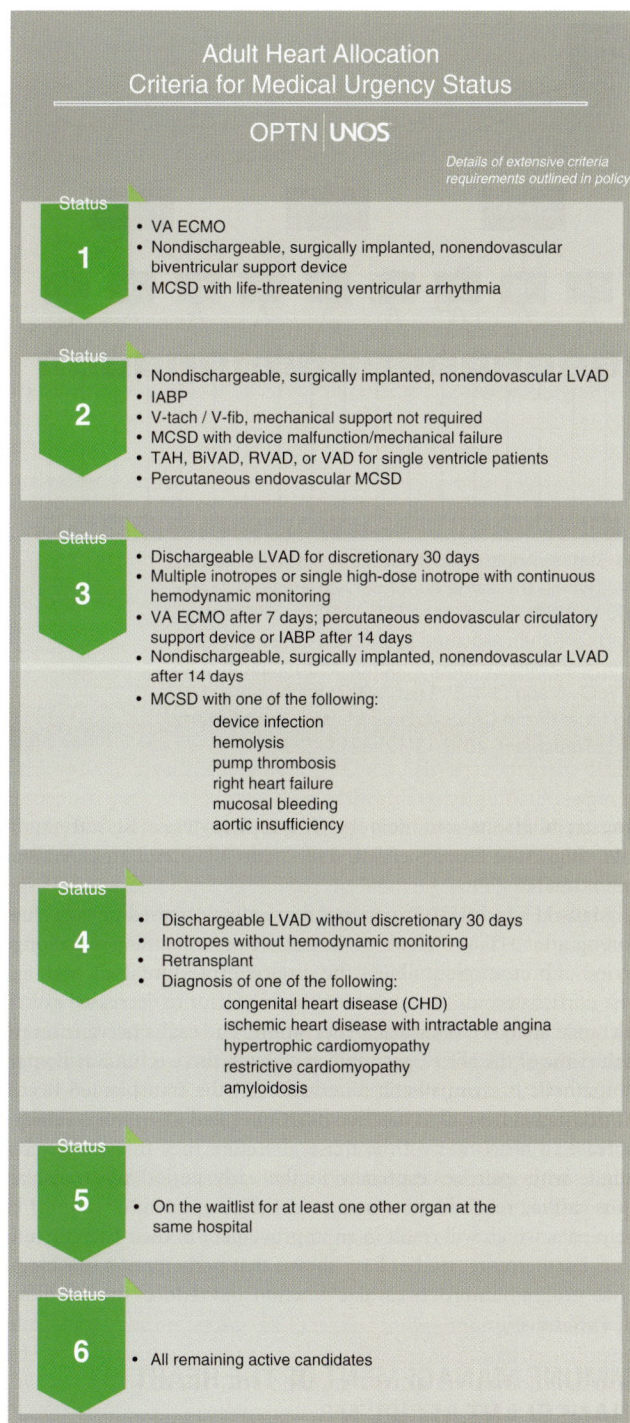

**Adult Heart Allocation
Criteria for Medical Urgency Status**

OPTN | UNOS

*Details of extensive criteria
requirements outlined in policy*

Status 1
- VA ECMO
- Nondischargeable, surgically implanted, nonendovascular biventricular support device
- MCSD with life-threatening ventricular arrhythmia

Status 2
- Nondischargeable, surgically implanted, nonendovascular LVAD
- IABP
- V-tach / V-fib, mechanical support not required
- MCSD with device malfunction/mechanical failure
- TAH, BiVAD, RVAD, or VAD for single ventricle patients
- Percutaneous endovascular MCSD

Status 3
- Dischargeable LVAD for discretionary 30 days
- Multiple inotropes or single high-dose inotrope with continuous hemodynamic monitoring
- VA ECMO after 7 days; percutaneous endovascular circulatory support device or IABP after 14 days
- Nondischargeable, surgically implanted, nonendovascular LVAD after 14 days
- MCSD with one of the following:
    device infection
    hemolysis
    pump thrombosis
    right heart failure
    mucosal bleeding
    aortic insufficiency

Status 4
- Dischargeable LVAD without discretionary 30 days
- Inotropes without hemodynamic monitoring
- Retransplant
- Diagnosis of one of the following:
    congenital heart disease (CHD)
    ischemic heart disease with intractable angina
    hypertrophic cardiomyopathy
    restrictive cardiomyopathy
    amyloidosis

Status 5
- On the waitlist for at least one other organ at the same hospital

Status 6
- All remaining active candidates

Fig. 44.5 Medical urgency tiers in the heart allocation system. Extracorporeal membrane oxygenation largely constitutes status 1. Patients with temporary intra-aortic balloon pumps or temporary mechanical circulatory support compose the bulk of status 2. There is regional sharing of these upper tiers. Candidates requiring multiple inotropes or a durable left ventricular assist device for 30 days constitute status 3. Candidates with single/low-dose inotropic support without hemodynamic monitoring or a durable left ventricular assist device after 30 days constitute status 4. Candidates for dual-organ transplant constitute status 5. All other candidates constitute status 6. *BiVAD*, Biventricular assist device; *IABP*, intra-aortic balloon pump; *LVAD*, left ventricular assist device; *MCSD*, mechanical circulatory support device; *TAH*, total artificial heart; *VAD*, ventricular assist device; *VA ECMO*, venoarterial extracorporeal membrane oxygenation. (From Organ Procurement and Transplantation Network Adult heart allocation. UNOS Transplant Pro. Available at: https://optn.transplant.hrsa.gov/learn/professional-education/adult-heart-allocation.)

Surgical Procedure

The HT procedure requires two surgeons. One surgeon travels to the hospital where the deceased donor is located and procures the donor heart. This surgeon performs an assessment of quality of the donor heart on arrival by first reviewing the echocardiogram, hemodynamics, and coronary angiogram (if performed). If the organ is acceptable, the procurement surgery proceeds. Once the heart has been surgically exposed, the surgeon makes a final check of the coronary arteries via palpation. If there are no abnormalities, the heart is arrested using cardioplegia solution, explanted, and placed in cold storage on ice. This marks the beginning of the cold ischemic time. The procurement team then travels back to the hospital, where the recipient has already been prepared for surgery.

Upon hearing that the donor heart is acceptable, the second surgeon proceeds with the recipient cardiectomy. A sternotomy is performed. The recipient is placed on cardiopulmonary bypass via placement of cannulas in the aorta and superior and inferior vena cavae. The aorta is cross-clamped and the recipient's heart is removed. Then the donor heart is brought onto the surgical field and the left atrial anastomosis is made, followed by the inferior vena cava, pulmonary artery, and aortic anastomoses (**Fig. 44.7**). The aortic cross-clamp is released and the heart begins to be perfused with blood. It will typically start to beat spontaneously. Inotropic and vasopressor support is initiated. Then then the patient is weaned from cardiopulmonary bypass. Hemostasis is achieved and the chest is closed. The recipient is then transported to the intensive care unit (ICU) for ongoing care.

Postoperative Care

During the initial phase the recipient is cared for in the ICU, where the focuses of care are hemodynamic support of the recently transplanted heart and the usual requirements after cardiothoracic surgery such as mechanical ventilation and chest tube drainage. Once the recipient's hemodynamic status has stabilized, he or she is transferred to the cardiac floor, where the main focus of care is on physical strengthening and learning the complex medical regimen that will be required at discharge.

While in the ICU, the recipient may be maintained on multiple inotropic and vasopressor medications. In general, inotropic support is needed to combat the effects of ischemia-reperfusion injury which affects the donor heart early posttransplant. Vasopressor support is also frequently needed, and up to 35% of HT recipients will experience vasoplegia after HT.[23] Vasoplegia is more common in patients who have previously undergone thoracic surgery or were supported with MCS.

Primary graft dysfunction (PGD) is an important cause of morbidity and mortality that presents immediately or within the first few hours after HT. PGD occurs when the recently implanted donor heart displays dysfunction of the left ventricle, right ventricle, or both in the absence of discernible secondary causes such as pulmonary hypertension or hyperacute rejection.[24] Dysfunction frequently manifests as hypotension, low cardiac output/index, and high filling pressures. The incidence of PGD varies by institution from around 5% to 25% of all HT. Risk factors for PGD include amiodarone use, African American ethnicity, diabetes mellitus, donor age, high right atrial pressure, increasing ischemic time, inotrope dependence, and recipient age.[25,26] When severe PGD is present, the use of MCS with an IABP or ECMO is frequently needed. Even with aggressive management of PGD, mortality remains high.

Immunosuppression is another important consideration of early posttransplant care, as "induction" immunosuppression is administered shortly after HT. Induction immunosuppression agents include antithymocyte globulin (ATG) as well as the interleukin-2

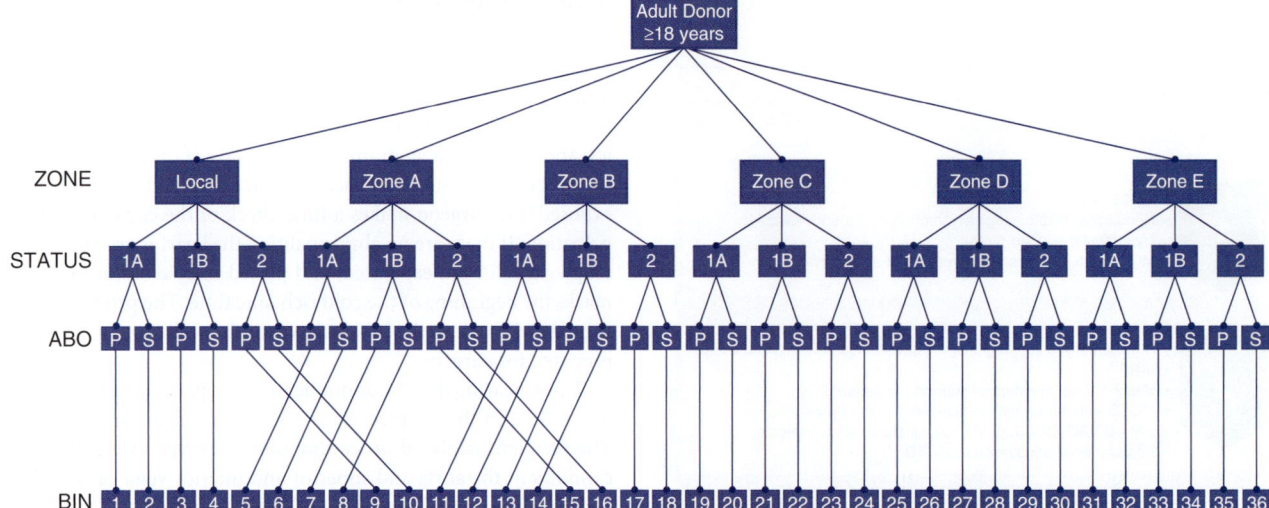

Fig. 44.6 Algorithm for donor heart allocation in the United States. Adult donor hearts are first allocated by geographic zone according to the location of the donor: local (within the same donor service area/organ procurement organization), zone A (0–500 miles), zone B (>500 to 1000 miles), zone C (>1000 to 1500 miles), zone D (>1500 to 2500 miles) and zone E (>2500 miles). Hearts are then allocated by medical urgency (status 1A, then 1B, then 2). Then hearts are allocated by ABO compatibility (primary = donor and recipient with identical ABO as well as O→B, A→AB and B→AB; secondary = O→A and O→AB). Last, within each priority bin, donor hearts are allocated by the accumulated active waiting time. (From Colvin-Adams M, Valapour M, Hertz M, et al. Lung and heart allocation in the United States. *Am J Transplant.* 2012;12[12]:3213–3234.)

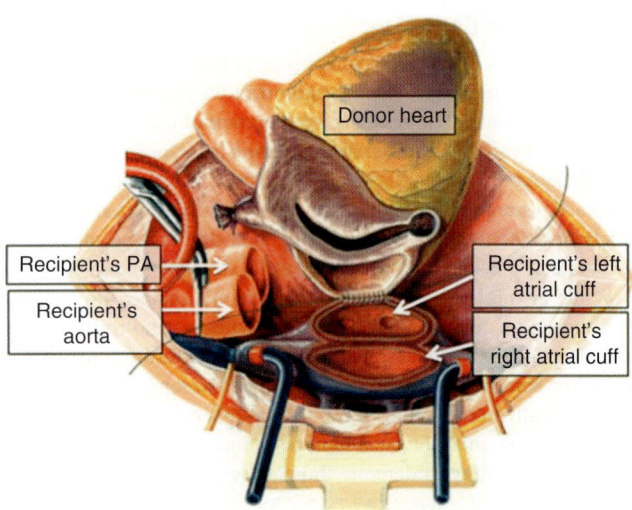

Fig. 44.7 Schematic of the orthotopic heart transplant procedure. After the sternotomy has been completed, the recipient is placed on cardiopulmonary bypass and the aorta is cross-clamped. The recipient's heart is removed. Then the donor heart is brought onto the surgical field and the left atrial anastomosis is made, followed by the inferior vena cava, pulmonary artery, and aortic anastomoses. (From Reichart B, Rose AG, Reichenspurner H. *Herz- und Herz-Lungen. Transplantation.* Percha, Germany: RS Schulz Verlag; 1987.)

antagonist basiliximab. Although induction immunosuppression has not been proven to be of benefit via a randomized clinical trial, it is used routinely by half of HT programs in the United States with the intent of enhancing tolerance to the donor graft. The use of induction immunosuppression has been used in two other circumstances as well: for recipients with renal dysfunction in whom induction immunosuppression is used to delay introduction of a calcineurin inhibitor and for recipients at an elevated immunologic risk in whom induction immunosuppression is used for its

long-term effects on memory T lymphocytes.[27] Recent studies have suggested improved survival with ATG as compared with basiliximab.[28]

Many HT recipients experience markedly decreased physical functioning after HT as a result of several factors, including a prolonged period of pretransplant illness, the surgical procedure itself, and high-dose corticosteroids. Another contributing factor to decreased exercise tolerance after HT is cardiac denervation. The vagus nerve is severed at the time of the HT surgery and, as a result, there is initially no parasympathetic or sympathetic innervation of the transplanted heart.[29] HT recipients have high baseline heart rates and experience a delayed increase in heart rate with exercise; therefore they frequently report fatigue with exercise, especially in the early period posttransplant. Thus cardiac rehabilitation is an essential component of care for HT recipients, which will result in an improvement in their exercise tolerance. Furthermore, studies have shown that participation in a cardiac rehab program improves cardiac function and reduces the risk of hospital readmission.[30,31]

IMMUNE MANAGEMENT OF THE HEART TRANSPLANT RECIPIENT

Overview

HT recipients must be maintained on immunosuppressive medications for life in order to keep their immune systems in a quiescent state. Without this immune quiescence, the recipient's immune system will mount a cellular and humoral response against the donor heart, leading to allograft dysfunction and failure. The clinical syndrome caused by this immune response is termed allograft rejection (AR). The primary goal of care of the HT recipient is to prevent AR. On the other hand, immunosuppression predisposes HT recipients to infections with typical as well as atypical pathogens. Thus the modus operandi in caring for HT recipients is to monitor and adjust the level of immunosuppressive medications to maintain a balance between "enough" and "too much" (**Fig. 44.8**).

From the early days of HT it was recognized that the risk of rejection was highest early after transplant, usually in the first year post-transplant, and that it decreases over time.[32] It is worth noting that diminution of immunosuppression below a certain threshold or augmentation of the recipient's immune system—for example due to subtherapeutic immunosuppressive drug levels or infection, can lead to rejection even long after HT. As a consequence of this, the clinical approach to immunosuppression is to apply a high level of immunosuppression early after transplant and gradually decrease this level over time while monitoring for the development of AR.

The initially universal incidence of rejection led to the practice of performing surveillance for rejection in asymptomatic patients via percutaneous endomyocardial biopsy (EMB)[33] in an effort to identify rejection earlier and thus treat it before hemodynamic sequelae developed. Although in the current era the incidence of rejection within the first year of HT is substantially lower, at 15%,[34] the importance of identifying rejection before severe clinical sequelae develop has led to persistence of the practice of performing routine surveillance EMB.

Clinical and Pathologic Subtypes of Cardiac Allograft Rejection

For HT recipients presenting with a clinical syndrome consistent with rejection, the three immediate goals should be to assess cardiac function, achieve hemodynamic stability, and initiate treatment of rejection via immunomodulation. As part of the assessment process, an echocardiogram and EMB should be performed for all patients with symptoms possibly consistent with rejection.

Patients with rejection present along a clinical spectrum, varying from an asymptomatic patient to a patient with fulminant cardiogenic shock (**Table 44.2**). Asymptomatic patients usually come to clinical attention at the time of a surveillance EMB showing rejection. Factors affecting the severity of hemodynamic perturbations in rejection have not been fully elucidated, but predictors of severity include right ventricular involvement,[35] as well as the physiologic inability to respond to the decreased allograft function with an increased systemic vascular resistance.[36] Arrhythmias can also occur, including atrial fibrillation in symptomatic rejection and polymorphic ventricular tachycardia/ventricular fibrillation in hemodynamic compromise rejection.[37]

The major pathologic types of rejection are acute cellular rejection (ACR) and antibody-mediated rejection (AMR), the features of which are discussed here. Mixed rejection, where both ACR and AMR coexist on the biopsy, is not uncommon but is not felt to be a distinct type of rejection. Similarly, a patient can present with clinical rejection and the EMB may show no evidence of rejection. This situation is termed biopsy-negative rejection and may be due to sampling error of the EMB or possibly to an atypical form of AMR (e.g., non-HLA antibody-mediated AMR).[38]

ACR is the most common form of rejection; in a large analysis by Kfoury et al. of patients undergoing HT between 1985 and 2014, it was found in 24% of biopsies.[39] Mechanistically, ACR is due to direct and indirect allorecognition, which leads to T-cell activation and infiltration of the allograft.[40] Histopathology shows infiltration of lymphocytes and macrophages, with the grade of rejection corresponding to the extent of cellular infiltration and myocyte injury. EMB samples are graded according to a common set of criteria developed by the ISHLT (**Table 44.3; Fig. 44.9A and B**).[41]

AMR is the next most common form of rejection, occurring in 9% of biopsies.[39] AMR is due predominantly to the binding of antibodies against HLA antigens to cardiac tissue, leading to complement activation and tissue injury. The ISHLT formulation for the diagnosis of AMR involves both an immunological and a histological component (see Table 44.3).[42] Immunologically, complement components C3d or C4d are seen in a capillary pattern. Histological findings suggestive of AMR include endothelial cell activation, intravascular macrophage accumulation and interstitial edema (see Fig. 44.9C and D).

Mixed rejection is the situation where an EMB displays both ACR and AMR, which has been found to occur in 8% of biopsies.[39] About 50% of mixed rejection biopsies show mild ACR and AMR (ACR grade 1R and AMR grade 1I/1H), and another 30% show mild CR but more severe AMR (ACR grade 1R and AMR grade 2). The pathological findings of each rejection type in mixed rejection are similar to the findings of each type when present individually, so mixed rejection is most likely a coexistence of the two rejection types.

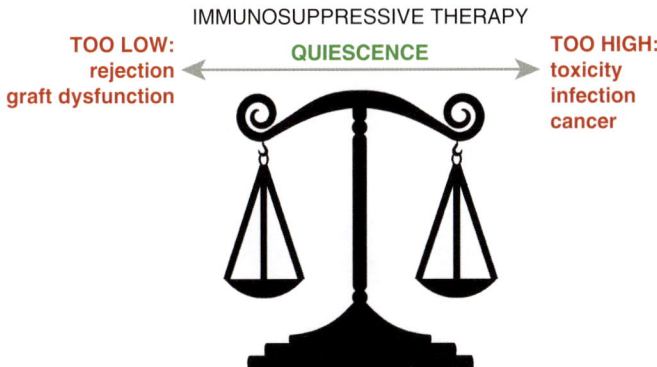

IMMUNOSUPPRESSIVE THERAPY

TOO LOW: rejection graft dysfunction

QUIESCENCE

TOO HIGH: toxicity infection cancer

Fig. 44.8 The primary goal of care of the heart transplant recipient is to use immunosuppressive therapy to prevent allograft rejection by inducing a state of immune quiescence. This requires achieving a delicate balance between immunosuppression in excess of what is required, referred to as "overimmunosuppression," and immunosuppression below what is required. Inadequate immunosuppression can lead to rejection/graft dysfunction, and overimmunosuppression can cause infection, drug toxicities, and cancer (over long periods of time). (Modified from Patel J, Kobashigawa JA. Minimization of immunosuppression: transplant immunology. *Transpl Immunol.* 2008;20[1–2]:48–54.)

TABLE 44.2	**Clinical Presentation of Transplant Rejection**		
	Asymptomatic	**Symptomatic**	**Hemodynamic Compromise**
Symptoms	None	Dyspnea, orthopnea, abdominal pain, weight gain	
Physical examination		↑JVP	↑JVP, +S3, cool extremities
Echo findings	Normal function	↓ RV and LV function (EF ~40%)	↓↓ RV and LV function (EF ~20%)
Hemodynamics	Normal	↑JVP, ↑PCWP, ↓CI	↑↑JVP, ↑↑PCWP, ↓↓CI
Hemodynamic management	None	Inotropes	Inotropes, MCS

CI, Cardiac index; *JVP,* jugular venous pulsation; *MCS,* mechanical circulatory support; *PCWP,* pulmonary capillary wedge pressure.

The risk of rejection varies significantly between individuals. The basis for this variability has not yet been fully elucidated, but several clinical and genetic factors have been identified as contributory. Clinical risk factors for rejection include medication non-compliance, younger age of the recipient, African American ethnicity, and circulating anti-HLA antibodies.[43] Genetic risk factors include increasing donor to recipient HLA mismatch[44] and genetic polymorphisms within the cytokine genes.[45]

Noninvasive Monitoring for Allograft Rejection

The EMB has several important limitations that have encouraged the development of alternative methods of diagnosis for rejection. First and foremost, the EMB is an invasive procedure that has potential to cause complications, albeit rarely, including tricuspid valve injury and tamponade.[46] Second, because the site for an EMB is chosen at random, sampling error is frequently known to occur. Biopsy-negative rejection, where rejection is suspected clinically but the biopsy shows no histological evidence of rejection, is not uncommon.[38] Finally, evaluation of the EMB for rejection by expert pathologists has significant inter-observer variability due to the presence of artifacts, which can include previous biopsy site, infection, and the Quilty effect (subendocardial lymphocyte infiltration that is felt to be benign).[47]

Gene expression profiling was established as a potentially clinically useful, noninvasive method for the diagnosis of ACR via the Cardiac Allograft Rejection Gene Expression Observational (CARGO) study.[48] The CARGO study tested the hypothesis that gene expression profiling, performed using a sample of mononuclear cells isolated from the peripheral blood, could discriminate significant ACR (ISHLT grade 2R and above) from immune quiescence. In this study, gene discovery was first performed using 247 samples from patients with ACR and 38 control samples. This led to the identification of 252 candidate genes, which were then individually

TABLE 44.3 Grading and Pathologic Findings for Cellular Rejection and Antibody-Mediated Rejection

Type	Grade	Pathologic Findings
Cellular rejection	0R	None
	1R	Interstitial and/or perivascular infiltrate with up to one focus of myocyte damage
	2R	Two or more foci of infiltrate with associated myocyte damage
	3R	Diffuse cellular infiltrate with multifocal myocyte damage with or without edema, hemorrhage, and vasculitis
Antibody-mediated rejection	0	None
Rejection	1I or 1H	Immunopathology (I) or histology (H) positive
	2	Immunopathology and histology positive
	3	Interstitial hemorrhage, capillary fragmentation and marked edema

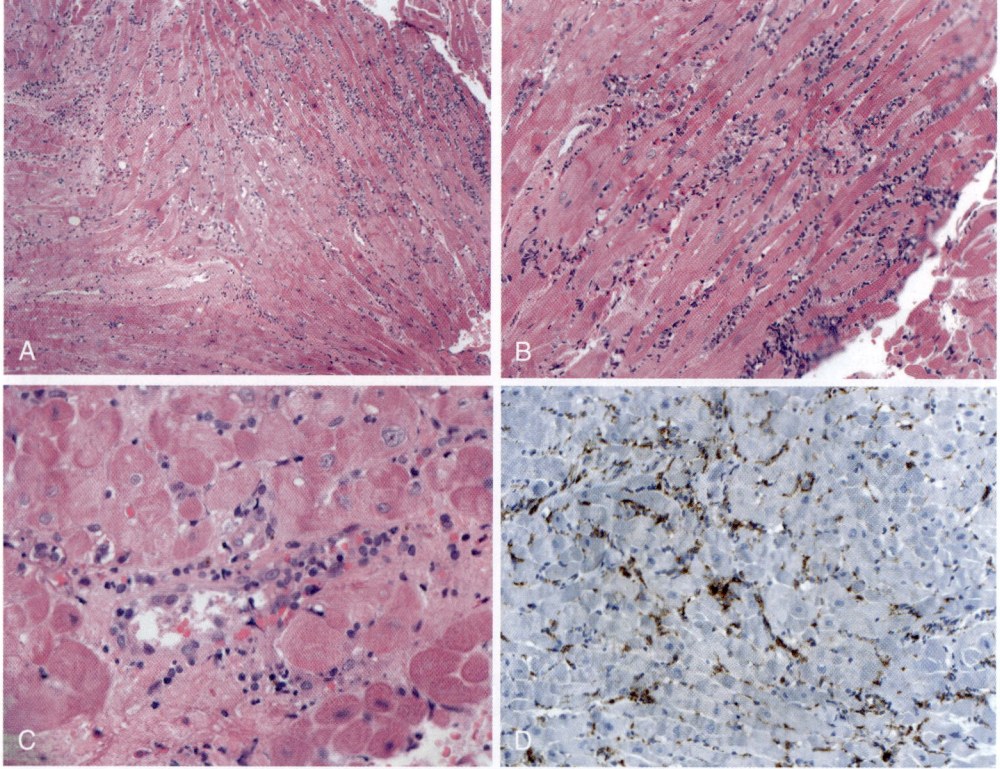

Fig. 44.9 Photomicrographs of endomyocardial biopsy samples showing cellular and antibody-mediated rejection. (A) Myocardium with lymphocytic infiltrate consistent with International Society for Heart and Lung Transplantation grade 2R cellular rejection (100× magnification). (B) Sample as in (A) at a higher magnification (200× magnification). (C) Sample showing capillaries with activated endothelial cells and intravascular macrophages consistent with antibody-mediated rejection (400× magnification). (D) Immunoperoxidase staining positive for CD68, highlighting intravascular macrophages (brown) in antibody-mediated rejection (400× magnification). (From Kransdorf EP, Kobashigawa JA. Genetic and genomic approaches to the detection of heart transplant rejection. *Per Med.* 2012;9[7]:693–705.)

analyzed in 109 samples from patients with rejection and 36 control samples. Ultimately, 11 genes were selected that provided the best discrimination between ACR and quiescence. In practice, the levels of these 11 genes are measured and combined to yield an expression score with a value between 0 and 40. Lower scores suggest immune quiescence and higher scores suggest immune activity potentially compatible with ACR.

This assay became available for clinical use as the AlloMap test (CareDx, Brisbane, CA) in 2005. The clinical experience with AlloMap showed that using a threshold score of 34, the negative predictive value for significant ACR approached 99%, while the positive predictive value is only 7%.[49] As such, AlloMap can serve as a test to indicate a quiescent state with the presence of significant ACR (ISHLT grade 2R or higher) being very unlikely, and thus avoiding the need for an EMB. However, the test is not sufficiently specific to serve as a stand-alone test for rejection. Patients with elevated scores require an EMB to confirm the presence of rejection. It is important to remember that AlloMap was developed to assess only for ACR. There are several important contraindications to the use of AlloMap, which are detailed in **Table 44.4**.

The clinical utility of the AlloMap was demonstrated through two clinical trials, the Invasive Monitoring Attenuation through Gene Expression (IMAGE) and Early Invasive Monitoring Attenuation through Gene Expression (EIMAGE) trials. In the IMAGE trial, a total of 602 adult patients between 6-months and 5-years posttransplant were randomized to a rejection surveillance protocol using primarily AlloMap or EMB.[49] In the AlloMap arm of the trial, a threshold score of 34 or above triggered an EMB, as did symptoms or signs of AR or a decrease in ejection fraction of ≥25% from baseline. Over a median duration of 19 months, the primary composite outcome of rejection with hemodynamic compromise, graft dysfunction due to non-rejection causes, death

or retransplantation, was similar between the AlloMap and EMB arms (14.5% and 15.3%, respectively). Patients in the AlloMap group had 67% fewer EMBs. Interestingly, there was a higher number of treated rejection episodes in the EMB arm, but given that there was a similar number of adverse events in both groups, a small number of rejection events are not detected by AlloMap but are clinically insignificant.

Since HT recipients are more likely to develop rejection early after HT and because most patients in the IMAGE trial were between 1 and 3 years posttransplant, the EIMAGE trial was performed to confirm the utility of AlloMap in monitoring for rejection early after HT.[50] In this trial, HT recipients ≥55 days but less than 185 days posttransplant were randomized to rejection surveillance via AlloMap or EMB. A similar primary composite outcome was used in EIMAGE and IMAGE. The trial showed a slightly higher percentage of endpoints in the EMB arm compared to the AlloMap arm (17% vs. 10%) that was not statistically significant. Thus, AlloMap is safe and effective for ACR monitoring in HT recipients starting as early as 55 days posttransplant and can reduce the number of invasive EMB required for rejection surveillance.

Treatment of Allograft Rejection

Once rejection has been confirmed by clinical and pathological evaluation, hemodynamic stabilization and immunomodulation should be initiated immediately. If the patient displays evidence of cardiogenic shock as evidenced by laboratory and/or hemodynamic parameters, inotropic support should be initiated and consideration should be given to placement of MCS. The use of both temporary (as a bridge to recovery) and permanent (as a bridge to retransplant) MCS have been reported in AR. ECMO may be especially useful for hemodynamic compromise rejection as it can be implemented quickly and provides biventricular support while treatment for rejection is provided. If ECMO is to be initiated, better outcomes occur when it is initiated at the time of worsening hemodynamic status, as compared to salvage therapy (at the time of cardiac arrest).[51]

The treatment regimen for rejection depends on both the clinical status of the patient and the pathological evaluation of the EMB. For patients hospitalized with symptomatic or hemodynamic compromise rejection, a bolus dose of corticosteroids and ATG are frequently administered. In addition to immunosuppression, we administer intravenous heparin, as coronary microvascular thrombosis occurs in severe rejection and heparin has been shown to improve coronary microvascular endothelial function in this setting.[52] For patients with AMR, plasma exchange and intravenous immunoglobulin are frequently administered. The Cedars-Sinai protocol for management of rejection is presented in **Table 44.5**. If the initial EMB shows AR, we repeat an EMB 2 weeks later to

---

TABLE 44.4 Clinical Contraindications to the Use of AlloMap for Cellular Rejection Monitoring

Active cardiac allograft dysfunction
Hemodynamic rejection in the last 6 months
Antibody-mediated rejection in last 12 months
Pregnancy
Blood transfusion in last 30 days
Hematopoietic growth factors in last 30 days
Patient less than 15 years of age
High-dose steroids in the last 21 days
Daily prednisone administration >20 mg
Dual organ transplant recipient (e.g., heart and kidney)

TABLE 44.5 Protocol for Management of Allograft Rejection

EMB Pathology	CLINICAL PRESENTATION OF REJECTION		
	Asymptomatic	Symptomatic	Hemodynamic Compromise
Cellular rejection	ACR1	All Grades	All Grades
	• No treatment needed	• Hemodynamic stabilization	• IV CS bolus
	• ACR2	• IV CS bolus	• ATG
	• Oral CS bolus	• ATG	• PLEX
	• Target higher CNI levels		• IV IG
Antibody-mediated rejection	AMR1/AMR2	AMR1/AMR2	• IV heparin
	• Oral CS bolus	• IV CS bolus	
	• IV IG/rituximab	• IV IG/rituximab	
	• Conversion to mTOR inhibitor	• Conversion to a mTOR inhibitor	

ACR, Acute cellular rejection grade; *AMR*, antibody-mediated rejection grade; *ATG*, antithymocyte globulin; *CS*, corticosteroid; *IG*, immunoglobulin; *IV*, intravenous; *mTOR*, mammalian target of rapamycin; *PLEX*, plasma exchange.

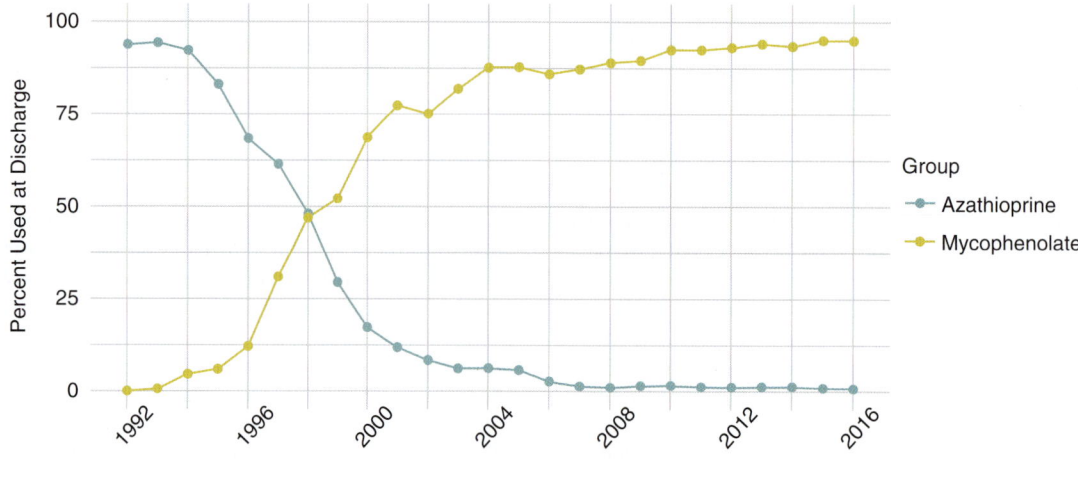

Fig. 44.10 Utilization of the antimetabolites azathioprine *(blue)* and mycophenolate mofetil *(yellow)* at discharge in heart transplants occurring in the United States between 1992 and 2016. Because of a series of clinical trials showing superiority of mycophenolate mofetil over azathioprine in preventing rejection, the use of azathioprine decreased and the use of mycophenolate mofetil increased during the 1990s. (Unpublished data from United Network for Organ Sharing.)

confirm that the augmented immunosuppression regimen has been effective at eradicating the AR. For patients that do not respond fully to medical treatment and display continued allograft dysfunction, extracorporeal photopheresis is frequently initiated with the hopes of improving allograft function. For patients with no response to treatment who display fulminant graft failure, retransplantation is not advisable, as it is associated with poor outcomes in the setting of AR.

Immunosuppression in Heart Transplantation
Historical Perspective

The improvement in posttransplant survival that has been seen over the 50-year history of HT is due in no small part to the availability of better immunosuppressive medications. In the early days of HT, immunosuppression was achieved with corticosteroids and the antimetabolite azathioprine (AZA), the only immunosuppressive agents that were available at the time. Survival after HT was poor until the arrival of the calcineurin inhibitor cyclosporine in the 1980s. The improved immunosuppression that was achieved led to lower rates of rejection and thus overall improved survival. During the 1990s, the most common maintenance immunosuppression regimen consisted of cyclosporine, AZA, and a corticosteroid.[53] The next antimetabolite agent, mycophenolate mofetil (MMF), which is a more selective inhibitor of T and B lymphocytes, became available in the late 1990s. A series of clinical trials, discussed later, showed that the use of MMF was associated with a lower risk of rejection as compared to AZA. As a result, the percentage of HT recipients prescribed MMF at discharge rapidly increased and the percentage of HT recipients prescribed AZA at discharge rapidly decreased from 1996 to 2000 (**Fig. 44.10**). The calcineurin inhibitor tacrolimus became available in the mid 1990s. Between 2000 and 2010 the percentage of HT recipients prescribed cyclosporine at discharge steadily decreased and the percentage of HT recipients prescribed tacrolimus at discharge steadily increased (**Fig. 44.11**). The other group of maintenance immunosuppressive agents used in HT, the mechanistic target of rapamycin (mTOR) inhibitors, sirolimus and everolimus, became used increasingly in the 2000s, although they remain less frequently used due to their side effect profile.

The Pharmacology of Immunosuppression

An understanding of the basic pharmacology and side effects of the major immunosuppressive agents is essential for the proper management of HT recipients (**Table 44.6**). Indeed, a substantial portion of posttransplant care is devoted to selecting the optimal immunosuppressive agent combination for each HT recipient, maintaining those agents within the therapeutic range and management of any side effects that develop during treatment.

The immunosuppressive regimen most commonly used in HT recipients in the 1990s was cyclosporine, AZA, and corticosteroids. In the current era, the most common regimen is tacrolimus and MMF, with or without prednisone. Cyclosporine and tacrolimus inhibit calcineurin, which is a signaling protein required for the activation and proliferation of T lymphocytes.[54] MMF inhibits the enzyme inosine monophosphate dehydrogenase which is required for nucleotide production, thus blocking the production of nucleic acids and ultimately inhibiting T and B lymphocyte proliferation.[54] Corticosteroids bind to the glucocorticoid receptor, which leads to downstream changes in the expression levels of multiple genes (an increase in anti-inflammatory gene transcription and a decrease in pro-inflammatory gene transcription). The mTOR inhibitors act by blocking the action of the mTORC1 complex, thus inhibiting T lymphocyte activation and proliferation.

The most important side effect of immunosuppressive agents is infection. Unfortunately, it remains difficult to quantitate the level of immunosuppression that individual HT recipients require to maintain their immune system in a quiescent state. Thus, the level of immunosuppression in individual HT recipients may be in excess of what is required, and they may develop infection. This situation is referred to as "over-immunosuppression."

Typically, over-immunosuppression is diagnosed when a transplant recipient presents with a significant infection. There are two laboratory tests that can provide information on the level of immunosuppression. First, the immune monitoring assay (ImmuKnow or Cylex) works by measuring adenosine triphosphate from CD4 T lymphocytes in peripheral blood.[55] In a retrospective study, patients with infections in the 30 days following an ImmuKnow assay were found to have significantly lower immune monitoring values. Next, quantitative measurement of immunoglobulin G levels can reveal

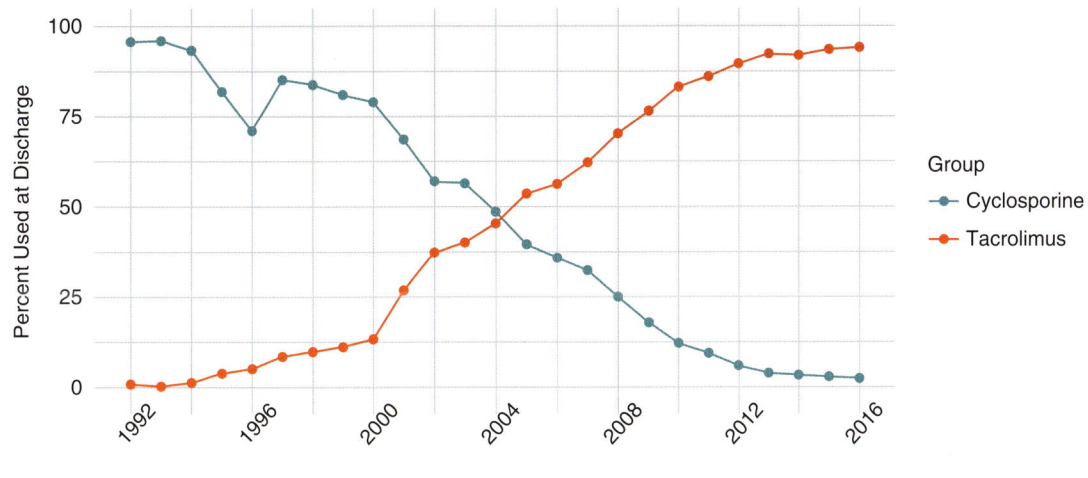

Fig. 44.11 Utilization of the calcineurin-inhibitors cyclosporine *(blue)* and tacrolimus *(red)* at discharge in heart transplants occurring in the United States between 1992 and 2016. Initial clinical trials of tacrolimus as compared with cyclosporine, performed in the late 1990s showed fewer side effects with cyclosporine but no difference in the incidence of rejection, likely owing to the small number of patients enrolled in these trials. In the 2000s, two trials showed that the use of tacrolimus was associated with a lower incidence of rejection compared with cyclosporine, leading to the decreased use of cyclosporine and increased use of tacrolimus. (Unpublished data from United Network for Organ Sharing.)

TABLE 44.6 Pharmacology and Side Effects of Immunosuppressive Agents for Heart Transplant Patients

Agent	Mechanism	Side Effects	Toxicities
Antimetabolite Agents			
Azathioprine	Inhibits proliferation of T and B lymphocytes via blocking nucleotide synthesis		• Leukopenia • Pancytopenia • Hepatotoxicity
Mycophenolate		• Dyspepsia • Diarrhea	• Leukopenia • Pancytopenia • Enterocolitis
Calcineurin Inhibitors			
Cyclosporine	Inhibits T-cell activation and proliferation via blocking action of calcineurin	• Hypertrichosis • Gingival hyperplasia • Hypertension	• Renal dysfunction • Seizures • Encephalopathy
Tacrolimus		• Tremor • Headaches • Hypertension	• Renal dysfunction • Seizures • Encephalopathy
mTOR Inhibitors			
Sirolimus	Inhibits T-cell activation and proliferation by blocking the action of the mTOR C1 complex	• Abdominal pain • Peripheral edema • VTE • HyperTG	• Leukopenia • Pneumonitis • Proteinuria
Everolimus		• Abdominal pain • Peripheral edema • VTE • HyperTG	• Leukopenia • Proteinuria
Corticosteroids			
Prednisone	Binds to glucocorticoid receptor leading to changes in gene transcription	• Weight gain • Emotional lability • Insomnia	• Hyperglycemia • Psychosis

HyperTG, Hypertriglyceridemia; *VTE*, venous thromboembolism.

TABLE 44.7 **Results of Major Clinical Trials of Different Immunosuppression Regimens in New Heart Transplant Recipients**

Study	Size	Rejection	CAV	Survival
AZA vs. MMF[57]	650	↓ with MMF	↓ with MMF	↑ with MMF
CSA vs. TAC[58]	82	NS	NS	
CSA vs. TAC[59]	85	NS	NS	
AZA vs. EVR[61]	634	↓ with EVR	↓ with EVR	NS
AZA vs. SIR[62]	136	↓ with SIR	↓ with SIR	NS
CSA vs. TAC[60]	314	↓ with TAC		NS
TAC/MMF vs. TAC/SIR vs. CSA/MMF[63]	343	↓ with TAC/MMF		NS
CSA/MMF vs. EVR/CSA[64]	176	NS		NS
TAC vs. TAC/MMF[65]	150	NS	NS	NS
CSA/MMF vs. CSA/EVR[69]	721	NS	↓ with EVR	NS
CSA/MMF vs. EVR/MMF[70]	118	↑ with EVR	↓ with EVR	NS

AZA, Azathioprine; *CAV*, cardiac allograft vasculopathy; *EVR*, everolimus; *MMF*, mycophenolate mofetil; *NS*, no significant difference; *SIR*, sirolimus.

the presence of hypogammaglobulinemia (IgG level <600 mg/dL). Hypogammaglobulinemia has been identified as a powerful predictor of posttransplant infection.[56] In our program, the identification of a low ImmunoKnow level or hypogammaglobulinemia prompts a reassessment of the immunosuppression regimen. If the patient is felt to be over-immunosuppressed, the trough level of calcineurin inhibitor or the dose of MMF can be attenuated, with close follow up.

Clinical Trials of Immunosuppressive Agents

The paucity of markers of immunosuppression intensity as well as the potential for significant side effects of immunosuppressive agents makes clinical trials of immunosuppression of paramount importance to establish the efficacy and safety of different immunosuppression regimens. Here we will present the results of the major clinical trials of different immunosuppression regimens in de novo HT recipients (summarized in **Table 44.7**).

The results of the first multicenter immunosuppression trial were reported in 1998.[57] This trial compared AZA and MMF and showed several benefits of MMF in the as-treated groups, including a decreased incidence of rejection and an attenuation in the decrease in coronary artery luminal area over time, which is a marker of cardiac allograft vasculopathy (CAV) development. Overall, a 45% relative reduction in mortality was seen in the MMF group, thus establishing MMF as the antimetabolite of choice in HT.

Once tacrolimus became available, two trials were performed to compare cyclosporine and tacrolimus.[58,59] These did not show a difference in survival or rejection between the groups, although both trials were small (less than 100 patients in each trial). However, a higher incidence of hypertension and hyperlipidemia was seen in the cyclosporine groups. Then in 2006 Grimm et al. published a larger study of cyclosporine versus tacrolimus, which showed a significantly lower incidence of rejection of grade 2R or greater with tacrolimus (56% vs. 71%).[60] No difference in survival was seen among the groups.

The mTOR inhibitors everolimus and sirolimus were then assessed in individual trials. Everolimus at two different doses (0.75 mg twice daily or 1.5 mg twice daily) was compared with AZA on a background of cyclosporine and corticosteroids in the "B253" study.[61] While survival was comparable between the groups, treatment with everolimus at either dose was associated with a decreased incidence of rejection as well as a smaller increase in maximal intimal thickness from baseline (a marker of CAV). Interestingly, patients treated with everolimus experienced fewer cytomegalovirus (CMV) infections (15% with AZA vs. 30% with everolimus) but more bacterial infections (25% with AZA

vs. 35% with everolimus). There was a higher rate of discontinuation of study medication in the everolimus groups (30% in the 0.75 mg twice daily group, 40% in the 1.5 mg twice daily group, and 29% in the AZA group).

Shortly thereafter the results of a trial comparing AZA to sirolimus on a similar background of cyclosporine and corticosteroids was published.[62] Once again a significantly lower incidence of rejection as well as a significant attenuation in first-year intravascular ultrasound parameters that predict the development of CAV was seen. These two trials established that mTOR inhibitors, used on a background of calcineurin inhibitors, reduce the progression of CAV.

Given the potential benefits of the mTOR inhibitors seen in the above trials, the specific combination of agents associated with the best rejection and survival outcomes, with the fewest adverse effects, was unclear. The "Triple Study" was thus undertaken, which compared three different regimens: tacrolimus plus sirolimus, tacrolimus plus MMF, or cyclosporine plus MMF.[63] A total of 343 patients at 28 centers in the United States were randomized. There was no difference in the incidence of rejection amongst the three groups, however when comparing groups against each other, there was a significantly lower incidence of rejection in the tacrolimus plus MMF group as compared to the cyclosporine plus MMF group (but not the tacrolimus plus sirolimus group). A higher serum creatinine was seen in the tacrolimus plus sirolimus group, especially amongst patients with elevated creatinine at baseline.

Given the increase in creatinine seen during cotreatment with calcineurin inhibitors and mTOR inhibitors, Lehmkuhl et al. assessed a regimen using reduced-dose cyclosporine with everolimus as compared to standard-dose cyclosporine with MMF.[64] No differences in rejection, survival, or renal function were seen between the groups in this trial.

In the quest to minimize side effects of immunosuppression, the question arose to whether chronic treatment with a calcineurin inhibitor by itself, that is without an antimetabolite or corticosteroid, would provide sufficient immunosuppression to prevent rejection. The TICTAC trial enrolled 150 HT recipients who were treated with tacrolimus and MMF for 2 weeks posttransplant, after which they were randomized to either wean off MMF over 2 weeks or to continue MMF treatment.[65] Corticosteroids were discontinued by 8 weeks posttransplant in all patients. Tacrolimus levels were maintained at moderate levels of 8 to 10 ng/dL, with a resultant rise in serum creatinine. The trial found no difference in the incidence of rejection at 1 year posttransplant. Importantly, survival was also not different between the groups at 1, 3, or 5 years posttransplant. Markers of CAV were also similar. The TICTAC trial established that monotherapy with tacrolimus is available for select patients.

The calcineurin inhibitors cyclosporine and tacrolimus are known to contribute to chronic renal dysfunction in HT recipients[66] and most patients will experience worsening of renal function over time while treated with these agents. Introduction of sirolimus and withdrawal of the calcineurin inhibitor was shown to be safe and to improve renal function in single-center studies of HT recipients at later times posttransplant.[67] Zuckermann et al. conducted the first multi-center clinical trial of a calcineurin inhibitor-free immunosuppression regimen for 116 HT recipients who were enrolled 1 to 8 years after HT.[68] They found an increased incidence of rejection events in the sirolimus group, although the difference was not statistically significant. Renal function, as measured by GFR, was significantly better at all time points starting at 4 weeks after trial enrollment. A secondary analysis of this trial showed that a MMF dose of 1000 mg per day or less and African American ethnicity were strong predictors of the development of rejection.[68] Taken together, these data suggest that a calcineurin inhibitor-free immunosuppression regimen containing sirolimus and MMF is a reasonable option for HT recipients with renal dysfunction as well as other indications as discussed below, but care must be taken to optimize the dose of MMF. Furthermore, alternative regimens should be considered for African American patients.

In 2013 the "A2310" study of cyclosporine with MMF versus everolimus was published.[69] Everolimus was used at two different doses (0.75 mg twice daily or 1.5 mg twice daily) in conjunction with reduced-dose cyclosporine and was compared with MMF in conjunction with standard-dose cyclosporine. The everolimus 1.5 mg twice daily group was terminated early due to increased mortality. However, the everolimus 0.75 mg twice daily group was associated with similar outcomes to the MMF group as far as rejection and survival. Similar to other trials utilizing mTOR inhibitors, a significant decrease in the progression of CAV by intravascular ultrasound was noted in the everolimus group. Patients treated with everolimus experienced a higher incidence of nonfatal serious events, driven by a significantly higher rate of pericardial effusion and bacterial infection, but a lower incidence of leukopenia/neutropenia and CMV infections.

The Scandinavian Heart Transplant Everolimus De Novo Study with Early Calcineurin Inhibitor Avoidance (SCHEDULE) trial randomized patients to standard-dose cyclosporine and MMF/corticosteroids or reduced-dose cyclosporine plus everolimus and MMF/corticosteroids, with withdrawal of cyclosporine between posttransplant weeks seven to 11.[70,71] At 1 year, there was a significantly higher incidence of asymptomatic rejection in the everolimus group but also improved renal function and lower progression of CAV by intravascular ultrasound.

Putting these data together, therapy with tacrolimus, MMF, and prednisone is the immunosuppression regimen for de novo HT recipients which provides the lowest risk of rejection and the best renal function. Cyclosporine should be used in place of tacrolimus if severe side effects of tacrolimus develop, such as seizures or encephalopathy. A regimen that uses an mTOR inhibitor, either sirolimus or everolimus (at a starting dose of 0.75 mg twice daily) in place of MMF, is appropriate in patients at high risk of CAV or CMV infection, with the following caveats: (1) renal function may be decreased on this regimen in the presence of a calcineurin inhibitor, and (2) patients will be at an increased risk of side effects of mTOR inhibitors such as pericardial effusion, proteinuria and fungal/bacterial infection. The use of calcineurin inhibitor-free regimens later after HT may be helpful in patients with cancer or renal dysfunction who are at low risk of rejection.

COMPLICATIONS IN THE HEART TRANSPLANT RECIPIENT

Overview of Outcomes After Heart Transplant

HT remains the therapy of choice for patients with end-stage heart failure, not only because of the excellent median survival, which now approaches 11 years,[2] but also because of the functional status that patients regain after HT. HT recipients have climbed mountains and completed marathons.[72] Beyond these successes are the inevitable medical complications of transplantation that all recipients will face.

The two main cardiac complications of HT include rejection and CAV. The three main non-cardiac complications are infection, renal failure and malignancy. Age at the time of HT is strongly related to the likelihood of each outcome. In a recent study utilizing the ISHLT Transplant Registry, the overall incidence of death due to rejection was 2% at 10 years.[73] There was a strong inverse relationship between increasing age and decreased risk of death due to AR, with recipients between the ages of 18 to 29 at the highest risk of rejection (**Fig. 44.12**). The overall incidence of death due to CAV was 3% at 10 years, again with a strong inverse relationship between increasing age and decreased risk of death due to CAV. Graft failure, which is not a specific cause of death and is likely to be a consequence of rejection or CAV, was the cause of death in 8% of patients and showed a similar trend.

The noncardiac complications of infection, renal failure and malignancy show a different trend as compared to the cardiac complications. The overall incidence of death due to infection, renal failure and malignancy are 6%, 10%, and 4%, respectively. For these outcomes, the risk of death due to each cause is directly proportional to the age at the time of HT.

Cardiac Allograft Vasculopathy

CAV is a major cause of morbidity and mortality after HT, occurring in 50% of HT recipients by 5 years and 65% of recipients by 10 years after HT (**Fig. 44.13**).[74] CAV is a major cause of allograft failure and is the primary indication for redo HT. Although both traditional CAD and CAV are characterized by coronary lesions, CAV has clinical and pathological characteristics quite distinct from CAD (**Table 44.8**).[75] CAV develops rapidly after HT, coming to clinical attention within years, whereas CAD takes decades after birth to present clinically. Risk factors for CAV include the traditional coronary disease factors such as age (in this case, increasing age of the donor) and hyperlipidemia,[16] in addition to immunologic risk factors such as previous episodes of cellular rejection[76] and donor specific antibodies.[77] Patients with CAD commonly present with angina or acute coronary syndromes, whereas HT recipients are identified as having significant CAV most frequently after routine surveillance studies.

The pathology of CAV is also distinct from CAD (see Table 44.8). The lesions of CAV are due to concentric fibromuscular hyperplasia of the intima which often leads to diffuse disease of the vessel,[78] whereas CAD lesions are typically focal. The term "vasculopathy" is used for CAV because it affects all parts of the cardiac vascular tree (i.e., epicardial arteries, intramyocardial arteries, and veins),[78] whereas CAD is limited to the epicardial arteries. As a result, patients with CAV can present with disease that is predominantly microvascular (i.e., predominantly affecting small arterioles and sparing the larger epicardial arteries), predominantly macrovascular (i.e., predominantly affecting the larger epicardial arteries), or with components of both (**Fig. 44.14**).[79] Myocardial fibrosis is commonly seen with severe forms of this disease.[80]

Due to the lack of innervation of the cardiac allograft, patients with CAV are usually asymptomatic until severe sequelae occur, such as allograft dysfunction, acute coronary syndromes,[81] or sudden cardiac

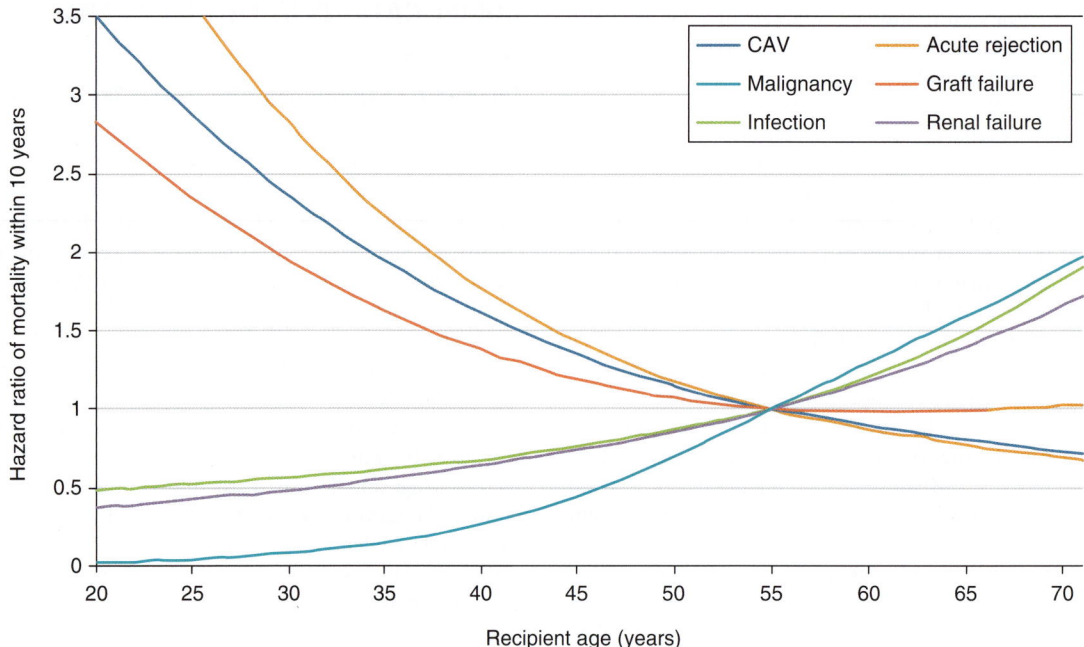

Fig. 44.12 The types of complications that occur after heart transplant (HT) are related to recipient age at the time of transplantation. The two main cardiac complications are acute rejection and cardiac allograft vasculopathy (CAV). There is a strong inverse relationship between increasing age and decreasing risk of death due to rejection and CAV, such that younger recipients are at much higher risk. The noncardiac complications of heart transplantation include infection, renal failure, and malignancy. For these outcomes, the risk of death due to each cause is directly proportional to the patient's age at the time of HT, such that older recipients are at much higher risk of these outcomes. (From Wever-Pinzon O, Edwards LB, Taylor DO, et al. Association of recipient age and causes of heart transplant mortality: Implications for personalization of posttransplant management—an analysis of the International Society for Heart and Lung Transplantation Registry. *J Heart Lung Transplant.* 2017;36[4]:407–417.)

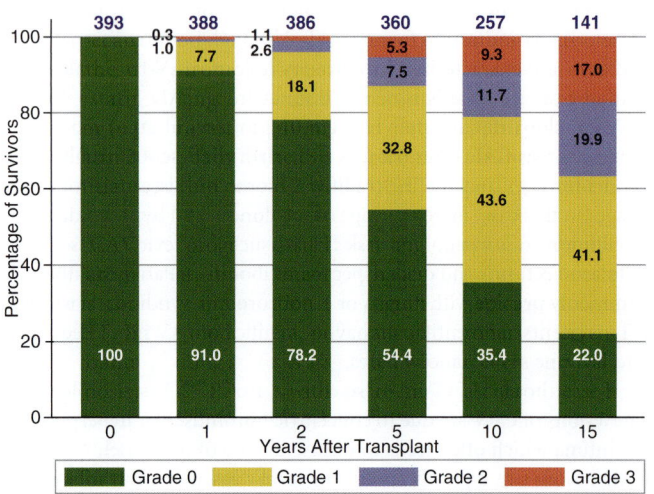

Fig. 44.13 Distribution of the severity of cardiac allograft vasculopathy (CAV), using the International Society for Heart and Lung Transplantation nomenclature, in a study of 393 patients who underwent heart transplantation. The blue number at the top of each bar indicates the number of survivors at that time point. The number inside the stacked bar indicates the percentage of patients with the respective CAV grade (by color). The prevalence and severity of CAV increases with time after transplant, with approximately 50% and 66% of patients having CAV at 5 and 10 years posttransplant, respectively. (From Agarwal S, Parashar A, Kapadia SR, et al. Long-term mortality after cardiac allograft vasculopathy: implications of percutaneous intervention. *JACC: Heart Fail.* 2014;2[3]:281–288.)

TABLE 44.8	Clinical and Pathologic Characteristics of Cardiac Allograft Vasculopathy and Coronary Artery Disease	
	CAV	**CAD**
Clinical Characteristics		
Presentation	Usually years after HT	Decades after birth
Risk factors	Traditional as well as immunologic	Traditional: age, hyperlipidemia
Symptoms at presentation	Asymptomatic, graft failure	Angina or ACS
Pathologic Characteristics		
Involved vessels	Epicardial arteries, intramyocardial arteries, veins	Epicardial arteries
Stenosis	Concentric	Eccentric
Distribution	Diffuse, from proximal to distal	Focal, proximal > distal
Calcification	Usually not present	Present
Inflammation	Seen in intima, media, adventitia	Intima

ACS, Acute coronary syndrome; *CAD,* coronary artery disease; *CAV,* cardiac allograft vasculopathy; *HT,* heart transplant.
Bottom panel modified from Seki A, Fishbein MC. Predicting the development of cardiac allograft vasculopathy. *Cardiovasc Pathol.* 2014;23[5]:253–260.

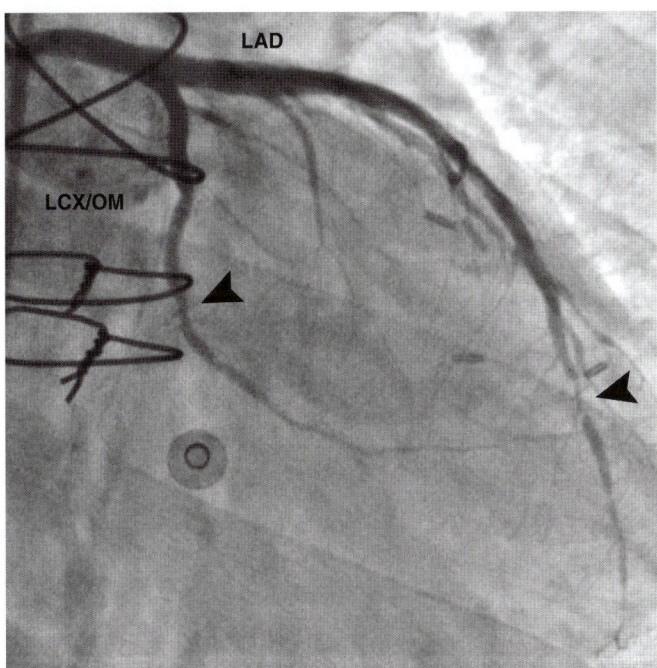

Fig. 44.14 Angiogram in the right anterior oblique projection showing macrovascular (discrete stenoses of the left circumflex and left anterior descending coronary arteries, indicated by the *arrowheads*) as well as microvascular (distal "pruning" of the left circumflex and left anterior descending coronary arteries) cardiac allograft vasculopathy in a 40-year-old male patient 10 years after heart transplantation.

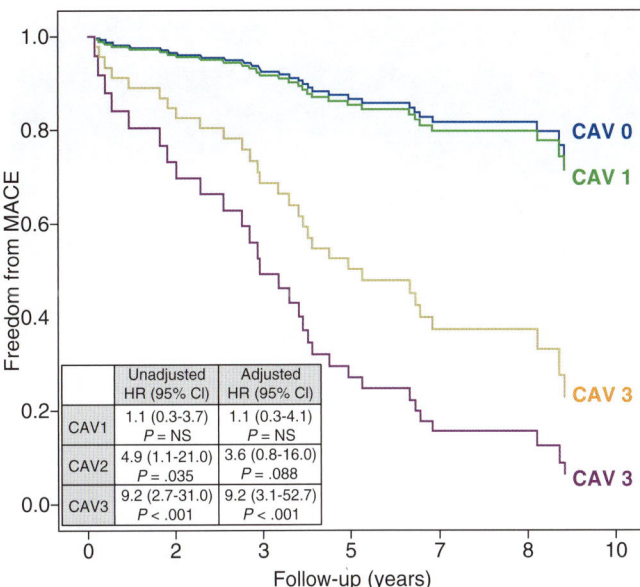

Fig. 44.15 Freedom from major adverse cardiac events in patients with and without cardiac allograft vasculopathy according to the grade of their disease (using the International Society for Heart and Lung Transplantation nomenclature). Patients with grade 2 and 3 disease have a significantly decreased freedom from major adverse cardiac events. (From Prada-Delgado O, Estévez-Loureiro R, Paniagua-Martín MJ, López-Sainz A, Crespo-Leiro MG. Prevalence and prognostic value of cardiac allograft vasculopathy 1 year after heart transplantation according to the ISHLT recommended nomenclature. *J Heart Lung Transplant.* 2012;31[3]:332–333.)

TABLE 44.9	Grading for Cardiac Allograft Vasculopathy
CAV Grade	**Description**
0: Not significant	No detectable angiographic lesion
1: Mild	Angiographic LM <50%, or primary vessel with maximum lesion of <70%, or any branch stenosis <70% (including diffuse narrowing) without allograft dysfunction
2: Moderate	Angiographic LM ≥50%; a single primary vessel ≥70%, or isolated branch stenosis ≥70% in branches of 2 systems, without allograft dysfunction
3: Severe	Angiographic LM ≥50%, or two or more primary vessels ≥70% stenosis, or isolated branch stenosis ≥70% in all 3 systems; or ISHLT CAV1 or CAV2 with allograft dysfunction (defined as LVEF ≤45% usually in the presence of regional wall motion abnormalities) or evidence of significant restrictive physiology

CAV, Cardiac vasculopathy; *LM,* left main; *ISHLT,* International Society for Heart and Lung Transplantation; *LVEF,* left ventricular ejection fraction.
Adapted from Mehra MR, Crespo-Leiro MG, Dipchand A, et al. International Society for Heart and Lung Transplantation working formulation of a standardized nomenclature for cardiac allograft vasculopathy—2010. *J Heart Lung Transplant.* 2010;29(7):717–727. https://doi.org/10.1016/j.healun.2010.05.017.

death.[82] As a result, most HT programs perform routine screening at regular intervals for the development of CAV. Coronary angiography is the preferred technique for diagnosing CAV, as it allows for risk stratification according to the ISHLT nomenclature for CAV (**Table 44.9**).[83] The ISHLT nomenclature bases the severity of CAV on the number of vessels affected and the severity of stenosis of the affected vessels. This nomenclature has prognostic significance, as Prada-Delgado et al. found that major adverse cardiac events (defined as ACS, coronary revascularization, hospital admission, redo HT, and death) increased successively with higher CAV grades, even after adjusting for other covariates (**Fig. 44.15**).[84] The ISHLT recommends performing annual or biannual coronary angiography to assess for the development of CAV.[22]

Coronary angiography has poor sensitivity for CAV due to coronary arterial remodeling which accompanies CAV. This is especially true at early time points posttransplant. Intravascular ultrasound (IVUS) has been used since the 1990s to improve the identification of CAV. The finding of a change in the maximal thickness of the coronary arterial intima between 6 weeks and 1 year posttransplant of 0.5 mm or more was associated with a 3.5-fold higher risk of death or graft loss at 5 years and a higher incidence of angiographic disease.[85] Therefore, the change in first-year maximal intimal thickness (MIT) is an important prognostic marker of CAV. An example of intimal thickening by IVUS is shown in **Fig. 44.16**. Because IVUS requires specific equipment and training, IVUS is not utilized by all HT programs.

Given the severe sequelae of CAV, pharmacologic interventions should be initiated shortly after transplant to prevent its development and progression. Pharmacologic interventions include the use of ATG for induction immunosuppression,[86] the use of the mTOR inhibitors sirolimus and everolimus, statin therapy,[87] aspirin use,[88] as well as treatment with vitamins C and E.[89] If the recipient is not started on a regimen containing an mTOR inhibitor initially and needs to be switched, the timing of the switch is important. Matsuo et al. showed that early conversion to sirolimus (i.e., within 2 years of HT) was associated with less plaque volume progression, whereas late conversion was associated with a higher increase in plaque volume over time as well as lesion calcification.[90]

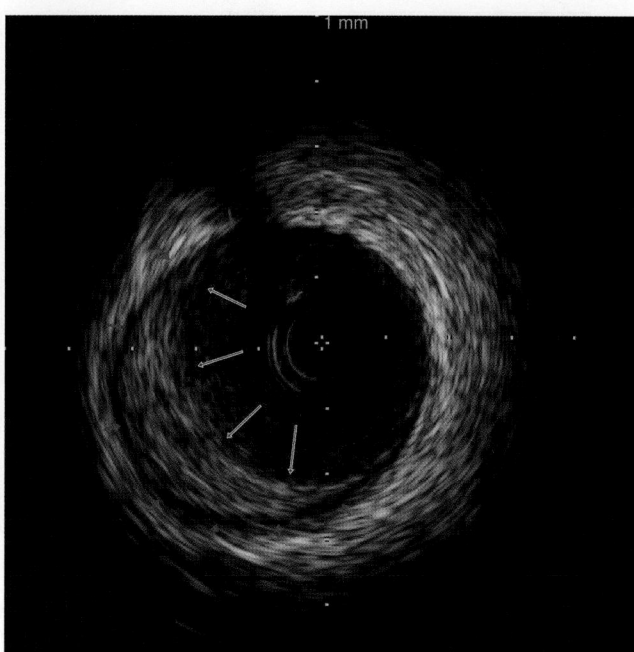

Fig. 44.16 Intravascular ultrasound image from the left anterior descending artery of a patient 1 year posttransplant showing intimal thickening. The lumen border is marked by the *small arrows*. The media/adventitia border is marked by the *large arrows*. The area between the *small* and *large arrows* is the area of intimal thickening, with a maximal intimal thickening of greater than 0.5 mm.

Statin therapy was first shown to be beneficial in HT in 1995.[91] A meta-analysis of nine studies has shown that statin use in HT recipients is associated with a reduction in all-cause mortality, a reduction in the risk of hemodynamically significant rejection and CAV.[87] Because both statins and calcineurin inhibitors are inhibitors of the cytochrome P450 isoform CYP3A, caution must be taken in statin dosing. In general, statin doses are kept to half of maximum (e.g., pravastatin 40 mg daily, atorvastatin 40 mg daily, rosuvastatin 20 mg daily). The ISHLT recommends that statin therapy be initiated within one to 2 weeks of HT, regardless of the lipid levels.[22]

Once CAV has progressed such that angiographically significant stenoses are present, its treatment is challenging and includes percutaneous coronary intervention (for significant epicardial disease) or redo HT. In the modern era, percutaneous coronary intervention with everolimus-eluting stents is associated with excellent survival and low restenosis rates.[92] Patients with severe microvascular disease have abundant myocardial fibrosis and clinically present with restrictive physiology.[80] For these patients, redo HT is associated with excellent survival for those patients who meet criteria to undergo a second HT.

INFECTION

Due to the use of immunosuppression, transplant patients are at a markedly increased risk of infection as compared to nonimmunosuppressed patients. This is especially true after treatment for rejection as massive augmentation of immunosuppression is administered. The type of infections that affect HT recipients range from typical infections such as bacterial pneumonia and urinary tract infections to atypical infections that are specific to immunocompromised hosts. Atypical infections can be caused by viruses such as CMV, bacteria such as *Nocardia* and fungi such as *Pneumocystis jirovecii* (PJP) and *Aspergillus*.

TABLE 44.10 Antibiotic Prophylaxis Protocol After Heart Transplant

Atypical Infection	Agent	Duration
Candida	Clotrimazole	3 months
Cytomegalovirus	Acyclovir	3 months
Donor negative/recipient negative	Valganciclovir	6 months
Donor negative/recipient positive	Valganciclovir	6 months
Donor positive/recipient negative	Valganciclovir	12 months
Donor positive/recipient positive		
Pneumocystis jirovecii	Bactrim Dapsone for sulfa allergy	12 months

Furthermore, transplant recipients are at risk of infections transmitted through the transplant itself, referred to as donor-transmitted infections.

The time that infections present with respect to the transplant is associated with the origin of the infection.[93] Donor-transmitted infections and those associated with the transplant surgery, for example wound infections and *Clostridium difficile*, tend to present within the first month after HT. After 1 month and lasting until 1 year after transplant, reactivation of latent pathogens or opportunistic infections are most common. CMV is an important pathogen in this time period, where reactivation can cause both acute infection and contribute to the development of long-term complications such as CAV. Several fungal pathogens can also be seen in this time period, such as PJP and *Aspergillus*. After one year, most pathogens are community acquired such as seasonal influenza.

The development of an atypical viral infection such as CMV or fungal infection such as PJP is associated with high morbidity and mortality. As such, prophylactic antibiotics are used to prevent these infections in all HT recipients within the first year after HT (**Table 44.10** for the Cedars-Sinai antibiotic prophylaxis protocol). Valganciclovir is used for CMV prophylaxis, with the duration of use tailored to the recipient's risk of CMV reactivation. This is in turn based on the donor and recipient's serological status, with donor positivity/recipient negativity for CMV at the highest risk of reactivation.[94] Clotrimazole is used for *Candida* prophylaxis. Bactrim or dapsone is used for PJP prophylaxis. Programs in regions where other fungal infections are endemic may utilize additional prophylaxis (e.g., *Coccidiomycosis* in the southwest).

Cancer

Solid organ transplant recipients are at a significantly increased risk of malignancy due to immunosuppression. HT recipients are at a particularly increased risk, due to the higher level of immunosuppression required as compared to other solid organ transplants. In an analysis of HT recorded in the UNOS database between 1999 and 2008, 11% of HT recipients developed a posttransplant malignancy, with an incidence of 14.3 cases per 1000 person-years.[95] Lung cancer and posttransplant lymphoproliferative disease were most common (3.2 cases and 2.2 cases per 1000-person years, respectively). In a multivariable regression model including age, sex, race, HLA mismatch, and immunosuppression regimen, increasing age was a strong risk factor for posttransplant malignancy, whereas Hispanic ethnicity was protective. Youn et al. had similar findings, noting a cumulative incidence of malignancy by 5 years post-HT of 7% for skin cancer, 4% for non-skin solid cancer, and 1% for lymphoproliferative disorders.[96] Survival in HT recipients with a diagnosis of malignancy was markedly reduced.

Given the increased incidence of malignancies in patients after HT, specialized management strategies are required. All HT recipients should be regarded as "at risk" for development of malignancy. This is especially true for patients with previously established risk factors for the development of posttransplant malignancy, such as those with a history of cancer or those with older age at the time of HT. Age- and sex-appropriate cancer screening recommendations should be followed. For patients with a diagnosis of cancer, switching the calcineurin inhibitor to an mTOR inhibitor may be of benefit. In the Efficacy of Rapamycin in Secondary Prevention of Skin Cancers in Kidney Transplant Recipients (TUMORAPA) study, conversion to a regimen containing sirolimus led to a 44% lower risk of recurrent squamous-cell carcinoma in 120 renal transplant recipients with a history of cutaneous squamous-cell carcinoma.[97] Statin use also appears to protect against malignancy.[87]

FUTURE INNOVATIONS

In this final section, we discuss ongoing innovations in the field of HT. We center on three areas of innovation: strategies to enlarge the number of donor hearts, strategies to improve access to transplantation and outcomes for allosensitized patients, and novel approaches to monitoring for rejection.

Novel Strategies to Enlarge the Donor Heart Pool

The number of HT that occur per year is limited by the number of donor hearts that become available. There are several strategies emerging to enlarge the pool of donor hearts. Currently, the vast majority of hearts used for HT in the United States are from donors with brain death (DBD), which has been declared according to specific criteria. Hearts obtained from donors after circulatory death (DCD) are emerging as an alternative source of hearts. In DCD, the donor has suffered advanced cranial or respiratory pathology but has not yet reached brain death according to the standard criteria.[98] Organs are procured for transplantation after the donor is removed from the ventilator and cessation of the donor's circulatory function occurs followed by a required observation period (usually 5 minutes). Messer et al. recently showed that DCD hearts were associated with comparable survival to DBD hearts in a study of 28 DCD HT.[99] The use of DCD hearts has the potential to increase the number of HTs by as much as 15%.[100] This procedure has yet to be performed in the United States.

Less than 50% of hearts offered for HT are accepted. This percentage has actually decreased over time, with only 32% of donor hearts accepted in 2010.[101] Donor characteristics associated with nonacceptance include age >50 years, female sex, hypertension, diabetes mellitus, cerebrovascular cause of death, and left ventricular ejection fraction <50%. These "extended criteria" donors have been associated with acceptable outcomes, especially when used at high-volume transplant centers.[102] Recently, the Organ Care System (TransMedics, Andover, MA) for ex vivo perfusion has been shown to have similar post-HT outcomes as compared to standard perfusion.[103] The Organ Care System is currently being tested in the International Trial to Evaluate the Safety and Effectiveness of the Portable Organ Care System Heart for Preserving and Assessing Expanded Criteria Donor Hearts for Transplantation (EXPAND Heart Trial). In this trial, extended criteria donor hearts or hearts with long expected Scross-clamp times will be supported with the Organ Care System. If lactate and perfusion pressures remain normal, the heart will be used for transplant. If this trial shows that these extended criteria donor hearts supported with the Organ Care System have outcomes similar to that of standard criteria donors, the donor heart pool could be significantly enlarged significantly using the Organ Care System.

A third strategy to increase the donor heart pool is the use of hearts from donors with hepatitis C viremia. Approximately 2% of the general population is chronically infected with hepatitis C virus (HCV), and of these persons, about 80% will have chronic HCV viremia. Traditionally, organs from HCV viremic donors have not been utilized due significantly worse posttransplant outcomes.[104] Recently, direct acting antiviral agents with high efficacy for HCV have become available. Schlendorf et al. have just published the first trial using HCV viremic donors for HCV seronegative recipients in HT[105] and have reported favorable short-term outcomes. Assessment of long-term outcomes is needed to ensure the safety of this strategy. If studies show that this strategy is safe, at least 100 additional HT per year could be performed.[106]

Improving Access and Outcomes for Allosensitized Patients

Allosensitized candidates have longer waiting times for HT due to the smaller compatible donor pool and are at an increased risk of rejection after HT. In addition to desensitization therapies, several novel approaches may improve access and outcomes for these patients. Recently, complement inhibitors including eculizumab (Soliris, Alexion Pharmaceuticals, New Haven, CT) and C1 inhibitor (Berinert, CSL Behring, Kankakee, IL) have become available for clinical use. These agents are being studied for use in transplants where a positive crossmatch is expected,[12] and the use of eculizumab or C1 inhibitor will abrogate the effect of the anti-HLA antibodies. Early results with these agents in kidney transplantation have been favorable.[107,108] In small series, combined heart-liver transplantation has also been shown to be an effective approach for transplantation of these patients,[109,110] as the liver is felt to act as an "immunologic sink" and adsorb deleterious HLA antibodies.

Novel Approaches to the Detection of Rejection

Despite being the "gold standard" method for the diagnosis of rejection, the EMB itself has significant limitations. The EMB can be negative in patients presenting with allograft dysfunction, likely due to sampling error or "patchy" infiltration of the allograft. More importantly, the EMB is limited by a high degree of variability between individual pathologist's interpretation of EMB findings.[47] Given these limitations, novel approaches to the detection of rejection would be extremely impactful.

Donor-derived cell-free DNA (dd-cfDNA) can be measured in the blood of HT recipients at the time of rejection.[111] This observation forms the basis for a novel, noninvasive test for HT rejection. De Vlaminck et al. compared dd-cfDNA at a threshold of 0.25% to EMB-proven ACR of grade 2R or higher and found that dd-cfDNA provided an area under the receiver operating characteristic curve of 0.83, with a sensitivity of 58% and a specificity of 93%.[112] Another benefit of dd-cfDNA is that it can be used to detect for ACR and AMR, as has recently been shown in kidney transplants.[113]

In addition to dd-cfDNA assays, gene expression profiling of tissue samples has also been shown to improve the diagnosis of rejection. Halloran et al. performed gene expression profiling of EMB samples followed by archetype analysis using rejection-associated transcripts identified in kidney transplant biopsy specimens[114]—a system termed the Molecular Microscope Diagnostic system (MMDx). They found that generally the histologic pathologic diagnosis correlated with the

EMB and with the MMDx diagnosis, but significant disparity was present—92% of the "no rejection" samples were assigned to the "no rejection" archetype but only 42% and 34% of AMR and ACR samples were assigned to the AMR and T cell–mediated rejection archetype, respectively. Thus further work is needed to clarify the molecular features of rejection that correlate with pathologic features and to determine their response to treatment and effect on prognosis.[115]

KEY REFERENCES

2. Lund LH, Khush KK, Cherikh WS, et al. The registry of the International Society for Heart and Lung Transplantation: thirty-fourth adult heart transplantation report—2017; focus theme: allograft ischemic time. *J Heart Lung Transplant.* 2017;36(10):1037–1046.

3. Mehra MR, Canter CE, Hannan MM, et al. The 2016 International Society for Heart Lung Transplantation listing criteria for heart transplantation: a 10-year update. *J Heart Lung Transplant.* 2016;35(1):1–23.

15. Kransdorf EP, Stehlik J. Donor evaluation in heart transplantation_ The end of the beginning. *J Heart Lung Transplant.* 2014;33(11):1105–1113.

39. Kfoury AG, Miller DV, Snow GL, et al. Mixed cellular and antibody-mediated rejection in heart transplantation_ In-depth pathologic and clinical observations. *J Heart Lung Transplant.* 2016;35(3):335–341.

63. Kobashigawa JA, Miller LW, Russell SD, et al. Tacrolimus with mycophenolate mofetil (MMF) or sirolimus vs. cyclosporine with MMF in cardiac transplant patients: 1-year report. *Am J Transplant.* 2006;6(6):1377–1386.

73. Wever-Pinzon O, Edwards LB, Taylor DO, et al. Association of recipient age and causes of heart transplant mortality: implications for personalization of post-transplant management-an analysis of the international society for heart and lung transplantation registry. *J Heart Lung Transplant.* 2017;36(4):407–417.

74. Agarwal S, Parashar A, Kapadia SR, et al. Long-term mortality after cardiac allograft vasculopathy: implications of percutaneous intervention. *JACC: Heart Fail.* 2014;2(3):281–288.

76. Raichlin E, Edwards BS, Kremers WK, et al. Acute cellular rejection and the subsequent development of allograft vasculopathy after cardiac transplantation. *J Heart Lung Transplant.* 2009;28(4):320–327.

96. Youn J-C, Stehlik J, Wilk AR, et al. Temporal trends of de novo malignancy development after heart transplantation. *J Am Coll Cardiol.* 2018;71(1):40–49.

115. Stehlik J, Kobashigawa J, Hunt SA, et al. Honoring 50 years of clinical heart transplantation in circulation: in-depth state-of-the-art review. *Circulation.* 2018;137(1):71–87.

The full reference list for this chapter is available on ExpertConsult.

Circulatory Assist Devices in Heart Failure

Gregory A. Ewald, Carmelo A. Milano, Joseph G. Rogers

OUTLINE

Management of advanced heart failure is often less evidence-based than earlier stages of the disease. By definition, these patients are typically failing evidence-based medical and electrical heart failure therapies, so there are few clinical trials to guide therapy. Professional societies have developed definitions of "advanced" heart failure, but all tend to share common data elements: objective evidence of ventricular dysfunction, marked functional limitations, evidence of volume overload and/or hypoperfusion, end-organ dysfunction, diminished responsiveness to diuretics, inability to tolerate standard heart failure therapies, and heart failure hospitalizations.[1] The size of the population that fulfills the definition of "advanced" heart failure is unknown but may exceed 250,000 patients in the United States (**see also Chapter 18**).[2] However, the morbidity and mortality associated with advanced heart failure are clear: 4-month readmission rates approximate 50% and the annualized mortality is 80% to 90%.[3-6]

In this chapter, we will discuss the role of mechanical therapies designed to improve cardiac output and lower cardiac filling pressures in patients with acute and chronic advanced systolic heart failure. In the past decade, this strategy has gained wide acceptance in the treatment of advanced heart failure patients.

ACUTE CARDIOGENIC SHOCK

During the past decade, the incidence of acute cardiogenic shock has doubled in the United States and remains an important cause of cardiovascular morbidity and mortality.[7] Most commonly, cardiogenic shock results from left ventricular (LV) failure after acute myocardial infarction (MI), or a mechanical complication following MI such as ventricular septal defect or mitral insufficiency (**see also Chapter 19**).[8] However, other conditions may present with similarly deranged hemodynamics, such as acute viral myocarditis (**see also Chapter 28**), giant cell myocarditis, or acute aortic insufficiency (AI) (**see also Chapter 26**). Postcardiotomy shock has been reported as a complication of cardiac surgery in 0.2% to 6% of cases and is associated with high short-term mortality risk without mechanically assisted circulation.[9]

Despite advances in coronary reperfusion, including a focus on early intervention, post-MI cardiogenic shock is associated with high short-term mortality. The SHOCK II-IABP trial examined the impact of the intra-aortic balloon pump (IABP) in patients with cardiogenic shock following acute MI. The 30-day mortality rate was 40% in both the IABP and medical therapy arms of the trial despite revascularization and contemporary medical therapy.[10]

The approach to acute cardiogenic shock requires rapid integration of clinical information targeted at determining the etiology, the severity of hemodynamic compromise, and the therapeutic options that address the physiologic needs of the individual patient (**Fig. 45.1**). A directed history, physical examination, and electrocardiogram (ECG) are critical elements of the initial evaluation. If the cause or severity of the heart failure is not evident following the aforementioned, echocardiography and/or coronary angiography should be performed to evaluate ventricular and valvular function. Endomyocardial biopsy should also be considered in new-onset, nonischemic cardiomyopathy but should probably be limited to centers with expertise in the performance of the procedure and interpretation of the histology.[11]

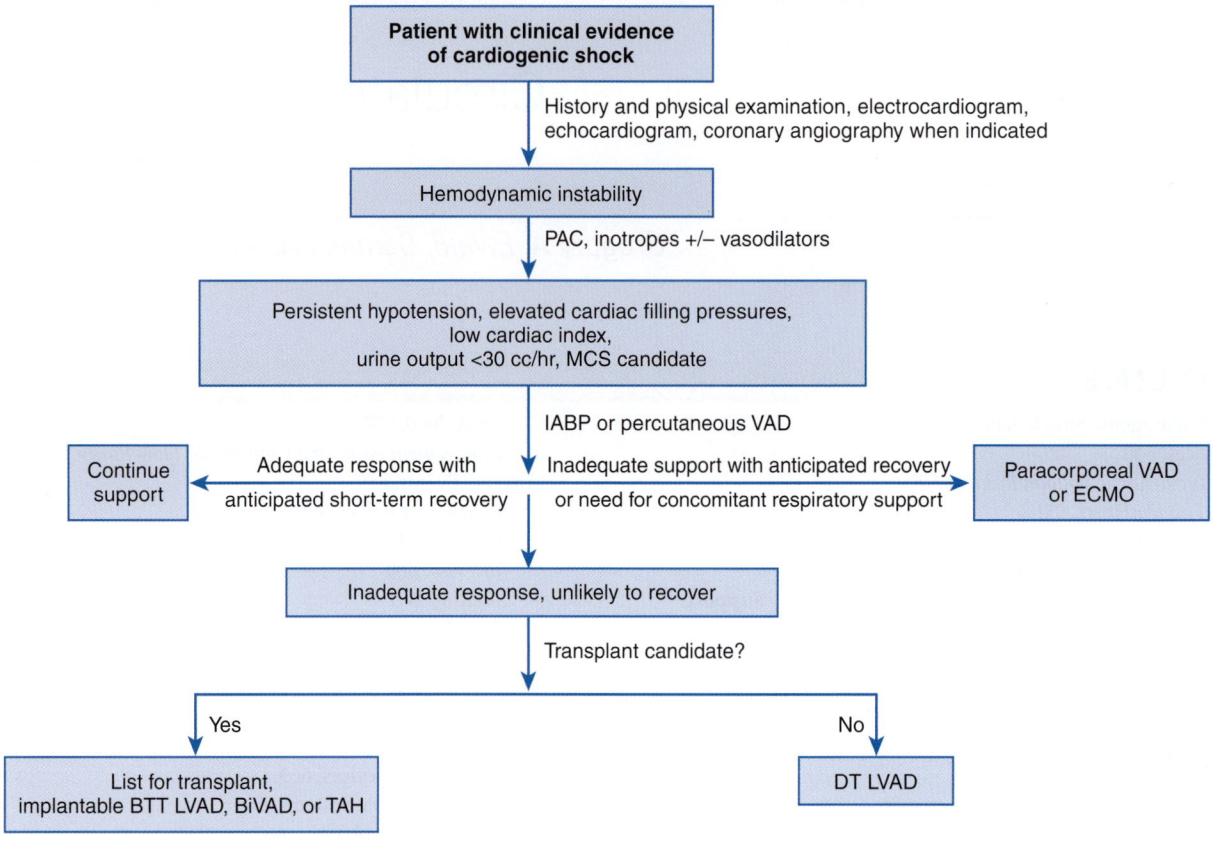

Fig. 45.1 Approach to the patient with cardiogenic shock using multimodality diagnostics and therapeutics. *BiVAD,* Biventricular assist device; *BTT,* bridge to transplant; *DT,* destination therapy; *ECMO,* extracorporeal membrane oxygenator; *IABP,* intra-aortic balloon pump; *LVAD,* left ventricular assist device; *MCS,* mechanically assisted circulation; *PAC,* pulmonary artery catheter; *TAH,* total artificial heart; *VAD,* ventricular assist device.

Initial interventions should include appropriate volume resuscitation, vasodilators in selected patients, and inotropic agents if the patient remains in shock. Placement of a pulmonary artery catheter (**see also Chapter 34**) has been advocated to guide volume administration and vasoactive drug therapy.[12] Mechanical circulatory support (MCS) should be considered in patients with persistent evidence of shock despite the aforementioned interventions. Device selection should be tailored to each patient's unique hemodynamic abnormalities and the need for respiratory support.

Devices

Intra-Aortic Balloon Pump

Over the past 50 years, the IABP has been the most commonly used MCS device. The IABP is generally inserted retrograde in the aorta via the femoral artery and positioned with the distal tip just beyond the left subclavian artery (**Fig. 45.2**). Balloon filling is triggered from the ECG or from the arterial pressure trace; the balloon inflates during diastole and deflates during systole. The favorable physiologic effects of diastolic augmentation include enhanced coronary blood flow and reduced left ventricular afterload.[13]

The effectiveness of the IABP is highly dependent on proper timing of the balloon inflation and deflation (**Fig. 45.3**).[14] Optimal timing results in IABP inflation just after the dicrotic notch in the aortic pressure tracing and deflation before the pressure upstroke of ventricular

systole. The hemodynamic and physiologic benefits of IABP support include elevation of systemic blood pressure relative to unassisted beats and reduction of LV afterload, LV wall stress, and myocardial oxygen demand.[13,15] Inappropriate timing with early inflation or late deflation results in balloon expansion during ventricular systole increasing the afterload against which the ventricle is ejecting. Late balloon inflation or early deflation limits the hemodynamic benefits of the therapy.[14] The hemodynamic effectiveness of the IABP may be limited by tachycardia, such as atrial fibrillation with rapid ventricular response. More than mild aortic valve insufficiency is likely to limit the hemodynamic benefits of IABP therapy by increasing LV loading and is a contraindication to therapy. Significant aortic or iliofemoral atherosclerotic disease is also a relative contraindication to IABP support and has led some to propose alternative insertion strategies, including subclavian artery or direct aortic access used in the context of cardiac surgery.[16]

The IABP has been used as an adjunctive therapy for many cardiac conditions, including acute MI, postinfarction VSD, acute mitral insufficiency with compromised hemodynamics, and cardiogenic shock.[17] However, improved outcomes with IABP therapy in clinical trials have been difficult to demonstrate. Perhaps the most validated use of the IABP is as adjunctive therapy for the treatment of acute MI treated with thrombolytic therapy. In this setting, the use of prophylactic IABP was associated with an 18% reduction in all-cause mortality.[18] However, the SHOCK II-IABP trial failed to demonstrate improved

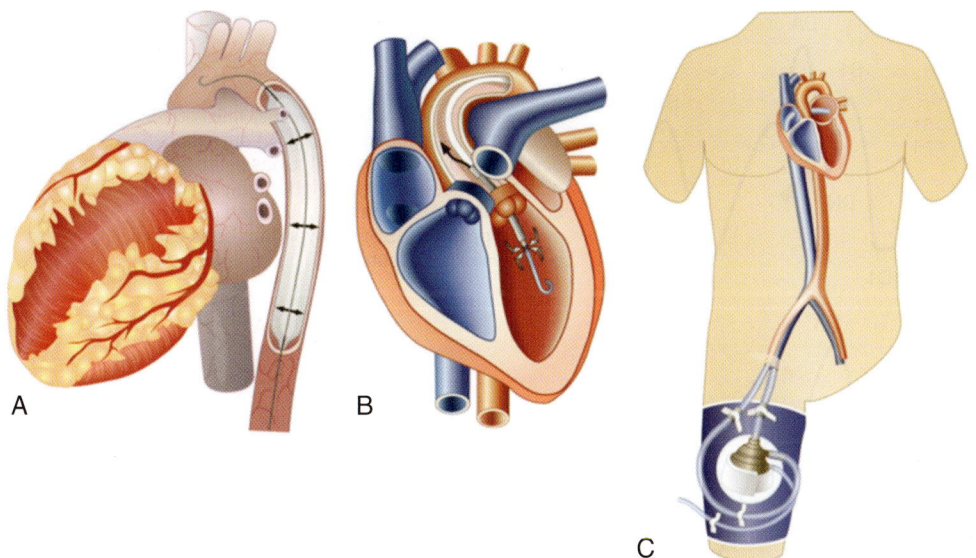

Fig. 45.2 **Percutaneous devices for mechanically assisted circulation.** The intra-aortic balloon pump (A) is inserted retrograde in the aorta and functions as a counterpulsation device with balloon inflation during diastole and deflation during systole. The Impella (B) is a microaxial flow device that is inserted across the aortic valve and withdraws blood from the left ventricle and delivers it in to the aortic root. The TandemHeart (C) is a paracorporeal centrifugal flow pump that withdraws blood from the left atrium via a transseptal catheter and returns blood to the iliofemoral system. (From Desai NR, Bhatt DL. Evaluating percutaneous support for cardiogenic shock: data shock and sticker shock. *Eur Heart J.* 2009;30[17]:2073–2075.)

survival in a more contemporary cohort of patients with acute MI and cardiogenic shock treated with IABP compared with those supported medically.[10]

The limitations of the IABP coupled with a lack of positive outcome studies has resulted in the proliferation of other percutaneous approaches for the treatment of cardiogenic shock and support of complex cardiac procedures, such as high-risk percutaneous coronary interventions and ventricular tachycardia ablations. These devices can be rapidly inserted and are approved for short-term (hours) support.

TandemHeart

The TandemHeart (CardiacAssist, Pittsburgh, PA) is an extracorporeal centrifugal continuous flow pump that receives blood from a 21-F cannula inserted in the femoral vein and passed into the left atrium via a transseptal puncture (see Fig. 45.2). The TandemHeart returns the blood to the arterial circulation via a 17-F catheter inserted in the iliofemoral system. In this configuration, the device can provide up to 5 L/min of flow and is approved for short-term support. The hemodynamic effects of the TandemHeart were compared with IABP in two small, randomized clinical trials that demonstrated superior improvements in cardiac index and the lowering of intracardiac filling pressures with the TandemHeart pump.[19,20] A nonrandomized, experiential series described the potential benefits of the TandemHeart in patients with cardiogenic shock. In this series, 117 patients with clinical evidence of shock (including almost 50% who were receiving or had just received cardiopulmonary resuscitation) were treated with the device. The median cardiac index increase from 0.5 to 3.0 L/min/m^2 was associated with improvement in serum lactate and creatinine. The 30-day survival in this cohort was 60% and largely dependent on candidacy for another treatment such as implantable left ventricular assist device (LVAD).[21] Limitations of the TandemHeart device include the transseptal puncture, which adds technical complexity and may require surgical closure if the patient is transitioned to surgical LVAD. In addition, the 17-F arterial cannula in the femoral artery can result in limb ischemia and often requires surgical closure. More recently,

the TandemHeart pump has been used in conjunction with a novel dual-lumen catheter (Protek Duo) that allows withdrawal of blood from the right atrium and delivery of blood to the pulmonary artery, providing isolated right heart support.[22] The TandemHeart systems for left and right heart support provide reasonable ventricular unloading and increased cardiac output without the need for major thoracic incisions that were previously necessary for temporary VAD applications. Importantly, these percutaneous systems use smaller cannulas relative to surgically placed devices, and this may result in limited flow and increased risk for hemolysis.

Impella

This miniaturized, microaxial flow pump is incorporated into a catheter-based technology and is available in several sizes capable of producing flows from 2.5 to 5.0 L/min (see Fig. 45.2). The smaller Impella (ABIOMED, Danvers, MA) pumps (9 F) can be inserted percutaneously via the femoral artery, whereas the larger device capable of greater blood flow requires surgical implantation techniques. Impella withdraws blood from the distal port in the LV and delivers it to the ascending aorta. This device has been demonstrated to improve cardiac output and reduce left ventricular filling pressures to a greater degree than IABP.[23] Impella 5.0 was studied in a prospective registry that included 16 patients with postcardiotomy shock.[24] Following implantation, the mean arterial pressure increased by 12 mm Hg and the mean cardiac index increased from 1.65 to 2.7 L/min/m^2. There were two primary safety events in this study, one stroke and one death, and the 30- and 180-day survival rates were 94% and 81%, respectively. The Impella EUROSHOCK Registry retrospectively examined 120 patients with cardiogenic shock following MI treated with Impella 2.5.[25] Less than half of the patients were able to be weaned from support, with an associated 30-day mortality rate of 64%. Furthermore, 15% of the patients experienced a major cardiac or cerebrovascular adverse event. Finally, a randomized trial of Impella CP versus IABP was conducted in patients with cardiogenic shock following acute MI.

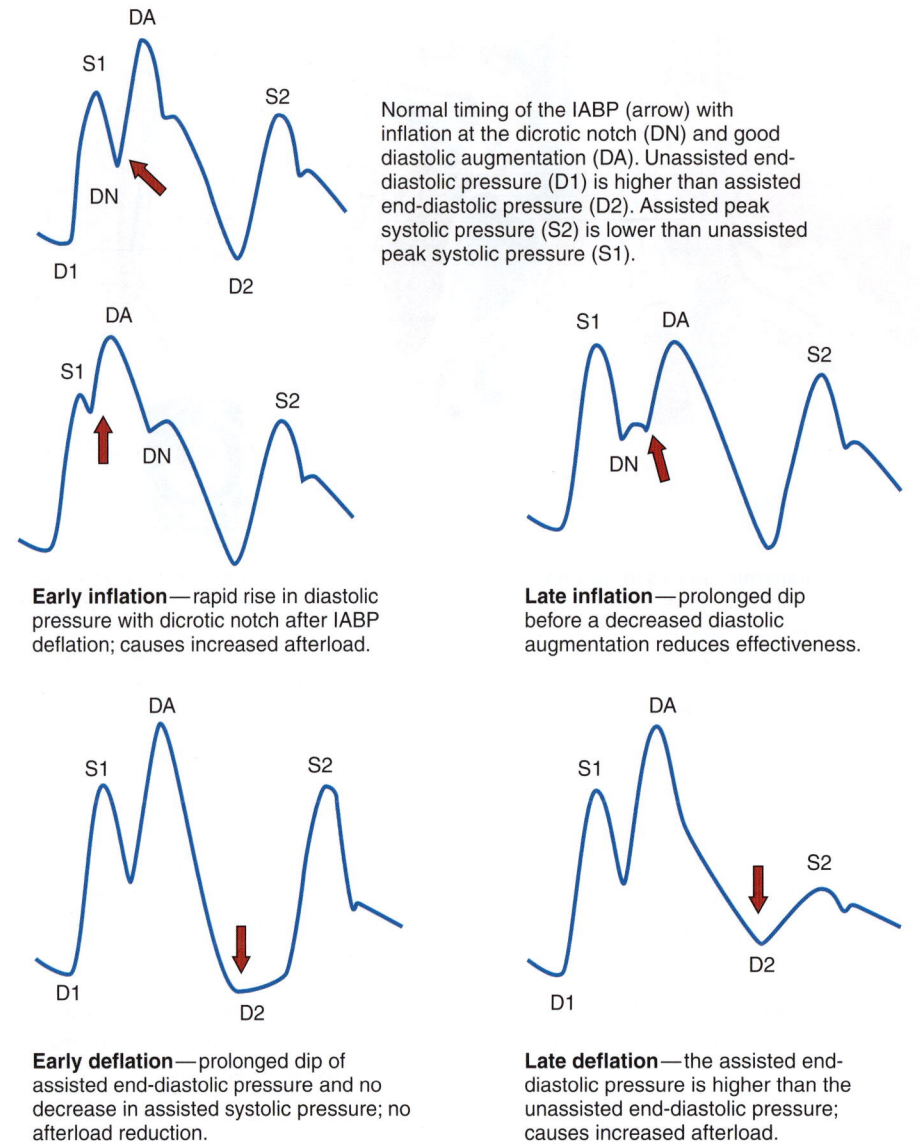

Normal timing of the IABP (arrow) with inflation at the dicrotic notch (DN) and good diastolic augmentation (DA). Unassisted end-diastolic pressure (D1) is higher than assisted end-diastolic pressure (D2). Assisted peak systolic pressure (S2) is lower than unassisted peak systolic pressure (S1).

Early inflation—rapid rise in diastolic pressure with dicrotic notch after IABP deflation; causes increased afterload.

Late inflation—prolonged dip before a decreased diastolic augmentation reduces effectiveness.

Early deflation—prolonged dip of assisted end-diastolic pressure and no decrease in assisted systolic pressure; no afterload reduction.

Late deflation—the assisted end-diastolic pressure is higher than the unassisted end-diastolic pressure; causes increased afterload.

Fig. 45.3 Appropriate and inappropriate timing of intra-aortic balloon pump *(IABP)*. (From Santa-Cruz RA, Cohen MG, Ohman EM. Aortic counterpulsation: a review of the hemodynamic effects and indications for use. *Catheter Cardiovasc Interv.* 2006;67[1]:68–77.)

No difference was observed between treatment group in either 30- or 60-day mortality rates.[26]

The design of Impella has been reconfigured to allow percutaneous right-sided support. The Impella RP features a 22-F pump mounted on an 11-F catheter that withdraws blood from the right atrial/inferior vena caval junction and delivers the blood to the pulmonary artery. The RECOVER RIGHT trial prospectively examined the outcomes of 30 patients with right heart failure following LVAD, cardiotomy, or an MI who were treated with Impella RP. The hemodynamic benefits of Impella RP support included clinically meaningful improvements in central venous pressure and cardiac output. The 30-day survival rate was 73% in this cohort.[27]

Extracorporeal Membrane Oxygenation

Extracorporeal membrane oxygenation (ECMO) is a temporary strategy to provide circulatory and/or respiratory support to critically ill patients. The ECMO circuit consists of a cannula inserted either percutaneously or centrally in the venous system for device inflow. (**Fig. 45.4**).

A centrifugal flow pump moves the blood through an oxygenator and returns it to the body via a cannula placed in the arterial system (venoarterial ECMO for cardiorespiratory failure) or to the venous system (venovenous ECMO for respiratory failure). Flow rates of 4 to 6 L/min are typical for most adult patients. ECMO can be initiated rapidly, and peripheral cannulation allows its use in many settings, including the cardiac catheterization laboratory, the intensive care unit, and the operating room. Overall, application of both venovenous (VV) ECMO and venoarterial (VA) ECMO has increased in the United States, related mainly to improvements in safety and durability of the oxygenators. In the setting of cardiogenic shock, establishing hemodynamic stability with ECMO allows time to assess cardiopulmonary recovery and improvement in end-organ function. ECMO is generally considered useful for short periods (days to weeks). An important complication of peripheral ECMO that limits longer-term benefit is a lack of direct LV unloading, with resultant ventricular distention and pulmonary venous hypertension. Furthermore, extended support is undesirable because the patient is typically confined to bed and the incidence of adverse events,

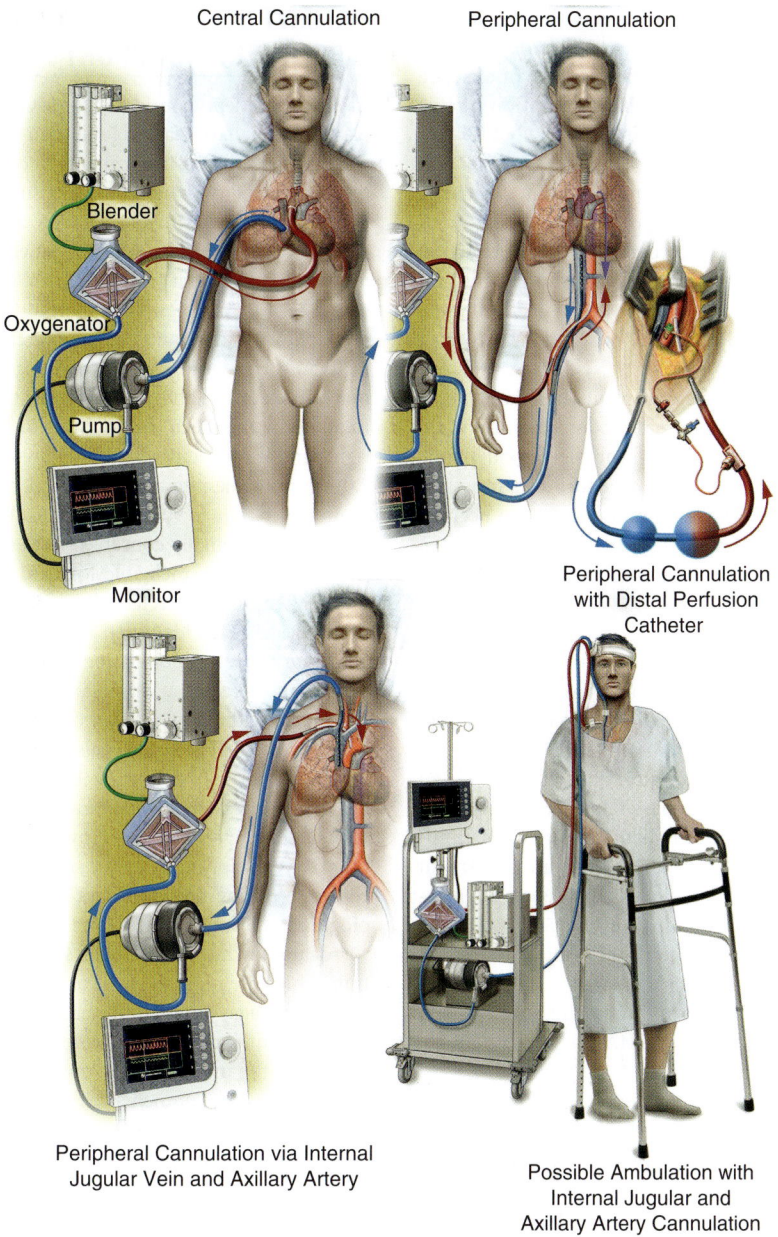

Central Cannulation

Peripheral Cannulation

Blender

Oxygenator

Pump

Monitor

Peripheral Cannulation
with Distal Perfusion
Catheter

Peripheral Cannulation via Internal
Jugular Vein and Axillary Artery

Possible Ambulation with
Internal Jugular and
Axillary Artery Cannulation

Fig. 45.4 Cannulation options for venoarterial extracorporeal membrane oxygenator are shown. (From Keebler ME, Haddad EV, Choi CW, et al. Venoarterial extracorporeal membrane oxygenation in cardiogenic shock. *JACC Heart Fail*, 2018;6[6]:503–516.)

including bleeding, hemolysis, thrombocytopenia, limb ischemia, vascular injury, and stroke, is related to the duration of support. Thus, after stabilization for a brief period, the clinical team must decide on the next step in the patient's care. In some cases, ECMO can be weaned and the patient separated from the system. In other cases, it serves as a bridge to another procedure such as permanent MCS or transplantation. There are limited outcomes data examining the role of ECMO for the treatment of heart failure and cardiogenic shock. Survival following ECMO support appears to be strongly related to the underlying cause of the ventricular dysfunction, as well as the timing of application, with patients placed on ECMO following cardiac arrest faring poorly. ECMO-supported patients still have a 50% in-hospital mortality, with 6-month survival rates as low as 30%.[28] ECMO has also been used to provide hemodynamic support during high-risk procedures such as percutaneous coronary interventions and ventricular tachycardia ablations.

INDICATIONS FOR IMPLANTABLE MECHANICAL CIRCULATORY SUPPORT DEVICES

Decision-making regarding implantation of durable MCS devices is dependent on the clinical status of the patient and the recognized indications for the therapy. Historically, there are two recognized indications for implantable LVADs: as a means to support critically ill patients until they can receive cardiac transplantation (bridge to transplant [BTT]) or as permanent therapy in non–transplant candidates (destination therapy [DT]). This narrowly focused paradigm is not aligned with contemporary use of these devices, and the following definitions are commonly used by clinicians:

Bridge to bridge is a strategy in which a short-term circulatory support device is used until a more definitive procedure can be performed. This is typically used for patients in cardiogenic shock who require rapid hemodynamic restoration to reverse the shock state and/or improve end-organ function. Device selection depends on the severity of hemodynamic compromise, the presence or absence of biventricular heart failure, and the anticipated duration of this approach. In many cases, percutaneous devices or ECMO are used.

Bridge to recovery may be used in disease processes anticipated to recover with a period of hemodynamic support, such as acute myocarditis, peripartum cardiomyopathy, cardiac transplant rejection with hemodynamic compromise, or postcardiotomy shock. Selection of the most appropriate device typically involves determination of the need to provide partial or full hemodynamic support and the projected duration of therapy.

Bridge to decision acknowledges that transplant candidacy is frequently confounded by potentially reversible comorbidities when the decision for durable MCS is made. The favorable hemodynamic impact of LVAD support commonly improves end-organ function, lowers pulmonary artery pressures, and allows the patient to become physically and nutritionally rehabilitated before consideration of transplantation. However, if the patient does not achieve these milestones, he or she may remain on mechanically assisted circulation for prolonged periods or indefinitely.

BTT is reserved for device implantation in patients listed for transplant at high priority who are failing optimal therapies. DT designates LVAD implantation in a patient with advanced heart failure who is currently ineligible for transplantation. The DT criteria are aligned with the inclusion criteria from clinical trials and include an ejection fraction less than 25%, NYHA class IIIb to IV symptoms, objective functional impairment with a maximal oxygen consumption of less than 14 mL/kg/min (or <50% predicted), and treatment with either optimal medical therapy for 45 of the past 60 days, intravenous inotropic support for 14 days, or an IABP for 7 days. During deliberations for LVAD financial coverage in the United States, the Centers for Medicare and Medicaid Services was unable to agree on the definition of NYHA class IIIb symptoms and subsequently supports only payment for patients with NYHA class IV functional limitations.

More recently, a clinical trial was completed that redefined LVAD implantation into either short- or long-term support.[29] This approach is more aligned with contemporary clinical practice because it is less dependent upon future events (such as transplantation).

PATIENT SELECTION FOR MECHANICAL CIRCULATORY SUPPORT

In general, patients considered for MCS have severely depressed ventricular function, have marked limitation in functional capacity, are treated with evidence-based medical and electrical therapies, and have a high residual mortality risk within the ensuing 1 to 2 years. Patient selection is critically important to achieving optimal postoperative outcomes. Selection criteria should identify patients with sufficient severity of illness to derive benefit from MCS while simultaneously avoiding those with a severity of illness or comorbidities that would compromise survival following implantation. Baseline characteristics of patients enrolled in LVAD trials demonstrated end-organ dysfunction with hyponatremia and elevated serum blood urea nitrogen and creatinine levels.[30,31] In addition, the mean ejection fraction was less than 0.20 with elevated right- and left-sided cardiac filling pressures and mean cardiac index of 2.0 L/min/m^2 despite treatment with continuous infusion intravenous inotropes in 80% to 90% of patients and IABP support in 20% to 40%.

DT was originally conceived as a treatment for patients with end-stage heart failure ineligible for cardiac transplantation. As a result, many of those being referred for DT LVAD are older than 65 years. Older age has been identified as an important predictor of adverse outcomes in the VAD population. The HeartMate II risk score demonstrated an increased postimplant mortality risk of 32% per decade.[32] Data from the Interagency Registry for Mechanically Assisted Circulation (INTERMACS) also described older age as a risk factor for early mortality following LVAD placement and highlighted the important interaction between age and other risk factors for mortality, such as severity of illness.[33] However, carefully selected patients older than 70 years appear to derive similar benefits with VAD as a younger cohort,[34] raising the important concept of chronologic versus physiologic age in patient selection. Chronologic age is likely an imperfect surrogate for the true predictors of adverse outcomes in this population, which are more likely measures of frailty and debilitation.[35]

Beyond age, other contraindications to implantable VAD therapy appear to influence short- and long-term outcomes and must be considered in the overall risk assessment of the candidate. INTERMACS developed a new nomenclature for classification of advanced heart failure that has been used to understand the impact of severity of illness on outcomes (**Table 45.1**).[36] Patients with INTERMACS profile 1 and 2 have a high early mortality hazard relative to MCS patients with

TABLE 45.1   INTERMACS Patient Profiles

Adult Profiles	Current CMS DT Indication?	IV Inotropes	Official Parlance	NYHA Class	Modifier Option
INTERMACS Level 1	Yes	Yes	"Crash and burn"	IV	A, TCS
INTERMACS Level 2	Yes	Yes	"Sliding fast" on inotropes	IV	A, TCS
INTERMACS Level 3	Yes	Yes	"Stable" on inotropes	IV	A, FF, TCS
INTERMACS Level 4	+peak V$_{O_2}$ ≤ 14	No	Resting symptoms on oral therapy at home	Ambulatory IV	A, FF
INTERMACS Level 5	+peak V$_{O_2}$ ≤ 14	No	"Housebound," comfortable at rest, symptoms with minimal activity or ADLs	Ambulatory IV	A, FF
INTERMACS Level 6	No	No	"Walking wounded," ADLs possible but meaningful activity limited	IIIb	A, FF
INTERMACS Level 7	No	No	Advanced class III	III	A, FF

A, Arrhythmia; *ADLs,* activities of daily living; *CMS,* Centers for Medicare and Medicaid Services; *DT,* destination therapy; *FF,* frequent flier; *INTERMAC,* interagency registry for mechanically assisted circulation; *IV,* intravenous; *NYHA,* New York Heart Association; *TCS,* temporary circulatory support; *V*$_{O_2}$, maximal oxygen consumption. From Stewart GC, Stevenson LW. Keeping left ventricular assist device acceleration on track. *Circulation.* 2011;123(14):1559–1568.

lesser degrees of hemodynamic compromise, leading many centers to be highly selective in the use of durable implantable LVADs in these patient cohorts.[33]

Right ventricular (RV) failure, defined as the need for prolonged inotropic therapy to support the right heart or a RV assist device, remains an Achilles heel of LVAD therapy and is associated with multisystem organ failure, prolonged hospitalization, and increased morbidity and mortality following LVAD implantation.[33] Unfortunately, prediction of post-LVAD RV failure is challenging despite identification of individual parameters and multivariable models that provide insights into the likelihood of RV failure in larger patient populations. Predictors of RV failure following LVAD fall into three general categories: (1) echocardiographic measurements; (2) hemodynamic parameters; and (3) clinical features before LVAD insertion. Increased RV size and severe RV systolic function are associated with post-LVAD RV failure.[37] Quantitative measures of RV performance, such as a tricuspid annular plane systolic excursion (TAPSE) of less than 7.5 mm, reduced RV peak longitudinal strain, and the severity of tricuspid insufficiency have been shown to be useful markers in the prediction of RV failure after LVAD.[37] Hemodynamic variables such as a central venous pressure to pulmonary capillary wedge pressure ratio of greater than 0.63 or an RV stroke work index of less than 250 to 300 mm Hg $\times$ mL/m^2 are linked to worse outcomes following LVAD placement.[38] Finally, general clinical features such as preoperative mechanical ventilation and abnormal renal and hepatic function have been identified as risk factors for RV failure.[38] A recent validation study of several published RV failure risk scores demonstrated only modest accuracy, highlighting the real clinical dilemma facing clinicians in the preimplant prediction of this important comorbidity.[39]

Renal failure requiring dialysis is considered a strong relative contraindication to durable MCS. Significant renal dysfunction was an exclusion criterion in the clinical trials, so the benefit and potential incremental complications of implanting an LVAD in dialysis patients are unknown. However, 1-year survival in LVAD patients requiring renal replacement therapy is approximately 50% and significantly reduced compared with nondialysis patients in the INTERMACS registry. Furthermore, support with newer-generation LVADs that provide continuous flow results in a minimal (and often imperceptible) pulse pressure, making measurement of blood pressure difficult during hemodialysis.

Active systemic infection is a strong relative contraindication to LVAD implantation. Patients with fever or unexplained leukocytosis should undergo thorough evaluation, including blood and urine cultures, chest x-ray, and other diagnostic testing directed at potential sites of infection. Hospitalized patients and those with chronic indwelling catheters should have intravenous cannulae removed. Patients with pacing systems and unexplained bacteremia may require chest wall or transesophageal echocardiography to rule out pacemaker-associated endocarditis.

An evaluation for cerebrovascular disease should be performed in at-risk patients using noninvasive imaging.[40] The presence of a prior stroke does not preclude implantation of an LVAD, but consideration must be given to the potential for meaningful rehabilitation and the patient's ability to interact with the device. For example, an individual with hemiparesis of a dominant arm may have difficulty making the electrical connections required to operate the VAD.

Other end-organ dysfunction may also limit favorable outcomes with VAD therapy and should be considered during the evaluation. Individuals with clinically significant chronic obstructive pulmonary disease whose FEV$_1$ is less than 1 L are likely to have residual dyspnea despite hemodynamic improvement and may have difficulty weaning from the ventilator postoperatively. A VE/MVV ratio of more than 80% on a preoperative cardiopulmonary exercise test suggests

a pulmonary component to dyspnea.[41] Patients with long-standing right heart failure or other conditions associated with liver injury should undergo an evaluation for hepatic insufficiency.[42] Serum transaminases, albumin, and imaging studies to examine the texture and contour of the liver may provide insights about the necessity for liver biopsy. The presence of an elevated model for end-stage liver disease (MELD) score has been linked to higher post-LVAD mortality.[43] Careful evaluation of the coagulation system is warranted in individuals with a history of a bleeding diathesis or in those with unexplained thrombotic or thromboembolic events. Patients with a history of gastrointestinal bleeding or intolerance to systemic anticoagulation with warfarin should be carefully evaluated because of their high risk of rebleeding following LVAD implantation. Patients with a low platelet count and exposure to heparin should be screened for heparin-induced thrombocytopenia with a PF4 antibody and a serotonin release assay.[44] To the extent possible, patients should have a normal coagulation profile before MCS surgery, because an elevated international normalized ratio (INR) at the time of LVAD implantation was identified as a risk factor for mortality.[32] Correction of coagulopathy will reduce the likelihood of bleeding complications and associated perioperative morbidity. Malnutrition is considered an important risk factor for adverse outcomes, including infection, prolonged debilitation, and mortality. However, the ability to favorably impact nutrition in a critically ill heart failure patient is unclear. Instead, nutrition management should be a primary focus of the entire VAD team following device implantation.[45] Supplemental enteral feedings may be required perioperatively, with additional support in the outpatient setting until nutritional deficits are corrected.

Disease processes with an anticipated survival of less than 3 years were an exclusion criterion in the DT clinical trials, so there are no data supporting the role for mechanically assisted circulation in the management of these patients.

Psychosocial factors also play a pivotal role in VAD outcomes. As part of the evaluation, patients should be seen by multiple health care providers, including those who focus primarily on prior history of compliance, substance use, health literacy, and the availability and abilities of family and friends who will participate in the ongoing outpatient management of the patient and the device. There is a high caregiver burden with MCS, including the need for device training, care of the percutaneous driveline, and companionship. These issues and expectations need to be clearly articulated by the team and agreed on by the patient and his or her caregivers prior to device implantation.

In an attempt to integrate large numbers of predictive clinical variables, the HeartMate II Risk Model was derived from a large clinical trials database and demonstrated that age, elevated INR, increased serum creatinine, and lower serum albumin were predictive of postimplant mortality.[32] Follow-up analyses in institutional datasets suggest only modest predictive accuracy (C-statistic 0.6) for short- and long-term outcomes.[46]

Recent successes in mechanically assisted circulation have resulted in acceptance of this approach as a useful therapy for the treatment of selected patients with advanced heart failure. The INTERMACS registry has captured almost all implants using FDA-approved MCS devices in the United States since 2006 and has carefully documented the growth of this field following the introduction of the new-generation continuous flow devices.[33] The number of centers implanting long-term devices is increasing and has expanded from traditional transplant centers to programs that do not perform transplantation. The impact of center volume on outcomes was recently reported from INTERMACS and showed that both very low volume and high volume programs had higher perioperative and long-term mortality rates.[47]

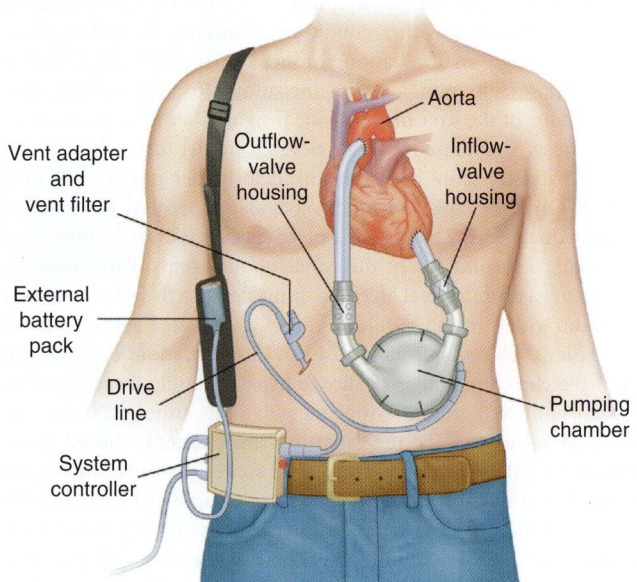

Fig. 45.5 The HeartMate XVE (Abbott, Abbott Park, IL) is an original electric, pulsatile device commercially available to support patients with the intent of bridging to transplantation or as permanent therapy. (From Wilson SR, Givertz MM, Stewart GC, Mudge GH Jr. Ventricular assist devices the challenges of outpatient management. *J Am Coll Cardiol.* 2009;54[18]:1647–1659.)

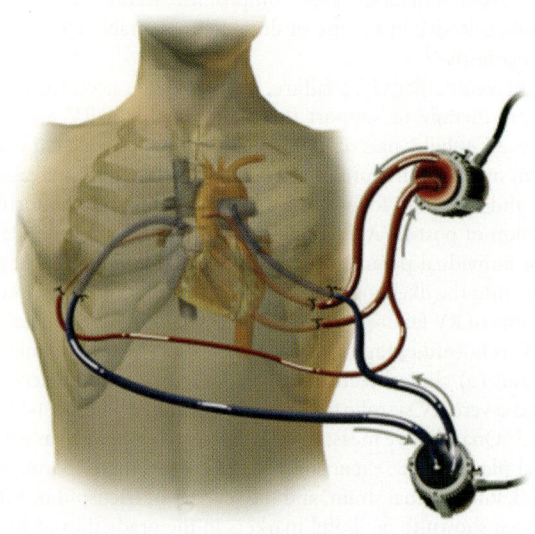

Fig. 45.6 CentriMag (Abbott, Abbott Park, IL) continuous flow ventricular assist devices (VADs). The CentriMag VAD is shown in a biventricular support strategy. In this figure, please note the cannulation of both the right superior pulmonary vein and the left ventricular apex in an attempt to more completely unload the left ventricle. (From cardiothoracicsurgery.org.)

MECHANICAL CIRCULATORY SUPPORT DEVICES

The mechanical blood pumps can be characterized in several ways: temporary versus permanent, intracorporeal versus extracorporeal, and pulsatile flow versus continuous flow. At present, the vast majority of clinically available pumps are continuous flow devices. Pulsatile flow pumps such as the ABIOMED 5000, Thoratec PVAD and IVAD, Novacor LVAD, and HeartMate XVE are of historical interest. However, their importance in supporting patients and forming the foundation of the principles of mechanically assisted circulation cannot be underestimated. For example, the HeartMate XVE (**Fig. 45.5**) and Novacor LVAD were the original electric, implantable LVADs that were tested in clinical trials and shown to be superior to optimal medical heart failure treatment in patients either awaiting transplantation or as DT.[5,6,48]

Temporary Continuous Flow Ventricular Assist Devices
CentriMag
The CentriMag (Abbott, Abbott Park, IL) pump is an extracorporeal device approved for short-term support in the United States and can be configured to provide univentricular (either right or left) or biventricular support (**Fig. 45.6**). It is a magnetically levitated centrifugal flow device capable of delivering 10 L/min, although the standard clinical flows are 4 to 6 L/min. PediaMag is a smaller version of the same device capable of flows to 1.5 L/min.

Rotaflow
Rotaflow (Maquet, Inc, Wayne, NJ) is an extracorporeal centrifugal flow pump with specifications that are similar to those of the Centrimag device. Rotaflow features a magnetically levitated rotor and has been used as an right ventricular assist device (RVAD), LVAD, or in ECMO circuits.

Durable Continuous Flow Pumps
A pivotal innovation in mechanically assisted circulation came with the observation that the human body did not require a "normal" pulse

pressure. This led to the development of LVAD pumps with rotary mechanisms that produced continuous rather than pulsatile blood flow. These devices are smaller nonvalved systems that draw blood from the LV apex and return the blood to the circulation via an outflow graft generally attached to the ascending aorta. The devices are electrically driven by external battery or AC power delivered to the pump via a subcutaneous driveline that exits the skin and is attached to a wearable controller that regulates and monitors pump function (**Fig. 45.7**). The blood-propelling mechanism in these devices rotates at a constant set speed and operates to maximally reduce LV size with minimal or no aortic valve opening. As a result, there may not be a detectable pulse in patients supported with a continuous flow device (**Fig. 45.8**), and most of the observed pulsatility is derived from the contribution of native ventricular systole to LVAD filling.

Cardiopulmonary bypass provided an extensive experience with short-duration nonpulsatile blood flow. The clinical trials of continuous flow LVADs provided the opportunity to explore the impact of chronic minimally pulsatile flow on end-organ function. Russell and colleagues were unable to demonstrate any decline in renal or hepatic function over a 6-month observation period.[49] Similarly, neurocognitive function was examined over 24 months of continuous flow support with no evidence of decline in executive cognitive function.[50] Finally, submaximal exercise performance was serially evaluated and shown to improve during the first 3 months following LVAD implantation and remain stable throughout a 24-month follow-up period, suggesting no detrimental impact on peripheral muscle function.[51] Thus there is no evidence from clinical trials to suggest a decline in end-organ function resulting from chronic circulatory support with minimal (or no) pulsatility.

HeartMate II
HeartMate II (HMII, Abbott, Abbott Park, IL) is an axial flow LVAD that is implanted in a preperitoneal pocket beneath the left costal margin. It is small, operates in a quiet mode, and is capable of flows

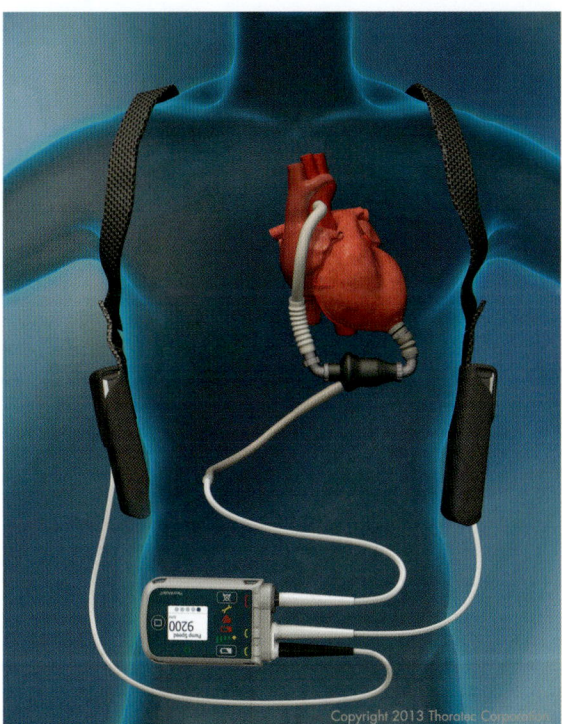

Fig. 45.7 Implant configuration of the HeartMate II left ventricular assist device (LVAD; Abbott Corp, Abbott Park, IL). The HeartMate II LVAD is implanted in a preperitoneal pocket with the inflow cannula attached to the LV apex and the outflow graft connected to the ascending aorta. A subcutaneous drive line connects the LVAD to the controller. Two batteries supply power to the controller. (HeartMate II is a trademark of St. Jude Medical, LLC, or its related companies. Reproduced with permission of St. Jude Medical, © 2018. All rights reserved.)

up to 10 L/min, although clinical flows are primarily 4 to 6 L/min. The HeartMate II is approved in the United States for BTT and DT. The pivotal HeartMate II BTT trial used a unique trial design that compared the outcomes of 133 patients supported on the device to objective performance criteria.[30] The primary composite end point of the study was survival on support to 180 days, transplant, or ventricular recovery that permitted device removal. Seventy-five percent of patients successfully achieved this end point with a 12-month actuarial survival of 68%. Following enrollment of the primary patient cohort, additional patients (n = 336) were enrolled in a continued access protocol. Evaluation of this extended population demonstrated improvement in the primary composite end point to 79% and a 12-month actuarial survival of 73%.[52]

The HeartMate II DT trial compared the rates of survival free from disabling stroke and reoperation to repair or replace the device in 200 patients randomized to either HeartMate II or HeartMate XVE.[31] There was a fourfold increase in successful achievement of the primary end point at 24 months in the HMII cohort. Actuarial survival at 24 months was 58% and 24% in the continuous flow and pulsatile flow cohorts, respectively. When the components of the primary end point were examined, device replacement and death were statistically less common in the HMII cohort and there was a trend toward fewer strokes. Quality of life and functional capacity were not different between study groups, suggesting that the hemodynamic benefits of MCS were more important determinants of these outcomes than the mode of circulatory support (pulsatile vs. continuous flow). Like the BTT trial, a continued access protocol allowed enrollment in the study, while the primary cohort completed follow-up. This resulted

in an expanded patient population of 281 patients. Analysis of the HeartMate II–treated patients in this cohort demonstrated a 2-year survival of 63%.[53]

HeartWare HVAD

HeartWare HVAD (Medtronic, Minneapolis, MN) is a bearingless centrifugal flow pump capable of providing up to 10 L of blood flow. Its small size and design allow placement in the pericardium (**Fig. 45.9**). The HVAD was studied as a BTT in a noninferiority trial that used concomitantly enrolled patients in the INTERMACS registry implanted with a commercially available device as a control group.[54] The primary end point was survival to 180 days on the originally implanted device, transplant, or device removal for recovery. Ninety-two percent of the HVAD population successfully achieved the primary end point compared with 90.7% of the control group (noninferiority, $P < .001$). On the basis of this trial, HVAD was approved as a BTT device by the FDA.

The HVAD was also evaluated in the DT application in a 446-patient randomized, noninferiority trial comparing the HVAD to the HMII. The primary end point, survival to 2 years on the originally implanted device without a disabling stroke, was not statistically different between the two groups.[55] However, there was a higher than anticipated stroke rate in the HVAD cohort. This led to the ENDURANCE Supplemental trial designed to test the impact of blood pressure control on the 12-month incidence of stroke. The HVAD cohort in the supplemental trial had an absolute stroke reduction of nearly 50% compared with the primary study but failed to reach its primary noninferiority end point.[56]

HeartMate 3

The HeartMate 3 (Abbott, Abbott Park, IL) is another intrapericardial centrifugal flow LVAD (**Fig. 45.10**) that incorporated several design features to reduce adverse events. Gaps between the rotor and the pump housing were increased to reduce shear force in the pump, hemolysis, and device thrombosis. In addition, an algorithm for speed increase and decrease every 2 seconds was used to improve device washing. The HeartMate 3 recently completed clinical trials with a novel adaptive design that focused on short-term (6 months) and long-term (24 months) support rather than BTT or DT. The comparator device in these studies was the HeartMate II, and the end point in both studies was survival without disabling stroke or the need to repair or replace the device. Both the short- and long-term trials demonstrated superiority of the HeartMate 3 device with important reductions in device thrombosis leading to device replacement as the key driver of the end point.[57,58]

Jarvik 2000

The Jarvik 2000 is a small axial flow device with several interesting innovations, including implantation of the pump directly into the left ventricle, variable speed control that can be manipulated by the patient, and novel power cord implantation. The BTT trial with this device has completed enrollment and is in the follow-up phase.

Management Issues of a Continuous Flow Pump

Beyond the unique physiology associated with continuous flow VADs, management of patients on these devices is nuanced. The minimally pulsatile blood flow can make standard blood pressure monitoring difficult. Doppler appears to be superior to auscultation or the use of automated blood pressure cuffs to assess blood pressure.[59] Hypertension is common following a period of support on a continuous flow LVAD. Careful assessment and management of hypertension may have a favorable impact on the risk of stroke and other adverse events in this patient population, particularly with the HVAD.

Systemic anticoagulation with warfarin and an antiplatelet agent is recommended with all commercially available devices. However, the

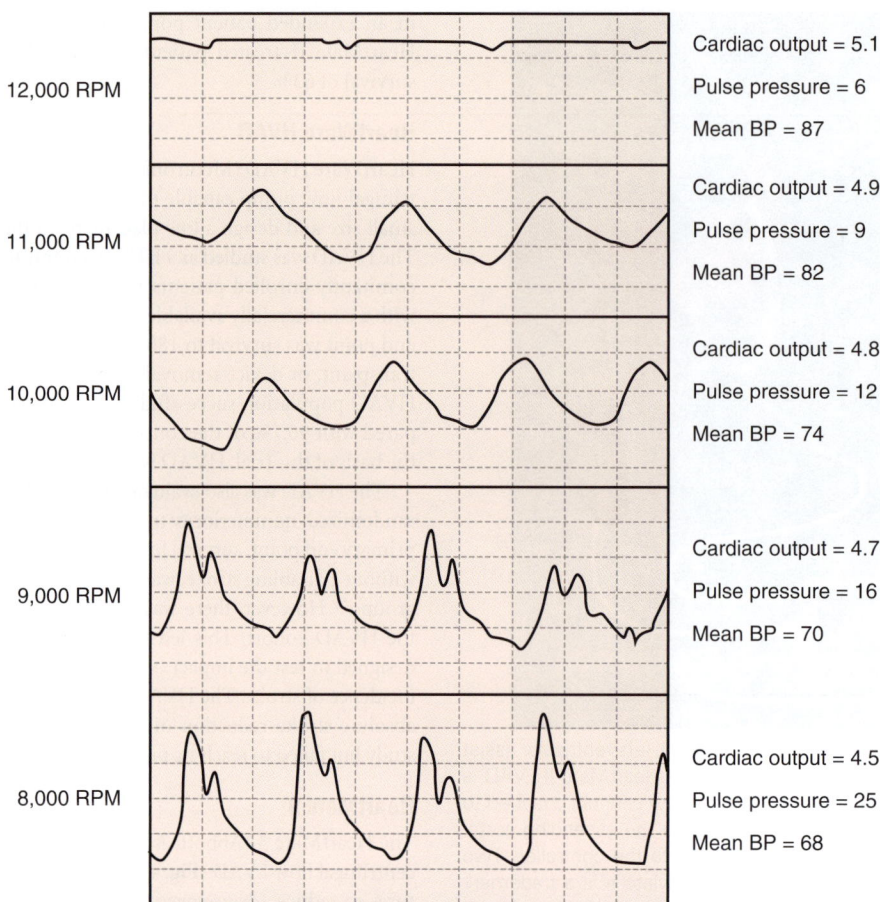

12,000 RPM — Cardiac output = 5.1 / Pulse pressure = 6 / Mean BP = 87

11,000 RPM — Cardiac output = 4.9 / Pulse pressure = 9 / Mean BP = 82

10,000 RPM — Cardiac output = 4.8 / Pulse pressure = 12 / Mean BP = 74

9,000 RPM — Cardiac output = 4.7 / Pulse pressure = 16 / Mean BP = 70

8,000 RPM — Cardiac output = 4.5 / Pulse pressure = 25 / Mean BP = 68

Fig. 45.8 Pulse Pressure in Continuous Flow Left Ventricular Assist Device (LVAD). The pulse pressure in a continuous flow LVAD is dependent on the speed. At slower speeds (8000–9000) a dicrotic notch can be seen in the arterial pressure tracing. As the ventricular assist device speed is increased further, the pulse pressure narrows as the cardiac output increases. These very low pulse pressures are often clinically imperceptible. (From Frazier OH, Jacob LP. Small pumps for ventricular assistance: progress in mechanical circulatory support. *Cardiol Clin.* 2007;25[4]:553–564.)

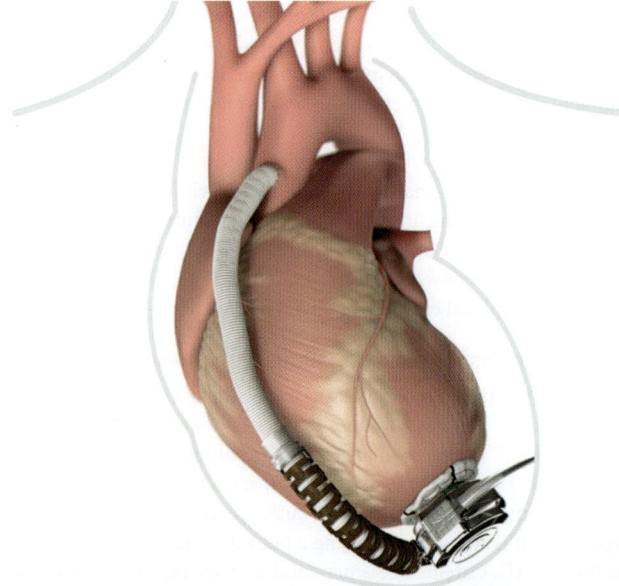

Fig. 45.9 HeartWare HVAD. The HeartWare HVAD (Medtronic, Minneapolis, MN) is a centrifugal flow pump with a size sufficiently small to be implanted in the pericardial space. The remainder of the implant configuration is similar to that shown in **Fig. 45.7**.

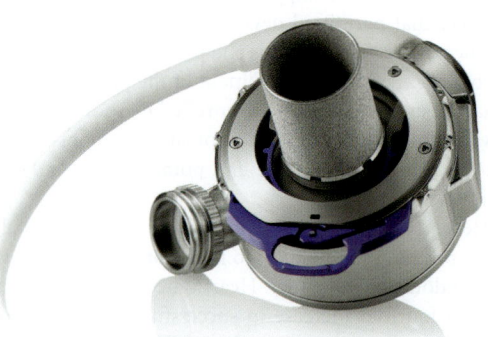

Fig. 45.10 HeartMate 3 left ventricular assist device (Abbott, Abbott Park, IL) is a fully magnetically levitated intrapericardial centrifugal flow device designed to improve hemocompatibility. Recent clinical trials show a significantly reduced incidence of device thrombosis relative to HeartMate II. (HeartMate 3 is a trademark of St. Jude Medical, LLC or its related companies. Reproduced with permission of St. Jude Medical, © 2018. All rights reserved.)

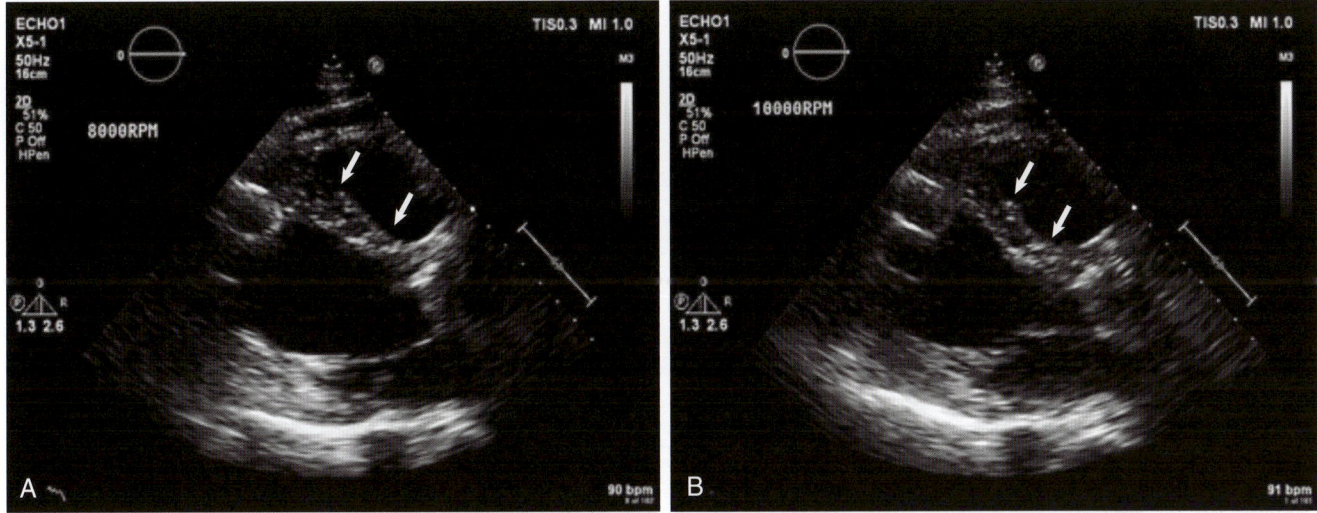

Fig. 45.11 The impact of excessive ventricular assist device speed on ventricular septal position. The impact of varying left ventricular assist device speed is demonstrated. At a pump speed of 8000 RPM (A) the ventricular septum (arrows) is positioned in the midline. When the speed is increased to 10,000 RPM (B), the ventricular septum is shifted toward the posterior wall.

target INR varies from device to device. A recent trial comparing dabigatran to a vitamin K antagonist in LVAD patients was stopped because of excess thromboembolic events in the dabigatran arm.[60] Thoughtful management of LVAD settings is also an important component of ongoing device care. The LVAD creates negative pressure at the LV apex. Excessive speed or intravascular volume depletion may result in the device pulling the ventricular septum toward the inflow cannula (**Fig. 45.11**). When this is severe, the myocardium may partially occlude flow into the VAD, causing a "suction" event. Contemporary devices will recognize this phenomenon and trigger an alarm or reduce the pump speed temporarily to allow LV filling that moves the inflow cannula away from the myocardium. Excessive pump speeds should be considered as a potential cause of ventricular tachycardia.

Multimodality imaging is a critical component of the ongoing care of LVAD patients (**Fig. 45.12**). Chest x-ray and echocardiography are useful tools to evaluate inflow cannula positioning, which should optimally be centered in the LV cavity, directed toward the mitral valve, and not in opposition to the ventricular myocardium. Chest wall echocardiography is also used to determine the most appropriate speed for the device.[37] The ramp study has been proposed as an objective test to determine optimal pump speed and to detect evidence of LVAD thrombosis.[61,62] In a ramp study, the VAD speed is decreased to a minimal level such that the LV dilates and the aortic valve opens, signifying inadequate left ventricular unloading. The LVAD speed is then incrementally increased with simultaneous monitoring of symptoms, vital signs, left ventricular size, and aortic valve movement using transthoracic echocardiography. The optimal speed results in maximal pump output and reduction of left ventricular diastolic diameter, maintenance of the ventricular septum in the "midline," and either intermittent or no aortic valve opening. Many programs perform the ramp study early after device implant and again with changes in the clinical status including worsening dyspnea, ventricular tachycardia, or evidence that the device is unloading the LV excessively. Cine CT can be useful to identify inflow cannula malposition when other imaging studies result in diagnostic uncertainty. CT is also useful to evaluate the outflow graft. Finally, cardiac catheterization may be particularly useful in patients presenting with dyspnea. An appropriately functioning LVAD will lower the LVEDP/PCWP into a normal or near normal range. Elevated left ventricular filling

pressures should raise the possibility of inadequate device speed, AI, or device malfunction.

Adverse Events

Adverse events following LVAD placement are common. A recent analysis demonstrated that 70% of patients have a major adverse event within 12 months of device implantation.[63] Most adverse events occur early after device implantation. However, some complications such as infections are time dependent, with progressive risk the longer the patient has an LVAD in place. One of the important challenges in understanding the rate of device-related complications was the lack of standardized definitions. The INTERMACS registry has developed standardized definitions for common adverse events that are now being used in the registry and in clinical trials.

Right Heart Failure

Right heart failure following LVAD implantation is associated with incremental morbidity and mortality. The need for continuous infusion inotropes to support RV performance for more than 2 weeks or an RV assist device following LVAD reduced 180-day survival from 87% to 66% in the HeartMate II BTT trial.[38] Furthermore, many events categorized as multisystem organ failure in the clinical LVAD trials can be traced back to RV failure. The clinical presentation is typically in the first hours following LVAD implantation and is characterized by systemic hypotension, elevated right atrial pressure, and poor VAD filling. Echocardiography may demonstrate a dilated and dysfunctional RV with or without tricuspid insufficiency and a small and underfilled left ventricle (**Fig. 45.13**). Prevention of RV failure by careful patient selection is desirable, but the available tools lack high predictive accuracy. Integration of clinical parameters, imaging measures of RV performance, and hemodynamic variables may assist the clinician in prognostication. Treatment of post-LVAD RV failure includes the use of pharmacologic agents that increase cardiac contractility such as dobutamine or milrinone, drugs that lower pulmonary artery pressures such as inhaled nitric oxide, prostacyclin, or oral phosphodiesterase-5 inhibitors such as sildenafil. If these agents are ineffective, an RV assist device may be required. Determination of significant right

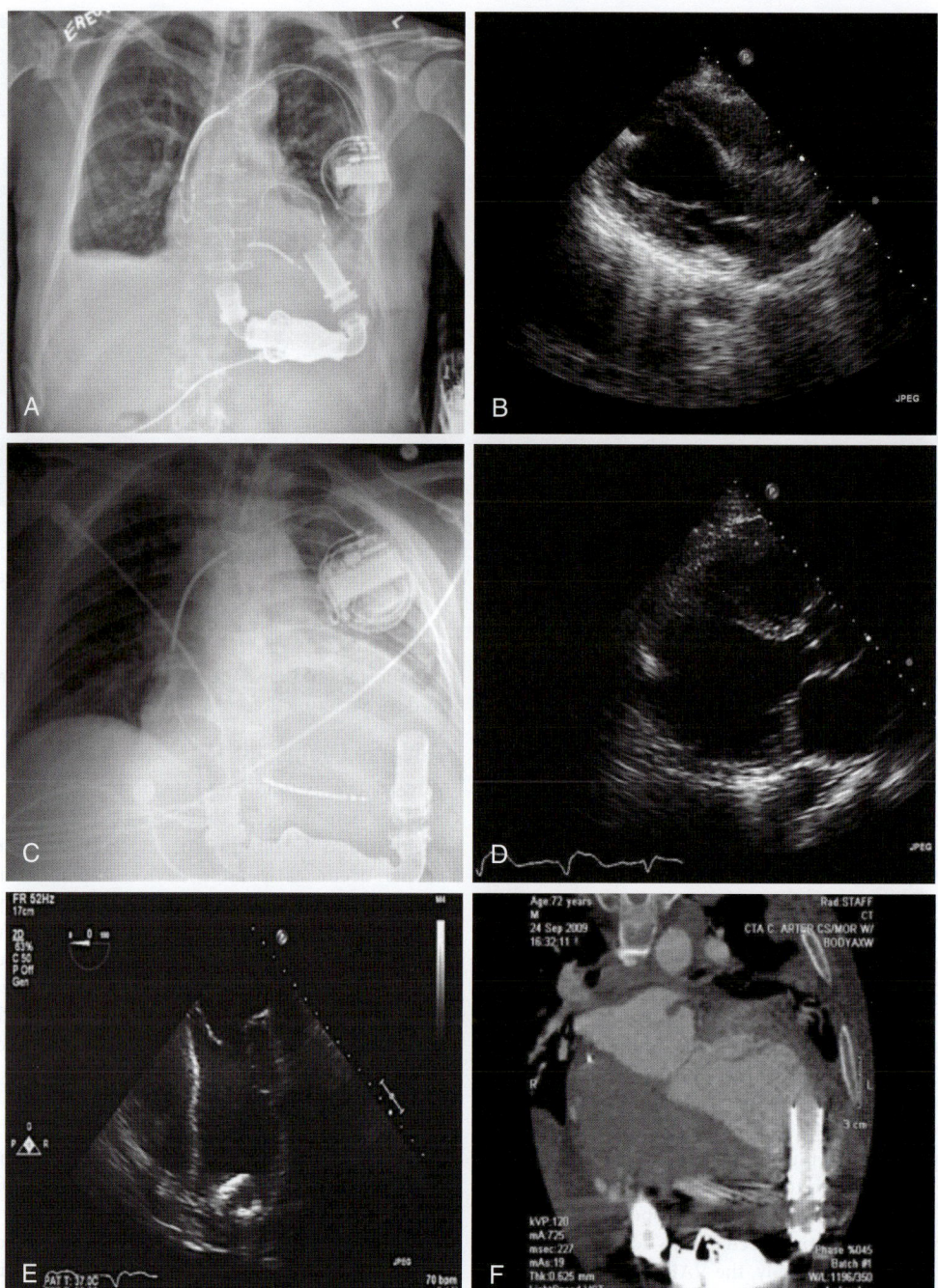

Fig. 45.12 The role of chest radiography, echocardiography, and chest computed tomography to evaluate proper left ventricular assist device positioning. A normally positioned inflow cannula is directed in the long axis of the ventricle at the mitral valve (A and B). Misdirected inflow cannulae are seen by chest x-ray (C), transthoracic echo (D), transesophageal echo (E), and cardiac computed tomography (F).

heart failure after LVAD should prompt the clinician to consider early transplantation in eligible patients.

Neurologic Events

In the clinical trials of MCS devices, neurologic event reporting has ranged in severity from metabolic encephalopathy to ischemic and hemorrhagic stroke. Hemorrhagic strokes have the highest associated mortality and result from the requisite use of anticoagulants and antiplatelet agents, the presence of acquired von Willebrand factor deficiency, and systemic hypertension (see later discussion). The stroke rate appears to be device

specific and has been reported as high as 29% in the first 24 months following implantation.[55]

Infection

The diagnosis and management of infections in patients supported on an MCS device can be challenging, relating to the complexity of intracorporeal foreign materials and their anatomic position, the presence of a percutaneous driveline, the surgical implant procedure, and the poor general health of many of the heart failure patients undergoing the procedure. Standardized definitions for device-specific,

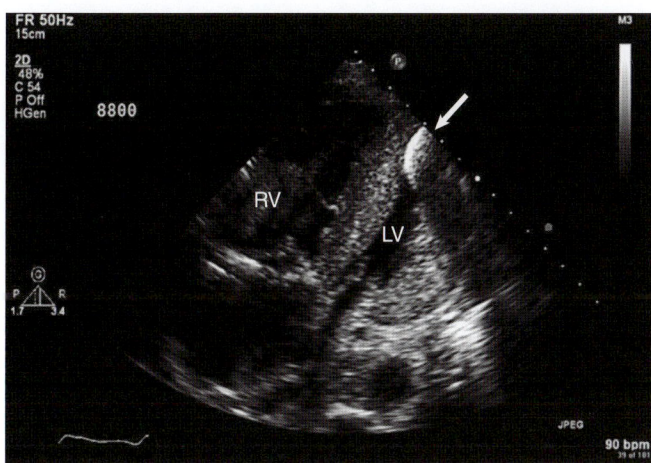

Fig. 45.13 Echocardiographic diagnosis of right ventricular failure. Apical four-chamber view from transthoracic echocardiography showing the left ventricular assist device cannula in the left ventricular apex *(arrow)*. The left ventricle *(LV)* is small and underfilled, whereas the right ventricle *(RV)* is markedly dilated.

device-related, and non-VAD infections in device-supported patients have been described.[64] During the early perioperative period, infectious complications are typically related to the surgical procedure and nosocomial infections, such as pneumonia, urinary tract infections, and wound infections.[65] Development of a sternal infection following VAD implantation can be a devastating complication because of the proximity of the VAD components. Infection of device components is almost impossible to correct without replacement of the pump. In many cases, long-term suppressive antibiotic therapy is used, and transplant should be considered if the infection is controlled and the patient is otherwise an acceptable candidate. Later infectious complications are more likely related to the percutaneous driveline. Trauma to the exit site can result in disruption of the driveline-tissue barrier, leading to an ascending infection that tracks proximally toward the device. The diagnosis is often made clinically by the identification of purulent drainage from the exit site coupled with erythema and tenderness along the driveline (which is commonly palpable). In some cases, CT imaging can identify areas along the driveline surrounded by fluid or stranding in the subcutaneous tissues. Antimicrobial therapy should be directed against the cultured organism. However, surgical débridement is often required with fashioning of a new exit site.

Bleeding

Bleeding is the most common, early adverse event early following LVAD implantation.[66,67] Early bleeding complications are primarily surgical and are treated with correction of operative coagulopathies, as well as identification and management of anastomotic bleeding sources. Late bleeding is more common with continuous flow LVADs than pulsatile pumps and is typically mucosal.[68-70] There appear to be at least three critical components to late bleeding following LVAD. First, many patients on contemporary continuous flow devices develop acquired von Willebrand disease caused by device-related shear stress applied to the von Willebrand molecules, resulting in exposure of a cleavage site for the ADAMTS13 enzyme.[69,71,72] Subsequent degradation of the large molecular weight von Willebrand multimers into smaller fragments that are less efficient at crosslinking platelets and clot stabilization increase bleeding risk. Second, small arteriovenous malformations (AVMs) occur primarily in the small intestine but may also be present in the large bowel or nasal mucosa.[73] Recent studies have demonstrated that continuous flow LVAD patients have elevated

levels of angiopoietin 2, a factor that promotes growth of abnormal blood vessels in the alimentary tract.[74] Finally, the requisite use of antiplatelet agents and anticoagulation associated with MCS use contributes to bleeding complications.

Valvular Heart Disease

Several valvular lesions can impact the performance of an LVAD. The presence of hemodynamically significant mitral stenosis will limit LVAD filling and should be addressed at the time of LVAD implantation. A previously implanted, undersized mitral annuloplasty ring may need to be removed at the time of LVAD implantation if it is causing significant limitation of flow across the mitral annulus. Mitral regurgitation (MR) is not typically thought to be an important valvular lesion in LVAD patients. In most cases a normally functioning LVAD will reduce the residual blood volume in the LV to such an extent that secondary mitral regurgitation will be significantly reduced. Residual MR following LVAD implantation is associated with persistent pulmonary hypertension, worse RV function, and shorter times to rehospitalization leading some to advocate for surgical correction at the time of implantation.[75,76] Aortic stenosis without insufficiency tends not to be a lesion that requires intervention as the LVAD circumvents this valve. De novo aortic stenosis has been reported in LVAD-supported patients and is thought to result from limited opening of the aortic valve with subsequent scarring and fusion of the aortic valve cusps.[77] As a result, some advocate setting the pump speed to allow intermittent opening of the aortic valve. The presence of greater than mild AI at the time of LVAD implantation should be corrected.[78] The optimal surgical technique has not been defined, but many surgeons favor the Park stitch that consists of a central oversewing of the three valve leaflets with sutures placed in the nodules of Arantius.[79] An alternative is replacement of the valve with a bioprosthesis. Development of clinically significant de novo AI following LVAD appears to be time dependent and may result in symptomatic heart failure if the regurgitant volume becomes sufficient.[80-82] To date, correction of AI in the LVAD population has typically required redo sternotomy with placement of an aortic bioprosthesis, but eventually catheter-based approaches may prove beneficial with less comorbidity.[83] Presence of a mechanical aortic prosthesis must be addressed at the time of LVAD implantation because of the risk of thrombus development with reduced leaflet movement. The surgical approach to these patients has been to either replace the valve with a bioprosthesis or alternatively occlude the valve with a circular felt patch.[84]

Hemolysis/Pump Thrombosis

Subtle alterations in the flow characteristics in the LVAD or its inflow or outflow cannulae may result in hemolysis. This can be caused by the development of thrombus on the blood-contacting components of the pump, twisting of the pliable outflow graft, or any other change in the VAD anatomy that alters the normal rheology. The clinical presentation is often asymptomatic and detected with serologic measures of red blood cell trauma, including elevated levels of serum lactate dehydrogenase (LDH) or plasma-free hemoglobin or a low serum haptoglobin. Recently, LDH level has been validated as a predictor of hemolysis, and elevated levels predate other manifestations of device thrombosis.[85,86] Patients are frequently asymptomatic, although they may complain of nausea and vomiting or abdominal pain.[87] In addition, hemoglobinuria may be seen in cases of more significant hemolysis. Paradoxically, the LVAD flow may appear elevated on the system monitor associated with high power consumption. Imaging of the device is a critical component of the evaluation. Transthoracic echocardiography should be performed to assess LV size and valvular function. Left ventricular enlargement, frequent opening of a previously closed aortic valve, and worsening mitral insufficiency all suggest increased left ventricular volume and pressure and abnormal LVAD function. A ramp study (previously described) may also be useful in establishing the diagnosis. Failure of the LV end-diastolic dimension to decrease with increasing pump speed is highly correlated with VAD thrombosis.[62] Cine CT of the chest allows determination of the LV inflow cannula position, as well as examination of the LV outflow graft. Finally, determination of invasive hemodynamics may provide useful information in some cases. Demonstration of elevated pulmonary capillary wedge pressure and a low cardiac output (that may be discrepant from the system monitor) are also suggestive of device malfunction. Treatment of hemolysis and LVAD thrombosis should be directed at the cause. If the inflow cannula is in continuity with the left ventricular myocardium, surgical repositioning may be required. If the outflow graft is twisted, surgical manipulation will be required to either untwist or replace the graft. Medical management of device thrombosis is more controversial. Some have advocated a stepped approach that includes the administration of unfractionated heparin, direct thrombin inhibitors, glycoprotein 2B/3A antagonists, or tissue plasminogen activator inhibitor.[88] If ineffective, LVAD replacement should be considered early if the patient is a suitable candidate. Two-year survival following device exchange for thrombosis is reduced relative to primary LVAD implant (56% vs. 69%, P < .0001).[89]

Support for Biventricular Heart Failure

Managing biventricular heart failure with MCS requires use of devices that were not intended for long-term, out-of-hospital use in the biventricular configuration, the use of continuous flow VADs implanted in both ventricles, or the total artificial heart (TAH). INTERMACS has provided important insights about the outcome of patients requiring biventricular support.[63] One-year survival in LVAD-treated patients was 80% versus 64%, and 48% in patients treated with a continuous flow or pulsatile biventricular assist devices (BiVADs), respectively (P < .0001).

The TAH can be used to support patients with severe biventricular failure and is approved as for BTT. The surgical approach requires a cardiectomy and attachment of the TAH to atrial cuffs and the great vessels. The SynCardia TAH (SynCardia Systems, Tucson, AZ) is available as both a 50-mL and 70-mL ventricle to accommodate a variety of patient sizes (**Fig. 45.14**). In a prospective clinical trial comparing TAH to optimal

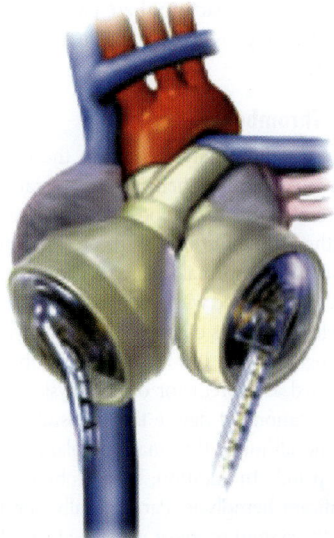

Fig. 45.14 SynCardia total artificial heart. The SynCardia total artificial heart replaces the function of both the right and left ventricles and requires a cardiectomy for implantation. The device is approved in the United States as a bridge to transplantation. (Reprinted with permission, syncardia.com.)

medical therapy and IABP, patients supported with TAH had a significantly improved survival to transplantation (79% vs. 46%, P < .001) than the control group.[90] Previously the SynCardia TAH was limited to use in the hospital because of the size of the pneumatic driver used to actuate the device. A smaller version of the driver has been developed that allows enhanced patient mobility and the ability to be managed outside the hospital. The CARMAT TAH features bioprosthetic valves and a bovine pericardial blood-contacting surface and is undergoing early phase clinical evaluation.[91]

Mechanical Circulatory Support in Children

The use of mechanical blood pumps in children poses several challenges beyond those encountered with adults. An array of devices must be available to accommodate body sizes from infant to adolescent. In addition, as body size increases, the need for higher device output may exceed the capabilities of an implanted pump. Many children with failing ventricles have structurally abnormal hearts or prior cardiac procedures that add technical limitations to MCS (**see also Chapter 27**). Furthermore, the daily interaction of a child with a VAD and the impact on physical and psychosocial growth is understudied. Finally, the paucity of small donor hearts for transplantation predictably results in relatively long support times.

The most commonly used mechanical device to support the circulation of children remains ECMO.[92] The versatility of ECMO, including its ability to support both cardiac and pulmonary systems, the ease and rapidity of implantation, and limited alternatives for mechanically assisted circulation in children, has resulted in the widespread adoption of this technology. The majority of pediatric patients are supported on ECMO for short durations, although a series of patients supported for more than 30 days has been reported.[93,94] Neurologic complications remain an important adverse event in ECMO-supported children. Twenty-four percent of children in the Extracorporeal Life Support Organization (ELSO) registry had a neurologic event.[95] Low birth weight, gestational age less than 34 weeks, the need for pre-ECMO cardiopulmonary resuscitation, systemic acidosis or the use of bicarbonate, and recurrent need for ECMO were important predictors of mortality. Age-dependent survival following ECMO in children has been demonstrated with neonates having lower survival rates than pediatric patients.[96]

An extracorporeal, pulsatile pump is also available for use in children. The Excor Pediatric VAD (Berlin Heart, Woodlands, TX) is manufactured in multiple sizes to accommodate children across a broad spectrum of body sizes (**Fig. 45.15**). This device was recently tested in a single-arm trial of children younger than 17 years who weighed 3 to 60 kg and had two-ventricle circulation and severe heart failure.[97] Study participants were enrolled in one of two cohorts based on body surface area (cohort 1 < 0.7 m^2; cohort 2 = 0.7–1.5 m^2) and compared with a historical control group supported with ECMO. The primary end point of the VAD-treated patients was death, withdrawal of support with an unacceptable neurologic outcome, or unsuccessful weaning from the device. The primary end point for the ECMO-treated control cohort was all-cause mortality. Both VAD-treated study cohorts had superior freedom from the primary end point compared with controls. Adverse events with the Excor device included bleeding, infection, stroke, and hypertension. In addition, pump exchange was common and most often resulted from device thrombosis. Based on the results of this clinical trial, the Excor was approved by the FDA as a BTT in children. An recent analysis of outcomes with the Excor device following FDA approval demonstrates lower rates of successful bridging to transplant or weaning the device in a "real world" cohort of patients compared with the clinical trial (77% vs. 90%, P = .05), with similar rates of bleeding and stroke.[98]

The DeBakey Child VAD is the other FDA-approved device for supporting children to transplant. Clinical application of this device has been limited by a relatively high risk of thrombosis.[99]

FUTURE DIRECTIONS

Partial Support Devices

An evolving innovation in the field of mechanically assisted circulation is the development and clinical assessment of partial support devices. Currently used VADs are designed to replace the entirety of the cardiac output. However, a larger patient population exists that would benefit from cardiac output augmentation and reduction in the left-sided filling pressures. The CircuLite Synergy (HeartWare) axial flow device was designed to be implanted in a pacemaker-like pocket fashioned in the infraclavicular subcutaneous tissues with pump inflow obtained through a minithoracotomy to access the right superior pulmonary vein and cannulation of the subclavian artery for device outflow. Eventually, inflow may be obtained by placing the cannula retrograde through the subclavian vein into the left atrium via a transseptal puncture. This device has been shown to augment cardiac index by 0.5 to 1.0 L/min/m^2 and reduce the left atrial pressure by 8 to 10 mm Hg.[100] Further development and clinical trials with this device are uncertain.

Totally Implantable Systems

Development of reliable totally implantable systems is anticipated to have an important impact on patient acceptance of the therapy, as well as to reduce the infection rates associated with these devices. As currently envisioned, patients would have a capacitor implanted in the soft tissue of the abdominal wall that would allow several hours of untethered use. Tethering would involve wearing a vest containing an energy transmission coil that would transfer energy from batteries to the subcutaneous capacitor. Other novel methods of battery charging are being explored, including the use of electrically charged rooms capable of charging battery-operated devices.

Novel Patient Populations

Approximately 80% of patients currently implanted with an LVAD have a severity of illness that requires treatment with intravenous inotropic therapy.[63] In this cohort, LVAD has been shown to provide important improvements in both quality of life and survival. The Risk Assessment and Comparative Effectiveness of Left Ventricular Assist Device and Medical Management (ROADMAP) study was a nonrandomized evaluation of the HeartMate II device compared with optimal medical therapy in patients ineligible for transplantation, who met current indications for DT and were not yet treated with inotropic therapy. LVAD-treated patients had a statistically better 12- and 24-month survival with improvement in submaximal exercise performance than the medically treated patients.[101,102]

Myocardial Recovery

An important promise of MCS is the opportunity to support the circulation sufficiently to allow recovery of native heart function, either by reversal of the process causing ventricular dysfunction, such as acute myocarditis, or allowing the use of adjuvant therapies that promote myocardial functional recovery. Contemporary registry data demonstrate a recovery rate with successful LVAD removal in approximately 1% to 2% of the implanted population.[103] Predictors of recovery include younger age, nonischemic cause, and shorter duration of heart failure before device implantation.[104] In general, the management strategy to promote myocardial recovery has included maintaining the device speed such that the heart size is maximally reduced and the use of standard heart failure therapies. Serial assessment of intrinsic myocardial function typically includes measurement of cardiac structure and function using echocardiography, submaximal and maximal exercise testing, and evaluation of hemodynamics. The aforementioned studies are performed with the pump speed turned down to achieve a net neutral flow such that there is no backflow through the outflow graft into the pump and left ventricle.

Preliminary results from the multicenter RESTAGE HF trial demonstrate that 40% to 45% of LVAD-supported patients with nonischemic cardiomyopathy treated with high doses of neurohormonal antagonists may have sufficient improvement in ventricular function to warrant device removal.[105] Stem cell therapy may also prove to be an important adjuvant to mechanically assisted circulation (**see also Chapter 41**). An NIH-sponsored clinical trial using allogeneic mesenchymal precursor cells was recently reported.[106] This safety trial included 30 patients randomized to administration of either 25 million allogeneic stem cells or control medium directly injected into the left ventricular myocardium during LVAD implantation. There were no safety events associated with direct myocardial injection of stem cells nor was there evidence of increased immunologic sensitization. Injection of mesenchymal precursor cells did not increase the likelihood of temporary VAD weaning at 90 days or 1 year, nor did it improve the ejection fraction in this small trial. A follow-up trial focused on efficacy using injection of 150 million cells is now underway.

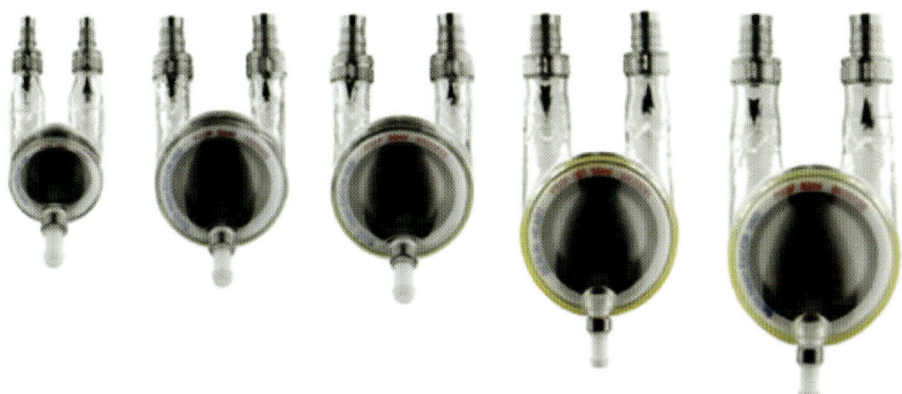

Fig. 45.15 The Berlin heart pediatric ventricular assist device (VAD). The Berlin heart VAD is an extracorporeal device that is manufactured with various chamber sizes (10, 25, 30, 50, and 60 mL) to accommodate a range of pediatric patients.

The field of mechanically assisted circulation is growing and evolving rapidly with proliferation of new devices designed for short- and long-term circulatory support. Clinical trials in the past several years have clearly demonstrated reduced mortality and quality-of-life improvements in patients with advanced heart failure. However, the persistently high mortality rates associated with cardiogenic shock following acute MI demands careful evaluation and innovative solutions that may require multiple devices to improve survival. The role of mechanically assisted circulation in expanded patient populations such as children, NYHA class III, and right heart failure will require new device design and thoughtful clinical trials. Moving forward, centers invested in mechanically assisted circulation will have clinical expertise with a broad array of VADs that can be tailored to the specific needs of the individual patient. Newer-generation continuous flow pumps with smaller size, more durable design, and novel blood-contacting surfaces are likely to have favorable and incremental impact on the long-term outcomes for MCS patients. Concerns that prolonged exposure to reduced pulsatility plays a role in some of the adverse events associated with these devices are likely to result in innovative device design and management strategies to restore a higher degree of pulsatility. Finally, there will be an even greater focus on the patient and caregiver experience as more patients live for prolonged periods of time on MCS devices.

KEY REFERENCES

7. Mandawat A, Rao SV. Percutaneous mechanical circulatory support devices in cardiogenic shock. *Circ Cardiovasc Intervent.* 2017;10: e004337.

28. Keebler ME, Haddad EV, Choi CW, et al. Venoarterial extracorporeal membrane oxygenation in cardiogenic shock. *J Am Coll Cardiol HF.* 2018. EPub ahead of print.

31. Slaughter MS, Rogers JG, Milano CA, et al. Advanced heart failure treated with continuous-flow ventricular assist device. *N Engl J Med.* 2009;361:2241–2251.

37. Stainback RF, Estep JD, Agler DA, et al. Echocardiography in the management of patients with left ventricular assist devices: recommendations from the American Society of Echocardiography. *J Am Soc Echocardiogr.* 2015;28:853–909.

40. Slaughter MS, Pagani FD, Rogers JG, et al. Clinical management of continuous-flow left ventricular assist devices in advanced heart failure. *J Heart Lung Transplant.* 2010;29:S1–S39.

55. Rogers JG, Pagani FD, Tatooles AJ, et al. Intrapericardial left ventricular assist device for advanced heart failure. *N Engl J Med.* 2017;376:451–460.

57. Mehra MR, Naka Y, Uriel N, et al. A fully magnetically levitated circulatory pump for advanced heart failure. *N Engl J Med.* 2017;376:440–450.

58. Mehra MR, Goldstein DJ, Uriel N, et al. Two year outcomes with a magnetically levitated cardiac pump in heart failure. *N Engl J Med.* 378:1386–1395.

88. Goldstein DJ, John R, Salerno C, et al. Algorithm for the diagnosis and management of suspected pump thrombus. *J Heart Lung Transplant.* 2013;32:667–670.

101. Estep JD, Starling RC, Horstmanshof DA, et al. Risk assessment and comparative effectiveness of left ventricular assist device and medical management in ambulatory heart failure patients. *J Am Coll Cardiol.* 2015;66:1747–1761.

The full reference list for this chapter is available on ExpertConsult.

Cardio-Oncology and Heart Failure

Joshua D. Mitchell, Douglas B. Sawyer, Daniel J. Lenihan

Heart failure (HF) as a consequence of cancer treatment is a well-known clinical challenge with a history as old as the earliest days of cytotoxic chemotherapies and radiation-based treatment. During the past several decades of advancement in cancer treatment with overall improvements in cancer survival, cardiovascular (CV) toxicities, specifically HF, have become increasingly recognized as a consequence of treatment with a diverse set of agents. Fortunately, a substantial amount of cardiotoxic effects may be preventable with careful control of known CV risk factors and the use of selected cardio-protective therapy. When left ventricular (LV) dysfunction does occur, prompt identification and treatment can lead to recovery, while delayed treatment is associated with much more limited benefit.

For patients who are still actively receiving chemotherapy or targeted therapy, decisions to hold or stop chemotherapy due to concern for cardiotoxicity are complex, with limited evidence for guidance but with obvious life and death implications. A close collaboration between the cardiology and oncology teams is therefore mandatory to optimize overall care. Differentiating between asymptomatic or mild LV dysfunction and more severe cardiomyopathy, as well as whether the HF is likely related to the chemotherapy, have major repercussions with regard to future treatment. For more in-depth coverage of this topic, recent consensus statements and recommendations by experts in this field are important resources.[1-3]

EPIDEMIOLOGY OF HEART FAILURE IN PATIENTS WITH CANCER

The population of patients who may have CV diseases, including HF, as well as cancer, increases each year. This is driven by several factors, most notably a direct result of the success of cancer therapies leading to greater survivorship, the age-associated risk of heart disease and malignancy in an aging population, the overlap in risk factors between heart disease and malignancy, and ultimately effects of targeted cancer therapy. Cancer survivors are at substantial increased risk compared to persons without malignancy for developing ischemic heart disease and HF throughout their lives.[4] Health behaviors, such as tobacco use and alcohol abuse, as well as obesity and associated metabolic disorders, increase the risk of developing both HF and certain cancers. In addition, CV disease and HF are known consequence of certain cancer therapies. The improvements in outcome for pediatric cancer patients have been tremendous and have resulted in a growing population of adults at risk for HF.[5] A striking example of unintended consequence of cancer treatment is the apparent rise in incidence of heart transplant patients with a history of anthracycline cardiomyopathy.[6] Additionally, although radiation therapy has improved over the decades, chest radiation remains an important cause of significant heart disease, including complex vascular and valvular disease, that may result in HF.[7,8] Newer emerging cancer therapies, which offer a great deal of hope for patients who have previously incurable malignancies, such as metastatic breast cancer and multiple myeloma, unfortunately do have direct and indirect deleterious effects on CV tissues in susceptible patients. The intertwining impact of cancer therapies in a myriad of CV tissues needs to be understood by both oncologists and cardiologists. In one study of Medicare patients over the age of 66 diagnosed with breast cancer, CV death was more prevalent than death due to the cancer itself.[9]

A growing number of agents are known to cause cardiac dysfunction and HF (**Table 46.1**). Thus, a patient being treated with potential cardiotoxic therapy should be considered a Stage A HF patient per American College of Cardiology (ACC)/American Heart Association (AHA) guidelines.[10] The risk of HF varies by chemotherapeutic regimen and individual risk factors, and there may be considerable time delay between exposure and clinical presentation. For some older chemotherapeutics, a great deal is known about CV safety and toxicity, while for newer therapies the risks may be largely unidentified. Moreover, many life-saving cancer therapies gain approval for treatment of cancer with relatively limited data regarding toxicity. Additionally, there may be an

TABLE 46.1 Common Cancer Treatments Known to Be Associated With the Development of Heart Failure

Class of Therapy	Generic Names	Timing	Risk Factors for HF
Anthracyclines	doxorubicin daunorubicin epirubicin idarubicin mitoxantrone	Concurrent and delayed	Cumulative dose Concurrent radiation therapy, cyclophos-phamide, or ErbB2 targeted therapies Age (young and old) Hypertension Known heart disease
Alkylating agent	cyclophospha-mide	Early	Dose, age, concurrent anthracyclines
HER2(ErbB2)-targeted therapies	trastuzumab pertuzumab lapatinib	Concurrent	Hypertension, age, low pre-treatment LVEF
VEGF/angiogen-esis targeted therapies	sunitinib sorafenib pazopanib bevacizumab	Concurrent	Hypertension
Bcr-Abl inhibitors	imatinib ponatinib	Concurrent	
Proteasome inhibitors	bortezomib carfilzomib	Concurrent	Prior anthracyclines
Mediastinal/chest radiation		Delayed	Cumulative dose Concurrent anthracy-clines Age (young) Hypertension
Check point inhibitors	ipilimumab nivolumab pembrolizumab	Concurrent	Combination therapy

Not an all-inclusive list of individual medications. Those listed are among the most frequently used from each class.
HF, Heart failure; *LVEF,* left ventricular ejection fraction; *VEGF,* vascular endothelial growth factor.

unpredictable lag time that occurs after the administration of chemotherapy before any development of the signs and symptoms of HF. As a result, if HF or other CV disease is detected in a patient with cancer during or after treatment with a novel therapy, some consideration should be given that the cancer treatment may be promoting CV disease.

There are also situations where HF may be a direct consequence of malignancy, rather than therapy. For instance, infiltrative cardiomyopathy secondary to primary amyloid light-chain (AL) amyloidosis occurs in the setting of multiple myeloma and plasma cell dyscrasia. The unique challenges this condition presents to the HF clinician are covered in detail elsewhere (**see Chapter 22**).

SPECIFIC CANCER THERAPIES, THEIR MECHANISMS OF CARDIOTOXICITY, AND IMPLICATIONS FOR CLINICAL PRACTICE

Anthracyclines

Anthracyclines are a mainstay of cancer treatment and a well-recognized cause of cardiomyopathy and HF. Anthracyclines' main antitumor effect is through the inhibition of topoisomerase II (topII),

an enzyme involved in uncoiling DNA. By inhibiting the enzyme, anthracyclines induce DNA strand breaks and apoptosis. In addition to the topIIα (topIIα) form of the enzyme that is predominant in cancer cells, there is also a topIIβ (topIIβ) form expressed in cardiac myocytes. Anthracyclines inhibit both, and the inhibition of the latter is plausibly culpable for a significant amount of the compound's cardiotoxicity. Mice lacking topIIβ are resistant to the cardiotoxicity of anthracyclines. Additional anthracycline toxic effects also have been linked to the generation of free radicals with the subsequent generation of reactive oxidant species that produce oxidative damage to lipids, proteins, and nucleic acids (**Fig. 46.1**).

It is well established that an individual's risk of HF secondary to anthracyclines is directly related to the cumulative drug exposure,[11] which is consistent with the concept that every anthracycline dose potentially causes some degree of irreversible cardiac damage. A combined analysis of three doxorubicin Phase III studies found a 7% incidence of cardiac events (LV dysfunction or heart failure) even at a lower dose of 150 mg/m² .[11] A dose threshold $\geq$250 mg/m² of doxorubicin ($\geq$600 mg/m² of epirubicin) has been identified, mainly from childhood cancer survivor studies, as being a threshold where the rate of HF increases substantially.[2] Other known risk factors for anthracycline HF include age (both young and elderly), hypertension, preexisting cardiac conditions, concurrent mediastinal radiation, and/or other therapies with cardiac effects including cyclophosphamide, paclitaxel, and trastuzumab (see later).[12]

Despite the likely immediate loss of myocardium during anthracycline treatment, patients with cancer frequently remain asymptomatic or only minimally symptomatic for months to years. Contractile reserve and compensatory mechanisms on the cellular and subcellular level presumably maintain cardiac function.[13] One of the survival factors implicated in the modulation of anthracycline cardiotoxicity is the neuregulin/ErbB signaling system, explaining the increased toxicity when anthracyclines are used concomitantly with ErbB2-targeted therapeutics.[14]

Genetic analysis of cohorts by genome-wide associations studies have identified a number of genetic loci that speak to the importance of cellular uptake mechanisms and carbonyl redox cycling in the cardiotoxicity of anthracyclines. Loci associated with genes encoding protein components of cellular transport systems including the ATP-cassette transporters in the multidrug resistance family are associated with the risk of cardiotoxicity.[15-17] Animal work supports the notion that these transporters regulate the uptake of anthracyclines. This purported mechanism has important implications for patients undergoing treatment with anthracyclines that are typically underappreciated by most practitioners. Commonly prescribed medications, including antihypertensives diltiazem and verapamil, are competitively transported by these same proteins, and concomitant treatment with these or other similarly transported pharmaceuticals, such as cyclosporine or digoxin, will raise the cytoplasmic anthracycline concentration.[18] Other antihypertensives such as beta-blockers (BBs), and angiotensin converting enzyme inhibitors (ACEIs) are not handled by this transporter and therefore will not alter intracellular anthracycline concentrations. Thus, all patients should have a careful review of their medication list with a focus on identifying substrates for the p-glycoprotein/MDR/ATP-cassette transporters, and consideration for a change in medication class if appropriate.

Radiation Therapy

Radiation therapy remains an important component of therapy for specific cancers. A history of mediastinal radiation may result in HF by a variety of mechanisms, and should be factored into the evaluation of any patient presenting with CV-based symptoms. The effects of mediastinal radiation on the heart are related to radiation dose, and

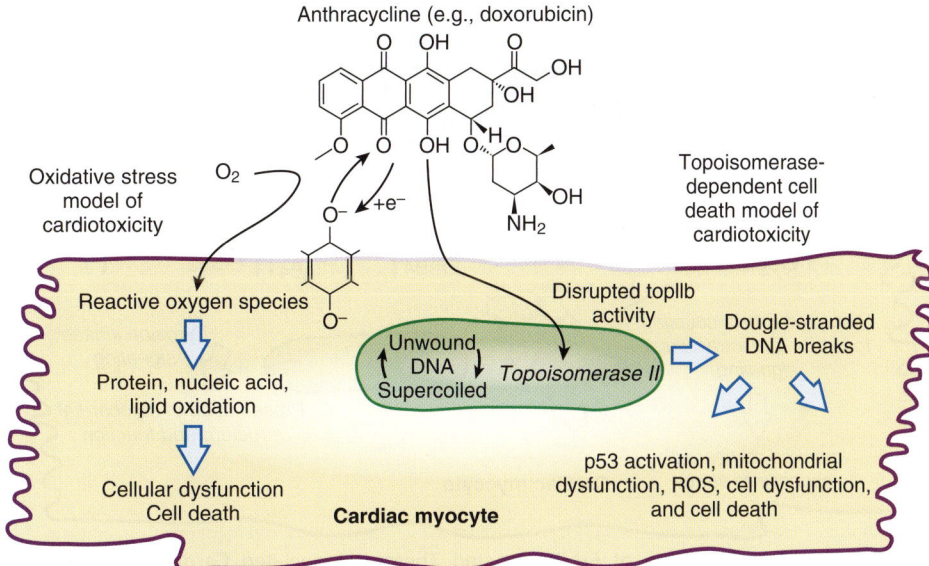

Fig. 46.1 Proposed Mechanisms of Anthracycline Cardiotoxicity. Anthracyclines are directly toxic to cardiac myocytes. The quinone moiety can redox cycle and reduce molecular oxygen to superoxide anion leading to an increase in reactive oxygen species, and resulting oxidant stress can lead to direct damage to cellular elements. Recent experimental studies in mice support a mechanism where alteration in topoisomerase IIβ (topIIβ) function leads to DNA damage upstream of mitochondrial function and oxidant stress.

can manifest anywhere between a few years after exposure to over two decades later.[8,19] A dose ≥30 Gy has been identified as a marker for significantly increased risk, being associated with a 2.8- to 4.7-fold risk of HF as a first event compared to no mediastinal radiation treatment (RT) after adjustment for anthracycline dose and other risk factors.[20]

Radiation can affect every part of the heart that is in the path of treatment, causing diffuse atherosclerosis, valvular disease, conduction disorders, pericardial disease, and myocardial disease with both diastolic and systolic dysfunction. Chest radiation is also associated with pulmonary hypertension,[21] and a 3% incidence of pacemaker or defibrillator malfunction in patients with preexisting devices.[22] The only known strategies to prevent cardiac disease during RT are to limit CV exposure, and to control CV risk factors optimally with the hopes of reducing the risk of subsequent CV injury. It is recommended that cardiologists are involved in patients with devices undergoing radiotherapy to help with appropriate planning and monitoring.

Cyclophosphamide

Acute cardiac injury in the form of myocarditis and pericarditis is a known complication of cyclophosphamide, particularly when used at high doses during induction therapy for some bone marrow transplant regimens. It is estimated that HF may occur in up to 7% to 28% of patients receiving high dose cyclophosphamide, but the exact incidence has not been established.[23] Pathologic examination shows disruption of endothelial cells, hemorrhagic myocarditis, and disrupted myocyte ultrastructure. Fulminant HF refractory to treatment has been reported in certain cases in which high dose cyclophosphamide was used. Risk factors identified for the development of cardiomyopathy include age, dose, and concurrent treatment with anthracyclines.[23] There are no current practice guidelines for monitoring cardiac function after cyclophosphamide induction therapy, nor any accepted practices for prevention. Careful monitoring by physical exam for signs of fluid retention, with maintenance of high suspicion for cardiac contribution to nonspecific symptoms of fatigue and malaise in the early weeks/months after induction therapy with cyclophosphamide is clinically prudent.

Targeted Therapies

Recent advances in cancer therapy have occurred through the discovery of specific signaling cascades contributing to cancer progression and the development of novel agents that target these processes. Several of these therapies have been associated with the development of HF and cardiomyopathy, and are highlighted below.

ErbB2 Targeted Therapies: Trastuzumab, Lapatinib, and Pertuzumab

Trastuzumab (Herceptin) and pertuzumab (Perjeta), are recombinant humanized monoclonal antibodies against the human epidermal growth factor receptor (EGFR) 2 (HER2, a.k.a. ErbB2) protein, an oncogene that when overexpressed in tumor cells promotes cell proliferation through constitutive activation of growth signaling pathways. Lapatinib (Tykerb/Tyverb) is a small molecule dual tyrosine kinase inhibitor (TKI) of the EGFR and the ErbB2 receptor, that blocks receptor activation of intracellular signaling. These therapies are used for the treatment of ErbB2-overexpressing tumors, including breast and gastric cancers. Cardiac side effects of ErbB2-targeted therapeutics were first detected in the pivotal trastuzumab breast cancer trials, where trastuzumab combined with anthracyclines showed greater cardiotoxicity compared to anthracycline alone.[14] The contemporary use of trastuzumab has expanded to include adjuvant therapy before and after surgery, potentially for longer than 1 year and for extended periods (more than 4 years). Risk factors for trastuzumab-associated cardiac dysfunction include older age, hypertension, diabetes mellitus, atrial fibrillation or flutter, adjuvant chemotherapy, renal failure, coronary artery disease, and weekly (more often) trastuzumab transfusion.[24,25] In contrast to delayed anthracycline cardiomyopathy, ErbB2-targeted therapy-related cardiac dysfunction generally occurs during treatment.[26] There is a reasonable likelihood of reversibility of LV dysfunction, especially when treated with typical HF therapy.[27] The cardiotoxic potential of lapatinib appears to be less than trastuzumab, perhaps due to the shorter half-life of this small molecule[28] Pertuzumab, on the other hand, has a similar rate of observed cardiotoxicity to that of

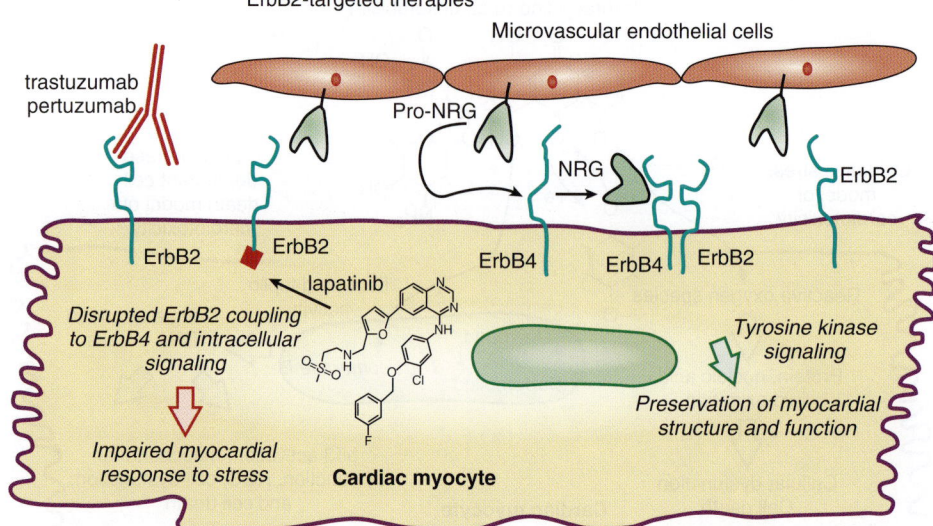

Fig. 46.2 Potential Mechanisms of ErbB2-targeted Therapy Associated Cardiac Dysfunction. The ErbB2 receptor tyrosine kinase is expressed in cardiac myocytes where it is activated by the ligand neuregulin *(NRG)* through heterodimerization with ErbB4 receptors. ErbB activation in cardiac myocytes is associated with a number of effects on cardiac myocytes including regulating cell structure, adaptations in Ca^{++} handling, and metabolism. ErbB2-targeted therapies interrupt NRG/ErbB signaling and prevent this stress-responsive pathway for regulating cardiac response to stress.

trastuzumab alone, but does not appear to have additive toxicity in large clinical trials.[29] While this may be due to differences in the biological properties of these ErbB2-targeted therapies, there has also been much greater scrutiny of cardiac function in patients being considered for treatment with ErbB2-targeted therapies since the initial trials.

The cardiac side effects of anti-ErbB2 therapeutics might be explained by studies examining the biology of the neuregulin, an EGF-family ligand and ErbB receptor in the CV system (**Fig. 46.2**). Neuregulin, ErbB2, and ErbB4 receptor tyrosine kinases play an important role in cell–cell crosstalk and mediate cellular responses to stress in the heart.[30] ErbB2 is expressed in the adult cardiomyocytes and disruption of its expression through genetic engineering in mice leads to progressive dilated cardiomyopathy.[31] Myocardial stress induced by ischemia activates neuregulin/ErbB signaling in the heart, and suppressing signaling prevents recovery from ischemic injury.[32,33]

Angiogenesis Inhibitors

Cancer treatments that target the signaling pathways for vascular endothelial growth factor (VEGF), and ultimately are intended to be angiogenic, are an important class of compounds that have been associated with development of HF. VEGF regulates angiogenesis, endothelial cell survival, vasodilatation, and cardiac contractile function.[34] The VEGF-targeted angiogenesis inhibitors, like ErbB2 targeted therapy, are either antibody-based, which bind and neutralize VEGF (e.g., bevacizumab), or small molecular inhibitors of VEGF tyrosine kinase receptors (TKIs; e.g., sunitinib, sorafenib). These are now used in the treatment of a variety of cancers.

A general CV class effect of these compounds is the augmentation of blood pressure.[35,36] Hypertension related to VEGF signaling pathway inhibition appears to occur through several mechanisms, including increased vascular stiffness, which may be mediated by increased activity of the renin–angiotensin system.[37] A preeclampsia-like syndrome with proteinuria and thrombotic microangiopathy has been reported in a subset of patients.[38,39] VEGF activates vascular eNOS via the PI-3kinase/PKB/Akt pathway, and this is one mechanism for VEGF-mediated vasorelaxation. Mice lacking VEGF demonstrate glomerular

pathology, with loss of podocytes and disruption of the basement membrane.[40] VEGF-targeted therapies are also associated with a 3-fold increase in risk for arterial thromboembolic events (stroke, transient ischemic attacks, myocardial infarction, angina, and other arterial events),[41,42] which appears to be an additional consequence of disrupting endothelial homeostasis.[43]

LV dysfunction and HF occurs in patients treated with bevacizumab (monoclonal antibody to the VEGF receptor), although HF appears to be more common in those treated with VEGF-targeted TKIs. VEGF signaling mediates the adaptation of the heart to pressure overload. Suppressing VEGF signaling in the setting of pressure overload leads to more rapid deleterious cardiac remodeling and HF in mice.[44]

Retrospective analyses of sunitinib-associated cardiac dysfunction report that up to 10% of patients receiving sunitinib experience some degree of HF,[45,46] although larger meta-analysis have reported an incidence of 4%.[47] Sunitinib induces mitochondrial injury and cardiomyocyte apoptosis in both mice and cultured rat cardiomyocytes.[48] Sunitinib inhibits several tyrosine kinases including AMP-activated kinase (AMPK) and platelet-derived growth factor receptors (PDGFR), which may explain the higher rate of clinical cardiac toxicity (**Fig. 46.3**). Mice lacking PDGF receptor expression respond to pressure overload induced by surgical aortic constriction with accelerated cardiac remodeling associated with impaired vascular growth and function.[49] Mice lacking AMPKa2 similarly are normal in the unstressed condition, but experience accelerated remodeling and LV dysfunction after pressure overload.[50] It is interesting that in each of these animals the phenotype of cardiac dysfunction is not manifested unless the animals are subjected to pressure overload. This would suggest that the hypertensive effect of VEGF-targeted TKIs may be requisite for the induction of contractile dysfunction.

It is yet unclear whether cardiac dysfunction induced by angiogenesis inhibitors is reversible. In early reports, patients with HF and LV dysfunction generally responded to temporary suspension of sunitinib and medical management.[48] However, the preclinical data in animals and cells supports a proapoptotic effect of sunitinib that would be associated with some degree of irreversible cardiac damage. Persistent

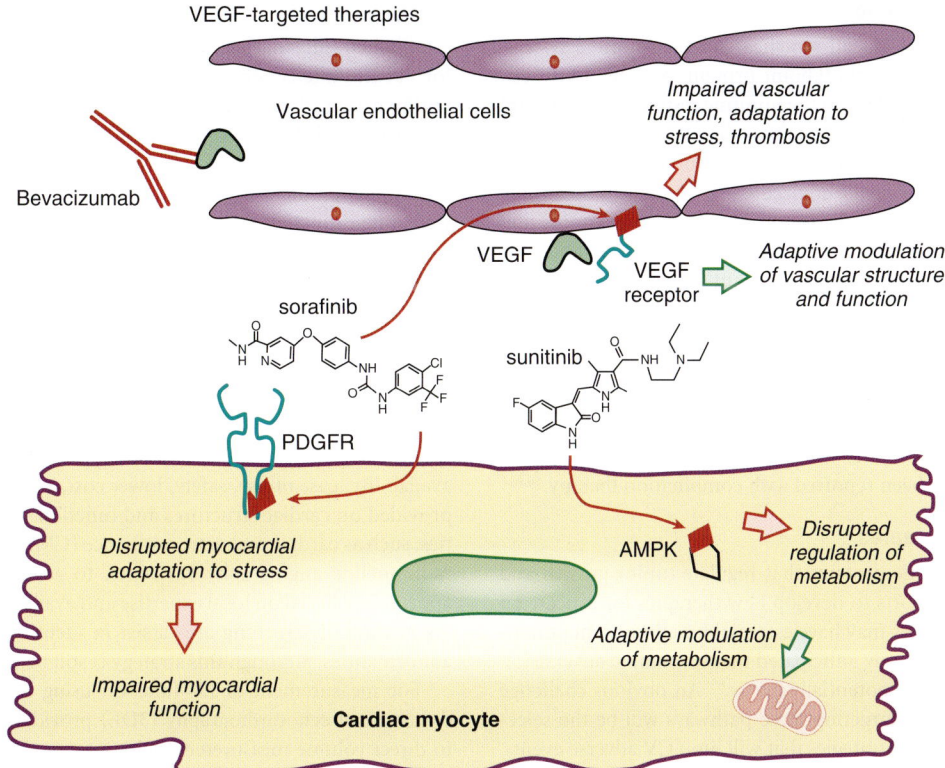

Fig. 46.3 Potential Mechanisms of Angiogenesis Inhibitor Associated Heart Failure. Bevacizumab, and other drugs that bind and inhibit vascular endothelial growth factor (VEGF) trap, block VEGF activity. Inhibition of VEGF receptor activation will reduce vascular reactivity as well as promote platelet activation. Sunitinib and sorafenib are small molecule inhibitors of tyrosine kinases that block the activity of not only the VEGF receptor, but also kinases such as platelet derived growth factor receptors (PDGFR) and AMP-activated kinase (AMPK). These other effects may explain why heart failure is more common in patients treated with these multityrosine kinase inhibitors.

cardiac dysfunction has been noted in some persons treated with sunitinib.[46] Predicting and preventing HF in these patients remains an important challenge for the future.

Bcr-Abl Inhibitors

Inhibitors of "Philadelphia Chromosome," Bcr-Abl, have become the first-line therapy for the ~90% of patients with chronic myelogenous leukemia, as well as other tumors with this oncogene. Imatinib (Gleevec) was the first Bcr-Abl inhibitor developed. Imatinib-associated LV systolic dysfunction has been reported,[51] and may occur due to the inhibition of Abl in cardiac myocytes where it regulates endoplasmic reticulum stress responses. Second- and third-generation Bcr-Abl inhibitors have been developed, which have distinct properties—most importantly the ability to overcome imatinib resistance via a number of strategies. Certain newer Bcr-Abl inhibitors have been linked to higher rates of peripheral arterial occlusive disease (nilotinib).[52] Most recently, a unique Bcr-Abl inhibitor that is able to block a specific mutant form of Bcr-Abl, ponatinib, has been linked to high rates of thromboemboli, arterial occlusion, and HF.[53]

Proteasome Inhibitors

The ubiquitin–proteasome system (UP-S) is a cellular protein degradation system that is vital to normal cellular function, and in some tumors critical for proliferation. Preclinical studies have shown that proteasome disruption inhibits proliferation, induces apoptosis, reverses chemoresistance, and enhances chemotherapy and radiation

efficacy in some tumors. The proteasome pathway is also critical for the maintenance of cardiac structure and function, and altered proteasome function is associated with cardiac pathophysiology.[54]

Bortezomib (Velcade) was the first proteasome inhibitor to be developed successfully as a cancer therapy. Bortezomib blocks proliferation and induces apoptosis of plasma cells,[55] and is therefore used for the initial treatment of patients with multiple myeloma. It also enhances sensitivity to conventional chemotherapy by inhibiting the proteasomal degradation of signaling molecules that regulate cell survival. The side effects reported include asthenia, peripheral neuropathy, gastrointestinal symptoms, and anorexia. There are a few reports of cardiac failure occurring in patients during treatment with bortezomib,[56] suggesting that under some circumstances inactivation of the cardiac proteasome can result in adverse effects on the heart.

Because of the success of generally well-tolerated bortezomib, newer proteasome inhibitors have been developed. Carfilzomib, an irreversible proteasome inhibitor, is approved as second-line therapy for relapsed multiple myeloma. Although this therapy appears to be more active in resistant myeloma cases than previous treatments, there may be a greater likelihood of cardiac events including HF, sudden cardiac death, and acute coronary syndrome.[57] It does seem apparent that there is a vascular component to the observed cardiotoxicity associated with carfilzomib, especially in combination with immune modulators ("imids").[58] The cardiac safety of carfilzomib and other proteasome inhibitors will become clearer as greater experience accumulates with these therapies.

Immune Checkpoint Inhibitors

Checkpoint proteins serve as "off switches" for the immune system. Tumor cells that bind to the checkpoint proteins are able to deactivate the associated T-cell and avoid the immune response. Checkpoint inhibitors block this interaction, maintaining the T cells in their activated form as they seek out and attack the tumor cells. This new class of chemotherapy has revolutionized the treatment of metastatic melanoma and is now approved for non–small cell lung cancer and renal cell cancer as well. The combination of ipilimumab, an antibody to anticytotoxic T-lymphocyte-associated antigen 4 (CTLA-4), and nivolumab, an antibody to programmed cell death protein 1 (PD-1), has achieved a substantial increase in 3-year survival in the treatment of melanoma.[59] Since checkpoint inhibitors inherently activate the immune system, immune-related adverse events are prevalent. Cardiac toxicity itself has been considered rare, but a growing number of case reports of fulminant myocarditis or serious conduction system issues, at times fatal, have now been reported with combination therapy.[60,61]

Emerging Cancer Therapies

There are many oncogenic proteins that regulate tumor growth and are targets of ongoing efforts to develop new therapies for cancer. To the extent that these targets may have essential functions in maintaining CV homeostasis, it is easily anticipated that substantial adverse CV effects (including HF) can potentially occur.[62] An obvious challenge for development of drugs targeting these pathways will be the selection of timing and delivery strategies that will limit CV adverse events. Mechanistically, it is apparent that normal myocardial tissue can be protected from brief interruptions in critical pathways regulating metabolism as long as fatty acid, oxygen, and glucose are in ready supply, allowing for adaptive changes in substrate utilization. However, longer interruptions of these essential cellular machinery cascades, and/or alterations during times of metabolic stress (e.g., ischemia, hemodynamic stress, or chronic increases in rate-pressure product) may increase the likelihood of CV dysfunction. Similarly, cancer therapies targeting proteins involved in regulating cell survival may have no deleterious effects in the absence of stressors promoting cell death.

One revolutionary new therapy that has recently been approved by the US Food and Drug Administration (FDA) for two types of leukemia and lymphoma is a type of immunotherapy referred to as chimeric antigen receptor (CAR) T-cell therapy. [63] The therapy works by collecting a patient's own T cells and engineering them to express a specific CAR that enables them to hone in on cancer cells. The modified T cells are then grown in the lab in significant quantities to be infused back into the patient. It remains to be seen to what degree this more targeted immune therapy may still lead to off-target immune-mediated toxicity.

RISK ASSESSMENT, SCREENING, AND MONITORING

Every patient preparing to undergo a potential cardio-toxic therapy should undergo an accurate CV risk assessment. Patients at higher CV risk include any patient with planned high-dose anthracycline therapy (doxorubicin $\geq$250 mg/m², epirubicin $\geq$600 mg/m²), treatment with high-dose radiotherapy ($\geq$ 30 Gy) where the heart is in the treatment field, or any patient with lower dose anthracycline therapy with concomitant radiation involving the heart.[2] In addition, patients receiving lower doses of anthracycline or trastuzumab alone are also at higher risk if they are older (>60 years), have compromised cardiac function (e.g., borderline LV ejection fraction [LVEF] 50%–54%, a history of cardiac dysfunction, a history of myocardial infarction, or $\geq$ moderate valvular disease), or multiple CV risk factors ($\geq$2 of smoking, hypertension, diabetes, dyslipidemia, or obesity).[2]

For patients at higher risk, the treatment team can consider established alternative regimens that pose decreased potential for cardiotoxicity; employ strategies that limit the toxicity of the regimen (e.g., liposomal formulation of doxorubicin, continuous doxorubicin infusion, or reduced radiation dose); or use prevention strategies such as coadministration of dexrazoxane or other potentially cardio-protective medications (see below). Patients also would be expected to benefit from the optimization of any baseline CV risk factors. Although TKIs are not included in the higher risk cohort detailed here, blood pressure control in patients receiving TKIs is an important clinical principle in reducing the likelihood for secondary LV dysfunction.

Pretreatment screening, including the measurement of LVEF, is recommended to help assess risk and to detect more advanced HF. Recent expert consensus statements and guidelines generally favor an echocardiogram over other modalities for baseline screening given the availability, ease of use, safety, lower cost, and additional information provided on cardiac structures and function. However, other modalities, such as cardiac magnetic resonance (CMR) imaging or multigated radionuclide angiography (MUGA), to assess LV function may be appropriate based on local expertise and availability. Cardiac biomarkers at time of screening also assist in identifying subclinical cardiac abnormalities, although this strategy is still being validated.

For measurement of LV function using echocardiography, three-dimensional echocardiography (3DE) provides superior accuracy due to direct volume measurement without geometric assumptions or significant influence from foreshortening (**see also Chapter 32**)(3). When 3DE is not available, quantitative two-dimensional (2D) echocardiography using Simpson's biplane method of discs is the most appropriate volume estimation for LVEF calculation, and contrast should be used when two contiguous endocardial segments cannot be adequately defined.[3] CMR and MUGA also provide accurate LV systolic function, though, for the reasons stated here, echocardiography is generally preferred as an initial test unless local expertise and availability dictate otherwise.

Routine monitoring of asymptomatic patients has been recommended during high-risk chemotherapy due to evidence that early identification and treatment of LV dysfunction leads to improved rates of recovery. However, an optimal monitoring frequency is not known. Patients who have received cancer treatments associated with delayed cardiac effects (e.g., anthracyclines, radiation) should generally receive some level of periodic assessment throughout their life.[5,64] As for initial screening, echocardiogram is considered the ideal modality for monitoring asymptomatic patients.[2] In the absence of signs and symptoms of HF, LV dysfunction—referred to as Cancer Therapeutics-Related Cardiac Dysfunction—has been defined as a drop of LVEF by more than 10% to a value less than 53%.[3]

Since the heart can initially adapt to substantial injury without a major change in LVEF, improved methods for earlier detection of cardiotoxicity have been sought. LV strain, a measure of the deformation of the myocardium, has been found to precede and predict changes in LVEF and has been recently incorporated into guidelines for cardiotoxicity monitoring.[3] A decrease in global longitudinal strain (GLS) at the 6-month visit greater than 15% performed optimally in identifying cardiac dysfunction in breast cancer patients at 12 months.[65] Cardiac biomarker-based strategies to screen for cardiac injury at the time of chemotherapy are also likely to lead to earlier diagnosis of cardiotoxicity, with early studies supporting the potential use of brain natriuretic peptide (BNP) and cardiac troponin for early detection of cardiotoxicity.[66,67] One randomized study of 114 patients showed that the use of enalapril in patients with elevated troponins soon after high-dose chemotherapy decreased the incidence of LV dysfunction and maladaptation.[68] A summary of cardiotoxicity screening methods is found in **Table 46.2**.

TABLE 46.2   Screening Methods for Diagnosis of Left Ventricular Dysfunction

Method	Timing[a]	Strengths	Limitations
Echocardiography: LVEF	Baseline Completion of 250 mg/m² of doxorubicin or equivalent Every 50 mg/m² thereafter 6 months after therapy[3] At the discretion of the provider 6–12 months after chemotherapy completion[2]	Low cost, widely available, low risk	LVEF reduction often a late manifestation Most accurate with 3D evaluation which is has reduced availability
Global longitudinal strain (GLS)	Same timing as LVEF above per ASE guidelines[3]	Earlier diagnosis of cardiotoxicity	Reduced availability compared to EF assessment
Global longitudinal strain rate	Unknown. Potentially same timing as GLS	More physiologic representation of contractility (rate of change of strain)	Requires higher frame rate for accuracy; not widely available, limited to research
CMR/MUGA: LV Ejection Fraction	Similar to LVEF assessment with echocardiography	Accurate assessment of volumes for LVEF estimation. CMR is the reference standard for volume assessment	Cost, availability, potential radiation with MUGA
CMR strain evaluation	Unknown. Potentially same as echocardiography GLS	Potentially rapid computation of reliable strain information from CMR images	Currently limited to research
Brain Natriuretic Peptide (BNP)/NT-proBNP	Immediately prior to or within 24 hours of completion of anthracycline[67] or cardiotoxic chemotherapy	Early diagnosis of LV dysfunction High sensitivity	Benefit currently limited to single center study of anthracyclines
Troponin	Same timing as LVEF above per ASE guidelines[3] Baseline and every 3 months during chemotherapy[66]	Early diagnosis of LV dysfunction High sensitivity Elevation potentially useful in selecting patients who will benefit from ACEI[68]	Limited evidence for widespread application or optimal screening timing.

[a]No firm evidence on optimal timing of any screening methods. Listed intervals are based on expert opinion or limited trial design.
3D, Three-dimensional; *ACEI*, angiotensin-converting enzyme inhibitors; *ASE*, American Society of Echocardiography; *CMR*, cardiac magnetic resonance; *EF*, ejection fraction; *LV*, left ventricle; *LVEF*, left ventricle ejection fraction; *MUGA*, multigated radionuclide angiography.

In patients who do develop clinical signs or symptoms of cardiomyopathy, an evaluation with an echocardiogram and cardiac biomarkers is recommended. A CMR can be useful if echo is not available. In addition, if myocarditis is of concern, CMR has the added ability of being able to evaluate for inflammation, fibrosis, and edema. If asymptomatic LV dysfunction or cardiomyopathy develop during treatment, cardio-protective strategies should be considered as well as a multidisciplinary discussion on the expected risk and benefit of continuing, holding, or altering treatment. There is still no strong evidence to guide the uniform alteration to the chemotherapy plan based on LVEF cutoffs or diagnosis of subclinical LV dysfunction by strain, and the decision must remain patient oriented.

PREVENTION OF HEART FAILURE DURING CANCER TREATMENT

Modification of Chemotherapeutic Regimens

For patients found to be at high cardiac risk during screening with plan for high-dose anthracyclines, established alternative chemotherapy regimens may be considered. Cardiotoxicity also can be limited through continuous infusion instead of bolus dosing of anthracyclines as well as the use of a liposomal formulation of doxorubicin.[69] For patients with planned radiation, adjustments to the dose and radiation field can potentially be made. Preventive therapies listed later also may be employed in patients deemed suitable. There is no current evidence that preventive therapies are useful or appropriate in all patients receiving chemotherapy. In all of these decisions, a close collaboration between the cardiology and oncology team will help to optimize the patient's risks and benefits of treatment.

Dexrazoxane

Dexrazoxane is the only approved agent for the prevention of anthracycline treatment-related HF and was developed with the concept that its iron-chelating properties will limit the generation of cytotoxic hydroxyl reactive oxygen species. However, subsequent research favors an alternative mechanism of action.[70] Both anthracycline and dexrazoxane interact with topII, enzymes that wind and unwind DNA to allow for packing and unpacking critical for normal cellular function. Dexrazoxane interacts with topII and prevents topIIβ-dependent anthracycline myocytotoxicity. There has been some theoretical concern that dexrazoxane could limit antitumor efficacy through its effects on topIIα, though a Cochrane meta-analysis found that dexrazoxane significantly reduced the incidence of clinical HF (RR 0.18, 95% CI 0.10 to 0.32, $P < .001$) with no difference in progression-free or overall survival.[71]

Beta-Blockers

There is emerging evidence that selected BBs can blunt or prevent LV dysfunction from cardiotoxic chemotherapy. The benefit is likely not a class effect. Carvedilol, but not propranolol, was shown to reduce mitochondrial toxicity from doxorubicin in an animal study.[72] Both carvedilol and nebivolol, two agents that also exhibit antioxidant activity, have been shown to reduce anthracycline induced LV dysfunction in their own small prospective human studies.[73-76] However, two human studies of 125 to 130 patients each have found no benefit from metoprolol.[77,78] Perindopril and bisoprolol protected against LVEF declines in a study of 74 breast cancer patients receiving trastuzumab, but they did not protect against the primary outcome of trastuzumab-mediated LV remodeling.[79]

Renin-Angiotensin-Aldosterone Axis Inhibition

There have been mixed results for the efficacy of ACEIs with one trial of lower dose anthracyclines showing no benefit for enalapril,[78] while another showed benefit when enalapril was given to patients at higher risk who exhibited troponin elevations.[68] Patients at highest risk would be expected to derive the most benefit theoretically, and studies in a lower risk population will certainly have power limitations due to lower event rates. Angiotensin receptor blockers (ARBs), including valsartan,[80] telmisartan,[81] and candesartan,[77] have all shown promise in smaller studies. Spironolactone, an aldosterone antagonist, was also found to be beneficial in a study of breast cancer patients receiving anthracyclines.[82] There is currently no evidence that spironolactone's antiandrogen effect, and the associated rise in estrogens, is any more than a theoretical concern. There are no data on the use of eplerenone, an aldosterone antagonist without an antiandrogen effect.

Statins

There is also emerging animal[83] and observational evidence[84] that statins—one of the most commonly prescribed CV medications—may limit anthracycline cardiotoxicity. The only prospective study to date was a study of 40 patients receiving anthracyclines and randomized to the use of atorvastatin 40 mg or no therapy. The study found no difference in the primary endpoint defined as prevention of the onset of LVEF <50%,[85] though it is likely the study was not sufficiently powered for this outcome. On further analysis, there was no difference in post-treatment in baseline in the statin group, while there was a significant drop in EF in the control group after treatment. Statins were associated with improved overall survival in a pooled retrospective analysis of renal cell cancer trial data, although patients were not randomized to statin treatment.[86] A prospective, randomized, controlled trial is currently underway to evaluate the ability of atorvastatin to reduce cardiac events in patients with breast cancer receiving anthracyclines (Preventing Anthracycline CV Toxicity with Statins).

MANAGING HEART FAILURE DURING CANCER TREATMENT

When prevention is unsuccessful and symptomatic HF develops, treatment should follow established ACC/AHA guidelines.[10,87] Guideline-directed medical therapy (**see also Chapter 37**) is associated with improvements in outcome, including improved cardiac function.[88] Yet, new onset HF in a patient who has begun chemotherapy, or preexisting HF in a patient newly diagnosed with cancer, is likely to change the treatment options offered by some medical and surgical oncologists. A careful cardiological assessment should be done, and there should be considerable discussion between the cardiology and oncology providers to ensure mutual understanding of the HF history and prognosis, cancer prognosis, and how the HF condition might influence oncologic treatment plans. In some patients, continued treatment with ErbB2-targeted therapy appears to be tolerated,[27] but in other patients a change in regimen may be necessary.

As cancer treatment ensues, cardiologists must be ready to manage the expected complications of cancer therapy that can include fluid retention, neurohormonal activation and changing hemodynamics, as well as increased thrombosis or bleeding risk (**Table 46.3**). Some familiarity with the medications used in oncology may improve the likelihood that a patient with HF can be managed effectively during cancer treatment without an HF exacerbation or discontinuation of cancer therapy. Typically, this requires more intensive attention to volume status and hemodynamics, with frequent HF clinic visits during active cancer treatment. Anticipating changes in fluid status induced from steroid-containing regimens in patients prone to fluid retention may

TABLE 46.3 Common Cancer Treatments and Treatment Effects That May Exacerbate Heart Failure

Class of Therapy	Effect	Strategy
Steroids	Subacute fluid retention	Careful monitoring of fluid status
		Adjustable diuretic dosing
Antiangiogenics	Hypertension	Adjust vasodilators/anti-hypertensives
Vomiting, diarrhea	Dehydration, Sensitivity to HF meds	Sliding scale diuretic plan, close monitoring by HF provider
Anemia, thrombocytopenia requiring transfusion	Volume load	Careful monitoring of fluid status
		Adjustable diuretic dosing
Sepsis syndrome	Sensitivity to HF meds	Careful hemodynamic monitoring and medication adjustment

HF, Heart failure.

help reduce the likelihood that acute HF becomes a complication of cancer treatment. Changes in blood pressure frequently occur during cancer treatment, requiring close monitoring and potential adjustment of HF medical therapy.

Standard therapy for CV disease and HF may interact with cancer outcomes based upon a number of observations, most of which were retrospective analyses of large cancer registry data sets. While further work is clearly needed before any firm conclusions should be drawn, or recommendations should be made, patients may be aware of these data. The use of BBs appears to improve cancer outcomes.[89,90] Aspirin and statins also have been associated with reduced likelihood of relapse for some malignancies,[91,92] and with statins there is a reduced likelihood of the patient developing HF.[84] Digoxin is a phytoestrogen, and its use has been associated with increased risk of estrogen-sensitive malignancies.[93,94]

ADVANCED THERAPIES IN THE CANCER PATIENT WITH HEART FAILURE

The efficacy of biventricular pacemakers in appropriate patients with anthracycline cardiomyopathy and HF has similarly been demonstrated in a very select group.[95] It certainly appears that the expected benefit of cardiac resynchronization in all HF patients who qualify is applicable to those cancer survivors who have typical clinical characteristics that warrant device implantation.

Advanced therapies, including electrophysiologic devices (**see Chapter 38**), mechanical circulatory support (**see Chapter 45**), and heart transplant (**see Chapter 44**), have been utilized with success in cancer survivors with HF refractory to medical therapy. The most experience is with cardiomyopathy secondary to anthracycline. Over 20 years of outcome data collected by the United Network of Organ Sharing (UNOS) reveal that heart transplant outcomes are similar for anthracycline cardiomyopathy patients as they are for other causes of HF.[6,96] Rates of infection and malignancy, as well as the likelihood of needing a right ventricular assist device were higher in chemotherapy-associated HF compared to nonischemic HF patients.[96] While this supports the use of heart transplant as a treatment in this group of patients, a disturbing trend was noted for increased numbers of heart transplants being done in cancer survivors,[6] suggesting that HF resulting from cancer treatment is potentially an emerging etiology of refractory HF.

KEY REFERENCES

1. Zamorano JL, Lancellotti P, Rodriguez Munoz D, et al. 2016 ESC Position Paper on cancer treatments and cardiovascular toxicity developed under the auspices of the ESC Committee for Practice Guidelines: the Task Force for cancer treatments and cardiovascular toxicity of the European Society of Cardiology (ESC). *Eur Heart J*. 2016;37:2768–2801.

2. Armenian SH, Lacchetti C, Barac A, et al. Prevention and monitoring of cardiac dysfunction in survivors of adult cancers: American Society of Clinical Oncology Clinical Practice Guideline. *J Clin Oncol*. 2017;35:893–911.

8. Darby SC, Ewertz M, McGale P, et al. Risk of ischemic heart disease in women after radiotherapy for breast cancer. *N Engl J Med*. 2013;368:987–998.

10. Yancy CW, Jessup M, Bozkurt B, et al. 2013 ACCF/AHA guideline for the management of heart failure: a report of the American College of Cardiology Foundation/American Heart Association Task Force on Practice Guidelines. *J Am Coll Cardiol*. 2013;62:e147–e239.

12. Armstrong GT, Oeffinger KC, Chen Y, et al. Modifiable risk factors and major cardiac events among adult survivors of childhood cancer. *J Clin Oncol*. 2013;31:3673–3680.

19. van Nimwegen FA, Schaapveld M, Cutter DJ, et al. Radiation dose-response relationship for risk of coronary heart disease in survivors of Hodgkin Lymphoma. *J Clin Oncol*. 2016;34:235–243.

60. Johnson DB, Balko JM, Compton ML, et al. Fulminant Myocarditis with combination immune checkpoint blockade. *N Engl J Med*. 2016;375:1749–1755.

71. van Dalen EC, Caron HN, Dickinson HO, Kremer LC. Cardioprotective interventions for cancer patients receiving anthracyclines. *Cochrane Database Syst Rev*. 2011:Cd003917.

77. Gulati G, Heck SL, Ree AH, et al. Prevention of cardiac dysfunction during adjuvant breast cancer therapy (PRADA): a 2 x 2 factorial, randomized, placebo-controlled, double-blind clinical trial of candesartan and metoprolol. *Eur Heart J*. 2016;37:1671–1680.

86. McKay RR, Lin X, Albiges L, et al. Statins and survival outcomes in patients with metastatic renal cell carcinoma. *Eur J Cancer*. 2016;52:155–162.

The full reference list for this chapter is available on ExpertConsult.

47

Disease Management and Telemedicine in Heart Failure

Anna Marie Chang, Loheetha Ragupathi, David Whellan

Heart failure (HF) currently affects more than 5 million Americans, and because of the aging population and the expected growth of the US population, the prevalence of HF is expected to increase to more than 8 million Americans by 2030 (**see also Chapter 18**).[1] Projections show that the total cost of HF will increase to almost $70 billion per year by 2030.[1] HF is the leading cause of hospitalization in patients older than 65 years of age.[2] Due to the high cost and increasing prevalence of HF hospitalizations, starting in 2012 the Centers for Medicare and Medicaid Services have implemented the Hospital Readmission Reduction Program, which reduces hospitals' Medicare payments up to 3% for higher-than-expected 30-day readmission rates for HF patients.[3] Many hospitals have responded to this potential financial penalty by initiating HF disease management and care coordination programs or processes that target high-risk HF patients.

Early studies demonstrate that HF disease management, defined as an integrative approach that aims to enhance quality of health care and its cost-effectiveness for patients with chronic conditions, decreases hospital readmission rates, improves quality of life (QOL), and decreases costs.[4-10] Rich and colleagues published a landmark multicenter randomized controlled trial examining HF disease management in 1995. The intervention consisted of intense education about HF and its treatment by an experienced cardiovascular team, including a geriatric cardiologist, clinic nurse, dietitian, case manager, and home care provider. The study demonstrated that survival for 90 days without readmission (the primary endpoint) occurred in 54% of the control group versus 64% in the treatment group ($P = .09$). However, when the analysis was restricted to survivors of the initial hospitalization, a significant difference in survival for 90 days without readmission was noted (risk ratio [RR] = 0.56, $P = .02$). The study also showed a significant improvement in the QOL and a decrease in the total cost of care in the treatment group versus the control group.[4] Common features of early studies on HF disease management are that they were based at health care systems, traditionally enrolled inpatients, and had small,

single-center trial designs. Because most HF patients receive their care in a community setting, it is unclear if trials performed at large health care centers can be replicated in a more "real-world" setting. There are many limitations to single-center trial designs, namely limited external validity (interventions tested in a single clinical environment are not necessarily generalizable to a broader population), implausible effect size, and unequal allocation of resources (often single-center trials are performed by an investigator with highly atypical expertise and commitment).[11] Along those lines, several meta-analyses were performed on disease management programs for HF.[12-19] Although these studies show favorable results for HF disease management programs, because these meta-analyses are based on small, single-center trials, caution must be used when interpreting these results.

Since then, several large, multicenter, randomized controlled trials have been published related to HF disease management programs.[20-31] The results of these trials have been mixed, with many being neutral. The reason for the lack of benefit in many of these HF disease management trials is unclear. There was significant heterogeneity among these trials; each targeted a different patient population, provided varying quality of usual care, and used different program designs and interventions. In this chapter, we will explore types of HF disease management program types and discuss how the approach to HF disease management may change in the future.

DEFINING DISEASE MANAGEMENT

Disease management is an approach to patient care that coordinates medical resources for patients across the entire health care delivery system.[32] A critical distinction between disease management and other approaches to traditional medical care is a shift in focus from treating patients during discrete episodes of care (i.e., hospital or clinic) to provisions of high-quality care across the continuum of care.[33] The goals of disease management are to (1) improve patients' knowledge about

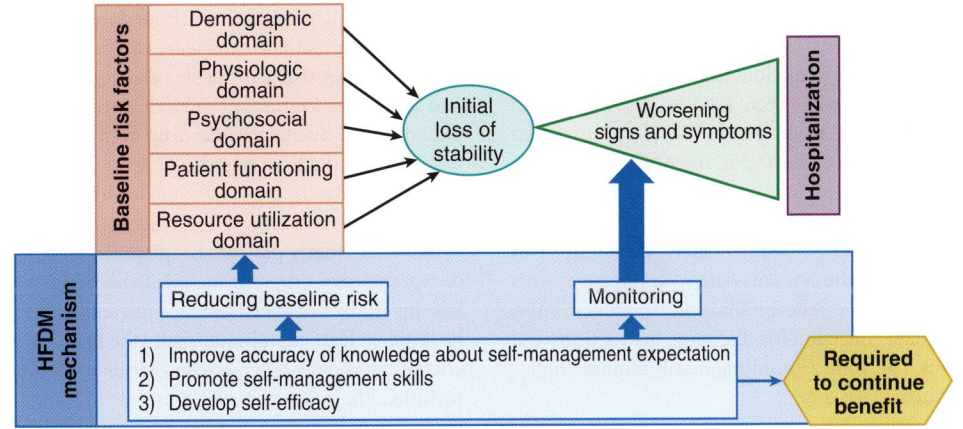

Fig. 47.1 Conceptual model for heart failure disease management *(HFDM)* and mechanisms by which HFDM interventions reduce hospitalizations. (From Andrikopoulou E, Abbate K, Whellan DJ. Conceptual model for heart failure disease management. *Can J Cardiol.* 2014;30[3]:304–311.)

their disease state; (2) facilitate health behavior change that improves self-care, including adherence to treatment and management of symptoms; and (3) improve clinical outcomes, including lower mortality and hospital readmissions.[34]

HF is a prime target for implementation of disease management programs because of its increasing prevalence, high costs to patients and society, high mortality and hospitalization rates, availability of evidence-based therapies, and need for timely identification of symptom progression and clinical deterioration. HF is often accompanied by a multitude of comorbidities and barriers to care, including advanced age, cognitive deficits, depression, low socioeconomic class, and low health literacy. HF patients also have multiple baseline risk factors such as medication or dietary nonadherence and propensity to ischemia, infection, and arrhythmias that may cause a perturbation of their already tenuous state and trigger deterioration that requires a hospitalization. These factors must be taken into account when conceptualizing an HF disease management program. HF disease management aims at detecting instability before the point of clinical deterioration severe enough to warrant admission to the hospital by (1) implementing strategies that modify patients' baseline risk; (2) monitoring for worsening signs and symptoms of decompensation; and (3) encouraging patient participation in their own care (**Fig. 47.1**).[35]

THE SELF-CARE PARADIGM

Self-care is the foundation upon which successful management of HF is built.[34] The self-care process includes both maintenance and management components.[36] Examples of self-care maintenance are adhering to prescribed medications, diets, exercise regimens, and doctor's appointments. Self-care management involves more complex skills, including monitoring symptoms and making decisions regarding their severity, identifying possible treatment options, and assessing whether the treatment implemented was effective. Since the initial symptoms of a HF exacerbation are often subtle, health care management is often difficult for patients to perform successfully, especially in situations involving cognitive deficits and depression. A major factor that influences patients' skills at self-care management activities is self-efficacy, or confidence in one's ability to perform self-care.[36] Most HF disease management programs involve a patient education component designed to provide knowledge so that patients can successfully perform self-care maintenance. In addition, HF disease management programs typically include a monitoring component in the outpatient setting, such as

specialized HF clinics, home visits by nurses, structured telephone support (STS), or telemonitoring (TM) to help patients with self-care management.

HEART FAILURE DISEASE MANAGEMENT CLASSIFICATION SCHEMES

Considerable variability exists among disease management programs in the literature. Significantly different populations have been targeted, and the spectrum of interventions studied has been wide. This heterogeneity has made comparison of HF disease management programs difficult. Grady and colleagues developed a classification scheme in an attempt to better categorize HF management programs. They identified the following settings for disease management: inpatient, specialty HF care outside the clinic setting (home visits, telephone calls, or TM), and primary care clinic.[37,38] In 2006, the American Heart Association's Disease Management Taxonomy Writing Group developed a system of classification that can be used both to categorize and compare disease management programs and to inform efforts to identify specific factors associated with effectiveness.[39] The taxonomy would include descriptions of eight domains: patient population, recipient, intervention content, delivery personnel, method of communication, intensity and complexity, environment, and outcome measures. The goal of this taxonomy is to establish a common language for evaluation of disease management. The authors hope that it will ultimately facilitate more rapid identification of effective program components.

HEART FAILURE DISEASE MANAGEMENT IN THE INPATIENT SETTING

Despite the opportunity to closely assess patients, modify therapy under observation, and provide intensive education during hospitalization for an acute exacerbation, the preponderance of evidence suggests that HF management during hospitalization is inadequate.[40] Approximately 20% of unplanned hospital readmissions for HF have been attributed to substandard inpatient care.[40]

In 1996, the Centers for Medicare and Medicaid Services (CMS) first implemented a program to track and improve the quality of HF care in hospitals. CMS subsequently aligned with The Joint Commission to create a national standardized "core" set of four HF performance metrics: measuring left ventricular function, using angiotensin-converting enzyme (ACE) inhibitors in patients with left ventricular systolic dysfunction, providing complete HF discharge instructions, and providing smoking cessation counseling in current or recent smokers. The original HF process measures have been modified only once since then by adding use of angiotensin II receptor blockers as an alternative to ACE inhibitors.[41] From 2002 to 2007, provision of discharge instructions improved from 31% to 78%, left ventricular function measures improved from 82% to 95%, use of ACE inhibitors or angiotensin II receptor blockers for left ventricular systolic dysfunction improved from 74% to 90%, and provision of smoking cessation advice improved from 42% to 96%.[41] Unfortunately, these improvements in performance measures did not correlate with improvements in 30-day or 1-year mortality or rehospitalization.[41,42] Since 2014, CMS no longer required data collection for discharge instructions and ACE inhibitors/ARB, but The Joint Commission still requires documentation of ACE inhibitors/ARB use.

It is unclear why an improvement in compliance with performance metrics did not correlate with improvement in clinical outcomes, but one hypothesis is that the perceived improvement in core metrics may simply have been better documentation of care that hospitals have been providing all along. Conversely, it may appear that hospitals have improved adherence with core metrics by "checking the appropriate boxes."[41] The reason for lack of clinically meaningful improvement could also be due to poorly chosen metrics. Of the four CMS-mandated HF performance measures, only prescription of an ACE inhibitor or ARB is supported by direct clinical trial evidence.[43] Data from the Organized Program to Initiate Lifesaving Treatment in Hospitalized Patients with Heart Failure (OPTIMIZE-HF), a registry and performance improvement program for patients hospitalized with HF, β-blockade at the time of hospital discharge, currently not a CMS performance measure, were strongly associated with reduced risk of mortality (hazard ratio [HR], 0.48; 95% confidence interval [CI], 0.30–0.79; $P = .004$) and mortality/rehospitalization during follow-up.[43] This performance measure was added to the AHA/ACC in 2011 Performance Measures (**Table 47.1**). In addition, rather than discharge instructions, the updated AHA/ACC Performance Measures also evaluates postdischarge appointments after HF hospitalization.

Although most evidence-based HF therapies are not represented by the CMS outcome metrics, an HF hospitalization is an opportune time to ensure patients are prescribed these potentially life-saving therapies. It is also an excellent time to initiate and/or reinforce patient education on topics such as dietary recommendations, medications, activity and exercise, risk factor modification, and symptom monitoring and recognition.[34] In 2005, the American Heart Association launched the Get With The Guidelines-HF (GWTG-HF) program. This is an in-hospital quality improvement program to ensure that every patient with HF receives the best care. The GWTG-HF module has a patient management tool that provides patient-specific guideline recommendations, allows for real-time data validation, and enables each institution to track its adherence to the guidelines individually and against national benchmarks.[44] The GWTG-HF program facilitates data collection and provides quality improvement tools to hospitals, including clinical decision support and dissemination of best practices, and regularly reports performance back to the participating hospitals.[44] Heidenreich and associates demonstrated that process of care, as defined by CMS performance measures, is higher in the GWTG-HF–participating hospitals than in other US hospitals. In addition, readmission rates, but not mortality, were lower in GWTG-HF hospitals.[44] In 2016, 637 hospitals were participating in GWTG-HF, and more than 86 publications had originated from the data.[45]

The process of disease management and self-care starts during an acute HF hospitalization. The transition of care from one health care venue (inpatient) to the next (outpatient: home, nursing home, etc.)

can be difficult in HF patients. Poor communication between inpatient teams and outpatient caregivers can result in medication errors and other mistakes that can result in adverse events for patients. Forster and associates found that 66% of untoward outcomes in discharged patients were due to adverse drug events.[46,47] Similarly, Gray and colleagues identified adverse drug events in 20% of patients discharged from hospital to home with home health care services.[47,48] Naylor et al. conducted a randomized controlled trial of a transitional care intervention for elderly patients hospitalized with acute HF. This 3-month comprehensive program included discharge planning and home follow-up led by advanced practice nurses (APN) with daily visits in the hospital, at least eight home visits (the first one within 24 hours of discharge), and daily telephone availability. Specifically, the intervention included the following components: (1) a standardized orientation and training program guided by a multidisciplinary team of HF for APNs; (2) use of care management strategies including identification of patients' and caregivers' goals, individualized plans of care developed and implemented by APNs in collaboration with patients' physicians, educational and behavioral strategies to address patients' and caregivers' learning needs, continuity of care, and care coordination across settings; and (3) APN implementation of an evidence-based protocol. This transitional care intervention decreased rehospitalizations or deaths at 1 year (56/118 [47.5%] vs. 74/121 [61.2%], adjusted $P = .01$).[49]

HEART FAILURE DISEASE MANAGEMENT IN THE OUTPATIENT SETTING

HF practice guidelines have a class I recommendation (level of evidence, A) to implement a multidisciplinary heart failure transitional care and disease management (HFDM) program for individuals at high risk for clinical decline or hospitalization. A variety of HFDM programs has been evaluated. These programs can be clinic based, home visit based, telephone/telehealth based, or a combination of the above. Many of these programs exist but are not properly used. Using GWTG-HF data, Gharacholou et al. showed that patients were not receiving regular referrals to specialized HFDM programs and referral occurred in only 19.2% of patients. The median rate of HFDM referral among all hospitals was 3.5% (25th–75th percentiles 0%–16.7%), and higher in hospitals who previously referred patients to HF management programs. In addition, it appeared that patients at higher risk of 90-day mortality were less likely referred to programs.[50] Thus there is a clear need to improve referrals to these programs, as HFDM programs have been shown to reduce hospitalizations, improve QOL, lower costs, and lower symptom burden, compared with patients not followed in HFDM.

Cardiac Rehabilitation for Heart Failure

One of the proven outpatient disease management programs is cardiac rehabilitation (CR). These programs comprise exercise counseling and training, risk factor and dietary education, and stress reduction. The efficacy and safety of exercise training among HF patients was testing the Heart Failure: A Controlled Trial Investigating Outcomes of Exercise Training (HF-ACTION) trial. This was a multicenter randomized controlled trial of 2331 medically stable outpatients with HFrEF of 35% or less, and NYHA class II to IV symptoms despite optimal medical therapy for at least 6 weeks, which evaluated 36 supervised exercise training sessions in addition to usual care versus usual care alone. There were nonsignificant improvements in the primary endpoints of all-cause mortality and hospitalization (HR, 0.93; 95% CI, 0.84–1.02; $P = .13$) with exercise training. After adjustment for highly

TABLE 47.1 ACC/AHA Heart Failure Performance Measures 2011

Performance Measure Name	Measure Description	Care Setting	Level of Measurement
1. LVEF Assessment	Percentage of patients aged ≥18 yr with a diagnosis of HF for whom the quantitative or qualitative results of a recent or prior (any time in the past) LVEF assessment is documented within a 12-mo period	Outpatient	Individual Provider
2. LVEF assessment	Percentage of patients aged ≥18 yr with a principal discharge diagnosis of HF with documentation in the hospital record of the results of an LVEF assessment performed either before arrival or during hospitalization, OR documentation in the hospital record that LVEF assessment is planned after discharge	Inpatient	Individual practitioner and facility
3. Symptom and activity assessment	Percentage of patient visits for those patients aged ≥18 yr with a diagnosis of HF with quantitative results of an evaluation of both current level of activity and clinical symptoms documented	Outpatient	Individual practitioner
4. Symptom management	Percentage of patient visits for those patients aged ≥18 yr with a diagnosis of HF and with quantitative results of an evaluation of both level of activity AND clinical symptoms documented in which patient symptoms have improved or remained consistent with treatment goals since last assessment, OR patient symptoms have demonstrated clinically important deterioration since last assessment with a documented plan of care	Outpatient	Individual practitioner
5. Patient self-care education	Percentage of patients aged ≥18 yr with a diagnosis of HF who were provided with self-care education on ≥3 elements of education during ≥1 visit within a 12-mo period	Outpatient	Individual practitioner
6. β-Blocker therapy for LVSD (outpatient and inpatient setting)	Percentage of patients aged ≥18 yr with a diagnosis of HF with a current or prior LVEF of <40% who were prescribed β-blocker therapy with bisoprolol, carvedilol, or sustained-release metoprolol succinate either within a 12-mo period when seen in the outpatient setting or at hospital discharge	Inpatient and outpatient	Individual practitioner and facility
7. ACE inhibitor (ACEI), or angiotensin receptor blocker (ARB) for LVS dysfunction (LVSD)	Percentage of patients aged ≥18 yr with a diagnosis of HF with a current or prior LVEF of <40% who were prescribed ACE inhibitor or ARB therapy either within a 12-mo period when seen in the outpatient setting or at hospital discharge	Inpatient and Outpatient	Individual practitioner and facility
8. Counseling about ICD implantation for patients with LVSD receiving combination medical therapy	Percentage of patients aged ≥18 yr with a diagnosis of HF with current LVEF ≤35% despite ACE inhibitor/ARB and β-blocker therapy for at least 3 mo who were counseled about ICD implantation as a treatment option for the prophylaxis of sudden death	Outpatient	Individual practitioner
9. Postdischarge appointment for HF patients	Percentage of patients, regardless of age, discharged from an inpatient facility to ambulatory care or home health care with a principal discharge diagnosis of HF for whom a follow-up appointment was scheduled and documented, including location, date, and time for a follow-up office visit or home healthcare visit (as specified)	Inpatient	Facility

ACE, Angiotensin-converting enzyme; HF, heart failure; ICD, implantable cardioverter-defibrillator; LVEF, left ventricular ejection fraction; LVSD, left ventricular systolic dysfunction. From Bonow RO, Ganiats TG, Beam CT, et al. ACCF/AHA/AMA-PCPI 2011 performance measures for adults with heart failure a report of the American College of Cardiology Foundation/American Heart Association Task Force on Performance Measures and the American Medical Association–Physician Consortium for Performance Improvement. J Am Coll Cardiol. 2012 59(20):1812–1832.

prognostic predictors of the primary endpoint, exercise training was associated with modest significant reductions for both all-cause mortality or hospitalization (HR, 0.89; 95% CI, 0.81–0.99; P = .03).[51]

Endurance-type exercise training is known to favorably affect peak VO_2, central hemodynamic function, autonomic function, peripheral vascular and muscle function, and exercise capacity in HF.[52] To summarize the studies on CR in HF, a Cochrane review was conducted in 2010 and updated in 2017 to include a total of 33 randomized controlled trials with 4740 patients with HF, predominantly HFrEF with NYHA class II to III symptoms.[52a] There was no difference seen in pooled mortality in exercise-based CR versus no exercise controls in trials with up to 1-year follow-up (25 trials, 1871 participants, RR 0.93; 95% CI 0.69–1.27, fixed-effect analysis). However, there was trend toward a reduction in mortality with exercise in trials with more than 1 year of follow-up (6 trials, 2845 participants: RR 0.88; 95% CI 0.75–1.02, fixed-effect analysis). In addition, compared with control, exercise training reduced the rate of overall (15 trials, 1328 participants: RR 0.75; 95% CI 0.62–0.92, fixed-effect analysis) and HF specific hospitalization (12 trials, 1036 participants: RR 0.61; 95% CI 0.46–0.80, fixed-effect analysis). Exercise also resulted in a clinically important improvement superior in the Minnesota Living with HF questionnaire (13 trials, 1270 participants: mean difference: −5.8 points; 95% CI −9.2 to −2.4, random-effects analysis). The 2013 ACCF/AHA guidelines for the management of HF provide a class I recommendation for the safety and efficacy of exercise training or regular physical exercise in patients with HF who are able to participate to improve functional status. CR is assigned a class IIa recommendation in clinically stable patients with HF to improve functional capacity, exercise duration, health-related quality of life (QOL), and mortality.[53]

On the basis of the accumulating evidence in favor of CR in HF, on February 18, 2014, the CMS expanded coverage for CR to include patients with stable, chronic HF with LVEF <35% and NYHA II-IV symptoms for 6 weeks despite being on optimal medical therapy and who have not had recent (<6 weeks) or planned (<6 months) major cardiovascular hospitalizations or procedures.[54]

Nevertheless, there are still several challenges to the use of CR in HF patients. The mean age of the HF-ACTION trial patients was 59 years. The incidence of HF increases with age, with incidence of 20 per 1000 in individuals 65 to 69 years of age to more than 80 per 1000 individuals in those older than 85 years of age.[53] The effect of CR in elderly patients is not known. Furthermore, the efficacy and safety of CR in the immediate post HF hospitalization period is not known. There is also a dearth of information on CR in HFpEF patients. Referral to CR overall, and specifically in HF patients, has been low; an estimate using the Get with the Guidelines HF registry reports a 10.4% referral rate between 2005 and 2014, although this has been increasing.[55] Furthermore, CR has a dose response relationship with mortality; therefore adherence to therapy is important, and this has been a challenge with CR overall.[56]

Clinic-Based Follow-Up

The data on outpatient follow-up for HF patients after hospital discharge have been mixed.[18,19,51,57-61] In a recent meta-analysis by McAlister and colleagues, the investigators determined that strategies incorporating follow-up by a specialized multidisciplinary team reduced mortality (RR 0.75, 95% CI 0.59–0.96), HF hospitalizations (RR 0.74, 95% CI 0.63–0.87), and all-cause hospitalizations (RR 0.81, 95% CI 0.71–0.92). Programs that focused on enhancing patient self-care activities reduced HF hospitalizations (RR 0.66, 95% CI 0.52–0.83) and all-cause hospitalizations (RR 0.73, 95% CI 0.57–0.93) but had no effect on mortality (RR 1.14, 95% CI 0.67–1.94). Strategies that employed telephone contact and advised patients to contact their primary care physician in the event of deterioration reduced HF

hospitalizations (RR 0.75, 95% CI 0.57–0.99) but not mortality (RR 0.91, 95% CI 0.67–1.29) or all-cause hospitalizations (RR 0.98, 95% CI 0.80–1.20). In 15 of 18 trials that evaluated cost, multidisciplinary strategies were cost saving.[18]

Phillips and et al. conducted a meta-analysis to determine the efficacy of interventions consisting of comprehensive discharge planning plus postdischarge support for older inpatients with HF. Eighteen studies with a total of 3304 patients were evaluated. During a pooled mean observation period of 8 months (range, 3–12 months), fewer intervention patients were readmitted compared with controls (555/1590 vs. 741/1714, number needed to treat = 12; RR 0.75; 95% CI 0.64–0.88). There was no statically significant difference in mortality between the control versus the intervention groups.[19]

Using GWTG-HF data, Hernandez et al. examined whether close outpatient follow-up after HF admission affected 30-day readmissions. Data from 225 hospitals, which included 30,136 patients, showed that there was substantial variation in rates of early outpatient follow-up. Those who were admitted to hospitals with the lowest quartile of early follow-up had higher readmission rates (30-day readmission rate, 23.3%) compared with those in higher quartiles: the rates of 30-day readmission were 20.5% among patients in the second quartile (risk-adjusted HR, 0.85; 95% CI, 0.78–0.93), 20.5% among patients in the third quartile (risk-adjusted HR, 0.87; 95% CI, 0.78–0.96), and 20.9% among patients in the fourth quartile (risk-adjusted HR, 0.91; 95% CI, 0.83–1.00).[62] HF patients with decreased mobility may find it difficult to frequently commute to the doctor's office, especially if they live in rural areas. Given these limitations, alternative HF disease management approaches have been studied, including visiting home nurses, telephone monitoring, and TM.

Home Nursing Visits

There are HF programs that deliver care primarily in patients' homes. Patients do not routinely go to a clinic or other outpatient setting to receive care; rather, the health care provider calls on the telephone or comes to the home.[37] There are many advantages to implementing a home-based HF disease management program. The home is the most important context of care for individuals with chronic HF. Patients often struggle to manage a complex regimen of medications, follow an unfamiliar diet, monitor weight and vital signs, and work to coordinate care among various providers who, in some cases, fail to communicate effectively.[63] Intuitively, it would seem that a home-based HF disease management approach would improve outcomes and reduce costs. It is unclear if a home-based approach is superior to other types of HF disease management programs.[47,64,65]

In 2012, Stewart and associates published the Which Heart Failure Intervention Is Most Cost-Effective and Consumer-Friendly in Reducing Hospital Care? (WHICH) trial, comparing a home-based intervention (HBI) with a clinic-based intervention (CBI). This was a prospective, multicenter, randomized controlled trial that enrolled 280 patients with HF being discharged from the hospital. The primary endpoint was all-cause, unplanned hospitalization or death during a 12- to 18-month follow-up. The primary endpoint occurred in 102 of 143 (71%) HBI versus 104 of 137 (76%) CBI patients (adjusted HR 0.97; 95% CI 0.73–1.30; P = .81). Ninety-six (67.1%) HBI versus 95 (69.3%) CBI patients had an unplanned hospitalization (P = .89), and 31 (21.7%) versus 38 (27.7%) died (P = .25).[47,64] Stewart and colleagues were able to follow 274 of these patients for more than 3 years, and found similar long-term results; that is, home-based interventions were not associated with prolonged event free survival compared with clinic-based interventions.[66]

Despite the merits of a home-based HF disease management program, it may not be feasible to conduct on a large scale due to limited nursing personnel and costs. Therefore, alternative methods of HF disease management have been explored, such as telephone-based interventions and TM.

Telephone Interventions and Telemonitoring

Another method of delivering care involves telephone and TM. STS consists of a health care provider, most often a nurse, calling patients after hospital discharge to confirm adherence to treatment, enhance patient education, and manage symptoms. TM is a digital, broadband, satellite, wireless, or Bluetooth transmission of physiologic data (e.g., electrocardiogram [ECG], blood pressure, weight, pulse oximetry, and respiratory rate). Both models of care have the potential to provide access to specialist care for a much larger number of patients across a much greater geography and might reduce the cost of care.[63] However, as in HF disease management trials of multidisciplinary clinics and home nursing visits, the results of trials in STS and TM are mixed.[21,61,67-81]

The Alere Trial (HF Home Care Trial), published in 2008, was a multicenter randomized controlled trial examining a computer-based home disease management program among older minority and female Medicare beneficiaries with HF receiving care in a community-based primary care setting. The study randomized 315 patients to examine the effect of the Alere DayLink Monitoring System in a resource-limited, diverse population. The HFMS system was compared with standard HF care, including enhanced patient education, education to clinicians, and follow-up. The primary endpoint of treatment failure, defined as the composite of cardiovascular death or rehospitalization within 6 months of enrollment, was compared between groups. No statistically significant difference was found between groups.[23]

The Home or Hospital in Heart Failure (HHH) study was a multinational, randomized controlled clinical trial, conducted in the United Kingdom, Poland, and Italy. Across these 11 centers, 461 HF patients were enrolled and randomized to either the usual outpatient care or HTM administered as three randomized strategies: (1) monthly telephone contact, (2) strategy 1 plus weekly transmission of vital signs, and (3) strategy 2 plus monthly 24-hour recording of cardiorespiratory activity.[61] Over a 12-month follow-up, there was no significant effect of HTM in reducing bed-days occupancy for HF or cardiac death plus HF hospitalization.[61] In 2012, the Interdisciplinary Network for Heart Failure (INH) study developed and evaluated in a randomized, controlled trial a nurse-coordinated disease management program (HeartNetCare-HF, HNC)[82]; 715 patients hospitalized for systolic HF were randomly assigned to HNC or usual care (UC). Besides telephone-based monitoring and education, HNC addressed individual problems raised by patients, pursued networking of health care providers, and provided training for caregivers. Endpoints were time to death or rehospitalization. Within 180 days, 130 HNC and 137 UC patients reached the primary endpoint (HR 1.02; 95% CI 0.81–1.30; $P = .89$), because more HNC patients were readmitted. Overall, 32 HNC and 52 UC patients died. Uncensored HR was 0.62 (0.40–0.96; $P = .03$). HNC patients improved more regarding NYHA class ($P = .05$), physical functioning ($P = .03$), and physical health component ($P = .03$).[82]

In 2010, Chaudhry and colleagues published the Tele-HF study,[28] a multicenter, randomized controlled trial to determine whether TM would reduce the combined endpoint of readmission or death from any cause among patients recently hospitalized for HF; 1653 patients were randomized to TM versus usual care. The intervention consisted of an interactive voice response system that collected data but did not provide education. Adherence with the system was poor, suggesting that patients did not engage with the service, perhaps because of the nature of the technology.[63] There was no significant difference between the two groups with respect to readmission for any cause or death.[28,63]

In 2011, Koehler and associates published Impact of Remote Telemedical Management (RTM) on Mortality and Hospitalization in Ambulatory Patients with Chronic Heart Failure: the Telemedical Interventional Monitoring in Heart Failure Study (TIM-HF).[29] This was a multicenter, randomized controlled trial designed to determine whether physician-led RTM compared with UC would result in reduced mortality in ambulatory patients with chronic HF; 710 stable HF patients (NYHA class II and III) were randomly assigned to RTM or UC. RTM used portable devices for ECG, blood pressure, and body weight measurements connected to a personal digital assistant that sent automated encrypted transmission via cell phones to the telemedical centers. The primary endpoint was death from any cause. The first secondary endpoint was a composite of cardiovascular death and hospitalization for HF. Compared with UC, RTM had no significant effect on all-cause mortality (HR 0.97; 95% CI 0.67–1.41; $P = .87$) or on cardiovascular death or HF hospitalization (HR 0.89; 95% CI 0.67–1.19; $P = .44$).[29] The lack of significant clinical improvement in TIM-HF may be related to the target population. Stable patients who are exceptionally well managed may not obtain as much benefit from TM as a group of patients who may not have exposure to such high-quality care at baseline. The Weight Monitoring in Patients with Severe Heart Failure (WISH) Trial was published in 2012.[83] This was a multicenter, randomized controlled trial designed to determine if daily electronic transmission of body weight to a HF clinic would reduce cardiac hospitalization in patients recently hospitalized with HF. A total of 344 patients were randomized to the intervention group versus the control group. No significant differences were found for the primary endpoint, cardiac rehospitalization (HR 0.90; 95% CI 0.65–1.26; $P = .54$), or for the secondary endpoints, which included all-cause hospitalization (HR 0.83; 95% CI 0.61–1.13; $P = .24$), death from any cause (HR 0.57; 95% CI 0.19–1.73; $P = .32$), or the composite endpoint of cardiac hospitalization and death from any cause (HR 0.90; 95% CI 0.65–1.26; $P = .54$).[83]

Bekelman et al. conducted a randomized controlled trial comparing a collaborative patient-centered disease management program of HF patients at four Veterans Affairs centers. Each intervention team consisted of a local primary care provider, cardiologist, psychiatrist, and nurse coordinator (registered nurse). The team assessed each intervention patient through a review of the VA electronic health record and baseline depression scores. In addition, the intervention patients received daily TM which collected biometric data and self-reported symptoms. After 1 year, there was significant improvement in the Kansas City Cardiomyopathy Questionnaire (KCCQ) overall summary scores in both groups. There were fewer deaths at 1 year in the intervention arm (8 of 187 [4.3%]) than in the usual care arm (19 of 197 [9.6%]) ($P = .04$). There was no significant difference in 1-year hospitalization rates between the intervention arm and the usual care arm (29.4% vs. 29.9%, $P = .87$).[84]

A Cochrane Review evaluating the effectiveness of STS and TM as a primary component of a chronic HF disease management program was published in 2011.[63,67] They included randomized controlled trials comparing TM or STS to UC in patients with HF. The primary outcomes analyzed were mortality and hospitalizations. Twenty-five peer-reviewed studies were included (11 evaluated TM and 16 evaluated STS, with 2 studies testing both TM and STS). Tele-HF, TIM-HF, and WISH were not included, because they were reported after the meta-analysis was completed. TM reduced all-cause mortality (RR 0.66; 95% CI 0.54–0.81; $P < .0001$). STS showed a similar but nonsignificant trend (RR 0.77; 95% CI 0.76–1.01; $P = .08$) (**Fig. 47.2**). Both TM (RR 0.79; 95% CI 0.76–0.940; $P = .008$) and STM (RR 0.77; 95% CI 0.68–0.87; $P < .0001$) reduced HF-related hospitalizations.[63,67] The quality of the methods used in the studies was variable, and many of the studies were small.[28]

STRUCTURED TELEPHONE SUPPORT

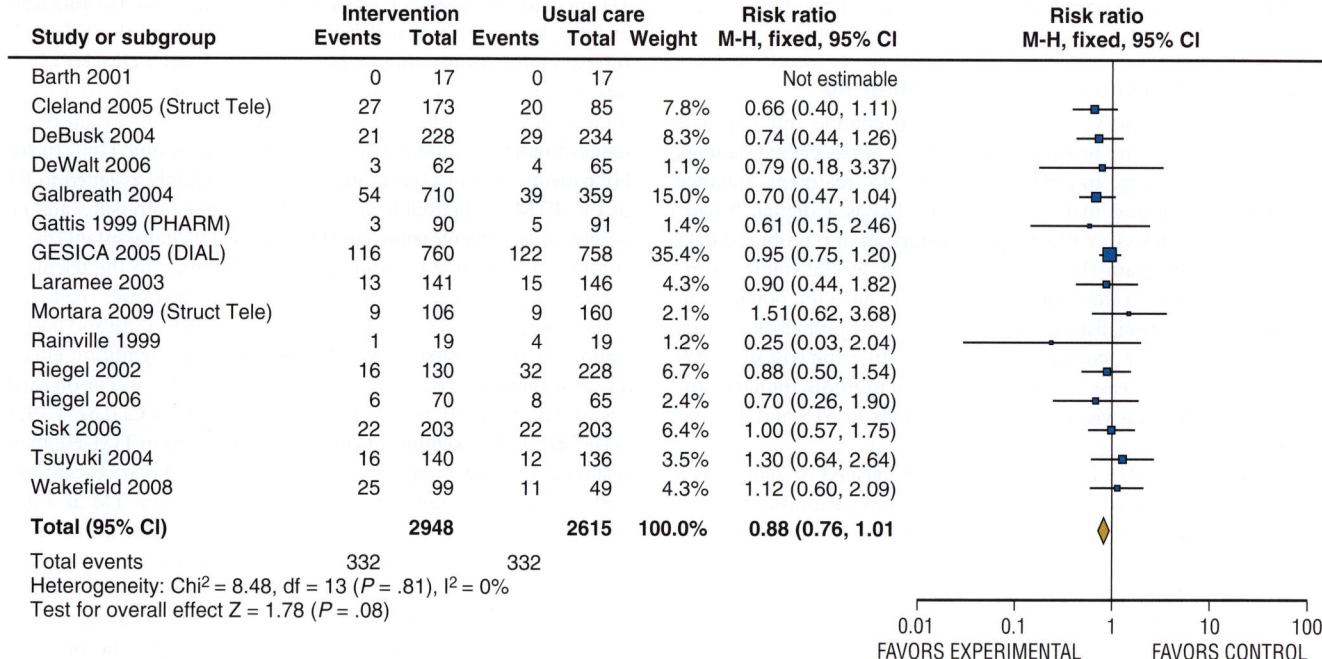

Study or subgroup	Intervention Events	Total	Usual care Events	Total	Weight	Risk ratio M-H, fixed, 95% CI
Barth 2001	0	17	0	17		Not estimable
Cleland 2005 (Struct Tele)	27	173	20	85	7.8%	0.66 (0.40, 1.11)
DeBusk 2004	21	228	29	234	8.3%	0.74 (0.44, 1.26)
DeWalt 2006	3	62	4	65	1.1%	0.79 (0.18, 3.37)
Galbreath 2004	54	710	39	359	15.0%	0.70 (0.47, 1.04)
Gattis 1999 (PHARM)	3	90	5	91	1.4%	0.61 (0.15, 2.46)
GESICA 2005 (DIAL)	116	760	122	758	35.4%	0.95 (0.75, 1.20)
Laramee 2003	13	141	15	146	4.3%	0.90 (0.44, 1.82)
Mortara 2009 (Struct Tele)	9	106	9	160	2.1%	1.51 (0.62, 3.68)
Rainville 1999	1	19	4	19	1.2%	0.25 (0.03, 2.04)
Riegel 2002	16	130	32	228	6.7%	0.88 (0.50, 1.54)
Riegel 2006	6	70	8	65	2.4%	0.70 (0.26, 1.90)
Sisk 2006	22	203	22	203	6.4%	1.00 (0.57, 1.75)
Tsuyuki 2004	16	140	12	136	3.5%	1.30 (0.64, 2.64)
Wakefield 2008	25	99	11	49	4.3%	1.12 (0.60, 2.09)
Total (95% CI)		**2948**		**2615**	**100.0%**	**0.88 (0.76, 1.01**

Total events: 332   332
Heterogeneity: Chi² = 8.48, df = 13 (*P* = .81), I² = 0%
Test for overall effect Z = 1.78 (*P* = .08)

TELEMONITORING

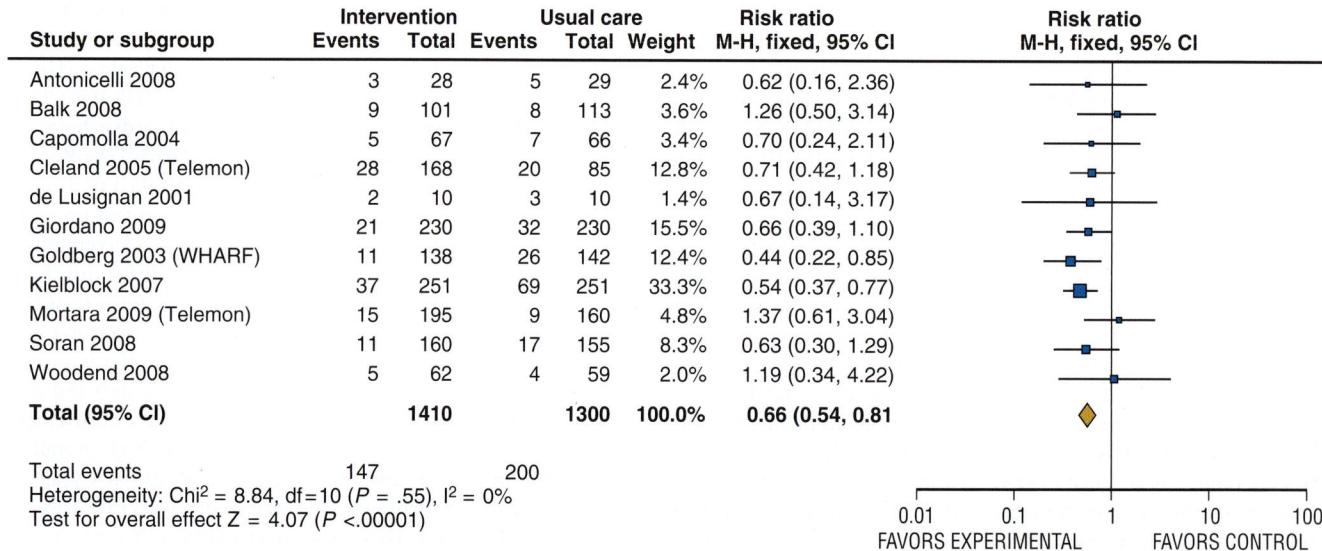

Study or subgroup	Intervention Events	Total	Usual care Events	Total	Weight	Risk ratio M-H, fixed, 95% CI
Antonicelli 2008	3	28	5	29	2.4%	0.62 (0.16, 2.36)
Balk 2008	9	101	8	113	3.6%	1.26 (0.50, 3.14)
Capomolla 2004	5	67	7	66	3.4%	0.70 (0.24, 2.11)
Cleland 2005 (Telemon)	28	168	20	85	12.8%	0.71 (0.42, 1.18)
de Lusignan 2001	2	10	3	10	1.4%	0.67 (0.14, 3.17)
Giordano 2009	21	230	32	230	15.5%	0.66 (0.39, 1.10)
Goldberg 2003 (WHARF)	11	138	26	142	12.4%	0.44 (0.22, 0.85)
Kielblock 2007	37	251	69	251	33.3%	0.54 (0.37, 0.77)
Mortara 2009 (Telemon)	15	195	9	160	4.8%	1.37 (0.61, 3.04)
Soran 2008	11	160	17	155	8.3%	0.63 (0.30, 1.29)
Woodend 2008	5	62	4	59	2.0%	1.19 (0.34, 4.22)
Total (95% CI)		**1410**		**1300**	**100.0%**	**0.66 (0.54, 0.81)**

Total events: 147   200
Heterogeneity: Chi² = 8.84, df = 10 (*P* = .55), I² = 0%
Test for overall effect Z = 4.07 (*P* < .00001)

Fig. 47.2 Effect of structured telephone support and telemonitoring on all-cause mortality. (From Inglis SC, Clark RA, McAlister FA, Stewart S, Cleland JG. Which components of heart failure programmes are effective? A systematic review and meta-analysis of the outcomes of structured telephone support or telemonitoring as the primary component of chronic heart failure management in 8323 patients: abridged Cochrane Review. *Eur J Heart Fail.* 2011;13[9]:1028–1040.)

A recent meta-analysis specifically evaluated how telemedicine interventions impacted patients' QOL, and the authors included 26 studies with 7066 participants. Three separate, random effects meta-analyses were conducted for mental, physical, and overall QoL. Telemedicine was not significantly more effective than usual care on mental and physical QoL, but was associated with a small significant increase in overall QoL and was more beneficial with long duration (≥52 weeks) and via TM.[85] Another recent meta-analysis directly compared different types of telemedicine, including STS, TM, and ECG monitoring; 30 randomized controlled trials (RCTs) (*N* = 10,193

patients) were included. Compared with usual care, STS and TM were both found to reduce the odds of mortality and hospitalizations. Video monitoring did not reduce outcomes.[86] More recently, an assessment of systematic reviews was published by Bashi et al. The authors included 19 systematic reviews of remote patient monitoring in HF. These reviews comprised between 4 and 56 studies each. Overall, 9 of the 19 systematic reviews indicated that these programs showed a reduction in all-cause mortality; 5 showed a reduction in all-cause hospitalizations. In another systematic review by Yun et al., 37 randomized controlled trials including 9582 patients comparing TM to

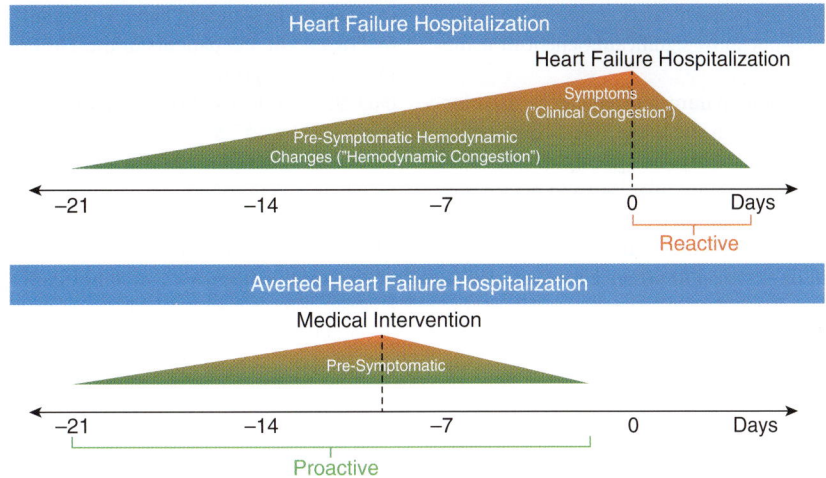

Fig. 47.3 The concept of pressure-guided heart failure therapy. (From Abraham WT, Perl L. Implantable hemodynamic monitoring for heart failure patients. *J Am Coll Cardiol.* 2017;70[3]:389–398.)

usual care were evaluated.[87] The authors found that all-cause mortality (RR 0.81, 95% CI 0.70–0.94) and HF-related mortality (RR 0.68, 95% CI 0.50–0.91) were significantly lower in the TM group than in the usual care group. In addition, the authors found that TM showed a significant benefit when ≥3 biologic data are transmitted or when transmission occurred daily. TM also reduced mortality risk in studies that monitored patients' symptoms, medication adherence, or prescription changes (**Fig. 47.3**).

Cardiac Telerehabilitation

More recently, there has also been interest in cardiac telerehabilitation as an adjunct or alternative to conventional CR to be able to improve the long-term success of cardiac rehab in a cost-effective manner. Some studies showed telerehabilitation to be noninferior when compared with standard CR. Frederix et al. studied a group of cardiac patients in the Telerehab III study, and then conducted a follow-up study up to 2 years later. The telerehabilitation program would start 6 weeks after the initiation of ambulatory rehabilitation. Patients would receive semiautomatic telecoaching via email and SMS text message regarding exercise, diet, and smoking cessation (70 patients in each arm). Both mean VO_2 peak and self-reported physical activity were increased in the intervention group[88] (mean VO_2 peak 22.46, SD 0.78 mL/[min × kg]) to 24 weeks (mean 24.46, SD 1.00 mL/[min × kg], $P < .01$) versus control group patients ($n = 70$), who did not change significantly (baseline: mean 22.72, SD 0.74 mL/[min × kg]; 24 weeks: mean 22.15, SD 0.77 mL/[min × kg], $P = .09$). While some of these changes, such as mean VO_2 peak, declined by 2 years, the patients in the tele-intervention group still had better results than the control group.[89]

Invasive Telemonitoring

In the noninvasive TM schemes discussed previously, the identification of risk factors for impending HF exacerbation relies upon identifying worsening of clinical signs and symptoms of HF. However, these signs and symptoms occur late in the natural history of HF exacerbation. These signs and symptoms are preceded by hemodynamic changes of increases in ventricular filling pressures.[90] The goal of invasive TM in HF, then, is to recognize impending HF exacerbation earlier, in order to initiate changes in medical therapy with the goal of averting hospitalization.[91]

From the 1990s onward, cardiac implantable electronic devices (CIED) with remote sensors have been developed to further this goal. Various iterations of these devices have included invasive TM measurements of intrathoracic impedance, right ventricular oxygen saturation,

right-sided cardiac pressure, left atrial pressure, and pulmonary artery pressure. Some devices have been standalone devices, whereas others have been incorporated into pacing and ICD technologies due to the high prevalence of their use in the HF population.

The Chronicle device (Medtronic Inc., Minneapolis, MN) was an implanted monitor designed to continuously record and store hemodynamic information, including right ventricular systolic, diastolic, pulse pressure, and estimated pulmonary arterial diastolic pressure. In addition, it also stored heart rate, patient activity levels, and central venous temperature.[92] It was tested in the landmark COMPASS-HF (Chronicle Offers Management to Patients with Advanced Signs and Symptoms of HFe) Trial[30] to determine the clinical impact of an invasive hemodynamic monitor-based management strategy in patients with advanced HF already receiving optimal medical care. The study was a prospective, multicenter, randomized, single-blinded, parallel-controlled trial of 274 New York Heart Association functional class III or IV HF patients who underwent the successful implant of the Chronicle device. Patients were randomized to the Chronicle group ($n = 134$) or the control group ($n = 140$). All patients received optimal medical therapy, but the hemodynamic information from the monitor was used to guide patient management only in the Chronicle group. Primary endpoints included freedom from system-related complications (DSRC), freedom from pressure-sensor failure, and reduction in the rate of HF-related events (hospitalizations and emergency or urgent care visits requiring intravenous therapy). The two safety endpoints were achieved, but the primary efficacy endpoint was not met because the Chronicle group had a nonsignificant 21% lower rate of all HF-related events compared with the control group ($P = .33$).[30]

As a result, in March 2007, the FDA's Circulatory System Devices Panel voted against the approval of Medtronic's implantable hemodynamic monitor because its use did not significantly improve clinical outcomes for HF patients. The COMPASS-HF study did, however, demonstrate chronically elevated filling pressures in many patients that increased the risk of HF events. In addition, patients enrolled had a progressive increase in risk for HF events with higher chronic 24-hour estimated pulmonary artery pressure (event risk 20% at 18 mm Hg, 34% at 25 mm Hg, and 56% at 30 mm Hg).[30,93]

Reducing Events in Patients with Chronic Heart Failure (REDUCEhf)[94] evaluated the use of the Chronicle device that was attached to an ICD to monitor right-sided intracardiac pressures. Endpoints were the same as for COMPASS-HF. REDUCEhf was designed to enroll 1300 patients, but was prematurely stopped with

400 patients due to lead failures. The primary safety endpoint was met, but analysis of available data did not show significant benefit in using invasive hemodynamic monitoring.[95]

Intrathoracic impedance is another parameter that can be used for invasive TM. When fluid accumulates in the lungs, this decreases the impedance to electrical current. In patients with pacing or ICD systems, the impedance between the right ventricular lead and device box has been shown to correlate with the pulmonary capillary wedge pressure in hospitalized patients.[96] The OptiVol feature (Medtronic Inc.) performs a daily measurement of electrical impedance between device box and the right-ventricular electrode, and derives variables for monitoring fluid status. The SENSEHF trial (Sensitivity and Positive Predictive Value of Implantable Intrathoracic Impedance Monitoring as a Predictor of Heart Failure Hospitalizations)[97] evaluated the performance of OptiVol intrathoracic fluid monitoring for the prediction of HF events in chronic HF patients newly implanted with an ICD. This was a prospective, multicenter study that enrolled 501 patients. The authors concluded that an intrathoracic impedance-derived fluid index had low sensitivity and positive predictive value (PPV) in the early period after implantation of a device in chronic HF patients. Sensitivity improved within the first 6 months after implant.[97]

In the PARTNERS HF (Program to Access and Review Trending Information and Evaluate Correlation to Symptoms in Patients with Heart Failure) Study,[27] Whellan and associates sought to determine the utility of combined HF device diagnostic information to predict clinical deterioration of HF in patients with systolic left ventricular dysfunction. This was a prospective, multicenter observational study in patients receiving cardiac resynchronization therapy (CRT) implantable cardioverter-defibrillators. A combined HF device diagnostic algorithm was developed on an independent dataset. The algorithm was considered positive if a patient had two of the following abnormal criteria during a 1-month period: long atrial fibrillation duration, rapid ventricular rate during atrial fibrillation, high (≥60) fluid index, low patient activity, abnormal autonomics (high night heart rate or low heart rate variability), or notable device therapy (low CRT pacing or implantable cardioverter-defibrillator shocks), or if they only had a very high (≥100) fluid index. The authors found that patients with positive combined HF device diagnostics had a 5.5-fold increased risk of HF hospitalization with pulmonary signs or symptoms within the next month (HR 5.5; 95% CI 3.4–8.8; $P < .0001$), and the risk remained high after adjusting for clinical variables (HR 4.8; 95% CI 2.9–8.1; $P < .0001$). The authors concluded that monthly review of HF device diagnostic data identifies patients at a higher risk of HF hospitalizations within the subsequent month.[27]

Two additional trials, MultiSENSE (Multisensor Chronic Evaluation in Ambulatory Heart Failure Patients) and IN-TIME, evaluated CIED based TM. The MultiSENSE study enrolled 900 patients with CRT-D devices and followed them for up to 1 year. A composite index and alert algorithm (HeartLogic) was developed that combined heart sounds, respiration, thoracic impedance, heart rate, and activity. The two coprimary endpoints were sensitivity to detect HF exacerbation greater than 40% and unexplained alert rate more than 2 alerts per patient-year. Both endpoints were significantly exceeded, with sensitivity of 70% (95% CI: 55.4%–82.1%) and an unexplained alert rate of 1.47 per patient-year (95% CI: 1.32–1.65). The median lead time before HFE was 34.0 days (interquartile range: 19.0–66.3 days).[98] In the IN-TIME (Implant-Based Multiparameter Telemonitoring of Patients with Heart Failure) study, patients with HF, NYHA class II–III symptoms, EF of no more than 35%, on guideline directed medical therapy (GDMT), no permanent atrial fibrillation, and a recent dual-chamber ICD or CRT-D implantation were enrolled. Patients were randomly assigned (1:1) to automatic, daily, implant-based, multiparameter TM,

in addition to standard care or standard care without TM. At 1 year, 63 (18.9%) of 333 patients in the TM group versus 90 (27.2%) of 331 in the control group ($P = .013$) had a worsened composite score (OR 0·63, 95% CI 0·43–0·90).[99] Both of these trials supported multiparameter CIED based TM.

The next iteration of CIED for invasive TM was the CardioMEMS, which is a pulmonary artery pressure sensor that is passive, wireless, uses radiofrequency sensing, and is without batteries or leads. The CHAMPION (CardioMEMS Heart Sensor Allows Monitoring of Pressure to Improve Outcomes in NYHA Class III HF Patients)[31] trial was a prospective, multicenter, randomized, single-blinded study designed to evaluate whether pulmonary artery pressure–guided treatment of HF was better than usual care. All patients underwent implantation of the device, but no pulmonary artery pressure measurements were performed in the control group. In the treatment group, clinicians used daily measurement of pulmonary artery pressures in addition to standard of care versus standard of care alone in the control group. The primary efficacy endpoint was the rate of HF–related hospitalizations at 6 months. The safety endpoints assessed at 6 months were freedom from device-related or DSRC and freedom from pressure-sensor failures. At 6 months, 84 HF–related hospitalizations were reported in the treatment group ($n = 270$) compared with 120 in the control group ($n = 280$; rate 0.32 vs. 0.44; HR 0.72; 95% CI 0.60–0.85; $P = .0002$; **Fig 47.4**). During the entire follow-up (mean 15 months [SD 7]), the treatment group had a 37% reduction in HF–related hospitalization compared with the control group (158 vs. 254; HR 0.63; 95% CI 0.52–0.77; $P < .0001$). Eight patients had DSRC, and overall freedom from DSRC was 98.6% (97.3–99.4), compared with a prespecified performance criterion of 80% ($P < .0001$), and overall freedom from pressure-sensor failures was 100% (99.3–100.0). The authors concluded that wireless, implantable hemodynamic monitors in patients with NYHA class III HF significantly improved HF management.[31]

Despite the apparent benefit of the CardioMEMS device based on results of the CHAMPION trial, in December 2011 the FDA decided that there was not reasonable assurance that the CardioMEMS monitoring system was effective and decided not to approve the device.[100] The FDA committee members based their decision not to approve the device on concerns regarding analysis of the primary endpoint, differential interaction between the sponsor and principal investigator (PI) with centers regarding management of enrolled patients, and concerns regarding efficacy in subpopulations.[100] The device has undergone further evaluation in response to the FDA review. Following a review to determine the effect of the differential interaction and an independent statistical analysis plan, the device was approved after a second review in 2014. Revised analyses confirmed a 28% lower rate of HF hospitalizations between the treatment and control groups during the first 6 months of the trial (84 vs. 120; $P = .0002$), and a 33% lower rate of HF hospitalizations during the entire randomized access part of the trial (182 vs. 279; $P = .0002$).[101]

A subsequent subgroup analysis of the 456 patients in the CHAMPION trial with HFrEF confirmed the reduction in morbidity and mortality of these patients on GDMT.[102] An analysis of post approval remote monitoring data from the first 2000 U.S. patients implanted with the device showed a slightly higher (34.9 ± 10.2 mm Hg) initial mean pulmonary artery pressure compared with CHAMPION treatment (31.3 ± 10.9 mm Hg) and CHAMPION control (32.0 ± 10.5 mm Hg) groups. They additionally experienced a greater reduction in PA pressure over time compared with the CHAMPION trial.[103] A cost effectiveness analysis found that CardioMEMS incurs a cost per quality adjusted life year of $82,301 in patients with HFrEF and $47,768 in HFpEF,[104] confirming an efficacious, but costly, addition to HF therapy. The use of CardioMEMS has been incorporated into the 2016 ESC

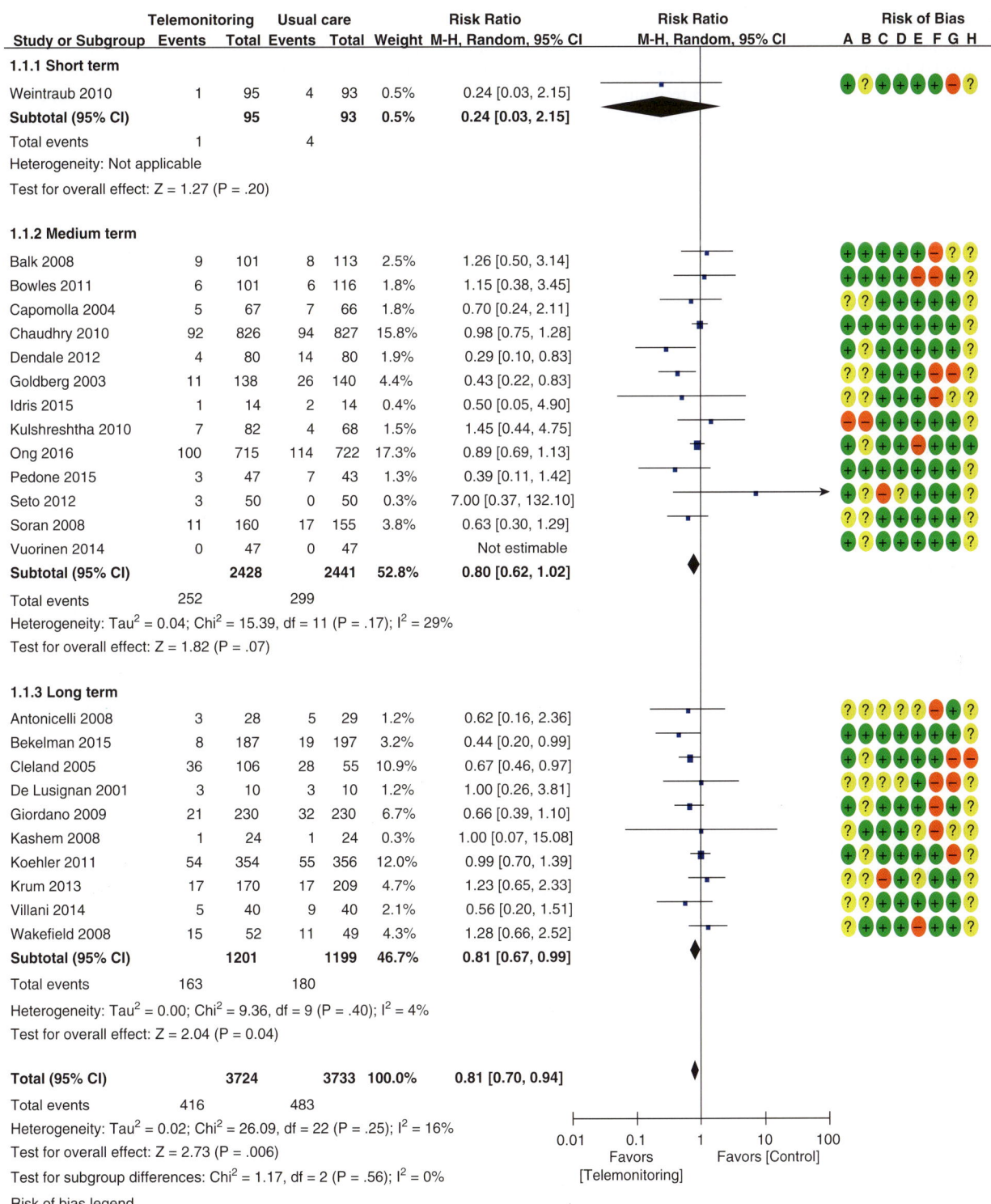

Fig. 47.4 Meta-analyses and forest plot of short-, medium-, and long-term outcomes comparing telemonitoring to usual care for heart failure patients. (From Yun JE, Park JE, Park HY, Lee HY, Park DA. Comparative effectiveness of telemonitoring versus usual care for heart failure: a systematic review and meta-analysis. *J Card Fail.* 2018;24[1]:19–28.)

HF guidelines, which report that monitoring of PA pressures using CardioMEMS may be considered in symptomatic patients with HF with previous HF hospitalization, to reduce the risk of recurrent HF hospitalization. A Class IIb level of evidence B recommendation has been assigned to this statement.[105] Thus far, invasive hemodynamic monitoring has not been addressed in the American HF guidelines.

Wearables and mHealth in Heart Failure

The advent of wearable technology to collect biometric data has been described as a disruptive innovation in medicine, as they have the potential to change the constructs of the systems in which we practice. These devices employ sensors to calculate various parameters, and then transmit this data to a platform such as a smartphone, computer, or the internet. mHealth, or mobile health, refers to the use of mobile or wireless technology in healthcare. Currently there are no professional society guidelines on the use of these devices, and they are not formally classified by the Food and Drug Administration as medical devices.[106] Nevertheless, their presence in the marketplace is increasing, including in the HF space, and therefore a discussion of these devices is warranted.

One of the most ubiquitous technologies comes in the form of mobile phones; mobile apps may offer a solution for symptom monitoring and self-care. A recent analysis identified 34 commercially available mobile applications for HF across Android Google Play, Amazon, and Apple iTunes stores.[107] The authors found they were heterogeneous in nature and the most common functionality was the ability to record information; only three peer-reviewed articles evaluated any of these mobile applications. Thus, although there is much excitement for mobile apps for symptom management in HF, they have not been well studied and have not consistently demonstrated positive effects on patient outcomes.

In 2015, a meta-analysis was done that assessed 31 randomized controlled trials with 25 wearable devices encompassing more than 7000 patients. The monitoring devices (weight, BP, oximetry, ECG heart rate/rhythm) were compared with usual care in HF patients with reduced or preserved EF. In meta-analyses, patients demonstrate that the use of wearable mHealth devices is associated improved outcomes: wearable devices were associated with decreased mortality (RR [95% CI] = .76 [0.63, 0.92]) and the risk of hospitalizations (0.81 [0.72, 0.91]) and appears to improve outcomes among younger (<70 years old) patients with recent hospitalizations.[108] Cajita et al. also performed a review of trials of mHealth based HF interventions.[109] The studies were limited to those that utilized a mobile device paired with ECG, BP, and scales, and the authors found nine studies that fit into these criteria. The results were heterogeneous, with some studies showing lowered mortality while others showed no difference.

The LINK-HF study reported on the use of a small, disposable chest adhesive multisensor patch to predict rehospitalization after HF admission. The patch recorded heart rate, heart rate variability, accelerometry, respiratory rate, and temperature. The data was continuously uploaded via smartphone to a cloud analytics platform. The study enrolled 100 patients from four Veteran's Affairs Hospitals in the United States. The platform analytics for prediction of HF achieved an ROC AUC of 0.88, specificity of 85.9%, sensitivity of 84.2%. Mean and median time between initial alert and readmission was 10.8 ± 9.7 days and 6.0 (4.2; 13.7) days.[110]

The SMILE (Sensible Medical Innovations Lung Fluid Status Monitor Allows Reducing Readmission Rate of Heart Failure Patients) trial evaluated the efficacy of the SensiVest, a product developed by Sensible Medical Innovations, headquartered in Israel. The system is composed of a wearable vest containing two embedded sensors, one in front and one behind the patient, and a bedside console. The vest uses radar technology to "see through" the chest and accurately detect the amount of fluid in the lungs. A patient wears the vest for 90 seconds a day, and the information is collected and automatically uploaded to a cloud server. The patient's cardiologist can review the data to determine if any treatment adjustments need to be made to restore the lungs to healthy fluid levels. The study enrolled 50 patients over 3 years, and found that during the active management period, there were 0.04 readmission/patient per 3 months.[111] This readmission rate was compared to the pre- and postmanagement periods for which readmission rates were 0.30 and 0.19 events/patient per 3 months, respectively. Clinician-investigators received 255 readings from the vest in 41 patients (82% of study participants) for measurements "out of range." In 73% of the notifications (n = 187), the physicians chose to change patient management, mainly by changing medications, and in almost 90% of cases, it involved increasing diuretic dose. Other interventions included counseling the patient to encourage dietary compliance, reinforcing compliance with prescribed medications, and adjustment of thresholds for persistent out-of-range readings despite the optimization of other therapies. Over three-quarters of these actions helped return the vest readings to baseline. While there is excitement and potential for mHealth technologies and wearables, both clinicians and patients will need these tools to be studied and validated before they can be effectively used.

WHY HAVE WE NOT SEEN CLEAR BENEFIT WITH HEART FAILURE DISEASE MANAGEMENT PROGRAMS?

Are We Targeting the Correct Patient Population?

Many of the recent multicenter, randomized, controlled trials on HF disease management programs have been neutral. There are several theories as to why these high-quality studies failed to demonstrate benefit. It is possible that some trials have targeted patient populations that may not necessarily benefit from a structured disease management program. The optimum acuity of illness to target may be NYHA class II and III, or other subpopulations with comorbid illnesses, though further research is needed in this area. In the era of limited health care dollars, it is imperative that we focus our resources in areas where we will derive the most benefit.

Do We Have the Correct Health Care Providers on the Team?

Generalists rather than cardiologists manage most patients with HF.[112] However, HF is a complex problem, with a high rate of treatment failures and rehospitalizations, and therefore may be more optimally managed with the guidance of specialists or subspecialists.[107] Edep and associates conducted a study designed to characterize physician practices in the management of HF and to determine whether these practices vary by specialty and how they relate to guideline recommendations. They found that cardiologists report practices more in conformity with published guidelines for HF than internists and family practitioners. Because of the large numbers of patients with HF and their substantial mortality, morbidity, and cost of care, these differences may have a major impact on outcomes and health care costs.[113]

A barrier to effective care in HF disease management is the time delay between identification of a problem and initiation of a treatment. The requirement that HF coordinators review data with physicians can introduce delays in care. Small studies have suggested that the team member receiving the data should be empowered to contact the patient directly with a treatment plan, without having to "triangulate" the discussion with a physician before recommending a plan to the patient (**Fig. 47.5**).[114]

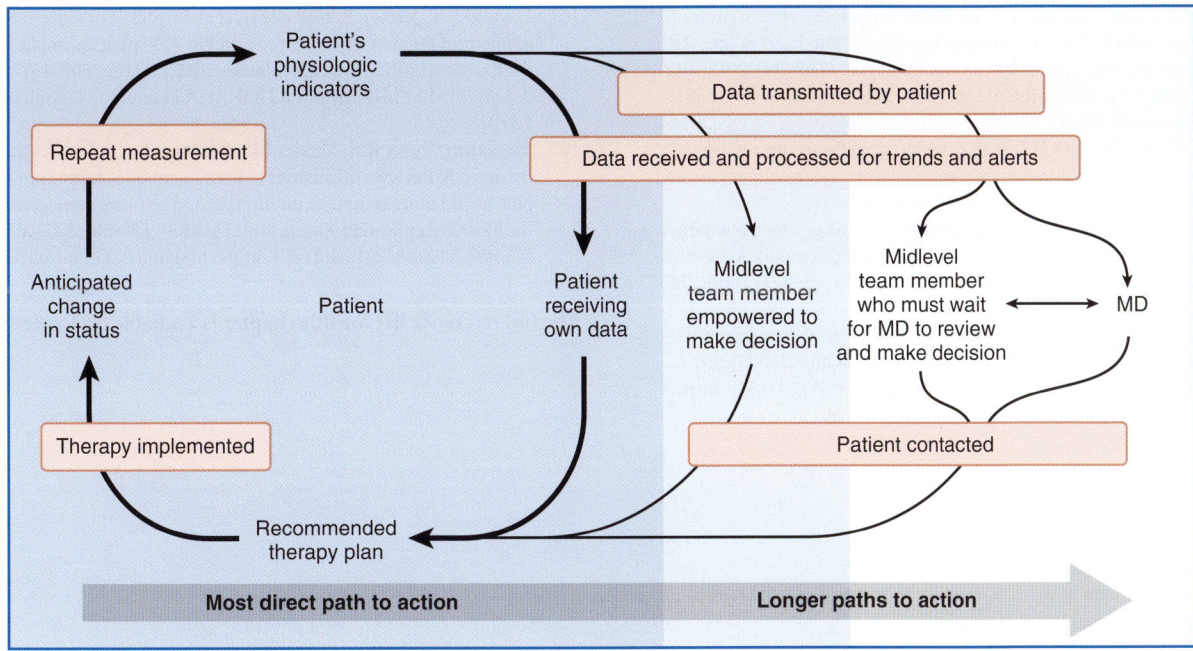

Fig. 47.5 The circle of home management of heart failure. (From Desai AS, Stevenson LW. Connecting the circle from home to heart failure disease management. *N Engl J Med.* 2010;363[24]2364–2367.)

Are We Measuring the Right Parameters?

Remote-monitoring approaches rely on the premise that routine surveillance of selected physiologic indicators will facilitate early detection of clinical deterioration and direct timely intervention to prevent adverse outcomes.[114] In regard to the Tele-HF trial, Desai and Stevenson hypothesize that an increase in weight and symptoms (the parameters monitored in the study) may not provide adequate warning. Results from trials of ambulatory hemodynamic monitoring in patients with HF suggest that weight is a poor surrogate for filling pressures and may be inadequate to anticipate the onset of decompensation.[90] The association between body weight and volume status lessens as the time since hospital discharge increases, because the target dry weight changes on the basis of caloric intake.[114] Although thoracic impedance alone was shown to be insensitive at predicting HF decompensation in patients with newly implanted ICDs, this parameter has been demonstrated to predict hospital readmission in PARTNERS-HF when viewed in combination with other parameters or when the threshold was set at a very high fluid index.[27] Although as clinicians we have been trained to treat the patients' symptoms and not a set of numbers or laboratory values, if markers are identified that predict decompensation before symptoms occur, early initiation of treatment may ward off deterioration and the need for hospitalization.

FUTURE DIRECTION OF HEART FAILURE DISEASE MANAGEMENT PROGRAMS

The most expensive aspect of health care in high-income countries is staff to run services and deliver care. Delivering care by increasing direct one-to-one interactions is likely to be an expensive long-term strategy.[63] Therefore, telemedicine and TM is likely to become a more prevalent component of HF disease management programs. However, there seems to be no standardization across the programs and interventions. In contrast, diabetes is successfully managed by empowering patients to use technology to monitor and treat their conditions. In the future, patients may be able to adjust their own diuretic regimen on the basis of daily readings from internal monitors. Similar to the insulin pump, "smart" drug-delivery systems can perhaps be developed to trigger the automated release of medications in response to cardiorenal indicators.[114] Further research is needed to develop accurate, user-friendly technology to provide patients with real-time feedback regarding their clinical status. We also need to develop mechanisms to allow relevant data to be transmitted to health care providers in a timely manner so that appropriate treatments can be initiated quickly. A downside to TM is the daily generation of reams of data, most of which is irrelevant to patient care. Managing this volume of information will likely increase the need for midlevel personnel specialized in HF management and may also create new concerns about liability for unread transmissions.[114] Data management will be an important component of HF disease management in the future. Until we determine the most efficacious way of delivering HF disease management to all patients, we must be judicious and use it in patients who will likely derive the most benefit, such as elderly, vulnerable, and underserved populations.

KEY REFERENCES

22. Ferrante D, Varini S, Macchia A, et al. Long-term results after a telephone intervention in chronic heart failure: DIAL (Randomized Trial of Phone Intervention in Chronic Heart Failure) follow-up. *J Am Coll Cardiol.* 2010;56(5):372–378.
28. Chaudhry SI, Mattera JA, Curtis JP, et al. Telemonitoring in patients with heart failure. *N Engl J Med.* 2010;363(24):2301–2309.
63. Inglis SC, Clark RA, McAlister FA, et al. Which components of heart failure programmes are effective? A systematic review and meta-analysis of the outcomes of structured telephone support or telemonitoring as the primary component of chronic heart failure management in 8323 patients: abridged Cochrane review. *Eur J Heart Fail.* 2011;13(9):1028–1040.
84. Bekelman DB, Plomondon ME, Carey EP, et al. Primary results of the Patient-Centered Disease Management (PCDM) for heart failure study: a randomized clinical trial. *JAMA Intern Med.* 2015;175(5):725–732. https://doi.org/710.1001/jamainternmed.2015.0315.

86. Kotb A, Cameron C, Hsieh S, Wells G. Comparative effectiveness of different forms of telemedicine for individuals with heart failure (HF): a systematic review and network meta-analysis. *PLoS One.* 2015;10(2). e0118681. https://doi.org/10118610.0111371/journal.pone.0118681. eCollection:0112015.

87. Yun JE, Park JE, Park HY, et al. Comparative effectiveness of telemonitoring versus usual care for heart failure: a systematic review and meta-analysis. *J Card Fail.* 2018;24(1):19–28.

89. Frederix I, Solmi F, Piepoli MF, Dendale P. Cardiac telerehabilitation: a novel cost-efficient care delivery strategy that can induce long-term health benefits. *Eur J Prev Cardiol.* 2017;24(16):1708–1717. https://doi.org/1710.1177/2047487317732274.

99. Hindricks G, Taborsky M, Glikson M, et al. Implant-based multiparameter telemonitoring of patients with heart failure (IN-TIME): a randomised controlled trial. *Lancet.* 2014;384(9943):583–590. https://doi.org/510.1016/S0140-6736(1014)61176-61174.

103. Heywood JT, Jermyn R, Shavelle D, et al. Impact of practice-based management of pulmonary artery pressures in 2000 patients implanted with the CardioMEMS Sensor. *Circulation.* 2017;135(16):1509–1517. https://doi.org/71510.1161/CIRCULATIONAHA.1116.026184. Epub 022017 Feb 026120.

107. Masterson Creber RM, Maurer MS, Reading M, Hiraldo G, Hickey KT, Iribarren S. Review and analysis of existing mobile phone apps to support heart failure symptom monitoring and self-care management using the Mobile Application Rating Scale (MARS). Eysenbach G, ed. *JMIR Mhealth Uhealth.* 2016;4(2):e74. https://doi.org/710.2196/mhealth.5882.

The full reference list for this chapter is available on ExpertConsult.

48

Management of Comorbidities in Heart Failure

Justin A. Ezekowitz

Patients with heart failure (HF) often have multiple comorbid conditions that may interact with the syndrome of HF and/or the choice of therapies. Research into the common comorbid conditions has furthered the understanding of the pathophysiologic basis for symptoms or structural abnormalities of HF, aided in the refinement of the often-complicated management because of the competing therapies, and provided clarity regarding the diagnostic certainty (or uncertainty) as a result of competing causes for signs and symptoms of disease. In clinical practice, this is seen on a day-to-day basis, and thus understanding the management of HF requires consideration of all aspects of human health.

In most chronic HF registry, administrative, or trial data, the number of comorbid conditions exceeds five (including other related components of cardiovascular disease [e.g., atrial fibrillation]) for many patients.[1] From the major registry data, the most common comorbid conditions and their approximate prevalence are depression (22%),[2] chronic obstructive pulmonary disease (COPD) (20%–30%),[1,2] diabetes (30%),[3] and sleep-disordered breathing (40%).[4] Other important cardiovascular conditions that interact with HF, such as atrial fibrillation (**see Chapter 38**) or coronary artery disease (**see Chapter 19**), are discussed elsewhere.

Importantly, although all of these comorbid conditions have a significant impact on prognosis, the specific treatment of the comorbid condition has generally not been shown to improve major clinical outcomes. For example, treating depression with sertraline did not lead to a reduction in cardiovascular events.[7] This creates a unique situation for clinicians caring for patients with HF because they require expert management beyond the disease-disease and drug-drug interactions. Each disease (HF and a comorbid condition) can exacerbate or be a trigger for the other, or complicate the treatment course because therapies typically used for the comorbid condition of interest may indeed exacerbate HF (e.g., etanercept for rheumatoid arthritis). Likewise, some therapies can be used for both, allowing for rational selection of therapy (e.g., angiotensin-converting enzyme [ACE] inhibitors for HF and diabetes) or potentially synergistic effects (continuous positive airway pressure [CPAP] for sleep apnea may induce better control of atrial fibrillation and HF symptoms). Thus the interaction is often far more complex than first anticipated, and clinicians should be aware and ask five simple questions when faced with this situation (**Table 48.1**). However, each situation will be unique, and where possible, an informed choice can be made by integrating information from the published literature, patient preferences, and in consultation with other health professionals.

ANEMIA AND IRON DEFICIENCY

Definitions, Prevalence, and Outcomes

Anemia is defined by the World Health Organization as a hemoglobin less than 13.0 g/dL in men and less than 12.0 g/dL in women. Additional other definitions are available, including those of the Centers for Disease Control and Prevention (<13.0 g/dL in men and <12.5 g/dL in women)[5] and National Kidney Foundation (<13.5 g/dL in males and <12.0 g/dL in females)[6] or by diagnosis (chart abstract coding) of anemia.[7] Using these definitions, the prevalence of anemia in patients with chronic HF has been found to be vary substantially based on the location or context surveyed, severity of illness, age, gender, race, and whether or not they were patients with acute or chronic HF. Given the limitations listed previously, the prevalence is approximately 15% to 20%[7,8] and approximately 30% to 50% in either acute HF populations or specialized clinics,[9,10] summarized elsewhere.[11]

More recently, there has been a better understanding that iron deficiency may be more important than the hemoglobin itself. **Table 48.2** highlights the definitions for iron deficiency, with a recognition that the most common definition in clinical trials is a ferritin less than 100 ng/mL, or iron saturation less than 20% if the ferritin ranges from 100 to 300 ng/mL.

Anemia has been associated with poor clinical outcomes. The within-person changes to hemoglobin over time may have additional

TABLE 48.1 Five Questions to Ask When Reviewing the Comorbid Condition in a Patient With Heart Failure

	Question	Considerations	Example
1.	Does the comorbid condition affect the characteristics of a test used to diagnosis or manage HF?	Test sensitivity or specificity modified due to known or unknown confounders because of the comorbid condition.	BNP levels in patients who are obese are lower than nonobese patients.
2.	Does HF affect the characteristics of a test used to diagnosis or manage a comorbid condition?	HF may modify the underlying pathophysiology upon which the test is based.	Pulmonary function tests can be abnormal for patients with HF even in the absence of COPD.
3.	Did this comorbid condition or its related therapies "cause" or exacerbate HF in this patient?	Some disease-disease links are strong, whereas others are putative.	Diabetic cardiomyopathy; anthracyclines for cancer
4.	Does the comorbid condition modify the options for treatment of HF?	Some therapies used in HF need to be carefully selected so as not to worsen a comorbid condition.	The risk/benefit of ACE inhibitors in end-stage renal disease; volume management with diuretics in COPD; appropriateness of cardiac resynchronization therapy in advanced COPD
5.	Should we modify the management of the comorbid condition due to the presence of HF?	Known risks for some therapies may include exacerbating HF.	Etanercept for rheumatoid arthritis; Herceptin for breast cancer

ACE, Angiotensin-converting enzyme; *BNP,* B-type natriuretic peptide; *COPD,* chronic obstructive pulmonary disease; *HF,* heart failure.

TABLE 48.2 Diagnostic Assays of Clinical Use for the Cause of Anemia

Category	Etiology	Test	Possible Results	Other Notes
General		Peripheral smear	Microcytic, normocytic, or macrocytic	Nondiagnostic but helpful for further testing
		Reticulocyte count/index	RI 1%–2% = normal; RI <2% with anemia = blood loss or inadequate bone marrow response; RI >3% bone marrow compensation	Helpful for determining bone marrow response to therapy
		Bone marrow biopsy	Variable	Invasive; often used for diagnosis in selected diseases
Blood loss	Gastrointestinal	Endoscopy	Ulcers, erosions, masses, polyps	Consider all antiplatelet, anticoagulant, and NSAID use
		Fecal occult blood	Positive compatible with IDA or blood loss	Consider further testing to identify source
Nutritional deficiency	Folate	Serum folate	<4 ng/mL	Can drop in acute illness
		RBC folate	Variable based on assay	Indicative of folate deficiency
		Serum B$_{12}$	<200 pg/mL	May need additional testing for pernicious anemia
	Iron	Serum transferrin saturation	<20% compatible with IDA	
		Ferritin	<50 ng/mL compatible with IDA	Can be elevated due to inflammation in HF
Sickle cell		Hemoglobin electrophoresis	HbSS, HbSC	
Thalassemia		Hemoglobin electrophoresis	% αβδ Hb	
Other		Ultrasound of kidneys, liver, spleen	Medicorenal disease; cirrhosis; splenomegaly	

Hb, Hemoglobin; *HF,* heart failure; *IDA,* iron deficiency anemia; *NSAID,* nonsteroidal antiinflammatory drug; *RBC,* red blood cell; *RI,* reticulocyte index.

importance. In the Valsartan Heart Failure trial (Val-HEFT), 16.9% of patients developed new-onset anemia, and a decline in hemoglobin over 12 months was strongly related to subsequent clinical outcomes even after adjusting for prognostic markers such as B-type natriuretic peptide (BNP) and estimated glomerular filtration rate (eGFR).[12] Most of the studies of patients with anemia and HF highlight a 1.5- to 2-fold increase in short- and long-term mortality even after adjustment for other clinical variables.

Diagnosis of Anemia

The diagnosis of anemia is a combination of symptoms, signs, and biomarkers related to the hematopoietic system. Given the substantial overlap of symptoms of HF and anemia (e.g., fatigue, shortness of breath), there are no specific symptoms that appear to aid diagnosis.

Similarly, given the lack of specificity of physical signs of anemia, there are no additional signs to aid in the diagnosis of anemia in a patient with HF.

The biomarkers for diagnosing and exploring the cause or subtype of anemia are multiple and well developed (see Table 48.2). They are aimed at diagnosing the most common conditions (nutritional deficiency or blood loss), ruling out other related diseases (bone-related malignancy, thyroid disease, sickle cell anemia, thalassemia), or establishing a diagnosis of anemia of chronic disease related to HF. Most patients will require some combination of the testing and repeat testing if an intervention is done (e.g., iron therapy should be followed by a repeat hemoglobin, iron saturation, and ferritin).

Given the variety of causes for anemia, targeted diagnosis and therapy are important (**Fig. 48.1**). However, many patients (up to 46%

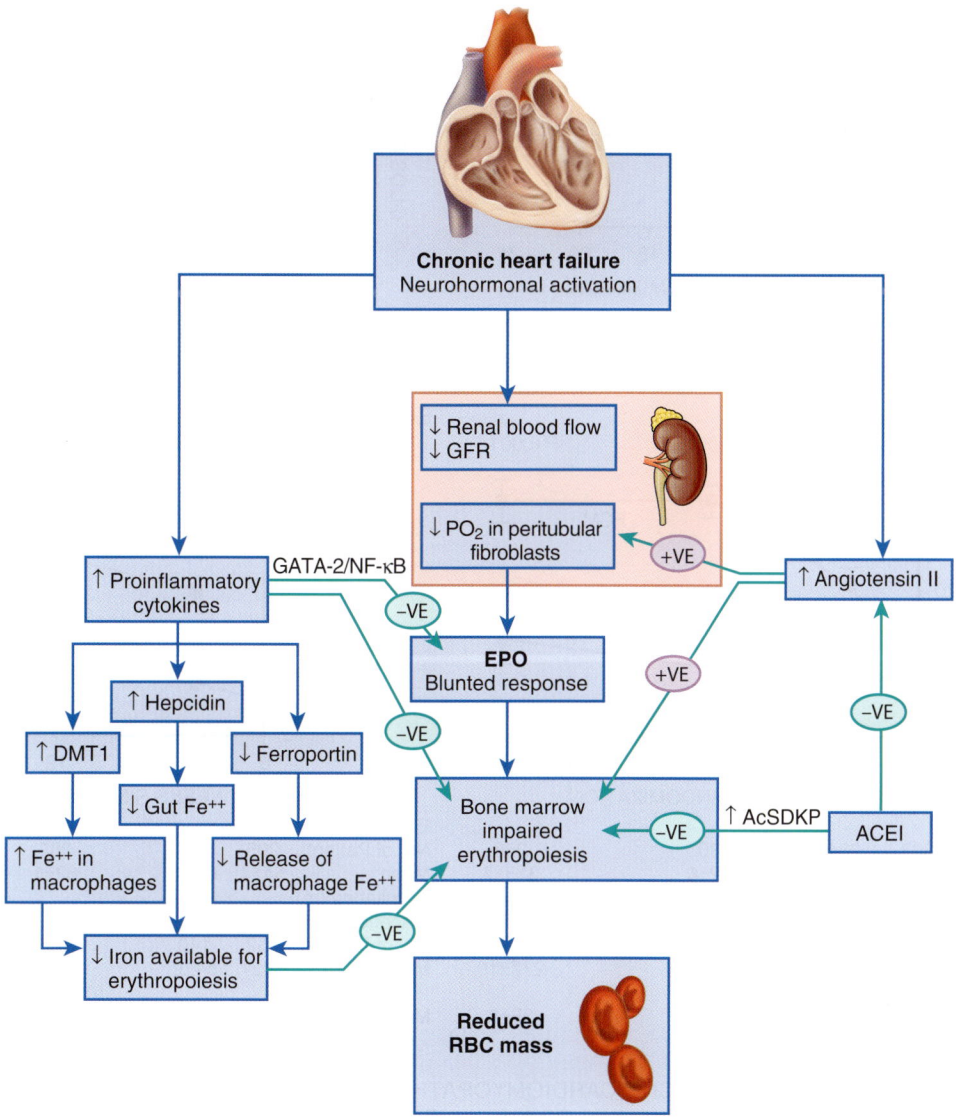

Fig. 48.1 Possible mechanisms involved in the genesis of anemia in heart failure. Shown is a diagram of the possible mechanisms of anemia in patients with heart failure. *ACEI,* Angiotensin-converting enzyme inhibitor; *AcSDKP, N*-acetyl-seryl-aspartyl-lysyl-proline; *DMT1,* divalent metal transporter 1; *EPO,* epoetin; *GFR,* glomerular filtration rate; *NF-κB,* nuclear factor-kappa B; *RBC,* red blood cell mass. (From Anand IS. Anemia and chronic heart failure implications and treatment options. *J Am Coll Cardiol.* 2008;52[7]:501–511. Illustration by Rob Flewell.)

in one series[13]) may have hemodilution as a cause of their anemia, so judicious measurement of hemoglobin after euvolemia is attained is essential when evaluating patients with anemia.

Treatment

Once a clear or working diagnosis is obtained, therapy will be targeted to the potential cause. The general approach to the treatment of anemia is beyond the scope of this chapter; thus the remainder of this section will focus on the results of randomized controlled trials (RCTs) that specifically enrolled patients with HF.

Iron therapy has remained the mainstay of therapy for iron deficiency anemia. Many guidelines recommend a trial of oral iron therapy, although this had not been subjected to rigorous study in patients with cardiovascular disease until the Iron Repletion Effects on Oxygen Uptake in Heart Failure (IRONOUT-HF) trial.[14] In this trial, 225 patients with left ventricular ejection fraction (LVEF) less than 40% and iron deficiency were randomized to 150 mg of iron polysaccharide

or placebo for 16 weeks. There was no difference between groups in 6-minute walk test, quality of life, N-terminal pro–B-type natriuretic peptide (NT-proBNP), or exercise capacity. Intravenous iron injections have recently been the subject of RCTs. The Ferinject Assessment in Patients with Iron Deficiency and Chronic Heart Failure (FAIR-HF) trial assessed patients with New York Heart Association (NYHA) class II or III, LVEF of less than or equal to 45%, and a hemoglobin between 95 and 135 g/dL, with iron deficiency anemia (ferritin <100 μg/L or was between 100 and 299 μg/L and transferrin saturation <20%).[15] For the primary end point at 24 weeks of Patient Global Assessment (PGA) and compared with a placebo, patients randomized to intravenous iron (and titrated to iron indices) had a twofold chance of improving (by PGA or one NYHA class). Similar positive outcomes were seen for the EQ-5D, KCCQ (Kansas City Cardiomyopathy Questionairre), and 6-minute walk test without any significant safety signal (or efficacy for clinical events) (**Fig. 48.2**). Three other trials have had similar results, summarized elsewhere,[16] and there are ongoing studies

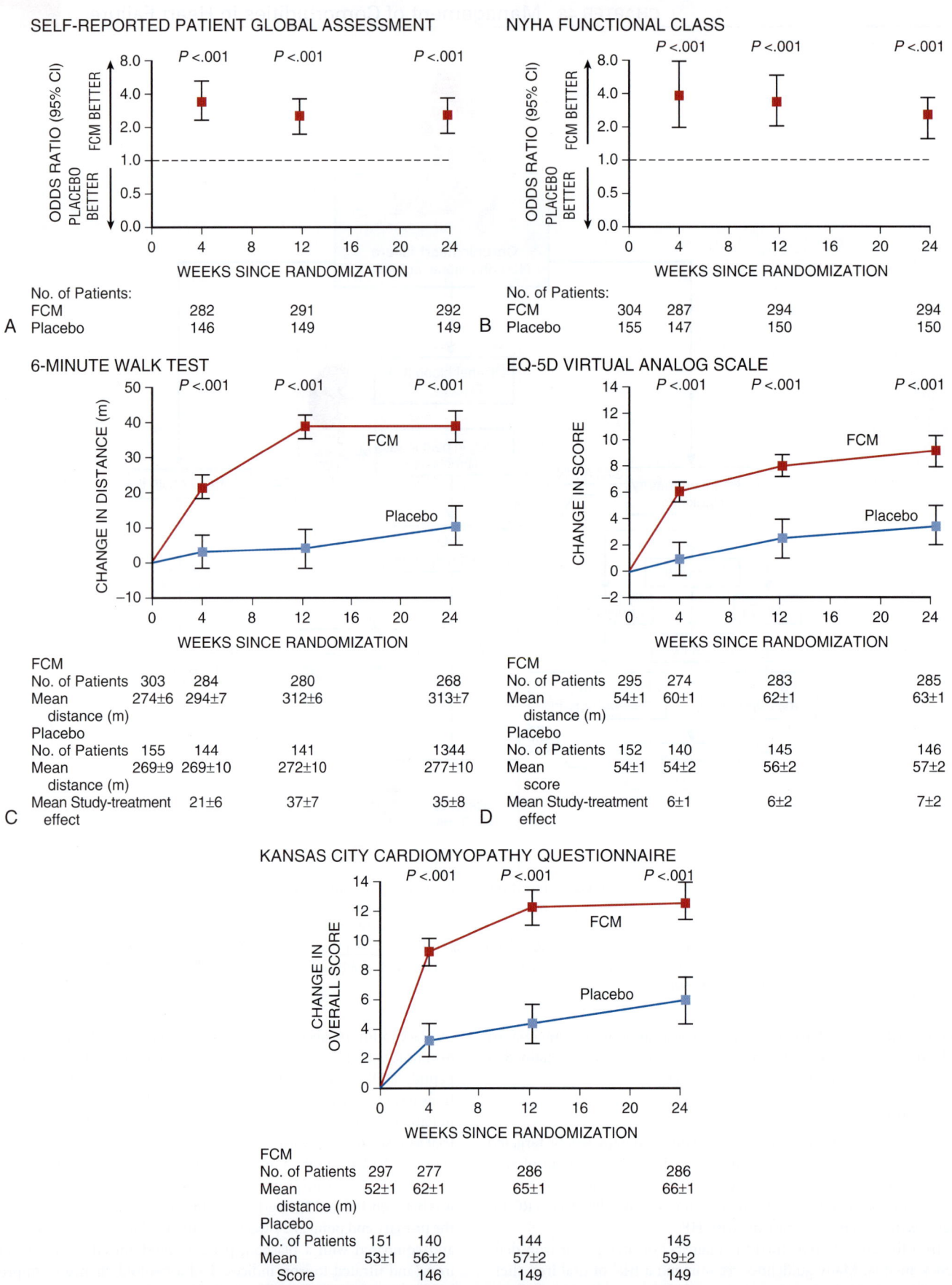

Fig. 48.2 Ferinject assessment in patients with iron deficiency and chronic heart failure trial results. The effects of ferric carboxymaltose on (A) patient global assessment, (B) New York Heart Association functional class, (C) 6-minute walk test, (D) EQ-5D, and (E) Kansas City Cardiomyopathy Questionnaire. *FCM*, Ferric carboxymaltose; *NYHA*, New York Heart Association. (From Anker SD, Comin Colet J, Filippatos G, et al. Ferric carboxymaltose in patients with heart failure and iron deficiency. *N Engl J Med*. 2009;361[25]:2436–2448.)

(clinicaltrials.gov: NCT00384657, NCT01453608, NCT03037931). Adequately powered RCTs such HEART-FID are required to assess if important clinical outcomes are altered. In the interim, it appears that intravenous iron is a reasonable therapeutic choice for carefully selected patients with the goal of improving symptoms.

Erythropoiesis-stimulating agents (ESAs), including erythropoietin and darbepoetin, are used in patients with chronic kidney disease to increase the hemoglobin level. In the RED-HF trial, 2278 patients with a LVEF less than or equal to 40%, NYHA II-IV, and a hemoglobin between 9.0 and 12.0 g/dL were randomized to darbepoetin or a placebo and a target hemoglobin of 13.0 g/dL and followed for a median of 28 months.[17] Overall, there was no meaningful difference between the groups for important clinical outcomes, including quality of life, symptoms, death, or rehospitalization; thus there was no additional benefit in a strategy of increasing hemoglobin via an ESA for clinical outcomes.

Summary/Conclusions

Ongoing trials of intravenous iron replacement for anemic patients or as an agent to improve clinical outcomes even in nonanemic patients are key steps in understanding if the correction of anemia can alter clinical outcomes. Key interactions between the bone marrow, the hematologic system, and the vasculature have both shed light on the mechanisms of anemia and helped in the understanding of other pathophysiologic roles of new molecules (e.g., hepcidin),[18] "old" systems (e.g., renin-angiotensin-aldosterone), or new targets (iron receptors).[19]

CHRONIC OBSTRUCTIVE PULMONARY DISEASE

Definitions, Prevalence, and Outcomes

The diagnosis of COPD is done by a combination of clinical history and physical examination findings and is confirmed by spirometry. The most commonly used criteria are the Global Initiative for Chronic Obstructive Lung Disease (GOLD) criteria that define COPD as a post-bronchodilator fixed ratio of FEV_1/FVC of 0.70 or less (**Table 48.3**).[20] Both obstructive and restrictive components of COPD are recognized as important and can coexist.

Given the significant overlap in symptoms, such as shortness of breath, fatigue, and other descriptors, studies have not shown that the two diseases can be distinguished based on symptoms.[21] Studies using the Framingham or other diagnostic symptom-based criteria are less useful given this overlap and can provide erroneous estimates of incidence, prevalence, or outcome relationships.[22] Similarly, the physical signs of HF may overlap, and specifically right ventricular failure

TABLE 48.3 Classification of Chronic Obstructive Lung Disease

Stage	FEV_1/FVC	Predicted FEV_1
Stage I: mild	<0.70	>80%
Stage II: moderate	<0.70	50%–79%
Stage III: severe	<0.70	30%–49%
Stage IV: very severe	<0.70	<30% or <50% plus chronic respiratory failure[a]

[a]Respiratory failure: arterial partial pressure of oxygen (Pao_2), 8.0 kPa (60 mm Hg) with or without arterial partial pressure of CO_2 ($Paco_2$). 6.7 kPa (50 mm Hg) while breathing air at sea level.
Adapted from Rabe KF, Hurd S, Anzueto A, et al. Global strategy for the diagnosis, management, and prevention of chronic obstructive pulmonary disease: GOLD executive summary. *Am J Respir Crit Care Med.* 2007;176(6):532–555.
FEV_1, Forced expiratory volume in 1 second; *FVC,* forced vital capacity.

signs may be evident in both diseases related to secondary pulmonary hypertension and direct myocardial effects. The overlap is summarized elsewhere.[23]

As a comorbidity in community-based surveys, COPD is present in up to one-third of outpatients,[1,2] distributed relatively between those with a reduced or preserved ejection fraction.[24] Importantly, many RCTs of current evidence-based therapy excluded COPD or other respiratory disorders, so estimates of prevalence from RCTs should be evaluated cautiously. Hence, establishing the diagnosis of COPD in a patient with HF, or HF in a patient with COPD, requires clinical vigilance, understanding the overlapping risk factors (e.g., smoking), and testing for both diseases.

Pulmonary Function Tests and Heart Failure

Pulmonary function tests (PFTs) and spirometry involve establishing the key parameters of FEV_1, FVC, lung diffusion of carbon monoxide (DLCO), and peak expiratory flow rate. As discussed previously, the diagnosis of COPD may be evident as per the GOLD criteria, but there are limitations to consider. For example, interstitial edema may cause partial obstruction and increased bronchial sensitivity leading to an obstructive pattern on PFTs.[25] This may partially or fully resolve after a patient diuresis if they were acutely ill.[26] Interestingly, peak expiratory flow has recently been assessed for its use as a clinical end point for RCTs of acute HF therapy given the relatively dynamic change seen over the first 24 hours of therapy.[27] Restrictive defects are also commonly evident[28] and may be caused by underlying lung disease, respiratory muscle weakness, secondary drug effects (e.g., amiodarone), or concomitant diseases (e.g., sarcoidosis).

The diffusion capacity is measured by the DLCO and reflects both the ability of gases to go across the membrane and the volume of blood in the capillary bed. It can change acutely and is linked to abnormal lung mechanics and severity of HF and should be interpreted with caution.[29] Nevertheless, PFTs should be done once the patient is clinically stable and preferably once adequately diuresed if the comorbid condition of COPD is being considered.

Treatment

Heart Failure–Related Treatment in Patients With COPD

The mainstay of therapy, including renin-angiotensin-aldosterone axis agents (e.g., ACE inhibitors, angiotensin receptor blockers [ARBs], mineralocorticoid receptor antagonists [MRAs]), have all been shown to be effective in patients with lung disease in the large RCTs and should be initiated and titrated accordingly. Other therapies, including defibrillators, cardiac resynchronization therapy, digoxin, nitrates, and diuretics, have limited data because of the limited enrollment in trials, and thus the results of RCTs should be applied with that caveat.

Beta-blockers and COPD have been controversial in terms of their use, effect on respiratory function, and clinical outcomes. Most of the earlier beta-blocker RCTs excluded patients with known COPD, given the concern of beta-receptor stimulation versus blockade in patients with reactive airways disease. As such, the RCT experience is limited, but no overt "risk" has been seen,[30] and the small subgroups have shown a preserved (although underpowered) treatment effect in the larger RCTs. Large population-based analyses have shown that, after propensity matching,[31] beta-blockers were associated with a reduced risk of mortality when used in patients with COPD and concomitant HF.

A small mechanistic trial of patients with severe COPD (baseline FEV_1 = 1.3 L) tested the beta_1-selective beta-blocker bisoprolol versus a placebo on the FEV_1 and noted a significant, small reduction in FEV_1 but no alteration of the reversibility following beta-agonists and overall lung volumes and no negative symptoms, impairment of quality of life, or clinical events.[32] One conclusion, given the limited sample

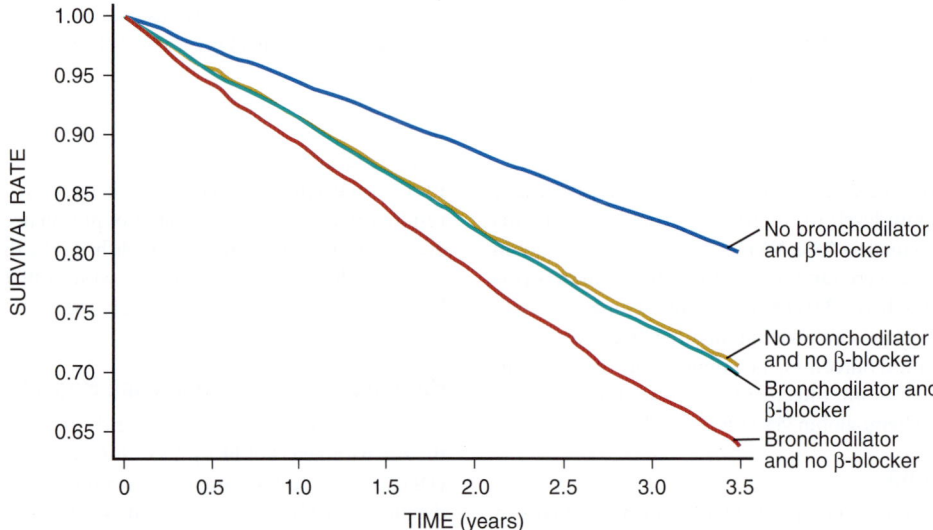

Fig. 48.3 Characteristics and outcomes of patients with heart failure receiving bronchodilators. (Adapted from Hawkins NM, Wang D, Petrie MC, et al. Baseline characteristics and outcomes of patients with heart failure receiving bronchodilators in the CHARM programme. *Eur J Heart Fail.* 2010;12[6]:557–565.)

size and large treatment effect in other populations, is that this reduction in FEV$_1$ is of minimal clinical importance and overweighed by the potential reduction in clinical events related to HF. Thus selection of a beta$_1$-selective beta-blocker with clinical trial evidence is limited to that of bisoprolol[32,33] and metoprolol succinate,[34] and could be considered in preference to carvedilol in this select population.

New agents such as ivabradine may be an option for patients with concomitant COPD who are unable to tolerate a beta-blocker. In the SHIFT trial, 10% of patients with a clear indication for a beta-blocker were not on any beta-blocker, and of these, one-third identified COPD as the principal reason.[35] In addition, in multivariable analysis, COPD was associated with being on a beta-blocker at less than 50% of target dose (odds ratio 0.67; 95% confidence interval [CI] 0.55–0.80),[36] and the effects of ivabradine versus placebo were still preserved. This indicates that for many patients with concomitant COPD and HF, ivabradine may be an option for reducing morbidity or mortality.

Chronic Obstructive Pulmonary Disease Treatment in Patients With Heart Failure

Concomitant inhaled bronchodilators, anticholinergic agents, and steroids form the therapeutic strategy for most patients with COPD. The controversy and an updated systematic review have summarized this elsewhere.[37] Bronchodilators, specifically the beta$_2$-agonists (e.g., formoterol, salbutamol, salmeterol, terbutaline), have efficacy in patients with COPD, but the trials have systematically excluded patients with HF.[38] Whether or not the association of harm for the use of these agents in patients with HF seen in observational studies is replicated in prospective RCTs is uncertain (**Fig. 48.3**).[41] Given the overlap in symptoms and difficulty in separating out the shared risk factors and similarity in patterns for hospitalization along with the confounding by indication of the use of beta-agonists, caution should be exercised before restricting the use of beta-agonists for patients with concomitant COPD and HF. Nevertheless, it would appear, given there are choices for initial therapy, that an anticholinergic may be a better first line choice. The anticholinergic agents (ipratropium, tiotropium) principally act via the cholinergic system. Tiotropium has been tested versus salmeterol and appears to have better efficacy in patients with at least moderate COPD to prevent exacerbations of COPD and has demonstrated relatively neutral safety outcomes.[39] Thus the strategy of

a long-acting anticholinergic agent would appear to be the appropriate strategy for patients with HF until further clinical trial information is available.

Inhaled steroids appear to have a relatively neutral safety profile and positive effect for clinical outcomes; however, oral steroids should be considered carefully. Oral steroids can produce intense sodium (and fluid) retention and thus should be used with caution.

Summary/Conclusions

The diagnosis of COPD in a patient with HF and vice versa is challenging despite clinical acumen, chest x-rays, and standard biomarkers. When COPD is present in a patient with HF, it conveys a negative prognosis and treatment should be targeted toward maximizing evidence-based therapies for HF and encouraging appropriate use of COPD therapies where applicable.

SLEEP-DISORDERED BREATHING

Definitions, Prevalence, and Outcomes

Sleep-disordered breathing is a complex interaction of neurologic, respiratory, cardiac, and mechanical events that create "apneic episodes." Apnea is typically defined as cessation of air flow for more than 10 seconds, whereas hypopnea is a 50% reduction in air flow.[40] The diagnosis of either obstructive sleep apnea (OSA) or central sleep apnea (CSA) involves quantifying the apnea-hypopnea index (AHI), typically expressed as a ratio of events per hour: mild (5–15 events), moderate (15–30 events), or severe (>30 events). Typically, to diagnose OSA or CSA, a full laboratory-based polysomnography study is needed and ambulatory methods considered best for areas where access is limited or for screening in patients at risk.

OSA is often a combination of reduced muscle tone, complemented by fluid shifts and increased tissue in the oropharynx (**Fig. 48.4A**).[41] CSA is a complex interaction of a reduction in Paco$_2$, leading to loss of the central drive for breathing, and involves the chemoreceptors, changes in venous blood flow, and vagal nerve activity in addition to other elements (see Fig. 48.4B).[42]

Up to 50% of patients with systolic HF have either CSA or OSA when formally assessed by laboratory-based polysomnography.[4] Importantly, most of these patients have moderate to severe OSA or

CSA, and the diagnosis tracks with the severity of illness. Patients with HF who are older than 60 years, are male, and have atrial fibrillation have been consistently shown to be at risk for CSA.[4,43] In patients with HF and preserved systolic function, 69% were found to have OSA (40%) or CSA (29%), and this was related to the diastolic function by echocardiogram, performance on a 6-minute walk test, or cardiopulmonary exercise test and higher NT-proBNP levels.[44] When present, OSA or CSA was found to be a risk factor for ventricular arrhythmias in 472 patients with a cardiac resynchronization therapy–defibrillator (CRT-D) device, and as the AHI increased the risk also increased, thus postulating the cause behind the relationship between OSA or CSA and mortality.[45]

Treatment

The treatment of OSA and CSA remain controversial. OSA is typically treated with nasal CPAP, and surrogate outcomes show general improvement in smaller RCTs testing this hypothesis for patients with HF.[46-48] No longer-term studies have shown a reduction in the morbidity or mortality, and indeed, signals of harm are evident.

Early trials showed promise for nasal CPAP to effectively improve LVEF in patients with HF and Cheyne-Stokes respiration,[49] but a larger and longer duration trial did not demonstrate a significant reduction in clinical events.[50] However, patients randomized to CPAP had a lower resultant AHI and a higher nocturnal oxygen level, LVEF, and 6-minute walk test. Those who had suppression of the AHI by CPAP had improved outcomes.[51] This would suggest that if CPAP is to be used for patients with CSA, a repeat sleep study 3 months after therapy initiation may help to identify those patients who will get a sustained benefit. Adaptive servoventilation (ASV) was developed for use in CSA. The Central Sleep Apnea by Adaptive Servo Ventilation in Patients with Heart Failure (SERVE-HF) trial,[52] patients with an EF less than or equal to 45%, AHI greater than or equal to 15, and a predominance of CSA were randomized to receive medical treatment with or without ASV. The primary end point of death, cardiovascular interventions and HF hospitalization, was not altered; however, all-cause mortality and cardiovascular mortality were significantly higher in the ASV group compared with the control group. The ongoing Effect of Adaptive Servo Ventilation on Survival and Hospital Admissions in

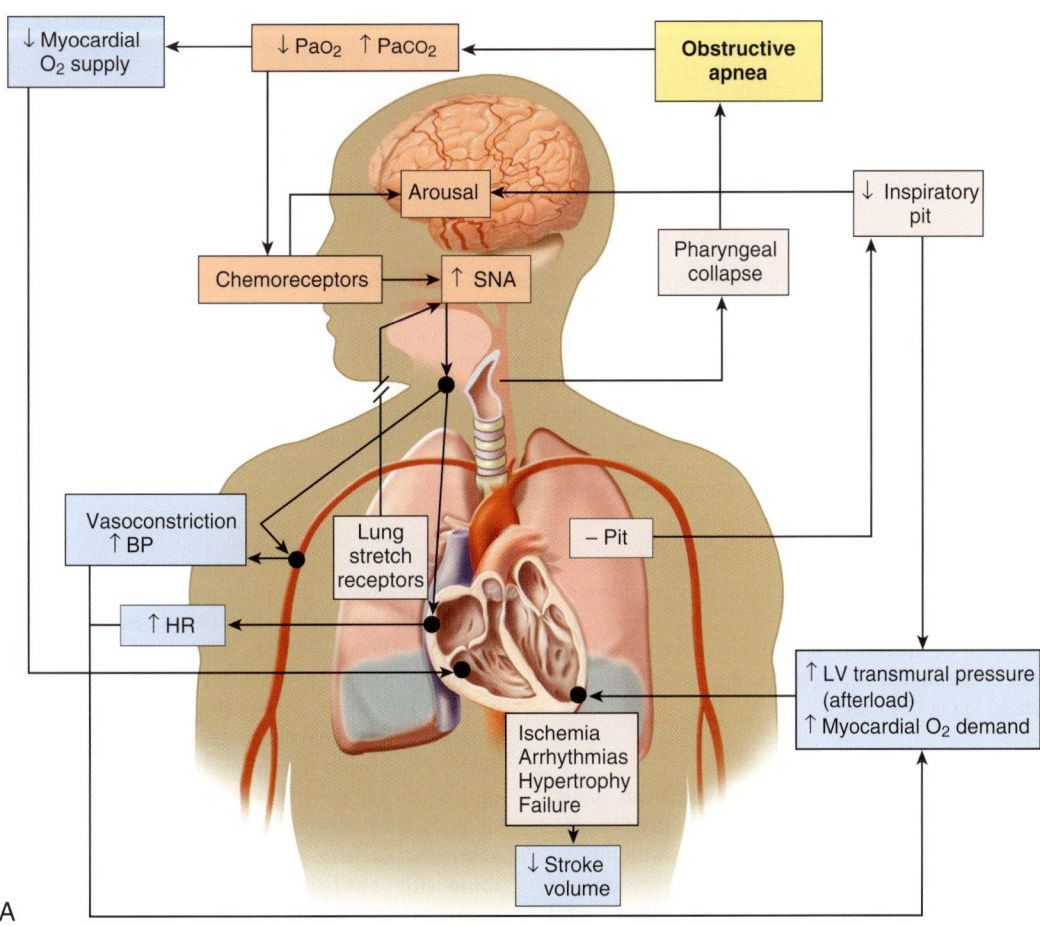

Fig. 48.4A (A) Pathophysiologic effects of obstructive sleep apnea on the cardiovascular system. Obstructive apneas increase left ventricular (LV) transmural pressure (i.e., afterload) through the generation of negative intrathoracic pressure (Pit) and elevations in systemic blood pressure (BP) secondary to hypoxia, arousals from sleep, and increased sympathetic nervous system activity (SNA). Apnea also suppresses the sympathetic inhibitory effects of lung stretch receptors, further enhancing SNA. The combination of increased LV afterload and increased heart rate (HR) secondary to increased SNA increases myocardial O_2 demand in the face of a reduced myocardial O_2 supply. These conditions predispose a patient acutely to cardiac ischemia and arrhythmias and chronically could contribute to LV hypertrophy and, ultimately, failure. The resultant fall in stroke volume will further augment SNA.

Continued

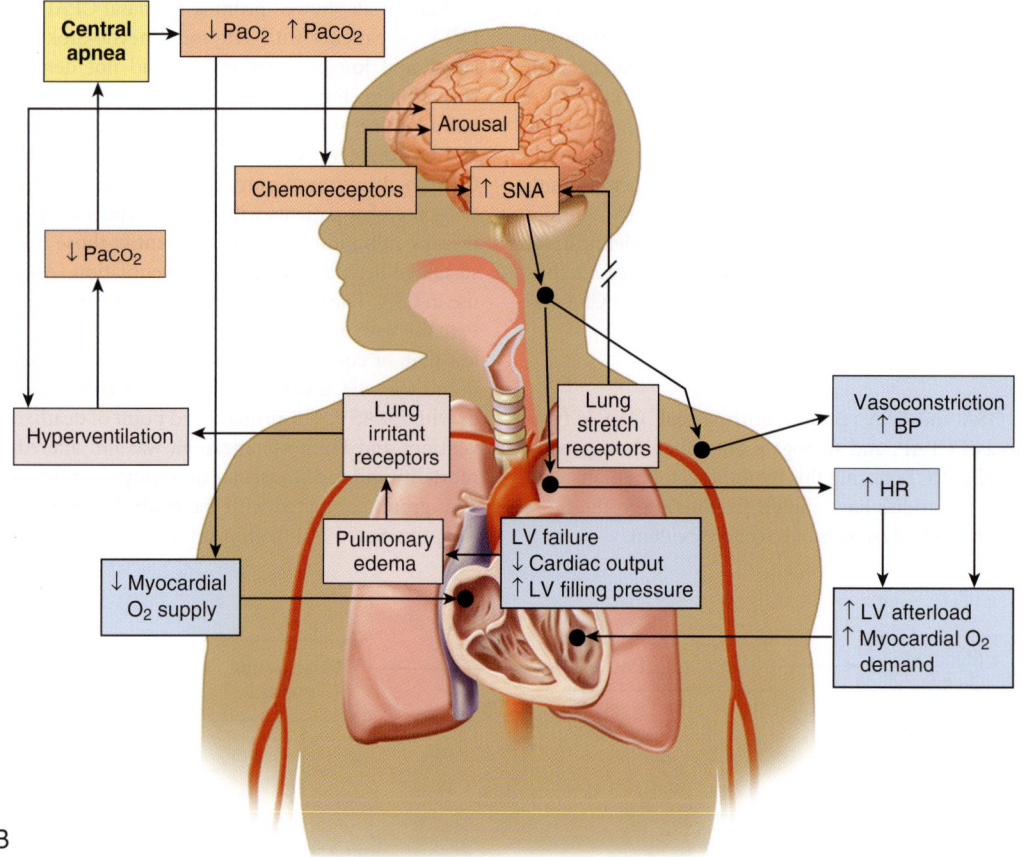

Fig. 48.4B, cont'd (B) Pathophysiology of central sleep apnea in heart failure *(HF)*. HF leads to increased LV filling pressure. The resulting pulmonary congestion activates lung vagal irritant receptors, which stimulate hyperventilation and hypocapnia. Superimposed arousals cause further abrupt increases in ventilation and drive $PaCO_2$ below the threshold for ventilation, triggering a central apnea. Central sleep apneas are sustained by recurrent arousals resulting from apnea-induced hypoxia and the increased effort to breathe during the ventilatory phase because of pulmonary congestion and reduced lung compliance. Although central apneas have a different pathophysiology than obstructive apneas and are not associated with the generation of exaggerated negative intrathoracic pressure, they both increase sympathetic SNA. The consequent increases in BP and HR increase myocardial O_2 demand in the face of reduced supply. This chain of events contributes to a pathophysiologic vicious cycle. (From Bradley TD, Floras JS. Sleep apnea and heart failure: Part I: obstructive sleep apnea. *Circulation.* 2003;107(12):1671–1678; and Bradley TD, Floras JS. Sleep apnea and heart failure: Part II: central sleep apnea. *Circulation.* 2003;107[13]:1822–1826.)

Heart Failure (ADVENT-HF) trial (NCT01128816) may provide more insight onto the role of ASV in HF.

Other therapies such as nocturnal or 24-hour oxygen, dental or mandibular devices or manipulation, atrial pacing, or CRT have not shown to be beneficial in OSA or CSA.

Summary/Conclusions

OSA or CSA may be present in patients with HF, and patients should be screened and tested appropriately. Specific subgroups to pay particular attention to include those unresponsive to therapy, with pulmonary hypertension, increased body mass index and hypertension, and those at risk on sleepiness scales. Treatment of patients with a formal diagnosis from a laboratory-based polysomnography test is best introduced and titrated by those with formal training and expertise in sleep medicine and caring for patients with HF.

DIABETES

Definitions, Prevalence, and Outcomes

Diabetes and HF share a number of features: they are both common, chronic, and increasing in prevalence. Worldwide, an estimated 10% of the adult population has diabetes,[53] and it is a well-established risk factor for coronary artery disease, a major cause of HF. In addition, diabetes alone can produce a "diabetic cardiomyopathy," and 6% of patients with new-onset diabetes will develop HF within 5 years (**Fig. 48.5**).[3] Accordingly, up to 30% of patients with HF have diabetes, making it one of the most common chronic comorbid conditions that a cardiovascular practitioner will deal with over the life span of a patient. Regardless of the definitions used by various guidelines across the world, the presence or absence of diabetes or the risk factors for diabetes is important for those with or at risk for HF.

Treatment
Treatment of Heart Failure for Patients With Diabetes

Patients with diabetes should be afforded the same options for treatment as those without diabetes, given the similarities in efficacy and safety of commonly used HF therapies between those with and without diabetes. Patients should be treated with HF guideline-endorsed therapies, including blockade of the renin-angiotensin-aldosterone axis, beta-blockers, implantable devices, and other therapies where appropriate.

Treatment of Diabetes for Patients With Heart Failure

There are many established and novel medications available to treat diabetes. It is unclear that treatment of diabetes itself modifies the natural history of HF or what targets (e.g., hemoglobin A_{1c} <7%) are both realistic and will modify clinical outcomes. Nevertheless, the medications listed next have been tested typically in a non-HF population, and it is reasonable (although not ideal) to consider each of the following for a patient with diabetes (**Table 48.4**). Future trials will inform the gaps in prevention and treatment of HF.

Biguanides (Metformin). Biguanides are the first-line therapy for many patients with diabetes, given their established efficacy and safety. They act by increasing insulin sensitivity in tissues and reduce gluconeogenesis. For patients with HF, most guidelines support this strategy despite the lack of RCT evidence.[54] Earlier concerns regarding the risk of lactic acidosis have not been borne out by thorough population-based analysis and systematic review.[55,56]

Sulfonylureas and meglitinides (e.g., Gliclazide, Glimepiride, Glyburide, Repaglinide). These agents stimulate the release of preformed insulin by binding to the potassium andenosine triphosphate (ATP) channel on the beta cell and therefore may induce hypoglycemia, a significant limitation in clinical practice considering the older population with HF. These also can induce weight gain from

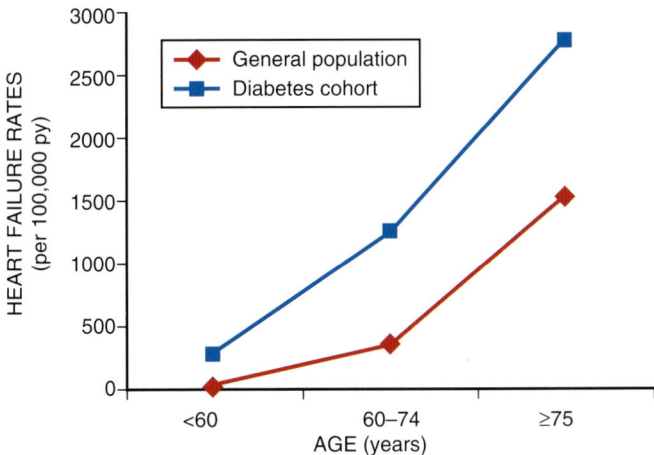

Fig. 48.5 Age and sex standardized rates of incident heart failure in patients with recent-onset type 2 diabetes compared with a general population. *py,* Person-years. (Adapted from Leung AA, Eurich DT, Lamb DA, et al. Risk of heart failure in patients with recent-onset type 2 diabetes: population-based cohort study. *J Card Fail.* 2009;152:152–157.)

uncertain mechanisms that may provide additional challenges to assessing a HF patient in terms of the cause of weight gain.

Thiazolidinediones (e.g., Rosiglitazone). These agents act by increasing insulin sensitivity, especially in skeletal muscle and adipose tissue. These agents are also responsible for significant fluid retention and thus have been associated with an increase in HF incidence.[57,58] Most guidelines are now recommending against using these agents in patients with known HF or at risk for HF.

DPP-IV inhibitors (e.g., Sitagliptin, Saxagliptin, Vidagliptin). These agents block the breakdown of GLP-1 via blocking the breakdown via DPP-IV, which in turn increases insulin secretion while suppressing glucagon secretion, all in response to the presence of glucose. These agents have not been extensively studied in HF, but large-scale trials are ongoing to test if new-onset HF and/or cardiovascular outcomes can be improved by these agents. Indeed, in the Trial Evaluating Cardiovascular Outcomes with Sitagliptin (TECOS) study, an RCT of 14,671 patients comparing sitagliptin with placebo showed no increase in HF hospitalization.[59] A similar result was not seen in the Saxagliptin Assessment of Vascular Outcomes Recorded in Patients with Diabetes Mellitus–Thrombolysis in Myocardial Infarction (SAVOR-TIMI) 53 trial, which randomized patients with type 2 diabetes who had a history of, or were at risk for, cardiovascular events to saxagliptin or placebo and followed them for a median of 2.1 years.[60] The primary end point was a composite of cardiovascular death, myocardial infarction, or ischemic stroke and was similar between groups; however, hospitalization for HF was higher with saxagliptin compared with placebo. In one RCT involving patients with HF and LVEF less than 40%, vildagliptin was associated with no change in LVEF compared with placebo over 1 year but did increase (worsen) end-diastolic and end-systolic ventricular volumes.[61]

Incretin mimetics (GLP-1 "Agonists" [e.g., Exanatide, Liraglutide]). These agents act as GLP agonists by mimicking the effect of naturally occurring GLP-1. GLP-1 are the subject of large ongoing clinical trials, and, as of yet, the clinical HF experience is limited; safety concerns have been raised in one trial.[62,63] In the FIGHT (Functional Impact of GLP-1 for Heart Failure Treatment) trial, there was no additional benefit on short-term clinical outcomes of using liraglutide in patients with or without diabetes with HF who recently hospitalized.[64]

SGLT-2 inhibitors. The sodium-glucose cotransporter-2 inhibitors are a unique class of medications that hold promise, supported principally by the Empagliflozin Cardiovascular Outcome Event Trial in Type 2 Diabetes Mellitus Patients–Removing Excess Glucose (EMPA-REG) trial.[65] This trial, which enrolled patients with diabetes and established cardiovascular disease (and approximately 10% had established HF), demonstrated a relative risk reduction

TABLE 48.4	Diabetes-Related Medications in Patients With Heart Failure		
Drug Class	**Specific Drug Example**	**General Guidance**	**Other Considerations**
Biguanides	Metformin	Safe	First line therapy for most patients
Sulfonylureas	Gliclazide, glyburide	Uncertain	Caution regarding hypoglycemia and weight gain
Meglitinides	Repaglinide	Uncertain	Caution regarding hypoglycemia and weight gain
Thiazolidinediones	Rosiglitazone, pioglitazone	Avoid	Fluid retention and increased HF-related events
DPP-IV inhibitors	Sitagliptin	Safe	Not tested directly in HF population
	Saxigliptin	Uncertain	Increased HF-related events in patients without known HF
	Vildagliptin	Uncertain	May worsen ventricular volumes
Incretin mimetics (GLP-1 agonists)	Exanatide, Liraglutide	Uncertain	May increase HF-related events
SGLT-2 inhibitors	Empagliflozin, dapagliflozin, canagliflozin, sotagliflozin	Uncertain	Reduces HF-related events in patients without HF
Insulin	Insulin and analogues	Uncertain	May increase weight gain and risk of hypoglycemia

DPP-IV, Dipeptidyl peptidase IV; *HF,* heart failure.

in all-cause mortality of 32% and of HF hospitalization of 35%. A similar result was seen in another trial using canagliflozin.[66] Ongoing trials enrolling patients with HF with or without diabetes and with preserved or reduced EF are ongoing (NCT03057951, NCT03036124, NCT03030235, NCT03057977) and will provide clear guidance as to their place in the treatment of patients with HF.

Insulin. Insulin is the mainstay of therapy for patients with poorly controlled diabetes. There are no large-scale trials supporting the use (or calling into question safety). Some observational analyses have highlighted the use of insulin as an independent predictor of poor outcomes, but this may indeed be a risk marker instead of a causal factor.

Summary/Conclusions

Diabetes and HF are two highly prevalent diseases, and their intersection complicates both diseases. Further work on the best strategies for treatment and targets for both day-to-day glucose management and long-term vascular prevention are clearly needed.

OVERALL SUMMARY

Patients with HF carry with them significant comorbid conditions and the risk for developing new medical problems that will require diagnosis and management. Given the high prevalence of anemia, diabetes, COPD, sleep-disordered breathing, and dyslipidemia, the clinician caring for this population requires expertise in many fields. Concomitant medications such as bronchodilators or diabetes therapies may improve or worsen HF, and much remains to be learned. Newer therapies hold promise for improving the outcomes of these patients with complex heart disease.

KEY REFERENCES

2. Ather S, Chan W, Bozkurt B, et al. Impact of noncardiac comorbidities on morbidity and mortality in a predominantly male population with heart failure and preserved versus reduced ejection fraction. *J Am Coll Cardiol.* 2012;59:998–1005.

7. Ezekowitz JA. Anemia is common in heart failure and is associated with poor outcomes: insights from a cohort of 12,065 patients with new-onset heart failure. *Circulation.* 2003;107:223–225.

15. Anker SD, Comin Colet J, Filippatos G, et al. Ferric carboxymaltose in patients with heart failure and iron deficiency. *N Engl J Med.* 2009;361:2436–2448.

16. Avni T, Leibovici L, Gafter-Gvili A. Iron supplementation for the treatment of chronic heart failure and iron deficiency: systematic review and meta-analysis. *Eur J Heart Fail.* 2012;14:423–429.

24. Hawkins NM, Petrie MC, Jhund PS, Chalmers GW, Dunn FG, McMurray JJV. Heart failure and chronic obstructive pulmonary disease: diagnostic pitfalls and epidemiology. *Eur J Heart Fail.* 2009;11:130–139.

35. Swedberg K, Komajda M, Böhm M, et al. Ivabradine and outcomes in chronic heart failure (SHIFT): a randomised placebo-controlled study. *Lancet.* 2010;376:875–885.

37. Hawkins NM, Petrie MC, MacDonald MR, et al. Heart failure and chronic obstructive pulmonary disease the quandary of Beta-blockers and Beta-agonists. *J Am Coll Cardiol.* 2011;57:2127–2138.

52. Cowie MR, Woehrle H, Wegscheider K, et al. Adaptive servo-ventilation for central sleep apnea in systolic heart failure. *N Engl J Med.* 2015;373:1095–1105.

53. Mathers CD, Loncar D. Projections of global mortality and burden of disease from 2002 to 2030. *PLoS Med.* 2006;3:e442.

56. Eurich DT, Weir DL, Majumdar SR, et al. Comparative safety and effectiveness of metformin in patients with diabetes mellitus and heart failure: systematic review of observational studies involving 34,000 patients. *Circ Heart Fail.* 2013;6:395–402.

The full reference list for this chapter is available on ExpertConsult.

Quality and Outcomes in Heart Failure

Adam D. DeVore, Adrian F. Hernandez

OUTLINE

Due to the prevalence and major morbidity of heart failure (HF), as well as its associated public health burden with regard to total health care expenditures, HF serves as one of the top conditions targeted for quality of care improvement.[1,2] Randomized clinical trials have established the efficacy of several therapies to reduce all-cause mortality and to reduce the risk of other adverse outcomes for patients with HF with reduced ejection fraction (HFrEF).[3] This evidence has been translated into professional society guideline recommendations including many class I recommendations for HF treatments, such as the use of angiotensin-converting enzyme inhibitors (ACEIs)/angiotensin receptor blockers (ARBs)/angiotensin receptor neprilysin inhibitors (ARNI), beta (β)-blockers, aldosterone antagonists, implantable cardioverter defibrillators (ICDs), and resynchronization therapy. However, there has been wide variation in the implementation of evidence into practice; often years go by before guideline recommended therapies are routinely applied to clinical practice.[4] This 15- to 20-year gap between evidence and routine practice is often referred to as the "Quality Chasm," which received national attention in a landmark report published by the influential Institute of Medicine (IOM).[5] Beyond the gap between evidence and care, there are also substantial disparities in care based on age, sex, race, ethnicity, and socioeconomic backgrounds.[6,7] While there are multiple reasons for this quality gap, clinical inertia has most often been noted as a major barrier.[8] In order to overcome inertia and other barriers, attention has increasingly turned toward aligning incentives in the delivery of health care by measuring and improving quality of care.

Historically, the pursuit of high-quality care has been challenging. Until receiving scrutiny from the IOM, payers, and government agencies, the need to translate life-prolonging therapies into practice did not receive due attention. Systems and strategies for improving quality of care were not routinely in place until early- to mid-2000. Unfortunately, the lack of systematic efforts for improving quality of care leaves a substantial proportion of patients at risk for hospitalizations and deaths, which could be prevented by better implementation of evidence-based therapies.[9] For example, if ARNI therapy was comprehensively used in eligible patients with chronic HFrEF, approximately 28,000 deaths per year could be prevented in the United States alone.[10] This chapter will review the existing framework for quality of care and how to integrate it into everyday practice through performance improvement systems that are designed to facilitate the use of evidence-based therapy and to improve outcomes for patients with HF in the inpatient and outpatient setting.

GENERAL PRINCIPLES OF QUALITY MEASUREMENT

Defining Quality

Defining quality of care is often controversial. While stakeholders such as patients, clinicians, and payers agree that quality is an important value for health care, it is often difficult to precisely define how quality is measured and what its limits may be. Recognizing that quality is a difficult value to conceptualize, the IOM proposed a definition of quality health care based on six dimensions. This definition is now widely accepted as the means by which health care quality can be characterized.[5]

Institute of Medicine Principles

The IOM defines health care quality as the degree to which health care services increase the likelihood of desired health outcomes and are consistent with current professional knowledge. Put simply, high quality health care involves the delivery of appropriate care, from which patients benefit.

TABLE 49.1	Institute of Medicine Aims for Health Care
1. Safe	Avoiding injuries to patients from the care that is intended to help them
2. Effective	Providing services based on scientific knowledge to all who could benefit and refraining from providing services to those not likely to benefit (avoiding underuse and overuse, respectively)
3. Patient-centered	Providing care that is respectful of and responsive to individual patient preferences, needs, and values, and ensuring that patient values guide all clinical decisions
4. Timely	Reducing waits and sometimes harmful delays for both those who receive and those who give care
5. Efficient	Avoiding waste, including waste of equipment, supplies, ideas, and energy
6. Equitable	Providing care that does not vary in quality because of personal characteristics such as gender, ethnicity, geographical location, and socioeconomic status

Institute of Medicine (US) Committee on Quality of Health Care in America. *Crossing the quality chasm: a new health system for the 21st century.* Washington, DC: The National Academies Press; 2001.

In the influential IOM report, *Crossing the Quality Chasm: A New Health System for the 21st Century*, six aims are outlined for health care improvement.[5] Health care should be safe, effective, patient-centered, timely, efficient, and equitable. As a result, efforts for improving quality of care generally target these six aims (**Table 49.1**).

Framework

While the goal of high quality care is directed toward having optimal outcomes, there needs to be a supportive framework capable of evaluating the steps towards these ideal outcomes. Most often referenced is the Donabedian Model, which is a conceptual model that provides a framework for examining health services and evaluating quality of care.[11] This model highlights three specific areas that may be targeted for quality measurement and improvement: structure, process, and outcomes.

Structure

Structure generally includes the context in which the care is delivered, such as the physical facility and organizational characteristics (i.e., staff, equipment, and human resources). While these structural factors of a health system, such as number of critical care beds or access to invasive procedures, are easy to measure and observe, they are often more difficult to change. Structure may represent the overall ability to provide quality of care and sometimes can be identified as a potential problem upstream for an adequate process of care. An example of a potential structural problem is the financial ability of a health system to leverage health information technology or other resource intensive services. This can be particularly troublesome for health systems that serve socioeconomic disadvantageous populations where health policy may penalize organizations that have high readmission rates.[12,13] In health systems that serve vulnerable populations, there are many different factors that need to be overcome for high quality care, one of which is access to financial resources, staff, clinical access, and other structural improvements that will prevent readmission for worsening HF. Procedural volume is a classic example of a structural relationship with outcome. Implantation and care for patients with left ventricular assist devices is quite complex for health systems. In general, hospitals

with higher procedural volume have better survival outcomes, which may represent the overall ability of the health system to deliver the service, as well as having the infrastructure to support care demands.[14] Despite their intimate relationship, the connection between structure and optimal outcomes is often difficult to demonstrate, given that the observed relationship is often modest, if observed at all. In the case of left ventricular assist devices, there appears to be a modest volume–outcome relationship for mortality but not readmission, making it difficult to determine what volume may be most appropriate for optimal outcomes. This is particularly difficult for structural relationships, such as procedural volumes with readmission, an outcome putatively expected to be influenced by infrastructural support.

Process

Process is the second area highlighted by the Donabedian Model as a target for quality measurement and improvement, and is most often the focus of development. In general, process represents the transactions or services that sum up health care, such as diagnosis, treatment, or other actions of care delivery. Measuring process is common, due to the difficulty of using outcome measures for quantifying quality of care. For most processes of care to be considered a measure of quality care, they typically must have a strong link to an important health outcome. Nevertheless, there are some process measures that are so fundamental to care (e.g., defining an HF patient's left ventricular ejection fraction [LVEF]), that they serve as a means to systematically define potential patient populations in which evidence-based therapies are targeted. Perhaps most importantly, a process measure must be actionable by a health care clinician or a health system.

Process measures are defined by the percentage of eligible patients receiving a given treatment or service, with the numerator indicating which patients received the treatment or service, and the denominator defining the eligible population. Typically, for a process measure to be considered important for defining quality of care as a performance measure, the measure usually needs to undergo a thorough review and endorsement by national bodies. The criteria for selecting quality evaluation process measures includes whether the measure is easily interpretable, actionable, and feasible. Professional societies (i.e., American Heart Association [AHA], American College of Cardiology [ACC], etc.) have traditionally formed a task force dedicated to defining process measures that may be considered quality performance measures. Programs such as the AHA's Get With The Guidelines (GWTG) will define process measures from Class I recommendations of care guidelines.[3] For process measures to be tied to either payment or public reporting, they normally must meet approval by national organizations that are dedicated to quality, such as the National Quality Forum or the Joint Commission. These quality-focused organizations review a proposed measure based on its importance, feasibility, and evidence as a best care allotment. Payers like the Centers for Medicare & Medicaid Services (CMS), ultimately impact health care once a process measure is implemented for performance of a health care system.

Challenges for defining process measures as a measure of quality of care include the link to outcome, the trade-off between specificity and sensitivity, and how to combine measures for an overall quality measure. Ideally, the definition yields a strong link to outcome, but as noted earlier, there are some fundamental process measures that may be important for quality of care that have high variability in delivery (e.g., measurement of LVEF). These basic measures may be difficult to link to outcome, due to confounding factors or ceiling effects. For example, certain basic measures of HF quality (LVEF assessment, smoking cessation counseling, ACEI/ARB use in left ventricular systolic dysfunction [LVSD], and discharge summaries) do not have a strong link to short- or long-term outcomes.[15] In contrast, other measures such as prescribing a β-blocker for patients with LVSD, have a strong link to outcomes.[16]

For any process measure, there will be a trade-off between sensitivity and specificity. For example, the evidence and guidelines strongly support the use of ACEIs, ARBs, or ARNIs due to the risk reduction for mortality and other important outcomes among patients with HFrEF. One could apply this evidence across all patients with HFrEF, thereby creating a very sensitive process measure. In order to be more specific and undeniable, a measure with widespread endorsement and used by payers should include absolute contraindications for ACEIs, ARBs, or ARNIs. To be even more specific, then further restriction of the eligible population to precisely those patients studied in clinical trials could be considered; however, applying such stringent standards would limit the general applicability of a process measure, as well as its potential impact on quality of care.

Another area of debate is how to measure the overall quality of health systems, particularly when multiple process measures may be available for evaluation. While outcome measures can provide an overall assessment of quality, they are often difficult to use due to their inability to fully address potential confounding factors, such as patient case mix or severity of illness. Furthermore, there is a need to summarize process measures that are considered more actionable. To address this need, an alternative approach to quantifying overall quality is to use composite measures that combine two or more measures, most often process measures.[17] These composite performance measures allow data reduction when there is a large array of individual indicators. They also allow for combining measures into a summary measure to better profile or inform decisions on clinician performance, such as pay-for-performance programs.

The most commonly used composite measures are "opportunity" scoring and "any-or-none" scoring. Opportunity scoring counts the number of times a given care process was actually performed (numerator), divided by the number of chances a clinician had to give this care correctly (denominator). Unlike simple averaging, each item is based on the percentage of eligible patients, which may vary from clinician to clinician. Any-or-none scoring is similar to composite outcomes for a clinical trial where a patient counts once towards the primary endpoint as an event regardless of how many events the patient may have had during the observation period. In this method, a patient is counted as failing if he or she experiences at least one missed process from a list of two or more processes. The use of any-or-none composites may be misleading, since this method is driven by the processes most commonly failed and, therefore, may not be representative of the overall number and range of processes that can occur during the health care process.[18]

Outcomes

Outcomes are the third area highlighted by the Donabedian Model as a target for quality measurement and improvement. Outcomes are easily understood as the all-encompassing measure of quality and represent the end-effects of health care on patients or populations. Outcome measures for HF may include mortality, morbidity, readmission, home-time, and quality of life. The rationale behind outcome measures such as 30-day mortality or 30-day readmission after a hospital stay for HF is three-fold. First, process measures typically focus on narrow aspects of care; the number of process measures that can be feasibly measured is finite. Second, due to eligibility criteria, process measures may only apply to a small segment of the population, yet there remains the need to fully assess the overall quality of the health system. Finally, the existing or typical process measures may have a limited relationship to the most meaningful outcomes that matter most to patients. Therefore outcome measures can provide a broad

perspective on health system performance and spur local innovation to improve the end results desired for quality of care.

Accurately measuring outcomes in a manner that is fair across health systems for performance profiling is challenging due to measured and unmeasured confounding factors such as patient case mix. Making conclusions on quality due to outcomes measurements requires large sample sizes, as well as rigorous adjustment methods for case mix and other factors. The challenge of using outcome as a quality measure may be best illustrated by considering HF mortality. At face value, mortality is an important outcome; however, for a group of patients under a single health care clinician who has different referral patterns (e.g., a cardiac transplant physician), mortality comparisons would be generally unfair. At the health system level, case mix may still be a factor, but it is more easily addressable due to a larger sample size and analytic methods that provide greater ability to conservatively draw comparisons between health systems, particularly when considering outliers.

Selecting the duration of exposure for an outcome also can be difficult and depends on the overall goal. For example, how far out from an admission should a hospital be accountable for a patient's outcome? While 30 days may seem like a reasonable amount of time to hold a hospital accountable, there is increasing pressure for health systems to be held accountable for outcomes up to 1 year. The more time that passes after a hospital admission, the more that actionable factors become difficult to define. Long-term outcomes more than 1-year post–hospital admission are unlikely affected by care during the index hospitalization. On the other hand, shorter observation periods may not allow enough time to accurately assess the potential benefit of a given process, such as ICD implantation or β-blocker therapy.

Notably, measuring outcomes is generally an insufficient means of improving quality, as efforts often have to be isolated into discrete processes or segments of care such as admission, discharge, and transitional care. Another challenge with measuring outcomes is that organizations using continuous quality improvement techniques need to assess performance measures at relatively frequent intervals since some outcome measures may be too small, occurring over short periods of time, or varying considerably (similar to day-to-day changes in the stock market). Receiving reliable outcomes data in a timely fashion may also be a challenge, especially for health systems that are not integrated or have patient care spread across disparate organizations.

In the end, quality is measured in a variety of ways. For many, quality needs to be summarized across different domains into a composite measure. The most publicized example of a composite measure that includes structural, process, and outcome measures is the annual US News & World Report Annual Index of Hospital Quality, yet whether this report reflects "true" quality is of considerable debate.[19] Looking toward the future, value of care will also become increasingly emphasized, and for some measures, value of care will be directly incorporated depending on the cost effectiveness of a given therapy.[20]

KEY COMPONENTS FOR QUALITY: INTEGRATIVE MODEL FOR QUALITY

The "cycle of quality" has been proposed, as attention to quality of care has evolved, along with the recognition of the need for a continuous cycle of quality improvement that considers the roles of different stakeholders including public, private, and governmental organizations. The cycle of quality model connects the innovation of initial scientific discovery with validated methods of translating research into effective care delivery (Fig. 49.1).[21] This model serves as a basis for accelerating development, encouraging appropriate adoption of new treatments, and achieving greater penetration of effective behavioral

THE CYCLE OF QUALITY

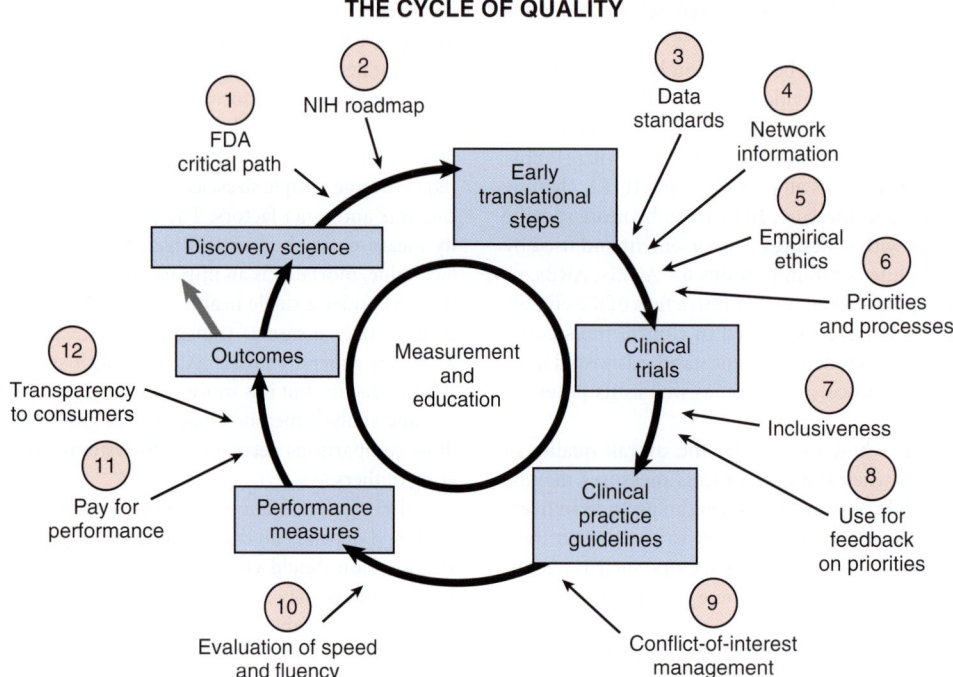

Fig. 49.1 The cycle of quality. This figure displays the cycle of quality and the consequent relationship between early translational steps, clinical trials, clinical practice guidelines, performance measures, outcomes, and discovery science. FDA, US Food & Drug Administration; NIH, National Institutes of Health. (Adapted with permission from Califf RM, Peterson ED, Gibbons RJ, et al. Integrating quality into the cycle of therapeutic development. J Am Coll Cardiol. 2002;40[11]:1895–1901.)

therapies and established technologies, with the ultimate goal being major improvements in patient health. The cycle of quality is a model that has been built upon the traditional quality framework that was first proposed by Donabedian. Key components for a cycle of quality include the roles of the health care system and health information technology accompanied by a learning environment.[22]

Health Care System

Health care systems are often characterized by how well the different service components are integrated. The fragmented nature of the US health care system serves as a prime example of the difficulties in enacting high-quality affordable care. Our health system is comprised of a variety of different systems responsible for care with and without direct links to payment. Furthermore, in most settings, no single group (whether it be physicians, hospitals, public payers, or private payers) has the full responsibility of a population's health. Patients often encounter many groups inside and outside of a health care system. Even within a single health care system, integration is challenging, as there are barriers with regard to information exchange for the most basic functions between inpatient and outpatient care, which leads to waste, duplication, and inevitably, higher costs. This fragmentation of information has highlighted the need for more accountable care organizations.[23]

While there are examples of integrated health care delivery systems, the pressure for all health care systems to be more integrated has generated consolidation, with hospitals purchasing clinician practices and strategic alliances across different components of health care delivery. For example, primary care physicians and cardiologists frequently deliver HF care, but they may not have access to common medical records or other functions. Often, the care of patients hospitalized with HF covers the full spectrum of clinicians, from hospitalists to consulting cardiologists to outpatient clinicians.[24] These clinicians and their affiliated hospitals may not be associated with each other, so follow-up after a hospital admission is often quite different than the care provided during a hospital episode.[25] Other components of the health system add to the complexity of care, including pharmacies, home health agencies, rehabilitation services, and skilled nursing facilities. Patients navigating these systems—particularly those that have frequent comorbidities—present enormous difficulties in ensuring that the right care is delivered at the right time. With such a diffuse system, comprised of so many different components in action, it is difficult to discern who is actually responsible for quality. HF care uses a variety of health care system components, thereby serving as a prime example of policy development to align incentives under an accountable care organization. For example, a bundled payment across the inpatient to outpatient care environment is an incentive intended to force individual components to become more integrated and efficient. Whether or not this emphasis on improved health system accountability actually leads to higher quality of care remains to be seen, especially if cost reduction is a key component.

Health Information Technology

Data drive the decisions and actions for improving quality of care. In order to be as close to real-time as possible, health information technology and its associated analytics become central to driving quality improvement. As described previously, process measures require data collection to define an eligible population, as well as those who receive a given care process. Collection of such data is necessary, but can be labor intensive if it is not integrated into the normal workflow or through the health record. With the requirement that health systems use electronic health records, health information technology becomes a platform to measure, evaluate, and act on key processes of care. More importantly, health information technology may allow for the development of real-time tools, such as integrated risk assessment models for outcome measures.[26]

TABLE 49.2 Heart Failure Performance Measures Over Time

2001 THE JOINT COMMISSION[33]	2005 ACCF/AHA[2]		2011 ACCF/AHA[34]	
Inpatient	Inpatient	Outpatient	Inpatient	Outpatient
1. LVEF assessment	1. LVEF assessment	1. LVEF assessment	1. LVEF assessment	1. LVEF assessment
2. ACE-I use for LVSD[a]	2. ACE-I/ARB use for LVSD	2. ACE-I/ARB use for LVSD	2. ACE-I/ARB use for LVSD	2. ACE-I/ARB use for LVSD
3. Discharge instructions	3. Discharge instructions	3. β-blocker use for LVSD	3. β-blocker use for LVSD	3. β-blocker use for LVSD
4. Smoking cessation counseling	4. Smoking cessation counseling	4. Symptom assessment	4. Follow-up after discharge	4. Symptom and activity assessment
	5. Anticoagulant for patients with a-fib	5. Activity assessment		5. Symptom management
		6. Patient education		6. Patient education
		7. Anticoagulant for patients with a-fib		7. ICD counseling for LVSD
		8. Physical exam for volume status		
		9. Laboratory testing with new diagnosis		
		10. BP measurement		
		11. Weight measurement		

[a]ARB later added as an acceptable alternative. *ACCF,* American College of Cardiology Foundation; *ACEI,* angiotensin-converting enzyme inhibitor; *a-fib,* atrial fibrillation; *AHA,* American Heart Association; *ARB,* angiotensin receptor blocker; *BP,* blood pressure; *ICD,* implantable cardioverter defibrillator; *LVEF,* left ventricular ejection fraction; *LVSD,* left ventricular systolic dysfunction.

Despite the promise of health information technology, the impact on electronic health records on HF outcomes is still evolving with significant challenges to improve health outcomes. That is, in the early development of electronic health records, the Veterans Administration demonstrated improved quality for the entire health system through a variety of tools, such as computerized order entry.[27] However, a large outpatient quality improvement intervention implemented as part of the Registry to Improve the Use of Evidence-Based Heart Failure Therapies in the Outpatient Setting (IMPROVE HF) program found that the use of electronic health records was not associated with improved quality of HF care compared to paper systems.[28] Similarly, an analysis of the AHA's GWTG-HF found no association between a hospital's adoption of electronic health records and the inpatient quality of care or inpatient/early postdischarge outcomes.[29] As electronic health records and advances in digital technology bridge the gap between home and clinic, there may be better models for improving quality of care. In the future, virtual clinical visits reliant on a combination of electronic health records from the clinic or the hospital, plus other digital data derived from the patient's daily activities, social interactions, or other information outside the health care system may be integrated to improve decision making for patients and clinicians.

STATUS OF HEART FAILURE QUALITY MEASURES AND PROGRAMS

Public Reporting

Public reporting of health care quality began as an attempt to not only incentivize health care systems to improve performance on quality metrics, but to increase transparency for patients and to empower them as consumers in the health care marketplace. Public reporting in HF care began shortly after individual states started reporting outcomes for patients undergoing coronary artery bypass surgery and percutaneous coronary intervention.

The first large-scale HF reporting effort began with the launch of Hospital Compare, a public reporting database founded by CMS.

In 2005, Hospital Compare began reporting information on quality process measures related to the care of patients with HF, as well as acute myocardial infarction and pneumonia. This later extended to outcome measures. In June of 2007, the database began reporting risk-adjusted mortality, and in July 2009, CMS began publicly reporting risk-standardized readmission rates.

Evaluating the impact of public reporting of process measures and outcomes is a challenge. Nearly all hospitals in the United States participated in the Hospital Compare program, and thus there are a limited number of available control groups for comparison purposes. One analysis specifically evaluated the impact of public reporting of process measures. Using data from 2000 to 2008, the investigators observed a modest improvement in the adjusted relative risk of 30-day mortality for Medicare patients with HF, 0.97 (95% confidence interval [CI] 0.95–0.99), but observed no improvement over time for acute myocardial infarction or pneumonia.[30] Another analysis evaluated the impact of public reporting of hospital readmission rates. The investigators observed no change in the trends of 30-day readmission or mortality before and after the implementation of CMS public reporting for acute myocardial infarction, pneumonia, or HF.[31]

Process Measures

In an attempt to improve outcomes for patients with HF, stakeholders developed specific process measures that could be quantified and modified. These process measures cover both the inpatient and outpatient domains of HF care and have been modified over time (**Table 49.2**). In 2002, the Joint Commission began providing quarterly feedback to sites on specific quality metrics and allowed sites to compare individual performance to national rates.[32] This process has also been utilized in HF-specific registries, including the Organized Program to Initiate Lifesaving Treatment in Hospitalized Patients with HF (OPTIMIZE-HF)[33] and most recently, the GWTG-HF program.[34] Improvement in these process measures has been a remarkable achievement in HF care, but the association between improvement in process measures and improved outcomes for patients with HF is modest.

The first large analysis of the process-outcome link examined the association between hospital-level performance in CMS's Hospital Compare program and risk-adjusted mortality.[35] The authors looked at differences in risk-adjusted mortality rates (inpatient, 30 days, and 1 year) for hospitals performing in the 25th and 75th percentile for assessment of LVSD and ACEI use for LVSD and found little to no differences between the hospital mortality rates. An analysis of data from OPTIMIZE-HF, which was a national quality improvement initiative designed to enhance guideline adherence in patients hospitalized with HF[33] examined outcomes associated with specific HF performance measures. This analysis specifically examined conformity to the 2005 ACC/AHA HF inpatient performance measures (see Table 49.2),[2] β-blocker use for LVSD, and associated mortality or all-cause rehospitalization 60 to 90 days postdischarge.[36] β-blocker use was associated with a reduced risk of mortality and mortality/rehospitalization, while ACEI/ARB use in eligible patients was only associated with reduced mortality/rehospitalization. There was no association with improved outcomes for the other individual measures.

Another analysis compared hospitals participating in the AHA's GWTG-HF program to those who were not.[37] Hospitals participating in the program had improved process of care performance on four measures (discharge instructions, assessment of LVSD, smoking cessation, and ACEI/ARB use in eligible patients); for every 10% increase in a composite of these four measures, there was an associated 0.1% decrease in all-cause 30-day readmission with no associated change in 30-day mortality.

Similar findings were seen in outpatients. An analysis of data from the registry to IMPROVE HF found an association between various performance measures (ACEI/ARB use, β-blocker use, aldosterone antagonist use, anticoagulant for atrial fibrillation, cardiac resynchronization therapy [CRT], ICD, and HF education) and reduced adjusted mortality.[38] The authors specifically noted that for every 10% increase in a composite score of the eligible measures, there was an associated 13% lower adjusted odds of 24-month mortality (adjusted odds ratio [OR] 0.87, 95% CI 0.84–0.90).

Perhaps the best evidence of a link between an association between improvement in process measures and improved HF outcomes comes from the Swedish HF Registry (SwedeHF).[39] In a study of 234,437 Swedish patients with incident HF diagnosed from 2006 to 2013, 21,888 (9.5%) patients were enrolled in SwedeHF. Patients enrolled in the registry were much more likely to receive medical therapy for chronic HFrEF compared with patients not enrolled in the registry (e.g., β-blockers were used in 84% of SwedeHF patients compared with 60% in non-SwedeHF patients). They also had a significantly lower hazard of all-cause mortality compared with non-SwedeHF patients, unadjusted hazard ratio (HR) 0.65 (95% CI 0.63–0.66), though the hazard attenuated with adjustment for baseline differences and there was no difference after adjusting for the observed differences in medical therapy for chronic HFrEF.

Outcome Measures

Mortality is the most commonly analyzed outcome in the attempt to understand the impact of a quality intervention on HF patients. Mortality analyses are appropriate given the high associated mortality[40] of HF, as well as the fact that mortality is an outcome that most clinical trial and observational databases can accurately quantify. There is also a growing interest in reporting the impact of quality interventions on hospitalization rates. Nonetheless, mortality and readmission rates may not be the best measures to evaluate quality of care, as outcome measurements do not provide information on the modifiable steps in the process of care. Analyzing individual components of care (process measures or leading indicators) allows for quantifiable and actionable

changes, and focusing only on mortality and hospitalization (outcomes or lagging indicators) rates may underrecognize patient-centered outcomes and values in health care.[41]

Pay-for-Performance

Initial programs for pay-for-performance incentives began at the state level. The first nationwide program, the CMS Premier Hospital Quality Incentives Demonstration, began in 2003. The program incentivized participating hospitals through bonus payments for process measure performance for a number of conditions including HF. The highest performing hospitals for these measures (LVEF assessment, ACEI/ARB use for LVSD, discharge instructions, and smoking cessation counseling) receive a financial bonus while the lowest performing hospital receives a financial penalty. The impact on outcomes was not well assessed.

In October 2012, CMS began imposing cuts on total Medicare reimbursements for higher-than-predicted readmission rates for HF and other chronic conditions. This program is better characterized as a penalty-for-performance program and is referred to as the Hospital Readmissions Reduction Program (HRRP). The impact of the HRRP on HF outcomes is unclear. Some analyses have highlighted an important decrease in 30-day readmissions. For example, an analysis of Medicare fee-for-service beneficiaries between October 2007 and May 2015 revealed a decrease in readmission rates starting in 2010 (the year of the HRRP's announcement) for conditions (HF, acute myocardial infarction, and pneumonia) targeted by HRRP (decrease from 21.5% to 17.8%) that was greater than that for conditions not targeted by HRRP (decrease from 15.3% to 13.1%).[42] HF-specific declines in 30-day readmission were also observed in a smaller analysis of hospitals participating in the AHA's GWTG-HF Registry.[43] The 30-day risk-adjusted readmission rate declined from 20.0% before HRRP implementation to 18.4% in the HRRP penalties phase (HR after vs. before HRRP implementation, 0.91; 95% CI, 0.8–0.95). However, the 30-day risk-adjusted mortality rate increased from 7.2% before HRRP implementation to 8.6% in the HRRP penalties phase (HR after vs. before HRRP implementation, 1.18; 95% CI, 1.10–1.27), suggesting a very concerning unintended consequence of the policy. Others have noted that HF 30-day postdischarge mortality rates have increased steadily over time, preceding the HRRP.[44] Additional analyses are necessary to understand the drivers of increased HF 30-day postdischarge mortality rates as well as the full impact of the HRPP. As previously noted, evaluating the policy programs that impact all hospitals simultaneously is essential but is limited by lack of adequate control groups.

Effectiveness

One measure of the evidence base supporting HF treatment comes from clinical practice guidelines. The 2013 ACC/AHA guidelines recognize 22.1% of recommendations at Level of Evidence A,[45] whereas in 2005, it was 26.4%[46]; this lack of improvement highlights the need for an evidence base for this common and expensive medical condition.

In addition to high-quality evidence from clinical trials, disease-specific registries have afforded the opportunity to examine the real-world effectiveness of therapies outside of trial settings. For patients not included in trials, this is an important step in integrating quality in the development cycle.[47] An analysis of the National Cardiovascular Data Registry ICD Registry demonstrated that survival after primary prevention ICD was similar in a real-world setting compared to the findings from the Multicenter Automatic Defibrillator Implantation Trial (MADIT-II) and the Sudden Cardiac Death in Heart Failure Trial (SCD-HeFT).[48] An analysis of the OPTIMIZE-HF registry linked with Medicare claims data also showed that β-blockers improved outcomes in elderly patients with LVSD.[49]

Patient-Centeredness

Clinical trials in cardiology have largely focused on mortality as a primary outcome. While using mortality as a primary outcome is both necessary and scientifically appropriate, it often compromises our understanding of the impact of cardiovascular care on patient-reported outcomes. In the field of HF, the Kansas City Cardiomyopathy Questionnaire is one of many disease-specific tools validated for the purposes of understanding the cardiovascular care impact on patient-reported outcomes,[50] yet this tool is rarely used in clinical practice. Since the application of HF therapies to treat patient symptoms is poorly understood, we are hopeful that current initiatives, such as the Patient-Centered Outcomes Research Institute (PCORI), may help address some of these gaps for patients with HF.[41]

Equity

Equitable care for patients with HF implies that care is at least offered to all eligible patients regardless of gender, ethnicity, geographical location, or socioeconomic status.[5] Previous variations in HF practice and outcomes have been well documented,[7,51-58] and while these differences are striking, not all variations in care are due to health care disparities. Unfortunately, the United States is currently lacking the research platform that would enable us to better understand these differences and address treatment disparities. Disease-based registries are typically voluntary, so limited information is available on patients treated at hospitals not participating in these registries, as well as patients without Medicare insurance. Nevertheless, there is hope that national efforts to address disparities in HF treatment may be effective. A previous analysis of the OPTIMZE-HF program suggested that African-Americans received evidence-based HF care in the setting of a quality improvement intervention.[59]

IMPROVING QUALITY OF CARE (IMPLEMENTATION)

Measuring quality of care is not, in and of itself, an end result; rather, it is necessary to improve care via evidence implementation through a variety of methods. **Table 49.3** describes different care goals and the quality improvement tools that are often available.[60] A variety of reports and tools can be used. In programs focusing on quality of care, there has been remarkable success in improving quality of care over time.[34]

Quality Improvement Registries

HF has been a leading example of registry-based systems delivering clinician feedback guideline recommended therapies, educational materials oriented to patients and clinicians, and abilities to benchmark against local, regional, and national norms. Through clinical decision support tools, patients receive more consistent delivery of care and also identify opportunities for standardizing care. Examples of registries include the Acute Decompensated HF National Registry (ADHERE), OPTIMIZE-HF, and the AHA's GWTG-HF Registry. Data from GWTG-HF has helped define disparities in care, gaps in transitional care, and potential methods for systematically improving readmission rates.

Health Care Delivery Models

Due to the attention towards more integrated or accountable care, health systems are developing new care models. The current transition from traditional fee for service, volume-based payment system to a value-based health care system is shown in **Fig. 49.2**.[61] These new models will need to be formally evaluated as prior studies have found that depending on the size, design, and intensity of the program, the improvement in outcomes may vary significantly.[62]

Future Directions for Quality of Care

Patients, clinicians, and payers all agree that evaluating and improving quality of care is an essential goal for health care, yet key questions for the future include: (1) Which measures should be used? (2) How should these measures be enforced or how should incentives be tied to improvement? (3) What are the most effective strategies for improving quality of care? and (4) Do the measures improve the value of care? In some cases, randomized trials should be considered to evaluate the positive or negative implications for policies designed to improve quality, particularly when there are potential financial rewards or penalties.

TABLE 49.3 Potential Methods for Quality Improvement

Major Quality Goal	QI Tool	Description
Care delivery and coordination	Patient lists	Lists of patients with a particular condition who may be due for an exam, procedure, etc.
	Patient-level reports	Summarize data on an individual patient (e.g., longitudinal data on blood pressure readings)
	Automated notifications	Prompts clinician or patient when an exam or other action is needed
	Automated communications	Summarizes patient information in a format that can be shared with the patient or other clinicians
	Decision support tools	Provide recommendations for care for an individual patient using evidence-based guidelines
Population measurement	Population-level standardized reports	Provides an analysis of population-level compliance with QI measures or other summaries (e.g., patient outcomes across the population)
	Benchmarking reports	Compares population-level data for various types of clinicians
	Ad-hoc reports	Enables participants to analyze registry data to explore their own questions
	Population-level dashboards	Provides snapshot look at QI progress and areas for continued improvement
	Third-party quality reporting	Enables registry data to be leveraged for reporting to third-party quality reporting initiatives

QI, Quality improvement.
From Gliklich RE, Dreyer NA, Matchar D, et al. *Registries for evaluating patient outcomes: a user's guide.* 3rd ed. Prepared by Outcome DEcIDE Center (Outcomes Sciences, Inc. dba Outcome) under Contract No. HHSA29020050035I TO1. AHRQ Publication No. 07-EHC001-1. Rockville, MD: Agency for Healthcare Research and Quality; 2014.

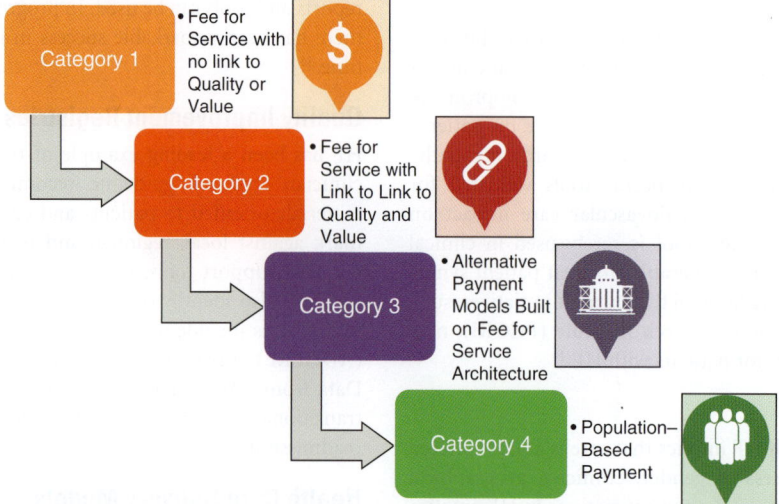

Fig. 49.2 Transitioning to a value-based health care system in the United States. This figure summarizes the transition from a fee for service, volume-based payment system to a value-based health care system. This framework was put forth by the Health Care Payment and Learning Network, created through the Department of Health and Human Services and the Centers for Medicare & Medicaid Services. Modified from Alternative Payment Model Framework and Progress Tracking [APM FPT] Work Group. Alternative payment model [APM] framework: final white paper. January 2016. MITRE corp.

Understanding the best method for improving quality via public reporting or pay-for-performance still remains an unknown. For example, initial reports of outcomes public reporting after coronary artery bypass graft surgery in New York state were encouraging,[63] but these outcomes were later attributed to secular trends unrelated to the intervention of public reporting.[64] This cautionary tale highlights the need for rigorous scientific investigations of quality metrics and improvement initiatives.

The stakes are large for translating evidence into practice. As many as 68,000 deaths could be delayed or prevented annually if all six guideline Class I evidence-based therapies were utilized optimally.[9] Achieving optimal implementation of these therapies will require substantial commitment towards improving quality in HF, including the application and evaluation of collaborative performance improvement systems that report on quality of care, providing clinical decision support, and supplying data feedback. Developing and expanding technologies to better implement practice standards, providing better patient interfaces, and supplying a learning environment focused on improving quality in HF will especially be needed as patients turn to easily accessible resources using mobile technology.

KEY REFERENCES

2. Bonow RO, Bennett S, Casey DE, et al. ACC/AHA clinical performance measures for adults with chronic heart failure: a report of the American College of Cardiology/American Heart Association Task Force on Performance Measures (Writing Committee to Develop Heart Failure Clinical Performance Measures) endorsed by the Heart Failure Society of America. *J Am Coll Cardiol.* 2005;46:1144–1178.

5. Institute of Medicine. *Crossing the Quality Chasm: A New Health System for the 21st Century.* Washington, DC: The National Academies Press; 2001.

11. Donabedian A. The quality of medical care. *Science.* 1978;200:856–864.

17. Hernandez AF, Fonarow GC, Liang L, et al. The need for multiple measures of hospital quality: results from the Get with the Guidelines-Heart Failure Registry of the American Heart Association. *Circulation.* 2011;124:712–719.

18. Peterson ED, DeLong ER, Masoudi FA, et al. ACCF/AHA 2010 position statement on composite measures for healthcare performance assessment: a report of American College of Cardiology Foundation/American Heart Association Task Force on Performance Measures (Writing Committee to Develop a Position Statement on Composite Measures). *J Am Coll Cardiol.* 2010;55:1755–1766.

36. Fonarow GC, Abraham WT, Albert NM, et al. Association between performance measures and clinical outcomes for patients hospitalized with heart failure. *JAMA.* 2007;297:61–70.

41. Selby JV, Beal AC, Frank L. The Patient-Centered Outcomes Research Institute (PCORI) national priorities for research and initial research agenda. *JAMA.* 2012;307:1583–1584.

43. Gupta A, Allen LA, Bhatt DL, et al. Association of the hospital readmissions reduction program implementation with readmission and mortality outcomes in heart failure. *JAMA Cardiol.* 2018;3(1):44–53.

44. Khera R, Dharmarajan K, Krumholz HM. Rising mortality in patients with heart failure in the United States: facts versus fiction. *JACC Heart Fail.* 2018 Jun 6.

47. Califf RM, Peterson ED, Gibbons RJ, et al. Integrating quality into the cycle of therapeutic development. *J Am Coll Cardiol.* 2002;40:1895–1901.

The full reference list for this chapter is available on ExpertConsult.

Decision Making and Palliative Care in Advanced Heart Failure

Larry A. Allen, Daniel D. Matlock

Existing therapies slow, but rarely reverse, heart failure disease progression.[1,2] As a result, the prevalence of symptomatic heart failure has increased,[3] as has the length of time that people spend in later stages of the disease.[4-6] At the far end of the heart failure spectrum are a group of patients with advanced (Stage D) heart failure for whom symptoms limit daily life despite the usual recommended therapies, and lasting remission into less symptomatic disease is unlikely.[7,8] Once hospitalized, regardless of etiology or left ventricular ejection fraction (LVEF), outcomes are poor, with frequent readmissions and median survival worse than for most cancers.[9] This is further complicated by multimorbidity (the average patient has more than four other diagnoses),[10] frailty (the median age of a patient hospitalized with heart failure is now over 77 years),[11] and psychosocial limitations (costs of care are not only increasing, but increasingly being shifted to patients).[12] This increasing prevalence and high symptom burden of advanced heart failure have broadened the need for palliative care services.[13,14] Simultaneously, the possibility of high-intensity therapies with complex trade-offs mandate a systematic and thoughtful approach to medical decision making.[15] This mandate is increasingly taking the form of requirements for shared decision making and palliative care involvement as part of payment policies for common heart failure devices: implantable cardioverter-defibrillators (ICDs), left ventricular assist devices (LVAD), and left atrial appendage occlusion.[16]

This chapter highlights how decision making and palliative care play a central role in the care of patients with advanced heart failure. Specifically, the chapter aims to describe theoretical foundations of medical decision making, to summarize issues around risk assessment, to outline a framework for major medical decisions faced by advanced heart failure patients and their clinicians, and to detail how palliative measures and communication can be better integrated into the care of these complex patients. The goals are to both emphasize the inclusion of formal palliative care services into the management of patients with symptomatic heart failure, and to help health care providers of all types incorporate these concepts into routine practice. The chapter draws from the prior work of researchers, clinicians, and policy experts in the fields of heart failure, palliative care, and medical decision making, with particular benefit from the Writing Group that crafted the American Heart Association's Scientific Statement on "Decision Making in Advanced Heart Failure."[15]

MEDICAL DECISION MAKING

Health care decisions nearly always involve uncertainty and are made within the context of incomplete knowledge of the future. Generally, we compare reasonable options to make treatment decisions. However, how potential benefits, risks, burdens, and costs of various options are weighed depends on the perspective of the decision maker. With growing emphasis on evidence-based medicine, shared decision making, and patient-centered care, improving processes for making complex decisions with difficult tradeoffs has garnered increasing attention, particularly in disease states like advanced heart failure.[17]

Health care providers have an ethical and legal mandate to involve patients in medical decisions. Judicial decisions (e.g., *Cruzan v Missouri Department of Health*)[18] and legislative actions (e.g., the Patient

Self-Determination Act)[19] have repeatedly affirmed the rights of patients, or duly-appointed surrogates, to choose their medical therapy from among reasonable options. The process of informed consent prior to procedural interventions is an embodiment of the ethical principal of autonomy in that it underscores the clinician's obligation to ensure that the patient is aware of the diagnosis and prognosis, the nature of the proposed intervention, the risks and benefits of that intervention, and all reasonable alternatives and their associated risks and benefits.[20] A gold standard for informed consent would entail a high-functioning health care system that is able to provide the resources with which an activated, informed patient can engage in productive discussions with a proactive, prepared health care team.

Shared decision making builds upon the principles that guide informed consent. It asks that clinicians and patients *share information with each other* and *work toward patient-centered decisions* about treatment.[21] Shared decision making incorporates the perspective of the patient, who is responsible for articulating goals, values, and preferences as they relate to his or her health care. Shared decision making also incorporates the perspective of the clinician, who is responsible for narrowing the diagnostic and treatment options to those that are medically reasonable and then communicating expected outcomes. Shared decision making aims to uphold the ideal that patients' values, goals, and preferences should guide the medical decision-making process. It should be assumed that discussions and decision making with patients also include, when appropriate, the family and other individuals involved, such as caregivers and companions. Thus, shared decision making puts into practice the principle of "patient-centered care," which the United States Institute of Medicine has identified as one of the six pillars of quality.[22]

Shared decision making is most naturally applied to preference-sensitive decisions, where both clinicians and patients generally agree that equipoise exists, and decision support helps patients think through, forecast, and deliberate their options; however, even seemingly one-sided medical decisions, such as tobacco cessation and medication adherence, remain dominated by patient choice. In situations where clinicians hold the view that scientific evidence for benefit strongly outweighs harm, behavioral support designed to describe, justify, and recommend may be appropriate.[23] Separately, certain therapeutic options may be considered unreasonable (transplantation or permanent mechanical circulatory support above a certain age or comorbidity burden) and therefore independent of patient demands. Situations of medical futility can be difficult to define but have standardized definitions and legal precedent.[24]

Finally, it should also be noted that health policy makers and societal considerations also play a role in medical decision making. Rules and regulations often help promote distributive justice and optimal resource allocation. Patient-clinician discussions regarding treatment options occur within the context of these societal rules and regulations. With the costs of care rising, these policy discussions will almost certainly become more common.[24] While clinicians should play a crucial role in these broader policy decisions, clinicians should simultaneously avoid allowing their own interpretation of societal considerations around cost in the absence of policy to dictate individual decisions at the bedside.

RISK ASSESSMENT AND EXPECTATIONS FOR THE FUTURE

Medical therapies tend to derive their indications and risk-benefit ratios from the nature and severity of the disease for which they are being considered. Therefore, assessment of prognosis provides the context for selecting among therapies for life-threatening disease.

TABLE 50.1   Criteria for Advanced Chronic Heart Failure, as Defined by the European Society of Cardiology

1. Moderate to severe symptoms of dyspnea and/or fatigue at rest or with minimal exertion (NYHA functional class III or IV)
2. Episodes of fluid retention and/or reduced cardiac output
3. Objective evidence of severe cardiac dysfunction demonstrated by at least one of the following:
   - left ventricular ejection fraction <30%;
   - pseudo-normal or restrictive mitral inflow pattern by Doppler;
   - high left and/or right ventricular filling pressures; or
   - elevated B-type natriuretic peptide
4. Severe impairment of functional capacity as demonstrated by either inability to exercise, 6-minute walk distance <300 m, or peak oxygen uptake <12–14 mL/g/min
5. History of at least one hospitalization in the past 6 months
6. Characteristics should be present despite optimal medical therapy

NYHA, New York Heart Association.
From Fang JC, Ewald GA, Allen LA, et al. Advanced (stage D) heart failure: a statement from the Heart Failure Society of America Guidelines Committee. *J Card Fail.* 2015;21(6):519–534; and Metra M, Ponikowski P, Dickstein K, et al. Advanced chronic heart failure: a position statement from the Study Group on Advanced Heart Failure of the Heart Failure Association of the European Society of Cardiology. *Eur J Heart Fail.* 2007;9(6–7):684–694.

Frequent reappraisal of a patient's clinical trajectory helps to calibrate future expectations, to guide communication, and to inform rational decisions. Recognizing when patients have entered into a state of advanced heart failure—American Heart Association Stage D "refractory end-stage heart failure" (**Table 50.1**)[7,8]—is important for considering and applying advanced therapies in an appropriate and timely manner. The INTERMACS profiles were designed to help clinicians quickly map disease severity with timely treatment approaches.[25]

Unfortunately, estimating prognosis is particularly challenging for heart failure. The clinical course varies dramatically across the spectrum of disease severity and is relatively unpredictable for individual patients (**Fig. 50.1**).[15] This contrasts with the more linear decline of patients with advanced cancer, which has traditionally been the model for decision making and palliative care in end-stage disease. Even late in heart failure, patients often enjoy "good days" and brief interludes of apparent stability, which can lull them and their care providers into postponing vital decisions. Prognosis is further clouded by the unique contrast between unexpected sudden death (i.e., lethal arrhythmia) and lingering death with congestive symptoms (i.e., progressive pump failure).

Hundreds of factors have been shown to predict mortality and hospitalization in heart failure, and multivariable risk models have been developed to integrate risk factors into useful prognostic tools for both ambulatory and hospitalized settings (**Table 50.2**). Such models can objectively ground prognostic estimates, which is important as physicians, nurses, and patients tend to significantly over-estimate survival.[26,27] However, such models rarely identify individual patients who will die in the next year[28] and, in the advanced heart failure population models, often underestimate absolute risk.[29] As a practical alternative for routine prognosis in day-to-day care, a number of clinical events are known to herald worsening disease (**Table 50.3**), which should prompt reassessment of patient goals of care as well as consideration of therapy options for advanced heart failure

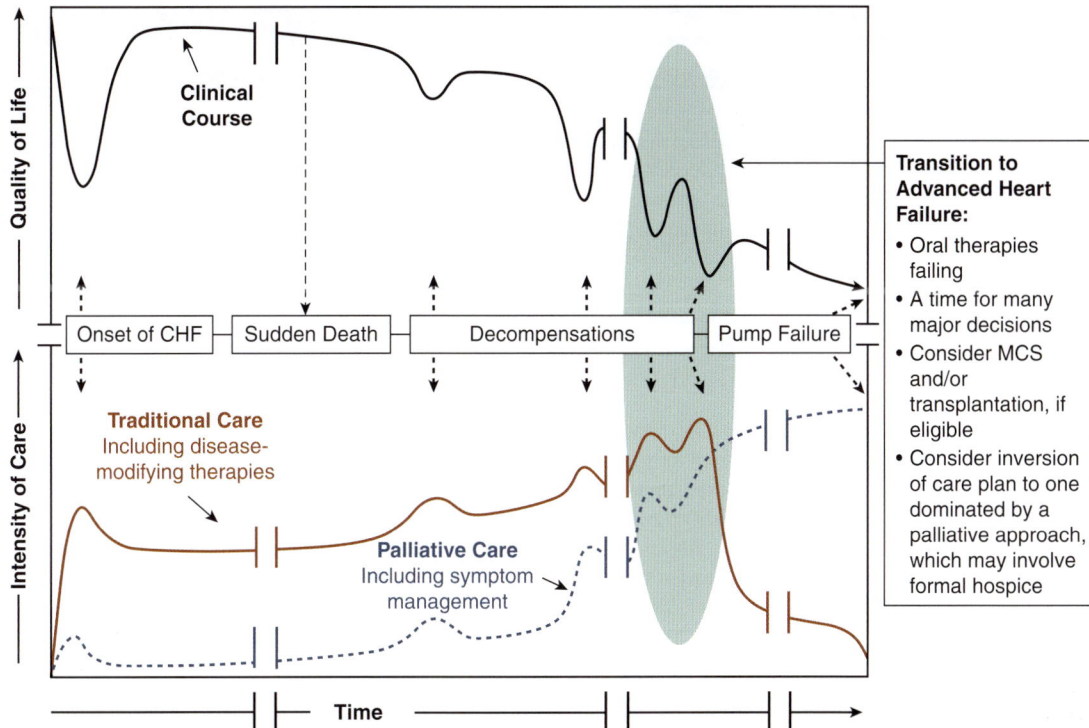

Fig. 50.1 A depiction of the clinical course of heart failure with associated types and intensities of available therapies. *(Black line)* Patients tend to follow a progressive, albeit nonlinear, decline in health-related quality of life as the disease progresses; this course can be interrupted by sudden cardiac death from arrhythmia or can end in a more gradual death from progressive pump failure. *(Gray line)* At disease onset, multiple oral therapies are prescribed for cardiac dysfunction and/or treatment of comorbidities. As disease severity increases, the intensity of care may increase in parallel with the intensification of diuretics, the addition of implantable cardioverter-defibrillators/cardiac resynchronization therapy (ICD/CRT) for those eligible, and the increasing interaction with the medical system through ambulatory visits and hospitalizations, until the time when standard therapies begin to fail *(transition to advanced heart failure)*. *(Dotted line)* Palliative therapies to control symptoms, address quality of life, and enhance communication are relevant throughout the course of heart failure, not just in advanced disease; palliative therapies work hand in hand with traditional therapies designed to prolong survival. The critical transition into advanced heart failure from the medical perspective is often followed with a transition in goals of care from the patient and family perspective, wherein palliative therapies may become the dominant treatment paradigm (for the majority of patients in whom transplantation and mechanical circulatory support are not an option). Clinicians must recognize the transition to advanced heart failure so that therapeutic options can be considered in a timely fashion and patients are able to proactively match medical decisions to clinical realities. *CHF*, Chronic heart failure; *MCS*, mechanical circulatory support. (From Allen LA, Stevenson LW, Grady KL, et al. Decision making in advanced heart failure: a scientific statement from the American Heart Association. *Circulation.* 2012;125(15):1928–1952.)

Prognostic considerations tend to focus on the singular outcome of mortality. However, other clinical outcomes also rank high in importance to individual patients (**Fig. 50.2**). Multiple studies have documented patients' willingness to sacrifice survival in exchange for symptom relief, a trade-off that varies between patients[30] and even within the same patient over time,[31] is correlated loosely with disease severity but strongly with do not resuscitate (DNR) status.[32] A full discussion of prognosis therefore includes not only the risks of death but also the patient's goals and values including potential burdens of worsening symptoms, limited functional capacity, loss of independence, reduced social functioning, decreased quality of life, and increased caregiver commitment. Unfortunately, even less is known about risk prediction for these latter outcomes.[33]

Ultimately the stochastic nature of heart failure conveys a high level of prognostic uncertainty for most individual patients. It is therefore vital to acknowledge and incorporate uncertainty in discussions about future care.

CATEGORIES OF MAJOR TREATMENT DECISIONS

In the face of complex treatment options for heart failure, a framework for classifying various medical decisions can help clinicians and their patients better anticipate and manage those decisions most likely to occur as the disease progresses to an advanced stage (**Table 50.4**). Clinicians should take an active role in defining the set of interventions that are medically reasonable, and from these, clinicians and patients can work together to determine which option is most consistent with patient values, goals, and preferences. The more that clinicians can anticipate medical decisions in advance (see the section "Risk Assessment" earlier), the more they can help patients have adequate time to consider their likely options.

Low-Intensity Interventions That May Improve Quantity and Quality of Life

While anticipating and addressing new management options that accompany progressive heart failure, clinicians should work to

TABLE 50.2   Selected Prognostic Models in Heart Failure

	Key Covariates	Outcome
Ambulatory		
Heart Failure Survival Score[98]	Peak VO$_2$, LVEF, serum sodium, mean BP, HR, ischemic etiology, QRS duration/morphology	All-cause mortality
Seattle Heart Failure Model[99] (depts.washington.edu/shfm)	NYHA class, ischemic etiology, diuretic dose, LVEF, SBP, sodium, hemoglobin, percent lymphocytes, uric acid, and cholesterol	All-cause mortality, urgent transplantation, or LVAD implantation
MAGGIC Heart Failure Risk Score (http://www.heartfailurerisk.org/)	Age, LVEF, sBP, BMI, creatinine, NYHA class, gender, smoking, diabetes, COPD, HF diagnosis >18 months prior, BB, ACEI	All-cause mortality
Hospitalized		
ADHERE Risk Model[100]	BUN, SBP, serum creatinine	In-hospital mortality
ESCAPE Discharge Score[101]	BNP, cardiopulmonary resuscitation or mechanical ventilation during hospitalization, BUN, sodium, age >70 years, daily loop diuretic dose, lack of beta-blocker, 6-minute walk distance	6-month mortality
EVEREST Risk Model[33]	Age, diabetes, h/o stroke, h/o arrhythmia, beta-blocker use, BUN, sodium, BNP, KCCQ scores	Mortality or persistently poor quality of life (KCCQ <45) over the 6 months after discharge

ACEI, Angiotensin-converting enzyme inhibitor; *ADHERE,* Registry for Acute Decompensated Heart Failure Patients; *BB,* beta-blocker; *BNP,* B-type natriuretic peptide; *BP,* blood pressure; *BUN,* blood urea nitrogen; *COPD,* chronic obstructive pulmonary disease; *CVA,* cerebrovascular accident; *EFFECT,* enhanced feedback for effective cardiac treatment; *ESCAPE,* evaluation study of congestive heart failure and pulmonary artery catheterization effectiveness; *EVEREST,* efficacy of vasopressin antagonism in heart failure outcome study with tolvaptan; *h/o,* (medical) history of; *HR,* heart rate; *KCCQ,* Kansas city cardiomyopathy questionnaire; *LVAD,* left ventricular assist device; *LVEF,* left ventricular ejection fraction; *NYHA,* New York Heart Association; *SBP,* systolic BP; *VO$_2$,* oxygen consumption.

TABLE 50.3   The I-NEED-HELP Mnemonic for Advanced Heart Failure[a]

I	Inotropes: Previous or ongoing requirement for dobutamine, milrinone, dopamine, etc.
N	NYHA Class/Natriuretic Peptides: Persisting NYHA IIIB or IV and/or persistently high BNP or NT-proBNP.
E	End-Organ Dysfunction: Worsening renal or liver dysfunction in the setting of heart failure.
E	Ejection Fraction: LVEF <25%.
D	Defibrillator Shocks: Recurrent appropriate defibrillator shocks for VT/VF.
H	Hospitalizations: >1 Hospitalizations for worsening heart failure in last 12 months.
E	Edema/Escalating Diuretics: Persistent fluid overload, increasing diuretics, or need for ultrafiltration.
L	Low Blood Pressure: Consistently low BP with systolic <90–100 mm Hg and symptoms.
P	Prognostic Medication: Inability to up-titrate (or need to decrease/cease) ACEI, BB, ARNI, MRA

[a]The I-NEED-HELP mnemonic provides a useful guide to remember events that herald worsening disease, which should prompt reassessment of patient goals of care as well as consideration of therapy options for advanced heart failure.

ACEI, Angiotensin-converting enzyme inhibitors; *ARNI,* angiotensin receptor-neprilysin inhibitor; *BB,* beta-blocker; *BNP,* B-type natriuretic peptide; *LVEF,* left ventricular ejection fraction; *MRA,* mineralocorticoid receptor antagonist; *NT-proBNP,* N-terminal B-type natriuretic peptide; *NYHA,* New York Heart Association; *VF,* ventricular fibrillation; *VT,* ventricular tachycardia.

Adapted from Baumwol J. "I Need Help." A mnemonic to aid timely referral in advanced heart failure. *J Heart Lung Transplant.* 2017;36(5):593–594.

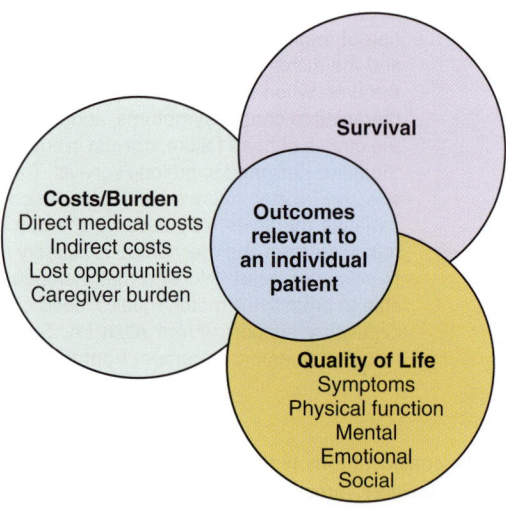

Fig. 50.2 Multiple outcomes that are of varying importance to individual patients. Discussions about the potential risks and benefits of therapy options should extend beyond survival to consider the full range of patient-centered outcomes. (From Allen LA, Stevenson LW, Grady KL, et al. Decision making in advanced heart failure: a scientific statement from the American Heart Association. *Circulation.* 2012;125[15]:1928–1952.)

optimize background medical therapy for heart failure and other comorbidities.[1,2] In order for patients to be defined as advanced Stage D heart failure, patients must have failed optimal medical therapy (see Table 50.1).[7] The need to decrease or discontinue neurohormonal antagonists (e.g., beta-blockers; Table 50.3) generally signals worsening disease.[34]

TABLE 50.4   Framework of Major Medical Decisions in Advanced Heart Failure Faced by Patients and their Clinicians

Types of Options	Examples of Interventions	Examples of Adverse Outcomes that Should Be Anticipated in High-Risk Patients
Low-Intensity Interventions That Might Improve Quantity and Quality of Life		
Medical therapy	Beta-blocker, ACEI/ARB, MRA, diuretics, control of hypertension and other comorbidities	• Hypotension, azotemia: threshold for accepting intolerance and considering advanced therapies?
High-Intensity Interventions That Might Improve Quantity and Quality of Life		
Procedures with the potential to improve cardiac function	CABG	• Inability to come off bypass: place mechanical circulatory support? • Ventilator dependence: tracheostomy versus extubate? • Stroke: feeding tube? institutional care?
	Valve surgery Pericardial stripping Percutaneous valve intervention	
	PCI	• Coronary occlusion: revert to CABG?
	CRT	• Unable to place coronary sinus lead: convert to thoracotomy?
Replacement of cardiac function	Transplantation	• Early graft failure or other serious postoperative complications: mechanical circulatory support or withdraw support? • Later graft failure: list for retransplantation?
	Permanent MCS/LVAD	• Stroke, infection, or recurrent bleeding: turn off device?
High-Intensity Interventions That Might Improve Quantity But Not Quality of Life		
Procedures to reduce the risk of sudden cardiac death	ICD	• Worsening pump failure disease: ICD deactivation?
Temporary Therapies to Stabilize Patients That Can Lead to Dependence		
Adjunctive therapies instituted during acute decompensation with potential chronic dependence	Temporary mechanical circulatory support devices (IABP, percutaneous VAD, ECMO)	• Unable to wean: convert to permanent LVAD or withdraw?
	IV inotropes	• Unable to wean: transition to home inotropes or discontinue?
	Renal replacement therapy (dialysis or ultrafiltration)	• Failure of acute kidney injury to resolve: initiate indefinite hemodialysis or discontinue?
Noncardiac Procedures With Increased Risk and Potentially Decreased Benefit		
	Joint replacement Hernia repair	• Worsening heart failure causing hemodynamic and/or respiratory collapse: continue ventilatory support and/or initiate circulatory support?
	Resection of pulmonary nodule, routine screening colonoscopy	• Not generally to be done, as risks are felt to outweigh potential benefit

ACEI, Angiotensin-converting enzyme inhibitor; *ARB*, angiotensin receptor blocker; *CABG*, coronary artery bypass grafting surgery; *CRT*, cardiac resynchronization therapy; *CRT-D*, CRT combined with ICD; *ECMO*, extracorporeal membranous oxygenation; *IABP*, intra-aortic balloon pump; *ICD*, implantable cardioverter-defibrillator; *LVAD*, left ventricular assist device *MCS*, mechanical circulatory support; *MRA*, mineralocorticoid receptor antagonist; *PCI*, percutaneous coronary intervention; *VAD*, ventricular assist device.

High-Intensity Interventions That May Improve Quantity and Quality of Life

A variety of invasive procedures exist that have the potential to improve cardiac function, thereby increasing both survival and quality of life. However, they also have the potential to cause harm and patient burden, particularly among patients with advanced heart failure who are older and have greater multimorbidity than patients studied in randomized trials. Therefore, decisions around such therapies should include detailed informed consent and shared decision making, even if the therapies are generally supported by a strong evidence base. Additionally, careful consideration of a range of potential complications should be addressed with patients pre-procedurally ("What if?") so that contingency plans are in place in case rare but serious events do occur.

Patients with heart failure may be considered for cardiac surgery for coronary, valvular, and pericardial disease. Cardiac surgeries involving general anesthesia, thoracic access, and cardiopulmonary bypass are higher risk as a consequence of underlying severe cardiac dysfunction. In order to consider cardiac surgery as an option, the surgery should be expected to convey significant long-term benefit. However, the benefit of many cardiac procedures in advanced chronic heart failure has been difficult to study.[35] The potential for residual cardiac dysfunction, perioperative death, protracted postoperative rehabilitation, and loss of independence must be considered and included thoughtfully in the shared decision, as surgery inherently increases short-term risk for the prospect of longer term benefit.

Less invasive percutaneous approaches for the treatment of coronary and valvular disease may be appealing in advanced heart failure. Catheter approaches to aortic, mitral, and even tricuspid disease have now been shown to be reasonable alternatives to surgery in certain populations (**see also Chapter 26**).[36,37] However, the benefits of valve repair or replacement are less well established in patients with significant heart failure, especially when treating functional (secondary) mitral regurgitation for patients with a dilated left ventricle.[38] Additionally, potential benefits may be diminished by noncardiac comorbidities, while risks of contrast-induced nephropathy, stroke, and 30-day mortality are increased in the advanced heart failure population. Patient-clinician discussions regarding percutaneous interventions should also include preprocedural consideration of whether emergency surgery would be appropriate and feasible.

Cardiac implantable electronic devices for bradycardia and cardiac resynchronization therapy (CRT) can improve cardiac function but require an invasive procedure, include the risk of infection, and necessitate long-term follow-up (**see also Chapter 38**).[39] Additionally, patients with advanced heart failure (New York Heart Association [NYHA] functional class IV) have represented a small fraction of patients included in randomized trials of CRT, creating uncertainty about the benefit in this population.[40] Regardless, the care team should plan for contingencies, such as consideration of an open thoracotomy for perforation or unsuccessful coronary sinus lead placement. Factors likely to modify the risk–benefit ratio of device implantation, such as noncardiovascular morbidity and acute decompensation, should also be recognized and incorporated into these discussions. Although CRT and ICDs are often packaged together, their purposes are quite different; CRT, like neurohormonal antagonist therapy, is designed to improve cardiac performance and can improve quality of life; ICDs do not. Therefore, the recommendation for CRT combined with ICD should prompt separate discussions around the indications for defibrillation versus cardiac resynchronization, as well as differences in the need for monitoring, the chances for inappropriate shocks and worsening heart failure, the risks for infection and lead malfunction, and the options for deactivation.

Cardiac transplantation and mechanical circulatory support offer the potential to fundamentally change the clinical course of heart failure by exchanging it for surgical therapy and a different set of benefits, risks, and burdens. In the case of transplantation, patients are asked to weigh their current clinical course against a posttransplant estimated mean survival of approximately 12 years as well as the risks of surgery, graft rejection, infection, and the other side effects of immunosuppression.[41] For permanently implanted LVADs in inotrope-dependent patients, 2-year survival is increased from less than 10% without LVAD to greater than 70% with LVAD, and a near doubling in quality of life measures among survivors, but at the risk of (1) reoperation to replace a malfunctioning pump (10%); (2) disabling stroke (11%); (3) device infection; (4) bleeding; and (5) recurrent hospitalizations.[42,43] Even in the setting of successful LVAD, patients must maintain a constant power source, perform vigilant driveline care, and manage other chronic diseases—and these issues spill over to caregivers. Thus, for eligible patients, whether to pursue transplantation and/or mechanical circulatory support involves complex tradeoffs and major uncertainties. For young patients dying from heart failure without other comorbidities and with adequate socioeconomic support, transplantation and LVAD are rarely declined. For older patients with significant noncardiac disease, declining an LVAD is not unusual.[44] For the majority of patients with heart failure these advanced therapies are not an option due to the predominance of heart failure with normal ejection fraction, multiple comorbidities, or very advanced age. Detailed clinical practice guidelines for transplantation and mechanical circulatory support—including detailed discussions of candidacy—are available,[45,46] and are covered in other chapters (**see also Chapters 44 and 45**). Medicare's 2013 decision memo requires the inclusion of palliative care service for programs to maintain certification for destination therapy implantation.[47]

High-Intensity Interventions That May Improve Quantity But Not Quality of Life

ICDs are fundamentally different than many life-saving therapies for patients with chronic heart failure with reduced ejection fraction.[48] ICDs improve survival by aborting lethal arrhythmias, but do not improve cardiac function or heart failure symptoms. At the same time, ICDs create an additional burden for patients including inappropriate shocks, increased risk of hospitalization, potential decrease in quality of life,[49] and higher likelihood of death from progressive pump failure, meticulous discussion of absolute risks with and without ICDs are particularly important for informed consent and shared decision making. Medicare's proposed 2018 changes to the national coverage determination for ICDs include "Requiring a patient-shared decision-making interaction prior to ICD implantation for certain patients."[50]

Temporary Therapies with Potential Dependence

Some therapies are intended for short-term use to stabilize patients, thereby allowing for recovery from potentially reversible insults or transition to more definitive therapy. Although initially intended as a temporary intervention, such stabilizing therapies can create indefinite dependence if the patient does not improve as hoped or develops an adverse event (e.g., stroke, progressive renal failure) that compromises previously anticipated options.

Short-term circulatory support with intra-aortic balloon pumps or percutaneous mechanical circulatory support devices may be initiated when acute hemodynamic instability requires urgent intervention to avoid permanent end-organ dysfunction and/or death. It may be instituted with the hope of supporting a reversible underlying condition, such as fulminate myocarditis or cardiogenic shock after acute myocardial infarction. It may also be initiated in patients who might be potential candidates for transplantation or permanent circulatory support in whom (1) there has not been opportunity to appropriately evaluate a patient's candidacy or preferences for more definitive high-dependence therapies, (2) reversibility of end-organ dysfunction is uncertain (INTERMACS profile 1), or (3) socioeconomic contraindications to more definitive therapies may resolve in the near future. If device dependency persists and contraindications to definitive therapies do not resolve, a decision will need to be made to discontinue therapy, which can be particularly challenging when patients or families are not in agreement with withdrawal. To whatever degree possible, these issues should be addressed prior to the initiation of short-term support.

Intravenous inotropic agents are commonly initiated in the acute setting for hemodynamic stabilization and to improve end-organ perfusion. Their use is most often anticipated to be temporary, with the hope of either clinical improvement or eligibility for more definitive therapies as above. Regardless of intent, the initiation of inotropic support for exacerbation of chronic heart failure should be considered a harbinger of severe heart failure (see Table 50.3). When patients fail to wean from intravenous inotropic support, decisions arise around continued chronic use. Therefore the goals of temporary inotrope use should be clearly established prior to initiation, and unexpected dependence on this therapy should prompt direct discussions about overall goals of care. High-quality evidence about the risks and benefits of ambulatory inotrope infusions in patients with advanced heart failure is limited, particularly when used for palliation (as opposed to bridge to transplantation). Available data suggest that outpatient inotrope infusions are associated with early improvement in NYHA functional class, fewer hospital days, and no major change in survival.[51] In a contemporary single-center experience of 197 patients discharged with continuous inotropes, 17% had ICD shocks, 29% had infections, and 57% were rehospitalized.[52] Thus inotropic infusion may offer a medical option to help end-stage patients leave the hospital and return home, but it must be recognized that their use is relatively expensive and only about half the hospice agencies will take patients on inotropes.[53] The decision to arrange for chronic continuous infusions should be offered only after checking availability and cost considerations, and should be subsequently guided by the patient's goals and preferences, including the need for symptom relief.

The prevalence of advanced kidney disease increases dramatically with worsening heart failure, and measures of renal dysfunction are strong predictors of adverse outcomes in patients with heart failure (see Tables 50.2 and 50.3). Dialysis in the setting of older age has been shown to add to patient burden, and in high-risk patients (e.g., those with heart failure) may not extend life.[54] Not surprisingly, ICDs may be less effective in heart failure patients on dialysis.[55] LVAD use in dialysis patients has a median survival of less than 3 weeks.[56] Therefore, the initiation of renal replacement therapies (e.g., hemodialysis, ultrafiltration) in patients with advanced heart failure or, conversely, the initiation of mechanical circulatory support in patients with severe chronic kidney disease should only be made after carefully assessing medical feasibility followed by a clear discussion with the patient about the risks and benefits of dialysis on the patient's quality of life and prognosis.[57]

Feeding tubes, placement of permanent peritoneal and pleural catheters for the control of volume status, and intensive care provide additional examples of therapies with questionable long-term value in patients with irreversible underlying disease. When such situations are anticipated, these types of near end-of-life interventions can be considered as part of a healthy discussion about end-of-life care, ideally prior to the occurrence of a near-terminal event.

Noncardiac Procedures in Patients with Advanced Heart Failure

The risks and benefits of interventions for noncardiac conditions may be significantly altered in patients with advanced heart failure. When the likelihood of meaningful recovery without the procedure is small, the increase in procedural risk in patients with advanced heart failure may be considered acceptable. Examples include both emergent (e.g., laparotomy for perforated viscous) and urgent (e.g., hip arthroplasty for fracture) surgical procedures. However, the majority of noncardiac procedures, such as knee replacement for degenerative joint disease, must be carefully considered in the context of patient preferences, as complications of the procedure may or may not outweigh the potential benefit. Major procedures should generally be discouraged when they do not offer a tangible improvement in quality of life (e.g., repair of asymptomatic abdominal aortic aneurysm). Routine screening tests (e.g., mammography, colonoscopy) are generally not appropriate in the context of a significant competing risk of mortality from advanced heart failure, yet such tests are frequently ordered at the end of life.[58]

PALLIATIVE CARE

Palliative care is interdisciplinary care aimed at preventing and relieving suffering.[14] The Centers for Medicare and Medicaid Services (CMS) defines palliative care as treatment for the relief of pain and other uncomfortable symptoms through the appropriate coordination of all aspects of care needed to maximize personal comfort and to relieve distress.[59] The World Health Organization provides an expanded definition, which includes the following: "provides relief from pain and other distressing symptoms; affirms life and regards dying as a normal process; intends neither to hasten or postpone death; integrates the psychological and spiritual aspects of patient care; offers a support system to help patients live as actively as possible until death; offers a support system to help the family cope during the patients illness and

in their own bereavement; uses a team approach to address the needs of patients and their families, including bereavement counselling, if indicated; will enhance quality of life, and may also positively influence the course of illness; is applicable early in the course of illness, in conjunction with other therapies that are intended to prolong life, such as chemotherapy or radiation therapy, and includes those investigations needed to better understand and manage distressing clinical complications."[60] Thus palliative care interventions are those in which the principal aim is to improve symptomatology and quality of life, in contrast to interventions that are primarily meant to be curative or prolong life. Palliative care can be offered simultaneously with other appropriate medical therapies and can be integrated at any point in the care of those afflicted with serious illness (**see Fig. 50.1**).

Types of Palliative Care
Primary Palliative Care

All clinicians caring for patients with advanced cardiovascular disease play a role to provide supportive and palliative interventions. This role is vital because (1) many of the therapies that improve symptoms and quality of life derive from treatment of the underlying cardiovascular disease; (2) prognosis and complex decisions are often best understood by the cardiovascular specialist; (3) integrated care is often preferable to further fragmentation through another consult team; and (4) there are not enough palliative care specialists to provide such services to everyone in need. Provision of supportive care by the usual care team has been designated as "primary" palliative care, to distinguish it from "secondary" or "subspecialty" palliative care. Clinicians supervising inpatient or longitudinal care for patients with heart failure should regard expertise in providing palliative care as integral to their professional competence.

Secondary (Specialty) Palliative Care

Palliative care clinicians receive specific training in the management of refractory symptoms and the facilitation of difficult care planning in life-threatening illnesses. Hospice and Palliative Medicine is a recognized medical subspecialty in the United States, Canada, England, Ireland, Australia, and New Zealand. Masters' degree programs have been developed for physicians, nurse practitioners, physician assistants, and nurses who are interested in becoming community palliative care specialists, and specialty certifications are also available for nurses, social workers, and chaplains. In most jurisdictions, specialty palliative care is provided by an interdisciplinary team who work with a patient's other clinicians to provide an "extra layer" of support.[61]

Indications for a Palliative Care Consultation

Various specialties may assume the central role in the coordination of patient care at different stages of disease progression, often with transition of leadership from primary care to cardiology to palliative care (**Fig. 50.3**).[62] Shared ownership and planning around palliative care needs can improve communication and understanding of patient goals and better end-of-life experiences. Formal consultation may be particularly helpful when symptoms remain intolerable or when medical decision making is particularly challenging. For example, since 2013, national standards require centers who offer permanent mechanical circulatory support to include palliative care specialists as part of the team from evaluation through to death.[63]

Data are mixed regarding the optimal use and effectiveness of specialty palliative care. A retrospective analysis of Medicaid patients in four New York hospitals from 2004 to 2007 indicated that palliative care consultation during hospitalization for the exacerbation of chronic fatal illness, including heart failure, was associated with a $4000 lower cost for discharged patients and $7000 lower cost for patients dying during that hospitalization.[64] The Palliative Care in Heart Failure (PAL-HF), single-center, randomized trial of 150 patients with advanced heart failure showed that randomization to a multidisciplinary palliative team intervention improved scores for quality of life and functional assessment of chronic illness therapy with palliative care (FACIT-Pal) at 6 months.[65] Yet, in a large randomized trial in intensive care settings, palliative care specialist supervision of at least two structured family meetings and written information did not decrease anxiety or depression and may have increased posttraumatic stress for families compared to similar intervention led by the intensive care unit teams.[66] To be effective, palliative care consultations need to be targeted to the right patients at the right time and integrated thoughtfully into the overall plan of medical care.

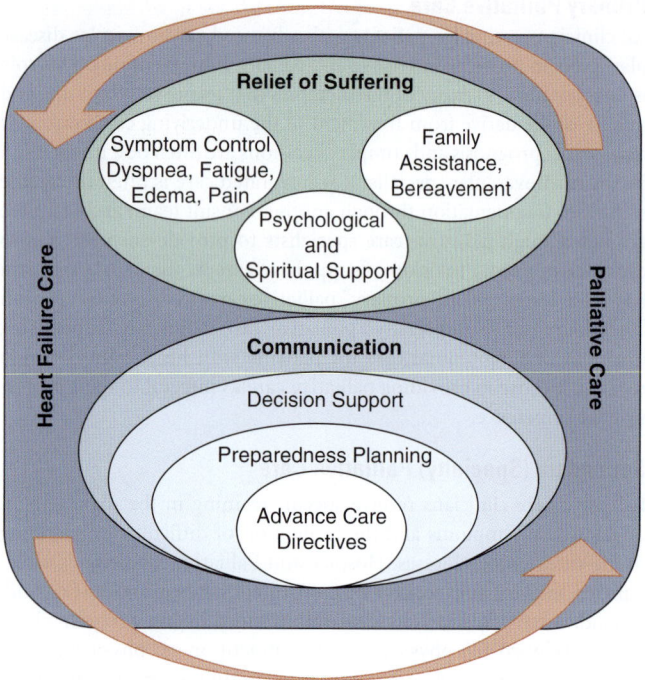

Fig. 50.3 Model of team-based palliative care for cardiovascular disease.

Hospice

The term hospice is used to describe a specific model of palliative care that is offered to patients who are at the end of life with a terminal disease when curative or life-prolonging therapy is no longer a focus of treatment. Historically, the hospice was developed for patients with cancer, but it is increasingly used for patients with cardiovascular disease, with 14.7% of admissions to US hospices in 2014 having a primary diagnosis of heart disease.[67] In practice, "hospice" describes a subset of palliative care services that have specific legal, administrative, and financial definitions. In the United States, referral is most often guided by the CMS hospice eligibility guidelines, which require that two physicians or a physician and a nurse practitioner (one of whom is often the hospice medical director) certify that the patient is expected to have 6 months or less to live, and the patient must be willing to forego usual medical services aimed at curing the underlying terminal diagnosis.[68] Which therapies are allowed to be continued is dependent upon individual hospice agencies, with about half capable of continuing inotropic infusion.[53] While the 6-month time period is rarely reached, patients who survive beyond it can usually continue to receive hospice benefits if the prognosis remains poor. Although hospice is provided in a variety of environments, it is most commonly provided for patients at home with the goal of keeping them in their home until death. Hospice can offer a number of benefits to enrollees and their families, including interdisciplinary team management, home visits, respite care, provision of medications and durable medical equipment, and a nurse who can always be contacted to advise on urgent symptom needs.

Less than half of all patients with heart failure receive hospice.[69] However, this is a marked increase from a decade ago (**Fig. 50.4**).[6,67] Appropriate timing of referral to hospice is important, as the family's perception of being referred "too late" is associated with greater dissatisfaction and unmet needs. One study of Medicare beneficiaries who received hospice demonstrated a longer survival compared to those heart failure patients who did not receive hospice, such that enrollment in hospice should not be equated with accelerated death or "giving up."[70] Families of those dying with hospice services tend to be more likely to rate their dying experience as "favorable or excellent" compared to those who died in an institution or at home with only home health services.[71]

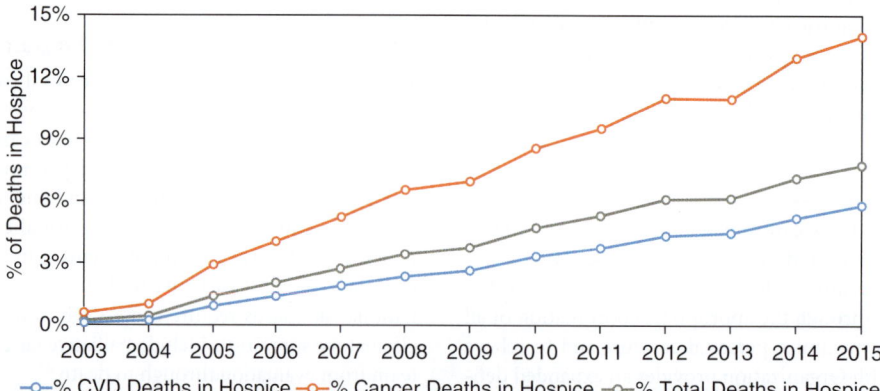

Fig. 50.4 Trends in the percentage of US total, cardiovascular disease (*CVD*), and cancer-related deaths occurring in hospice from 2003 to 2015. (From Warraich HJ, Hernandez AF, Allen LA. How medicine has changed the end of life for patients with cardiovascular disease. *J Am Coll Cardiol.* 2017;70[10]:1276–1289; and Centers for Disease Control and Prevention, National Center for Health Statistics. Underlying Cause of Death from 1999–2015 on CDC-WONDER Online Database. Released December; 2016. https://wonder.cdc.gov/ucd-icd10.html. Accessed February 19, 2018.)

Symptom Palliation

Even with expert cardiovascular management, symptoms are rarely completely relieved and often worsen as the disease becomes increasingly refractory to cardiovascular-focused therapies.[7] The basic principles, strategies, and expected benefits of palliative care approaches to symptoms pertain to severely symptomatic and functionally limited patients with end-stage cardiovascular disease.[72] The most prevalent complaints for patients with heart failure are dyspnea, pain, edema, depression, and fatigue. Other sources of suffering that have been identified include isolation, difficulty navigating the health care system, and the feeling of uncertainty surrounding prognosis and longevity. Because many of the symptomatic complaints expressed by patients with advanced heart failure are the result of the underlying cardiac dysfunction, heart failure therapies (e.g., diuretics) form the foundation of symptom palliation for patients with heart failure. Furthermore, cardiovascular disease rarely occurs in isolation, such that integrated approaches to care, which consider symptoms arising from multiple causes, apply to most patients with heart failure. Medications and nonpharmacologic therapies are generally added in a step-wise and complementary fashion, which generally involves first optimizing therapies for underlying disease, removing exacerbating factors, and then adding palliative treatments for specific symptomatology (**Fig. 50.5**). A palliative care specialist is rarely needed to prescribe the interventions; most clinicians can learn to provide these services.

Dyspnea

Dyspnea is the most common symptom experienced in advanced heart failure. The mainstay of therapy is diuresis and vasodilation to decrease pulmonary congestion.[1] However, patients with advanced heart failure may have hypotension, renal dysfunction, or other factors that may limit the effective use of these therapies to diminish dyspnea. For patients with dyspnea refractory to hemodynamic interventions (diuretics, afterload reduction, inotropes) and oxygen, international guidelines recommend the use of opioids[73]; although not all studies have been positive.[74] Low dosages of opioids are often sufficient to achieve relief of dyspnea. As the drug may accumulate in end-stage heart failure, only cautious dose increases should occur within the first week. Opioids must be accompanied by laxatives in time to prevent rather than reverse constipation. Renal function is impaired in many older patients with advanced cardiovascular disease so oxycodone may be preferred to morphine (as some metabolites of morphine can accumulate and cause confusion). Clinicians report fear of adverse respiratory effects and addiction as important barriers to opioid prescription,

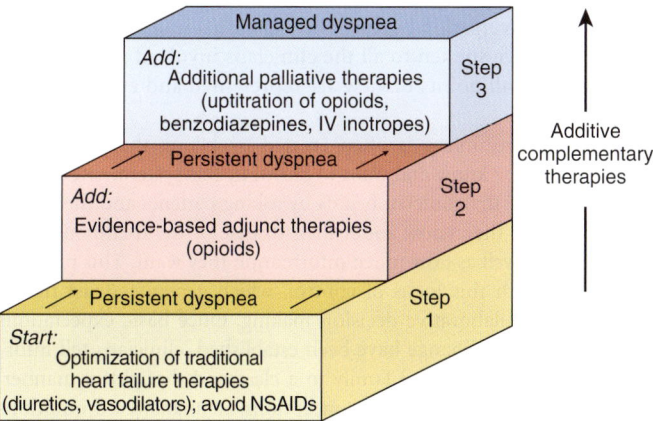

Fig. 50.5 A step-wise approach to the palliation of dyspnea in patients with heart failure. *NSAIDs,* Nonsteroidal antiinflammatory drugs.

despite studies showing limited adverse effects and low rates of dependence and addiction in appropriately treated patients.[75] Scopolamine is occasionally used to decrease secretions but should not be used routinely as it often causes disorientation and confusion. Benzodiazepines also have been tested for control of breathlessness, but have been found to be inferior to opiates.[76] Oxygen is only beneficial in reducing dyspnea in hypoxic patients and has no role in the nonhypoxic patient.[77,78]

Pain

The majority of patients with symptomatic heart failure report some form of pain, which increases with NYHA functional class. An estimated 69% of class III patients and 89% of class IV patients report pain.[79] Though pain syndromes in heart failure are not well described, it is thought that both heart failure itself and underlying medical comorbidities and psychosocial stressors contribute to the experience of pain. Unfortunately, there are little high-quality data to guide the management of pain in advanced heart failure. As a first step, providers should do all they can to treat heart failure and comorbidities, as well as screen for and treat coexistent depression and anxiety, as these can exacerbate pain. If pain persists, opiates should be considered and up-titrated. In choosing opiates, special caution should be given to methadone, which can prolong the QT interval. Nonsteroidal antiinflammatory drugs should be avoided in patients with heart failure due to their propensity to cause sodium and fluid retention.[80] Though there is a high prevalence of pain among the advanced heart failure population, the use of opiates appears to be disproportionately low among these patients. One study demonstrated that the usage of opiates was only 22% among patients with advanced heart failure compared to nearly 50% among patients with cancer.[81]

Depression

Depression is highly prevalent among patients with advanced heart failure. Approximately 20% of patients meet criteria for major depressive disorder, and a greater percentage report depressive symptoms. Even when adjusting for covariates, patients with worsening depression have worse clinical outcomes. Unfortunately, limited data are available on pharmacologic, cognitive, and exercise therapy for depression in patients with advanced cardiovascular disease. A trial of 469 patients with symptomatic heart failure found no significant difference in depression or cardiovascular status in the treatment group compared with placebo.[82] In another trial of 158 heart failure patients, cognitive behavioral therapy was effective in reducing depression compared with usual care (12.8% vs. 17.3%; $P = .008$), but did not influence self-care.[83] Despite these mixed data, many clinicians continue to try pharmacological therapy with selective serotonin reuptake inhibitors (SSRIs), psychostimulants (e.g., methylphenidate), or tricyclic antidepressants (i.e., nortriptyline, which has less significant anticholinergic effects such as orthostatic hypotension than other tricyclics). Medication side effects that may warrant monitoring in some patients include QT prolongation with tricyclic antidepressants and hyponatremia with SSRIs.[80]

Fatigue

As with other symptoms, the primary approach to fatigue is the identification and treatment of all potential secondary causes, such as depression, thyroid dysfunction, anemia, overdiuresis, electrolyte disturbances, and occult infection. Sleep apnea may contribute, although treatment of sleep apnea with positive pressure ventilation in advanced heart failure remains controversial.[84] Pharmacological options for primary fatigue can include stimulants, such as methylphenidate, but this may have negative cardiovascular effects.[80] Nonpharmacological techniques include aerobic exercise and training in energy conservation.

End-of-Life Care and Device Deactivation

Although the prognostic uncertainty inherent in heart failure makes it difficult to accurately anticipate the end of life, some patients enter a terminal phase of the disease that may be relatively apparent to the patients, caregivers, and/or clinicians. In such situations, where the goals of care often transition from a focus on survival to quality of life and assuring a good death, clinicians should take responsibility for initiating and coordinating a comprehensive plan of care consistent with patient values, preferences, and goals.

The option and ease of ICD deactivation should be discussed prior to implantation and again for major changes in clinical status or transitions in goals of care.[85] At present, this is done only rarely, thus leaving many patients vulnerable to inappropriate device discharge and unnecessary suffering.[86] A national survey of hospices found that less than 10% of hospices have a policy regarding deactivation of ICDs, and greater than 50% of hospices had at least one patient who had been shocked within the last year.[87] For a device near end-of-battery life, the generator should not be changed without careful review of whether or not active defibrillation is consistent with overall goals of care and anticipated duration of good quality survival.

Although the legal construct of patient autonomy does not recognize different degrees of dependence on therapies to be withdrawn, clinicians, patients, and caregivers/families may view scenarios in which proactive withdrawal leads to direct patient demise as unique and emotionally difficult. Examples include withdrawal of renal replacement therapy, feeding tubes, or pacemaker support for patients dependent on cardiac pacing.

An increasingly common scenario is the withdrawal of mechanical circulatory support devices, either temporary or durable, in patients who are not expected to recover to return to an acceptable quality of life.[88] With improvements in medical technology and associated outcomes, patients maintained with mechanical circulatory support may not only be susceptible to death from cardiovascular causes and pump complications, but also other life-limiting disease. The discussion regarding discontinuing device therapy should be part of the consent process prior to implantation. Device deactivation can be done in the hospital or at home, attended by a device-trained individual and others as requested (hospice nurse, chaplain, etc.). Discontinuation of power to valveless continuous flow devices typically results in an immediate and marked reduction in systemic blood flow, with most deaths occurring in less than 20 minutes. This clinical scenario has been likened to withdrawal of endotracheal intubation and ventilatory support, although patients with LVAD support are more likely to be awake and alert at the time of the decision to discontinue support.

DECISION-MAKING APPROACHES AND COMMUNICATION SKILLS

Advanced heart failure—with its high degree of prognostic uncertainty and complex trade-offs in the choice of medical care—demands a thoughtful approach to communication and medical decision making. Most patients and families want accurate and honest conversations with their clinicians. Ideally, these interactions are not one-time events but occur as an evolving series of discussions over time, particularly as a patient's condition changes. Clinicians must attend to the emotional nature of conversations with patients to build trust and clarify core values.

Timing of Discussions

Finding appropriate time to discuss preferences, prognosis, and medical options is a formidable challenge in routine clinical practice. Such discussions require a major commitment of time, focus,

and emotional energy. Current organizational and reimbursement structures tend to disincentivize encounters of this nature. As a result, formal discussions about prognosis and decision making are often deferred until more emergent occasions, when thoughtful decision making may be impaired. Instead, such discussions should occur both routinely and at the occurrence of major clinical events that herald a worsening prognosis (see Table 50.3). Some have argued for an "Annual Heart Failure Review," modeled after primary care annual wellness visits, to routinize decision making and ensure anticipatory guidance.[15] In addition to "voluntary advance care planning," including formal designation of a health care proxy and DNR status, such reviews could also include the clarification of the patient's values, a formal assessment of prognosis, a review of existing therapies, and discussions about possible future events. Understandably, such a review would require considerable face-to-face time between the patient, family, and physician, and thus requires a commitment by individual clinicians as well as the health care delivery system.

Optimal Communication Techniques

Open, clear, and accurate communication with patients with heart failure is important for several reasons.[15] First, the majority of patients with serious illness want information about their illness and to be included in the decision-making process. And as they understand more about their disease and options, they are progressively more likely to want an active role in medical decisions. Second, when clinicians have conversations with patients about their prognosis and desires, patients are more likely to receive care that is aligned with their goals and preferences. These conversations also improve the patient-clinician relationship. Finally, when conversations occur, families of deceased patients have better outcomes in terms of the manner in which they cope with loss of their loved one as well as their own psychological outcome. There is no single best way to have these conversations, and they must be tailored to individual patients under existing circumstances. However, there are practices that can help optimize communication. **Table 50.5** outlines specific tasks, steps, and phrases that can be used to facilitate better communication.

Before one can embark upon difficult conversations with patients and their families, it is important to establish the right context for the conversation. This includes asking if patients want to have the conversation by themselves or would like other individuals present, remembering that patients often define family in a myriad of ways. Creating the right setting also involves assuring that the right clinicians are present, or at least have been consulted, before the conversation begins. The individual leading the meeting ideally will have spoken to all the clinicians involved in the care of the patient so all points of view are represented and everyone is on the same page.

A helpful beginning is often created by asking the patient and family what they know and want to know. In this system, often called Ask-Tell-Ask,[89] the clinician begins by asking patients and their families both what they know about their disease or the treatment being considered as well as how much information they want. This provides the patient with this locus of control, which generates trust that is essential for collaborative decision making. Once basic expectations for information exchange have been established, clinicians tell information to the patient and family in a clear and thoughtful manner, while also clearing up any misconceptions or unanswered questions they might have. It is important to initially focus on the larger picture of the patient's health, as the ability to cognitively hear information, particularly in stressful situations, is limited. Finally, clinicians should

TABLE 50.5 Core Tasks, Skills, and Sample Phrases to Improve Clinician-Patient Communication in Advanced Heart Failure

Steps in the Roadmap	Elements of the Step	Sample Phrases
Establish the setting and participants	Determine who should be present and assure that all appropriate clinicians are present as well	"In preparation for our meeting tomorrow, I'm going to have the cardiothoracic surgeon there to be a part of our conversation. In terms of your family or support network, who is it important that we make sure is there?"
Determine what patients know and want to know	ASK what patients/families know	"Tell me about your heart disease; how have you been doing lately?" "What is your understanding of what is occurring now and why we are considering the treatment that we have been discussing?"
	ASK what patients/families want to know	"Sometime patients want to know all the details, whereas other times they just want to know a general outline. What kind of person are you?" "How much information would you like to know about what is happening with your heart disease?"
	TELL the patient/family the information in a sympathetic and thoughtful manner while also clearing up any misconceptions or unanswered questions	"I think you have a pretty good understanding of what is happening with your heart, but there are a few points I'd like to review and clarify."
	ASK the patient or family to repeat back the information that has been delivered	"Now that I've clarified a few things about your illness, I want to make sure you understand what I've said. Tell me in your own words what we've been talking about."
Establish goals and preferences	Use open-ended questions to gain understanding of the patient's values in order to determine what is most important to them	"Help me to understand what is important to you. Some patients say they want to live as long as possible, regardless of quality of life. Sometimes patients tell me they are worried that they will be in a great deal of pain or have other uncontrolled symptoms. What is important to you at this point in terms of your health care?" "What are you hoping for?" "What is important to you now?" "What is your biggest concern right now?" "When you think about the future, what are the things you want to avoid?" In cases where the patient is not involved in the conversation, a useful phrase might be, "What would your loved one say right now if he or she was hearing what we are discussing?"
Work with patient and family to tailor treatments and decisions to goals	Tailor explanation of benefits/ burdens of a particular therapy based on goals established	"I think I understand what is important to you now, and it helps me better explain to you the decisions and treatments at hand now. I'd like to take a moment to review the benefits and burdens of each of the treatments based on what you've said is important to you at this point…"
	Be willing to make a recommendation based on the patient's goals	"Would it be helpful if I made a recommendation based on what you've said the overall focus of care should be now?" "Based on what you have told me, if you get sicker and need to go back on a breathing machine again to stay alive, that is very unlikely to provide the kind of life you want to lead. Therefore, I think you should not go back on those machines."
	Acknowledge that there is uncertainty in the course of heart failure	"One of the most difficult things about heart disease is that we can never know for sure exactly what will happen in the next (hours, days, weeks, etc.). We must make our best guess and decide what to do based on that information. If things change, we can always readdress this discussion at any time in the future."

From Allen LA, Stevenson LW, Grady KL, et al. Decision making in advanced heart failure: a scientific statement from the American Heart Association. *Circulation.* 2012;125(15):1928–1952; and Havranek EP, Mujahid MS, Barr DA, et al. Social determinants of risk and outcomes for cardiovascular disease: a scientific statement from the American Heart Association. *Circulation.* 2015;132(9):873–898.

ask the patient or family to repeat back the information that has been delivered in order to assess their understanding and to clarify elements that may remain unclear.

One of the core elements of good communication is that it grounds discussions in patients' values, goals, and desired outcomes. Optimal communication with patients with advanced heart failure should not begin with questions about treatments. Open-ended questions to gain insight into the patient's life are useful: "What are you hoping for?" or "What is important outside of the hospital?" or "What is your biggest concern right now?" After

clarifying the patient's goals, it is often useful for the clinician to summarize what has been expressed: "Let me see if I understand what you are saying." Too often values are configured as mutually exclusive—"Do you want A or B?"—when in reality patients usually want both quantity and quality of life, and sometimes therapies can achieve both. The job of the clinician is to help patients and their families prioritize values when they may come into conflict. A common response from patients to a trusted clinician is "What would you do?" This question suggests that the patient feels she shares similar values as the clinician and feels the clinician understands the medical details better. While this deferential approach can be reasonable, once patients better understand the medical situation, they often feel empowered to take back agency.

After values and goals are clarified, the conversation can then move to discussing the role of specific treatments within the context of the desired outcomes. This involves working with the patient and family to (1) summarize the range of medically reasonable treatments for this particular patient at this particular time, and then (2) explain the risks and benefits of each treatment option within the context of the personalized goals and desires set forth by the patient and family. Working within this context, the clinician helps the patient understand which treatments are most appropriate, based upon their likelihood of getting the patient to the desired outcome. Uncertainty about outcomes of specific treatments should be communicated honestly and openly with patients and their families. A helpful way to recognize uncertainty and remain focused on goals of care is a "Best Case/Worst Case/Most Likely" framework.[90] Such scenario planning shifts the focus of decision-making conversations away from an isolated treatment to a discussion about treatment alternatives, their range of potential outcomes, and how those relate to goals of care.

Overcoming Barriers to Optimal Communication

Engaging patients in selecting treatments aligned with their informed goals and values requires that clinicians not only present the options clearly, but that they are also attentive to patients' emotional needs and impaired decision-making capacities. In such settings, cognitive information is often not accurately processed.

Responding empathetically has been shown to strengthen the patient-clinician relationship, increase patient satisfaction, and make patients more likely to disclose future worries. One useful device that can help clinicians respond empathetically in conversations is the mnemonic N-U-R-S-E: *N*aming the emotion expressed in the conversation, demonstrating *U*nderstanding of the emotion, *R*especting the emotion displayed by the patient or family, *S*upporting the patient/family, and *E*xploring the emotion in the context of the discussion.[91] This assists clinicians in demonstrating verbal empathy and assures that the complex emotional components of the conversation are addressed.

Cognitive impairments compound difficulties with communication, comprehension, and decision making. Mild cognitive decline is seen in 25% to 50% of adults with heart failure.[92] Heart failure patients tend to have poorer memory, psychomotor speed, and executive function; patients most likely to experience cognitive decline are those with the worst heart failure severity. Limitations in health literacy and numeracy further interfere with the understanding and integration of the information discussed as it relates to decision making. Nearly 10% of the US population is functioning at below basic literacy levels.

Sensitivity to cultural, religious, and language differences can facilitate understanding of patient choices when discussing treatment options. While clinicians are not expected to be experts in cultural or religious issues relating to decision making, it is important that they are aware of the influence of these elements on decision making.[93]

Decision Support to Assist With Particularly Difficult Conversations

In many cases, the decision at hand may be particularly complex or may require assistive methods to help patients and caregivers understand the potential risks and benefits. In these cases, a decision support intervention, such as a decision aid or a decision coach, can help enhance conversations between patients and clinicians.

"Patient decision aids" are tools that help patients and caregivers become involved in decision making by providing standardized information about the treatment options and how decisions relate to values, goals, and preferences. Decision aids come in various forms including booklets, pamphlets, videos, and web-based systems (see http://decisionaid.ohri.ca/), and are designed to complement, not replace, a clinical encounter. They can be used during or independently from a face-to-face encounter. Decision aids attempt to present probabilities of relevant risks and benefits in ways that patients can understand. A key difference between decision aids and a simple information pamphlet is that decision aids do not only provide data about the anticipated risks and benefits but also provide guidance to help patients clarify their personal values and make a decision. Decision aids can help patients clarify their values explicitly through a simple pro/con list or implicitly through an "imagined future" exercise. Decision aids improve patient knowledge, reduce decisional conflict, increase patients' participation in decision making, and reduce the number of people remaining undecided with no associated adverse health outcomes.[94]

UNMET NEEDS AND DIRECTIONS FOR THE FUTURE

The unique role of heart failure clinicians asks that they assume the primary responsibility for medical decision making and end-of-life care for many patients with advanced heart failure. Yet, the diverse tasks and clinical demands limit the capacity to conduct thorough prognostication, treatment, and shared decision making. As such, the routine conduct of these activities must be efficiently integrated into routine care. The more the clinicians perform shared decision making, the better they will be at making it a natural part of their routine practice of care. Ultimately, this approach to care can only occur within health systems that shift incentives from doing things to helping decide which things should and should not be done.[13]

Multiple studies have shown variation and deficiencies in the ability of clinicians to communicate with patients and address end-of-life issues. Given the important yet difficult task of communication in clinical practice, improving communication should be a core element of the "performance-based" training and certification processes. Several interventions have successfully improved communication skills for clinicians, particularly around end-of-life care.[95] Useful decision aids for commonly encountered medical decisions in heart failure are increasingly available and shown to improve decisional outcomes.[96] Public policy is increasingly requiring the use of formal decision aids for heart failure treatments.[16]

At a more basic level, our understanding of how patients with advanced heart failure make choices is limited. There is also no consensus in the literature on the best way to measure whether a medical decision was a "good" one. Decisional quality, defined as "the extent to which the implemented decision reflects the considered preferences of a well-informed patient," is emerging as another possible measure to assess the quality of decision making, but validated measures to quantify decisional quality tend to be decision specific and can be fluid over time.

Finally, our understanding of health-related quality of life for patients with advanced heart disease is limited. Although health-related quality of life measurements have been developed for patients with symptomatic heart failure, questions remain about their sensitivity in very advanced stages of disease and their relevance after major interventions, such as LVAD.[97] Our understanding of the burden and quality of life of caregivers of heart failure patients is even more limited, as is knowledge about how best to improve caregiver quality of life.[13]

CONCLUSIONS

The importance of decision making and palliative care in advanced heart failure cannot be overstated given the complex myriad of treatment options that confront patients and their caregivers. Although the promotion of shared decision making and the incorporation of palliative care into the management of patients with advanced heart failure may seem daunting to busy practicing clinicians, guiding principles and simple tools can help set future expectations, anticipate major decisions, and promote productive conversations.

KEY REFERENCES

6. Warraich HJ, Hernandez AF, Allen LA. How medicine has changed the end of life for patients with cardiovascular disease. *J Am Coll Cardiol.* 2017;70(10):1276–1289.
7. Fang JC, Ewald GA, Allen LA, et al. Advanced (stage D) heart failure: a statement from the Heart Failure Society of America Guidelines Committee. *J Card Fail.* 2015;21(6):519–534.
13. Braun LT, Grady KL, Kutner JS, et al. Palliative care and cardiovascular disease and stroke: a policy statement from the American Heart Association/American Stroke Association. *Circulation.* 2016;134(11):e198–e225.
15. Allen LA, Stevenson LW, Grady KL, et al. Decision making in advanced heart failure: a scientific statement from the American Heart Association. *Circulation.* 2012;125(15):1928–1952.
17. Fried TR. Shared decision making—finding the sweet spot. *N Engl J Med.* 2016;374(2):104–106.
28. Allen LA, Matlock DD, Shetterly SM, et al. Use of risk models to predict death in the next year among individual ambulatory patients with heart failure. *JAMA Cardiol.* 2017;2(4):435–441.
34. Baumwol J. "I Need Help"-A mnemonic to aid timely referral in advanced heart failure. *J Heart Lung Transplant.* 2017;36(5):593–594.
50. Proposed Decision Memo for Implantable Cardioverter Defibrillators (CAG-00157R4). https://www.cms.gov/medicare-coverage-database/details/nca-proposed-decision-memo.aspx?NCAId=288. Accessed January 1, 2018.
67. 2016 edition. *Nhpco Facts and Figures: Hospice Care in America.* Alexandria, VA: National Hospice and Palliative Care Organization; 2017. https://www.nhpco.org/sites/default/files/public/Statistics_Research/2016_Facts_Figures.pdf. Accessed February 19, 2018.
94. Stacey D, Legare F, Lewis KB. Patient decision aids to engage adults in treatment or screening decisions. *JAMA.* 2017;318(7):657–658.

The full reference list for this chapter is available on ExpertConsult.

Page numbers followed by *f* indicate figures; *t*, tables; *b*, boxes.